D1395038

BMA LIBRARY
WITHDRAWN FROM
LIBRARY
BRITISH MEDICAL ASSOCIATION

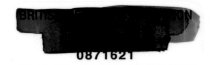
0871621

Congestive Heart Failure

THIRD EDITION

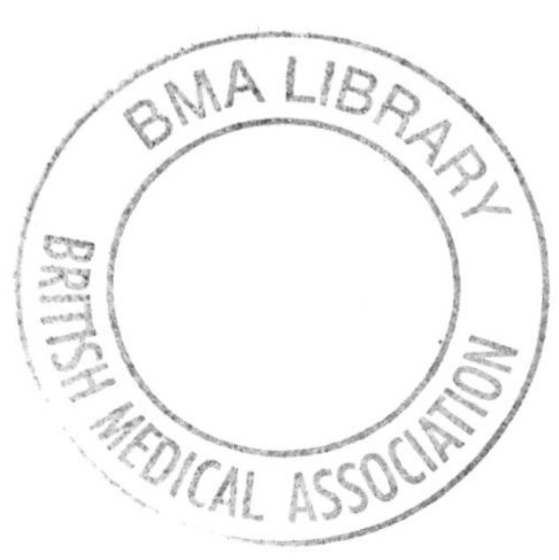

Congestive Heart Failure

THIRD EDITION

EDITORS

JEFFREY D. HOSENPUD, MD
Department of Transplantation
Mayo Clinic—Jacksonville
Jacksonville, Florida

BARRY H. GREENBERG, MD
Professor of Medicine
Director, Advanced Heart Failure Program
University of California, San Diego
UCSD Medical Center
San Diego, California

Lippincott Williams & Wilkins
a Wolters Kluwer business
Philadelphia • Baltimore • New York • London
Buenos Aires • Hong Kong • Sydney • Tokyo

Acquisitions Editor: Frances DeStefano
Managing Editor: Joanne Bersin
Project Manager: Fran Gunning
Marketing Manager: Angela Panetta
Manufacturing Coordinator: Kathleen Brown
Design Coordinator: Risa Clow
Production Services: SPi
Printer: Edwards Brothers

530 Walnut Street
Philadelphia, PA 19106 USA
www.LWW.com

Library of Congress Cataloging-in-Publication Data

Congestive heart failure / editors, Jeffrey D. Hosenpud, Barry H. Greenberg. — 3rd ed.
p. ; cm.
Includes bibliographical references and index.
ISBN: 0-7817-6285-5
1. Congestive heart failure. I. Hosenpud, Jeffrey D. II. Greenberg, Barry H.
[DNLM: 1. Heart Failure, Congestive—diagnosis. 2. Heart Failure, Congestive—physiopathology. 3. Heart Failure, Congestive—therapy. 4. Diagnosis, Diffrential. WG 370 C7513 2006]

RC685.C53C665 2006
616.1'29--dc22

2006018498

Care has been taken to confirm the accuracy of the information presented and to describe generally accepted practices. However, the authors, editors, and publisher are not responsible for errors or omissions or for any consequences from application of the information in this book and make no warranty, expressed or implied, with respect to the currency, completeness, or accuracy of the contents of the publication. Application of this information in a particular situation remains the professional responsibility of the practitioner.

The authors, editors, and publisher have exerted every effort to ensure that drug selection and dosage set forth in this text are in accordance with current recommendations and practice at the time of publication. However, in view of ongoing research, changes in government regulations, and the constant flow of information relating to drug therapy and drug reactions, the reader is urged to check the package insert for each drug for any change in indications and dosage and for added warnings and precautions. This is particularly important when the recommended agent is a new or infrequently employed drug.

Some drugs and medical devices presented in this publication have Food and Drug Administration (FDA) clearance for limited use in restricted research settings. It is the responsibility of the health care provider to ascertain the FDA status of each drug or device planned for use in their clinical practice.

To purchase additional copies of this book, call our customer service department at (800) 638-3030 or fax orders to (301) 223-2320. International customers should call (301) 223-2300.

Visit Lippincott Williams & Wilkins on the Internet: at LWW.com. Lippincott Williams & Wilkins customer service representatives are available from 8:30 am to 6 pm, EST.

Printed in the USA

10 9 8 7 6 5 4 3 2 1

Dedication

The authors are deeply grateful for the support given to them by their families over the course of the three editions of this text. Without this our work would not have been possible. We also wish to acknowledge the help and encouragement provided by our colleagues in San Diego, Milwaukee, and elsewhere for this edition of the text. Finally, we remain deeply indebted to our patients, who in a very real and immediate sense remain our teachers day in and day out.

Contents

Preface

Having first decided to organize and edit a book on heart failure in 1992 (with a 1994 publication date), we have been astounded at the changes in the field over a relatively brief 14-year period. It is with some amusement that we now look back at our first edition and note a combined chapter of beta agonists and antagonists, a separate chapter on phosphodiesterase inhibitors, and an extensive discussion of antiarrhythmic therapy in congestive heart failure (CHF) with only a brief mention of implantable defibrillators. On the other hand, it is somewhat disheartening to see that the majority of our advances over this period have come from very generic approaches to CHF, with much less progress in interfering with underlying etiologies. Nonetheless, we continue to move forward on a broad front with an expanded view of the genetics of primary cardiac muscle disease, better imaging techniques, routine screening blood testing, and standardization of medical management. We have the addition of new agents to the therapeutic armamentarium, widespread use of prophylactic defibrillators, and several novel approaches, including biventricular pacing, continuous flow ventricular assist technology, and cellular transplantation.

The fact that both our understanding and treatment of heart failure continue to evolve at a rapid rate is the real motivation that led us to move forward with the third edition of *Congestive Heart Failure*. As with the first two editions, the aim is to provide a comprehensive overview of heart failure and to point out areas where future advances are likely. Again, the text is geared to both the scientist and clinician with the hope that each will find the broad base of information valuable in some way in their respective daily activities.

We would like to acknowledge the excellent contributions of our authors, who not only supplied these chapters in a timely fashion but who were so responsive to editorial comments and revisions. Their professionalism, inquisitiveness, and enthusiasm made our role a joy rather than a burden. Finally, the loving support and encouragement of our families in this and all our other professional endeavors has been instrumental in whatever success we have achieved.

Jeffrey D. Hosenpud, MD
Barry H. Greenberg, MD

Contributors

William T. Abraham, MD Professor of Internal Medicine; Adjunct Professor of Physiology and Cell Biology; Chief, Division of Cardiovascular Medicine; Associate Director, Davis Heart and Lung Research Institute, The Ohio State University College of Medicine, Columbus, Ohio

Philip B. Adamson, MD, FACC Associate Professor of Medicine, Cardiovascular Disease; Associate Professor of Physiology; Director, Heart Failure Treatment Program, Oklahoma City, Oklahoma

Robert A. Ahokas, MD Department of Obstetrics and Gynecology, University of Tennessee Health Science Center, Memphis, Tennessee

Mouaz Al-Mallah, MD Cardiology Fellow, Henry Ford Hospital, Detroit, Michigan

David W. Baker, MD, MPH Associate Professor of Medicine; Chief, Division of General Internal Medicine, Feinberg School of Medicine, Northwestern University, Chicago, Illinois

Bradley A. Bart, MD, FACC Assistant Professor of Medicine, Division of Cardiology, University of Minnesota; Director, Nuclear Cardiac Imaging, Hennepin County Medical Center, Minneapolis, Minnesota

Syamal K. Bhattacharya, MD Department of Surgery, University of Tennessee Health Science Center, Memphis, Tennessee

Philip F. Binkley, MD Heart Failure Program, Division of Cardiovascular Medicine, Department of Medicine, University of Southern California, Keck School of Medicine, Los Angeles, California

Fahed Bitar, MD Heart Failure Program, Division of Cardiovascular Medicine, Department of Medicine, University of Southern California, Keck School of Medicine, Los Angeles, California

Javed Butler, MD Assistant Professor, Department of Medicine; Director, Heart Transplant Program, Vanderbilt University, Nashville, Tennessee

Blase A. Carabello, MD Professor of Medicine, General Medicine, Baylor College of Medicine; Medical Care Line Executive, Department of Medicine, Michael E. Debakey, VA Medical College, Houston, Texas

Kanu Chatterjee, MD Cardiology Division, San Francisco, California

Xiongwen Chen Postdoctoral Research Fellow, Cardiovascular Research Center, Department of Physiology, Temple University School of Medicine, Philadelphia, Pennsylvania

Wilson S. Colucci, MD Duke University, Durham, North Carolina

George Cooper, IV, MD Distinguished University Professor, Medical University of South Carolina; Chief, Cardiology Section, Department of Medicine, Ralph H. Johnson VA Medical Center, Charleston, South Carolina

Maria Rosa Costanzo, MD Heart Failure Specialist, Midwest Heart Foundation, Lombard, Illinois; Medical Director, Edward Hospital Center for Advanced Heart Failure, Department of Cardiology, Edward Hospital, Naperville, Illinois

Bart L. Cox, MD Cardiovascular Associates of Wisconsin, LLP, Milwaukee, Wisconsin

Mark A. Creager, MD Professor, Department of Medicine, Harvard Medical School; Director, Vascular Center, Simon C. Fireman Scholar in Cardiovascular Medicine, Cardiovascular, Brigham and Women's Hospital, Boston, Massachusetts

Reynolds M. Delgado, III, MD Assistant Clinical Professor, Department of Medicine, Baylor College of Medicine, Waco, Texas

Uri Elkayam, MD Division of Cardiovascular Medicine, Los Angeles County/University of Southern California Medical Center, Los Angeles, California

Gregory K. Feld, MD Cardiac Electrophysiology Program, Division of Cardiology, Department of Medicine, University of California, San Diego, California

Arthur Feldman, MD Farber Institute for Neurosciences, Thomas Jefferson University, Philadelphia, Pennsylvania

G. Michael Felker, MD DUMC 3850, Durham, North Carolina

Paul E. Fenster, MD Associate Professor, Department of Medicine, University of Arizona; Director of Adult Echocardiography, Department of Medicine, University Medical Center, Tucson, Arizona

Gregg C. Fonarow, MD Professor of Medicine, Department of Cardiology; Director, Ahmanson-UCLA Cardiomyopathy Center, UCLA Medical Center; Los Angeles, California

Shi Yin Foo, MD, PhD Instructor, MGH-Medicine, Harvard Medical School; Graduate Assistant in Medicine, Division of Cardiology, Massachusetts General Hospital, Boston, Massachusetts

Gary S. Francis, MD Professor of Medicine, Lerner College of Medicine, Case Western Reserve University; Head, Clinical Cardiology, Cleveland Clinic, Cleveland, Ohio

O. H. Frazier, MD Chief, Transplant Service; Director, Cardiovascular Surgical Research, Texas Heart Institute at St. Luke's Episcopal Hospital, Texas Medical Center, Houston, Texas

Ivan C. Gerling, MD Division of Endocrinology, University of Tennessee Health Science Center, Memphis, Tennessee

Steven Goldsmith, MD Associate Director, Cardiology Division, Hennepin County Medical Center, Minneapolis, Minnesota

Scott H. Goodnight, MD Professor of Medicine and Pathology, Oregon Health Sciences University, Portland, Oregon

Stephen S. Gottlieb, MD Professor, Department of Medicine, University of Maryland School of Medicine; Director, Department of Cardiomyopathy and Pulmonary Hypertension, Baltimore, Maryland

Barry H. Greenberg, MD Professor of Medicine, Director, Advanced Heart Failure Program, University of California, San Diego, UCSD Medical Center, San Diego, California

Swaminatha V. Gurudevan, MD Department of Cardiology, UCI Medical Center, University of California, Irvine, Irvine, California

Judith Karen Gwathmey, VMD, PhD, FACC, FAHA Gwathmey Inc.; Division of Cardiology, Beth Israel Deaconess Medical Center, Harvard Medical School, Cambridge, Massachusetts

Paul J. Hauptman, MD Internal Medicine, Division of Cardiology, Saint Louis University Hospital, St. Louis, Missouri

Roger Joseph Hajjar, MD Massachusetts General Hospital, Boston, Massachusetts

Parta Hatamizadeh, MD Heart Failure Program, Division of Cardiovascular Medicine, Department of Medicine, University of Southern California, Keck School of Medicine, Los Angeles, California

Tamara B. Horwich, MD Cardiology Fellow, Department of Medicine, Division of Cardiology, David Geffen School of Medicine at UCLA; UCLA Medical Center, Los Angeles, California

Jeffrey David Hosenpud, MD Department of Transplantation, Mayo Clinic—Jacksonville, Jacksonville, Florida

Steven R. Houser, PhD Director, Cardiovascular Research Center, Senior Associate Dean for Research, Department of Physiology, Temple University School of Medicine, Philadelphia, Pennsylvania

Susan Isakson, MD VA San Diego Medical Center, San Diego, California

Anantharam V. Kalya, MD The Care Group, LLC, Indianapolis, Indiana

Ralph A. Kelly, MD Associate Professor, Department of Medicine, Harvard Medical School; Department of Medicine, Brigham and Women's Hospital, Boston, Massachusetts

Sarkis Kiramijyian, MD Heart Failure Program, Division of Cardiovascular Medicine, Department of Medicine, University of Southern California, Keck School of Medicine, Los Angeles, California

Marvin A. Konstam, MD Professor of Medicine, Department of Medicine, Tufts University School of Medicine; Chief of Cardiology, Department of Cardiology, Tufts–New England Medical Center, Boston Massachusetts

Mikhail Kosiborod, MD Assistant Professor of Medicine, Department of Medicine, University of Missouri-Kansas City/Mid-America Heart Institute, Kansas City, Missouri

Henry Krum, MD Departments of Epidemiology and Preventative Medicine, Monash University Alfred Hospital, Monash University Central and Eastern Clinical School, Melbourne, Victoria, Australia

Harlan M. Krumholz, MD Professor of Medicine and EPI and Public Health, Yale University School of Medicine; Director, CTR for Outcomes, Research and Evaluations, Yale—New Haven Health, New Haven, Connecticut

David Krummen, MD Cardiac Electrophysiology Program, Division of Cardiology, Department of Medicine, University of California, San Diego, California

Jody L. Kujovich, MD Department of Medicine, Oregon Health Science, University and University Hospital, Portland, Oregon

Carolyn S. P. Lam, MD Cardiorenal Research Laboratory, Mayo Clinic College of Medicine, Rochester, Minnesota

Yuk M. Law, MD Assistant Professor, Department of Pediatrics, Oregon Health and Science University; Director of Heart Failure and Transplant Services, Department of Pediatrics, Doernbecher Children's Hospital, Portland, Oregon

Carl V. Leier, MD Davis Heart and Lung Research Institute, Ohio State University, Colombia, Ohio

Peng Li, MD University of California, Irvine; Shanghai Medical University, China

JoAnn Lindenfeld, MD Professor, Department of Medicine, University of Colorado Health Sciences Center; Medical Director, Cardiac Transplant Program, Department of Medicine, University of Colorado Hospital, Denver, Colorado

Niall G. Mahon, MD Professor of Cardiac Medicine, Department of Cardiological Sciences, St. George's Hospital Medical School; Consultant Cardiologist, Department of Cardiology, St. George's Hospital, London, United Kingdom

Alan Maisel, MD VA Sand Diego Medical Center, San Diego, California

Donna Mancini, MD Columbia Presbyterian Medical Center, Department of Medicine, New York, New York

Douglas L. Mann, MD Professor of Medicine, Molecular Physiology and Biophysics, Department of Medicine, Baylor College of Medicine; Chief of Cardiology, Department of Medicine, Texas Heart Institute and St. Luke's Episcopal Hospital, Houston, Texas

Barry M. Massie, MD Chief, Cardiology Division, San Francisco VAMC; Professor of Medicine, University of California, San Francisco, San Francisco, California

Patrick M. McCarthy, MD Cardiac Thoracic Surgery, Northwestern Memorial Hospital, Faculty Foundation, Chicago, Illinois

William J. McKenna, MD, FRCP, FESC, FACC Professor of Cardiac Medicine, Department of Cardiological Sciences, St. George's Hospital Medical School; Consultant Cardiologist, Department of Cardiology, St. George's Hospital, London, United Kingdom

Jean-Jacques Mercadier, MD, PhD Professor of Physiology and Medicine, Department of Physiology, Faculté de Médecine de l'Universiteé Denis Diderot (Paris 7); Head of Cardiovascular Division, Department of Physiology, Hôpital Bichat—Claude Bernard, Paris, France

Roger M. Mills, MD Henry Ford Hospital, Heart Failure, Cardiac Transplant, Detroit, Michigan

Frederica del Monte, MD Massachusetts General Hospital, Boston, Massachusetts

Timothy J. Myers, BS, CCRA Director, School for Cardiac Support, Center for Cardiac Support, Texas Heart Institute at St. Luke's Episcopal Hospital, Houston, Texas

Jagat Narula, MD University of California Irvine, Orange County, California

Alan S. Nies, MD MERCK Research Laboratories, Rahway, New Jersey

Anju Nohria, MD Instructor in Medicine, Internal Medicine, Harvard Medical School; Associate Physicians, Internal Medicine, Brigham and Young Women's Hospital, Boston, Massachusetts

Paul Nolan, MD Professor, Department of Pharmacy Practice & Science, College of Pharmacy, University of Arizona, Tucson, Arizona

Richard D. Patten, MD Assistant Professor of Medicine, Associate Medical Director, Cardiac Transplant Program, Division of Cardiology and Molecular Cardiology Research Institute, Tufts-New England Medical Center, Boston, Massachusetts

Denis Pellerin, MD Professor of Cardiac Medicine, Department of Cardiological Sciences, St. George's Hospital Medical School; Consultant Cardiologist, Department of Cardiology, St. George's Hospital, London, United Kingdom

Stephen D. Persell, MD Assistant Professor of Medicine, Division of General Internal Medicine, Feinberg School of Medicine, Northwestern University, Chicago, Illinois

Margaret M. Redfield, MD Mayo Clinic and Foundation, Cardiorenal Laboratory, Rochester, Minnesota

Howard A. Rockman, MD Duke University Medical Center, Durham, North Carolina

Anthony Rosenzweig, MD Director, Cardiovascular Research, BIDMC-Medicine, Harvard Medical School; Associate Chief of Cardiology, Division of Cardiology, Beth Israel Deaconess Medical Center, Boston, Massachusetts

David J. Sahn, MD Pediatric Cardiology, Portland, Oregon

Robert W. Schrier, MD Department of Medicine, University of Colorado Health Sciences Center, Denver, Colorado

Ralph Shabetai, MD Cardiology 111A, VA Health Care System, La Jolla, California

Marc A. Silver, MD Clinical Professor of Medicine, Department of Medicine, University of Illinois at Chicago; Chairman, Department of Medicine, Director, Heart Failure Institute, Advocate Christ Medical Center, Oak Lawn, Illinois

Ozlem Soran, MD Cardiovascular Institute, University of Pittsburgh School of Medicine, Pittsburgh, Pennsylvania

Sunny Srivastava, MD Department of Cardiology, Tufts–New England Medical Center, Boston Massachusetts

Rebecca P. Streeter, MD Division of Cardiology, Department of Medicine, Columbia University College of Physicians and Surgeons, New York, New York

Yao Sun, MD Division of Cardiovascular Diseases, University of Tennessee Health Science Center, Memphis, Tennessee

W. H. Wilson Tang, MD, FACC Assistant Professor in Medicine, Cleveland Clinic Lerner College of Medicine; Staff, Section of Heart Failure & Cardiac Transplant Medicine; Assistant Program Director, General Clinical Research Center (GCRC), Cleveland Clinic Foundation, Cleveland, Ohio

John R. Teerlink, MD Director of the Heart Failure Clinic, San Francisco VAMC; Assistant Professor of Medicine, University of California, San Francisco

James E. Udelson, MD Associate Professor of Medicine and Radiology, Department of Medicine, Tufts University School of Medicine; Associate Chief, Department of Cardiology, Tufts–New England Medical Center, Boston Massachusetts

Mani A. Vannan, MBBS, MRCP, MRCPI, FACC Professor of Medicine, University of California, Irvine, Orange, California

Emilio Vanoli, MD Associate Professor of Medicine, Cardiovascular Disease; Associate Professor of Physiology; Director, Heart Failure Treatment Program, Oklahoma City, Oklahoma

Karl T. Weber, MD Division of Cardiovascular Diseases, University of Tennessee Health Science Center, Memphis, Tennessee

Rachel Wilson, MD Cardiovascular Research Center, Department of Physiology, Temple University School of Medicine, Philadelphia, Pennsylvania

Epidemiology and Pathophysiology of Heart Failure

Epidemiology of Heart Failure

1

Mikhail Kosiborod *Harlan M. Krumholz*

The epidemic of heart failure (HF) is an important public health issue facing the health care system. The scope of the epidemic is profound, with 5 million Americans carrying the diagnosis, 600,000 incident cases, and 1 million hospitalizations occurring annually at a cost of more than $25 billion (1). With no clear evidence that the incidence of HF is decreasing, and with multiple reports of rising prevalence, recent studies project marked increases in the numbers of patients, hospitalizations, and costs associated with HF in the near future (2).

Several key factors need to be considered to better understand the reasons behind the current HF epidemic and its human and economic impact. These include recent trends in HF incidence, prevalence, survival, and hospitalization rates. A detailed review of these factors as well as other pertinent issues, including epidemiology and disease characteristics within special patient populations, will be provided in this chapter.

INCIDENCE

The American Heart Association estimates that there are 600,000 new HF cases diagnosed annually (1), yet analyzing HF incidence is inherently challenging. Most data about HF incidence come from prospective cohort studies, such as the Framingham Heart Study, which consistently apply well-defined criteria for HF diagnosis and account for both inpatient and outpatient cases. However, these studies analyze relatively small, homogeneous patient populations in geographically limited areas and their results are difficult to apply to a diverse population of HF patients in the United States. Although studies of large, administrative databases offer certain advantages, such as analyzing very large patient populations across geographic regions, they rely on hospital billing codes for HF diagnosis and usually do not include outpatients.

Nevertheless, several key investigations offer insight into trends in HF incidence. Most recent studies suggest that the incidence of HF has not changed substantially in the past 30 years. Although data from the Framingham Heart Study showed that the incidence of HF has decreased since the period of 1950–1969, whether any significant change in incidence occurred since 1970 is not as clear (Table 1-1) (3).

In fact, the Rochester Epidemiology Project from Olmsted County, Minnesota, shows that there has been a very modest (and not statistically significant) relative increase in HF incidence of 4% in men and 11% in women between the periods of 1979–1984 and 1996–2000 (4). The same lack of substantial change in incidence is supported by administrative data analysis from the Resource Utilization Among Congestive Heart Failure (REACH) study from the Henry Ford Health System (5).

There are several factors that may explain the lack of improvement in HF incidence. First, given the aging of the U.S. population (Fig. 1-1), the number of elderly persons is increasing. There is clear evidence from multiple sources (1,5,6) that HF incidence increases dramatically with age, reaching >40 per 1,000 people in the >85-year age group (Fig. 1-2).

Second, although data indicate that the control of hypertension has improved in recent decades, more than half of patients with a diagnosis of hypertension still have poor control (7,8). Since the prevalence of hypertension is on the rise (8), this could in part be contributing to the unchanged HF incidence rates.

TABLE 1-1
TEMPORAL TRENDS IN THE AGE-ADJUSTED INCIDENCE OF HEART FAILURE

	Men		Women	
Period	Incidence of Heart Failure Rate/100,000 Person-yr	Rate Ratio	Incidence of Heart Failure Rate/100,000 Person-yr	Rate Ratio
1950–1969†	627 (475–779)	1.00	420 (336–504)	1.00
1970–1979	563 (437–689)	0.87 (0.67–1.14)	311 (249–373)	0.63 (0.47–0.84)
1980–1989	536 (448–623)	0.87 (0.67–1.13)	298 (247–350)	0.60 (0.45–0.79)
1990–1999	564 (463–665)	0.93 (0.71–1.23)	327 (266–388)	0.69 (0.51–0.93)

All values were adjusted for age (<55, 55 to 64, 65 to 74, 75 to 84, and >85 years). Values in parentheses are 95% confidence intervals.
†This period served as the reference period.
From Levy D, Kenchaiah S, Larson MG, et al. Long-term trends in the incidence of and survival with heart failure. *N Engl J Med.* 2002;347:1397–1402, with permission.

Third, although mortality after acute myocardial infarction (AMI) is declining (9), the decrease in the incidence of AMI has been less impressive (10). As patients survive longer after AMI, their lifetime risk of HF may be increasing. Finally, the prevalence of diabetes and obesity—both major risk factors for the development of HF—is on the rise (11,12).

PREVALENCE

While the incidence of HF has been relatively stable during the past several decades, its prevalence has been rising dramatically and is the main factor underlying the current HF epidemic. It is estimated that the number of people with HF in the United States currently exceeds 5 million, a marked increase from the 1 to 2 million estimated in 1971 (1). This increase in prevalence has also been documented in studies of individual health care systems (5) (Fig. 1-3).

Similar to incidence, the prevalence of HF increases considerably with age. The Rotterdam study (14) demonstrates that while <1% of individuals aged 55 to 64 years are diagnosed with HF, this increases to >17% in the ≥85-year age group. These data are corroborated by findings from the Cardiovascular Health Study (Fig. 1-4) and the National Health and Nutrition Examination Survey (NHANES) (6,13,14).

There are several key reasons for the dramatic temporal increases in the prevalence of HF. As mentioned previously, the incidence rates have not declined in recent decades; they remain high. At the same time, recent evidence suggests that although long-term HF mortality remains high, innovations in the management of HF have resulted in slight improvements in survival (3,4,15,16). The rapid increase in the overall number as well as proportion of elderly persons (the group with the highest HF prevalence) in the United States, the lack of decline in incidence, and longer survival with the HF diagnosis are all likely contributors to the rapidly increasing prevalence of HF.

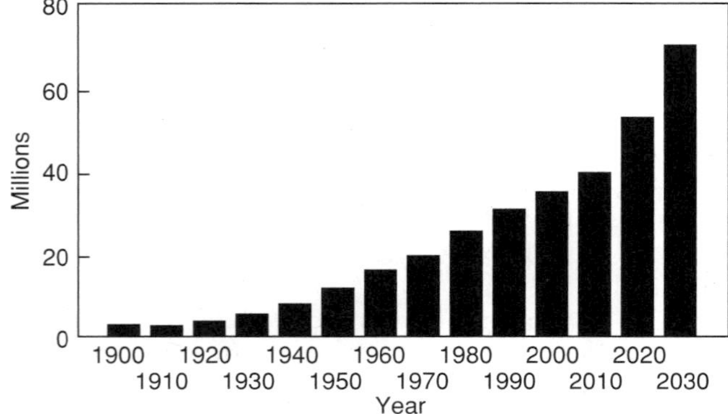

Figure 1-1 Growth of the elderly population (1900 to 2030). (Adapted from U.S. Bureau of the Census.)

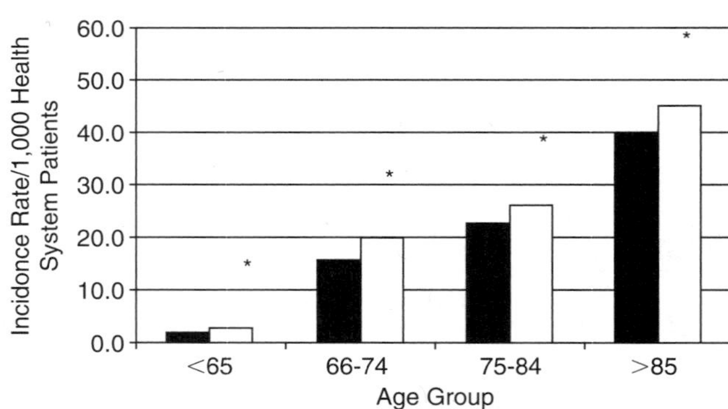

Figure 1-2 Incident cases of heart failure in men (white bars) and women (black bars) by age group in the Resource Utilization Among Congestive Heart Failure (REACH) study. $p < 0.0000001$ for all pairwise comparisons. (Reprinted from McCullough PA, Philbin EF, Spertus JA, et al. Confirmation of a heart failure epidemic: findings from the Resource Utilization Among Congestive Heart Failure [REACH] study. *J Am Coll Cardiol.* 2002;39:60–69, with permission.)

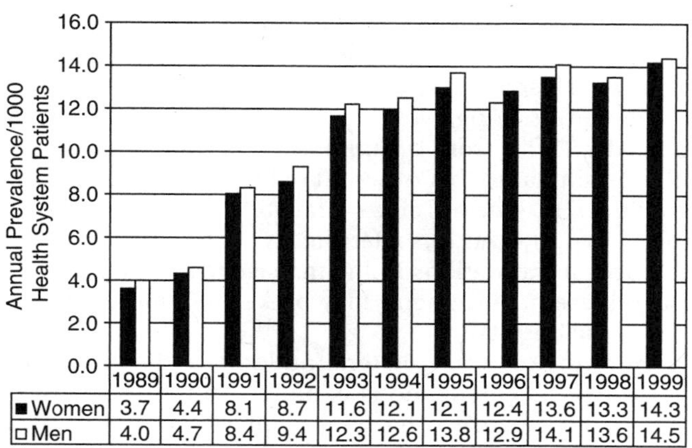

	1989	1990	1991	1992	1993	1994	1995	1996	1997	1998	1999
■ Women	3.7	4.4	8.1	8.7	11.6	12.1	12.1	12.4	13.6	13.3	14.3
□ Men	4.0	4.7	8.4	9.4	12.3	12.6	13.8	12.9	14.1	13.6	14.5

Figure 1-3 Age and gender-adjusted prevalence of congestive heart failure in an integrated health system from 1989 to 1999. For both men and women, the prevalence of congestive heart failure has tripled over the decade of the 1990s. $p < 0.0001$ for linear trend in women and men. (Reprinted from McCullough PA, Philbin EF, Spertus JA, et al. Confirmation of a heart failure epidemic: findings from the Resource Utilization Among Congestive Heart Failure [REACH] study. *J Am Coll Cardiol.* 2002;39:60–69, with permission.)

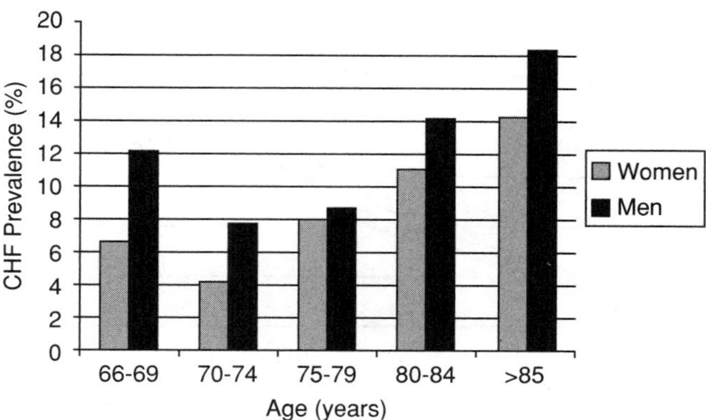

Figure 1-4 Prevalence (per 100) of CHF by age (years) and gender. (Reprinted from Kitzman DW, Gardin JM, Gottdiener JS, et al. Importance of heart failure with preserved systolic function in patients ≥65 years of age. CHS Research Group. Cardiovascular Health Study. *Am J Cardiol.* 2001;87:413–419, with permission.)

Substantial increases in prevalence are expected in the near future. A recent analysis from Scotland predicts that if current trends in HF incidence and mortality continue, there will be a 31% prevalence increase in men and a 17% increase in women by the year 2020 (2). These increases are likely to have a substantial economic impact, with a subsequent rise in hospitalizations and outpatient visits (Fig. 1-5).

HOSPITALIZATIONS AND ECONOMIC BURDEN

According to data from the National Hospital Discharge Survey, the total number of HF-related hospitalizations has increased from 377,000 in 1979 to 1,088,349 in 1999, a 289% relative increase (1) (Fig. 1-6). It is estimated by the National Heart, Lung, and Blood Institute that hospital charges alone for HF will total nearly $15 billion in 2005 (1).

Although hospitalization rates in both Europe and the United States rose dramatically during the 1980s and early 1990s, more current data on trends in hospitalization rates

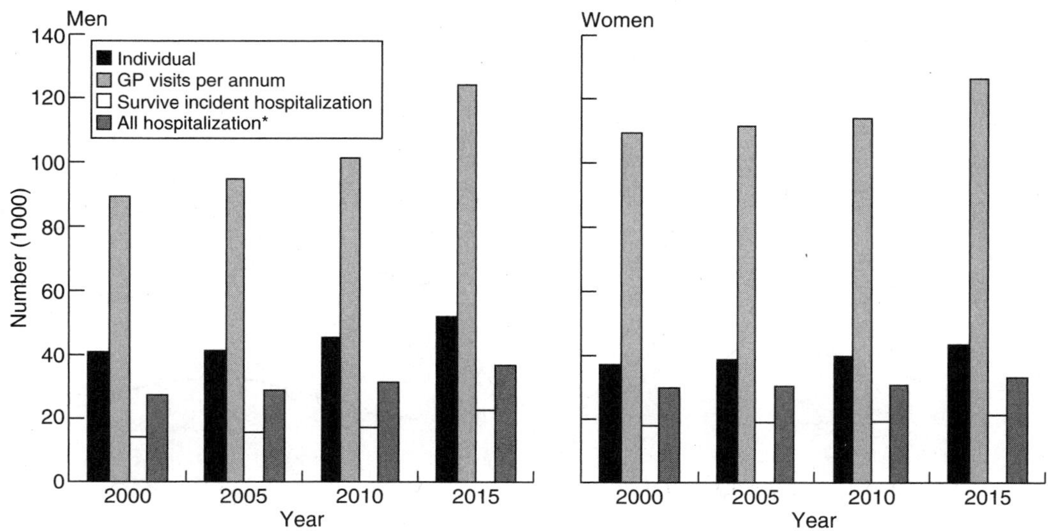

Figure 1-5 Summary of the projected burden of heart failure in Scotland, 2000 to 2020. Estimated individuals with heart failure and general practitioner visits specific to year. *Figures reflect accumulated number in the previous 5 years (for example, total number of patients who survived an incident hospital admission 2006 to 2010). "All hospitalization" refers to incident ("first ever") and other hospital discharges with heart failure as the principal coding. (Reprinted from Stewart S, MacIntyre K, Capewell S, et al. Heart failure and the aging population: an increasing burden in the 21st century? *Heart* [British Cardiac Society]. 2003;89:49–53, with permission.)

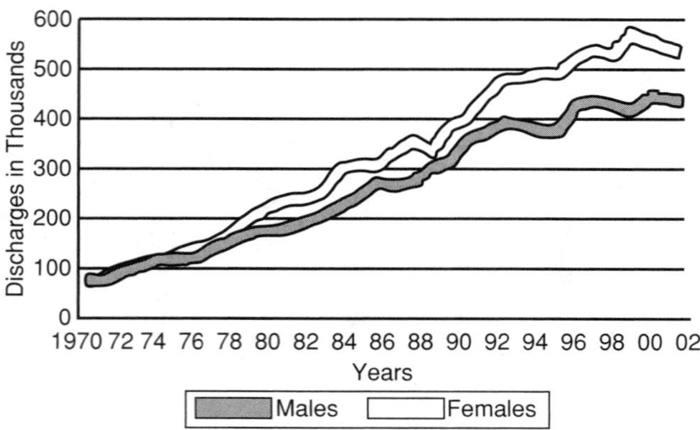

Figure 1-6 Hospital discharges for congestive heart failure by sex (United States: 1970–2002). (Adapted from American Heart Association Heart Disease and Stroke Statistics—2005 Update. http://www.americanheart.org/presenter.jhtml?identifier=3000090. Accessed June 6, 2005.)

have been conflicting. Analysis of national data from Scotland indicates that the total number of hospitalizations with a principal discharge diagnosis of HF peaked in 1993–1994 for both men and women, and has since leveled off (17) (Fig. 1-7). Trends in sex- and age-specific hospitalization rates revealed a similar pattern, with the only exception being men aged ≥85 years, where hospitalization rates continue to increase. Similar administrative database studies from both Sweden and Canada have also shown a relative decrease in HF hospitalization rates between 1993 and 2000 (18,19).

However, data from the U.S. National Hospital Discharge Survey indicate that the total number of hospitalizations with a primary discharge diagnosis of HF continued to rise during the 1990s; specifically, there has been a 34% relative increase between 1990 and 1999 (20) (Fig. 1-8). A close analysis of the sex-specific hospitalization rates revealed that most of the increase occurred in women, while the rates in men remained relatively stable. National Hospital Discharge Survey data from 1999–2002 are more reassuring, with the total number of hospitalizations decreasing from >1 million to 970,000, suggesting a plateau similar to that observed in Europe during the mid-1990s (1,21). One possible explanation for this leveling off in HF hospitalizations (despite rising HF prevalence) is that recent innovations in the management of HF, including disease management, may be keeping more patients out of the hospital.

Nevertheless, the long-term outlook for the total number of HF hospitalizations is not as optimistic. Most of the marked increases have taken place in patients aged ≥65 years (Fig. 1-9). Even if age-adjusted hospitalization rates remain stable, given the predicted dramatic aging of the U.S. population, the total number of HF-related hospitalizations will likely rise substantially. Despite the current plateau in HF hospitalizations in Scotland and Canada, considerable future increases in HF hospitalizations and associated costs are predicted in both countries (2,22).

OUTCOMES

The American Heart Association estimates that more than 50,000 patients die from HF each year. Although data come from a variety of sources, it is clear that despite innovations in the management of this condition, HF outcomes (e.g., mortality and readmissions) remain poor. The estimates for long-term mortality vary significantly, depending on the patient populations studied. Studies that include outpatients as well as inpatients of all age groups, such as the Framingham Heart Study and the Rochester Epidemiology Project, generally produce lower mortality rates than do administrative database investigations, which usually focus on hospitalized elderly patients with HF.

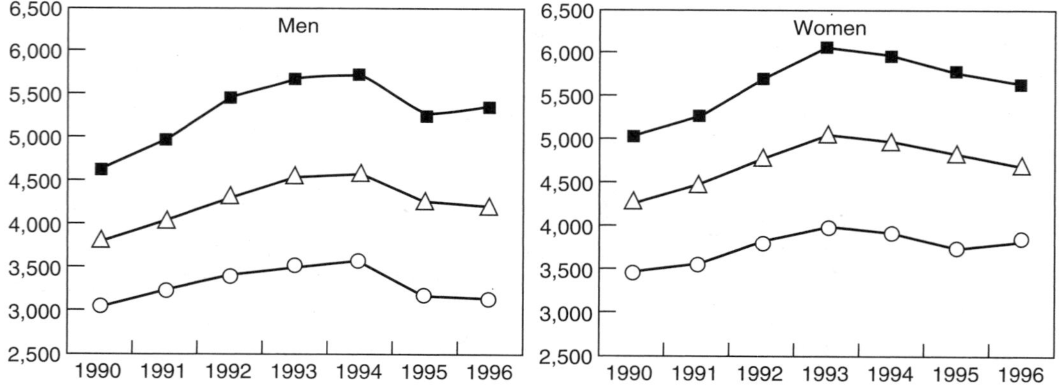

Figure 1-7 Sex-specific trends in the number of hospitalizations for heart failure as the principal diagnosis and the number of patients who contributed to these (including those with a "first ever" hospitalization, 1990–1996). ■ = total hospitalizations (principal diagnosis). Δ = number of individual patients hospitalized (principal diagnosis) and ○ = number of individual patients with a "first ever" hospitalization for heart failure (principal diagnosis). (Reprinted from Stewart S, MacIntyre K, MacLeod MM, et al. Trends in hospitalization for heart failure in Scotland, 1990–1996. An epidemic that has reached its peak? *Eur Heart J.* 2001;22:209–217, with permission.)

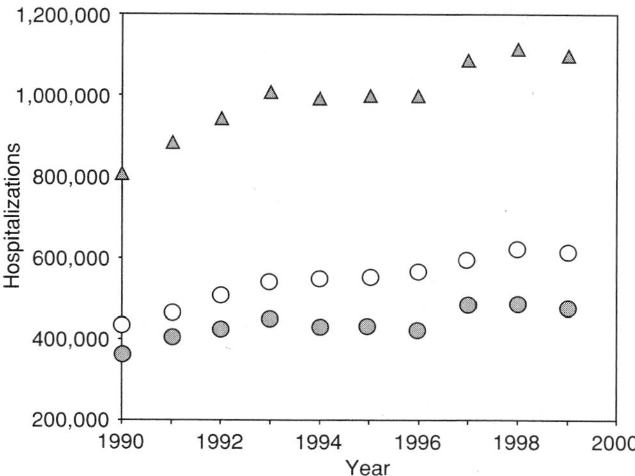

Figure 1-8 Annual hospitalizations for heart failure as a primary diagnosis. Triangles represent all hospitalizations; open circles represent females; filled-in circles represent males. (Reprinted from Koelling TM, Chen RS, Lubwama RN, et al. The expanding national burden of heart failure in the United States: the influence of heart failure in women. *Am Heart J.* 2004;147:74–78, with permission.)

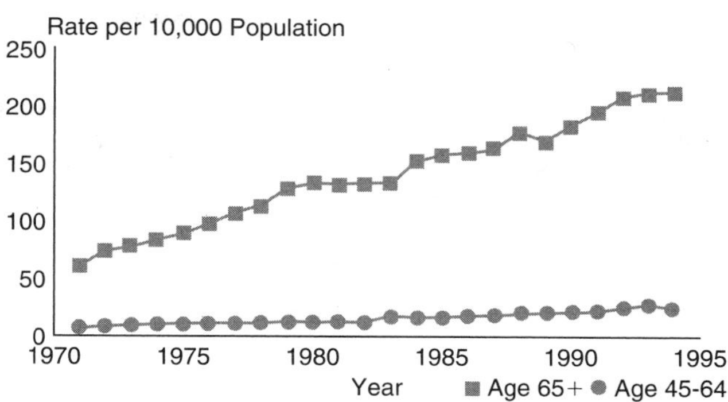

Figure 1-9 Hospitalization rates for CHF by age, 1971 to 1994. (Adapted from the National Hospital Discharge Survey, National Center for Health Statistics.)

SHORT-TERM MORTALITY

Most data for in-hospital and 30-day mortality come from administrative database studies in the United States and Canada, with recent estimates ranging between 4% to 5% for in-hospital and 9% to 11% for 30-day mortality (15,16). Although in-hospital mortality markedly declined during the 1990s according to most recent studies (with a 53% relative risk reduction between 1991 and 1997 in one study) (16), the data for 30-day mortality are less clear. In fact, data from Ontario, Canada (15) as well as a recent analysis of national Medicare data (25) both show no change in 30-day mortality from 1992–1999. These data, when considered together with the recent decline in hospital length of stay (23), suggest that although the proportion of patients dying of HF during hospitalization is decreasing, more patients are likely dying out-of-hospital shortly following discharge. Data from northeast Ohio confirm a higher post-discharge mortality in a sample of 23,505 Medicare beneficiaries (16).

LONG-TERM MORTALITY

Recent estimates from Framingham report 1- and 5-year age-adjusted mortality after the diagnosis of HF at 28% and 59% for men and 24% and 45% for women, respectively, from 1990–1999 (3) (Table 1-2). The Rochester Epidemiology Project reported slightly lower estimates for 1996–2000 [1- and 5-year age-adjusted mortality of 21% and 50% for men and 17% and 46% for women, respectively (4)], whereas REACH states an overall, crude 1-year case-fatality rate of 15.1% (5). The mortality rates in hospitalized, mostly elderly HF patients are considerably higher: >30% 1-year mortality in the United States, 35% in Canada, and 44% in Scotland (15,24). In fact, the elderly account for nearly 90% of all HF deaths.

The data on recent trends in long-term HF survival suggest improvement during the past 30 to 50 years (3,4). Specifically, in Framingham the long-term mortality rate declined by approximately one-third in both men and

TABLE 1-2

TEMPORAL TRENDS IN AGE-ADJUSTED MORTALITY AFTER THE ONSET OF HEART FAILURE AMONG MEN AND WOMEN 65 TO 74 YEARS OF AGE

	30-Day Mortality		1-Year Mortality		5-Year Mortality	
Period	**Men**	**Women**	**Men**	**Women**	**Men**	**Women**
1950–1969	12 (4–19)	18 (7–27)	30 (18–40)	28 (16–39)	70 (57–79)	57 (43–67)
1970–1979	15 (7–23)	16 (6–24)	41 (29–51)	28 (17–38)	75 (65–83)	59 (45–69)
1980–1989	12 (5–18)	10 (4–16)	33 (23–42)	27 (17–35)	65 (54–73)	51 (39–60)
1990–1999	11 (4–17)	10 (3–15)	28 (18–36)	24 (14–33)	59 (47–68)	45 (33–55)

All values were adjusted for age (<55, 55 to 64, 65 to 74, 75 to 84, and >85 years). Values in parentheses are 95% confidence intervals.
From Levy D, Kenchaiah S, Larson MG, et al. Long-term trends in the incidence of and survival with heart failure. *N Engl J Med.* 2002;347:1397–1402, with permission.

TABLE 1-3

RELATIVE RISK FOR DEATH AFTER ONSET OF HEART FAILURE DEFINED BY THE FRAMINGHAM CRITERIA (95% CI)

	Relative Risk			
Age, y	**1979–1984**	**1985–1990**	**1991–1995**	**1996–2000**
Men				
60	1.00	0.84 (0.69–1.02)	0.63 (0.50–0.80)	0.48 (0.36–0.64)
70	1.00	0.84 (0.73–0.97)	0.74 (0.63–0.88)	0.59 (0.49–0.71)
80	1.00	0.85 (0.72–1.00)	0.88 (0.76–1.04)	0.72 (0.61–0.87)
Women				
60	1.00	0.80 (0.63–1.03)	0.95 (0.73–1.24)	0.67 (0.48–0.92)
70	1.00	0.91 (0.77–1.06)	0.99 (0.83–1.18)	0.79 (0.64–0.98)
80	1.00	1.02 (0.90–1.15)	1.03 (0.90–1.17)	0.94 (0.82–1.09)

Values in parentheses are 95% confidence intervals.
From Roger VL, Weston SA, Redfield MM, et al. Trends in heart failure incidence and survival in a community-based population. *JAMA.* 2004;292:344–350, with permission.

women between the time periods of 1950–1969 and 1990–1999 (3). The Rochester Epidemiology Project investigators also demonstrated that the relative risk of long-term mortality (mean follow-up of 4.2 years) declined in both men and women when the time period of 1996–2000 was compared with the referent period of 1979–1984 (4) (Table 1-3). The magnitude of this improvement varied by age group, with younger HF patients (aged 60 to 70 years) experiencing the most benefit (relative risk decrease of 52% and 33% in men and women, respectively). In older patients, the magnitude of improvement was considerably more modest, and in women aged >80 years it was not statistically significant. An administrative database study from Scotland also showed a 15% to 18% reduction in 1-year case-fatality rates between the mid-1980s and mid-1990s (24).

It is less clear whether long-term mortality continued to improve within the decade of the 1990s. A study of Medicare beneficiaries from Northeast Ohio showed a 15% relative risk reduction in 1-year mortality from 1991 to 1997 (16). A recent administrative database study of elderly HF patients from Ontario, Canada, also showed an overall statistically significant trend toward better survival from 1992 to 1999; however, most of the change appears to have occurred from 1992 to 1993, with only an 0.3% absolute decrease in crude mortality during 1993–1999 (15). Similarly, analysis of a national sample of Medicare beneficiaries from 1992–1999 revealed a 7% relative risk reduction in 1-year mortality from 1993–1994; however, these data suggested that there was no continuous improvement after 1994 (25). Data from REACH also did not show a significant change in HF survival between the early and late 1990s (5) (Fig. 1-10).

HOSPITAL READMISSIONS

Readmission rates remain extremely high for hospitalized HF patients, with 30-day rates reaching 14% and 6-month rates exceeding 40% (26). This contributes substantially to the overall burden of HF hospitalizations and associated costs. National Medicare data show a 9% increase in the odds of hospital readmission at 30 days from 1993–1999,

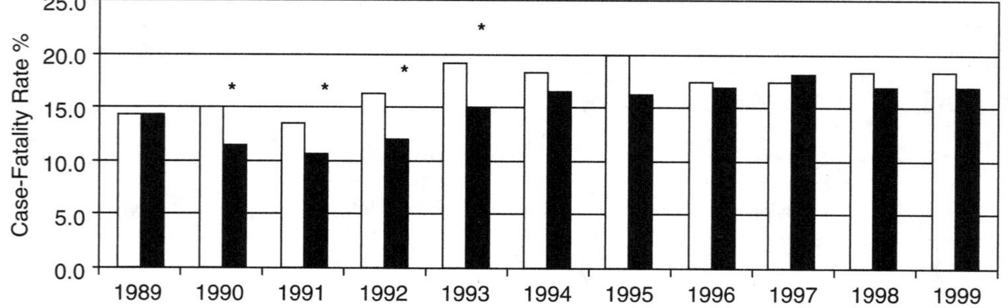

Figure 1-10 Case-fatality rate per year among incident (white bars) and prevalent (black bars) cases in the Resource Utilization Among Congestive Heart Failure (REACH) study. The higher mortality among incident cases relative to prevalent cases before 1994 most likely represents lead-time bias in the index case ascertainment algorithm. $p < 0.01$. (Reprinted from McCullough PA, Philbin EF, Spertus JA, et al. Confirmation of a heart failure epidemic: findings from the Resource Utilization Among Congestive Heart Failure [REACH] study. *J Am Coll Cardiol.* 2002;39:60–69, with permission.)

and no change in 6-month readmission rates during the same time period (Kosiborod M. et al., in print).

Overall, recent data suggest that despite innovations in HF care, improvements in HF outcomes over the past decade have been modest at best. There are several possible explanations for this phenomenon. As mentioned previously, the overwhelming and rising majority of HF patients are elderly. Due to the high burden of multiple comorbidities in this group (27), many such patients have contraindications to angiotensin-converting enzyme (ACE) inhibitors and/or beta-blockers. Furthermore, nearly half of elderly HF patients have preserved left ventricular ejection fraction (LVEF)—a condition in which the efficacy of ACE inhibitors and beta-blockers has not been definitively demonstrated (6,28). Even among ideal candidates, <70% of elderly HF patients are prescribed ACE inhibitors (29). Several studies reveal that ACE inhibitor utilization rates leveled off during the mid-1990s and did not improve from 1995 to 2000 (30,31). Data from the Cardiovascular Health Study show that <20% of elderly HF patients were receiving both a beta-blocker and an ACE inhibitor in the late 1990s (30). Finally, adherence with these therapies is an additional issue, even among those patients for whom medications are appropriately prescribed (32).

Since most of the data on HF mortality trends during the 1990s come from database studies of hospitalized patients, another possible explanation merits consideration. Data indicate that while the prevalence of HF is rising, hospitalization rates may have stabilized during the mid- and late 1990s. Furthermore, national Medicare data show that the proportion of patients with multiple comorbidities has increased considerably between the early and late 1990s, resulting in a sicker population of patients being hospitalized over time (25). This suggests that the introduction of ACE inhibitors and beta-blockers may have kept more patients out of the hospital, thus selecting sicker patients with higher disease severity and comorbidity burden into cohorts hospitalized during the late 1990s.

RISK FACTORS AND PROGNOSIS

According to data from Framingham, the lifetime risk of developing HF for someone who is currently aged 40 years in the United States is 21% in men and 20% in women (33). Although the epidemiology of predisposing conditions for HF has been evolving over the past several decades, coronary artery disease (CAD) and hypertension remain the main risk factors.

Several studies demonstrate a decline in mortality after acute myocardial infarction (AMI), which is likely due to advances in treatment. In a community-based study of patients hospitalized in Worcester, Massachusetts, investigators reported a decline in in-hospital mortality from 17.8% to 11.7% between the mid-1970s and the 1990s (9). Most of this decline was due to lower mortality among the patients with Q-wave AMI (10). However, change in the overall incidence of AMI has been minimal. According to data from Olmsted County, Minnesota, there has been a relative decrease of 3% in the incidence of AMI between 1988 and 1998, a change that was not statistically significant (34). Another community-based study from Worcester, Massachusetts, suggests that the changing epidemiology of AMI may be behind this lack of improvement. In that study, the incidence of Q-wave AMI declined significantly between 1975 and 1998 (from 0.17% to 0.10%), although the incidence of non-Q-wave AMI more than doubled during the same time period (from 0.06% to 0.13%) (10).

The incidence of CAD overall has also remained relatively stable. Data from Olmsted County, Minnesota, indicated a 9% relative risk decline between 1988 and 1998, which did not reach statistical significance (34). Recent data from Framingham indicates that the lifetime risk of CAD at age 40 years is quite high—49% in men and 32% in women (35). Due to high lifetime risk of incident CAD, no significant decline in either AMI or CAD incidence during recent decades, and better survival after AMI, the overall number of patients living with CAD may be increasing. This is the most likely reason that CAD continues to be one of the highest-impact risk factors for developing HF in the United States, with a population-attributable risk of 68% (36).

Hypertension remains another major risk factor for developing HF. Framingham has shown that hypertension antedates HF in 91% of patients and has a 39% population-attributable risk of HF in men and a 59% population-attributable risk in women (37). The lifetime risk of HF doubles in patients with a blood pressure ≥160/100 mm Hg compared with those who have blood pressure <140/90 (33). Data from NHANES demonstrates that the prevalence of hypertension has risen by 3.7% between 1988–1991 and 1999–2000, with no change in the awareness of hypertension during this time period (8). Although the treatment rates and control of hypertension have both slightly improved by 6%, over two-thirds of hypertensive patients still did not have adequate control of their blood pressure. These data are corroborated by the Cardiovascular Health Study, which reported that despite improved hypertension treatment and control rates, more than half of elderly HF patients did not have adequate hypertension control in the late 1990s (38). According to Framingham, suboptimal hypertension control is mainly explained by poor control of systolic hypertension (39). This is an important finding, since Framingham data also indicate that systolic blood pressure and pulse pressure are more important predictors of future HF than diastolic blood pressure (40).

The obesity and diabetes epidemics are also included among the most important current public health threats. The prevalence of diabetes and obesity has been on the rise in the United States (11,41–48). Both conditions are significant risk factors for developing HF, according to data from NHANES and Framingham (36,49–52). With regard to obesity, Framingham revealed a 5% increase in the risk of developing HF for every 1 point of body mass index increase in men, and a 7% increase in women (52). Obese patients had twice the risk of developing HF compared with those with a normal body mass index (52). The control of glucose, hypertension, and lipids in patients with diabetes did not improve substantially between 1988–1994 and 1999–2000 (53). Given the rising prevalence of diabetes and poor risk-factor control in diabetic patients, this condition may become an even more prominent risk factor for future development of HF.

There are a number of other important risk factors for the development of HF. Although the data for temporal population trends in valvular heart disease are limited, the NHANES 19-year follow-up study showed that it has a population-attributable risk of 2.2% for the development of HF (36). Framingham also showed valvular disease to be a strong and independent risk factor for the development of HF in both men and women (50,54).

More than 25 years ago, Framingham showed electrocardiographic left ventricular hypertrophy to be a predictor of future HF independent of hypertension (55). Recently, increased left ventricular mass, as assessed by transthoracic echocardiography, was demonstrated to be independently predictive of future cardiovascular events (including HF) in the Rochester Epidemiology Project; specifically, there was a 1% relative risk increase for every 10 g/m increase in the left ventricular mass/height (56). Left ventricular mass was also a predictor of left ventricular systolic dysfunction (LVSD) in the Cardiovascular Health Study; 14.1% of patients in the highest left ventricular mass quartile developed LVSD versus 4.8% in the lowest quartile (57).

Finally, inflammatory markers such as C-reactive protein (CRP) homocysteine, and IL-6 (interleukin-6) have been shown to be independently predictive of future HF. In Framingham, the relative risk of developing HF increased by 68% per tertile increase in concentration of IL-6, and 60% per tertile increase in concentration of TNF-α (tumor necrosis factor alpha). Patients with elevated C-reactive protein (CRP) levels (≥5 mg/dL) were also at increased risk of HF (HR 2.81; 95% CI 1.22–6.50) (58). Patients with elevation of all three proinflammatory cytokines had a markedly increased risk of HF (HR 4.07; 95% CI 1.34–12.37) (58). Framingham also showed that women, but not men, in quartiles with higher homocysteine levels were at greater risk than those in the quartile with the lowest homocysteine levels (HR 1.47 per quartile; p for trend = 0.008) (59).

Several other risk factors for developing HF also deserve mention. Data from the Cardiovascular Health Study and the Established Populations for Epidemiologic Studies of the Elderly (EPESE) showed that chronic kidney disease was an independent risk factor for developing HF (60,61). Smoking was shown to be an important predictor of HF, as well, with a population-attributable risk of 17.1% in NHANES (36). Another study based on data from NHANES showed that dietary sodium intake predisposes to development of HF, with a 26% relative risk increase for every 100 mmol per day of sodium in obese persons (62). However, despite prior belief that alcohol intake may predispose to HF, data from both Framingham and a prospective cohort from New Haven, Connecticut, showed that increasing levels of alcohol consumption are associated with lower risk of developing HF, with a relative risk reduction between 47% and 59% (63,64).

SPECIAL POPULATIONS

Women with Heart Failure

Data from Framingham (3) and the Rochester Epidemiology Project (4) as well as the REACH study (5), the Cardiovascular Health Study (6), and the Rotterdam study (14) provide recent estimates for age-adjusted HF incidence among men and women. Generally, HF incidence is lower in women than men (5,61). Data from the Cardiovascular Health Study show that male gender confers a 2.08 risk ratio (1.57–2.75) for incident HF among the 65-and-older age group (61).

Data from multiple sources indicate that women have lower age-adjusted, long-term mortality compared with men. Framingham showed that age-adjusted, 5-year mortality during the decade of 1990–1999 was 59% in men and 45% in women (3), while in the Rochester Epidemiology Project, age-adjusted, 5-year mortality from 1996–2000 was 50% and 46% in men and women, respectively (4). Similar age-based differences in survival were seen in the REACH study (5). Finally, data from the National Heart Care Project, which analyzed elderly Medicare beneficiaries hospitalized with HF, also showed lower 30-day (9.2% versus 11.4%) and 1-year (36% versus 43%) mortality in women compared with men (65).

The reason for this sex-based difference in survival is unclear. The survival advantage in women is unlikely to be due to differences in the etiology of HF and other clinical characteristics. Although elderly women are more likely than men to have HF with preserved left ventricular ejection fraction (LVEF) (43% versus 23%), the National Heart Care Project demonstrated that women continued to have a 25% lower relative risk of death at 30 days and a 15% lower risk of death at 1 year after adjustment for multiple other demographic and clinical characteristics, including LVEF (65). This survival advantage persisted despite women receiving slightly lower quality of care during hospitalization; specifically, women were less likely than men to receive assessment of LVEF and be prescribed ACE inhibitors during hospitalization (65).

Minority Populations

Population studies suggest that although younger African-American patients with HF have higher mortality compared with whites, this relationship reverses after the age of 65 years (66). In fact, data from the National Heart Care Project indicate that although African-American patients had higher rates of readmission than white patients (68.2% versus 63.0%; p <0.001), they had lower 30-day (6.3% versus 10.7%; p <0.001) and 1-year (31.5% versus 40.1%; p <0.001) mortality rates (67). These differences persisted after adjustment for other demographic and clinical characteristics (including LVEF), with African-American patients having a 9% higher relative risk of readmission at 1 year, but a 22% lower relative risk of 30-day mortality and a 7% lower relative risk of 1-year mortality (67).

In addition, data from this study revealed that African-American and white HF patients received similar quality of care during hospitalization, with similar rates of LVEF assessment (67.8% versus 66.7%, respectively; p = 0.29) and ACE inhibitor or angiotensin receptor blocker use (85.7% versus 82.5%, respectively; p = 0.08) (67). These findings were unchanged after multivariable adjustment. Although the absence of racial differences in that study could be due to the survival effect among African-American HF patients, and/or the fact that all patients had medical insurance (Medicare) and demonstrated an ability to access the health care system by virtue of their hospitalization, these data nevertheless suggest absence of important racial disparities in quality of care and outcomes among elderly patients with HF.

Heart Failure with Preserved Systolic Function

According to data from the Rochester Epidemiology Project, 44% of patients with a confirmed HF diagnosis have preserved systolic function (68). Among patients aged ≥65 years, the prevalence of HF with preserved systolic function is even higher. The Cardiovascular Health Study shows that 63% of HF patients aged ≥65 years have normal left ventricular systolic function (LVSF), and 78% have either normal or mildly reduced (LVEF 45% to 54%) LVSF (69). Given the fact that the prevalence of HF with preserved LVSF is highest in the elderly, a group that represents the fastest-growing segment of both the U.S. general population as well as the HF patient population, the numbers of HF patients with preserved LVSF will likely rise substantially in the near future.

Data from the National Heart Care Project also show that female gender was an even more powerful predictor of HF with preserved LVSF than age. In that study, women had a 71% higher relative risk of HF with preserved LVSF than men (28). Other important predictors of HF with preserved LVSF included hypertension, chronic obstructive pulmonary disease, atrial fibrillation, and aortic stenosis.

Several studies have demonstrated that long-term mortality is lower in patients with preserved versus reduced LVSF. In Framingham, mortality during a median follow-up of 6.2 years was 9% in those with normal versus 19% in those with impaired LVSF (70). Similar results were seen in the Cardiovascular Health Study (Fig. 1-11). There were 87 deaths per 1,000 person-years in HF patients with preserved LVSF versus 154 deaths per 1,000 person-years in those with impaired LVSF. However, mortality among those patients with preserved LVSF was markedly higher than in healthy controls. Most important, the majority of deaths among HF patients were among those with preserved LVSF, mainly due to their higher overall numbers (69). Furthermore, another study demonstrated that although HF patients with preserved LVSF have lower mortality, they experience similar rates of hospital readmission and functional decline (71). Thus, the overall economic impact of this condition is substantial and likely overshadows that of HF patients with impaired LVSF. Unfortunately, the efficacy of therapies that have been shown to be lifesaving in patients with impaired LVSF (such as ACE inhibitors and beta-blockers) has not been definitively demonstrated in HF with preserved LVSF. Thus, evidence-based treatment strategies for this large patient population have not been established.

Asymptomatic Left Ventricular Dysfunction

Both asymptomatic systolic and diastolic left ventricular dysfunction have been strongly associated with development of clinical HF. In Framingham, patients with asymptomatic left ventricular systolic dysfunction (ALVD) were at higher risk of developing HF than patients without ALVD, and the risk increased with greater severity of ALVD (Fig. 1-12). After multivariable adjustment, there was a gradient of rising HF risk with increasing degrees of ALVD (HR 3.3, 95% CI 1.65–6.64 for mild ALVD; HR 7.77, 95% CI 3.86–15.63 for moderate-to-severe ALVD; no ALVD: referent) (72). Presence of both systolic and diastolic dysfunction in patients who did not have symptoms of HF

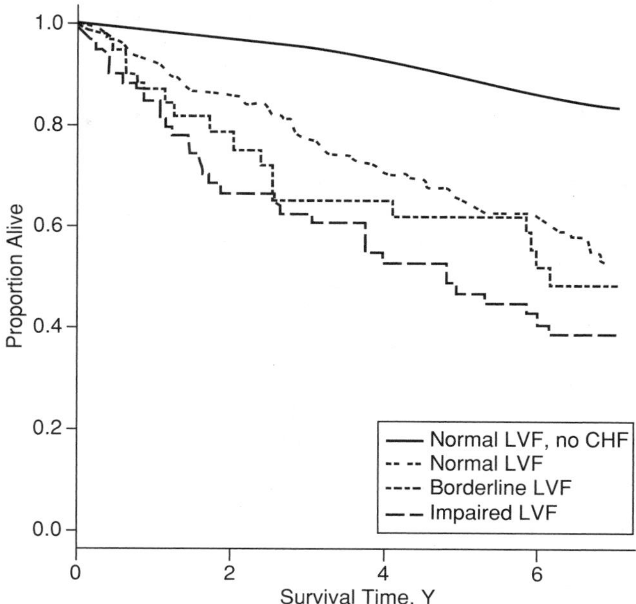

Figure 1-11 Unadjusted Kaplan-Maier survival curves for participants with CHF based on left ventricular function (LVF). (Reprinted from Gottdiener JS, McClelland RL, Marshall R, et al. Outcome of congestive heart failure in elderly persons: influence of left ventricular systolic function. The Cardiovascular Health Study. *Ann Intern Med.* 2002;137:631–639, with permission.)

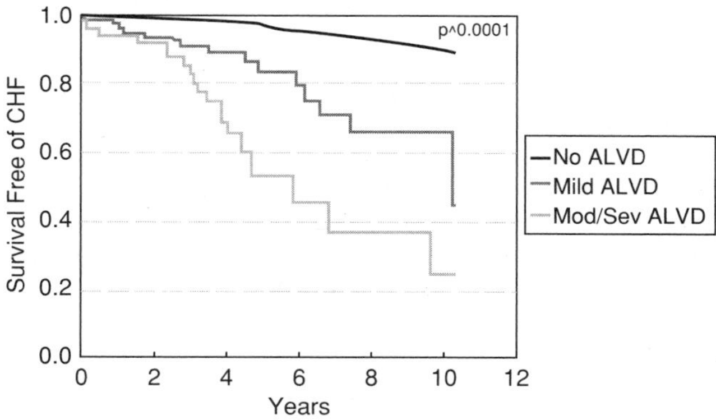

Figure 1-12 Kaplan-Meier curves for survival free of CHF. Referent group consists of subjects with normal left ventricular systolic function (EF >50%). Mild ALVD indicates an EF of 40% to 50%; Mod/Sev ALVD, moderate-to-severe asymptomatic left ventricular systolic dysfunction (EF <40%). (Reprinted from Wang TJ, Evans JC, Benjamin EJ, et al. Natural history of asymptomatic left ventricular systolic dysfunction in the community. *Circulation.* 2003;108:977–982, with permission.)

at baseline was independently predictive of future HF in the Cardiovascular Health Study (73).

PREDICTION MODELS FOR HEART FAILURE OUTCOMES

Several prediction models of mortality have been developed to improve risk stratification, counseling, and management of patients with HF. Lee et al. (74) studied 4,031 community-based patients hospitalized with HF in Ontario, Canada. Multivariable predictors of mortality at 30 days and 1 year included older age, lower systolic blood pressure, higher respiratory rate, higher blood urea nitrogen (BUN) level, hyponatremia, and comorbidities (such as cerebrovascular disease, chronic obstructive pulmonary disease, cirrhosis, dementia, and cancer). A risk index was subsequently developed, which stratified patients as low-, intermediate-, and high-risk. Patients with very high-risk scores (>150) had a mortality rate of 59% at 30 days and 78.8% at 1 year, whereas patients with very low-risk scores had corresponding rates of 0.8% and 9.0%, respectively.

Another prediction model for 1-year, event-free survival, the HF survival score, was developed by Aaronson et al. (75) by analyzing data from 268 outpatients with severe HF, and then was prospectively validated in a cohort of 199 patients with similar characteristics. In this model, predictors of survival or urgent heart transplantation included presence of CAD, resting heart rate, LVEF, mean arterial pressure, interventricular conduction delay on electrocardiogram, serum sodium, and peak VO_2. The model effectively separated patients into low-, high-, and intermediate-risk categories, with 1-year survival ranging between 93% and 43% in low- and high-risk groups, respectively.

Another study that utilized data from the Digitalis Investigation Group analyzed factors predictive of mortality in 4,277 HF outpatients with reduced LVEF (<45%) who were in sinus rhythm and taking ACE inhibitors. In that study, LVEF, renal function, cardiomegaly, functional class, signs or symptoms of HF, blood pressure, and lower body mass index were associated with reduced 12-month survival. In addition to these variables, age and the use of nitrates at baseline were also predictive of 36-month mortality (76).

There are several prediction models for short-term mortality. Data from 949 patients who participated in the Outcomes of a Prospective Trial of Intravenous Milrinone for Exacerbations of Chronic Heart Failure (OPTIME-HF) study identified age, systolic blood pressure, New York Heart Association class, BUN, and serum sodium as predictors of 60-day mortality following hospitalization for decompensated HF (77). Recently published data from the Acute Decompensated Heart Failure National Registry (ADHERE) again identified factors associated with in-hospital mortality by analyzing 33,046 hospitalizations from 263 hospitals in the United States, and then validating the model with data from 32,229 additional hospitalizations (78). In this study, BUN, systolic blood pressure, and serum creatinine were most predictive of in-hospital mortality.

Several studies attempted to identify factors associated with increased mortality in HF patients with preserved systolic function. Data from 988 outpatients with HF and preserved systolic function who participated in the Digitalis Investigation Group study showed that glomerular filtration rate, New York Heart Association class, male gender, and older age were the strongest predictors of survival during 3.1 years of follow-up (79). Another study evaluated 2,498 patients with class 2 to 4 HF symptoms and LVEF >40% who underwent cardiac catheterization at Duke University. In addition to variables already identified in the Digitalis Investigation Group study, ejection fraction, CAD index, diabetes, peripheral vascular disease, and minority ethnic group were also predictive of 5-year mortality (80).

Studies have also developed prediction models for the outcome of hospital readmission. One study evaluated 1,129 elderly patients hospitalized with HF in 18 Connecticut hospitals who comprised the derivation cohort, and 1,047 similar patients in the validation cohort. Four factors were significantly associated with hospital readmission within 6 months: prior admission within 1 year, prior HF, diabetes, and creatinine >2.5 mg/dL. The readmission rates ranged between 26% in patients with no risk factors and 59% in patients with three or more risk factors (81). In another administrative database study of 17,448 survivors of hospitalization with HF, male sex, at least one prior admission within 6 months of the index admission, Deyo comorbidity score >1, and length of stay in the index hospitalization >7 days were predictive of hospital readmission within 6 months (26).

Although a multitude of other factors have been shown to be important predictors of mortality and hospital readmission in patients with HF, they have not been incorporated into clinical prediction models.

REFERENCES

1. American Heart Association. Heart disease and stroke statistics—2005 update. http://www.americanheart.org/presenter.jhtml?identifier=3000090. Accessed June 6, 2005.
2. Stewart S, MacIntyre K, Capewell S, et al. Heart failure and the aging population: an increasing burden in the 21st century? *Heart* (British Cardiac Society) 2003;89:49–53.
3. Levy D, Kenchaiah S, Larson MG, et al. Long-term trends in the incidence of and survival with heart failure. *N Engl J Med.* 2002;347:1397–1402.
4. Roger VL, Weston SA, Redfield MM, et al. Trends in heart failure incidence and survival in a community-based population. *JAMA.* 2004;292:344–350.
5. McCullough PA, Philbin EF, Spertus JA, et al. Confirmation of a heart failure epidemic: findings from the Resource Utilization Among Congestive Heart Failure (REACH) study. *J Am Coll Cardiol.* 2002;39:60–69.
6. Kitzman DW, Gardin JM, Gottdiener JS, et al. Importance of heart failure with preserved systolic function in patients ≥65 years of age. CHS Research Group. Cardiovascular Health Study. *Am J Cardiol.* 2001;87:413–419.
7. Psaty BM, Koepsell TD, Yanez ND, et al. Temporal patterns of antihypertensive medication use among older adults, 1989 through 1992. An effect of the major clinical trials on clinical practice? *JAMA.* 1995;273:1436–1438.
8. Hajjar I, Kotchen TA. Trends in prevalence, awareness, treatment, and control of hypertension in the United States, 1988–2000. *JAMA.* 2003;290:199–206.

9. Goldberg RJ, Yarzebski J, Lessard D, et al. A two-decades (1975 to 1995) long experience in the incidence, in-hospital and long-term case-fatality rates of acute myocardial infarction: a community-wide perspective. *J Am Coll Cardiol.* 1999;33:1533–1539.
10. Furman MI, Dauerman HL, Goldberg RJ, et al. Twenty-two-year (1975 to 1997) trends in the incidence, in-hospital and long-term case fatality rates from initial Q-wave and non-Q-wave myocardial infarction: a multi-hospital, community-wide perspective. *J Am Coll Cardiol.* 2001;37:1571–1580.
11. Gregg EW, Cadwell BL, Cheng YJ, et al. Trends in the prevalence and ratio of diagnosed to undiagnosed diabetes according to obesity levels in the U.S. *Diabetes Care.* 2004;27:2806–2812.
12. Okosun IS, Chandra KM, Boev A, et al. Abdominal adiposity in U.S. adults: prevalence and trends, 1960–2000. *Prev Med.* 2004;39:197–206.
13. Schocken DD, Arrieta MI, Leaverton PE, et al. Prevalence and mortality rate of congestive heart failure in the United States. *J Am Coll Cardiol.* 1992;20:301–306.
14. Bleumink GS, Knetsch AM, Sturkenboom MC, et al. Quantifying the heart failure epidemic: prevalence, incidence rate, lifetime risk and prognosis of heart failure. The Rotterdam study. *Eur Heart J.* 2004;25:1614–1619.
15. Lee DS, Mamdani MM, Austin PC, et al. Trends in heart failure outcomes and pharmacotherapy: 1992 to 2000. *Am J Med.* 2004;116:581–589.
16. Baker DW, Einstadter D, Thomas C, et al. Mortality trends for 23,505 Medicare patients hospitalized with heart failure in Northeast Ohio, 1991 to 1997. *Am Heart J.* 2003;146:258–264.
17. Stewart S, MacIntyre K, MacLeod MM, et al. Trends in hospitalization for heart failure in Scotland, 1990–1996. An epidemic that has reached its peak? *Eur Heart J.* 2001;22:209–217.
18. Schaufelberger M, Swedberg K, Koster M, et al. Decreasing one-year mortality and hospitalization rates for heart failure in Sweden; data from the Swedish Hospital Discharge Registry 1988 to 2000. *Eur Heart J.* 2004;25:300–307.
19. Hall RE, Tu JV. Hospitalization rates and length of stay for cardiovascular conditions in Canada, 1994 to 1999. *Can J Cardiol.* 2003;19:1123–1131.
20. Koelling TM, Chen RS, Lubwama RN, et al. The expanding national burden of heart failure in the United States: the influence of heart failure in women. *Am Heart J.* 2004;147:74–78.
21. Kozak LJ, Owings MF, Hall MJ. National Hospital Discharge Survey: 2001 annual summary with detailed diagnosis and procedure data. *Vital Health Stat.* 2004;13:1–198.
22. Johansen H, Strauss B, Arnold JM, et al. On the rise: the current and projected future burden of congestive heart failure hospitalization in Canada. *Can J Cardiol.* 2003;19:430–435.
23. Baker DW, Einstadter D, Husak SS, et al. Trends in postdischarge mortality and readmissions: has length of stay declined too far? *Arch Intern Med.* 2004;164:538–544.
24. MacIntyre K, Capewell S, Stewart S, et al. Evidence of improving prognosis in heart failure: trends in case fatality in 66,547 patients hospitalized between 1986 and 1995. *Circulation* 2000;102:1126–1131.
25. Kosiborod M, Lichtman JH, Wang Y, et al. National mortality trends in elderly patients hospitalized with heart failure between 1992 and 1999. *J Am Coll Cardiol.* 2004;43:239A–240A.
26. Krumholz HM, Parent EM, Tu N, et al. Readmission after hospitalization for congestive heart failure among Medicare beneficiaries. *Arch Intern Med.* 1997;157:99–104.
27. Braunstein JB, Anderson GF, Gerstenblith G, et al. Noncardiac comorbidity increases preventable hospitalizations and mortality among Medicare beneficiaries with chronic heart failure. *J Am Coll Cardiol.* 2003;42:1226–1233.
28. Masoudi FA, Havranek EP, Smith G, et al. Gender, age, and heart failure with preserved left ventricular systolic function. *J Am Coll Cardiol.* 2003;41:217–223.
29. Masoudi FA, Rathore SS, Wang Y, et al. National patterns of use and effectiveness of angiotensin-converting enzyme inhibitors in older patients with heart failure and left ventricular systolic dysfunction. *Circulation.* 2004;110:724–731.
30. Smith NL, Chan JD, Rea TD, et al. Time trends in the use of beta-blockers and other pharmacotherapies in older adults with congestive heart failure. *Am Heart J.* 2004;148:710–717.
31. Stafford RS, Radley DC. The underutilization of cardiac medications of proven benefit, 1990 to 2002. *J Am Coll Cardiol.* 2003;41:56–61.
32. Struthers AD, MacFadyen R, Fraser C, et al. Nonadherence with angiotensin-converting enzyme inhibitor therapy: a comparison of different ways of measuring it in patients with chronic heart failure. *J Am Coll Cardiol.* 1999;34:2072–2077.
33. Lloyd-Jones DM, Larson MG, Leip EP, et al. Lifetime risk for developing congestive heart failure: the Framingham Heart Study. *Circulation.* 2002;106:3068–3072.
34. Arciero TJ, Jacobsen SJ, Reeder GS, et al. Temporal trends in the incidence of coronary disease. *Am J Med.* 2004;117:228–233.
35. Lloyd-Jones DM, Larson MG, Beiser A, et al. Lifetime risk of developing coronary heart disease. *Lancet.* 1999;353:89–92.
36. He J, Ogden LG, Bazzano LA, et al. Risk factors for congestive heart failure in US men and women: NHANES I epidemiologic follow-up study. *Arch Intern Med.* 2001;161:996–1002.
37. Levy D, Larson MG, Vasan RS, et al. The progression from hypertension to congestive heart failure. *JAMA.* 1996;275:1557–1562.
38. Psaty BM, Manolio TA, Smith NL, et al. Time trends in high blood pressure control and the use of antihypertensive medications in older adults: the Cardiovascular Health Study. *Arch Intern Med.* 2002;162:2325–2332.
39. Lloyd-Jones DM, Evans JC, Larson MG, et al. Differential control of systolic and diastolic blood pressure: factors associated with lack of blood pressure control in the community. *Hypertension.* 2000;36:594–599.
40. Haider AW, Larson MG, Franklin SS, et al. Systolic blood pressure, diastolic blood pressure, and pulse pressure as predictors of risk for congestive heart failure in the Framingham Heart Study. *Ann Intern Med.* 2003;138:10–16.
41. Gregg EW, Cheng YJ, Cadwell BL, et al. Secular trends in cardiovascular disease risk factors according to body mass index in US adults. *JAMA.* 2005;293:1868–1874.
42. Ford ES, Mokdad AH, Giles WH. Trends in waist circumference among U.S. adults. *Obes Res.* 2003;11:1223–1231.
43. Mokdad AH, Ford ES, Bowman BA, et al. Prevalence of obesity, diabetes, and obesity-related health risk factors, 2001. *JAMA.* 2003;289:76–79.
44. Mokdad AH, Ford ES, Bowman BA, et al. Diabetes trends in the U.S.: 1990–1998. *Diabetes Care.* 2000;23:1278–1283.
45. Mokdad AH, Serdula MK, Dietz WH, et al. The spread of the obesity epidemic in the United States, 1991–1998. *JAMA.* 1999;282:1519–1522.
46. Mokdad AH, Serdula MK, Dietz WH, et al. The continuing epidemic of obesity in the United States. *JAMA.* 2000;284:1650–1651.
47. Mokdad AH, Bowman BA, Ford ES, et al. The continuing epidemics of obesity and diabetes in the United States. *JAMA.* 2001;286:1195–1200.
48. Greenlund KJ, Zheng ZJ, Keenan NL, et al. Trends in self-reported multiple cardiovascular disease risk factors among adults in the United States, 1991–1999. *Arch Intern Med.* 2004;164:181–188.
49. Haldeman GA, Croft JB, Giles WH, et al. Hospitalization of patients with heart failure: National Hospital Discharge Survey, 1985 to 1995. *Am Heart J.* 1999;137:352–360.
50. Ho KK, Pinsky JL, Kannel WB, et al. The epidemiology of heart failure: the Framingham study. *J Am Coll Cardiol.* 1993;22:6A–13A.
51. Kannel WB, Hjortland M, Castelli WP. Role of diabetes in congestive heart failure: the Framingham study. *Am J Cardiol.* 1974;34:29–34.
52. Kenchaiah S, Evans JC, Levy D, et al. Obesity and the risk of heart failure. *N Engl J Med.* 2002;347:305–313.
53. Saydah SH, Fradkin J, Cowie CC. Poor control of risk factors for vascular disease among adults with previously diagnosed diabetes. *JAMA.* 2004;291:335–342.
54. Kannel WB, D'Agostino RB, Silbershatz H, et al. Profile for estimating risk of heart failure. *Arch Intern Med.* 1999;159:1197–1204.
55. Kannel WB, Levy D, Cupples LA. Left ventricular hypertrophy and risk of cardiac failure: insights from the Framingham study. *J Cardiovasc Pharmacol.* 1987;10 (Suppl 6):S135–S140.
56. Tsang TS, Barnes ME, Gersh BJ, et al. Prediction of risk for first age-related cardiovascular events in an elderly population: the incremental value of echocardiography. *J Am Coll Cardiol.* 2003;42:1199–1205.

57. Drazner MH, Rame JE, Marino EK, et al. Increased left ventricular mass is a risk factor for the development of a depressed left ventricular ejection fraction within five years: the Cardiovascular Health Study. *J Am Coll Cardiol.* 2004;43:2207–2215.
58. Vasan RS, Sullivan LM, Roubenoff R, et al. Inflammatory markers and risk of heart failure in elderly subjects without prior myocardial infarction: the Framingham Heart Study. *Circulation.* 2003;107:1486–1491.
59. Vasan RS, Beiser A, D'Agostino RB, et al. Plasma homocysteine and risk for congestive heart failure in adults without prior myocardial infarction. *JAMA.* 2003;289:1251–1257.
60. Chae CU, Albert CM, Glynn RJ, et al. Mild renal insufficiency and risk of congestive heart failure in men and women ≥70 years of age. *Am J Cardiol.* 2003;92:682–686.
61. Gottdiener JS, Arnold AM, Aurigemma GP, et al. Predictors of congestive heart failure in the elderly: the Cardiovascular Health Study. *J Am Coll Cardiol.* 2000;35:1628–1637.
62. He J, Ogden LG, Bazzano LA, et al. Dietary sodium intake and incidence of congestive heart failure in overweight U.S. men and women: first National Health and Nutrition Examination Survey Epidemiologic Follow-up Study. *Arch Intern Med.* 2002;162: 1619–1624.
63. Walsh CR, Larson MG, Evans JC, et al. Alcohol consumption and risk for congestive heart failure in the Framingham Heart Study. *Ann Intern Med.* 2002;136:181–191.
64. Abramson JL, Williams SA, Krumholz HM, et al. Moderate alcohol consumption and risk of heart failure among older persons. *JAMA.* 2001;285:1971–1977.
65. Rathore SS, Foody JM, Wang Y, et al. Sex, quality of care, and outcomes of elderly patients hospitalized with heart failure: findings from the National Heart Failure Project. *Am Heart J.* 2005;149:121–128.
66. Gillum RF. Epidemiology of heart failure in the United States. *Am Heart J.* 1993;126:1042–1047.
67. Rathore SS, Foody JM, Wang Y, et al. Race, quality of care, and outcomes of elderly patients hospitalized with heart failure. *JAMA.* 2003;289:2517–2524.
68. Redfield MM, Jacobsen SJ, Burnett JC, Jr., et al. Burden of systolic and diastolic ventricular dysfunction in the community: appreciating the scope of the heart failure epidemic. *JAMA.* 2003;289: 194–202.
69. Gottdiener JS, McClelland RL, Marshall R, et al. Outcome of congestive heart failure in elderly persons: influence of left ventricular systolic function. The Cardiovascular Health Study. *Ann Intern Med.* 2002;137:631–639.
70. Vasan RS, Larson MG, Benjamin EJ, et al. Congestive heart failure in subjects with normal versus reduced left ventricular ejection fraction: prevalence and mortality in a population-based cohort. *J Am Coll Cardiol.* 1999;33:1948–1955.
71. Smith GL, Masoudi FA, Vaccarino V, et al. Outcomes in heart failure patients with preserved ejection fraction: mortality, readmission, and functional decline. *J Am Coll Cardiol.* 2003;41:1510–1518.
72. Wang TJ, Evans JC, Benjamin EJ, et al. Natural history of asymptomatic left ventricular systolic dysfunction in the community. *Circulation.* 2003;108:977–982.
73. Aurigemma GP, Gottdiener JS, Shemanski L, et al. Predictive value of systolic and diastolic function for incident congestive heart failure in the elderly: the Cardiovascular Health Study. *J Am Coll Cardiol.* 2001;37:1042–1048.
74. Lee D, Austin P, Rouleau J, et al. Predicting mortality among patients hospitalized for heart failure: derivation and validation of a clinical model. *JAMA.* 2003;290:2581–2587.
75. Aaronson KD, Schwartz JS, Chen TM, et al. Development and prospective validation of a clinical index to predict survival in ambulatory patients referred for cardiac transplant evaluation. *Circulation.* 1997;95:2660–2667.
76. Brophy JM, Dagenais GR, McSherry F, et al. A multivariate model for predicting mortality in patients with heart failure and systolic dysfunction. *Am J Med.* 2004;116:300–304.
77. Felker GM, Leimberger JD, Califf RM, et al. Risk stratification after hospitalization for decompensated heart failure. *J Card Fail.* 2004;10:460–466.
78. Fonarow GC, Adams KF, Jr., Abraham WT, et al. Risk stratification for in-hospital mortality in acutely decompensated heart failure: classification and regression tree analysis. *JAMA.* 2005;293:572–580.
79. Jones RC, Francis GS, Lauer MS. Predictors of mortality in patients with heart failure and preserved systolic function in the Digitalis Investigation Group trial. *J Am Coll Cardiol.* 2004;44: 1025–1029.
80. O'Connor CM, Gattis WA, Shaw L, et al. Clinical characteristics and long-term outcomes of patients with heart failure and preserved systolic function. *Am J Cardiol.* 2000;86:863–867.
81. Krumholz HM, Chen YT, Wang Y, et al. Predictors of readmission among elderly survivors of admission with heart failure. *Am Heart J.* 2000;139:72–77.

Cellular and Molecular Abnormalities in Failing Cardiac Myocytes

2

Rachel Wilson *Xiongwen Chen* *Steven R. Houser*

Congestive heart failure (CHF) is a syndrome characterized by poor pump performance of the heart, which initially leads to decreased exercise tolerance but eventually progresses to involve pulmonary and systemic congestion. It is the ultimate outcome of many cardiovascular diseases, including hypertension, ischemic coronary disease, idiopathic myopathies, and valvular disorders. Remodeling of the failing heart at the organ, cellular, and molecular levels leads to progressive deterioration of cardiac pump function and arrhythmia, the major causes of morbidity and mortality in heart failure (HF) patients. In this chapter, we will focus on changes that occur in individual cardiac myocytes at the cellular and molecular levels that cause depressed cardiac contractility (the ability of the muscle to develop force and shorten) and lethal arrhythmias. The knowledge on this topic is substantial and has been obtained from studies of failing human myocytes and tissues and from failing myocytes from animal models in which heart failure was induced by increasing hemodynamic stress (pressure and volume overload), occlusion of coronary arteries (myocardial infarction), rapid pacing, or transgenetic approaches (gene overexpression or knockout) in mice. Throughout the chapter we will identify areas of consensus and those that still are unresolved. In addition, we will briefly discuss the most recent advances on the idea that CHF can result from excess myocyte death and cardiac repair may be possible by generating new myocardium.

DECREASED MYOCYTE CONTRACTILITY RESERVE IS CENTRALLY INVOLVED IN HEART FAILURE

Depressed contractility of cardiac myocytes plays a critical role in heart failure. In the mildest early stages of HF, slowing of myocyte contraction and relaxation rates and prolongation of the action potential duration have been consistently observed (1). In advanced HF, force production and shortening magnitude are normal or even greater than normal (2) at slow beating rates (<30 per minute), but decrease (or remain constant) when heart rate increases (negative force-frequency relationship). This is contrary to the relationship in nonfailing myocytes, where increasing the heart rate causes force production and shortening magnitude to increase (positive force-frequency relationship) (2). The responses of failing myocytes to high extracellular Ca^{2+} and adrenergic stimulation are also significantly reduced. These studies show that the fundamental cellular alterations of failing myocytes allow for contractile function to be maintained at rest, when the heart rate is slow, but lead to the inability of the myocytes to increase their contractile performance (contractility) when demand for additional cardiac output is increased. We and others have termed this phenomenon *depressed contractility reserve*.

ABNORMAL CA^{2+} HANDLING IS PRIMARILY RESPONSIBLE FOR DECREASED MYOCYTE CONTRACTILITY

With each heartbeat, depolarization of the myocyte surface membrane causes opening of Ca^{2+} channels that reside in the transverse tubules. The subsequent Ca^{2+} influx induces Ca^{2+} release from the sarcoplasmic reticulum (SR). The resultant increase in cytosolic $[Ca^{2+}]$ (the so-called Ca^{2+} transient) activates myofibrillar proteins to cause contraction. The force and speed of contraction are regulated by varying these Ca^{2+}-dependent processes.

Myocyte contractility is depressed in CHF, with the fundamental defect being an inability to increase force much beyond that exhibited at resting levels. By studying animal models and explanted failing human hearts, multiple causes of depressed myocyte contractility in heart failure have been revealed, including altered cytoskeleton (3); changes in myofilament function human CHF (4); animal CHF (5); altered β-adrenergic signaling (6); and abnormal myocyte Ca^{2+} regulation and excitation-contraction coupling (ECC) (1). In this chapter, we will focus on alterations in myocyte electrophysiological and contractile function in CHF, with a concentration on those factors producing alterations in Ca^{2+} regulation.

One of the common observations made in failing cardiac myocytes from both human patients and animal models is that the action potential (AP) is prolonged (Fig. 2-1). There are multiple contributors to AP prolongation, with reduced repolarizing potassium (K^+) currents playing a central role, as discussed later. Parallel to the prolonged APs, the Ca^{2+} transient is also prolonged in myocytes from explanted hearts of human HF patients (7) and animal CHF models. At very slow pacing frequencies, the relatively normal contractility seen in cardiac myocytes from human patients with end-stage cardiac disease corresponds with a maintained amplitude of the Ca^{2+} transient similar to that seen in nonfailing human myocytes. However, the amplitude of the Ca^{2+} transient is decreased [in human (7) and animal models (8)] at physiological pacing rates. In addition, diastolic Ca^{2+} concentration becomes elevated (9) and the decay of the Ca^{2+} transient is slowed (7,9). These changes contribute to diastolic dysfunction and eventually to poor systolic (pump) performance.

The regulation of the Ca^{2+} transient is abnormal in failing cardiac myocytes. In normal cardiomyocytes, increasing the beating rate causes an increase in the amplitude of the Ca^{2+} transient and the force of contraction (positive force-frequency relationship) (Fig. 2-2). In myocytes with mild to moderate hypertrophy, the peak systolic Ca^{2+} is normal under basal conditions (e.g., low stimulation frequency), but becomes depressed when conditions that increase cellular Ca^{2+} loading are imposed (faster pacing rates, high extracellular Ca^{2+} or catecholamine exposure). In severely failing myocytes (e.g., myocytes from end-stage human heart failure), peak systolic Ca^{2+} and force (or shortening) are both close to normal at very slow pacing rates. However, when the beating rate is increased there is

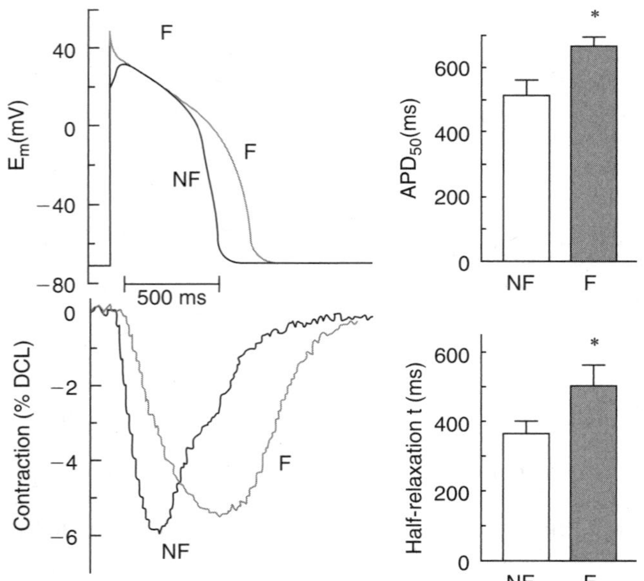

Figure 2-1 Action potential and contraction changes in heart failure. Representative action potentials **(top)** and contraction **(bottom)**, measured as % of diastolic cell length from nonfailing (NF) and failing (F) myocytes. Action potential duration and contraction duration were significantly longer in failing (F) than nonfailing (NF) myocytes. All myocytes were paced at 0.5 Hz.

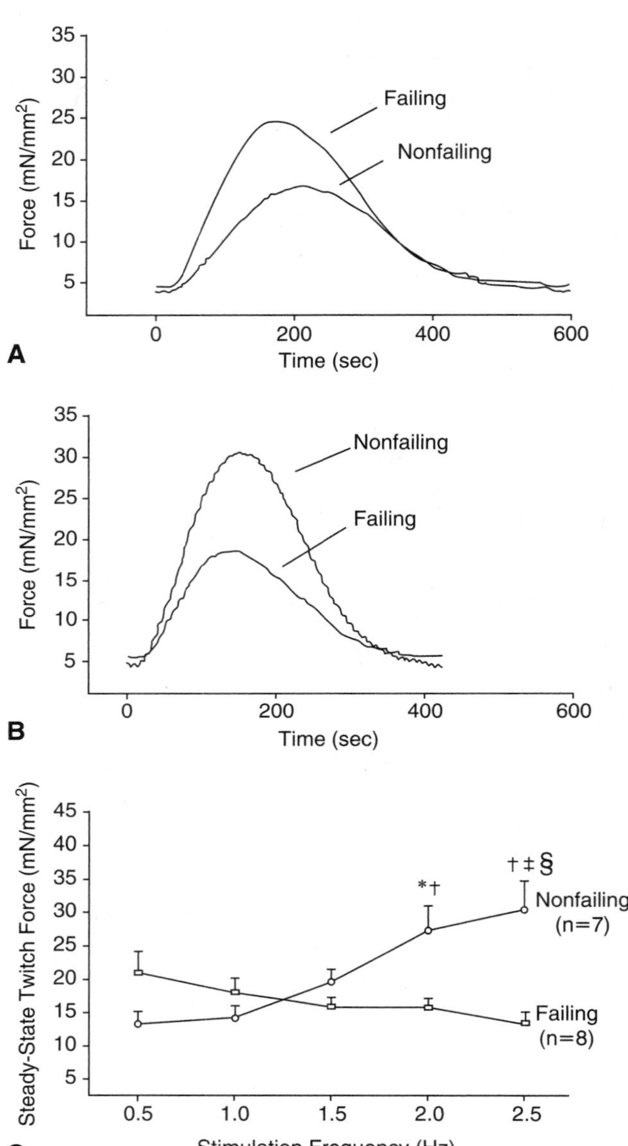

Figure 2-2 Force-frequency relationship in nonfailing and failing myocardium. Steady-state twitch tracings (1.75 mM Ca^{2+}) of trabeculae from failing and nonfailing human hearts at **(A)** 0–5 Hz and **(B)** 2.5 Hz are represented. **(C)** Average steady-state twitch force as a function of stimulation frequency in failing and nonfailing myocardium. The positive relationship in nonfailing human ventricular muscle is reversed in failing muscle.
* $p < 0.05$ when compared to within-group twitch force at 1.0 Hz; † $p < 0.01$ when compared to within-group twitch force at 0.5 Hz; ‡ $p < 0.01$ when compared to within-group twitch force at 1.0 Hz; § $p < 0.05$ when comparing between-groups twitch force.

either no change or a decrease in peak systolic Ca^{2+} and force of contraction (negative force-frequency relationship). Furthermore, diastolic Ca^{2+} in failing myocytes increases more than in nonfailing myocytes. These results strongly support the idea that changes in myocyte Ca^{2+} handling are a final common pathway for progressive deterioration of cardiac pump function in CHF. More support for this notion comes from studies that show that the transition from compensated hypertrophy to the early stages of CHF occurs when myocytes first lose their ability to normally maintain Ca^{2+} balance, and correction of Ca^{2+} handling defects is able to delay or prevent this transition (10).

ABNORMAL EXCITATION-CONTRACTION COUPLING IN FAILING MYOCYTES

Ca^{2+} transients (dynamic cytosolic Ca^{2+} changes) are brought about by a combination of Ca^{2+} influx and SR Ca^{2+} release. When a cardiac myocyte is depolarized, an action potential is elicited and Ca^{2+} enters the myocyte down its transmembrane electrochemical gradient through the L-type calcium channel (LTCC). This Ca^{2+} influx, termed the *Ca^{2+} current*, I_{Ca}, then triggers a larger amount of Ca^{2+} to be released from the SR by activating the Ca^{2+} release channel (ryanodine receptor, RyR) through a mechanism termed *calcium-induced calcium release (CICR)* (11,12). The efficacy of I_{Ca} as a trigger to induce SR Ca^{2+} release is termed the ECC gain. These processes cause the free cytosolic Ca^{2+} concentration to increase rapidly and Ca^{2+} binds to the thin filament protein troponin C to induce contraction. The rate and magnitude of myocyte contraction (force and shortening) are largely determined by the amount of Ca^{2+} entering the cytoplasm with each systole. The duration of contraction and the rate of relaxation are primarily determined by processes that reduce cytosolic $[Ca^{2+}]$. Cytosolic Ca^{2+} is lowered by three principal processes: sequestration back into the SR via SR Ca^{2+}-ATPase (SERCA), transport out of the cell via the sarcolemmal Ca^{2+}-ATPase, and transport out of the cell by the Na^+/Ca^{2+} exchanger (NCX) (Fig. 2-3, ECC). In a steady state, the Ca^{2+} that enters with each action potential is removed from the cell primarily by the NCX, and the Ca^{2+} that is released from the SR is resequestered there via SERCA. The amplitude and duration of the Ca^{2+} transient are regulated in the normal heart to orchestrate changes in myocyte contractility. In CHF this regulation is abnormal and results in Ca^{2+} transients of reduced size and prolonged duration. Decreased SR Ca^{2+} release is now known to be the principal reason for the reduced size of the Ca^{2+} transient in HF. Significantly, it appears that multiple cellular defects can contribute to the reduced SR Ca^{2+} release of the failing myocyte.

The ECC process is abnormal in failing myocytes from human and most animal models and contributes to the reduced size of the Ca^{2+} transient. In a rat hypertrophy/HF model, it has been shown that $I_{Ca\text{-}L}$ is a less effective trigger of SR Ca^{2+} release in hypertrophied and failing myocytes. This defective signaling could be rescued in hypertrophied (but not failing) myocytes by exposure to β-adrenergic agonists, which increase I_{Ca} and SR Ca^{2+} load. We and others have also shown that Ca^{2+} release from the SR in failing cardiomyocytes is disorganized and this contributes to reduced Ca^{2+} transient size (13,14). Furthermore, in some animal CHF models where there is no change of SR Ca^{2+} load, the Ca^{2+} transients are smaller than in normal cardiac myocytes (8). Cannell et al. (15) and Gomez et al. (8) found that in spontaneously hypertensive rats (SHRs) the ability of $I_{Ca\text{-}L}$ to trigger calcium release from the SR in both hypertrophied and failing hearts was reduced (a reduction in ECC gain). Several models were proposed to explain these ECC defects. These include a decreased density of T-tubules, an increased distance between the sarcolemmal LTCC and RyR on the face of the junctional SR membrane, and mismatch of the numbers or properties of the LTCC and RyR. He et al. (16) reported a decrease in T-tubule density in tachycardia-induced failing canine myocytes. However, this is not supported by a recent, preliminary report in failing human myocytes. In addition, reduced ECC gain does not adequately explain the fact that Ca^{2+} transients are similar in normal and failing human myocytes at slow pacing rates and only become significantly different when the pacing rate increases. In this regard, a frequency-dependent abnormality in ECC, decrease in the size of $I_{Ca\text{-}L}$, or its efficacy as a trigger of SR Ca release could be responsible for the reduction in SR Ca^{2+} release at fast heart rates in failing human myocytes. The respective roles of the SR Ca^{2+} load and the L-type calcium current in abnormal ECC in failing myocytes will be discussed in some detail below.

β-Adrenergic Signaling

Physiologically, ECC is primarily regulated via the sympathetic neurohormones norepinephrine and epinephrine, which increase cardiac myocyte force-generating capacity and heart rate. Catecholamines mediate their chronotropic and inotropic effects by binding to the seven transmembrane spanning β-adrenergic receptors ($\beta\text{-AR}_S$) (primarily β_1 and β_2 subtypes), which couple to adenylyl cyclase via stimulatory G-proteins to produce cAMP (Fig. 2-3). There is some evidence that β_2-AR can couple to inhibitory G-proteins, but this topic will not be discussed in this chapter. Increased intracellular cAMP activates protein kinase A (PKA), which phosphorylates multiple proteins to induce increased myocyte force-generating capacity, while decreasing the duration of contraction. PKA phosphorylation of the LTCC causes an increased channel open probability and an increased Ca^{2+} influx ($I_{Ca\text{-}L}$) with each action potential. This Ca^{2+} increases the efficacy of EC coupling and supplies the Ca^{2+} needed to increase SR Ca^{2+} stores. Phosphorylation of phospholamban (PLB, an inhibitor of SERCA) removes its inhibition of SERCA, thereby increasing SERCA activity and causing more Ca^{2+} to be transported into the SR, again causing the SR Ca^{2+} load to increase. PKA also phosphorylates the SR Ca^{2+} release channel (RyR), causing an increase in RyR open probability and contributing to increased SR Ca^{2+} release. PKA also phosphorylates troponin C and the pacemaker-related so-called funny channel to modulate myofilament Ca^{2+} binding affinity and the rate of firing of pacemaker cells,

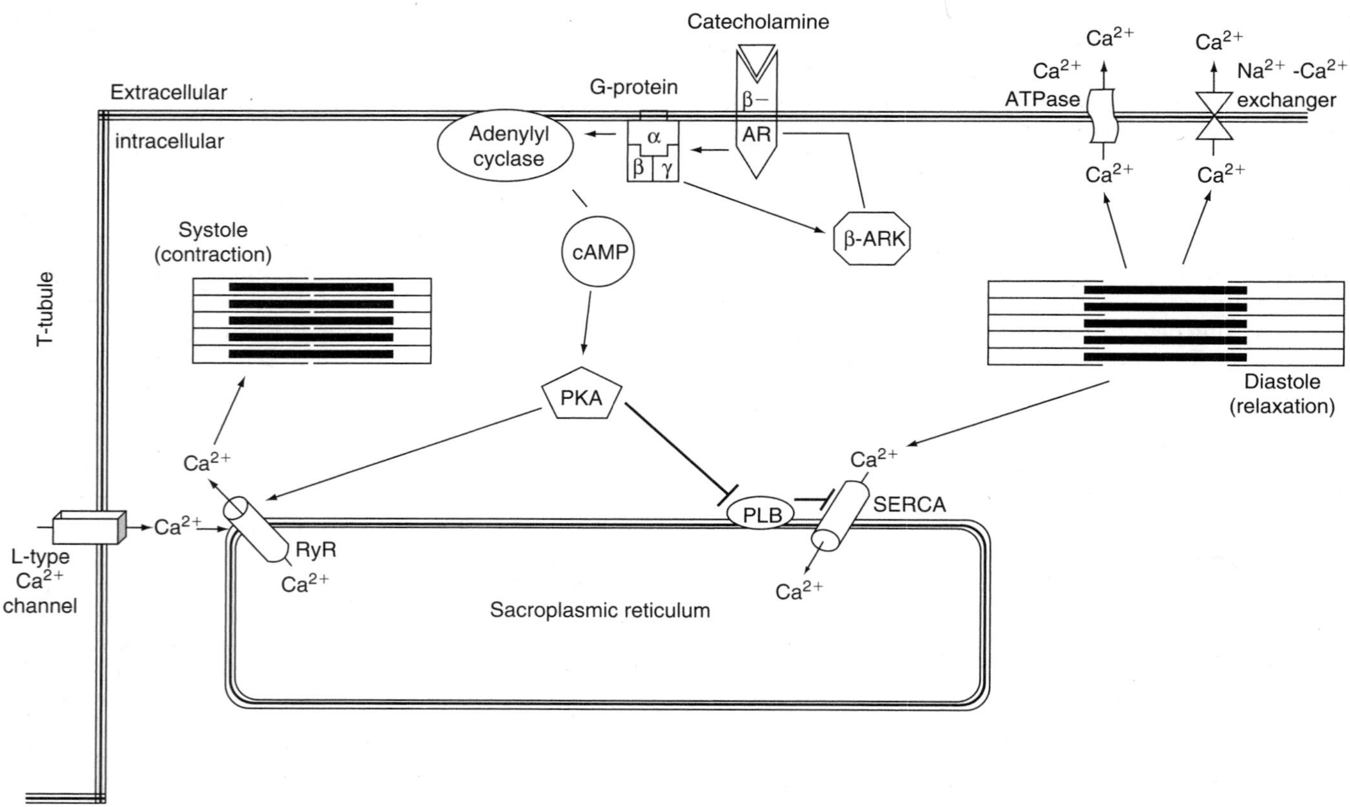

Figure 2-3 Excitation-contraction coupling and adrenergic pathway. Cardiac contraction is initiated by the influx of extracellular calcium through L-type calcium channels (LTCCs) in response to electric stimulation. The rise in intracellular calcium triggers calcium release from the sarcoplasmic reticulum (SR) via the ryanodine receptor (RyR). Calcium then associates with troponin C in the sarcomere and stimulates contraction (systole). Calcium is released from the sarcomere (diastole) and removed the cytoplasm by resequestration into the SR by the SR calcium ATPase (SERCA), extrusion from the cell by the sarcolemmal sodium-calcium exchanger (NCX), or extrusion from the cell by the sarcolemmal calcium ATPase. Activation of the β-adrenergic receptor (β-AR) by catecholamine binding activates adenylyl cyclase through a G-protein, generating cAMP, which activates protein kinase A (PKA). PKA phosphorylates the RyR and phospholamban (PLB), which modulates the activity of SERCA. Activation of β-AR kinase (β-ARK) by β-AR signaling creates a negative feedback loop.

respectively. The net effect of sympathetic stimulation is to enhance myocyte contractility and relaxation by increasing the size of the Ca^{2+} transient and hastening the rate of its decay.

In conditions of sustained pathological hemodynamic stress that lead to HF, the sympathetic nervous system is chronically upregulated in an attempt to maintain cardiac output. This persistent sympathetic activation produces abnormalities in adrenergic signaling that reduce contractility reserve in failing cardiac myocytes. β-adrenergic signaling pathways can activate β-adrenergic receptor kinases (β-ARKs, members of the G-protein coupled receptor kinase family, GRKs), which act on the β-AR to decrease its activity in a negative feedback mechanism (17) (Fig. 2-3). Sustained exposure to β-agonists results in attenuation of signaling through this pathway by a combination of receptor phosphorylation, receptor internalization, reduced receptor protein synthesis, and increased receptor degradation (18). Phosphorylation of β-ARs by PKA or GRKs (19–21) induces endocytosis of agonist-bound receptors (22). For GPCRs, this can occur via two pathways: clathrin-coated pits or caveolae. β_2-adrenergic receptors are internalized preferentially by the clathrin-coated pit pathway (23), though there is evidence that localization to caveolae is necessary for the physiological activity of the β_2-AR (24).

β-Adrenergic Signaling in Hypertrophy and Heart Failure

A variety of disruptions in the β-adrenergic signaling pathways have been observed in heart failure. Chronic upregulation of sympathetic nervous system activity in CHF causes increased circulating catecholamines (25,26). This leads to one of the prominent features of the failing heart—desensitization and downregulation of β-ARs

(27,28). Many studies have shown that β_1-AR mRNA and receptor number decrease by approximately 50% in human heart failure (29), but no change in either parameter for β_2-ARs occurs (29).

Studies employing transgenic mouse models have further emphasized the important role in β_1-ARs in heart failure. Overexpression of β_1-ARs in mouse myocardium causes hypertrophy and interstitial fibrosis, leading to cardiac dysfunction with aging (30,31). Functional studies of these mice indicated that contractility and rate of isovolumic relaxation are initially increased in young animals. However, both systolic and diastolic function were impaired and contractility and relaxation declined steadily with age (32). It is clear that persistent overstimulation of the β_1-AR in healthy mouse hearts is maladaptive, and evidence from some studies indicates that the mechanism involves apoptosis (33,34).

In contrast to the significant downregulation of β_1-ARs in heart failure, there is no major change in the number of β_2-ARs, though their activity is depressed due to uncoupling from adenylyl cyclase (27). The change in the β_1/β_2-AR ratio may point to an increased role of β_2-AR activity in conditions where β_1-ARs are suppressed. This is supported by studies in which β_2-ARs were overexpressed. At lower levels (60- to 100-fold increase above endogenous levels), cardiac function was enhanced independent of ligand binding: contraction amplitude increased, calcium transients were greater, and relaxation times were faster in the transgenic mice than their nontransgenic littermates (35,36). However, in transgenic mice with higher myocardial β_2-AR transgenic overexpression (200- to 350-fold increase above endogenous levels), there was an age-dependent progression to cardiac myopathy (35,37).

Because of the dose-dependent disparities in β_2-AR, several studies have examined whether β_2-AR overexpression is advantageous or deleterious in cardiac hypertrophy and failure. β_2-AR-overexpressing mice subjected to transverse aortic constriction (TAC) to induce chronic pressure overload exhibited more severe heart failure than did sham-operated control animals (38), and also showed a decrease in transgene expression and in β_2-AR-ligand binding (39). However, cardiac-specific β_2-AR overexpression was beneficial in transgenic mice subjected to coronary ligation (myocardial infarction, MI). Infarct size and hypertrophy were comparable in transgenic and wild-type mice, but the β_2-AR-overexpressing animals exhibited higher contractility, lower left ventricular end diastolic pressure (LVEDP), and a lower incidence of pleural effusion after 9 weeks of infarction (40). Our view of these data is that β_2-AR signaling is cardioprotective, at least at normal or modestly increased levels of activity. The data suggesting that persistent β_1 activity is ultimately harmful while β_2 signaling is protective imply that these adrenergic receptors are coupled to different downstream signaling pathways. There is some evidence suggesting that β_2 activity is antiapoptotic and this could be related to its beneficial role in cardiac stress states (41).

The desensitization of β-ARs in heart failure is due in part to the actions of β-AR kinase 1 (βARK1, also known as GRK2) (20–22,42). Cytosolic βARK binds to the $G_{\beta}\gamma$ subunit freed by β-AR activation of the G-protein, which allows it to translocate to the plasma membrane and phosphorylate the agonist-bound β-AR (42). In the heart, βARK forms a stable cytosolic complex with phosphoinositide 3-kinase (PI3K). Translocation of βARK to the plasma membrane has been shown to facilitate PI3K movement to the membrane as well, which appears to play an important role in the internalization of the β-AR in response to catecholamine stimulation (43,44).

Many studies have supported the role of PI3K in cardiac hypertrophy and failure (45). Cardiac-specific constitutive activation of the p110α subunit of PI3K caused a significant increase in heart size, and constitutive activation of a downstream effector of PI3K, Akt, also increased cardiac hypertrophy (45). In response to short-term transverse aortic constriction (TAC) in the mouse, the subunit p110γPI3K (PI3Kγ) was activated without an increase in protein levels, and this activation was shown to be βARK-dependent (46,47). Cardiac-specific overexpression of an inactive PI3Kγ mutant prevented β-AR desensitization and internalization, but there is evidence that other isoforms can compensate for the loss of PI3Kγ (48).

Another characteristic of the β-adrenergic pathway in heart failure is that persistent elevation in circulating catecholamines causes a disruption in the binding of β-ARs to their respective G-proteins (27). In normal myocardium, β_2-AR/G_i coupling appears to act as a brake on the β-AR/G_s/adenylyl cyclase pathway (49–53). $G_{\alpha i}$ levels are increased in failing hearts (50), which, combined with the altered ratio of β_1/β_2-ARs as discussed earlier, indicates a prominent role in β_2-AR/$G_{\alpha i}$ signaling in heart failure. This has been further supported by studies crossing transgenic mice overexpressing β_2-AR with mice overexpressing an inactivated $G_{\alpha i}$ subunit. The β_2-AR/heterozygous $G_{\alpha i2}$ knockout mice developed earlier and more robust cardiac hypertrophy and earlier heart failure, and the β_2-AR/homozygous $G_{\alpha i2}$ knockout mice died within 4 days of birth (51). These data indicate an essential role for $G_{\alpha i2}$ in protection from chronically increased β_2-AR signaling (53).

There is now ample evidence that β_2-AR can couple promiscuously to multiple signaling pathways (including $G_{\alpha i}$ and $G_{\alpha s}$) and is involved in the regulation of cardiac contractility, hypertrophy, and heart failure. β_2-AR activation has been shown to activate a G_i-$G_{\beta\gamma}$-PI3K–mediated survival pathway (41). The factors that regulate how, why, and when β_2-ARs switch their coupling from G_s to G_i in myocytes are not well known at present but could involve signaling involving L-type Ca^{2+} channels and MAP kinase pathways (54,55).

β-Blockers as Therapy for Heart Failure

As previously elucidated, multiple steps in the β-adrenergic signaling pathway are disrupted in the hypertrophied and failing heart, primarily involving the downregulation and desensitization of the β-ARs. Paradoxically, however, inhibitors of the β-ARs (β-blockers), which might exacerbate the disruption of β-adrenergic signaling in heart failure and are known to precipitate negative inotropy at sufficiently high concentrations, have demonstrated a noteworthy efficiency in preventing pathological remodeling in heart failure, improving cardiac function, and even improving survival in heart failure patients (6,56). Though the mechanisms for the improvement seen with β-blockers have not yet been completely elucidated, recent studies have provided insight into possible mechanisms (57,58).

One of many possible mechanisms for improving cardiac function in CHF is the reduction of persistently activated adenylyl cyclase, thereby decreasing cAMP levels and PKA activity and correcting the phosphorylation defects of Ca^{2+} regulatory proteins. One of the downstream effectors of PKA is the RyR, and hyperphosphorylation of the RyR is thought to be involved in dysregulated Ca^{2+} in heart failure (58). Reducing the hyperphosphorylation of the RyR restores RyR function toward normal, which may partially explain the beneficial effects of β-blockers on contractility and adrenergic responsiveness in CHF patients (59). β-blockers may also help restore the energy balance in failing hearts, which are typically energy-deficient and starved for high-energy phosphates (59). Also, β-blockers have been shown to reverse some HF-specific alterations in cardiac gene expression, another possible mechanism of the beneficial effects of β-blockers (59). While the mechanisms for the beneficial effects of β-blockers are still not clear, this represents a major area for exploration for novel CHF therapies.

THE L-TYPE CA^{2+} CURRENT (I_{CA-L}) IN FAILING MYOCYTES

The LTCC plays multiple critical roles in the function of cardiac myocytes. The LTCC is responsible for the upstroke of the action potential (AP) in the sinoatrial node (SA) cells and contributes to the pacemaker activity of these cells. The current through the LTCC is also responsible for the conduction of the AP through the AV node and the plateau phase of the AP in the atrial, ventricular, and His-Purkinje systems (60). The major function of the LTCC in cardiac myocytes is to control the influx of Ca^{2+} ions that serve as the trigger for SR Ca^{2+} release (ECC). Ca^{2+} influx through the LTCC elevates the $[Ca^{2+}]$ in a diffusion-limited subsarcolemmal space between the T-tubules and junctional SR, which are in close proximity. Accumulation of subsarcolemmal Ca^{2+} promotes Ca^{2+} binding to and opening of the Ca^{2+} release channel (RyR) in the junctional SR. The Ca^{2+} influx through LTCC must be balanced by Ca^{2+} efflux through the NCX and sarcolemmal Ca^{2+}-ATPase. Unbalanced fluxes either load or unload the SR until flux balance is restored in a new steady state.

Changes in the abundance, isoform type, regulation, or localization of the LTCC could cause abnormal Ca^{2+} handling in CHF. These topics have been well-studied, but the results are far from conclusive. In general, the consensus of these studies is that in mild to moderate hypertrophy, LTCC abundance and Ca^{2+} influx are either increased or unchanged (61–63). These changes are associated with a transient increase in myocyte contractility and the initiation of pathological cardiac hypertrophy. In severe left ventricular hyperthrophy (LVH) and CHF, available evidence suggests that LTCC abundance and Ca^{2+} influx are either unchanged (64–66) or reduced (67). These changes are associated with a progressive reduction in cardiac contractility and dilation of the ventricular wall. The data from animal models fall into this generalized scheme very well, but the data from terminal human heart failure patients are less uniform, possibly due to a larger variation in disease etiology and to the fact that some human studies have been performed using very poor-quality isolated myocyte preparations. Supporting our hypothesis are studies showing that dihydropyridine (DHP) binding is unchanged in idiopathic dilated hearts but is decreased in ischemic cardiomyopathy. A study performed by Takahashi et al. (67) examined DHP binding sites in CHF myocardium with four etiologies (ischemic, idiopathic, hypertensive, and congenital) and found that LTCC expression was down by ~47% at both mRNA and DHP binding (protein) levels in all groups. These results are consistent with a study in which I_{Ca} was measured in nonfailing and failing human myocytes from our group, in which we suggest a significant reduction in LTCC density in end-stage human heart failure (68).

One study in human myocardium has explored the idea that LTCC isoform shifts occur in CHF. This study revealed the switching of splicing isoforms at segment 3 in domain IV in failing human hearts using competitive RT-PCR (69). The functional significance of these isoform shifts is largely unknown and deserve further study.

In our view, the most reliable approach to determine the density of functional LTCCs is with biophysical techniques. LTCC abundance and function have been studied at the whole-cell and single-channel levels (61–63). These studies suggest that in mild to moderate hypertrophy, I_{Ca-L} increases or remains constant and I_{Ca-L} kinetics do not change, whereas in severe cardiac hypertrophy and heart failure I_{Ca-L} density decreases but there are few, if any, changes of channel properties (61–63). In this regard, a few studies have found that I_{Ca-L} decay is slowed in HF and have suggested that this slower decay might result in larger Ca^{2+} influx and contribute to the prolongation of action potentials in failing cardiac myocytes (70). In a pacing-induced dog model of CHF, I_{Ca-L} density was not changed but the inactivation at positive potentials was slowed, which resulted in a higher plateau of APs (71). These ideas need further study.

There are fewer studies on I_{Ca-L} in human cardiac myocytes, in part because of inherent difficulties in obtaining suitable samples of viable cardiac tissue. Some studies did not find significant difference of I_{Ca-L} density between failing and nonfailing ventricular myocytes (9,68,72,73). However, these experiments were all performed at very slow pacing frequencies. At slow pacing rates, even with impaired mechanics, the LTCC will be able to reset itself before a subsequent stimulation, regardless of resting (diastolic) membrane potential. This is relevant because Shin et al. (74) found that diastolic membrane voltage (e.g., −80 to −50 mV) modifies the decay of I_{Ca-L} and this modification is impaired in failing myocytes at or near physiological pacing rates. Therefore, I_{Ca-L} decreases when the beating frequency is increased in failing human myocytes (75). These results suggest that the negative force-frequency relationship seen in CHF involves a frequency-dependent depression of Ca^{2+} influx through the LTCC.

More recent studies of failing human myocytes have suggested that LTCC density is reduced and that basal properties of the LTCC are altered. Schroder et al. (76) found that the LTCC current density was not altered in failing myocytes (whole-cell measurements), but the open probability of individual LTCCs in failing human cardiac myocytes was increased. These results strongly support the idea that LTCC number is reduced in terminal HF but LTCC activity is increased to maintain $I_{Ca\text{-}L}$ density. Another indication that LTCC number is reduced in CHF comes from studies from He et al. (16), who reported a decreased gating current in failing cardiac myocytes from a pacing-induced canine heart failure model, even though $I_{Ca\text{-}L}$ density was not altered. The most definitive study on this topic by Chen et al. (68) found no differences in basal I_{Ca} density in human HF myocytes. However, the maximal $I_{Ca\text{-}L}$ density after exposure either to the LTCC agonist Bay K 8644 or maximally effective concentrations of β-adrenergic agonist (isoproterenol) was significantly smaller in failing myocytes (Fig. 2-4). These experiments provide strong support for the idea that the reduction in LTCC number in heart failure is accompanied by an increase in basal LTCC phosphorylation, which maintains LTCC density under normal conditions but limits the capacity for phosphorylation-mediated regulation of $I_{Ca\text{-}L}$. This is undoubtedly involved in the inability of the failing human heart to increase contractility much beyond that seen in the basal state, as further discussed later.

The electromechanical defects of the failing heart are caused by alterations in the abundance and isoform type of Ca^{2+} regulatory proteins as well as by posttranslational modifications. Many studies have shown that in failing myocardium, the responsiveness of $I_{Ca\text{-}L}$ to β-adrenergic stimulation is diminished (9,73). This is a critical defect since β-adrenergic–mediated increases in Ca^{2+} influx

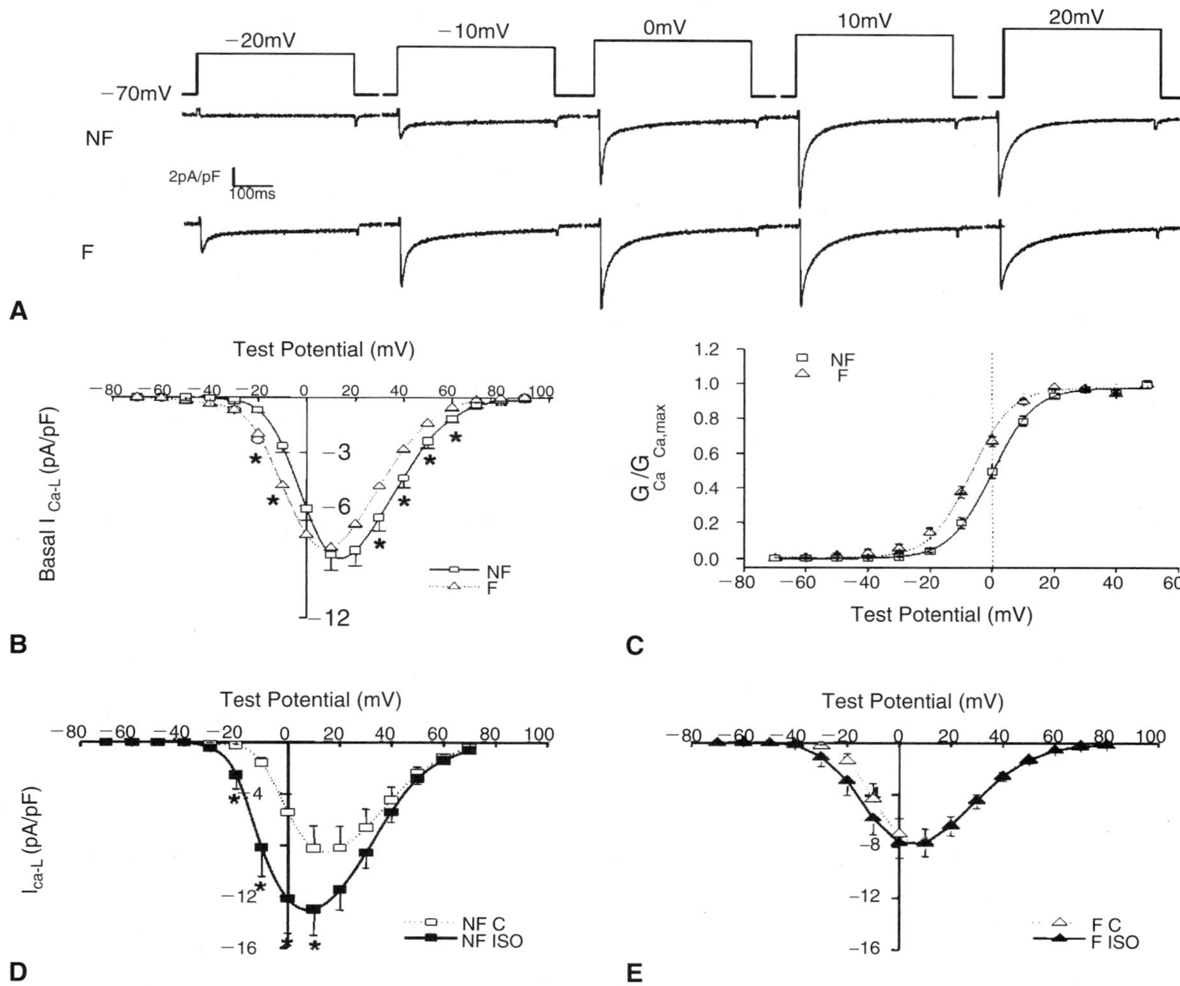

Figure 2-4 L-type Ca^{2+} current properties in nonfailing and failing human left ventricular myocytes. **(A)** Representative L-type Ca^{2+} currents. Note that the $I_{Ca\text{-}L}$ densities are not similar in these cells but the voltage dependence of activation is shifted to negative voltages in the failing myocytes. **(B)** $I_{Ca\text{-}L}$-voltage relationships in nonfailing (NF) and failing (F) myocytes. Maximal $I_{Ca\text{-}L}$ density is not significantly different between groups. **(C)** Voltage dependency of $I_{Ca\text{-}L}$ activation in nonfailing and failing myocytes fit with the Boltzmann equation. Voltage at which G_{Ca} is half of its maximally activated value (V = 0.5) in nonfailing myocytes is significantly more positive (p = 0.001) than in failing myocytes. **(D)** and **(E)** Effect of 1 μM isoproterenol (ISO) on the $I_{Ca\text{-}L}$-voltage relationship in nonfailing and failing myocytes. ISO increases $I_{Ca\text{-}L}$ significantly in nonfailing myocytes but has little effect in failing myocytes. Significant differences ($p < 0.05$, repeated ANOVA) between NF versus F (*) as indicated.

through the LTCC is a major mechanism for increasing SR Ca^{2+} stores and contractility. Ming et al. (77) showed a diminished responsiveness of I_{Ca-L} to adrenergic stimulation in hypertrophied/failing guinea pig hearts, and Laurent et al. (78) observed similar defects in ventricular myocytes from a pacing-induced canine HF model. The defects in I_{Ca-L} regulation by adrenergic signaling pathways are multifactorial and include reductions in β-AR density and uncoupling of agonist binding from activation of adenylyl cyclase. There are a few studies that are not consistent with the idea of blunted adrenergic effects on cardiac Ca^{2+} channels in failing myocytes. For example, Mewes and Ravens (72) did not find any difference in response of I_{Ca-L} to forskolin (an adenylyl cyclase activator) between failing and nonfailing ventricular myocytes. In another study, stimulation of I_{Ca-L} by the β_2 adrenergic system was enhanced in failing ventricular myocytes (79). This last observation suggests that β-receptor subtype signaling may be altered in HF, as discussed earlier in this chapter.

THE NA^+/CA^{2+} EXCHANGER IN THE FAILING HEART

The NCX is the major route for Ca^{2+} efflux in ventricular myocytes (80). The NCX removes Ca^{2+} from the cytoplasm at normal resting potentials (−80 mV) and during all but the earliest portion of the AP. The energy for this transport is derived from the Na^+ electrochemical gradient. This Na^+-mediated Ca^{2+} efflux is termed *forward-mode NCX*. This represents the Ca^{2+} efflux that balances Ca^{2+} influx through the L-type Ca^{2+} channel.

When the membrane potential is depolarized and/or intracellular Na^+ increases, the changes in the Na^+ and Ca^{2+} electrochemical gradients can be sufficient to produce Ca^{2+} entry via what has been termed *reverse-mode NCX* (81–83). This Ca^{2+} influx through reverse mode NCX can be sufficient to increase intracellular Ca^{2+} during systole and contribute to contraction (83,84). In addition, Ca^{2+} influx through reverse mode NCX can be a significant source of Ca^{2+} to load the SR, especially in CHF (83). Finally, even though Ca^{2+} influx through reverse mode NCX is not an independent trigger of SR Ca^{2+} release, it appears to work in concert with I_{Ca-L} to modulate ECC.

The idea that a change in the activity of the NCX contributes to the altered contractility (Ca^{2+} regulation) of the failing myocyte has been studied. Unfortunately, the results of studies in which NCX abundance and/or activity has been measured in failing myocytes have been inconsistent (85). An increase in NCX function coupled with a decrease in SERCA function have been observed in hypertrophied/failing rat (86), mouse, rabbit, canine (87), and human (84,88–90) ventricular myocytes. These changes unload the SR of stored Ca^{2+} and thereby depress systolic function. Detailed examination of ventricular myocytes from advanced end-stage human heart failure has not revealed changes in either NCX activity or abundance (91).

One possible explanation for the disparity is that some measurements of NCX activity are performed with a fixed intracellular Na^+ concentration applied through patching pipettes. It has been reported that intracellular Na^+ in failing myocytes may be higher than in nonfailing myocytes (92). Higher intracellular Na^+ reduces forward-mode NCX activity. Since $[Na^+]_i$ is elevated in HF, fixing the $[Na^+]_i$ would impact the results significantly. Another possible explanation for the apparent differences in the literature is that at the early stages of hypertrophy/heart failure, NCX activity is increased, in conjunction with the increased Ca^{2+} signaling that appears to be present at this time. In end-stage HF failure, Ca^{2+} influx may actually decrease (or return to normal levels) and the NCX activity may also return to that seen in normal myocytes. These ideas would best be pursued in an animal model with progressive deterioration of cardiac function.

The functional role of these changes in NCX activity in CHF is still not entirely clear. It has been suggested that the increased NCX activity in hypertrophy and CHF is a compensation for the associated reduction in SERCA2 function and serves to remove cytosolic Ca^{2+} (93). This seems unlikely because myocytes from large mammals have long action potentials and high plateau voltages, and SR Ca^{2+} release and reuptake occur during the AP plateau when forward-mode NCX is more modest (80). Forward-mode NCX and SERCA2 work in concert to produce the decay of the Ca^{2+} transient in small mammals (rats and mice) because the AP duration is much shorter than the Ca^{2+} transient in these animals (94). Even in these species, however, Ca^{2+} efflux via the NCX only contributes slightly (<5%) to the decay of the Ca^{2+} transient, even when the NCX is overexpressed (95).

Alterations in the activity of the NCX are likely to be more critically linked to changes in diastolic $[Ca^{2+}]$ and the overall maintenance of Ca^{2+} homeostasis, rather than to the decay of the systolic Ca^{2+} transient. Diastolic Ca^{2+} has been found to be increased in failing myocytes (96), especially as heart rate increases. These changes in diastolic $[Ca^{2+}]$ are produced by the NCX and are partially related to the associated increase in cell $[Na^+]_i$ in these cells (92,96). While this increase in diastolic $[Ca^{2+}]$ might help maintain SR Ca^{2+} loading, it can produce alterations in diastolic stiffness that contribute to filling disorders. Elevated diastolic $[Ca^{2+}]$ could also cause diastolic SR Ca^{2+} release via effects on the Ca^{2+} release channel (RyR), as discussed later.

THE SARCOPLASMIC RETICULUM IN THE FAILING HEART—ABNORMALITIES OF SR CA^{2+}-ATPASE, PHOSPHOLAMBAN, AND RYANODINE RECEPTOR

The decreased $[Ca^{2+}]_i$ transient amplitude of the failing myocyte is primarily due to a decreased amount of Ca^{2+} released from the SR. This could result from reduced SR Ca^{2+} uptake and storage and/or altered EC coupling with reduced release from a normally loaded SR. The SR Ca^{2+} load is determined by the Ca^{2+} available for loading, the activity of SERCA, the activity of the sodium-calcium exchanger (NCX); the buffering capacity of the SR, and the rate of SR Ca^{2+} leak during diastole. All of these factors have been evaluated and are likely to play some role in abnormalities in Ca^{2+} regulation in CHF, as discussed later.

The major source of Ca^{2+} for loading the SR is the Ca^{2+} influx through the LTCC, the L-type calcium current. This topic was discussed in detail previously. In early hypertrophy the Ca^{2+} current is increased and this supports increased SR Ca^{2+} loading. After the transition to decompensated CHF, the Ca^{2+} current density is reduced. However, the AP duration is prolonged and this gives additional time for Ca^{2+} entry. Therefore, it is not clear if Ca^{2+} flux is altered significantly in CHF, a topic that needs further investigation. Another potential source for Ca^{2+} entry is via reverse-mode NCX. This is a very small source of Ca^{2+} for SR loading in the normal heart, but appears to be more important in CHF (84). The consensus from studies performed to date is that SR Ca^{2+} loading alterations in CHF are not primarily due to abnormalities in Ca^{2+} influx.

A large number of studies link depressed cardiac function in CHF with alterations in the abundance and activity of SERCA2, the transporter primarily responsible for transporting Ca^{2+} into the SR. Reduced SERCA function in CHF can explain the reduced amplitude and decay kinetics of the Ca^{2+} transient in failing cardiomyocytes. The decrease in function and/or expression of SERCA2 results in a smaller amount of Ca^{2+} stored in the SR (91), especially when the competing cytosolic Ca^{2+} removal by the Na^+-Ca^{2+} exchanger is upregulated in failing cardiomyocytes (88,97). In addition, some studies suggest that the RyR is hyperphosphorylated in failing myocytes, which is thought to induce abnormal channel opening (a so-called leaky SR), which further decreases the SR Ca^{2+} content (98).

Some studies have failed to detect reduced SERCA2 protein abundance or Ca^{2+} uptake rates in failing human hearts (99,100), suggesting that the routinely observed derangements in cellular Ca^{2+} handling in human myocytes are not always caused by a reduction in the abundance of SERCA2 protein. It is well-known that the function of SERCA is tightly regulated by its associated protein phospholamban (PLB), which inhibits SERCA activity when not phosphorylated under basal condition. Phosphorylation of PLB causes its dissociation from SERCA and removes its inhibitory effect (101). PLB can be phosphorylated at serine^{16} by protein kinase A and at threonine^{17} by Ca^{2+}/calmodulin-dependent kinases (101–103) to produce these effects. PLB phosphorylation is essential for β-adrenergic-mediated increases in cardiac contractility in normal myocytes (104). In failing cardiomyocytes, some studies have shown an increased PLB/SERCA ratio without changes in SERCA abundance (105,106). In addition, reduced PLB phosphorylation has been reported and linked to increased phosphatase activity in failing myocytes (107–109). These studies suggest that PLB hypophosphorylation contributes to the depressed β-adrenergic responsiveness in CHF (109). In a model of CHF in mice in which the muscle LIM protein (MLP)—a Z disk structural component—is knocked out ($MLP^{-/-}$), contractile reserve can be restored by crossing the knockout animal either the PLB knockout ($PLB^{-/-}$) mouse (110) or a βARK-CT transgenic mouse (111). Transcoronary arterial delivery of a pseudophosphorylated human PLB has been shown to prevent CHF progression in a hamster CHF model (112). In addition, the contractility of isolated failing human myocytes is improved when SERCA2 expression is increased via adenoviral gene transfer techniques (113). Together, these studies show that (at least in certain animal models) rescuing deranged Ca^{2+} regulation can slow or stop the progression of CHF. However, studies in small animals such as mice must be viewed cautiously because it is now clear that humans with a PLB null defect develop lethal dilated cardiomyopathy (114). Why PLB knockout is advantageous in small animals but causes cardiomyopathy in humans is currently being explored in a number of laboratories.

Recent successes in rescuing animal models of CHF by manipulation of contractility reserve have fostered enthusiasm in targeting key molecules on the SR, including SERCA2, PLB, and RyR, with more specific approaches (gene transfer or novel molecule-specific drugs) for heart failure therapy (97). The transition of the compensated hypertrophic state to decompensated heart failure is usually temporally parallel with the inability of myocytes to regulate Ca^{2+} handling (10), and preventing Ca^{2+} handling defects from evolving could avert or delay the onset of heart failure (115). Feldman et al. (10) found that reduced SR function is involved in the transition from compensated hypertrophy to early CHF. Increasing SERCA2 expression with adenoviral gene transfer can improve the contractility of the hypertrophied (116,117) or senescent (117) rat heart and delay the onset of CHF. These studies are likely to lead to clinical trials that will ultimately determine if these approaches will have therapeutic benefits in CHF patients.

In recent years, abnormalities of the RyR in failing cardiomyocytes have been defined (59,98). Marx et al. reported that the RyR is hyperphosphorylated by PKA in failing cardiomyocytes and this causes the displacement of the associated stabilizing protein FKBP 12.6, resulting in RyR subconductance states that allow for abnormal Ca^{2+} efflux from the SR (98,118). Stabilizing hyperphosphorylated RyR with genetically altered calstabin2 protein (118) or JTV519, a 1,4-benzothiazepine derivative, can improve the contractile function of failing canine hearts (119) and repress arrhythmia in a rat heart failure model (120). There is ample evidence that cardiac contractility is depressed in CHF and that alterations in myocyte Ca^{2+} regulation are involved. Novel methods for altering Ca^{2+} regulation have been developed and have been shown to be beneficial in animal models. The next step will be to test these approaches in humans with CHF.

ALTERATIONS OF POTASSIUM CURRENTS IN FAILING CARDIOMYOCYTES

Potassium currents are largely responsible for repolarization of cardiomyocytes and are the key determinants of the AP duration. They also modulate the profile of the AP, which has profound effect on Ca^{2+} influx. In cardiomyocytes from humans and other large mammals, there are multiple types of potassium currents that contribute to the AP wave shape. The transient outward K^+ current (I_{to}), delayed rectifying K^+ current, inward rectifying K^+ currents, and ligand gated K^+ channels ($I_{K(Ach)}$ and $I_{K\ (ATP)}$) are the major types in human myocytes. I_{to} is involved in early repolarization of the AP during phase 1. It is mediated by a number of different genes, including Kv1-4, Kv4-2, and Kv4-3. Delayed rectifiers, which are involved in final repolarization during phase 3, end the AP. Multiple genes, including I_{kr} (HERG), I_{Ks} (KvLQT1), and I_{Kur} (Kv1-5), encode delayed rectifier channel proteins. Mutations in these channels in humans cause long QT syndrome and are proarrhythmic. Inward rectifier channels are involved in the generation of the resting potential and final phases of AP repolarization. Kir2-1 is the principal gene in this regard.

The most consistent change in K^+ currents in failing myocytes from large and small animals and in humans is a reduction in the density of the transient outward current. The effect of the decrease of I_{to} on the duration of the AP remains controversial (121–123) in large animals but in small mammals it increases the duration of the AP. What is very clear is that phase 1 of the AP is affected by I_{to} (a positive voltage shift) and this reduces Ca^{2+} influx through the LTCC (124). Recently, our group has shown that the alterations in phase 1 repolarization in failing myocytes decreases peak $I_{Ca\text{-}L}$ and reduces the trigger for SR Ca release, which causes dyssynchronous Ca^{2+} release (14). These studies strongly support a role for altered expression of K^+ currents in contractility defects in the failing heart.

Changes of other K^+ currents in hypertrophied and failing cardiomyocytes are less well-studied. There are limited studies on delayed rectifier K^+ currents in hypertrophied and failing cardiomyocytes (125). Our group was the first to show reduced delayed rectifier K^+ currents in diseased myocytes and the linkage to prolongation of the AP duration. Reduced I_{Kr} density and HERG mRNA levels have also been reported in myocytes from infarcted canine ventricles (126). However, I_{Kr} density increases in subendocardial Purkinje cells in the infarcted heart. I_{Ks} has been reported to be decreased in hypertrophied feline (125,127), rabbits (128) and human ventricular myocytes, with slowed activation and accelerated deactivation. Similar changes have been observed in myocytes from infarcted canine ventricles (126). In contrast, I_{Ks} does not change in ventricular myocytes from pressure-overloaded guinea pigs (129) and spontaneously hypertensive rats (130). Significantly, changes in I_{Kr} and I_{Ks} are not always consistent with the alterations in the mRNA and protein abundance (131).

Generally, the inward rectifier I_{k1} is reduced in hypertrophied and failing cardiomyocytes (87,131–133), including myocytes from terminally failing human hearts (133). Decreased I_{K1} results in longer AP duration and lower resting membrane potential, and predisposes the myocyte to early and delayed afterdepolarizations (EAD and DAD, respectively) (87,132). In infarcted hearts, I_{K1} is reduced in canine Purkinje cells (134) and in myocytes from the border zone of infarcted rat hearts (135). The open probability of the I_{K1} channel is greater in myocytes from idiopathic dilated hearts than in those from ischemic hearts (136).

Our view of the studies performed to date is that there is a reduction in the abundance and activity of K^+ channels that regulate the early and late portions of the AP. The positive voltage shift in the early portion of the AP reduces Ca^{2+} influx and can cause EC coupling defects. The decreased K^+ currents during the AP plateau phase cause AP prolongation and acquired long QT syndrome, and predispose the heart to arrhythmias.

Arrhythmia in Hypertrophy and Heart Failure

The electrical activity of the heart is propagated throughout the heart via direct cell–cell coupling and via the cardiac conduction system. One common facet of cardiac pathology is arrhythmia, the endpoint of several possible mechanisms. In many forms of heart failure, ventricular remodeling occurs and the increased fibrosis seen contributes to arrhythmogenesis by direct physical interference with normal electrical conduction throughout the myocardium. Physical disruption of cell–cell coupling proteins and cell–matrix proteins such as connexins or integrins may also contribute to arrhythmogenesis in hypertrophy and failure (137). Arrhythmias can develop in response to the alterations in ion channel mechanics and calcium handling discussed earlier in this chapter. Alterations in expression of the gene SCN5A, which encodes a sodium channel in humans, have been linked to early-onset cardiomyopathies and arrhythmias (138). This gene may be partially responsible for the increased AP duration commonly seen in hypertrophy and heart failure, as discussed previously. Other ion channel irregularities seen in heart failure that may contribute to arrhythmogenesis were discussed in detail earlier in the chapter.

Another possible mechanism for arrhythmia involves calcium handling proteins. As discussed previously, the sarcoplasmic reticulum Ca^{2+} release channel, or RyR, is hyperphosphorylated in heart failure (119,120,139), increasing the probability of Ca^{2+} leaking from the SR. This in turn increases the cytosolic Ca^{2+} concentration, creating an increased chance of spontaneous arrhythmic contractions. Changes in other calcium-handling proteins (including phospholamban, SERCA, the Na^+/Ca^{2+} exchanger, and L-type Ca^{2+} channel) are also potential substrates for arrhythmogenesis.

UNBALANCED MYOCYTE LOSS AND NEW MYOCYTE REGENERATION IN THE FAILING HEART

The conventional view of the heart is that it is a postmitotic organ without the capacity for generation of new cardiac myocytes. Therefore, any myocyte death reduces the number of myocytes and could eventually lead to CHF. The idea that new myocytes can be formed from a cardiac stem cell has recently been proposed; this has dramatically changed our view of the adult heart and opened the door to novel therapies for cardiac regeneration. This topic is discussed in the next section of this chapter.

Many recent studies show that myocyte death is a major factor contributing to the initiation and progression of heart disease. Loss of functional myocardium will reduce the contractile potential of the heart, independent of defects in the surviving myocytes as previously discussed. Recent studies show that both apoptosis and necrosis contribute to cell death during MI (33) and ischemia/reperfusion injury (140–144). Necrosis is the major form of cell death when long-lasting ischemia occurs, whereas apoptosis plays more a important role in cell death after reperfusion (140–144) and in the infarct border zone.

In chronic hemodynamic stress states such as pressure overload-induced hypertrophy, the role of apoptosis in the progress of hypertrophy is not as clear (145). Increased apoptosis has been reported in the hypertrophied heart of spontaneously hypertensive rats (146–148), rats with angiotensin II-induced hypertension (149), and patients with hypertension (145,150). Nediani et al. (151) showed that in volume-overloaded swine hearts, apoptotic cells were apparent 2 days after the establishment of volume overload. In rat hearts after healing of myocardial infarction, cardiac hypertrophy developed and apoptosis was increased (152).

There is accumulating evidence to show that apoptosis plays an important role in the transition from hypertrophy to HF (146,153). Studies show that apoptosis is increased in patients with idiopathic (154), ischemic, or hypertrophic cardiomyopathy (33,34). Akyurek et al. (154) found that expression of the proapoptotic protein *Bax* negatively correlated with the severity of heart failure (i.e., more apoptosis occurred during the early stage of heart failure). Wencker et al. (155) demonstrated that conditional overexpression of caspase-8 (a protease involved in apoptosis) in mice was able to induce dilated cardiomyopathy with a very low apoptotic rate (23 per 10^5 myocytes).

CARDIAC REGENERATION

The heart has traditionally been regarded as a postmitotic organ. Recent evidence from a number of laboratories, however, has suggested that stem cells derived from a variety of sources are capable of differentiating into cardiac myocytes (156–166). Stem cells derived from adult myocardium have been described in human and animal studies. These cells are present in low numbers in healthy myocardium, indicating a possible endogenous repair mechanism in the adult heart. The number of these cells appears to be reduced in aging and heart failure (167–170), and early data imply that injection of stem cells derived from various sources may contribute to myocardial repair after injury (158,161,166,169,171). Of the possible sources of stem cells for cardiac repair (including embryonic, bone marrow-derived, skeletal muscle-derived, and mesenchymal stem cells), cells derived from the adult heart seem the most promising. They are autologous, removing the possibility of immune reaction; they also are clonogenic, self-renewing, and capable of differentiating into multiple cardiac cell types (156,162,164). It is clear, however, that the endogenous repair mechanism in the heart is not sufficient to restore function to a failing heart. Thus, strategies for modulating the division, differentiation, and integration of these native cardiac stem cells into new myocardium in regions of cardiac damage are clearly necessary.

The potential hurdles to overcome before stem cell therapy becomes a viable clinical target are varied and numerous. New cardiac myocytes must integrate completely into the electromechanical milieu of the myocardium in order to avoid arrhythmogenesis. New tissue must consist of not only functional myocytes but also new blood vessels functionally connected to the preexisting vasculature. Undifferentiated embryonic stem cells injected into the heart in animal studies have developed teratomas (172), an obvious source of concern. This is a young field with a great deal of potential for future therapies in all forms of cardiac disease, but a great deal of work remains to be done before universal clinical applications are viable.

ACKNOWLEDGMENTS

The authors are supported by the following research grants from the National Heart Lung and Blood Institute: NHLBI HL61495, NHLBI HL33921, and NHLBI AG17022.

REFERENCES

1. Houser SR, Piacentino V, 3rd, Weisser J. Abnormalities of calcium cycling in the hypertrophied and failing heart. *J Mol Cell Cardiol.* 2000;32:1595–1607.
2. Rossman EI, Petre RE, Chaudhary KW, et al. Abnormal frequency-dependent responses represent the pathophysiologic signature of contractile failure in human myocardium. *J Mol Cell Cardiol.* 2004;36:33–42.
3. Tagawa H, Wang N, Narishige T, et al. Cytoskeletal mechanics in pressure-overload cardiac hypertrophy [see comments]. *Circ Res.* 1997;80:281–289.
4. Schwartz K, Carrier L, Lompre AM, et al. Contractile proteins and sarcoplasmic reticulum calcium-ATPase gene expression in the hypertrophied and failing heart. *Basic Res Cardiol.* 1992;87(Suppl 1):285–290.
5. Li P, Hofmann PA, Li B, et al. Myocardial infarction alters myofilament calcium sensitivity and mechanical behavior of myocytes. *Am J Physiol.* 1997;272:H360–H370.
6. Olson EN. A decade of discoveries in cardiac biology. *Nat Med.* 2004;10:467–474.
7. Beuckelmann DJ, Nabauer M, Erdmann E. Intracellular calcium handling in isolated ventricular myocytes from patients with terminal heart failure. *Circulation.* 1992;85:1046–1055.
8. Gomez AM, Valdivia HH, Cheng H, et al. Defective excitation-contraction coupling in experimental cardiac hypertrophy and heart failure. *Science.* 1997;276:800–806.
9. Beuckelmann DJ, Erdmann E. Ca (2^+)-currents and intracellular [Ca 2^+]i-transients in single ventricular myocytes isolated from terminally failing human myocardium. *Basic Res Cardiol.* 1992;87(Suppl 1):235–243.
10. Feldman AM, Weinberg EO, Ray PE, et al. Selective changes in cardiac gene expression during compensated hypertrophy and the transition to cardiac decompensation in rats with chronic aortic banding. *Circ Res.* 1993;73:184–192.
11. Fabiato A. Calcium-induced release of calcium from the cardiac sarcoplasmic reticulum. *Am J Physiol.* 1983;245:C1–14.
12. Fabiato A. Time and calcium dependence of activation and inactivation of calcium-induced release of calcium from the sarcoplasmic reticulum of a skinned canine cardiac Purkinje cell. *J Gen Physiol.* 1985;85:247–289.
13. Litwin SE, Zhang D, Bridge JH. Dyssynchronous Ca (2^+) sparks in myocytes from infarcted hearts. *Circ Res.* 2000;87:1040–1047.
14. Harris DM, Mills GD, Chen X, et al. Alterations in early action potential repolarization causes localized failure of sarcoplasmic reticulum Ca2+ release. *Circ Res.* 2005;96:543–550.
15. Cannell MB. New insights into cardiac excitation-contraction coupling in normal and hypertension/failure animal models. *J Human Hyper.* 1997:555–558.
16. He J, Conklin MW, Foell JD, et al. Reduction in density of transverse tubules and L-type Ca (2^+) channels in canine tachycardia-induced heart failure. *Cardiovasc Res.* 2001:298–307.
17. Rockman HA, Koch WJ, Lefkowitz RJ. Seven-transmembrane-spanning receptors and heart function. *Nature.* 2002;415:206–212.

18. Ferguson SS. Evolving concepts in G protein-coupled receptor endocytosis: the role in receptor desensitization and signaling. *Pharmacol Rev.* 2001;53:1–24.
19. Hausdorff WP, Bouvier M, O'Dowd BF, et al. Phosphorylation sites on two domains of the beta 2-adrenergic receptor are involved in distinct pathways of receptor desensitization. *J Biol Chem.* 1989;264:12657–12665.
20. Penn RB, Pronin AN, Benovic JL. Regulation of G protein-coupled receptor kinases. *Trends Cardiovasc Med.* 2000;10:81–89.
21. Pitcher JA, Freedman NJ, Lefkowitz RJ. G protein-coupled receptor kinases. *Ann Rev Biochem.* 1998;67:653–692.
22. Claing A, Laporte SA, Caron MG, et al. Endocytosis of G protein-coupled receptors: roles of G protein-coupled receptor kinases and beta-arrestin proteins. *Prog Neurobiol.* 2002;66:61–79.
23. Luttrell LM, Lefkowitz RJ. The role of beta-arrestins in the termination and transduction of G-protein-coupled receptor signals. *J Cell Sci.* 2002;115:455–465.
24. Xiang Y, Rybin VO, Steinberg SF, et al. Caveolar localization dictates physiologic signaling of beta 2-adrenoceptors in neonatal cardiac myocytes. *J Biol Chem.* 2002;277:34280–34286.
25. Dorn GW, 2nd. Adrenergic pathways and left ventricular remodeling. *J Card Fail.* 2002;8:S370–S373.
26. Packer M. The neurohormonal hypothesis: a theory to explain the mechanism of disease progression in heart failure. *J Am Coll Cardiol.* 1992;20:248–254.
27. Bristow MR. Why does the myocardium fail? Insights from basic science. *Lancet.* 1998;352(Suppl 1):SI8–SI14.
28. Bristow MR, Ginsburg R, Minobe W, et al. Decreased catecholamine sensitivity and beta-adrenergic-receptor density in failing human hearts. *N Engl J Med.* 1982;307:205–211.
29. Ungerer M, Bohm M, Elce JS, et al. Altered expression of beta-adrenergic receptor kinase and beta 1-adrenergic receptors in the failing human heart. *Circulation.* 1993;87:454–463.
30. Engelhardt S, Hein L, Wiesmann F, et al. Progressive hypertrophy and heart failure in beta1-adrenergic receptor transgenic mice. *Proc Natl Acad Sci USA.* 1999;96:7059–7064.
31. Bisognano JD, Weinberger HD, Bohlmeyer TJ, et al. Myocardial-directed overexpression of the human beta(1)-adrenergic receptor in transgenic mice. *J Mol Cell Cardiol.* 2000;32:817–830.
32. Engelhardt S, Boknik P, Keller U, et al. Early impairment of calcium handling and altered expression of junctin in hearts of mice overexpressing the beta1-adrenergic receptor. *Faseb J.* 2001; 15:2718–2720.
33. Gill C, Mestril R, Samali A. Losing heart: the role of apoptosis in heart disease—a novel therapeutic target? *Faseb J.* 2002;16: 135–146.
34. Yamamoto S, Sawada K, Shimomura H, et al. On the nature of cell death during remodeling of hypertrophied human myocardium. *J Mol Cell Cardiol.* 2000;32:161–175.
35. Liggett SB, Tepe NM, Lorenz JN, et al. Early and delayed consequences of beta(2)-adrenergic receptor overexpression in mouse hearts: critical role for expression level. *Circulation.* 2000;101: 1707–1714.
36. Milano CA, Allen LF, Rockman HA, et al. Enhanced myocardial function in transgenic mice overexpressing the beta 2-adrenergic receptor. *Science.* 1994;264:582–586.
37. Du XJ, Gao XM, Wang B, et al. Age-dependent cardiomyopathy and heart failure phenotype in mice overexpressing beta(2)-adrenergic receptors in the heart. *Cardiovasc Res.* 2000;48:448–454.
38. Schwarz B, Percy E, Gao XM, et al. Altered calcium transient and development of hypertrophy in beta2-adrenoceptor overexpressing mice with and without pressure overload. *Eur J Heart Fail.* 2003;5:131–136.
39. Sheridan DJ, Autelitano DJ, Wang B, et al. Beta(2)-adrenergic receptor overexpression driven by alpha-MHC promoter is downregulated in hypertrophied and failing myocardium. *Cardiovasc Res.* 2000;47:133–141.
40. Du XJ, Gao XM, Jennings GL, et al. Preserved ventricular contractility in infarcted mouse heart overexpressing beta(2)-adrenergic receptors. *Am J Physiol Heart Circ Physiol.* 2000;279:H2456–H2463.
41. Zhu WZ, Zheng M, Koch WJ, et al. Dual modulation of cell survival and cell death by beta(2)-adrenergic signaling in adult mouse cardiac myocytes. *Proc Natl Acad Sci USA.* 2001;98:1607–1612.
42. Petrofski JA, Koch WJ. The beta-adrenergic receptor kinase in heart failure. *J Mol Cell Cardiol.* 2003;35:1167–1174.
43. Naga Prasad SV, Laporte SA, Chamberlain D, et al. Phosphoinositide 3-kinase regulates beta2-adrenergic receptor endocytosis by AP-2 recruitment to the receptor/beta-arrestin complex. *J Cell Biol.* 2002;158:563–575.
44. Naga Prasad SV, Barak LS, Rapacciuolo A, et al. Agonist-dependent recruitment of phosphoinositide 3-kinase to the membrane by beta-adrenergic receptor kinase 1. A role in receptor sequestration. *J Biol Chem.* 2001;276:18953–18959.
45. Prasad SV, Perrino C, Rockman HA. Role of phosphoinositide 3-kinase in cardiac function and heart failure. *Trends Cardiovasc Med.* 2003;13:206–212.
46. Naga Prasad SV, Esposito G, Mao L, et al. Gβγ-dependent phosphoinositide 3-kinase activation in hearts with in vivo pressure overload hypertrophy. *J Biol Chem.* 2000;275:4693–4698.
47. Koch WJ, Rockman HA, Samama P, et al. Cardiac function in mice overexpressing the beta-adrenergic receptor kinase or a beta ARK inhibitor. *Science.* 1995;268:1350–1353.
48. Nienaber JJ, Tachibana H, Naga Prasad SV, et al. Inhibition of receptor-localized PI3K preserves cardiac beta-adrenergic receptor function and ameliorates pressure overload heart failure. *J Clin Invest.* 2003;112:1067–1079.
49. Iwase M, Bishop SP, Uechi M, et al. Adverse effects of chronic endogenous sympathetic drive induced by cardiac GS alpha overexpression. *Circ Res.* 1996;78:517–524.
50. Feldman AM, Cates AE, Veazey WB, et al. Increase of the 40,000-mol wt pertussis toxin substrate (G protein) in the failing human heart. *J Clin Invest.* 1988;82:189–197.
51. Foerster K, Groner F, Matthes J, et al. Cardioprotection specific for the G protein Gi2 in chronic adrenergic signaling through beta 2-adrenoceptors. *Proc Natl Acad Sci U* SA. 2003;100:14475–14480.
52. Xiao RP, Ji X, Lakatta EG. Functional coupling of the beta 2-adrenoceptor to a pertussis toxin-sensitive G protein in cardiac myocytes. *Mol Pharmacol.* 1995;47:322–329.
53. Barki-Harrington L, Perrino C, Rockman HA. Network integration of the adrenergic system in cardiac hypertrophy. *Cardiovasc Res.* 2004;63:391–402.
54. Lohse MJ, Engelhardt S, Eschenhagen T. What is the role of beta-adrenergic signaling in heart failure? *Circ Res.* 2003;93:896–906.
55. Xiao RP, Cheng H, Zhou YY, et al. Recent advances in cardiac beta(2)-adrenergic signal transduction. *Circ Res.* 1999;85: 1092–1100.
56. Bristow M. Antiadrenergic therapy of chronic heart failure: surprises and new opportunities. *Circulation.* 2003;107:1100–1102.
57. Lowes BD, Gilbert EM, Abraham WT, et al. Myocardial gene expression in dilated cardiomyopathy treated with beta-blocking agents. *N Engl J Med.* 2002;346:1357–1365.
58. Reiken S, Wehrens XH, Vest JA, et al. Beta-blockers restore calcium release channel function and improve cardiac muscle performance in human heart failure. *Circulation.* 2003;107: 2459–2466.
59. Wehrens XH, Marks AR. Novel therapeutic approaches for heart failure by normalizing calcium cycling. *Nat Rev Drug Discov.* 2004;3:565–573.
60. Wang Y, Rudy Y. Action potential propagation in inhomogeneous cardiac tissue: safety factor considerations and ionic mechanism. *Am J Physiol Heart Circ Physiol.* 2000:H1019–H1029.
61. Houser SR. Reduced abundance of transverse tubules and L-type calcium channels: another cause of defective contractility in failing ventricular myocytes. *Cardiovasc Res.* 2001:253–256.
62. Mukherjee R, Spinale FG. L-type calcium channel abundance and function with cardiac hypertrophy and failure: a review. *J Mol Cell Card.* 1998:1899–1916.
63. Tomaselli GF, Marban E. Electrophysiological remodeling in hypertrophy and heart failure *Cardiovasc Res.* 1999:270–283.
64. Gruver EJ, Morgan JP, Stambler BS, Gwathmey JK. Uniformity of calcium channel number and isometric contraction in human right and left ventricular myocardium. *Basic Res Cardiol.* 1994:139–148.
65. Rasmussen RP, Minobe W, Bristow MR. Calcium antagonist binding sites in failing and nonfailing human ventricular myocardium. *Biochem Pharmacol.* 1990:691–696.
66. Schwinger RH, Hoischen S, Reuter H, et al. Regional expression and functional characterization of the L-type Ca^{2+}-channel in myocardium from patients with end-stage heart failure and in non-failing human hearts. *Am J Cardiol.* 1999:507–514.

67. Takahashi T, Allen PD, Lacro RV, et al. Expression of dihydropyridine receptor (Ca^{2+} channel) and calsequestrin genes in the myocardium of patients with end-stage heart failure. *J Clin Invest.* 1992:927–935.
68. Chen X, Piacentino V, 3rd, Furukawa S, et al. L-type Ca^{2+} channel density and regulation are altered in failing human ventricular myocytes and recover after support with mechanical assist devices. *Circ Res.* 2002;91:517–524.
69. Yang Y, Chen X, Houser S. L-type calcium channel alpha1c sununit N-terminal isoform expression in human ventricular myocytes. *Biophys J.* 1999:A341.
70. Yatani A, Honda R, Tymitz KM, et al. Enhanced Ca^{2+} channel currents in cardiac hypertrophy induced by activation of calcineurin-dependent pathway. *J Mol Cell Cardiol.* 2001:249–259.
71. Han W, Chartier D, Li D, et al. Ionic remodeling of cardiac Purkinje cells by congestive heart failure. *Circulation.* 2001:2095–2100.
72. Mewes T, Ravens U. L-type calcium currents of human myocytes from ventricle of non-failing and failing hearts and from atrium. *J Mol Cell Cardiol.* 1994;26:1307–1320.
73. Ouadid H, Albat B, Nargeot J. Calcium currents in diseased human cardiac cells. *J Cardiovasc Pharmacol.* 1995;25:282–291.
74. Shin HM, Je HD, Gallant C, et al. Differential association and localization of myosin phosphatase subunits during agonist-induced signal transduction in smooth muscle. *Circ Res.* 2002:546–553.
75. Sipido KR, Stankovicova T, Flameng W, et al. Frequency dependence of Ca^{2+} release from the sarcoplasmic reticulum in human ventricular myocytes from end-stage heart failure. *Cardiovasc Res.* 1998:478–488.
76. Schroder F, Handrock R, Beuckelmann DJ, et al. Increased availability and open probability of single L-type calcium channels from failing compared with nonfailing human ventricle. *Circulation.* 1998:969–976.
77. Ming Z, Nordin C, Siri F, et al. Reduced calcium current density in single myocytes isolated from hypertrophied failing guinea pig hearts. *J Mol Cell Cardiol.* 1994:1133–1143.
78. Laurent CE, Cardinal R, Rousseau G, et al. Functional desensitization to isoproterenol without reducing cAMP production in canine failing cardiocytes. *Am J Physiol Regul Integr Comp Physiol.* 2001:R355–R364.
79. Zhang ZS, Cheng HJ, Ukai T, et al. Enhanced cardiac L-type calcium current response to beta2-adrenergic stimulation in heart failure. *J Pharmacol Exp Ther.* 2001:188–196.
80. Bers DM, Bridge JH. Relaxation of rabbit ventricular muscle by Na-Ca exchange and sarcoplasmic reticulum calcium pump. Ryanodine and voltage sensitivity. *Circ Res.* 1989;65:334–342.
81. Eisner DA, Lederer WJ, Vaughan-Jones RD. The quantitative relationship between twitch tension and intracellular sodium activity in sheep cardiac Purkinje fibres. *J Physiol.* 1984;355: 251–266.
82. Bers DM, Christensen DM, Nguyen TX. Can Ca entry via Na-Ca exchange directly activate cardiac muscle contraction? *J Mol Cell Cardiol.* 1988;20:405–414.
83. Nuss HB, Houser SR. Sodium-calcium exchange-mediated contractions in feline ventricular myocytes. *Am J Physiol.* 1992;263: H1161–H1169.
84. Gaughan JP, Furukawa S, Jeevanandam V, et al. Sodium/calcium exchange contributes to contraction and relaxation in failed human ventricular myocytes. *Am J Physiol.* 1999;277:H714–H724.
85. Barry WH. $Na(^+)$-$Ca(^{2+})$ exchange in failing myocardium: friend or foe? *Circ Res.* 2000;87:529–531.
86. Wasserstrom JA, Holt E, Sjaastad I, et al. Altered E-C coupling in rat ventricular myocytes from failing hearts 6 weeks after MI. *Am J Physiol Heart Circ Physiol.* 2000;279:H798–H807.
87. O'Rourke B, Kass DA, Tomaselli GF, et al. Mechanisms of altered excitation-contraction coupling in canine tachycardia-induced heart failure. I: experimental studies. *Circ Res.* 1999;84: 562–570.
88. Pieske B, Maier LS, Bers DM, et al. Ca^{2+} handling and sarcoplasmic reticulum Ca^{2+} content in isolated failing and nonfailing human myocardium. *Circ Res.* 1999;85:38–46.
89. Studer R, Reinecke H, Bilger J, et al. Gene expression of the cardiac Na^+-Ca^{2+} exchanger in end-stage human heart failure. *Circ Res.* 1994;75:443–453.
90. Hasenfuss G, Schillinger W, Lehnart SE, et al. Relationship between Na^+-Ca^{2+}-exchanger protein levels and diastolic function of failing human myocardium. *Circulation.* 1999;99:641–648.
91. Piacentino V, 3rd, Weber CR, Chen X, et al. Cellular basis of abnormal calcium transients of failing human ventricular myocytes. *Circ Res.* 2003;92:651–658.
92. Pieske B, Houser SR, Hasenfuss G, et al. Sodium and the heart: a hidden key factor in cardiac regulation. *Cardiovasc Res.* 2003;57: 871–872.
93. Hasenfuss G, Meyer M, Schillinger W, et al. Calcium handling proteins in the failing human heart. *Basic Res Cardiol.* 1997;92(Suppl 1):87–93.
94. Bridge JH, Ershler PR, Cannell MB. Properties of Ca^{2+} sparks evoked by action potentials in mouse ventricular myocytes. *J Physiol.* 1999:469–478.
95. Yao A, Su Z, Nonaka A, et al. Effects of overexpression of the Na^+-Ca^{2+} exchanger on $[Ca^{2+}]_i$ transients in murine ventricular myocytes. *Circ Res.* 1998:657–665.
96. Weber CR, Piacentino V, 3rd, Houser SR, et al. Dynamic regulation of sodium/calcium exchange function in human heart failure. *Circulation.* 2003;108:2224–2229.
97. Dipla K, Mattiello JA, Margulies KB, et al. The sarcoplasmic reticulum and the Na^+/Ca^{2+} exchanger both contribute to the Ca^{2+} transient of failing human ventricular myocytes. *Circ Res.* 1999;84:435–444.
98. Marx SO, Reiken S, Hisamatsu Y, et al. PKA phosphorylation dissociates FKBP12-6 from the calcium release channel (ryanodine receptor): defective regulation in failing hearts. *Cell.* 2000;101: 365–376.
99. Schwinger RH, Bohm M, Schmidt U, et al. Unchanged protein levels of SERCA II and phospholamban but reduced Ca^{2+} uptake and $Ca(^{2+})$-ATPase activity of cardiac sarcoplasmic reticulum from dilated cardiomyopathy patients compared with patients with nonfailing hearts. *Circulation.* 1995;92:3220–3228.
100. Movsesian MA, Bristow MR, Krall J. Ca^{2+} uptake by cardiac sarcoplasmic reticulum from patients with idiopathic dilated cardiomyopathy. *Circ Res.* 1989;65:1141–1144.
101. Kirchberger MA, Tada M, Katz AM. Adenosine 3':5'-monophosphate-dependent protein kinase-catalyzed phosphorylation reaction and its relationship to calcium transport in cardiac sarcoplasmic reticulum. *J Biol Chem.* 1974;249:6166–6173.
102. Simmerman HK, Collins JH, Theibert JL, et al. Sequence analysis of phospholamban. Identification of phosphorylation sites and two major structural domains. *J Biol Chem.* 1986;261: 13333–13341.
103. Le Peuch CJ, Haiech J, Demaille JG. Concerted regulation of cardiac sarcoplasmic reticulum calcium transport by cyclic adenosine monophosphate-dependent and calcium-calmodulin-dependent phosphorylations. *Biochemistry.* 1979;18:5150–5157.
104. McIvor ME, Orchard CH, Lakatta EG. Dissociation of changes in apparent myofibrillar Ca^{2+} sensitivity and twitch relaxation induced by adrenergic and cholinergic stimulation in isolated ferret cardiac muscle. *J Gen Physiol.* 1988;92:509–529.
105. Koss KL, Grupp IL, Kranias EG. The relative phospholamban and SERCA2 ratio: a critical determinant of myocardial contractility. *Basic Res Cardiol.* 1997;92(Suppl 1):17–24.
106. Meyer M, Bluhm WF, He H, et al. Phospholamban-to-SERCA2 ratio controls the force-frequency relationship. *Am J Physiol.* 1999;276:H779–H885.
107. Simmerman HK, Jones LR. Phospholamban: protein structure, mechanism of action, and role in cardiac function. *Physiol Rev.* 1998;78:921–947.
108. Schwinger RH, Munch G, Bolck B, et al. Reduced $Ca(^{2+})$-sensitivity of SERCA 2a in failing human myocardium due to reduced serin-16 phospholamban phosphorylation. *J Mol Cell Cardiol.* 1999;31:479–491.
109. Huang B, Wang S, Qin D, et al. Diminished basal phosphorylation level of phospholamban in the postinfarction remodeled rat ventricle: role of beta-adrenergic pathway, G(i) protein, phosphodiesterase, and phosphatases. *Circ Res.* 1999;85:848–855.
110. Minamisawa S, Hoshijima M, Chu G, et al. Chronic phospholamban-sarcoplasmic reticulum calcium ATPase interaction is the critical calcium cycling defect in dilated cardiomyopathy. *Cell.* 1999;99:313–322.

111. Rockman HA, Chien KR, Choi DJ, et al. Expression of a beta-adrenergic receptor kinase 1 inhibitor prevents the development of myocardial failure in gene-targeted mice. *Proc Natl Acad Sci USA*. 1998;95:7000–7005.
112. Hoshijima M, Ikeda Y, Iwanaga Y, et al. Chronic suppression of heart-failure progression by a pseudophosphorylated mutant of phospholamban via in vivo cardiac rAAV gene delivery. *Nat Med.* 2002;8:864–871.
113. del Monte F, Harding SE, Schmidt U, et al. Restoration of contractile function in isolated cardiomyocytes from failing human hearts by gene transfer of SERCA2a. *Circulation* 1999;100:2308–2311.
114. Haghighi K, Kolokathis F, Pater L, et al. Human phospholamban null results in lethal dilated cardiomyopathy revealing a critical difference between mouse and human. *J Clin Invest.* 2003;111: 869–876.
115. Dorn GW, 2nd, Molkentin JD. Manipulating cardiac contractility in heart failure: data from mice and men. *Circulation* 2004;109: 150–158.
116. Miyamoto MI, del Monte F, Schmidt U, et al. Adenoviral gene transfer of SERCA2a improves left-ventricular function in aortic-banded rats in transition to heart failure. *Proc Natl Acad Sci USA*. 2000;97:793–798.
117. Schmidt U, del Monte F, Miyamoto MI, et al. Restoration of diastolic function in senescent rat hearts through adenoviral gene transfer of sarcoplasmic reticulum Ca($^{2+}$)-ATPase. *Circulation* 2000;101:790–796.
118. Most P, Koch WJ. Sealing the leak, healing the heart. *Nat Med.* 2003;9:993–994.
119. Yano M, Kobayashi S, Kohno M, et al. FKBP12-6-mediated stabilization of calcium-release channel (ryanodine receptor) as a novel therapeutic strategy against heart failure. *Circulation* 2003;107:477–484.
120. Wehrens XH, Lehnart SE, Reiken SR, et al. Protection from cardiac arrhythmia through ryanodine receptor-stabilizing protein calstabin2. *Science.* 2004;304:292–296.
121. Beuckelmann DJ, Nabauer M, Erdmann E. Alterations of K^+ currents in isolated human ventricular myocytes from patients with terminal heart failure. *Circ Res.* 1993;73:379–385.
122. Winslow RL, Rice J, Jafri S, et al. Mechanisms of altered excitation-contraction coupling in canine tachycardia-induced heart failure, II: model studies. *Circ Res.* 1999;84:571–586.
123. Hoppe UC, Johns DC, Marban E, et al. Manipulation of cellular excitability by cell fusion: effects of rapid introduction of transient outward K^+ current on the guinea pig action potential. *Circ Res.* 1999;84:964–972.
124. Sah R, Ramirez RJ, Oudit GY, et al. Regulation of cardiac excitation-contraction coupling by action potential repolarization: role of the transient outward potassium current(I (to)). *J Physiol.* 2003;546:5–18.
125. Kleiman RB, Houser SR. Outward currents in normal and hypertrophied feline ventricular myocytes. *Am J Physiol.* 1989;256: H1450–H1461.
126. Jiang M, Cabo C, Yao J, et al. Delayed rectifier K currents have reduced amplitudes and altered kinetics in myocytes from infarcted canine ventricle. *Cardiovasc Res.* 2000;48:34–43.
127. Furukawa T, Bassett AL, Furukawa N, et al. The ionic mechanism of reperfusion-induced early after depolarizations in feline left ventricular hypertrophy. *J Clin Invest.* 1993;91:1521–1531.
128. Tsuji Y, Opthof T, Kamiya K, et al. Pacing-induced heart failure causes a reduction of delayed rectifier potassium currents along with decreases in calcium and transient outward currents in rabbit ventricle. *Cardiovasc Res.* 2000;48:300–309.
129. Ahmmed GU, Dong PH, Song G, et al. Changes in Ca($^{2+}$) cycling proteins underlie cardiac action potential prolongation in a pressure-overloaded guinea pig model with cardiac hypertrophy and failure. *Circ Res.* 2000;86:558–570.
130. Brooksby P, Levi AJ, Jones JV. The electrophysiological characteristics of hypertrophied ventricular myocytes from the spontaneously hypertensive rat. *J Hypertens.* 1993;11:611–622.
131. Akar FG, Wu RC, Juang GJ, et al. Molecular mechanisms underlying potassium current down-regulation in canine tachycardia-induced heart failure. *Am J Physiol Heart Circ Physiol.* 2005;288(6): H2887–2896.
132. Nabauer M, Kaab S. Potassium channel down-regulation in heart failure. *Cardiovasc Res.* 1998;37:324–334.
133. Kaab S, Dixon J, Duc J, et al. Molecular basis of transient outward potassium current downregulation in human heart failure: a decrease in Kv4-3 mRNA correlates with a reduction in current density. *Circulation.* 1998;98:1383–1393.
134. Pinto JM, Boyden PA. Electrical remodeling in ischemia and infarction. *Cardiovasc Res.* 1999;42:284–297.
135. Yao JA, Jiang M, Fan JS, et al. Heterogeneous changes in K currents in rat ventricles three days after myocardial infarction. *Cardiovasc Res.* 1999;44:132–145.
136. Koumi S, Backer CL, Arentzen CE. Characterization of inwardly rectifying K^+ channel in human cardiac myocytes. Alterations in channel behavior in myocytes isolated from patients with idiopathic dilated cardiomyopathy. *Circulation.* 1995;92:164–174.
137. Saffitz JE, Kleber AG. Effects of mechanical forces and mediators of hypertrophy on remodeling of gap junctions in the heart. *Circ Res.* 2004;94:585–591.
138. Olson TM, Michels VV, Ballew JD, et al. Sodium channel mutations and susceptibility to heart failure and atrial fibrillation. *JAMA.* 2005;293:447–454.
139. Brillantes AM, Allen P, Takahashi T, et al. Differences in cardiac calcium release channel (ryanodine receptor) expression in myocardium from patients with end-stage heart failure caused by ischemic versus dilated cardiomyopathy. *Circ Res.* 1992;71:18–26.
140. Gottlieb RA, Burleson KO, Kloner RA, et al. Reperfusion injury induces apoptosis in rabbit cardiomyocytes. *J Clin Invest.* 1994:1621–1628.
141. Kajstura J, Cheng W, Reiss K, et al. Apoptotic and necrotic myocyte cell deaths are independent contributing variables of infarct size in rats. *Lab Invest.* 1996:86–107.
142. James TN. The variable morphological coexistence of apoptosis and necrosis in human myocardial infarction: significance for understanding its pathogenesis, clinical course, diagnosis and prognosis. *Coron Artery Dis.* 1998:291–307.
143. Zhao ZQ, Nakamura M, Wang NP, et al. Reperfusion induces myocardial apoptotic cell death. *Cardiovasc Res.* 2000:651–660.
144. Freude B, Masters TN, Robicsek F, et al. Apoptosis is initiated by myocardial ischemia and executed during reperfusion. *J Mol Cell Cardiol.* 2000:197–208.
145. Yamamoto S, Sawada K, Shimomura H, et al. On the nature of cell death during remodeling of hypertrophied human myocardium. *J Mol Cell Cardiol.* 2000:161–175.
146. Bailey BA, Dipla K, Li S, Houser SR. Cellular basis of contractile derangements of hypertrophied feline ventricular myocytes. *J Mol Cell Cardiol.* 1997;29:1823–1835.
147. Diez J, Panizo A, Hernandez M, et al. Cardiomyocyte apoptosis and cardiac angiotensin-converting enzyme in spontaneously hypertensive rats. *Hypertension.* 1997;30(5):1029–1034.
148. Liu JJ, Peng L, Bradley CJ, et al. Increased apoptosis in the heart of genetic hypertension, associated with increased fibroblasts. *Cardiovasc Res.* 2000; 45(3):729–735.
149. Diep QN, El Mabrouk M, Yue P, et al. Effect of AT(1) receptor blockade on cardiac apoptosis in angiotensin II-induced hypertension. *Am J Physiol Heart Circ Physiol.* 2002;282(5): H1635–H1641.
150. Gonzalez A, Lopez B, Ravassa S, et al. Stimulation of cardiac apoptosis in essential hypertension: potential role of angiotensin II. *Hypertension.* 2002;39(1):75–80.
151. Nediani C, Celli A, Formigli L, et al. Possible role of acylphosphatase, Bcl-2 and Fas/Fas-L system in the early changes of cardiac remodeling induced by volume overload. *Biochem Biophys Acta.* 2003;1638(3):217–226.
152. Sam F, Sawyer DB, Chang DL, et al. Progressive left ventricular remodeling and apoptosis late after myocardial infarction in mouse heart. *Am J Physiol Heart Circ Physiol.* 2000;279(1): H422–H428.
153. Hein S, Arnon E, Kostin S, et al. Progression from compensated hypertrophy to failure in the pressure-overloaded human heart: structural deterioration and compensatory mechanisms. *Circulation.* 2003;107(7):984–991.
154. Akyurek O, Akyurek N, Sayin T, et al. Association between the severity of heart failure and the susceptibility of myocytes to apoptosis in patients with idiopathic dilated cardiomyopathy. *Int J Cardiol.* 2001;80(1):29–36.
155. Wencker D, Chandra M, Nguyen K, et al. A mechanistic role for cardiac myocyte apoptosis in heart failure. *J Clin Invest.* 2003;111(10):1497–1504.

156. Beltrami AP, Barlucchi L, Torella D, et al. Adult cardiac stem cells are multipotent and support myocardial regeneration. *Cell.* 2003;114:763–776.
157. Dimmeler S, Zeiher AM. Wanted! The best cell for cardiac regeneration. *J Am Coll Cardiol.* 2004;44:464–466.
158. Jackson KA, Majka SM, Wang H, et al. Regeneration of ischemic cardiac muscle and vascular endothelium by adult stem cells. *J Clin Invest.* 2001;107:1395–1402.
159. Kajstura J, Zhang X, Reiss K, et al. Myocyte cellular hyperplasia and myocyte cellular hypertrophy contribute to chronic ventricular remodeling in coronary artery narrowing-induced cardiomyopathy in rats. *Circ Res.* 1994;74:383–400.
160. Kocher AA, Schuster MD, Szabolcs MJ, et al. Neovascularization of ischemic myocardium by human bone marrow-derived angioblasts prevents cardiomyocyte apoptosis, reduces remodeling and improves cardiac function. *Nat Med.* 2001;7:430–436.
161. Liu J, Hu Q, Wang Z, et al. Autologous stem cell transplantation for myocardial repair. *Am J Physiol Heart Circ Physiol.* 2004;287: H501–H511.
162. Nadal-Ginard B, Kajstura J, Leri A, et al. Myocyte death, growth, and regeneration in cardiac hypertrophy and failure. *Circ Res.* 2003;92:139–150.
163. Oh H, Bradfute SB, Gallardo TD, et al. Cardiac progenitor cells from adult myocardium: homing, differentiation, and fusion after infarction. *Proc Natl Acad Sci USA.* 2003;100:12313–12318.
164. Quaini F, Urbanek K, Graiani G, et al. The regenerative potential of the human heart. *Int J Cardiol.* 2004;95(Suppl 1):S26–S28.
165. Tomita S. Cell-based therapy to regenerate myocardium: from bench to bedside. *Artif Organs.* 2004;28:40–44.
166. Sunkomat JN, Gaballa MA. Stem cell therapy in ischemic heart disease. *Cardiovasc Drug Rev.* 2003;21:327–342.
167. Scheubel RJ, Zorn H, Silber RE, et al. Age-dependent depression in circulating endothelial progenitor cells in patients undergoing coronary artery bypass grafting. *J Am Coll Cardiol.* 2003;42: 2073–2080.
168. Sussman MA, Anversa P. Myocardial aging and senescence: where have the stem cells gone? *Ann Rev Physiol.* 2004;66:29–48.
169. Torella D, Rota M, Nurzynska D, et al. Cardiac stem cell and myocyte aging, heart failure, and insulin-like growth factor-1 overexpression. *Circ Res.* 2004;94:514–524.
170. Capogrossi MC. Cardiac stem cells fail with aging: a new mechanism for the age-dependent decline in cardiac function. *Circ Res.* 2004;94:411–413.
171. Kudo M, Wang Y, Wani MA, et al. Implantation of bone marrow stem cells reduces the infarction and fibrosis in ischemic mouse heart. *J Mol Cell Cardiol.* 2003;35:1113–1119.
172. Trounson A. Human embryonic stem cells: mother of all cell and tissue types. *Reprod Biomed Online.* 2002;4(Suppl 1):58–63.

Determinants of Cardiac Remodeling and Progression to Heart Failure

3

Jean-Jacques Mercadier

The pathways and mechanisms of cardiac hypertrophy and progression to heart failure (HF) have been for decades (if not centuries) questions challenging the intelligence of physiologists and physicians around the world (1–5). The question of the adaptive nature of cardiac hypertrophy arose logically when its etiologies (mainly hypertension and other causes of chronic mechanical overload of the heart such as valvular heart diseases) were progressively deciphered and when Laplace's law was transposed to cardiac physiology and pathophysiology. According to Laplace's law, the increase in wall thickness of the left ventricle (LV) allows normalization of LV wall stress during both systole and diastole, thus allowing each cardiac myocyte to operate under a normal load (i.e., normal working conditions). This concept allowed Meerson (1) to describe the time course of heart diseases due to LV chronic hemodynamic overload as three successive phases according to the degree of normalization of this load and what was considered at that time as the resulting LV function. During the first phase that immediately follows the imposition of the overload to the LV, the load by definition exceeds LV muscle mass, resulting in decreased LV output and the activation of a number of local and systemic processes recruited that emergently maintain mean blood pressure in the short term, and to normalize LV working conditions (i.e., ventricular wall stress) in the long term. If these mechanisms are successful, the patient (or animal in the experimental setting) survives, allowing the occurrence of the second phase of compensated/compensatory LV hypertrophy (LVH) during which the development of myocardial hypertrophy serves to normalize LV wall stress (i.e., has more or less exactly compensated the increase in load, allowing normalization of LV function and therefore, cardiac output) (6). The third phase returns full circle to the first one, during which LV load again progressively exceeds its contractile capacities allowed by a given myocardial mass and contractile performance that progressively declines. This results in decreased cardiac output and marks the entry to the chronic HF phase.

In this scheme, LVH is, by definition, adaptive. Decompensation occurs when the progression of load due to causative disease leads to deterioration of LV contractile function and to the increasing activation of the neurohumoral systems that surpass the growth capacity of the myocardium. This has been the dominating paradigm for almost four decades (Fig. 3-1).

However, since the beginning of the 1980s the adaptive nature of the second phase of compensated LVH has been challenged by two sets of concepts. The first arose from the demonstration that, beyond the increase in LV mass and an apparently conserved LV contractile function, the LV undergoes a profound tissular, cellular, and molecular remodeling. The latter is characterized by the expression of a protein phenotype typical of the embryonic/fetal stages of cardiac development [expression of β-MHC (Myosin Heavy Chain) instead of α-MHC, high levels of expression of natriuretic peptides, low level of expression of the Ca^{2+}-ATPase of the sarcoplasmic reticulum (SERCA), etc.] known as the re-expression of the fetal gene program (FGP) (7). Although the α- to β-MHC transition could be considered, from an energetic perspective, as an adaptive process at the myocyte level, and the ventricular recruitment for the production of natriuretic peptides as an adaptation of the LV pump in face of an increased preload, the truly adaptive and beneficial nature of other changes such as decreased SERCA expression and pump function, cardiac myocyte apoptosis, or LV interstitial fibrosis were obviously questionable. The second set of concepts arose

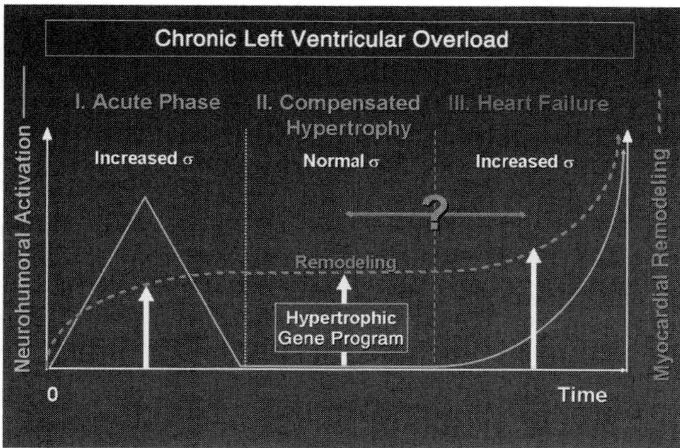

Figure 3-1 Progression of chronic work overload of the left ventricle from the onset of overload to chronic heart failure. This scheme is best-suited for myocardial infarction or experimental animal models in which the onset of the overload is sudden. During the acute initial phase, alteration of LV pump function results in activation of systemic neurohumoral systems aimed at maintaining mean blood pressure as normal as possible. Together with LV mechanical overload (mainly diastolic stretch), neurohumoral activation immediately triggers myocardial cellular and molecular remodeling characterized by the expression of the hypertrophic (fetal) gene program. Such a process persists during the second phase of compensated hypertrophy despite possible normalization of wall stress (sigma) and disappearance of systemic neurohumoral activation. This may be due, at least in part, to incomplete normalization of wall stress and to tissular neurohumoral activation. A strict limit between the second and third phases is hypothetical (?), progression to heart failure being progressive with gradual reappearance of decreased LV pump function. This decrease, associated with progressive increase in LV dimensions, reactivates mechanical overload and systemic neurohumoral systems, futher boosting myocardial remodeling.

from clinical research demonstrating that cardiac hypertrophy, even during its so-called compensated/compensatory phase, is a risk factor for HF and sudden death (8,9).

Finally, owing to the availability of more and more sophisticated transgenic (TG) mouse models and new tools to decipher the complexity of intracellular signaling, the last 10 years have been a time of a profound conceptual revolution regarding cardiac hypertrophy, its determinants, pathways, and biological significance. In particular, it has become progressively clearer that besides the adaptive nature of LVH, detrimental processes occurring from the very beginning of the overload and worsening during the phase of compensated/compensatory hypertrophy were, at least in part, responsible for the progression to HF. Thus, modification of the initial paradigm allows one to describe a continuum of myocardial, cellular, and molecular remodeling processes and pathways operating from the very beginning of LV reaction to biomechanical stress. It also sets the stage to distinguish between those processes governing physiological, beneficial, and/or adaptive responses from pathological, detrimental, and/or maladaptive hypertrophy. The purpose of this chapter is to review the determinants of this paradigm, with a special focus on the processes involved in the essentially pathological, detrimental, and/or maladaptive hypertrophy governing the progression to HF and the possible new therapeutic targets thus revealed.

EXPERIMENTAL MODELS AND INITIATORS OF CARDIAC HYPERTROPHY

Experimental Models

It is classical to distinguish between two different LV hypertrophic phenotypes with distinct triggers: concentric hypertrophy due to pressure overload (PO) and eccentric hypertrophy due to volume overload. The latter is also seen after large myocardial infarction (MI). Accordingly, experimental models of hypertension/PO of the LV are used to reproduce concentric hypertrophy and models of valvular regurgitation, or high-output arteriovenous fistula are used to reproduce eccentric LV hypertrophy (10). A detailed description of the various models of hypertension has been produced recently by Pinto et al. (11), who elegantly compared the advantages and disadvantages of each model regarding end-organ damage, among which is LVH, eventually followed by HF. It should be emphasized that despite a number of common features (hypertension, LVH, and impaired endothelium-dependent vascular relaxation), each model also more or less specifically imprints LV remodeling, leading to more- or less-specific cardiac phenotypes. It must also be pointed out that the models used for hypertension research are not necessarily the same as those used for research on cardiac hypertrophy and the mechanisms of its development. In the latter context, most of the studies carried out during the 1980s and early 1990s have used (probably because of the simplicity of its performance) the model of constriction of the abdominal aorta (AAC). This utilizes a metal clip or a thread placed around the abdominal aorta, usually between the renal arteries (10), making it a model similar to the 2K1C Goldblatt model because of its early activation of the renin-angiotensin system (RAS) (12). But constriction of the thoracic aorta (TAC) has also been used, although with some differences with AAC regarding pattern of molecular remodeling (13). Around the mid-1990s transgenesis opened new avenues for research in the mechanisms of LVH and progression to HF. Since that time, each model has been developed to address a specific question related to the role of proteins involved either in myocyte function (such as phospholamban) (14) or to signaling pathways involved in the development of LVH (15). The extremely numerous transgenic mouse models cannot be detailed here but, rather, specific models will be referenced throughout this chapter, wherever necessary.

At this stage, it is important to distinguish between two different types of models: those spontaneously exhibiting a clear cardiac phenotype such as occurs with Gαq (15) or calcineurin (16) overexpression, and those with no cardiac phenotype, for which a mechanical stress (usually TAC-induced PO) is necessary to unmask a cardiac phenotype or to induce progression from compensated LVH to HF (17–19). Both types of models have markedly contributed to the elucidation of molecular mechanisms responsible for LVH and progression to HF. It is important to note that with the transition from rat to mouse, AAC has been progressively abandoned in favor of TAC. Except for when the clip is placed in young animals with little or no initial aortic constriction (but with constriction developing progressively with time as animals grow), the mechanical component of the load imposed to the LV is much greater in the latter model than in the former, in which activation of the RAS seems to play a more important role (13,20). Therefore, it is clear that data obtained during the 1980s and 1990s using AAC in rats cannot be directly compared with data obtained more recently using TAC in mice.

Finally, the model of MI must be considered in the context of HF. Even if MI is an invaluable model to reproduce chronic HF (which is most often congestive in the setting of experimental models), allowing studies of peripheral adaptation or maladaptation or pharmacological studies, MI is not an appropriate model to identify the determinants of myocardial hypertrophy and the progression to HF. Indeed, LV remodeling following MI is more complex than that seen in models of pure pressure or volume overload, as the increase in systolic and diastolic stress on the noninfarcted myocardium depends on scar size and associated LV shape changes (21–24). This results in a complex pattern of tissular, cellular, and molecular remodeling (25), highly variable within an experimental group depending on the scar size. On the other hand, MI is a very useful model to test new therapies aimed at preventing HF. For instance, it has recently been demonstrated that blocking the calmodulin kinase II (CaMKII) can substantially prevent maladaptive remodeling post-MI (see Ca^{2+} Calmodulin-Dependent Protein Kinase IL).

Ca^{2+}/Calmodulin-Dependent Protein Kinase II)

Because adult cardiac myocytes are terminally differentiated cells that have lost most of their capacity to undergo complete cell division, cardiac hypertrophy is characterized by myocyte hypertrophy associated with hyperplasia of the nonmuscle cells (26). Indeed, if LV dysfunction is not present and the ventricle is hemodynamically compensated, myocyte hypertrophy is the predominant form of cell growth and myocyte proliferation (which is very low) is not significantly greater than that in control hearts (27). During LV concentric hypertrophy, myocyte growth is characterized by parallel addition of sarcomeres that induces lateral growth of the cell. This contrasts with volume overload during which myocytes increase in length due to the addition of sarcomeres in series, and points to the existence of different triggers and signaling pathways between the two types of LVH (28).

Although it is usual to contrast mechanical to neurohumoral triggers of LVH, in reality these two components probably cooperate in most models of chronic hemodynamic overload. This is all the more evident due to the existence of an active RAS in the heart (29), since it has been established that mechanical signals such as myocardial and myocyte stretch trigger myocyte hypertrophy through the involvement of many neurohumoral factors (see Neurohumoral Inhibitors). Nonetheless, recent data have clearly shown that, in contrast to what was postulated earlier (30), myocyte stretch can trigger myocyte hypertrophy directly through the involvement of integrins, myocyte costamere, and cytoskeleton, without the apparent contribution of neurohormones (19,31).

The question of triggers and pathways leading to cardiac myocyte hypertrophy is best understood in its historical context. This approach stresses the importance of cell culture, pioneered by the work of Simpson (32) in demonstrating the prohypertrophic effect of norepinephrine and in identifying, during the 1980s, the vast number of neurohumoral agents, growth factors, and cytokines associated with inducing hypertrophy of isolated neonatal or adult cardiac myocytes. Although isolated myocytes and cell culture systems remain invaluable tools for specific purposes [e.g., in the context of in vivo animal models (19,31)], the technology was surpassed around the mid-1990s by transgenesis, which most often permits similar questions to be addressed in the invaluable in vivo setting. Therefore, this chapter will focus on in vivo and, especially, transgenic models.

Mechanical Initiators

In the context of PO-induced LVH, the existence of a mechanical trigger is obvious. However, identification of the precise trigger responsible for LVH in this setting is not as easy. According to the hypothesis that concentric LVH is aimed at normalizing systolic wall stress, the trigger would be the increased systolic load imposed on cardiac myocytes during their contraction. However, the scientific proof of such a trigger remains elusive since such a pure systolic overload is difficult to reproduce in vitro as well as in experimental models. In fact, most in vitro and in vivo studies have focused on the role of passive (diastolic) stretch. We have shown that following AAC in the rat, hypertension and the associated LVH are delayed and preceded by a phase of volume overload due to RAS activation, which triggers gene reprogramming (most probably through the volume overload-induced stretch of the LV wall) (12). Such a mechanism is probably also involved when a tight TAC abruptly increases LV afterload, resulting in decreased ejection fraction and increased end-systolic volume that stretches the LV both during diastole and systole. It should be emphasized that most experimental models poorly reproduce what actually takes place in humans, especially in the setting of genetic hypertension. However, these models have been invaluable for identifying the triggers and pathways of LVH and progression to HF.

Myocyte Stretch

As discussed previously, whether the stretch signal can be transmitted to the nucleus and genes without the intervention of a neurohumoral signal has been questioned for a long time, especially since the study by Sadoshima et al. that demonstrated that growth of neonatal rat ventricular myocytes (NRVM) following stretch necessitated the autocrine activation of AT1 receptors following the release of angiotensin II (Ang II) (30). At the same time, Yamazaki et al. showed that myocyte stretch induces cardiac myocyte hypertrophy through a mechanism implying, at least in part, an increased synthesis and secretion of Ang II and endothelin-1 (ET-1) (33,34). However, a large amount of data has accumulated during the past few years to suggest that stimulation of Ang II receptors by the peptide is not a mandatory step in the cascade of events linking myocyte stretch to gene reprogramming. For instance, the Rho family of small

G-proteins plays a critical role in mediating hypertrophic responses to myocyte stretch, independent of Ang II stimulation (35). Moreover, AT1 receptors can be activated by stretch through an Ang II-independent mechanism (36).

Reactive oxygen species (ROS)-mediated extracellular signal-regulated kinase (ERK)1/2 activation also seems to be involved in cardiac myocyte hypertrophy induced by cyclic stretch of low amplitude (5%), and ROS production is greatly stimulated by Ang II-mediated NAD(P)H stimulation. In contrast, cyclic stretch of high amplitude (25%), which activates both extracellular signal-regulated kinase 1/2 and c-Jun N-terminal kinase (JNK), is associated with myocyte apoptosis (37) (Table 3-1).

Another important activation of the upstream mechanism that may be involved in stretch-induced cardiac myocyte hypertrophy is the Na^+-H^+ exchanger. Gene expression and activity of the Na^+-H^+ exchanger is increased in stretched cardiac myocytes (38) as well as in several models of LVH, including PO (39). The resulting increase in intracellular Na^+ concentration decreases the transmembrane Na^+ gradient, in turn promoting a rise in intracellular Ca^{2+} concentration via decreased Na^+-Ca^{2+} exchange. The resulting increase in intracellular Ca^{2+} may activate a number of signaling pathways, including calcineurin–NFAT, CaMK, PKC, and MAPK cascades, thus providing mechanisms by which the Na^+-Ca^{2+} exchanger can promote hypertrophy. Accordingly, HOE 694, an inhibitor of the exchanger, markedly attenuates stretch-induced activation of Raf-1 and MAPK and increase in protein synthesis, although this compound has no effect on Ang II- and ET-1-induced Raf-1 and MAPK activation (38). NHE inhibition is also able to attenuate LVH and fibrosis in spontaneously hypertensive rats (SHRs) (40) and the cardiomyopathic phenotype and, especially, LV dysfunction and fibrosis in mice overexpressing the β1-adrenergic receptor (41).

Regardless of what the upstream transducer is, a number of downstream effectors such as ERK1/2, p90RSK, p38 kinase (p38), Src, and BMK1 are activated by acute myocyte stretch as well as during chronic PO (42). A recent study indicates that PKC-α and -δ are important regulators in mediating activation of Rho GTPases and MAPKs in the cyclic stretch-induced hypertrophic process (43). However, it must be pointed out that most of these studies have been performed using myocytes isolated from neonatal ventricles, thus raising doubts about the possibility of directly extrapolating the results to adult myocytes and the in vivo setting.

Despite the interest of the aforementioned studies, it is clear that a conceptual leap has been accomplished with the recent identification of important transducers of stretch signaling. Mice deleted of the muscle Lim protein (MLP) gene (a gene that encodes a protein of the Z band of the sarcomere that associates with titin and T-cap/telethonin) exhibit dilated cardiomyopathy (DCM) with no hypertrophy when submitted to PO (31). Myocytes isolated from the ventricle of these mice are unable to express FGP when stretched, whereas they are fully responsive to phenylephrine (PE) or ET-1 stimulation. Similarly, mice deficient for melusin, a muscle-specific protein that interacts with the integrin β1 cytoplasmic domain, exhibit DCM with no LVH when submitted to PO, whereas LVH in these mice is perfectly induced by chronic administration of Ang II or PE at doses that do not increase blood pressure (19).

Extra- and Intra-Cellular Signaling

The previously-mentioned studies have generated a renewal of interest in the signals mediated through the cell membrane via the integrins and associated proteins. Integrins are a large family of heterodimeric cell surface receptors that link the extracellular matrix to the intracellular cytoskeleton and signal bidirectionally across the cell membrane of cardiac myocytes and fibroblasts. Most interestingly from the cardiovascular viewpoint, they have been shown to function as mechanotransducers. The repertoire of integrins present on cells is modulated in the remodeled myocardium. Furthermore, hemodynamic loading may alter key integrin-mediated signaling events (44,45). The importance of integrins in the hypertrophic process is strengthened by the observation that β1 integrin knockout mice are intolerant to TAC (46). Other important proteins involved in extra- and intra-cellular signaling are discoidin domain receptors (DDRs), which are transmembrane complexes that attach specifically to collagen which have tyrosine kinase motifs in the cytoplasmic domain, and the cadherins, which regulate cell–cell interaction. The arrangement and localization of these proteins on the surface of myocytes and fibroblasts suggest that they may play an important role not only in force transmission but also in cell signaling (45).

It is important to note that cardiac fibroblasts also have the ability to sense, integrate, and functionally respond to mechanical stimuli through the secretion of autocrine/paracrine factors such as Ang II, ET-1, or tumor necrisos factor-α (TNF-α) that are released in response to mechanical stimulation and exert their effect on both fibroblasts and cardiac myocytes (45). These neurohumoral factors and cytokines activate intracellular pathways through their binding to their respective receptors. For instance, osteopontin (OPN), a protein secreted by both fibroblasts and cardiac myocytes that binds to integrins, also seems to play an important role in LVH. It plays an important role in cardiac fibrosis, probably through the modulation of cellular adhesion and proliferation of fibroblasts. Its expression is increased in cardiac hypertrophy and its absence attenuates fibrosis (47). Moreover, increased phosphorylation of JNK, p38, Akt, and GSK-3β is significantly lower in the heart of OPN knockout mice submitted to TAC than in their wild type (WT) controls, suggesting that increased OPN expression may play an important role in modulating PO-induced LVH (48).

Neurohumoral Initiators

Catecholamines

Intuitively, the increase in sympathetic tone and activation of the RAS that occurs at the acute phase of MI should play an important role in the subsequent hypertrophy of the noninfarcted myocardial area. It is less clear whether α- and/or β-adrenoceptor activation should play an important role in the development of PO-induced LVH. As previously mentioned, the prohypertrophic effect of α-adrenergic stimulation was the first demonstrated prohypertrophic effect of a neurohumoral agent on isolated cardiac myocytes (32). A similar observation was done for β-adrenoceptor

TABLE 3-1
SIGNALING MECHANISMS THAT INITIATE MYOCYTE/MYOCARDIAL REMODELING IN VITRO AND/OR IN VIVO

Experimental Model	Nature of the Initiating Stress	Neurohumoral Mediator(s)	Cell Target	Downstream Pathway(s)	References
Stretch of NRVM	Mechanical	Ang II ± ET-1? (± influx of Ca^{2+})	AT1R/ET-1AR	Raf-1 – MAPK	30,33,34,36,60,61
Stretch of NRVM	Mechanical	—	NAD(P)H oxidase	ROS – ERK1/2 – (JNK)	37
Stretch of NRVM	Mechanical	—	Na^+-H^+ exchanger	Raf-1 – MAPK	38
PO–rabbit	Mechanical (±NH?)	?	Na^+-H^+ exchanger	—	39
PO–SHR	Mechanical (±NH?)	?	Na^+-H^+ exchanger	—	40
Cardiac overexpression of the β1-adrenergic receptor	—	—	Na^+-H^+ exchanger	—	41
Stretch of NRVM	Mechanical	—	MLP	MLP – (Calsarcin – Calcineurin?)	31
PO inmice KO for MLP	Mechanical (±NH?)	?			
PO in mice KO for melusin	Mechanical (±NH?)	?	Melusin	Melusin – GSK-3β	19
PO in mice KO for β-1 integrin	Mechanical (±NH?)	?	β1-integrin	-	46
PO in mice KO for osteopontin	Mechanical (±NH?)	?	Osteopontin	JNK, p38K, Akt – GSK-3β	48
N(A)RVM	Neurohumoral	Catecholamines	α1-adrenergic receptors β-adrenergic receptors	Gαq/11 – PLC – IP3/DAG Gαs – AC -cAMP	32,49,50§
PO in mice KO for dopamine β-hydroxylase	Mechanical (±NH?)	Catecholamines	α1-adrenergic receptors β-adrenergic receptors	Idem + ERK1/2, JNK, p38K	51
PO in mice KO for AT1(A)R	Mechanical (±NH?)	Ang II?	AT2R?	—	53,54,52, 55§
PO in mice KO for AT2R	Mechanical (±NH?)	Ang II?	AT1R?	p70 (S6k)	57,58
Nephrectomy + 1%NaCl diet + aldosterone	Neurohumoral ± mechanical	Aldosterone	MR	Calcineurin – NFAT?	69
Cardiac overexpression of the mineralocorticoid receptor	—	—	MR	Calcineurin – NFAT?	67
PO in rat–TGF-β1 overexpression – mice KO for TGF-β1	Mechanical (±NH?)	TGF-β1	TGB-βR (RTK family)	TAK1 – p38	72,73,74,75,71§
PO in mice KO for FGF-2	Mechanical (±NH?)	FGF-2	FGFR (RTK family)	—	78,79
PO–physical training	Mechanical (±NH?)	IGF-1	IGF-1R	PI3K -Akt	80,81,4§
NRVM and fibroblasts, overexpression of IL-6 and its receptor	Neurohumoral	IL-6/11, LIF, CT-1	gp130/gp80	MAPK – Jak/STAT	82,83
PO in mice overexpressing a DN gp130 mutant	Mechanical (±NH?)	IL-6/11, LIF, CT-1?	gp130/gp80	—	84,18
PO inmice KO for gp130					

This table gives examples of studies aimed at identifying upstream initiating mechanisms. Downstream signal transducers and signaling cascades are given when identified or hypothesized in the corresponding articles. § refers to recent review articles. ? indicates uncertainity about the involvement of the factor.

stimulation (49). The role of α- and β-adrenergic signaling during cardiac hypertrophy and failure has been reviewed in detail recently (50) and will not be detailed here, with the exception of the downstream signaling cascades involved (see Gg/G11 Signaling and Gs/Gi signaling). There are numerous studies of transgenic mice demonstrating both the requirement of norepinephrine and epinephrine for the induction of in vivo PO-induced LVH and the detrimental effects of such an activation; the LVH associated with activation of these receptors and downstream pathways most often results in maladaptive hypertrophy progressing to HF. More interesting is the demonstration of an apparently almost universal requirement of endogenous catecholamines for the induction of in vivo PO-induced cardiac hypertrophy and for the activation of hypertrophic signaling pathways (51).

Angiotensin II and Endothelin-1

As already mentioned, Ang II of systemic or tissular origin is probably the most important humoral agent involved in LVH, especially its maladaptive aspects. Ang II acts through binding to its specific receptors, the type 1 and type 2 Ang II receptors (AT1R and AT2R, respectively). AT1R is probably the most important receptor involved in LVH induced by mechanical and/or neurohumoral stimulation. Its level of expression is also influenced by PO. In the long term, AT1R protein and mRNA levels have been found to be consistently increased in all models of PO-induced LVH in the rat (52). However, although subpressor doses of Ang II failed to increase LV mass in mice deleted of the AT1R, PO fully induced LVH in these mice with myocyte hypertrophy, myocardial fibrosis, and expression of FGP, suggesting that AT1-mediated Ang II signaling is not necessary for the development of PO-induced LVH (53,54).

Despite its demonstrated involvement in cardiac development, the role of AT2R in LVH has remained elusive until recently. More precisely, many in vitro and in vivo studies have suggested that AT2R stimulation exerts counterbalancing suppressant effects against the growth-promoting, profibrotic, and hypertrophic effects of AT1R stimulation (55). For instance, lentivirus-mediated overexpression of AT2R in the heart of 5-day-old SHRs led to decreased LV wall thickness and decreased heart weight-to-body weight ratio (HW/BW), indicating that early AT2R overexpression attenuates the development of cardiac hypertrophy in this context (56).

Recent data, however, have suggested a possible different role in which AT2R would support rather than oppose the effects of AT1R stimulation (55). For instance, targeted deletion of mouse AT2R prevented AAC-induced LVH (57), and LVH and fibrosis induced by infusion of a hypertensive dose of Ang II were eliminated in mice lacking the AT2R, indicating that this receptor is essential for LVH and fibrosis in chronic, Ang II-induced hypertension (58). In the same experimental setting in rats, AT2R blockade with PD123319 had no influence on LVH, α-skeletal actin, and β-MHC expression but did increase the expression of c-fos, ET-1, IGF-1, and atrial natriuretic peptides and decreased vascular endothelial growth factor (VEGF) and fibroblast growth factor-1 (FGF-1) expression. This suggests that AT2R plays a functional role in the hypertrophic process by selectively regulating the expression of growth-promoting and growth-inhibiting factors (59).

Endothelin-1 (ET-1) has long been known to be a possible mediator of hypertrophy, both independently and in response to other growth factors, especially Ang II. Both exposure to Ang II and stretching of NRVM induce ET-1 mRNA and secretion of ET-1 in the culture medium. In these cells, the Ang II-induced increase in protein synthesis is blocked by ET-1 antisense oligonucleotides, suggesting that autocrine/paracrine synthesis of ET-1 is an obligatory intermediate step in Ang II-induced myocyte hypertrophy (60). In addition, stretch-induced activation of MAPK and increase in protein synthesis are inhibited by the ET-1 antagonist BQ123 (61). Co-culture of NRVM with cardiac fibroblasts has enabled the demonstration of the interaction between the two cell types, with Ang II stimulating cardiac myocyte hypertrophy, at least in part, via paracrine release of TGF-β1 and ET-1 from fibroblasts (62).

Mineralocorticoid

The role of aldosterone and mineralocorticoid receptor (MR) stimulation, independent of the role of Ang II, in the development of LVH has been a matter of debate. Indeed, if mineralocorticoids are used to induce hypertension and LVH in the deoxycorticosterone acetate (DOCA)-salt model, the actual role of mineralocorticoids on myocyte hypertrophy is unclear; aldosterone is better-known for its profibrotic effects than as an important mediator of myocyte hypertrophy. In fact, aldosterone induces cardiac fibrosis through an increase of cardiac AT1R receptor levels, thereby potentiating the profibrotic effect of Ang II (63). However, small amounts of aldosterone are also produced in the heart and this production is increased by Ang II, suggesting that the heart contains a steroidogenic system that is regulated similarly to the adrenal one (64).

In rats that are double-transgenic for the human renin and angiotensinogen genes (dTGR) and that develop hypertension, vasculopathy, LVH, and fibrosis, both spitonolactone and the AT1R blocker valsartan prevented death and vasculopathy and reversed LVH, while only valsartan normalized blood pressure. This suggests that aldosterone promotes LVH and fibrosis by a mechanism independent of increased blood pressure (65). Transcription factors AP-1 and nuclear factor kappa B (NF-κB) were activated in dTGR compared with controls. MR blockade downregulated these effectors and reduced Ang II-induced cardiac damage (65). Similarly, mice with cardiac-specific overexpression of 11β–hydroxysteroid dehydrogenase type 2 (which converts glucocorticoids to receptor-inactive metabolites, thus allowing aldosterone to occupy and activate MRs) spontaneously develop LVH, fibrosis, and HF—all effects mitigated by the MR blocker eplerenone (66). Mice with cardiac-specific conditional overexpression of the human MR exhibit a high rate of death associated with severe ventricular arrhythmias (67). Such alterations are prevented by spironolactone, suggesting novel opportunities for prevention of arrhythmia-related, sudden cardiac death. Unexpectedly, spironolactone also reversed interstitial fibrosis, attenuated myocyte disarray, and improved diastolic function in the cardiac troponin-T (cTnT)-Q92 transgenic mouse model of human hypertrophic cardiomyopathy (HCM), suggesting aldosterone as an important pathophysiological link between sarcomeric mutations and cardiac phenotype in HCM (68).

The prohypertrophic/profibrotic effects of mineralocorticoids on the heart are likely mediated, at least in part, by stimulation of the calcineurin/NFAT pathway, since FK506 or cyclosporine partially prevented LVH and fibrosis in uninephrectomized rats placed on a 1.0% NaCl diet and treated with aldosterone (69). In vitro data suggest that aldosterone also potentiates the effects of Ang II on ROS generation, EGFR transactivation, and ERK1/2 phosphorylation (70). This may explain, at least in part, why MR blockade decreases end-organ damage in dTGR (65).

Peptide Growth Factors and Receptor Tyrosine Kinases

Receptor tyrosine kinases (RTKs) transmit signals from many peptide growth factors, including fibroblast growth factor (FGF), nerve growth factor (NGF), epidermal growth factor (EGF), platelet-derived growth factor (PDGF), transforming growth factor-β (TGF-β), insulin, and insulin-like growth factor-1 (IGF-1). The mechanism of receptor activation includes ligand-induced dimerization and mutual autophosphorylation on tyrosine residues of the cytoplasmic tail. This allows recruiting signaling molecules to the membrane, where they form transient complexes that transmit signals downstream in the cell.

TGF-β and the RAS play a pivotal role in the development of LVH and HF. Recent studies indicate that Ang II and TGF-β do not act independently from one another but, rather, act as part of a signaling network in order to promote cardiac remodeling (71). As previously described, Ang II stimulates cardiac myocyte hypertrophy through paracrine release of TGF-β1 and ET-1 from fibroblasts (62). Ang II upregulates TGF-β expression via activation of the AT1R in cardiac myocytes and fibroblasts, and induction of this cytokine seems necessary for Ang II-induced cardiac hypertrophy in vivo. In the rat, AAC is associated with early myocardial fibroblast activation (proliferation and phenotype transition to myofibroblasts) followed by myocyte hypertrophy and fibrosis. This is associated with early induction of myocardial TGF-β mRNA expression. An anti-TGF-β neutralizing antibody inhibits fibroblast activation and subsequently prevents collagen mRNA induction and myocardial fibrosis, but not myocyte hypertrophy (72). Whether TGF-β is directly involved in myocyte hypertrophy, fibrosis, or both remained a matter of debate until the development of TG mice. TG mice with elevated levels of activated TGF-β1 in the heart show overt fibrosis only in the atria and an inhibition of ventricular fibroblast DNA synthesis, suggesting that TGF-β1 alone is insufficient to promote ventricular fibrosis (73). Although WT mice subjected to chronic subpressor doses of Ang II showed LVH and impaired LV function, TGF-β1-deficient mice showed no significant changes in LV mass and percent LV fractional shortening. Cardiomyocyte cross-sectional area was also markedly increased in Ang II-treated WT mice but was unchanged in Ang II-treated, TGF-β-deficient mice. Atrial natriuretic peptide (ANP) expression was increased sixfold in Ang II-treated WT, but not in TGF-β1-deficient mice. Taken together, these results indicate that TGF-β1 is an important mediator of the hypertrophic growth response of cardiac myocytes to Ang II in vivo (74).

An important downstream effector of TGF–β is the TGF-β-activated kinase TAK1, a member of the MAP kinase kinase kinase family (see Intracellular Signaling Pathways and Mitogen-Activated Protein Kinases). Indeed, TAC-induced LVH in mice is associated with TGF-β upregulation and a sevenfold increase of TAK1 kinase activity. Moreover, an activating mutation of TAK1 expressed in the myocardium of TG mice is sufficient to produce p38 phosphorylation, LVH, interstitial fibrosis, severe LV dysfunction, induction of FGP, apoptosis, and early mouse lethality (75). Another important downstream mediator of TGF-β is connective tissue growth factor (CTGF). This secreted protein binds to cell surface and possesses a broad spectrum of biological effects, including stimulation of fibroblast proliferation, extracellular matrix (ECM) production, and myocyte hypertrophy (76). CTGF is rapidly upregulated in NRVM exposed to phenylephrine or ET-1, suggesting that this growth factor is involved in cardiac hypertrophy and fibrosis (77).

Whether FGF-2 is involved in the development of PO-induced LVH has also been a matter of debate. In one study, mice lacking FGF-2 developed significantly less LVH in response to TAC than did their WT controls (78). In another study, normotensive mice lacking FGF-2 developed DCM and exhibited impaired cardiac growth in response to 2K1C-induced hypertension (79). In vitro experiments from the same study indicated that FGF-2 of fibroblast origin is a crucial mediator of LVH via autocrine/paracrine actions on cardiac myocytes.

Insulin-like growth factor 1, the main mediator of the growth effects of growth hormone (GH), is expressed in the myocardium in response to PO (80). However, evidence is accumulating to suggest that IGF-1 signaling through the recruitment of PI3K/Akt (see Intracellular Signaling Pathways) is involved in physiological/adaptive LVH seen during exercise conditioning or pregnancy rather than in PO-induced pathological/maladaptive LVH (4,81). However, in the latter context, IGF-1 expression may serve as an important cardioprotective mechanism.

Cardiotrophin-1, Leukemia Inhibitory Factor, and the Interleukin-6 Receptor

Following binding of interleukin-6 (IL-6), leukemia inhibitory factor (LIF), or cardiotrophin-1 (CT-1), the transmembrane receptor gp130 is activated by several mechanisms, including heterodimerization with gp80—a process that rapidly activates the Janus kinase/signal transducer and activator of transcription (JAK/STAT) and the extracellular signal-regulated kinase (ERK) pathways. Ang II induces IL-6, LIF, and CT-1 in cardiac fibroblasts, and these cytokines (particularly LIF and CT-1) activate gp130-linked signaling and contribute to Ang II-induced cardiac myocyte hypertrophy (82). Mice double-transgenic for IL-6 and its receptor develop myocardial hypertrophy (83), and mice with cardiac-specific expression of a dominant-negative mutant of gp130 develop less LVH when submitted to TAC than do their WT controls (84). More interestingly in the context of PO-induced LVH, mice with deleted gp130 develop severe DCM and HF associated with massive myocyte apoptosis when submitted to TAC, indicating an obligatory activation of the gp130 pathway to prevent myocyte apoptosis and HF following PO of the LV (18).

INTRACELLULAR SIGNALING PATHWAYS

Gq/G11 Signaling

α1-adrenergic, Ang II, and ET-1 receptors are coupled to heterotrimeric Gq/G11 proteins that activate phospholipase C (Fig. 3-2). Stimulation of all has been shown to be sufficient to induce hypertrophy of NRVM in culture. The role of G-proteins in this process was clarified during the second half of the 1990s with the development of important TG mouse models (4,85). TG overexpression of these receptors, as well as Gq/G11, results in cardiac hypertrophy, which possibly leads to cardiomyopathy with depressed cardiac function depending on the degree of overexpression of the transgene (15). More interesting are the effects of TAC in mice overexpressing Gαq (17). Although nontransgenic mice developed concentric LVH associated with the typical re-expression of FGP, Gαq-overexpressing mice developed excentric hypertrophy leading to HF with no further increase in FGP expression. This study is of special importance because it indicated for the first time that the sole stimulation of a signaling pathway, without mechanical overload, is able to reproduce the ventricular phenotype produced by PO, thereby demonstrating the importance of Gαq stimulation in the development of PO-induced LVH. Also, because HF occurred rapidly after TAC in TG mice with LVs already exhibiting all the features of PO-induced LVH, the study demonstrated the limits of adaptation due to LVH and re-expression of FGP. Moreover, it was also one of the first studies suggesting that the phenotypical changes resulting from PO/Gαq overstimulation may be maladaptive rather than adaptive.

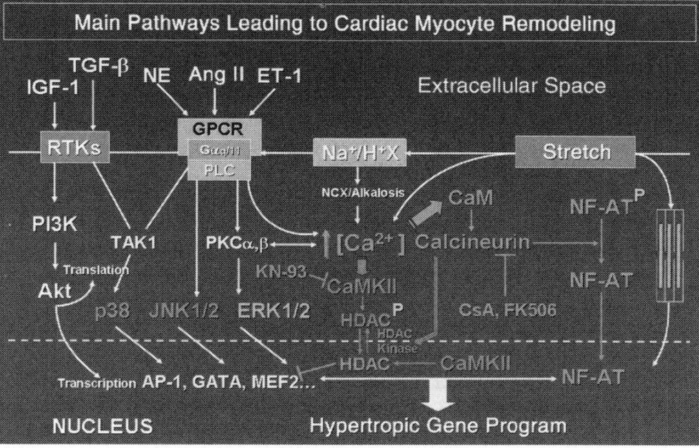

Figure 3-2 Simplified overview of the main pathways leading from biomechanical stress to cardiomyocyte gene reprogramming. Myocyte stretch and stimulation of the Gq protein coupled receptors (GPCR) by norepinephrine (NE), angiotensin II (Ang II) and endothelin (ET-1) are the main upstream initiators of a number of intracellular cascades [MAPK (p38, JNK, ERK), calcineurin–NFAT, CaMK-HDAC, and so forth] whose downstream effectors act on transcription factors and genes to induce the expression of the hypertrophic gene program. Increased cytosolic free calcium concentration plays a central role in this process. On the **left**, the PI-3K–Akt pathway is the main signaling pathway responsible for physiological LVH resulting from exercise conditioning or pregnancy, with effects on both gene transcription and mRNA translation.

Conversely, when TAC was performed in mice in which Gq signaling had been blocked by the expression of a specific peptide that uncouples Gq from its coupled receptors, TG mice developed less LVH than did WT controls, further demonstrating the role of Gq in the initiation of myocardial hypertrophy (86). Interestingly, cardiac contractility was preserved in these mice despite the lack of normalization of the LV wall stress, and the animals displayed a slower pace of deterioration of systolic function compared with WT controls. This indicates that LVH is not a mandatory adaptive mechanism, at least in this model and for the time period considered (87). Similarly, in TG mice with cardiac-specific overexpression of RGS4, a protein which inactivates signaling through heterotrimeric G-proteins by increasing the GTPase activity of Gαq/Gαi (88), PO failed to induce LVH (89). Similarly, cross-breeding RGS4-overexpressing mice with Gq-overexpressing mice delayed the LV contractile dysfunction and FGP induction seen in the latter (90). The importance of Gq/G11 signaling in the development of LVH was strengthened by the combined ablation of Gq and G11 (91). Such an approach resulted in an almost complete lack of LVH and activation of FGP in response to TAC, demonstrating the requirement for Gq/G11 for most (if not all) features of PO-induced LVH (91).

An intriguing mechanism has been suggested from in vitro studies that the prohypertrophic effect of norepinephrine, Ang II, and ET-1 would necessitate the activation of the myocardial heparin-binding epidermal growth factor receptor (HB-EGFR), a member of the ErbB family of receptor tyrosine kinases. The process would require the cell surface cleavage and shedding of the ectodomain of HB-EGF by a disintegrin and metalloproteinase (ADAM12), likely activated by PKCδ, which cleaves membrane-bound HB-EGF, allowing HB-EGFR activation in response to GqPCR stimulation or PO (92). In vivo, KBR-7785, an inhibitor of ADAM12, attenuated LVH induced by TAC or PE or Ang II infusion. An antisense oligodesoxynucleotide to EGFR prevented LVH in Ang II-infused rats and attenuated Ang II-enhanced EGFR expression and ERK activation, reinforcing the concept that Ang II requires EGFR to mediate ERK activation in the heart (93). Similar findings were observed with young but not adult SHRs, suggesting a critical role of the EGFR-activated ERK pathway in cardiovascular development but not in the maintenance of established LVH (94).

The role of the ErbB receptor family for maintaining normal cardiac trophicity and contractile function is further supported by conditional ErbB2 knockout in mice, which leads to DCM (95,96). Similarly, mice expressing an uncleavable or a transmembrane domain truncated form of HB-EGF instead of the WT form develop severe heart failure (97,98). It has been shown that transactivation of the EGFR by the AT1R can also be mediated by ROS and inhibited by antioxidants such as N-acetyl cysteine (99). Finally, the dihydropyridine calcium-channel-blocker amlodipine reduced TAC-induced LVH, a reduction associated with inhibition of EGFR phosphorylation (100). Future studies will tell us the actual importance of HB-EGF shedding in the development of LVH and progression to HF.

Gs/Gi Signaling

Whereas the β1-adrenoceptor couples to Gs, which in turn activates adenylyl cyclase (AC), the β2-receptor couples to both Gs and Gi. β-adrenergic stimulation activates protein synthesis of adult rat ventricular myocytes in culture (49). In vivo, overexpression of β1-receptors, despite the expected positive inotropic effect, results in progressive deterioration of cardiac performance, myocyte hypertrophy, and myocardial fibrosis (101). Similar findings were found with Gαs overexpression, which results in myocardial damage characterized by cellular degeneration, necrosis, and replacement fibrosis, with the remaining cells undergoing hypertrophy (102,103). Interestingly, these effects do not seem to depend on AC activation (103). Indeed, overexpression of AC type V (104) or type VI (105,106) [the main AC isoforms expressed in the heart (107,108)] had no adverse effects on cardiac structure and function and even attenuated the deleterious effects of Gq overexpression (106,109). However, disruption of AC type V protected the LV from TAC-induced dysfunction, probably by preventing cardiac myocyte apoptosis (110). Interestingly, recent findings implicate cyclic adenosine monophosphate (cAMP) as an inhibitor of ECM formation by means of blockade of the transformation of cardiac fibroblasts to myofibroblasts, and suggest that increasing AC expression (thereby enhancing cAMP generation through stimulation of receptors expressed on cardiac fibroblasts) could provide a means to attenuate and prevent cardiac fibrosis (111).

Both β_2-adrenergic and muscarinic receptors couple to Gi, thus inhibiting AC and opposing Gs-dependent signaling. Gi upregulation is an important mechanism in the downregulation of the β-adrenergic signaling pathway during HF (112). Interestingly, Gi is upregulated in hypertensive LVH before the development of heart failure, suggesting that it is involved in the progression to HF (113). Overexpression of β_2-receptors is deleterious only when high levels are expressed. In contrast, moderate levels of expression are able to rescue the cardiomyopathic phenotype of mice with Gq overexpression (114). This could be due, at least in part, to the antiapoptotic effect of moderate β-adrenergic stimulation (115).

Mitogen-Activated Protein Kinases

Mitogen-activated protein kinase (MAPK) signaling pathways consist of a sequence of successively active kinases (cascades) that ultimately result in the phosphorylation and activation of terminal kinases such as ERKs, JNKs, and p38s. The latter two groups are also categorized as stress-responsive MAPKs because they are not only activated by anabolic stimuli and GPCRs, but also by pathological stress such as ischemia and cytotoxic agents (116,117). The various cascades are activated in cardiac myocytes by ligand binding to GPCR, receptor tyrosine kinases, IL-6 receptor, and stress stimuli. Once activated, the terminal kinases each phosphorylate a number of targets that include transcription factors, resulting in the reprogramming of cardiac myocyte gene expression (Fig. 3-3).

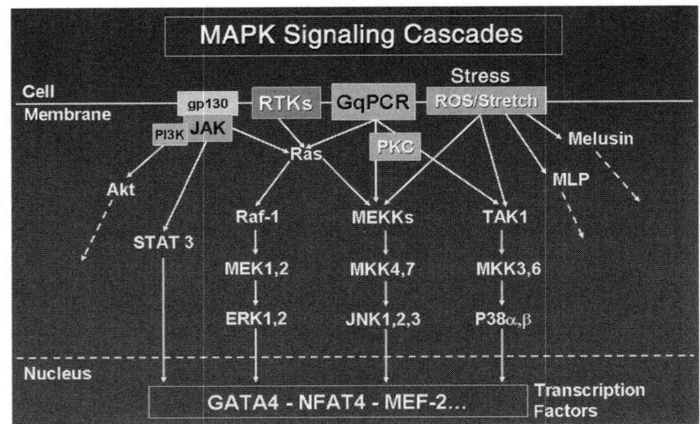

Figure 3-3 Simplified overview of the three best-characterized MAPK signaling cascades: ERK, JNK, and p38. On the **left**, the gp130-JAK are upstream activators of ERK1/2 through Ras activation. On the **right**, ROS and myocyte stretch activate MAPK cascades, the latter also activating a number of other proteins/pathways such as MLP and melusin.

ERKs are directly phosphorylated by MEK1 or MEK2 which, in turn, are phosphorylated by Raf-1 (118). Among at least five different ERK proteins, ERK 1 and 2 (ERK1/2) are the more abundantly expressed and best-studied in the heart. ERK1/2 are activated downstream of a cascade involving Ras, Raf-1, and MEK1/2 (119). They are activated in cultured cardiac myocytes in response to agonist stimulation and cell stretching. They are also activated by acute PO in mice (42,51). A large number of studies strongly support the concept that ERK1/2 activation is a prerequisite in the initiation or effective progression of myocyte hypertrophy in culture. However, a number of similarly designed studies have disputed such a conclusion. One study even suggested that, in the very specific context of ANP stimulation (see Negative Regulators of Cardiac Hypertrophy), ERK activation was associated with prevention of myocyte hypertrophy (120).

Experiments using TG mice have helped to somewhat clarify the situation. Although Gq cardiac overexpression is not associated with ERK1/2 activation (15), MEK1 overexpression is associated with moderate LVH with few (if any) signs of histopathology and interstitial fibrosis up to 6 months of age. Interestingly, MEK1-overexpressing mice demonstrated enhanced LV contractile performance and resistance to ischemia/reperfusion-induced myocytes apoptosis (121). Importantly, overexpression of the muscle-specific β-1 integrin interacting protein melusin increased basal phosphorylation of ERK1/2 and GSK-3β, and ERK1/2 was hyperphosphorylated together with Akt and GSK-3β in melusin-overexpressing mice submitted to PO (122). This was associated with a delayed transition to HF, probably due to a decreased level of cardiomyocyte apoptosis and ECM deposition as well as increased capillary density compared with WT mice. In contrast, mice overexpressing Ras showed a cardiomyopathic phenotype, possibly due to the fact that Ras can also activate the JNK branch of the MAPK cascades as well as other signaling pathways (123). Moreover, it has been suggested that activation of the Raf–MEK–ERK cascade represents a common pathway for alteration in intracellular Ca^{2+} homeostasis induced by Ras and PKC in cardiac myocytes (124) (Fig. 3–3).

JNKs are directly phosphorylated by MKK4 or MKK7, which, in turn, are activated by MEKK1 (118). In vitro, agonist stimulation by PE, Ang II, and ET-1, as well as cell stretching results in rapid phosphorylation of JNK (2). A dominant-negative MKK4 mutant attenuates the hypertrophic response to ET-1 in vitro (125) and to PO in vivo (126). In mice both overexpressing Gq and deficient for MEKK1, the hypertrophic phenotype and JNK activation seen in the former model are both abrogated, an effect associated with improved systolic function (127). This suggests that MEKK1 activation (and the resulting JNK activation) is necessary for most, if not all, adverse consequences of chronic Gq activation in the heart. Surprisingly, loss of cardiac JNK activity leads to spontaneous cardiac hypertrophy that is greatly exacerbated by PO (128). This is due to the cross-talk between MAPK cascades and Ca^{2+} activated signaling through calcineurin (see Clacineurin—Nuclear Factor of Activated T Cells), with JNK phosphorylating the calcineurin target NFAT, thus leading to its nuclear export and inactivation.

MAPKs of the p38 family are activated by MKK3 and MKK6 which, in turn, are activated by TAK1 (118). The p38 MAPK branch is activated by the same agonists that activate the other MAPK branches, as well as by PO (75). In vitro, p38β seems to mediate cardiac hypertrophy while p38α seems to protect against cardiac myocyte apoptosis (129). However, the role of p38 MAPK in the development of TAC-induced LVH has been controversial (116). A constitutively active TAK1 mutant results in cardiac hypertrophy and subsequent HF (75), suggesting that stimulation of this MAPK branch results in maladaptive growth of the myocardium. Targeted activation of p38 MAPK in mice using activated mutants of upstream kinases (MKK 3 and 6) induces marked LV interstitial fibrosis with expression of the FGP characteristic of PO-induced LVH, but with no LVH (130,131). The hemodynamic profile consists in LV systolic dysfunction and increased passive chamber stiffness, the negative inotropic effect of p38 MAPK being mediated by decreased myofilament sensitivity to Ca^{2+} (131).

Cardiac-specific p38α knockout mice displayed normal global cardiac structure and function. In response to PO, they developed significant levels of LVH, as seen in controls, but also developed LV dysfunction and heart dilatation. This abnormal response to PO was accompanied by massive cardiac fibrosis and the appearance of apoptotic myocytes (132). These results confirm in vitro data (129) and demonstrate that p38α plays a critical role in myocyte survival in response to PO, and no role in PO-induced LVH. TG mice expressing dominant-negative p38α, MKK3, or MKK6 each showed enhanced LVH following TAC, or 14-day infusion of Ang II, isoproterenol, or PE through a mechanism involving enhanced calcineurin–NFAT signaling (133). Important downstream targets of p38 MAPK seem to be the myocyte enhancer factor-2 (MEF2) transcription factor family, an important family of transcription factors involved in cardiac development and regulators of cardiac gene expression (134), and NFATc4, the downstream effector of calcineurin (135).

It must be pointed that MAPK cascades can also be activated by ROS (99). JNK and p38 are strongly activated by ROS or by a mild oxidative shift of the intracellular thiol/disulfide redox state. Ang II induces the production of ROS and activates ERK1/2 and p38, and JNK and p38 were shown to be activated by hydrogen peroxide in perfused rat hearts (136).

Clacineurin—Nuclear Factor of Activated T Cells

With the publication of a seminal paper by Olson et al. (16), calcineurin burst into the field of molecular cardiology in 1998, at a moment when research attention was focused on Gq/G11 coupled receptors and MAPKs cascades (137). This paper demonstrated that this Ca^{2+}-sensitive phosphatase is a critical mediator of cardiac hypertrophy and HF. The physiological role of this serine-threonine phosphatase [consisting of a catalytic A subunit and a regulatory B subunit, whose activity is inhibited by cyclosporine A (CsA) and FK505 (tacrolimus)] was first elucidated in T-lymphocytes in which elevations in cytoplasmic Ca^{2+} concentrations promote its association with calmodulin and consequent activation of the enzyme (138). Calcineurin then dephosphorylates transcription factors of the NFAT (nuclear factor of activated T-cells) family, which results in the translocation of these factors in the nucleus. In the heart, NFATc4 binds to the transcription factor GATA-4, where they activate the transcription of hypertrophic genes. The activity of calcineurin is modulated by a family of cofactors, referred to as modulatory calcineurin-interacting proteins (MCIPs). In the heart, the MCIP1 gene is activated by calcineurin and has been proposed to fulfill a negative feedback loop that limits calcineurin signaling, which would otherwise lead to excessive or pathological/maladaptive cardiac growth (139).

Although a large number of studies have clearly demonstrated that activation of the calcineurin–NFAT pathway is sufficient to induce massive LVH that possibly turns into HF, the question rapidly arose of whether calcineurin activation is also necessary for this process to occur (139). The answer has been controversial because of the conflicting results of studies using cyclosporin and/or FK506 to prevent hypertrophy (140); most of them showed clear inhibition or attenuation but others failed to do so [reviewed in (2)]. The possible unspecific effects of these immunosuppressive agents have also contributed to this controversy.

The issue was somewhat clarified by the use of TG mice overexpressing endogenous calcineurin inhibitors (Cabin/Cain, AKAP79, MCPI1), which clearly validated the role of calcineurin–NFAT as a major signaling pathway for cardiac hypertrophy (141,142). For instance, mice deficient in calcineurin-Aβ (which display a 80% decrease in calcineurin activity) showed a resistance to diverse hypertrophic stimuli such as PO, Ang II, and isoproterenol (143), suggesting that calcineurin functions as a central regulator of cardiac hypertrophy resulting from these stressors. However, some uncertainty still persists regarding its necessary role. Of interest are studies that suggest that the degree of stimulation of the calcineurin–NFAT pathway may play a role in the resulting phenotype. For instance, although data suggest that stimulation of the calcineurin–NFAT pathway leads to maladaptive/pathological hypertrophy but is not involved in exercise-induced physiological hypertrophy (81), it was shown that cardiac-specific expression of the calcineurin inhibitor MCIP1 inhibited LVH, reinduction of FGP, and progression to HF that otherwise result from expression of a constitutively active form of calcineurin, but also attenuated exercise-induced physiological hypertrophy (141). Moreover, mice with MCIP1 overexpression showed a 5% to 10% decline in cardiac mass relative to WT littermates, suggesting that a baseline level of calcineurin activity is required to maintain normal trophicity of the heart (141). Therefore, a baseline calcineurin–NFAT tone would lead to cardiac eutrophy, moderate stimulation would lead to physiological/adaptive hypertrophy, and strong stimulation would lead to pathological/maladaptive hypertrophy.

The calcineurin-interacting protein calsarcin has been suspected to be an important intermediate between mechano-sensing at the sarcomere level and calcineurin since calsarcin tethers calcineurin to α-actinin at the z-line (144). In fact, calsarcin-1 negatively modulates the function of calcineurin, since the absence of calsarcin-1 is associated with an activation of the FGP (despite the absence of hypertrophy) and a enhanced cardiac growth response to PO (145).

Recently, a series of data have pointed to the interconnection between the MAPK and calcineurin–NFAT cascades (146). For instance, as already mentioned, reduced p38 signaling promotes myocyte growth through a mechanism involving enhanced calcineurin–NFAT signaling, thus demonstrating the inhibitory effect that p38 exerts on the calcineurin–NFAT cascade (133). Similarly, it appears that calcineurin–NFAT and MEK1-ERK1/2 pathways constitute a codependent signaling module that in a coordinated manner regulates the growth response in cardiac myocytes (147).

Ca^{2+}/Calmodulin-Dependent Protein Kinase II

The Ca^{2+}/calmodulin-dependent protein kinases (CaMKs) are serine/threonine kinases that are regulated by Ca^{2+} bound to calmodulin (CaM) (148). Among the four CaMK family members (CaMKI to IV), only CaMKII seems relevant to signalization of cardiac hypertrophy. The δ isoform is the predominant CaMKII isoform in the heart and two splice variants, δB and δC, are present in adult myocardium. The δB isoform contains a nuclear localization signal that is absent from δC. Because of this difference, CaMKII consisting predominantly of δB subunits localize primarily to the nucleus, while isoforms composed of δC subunits localize to the cytoplasm. A growing body of evidence indicates that CaMKII is an important integrator linking altered intracellular Ca^{2+} signals to transcriptional responses, with a prominent role in the development of cardiac hypertrophy, arrhythmias, and progression to HF. CaMKII expression and activity are increased in the ventricles of SHRs and of mice following TAC [reviewed in (148)]. Importantly, it seems that δB and δC isoforms play distinct roles in LVH and HF. Following TAC, both δB and δC isoforms show increased expression and activation, but only the latter is sustained for at least 7 days. This supports the concept that CaMKδB would participate in the development of LVH through the activation of a number of transcription factors, especially MEF2 through the phosphorylation of HDAC (see Transcriptional and Posttranscriptional Regulation).

TRANSCRIPTIONAL AND POSTTRANSCRIPTIONAL REGULATION

CaMKδC on its side, would participate in the development of HF through phosphorylation of the ryanodine receptor (RyR), responsible for the SR Ca^{2+} leakage and the resulting ventricular arrhythmias, and the induction of cardiac myocyte apoptosis seen during HF (148). This is supported by the fact that mice overexpressing CaMKδC develop DCM with markedly depressed cardiac function and die prematurely (149,150), as compared to mice overexpressing CaMKδB, which developed a less-severe DCM (151). Moreover, maladaptive LV remodeling following excessive β-adrenergic stimulation or MI was substantially prevented in transgenic mice with CaMKII inhibition (26). Studies using CaMKII knockout mouse models should allow to precise the role for each CaMKII isoform in adaptive versus maladaptive LVH.

Gp130/STAT3 Signaling

Gp130, in association with gp80, is the receptor of several cytokines including IL-6/11, LIF, and CT-1 known to promote survival of a number of cell types. CT-1 induces cardiac myocyte hypertrophy in vitro, and mice double-transgenic for IL-6 and its receptor exhibit marked cardiac hypertrophy (83). Activation of gp130 is transient after TAC and the mechanisms of gp130 inactivation during PO-induced LVH remain unclear. Binding of ligands to the gp130 receptor complex results in the activation of Janus kinase (JAK). In turn, activated JAK rapidly phosphorylates tyrosine residues of these receptors and induces the subsequent recruitment of various signaling molecules, including MEK1-ERK1/2, Akt, and the signal transducer and activator of transcription 3 (STAT3) to the receptor complex. Activated STAT3 forms dimers and translocates to the nucleus where it leads to transcriptional activation of genes involved in both myocyte growth and survival (152). Among these genes, the suppressor of cytokine signaling 3 (SOCS3), an intrinsic inhibitor of JAK, is induced in response to TAC and serves as a key molecular switch for a negative feedback mechanism that blocks myocyte hypertrophy and survival (153).

Overexpression of STAT3 in mice is sufficient to induce cardiac hypertrophy (154), while overexpression of a dominant-negative mutant of gp130 attenuates cardiac hypertrophy induced by TAC through the suppression of STAT3, but not ERK, activation (84). The JAK/STAT pathway can also be activated by Ang II through AT1R and/or AT2R (155), and plays a role in autocrine activation and maintenance of the local RAS in cardiac hypertrophy since the promoter of the angiotensinogen gene is a target for STAT3 and STAT5A activated during hypertrophy (82,155,156). Altogether, it seems that this pathway plays a more important role in protecting myocytes against stress-induced apoptosis than in signaling cardiac myocyte hypertrophy.

Protein Kinase C

Protein kinase C (PKC) is a ubiquitous serine/threonine kinase activated predominantly by Gq/G11 coupled receptors and the subsequent activation of phospholipase C that hydrolyzes phosphatidylinositol 4,5 biphosphate (PIP2) to produce diacylglycerol (DAG) and inositol 1,4,5-triphosphate (IP3). Phorbol esters such as PMA activate PKC and mimic the prohypertrophic effects of PE on cultured NRVM. PKC- and IP3-mediated Ca^{2+} release were considered to be the major effectors of Gq/G11 signaling until the discovery of the activation of the PI3K/Akt pathway by βγ subunits of activated Gq/G11 (4) and see Phosphoinositide 3-kinase/Akt/Glycogen Sythase Kinase-3.

Phosphoinositide-3 Kinase/Akt/Glycogen Synthase Kinase-3

At least 12 different PKC isoforms exist; the activity of each isoform depends on its level of expression, localization within the cell, and degree of phosphorylation (157). The so-called conventional PKC isoforms (PKCα and β) are activated by Ca^{2+} and DAG, whereas activation of the so-called novel isoforms (PKCδ and ε) is DAG-dependent but not require Ca^{2+}. A number of these isoforms (PKCα, PKCβ, and PKCε) were shown to be activated and/or upregulated during cardiac hypertrophy and progression to HF, but the role of each isoform remained unclear until the development of specific TG mouse models (4). Interestingly, mice that are null for PKCα, β, δ, or ε exhibited no baseline cardiac phenotype and exhibited only subtle phenotypes provoked by various types of cardiac stress (probably due to compensatory mechanisms involving other PKC isoforms that have occurred during development), masking the effects of specific PKC isoform inactivation.

These problems have been solved, at least partially, by the development of models of inhibition of PKC translocation. Although PKCα has been considered from in vitro studies to be a key regulator of cardiomyocyte hypertrophic growth (158), transgenic models showed no effect of PKCα overexpression on cardiac growth and no effect of PKCα inhibition on the hypertrophic response to PO (159). Instead, PKCα appears to be more of a regulator of cardiac contractility. Indeed, chronic PKCα activation in mice with Gq-mediated cardiac hypertrophy decreased ventricular performance and led to lethal cardiomyopathy (15). In contrast, chronic inhibition of PKCα improved LV contractility in these mice whereas further activation caused a lethal restrictive cardiomyopathy with marked interstitial fibrosis (160). PKCβ is sufficient to produce cardiac hypertrophy in mice but is not necessary for hypertrophy in response to α-adrenergic stimulation or PO. It seems that PKCδ can also participate in cardiac growth but its role as an inductor of cardiac myocyte apoptosis during ischemia seems more important (161).

PKCε is the best-characterized PKC isoform in cardiac hypertrophy, being activated by many hypertrophic stimuli. Its role seems essential for eutrophic cardiac growth, since high expression of a PKCε translocation inhibitor results in myocardial hypoplasia and lethal perinatal heart failure (162). The role of PKCε has been controversial in that it has been considered a key mediator of either maladaptive hypertrophy (163), or hypertrophy with minor alteration of cardiac function (164), or no hypertrophy at all (165); considerable data now argue for its having a role in adaptive physiological hypertrophy (4). In PKCε knockout mice, TAC induced LVH similar to that seen in WT controls. However, knockout mice developed more interstitial fibrosis with an increased expression of collagen I and III. This was associated with an upregulation of PKCδ and activation of the p38 and JNK pathways (166).

Finally, the physiological substrates of these kinases and the downstream effects of each PKC isoform is not totally elucidated (4,167). It is clear, however, that specific PKC isoforms couple to MAPK pathways to regulate myocyte function and growth (167). ET-1 stimulation of ERKs is mediated by PKCε and leads to cardiac myocyte hypertrophy. PKCδ preferentially activates JNKs and p38 MAPKs with minimal activation of ERKs (165). In summary, it seems that PKCε activity is beneficial, whereas PKCα activity is detrimental (at least in the context of Gq/G11-mediated LVH). Surprisingly, in SHRs prone to HF whose LVH is associated with a 10-fold increased expression of phosphoactive PKCα, a fourfold increase of PKCδ, and a threefold increase of PKCε, an AT1R blocker normalized blood pressure and reduced heart mass without affecting PKC expression or activity (168).

Phosphoinositide-3 Kinase/Akt/Glycogen Synthase Kinase-3

Phosphoinositide-3 kinases (PI-3Ks) are a family of lipid kinases that mediate many cellular responses in both physiologic and pathophysiologic states (4,169). Cardiac eutrophy and physiological hypertrophy seen during physical training or during pregnancy are largely mediated by signaling through GH and its main effector, IGF-1. When IGF-1, insulin, and other growth factors bind to their membrane tyrosine kinase receptors, a 110-kDa PI-3K of the Iα subtype (p110α) is activated and translocates to the membrane; this process is triggered by the interaction of the p85 subunit of PI-3K with the growth factor receptor. p110α then phosphorylates PIP2 at the 3′ position of the inositol ring, which produces PIP3 and leads to the recruitment of the protein kinase Akt, also known as PKB (4,119). Full activation of Akt needs successive phosphorylations by two kinases, PDK1 and PDK2, leading to the phosphorylation and activation of the mammalian target of rapamycin (mTOR), and phosphorylation (and thereby inhibition) of glycogen synthase kinase (GSK-3). mTOR is a central regulator of protein synthesis via its effects on both ribosome biogenesis and activation of the protein translation machinery (4). The immunosuppressive drug rapamycin, via its binding to its intracellular receptor FKBP12 and the resulting inhibition of mTOR and downstream effector p70 ribosomal S6 kinase (p70S6K), attenuates TAC-induced LVH in mice (170). GSK-3 is known to inhibit protein translation and a number of transcription factors involved in the expression of the hypertrophic gene program. Therefore, the phosphorylation-mediated inhibition of GSK-3 by Akt promotes both gene transcription and protein synthesis. Interestingly, Fas receptor signaling through GSK-3β inhibition seems to be necessary for the development of cardiac hypertrophy following PO (171).

Accumulated data support the concept that the p110α/Akt pathway is involved in IGF-1-induced cardiac growth and exercise-induced cardiac hypertrophy, and that this hypertrophy does not progress to HF (172,173). For instance, cardiac-specific expression of a dominant-negative p110α mutant in mice impaired normal heart growth and prevented exercise-induced but not PO-induced LVH (173). Moreover, LVs hypertrophied in response to PO showed significant dilation and dysfunction, suggesting that p110α is also essential for maintaining contractile function in response to PO. Cardiac-specific overexpression of H11 kinase, the eukaryotic homolog of the viral protein kinase ICP10, a kinase involved in the so-called immortalization of cells infected with herpes simplex virus 2, exhibits concentric LVH with preserved contractile function associated with Akt/p70S6K activation and no activation of MAPK cascades (174). However, overexpression of constitutively active Akt mutants stimulates heart growth that may (175) or may not (176,177) culminate in HF, likely depending on the degree of overexpression (4). In contrast, p110α is not necessary for the hypertrophic response to PO, although it may be important to maintain LV function in this setting (173).

In sharp contrast to what results from stimulation of tyrosine kinase receptors, upon stimulation of GqPCR, the PI-3K isoform p110γ associates with the βγ subunits of Gq and phosphorylates PIP2, which leads to the membrane recruitment of PDK1 and Akt. p110γ activity is increased in TAC-induced LVH (178), whereas mice deficient of this kinase are protected from hypertrophy, fibrosis, and cardiac dysfunction evoked by long-term exposure to the β-adrenoceptor agonist isoproterenol (179). In mice, comparison of the effects of a targeted mutation in the p110γ gene that induces loss of kinase activity and of p110γ knockout reveals that p110γ has a dual activity in the heart: (a) owing to its kinase activity, it activates Akt, thereby participating in TAC-induced LVH remodeling, and (b) owing to protein interaction with phosphodiesterase 3B, it reduces myocyte cAMP level, thereby decreasing cardiac contractility (180). In summary, p110α is required for normal and exercise-induced cardiac growth (173), whereas p110γ is required for PO-induced and/or Gq/G11-mediated LVH, but not for normal cardiac growth (4,180,181).

Of note, activity of mTOR and GSK-3 can also be regulated by GqPCR agonists through a mechanism that does not involve Akt but rather, Ras and MEK/ERK activation (182,183). Finally, PIP3 can be inactivated by dephosphorylation by the phosphatase and tensin homolog on chromosome 10 (PTEN), resulting in the inactivation of the whole PI-3K/Akt pathway. Accordingly, cardiac-specific inactivation of PTEN results in cardiac hypertrophy (181,184).

Small G-Proteins

Small G-proteins provide another type of functional link between cell membrane receptors and various signaling pathways. They are activated by GTP binding and their GTPase activity hydrolyzes GTP to GDP, which brings them back to the inactive state. At least five families of small G-proteins have been described, each consisting of several members (185). The first small G-protein shown to be implicated in cardiac hypertrophy was Ras, the overexpression of a constitutively activated mutant of which in mice is associated with cardiac hypertrophy, LV diastolic dysfunction, and premature death (186). Ras signaling is coupled to multiple downstream effectors, including Raf, PI-3K, and the MAPK pathways. Regarding the latter, although Ras can directly activate Raf-1 leading to ERK1/2 activation (118,119), it can also activate the JNK branch as well as other signaling pathways which participate in the hypertrophic response (123). Interestingly, it appears that Ras also functions in the calcineurin–NFAT signaling pathway in cardiac myocytes since activated Ras is associated with nuclear NFAT translocation (a process blocked by cyclosporin A), while a dominant-negative Ras mutant blunts PE-stimulated calcineurin activity and NFAT-dependent transcription and nuclear localization (187).

The Rho family of small G-proteins (RhoA, Rac, and Cdc42 subfamilies) regulates the cytoskeletal organization in nonmuscle cells and in cardiac myocytes. Dominant-negative RhoA mutants, as well as inhibitors of its downstream effector Rho-kinase (ROCK), prevent PE-, ET-1-, or Gq-stimulated cardiac myocyte hypertrophy in vitro, suggesting a prohypertrophic effect of RhoA activation in vivo (188).

A number of the prohypertrophic effects of Ang II on NRVM are attenuated by antagonists of the Rho family of small G-proteins, suggesting that these proteins and downstream effectors play important roles in Ang II-induced hypertrophic responses (189). Indeed, long-term infusion of Ang II in the rat causes hypertrophy of vascular smooth muscle and cardiac myocytes, associated with Rho-kinase activation, vascular NAD(P)H oxidase expression (nox1, nox4, gp91^{phox}, and p22^{phox}), and endothelial production of superoxide anions. These effects are significantly suppressed by fasudil, which is metabolized to a specific Rho-kinase inhibitor, hydroxyfasudil, indicating that Rho-kinase is substantially involved in Ang II-induced cardiovascular remodeling (190). Similarly, during the compensated LVH stage of Dahl salt-sensitive hypertensive rats, LVH is significantly attenuated by Y-27632, a specific Rho-kinase inhibitor (191). In parallel, Y-27632 upregulated decreased eNOS expression. This both confirms the role of small G-proteins of the Rho family and Rho-kinase pathway in hypertensive cardiovascular remodeling, and points to a new potential therapeutic strategy for hypertension-associated LVH. Surprisingly, however, transgenic overexpression of RhoA in mice was not associated with cardiac hypertrophy but, rather, with conduction abnormalities and bradycardia that ultimately led to cardiac dilation and HF (192). Similarly, constitutive activation of Rac in cardiac myocytes results in cardiomyopathy associated with alterations in focal adhesions (193).

OXIDATIVE STRESS AND CARDIAC HYPERTROPHY

Small G-proteins of the Rho family are also involved in the generation of reactive oxygen species (ROS), through their participation in the structure and function of NAD(P)H oxidases. The production of baseline levels of ROS by

NAD(P)H oxidases is involved in a number of physiological functions. In disease states, excessive amounts of ROS may arise either from excessive stimulation of NAD(P)H oxidases or from less well-regulated sources such as the electron-transport chain of mitochondria (99). A number of recent animal studies have suggested that (a) a phagocyte-type NAD(P)H oxidase may be a relevant source of ROS in the myocardium, and (b) that NAD(P)H oxidase-dependent ROS production is involved in LVH induced by PO (194,195), stretch (35), Ang II (196,197), and α-adrenergic stimulation (198).

In cardiac myocytes, NAD(P)H oxidase consists of a membrane-bound complex (cytochrome b_{558}) comprising $gp91^{phox}$ and $p22^{phox}$, and a cytosolic complex comprising $p40^{phox}$, $p47^{phox}$, and $p67^{phox}$ (99). Various stimuli lead to the phosphorylation of the cytosolic components and the entire complex then migrates to the membrane. This necessitates the participation of two small G-proteins, Rac1 and Rap. Upon activation, Rac1 binds GTP and migrates to the membrane together with the cytosolic complex. This requires the covalent attachment of geranylgeranyl pyrophosphate (GGPP), an isoprenoid intermediate of the cholesterol biosynthetic pathway that serves as lipid attachment for a number of signaling molecules (199) (Fig. 3-4).

By inhibiting L-mevalonic acid synthesis, statins also prevent the synthesis of GGPP and inhibit Rac1 and Rho isoprenylation, leading to the accumulation of inactive Rac1 and Rho in the cytoplasm (199). Because Rac1 is required for NAD(P)H oxidase activity and cardiac hypertrophy is mediated, in part, by myocardial oxidative stress, it could be hypothesized that statins, which inhibit Rac1 geranylgeranylation, would also inhibit cardiac hypertrophy. In fact, treatment with simvastatin decreases both oxidative stress and the degree of LVH following TAC in mice (200). Interestingly, statins are also able to prevent LVH in transgenic rabbits expressing the β-myosin heavy chain mutation Q403 (a model of human hypertrophic cardiomyopathy), suggesting a role for ROS in the development of familial hypertrophic cardiomyopathies (201).

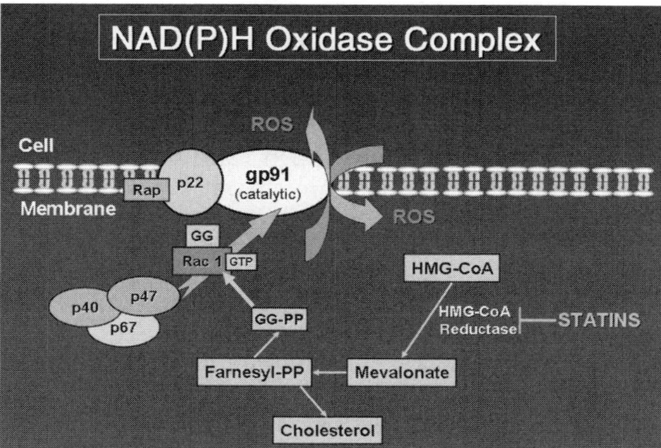

Figure 3-4 Upon activation, the cytosolic complex (p40, p47, and p67) migrates to the membrane to join the membrane-bound gp91 catalytic and p22 subunits. This requires the cooperation of Rap and Rac1. The latter necessitates the binding of geranylgeranylpyrophosphate (GGPP) that is synthesized on the pathway of cholesterol synthesis. Inhibition of HMG-CoA reductase by statins blocks both cholesterol production and activation of the NAD(P)H oxidase complex.

Surprisingly, although the increase in NAD(P)H oxidase activity and LVH induced by chronic Ang II infusion were blunted in $gp91^{phox}$-deficient mice (202), this was not the case in mice submitted to TAC (202,203), probably because of the induction of an alternative $gp91^{phox}$ isoform, Nox4. This suggests a differential response of the cardiac Nox isoforms $gp91^{phox}$ and Nox4, to Ang II versus PO (202). In the same line, cross-breeding TG mice with Ang II-dependent hypertension due to high production of active human renin in the liver (TTRhRen) with $gp91^{phox}$-deficient mice reduced cardiac NAD(P)H activity, ROS generation, and interstitial fibrosis; however, this had no effect on development of hypertension or LVH (204). Interestingly, the antioxidant N-acetylcysteine inhibited TAC-induced LVH in both $gp91^{phox}$ null and WT mice (202). Thus, eliminating $gp91^{phox}$ does not seem to prevent the development of hypertension and LVH in a model in which the endogenous RAS is chronically upregulated, probably because of the induction of other Nox isoform(s) that substitute for $gp91^{phox}$.

ROS may also originate from other cellular sources such as mitochonrdrial electron-transport leakage, xanthine oxidase, and nitric oxide synthase (NOS). Indeed, instead of producing NO, NOS can be converted in a ROS generator as demonstrated in vascular endothelium exposed to increased oxidant or hemodynamic stress. NOS 3 is the dominant NOS isoform in cardiac myocytes and functions as a homodimer that produces NO and L-citrulline from L-arginine. When exposed to oxidant stress or when deprived of its reducing cofactor tetrahydrobiopterin (BH4) or substrate L-arginine, NOS 3 uncouples to the monomeric form that generates O_2^- rather than NO. A recent study indicates that such uncoupling occurs in myocardium exposed to chronic PO and that this serves as a major source for myocardial ROS, a mechanism which participates in LVH and (especially) LV dilative remodeling—a hallmark of progression to HF (205).

MISCELLANEOUS

Because the transcription factor NF-κB regulates expression of a variety of genes involved in immune responses, inflammation, proliferation, and apoptosis, it may play an important role in LVH and progression to HF (206). Indeed, the nuclear translocation of NF-κB and its transcriptional activity in NRVM are stimulated by several hypertrophic agonists, including PE, ET-1, and Ang II (207). Activation of NF-κB is involved in the hypertrophic response to myotrophin, a hypertrophic activator identified from SHR hearts and cardiomyopathic human hearts (208). The small G-protein Rac1 induces cardiac myocyte hypertrophy through stimulation of the apoptosis signal-regulating kinase 1 (ASK1) and NF-κB (209). The inhibitor of NF-κB signaling, A20, is dynamically regulated during acute biomechanical stress in the heart and functions to attenuate cardiac hypertrophy without sensitizing cardiac myocytes to apoptosis (210).

Cardiac hypertrophy is classically associated with a suppression of fatty acid oxidation that is accompanied by an increase in glucose utilization. Genes involved in fatty acid oxidation are regulated primarily by the peroxisome proliferator-activated receptor (PPAR) family of transcription factors that can be activated by a number of ligands, including unsaturated fatty acids, and isoform-specific drugs such as fibrates (PPARα) and the antidiabetic drugs of the thiazolidinedione class (PPARγ). ET-1-induced cardiac myocyte hypertrophy is inhibited by fenofibrate-mediated activation of PPARα (211). Expression of PPARα, the predominant PPAR isoform in the heart, is decreased in PO-induced LVH (212), and overexpression of PPARα leads to cardiomyopathy with cardiac dysfunction (213). In contrast, mice lacking the PPARα gene are protected from diabetes-associated LV hypertrophy and dysfunction (214). Drugs of the thiazolidinedione class that activate PPARγ attenuate Ang II-induced hypertrophy of NRVM (215,216), and heterozygous PPARγ-deficient mice display exaggerated TAC-induced LVH; the PPARγ agonist pioglitazone mitigates LVH in WT mice (216).

TRANSCRIPTIONAL AND POSTTRANSCRIPTIONAL REGULATION

Cardiac transcription factors play a determining role in the expression of the cardiac gene program during embryogenesis. Similarly, they play a key role in the process of myocardial hypertrophy because, being located at the end of signal transduction pathways that are activated by the large variety of molecules previously described, they integrate these signals in a specific and subtle way that leads to gene expression reprogramming, possibly leading to cardiac hypertrophy. These transcription factors and their role in cardiac hypertrophy have been the subject of a recent review (217). NFAT has been previously described as the downstream effector of calcineurin. Only GATA4 and MEF2 will be briefly described next.

GATA4 directly regulates basal expression of a spectrum of cardiac-specific genes (α-MHC, ANP, BNP, NCX1, and so forth) (218). GATA-binding elements in the promoter region of a number of genes are required for the upregulation of these genes in response to a number of hypertrophic stimuli. GATA4 is activated through serine phosphorylation by the ERK and p38 pathways. Similarly to NFAT, the transcriptional activity of GATA4 is regulated through the nucleocytoplasmic shuttling mechanism controlled by GSK-3β. Direct phosphorylation of GATA4 by GSK-3β leads to its export from the nucleus, thus negatively regulating its transcriptional activity. GATA4 is also regulated through interaction with other transcription factors such as NFAT. Mice with cardiac GATA4 overexpression exhibit cardiac hypertrophy (219).

MEF2-binding DNA sequences are present in the promoter region of a number of genes expressed in the heart (α-MHC, MLC, troponins, SERCA, and so forth). MEF2 transcriptional activity is regulated by multiple mechanisms, including calcineurin dephosphorylation, p38 phosphorylation, or by association with activators or repressors. Of special importance is its association with class II histone deacetylases (HDACs). By deacetylating nucleosomal histones, HDACs promote chromatin condensation, leading to transcriptional repression when they are recruited to target genes via binding with specific transcription factors such as MEF2. HDACs are opposed by histone acetyltransferases (HATs), which relax chromatin, thereby activating target genes. PO and calcineurin activate an HDAC kinase that phosphorylates HDAC favoring its nuclear export, thus relieving its inhibitory effect on MEF2-mediated activation of transcription. (see Fig. 3-2). HDAC9-deficient mice show increased MEF2 activity, develop spontaneous cardiac hypertrophy with aging, and exhibit an even more severe LVH after TAC (220).

A number of signaling pathways, the stimulation of which leads to the activation of transcription factors, also have an influence on protein translation. This is especially the case of the PI-3K/Akt pathways and their downstream targets, GSK-3 and mTOR. Activation of Akt both activates mTOR (which activates protein synthesis via its effects on both ribosome biogenesis and activation of the protein translation machinery) and inhibits GSK-3. Since GSK-3 inhibits protein translation and a number of transcription factors, its inhibition promotes both protein synthesis and gene transcription (4).

NEGATIVE REGULATORS OF CARDIAC HYPERTROPHY

Negative regulators of cardiac hypertrophy have been the subject of a recent review (221) and will not be detailed here. Only the role of major transcription regulators considered previously, and that of natriuretic peptides, will be summarized here. Negative regulators of cardiac hypertrophy can be classified into two categories (221). The first comprises those that are activated in basal conditions and whose activity is decreased by hypertrophic stimuli. The second comprises those whose activity is nil or minimal in basal conditions and which are activated upon induction of hypertrophy, thereby acting as negative feedback regulators. GSK-3β and HDAC fall into the first category; natriuretic peptides fall into the second. As previously indicated, GSK-3β acts as a negative regulator of both transcription and protein synthesis. It neutralizes the positive action of a number of transcription factors such as GATA4 and NFAT via their phosphorylation, which leads to their nuclear export. GSK-3β also inhibits protein translation, especially through phosphorylation of the translation initiator eIF2Bε (222). GSK-3β is strongly inhibited via its phosphorylation by Akt following TAC in mice (19). Similarly, Fas receptor signaling is involved in PO-induced LVH through inhibition of GSK-3β (171). By contrast, cardiac-specific overexpression of GSK-3β inhibits cardiac hypertrophy (223). In melusin-null mice, TAC-induced Akt and GSK-3β phosphorylation are markedly attenuated while kinase activity is enhanced, in keeping with the inhibitory effect of GSK-3β phosphorylation, thereby abrogating TAC-induced activation of transcription factors and leading to cardiomyopathy (19). Taken together, these data indicate that GSK-3β phosphorylation is induced by PO, relieving the negative effect of GSK-3β on gene transcription and protein synthesis, thereby promoting hypertrophy. This process is abrogated in melusin-null mice submitted to

TAC, which may explain why the LV of these mice cannot hypertrophy adequately and rapidly progresses to LV dilation and HF. By contrast, TAC in mice with cardiac melusin overexpression is associated with Akt, GSK-3β, and ERK hyperphosphorylation and protection against progression to HF (122).

The natriuretic peptides ANP and BNP belong to the second group of negative regulators of hypertrophy which are activated and/or upregulated upon induction of hypertrophy (12). As revealed in cell culture models with enhanced cGMP synthesis (224) or in models resulting from genetic manipulation of natriuretic peptide receptor signaling, inhibition of this pathway worsens hypertrophy (225), whereas hyperstimulation of this pathway can blunt LVH despite sustained PO. ERK activation is required for the antihypertrophic effect of ANP in NRVM (120). Similarly, preventing cGMP catabolism by chronic inhibition of cGMP phosphodiesterase 5A by sildenafil prevents TAC-induced LVH in mice and even reverses pre-established, TAC-induced LVH and LV dysfunction through deactivation of multiple hypertrophy signaling pathways triggered by PO (calcineurin/NFAT, PI-3K/Akt, ERK1/2) (226).

Adenosine is known to protect the heart from excessive catecholamine exposure, reduce production of ET-1, and attenuate RAS activation. Stimulation of adenosine receptors attenuates both TAC-induced LV hypertrophy and dysfunction via adenosine A1-receptor-mediated mechanisms (227). Leptin, the product of the ob-gene, regulates cellular homeostasis and glycemic control. While initially described as an adipocyte-derived protein with expression and secretion restricted to adipose tissue, recent reports have shown expression of leptin in several tissues, including the heart. Mice lacking leptin or functional leptin receptor develop progressive LVH, a process that can be reversed by leptin infusion and, to a much lesser extent, by caloric restriction, pointing to an antihypertrophic effect of leptin on the heart (228). In general, human obesity is associated with hyperleptinemia and apparent leptin resistance (229), suggesting that LVH observed in these patients is in part due to the lack of leptin-attenuating effect on LVH. Interestingly, leptin levels are also elevated in hypertension (230) and HF (231), suggesting the existence of leptin resistance in these disorders. The adipocytokine adiponectin is decreased in patients with obesity-linked diseases. PO-induced LVH is enhanced in mice deficient in adiponectin with increased ERK and decreased AMPK signaling (232,233). Together with in vitro experiments, this suggests that adiponectin inhibits hypertrophic signaling in the myocardium through activation of AMPK signaling.

ADAPTATION, MALADAPTATION, AND PROGRESSION TO HEART FAILURE

Observational evidence suggests that, except in specific settings (e.g., the acute phase of MI or acute myocarditis), HF is an ultimate condition that results from a chronic disease process with a more or less continuous slow progression from a compensated state to the state of chronic HF. This progression of the pathological process is reflected by the stages of the New York Heart Association (NYHA) classification resulting from the fact that LV dysfunction is mild and masked before being severe and symptomatic. Through a conceptual process that mirrors disease progression, the therapeutic approach to HF has moved from the purely symptomatic treatment of an advanced disease to prevention of the progression from a less severe to a more severe stage of the disease and, finally, now to prevention from the very onset of the disease such as is done at the acute phase of MI. This means that, at least in this context, the concept is now well-accepted that pathological or detrimental or maladaptive remodeling processes are operating from the onset of the disease and need to be blocked as early as possible.

Things are more controversial in other pathophysiological settings, such as those in which the heart has to adapt to (or to cope with) chronically abnormal working conditions most often coming from outside (e.g., hypertension) as well as from inside the cardiac myocyte (e.g., mutations in sarcomeric or other myocyte proteins). Articles have been published addressing the questions of whether LVH is good, bad, or ugly (2); is adaptive or maladaptive (4); or whether load-induced LVH progresses to systolic failure; or whether LVH and systolic dysfunction develop in parallel; or whether LVH is a reaction to pre-existing systolic dysfunction (5). Others seek to clarify the terminology used and propose criteria for classifying the different types of cardiac hypertrophy (3). The obfuscation, mainly due to a problem of definition (3), has been recently worsened by the demonstration that, at least in the short term, LVH should no longer be regarded as a mandatory compensatory mechanism in response to PO and that as a consequence, LVH and alteration in LV function need to be dissociated as independent processes (87,234). Even if the mandatory/indispensable nature of LVH as an adaptation (and not adaptive) process to sustained PO is clearly questioned by the above-mentioned studies, hypertrophy will remain a reaction of adaptation of the LV in response to a sustained workload that helps to normalize wall stress (i.e. the load carried by cardiac myocytes). In this respect, LVH is only an adaptation of the LV pump. This adaptation does not prejudge either the intrinsic quality of the myocardium and its constitutive myocytes, or the short- or long-term prognosis associated with a probably infinite variety of distinct phenotypes, at least when humans instead of mice are concerned. LV hypertrophy (and LV dilation in specific settings) simply participates in the adaptation of the heart to unusual functional requirements. However, adaptation does not mean that all the associated processes are beneficial. Adaptation is, in general, associated with the loss of degrees of freedom. LVH is only one aspect of the overall remodeling process (others are tissular, cellular, and molecular remodeling); remodeling is sometimes physiological/beneficial and well-adapted to the situation, even allowing active maintenance of normal function without detrimental consequences or outcome. Examples would be the remodeling that occurs during gestation or physical training. It is more often pathological or detrimental or deleterious, and negatively impacts the prognosis, when it is triggered by chronic biomechanical stress associated with various degrees of abnormal diastolic stretch, increased systolic load, sustained excessive AT1R and β1-adreoceptor stimulation, and oxidative stress of cardiac myocytes and other myocardial cells.

The triggers, signaling pathways, and mechanisms described throughout this chapter clearly establish that adaptation to biomechanical stress comprises the activation of an enormous number of parallel (but also overlapping and redundant) signaling pathways that lead to alterations in cardiac phenotype, including LVH and alterations in LV contractility. Some of these triggers and pathways, such as the ERK (121) and PI-3K/Akt (172,173,176) pathways, and mild activation of the calcineurin–NFAT pathway are clearly beneficial, leading to the so-called adaptive phenotype with no deleterious consequences (perhaps even providing a cardioprotective effect). Others, such as JNK and p38 (75,130), CaMKII (148), and strong calcineurin–NFAT activation (81), are clearly deleterious, leading to the so-called maladaptive phenotype. Some molecules such as MLP (31) or melusin (19) are indispensable for the adaptation process to PO to occur, and others such as gp130 (18) are necessary to block the activation of deleterious PO-induced processes such as myocyte apoptosis. Thus, the whole myocyte signaling triggered by biomechanical stress functions as a gigantic web that integrates a large number of signals acting through pathways that are as important through their direct effect as by modulating the activation of other pathways. In such a scheme, the final phenotype depends on the delicate balance between the stimulation of beneficial versus deleterious or detrimental pathways and the strength of stimulation of each. The importance of the strength of stimulation is especially well-illustrated by Gq/G11 overexpression (15) and activation of the calcineurin–NFAT pathway. Intracellular signaling pathways, *Gq/G11 signaling* and *clacineurin*, and nuclear factor of activated T cells, also result in compensated LVH or rapid progression to HF depending on the degree of the overexpression or activation (4) (Fig. 3-5).

From the previous discussion it appears that the terms adaptive and maladaptive are probably not best-suited to characterize LVH, especially since we know now that hypertrophy may be lacking in the adaptation process. In French, the term maladaptive does not exist, which both simplifies things and makes the communication with our English-speaking colleagues complicated. This is why I agree with the proposal of Dorn, Robbins, and Sugden to banish the terms physiological and pathological to characterize LVH (3). I disagree, however, with their proposal to use the terms adaptive and maladaptive to quality LVH (surprisingly, based on the contractile function of hypertrophic cardiac myocytes) and propose to banish these two terms as well as any other adjective dichotomously describing LVH. This is because mechanical overload-induced LV remodeling is associated with various degrees of LV hypertrophy—an adaptation mechanism of the LV pump—*and* the development of various degrees of more or less interdependent beneficial and detrimental processes. Owing to the progress of cardiac research during the last 10 years, such processes are now described ever-more precisely and may serve as many targets for future therapies preventing progression to HF (26,235,236).

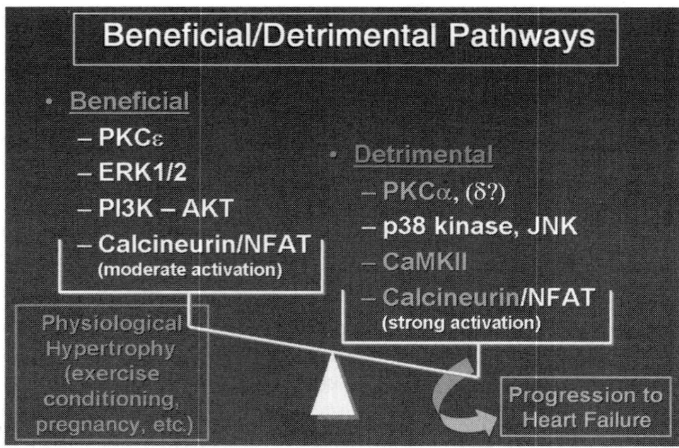

Figure 3-5 Pathways whose activation during cardiac myocyte growth or remodeling is either beneficial or detrimental to myocyte contractile function and survival. Stimulation of beneficial pathways is seen in physiological hypertrophy resulting from physiological biomechanical stimulation, as seen in the athlete's heart or the mother's heart during pregnancy. Stimulation of detrimental pathways predominates following sustained biomechanical stress, as seen in most (if not all) cases of cardiovascular diseases.

CONCLUSION

The understanding of progression to HF has enlarged incredibly during the last decade owing to the progress in functional genomics and the development of innovative research tools, including ever-more sophisticated TG mouse models. This will certainly continue with the development of sophisticated models of conditional gene expression or inactivation. Reaction of the heart to biomechemical stress through a complex web of beneficial and detrimental influences offers a broad, open field for future pathophysiological research and the development of new therapies to prevent the progression to HF. The finding of integrators or central check points that would be responsible for most (if not all) of the detrimental or beneficial processes affecting the heart submitted to stress, and that could ideally offer simple targets for the development of new therapies seems, at least to me, to be another Rosetta stone in the field of cardiac hypertrophy/failure investigation. More likely, gene profiling (including the most important genes and discovery of important functional polymorphisms of the signaling pathways previously described), together with the discovery of intermediate markers should allow the profiles of individual patients to be better characterized. This could better delineate a patient's position in the course of progression to HF and enable, together with the treatment of the causative disease, an à la carte therapy to prevent his or her progression to HF.

REFERENCES

1. Meerson FZ. Compensatory hyperfunction of the heart and cardiac insufficiency. *Circ Res*. 1962;10:250–258.
2. Frey N, Olson EN. Cardiac hypertrophy: the good, the bad, the ugly. *Annu Rev Physiol*. 2003;65:45–79.
3. Dorn GW, Jr., Robbins J, Sugden PH. Phenotyping hypertrophy: eschew obfuscation. *Circ Res*. 2003;92:1171–1175.

4. Dorn GW, Jr., Force T. Protein kinase cascades in the regulation of cardiac hypertrophy. *J Clin Invest.* 2005;115:527–537.
5. Berenji K, Drazner MH, Rothermel BA, et al. Does load-induced ventricular hypertrophy progress to systolic heart failure? *Am J Physiol.* (*Heart Circ Physiol.*) 2005;289:H8–H16.
6. Grossman W, Jones D, McLaurin LP. Wall stress and patterns of hypertrophy in the human left ventricle. *J Clin Invest.* 1975;56: 56–64.
7. Mercadier JJ. Progression from cardiac hypertrophy to heart failure. In: Hosenpud JD, Greenberg BH, eds. *Congestive Heart Failure,* Philadelphia: Lippincott Williams & Wilkins; 2000: 41–65.
8. Levy D, Garrison RJ, Savage DD, et al. Prognostic implications of echocardiographically determined left ventricular mass in the Framingham Heart Study. *N Engl J Med.* 1990;322:1561–1566.
9. Koren MJ, Devereux RB, Casale PN, et al. Relation of left ventricular mass and geometry to morbidity and mortality in uncomplicated essential hypertension. *Ann Intern Med.* 1991;114: 345–352.
10. Mercadier JJ, Lompre AM, Wisnewsky C, et al. Myosin isoenzyme changes in several models of rat cardiac hypertrophy. *Circ Res.* 1981;49:525–532.
11. Pinto YM, Paul M, Ganten D. Lessons from rat models of hypertension: from Goldblatt to genetic engineering. *Cardiovasc Res.* 1998;39:77–88.
12. Mercadier JJ, Samuel JL, Michel JB, et al. Atrial natriuretic factor gene expression in rat ventricle during experimental hypertension. *Am J Physiol.* 1989;257:H979–H987.
13. Wiesner RJ, Ehmke H, Faulhaber J, et al. Dissociation of left ventricular hypertrophy, beta-myosin heavy chain gene expression, myosin isoform switch in rats after ascending aortic stenosis. *Circulation.* 1997;95:1253–1259.
14. Luo W, Grupp IL, Harrer J, et al. Targeted ablation of the phospholamban gene is associated with markedly enhanced myocardial contractility and loss of beta-agonist stimulation. *Circ Res.* 1994;75:401–409.
15. D'Angelo DD, Sakata Y, Lorenz JN, et al. Transgenic Galphaq overexpression induces cardiac contractile failure in mice. *Proc Natl Acad Sci USA.* 1997;94:8121–8126.
16. Molkentin JD, Lu JR, Antos CL, et al. A calcineurin-dependent transcriptional pathway for cardiac hypertrophy. *Cell* 1998;93:215–228.
17. Sakata Y, Hoit BD, Liggett SB, et al. Decompensation of pressure-overload hypertrophy in G alpha q-overexpressing mice. *Circulation.* 1998;97:1488–1495.
18. Hirota H, Chen J, Betz UA, et al. Loss of a gp130 cardiac muscle cell survival pathway is a critical event in the onset of heart failure during biomechanical stress. *Cell* 1999;97:189–198.
19. Brancaccio M, Fratta L, Notte A, et al. Melusin, a muscle-specific integrin beta1-interacting protein, is required to prevent cardiac failure in response to chronic pressure overload. *Nat Med.* 2003;9:68–75.
20. Kobayashi S, Yano M, Kohno M, et al. Influence of aortic impedance on the development of pressure-overload left ventricular hypertrophy in rats. *Circulation.* 1996;94:3362–3368.
21. Pfeffer MA, Pfeffer JM, Fishbein, MC, et al. Myocardial infarct size and ventricular function in rats. *Circ Res.* 1979;44:503–512.
22. Picard MH, Wilkins GT, Ray PA, et al. Natural history of left ventricular size and function after acute myocardial infarction. Assessment and prediction by echocardiographic endocardial surface mapping. *Circulation.* 1990;82:484–494.
23. Pfeffer MA, Braunwald E. Ventricular remodeling after myocardial infarction. Experimental observations and clinical implications. *Circulation.* 1990;81:1161–1172.
24. Michel JB, Nicolletti A, Arnal JF. Left ventricular remodelling following experimental myocardial infarction. *Eur Heart J.* 1995; (16 Suppl I):49–57.
25. Prunier F, Chen Y, Gellen B, et al. Left ventricular SERCA2a gene down-regulation does not parallel ANP gene up-regulation during post-MI remodelling in rats. *Eur J Heart Fail.* 2005;7:739–747.
26. Zhang R, Khoo MS, Wu Y, et al. Calmodulin kinase II inhibition protects against structural heart disease. *Nat Med.* 2005;11:409–417.
27. Nadal-Ginard B, Kajstura J, Leri A, et al. Myocyte death, growth, regeneration in cardiac hypertrophy and failure. *Circ Res.* 2003;92:139–150.
28. Miyamoto T, Takeishi Y, Takahashi H, et al. Activation of distinct signal transduction pathways in hypertrophied hearts by pressure and volume overload. *Basic Res Cardiol.* 2004;99: 328–337.
29. Lindpaintner K, Jin MW, Niedermaier N, et al. Cardiac angiotensinogen and its local activation in the isolated perfused beating heart. *Circ Res.* 1990;67:564–573.
30. Sadoshima J, Xu Y, Slayter HS, et al. Autocrine release of angiotensin II mediates stretch-induced hypertrophy of cardiac myocytes in vitro. *Cell.* 1993;75:977–984.
31. Knoll R, Hoshijima M, Hoffman HM, et al. The cardiac mechanical stretch sensor machinery involves a Z disc complex that is defective in a subset of human dilated cardiomyopathy. *Cell.* 2002;111:943–955.
32. Simpson, P. Norepinephrine-stimulated hypertrophy of cultured rat myocardial cells is an alpha 1 adrenergic response. *J Clin Invest.* 1983;72:732–738.
33. Yamazaki T, Tobe K, Hoh E, et al. Mechanical loading activates mitogen-activated protein kinase and S6 peptide kinase in cultured rat cardiac myocytes. *J Biol Chem.* 1993;268: 12069–12076.
34. Yamazaki T, Komuro I, Kudoh S, et al. Mechanical stress activates protein kinase cascade of phosphorylation in neonatal rat cardiac myocytes. *J Clin Invest.* 1995;96:438–446.
35. Aikawa R, Komuro I, Yamazaki T, et al. Rho family small G proteins play critical roles in mechanical stress-induced hypertrophic responses in cardiac myocytes. *Circ Res.* 1999;84:458–466.
36. Zou Y, Akazawa H, Qin Y, et al. Mechanical stress activates angiotensin II type 1 receptor without the involvement of angiotensin II. *Nat Cell Biol.* 2004;6:499–506.
37. Pimentel DR, Amin JK, Xiao L, et al. Reactive oxygen species mediate amplitude-dependent hypertrophic and apoptotic responses to mechanical stretch in cardiac myocytes. *Circ Res.* 2001;89:453–460.
38. Yamazaki T, Komuro I, Kudoh S, et al. Role of ion channels and exchangers in mechanical stretch-induced cardiomyocyte hypertrophy. *Circ Res.* 1998;82:430–437.
39. Takewaki S, Kuro-o M, Hiroi Y, et al. Activation of Na(+)-H+ antiporter (NHE-1) gene expression during growth, hypertrophy and proliferation of the rabbit cardiovascular system. *J. Mol Cell Cardiol.* 1995;27:729–742.
40. Cingolani HE, Rebolledo OR, Portiansky EL, et al. Regression of hypertensive myocardial fibrosis by Na(+)/H(+) exchange inhibition. *Hypertension.* 2003;41:373–377.
41. Engelhardt S, Hein L, Keller U, et al. Inhibition of Na(+)-H(+) exchange prevents hypertrophy, fibrosis, heart failure in beta(1)-adrenergic receptor transgenic mice. *Circ Res.* 2002; 90:814–819.
42. Takeishi Y, Huang Q, Abe J, et al. Src and multiple MAP kinase activation in cardiac hypertrophy and congestive heart failure under chronic pressure-overload: comparison with acute mechanical stretch. *J Mol Cell Cardiol.* 2001;33:1637–1648.
43. Pan J, Singh US, Takahashi T, et al. PKC mediates cyclic stretch-induced cardiac hypertrophy through Rho family GTPases and mitogen-activated protein kinases in cardiomyocytes. *J Cell Physiol.* 2005;202:536–553.
44. Ross, RS. The extracellular connections: the role of integrins in myocardial remodeling. *J Card Fail.* 2002;8:S326–S331.
45. Sussman MA, McCulloch A, Borg TK. Dance band on the Titanic: biomechanical signaling in cardiac hypertrophy. *Circ Res.* 2002;91:888–898.
46. Shai SY, Harpf AE, Babbitt CJ, et al. Cardiac myocyte-specific excision of the beta1 integrin gene results in myocardial fibrosis and cardiac failure. *Circ Res.* 2002;90:458–464.
47. Collins AR, Schnee J, Wang W, et al. Osteopontin modulates angiotensin II-induced fibrosis in the intact murine heart. *J Am Coll Cardiol.* 2004;43:1698–1705.
48. Xie Z, Singh M, Singh, K. Osteopontin modulates myocardial hypertrophy in response to chronic pressure overload in mice. *Hypertension.* 2004;44:826–831.
49. Dubus I, Samuel JL, Marotte F, et al. Beta-adrenergic agonists stimulate the synthesis of noncontractile but not contractile proteins in cultured myocytes isolated from adult rat heart. *Circ Res.* 1990;66:867–874.
50. Barki-Harrington L, Perrino C, Rockman HA. Network integration of the adrenergic system in cardiac hypertrophy. *Cardiovasc Res.* 2004; 63:391–402.

51. Rapacciuolo A, Esposito G, Caron K, et al. Important role of endogenous norepinephrine and epinephrine in the development of in vivo pressure-overload cardiac hypertrophy. *J Am Coll Cardiol.* 2001;38:876–882.
52. Matsubara H. Pathophysiological role of angiotensin II type 2 receptor in cardiovascular and renal diseases. *Circ Res.* 1998;83:1182–1191.
53. Harada K, Komuro I, Shiojima I, et al. Pressure overload induces cardiac hypertrophy in angiotensin II type 1A receptor knockout mice. *Circulation.* 1998;97:1952–1959.
54. Harada K, Komuro I, Zou Y, et al. Acute pressure overload could induce hypertrophic responses in the heart of angiotensin II type 1a knockout mice. *Circ Res.* 1998;82:779–785.
55. Levy BI. Can angiotensin II type 2 receptors have deleterious effects in cardiovascular disease? Implications for therapeutic blockade of the renin-angiotensin system. *Circulation.* 2004;109:8–13.
56. Metcalfe BL, Huentelman MJ, Parilak LD, et al. Prevention of cardiac hypertrophy by angiotensin II type-2 receptor gene transfer. *Hypertension.* 2004;43:1233–1238.
57. Senbonmatsu T, Ichihara S, Price E, Jr., et al. Evidence for angiotensin II type 2 receptor-mediated cardiac myocyte enlargement during in vivo pressure overload. *J Clin Invest.* 2000; 106:R25–R29.
58. Ichihara S, Senbonmatsu T, Price E, Jr., et al. Angiotensin II type 2 receptor is essential for left ventricular hypertrophy and cardiac fibrosis in chronic angiotensin II-induced hypertension. *Circulation.* 2001;104:346–351.
59. Lako-Futo Z, Szokodi I, Sarman B, et al. Evidence for a functional role of angiotensin II type 2 receptor in the cardiac hypertrophic process in vivo in the rat heart. *Circulation.* 2003;108:2414–2422.
60. Ito H, Hirata Y, Adachi S, et al. Endothelin-1 is an autocrine/paracrine factor in the mechanism of angiotensin II-induced hypertrophy in cultured rat cardiomyocytes. *J Clin Invest.* 1993;92:398–403.
61. Yamazaki T, Komuro I, Kudoh S, et al. Endothelin-1 is involved in mechanical stress-induced cardiomyocyte hypertrophy. *J Biol Chem.* 1996;271:3221–3228.
62. Gray MO, Long CS, Kalinyak JE, et al. Angiotensin II stimulates cardiac myocyte hypertrophy via paracrine release of TGF-beta 1 and endothelin-1 from fibroblasts. *Cardiovasc Res.* 1998;40: 352–363.
63. Robert V, Heymes C, Silvestre JS, et al. Angiotensin AT1 receptor subtype as a cardiac target of aldosterone: role in aldosterone-salt-induced fibrosis. *Hypertension* 1999;33:981–986.
64. Delcayre C, Silvestre JS, Garnier A, et al. Cardiac aldosterone production and ventricular remodeling. *Kidney Int.* 2000;57: 1346–1351.
65. Fiebeler A, Schmidt F, Muller DN, et al. Mineralocorticoid receptor affects AP-1 and nuclear factor-kappab activation in angiotensin II-induced cardiac injury. *Hypertension* 2001;37:787–793.
66. Qin W, Rudolph AE, Bond BR, et al. Transgenic model of aldosterone-driven cardiac hypertrophy and heart failure. *Circ Res.* 2003;93:69–76.
67. Ouvrard-Pascaud A, Sainte-Marie Y, Benitah JP, et al. Conditional mineralocorticoid receptor expression in the heart leads to life-threatening arrhythmias. *Circulation* 2005;111:3025–3033.
68. Tsybouleva N, Zhang L, Chen S, et al. Aldosterone, through novel signaling proteins, is a fundamental molecular bridge between the genetic defect and the cardiac phenotype of hypertrophic cardiomyopathy. *Circulation* 2004;109:1284–1291.
69. Takeda Y, Yoneda T, Demura M, et al. Calcineurin inhibition attenuates mineralocorticoid-induced cardiac hypertrophy. *Circulation* 2002;105:677–679.
70. Mazak I, Fiebeler A, Muller DN, et al. Aldosterone potentiates angiotensin II-induced signaling in vascular smooth muscle cells. *Circulation* 2004;109:2792–2800.
71. Rosenkranz S. TGF-beta1 and angiotensin networking in cardiac remodeling. *Cardiovasc Res.* 2004;63:423–432.
72. Kuwahara F, Kai H, Tokuda K, et al. Transforming growth factor-beta function blocking prevents myocardial fibrosis and diastolic dysfunction in pressure-overloaded rats. *Circulation* 2002;106:130–135.
73. Nakajima H, Nakajima HO, Salcher O, et al. Atrial but not ventricular fibrosis in mice expressing a mutant transforming growth factor-beta(1) transgene in the heart. *Circ Res.* 2000; 86:571–579.
74. Schultz Jel J, Witt SA, Glascock BJ, et al. TGF-beta1 mediates the hypertrophic cardiomyocyte growth induced by angiotensin II. *J Clin Invest.* 2002;109:787–796.
75. Zhang D, Gaussin V, Taffet GE, et al. TAK1 is activated in the myocardium after pressure overload and is sufficient to provoke heart failure in transgenic mice. *Nat Med.* 2000;6:556–563.
76. Matsui Y, Sadoshima J. Rapid upregulation of CTGF in cardiac myocytes by hypertrophic stimuli: implication for cardiac fibrosis and hypertrophy. *J Mol Cell Cardiol.* 2004;37:477–481.
77. Kemp TJ, Aggeli IK, Sugden PH, et al. Phenylephrine and endothelin-1 upregulate connective tissue growth factor in neonatal rat cardiac myocytes. *J. Mol Cell Cardiol.* 2004;37:603–606.
78. Schultz JE, Witt SA, Nieman ML, et al. Fibroblast growth factor-2 mediates pressure-induced hypertrophic response. *J Clin Invest.* 1999;104:709–719.
79. Pellieux C, Foletti A, Peduto G, et al. Dilated cardiomyopathy and impaired cardiac hypertrophic response to angiotensin II in mice lacking FGF-2. *J Clin Invest.* 2001;108:1843–1851.
80. Donohue TJ, Dworkin LD, Lango MN, et al. Induction of myocardial insulin-like growth factor-I gene expression in left ventricular hypertrophy. *Circulation.* 1994;89:799–809.
81. Wilkins BJ, Dai YS, Bueno OF, et al. Calcineurin/NFAT coupling participates in pathological, but not physiological, cardiac hypertrophy. *Circ Res.* 2004;94:110–118.
82. Sano M, Fukuda K, Kodama H, et al. Interleukin-6 family of cytokines mediate angiotensin II-induced cardiac hypertrophy in rodent cardiomyocytes. *J Biol Chem.* 2000;275:29717–29723.
83. Hirota H, Yoshida K, Kishimoto T, et al. Continuous activation of gp130, a signal-transducing receptor component for interleukin 6-related cytokines, causes myocardial hypertrophy in mice. *Proc Natl Acad Sci USA.* 1995;92:4862–4866.
84. Uozumi H, Hiroi Y, Zou Y, et al. gp130 plays a critical role in pressure overload-induced cardiac hypertrophy. *J Biol Chem.* 2001;276:23115–23119.
85. Dorn GW, Jr., Brown JH. Gq signaling in cardiac adaptation and maladaptation. *Trends Cardiovasc Med.* 1999;9:26–34.
86. Akhter SA, Luttrell LM, Rockman HA, et al. Targeting the receptor-Gq interface to inhibit in vivo pressure overload myocardial hypertrophy. *Science.* 1998;280:574–577.
87. Esposito G, Rapacciuolo A, Naga Prasad SV, et al. Genetic alterations that inhibit in vivo pressure-overload hypertrophy prevent cardiac dysfunction despite increased wall stress. *Circulation.* 2002;105:85–92.
88. Sugden PH. RGS proteins to the rescue. *J Mol Cell Cardiol.* 2001;33:189–195.
89. Rogers JH, Tamirisa P, Kovacs A, et al. RGS4 causes increased mortality and reduced cardiac hypertrophy in response to pressure overload. *J Clin Invest.* 1999;104:567–576.
90. Rogers JH, Tsirka A, Kovacs A, et al. RGS4 reduces contractile dysfunction and hypertrophic gene induction in Galpha q overexpressing mice. *J Mol Cell Cardiol.* 2001;33:209–218.
91. Wettschureck N, Rutten H, Zywietz A, et al. Absence of pressure overload induced myocardial hypertrophy after conditional inactivation of Galphaq/Galpha11 in cardiomyocytes. *Nat Med.* 2001;7:1236–1240.
92. Asakura M, Kitakaze M, Takashima S, et al. Cardiac hypertrophy is inhibited by antagonism of ADAM12 processing of HB-EGF: metalloproteinase inhibitors as a new therapy. *Nat Med.* 2002;8: 35–40.
93. Kagiyama S, Eguchi S, Frank GD, et al. Angiotensin II-induced cardiac hypertrophy and hypertension are attenuated by epidermal growth factor receptor antisense. *Circulation.* 2002;106:909–912.
94. Kagiyama S, Qian K, Kagiyama T, et al. Antisense to epidermal growth factor receptor prevents the development of left ventricular hypertrophy. *Hypertension.* 2003;41:824–829.
95. Crone SA, Zhao YY, Fan L, et al. ErbB2 is essential in the prevention of dilated cardiomyopathy. *Nat Med.* 2002;8:459–465.
96. Ozcelik C, Erdmann B, Pilz B, et al. Conditional mutation of the ErbB2 (HER2) receptor in cardiomyocytes leads to dilated cardiomyopathy. *Proc Natl Acad Sci USA.* 2002;99:8880–8885.
97. Yamazaki S, Iwamoto R, Saeki K, et al. Mice with defects in HB-EGF ectodomain shedding show severe developmental abnormalities. *J Cell Biol.* 2003;163:469–475.
98. Iwamoto R, Yamazaki S, Asakura M, et al. Heparin-binding EGF-like growth factor and ErbB signaling is essential for heart function. *Proc Natl Acad Sci USA.* 2003;100:3221–3226.

99. Droge W. Free radicals in the physiological control of cell function. *Physiol Rev*. 2002;82:47–95.
100. Liao Y, Asakura M, Takashima S, et al. Amlodipine ameliorates myocardial hypertrophy by inhibiting EGFR phosphorylation. *Biochem Biophys Res Commun*. 2005;327:1083–1087.
101. Bisognano JD, Weinberger HD, Bohlmeyer TJ, et al. Myocardial-directed overexpression of the human beta(1)-adrenergic receptor in transgenic mice. *J Mol Cell Cardiol*. 2000;32:817–830.
102. Iwase M, Bishop SP, Uechi M, et al. Adverse effects of chronic endogenous sympathetic drive induced by cardiac GS alpha overexpression. *Circ Res*. 1996;78:517–524.
103. Gaudin C, Ishikawa Y, Wight DC, et al. Overexpression of Gs alpha protein in the hearts of transgenic mice. *J Clin Invest*. 1995;95:1676–1683.
104. Tepe NM, Lorenz JN, Yatani A, et al. Altering the receptor-effector ratio by transgenic overexpression of type V adenylyl cyclase: enhanced basal catalytic activity and function without increased cardiomyocyte beta-adrenergic signalling. *Biochemistry* 1999;38:16706–16713.
105. Gao MH, Lai NC, Roth DM, et al. Adenylylcyclase increases responsiveness to catecholamine stimulation in transgenic mice. *Circulation*. 1999;99:1618–1622.
106. Roth DM, Gao MH, Lai NC, et al. Cardiac-directed adenylyl cyclase expression improves heart function in murine cardiomyopathy. *Circulation*. 1999;99:3099–3102.
107. Espinasse I, Iourgenko V, Defer N, et al. Type V, but not type VI, adenylyl cyclase mRNA accumulates in the rat heart during ontogenic development. Correlation with increased global adenylyl cyclase activity. *J Mol Cell Cardiol*. 1995;27:1789–1795.
108. Espinasse I, Iourgenko V, Richer C, et al. Decreased type VI adenylyl cyclase mRNA concentration and Mg(2+)-dependent adenylyl cyclase activities and unchanged type V adenylyl cyclase mRNA concentration and Mn(2+)-dependent adenylyl cyclase activities in the left ventricle of rats with myocardial infarction and longstanding heart failure. *Cardiovasc Res*. 1999;42:87–98.
109. Roth DM, Bayat H, Drumm JD, et al. Adenylyl cyclase increases survival in cardiomyopathy. *Circulation*. 2002;105:1989–1994.
110. Okumura S, Takagi G, Kawabe J, et al. Disruption of type 5 adenylyl cyclase gene preserves cardiac function against pressure overload. *Proc Natl Acad Sci USA*. 2003;100:9986–9990.
111. Swaney JS, Roth DM, Olson ER, et al. Inhibition of cardiac myofibroblast formation and collagen synthesis by activation and overexpression of adenylyl cyclase. *Proc Natl Acad Sci USA*. 2005;102:437–442.
112. Eschenhagen T, Mende U, Nose M, et al. Increased messenger RNA level of the inhibitory G protein alpha subunit Gi alpha-2 in human end-stage heart failure. *Circ Res*. 1992;70:688–696.
113. Bohm M. Alterations of beta-adrenoceptor-G-protein-regulated adenylyl cyclase in heart failure. *Mol Cell Biochem*. 1995; 147:147–160.
114. Dorn GW, Jr., Tepe NM, Lorenz JN, et al. Low- and high-level transgenic expression of beta2-adrenergic receptors differentially affect cardiac hypertrophy and function in Galphaq-overexpressing mice. *Proc Natl Acad Sci USA*. 1999;96:6400–6405.
115. Henaff M, Hatem SN, Mercadier, JJ. Low catecholamine concentrations protect adult rat ventricular myocytes against apoptosis through cAMP-dependent extracellular signal-regulated kinase activation. *Mol Pharmacol*. 2000;58:1546–1553.
116. Petrich BG, Wang Y. Stress-activated MAP kinases in cardiac remodeling and heart failure; new insights from transgenic studies. *Trends Cardiovasc Med*. 2004;14:50–55.
117. Sugden PH, Clerk A. "Stress-responsive" mitogen-activated protein kinases (c-Jun N-terminal kinases and p38 mitogen-activated protein kinases) in the myocardium. *Circ Res*. 1998;83:345–352.
118. Bueno OF, Molkentin JD. Involvement of extracellular signal-regulated kinases 1/2 in cardiac hypertrophy and cell death. *Circ Res*. 2002;91:776–781.
119. Sugden PH. Ras, Akt, mechanotransduction in the cardiac myocyte. *Circ Res*. 2003;93:1179–1192.
120. Silberbach M, Gorenc T, Hershberger RE, et al. Extracellular signal-regulated protein kinase activation is required for the anti-hypertrophic effect of atrial natriuretic factor in neonatal rat ventricular myocytes. *J Biol Chem*. 1999;274:24858–24864.
121. Bueno OF, De Windt LJ, Tymitz KM, et al. The MEK1-ERK1/2 signaling pathway promotes compensated cardiac hypertrophy in transgenic mice. *Embo J*. 2000;19:6341–6350.
122. De Acetis M, Notte A, Accornero F, et al. Cardiac overexpression of melusin protects from dilated cardiomyopathy due to long-standing pressure overload. *Circ Res*. 2005;96:1087–1094.
123. Molkentin JD, Dorn GW, Jr. Cytoplasmic signaling pathways that regulate cardiac hypertrophy. *Annu Rev Physiol*. 2001;63:391–426.
124. Ho PD, Zechner DK, He H, et al. The Raf-MEK-ERK cascade represents a common pathway for alteration of intracellular calcium by Ras and protein kinase C in cardiac myocytes. *J Biol Chem*. 1998;273:21730–21735.
125. Choukroun G, Hajjar R, Kyriakis JM, et al. Role of the stress-activated protein kinases in endothelin-induced cardiomyocyte hypertrophy. *J Clin Invest*. 1998;102:1311–1320.
126. Choukroun G, Hajjar R, Fry S, et al. Regulation of cardiac hypertrophy in vivo by the stress-activated protein kinases/c-Jun NH(2)-terminal kinases. *J Clin Invest*. 1999;104:391–398.
127. Minamino T, Yujiri T, Terada N, et al. MEKK1 is essential for cardiac hypertrophy and dysfunction induced by Gq. *Proc Natl Acad Sci USA*. 2002;99:3866–3871.
128. Liang Q, Bueno OF, Wilkins BJ, et al. c-Jun N-terminal kinases (JNK) antagonize cardiac growth through cross-talk with calcineurin-NFAT signaling. *Embo J*. 2003;22:5079–5089.
129. Wang Y, Huang S, Sah VP, et al. Cardiac muscle cell hypertrophy and apoptosis induced by distinct members of the p38 mitogen-activated protein kinase family. *J Biol Chem*. 1998;273:2161–2168.
130. Liao P, Georgakopoulos D, Kovacs A, et al. The in vivo role of p38 MAP kinases in cardiac remodeling and restrictive cardiomyopathy. *Proc Natl Acad Sci USA*. 2001;98:12283–12288.
131. Liao P, Wang SQ, Wang S, et al. p38 Mitogen-activated protein kinase mediates a negative inotropic effect in cardiac myocytes. *Circ Res*. 2002;90:190–196.
132. Nishida K, Yamaguchi O, Hirotani S, et al. p38alpha mitogen-activated protein kinase plays a critical role in cardiomyocyte survival but not in cardiac hypertrophic growth in response to pressure overload. *Mol Cell Biol*. 2004;24:10611–10620.
133. Braz JC, Bueno OF, Liang Q, et al. Targeted inhibition of p38 MAPK promotes hypertrophic cardiomyopathy through upregulation of calcineurin-NFAT signaling. *J Clin Invest*. 2003;111:1475–1486.
134. Han J, Molkentin JD. Regulation of MEF2 by p38 MAPK and its implication in cardiomyocyte biology. *Trends Cardiovasc Med*. 2000;10:19–22.
135. Yang TT, Xiong Q, Enslen H, et al. Phosphorylation of NFATc4 by p38 mitogen-activated protein kinases. *Mol Cell Biol*. 2002;22:3892–3904.
136. Clerk A, Fuller SJ, Michael A, et al. Stimulation of "stress-regulated" mitogen-activated protein kinases (stress-activated protein kinases/c-Jun N-terminal kinases and p38-mitogen-activated protein kinases) in perfused rat hearts by oxidative and other stresses. *J Biol Chem*. 1998;273:7228–7234.
137. Sugden PH. Signaling in myocardial hypertrophy: life after calcineurin? *Circ Res*. 1999;84:633–646.
138. Clipstone NA, Crabtree, GR. Identification of calcineurin as a key signalling enzyme in T-lymphocyte activation. *Nature*. 1992;357:695–697.
139. Wilkins BJ, Molkentin JD. Calcium-calcineurin signaling in the regulation of cardiac hypertrophy. *Biochem Biophys Res Commun*. 2004;322:1178–1191.
140. Sussman MA, Lim HW, Gude N, et al. Prevention of cardiac hypertrophy in mice by calcineurin inhibition. *Science*. 1998;281:1690–1693.
141. Rothermel BA, McKinsey TA, Vega RB, et al. Myocyte-enriched calcineurin-interacting protein, MCIP1, inhibits cardiac hypertrophy in vivo. *Proc Natl Acad Sci USA*. 2001;98:3328–3333.
142. Fiedler B, Wollert KC. Interference of antihypertrophic molecules and signaling pathways with the Ca2+-calcineurin-NFAT cascade in cardiac myocytes. *Cardiovasc Res*. 2004;63:450–457.
143. Bueno OF, Wilkins BJ, Tymitz KM, et al. Impaired cardiac hypertrophic response in calcineurin Abeta -deficient mice. *Proc Natl Acad Sci USA*. 2002;99:4586–4591.
144. Frey N, Richardson JA, Olson EN. Calsarcins, a novel family of sarcomeric calcineurin-binding proteins. *Proc Natl Acad Sci USA*. 2000;97:14632–14637.
145. Frey N, Barrientos T, Shelton JM, et al. Mice lacking calsarcin-1 are sensitized to calcineurin signaling and show accelerated cardiomyopathy in response to pathological biomechanical stress. *Nat Med*. 2004;10:1336–1343.

146. Molkentin JD. Calcineurin-NFAT signaling regulates the cardiac hypertrophic response in coordination with the MAPKs. *Cardiovasc Res*. 2004;63:467–475.
147. Sanna B, Bueno OF, Dai YS, et al. Direct and indirect interactions between calcineurin-NFAT and MEK1-extracellular signal-regulated kinase 1/2 signaling pathways regulate cardiac gene expression and cellular growth. *Mol Cell Biol*. 2005;25:865–878.
148. Zhang T, Brown JH. Role of Ca2+/calmodulin-dependent protein kinase II in cardiac hypertrophy and heart failure. *Cardiovasc Res*. 2004;63:476–486.
149. Zhang T, Maier LS, Dalton ND, et al. The deltaC isoform of CaMKII is activated in cardiac hypertrophy and induces dilated cardiomyopathy and heart failure. *Circ Res*. 2003;92:912–919.
150. Maier LS, Zhang T, Chen L, et al. Transgenic CaMKIIdeltaC overexpression uniquely alters cardiac myocyte Ca2+ handling: reduced SR Ca2+ load and activated SR Ca2+ release. *Circ Res*. 2003;92:904–911.
151. Zhang T, Johnson EN, Gu Y, et al. The cardiac-specific nuclear delta(B) isoform of Ca2+/calmodulin-dependent protein kinase II induces hypertrophy and dilated cardiomyopathy associated with increased protein phosphatase 2A activity. *J Biol Chem*. 2002;277:1261–1267.
152. Yamauchi-Takihara K, Kishimoto T. A novel role for STAT3 in cardiac remodeling. *Trends Cardiovasc Med*. 2000;10:298–303.
153. Yasukawa H, Hoshijima M, Gu Y, et al. Suppressor of cytokine signaling-3 is a biomechanical stress-inducible gene that suppresses gp130-mediated cardiac myocyte hypertrophy and survival pathways. *J Clin Invest*. 2001;108:1459–1467.
154. Kunisada K, Negoro S, Tone E, et al. Signal transducer and activator of transcription 3 in the heart transduces not only a hypertrophic signal but a protective signal against doxorubicin-induced cardiomyopathy. *Proc Natl Acad Sci USA*. 2000;97:315–319.
155. Mascareno E, Siddiqui MA. The role of Jak/STAT signaling in heart tissue renin-angiotensin system. *Mol Cell Biochem*. 2000;212:171–175.
156. Booz GW, Day JN, Baker KM. Interplay between the cardiac renin angiotensin system and JAK-STAT signaling: role in cardiac hypertrophy, ischemia/reperfusion dysfunction, heart failure. *J Mol Cell Cardiol*. 2002;34:1443–1453.
157. Malhotra A, Kang BP, Opawumi D, et al. Molecular biology of protein kinase C signaling in cardiac myocytes. *Mol Cell Biochem*. 2001;225:97–107.
158. Braz JC, Bueno OF, De Windt LJ, et al. PKC alpha regulates the hypertrophic growth of cardiomyocytes through extracellular signal-regulated kinase1/2 (ERK1/2). *J Cell Biol*. 2002;156: 905–919.
159. Braz JC, Gregory K, Pathak A, et al. PKC-alpha regulates cardiac contractility and propensity toward heart failure. *Nat Med*. 2004;10:248–254.
160. Hahn HS, Marreez Y, Odley A, et al. Protein kinase Calpha negatively regulates systolic and diastolic function in pathological hypertrophy. *Circ Res*. 2003;93:1111–1119.
161. Chen L, Hahn H, Wu G, et al. Opposing cardioprotective actions and parallel hypertrophic effects of delta PKC and epsilon PKC. *Proc Natl Acad Sci USA*. 2001;98:11114–11119.
162. Mochly-Rosen D, Wu G, Hahn H, et al. Cardiotrophic effects of protein kinase C epsilon: analysis by in vivo modulation of PKCepsilon translocation. *Circ Res*. 2000;86:1173–1179.
163. Pass JM, Zheng Y, Wead WB, et al. PKCepsilon activation induces dichotomous cardiac phenotypes and modulates PKCepsilon-RACK interactions and RACK expression. *Am J Physiol*. (*Heart Circ Physiol*.) 2001;280:H946–H955.
164. Takeishi Y, Ping P, Bolli R, et al. Transgenic overexpression of constitutively active protein kinase C epsilon causes concentric cardiac hypertrophy. *Circ Res*. 2000;86:1218–1223.
165. Heidkamp MC, Bayer AL, Martin JL, et al. Differential activation of mitogen-activated protein kinase cascades and apoptosis by protein kinase C epsilon and delta in neonatal rat ventricular myocytes. *Circ Res*. 2001;89:882–890.
166. Klein G, Schaefer A, Hilfiker-Kleiner D, et al. Increased collagen deposition and diastolic dysfunction but preserved myocardial hypertrophy after pressure overload in mice lacking PKCepsilon. *Circ Res*. 2005;96:748–755.
167. Clerk A, Sugden PH. Untangling the web: specific signaling from PKC isoforms to MAPK cascades. *Circ Res*. 2001;89:847–849.
168. Johnsen DD, Kacimi R, Anderson BE, et al. Protein kinase C isozymes in hypertension and hypertrophy: insight from SHHF rat hearts. *Mol Cell Biochem*. 2005;270:63–69.
169. Oudit GY, Sun H, Kerfant BG, et al. The role of phosphoinositide-3 kinase and PTEN in cardiovascular physiology and disease. *J Mol Cell Cardiol*. 2004;37:449–471.
170. Shioi T, McMullen JR, Tarnavski O, et al. Rapamycin attenuates load-induced cardiac hypertrophy in mice. *Circulation*. 2003;107:1664–1670.
171. Badorff C, Ruetten H, Mueller S, et al. Fas receptor signaling inhibits glycogen synthase kinase 3 beta and induces cardiac hypertrophy following pressure overload. *J Clin Invest*. 2002;109:373–381.
172. Shioi T, Kang PM, Douglas PS, et al. The conserved phosphoinositide 3-kinase pathway determines heart size in mice. *Embo J*. 2000;19:2537–2548.
173. McMullen JR, Shioi T, Zhang L, et al. Phosphoinositide 3-kinase(p110alpha) plays a critical role for the induction of physiological, but not pathological, cardiac hypertrophy. *Proc Natl Acad Sci USA*. 2003;100:12355–12360.
174. Depre C, Hase M, Gaussin V, et al. H11 kinase is a novel mediator of myocardial hypertrophy in vivo. *Circ Res*. 2002;91: 1007–1014.
175. Shioi T, McMullen JR, Kang PM, et al. Akt/protein kinase B promotes organ growth in transgenic mice. *Mol Cell Biol*. 2002;22:2799–2809.
176. Condorelli G, Drusco A, Stassi G, et al. Akt induces enhanced myocardial contractility and cell size in vivo in transgenic mice. *Proc Natl Acad Sci USA*. 2002;99:12333–12338.
177. Matsui T, Li L, Wu JC, et al. Phenotypic spectrum caused by transgenic overexpression of activated Akt in the heart. *J Biol Chem*. 2002;277:22896–22901.
178. Naga Prasad SV, Esposito G, Mao L, et al. Gbetagamma-dependent phosphoinositide 3-kinase activation in hearts with in vivo pressure overload hypertrophy. *J Biol Chem*. 2000;275:4693–4698.
179. Oudit GY, Crackower MA, Eriksson U, et al. Phosphoinositide 3-kinase gamma-deficient mice are protected from isoproterenol-induced heart failure. *Circulation*. 2003;108:2147–2152.
180. Patrucco E, Notte A, Barberis L, et al. PI3Kgamma modulates the cardiac response to chronic pressure overload by distinct kinase-dependent and -independent effects. *Cell*. 2004;118:375–387.
181. Crackower MA, Oudit GY, Kozieradzki I, et al. Regulation of myocardial contractility and cell size by distinct PI3K-PTEN signaling pathways. *Cell*. 2002;110:737–749.
182. Wang L, Proud CG. Ras/Erk signaling is essential for activation of protein synthesis by Gq protein-coupled receptor agonists in adult cardiomyocytes. *Circ Res*. 2002;91:821–829.
183. Proud CG. Ras, PI3-kinase and mTOR signaling in cardiac hypertrophy. *Cardiovasc Res*. 2004;63:403–413.
184. Schwartzbauer G, Robbins J. The tumor suppressor gene PTEN can regulate cardiac hypertrophy and survival. *J Biol Chem*. 2001;276:35786–35793.
185. Clerk A, Sugden PH. Small guanine nucleotide-binding proteins and myocardial hypertrophy. *Circ Res*. 2000;86:1019–1023.
186. Hunter JJ, Tanaka N, Rockman HA, et al. Ventricular expression of a MLC-2v-ras fusion gene induces cardiac hypertrophy and selective diastolic dysfunction in transgenic mice. *J Biol Chem*. 1995;270:23173–23178.
187. Ichida M, Finkel T. Ras regulates NFAT3 activity in cardiac myocytes. *J Biol Chem*. 2001;276:3524–3530.
188. Hoshijima M, Sah VP, Wang Y, et al. The low molecular weight GTPase Rho regulates myofibril formation and organization in neonatal rat ventricular myocytes. Involvement of Rho kinase. *J Biol Chem*. 1998;273:7725–7730.
189. Aikawa R, Komuro I, Nagai R, et al. Rho plays an important role in angiotensin II-induced hypertrophic responses in cardiac myocytes. *Mol Cell Biochem*. 2000;212:177–182.
190. Higashi M, Shimokawa H, Hattori T, et al. Long-term inhibition of Rho-kinase suppresses angiotensin II-induced cardiovascular hypertrophy in rats in vivo: effect on endothelial NAD(P)H oxidase system. *Circ Res*. 2003;93:767–775.
191. Mita S, Kobayashi N, Yoshida K, et al. Cardioprotective mechanisms of Rho-kinase inhibition associated with eNOS and oxidative stress-LOX-1 pathway in Dahl salt-sensitive hypertensive rats. *J Hypertens*. 2005;23:87–96.

192. Sah VP, Minamisawa S, Tam SP, et al. Cardiac-specific overexpression of RhoA results in sinus and atrioventricular nodal dysfunction and contractile failure. *J Clin Invest.* 1999;103:1627–1634.
193. Sussman MA, Welch S, Walker A, et al. Altered focal adhesion regulation correlates with cardiomyopathy in mice expressing constitutively active rac1. *J Clin Invest.* 2000;105:875–886.
194. Li JM, Gall NP, Grieve DJ, et al. Activation of NADPH oxidase during progression of cardiac hypertrophy to failure. *Hypertension.* 2002;40:477–484.
195. MacCarthy PA, Grieve DJ, Li JM, et al. Impaired endothelial regulation of ventricular relaxation in cardiac hypertrophy: role of reactive oxygen species and NADPH oxidase. *Circulation.* 2001;104:2967–2974.
196. Bendall JK, Cave AC, Heymes C, et al. Pivotal role of a gp91(phox)-containing NADPH oxidase in angiotensin II-induced cardiac hypertrophy in mice. *Circulation.* 2002;105:293–296.
197. Nakagami H, Takemoto M, Liao JK. NADPH oxidase-derived superoxide anion mediates angiotensin II-induced cardiac hypertrophy. *J Mol Cell Cardiol.* 2003;35:851–859.
198. Xiao L, Pimentel DR, Wang J, et al. Role of reactive oxygen species and NAD(P)H oxidase in alpha(1)-adrenoceptor signaling in adult rat cardiac myocytes. *Am J Physiol.* (*Cell Physiol.*) 2002;282:C926–C934.
199. Liao JK, Laufs U. Pleiotropic effects of statins. *Annu Rev Pharmacol Toxicol.* 2005;45:89–118.
200. Takemoto M, Node K, Nakagami H, et al. Statins as antioxidant therapy for preventing cardiac myocyte hypertrophy. *J Clin Invest.* 2001;108:1429–1437.
201. Senthil V, Chen SN, Tsybouleva N, et al. Prevention of cardiac hypertrophy by atorvastatin in a transgenic rabbit model of human hypertrophic cardiomyopathy. *Circ Res.* 2005;97(3):285–292.
202. Byrne JA, Grieve DJ, Bendall JK, et al. Contrasting roles of NADPH oxidase isoforms in pressure-overload versus angiotensin II-induced cardiac hypertrophy. *Circ Res.* 2003;93:802–805.
203. Maytin M, Siwik DA, Ito M, et al. Pressure overload-induced myocardial hypertrophy in mice does not require gp91phox. *Circulation.* 2004;109:1168–1171.
204. Touyz RM, Mercure C, He Y, et al. Angiotensin II-dependent chronic hypertension and cardiac hypertrophy are unaffected by gp91phox-containing NADPH oxidase. *Hypertension.* 2005;45: 530–537.
205. Takimoto E, Champion HC, Li M, et al. Oxidant stress from nitric oxide synthase-3 uncoupling stimulates cardiac pathologic remodeling from chronic pressure load. *J Clin Invest.* 2005;115:1221–1231.
206. Purcell NH, Molkentin JD. Is nuclear factor kappaB an attractive therapeutic target for treating cardiac hypertrophy? *Circulation.* 2003;108:638–640.
207. Purcell NH, Tang G, Yu C, et al. Activation of NF-kappa B is required for hypertrophic growth of primary rat neonatal ventricular cardiomyocytes. *Proc Natl Acad Sci USA.* 2001;98:6668–6673.
208. Gupta S, Purcell NH, Lin A, et al. Activation of nuclear factor-kappaB is necessary for myotrophin-induced cardiac hypertrophy. *J Cell Biol.* 2002;159:1019–1028.
209. Higuchi Y, Otsu K, Nishida K, et al. The small GTP-binding protein Rac1 induces cardiac myocyte hypertrophy through the activation of apoptosis signal-regulating kinase 1 and nuclear factor-kappa B. *J Biol Chem.* 2003;278:20770–20777.
210. Cook SA, Novikov MS, Ahn Y, et al. A20 is dynamically regulated in the heart and inhibits the hypertrophic response. *Circulation.* 2003;108:664–667.
211. Irukayama-Tomobe Y, Miyauchi T, Sakai S, et al. Endothelin-1-induced cardiac hypertrophy is inhibited by activation of peroxisome proliferator-activated receptor-alpha partly via blockade of c-Jun NH2-terminal kinase pathway. *Circulation.* 2004;109:904–910.
212. Lehman JJ, Barger PM, Kovacs A, et al. Peroxisome proliferator-activated receptor gamma coactivator-1 promotes cardiac mitochondrial biogenesis. *J Clin Invest.* 2000;106:847–856.
213. Finck BN, Lehman JJ, Leone TC, et al. The cardiac phenotype induced by PPARalpha overexpression mimics that caused by diabetes mellitus. *J Clin Invest.* 2002;109:121–130.
214. Finck BN, Han X, Courtois M, et al. A critical role for PPARalpha-mediated lipotoxicity in the pathogenesis of diabetic cardiomyopathy: modulation by dietary fat content. *Proc Natl Acad Sci USA.* 2003;100:1226–1231.
215. Yamamoto K, Ohki R, Lee RT, et al. Peroxisome proliferator-activated receptor gamma activators inhibit cardiac hypertrophy in cardiac myocytes. *Circulation.* 2001;104:1670–1675.
216. Asakawa M, Takano H, Nagai T, et al. Peroxisome proliferator-activated receptor gamma plays a critical role in inhibition of cardiac hypertrophy in vitro and in vivo. *Circulation.* 2002;105:1240–1246.
217. Akazawa H, Komuro, I. Roles of cardiac transcription factors in cardiac hypertrophy. *Circ Res.* 2003;92:1079–1088.
218. Pikkarainen S, Tokola H, Kerkela R, et al. GATA transcription factors in the developing and adult heart. *Cardiovasc Res.* 2004;63:196–207.
219. Liang Q, De Windt LJ, Witt SA, et al. The transcription factors GATA4 and GATA6 regulate cardiomyocyte hypertrophy in vitro and in vivo. *J Biol Chem.* 2001;276:30245–30253.
220. Zhang CL, McKinsey TA, Chang S, et al. Class II histone deacetylases act as signal-responsive repressors of cardiac hypertrophy. *Cell* 2002;110:479–488.
221. Hardt SE, Sadoshima J. Negative regulators of cardiac hypertrophy. *Cardiovasc Res.* 2004;63:500–509.
222. Hardt SE, Tomita H, Katus HA, et al. Phosphorylation of eukaryotic translation initiation factor 2Bepsilon by glycogen synthase kinase-3beta regulates beta-adrenergic cardiac myocyte hypertrophy. *Circ Res.* 2004;94:926–935.
223. Antos CL, McKinsey TA, Frey N, et al. Activated glycogen synthase-3 beta suppresses cardiac hypertrophy in vivo. *Proc Natl Acad Sci USA.* 2002;99:907–912.
224. Calderone A, Thaik CM, Takahashi N, et al. Nitric oxide, atrial natriuretic peptide, cyclic GMP inhibit the growth-promoting effects of norepinephrine in cardiac myocytes and fibroblasts. *J Clin Invest.* 1998;101:812–818.
225. Lopez MJ, Wong SK, Kishimoto I, et al. Salt-resistant hypertension in mice lacking the guanylyl cyclase-A receptor for atrial natriuretic peptide. *Nature.* 1995;378:65–68.
226. Takimoto E, Champion HC, Li M, et al. Chronic inhibition of cyclic GMP phosphodiesterase 5A prevents and reverses cardiac hypertrophy. *Nat Med.* 2005;11:214–222.
227. Liao Y, Takashima S, Asano Y, et al. Activation of adenosine A1 receptor attenuates cardiac hypertrophy and prevents heart failure in murine left ventricular pressure-overload model. *Circ Res.* 2003;93:759–766.
228. Barouch LA, Berkowitz DE, Harrison RW, et al. Disruption of leptin signaling contributes to cardiac hypertrophy independently of body weight in mice. *Circulation.* 2003;108:754–759.
229. Flier JS. Clinical review 94: what's in a name? In search of leptin's physiologic role. *J Clin Endocrinol Metab.* 1998;83:1407–1413.
230. Aizawa-Abe M, Ogawa Y, Masuzaki H, et al. Pathophysiological role of leptin in obesity-related hypertension. *J Clin Invest.* 2000;105:1243–1252.
231. Leyva F, Anker SD, Egerer K, et al. Hyperleptinaemia in chronic heart failure. Relationships with insulin. *Eur Heart J.* 1998;19: 1547–1551.
232. Shibata R, Ouchi N, Ito M, et al. Adiponectin-mediated modulation of hypertrophic signals in the heart. *Nat Med.* 2004;10: 1384–1389.
233. Liao Y, Takashima S, Maeda N, et al. Exacerbation of heart failure in adiponectin-deficient mice due to impaired regulation of AMPK and glucose metabolism. *Cardiovasc Res.* 2005;67:705–713.
234. Hill JA, Karimi M, Kutschke W, et al. Cardiac hypertrophy is not a required compensatory response to short-term pressure overload. *Circulation.* 2000;101:2863–2869.
235. Force T, Kuida K, Namchuk M, et al. Inhibitors of protein kinase signaling pathways: emerging therapies for cardiovascular disease. *Circulation.* 2004;109:1196–1205.
236. Pathak A, del Monte F, Zhao W, et al. Enhancement of cardiac function and suppression of heart failure progression by inhibition of protein phosphatase 1. *Circ Res.* 2005;96:756–766.

Cytoskeletal Abnormalities in Cardiocytes During Heart Failure

4

George Cooper, IV

The cytoskeleton as classically defined for eukaryotic cells consists of three systems of protein filaments. These are the microtubules, the intermediate filaments, and the microfilaments. In mature striated muscle such as the heart of the adult mammal, these three types of cytoskeletal filaments are superimposed spatially on the specialized system of contractile protein filaments, the myofilaments. A very useful classification of these and the other structural proteins of the cardiac muscle cell has been provided by Schaper et al. in terms of five families of structurally related proteins (1), and an equally useful review of the functional significance of each class of proteins has been provided by White et al. (2). The first of these groupings consists of the contractile proteins of the sarcomere, actin and myosin, and their regulatory proteins, including the troponins and tropomyosin. The second of these groupings consists of noncontractile sarcomeric structural proteins such as α-actinin and titin. The third group consists of membrane-associated proteins such as dystrophin, vinculin, talin, and spectrin. The fourth group comprises the proteins of the intercalated disk, of the adheren junctions, and of the gap junctions. The fifth group, which is the subject of this chapter, consists of the classical cytoskeletal proteins. These are tubulin, the predominant protein of the microtubules; desmin, the predominant protein of the intermediate filaments in muscle; and actin, the predominant protein of the microfilaments. As a general statement, the protein filaments that comprise the classical cytoskeleton interrelate the other four groupings of structural proteins as well as the cellular organelles and thus maintain the structural and functional integrity of the cardiac muscle cell.

During the progression from cardiac normality through compensated cardiac hypertrophy to decompensated cardiac failure, there are a number of changes within the cardiac muscle cell, or cardiocyte, in the microtubule network and in the intermediate filament network, without apparent changes in the microfilaments (3,4). For the microtubules, the changes are solely secondary (i.e., they occur only in response to imposed pathological challenges) (5–8). For the intermediate filaments, there are some similarly reactive secondary changes (7–10), but there are also primary abnormalities of the intermediate filaments which can themselves lead to cardiac failure (11–13). For the microfilaments, neither primary nor specific secondary changes have been described in response to or causative of cardiac hypertrophy and failure (1).

MICROTUBULES

Microtubules, which are hollow protein cylinders about 25 nm in diameter, are composed primarily of α-tubulin and β-tubulin. Each of these proteins is encoded by a multigene family and they form the αβ-tubulin heterodimer immediately after protein translation (14). These heterodimers form filaments that nucleate in the cardiocyte along the nuclear membranes (the minus end of the microtubule) and then extend outward toward the cell periphery (the plus end of the microtubule) (15). They are quite dynamic—constantly undergoing cycles of polymerization, abrupt depolymerization, and repolymerization (16).

In the mature cardiocyte, where the mitotic spindle does not form since cell division has ceased, the normal role for the microtubules is to subserve intracellular trafficking (17–19). Here, the microtubule network can be thought of as a railroad yard within which locomotives pull cargos along microtubule tracks. There are two classes of these locomotives. The first of these is the dyneins, which move cargos along microtubules toward their minus end (i.e., from the cell periphery toward the cell center). The second class is the kinesins, which move cargos along microtubules toward their plus end (i.e., from the center of the cell toward the periphery). Given the fact that the mature striated muscle cell is packed with structural proteins, it is a very diffusion-restricted space, such that long-range movement of macromolecules and particles within these very large cells is virtually impossible. Because of this, movement of membrane vesicles, organelles, and macromolecular complexes by these motor proteins along microtubule tracks is essential to cellular homeostasis. Examples of how this railway system operates include the movement of membrane vesicles to enable the recycling of activated G protein-coupled receptors (18,19) and the movement of mRNA (20) as a component of ribonucleoprotein particles to sites of structural protein synthesis such as the sarcomere.

Microtubules in Cardiac Pathology

As indicated earlier, there are no reports of primary microtubule defects that are responsible for cardiac pathology. This may be due to the fact that the isoforms comprising each member of the tubulin heterodimer pair are encoded by one or more members of a multigene family rather than by alternative splicing of a single gene (14). Thus, there is much more plasticity and redundancy for the expression of these proteins than would be the case were each of them encoded by a single gene (see the section on desmin, later). Indeed, different isoforms of β-tubulin are expressed in the heart developmentally and there is no evidence that these isoforms differ functionally in mammals (21).

There are, however, alterations of the microtubule portion of the cytoskeleton that occur secondary to pathophysiological insults to the heart and that may contribute to a poor outcome. In some cases described later for animal models of human disease, this may take the form of a vicious cycle wherein changes in the cardiocyte microtubule network may interfere with the compensatory response of the heart to pathological challenges in terms of both contractile function and hypertrophic growth.

Cardiac Hypertrophy and Failure Induced by Ventricular Pressure Overloading

An association between pressure overload cardiac hypertrophy and densification of the cardiocyte microtubule network was initially reported as a transient change affecting a minority of the cardiocytes from the overloaded ventricle during the early stages of this growth process (16). An increase in cardiocyte microtubules was later found to be a persistent feature of cardiac hypertrophy in response to a substantial pressure overload that affected all of the cardiocytes in the overloaded ventricle (3,4); this cytoskeletal change was associated with contractile dysfunction and the eventual development of congestive heart failure (22,23). This finding in right ventricular myocardium was not present at any stage of the hypertrophic process for an equivalent degree and duration of right ventricular hypertrophy in response to a volume overload that did not result in cardiac dysfunction (3,24). Taken together, these findings suggested that for hemodynamic overloads microtubule network densification is a persistent and relatively specific feature of the cardiac cytoskeletal response to severe pressure overloading. Of most interest, however, was the fact that depolymerization of this dense microtubule network, which imposes a viscous load on the contracting myofilaments (25), restored the initially abnormal cellular contractile function characteristic of severe right ventricular pressure overload hypertrophy to normal (3,4,22,26).

In attributing the improvement in contractile function to removal of this viscous load, it was important to be sure that this effect was not due to unrecognized side effects of colchicine, the drug used for this purpose, or the resultant increased concentration of αβ-tubulin heterodimers, since there are data to suggest that this heterodimer may act as a functional analog of G proteins to activate adenyl cyclase and increase calcium transients when the αβ-tubulin concentration is increased by colchicine (27). However, the restoration of normal contractile function was seen regardless of whether the microtubules were depolymerized using the chemical agent colchicine or, instead, by using the physical modality of transient hypothermia (3,4,28); colchicine did not augment either cardiocyte cyclic adenosine monophosphate (cAMP) levels or their calcium transients (29). Furthermore, microtubule depolymerization via vincristine, which decreases the soluble αβ-tubulin heterodimer concentration, duplicates the mechanical effects on cardiocytes of microtubule depolymerization via colchicine, which increases the soluble αβ-tubulin heterodimer concentration (30). Thus, a positive inotropic effect of αβ-tubulin heterodimers (independent of the direct physical consequences of microtubule depolymerization) was excluded as an explanation for the ameliorative effects of this intervention on the contractile dysfunction of pressure-hypertrophied myocardium.

In the clinically more important setting of left ventricular pressure overload hypertrophy, the findings were very similar to those for right ventricular hypertrophy, but it was also possible to assign more specificity to the setting in which the cytoskeletal abnormality occurs (23). Thus, Figure 4-1 shows that when mongrel dogs of random sex are submitted to a gradually increasing pressure overload on the left ventricle, with aortic pressure gradients as high as 180 mm Hg, the animals tend to segregate into two groups in terms of the extent of compensatory hypertrophy which is produced. Figure 4-2 shows that this has clear consequences in terms of left ventricular function. In the "Hypertrophy" group of dogs (which had compensated left ventricular hypertrophy), the relationship between mean normalized systolic ejection rate and mean systolic stress remained normal throughout the hypertrophic process. In the "Failure" group of dogs (which developed left ventricular failure), there was a progressive reduction in left ventricular function during the process of noncompensatory hypertrophy and, at the time of final study, there was a very significant increase in left ventricular wall stress.

A comparison of the feline right ventricular pressure overload model to the canine left ventricular pressure overload model provided an initial insight into the specific setting in which hemodynamically driven microtubule

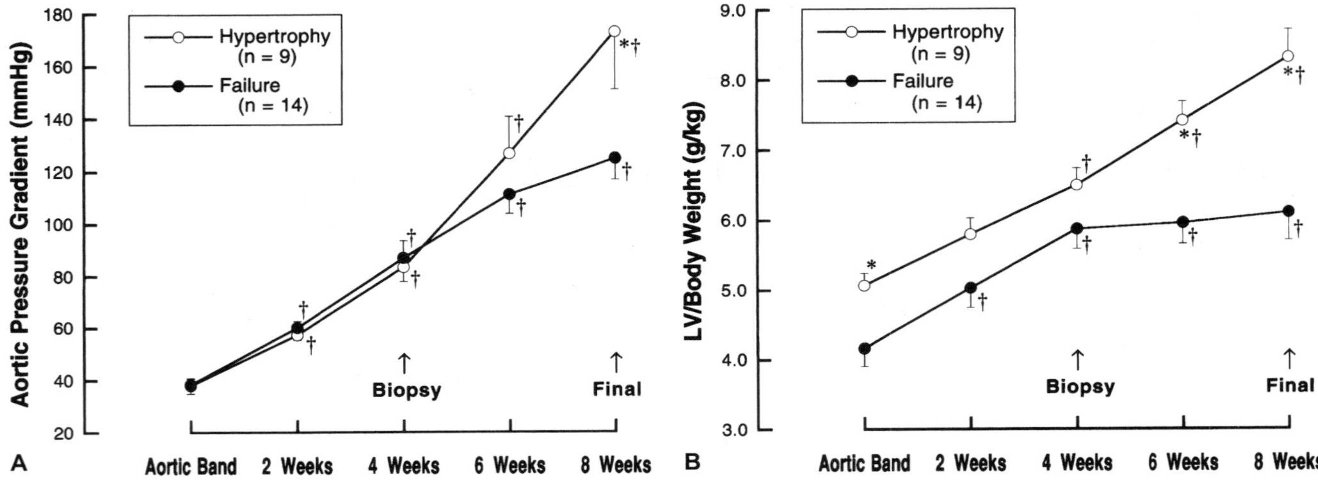

Figure 4-1 Canine left ventricular (LV) afterload increases and resultant LV mass increments with progressive stenosis of the ascending aorta. The group of dogs denoted as "Hypertrophy" maintained normal LV function throughout the course of the study; the group of dogs denoted as "Failure" developed LV systolic dysfunction as the afterload became more severe. **Both panels**: The times at which the animals were studied and the aortic band was tightened are indicated on the abscissa; the **vertical arrows** indicate the times of LV biopsy and of final study. **A,** The aortic pressure gradient as measured by cardiac catheterization is indicated on the ordinate. **B,** The LV to body weight ratio as measured by ventriculography is indicated on the ordinate. Statistical comparisons, which considered all dogs from a given experimental group together, were by two-way ANOVA and a means comparison contrast, where n = number of dogs. (Reproduced from Tagawa H, Koide M, Sato H, et al. Cytoskeletal role in the transition from compensated to decompensated hypertrophy during adult canine left ventricular pressure overloading. *Circ Res.* 1998;82:751–761, with permission.)
* $p < 0.01$ for difference between the two groups of dogs at matched time points.
† $p < 0.01$ for difference from the initial aortic band value within a group.

network densification occurs. In the right ventricular pressure overload hypertrophy and failure model there is a uniform increase in microtubule network density in all cardiocytes from these ventricles; as discussed elsewhere (5), it is likely but not known that these right ventricles had high wall stress from the onset of pressure overloading. Indeed, Figure 4-3 shows that increased tubulin polymer and total tubulin, as well as microtubule network densification, are confined to failing left ventricles where high wall stress can be accurately documented in the intact animal. Figure 4-2 shows that this has a clear functional consequence at the level of ventricular contraction, and Figure 4-4 shows that this has an equally clear functional consequence at the level of sarcomere contraction in the cells from these same ventricles. That is, in the animals with compensated left ventricular hypertrophy, contractile function at the level of the cardiocyte sarcomeres is well-preserved both at the midpoint of the study when a biopsy was done and at the end of the study. However, in the animals with decompensated left ventricular hypertrophy, while sarcomere contractile function was normal at the midpoint of the study when the biopsy was taken, it had become distinctly abnormal at the end of the study when wall stress was very high. However, Figure 4-4D shows that even in cardiocytes from failing left ventricles, microtubule depolymerization restores grossly abnormal sarcomere contractile function to normal, strongly suggesting that microtubule network densification has an important role to play in the contractile dysfunction seen in this particular form of hypertrophy. Thus, the phenomenon of microtubule network densification with an associated contractile dysfunction apparently specific to this cytoskeletal alteration was originally observed in the pressure overloaded right ventricle. Figures 4-1 through 4-4 confirm this finding in the pressure overloaded left ventricle but assign much more specificity to this pathophysiology in that the linked cytoskeletal and contractile abnormalities are found only with severe pressure overloaded hypertrophy wherein the hypertrophic response had not been sufficient to maintain normal left ventricular wall stress.

When the effect of microtubule depolymerization by colchicine was assessed in vivo, similar results were found at the level of left ventricular function in the intact dog (28) and mouse (30). Figure 4-5A shows that when dogs having the same characteristics as the "Failure" dogs shown in Figure 4-1 were studied in the cardiac catheterization laboratory, they initially showed depressed left ventricular function and elevated left ventricular wall stress, much like that shown for this group of dogs at final study in Figure 4-2. When the aortic pressure gradient was relieved, there was, as expected, a marked reduction in left ventricular wall stress (Fig. 4-5A, 1→2). There was then no immediate effect of intravenous colchicine on left ventricular wall stress or function (Fig. 4-5A, 2→3), since it takes ~45 minutes for the microtubules to depolymerize after colchicine administration (3). However, 1 hour after intravenous colchicine, when virtually complete depolymerization of the myocardial microtubules had occurred, there was a marked increase in the function of the left ventricle in vivo (Fig. 4-5A, 3→4). This occurred despite the fact that, as

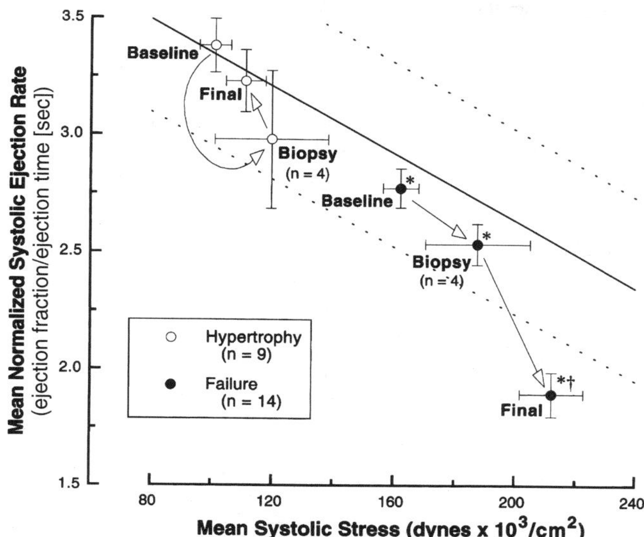

Figure 4-2 The relationship between mean normalized systolic ejection rate and mean systolic stress for the same two groups of dogs whose data are given in Figure 4-1. The solid and parallel dashed lines define this relationship and its 95% confidence interval, calculated using a least-squares linear regression analysis, for 40 β-blocked normal dogs studied in this laboratory. The **arrows** indicate for each group (separately) the progression through the indicated time points of this study. Statistical comparisons, which considered all dogs from a given experimental group together, were by two-way ANOVA and a means comparison contrast, where n = the number of dogs in each group and the number of dogs in the subset of each group submitted to LV biopsy. (Reproduced from from Tagawa H, Koide M, Sato H, et al. Cytoskeletal role in the transition from compensated to decompensated hypertrophy during adult canine left ventricular pressure overloading. *Circ Res.* 1998;82:751–761, with permission.)
*$p<0.01$ for difference between the two groups of dogs at matched time points.
†$p<0.01$ for difference from the initial baseline value within a group.

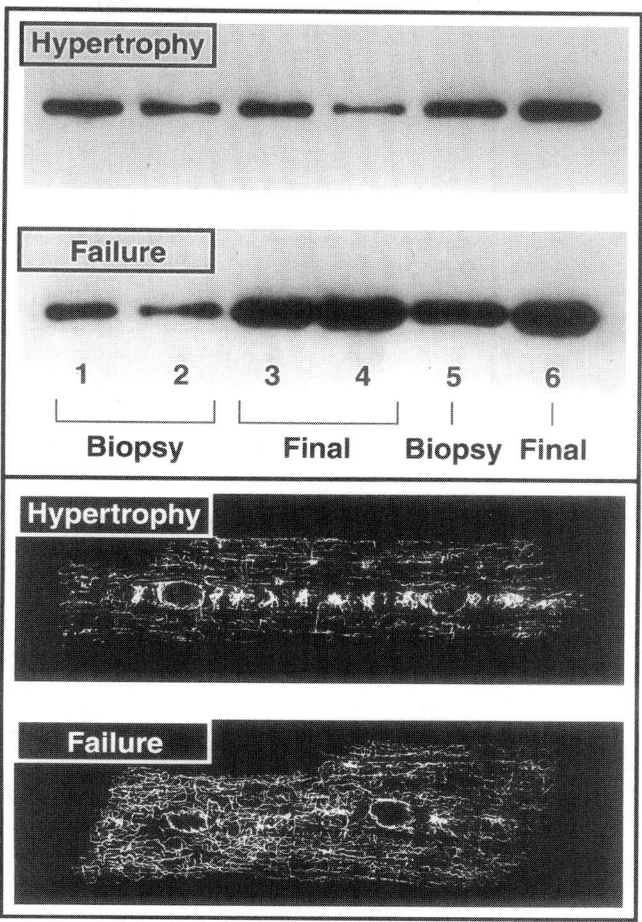

Figure 4-3 Free and polymerized myocardial β-tubulin and immunofluorescence confocal micrograph analysis of microtubules in isolated cardiocytes; the antibody was to β-tubulin in both cases. **Upper panel**: Immunoblot analysis of dogs from the same hypertrophy and failure groups as those shown in Figures 4-1 and 4-2. Lanes 1 and 3 represent free β-tubulin, lanes 2 and 4 represent polymerized β-tubulin, and lanes 5 and 6 represent total β-tubulin. Lanes 1, 2, and 5 of the immunoblots are from the LV biopsy of a given dog, and lanes 3,4, and 6 of the immunoblot are from the same LV at final study. **Lower panel**: Immunofluorescence confocal micrograph analysis of microtubules in isolated cardiocytes. The LV cardiocyte obtained from a hypertrophy dog at the time of final study is labeled "Hypertrophy," and the LV cardiocyte obtained from a failure dog at the time of final study is labeled "Failure." Each micrograph is a single 0- to 0.7-μm confocal section taken at the level of the nuclei. (Reproduced from Tagawa H, Koide M, Sato H, et al. Cytoskeletal role in the transition from compensated to decompensated hypertrophy during adult canine left ventricular pressure overloading. *Circ Res.* 1998;82:751–761, with permission.)

shown in Figure 4-5B, in normal dogs colchicine is, if anything, an intrinsically negative inotropic agent.

As had been done for the isolated cardiocytes from the feline right ventricle, microtubule depolymerization by hypothermia was used in our study of the intact dog (28) in order to be sure that any effects of microtubule depolymerization on left ventricular function were not due to unrecognized secondary effects of colchicine. As is seen in Figure 4-6A, when a dog with severe aortic stenosis and heart failure corresponding to the "Failure" group in Figure 4-1 was studied, there was at baseline a shift in the ratio of free to polymerized tubulin toward the polymerized form, reflecting greater microtubule network density. When the aortic stenosis was relieved such that the wall stress was reduced (Fig. 4-6A, 1→2) and the dog was then submitted to cold cardioplegia for 1 hour, the immunoblot shows that the microtubules fully depolymerized. When the dog was then allowed to recover and the microtubules repolymerized in a normal loading environment, there was a clear improvement in left ventricular function (Fig. 4-6A, 2→3). In contrast, the dog shown in Figure 4-6B had much less aortic stenosis, left ventricular wall stress, and resultant left ventricular hypertrophy. Here, the immunoblot shows that both the initial and the final ratio of free to polymerized tubulin had the normal value of ~2:1, reflecting normal microtubule network density. In this dog, the balloon deflation—cold cardioplegia—rewarming sequence actually produced a negative inotropic effect (Fig. 4-6B, 1→2).

As a final step, the question of whether microtubule network densification is seen in severe pressure overload hypertrophy and failure was taken to the clinical setting (31). Figure 4-7 shows that patients with aortic stenosis can be classified into four groups in terms of the relationship between midwall left ventricular fractional shortening and mean systolic stress. When biopsy samples from these four

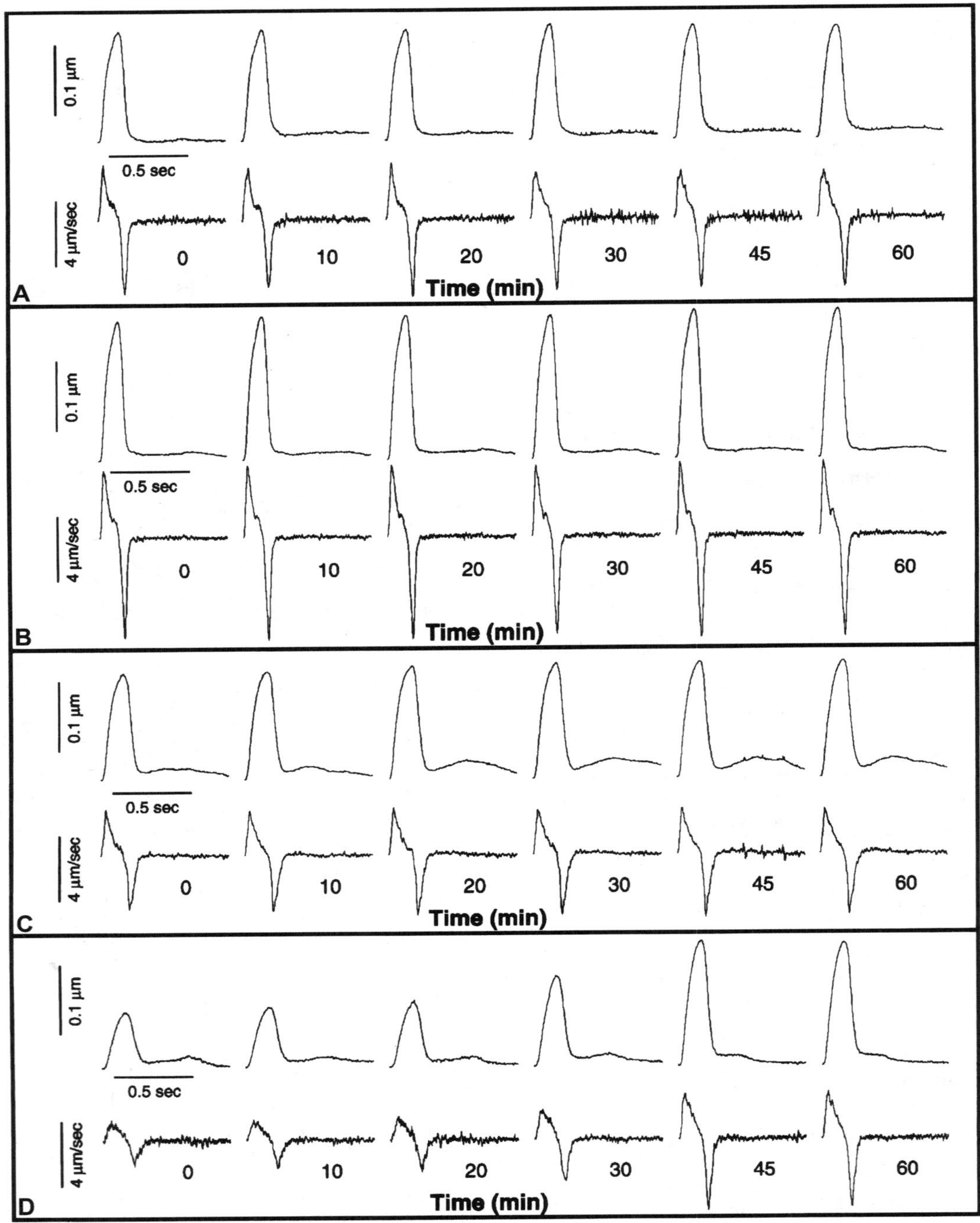

Figure 4-4 Single cardiocytes from dogs from the same hypertrophy and failure groups as those shown in Figures 4-1 through 4-3. Each panel shows sequential samples from a single LV cardiocyte, where for each contraction sarcomere length versus time is given above, and the rate of length change versus time is given below. The time in minutes after the addition of 10^{-6} M colchicine, which results in virtually complete microtubule depolymerization in 45 minutes, is indicated. **A,** LV cardiocyte obtained by biopsy from a "Hypertrophy" dog at 4 weeks after aortic banding. **B,** LV cardiocyte obtained from the same dog at final study. **C,** LV cardiocyte obtained by biopsy from a "Failure" dog at 4 weeks after aortic banding. **D,** LV cardiocyte obtained from the same dog at final study. (Reproduced from Tagawa H, Koide M, Sato H, et al. Cytoskeletal role in the transition from compensated to decompensated hypertrophy during adult canine left ventricular pressure overloading. *Circ Res.* 1998;82:751–761, with permission.)

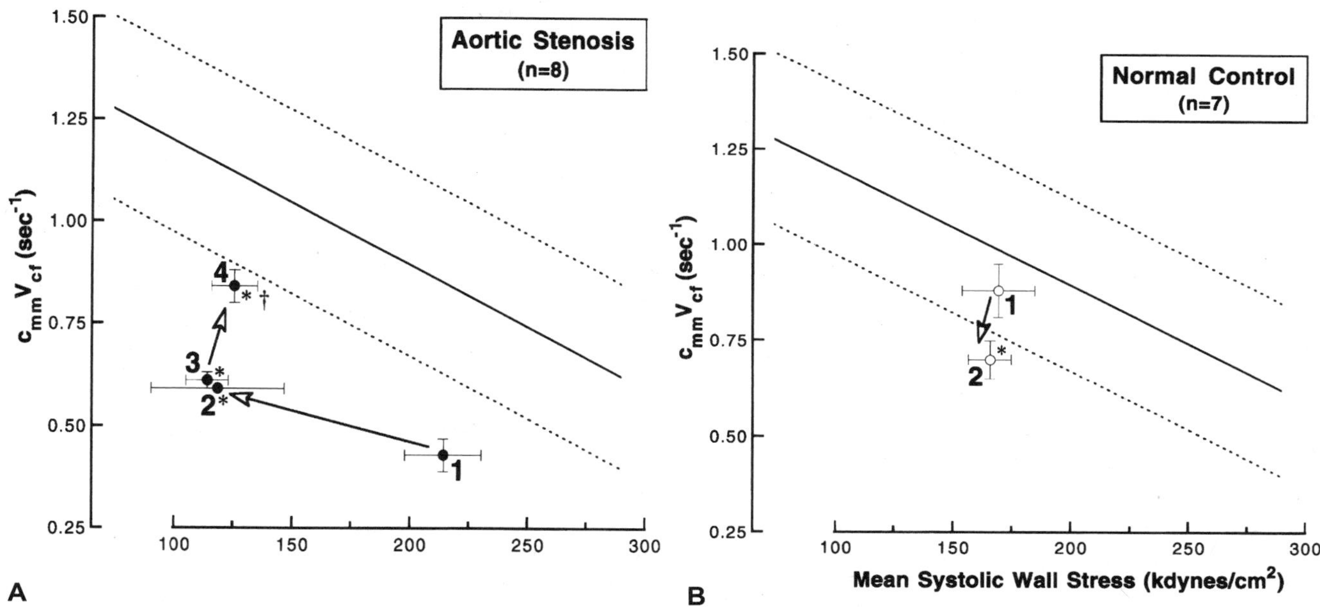

Figure 4-5 LV systolic function assessed by the relationship of $c_{mm}V_{cf}$ to mean systolic wall stress in aortic stenosis dogs at 8 weeks after initial aortic banding **(A)** and in normal control dogs **(B)**. For the aortic stenosis dogs in **(A)**, data are shown at baseline (1), after reducing the aortic pressure gradient via band release (2), 1 hour later before administering colchicine (3), and one further hour later after administering colchicine (4). Colchicine caused a clear increase in LV contractility (line 3→4). For the normal control dogs in **(B)**, data are shown at baseline (1) and one hour later after administering colchicine (2). In direct contrast to the data for the aortic stenosis dogs, colchicine caused here a clear decrease in LV contractility (line 1→2). Statistical comparisons were by one-way ANOVA followed by Scheffé's S procedure. (Reproduced from Koide M, Hamawaki M, Narishige T, et al. Microtubule depolymerization normalizes in vivo myocardial contractile function in dogs with pressure-overload left ventricular hypertrophy. *Circulation.* 2000;102:1045–1052, with permission.)
* $p < 0.05$ for difference from "1" value.
† $p < 0.05$ for difference from "3" value.

groups of patients were used to prepare immunoblots, it was found (as shown in Fig. 4-8) that there was a minor increase in microtubule protein in the borderline abnormal aortic stenosis patients, but there was a striking increase in the microtubule protein in patients with distinctly abnormal left ventricular function and elevated mean systolic stress. Thus, increased myocardial microtubules are found consistently in severe pressure overload cardiac hypertrophy and failure in the right and left ventricles of experimental animal models, as well as in the left ventricles of patients.

It is nonetheless important to note that not all investigators who have looked for this cytoskeletal alteration in experimental models of pressure overload cardiac hypertrophy have replicated these findings (32,33). As reviewed elsewhere, there are many factors that might be responsible for this variation (5). Briefly, since microtubule network densification as evidenced by Cooper et al. (5) is neither species- nor chamber-specific, an underlying and unifying reason for interlaboratory variation may well be that, as shown above, this cytoskeletal change does not happen with modest pressure overload hypertrophy but, instead, only happens with very substantial pressure overloading leading to increased wall stress and an approximate doubling of ventricular mass. Furthermore, several other investigators have confirmed the basic finding of increased tubulin and microtubules in animal models of cardiac pressure loading (6,34–40), with an extraordinary increase in microtubule protein seen with severe pressure overloading (38).

Cardiomyopathy and End-Stage Heart Disease

In addition to the findings previously summarized for pressure overload cardiac hypertrophy and failure, increased cardiocyte microtubules have been documented during cardiac transplantation in hearts explanted from patients with end-stage cardiac disease of this and various other etiologies. Several such studies have shown increased tubulin protein and increased microtubule network density in these explanted hearts (1,7–10). As was the case for the study of clinical aortic stenosis (Figs. 4-7 and 4-8), this increase in microtubules was found to correlate with the degree of contractile dysfunction in these patients. In parallel with the studies of pressure overload cardiac hypertrophy, similar findings have been reported in an experimental animal model of dilated cardiomyopathy (41).

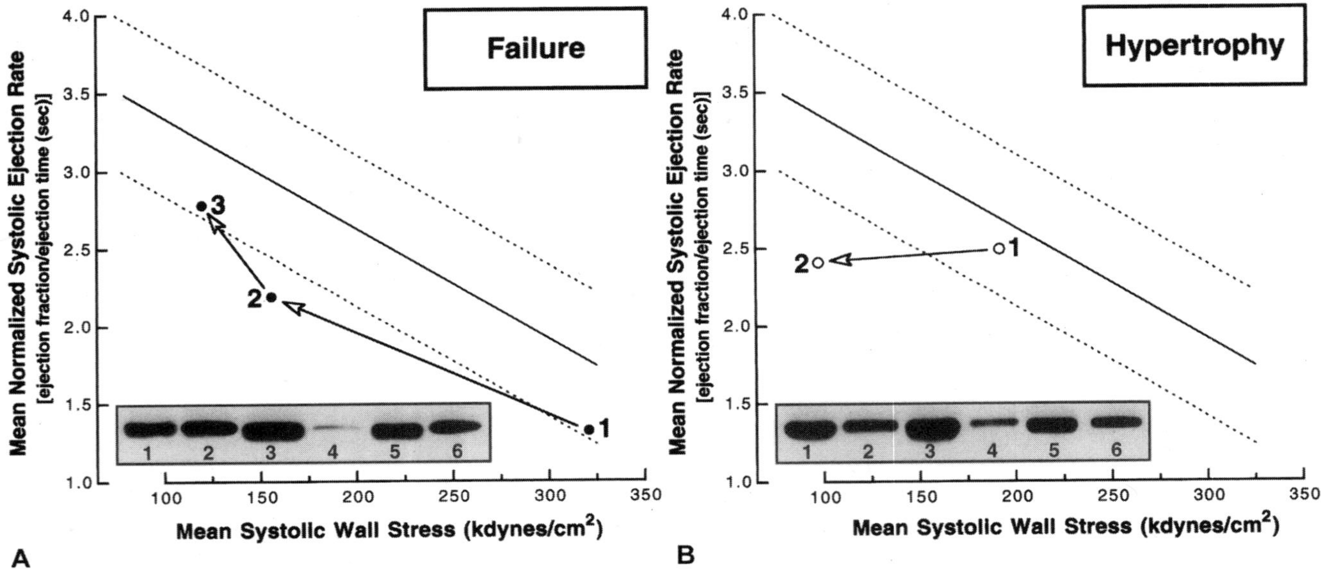

Figure 4-6 Effects of myocardial hypothermia and consequent microtubule depolymerization on canine LV microtubule polymerization state and in vivo contractile function for two dogs with aortic stenosis. LV systolic function was assessed by the relationship of mean normalized systolic ejection rate to mean systolic wall stress. **A,** Dog with severe aortic stenosis (LV mass = 7 to 9 g/kg); **B,** Dog with moderate aortic stenosis (LV mass = 5 to 9 g/kg), both at 8 weeks after initial aortic banding. **A** shows data first during normothermia at baseline (1), after reducing the aortic pressure gradient via balloon deflation (2), and then 3 hours after the myocardial rewarming that followed 1 hour of cold blood coronary artery perfusion (3). The latter intervention caused a clear increase in LV contractility (line 2→3). **B** shows data at baseline (1) and after the balloon deflation (cold) rewarming sequence used for the first dog (2). In direct contrast to the data for the severe aortic stenosis dog, here cold cardioplegia caused a clear decrease in the initially normal LV contractility (line 1→2). For both dogs, the $c_{mm}V_{cf}$ versus mean systolic wall stress relationship was confirmatory. In the myocardial immunoblots for the same two dogs, lanes 1, 3, and 5 are free β-tubulin and lanes 2, 4, and 6 are polymerized β-tubulin. For each dog, the sample for lanes 1 and 2 was obtained at baseline, the sample for lanes 3 and 4 was obtained immediately after 1 hour of cold cardioplegia, and the sample for lanes 5 and 6 was obtained immediately after the final ventriculogram. The initial ratio of free to polymerized tubulin (lanes 1 and 2) is normal at ~2:1 in the "Hypertrophy" dog but has shifted to ~1:1 in the "Failure" dog, reflecting an increase in myocardial microtubules. Cold cardioplegia caused virtually complete microtubule depolymerization in both dogs (lanes 3 and 4). Microtubule repolymerization in a setting on normal ventricular wall stress returned the ratio of free to polymerized tubulin to the normal ~2:1 value in both dogs (lanes 5 and 6). (Reproduced from Koide M, Hamawaki M, Narishige T, et al. Microtubule depolymerization normalizes in vivo myocardial contractile function in dogs with pressure-overload left ventricular hypertrophy. *Circulation.* 2000;102:1045–1052, with permission.)

Etiology and Noncontractile Effects of Cardiac Microtubule Network Densification

Apart from considering the microtubule-associated contractile dysfunction of hypertrophied myocardium, it is interesting to consider both the etiology of this cytoskeletal alteration and what effects it might have in terms of normal microtubule functions in the interphase cardiac muscle cell. In terms of etiology, the hypertrophic induction of increases in total tubulin protein and microtubules is caused by increased expression of α-tubulin and β-tubulin on the mRNA and protein levels (26). But the upregulated β-tubulin is not β-4 tubulin, the predominant β-tubulin isoform of the adult heart. Instead, the increase in β-tubulin is caused by re-expression of β-1 tubulin, the predominant β-tubulin expressed in the fetal heart (14). More interesting with respect to etiology, however, is the fact that (as seen in Fig. 4-9) there is increased expression during hypertrophy not only of tubulin but also of a fibrous microtubule-associated protein, MAP4 (24). Binding of this protein to microtubules, which has been found to occur extensively in pressure overload-hypertrophied myocardium (21), stabilizes these microtubules (24). Thus, increased tubulin expression and stabilization of the microtubules (once formed) may well play a very important role in the increased density of the microtubule network seen in cardiac disease states.

In terms of microtubule functions, there are potentially critical effects of extensive binding of MAP4 to the microtubules of hypertrophied cardiocytes. Since microtubules serve as "railroad tracks" along which cargos are transported by dynein and kinesin "locomotives" (42), a reasonable question is: What is the effect of having these tracks covered extensively by MAP4, a large (~220 kDa)

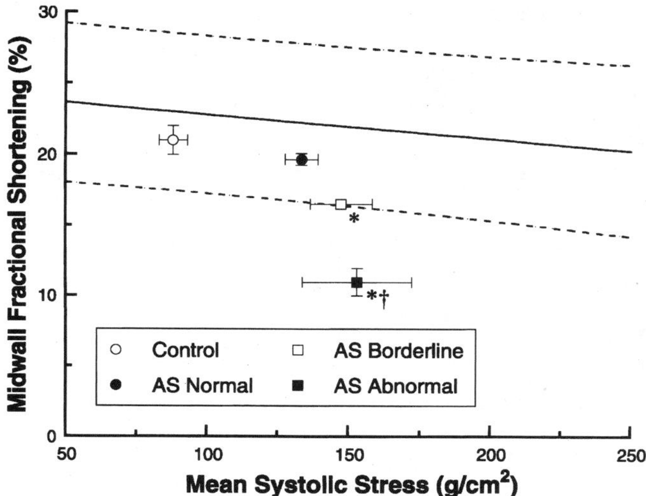

Figure 4-7 LV function in control patients and in patients with aortic stenosis. The solid and parallel dashed lines define the relationship between midwall fractional shortening and mean systolic stress, as well as its 95% prediction interval, for 84 patients found not to have cardiac pathology. The two control patients had Marfan syndrome; 13 patients with aortic stenosis were grouped according to LV functional status, with four in the normal function group, three in the borderline function group, and six in the abnormal function group. (Reproduced from Zile MR, Green GR, Schuyler GT, et al. Cardiocyte cytoskeleton in patients with left ventricular pressure overload hypertrophy. *J Am Coll Cardiol.* 2001;37:1080–1084, with permission.)

fibrous protein? It turns out that in a number of cell types the effect is to impede forward progress of the locomotives and thus of their cargos. This is because adherent MAPs cause steric inhibition of the association of the motor proteins with their microtubule tracks (42).

As an example of one pathophysiological consequence of this situation, one can consider the impact of microtubule-bound MAPs on β-adrenergic receptor function. It is well-established that β-receptor downregulation occurs during cardiac hypertrophy and failure. An important mechanism regulating the availability of previously activated β-adrenergic receptors is their recycling back to the sarcolemma via microtubules after agonist-induced internalization (18,19). It has been known for some time that microtubules are required for cardiocyte β-adrenergic receptor transport (43). It has now been found that binding of MAP4 to cardiocyte microtubules leads to β-adrenergic receptor downregulation by inhibiting microtubule-based transport (19), and it will be interesting in the future to see if this is one of the mechanisms responsible for β-adrenergic receptor downregulation in cardiac hypertrophy and failure.

A more general question having potentially much more important clinical significance is whether the difference between the compensated hypertrophy and failure groups seen in Figure 4-1 might be related to the MAP4 upregulation that is seen along with tubulin upregulation in high-wall-stress cardiac hypertrophy and failure. That is, the translation and assembly of structural proteins in the cardiocyte very likely require that translation-competent mRNAs be transported by kinesin motors as part of

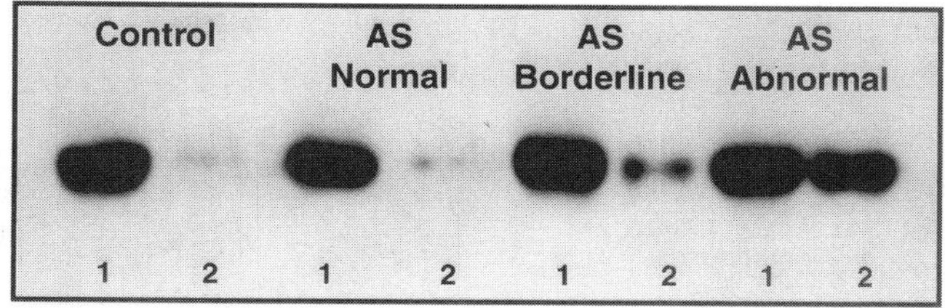

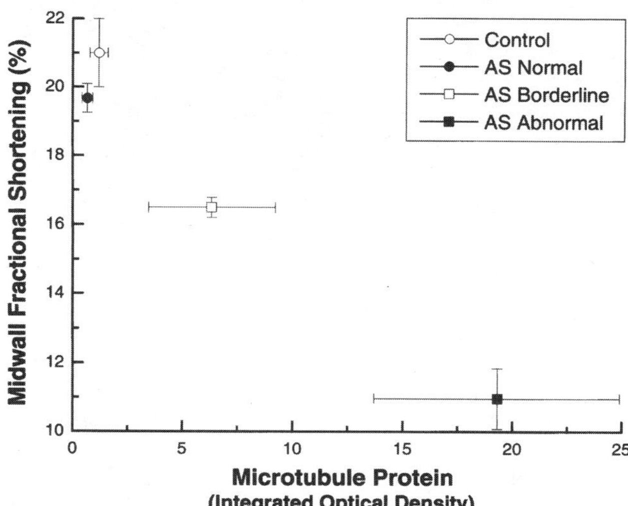

Figure 4-8 Myocardial tubulin in normal and aortic stenosis patients. The immunoblot was prepared from LV biopsies from one patient from each of the four study groups defined in Figure 4-7. Free tubulin is in lane 1 and polymerized tubulin (microtubules) is in lane 2. An equal amount of tubulin protein was loaded in each of the free tubulin lanes, and an equal volume of the polymerized tubulin (microtubule) fraction was loaded in each of the polymerized tubulin lanes. The summary data in the **lower panel** show the relationship of LV contractile function to LV microtubule protein for all of the patients in the four groups defined in Figure 4-7. (Reproduced from Zile MR, Green GR, Schuyler GT, et al. Cardiocyte cytoskeleton in patients with left ventricular pressure overload hypertrophy. *J Am Coll Cardiol.* 2001;37:1080–1084, with permission.)

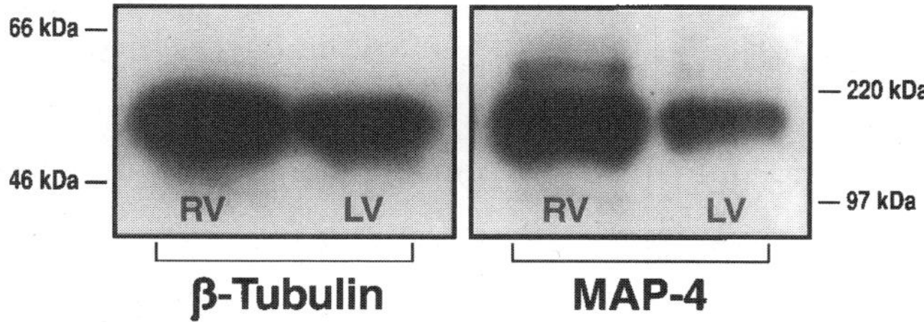

Figure 4-9 Immunoblots showing upregulation of β-tubulin versus MAP4 protein in pressure overload-hypertrophied right ventricular (RV) myocardium. While both β-tubulin and MAP4 were greater in the hypertrophied RV than in the same-animal normally loaded LV, densitometric analysis of immunoblots from four such cats RV-pressure-overloaded 2 weeks earlier via pulmonary artery banding showed that the RV/LV ratio of MAP4 was threefold ± 0.5-fold greater than the RV/LV ratio of β-tubulin. (Reproduced from Sato H, Nagai T, Kuppuswamy D, et al. Microtubule stabilization in pressure overload cardiac hypertrophy. *J Cell Biol.* 1997;139:963–973, with permission.)

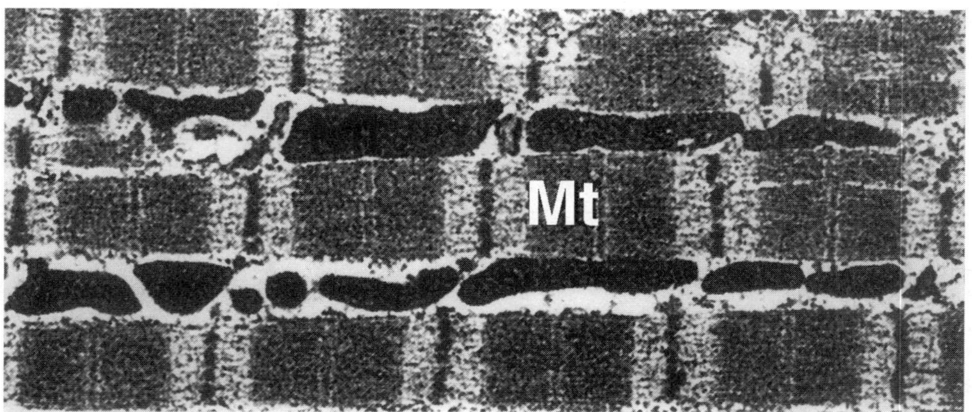

Figure 4-10 Electron micrograph of a longitudinal section of normal feline myocardium. The cytoplasm is packed full of contractile myofibrils (Mf) with rows of interposed mitochondria (Mt). (Reproduced from Thompson EW, Marino TA, Uboh CE, Kent RL, Cooper G. Atrophy reversal and cardiocyte redifferentiation in reloaded cat myocardium. *Circ Res.* 1984;54:367–377, with permission.)

ribonucleoprotein particles along microtubules to the requisite polysomes at the sites where the proteins are to be made and assembled. This transport mechanism would be required because, as noted earlier and seen in Figure 4-10, the cardiocyte cytoplasm is an extremely diffusion-restricted volume of space, since it is tightly packed with myofilaments and mitochondria (44). Thus, it is entirely possible that the cessation of compensatory hypertrophic growth seen in the failure group of dogs in Figure 4-1, and the consequent progressive increase in left ventricular wall stress, are a function of the inhibition of mRNA transport to the polysomes because of MAP4 decoration of microtubules. While this is a speculative idea for explaining the transition from compensated hypertrophy to decompensated heart failure, it might well represent an interesting area for future investigation.

INTERMEDIATE FILAMENTS

Desmin

Intermediate filaments are composed of parallel protein chains intertwined in a coiled-coil rod about 10 nm in diameter. In mature mammalian muscle, including cardiac muscle, the constitutive protein of the intermediate filaments is desmin. This protein is encoded by a single copy gene that is evolutionarily conserved. The relatively inextensible desmin filaments form a structural lattice that surrounds the Z-disks of the sarcomeres and connects them to one another (both side-to-side and end-to-end) along the length of the myofilament. They also link the myofilaments to the cardiocyte membrane-associated proteins, to the nucleus, to cytoplasmic organelles such as mitochondria, and to other cytoskeletal polymers via cytolinker proteins such as plectin and the plakins (12,45,46).

Figure 4-11 shows the microtubule network and the intermediate filament network in the same cardiac muscle cell (23). While there is no apparent physical relationship of the microtubules to other cellular structures, the intermediate filaments show a clear aggregation at the level of the Z-disks. Thus, while the extensive microtubule network is physically well-suited to subserve the intracellular transport processes, the intermediate filaments can be thought of as forming the structural backbone of contracting striated muscle, keeping the various components in their proper spatial locations and properly related to one another for efficient mechanical output.

The fact that desmin is one of the first muscle-specific proteins to appear during myogenesis (11,13) had led to the idea that it was essential for this process. However, experiments using desmin knockout mice have shown that this is not the case, since these mice are born with normal cardiocyte architecture (13). However, the lack of desmin eventually causes dilated cardiomyopathy in desmin-null mice (11–13,47–51). Indeed, the fate of the skeletal and cardiac muscles in these mice reinforces the role of desmin intermediate filaments as mechanical linkers of the various intracellular components of the muscle cell. What is found is that the cells of both the heart and active skeletal muscles essentially fall apart (i.e., because they cannot resist externally imposed or internally generated physical stress, they become mechanically unstable and degenerate) (47).

This is probably the basis for the dilated cardiomyopathy that is the common endpoint phenotype for the different mutations of desmin and a missense mutation of αβ-crystallin that are observed clinically, where the latter protein normally acts as a chaperone that stabilizes desmin structure and prevents its aggregation (48,49). These rather unusual cardiomyopathies, which sometimes have a familial occurrence, have heart failure as their most common feature (11,13). However, the cardiac phenotype also varies somewhat, depending on the specific structural change in the desmin molecule caused by a particular mutation, such that diastolic dysfunction or conduction abnormalities may sometimes predominate (11). Thus, in contrast to the lack of known primary cardiac defects caused by tubulin mutations, there are primary cardiac defects, sometimes called desminopathies, caused by desmin and αβ-crystallin mutations.

Apart from these primary cardiac abnormalities caused by desmin mutations, there are secondary abnormalities of the intermediate filament network that arise during cardiac disease states in a manner analogous to the abnormalities of the microtubule network that are secondary to cardiac diseases. Thus, it is found both in experimental animal

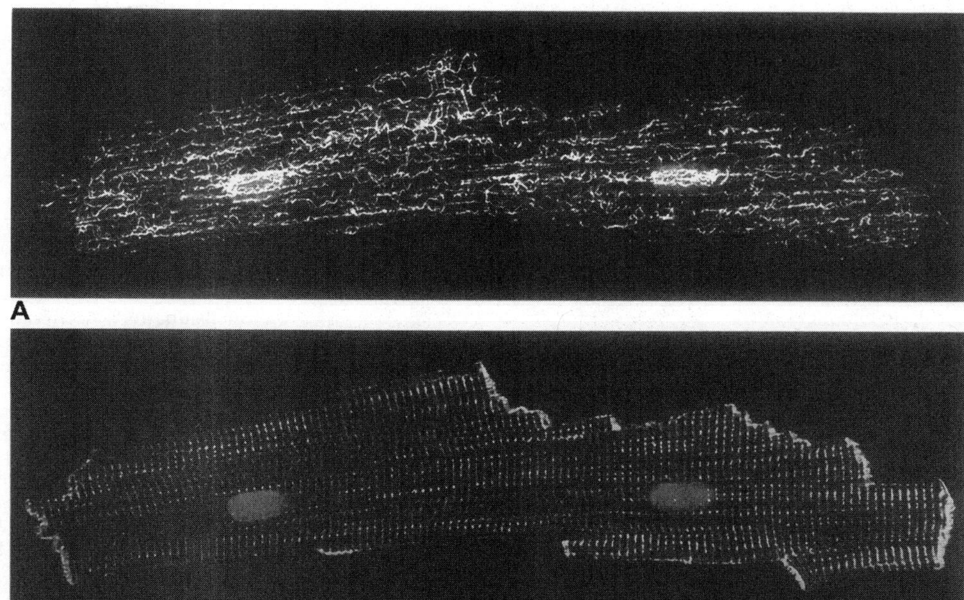

Figure 4-11 Structure of the microtubules and intermediate filaments in the same hypertrophied LV cardiocyte from a dog with aortic stenosis. **A**, Where the primary antibody was to β-tubulin, shows the dense microtubule network characteristic of hypertrophied and failing severely pressure-overloaded myocardium. **B**, Where the same cardiocyte was stained with a desmin antibody, shows the immunolocalization of desmin at the Z-disks of the sarcomeres. In this study, the intermediate filament architecture appears to be normal. The nuclei were stained with TO-PRO-3. Each micrograph is a single 0- to 0.7-μm confocal section. (Reproduced from Tagawa H, Koide M, Sato H, et al. Cytoskeletal role in the transition from compensated to decompensated hypertrophy during adult canine left ventricular pressure overloading. *Circ Res.* 1998;82: 751–761, with permission.)

models (6,37) and in clinical material (1,7–10) that during hemodynamic cardiac overloading and end-stage dilated cardiomyopathy both desmin and tubulin are upregulated on the mRNA and protein levels, and both intermediate filaments and microtubules are increased in quantity and quite disorganized.

MICROFILAMENTS

Because both the microfilaments and the sarcomeric thin filaments are composed of actin, it is very difficult in mature striated muscle either to visualize the microfilaments or to selectively affect them experimentally in an effort to determine their function (4). Thus, in terms of a structural role it is not clear that the microfilaments are an important component of the normal cardiocyte cytoskeleton or that they are involved in cardiac disease in either a primary (4) or a secondary (1) manner.

The cardiocyte microfilaments may, instead, have their most important role in cell signaling, as reviewed by White et al. (2). Here, their close association with the transsarcolemmal integrins, the adjacent costameres, and a number of actin-binding and membrane-associated proteins positions the microfilaments to have a major role in both integrin-mediated signaling and mechanically mediated signaling (52–54). An example of the former is the role that nonreceptor tyrosine kinases such as c-Src may play in hypertrophic cardiac growth regulation by their association with cytoskeletal structures via load activation of integrin-mediated signaling (55). An example of the latter is the anabolic effect during load-induced hypertrophy of sodium entry through stretch-activated ion channels (56).

SUMMARY

Since the primary function of the heart is to serve as a motor, almost all of our efforts to understand it in health and disease have focused on the structure, function, and regulation of this motor at the levels of cardiac function in the intact organism through molecular function in the sarcomere. More recently, cytoskeletal elements other than the myofilament motors have begun to receive attention. Of these, the three filament systems of the classical cytoskeleton have major roles in the normal cardiocyte. These roles are trafficking in the case of the microtubules, structural support in the case of the intermediate filaments, and signal transduction in the case of the microfilaments. In cardiac disease, primary causative abnormalities appear (so far) to be a feature only of alterations in the desmin intermediate filaments. Changes secondary to cardiac diseases that are initiated by other causes, but which compound them, are a feature of both microtubules and intermediate filaments. Finally, this is a very new area of interest in the study of heart failure. As such, far less is known at present than will be known in the near future.

ACKNOWLEDGMENTS

The work from the laboratories of myself and my colleagues that is described in this chapter was supported by Program Project Grant HL-48788 from the National Heart, Lung, and Blood Institute and by Merit Awards from the Research Service of the Department of Veterans Affairs.

REFERENCES

1. Kostin S, Heling A, Hein S, et al. The protein composition of the normal and diseased heart. *Heart Fail Rev.* 1998;2:245–260.
2. Calaghan SC, Le Guennec J-Y, White E. Cytoskeletal modulation of electrical and mechanical activity in cardiac myocytes. *Prog Biophys Mol Biol.* 2004;84:29–59.
3. Tsutsui H, Ishihara K, Cooper G. Cytoskeletal role in the contractile dysfunction of hypertrophied myocardium. *Science* 1993;260:682–687.
4. Tsutsui H, Tagawa H, Kent RL, et al. Role of microtubules in contractile dysfunction of hypertrophied cardiocytes. *Circulation.* 1994;90:533–555.
5. Cooper G. Cardiocyte cytoskeleton in hypertrophied myocardium. *Heart Fail Rev.* 2000;5:187–201.
6. Wang X, Li F, Campbell SE, et al. Chronic pressure overload cardiac hypertrophy and failure in guinea pigs: II. Cytoskeletal remodeling. *J. Mol Cell Cardiol.* 1999;31:319–331.
7. Schaper J, Froede R, Hein S, et al. Impairment of the myocardial ultrastructure and changes of the cytoskeleton in dilated cardiomyopathy. *Circulation.* 1991;83:504–514.
8. Heling A, Zimmermann R, Kostin S, et al. Increased expression of cytoskeletal, linkage, and extracellular proteins in failing human myocardium. *Circ Res.* 2000;86:846–853.
9. Hein S, Kostin S, Heling A, et al. The role of the cytoskeleton in heart failure. *Cardiovasc Res.* 2000;45:273–278.
10. Kostin S, Hein S, Arnon E, et al. The cytoskeleton and related proteins in the human failing heart. *Heart Fail Rev.* 2000;5: 271–280.
11. Capetanaki Y. Desmin cytoskeleton in healthy and failing heart. *Heart Fail Rev.* 2000;5:203–220.
12. Samuel J-L, Corda S, Chassagne C, et al. The extracellular matrix and the cytoskeleton in heart hypertrophy and failure. *Heart Fail Rev.* 2000;5:239–250.
13. Carlsson L, Thornell LE. Desmin-related myopathies in mice and man. *Acta Physiol Scand.* 2001;171:341–348.
14. Narishige T, Blade KL, Ishibashi Y, et al. Cardiac hypertrophic and developmental regulation of the β-tubulin multigene family. *J Biol Chem.* 1999;274:9692–9697.
15. Ishibashi Y, Hazen-Martin DJ, Cooper G. Existence and localization of microtubule organizing center in terminally differentiated cardiocytes. *J Histochem Cytochem.* 1999;47:1646.
16. Rappaport L, Samuel JL. Microtubules in cardiac myocytes. *Int Rev Cytol.* 1988;113:101–143.
17. Webster DR. Microtubules in cardiac toxicity and disease. *Cardiovasc Toxicol.* 2002;2:75–89.
18. Cheng G, Iijima Y, Ishibashi Y, et al. Inhibition of G protein-coupled receptor trafficking in neuroblastoma cells by MAP 4 decoration of microtubules. *Am J Physiol.* (*Heart Circ Physiol.*) 2002;283:H2379–H2388.
19. Cheng G, Qiao F, Gallien TN, et al. Inhibition of β-adrenergic receptor trafficking in adult cardiocytes by MAP4 decoration of microtubules. *Am J Physiol.* (*Heart Circ Physiol.*) 2005;288: H1193–H1202.
20. Perhonen M, Sharp WW, Russell B. Microtubules are needed for dispersal of α-myosin heavy chain mRNA in rat neonatal cardiac myocytes. *J. Mol Cell Cardiol.* 1998;30:1713–1722.
21. Takahashi M, Shiraishi H, Ishibashi Y, et al. Phenotypic consequences of β1-tubulin expression and MAP4 decoration of microtubules in adult cardiocytes. *Am J Physiol.* (*Heart Circ Physiol.*) 2003;285:H2072–H2083.
22. Tagawa H, Koide M, Sato H, Cooper G. Cytoskeletal role in the contractile dysfunction of cardiocytes from hypertrophied and failing right ventricular myocardium. *Proc Assoc Am Physicians.* 1996;108:218–229.
23. Tagawa H, Koide M, Sato H, et al. Cytoskeletal role in the transition from compensated to decompensated hypertrophy during adult canine left ventricular pressure overloading. *Circ Res.* 1998;82:751–761.
24. Sato H, Nagai T, Kuppuswamy D, et al. Microtubule stabilization in pressure overload cardiac hypertrophy. *J Cell Biol.* 1997;139: 963–973.
25. Tagawa H, Wang N, Narishige T, et al. Cytoskeletal mechanics in pressure-overload cardiac hypertrophy. *Circ Res.* 1997;80:281–289.
26. Tagawa H, Rozich JD, Tsutsui H, et al. Basis for increased microtubules in pressure-hypertrophied cardiocytes. *Circulation.* 1996;93:1230–1243.
27. Gomez AM, Kerfant BG, Vassort G. Microtubule disruption modulates Ca^{2+} signaling in rat cardiac myocytes. *Circ Res.* 2000;86: 30–36.
28. Koide M, Hamawaki M, Narishige T, et al. Microtubule depolymerization normalizes in vivo myocardial contractile function in dogs with pressure-overload left ventricular hypertrophy. *Circulation.* 2000;102:1045–1052.
29. Zile MR, Koide M, Sato H, et al. Role of microtubules in the contractile dysfunction of hypertrophied myocardium. *J Am Coll Cardiol.* 1999;33:250–260.
30. Ishibashi Y, Takahashi M, Isomatsu Y, et al. Role of microtubules versus myosin heavy chain isoforms in contractile dysfunction of hypertrophied murine cardiocytes. *Am J Physiol.* (*Heart Circ Physiol.*) 2003;285:H1270–H1285.
31. Zile MR, Green GR, Schuyler GT, et al. Cardiocyte cytoskeleton in patients with left ventricular pressure overload hypertrophy. *J Am Coll Cardiol.* 2001;37:1080–1084.
32. Bailey BA, Dipla K, Li S, et al. Cellular basis of contractile derangements of hypertrophied feline ventricular myocytes. *J Mol Cell Cardiol.* 1997;29:1823–1835.
33. Palmer BM, Valent S, Holder EL, et al. Microtubules modulate cardiomyocyte β-adrenergic response in cardiac hypertrophy. *Am J Physiol.* (*Heart Circ Physiol.*) 1998;275:H1707–H1716.
34. Watson PA, Hannan R, Carl LL, et al. Contractile activity and passive stretch regulate tubulin mRNA and protein content in cardiac myocytes. *Am J Physiol.* (*Cell Physiol.*) 1996;271:C684–C689.
35. Ishibashi Y, Tsutsui H, Yamamoto S, et al. Role of microtubules in myocyte contractile dysfunction during cardiac hypertrophy in the rat. *Am J Physiol.* (*Heart Circ Physiol.*) 1996;271:H1978–H1987.
36. Takahashi M, Tsutsui H, Tagawa H, et al. Microtubules are involved in early hypertrophic responses of myocardium during pressure overload. *Am J Physiol.* (*Heart Circ Physiol.*) 1998;275:H341–H348.
37. Wang X, Li F, Gerdes AM. Chronic pressure overload cardiac hypertrophy and failure in guinea pigs: I. Regional hemodynamics and myocyte remodeling. *J. Mol Cell Cardiol.* 1999;31:307–317.
38. Lemler MS, Bies RD, Frid MG, et al. Myocyte cytoskeletal disorganization and right heart failure in hypoxia-induced neonatal pulmonary hypertension. *Am J Physiol.* (*Heart Circ Physiol.*) 2000;279: H1365–H1376.
39. Scopacasa BS, Teixeira VP, Franchini KG. Colchicine attenuates left ventricular hypertrophy but preserves cardiac function of aortic-constricted rats. *J Appl Physiol.* 2003;94:1627–1633.
40. Davis FJ, Pillai JB, Gupta M, et al. Concurrent opposite effects of trichostatin A, an inhibitor of histone deacetylases, on expression of α-MHC and cardiac tubulins: implication for gain in cardiac muscle contractility. *Am J Physiol.* (*Heart Circ Physiol.*) 2005;288: H1477–H1490.
41. Eble DM, Spinale FG. Contractile and cytoskeletal content, structure, and mRNA levels with tachycardia-induced cardiomyopathy. *Am J Physiol.* (*Heart Circ Physiol.*) 1995;268:H2426–H2439.
42. Sheetz MP. Motor and cargo interactions. *Eur J Biochem.* 1999;262:19–25.
43. Limas CJ, Limas C. Rapid recovery of cardiac β-adrenergic receptors after isoproterenol-induced "down"-regulation. *Circ Res.* 1984;55:524–531.
44. Thompson EW, Marino TA, Uboh CE, et al. Atrophy reversal and cardiocyte redifferentiation in reloaded cat myocardium. *Circ Res.* 1984;54:367–377.
45. Leung CL, Green KJ, Liem RK. Plakins: a family of versatile cytolinker proteins. *Trends Cell Biol.* 2002;12:37–45.
46. Wiche G. Role of plectin in cytoskeleton organization and dynamics. *J Cell Sci.* 1998;111:2477–2486.
47. Galou M, Gao J, Humbert J, et al. The importance of intermediate filaments in the adaptation of tissues to mechanical stress: evidence from gene knockout studies. *Biol Cell.* 1997;89:85–97.
48. Wang X, Osinska H, Gerdes AM, et al. Desmin filaments and cardiac disease: establishing causality. *J Card Fail.* 2002;8:S287–S292.
49. Goldfarb LG, Vicart P, Goebel HH, et al. Desmin myopathy. *Brain.* 2004;127:723–734.
50. Haubold K, Herrmann H, Langer SJ, et al. Acute effects of desmin mutations on cytoskeletal and cellular integrity in cardiac myocytes. *Cell Motil Cytoskeleton.* 2003;54:105–121.

51. Paulin D, Li Z. Desmin: a major intermediate filament protein essential for the structural integrity and function of muscle. *Exp Cell Res*. 2004;301:1–7.
52. Kaprielian RR, Severs NJ. Dystrophin and the cardiomyocyte membrane cytoskeleton in the healthy and failing heart. *Heart Fail Rev*. 2000;5:221–238.
53. Wu C, Dedhar S. Integrin-linked kinase (ILK) and its interactors: a new paradigm for the coupling of extracellular matrix to actin cytoskeleton and signaling complexes. *J Cell Biol*. 2001;155: 505–510.
54. Ross RS. The extracellular connections: the role of integrins in myocardial remodeling. *J Card Fail*. 2002;8:S326–S331.
55. Kuppuswamy D, Kerr C, Narishige T, et al. Association of tyrosine-phosphorylated c-Src with the cytoskeleton of hypertrophying myocardium. *J Biol Chem*. 1997;272:4500–4508.
56. Kent RL, Hoober JK, Cooper G. Load responsiveness of protein synthesis in adult mammalian myocardium: role of cardiac deformation linked to sodium influx. *Circ Res*. 1989;64:74–85.

Abnormalities in Calcium Cycling in Heart Failure

5

Judith Karen Gwathmey *Federica del Monte* *Roger Joseph Hajjar*

The major abnormality in the failing heart is loss of contractility. The seemingly logical corollary that an increase in intracellular calcium concentration would benefit patients with chronic heart failure stimulated the development of inotropic agents. The premise was that myocardial contractility would be restored by increasing myocardial calcium concentration.

Supporting this concept was the observation that adaptive/maladaptive changes that occurred in failing myocardium, such as altered sarcoplasmic reticulum (SR) calcium ATPase activity, isoform replacement of proteins involved in adenosine triphosphate (ATP) supply and demand, as well as isoform shifts in contractile proteins, impacted myofilament activation and calcium concentration/mobilization. The proteins essential for calcium sequestration and release, myofilament activation, and energy production are now known to not only be altered but also to have functional consequences. In this chapter we will address the question of whether changes in structure and/or function of calcium cycling proteins alone or in combination with deprivation of energy supply (e.g., ATP and phosphocreatine [PCr]), and/or changes at the level of the myofilaments, and/or accumulation of metabolites are sufficient to alter calcium-regulated contractile activation and contribute to impaired contractility in the failing human heart.

EXCITATION–CONTRACTION COUPLING IN THE HEART

Figure 5-1 demonstrates a simplistic schematic of excitation–contraction in the heart. The heart rhythmically goes through each beat, which is governed by the contraction and relaxation cycle of individual cardiac myocytes and the heart as a whole. The process begins with electrical signals on the membrane of the cardiac cell that eventually end in activation of the myofilaments and cross-bridge cycling, resulting in force production (1). The cardiac action potential is produced by the coordinated interaction of several ion channels that transduce physiological signals within and between cardiac myocytes.

Action potential conduction in the heart depends on ion conductance through specific voltage-gated ion channels that mediate rapid, voltage-dependent changes in ion permeability, which causes a change in the membrane potential. In the human heart, depolarization of the cell membrane leads to the opening of voltage-gated L-type calcium channels, located in the T-tubular regions of the cardiac myocyte, allowing the trans-sarcolemmal influx of a small amount of calcium into the cell (Fig. 5-1) (1–8). The L-type calcium channels are located in close proximity to the calcium release channels, known as ryanodine receptors, which are located on the SR (the major calcium-storing organelle in the cardiac myocyte). Calcium entering the cells through a single L-type calcium channel triggers the opening of one or a cluster of ryanodine receptors, resulting in the local release of calcium from the SR (1–5,8). During membrane depolarization, a large number of L-type calcium channels are opened, resulting in a large release of calcium from the SR through the ryanodine receptors, raising cytosolic calcium from 0.1–0.2 μmol/L to 2–10 μmol/L.

The calcium spark has been identified as a functional calcium signaling and releasing unit (4). Functionally, calcium sparks are calcium releases from the SR through the opening of the ryanodine receptors. Calcium sparks are depicted and measured by their morphology and the

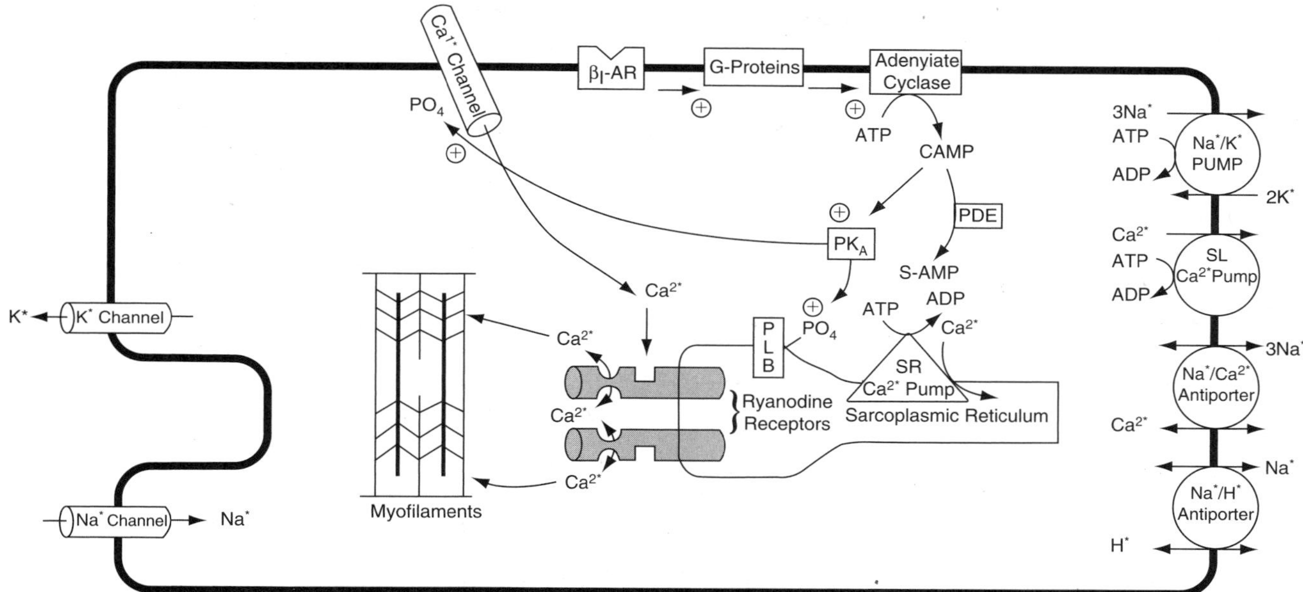

Figure 5-1 In the scheme of excitation–contraction coupling, there are two competing mechanisms for removing calcium from the cytoplasm: SERCA2a and the sodium–calcium exchanger. SERCA2a is inhibited by phospholamban when this protein is unphosphorylated. Phosphorylation of phospholamban through protein kinase A, calmodulin, and protein kinase C is balanced by dephosphorylation through protein phosphatases. (From Gwathmey JK, Hajjar RJ. The complexity of simplicity: the pathopysiology of heart failure. Hype or hope? *Res Phys.* 1993;39(4):45–49, with permission.)

frequency of occurrence. Morphology of the calcium sparks refers to the amplitude, width, and duration of the spark. The more active the calcium release channels are, the more calcium is released from the SR. Therefore, adaptive modifications that change ryanodine receptor activity or the modulators that regulate ryanodine receptor activity will have an impact on the size and frequency of calcium sparks and the subsequent release of calcium into the cytosol.

Calcium content of the SR also regulates calcium sparks. SR luminal calcium concentration plays a critical role in regulating ryanodine receptors by increasing the activity of the receptors and by sensitizing the threshold of receptor activation by signaling between L-type calcium channels and ryanodine receptors. Calcium sparks can be directly triggered by the influx of calcium through the L-type calcium channels. Thus, the kinetics, fidelity, and stoichiometry of coupling between L-type calcium channels and ryanodine receptors may play a critical role in the determination of signal transduction during excitation-contraction coupling. Although the number of calcium channels in failing human hearts has been reported to not be changed, the ryanodine receptors have been reported to be leaky, suggesting possible uncoupling or structural changes (9–15). The distance of the cleft between the cell membrane and the SR membrane, which is roughly 12 nm in normal cardiac myocytes, is thought to be critical for proper coupling and signal transduction between the L-type calcium channels and the ryanodine receptors. Expansion of the distance between L-type calcium channels and ryanodine receptors can therefore decrease or abolish the signaling reliability. This potential structural uncoupling may therefore impact the amount of calcium released from the SR. Furthermore, the amount of calcium stored in the SR may be reduced, thereby resulting in less calcium being available upon release for contractile activation at higher rates of contraction.

The rise of calcium in the myofibrillar space in turn results in cross-bridge formation and contraction (16–17). The contractile elements consists of an array of thick and thin filaments. The thick filaments consist mainly of myosin heavy chains (MHCs) and two pairs of light chains (16). Each myosin head has an ATP-binding area in close proximity to myosin ATPase, which cleaves ATP. Two MHC isoforms exist in human myocardium, alpha- and beta-MHC. In human ventricular myocardium only 10% to 20% is alpha-MHC, while the beta-MHC is more abundant (18). The thin filaments are composed of actin and the troponin complex. These regulatory proteins are carried on a long, helical molecule called tropomyosin. The troponin complex is made up of troponin C, troponin I, and troponin T. Troponin C is the calcium-binding protein. The strength of the bond linking troponin I (an inhibitory protein) and actin varies depending on the intracellular calcium concentration.

When cytosolic calcium is in the nanomolar range, the tropomyosin–troponin complex is positioned in such a way that the myosin heads cannot interact with actin. When cytosolic calcium increases to micromolar ranges, actin binds to troponin C, strengthening the bond between troponin C and troponin I and weakening the bond linking troponin I to actin. This leads to a conformational change of the tropomyosin–troponin C complex that allows the myosin head to interact with actin (Fig. 5-2).

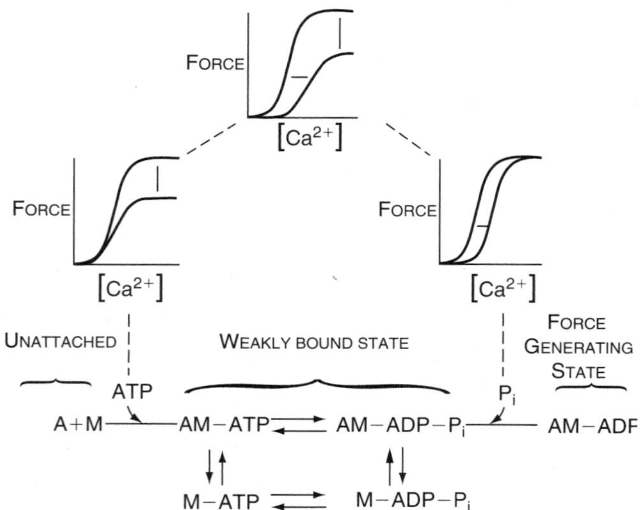

Figure 5-2 When cytosolic calcium increases to micromolar ranges, actin binds to troponin C, strengthening the bond between troponin C and troponin I and weakening the bond linking troponin I to actin. This leads to a conformational change of the tropomyosin–troponin C complex that allows the myosin head to interact with actin. When calcium binds to troponin C, it exposes the active site on the thin filament, permitting the myosin head to bind weakly to actin filaments. Subsequent ATP hydrolysis allows a strong binding of the myosin head to actin, which is followed by a power stroke that produces the force of contraction. Relaxation occurs when ATP binds to the myosin head, causing a dissociation of the thin from the thick filaments. Calcium is detached from troponin C and is resequestered into the SR by the calcium ATPase pump (SERCA2a) and is extruded from the cell by the sarcolemmal sodium–calcium exchanger. As shown in this figure, there are three types of changes that can decrease force production. (From Gwathmey JK, Hajjar RJ, Solaro RJ. Contractile deactivation and uncoupling of cross-bridges: effects of 2, 3-butanediene monoxine on mammalian myocardium. *Circ Res.* 1991;69: 1280–1292, with permission.)

When calcium binds to troponin C, it exposes the active site on the thin filament, permitting the myosin head to bind weakly to actin filaments. Subsequent ATP hydrolysis allows a strong binding of the myosin head to actin, which is followed by a power stroke that produces the force of contraction (16). Relaxation occurs when ATP binds to the myosin head, causing a dissociation of the thin from the thick filaments. Calcium is detached from troponin C and is resequestered into the SR by the calcium ATPase pump (SERCA2a) and is extruded from the cell by the sarcolemmal sodium–calcium exchanger.

As shown in Figure 5-2, there are three types of changes that can decrease force production (16). There can be a depression of maximal force (F_{max}) that constitutes a change in the intracellular calcium concentration–force relationship. A decrease in F_{max} can be the result of uncoupling of cross-bridges. However, it is known that the maximal calcium activated force in human failing myocardium is not diminished (2,19–21). This has also been demonstrated in an avian model of heart failure (22,23). Accumulation of inorganic phosphate (as can be possibly seen as a result of ATP splitting) is known to affect the responsiveness of the contractile proteins in this manner (e.g., inorganic phosphate increases during hypoxia).

A decrease in intracellular calcium concentration, resulting in a decrease in force production along with an unaltered intracellular calcium concentration–force relationship, is another mechanism to be considered. As depicted in Figure 5-2, a rightward shift of the intracellular calcium concentration–force relationship can result from a decrease in the sensitivity of troponin C to calcium. A decrease in intracellular pH is known to produce this effect (e.g., during ischemia). Also, an increase in inorganic phosphate can result in a decrease in the sensitivity of the myofilaments to calcium, along with a decrease in maximal force. We will take a more in-depth look at the relationship between calcium availability, the myofilaments, and contractility.

The extent of contribution of the SR and the sodium–calcium exchanger to lowering cytosolic calcium concentrations varies among species. In humans, ~75% of the calcium is removed from the cytosol by SERCA2a and ~25% by the sodium–calcium exchanger. SERCA2a transports calcium back to the luminal space of the SR against a calcium gradient by an energy-dependent mechanism (one molecule of ATP is hydrolyzed for the transport of two molecules of calcium), where it binds to a calcium-buffering protein, calsequestrin.

The calcium-pumping activity of SERCA2a is regulated by phospholamban. In its unphosphorylated state, phospholamban inhibits the SR calcium-ATPase, whereas phosphorylation of phospholamban by cyclic adenosine monophosphate (cAMP)-dependent protein kinase A (PKA) and by calcium-calmodulin-dependent PKA reverses this inhibition (24,25).

In the heart there are also a number of endogenous and exogenous factors that regulate the strength of contraction. Circulating and locally released catecholamines bind to myocardial β-1 and β-2 adrenoreceptors (26). β-3 receptors have been recently identified in the heart but their primary role appears to be an inhibitory effect on contractility. On the other hand, both β-1 and β-2 adrenoreceptors activate adenylate cyclase through stimulatory G proteins (Gs alpha), which results in the production of cAMP (Fig. 5-1). Binding of cAMP to the regulatory subunit of PKA triggers a conformational change that allows the catalytic subunits of the enzyme to dissociate and phosphorylate protein substrates. PKA phosphorylates (a) L-type calcium channels, resulting in increased calcium entry; (b) phospholamban, resulting in enhanced calcium uptake into the SR; and (c) troponin I, resulting in enhanced detachment of calcium from troponin C and decreased myofilament calcium sensitivity. The effects of PKA phosphorylation therefore increase the strength of the contraction while also enhancing relaxation.

Cardiac ryanodine receptors are also regulated by the beta-adrenergic receptor (beta-AR) signaling pathway. The ryanodine receptor has a delicate balance between PKA phosphorylation and phosphatases (i.e., protein phosphatase 1 [PP1] and 2 [PP2A]) (27). Activation of the sympathetic nervous system results in binding of norepinephrine to the beta-AR and an elevation of cAMP levels with resultant activation of PKA. In addition, there are other molecules such as FKB 12–6, which bind the L-type calcium channel receptor to the ryanodine receptor and stabilize the interaction. Upon activation of the beta-AR, PP1 and PP2A levels in the ryanodine receptor decrease and the ryanodine receptors become phosphorylated. This pathologically increases calcium-dependent activation of the ryanodine calcium release channels and results in deletion of SR calcium stores. This results in an uncoupling of ryanodine receptors from each other, thereby reducing excitation–contraction coupling gain. This is important in that the ryanodine calcium release channels have been shown to become leaky in failing human hearts (9,12–14).

One can readily understand how depleted SR calcium stores can result in reduced contractile activation, a negative force–interval relationship (i.e., negative treppe), thereby negatively impacting myocardial contractility (Fig. 5-3) (12,14). The force–frequency relationship significantly contributes to the beat-to-beat regulation of the contractile strength in the heart. In a normal heart, increasing heart rate results in enhanced trans-sarcolemmal calcium influx, resulting in more calcium being stored in the SR for subsequent release and stronger contraction. However, in the failing human heart a negative force–interval relationship has been reported (28–34). At higher rates of contraction there is a decline in force as well as an increase in diastolic force (Fig. 5-3) (28–34). This negative treppe is associated with a dramatic increase in diastolic calcium concentrations and a reduction in the amplitude of the peak calcium transient. Also, there is evidence that at higher contraction rates there is likely an accumulation of metabolites (e.g., inorganic phosphate) or possibly a change in intracellular pH; this appears to result in a rightward shift on the calcium axis, resulting in diminished force for any given intracellular calcium concentration in the cell (Fig. 5-4) (29).

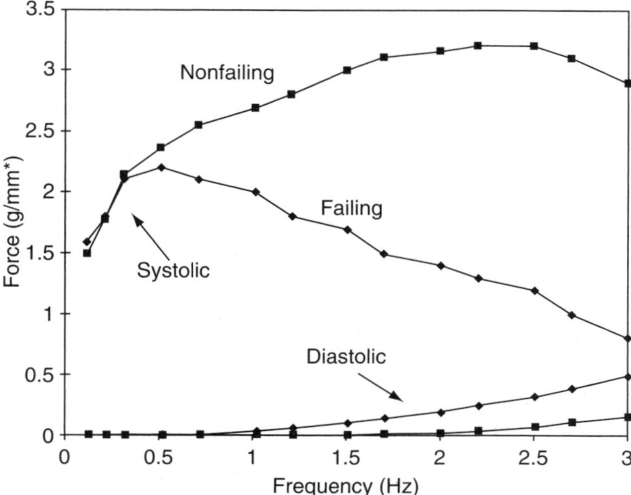

Figure 5-3 Force–interval relationship. There is no difference in the force of contraction in isolated muscle preparations from nonfailing and failing human hearts at slower stimulation rates. However, at higher rates of stimulation there is a decrease in the force of contraction seen in muscles isolated from failing human hearts, unlike the continued increase in force noted in muscles from nonfailing human hearts. Also noted in muscles from failing human hearts associated with the decline in systolic force of contraction was an increase in diastolic force at higher rates of contraction. This observation has been shown to be associated with a rise in intracellular diastolic calcium concentration. (From Schmidt U, Hajjar RJ, Gwathmey JK. The force-interval relationship in human myocardium. *J Card Fail.* 1995;1(4):311–321, with permission.)

As demonstrated in Figure 5-4, with delays after high rates of stimulation before tetanization in isolated muscle strips from the hearts of patients with heart failure, there is an increase in calcium-activated force with no change in extracellular calcium concentration. Similarly, it was demonstrated that despite having the same intracellular calcium concentration as a muscle subjected to lower rates of contraction, muscles stimulated at higher rates of contraction and then tetanized generated less force. This dramatic example suggests that changes in myofilament calcium activation and contractility may change in a dynamic manner, possibly on a beat-to-beat basis, and might partly explain why, at lower rates of stimulation, peak twitch force is similar for muscle strips from nonfailing and failing human hearts (Fig. 5-3).

HYPOTHESES FOR DECREASED CONTRACTILE PERFORMANCE IN THE FAILING HEART

Calcium Mobilization Versus Availability: Impact on Contractile Performance

It has been proposed that the diminished contractility seen in the failing heart is due to diminished intracellular calcium. Using the calcium indicator Indo in isolated myocytes from failing human hearts, it was reported that peak SR calcium release was 1 μmol/L, a value similar to that observed for normal mammalian myocardium (35). Furthermore, a significantly higher resting calcium concentration has been demonstrated, particularly with increased rates of stimulation and contraction. These experimental findings have been confirmed in multicellular preparations using aequorin and Fura-2 (28,29).

Experiments using aequorin have reported an increased diastolic calcium concentration associated with an increase in diastolic force in multicellular preparations similar to that reported in isolated cardiac myocytes (28,29). Only at higher stimulation rates was there a decrease in peak cytosolic calcium concentration detected with aequorin. Del Monte et al. also reported that there was a decrease in peak systolic calcium at high stimulation rates, with an associated elevated diastolic calcium concentration in cardiac myocytes from failing human hearts (28). The peak calcium concentration at basal stimulation rates for myocytes from nonfailing human hearts versus myocytes from failing human hearts was 551±32 nmol/L, versus 508±25 ($p > 0.05$) nmol/L, respectively. As reported with aequorin in multicellular preparations, with higher frequencies of contraction there was a disproportionate rise in the diastolic calcium concentration, a reduced peak systolic calcium transient, and slowed relaxation (29,36) (Fig. 5-5). Despite the controversy as to whether or not the peak of the calcium transient is diminished at lower rates of contraction, one must take into consideration the effect of a longer duration of calcium availability, which has been demonstrated with all calcium indicators (Figs. 5-5 and 5-6)

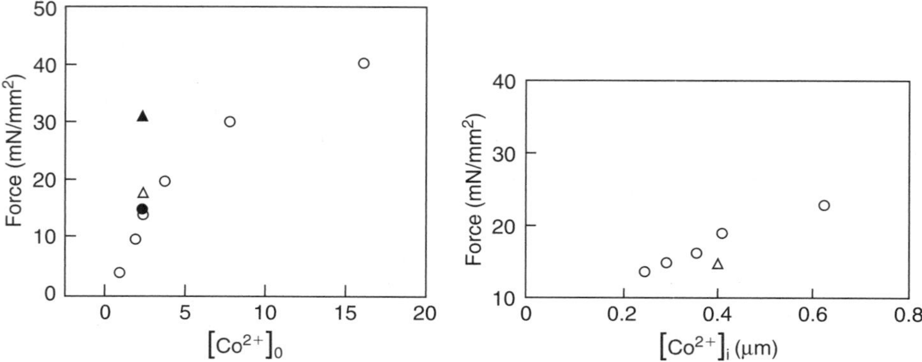

Figure 5-4 **Left panel** steady-state force–calcium relationship in myopathic tissue in the presence of increasing extracellular calcium concentrations at a basal stimulation rate of 0.33 Hz (o). Tetanization basal frequency of 1 Hz (●) without delay; 5-second delay (Δ); 20-second delay (▲). **Right panel** is the steady-state force–intracellular calcium relationship at varying intracellular calcium concentrations at 0.33 Hz (o) compared to basal frequency of 1 Hz in 2.5-mmol/L extracellular calcium without delay (Δ). The **left panel** demonstrates that with delays, despite no change in intracellular calcium, the force increases. The **right panel** shows that despite having the same intracellular calcium at 1 Hz as at 0.33 Hz, the force is less. These data suggest a change in myofilament calcium responsiveness. (From Gwathmey JK, Slawsky MT, Hajjar RJ, et al. Role of intracellular calcium handling in force-interval relationships of human ventricular myocardium. *J Clin Invest.* 1990;85(5):1599–1628, with permission.)

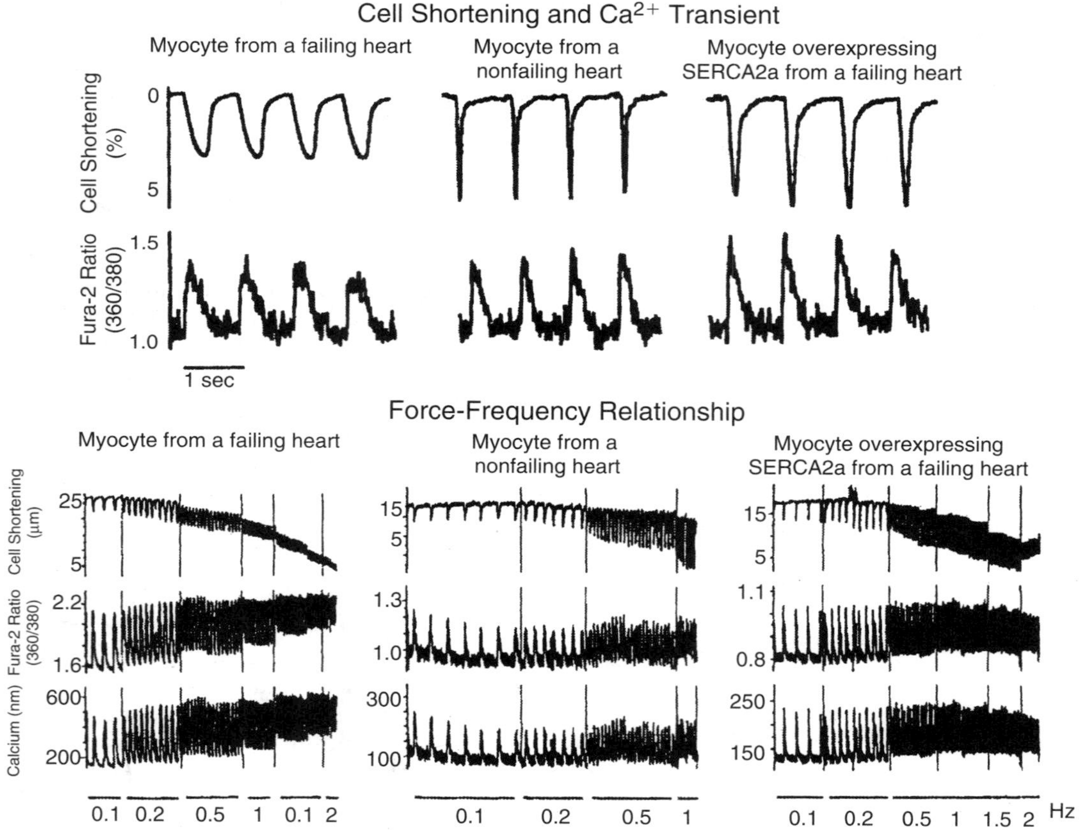

Figure 5-5 The **top panel** demonstrates cell shortening and associated calcium transient in an isolated cardiac myocyte from a nonfailing human heart and a failing human heart. The **far right panel** demonstrates how transfection with SERCA2a restores cell shortening and abbreviates the time course of the calcium transient. The **lower panels** demonstrate the impact of increasing the frequency of shortening in an isolated myocyte from nonfailing and failing hearts. Myocyte overexpressing SERCA2a has a more normal force interval relationship. There was a significant reduction in the increase in diastolic calcium concentrations and reduced shortening noted in a myocyte isolated from a failing human heart with SERCA2a transfection. The same hearts were shown to have a significant reduction in SERCA2a protein content. (From del Monte F, Harding S, Schmidt U, et al. Restoration of contractile function in isolated cardiomyocytes from failing human hearts by gene transfer of SERCA2a. *Circulation* 1999; 100(23):2308–2313, with permission.)

(28,36). Time course and duration of calcium availability can be key factors in determining "apparent myofilament calcium sensitivity and calcium responsiveness" (37).

Myofilament Calcium Responsiveness and Heart Failure

Contractility is determined not only by the amount of calcium that is available in the cytosol, but also by the duration and time course of calcium availability and the duration of troponin C–calcium interaction (5,37). The first report of intracellular calcium signals in nonfailing and failing human myocardium demonstrated a slowed time course to the decay from the peak calcium transient to diastolic levels (Fig. 5-6) (36). An elevated diastolic calcium concentration was also clearly demonstrated (28,29,36). These first images that captured calcium handling in nonfailing and failing human myocardium challenged the then-current dogma that more calcium was needed in the failing heart. They also raised the question of whether better mobilization of calcium was needed, as opposed to the use of inotropes that acted by increasing intracellular calcium concentrations.

In response to this unexpected observation, many investigators attempted to make inferences about changes in calcium responsiveness and force of contraction by using the peak twitch force–peak light or calcium relationship. This was then extended to the use of fluorescence indicators in isolated myocytes and became the peak fluorescence–peak shortening relationship. We, as well as other investigators, have discussed the limitations of the use of this technique and the fact that the relationship can be artifactually shifted by alterations in the duration of the calcium transient, time course of contraction, as well as changes in the cross-bridge cycling kinetics (17). To make this point clearer and to demonstrate the impact of changes in the time course of calcium mobilization and time course of contraction on contractility, we performed several studies using intracellular calcium signals as well as skinned fiber preparations. The advantage of using skinned fibers is that the exact amount of calcium delivered to the contractile elements is known and can be studied under steady-state conditions.

We compared peak twitch force–peak calcium relationships to skinned fiber force–calcium relationships in muscles from the same experimental animal. We established two models of disease: pressure-overload hypertrophy (POH) and hyperthyroidism in the ferret. We were motivated to do this for several reasons. With ventricular POH, isolated muscles demonstrate an isometric twitch and associated intracellular calcium transient that are prolonged (38–40). In contrast, ferrets made hyperthyroid by injection of thyroxine have abbreviated time courses of the isometric twitch and intracellular calcium (41). In both situations (POH and hyperthyroidism) there are no significant differences in diastolic or peak intracellular calcium concentration. These two models, therefore, provide an opportunity to study the effects of changes in time course of the intracellular calcium transient and isometric twitch in the presence of similar amounts of peak and diastolic intracellular calcium concentrations. Therefore, we had a relatively simple system to investigate the effect of time course changes of the calcium transient and contraction on myocardial contractility and the apparent force–calcium relationship.

As mentioned earlier, there are two key players in the calcium signal reported with calcium indicators: (a) troponin C Ca^{2+} binding affinity and (b) SR function. Troponin C and the SR are the most important calcium sinks in myocardial cells. Troponin C binds Ca^{2+} immediately after the ion enters the myofibrillar space. Within 20 milliseconds in frog skeletal muscle at 0°C, troponin C is at least 90% saturated (42). Force does not begin to rise until after 10 milliseconds. Therefore, if the affinity of troponin C is altered it will affect the time course as well as amplitude of the calcium signal. Similar to placing a low-pass filter in an electronic circuit, as the affinity increases, the time course will become longer and the peak shorter. If the affinity decreases, the calcium signal will be briefer and taller. Therefore, the amplitude of the calcium transient is determined by the rate at which the SR releases

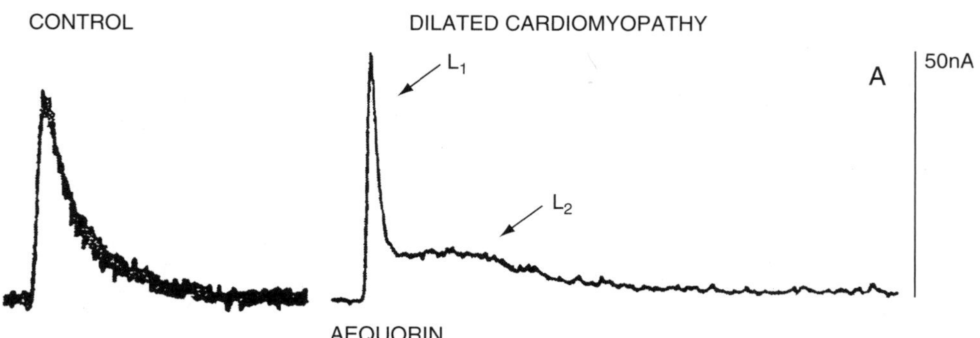

Figure 5-6 Intracellular calcium transients from isolated muscles from nonfailing and failing human hearts loaded with aequorin, a bioluminescent protein. The **left panel** is calcium transient from a nonfailing human heart and the **right panel** is from a patient who had undergone cardiac transplantation for dilated cardiomyopathy. (From Gwathmey JK, Copelas L, Mackinnon R, et al. Abnormal intracellular cacium handling in myocardium from patients with end-stage heart failure. *Circ Res.* 1987;61:70–76, with permission.)

calcium and the rate at which troponin C binds the free calcium.

The time course of the intracellular calcium signal is therefore regulated by the balance between the release of calcium and its uptake by the SR. Thus, one would anticipate that interventions that increase the affinity of troponin C to calcium would decrease the amplitude of the intracellular calcium signal. They would also be expected to decrease the decline of intracellular calcium signal since calcium would be released more slowly from troponin C. On the other hand, a decrease in the affinity of troponin C to calcium would result in an elevated peak intracellular calcium concentration and a shorter time course. Agents that increase the rate of calcium uptake by the SR would be expected to shorten the time course of the calcium signal without affecting the peak intracellular calcium concentration, and agents that decrease the rate of calcium uptake by the SR would be expected to lengthen the time course of intracellular calcium transient without affecting the peak intracellular calcium concentration.

It is important to note that excluded in our discussions are the effects on the time course or amplitude of the calcium signal of cellular extrusion mechanisms (e.g., the sodium–calcium exchanger, as well as additional calcium buffers such as mitochondria). It is thought that the effects are relatively small compared to the key players and that these factors are less subject to large kinetic changes.

As shown in Figures 5-7 and 5-8, we can demonstrate shifts in the apparent calcium sensitivity for force calcium activation in the absence of a true change in myofilament calcium sensitivity. In the case of POH, one obtains a higher force for any given level of extracellular calcium. In contrast with hyperthyroidism, decreasing the time course of the intracellular calcium transient resulted in a rightward shift on the calcium axis (i.e., an apparent decrease in the sensitivity of the myofilaments despite having with no change in sensitivity of the myofilaments). Therefore, investigators must use caution when drawing conclusions regarding myocardial contractility and its relationship to intracellular calcium concentrations.

Our examples demonstrate that a slower calcium transient as well as a faster calcium transient alone can alter the apparent force–calcium relationship and myocardial contractility in a predictable direction (Fig. 5-9) (37,38–41). It is important to note that in skinned fibers from the same hearts with pressure overload or hyperthyroidism there is no change in the force–calcium relationship (37). This is similar to our observations in myocardial fibers from failing and nonfailing human hearts (Fig. 5-10) (20,21). In skinned fibers from nonfailing and failing human hearts, no differences in myofilament calcium sensitivity or maximal calcium activated force were detected (20,21). This observation has been confirmed by us at the level of a single isolated myocyte (Fig. 5-11) (unpublished data). These observations are identical to reports in an avian model of heart failure that we have demonstrated mimics subcellular as well as genomic changes seen in the failing human heart (22,23). However, if multicellular muscle preparations were challenged with changes in intracellular pH, phosphate, PKA, PKC, and cAMP, differences were

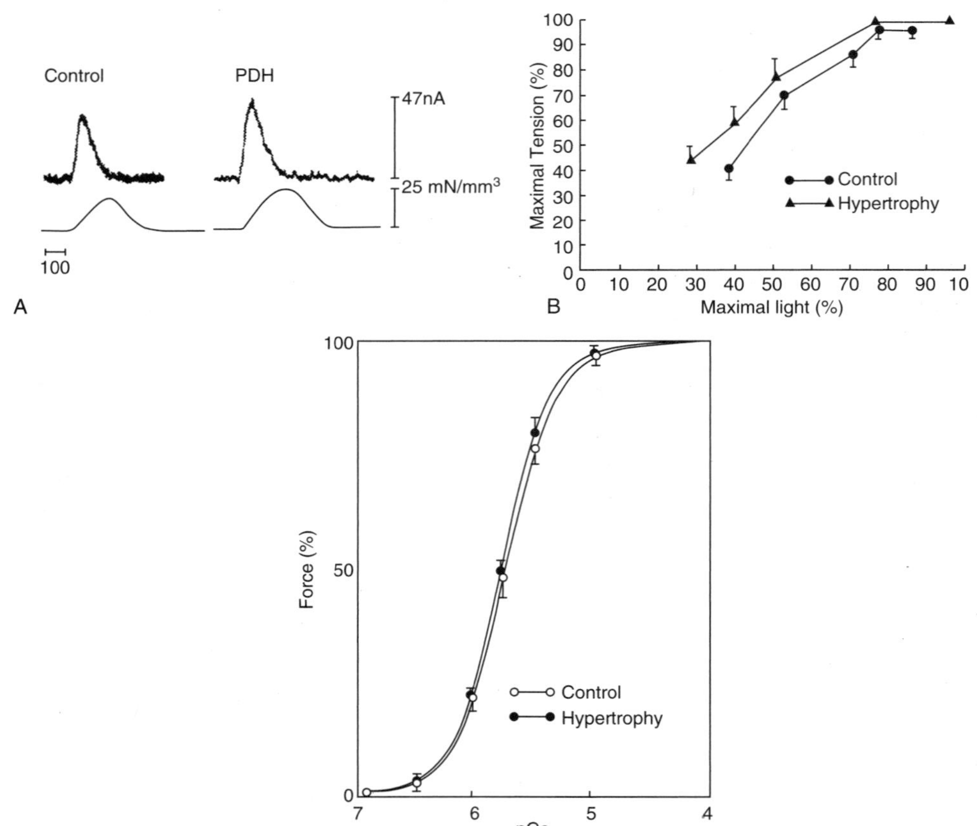

Figure 5-7 Force and calcium signals from a pressure-overload hypertrophy (POH) muscle (**A**). The calcium and force signals are prolonged compared to the control muscle. Plotting peak twitch force production versus peak light for increasing extracellular calcium concentrations in muscles from ferrets with POH and age-matched controls, we obtained the relationship in **B**. The relationship was shifted to the left in the case of POH, suggesting an increase in myofilament calcium sensitivity. Muscles from the same hearts were skinned with saponin. **C** shows the force–pCa relationships from POH and control animals. There were no significant differences in the Ca^{2+} sensitivity between POH and control muscles. (From Gwathmey JK, Hajjar RJ. Intracellular calcium related to force development in twitch contraction of mammalian myocardium. *Cell Calcium.* 1990;121:531–538, with permission.)

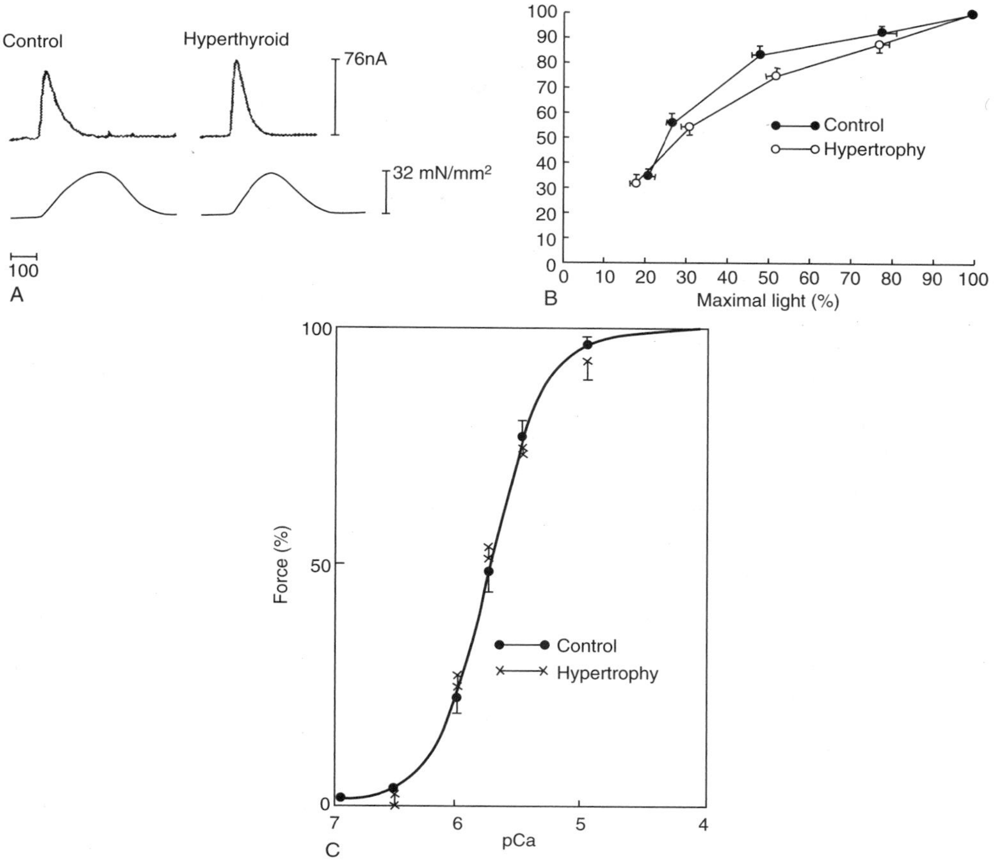

Control Hyperthyroid
76nA
32 mN/mm²
100
A

Control
Hypertrophy
Maximal light (%)
B

Force (%)
Control
Hypertrophy
pCa
C

Figure 5-8 Hyperthyroidism. **A** depicts the force and calcium measurements obtained from thyrotoxic hearts. The time course of the calcium and force signals is abbreviated in thyrotoxic muscles. The relationship between peak force and peak [Ca^{2+}] in the thyrotoxic hearts is shifted to the right as compared to the control, indicating a decrease in the calcium sensitivity of the myofilaments **(B)**. Muscles from the same hearts were skinned with saponin. **C** shows the force–pCa relationships from thyrotoxic and control animals. There were no significant differences in the Ca^{2+} sensitivity and maximal Ca^{2+} activated force production between thyrotoxic and control muscles. (From Gwathmey JK, Hajjar RJ. Intracellular calcium related to force development in twitch contraction of mammalian myocardium. *Cell Calcium.* 1990; 121:531–538, with permission.)

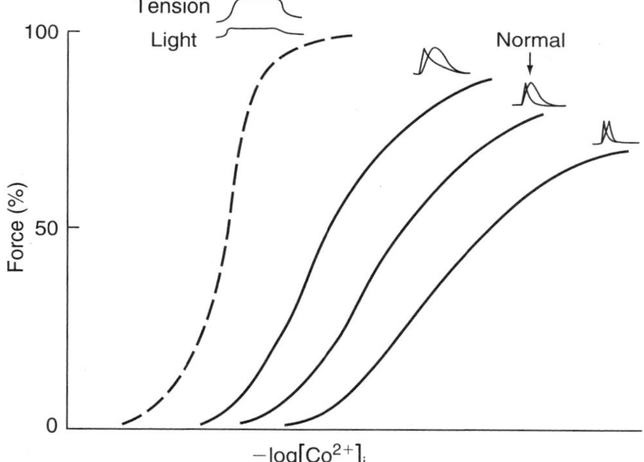

Figure 5-9 The effect of simply altering the time course of the calcium transient on the apparent force–calcium relationship with respect to steady-state force–calcium relationships. Steady-state force–calcium relationships are traditionally obtained using skinned fibers or steady-state muscle tetanizations. The sensitivity of the myofilaments to calcium are highest under steady-state conditions. Abbreviation of the time course of the contraction and time course of the calcium signal results in a rightward shift on the calcium axis to higher calcium concentrations. This means that a higher level of calcium is needed to obtain the same amount of force if the transient were of normal duration, longer duration, or at steady state. Prolongation of the calcium transient, as has been reported in failing human myocardium and the time course of contraction and relaxation results in a leftward shift on the calcium axis toward lower calcium concentrations and closer to the steady-state force–calcium relationship. (From Gwathmey JK, Hajjar RJ. Intracellular calcium related to force development in twitch contraction of mammalian myocardium. *Cell Calcium.* 1990;121:531–538, with permission.)

detected in the force–calcium relationship between fibers from nonfailing and failing human hearts, similar to our observations in an avian model of heart failure (20–23,43).

Figure 5-12 demonstrates experiments performed with an agent that acts at the level of the contractile elements (i.e., 12-deoxyphorbol 13-isobutyrate 20-acetate) (43). Again, under experimental conditions with agents targeted to act at the level of the myofilaments in intact muscle preparations, we found a difference in myofilament calcium responsiveness that might partially explain the differences seen in myocardial contractility in the failing human heart (20,43). Thus, it is important to consider phosphorylation/dephosphorylation of subcellular organelles in the relationship to myocardial contractility (24,44–49)

We must therefore conclude that failing human myocardium does not have a significant change in myofilament calcium activation under nonstress conditions, but does demonstrate a prolonged time course of the calcium transient, which in combination with a slower cross-bridge cycling rate or kinetics (Fig. 5-13) might allow it to demonstrate normal levels of myocardial force production under ideal physiological conditions (e.g., slower rates of contraction and better mobilization of intracellular calcium) (49). Physiological stresses on the heart may therefore result in the relationship between myocardial contractility and calcium concentration to be artifactually shifted. In fact, measured calcium transients most likely do not reflect true calcium availability or myofilament calcium sensitivity. These examples might explain, in part, how similar levels

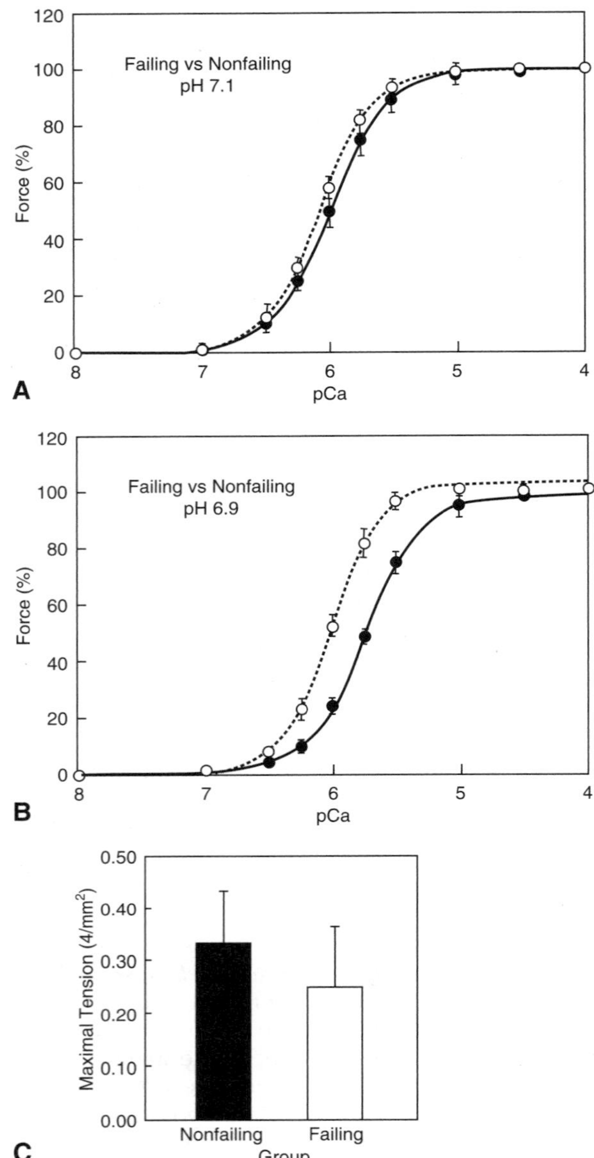

Figure 5-10 Change in intracellular pH in failing (o) and nonfailing (●) human myocardium. Notice the lack of difference in the force–calcium relationship at pH 7.1 (standard for skinned fiber experiments) **(A)**. **B** at pH 6.9 shows a rightward shift on the calcium axis by muscle from failing human hearts, indicating a strong decrease in myofilament calcium sensitivity and responsiveness. This suggests differences in sensitivity to changes in pH. Differences in the response of the myofilaments (calcium–force relationship) were also noted for inorganic phosphate as well as PKA and cAMP. **C** demonstrates there are no differences in maximal calcium-activated force. (Gwathmey JK, Liao R, Helm PA, et al. Cardiovascular Drugs and Therapy 1995;9:581–587 and Hajjar RJ, Schwinger RHG, Schmidt U, et al. Myofilament calcium regulation in human myocardium. *Circulation.* 2000;101:1679–1685, with permission.)

of force development can occur in muscles from failing human hearts when stimulated at slower rates (Fig. 5-13). Similarly, by lowering heart rate, myocardial contractility might paradoxically be improved (30,32,49).

One must keep in mind that human myocardium has a significant slowing of cross-bridge cycling rate, similar to other animal models (Fig. 5-13) (17,22). This allows for longer times for attachment and greater force at a reduced energy expenditure. A combination of longer troponin C calcium binding and longer duration of calcium availability (Figs. 5-5 and 5-6) can theoretically result in a higher force and better contractile performance despite a possible reduction in calcium available or peak amplitude of the calcium transient. As demonstrated in Figures 5-5 and 5-6, failing human hearts have a slowed return to baseline diastolic calcium concentrations, which nevertheless remain elevated compared to calcium levels in nonfailing muscle strips (28,29).

The only reasonable conclusion that can be made regarding the relationship between calcium availability and peak intracellular calcium concentrations to myocardial contractility is that a correlation is not straightforward, especially in the failing human heart. Factors can alter the apparent calcium sensitivity of the myofilaments and change the true myofilament calcium sensitivity and responsiveness (i.e., slope of the force–calcium relationship) as a result of higher work demands. ATP utilization, phosphorylation or dephosphorylation of the contractile elements, the amount as well as well functional integrity of the SR and phospholamban in combination with the accumulation of metabolites, coupled with changes in the time course of the calcium signal, must all be considered. Only then can one attribute a causative relation between calcium availability, a reduction in the peak amplitude of the calcium transient, and depressed contractile performance noted in patients with heart failure.

Nevertheless, current data suggest that the failing cardiac myocyte has sufficient free ionized intracellular calcium to support normal contractile activation. This is supported on several fronts. First, at low rates of contraction there is no difference between peak force in multicellular or isolated myocyte preparations (28,29–31). Skinned fibers and isolated cardiac myocytes, when exposed to increasing concentrations of calcium, demonstrate no difference in peak force or myofilament calcium sensitivity (19,20,22). Cardiac muscle tetanization demonstrates the same peak tetanic force with no shift on the calcium axis (19,43), and slowing the heart rate in patients with heart failure can improve systolic function.

Additional observations pointing to the presence of sufficient intracellular calcium are supported by observations that reducing intracellular calcium concentration via the sodium-calcium exchanger often has detrimental effects on contractile performance (50,51). Overexpression of the sodium-calcium exchanger in cardiac myocytes from failing human hearts has been shown to result in a paralysis of contractile function and depletion of intracellular calcium stores (unpublished observation). However, elevated sodium-calcium exchanger levels in a rabbit myocardial infarction model have been suggested to support contractility and offset the effects of lowered calcium influx (50). A recent study has correlated increases in the sodium–calcium exchanger with decreases in contraction and the appearance of delayed afterdepolarizations in a rabbit model of heart failure secondary to aortic insufficiency and aortic constriction (51).

Yet another important observation was made when an intracellular calcium buffer was overexpressed (52). It was

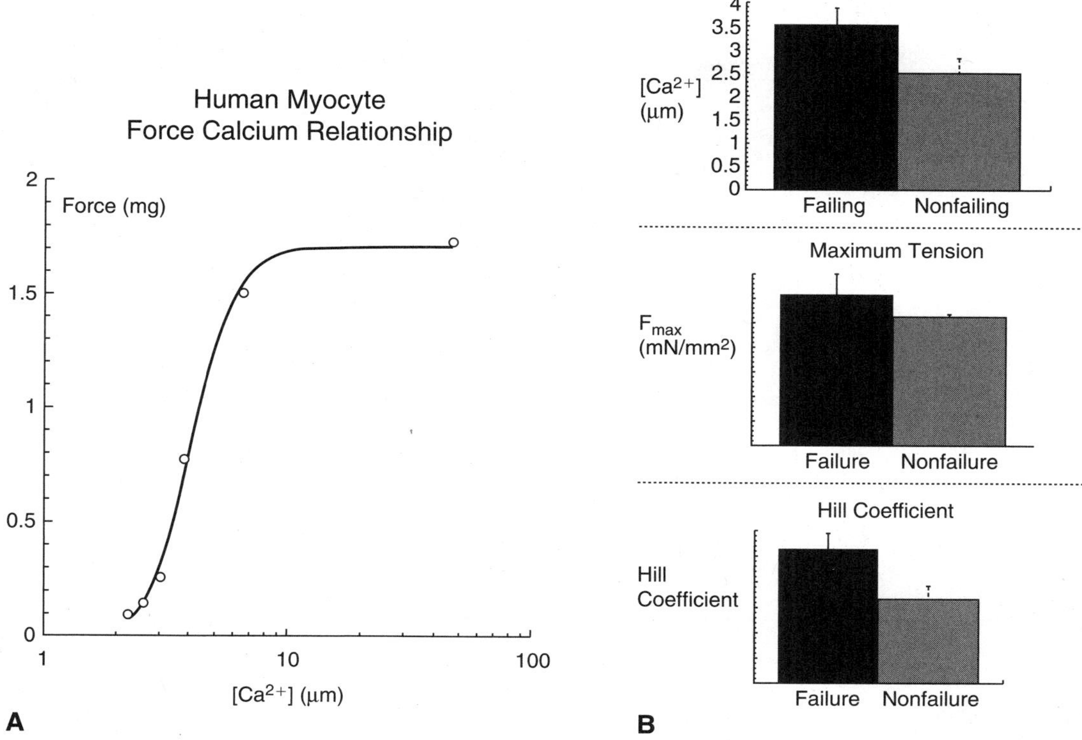

Figure 5-11 We isolated cardiac myocytes and skinned them using a detergent to generate force–calcium relations. **A** demonstrates a force-calcium relationship from a skinned single isolated cardiac myocyte from a nonfailing human heart. **B** demonstrates that even at the level of the isolated myocyte there are no differences in myofilament calcium responsiveness or sensitivity between myocytes isolated from failing and non-failing human hearts. Also, there is no difference in maximal calcium-activated force.

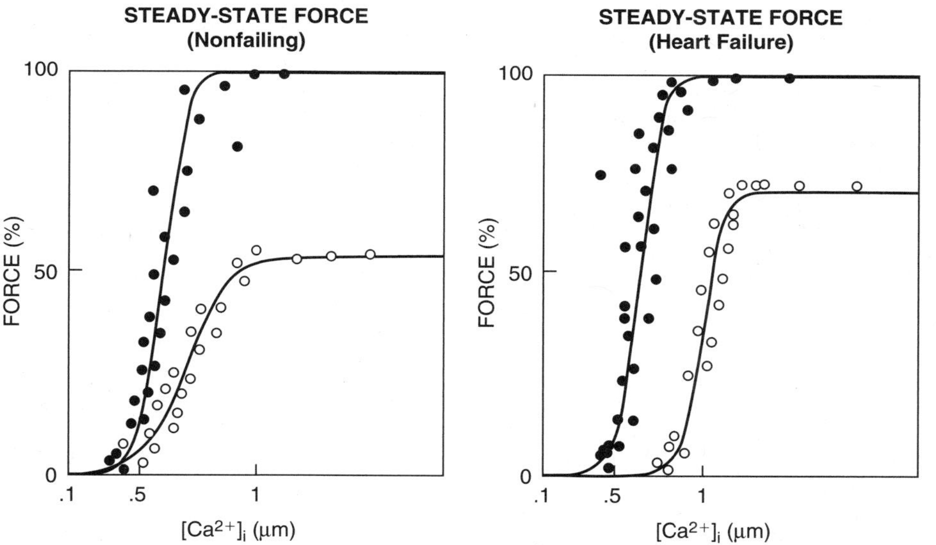

Figure 5-12 Intracellular calcium concentrations were measured using aequorin. Isolated muscles from nonfailing and failing human hearts were loaded with a bioluminescent indicator and then tetanized to obtain steady-state force–calcium relationships. 12-deoxyphorbol 13-isobutyrate 20-acetate (DPBA) was added. DPBA was shown to decrease myofilament calcium sensitivity. It was proposed that differential phosphorylation of troponin I and T (and/or isoforms), which later were confirmed would explain this observation. In muscle from failing human hearts there was a significant shift on the calcium axis to higher calcium concentrations with little change in the slope of the relationship. Maximal calcium-activated force, though reduced, was not as significantly depressed as in fibers from nonfailing human hearts. In the latter there was a greater impact on maximal calcium-activated force as opposed to a shift on the calcium axis. •, pre-DPBA; o, post-DPBA. (From Gwathmey JK, Hajjar RJ. Effect of protein kinase C activation on sarcoplasmic reticulum function and apparent myofibrillar Ca^{2+} sensitivity in intact and skinned muscles from normal and diseased human myocardium. *Circ Res.* 1990;67:744–752, with permission.)

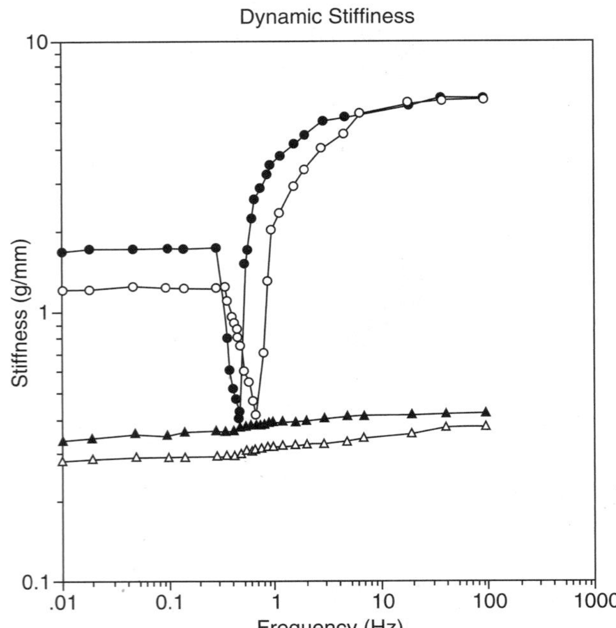

Figure 5-13 Dynamic stiffness curves in skinned fiber preparations from nonfailing (○) and failing human hearts (●) that are maximally activated. Thirty frequencies of oscillations were used. Also shown are stiffness measurements for the same nonfailing (△) and failing (▲) human heart muscles. Notice the fall in force at lower frequencies for muscles from failing human hearts, indicating a slower cross-bridge cycling rate. At higher frequencies of oscillation (when it is thought that all cross-bridges are attached) the maximal force is the same for muscles from nonfailing and failing human hearts. (From Hajjar RJ, Gwathmey JK. Cross-bridge dynamics in human ventricular myocardium: regulatory properties of contactility in the failing heart. *Circulation.* 1992;86:1819–1826, with permission.)

hypothesized that if an intracellular calcium buffer were increased, the rate of decline of the intracellular calcium transient would be abbreviated. This approach should also have an additional advantage in that the process would occur in a *non–ATP*-dependent fashion and should therefore improve contractile performance. SERCA2a, in contrast, requires ATP splitting for calcium removal and therefore might negatively impact myocardial energetics and diastolic function. Parvalbumin is a soluble, low–molecular-weight, intracellular binding protein that is highly expressed in skeletal muscle but not in the heart of mammalian species. This protein contains two sites that bind calcium, as well as magnesium, with even higher affinity than the calcium–magnesium sites of troponin-C. Parvalbumin's calcium-binding affinity is, however, lower than that of the SR calcium pump. Thus it has been suggested that parvalbumin might function as a so-called calcium shuttle, transporting calcium from troponin to the SR calcium pump during muscle relaxation. With its distinct features of calcium buffering, it was suggested that parvalbumin might therefore be effective for treating abnormalities in relaxation reported in heart failure. However, recent studies using overexpression of parvalbumin in an ischemia reperfusion model failed to show significant benefit in reducing the occurrence of arrhythmias (53) or improvement in cardiac performance. Similarly, we have observed that cardiac myocytes isolated from failing human hearts overexpressing paralbumin demonstrate a negative impact on function, as observed with overexpression of the sodium-calcium exchanger using adenoviral vectors (unpublished data).

In contrast to overexpression of the sodium-calcium exchanger, overexpression of SERCA2a resulted in a restoration of the time course of the calcium transient and peak amplitude associated with restoration in function at higher frequencies of stimulation (Fig. 5-5). Similarly, using antisense strategies to inhibit phospholamban results in a similar normalization of contractile function, as seen with overexpression of SERCA2a in cardiac myocytes isolated from failing human hearts (54). We therefore propose that enhancers of calcium mobilization (e.g., SERCA2a overexpression), as opposed to intracellular calcium buffers that lower diastolic calcium concentrations and likely impact SR calcium loading (e.g., sodium-calcium exchanger and parvalbumin), might be a better approach to restoring contractile function, regardless of the effects on hemodynamics and energy requirements.

It would appear that despite having sufficient intracellular calcium as well as an elevated diastolic calcium concentration, the myocyte must not only have a better way to mobilize the available calcium but must also be relatively selective in the *mechanism* by which it is mobilized.

Heart Failure: Role of SERCA2a and Phospholamban

In humans, ~75% of the calcium is removed by SERCA2a and ~25% by the sodium-calcium exchanger. The calcium pumping activity of SERCA2a is influenced by phospholamban. In the unphosphorylated state, phospholamban inhibits the calcium-ATPase, whereas phosphorylation of phospholamban by cAMP-dependent PKA and by calcium-calmodulin-dependent PKA reverses this inhibition. In the failing human heart, there is a decrease in the relative ratio of SERCA2a/phospholamban (25,34,54). Using transgenic and gene transfer approaches, increasing levels of phospholamban relative to SERCA2a in isolated cardiac myocytes are reported to significantly alter intracellular calcium mobilization and to prolong the relaxation phase of the calcium transient, decrease calcium release, and increase resting calcium concentration (56–65). These observations suggest that an abnormal ratio of phospholamban to SERCA2a contributes significantly to abnormalities in calcium mobilization and myocardial contractility in failing ventricular myocardium.

In neonatal rat myocytes in vitro, overexpression of SERCA2a has been demonstrated to rescue the phenotype created by increasing the phospholamban/SERCA2a ratio (57). More important, in human cardiac myocytes isolated from the left ventricles of patients with end-stage heart failure, gene transfer of SERCA2a resulted in an increase in both protein expression and pump activity and induced a faster contraction velocity and enhanced relaxation velocity (Fig. 5-5). Furthermore, diastolic calcium concentrations were decreased while systolic calcium was increased and the frequency response was normalized. However, these in vitro models may not reflect the behavior of intact hearts. In an animal model of POH in transition to failure (where SERCA2a protein levels and activity are decreased and severe contractile dysfunction is present), overexpression of SERCA2a by in vivo gene transfer restored both systolic and diastolic function to normal levels (66–68). In addition, overexpression of SERCA2a decreased left ventricular size and restored the slope of the end-systolic pressure–dimension relationship (a load-independent parameter of contractility) to control levels. In models of transgenic overexpression of SERCA2a and in overexpression experiments performed on isolated cardiac myocytes, contractility was increased (68–75), while decreases in SERCA2a expression accelerated pressure-overload–induced cardiac dysfunction and failure (46).

The SERCA2a/phospholamban ratio can also be normalized by decreasing phospholamban. This has been recently achieved by adenoviral gene transfer using antisense strategies with phospholamban (54,59). Overexpression of a dominant negative mutant of phospholamban or decreasing the steady-state level of phospholamban has been reported to enhance SERCA2 activity (54,59). This is consistent with the observation that genetic ablation of phospholamban rescues abnormalities in contractile function in a mouse model of dilated cardiomyopathy (49). However, it is not clear which strategy is preferable in terms of improving contractile function of the failing human heart: overexpression of SERCA2a or ablation of phospholamban activity.

More recently, two reports have revealed an association between phospholamban mutations and cardiomyopathy (76,77). The inheritance of the phospholamban mutation encoding Arg9Cys has been linked to the dominant inheritance of dilated cardiomyopathy in a large American family (77). The level of phospholamban phosphorylation is markedly reduced in persons with this muation. The effects of the mutation have been characterized by expression in a heterologous cell culture and by the creation of a transgenic mouse. The key effect of the mutation is reported to be an enhancement of the affinity of the Arg9Cys mutant phospholamban for cAMP-dependent PKA. In attempting to phosphorylate mutant phospholamban, PKA becomes trapped in a stabilized mutant phospholamban–PKA complex and can no longer dissociate to phosphorylate wild-type phospholamban molecules. The effect appears to be local and restricted to the SR, perhaps because a specific fraction of cAMP-dependent PKA is associated with the SR through A-kinase anchoring proteins. Affected individuals have a chronically inhibited SERCA2a and can never draw on their full cardiac reserve.

A second human phospholamban mutation, Leu39stop, has been discovered in two large Greek families (76). The heterozygous inheritance of the Leu39stop mutation in one family resulted in left ventricular hypertrophy in one-third of the older affected family members, without diminished contractile performance. However, the inheritance of two copies of the mutant phospholamban gene led to dilated cardiomyopathy and heart failure in two teenage siblings. In heterologous expression studies, the Leu39stop mutant protein was unstable or misrouted to other membranes and no protein was detected in the endoplasmic reticulum or in a cardiac explant from one of the affected individuals. As a result, there was no effect of the mutant protein in either the homozygous or heterozygous state on the calcium affinity of SERCA2a. We would suggest that the two homozygous mutant individuals can be considered to be equivalent to a phospholamban-null genotype with a phenotype of dilated cardiomyopathy. Therefore, in contrast to the benefits of phospholamban ablation in mice, humans who lack phospholamban develop lethal cardiomyopathy.

A caveat in these studies is that the number of affected individuals is very low and the lod score for linkage of the mutation to the disease is low. Our own results, however, have shown that ablation of phospholamban by gene transfer to cardiac myocytes isolated from failing human hearts results in increased contractility, improved calcium mobilization, and restoration of the frequency response (54). The reason for the discrepancy between the cardiac phenotypes in mice and humans has yet to be uncovered. This might reflect differences in isoform types (78).

Myocardial Energetics and Heart Failure

Another hypothesis that might explain heart failure and the relationship to intracellular calcium is that there is inadequate energy supply (77). Energetics have also been implicated in several animal models of heart failure (80–88). All cellular processes—maintaining membrane stability, ion homeostasis, macromolecular synthesis, as well as external work—depend on availability of ATP. Estimates of energy supply have been made from activities (maximum velocity, V_{max}) of key enzymes involved in ATP-producing pathways, namely the creatine kinase (CK) reaction, oxidative phosphorylation (which is estimated from oxygen consumption) and glycolysis, and from high-energy phosphate content and turnover rates. Estimates of energy demand use measures of cardiac performance, heat, and actomysin ATPase activity.

Whether there are changes in enzyme activity or in high-energy phosphate content in failing human myocardium has been controversial. Part of the problem has resided in the use of biopsy samples and the difficulty of obtaining appropriate controls. Using ^{31}P nuclear magnetic resonance (NMR) spectroscopy to measure relative ATP and PCr as well as biochemical approaches energy depletion has now been clearly demonstrated (89–91). The PCr/ATP ratio has been reported to be diminished in failing human myocardium. The characteristic of reduced PCr/ATP ratios has been reproduced in animal models of failure, as well (79–81,83,90,91).

Direct measurement of total creatine in failing human myocardium shows that the guanidino pool is lower (89). The majority of evidence now shows that the primary energy reserve molecule, PCr, is diminished in failing human myocardium. In addition, the tissue content of the enzyme that catalyzes phosphoryl transfer between ATP and PCr (namely, CK) has been demonstrated to be lower than in nonfailing myocardium. This has been observed by several groups. Because decreased CK activity (V_{max}) and substrate combine to reduce the velocity of the CK reaction, phosphoryl turnover rates *must* be lower in failing human myocardium. Direct measurements of the CK reaction velocity using ^{31}P magnetization transfer in animal models of heart failure have shown that the turnover of the primary high-energy phosphate compounds is indeed significantly slower in failing myocardium (83,90,91) (Tables 5-1 and 5-2).

On the utilization side, myofibrillar ATPase and myofibrillar protein content are lower in failing human

TABLE 5-1
CHANGES IN MYOCARDIAL ENERGETICS IN AN AVIAN MODEL

	Control (n = 5)	Fz-DCM (n = 5)	P*
$[Ca^{2+}]$ = 2.5 mmol/L (no pacing)			
RPP × 10^{-3}, mm Hg/min	23.4 ± 1.2	6.3 ± 0.7	<0.0001
MVO_2, μmol O_2 × min^{-1} × g^{-1}	21.1 ± 0.3	20.8 ± 0.3	0.34
ATP synthesis, (mmol/L)/s	0.92 ± 0.01	1.30 ± 0.02	<0.0001
$[Ca^{2+}]$ = 5.5 mmol/L (no pacing)			
RPP × 10^{-3}, mm Hg/min	32.3 ± 1.5	6.8 ± 0.5	<0.0001
MVO_2, μmol O_2 × min^{-1} × g^{-1}	34.6 ± 0.3	27.3 ± 0.7	<0.0001
p†	<0.0001	<0.0001	
ATP synthesis, (mmol/L)/s	1.51 ± 0.01	1.71 ± 0.05	0.003
$[Ca^{2+}]$ = 2.5 mmol/L (no pacing)			
RPP × 10^{3}, mm Hg/min	23.6 ± 0.7	6.1 ± 0.5	<0.0001
p†	0.91	0.83	
MVO_2. μmol O_2 × min^{-1} × g^{-1}	21.5 ± 0.4	22.3 ± 0.4	0.21
p†	0.45	0.017	
ATP synthesis, (nmol/L)/s	0.94 ± 0.02	1.39 ± 0.03	<0.0001
$[Ca^{2+}]$ = 2.5 mmol/L (paced at 300 bpm)			
RPP × 10^{-3}, mm Hg/min	20.7 ± 1.0	4.3 ± 0.6	<0.0001
p†	0.12	0.06	
MVO_2, μmol O_2 × min^{-1} × g^{-1}	18.3 ± 0.5	28.3 ± 0.7	<0.0001
p†	0.0011	<0.0001	
ATP synthesis, (mmol/L)/s	0.80 ± 0.02	1.79 ± 0.04	<0.0001

Values are mean ± SEM.
*Compared with control.
†Compared with baseline ($[Ca^{2+}]$ = 2.5 mmol/L and no pacing).
This table demonstrates changes in myocardial energetics in an avian model that has been demonstrated to be predictive of the human condition and clinical outcomes. Furazolidone induces dilated cardiomyopathy in turkey poults. Fz-DCM, furazolidine-fed turkey poults with dilated cardiomyopathy.
(From Liao R, Nascimben L, Friedrich DP, et al. Decreased energy reserve in an animal model of dilated cardiomyopathy. Relationship to contractile performance. *Circ Res.* 1996;78:893–902, with permission.)

TABLE 5-2
THE CK SYSTEM: ENZYME ACTIVITIES, SUBSTRATE CONCENTRATIONS, AND FLUX THROUGH THE CK REACTION IN CONTROL AND Fz-DCM HEARTS

	Control (n = 7)	Fz-DCM (n = 4)	P*
CK activity, (mmol/L)/s	58±4	38±2	0.006
[ATP], mmol/L	8.5±0.4	6.5±0.4	0.01
[PCr], mmol/L	10.5±0.4	6.1±0.3	0.0001
Free [Cr], mmol/L	7.4±1.1	7.3±1.0	0.97
Total [Cr], mmol/L	17.9±1.2	13.5±1.0	0.036
[ADP], mmol/L	0.047±0.008	0.062±0.011	0.27
k_{for}, s^{-1}	0.75±0.04	0.37±0.05	0.0003
V_{for}, (mmol/L)/s	7.8±0.4	2.3±0.4	0.0001

Values are mean ± SEM.
*Compared with control.
This table demonstrates the loss of contractile reserve in the presence of increased concentrations of extracellular calcium and increased heart rates in hearts from animals with heart failure. Furazolidine induces dilated cardiomyopathy in turkey poults. Fz-DCM, furazolidone-fed turkey poults with dilated cardiomyopathy.
(From Liao R, Nascimben L, Friedrich DP, et al. Decreased energy reserve in an animal model of dilated cardiomyopathy. Relationship to contractile performance. *Circ Res.* 1996;78:893–902, with permission.)

myocardium (44,92). As previously mentioned, cross-bridge cycling dynamics have been demonstrated to be slower in failing human myocardium compared with non-failing myocardium (17) (Fig. 5-13). It is tempting to speculate that this is an adaptive response. Nevertheless, the causal relationships between energy use and supply remains to be established.

Cardiac muscle contains a large amount of PCr and CK. The creatine kinase system acts as an energy reserve system, especially during high workloads. A decrease in CK (phamacologically or genetically) decreases the ability of cardiac muscle to increase work and myocardial contractility (Table 5-1).

In addition, impaired calcium mobilization may be due to a limited thermodynamic driving force for SERCA2a. Increasing extracellular calcium in Langendorff perfused hearts increases contractile performance in normal hearts, but not in CK-inhibited hearts (82). This suggests that failure to increase SR calcium stores during inotropic stimulation in hearts with low thermodynamic driving force blocks the heart from recruiting its contractile reserve. In animal models of heart failure we and others have shown that the PCr/ATP ratio is decreased. In fact, O'Donnell et al. (74) have shown that increasing inotropy with dobutamine even further decreases this ratio. It is therefore important to evaluate whether manipulation of SERCA2a or other calcium mobilization proteins will affect cardiac metabolism.

As demonstrated in Tables 5-1 and 5-2, hearts with depressed energy reserve have a reduced ability to increase their rate pressure product in response to an increase in extracellular calcium (e.g., being given an inotrope). Furthermore, the ΔG approaches the free energy for ATP hydrolysis required for the SR calcium ATPase pump. These data demonstrate that calcium homeostasis in failing hearts can be affected by decreased energy reserve and, more important, reduction in energy supply can negatively impact intracellular calcium concentration and mobilization (79). Prolonged inhibition of energy reserve caused by either decreasing CK activity or decreasing the tissue content of its substrate (creatine) can therefore potentially result in or exacerbate heart failure because there is a mechanistic relationship between myocardial energetics and calcium mobilization. This unexpected relationship has been demonstrated in our avian model of heart failure.

To maintain intracellular calcium concentrations within a fixed range (100 nmol/L to 10 μmol/L), energy is required to fuel calcium pumps. The by products of ATP hydrolysis (e.g., ADP, inorganic phosphate, Mg) inhibit calcium pump activity as well as impact the relationship between calcium, myofilament activation, and myocardial contractility (93). If energy is reduced and/or intracellular calcium levels are elevated, by products of ATP hydrolysis (and thereby energy use in the heart) can actually accumulate, at least transiently (Fig. 5-4). In this way, a vicious cycle coupling ATP hydrolysis and calcium movements may ensue. This scenario has practical clinical consequences for patients with heart failure. Failing hearts, as mentioned previously, have a slowed restoration of diastolic calcium levels and are energy-compromised. When these hearts attempt to increase work, further ATP hydrolysis is required, resulting in a mismatch between energy supply and demand, leading to cardiac decompensation. When stressed by increased work and/or further decreases in energy supply, even patients with compensated heart disease often demonstrate decompensation and contractile failure, likely in part as a result of the mismatch between energy supply and demand.

Although there is no controversy regarding the function of the CK system as an energy reserve system, whether or not there are physiological consequences to changes in the reaction velocity in failing hearts CK remains controversial. The CK system functions as an energy reserve system, especially during high-workload conditions. A link between energy reserve and contractile reserve can be clearly shown for the ATP supply–demand mismatch that occurs in hypoxia and ischemia when phosphoryl transfer from PCr to ADP slows the rate of tissue ATP depletion. The link also has been shown in experiments designed to selectively perturb the CK reaction in intact striated muscle.

First, in rats in which the myocardial PCr pool was replaced with a poorly hydrolyzable creatine analog, β-guanidinopropionic acid, PCr content, CK reaction velocity, and heart function all decreased under high-workload conditions (94). Second, acute selective chemical inhibition of CK activity in intact rodent hearts with iodoacetamide resulted in decreased contractile reserve when the heart was inotropically stressed with either high extracellular calcium concentrations or norepinephrine (95). Third, depleting the muscle isoform of CK using bioengineering technology reduces the ability of skeletal muscle to sustain burst activity (96). Each of these experiments demonstrated that decreased energy reserve from CK limits the ability of striated muscle to increase contractile performance. Our experiments in the failing avian heart were an attempt to address the consequence of chronic inhibition. Our experimental findings indicate that creatine-deficient hearts have decreased contractile performance.

An important consequence of decreased energy reserve that may impact intracellular calcium concentration and myocardial contractility is the occurrence of a lower calcium gradient across the SR and/or sarcolemma. Figure 5-14 plots the rate–pressure product (RPP) for two hearts perfused with normal (~1.75 mM) and then with elevated (3 mM) $[Ca^{2+}]_o$-containing buffer versus the absolute value of free energy available from ATP hydrolysis, ΔG. One heart had 100% CK activity, whereas in the other, CK activity was chemically inhibited to ~1% of control. Because the velocity of the CK reaction in these two hearts differed by a factor of 100, energy reserve also differed. Free energy available from ATP hydrolysis is proportional to the phosphorylation potential, ATP (ADP P_i), and is a measure of the driving force for ATP-using reactions. Because CK functions to maintain high ATP and low ADP and inorganic phosphate, the phosphorylation potential and, hence, the free energy available from ATP hydrolysis, are lower in CK-inhibited hearts. Also shown in Fig. 5-14 are the minimum values for the free energy needed to drive the SR Ca^{2+} ATPase, the Na^+/K^+ ATPase, and the myosin ATPase reactions. The plot shows that the heart, with depressed energy reserve, has a reduced ability to increase its RPP in response to increases in extracellular calcium concentrations (also seen in our avian model, Tables 5-1 and 5-2). It also shows that the value of ΔG for these hearts approaches the free energy of ATP hydrolysis

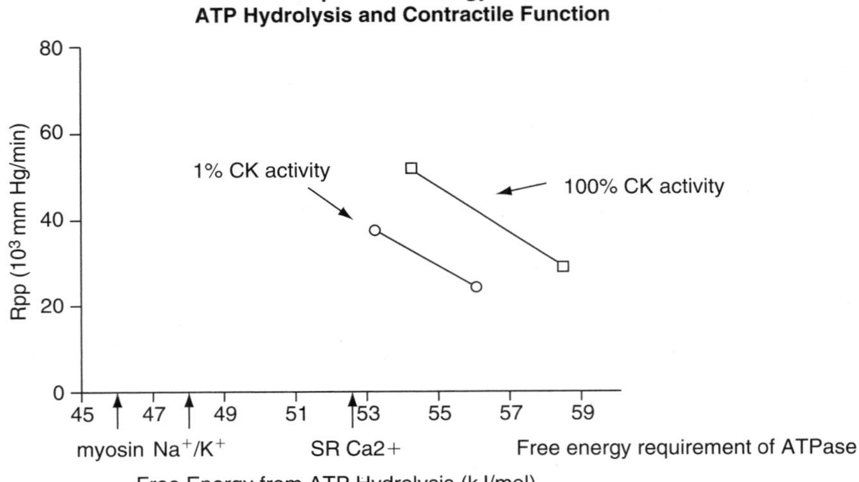

Figure 5-14 The relationship of free energy available from ATP hydrolysis and contractile function. Pressure product versus absolute value of free energy available from ATP hydrolysis for a rat heart with 100% CK activity was chemically inhibited to ~1% of conrol. Changes in RPP were made by increasing $(Ca^{2+})°$ perfusion buffer from 1.75 to 3.0 mM. Free energy from ATP hydrolysis is calculated from the equation: $\Delta G = \Delta G)° + RT$ in (ATP) (ADP) (P_1). ATP and P_1 were measured using ^{31}P nuclear magnetic resonance spectroscopy, and ADP was calculated using the creatine kinase equilibrium expression. Also shown are values for the free energy requirement for the SR Ca^{2+} ATPase and $Na+/K^+$ ATpase and myosin ATPase. The relationship of free energy available from ATP hydrolysis and contractile function. This figure demonstrates the point at which contractile function is significantly impaired and the free energy is reduced to an activity level that impacts contractile function that occurs at the ΔG free energy requirement for the SR Ca^{2+} ATPase activity (SERCA2a). (From Gwathmey JK, Ingwall JS. Basic pathophysiology of congestive heart failure. *Cardiol in Rev.* 1995;3(5):282–291, with permission.)

required for the SR Ca^{2+} ATPase pump. This calculation suggests that calcium homeostasis and the function of the SR Ca^{2+} ATPase pump in failing hearts can be affected by decreased energy reserve.

CONCLUSIONS

The role of calcium in myocardial contraction is not straightforward (97–100). Broad generalizations with regard to calcium concentrations measured intracellularly cannot be simply applied. It is not solely the amount of available calcium, but also the ability to mobilize the calcium that appear to be important. To effectively utilize the calcium that is available for contractile activation, multiple aspects of calcium homeostasis must be balanced. It remains to be determined whether the best approach would be through enhanced mobilization of intracellular calcium by ablating phospholamban using antisense or small-molecule strategies, or enhancing SR Ca^{2+} ATPase activity by overexpression of SERCA2a or small-molecule approaches. Another approach might be to simply alter myofilament calcium sensitivity in the systolic range while not negatively impacting force in the diastolic range in a nonenergy-requiring manner (e.g., calcium sensitizers) (101–103). It is, nevertheless, clear that significant reductions in intracellular calcium concentrations appear to be detrimental to myocardial contractility. The question then becomes what is enough and what is not enough. Too much calcium is known to be directly toxic to the heart; it can induce apoptosis and activate other signaling pathways (e.g., hypertrophy). Too little calcium is known to result in a significant reduction in myocardial contractility. Physicians and scientists are encouraged to not simply regard the calcium concentration in the heart in isolation but, rather, embrace its relationship to other subcellular events and signaling pathways within as well as external to the heart itself.

ACKNOWLEDGMENTS

This work is supported in part by grants to JKG from the National Institutes of Health, Heart, Lung, and Blood Institute (HL 67516) and the National Institute of Alcohol, Alcoholism and Alcohol Abuse (AA066758). Sandy Occil is thanked for preparing and editing this chapter.

REFERENCES

1. Dorn GW, 2nd, Mochly-Rosen D. Intracellular transport mechanisms of signal transducers. *Ann Rev Phys.* 2002;64:407–429.

2. Vahl CF, Bonz A, Limek T, et al. Intracellular calcium transient of working human myocardium of seven patients transplanted with congestive heart failure. *Circ Res*. 1994;74:952–958.
3. Koss KL, Kranias EG. Phospholamban: a prominent regulator of myocardial contractility. *Circ Res*. 1996;79:1059–1063.
4. Wier WG, Lopez-Lopez JR, Shacklock PS, et al. Calcium signaling in cardiac muscle cells. *Ciba Found Symp*. 1995;188:146–160.
5. Bers DM. Calcium fluxes involved in control of cardiac myocyte contraction. *Circ Res*. 2000;87:275–281.
6. Harigaya S, Schwartz A. Rate of calcium binding and uptake in normal animal and failing human cardiac muscle-membrane vesicles (relaxing system) and mitochondria. *Circ Res*. 1969;25: 781–794.
7. Lee KH, Hajjar RJ, Matsui T, et al. A. Cardiac signal transduction. *J Nucl Cardiol*. 2000;7:63–71.
8. Bers DM. Cardiac excitation-contraction coupling. *Nature*. 2002;415(6868):198–205.
9. Marks AR. Cardiac intracellular calcium release channels: role in heart failure. *Circ Res*. 2000;87:8–11.
10. Gruver EJ, Glass MG, Gwathmey JK, et al. An animal model of dilated cardiomyopathy: characterization of dihydropyridine receptors and contractile performance. *Am J Physiol*. 1993;265(34, *Heart Circ Physiol*.):H1704–H1711.
11. Gruver EJ, Morgan JP, Stambler BS, et al. Uniformity of calcium channel number and isometric contraction in human right and left ventricular myocardium. *Basic Res Cardiol*. 1994;89:139–148.
12. O'Brien PJ, Gwathmey, JK. Myocardial Ca^{2+}- and ATP-cycling imbalances in end-stage idiopathic dilated and ischemic cardiomyopathies. *Cardiovasc Res*. 1995;30:394–404.
13. Marks AR, Reiken S, Marx SO. Progression of heart failure: is protein kinase A hyperphosphorylation of the ryanodine receptor a contributing factor? *Circulation* 2002;105:272–275.
14. Bers DM, Eisner DA, Valdivia HH. Sarcoplasmic reticulum Ca^{2+} and heart failure: roles of diastolic leak and Ca^{2+} transport. *Circ Res*. 2003;93:487–490.
15. Li Y, Kranias EG, Mignery GA, et al. Protein kinase A phosphorylation of the ryanodine receptor does not affect calcium sparks in mouse ventricular myocytes. *Circ Res*. 2002;90:309–316.
16. Gwathmey JK, Hajjar RJ, Solaro RJ. Contractile deactivation and uncoupling of cross-bridges: effects of 2,3-butanedione monoxime on mammalian myocardium. *Circ Res*. 1991;69:1280–1292.
17. Hajjar RJ, Gwathmey JK. Cross-bridge dynamics in human ventricular myocardium: regulatory properties of contractility in the failing heart. *Circulation*. 1992;86:1819–1826.
18. Nakao K, Minobe W, Bristow MR, et al. Related articles, links myosin heavy chain gene expression in human heart failures. *J Clin Invest*. 1997;100(9):2362–2370.
19. Gwathmey JK, Hajjar RJ. Relation between steady state force and intracellular calcium concentration is intact human myocardium. Index of myofibrillar responsiveness to calcium. *Circulation*. 1990;82:1266–1278.
20. Hajjar RJ, Gwathmey JK, Briggs GM, et al. Differential effects of DPI 201-106 on the sensitivity of the myofilaments to Ca^{2+} in intact and skinned trabeculae from control and myopathic human hearts. *J Clin Invest*. 1988;82(5):1578–1584.
21. Hajjar RJ, Schwinger RHG, Schmidt U, et al. Myofilament calcium regulation in human myocardium. *Circulation*. 2000;101: 1679–1685.
22. Gwathmey, JK, Hajjar RJ. Calcium-activated force in a turkey model of spontaneous dilated cardiomyopathy: adaptive changes in thin myofilament Ca^{2+} regulation with resultant implications on contractile performance. *J Mol Cell Cardiol*. 1992;24:1459–1470.
23. Okafor CC, Li X, Saunders L, et al. Myofibrillar responsiveness to cAMP, PKA and caffeine in an animal model of heart failure. *Biochem Biophys Res Comm*. 2003;300:592–599.
24. Feldman MD, Copelas L, Gwathmey JK, et al. Deficient production of cyclic AMP: pharmacologic evidence of an important cause of contractile dysfunction in patients with end-stage heart failure. *Circulation*. 1987;75:331–339.
25. Schmidt U, Hajjar RJ, Kim CS, et al. Human heart failure: cAMP stimulation of SR Ca^{2+}- ATPase activity and phosphorylation level of phospholamban. *Am J Physiol*. 1999;277:H474–H480.
26. Dorn GW, 2nd, Tepe NM, Wu G, et al. Mechanisms of impaired beta-adrenergic receptor signaling in G(alphaq)-mediated cardiac hypertrophy and ventricular dysfunction. *Mol Pharmacol*. 2000;57:278–287.
27. Carr AN, Schmidt AG, Suzuki Y, et al. Type 1 phosphatase, a negative regulator of cardiac function. *Mol Cell Biol*. 2002;22:4124–4135.
28. del Monte F, Harding S, Schmidt U, et al. Restoration of contractile function in isolated cardiomyocytes from failing human hearts by gene transfer of SERCA2a. *Circulation*. 1999; 100(23):2308–2313.
29. Gwathmey JK, Slawsky MT, Hajjar RJ, et al. Role of intracellular calcium handling in force-interval relationships of human ventricular myocardium. *J Clin Invest*. 1990;85(5):1599–1611.
30. Feldman MD, Gwathmey JK, Phillips PJ, et al. Reversal of the force-frequency relationship in working myocardium from patients with end-stage heart failure. *J Applied Cardiol*. 1988;3:273–283.
31. Schmidt U, Hajjar RJ, Gwathmey JK. The force-interval relationship in human myocardium. *J Card Fail*. 1995;1(4):311–321.
32. Schmidt U, Hajjar RJ, Helm PA, et al. Contribution of abnormal sarcoplasmic reticulum ATPase activity to systolic and diastolic dysfunction in human heart failure. *J Mol Cell Card*. 1998;30: 1929–1937.
33. Hajjar RJ, DiSalvo TG, Schmidt U, et al. Clinical correlates of the myocardial force-frequency relationship in patients with end-stage heart failure. *J Heart Lung Transp*. 1997;16:1157–1167.
34. Meyer M, Bluhm WF, He H, et al. Phospholamban-to-SERCA2 ratio controls the force-frequency relationship. *Am J Physiol*. 1999;276:H779–H785.
35. Lederer WJ, Berlin JR, Cohen NM, et al. Excitation-contraction coupling in heart cells. *Ann NY Acad Sci*. 1990;588:190–206.
36. Gwathmey JK, Copelas L, MacKinnon R, et al. Abnormal intracellular calcium handling in myocardium from patients with end-stage heart failure. *Circ Res*. 1987;61:70–76.
37. Gwathmey JK, Hajjar RJ. Intracellular calcium related to force development in twitch contraction of mammalian myocardium. *Cell Calcium*. 1990;121:531–538.
38. Gwathmey JK, Morgan JP. Altered calcium handling in experimental pressure-overload hypertrophy in the ferret. *Circ Res*. 1985;57:836–843.
39. Gwathmey JK, Morgan JK. Sarcoplasmic reticulum calcium mobilization in right ventricular pressure-overload hypertrophy in the ferret: relationships to diastolic dysfunction and a negative treppe. *Pflugers Arch*. 1993;322:599–608.
40. Gwathmey JK, Liao R, Ingwall J. Comparison of twitch force and Ca^{2+} handling in papillary muscles from right ventricular pressure-overload hypertrophy in weanling and juvenile ferrets. *Cardiovasc Res*. 1995;29:475–481.
41. MacKinnon R, Gwathmey JK, Allen PD, et al. Modulation by the thyroid state of intracellular calcium and contractility in ferret ventricular muscle. *Circ Res*. 1988;63:1080–1089.
42. Blinks JR, Endoh M. Modification of myofibrillar responsiveness to Ca^{2+} as an inotrpic mechanism. *Circulation*. 1986;73(85):98.
43. Gwathmey JK, Hajjar RJ. Effect of protein kinase C activation on sarcoplasmic reticulum function and apparent myofibrillar Ca^{2+} sensitivity in intact and skinned muscles from normal and diseased human myocardium. *Circ Res*. 1990;67:744–752.
44. Okafor CC, Liao R, Perrault-Micale C, et al. Mg-ATPase and Ca^{2+}-activated myosin ATPase activity in ventricular myofibrils from non-failing and diseased human hearts: effects of calcium sensitizing agents MCI-154, DPI 201-106, and caffeine. *Mol Cellular Biochem*. 2003;245(1–2):77–89.
45. Wu G, Toyokawa T, Hahn H, et al. Epsilon protein kinase C in pathological myocardial hypertrophy. Analysis by combined transgenic expression of translocation modifiers and Galphaq. *J Biol Chem*. 2000;275:29927–29930.
46. Chen L, Hahn H, Wu G, et al. Opposing cardioprotective actions and parallel hypertrophic effects of delta PKC and epsilon PKC. *Proc Natl Acad Sci USA*. 2001;98:11114–11119.
47. Braz JC, Gregory K, Pathak A, et al. PKC-alpha regulates cardiac contractility and propensity toward heart failure. *Nature Med*. 2004;10:248–254.
48. Washington B, Butler K, Doye AA, et al. Heart function challenged with β-receptor agonism and antagonism in a heart failure model. *Cardiovasc Drugs Ther*. 2001;15:479–486.
49. Gwathmey JK, Kim CS, Hajjar RJ, et al. Cellular and molecular remodeling in a heart failure model treated with the β-blocker

carteolol. *Am J Physiol.* 1999; 276 (45, *Heart Circ Physiol.*): H1678–H1690.

50. Ranu K, Terracciano CMN, Davia K, et al. Effects of sodium/calcium-exchanger overexpression on excitation-contraction coupling in adult rabbit ventricular myocytes. 2000. In review.
51. Pogwizd SM, Qi M, Yuan W, et al. Upregulation of Na(+)/Ca($^{2+}$) exchanger expression and function in an arrhythmogenic rabbit model of heart failure [see comments]. *Circ Res.* 1999;85: 1009–1019.
52. Wahr PA, Michele DE, Metzger JM. Parvalbumin gene transfer corrects diastolic dysfunction in diseased cardiac myocytes. *Proc Natl Acad Sci USA.* 1999;96:11982–11985.
53. del Monte F, Lebeche D, Guerrero JL, et al. Abrogation of ventricular arrhythmias in a model of ischemia and reperfusion by targeting myocardial calcium cycling. *Proc Natl AcadSci USA.* 2004;101(15):5622–5627.
54. del Monte F, Harding SE, Dec GW, et al. Targeting phospholamban in human heart failure by gene transfer. *Circulation.* 2002; 105:904–907.
55. del Monte F, Dalal R, Tabchy A, et al. Transcriptional changes following restoration of SERCA2a levels in failing rat hearts. *Faseb J.* 2004;10.
56. Davia K, Hajjar RJ, Terracciano CMN, et al. Functional alterations in adult rat myocytes following overexpression of phospholamban using adenovirus. *Physiol Genomics.* 1999;1:41–50.
57. Hajjar RJ, Schmidt U, Kang JX, et al. Adenoviral gene transfer of phospholamban in isolated rat cardiomyocytes rescue effects by concomitant gene transfer of sarcoplasmic reticulum Ca^{2+} ATPase. *Circ. Res.* 1997;81:145–153.
58. Schultz Jel J, Glascock BJ, Witt SA, et al. Accelerated onset of heart failure in mice during pressure overload with chronically decreased SERCA2 calcium pump activity. *Am J Physiol Heart Circ Physiol.* 2004;286:H1146–H1153.
59. He H, Meyer M, Martin JL, et al. Effects of mutant and antisense RNA of phospholamban on SR Ca($^{2+}$)-ATPase activity and cardiac myocyte contractility. *Circulation.* 1999;100:974–980.
60. Minamisawa S, Hoshijima M, Chu G, et al. Chronic phospholamban-sarcoplasmic reticulum calcium ATPase interaction is the critical cycling defect in dilated cardiomyopathy. *Cell.* 1999;99:313–322.
61. Hajjar RJ, del Monte F, Matsui T, et al. Prospects for gene therapy for heart failure. *Circ Res.* 2000;86:616–621.
62. Luo W, Grupp IL, Harrer J, et al. Targeted ablation of the phospholamban gene is associated with markedly enhanced myocardial contractility and loss of beta-agonist stimulation. *Circ Res.* 1994;75:401–409.
63. Kadambi VJ, Ponniah S, Harrer JM, et al. Cardiac-specific overexpression of phospholamban alters calcium kinetics and resultant cardiomyocyte mechanics in transgenic mice. *J Clin Invest.* 1996;97:533–539.
64. Luo W, Wolska BM, Grupp IL, et al. Phospholamban gene dosage effects in the mammalian heart. *Circ Res.* 1996;78:839–847.
65. Eizema K, Fechner H, Bezstarosti K, et al. Adenovirus-based phospholamban antisense expression as a novel approach to improve cardiac contractile dysfunction: comparison of a constitutive viral versus an endothelin-1-responsive cardiac promoter. *Circulation.* 2000;101:2193–2199.
66. Miyamoto MI, del Monte F, Schmidt U, et al. Adenoviral gene transfer of SERCA2a improves left-ventricular function in aortic-banded rats in transition to heart failure. *Proc Natl Acad Sci USA.* 2000;97:793–798.
67. Bukhari, F, del Monte F, Hajjar RJ. Genetic maneuvers to ameliorate ventricular function in heart failure: therapeutic potential and future potentials. *Exp Rev Cardiovasc Ther.* 2005;3:85–97.
68. del Monte F, Lebeche D, Schmidt U, et al. Improvement in survival and cardiac metabolism following gene transfer of SERCA2a in a rat model of heart failure. *Circulation.* 2001.
69. Davia K, Bernobich E, Hardeep KR, et al. Protective effects of SERCA2a gene transfer into adult rabbit ventricular myocytes. 2000. In review.
70. Davia K, Davies CH, Harding SE. Effects of inhibition of sarcoplasmic reticulum calcium uptake on contraction in myocytes isolated from failing human ventricle. *Cardiovasc Res.* 1997;33:88–97.
71. Schmidt U, del Monte F, Miyamoto MI, et al. Restoration of diastolic function in senescent rat hearts by adenoviral gene transfer of sarcoplasmic reticulum Ca^{2+} ATPase. *Circulation.* 2000;101: 790–796.
72. He H, Giordano FJ, Hilal-Dandan R, et al. Overexpression of the rat sarcoplasmic reticulum Ca^{2+} ATPase gene in the heart of transgenic mice accelerates calcium transients and cardiac relaxation. *J Clin Invest.* 1997;100:380–389.
73. Baker DL, Hashimoto K, Grupp IL, et al. Targeted overexpression of the sarcoplasmic reticulum Ca^{2+}-ATPase increases cardiac contractility in transgenic mouse hearts. *Circ Res.* 1998;83: 1205–1214.
74. O'Donnell JM, Sumbilla CM, Ma H, et al. Tight control of exogenous SERCA expression is required to obtain acceleration of calcium transients with minimal cytotoxic effects in cardiac myocytes. *Circ Res.* 2001;88:415–421.
75. Hajjar RJ, Kang JX, Gwathmey JK, et al. Physiological effects of adenoviral gene transfer of sarcoplasmic reticulum calcium ATPase in isolated rat myocytes. *Circulation* 1997;95:423–429.
76. Schmitt JP, Kamisago M, Asahi M, et al. Dilated cardiomyopathy and heart failure caused by a mutation in phospholamban. *Science.* 2003;299(5611):1410–1413.
77. Haghighi K, Kolokathis F, Pater L, et al. Human phospholamban null results in lethal dilated cardiomyopathy revealing a critical difference between mouse and human. *J Clin Invest.* 2003;111(6): 869–876.
78. Cavagna M, O'Donnell JM, Sumbilla C, et al. Exogenous Ca^{2+}-ATPase isoform effects on Ca^{2+} transients of embryonic chicken and neonatal rat cardiac myocytes. *J Physiol.* 2000;528 (Pt 1): 53–63.
79. Gwathmey JK, Ingwall JS. Basic pathophysiology of congestive heart failure. *Cardiol Rev.* 1995;3(5):282–291.
80. Gwathmey JK, Davidoff AJ. Experimental aspects of cardiomyopathy. *Curr Opin Cardiol.* 1993;8:480–495.
81. Davidoff AJ, Gwathmey JK. Pathophysiology of cardiomyopathies: Part I. Animal models and humans. *Curr Opin Cardiol.* 1994;9:357–368.
82. Gwathmey JK, Davidoff AJ. Pathophysiology of cardiomyopathies: Part II. Drug-induced and other interventions. *Curr Opin Cardiol.* 1994;9:369–378.
83. Liao R, Nascimben L, Friedrich DP, et al. Decreased energy reserve in an animal model of dilated cardiomyopathy. Relationship to contractile performance. *Circ Res.* 1996; 78:893–902.
84. Tian R, Ingwall JS. Energetic basis for reduced contractile reserve in isolated rat hearts. *Am J Physiol.* 1996;270:H1207–H1216.
85. Tian R, Halow JM, Meyer M, et al. Thermodynamic limitation for Ca^{2+} handling contributes to decreased contractile reserve in rat hearts. *Am J Physiol.* 1998;275:H2064–H2071.
86. Tian R, Nascimben L, Kaddurah-Daouk R, et al. Dephospholambanetion of energy reserve via the creatine kinase reaction during the evolution of heart failure in cardiomyopathic hamsters. *J Mol Cell Cardiol.* 1996;28:755–765.
87. Tian R, Gaudron P, Neubauer S, et al. Alterations of performance and oxygen utilization in chronically infarcted rat hearts. *J Mol Cell Cardiol.* 1996;28:321–330.
88. Tian R. Thermodynamic limitation for the sarcoplasmic reticulum Ca($^{2+}$)-ATPase contributes to impaired contractile reserve in hearts. *Ann NY Acad Sci.* 1998;853:322–324.
89. Nascimben L, Ingwall JS, Pauletto P, et al. Creatine kinase system in failing and nonfailing human myocardium. *Circulation.* 1996;94:1894–1901.
90. McCune SA, O'Donnell MJ, Narayan P, et al. 31P-NMR analysis of congestive heart failure in the SHHF/Mcc-facp rat heart. *J Mol Cell Cardiol.* 1998;30:235–241.
91. Neubauer S, Horn M, Naumann A, et al. Impairment of energy metabolism in intact residual myocardium of rat hearts with chronic myocardial infarction. *J Clin Invest.* 1995:95(3): 1092–1100.
92. Pagani ED, Aousi AA, Grant AM, et al. Changes in myofibrillar content and Mg-ATPase activity in ventricular tissues from patients with heart failure caused by coronary artery disease, cardiomyopathy, or mitral valve insufficiency. *Circ Res.* 1988;63(2): 380–385.
93. Hajjar RJ, Gwathmey JK. Direct evidence of changes in myofilament responsiveness to Ca^{2+} during hypoxia and reoxygenation in myocardium. *Am J Physiol.* 1990;259(28, *Heart Circ Physiol.*) H784–H795.

94. Zweier JL, Jacobus WE, Korecky B, et al. Bioenergetic consequences of cardiac phosphocreatine depletion induced by creatine analogue feeding. *J Biol Chem*. 1991;266:20296–20304.
95. Hamman BL, Bittl JA, Jacobus WE, et al. Inhibition of creatine kinase decreases the contractile reserve of the isolated rat heart. *Proc 5th Annual Meeting of Society of Magnetic Resonance in Medicine*, Montreal, Canada. 19086. Works in progress:133.
96. Van Deursen J, Heerschap A, Oerlemans F, et al. Skeletal muscles of mice deficient in muscle creatine kinase lack burst activity. *Cell*. 1993;74:621–631.
97. Gwathmey JK, Hajjar RJ, Allen PD. Excitation-contraction coupling in human ventricular myocardium: relationship to the pathophysiology of heart failure. In: Gwathmey JK, Briggs GM, Allen PD, eds. *Heart Failure: Basic Science and Clinical Aspects*. New York: Marcel Dekker; 1993:121–144.
98. Ingwall JS, Nascimben L, Gwathmey JK. Heart failure: is the pathology due to calcium overload or to mismatch in energy supply and demand? In: Gwathmey JK, Briggs GM, Allen PD, eds. *Heart Failure: Basic Science and Clinical Aspects*. New York: Marcel Dekker; 1993:667–700.
99. Gwathmey JK, Briggs GM, Allen PD, eds. *Heart Failure: Basic Research and Clinical Aspects*. New York: Marcel Dekker; 1993.
100. Shorofsky SR, Balke CW, Gwathmey JK. Calcium channels in cardiac hypertrophy and heart failure. *Heart Fail Rev*. 1998;2(3): 163–171.
101. Hajjar RJ, Gwathmey JK. Calcium sensitizing inotropic agents in the treatment of heart failure: a critical view. *Cardiovasc Drugs and Ther*. 1991;5:961–996.
102. Hajjar RJ, Schmidt U, Helm P, et al. Ca^{2+}-sensitizers impair cardiac relaxation in failing human myocardium. *J Pharmacol Exp Ther*. 1997;280(1):247–254.
103. Liao R, Gwathmey JK. Effects of MCI-154 and caffeine on Ca^{2+}-regulated interactions between troponin subunits from bovine heart. *J Pharmacol Exper Ther*. 1994:270:831–839.

Abnormalities in Cardiac Contraction: Systolic Dysfunction

6

Blase A. Carabello

To sustain life, the heart must pump a cardiac output adequate to supply the tissues' needs for nutrients. In providing this perfusion, the ventricles must generate enough pressure to overcome the resistance offered by the systemic and pulmonary circulations. This vital function of the heart as a pump is best described by Ohm's law as it applies to the circulation, where BP = CO × TR (BP, blood pressure; CO, cardiac output; TR, total resistance). Cardiac output, in turn, is maintained by the cyclical contraction and relaxation of the ventricles, which generate pressure and propel blood forward. If the heart fails to perform its function, failure can only occur in three ways: (a) failure of proper cycle generation (i.e., arrhythmia), (b) failure to relax properly (diastolic dysfunction), or (c) failure to contract properly (systolic function). This chapter will address systolic dysfunction. It will define the components of systolic mechanics and ways of measuring abnormalities of these components in the overall assessment of systolic dysfunction.

Over the past 50 years there has been an often-repeated scenario consisting of interest in a new measure of systolic function followed by discoveries of its limitations followed by disuse. After scores of indexes have passed through this cycle, ejection fraction, despite its load dependencies and insensitivity to inotropic change, remains the most commonly used index of systolic function. However, the explosion of transgenic manipulations and the advent of cell and gene therapy for ventricular dysfunction necessitates accurate and sensitive methods for evaluating the success of such therapies. Thus, now more than ever, it is important to consider which forms of evaluation are best suited for assessing systolic function in the modern era.

DETERMINANTS OF CARDIAC OUTPUT

Cardiac output is the product of the volume ejected from either ventricle during one beat (stroke volume) and the heart rate. Stroke volume is obtained by measuring cardiac output using a variety of means (e.g., Fick, thermodilution) and dividing by the heart rate or by analyzing cardiac images to obtain end-diastolic and end-systolic volumes. Certainly maintenance of an adequate stroke volume is important to the patient, but obtaining the value for stroke volume gives little information about overall cardiac function or about whether systolic dysfunction exists. For instance, in hemorrhagic shock the underfilled ventricles have a greatly reduced stroke volume even though the ventricles themselves may be perfectly normal. Conversely, in dilated cardiomyopathy a left ventricle ejecting only 20% of an end-diastolic volume of 400 mL maintains a normal stroke volume (80 mL) despite what is obviously severe systolic dysfunction.

To evaluate systolic function, one must take into account the four basic properties that determine stroke volume: preload, afterload, contractility, and myocardial mass. Stroke volume varies directly with preload and contractility and, inversely, with afterload. Additionally, the innate size (mass) of the muscle composing the ventricle is a key determinant of stroke volume; that is, an elephant's heart produces a greater stroke volume than a rat's heart, regardless of preload, afterload, or contractility. Furthermore, when the myocardium is overloaded by requirements to generate excess pressure or volume, the major form of long-term compensation is the development of hypertrophy. When the stress is a volume overload, new sarcomeres are laid down in series, producing an increase in myocardial mass as well as chamber volume (eccentric hypertrophy). When the stress is a pressure overload, new sarcomeres are laid down in parallel, producing increased wall thickness (concentric hypertrophy), which increases myocardial mass but not chamber volume. In evaluating overall cardiac function, myocardial mass and hypertrophy must be considered together with preload, afterload, and contractility. For instance, in aortic stenosis, the left ventricle may be able to develop a systolic pressure of 270 mm Hg by a doubling of left ventricular mass. However, even though the pressure-generating ability of the entire chamber is increased, individual units of myocardium actually may have depressed contractility (1,2).

Preload and Measurement of Preload

The Frank-Starling law of the heart indicates that as end-diastolic volume and diastolic sarcomere stretch increase, force generation increases (3). According to the sliding filaments theory, increased force generation occurs with increased sarcomere stretch up to 2.2 μm. At this sarcomere length, the thin actin filaments are stretched to a configuration allowing maximal cross-bridge interaction with the thick myosin filaments (Fig. 6-1) (4,5). The term preload is intimately linked to the Frank-Starling concept, although no exact definition of preload is universally accepted. Most authorities define preload as the actual sarcomere stretch that exists at the end of diastole. However, others define preload as the force that causes this sarcomere stretch. This difference in definition can lead to real discrepancies in the concept of preload.

For instance, in hypertrophic states where ventricular compliance can be reduced, increased diastolic distending force actually may cause less than normal sarcomere stretch (6). In this case, is preload increased or decreased? Because it is the actual presystolic sarcomere stretch that affects systolic contraction, I favor end-diastolic sarcomere length as the most precise definition of preload. Thus, in the case above, preload is reduced despite increased filling pressure. Unfortunately, defined in this way, preload is difficult to evaluate except in research settings where actual sarcomere length can be obtained. In clinical practice, preload is inferred from end-diastolic pressure, end-diastolic stress, or end-diastolic dimension or volume. Each has its inherent limitations in the assessment of preload. For instance, an end-diastolic pressure of 15 mm Hg might cause near-maximum sarcomere stretch in one patient with a compliant ventricle and much less sarcomere stretch in another patient with a less compliant ventricle. In these two patients the same end-diastolic pressure produces a different preload (sarcomere stretch). End-diastolic stress that takes into account geometry and chamber thickness examines the force producing sarcomere stretch. Although more sophisticated, it shares the same limitations as end-diastolic pressure. A given end-diastolic stress will stretch the sarcomeres to a greater degree in more compliant ventricles than in less compliant ventricles. Fortunately, both end-diastolic pressure and end-diastolic stress may be used as relative indicators of preload if compliance in a given patient has not changed. Thus, although one cannot be certain what the sarcomere stretch is in a given patient, if

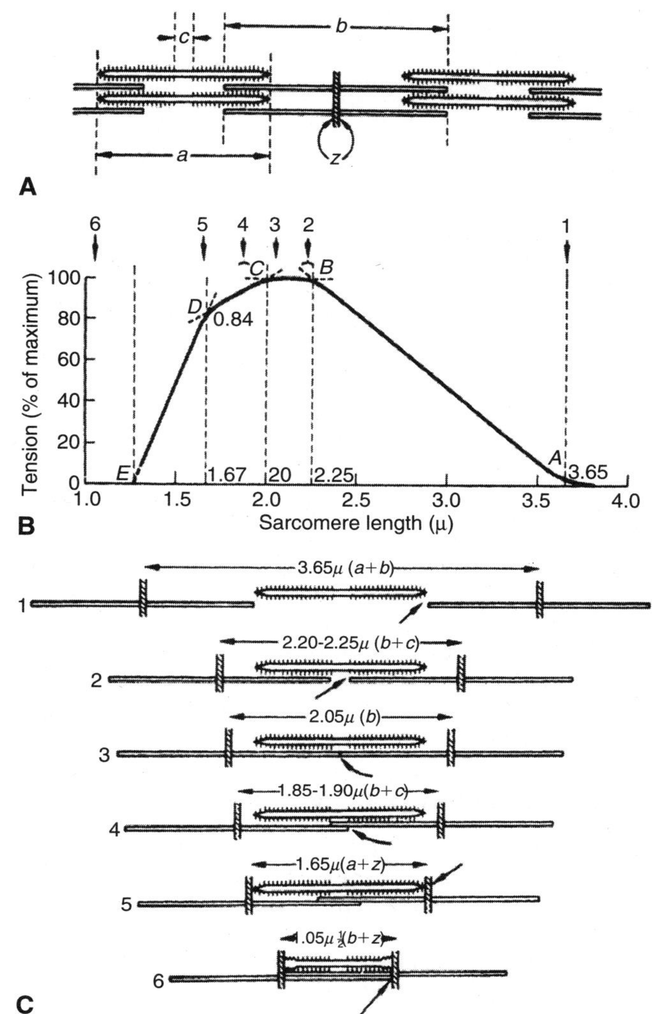

Figure 6-1 Top panel **(A)** is a schematic of a sarcomere. The thin filaments (actin) are attached at the Z band. The length of two actin filaments as they extend from the Z band is denoted by *b*. The length of a thick filament (myosin) is denoted by *a*. Tension is correlated with sarcomere stretch in panels **B** and **C**. Position number 1 shows extreme sarcomere stretch where neither actin filament can interact with the myosin filament; thus, tension production is zero. Positions 2 and 3 demonstrate situations of maximal actin myosin overlap; thus tension production is maximal. In positions 4 and 5, the sarcomere has been shortened such that the actin filaments overlap one another, preventing cross-bridge attachment in the overlapping areas, reducing tension development. In position 6 there is complete actin overlap, preventing any cross-bridging with the myosin, and the tension development again is zero. (Reproduced from Braunwald E, Ross J, Jr., Sonnenblick EH, eds. *Mechanisms of Contraction of the Normal and Failing Heart.* 2nd ed. Boston: Little, Brown; 1972:77, with permission.)

end-diastolic pressure is increased from 15 to 20 mm Hg, it is likely that preload has increased unless compliance has become reduced, as it might in acute ischemia.

End-diastolic dimension or volume is obviously in part dependent on sarcomere stretch. As stretch increases, end-diastolic dimension (or volume) must also increase. However, if eccentric cardiac hypertrophy has intervened, more sarcomeres stretched to a lesser degree produce the same end-diastolic dimension as fewer sarcomeres stretched to a greater degree in the normal heart. Thus, neither dimension nor volume is a precise measurement of preload. Like end-diastolic pressure and stress, end-diastolic dimension and volume can be used as relative indicators of preload. If end-diastolic dimension in a given patient is increased acutely, it is certain that preload has increased. On the other hand, if in the same patient a volume overload has been interposed and end-diastolic dimension is examined 3 months after volume overloading, an increased diastolic dimension could be due to either increased preload, eccentric hypertrophy (increased number of series sarcomeres), or both.

In summary, sarcomere stretch probably is the best definition for preload because it is this property that is one of the key determinants of systolic function. However, no precise, easily obtained method is available for determining this property. End-diastolic pressure, stress, dimension, and volume (if increased acutely in a given patient) usually indicate that preload is increased. Unfortunately, because compliance differs from ventricle to ventricle and because the presence of eccentric cardiac hypertrophy may alter end-diastolic length or volume independent of sarcomere stretch, none of these measures can be used as an absolute measure of preload when comparing one patient or one ventricle with another.

Afterload and Measures of Afterload

Afterload is the force that the myocardium must overcome in order to shorten; it is the force that resists contraction. As this force increases, a ventricle of given strength will be less capable of overcoming the force and will shorten less completely to a greater end-systolic dimension or volume. Thus, evaluation of afterload is important in assessing overall ventricular performance. For instance, under high afterload, a ventricle of normal strength may be unable to shorten normally and thus will appear to have depressed function. This situation has been termed *afterload mismatch* (7). It can cause the erroneous judgment that ventricular muscle strength is reduced when, in fact, excess afterload is the cause for the poor ventricular performance.

Peripheral resistance, systolic pressure, systolic stress, and systolic impedance all have been used to assess afterload. Total peripheral resistance has several limitations as an indicator of afterload. Mathematically, peripheral resistance = mean arterial pressure / cardiac output. In turn, mean arterial pressure = (2 × diastolic pressure + systolic pressure)/3.

Thus, mean arterial pressure is predominantly determined by a *diastolic* property. Consequently, total peripheral resistance makes a significant departure from the definition of afterload—the *systolic* force against which the heart contracts. Although flow occurs only during systole in the proximal aorta, in the periphery, flow is less pulsatile and is present during both systole and diastole. Because most of the peripheral resistance occurs distally at the arteriolar level, some of the flow opposed by this resistance occurs during diastole. Thus, total peripheral resistance is inherently limited as an indicator of afterload by dependence on a diastolic factor. This is probably a key reason why Lang et al. have demonstrated that there may be significant discrepancies between total peripheral resistance and other, more succinct indicators of afterload (8).

Systolic pressure also is used as an indicator of afterload. Because pressure is equal to force divided by area, systolic force is incorporated into the expression of pressure; thus, systolic pressure does reflect afterload. Pressure is an expression of the force that the ventricle must overcome; thus, systolic pressure represents chamber afterload. However, pressure is not normalized for the myocardial mass present. If ventricular hypertrophy is present, there is more muscle to bear the load. In this case, normalization for the amount of myocardium present is needed to examine afterload on individual muscle fibers in assessing myocardial strength. Here, examination of wall stress is a better indicator of myocardial load than pressure. Wall stress in its simplest definition is stated by the Laplace relationship: stress $= (p \times r)/2h$, where $p =$ pressure, $r =$ radius, and $h =$ thickness. Stress normalizes the pressure in the ventricle for its radius and thickness and, thus, examines the force that a unit of myocardium must generate during systole in order to shorten. Although wall stress examines forces occurring in the ventricle itself, stress neglects coupling with vasculature, which is the actual source of the resistance (afterload) against which the ventricle must contract.

In this respect, aortic impedance is a useful indicator of afterload. Descriptively, aortic impedance is the vascular resistance against which the ventricle contracts in systole; it differs from total peripheral resistance, which as previously noted is both a systolic and diastolic phenomenon. Impedance can be measured by examining the Fourier analysis of the instantaneous relationship between systolic aortic pressure and flow. Unfortunately, impedance loses its usefulness as a descriptor of afterload in aortic stenosis or in situations such as mitral regurgitation, where ejection from the left ventricle into more than one chamber occurs. During mitral regurgitation, ejection from the ventricle occurs both into the left atrium as well as into the aorta; thus, aortic impedance only examines partial afterload. In many severe cardiac diseases, ventricular dilatation leads to some mitral regurgitation and diminishes impedance as a useful tool for measuring afterload.

CONTRACTILITY

Contractility is the ability of the myocardium to develop force independent of loading conditions. In essence, it is the strength of the ventricle. It is this property that is best related to prognosis. Diseases that lead to a reduction in contractility lead to progressive cardiovascular deterioration and eventually to death. Thus, it is not surprising that there have been multiple attempts to measure this prognostic property in both experimental and clinical settings. However, no "contractilometer" exists; that is, there is no simple, precise way to measure ventricular contractility. The ideal index of contractility should be independent of preload, afterload, and myocardial mass but also should be sensitive to small changes in inotropic state and be easy to apply. No currently available index entirely fulfills these criteria. The following section reviews some of the indexes of contractility that have been used and examines their assets and limitations.

Isovolumic Indexes of Ventricular Contractility

As the name implies, isovolumic indexes examine ventricular contraction during the period of isovolumic systole (i.e., after the atrioventricular valves have closed but before the semilunar valves have opened). The cornerstone of the isovolumic indexes of contractile function is the rate of change of ventricular pressure (*P*) development (*dP/dt*). In theory, this rate of change reflects the velocity of contractile element shortening before the elastic elements are stretched to the point where they cause overall ventricular shortening (the point at which the semilunar valves open and volume is ejected from the ventricle). Examination of left ventricular *dP/dt/P* (velocity of shortening) at various pressures before the opening of the aortic valve can be used to extrapolate to the velocity that might have occurred if no pressure were present in the ventricle (9). This property, termed V_{max}, is equivalent to the maximum velocity of contractile element shortening if no load were present (Fig. 6-2); it was originally thought to be a good indicator of contractile function.

V_{max} is sensitive to changes in contractile state (10). However, some dependence on preload and the need to extrapolate to a theoretical, unconfirmable state has reduced enthusiasm for its use (11). Furthermore, the index was unable to separate patients with clear contractile dysfunction from normal subjects in two important clinical studies, obviously raising questions about the clinical usefulness of V_{max} as an accurate index of contractile function (12,13). Maximum *dP/dt* is also used as a measure of contractility. This index is sensitive to changes in inotropy (14). However, it is unreliable in comparing individuals to themselves over time or in comparing groups of individuals to each other because of a wide range of normal values (12).

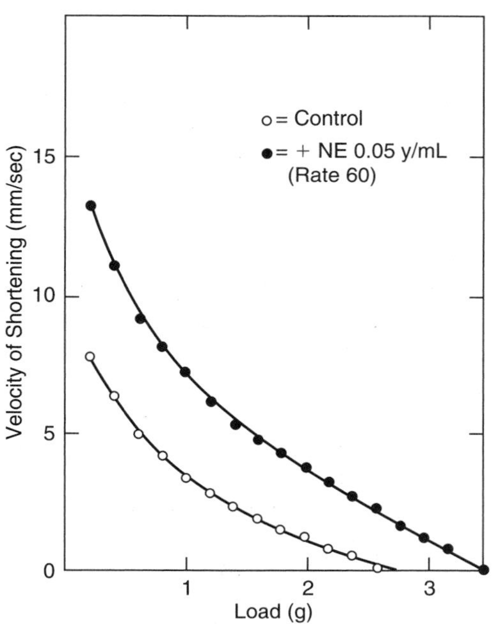

Figure 6-2 Velocity of shortening of a papillary muscle is plotted against load in the control state and in the presence of norepinephrine at several different loads. Extrapolation of these curves to zero load would give the velocity of shortening at zero load (V_{max}). Norepinephrine (NE) obviously increased V_{max}, indicating increased contractility. (Reproduced from Braunwald E, Ross J, Jr., Sonnenblick EH, eds. *Mechanisms of Contraction of the Normal and Failing Heart*. 2nd ed. Boston: Little, Brown; 1972:49, with permission.)

Ejection Phase Indexes of Contractile Function

The ejection phase indexes of contractile function examine ventricular performance from end-diastole to end-systole. The most popular of such indexes are ejection fraction and the mean velocity of circumferential fiber shortening. Ejection fraction is equal to the stroke volume divided by the end-diastolic volume. Descriptively, it is the percentage of the end-diastolic volume that is ejected during systole. As such, it does not examine force generation (which is part of the definition of contractility) but, rather, examines the global shortening performance of the ventricle.

Ejection fraction has two major advantages as an index of contractile function. First, in a large variety of clinical and experimental circumstances it has been an excellent prognostic indicator of outcome and thus has clinical relevance (15). Second, it is easy to obtain and is dimensionless; it can thus be applied to virtually any patient or experimental subject. Its major drawback (besides the theoretical consideration that it does not examine force generation) is that it is not dependent only on contractility (the property one wishes to measure); it is also dependent on preload, afterload, and cardiac mass (16–18). This fact may cause ejection fraction to lead to erroneous conclusions regarding contractility. For example, in mitral regurgitation, where preload is greatly increased and afterload is normal or reduced (19,20), ejection fraction is enhanced by these favorable loading conditions and will overestimate contractility (21). Conversely, in aortic stenosis, where afterload may be increased, ejection fraction may be reduced by afterload mismatch rather than by depressed contractility; thus, ejection fraction may underestimate contractile function in this disease (22).

The mean velocity of circumferential fiber shortening is defined as the shortening fraction divided by ejection time: [(EDD − ESD)/(EDD × ET), where EDD = end-diastolic dimension, ESD = end-systolic dimension, and ET = ejection time]. This index depends less on preload than does ejection fraction (23). However, like ejection fraction, the mean velocity of circumferential fiber shortening (V_{cf}) is also afterload-dependent.

Afterload-Corrected Ejection Phase Indexes

Because ejection fraction and V_{cf} are afterload-dependent, plotting them against existing afterload (Fig. 6-3) helps correct for the afterload present. As shown, ejection fraction and V_{cf} are inversely but linearly related to afterload (wall stress). A given individual can be plotted against the normal ejection fraction–end systolic stress or V_{cf}-end-systolic–stress relationship to examine contractile function (1,24). A patient whose plot is downward and to the left of this relationship demonstrates decreased ejection perfor-

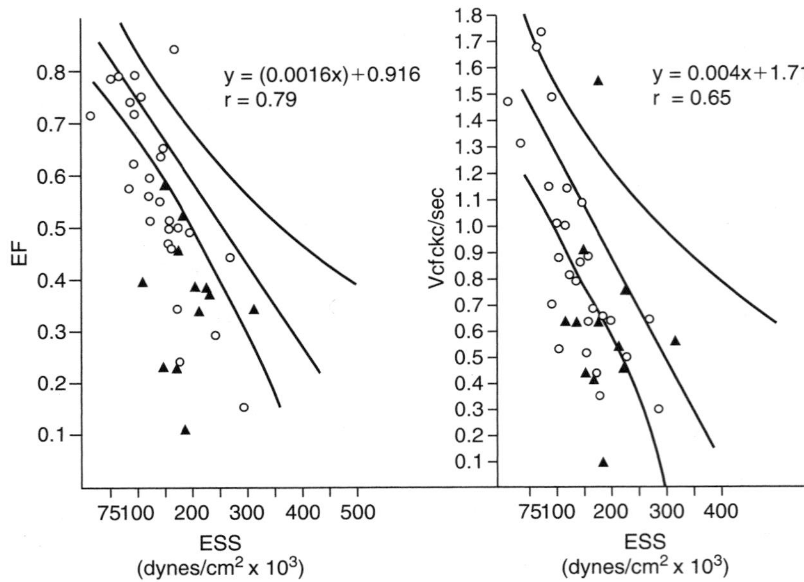

Figure 6-3 Ejection fraction (EF, **left panel**) and the mean velocity of circumferential fiber shortening (V_{cf}, **right panel**) are plotted against end-systolic stress (ESS). The slope of the normal relationship and the 95% confidence limits are demonstrated. Patients with valvular disease who had a satisfactory outcome at surgery (O) and those patients with a poor outcome (▲) are plotted against the normal relationships. As can be seen, most patients with a poor outcome fell down and to the left of the normal relationship, indicating that they had reduced contractile function prior to surgery. (Reproduced from Carabello BA, Williams H, Gash AK, et al. Hemodynamic predictors of outcome in patients undergoing valve replacement. *Circulation.* 1986;74:1309–1316, with permission.)

mance for a given amount of afterload. In this circumstance, excess afterload cannot explain reduced ejection performance (because excess afterload is not present or is modest) and the reduced ejection performance is thus likely due to reduced contractile function. This relationship has been used effectively in many studies to infer contractile function. However, to date no universal slope, intercept, and confidence intervals for these relationships have been agreed on. Therefore, each laboratory must develop its own relationship from normal subjects against which patients will be plotted.

END-SYSTOLIC INDEXES OF CONTRACILITY

End-Systolic Volume

End-systolic volume or dimension is dependent on contractile state, afterload, and left ventricular myocardial mass but is not dependent on preload (25). Therefore, by examining end-systolic dimension or end-systolic volume instead of the entire ejection phase, preload is removed as a confounding influence in the determination of contractile function. Not surprisingly, in disease states where preload is exaggerated, such as in aortic and mitral regurgitation, end-systolic volume and end-systolic dimension have been valuable indicators regarding the timing of surgery (26–29). As end-systolic dimension or volume increases there is a proportionately less favorable prognosis, presumably because contractile function is increasingly depressed. The implication of increased end-systolic volume is that the weaker ventricle is unable to contract as completely as a stronger ventricle and, thus, remains larger at the end of systole.

The End-Systolic Stress: Volume Ratio

As noted above, end-systolic volume is preload-independent but remains dependent on contractile function, afterload, and overall heart size. We, and others, have attempted to correct end-systolic volume by making a ratio of end-systolic stress to end-systolic volume index (21,30). The concept behind the ratio is that a stronger ventricle will contract to a smaller volume against the same afterload than will a weaker ventricle. Thus, the denominator of the ratio will be smaller and the ratio itself will be consequently larger. By incorporating afterload into the index, it seemed that this ratio might better assess contractility than end-systolic volume alone. Unfortunately, the index is still somewhat afterload-dependent (31).

Table 6-1 lists some of the studies in which the ratio of end-systolic stress to volume or end-systolic pressure to volume has been used and the relative success of the index (20,21). We have found it particularly useful in predicting the outcome of patients undergoing surgery for mitral regurgitation, where it has superior predictive accuracy to end-systolic volume alone (21,29).

Time-Varying Elastance and the Slope of End-Systolic Pressure–Volume Relationship

As afterload increases, a ventricle of given contractile function will be less able to overcome the afterload and thus will remain larger at a given time in systole (25). Progressive increases in afterload produce a nearly linear increase in volume. By matching the afterload–volume coordinates from multiple, variably loaded beats, one can develop the slope of the afterload–volume relationship (32–40). As demonstrated in Figure 6-4, beginning at the QRS and proceeding through systole, the slope (elastance) of the relationship of pressure (chamber afterload) and volume increases progressively until it reaches a maximum value (E_{max}) at the end of systole. Thus, elastance varies with time from the beginning of systole. Elastance also varies with contractile state. Maximum elastance increases as contractile function increases, indicating that for any given incremental change in pressure (Δy) the resultant increase in volume (Δx) is less, resulting in a steeper slope (41).

TABLE 6-1
PUBLISHED STUDIES COMPARING VARIOUS INDEXES OF CARDIAC FUNCTION

Reference	No. of Subjects	Index Examined	Disease	Conclusions
30	8 dogs ESS/ESVI	PSP/ESVI CMP	Pacing	Correlated well with resting EF, afterload independence an advantage over EF
29	7 dogs	MSVR	—	Ratio increased appropriately with inotropic state, but ratio was afterload-dependent, varying directly with afterload
31	11 patients	PSP/ESV	Status post-CABG	Ratio was preload-independent but increased if afterload increased
32	11 patients	ESS/ESVI	Sickle cell anemia	Ratio correlated well with slope of the ESPVR
33	11 patients	ESS/ESVI	Hypertension	Ratio correlated well with slope of the ESPVR
19	21 patients	ESS/ESVI	MR	Ratio was prognostic of outcome and superior to EF
27	37 patients	ESS/ESVI	Valvular HD	Ratio predictive of outcome in MR but not for AS or AR
34	76 patients	PSP/ESVI	MR	Low PSP/ESVI associated with increased mortality but EF was superior in predicting overall clinical outcome
35	33 patients	PSP/ESVI	CAD	Failure of ratio to increase with exercise correlated with the extent of CAD
36	30 patients	PSP/ESV	CAD	Ratio was depressed at rest in 71% of patients with CAD and depressed with exercise in 95%
37	243 patients	PSP/ESV	CAD	Ratio 84% sensitive to CAD during exercise but not superior to EF
38	20 patients	PSP/ESV	CAD	Ratio responded appropriately to increased inotropic state but was inferior to ESPVR in assessing contractility

AR, aortic regurgitation; AS, aortic stenosis; CABG, coronary artery bypass grafting; CAD, coronary artery disease; CMP, cardiomyopathy; EF, ejection fraction; ESPVR, end-systolic pressure-volume relationship; ESS, end-systolic stress; ESV, end-systolic volume; ESVI, end-systolic volume index; HD, heart disease; MR, mitral regurgitation; MSVR, maximum stress/volume ratio; PSP, peak systolic pressure.

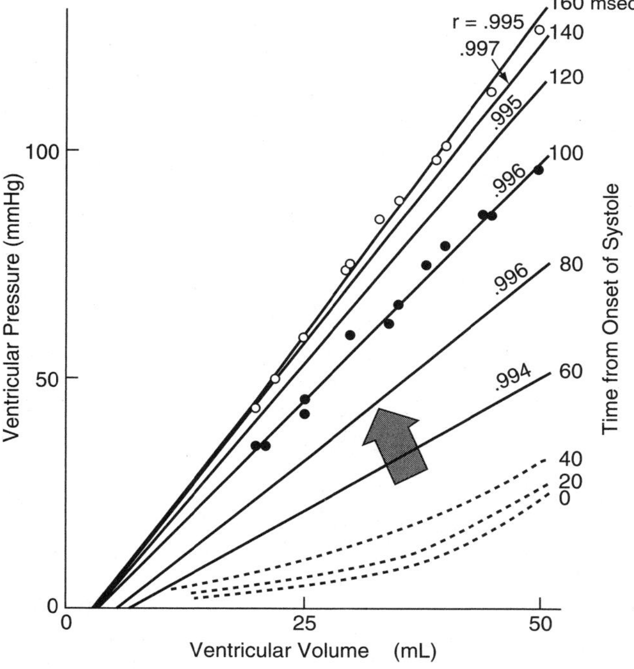

Figure 6-4 Ventricular pressure is plotted against ventricular volume in an isolated ventricle at several different afterloads (ventricular pressures) beginning at 60 milliseconds from the onset of systole to the point at which the slope of the relationship is maximal (E_{max}), at 160 milliseconds after the onset of systole. (Reproduced from Sagawa K, Suga H, Shoukas AA, et al. End-systolic pressure/volume ratio: a new index of ventricular contractility. *Am J Cardiol.* 1977;40:748, with permission.)

The time-varying method for assessing contractile function is cumbersome to develop because it requires the assessment of pressure and volume at multiple times during systole and synchronization of these times from multiple variably loaded beats. However, maximum elastance occurs at end-systole, where the pressure and volume coordinates are usually coincident with the upper left-hand corner of the ventricular pressure–volume curve (Fig. 6-5) (42). These coordinates are usually closely related to dicrotic notch pressure and end-ejection volume, which therefore often can be used to represent the values for pressure and volume at E_{max}, obviating the time variation analysis. By plotting the coordinates of the upper left-hand corners of the pressure–volume loops from multiple variably loaded beats as shown in Fig. 6-6, the slope of the end-systolic-pressure–volume relationship (ESPVR) can be obtained. As with maximum elastance, steeper slopes indicate increased contractile performance (Fig. 6-6).

It is clear that the slope of the ESPVR is accurate in assessing acute changes in contractility (25,31). However, this relationship has several limitations. First, although in general usage the relationship is considered linear, some curvilinearity of the relationships has been demonstrated (43,44). Furthermore, the curvilinearity may produce a relatively convex shape at high-contractility states and a relatively concave shape at low-contractility states (44). The effects of these changes of the slope on the predictability of the relationship have yet to be defined. Second, the pressure–volume relationship examines the performance of the chamber as a whole because the afterload (pressure) is

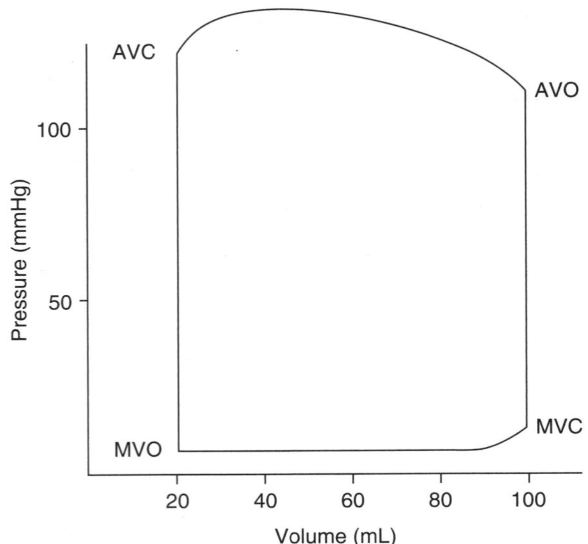

Figure 6-5 A left ventricular pressure–volume loop is demonstrated. MVO, mitral valve opening; MVC, mitral valve closure; AVO, aortic valve opening; AVC, aortic valve closure. End-systole defined as E_{max} usually corresponds with the upper left-hand corner (AVC), obviating the need for development of the entire time-varying elastance relationship to determine E_{max}. (Reproduced from Carabello BA. Cardiac catheterization. In: Parmley WW, Chatterjee K, eds. *Cardiology*. Vol. 1. Physiology, pharmacology, diagnosis. Philadelphia: JB Lippincott; 1990:11, with permission.)

the afterload on the chamber and is not normalized to the amount of myocardium present. To overcome this problem, the stress–volume relationship can be used. In this relationship, the term *fiber elastance* is indicative of the afterload-volume relationship normalized to the mass of myocardium available to generate force (31,45,46).

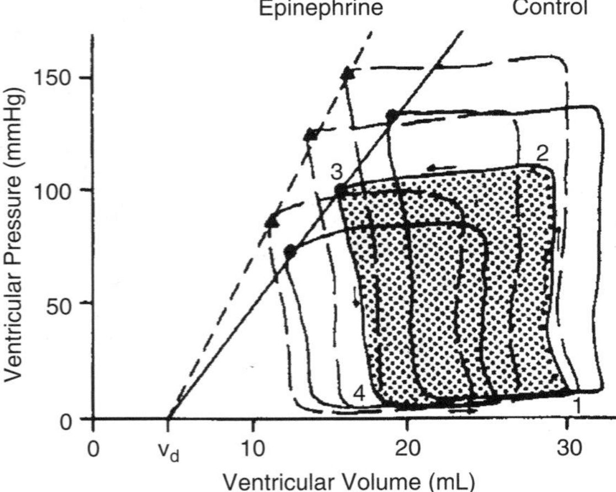

Figure 6-6 Pressure–volume loops from differently afterloaded beats are demonstrated in the isolated ventricle. As afterload increases, end-systolic volume increases as the ventricle shortens less completely against increasing load. The ESPVR is plotted using the coordinates of the upper left-hand corner of these loops in the control state (●) and during the presence of epinephrine (▲). Epinephrine increases the inotropic state, allowing the ventricle to shorten more completely at any given increase in afterload, producing a steeper slope of the ESPVR. (Reproduced from Suga H, Sagawa K, Shoukas AA. Load independence of the instantaneous pressure-volume ratio of the canine left ventricle and effects of epinephrine and heart rate on the ratio. *Circ Res*. 1973;32:314–323, with permission.)

Both the pressure–volume and stress–volume relationships, unfortunately, are dependent on ventricular size (47). The slope of any relationship is defined as a change in the y-axis term divided by the change in the x-axis term. In a rat, a change in end-systolic pressure of 10 mm Hg might yield a change in end-systolic volume of 0 to 1 mL. The slope of this relationship would then be 100 mm Hg/mL. In a human, a similar change in pressure might yield a 3-mL change in end-systolic volume, yielding a slope of 3 to 33 mm Hg/mL. It is unlikely that the contractile function of the rat is 30 times higher than that of the human but, rather, it is the small size of the rat compared with the human that causes a relatively smaller change in volume for any change in pressure.

Less dramatic but important differences exist within the same species (48). Thus, some method for normalizing this relationship for size is needed, but none has yet been agreed on. Some investigators have multiplied the slope by the end-diastolic volume present at the time the slope was obtained (45). However, end-diastolic volume is affected not only by the number of sarcomeres present but also by the stretch of those sarcomeres (preload). Thus, volume correction may lead to overcorrection. Other investigators have suggested normalizing for myocardial mass because the intended correction is to normalize for the number of sarcomeres present Finally, end-ejection may become uncoupled from end-systole in pathological states such as mitral regurgitation (49,50). In such instances, the upper left-hand corner of the pressure–volume loop may no longer represent end-systole, necessitating the more cumbersome isochronal assessment of E_{max}.

End-Systolic Stiffness

Recently, end-systolic stiffness has been proposed as a load- and size-independent index of contractility (17,51). Stiffness is defined as the change in strain (ε) produced by a change in stress (dσ/dε). Strain is the change in length, area, or volume in reference to some baseline length, area, or volume (e.g., $\Delta L/L_0$, where L = length) and thus is a dimensionless property. As such, it is not affected by heart size. By examining the relationship of change in stress to the change in strain, the constant k (stiffness constant) relating these two variables can be obtained (Fig. 6-7). Increased end-systolic stiffness indicates end-systolic contractility. Recently, this index has been demonstrated to be independent of preload and ventricular size (51). The exact place of this index in the armamentarium of contractility indexes has yet to be determined.

The previously discussed end-systolic relations require the definition of load and volume at multiple, different afterloads. This need makes them difficult to apply to sick patients and makes it unlikely that these measures will gain widespread clinical usage. However, they will continue to be useful in experimental investigations of contractility.

RECRUITABLE STROKE WORK

Stroke work is the area under the ventricular pressure volume curve during a cardiac cycle. Either increased ventricu-

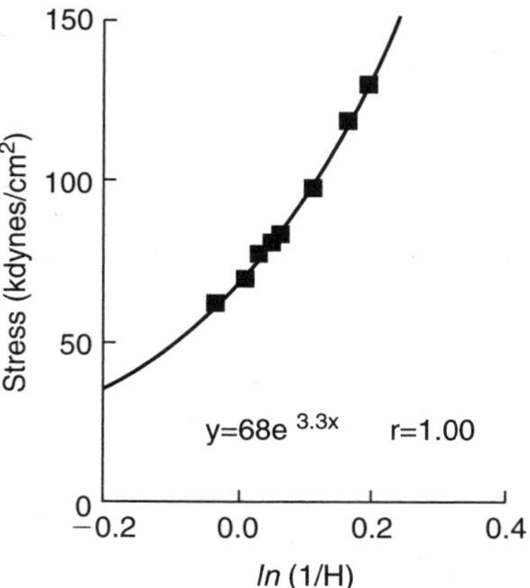

Figure 6-7 End-systolic stress is plotted against end-systolic strain [represented as *ln* (1/*H*), where *H* = wall thickness] from multiple, variably loaded beats. The exponential constant relating stress (*y*) to strain (*x*) is 3.3, which is the stiffness constant, the indicator of contractility. (Reproduced from Nakano K, Sugawara M, Ishihara K, et al. Myocardial stiffness derived from end-systolic wall stress and the logarithm of the reciprocal of wall thickness: a contractility index independent of ventricular size. *Circulation.* 1990;82:1352–1361, with permission.)

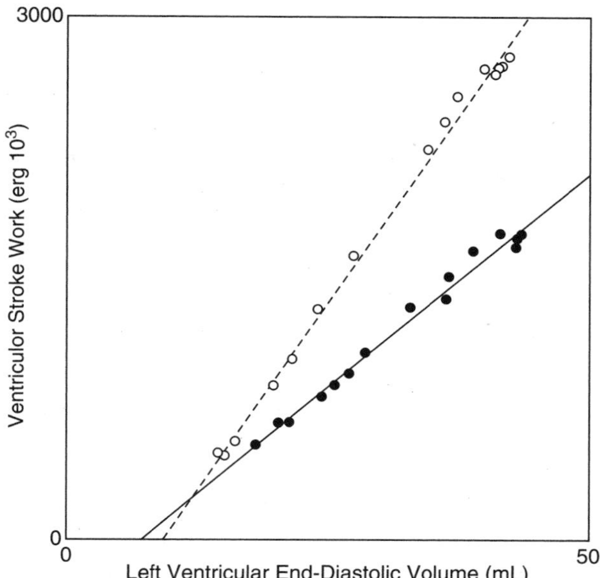

Figure 6-8 Ventricular stroke work is plotted against left ventricular end-diastolic volume in the control state (●) and after calcium infusion (O). The increased slope after calcium infusion indicates that more stroke work was performed at a lower preload (end-diastolic volume), consistent with increased contractility. (Reproduced from Glower DD, Spratt JA, Snow ND, et al. Linearity of the Frank-Starling relationship on the intact heart: the concept of preload recruitable stroke work. *Circulation.* 1985;71:994–1009, with permission.)

lar pressure or volume will increase stroke work. Thus, stroke work partially takes into account changes in preload and afterload. By increasing preload (here defined as end-diastolic volume), the amount of stroke work that the ventricle can perform is increased (52). The relationship of end-diastolic volume to stroke work has been proposed as an index of contractile function. As shown in Figure 6-8, a calcium-mediated increase in contractile state produced more recruitable stroke work for a relatively smaller increase in end-diastolic volume compared to a baseline. Thus, the relationship was able to detect an increase in inotropic state. This index has been demonstrated to be relatively load-insensitive and sensitive to changes in inotropic state. However, the effects of intervening left ventricular hypertrophy on recruitable stroke work have not yet been defined. Because hypertrophied ventricles should be able to do more stroke work than normal ventricles, it is not clear how myocardial contractility can be assessed using this relationship in hypertrophic states. It is likely that some correction for the presence of hypertrophy will need to be made, but this awaits further investigation. A relative comparison of the indexes of contractile function is shown in Table 6-2.

The foregoing discussion of contractility and indexes of contractility deal with the ventricle as if the disease processes affect it globally. However, some diseases (most notably, coronary disease) affect the ventricle segmentally,

TABLE 6-2
DEPENDENCIES OF VARIOUS INDEXES OF CONTRACTILITY

	Affected by Changes in			
Index	**Contractility**	**Preload**	**Afterload**	**Myocardial Mass**
dp/dt	+++	+	++	0
V_{max}	+++	+	+	0
Ejection fraction	++	++	+++	0
V_{cf}	++	+	+++	0
ESV	++	0	++	++
E/ESVI	++	0	+	++
ESPVR	++	+	0	++
dσ/dε	+++	0	0	0
Recruitable stroke work	++	0	0	?

0, no change; +−+++, level of change; ?, change undetermined.

severely disrupting contractile function in some areas while not affecting other areas. Sophisticated finite element models analyzing segmental contractile function have been used; however, their complexity precludes routine use. Clinically, segmental wall motion alone is generally used to determine regional contractile function. The assumption made in doing so is that afterload and preload are homogenous throughout the ventricle, and regional wall motion deficits can therefore be judged to reflect regional impairment of contractile function. Although this assumption is not always true, it is fair to say that impaired regional shortening fraction usually indicates impaired regional contractile function.

VALIDATION

As previously noted, the definition of contractility is the innate ability of the myocardium to generate force, and a variety of indexes have been derived to attempt to predict this ability. However, in most cases no independent gold standard exists against which to match the various indexes that have been derived. However, validation has been possible in some cases. In the laboratory we have been able to compare in vivo left ventricular contractile function with the contractile function of myocytes isolated from a given ventricle studied in vitro by investigators blinded to the in vivo data.

As shown in Figure 6-9, myocytes are studied using laser diffraction to project sarcomere register onto a photodiode, which in turn records sarcomere movement, allowing us to measure the extent and velocity of sarcomere contraction (53). Cells are studied both at baseline and during a graded increase in bath viscosity, imposing an afterload on the cells. This viscosity–velocity relationship is akin to the force–velocity relationship of classic muscle mechanics. As can be seen in Figure 6-10, the best in vivo correlation with myocyte function was obtained using end-systolic stiffness (k). The end-ejection-stress–volume relationship (EESVR) corrected for mass also had an excellent correlation. In another group of studies (Fig. 6-11), myocyte function was compared with afterload-corrected, mean normalized ejection rate (MNSER; ejection fraction divided by ejection time). MNSER is very similar to V_{cf} except that it uses volume rather than dimension (54). As shown in Figure 6-11B, in every case where afterload-corrected MNSER fell down and to the left of the normal relationship, myocyte function was also depressed. Thus, it seems that afterload-corrected MNSER, end-systolic stiffness, and mass-corrected EESVR correlate extremely well with an independent evaluation of muscle function, that of the myocytes isolated from the chambers themselves.

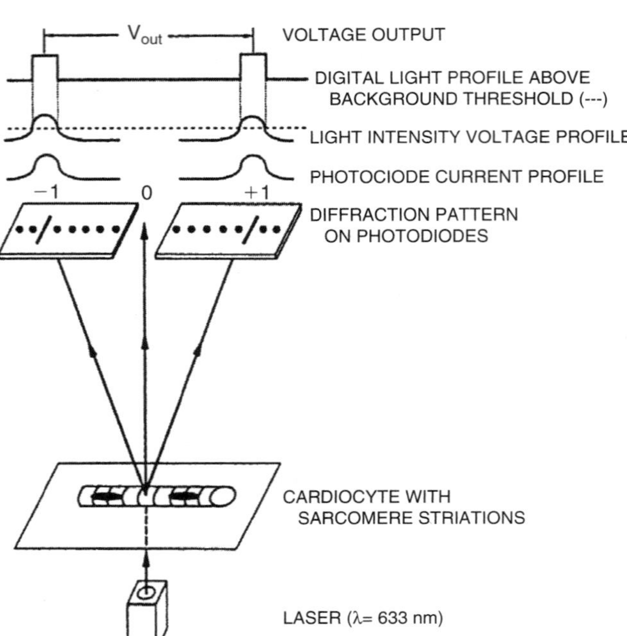

Figure 6-9 The laser diffraction device used for recording the sarcomere motion is shown. (Reproduced from Urabe Y, Mann DL, Kent RL, et al. Cellular and ventricular contractile dysfunction in experimental canine mitral regurgitation. *Circ Res.* 1992;70:131–147, with permission.)

NEWER INDEXES OF VENTIRCULAR FUNCTION

As noted at the beginning of this chapter, new indexes of ventricular function undergo a typical evolution of discovery, enthusiasm, realization of imperfections, and reduced enthusiasm or abandonment. Hopefully, this tradition can be avoided in the use of some newer indexes of function.

Tissue Doppler Imaging, Strain Rate Imaging and MR Tagging

Doppler interrogation of left ventricular movement (tissue Doppler imaging, TDI) can measure segmental differences in myocardial velocities addressing differences in regional function (55,56). However, in assessing viability TDI cannot distinguish between active contraction versus nonviable myocardium moved passively by tethering to adjacent viable tissue.

Strain is defined as a change in length/reference length (akin in some respects to regional shortening fraction). Strain rate imaging (SRI) is a refinement of TDI that employs an algorithm that calculates differences in velocities of adjacent areas of myocardium to derive strain and strain rate. SRI appears superior to TDI in assessing myocardial function (57). Mitral annular velocity seems particularly sensitive in detecting early ventricular dysfunction (58,62). Strain is both preload- and afterload-sensitive, while strain rate is primarily afterload-sensitive in a manner similar to V_{cf}. The advantages of strain imaging are the ease with which regional measurements can be made echocardiographically and the ability to examine regional function. It must be noted that this technique does not fulfill the criteria for the perfect index of contractility and its exact role in clinical medicine has not yet been established.

MRI tagging also affords rapid assessment of regional and global wall motion (63,64). In this process, specific portions of the myocardium are tagged using localized magnetic resonant frequency pulses placed perpendicular to the myocardium. Tagging is followed by an imaging

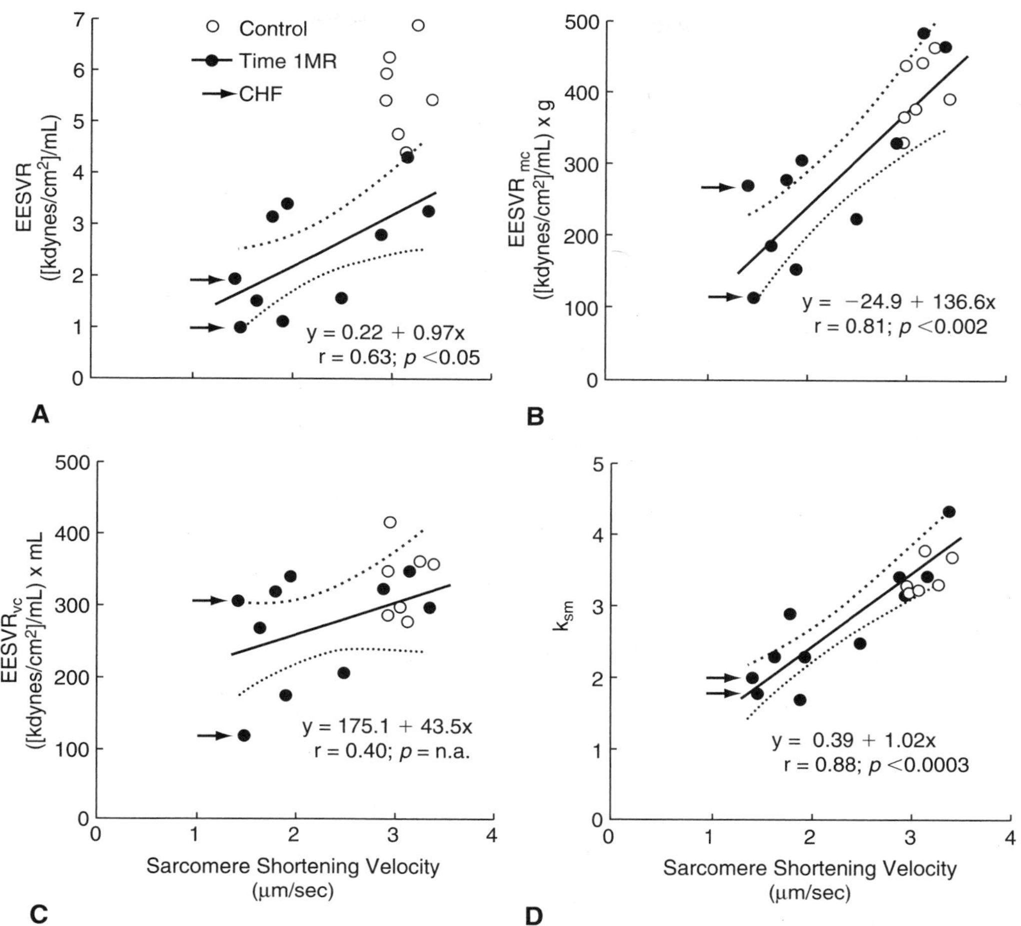

Figure 6-10 The slope of the EESVR **(A)**; EESVR corrected for mass ($EESVR_{mc}$) **(B)**; EESVR corrected for volume ($EESVR_{vc}$) **(C)**; and systolic stiffness (k_{sm}) **(D)** are indexes of chamber function and are correlated to sarcomere shortening velocity of myocytes taken from the respective ventricles. The subjects were controls in dogs with mitral regurgitation. As can be seen, there is an excellent correlation between end-systolic stiffness and mass-corrected EESVR with isolated myocyte function. (Reproduced from Urabe Y, Mann DL, Kent RL, et al. Cellular and ventricular contractile dysfunction in experimental canine mitral regurgitation. *Circ Res.* 1992;70:131–147, with permission.)

sequence that records wall motion in relation to a superimposed grid. The technique's major limitation compared to Doppler interrogation is cost.

Myocardial Performance Index

Recently Tei et al. have proposed an index that takes into account both systolic and diastolic Doppler time intervals shown in Figure 6-12 (65). Its key components are ejection period, isovolumic contraction time, and isovolumic relaxation time—somewhat reminiscent of the systolic time intervals of 4 decades ago. The index is essentially a ratio of isovolumic time to ejection time. Several studies have reported its usefulness (66) but its ultimate place in clinical medicine has yet to be determined.

INTEGRATION OF VENTRICULAR MECHANICS IN ASSESSING CARDIAC FUNCTION

Interpreting cardiac performance at any given time requires a cautious analysis of preload, afterload, contractile function, and intervening hypertrophy. No simple way exists to accomplish this. Left ventricular function curves that can be derived from data obtained using a Swan-Ganz catheter can be used to analyze overall cardiac function but do not give information about which components of function are involved. Two cardiac function curves plotting stroke volume against wedge pressure (as could be obtained from measurements made using a Swan-Ganz catheter) are demonstrated in Figure 6-13. An acute change from curve

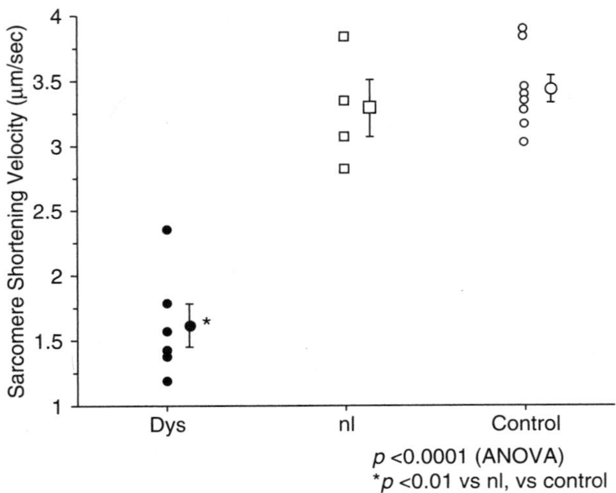

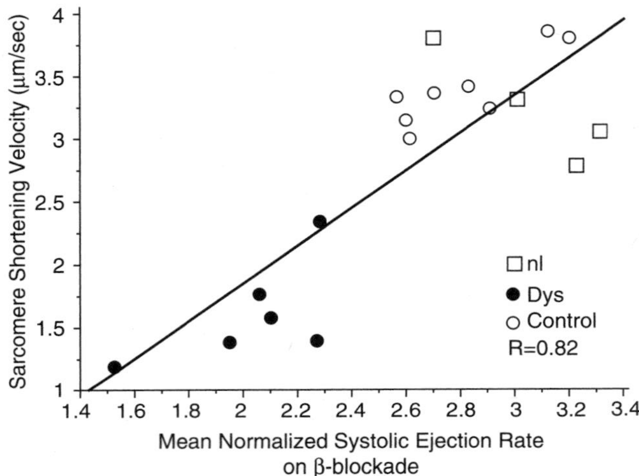

Figure 6-11 Sarcomere shortening velocity of myocytes taken from dogs with aortic stenosis and left ventricular dysfunction (*dys*), dogs with aortic stenosis and normal function (*nl*), and control animals is shown in the **upper panel**. Dysfunction was judged by the relationship between mean normalized systolic ejection rate and wall stress. As can be seen, when the in vivo index predicted dysfunction, the myocytes also demonstrated dysfunction. In the **lower panel**, the two indexes are correlated. (Reproduced from Koide M, Nagatsu M, Zile MR, et al. Premorbid determinants of left ventricular dysfunction in a novel model of gradually induced pressure overload in the adult canine. *Circulation*. 1997;95:1601–1610, with permission.)

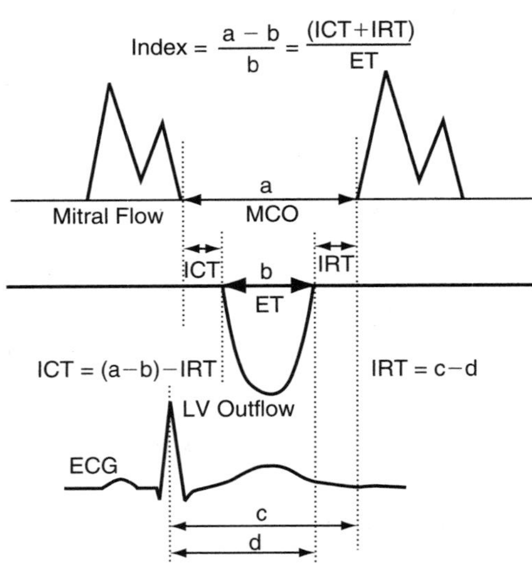

Figure 6-12 Schema for measurements of Doppler time intervals. The index is defined $(a - b)/b$, where a is the interval between cessation and onset of the mitral inflow, and b is the ejection time (ET) of left ventricular (LV) outflow. Isovolumetric relaxation time (IRT) is measured by subtracting the interval c between the R wave and the cessation of left ventricular outflow from the interval d between the R wave and the onset of mitral flow. Isovolumetric contraction time (ICT) is obtained by subtracting isovolumetric relaxation time from $a - b$. ECG, echocardiogram; MCO, interval from cessation to onset of mitral flow. (Reproduced from Yeon SB, Reichek N, Tallant BA, et al. Validation of in vivo myocardial strain measurement by magnet resonance tagging in sonomicrometry. *J Am Coll Cardiol*. 2001;38(2):55–61, with permission.)

A to curve B often is misinterpreted as an increase in contractile function. Although an increase in contractile function could cause this change, the same changes could be affected by several other mechanisms. An acute improvement in left ventricular compliance (as might occur with the relief of ischemia) would allow a greater end-diastolic volume at any wedge pressure, producing increased stroke volume at any given wedge pressure, and thereby causing the improvement from curve A to curve B. Likewise, a reduction in afterload would permit enhanced stroke volume (by reducing end-systolic volume) at any given wedge pressure, again producing the change from curve A to curve B without any change in contractile function. If these two curves were observed at points in time far removed from one another, the development of left ventricular hypertrophy also could effect the change in the curves from A to B without any change in contractile function. Thus, although left ventricular function curves are useful in assessing overall changes in cardiac function, referring to such curves as Frank-Starling curves or contractility curves is clearly not accurate.

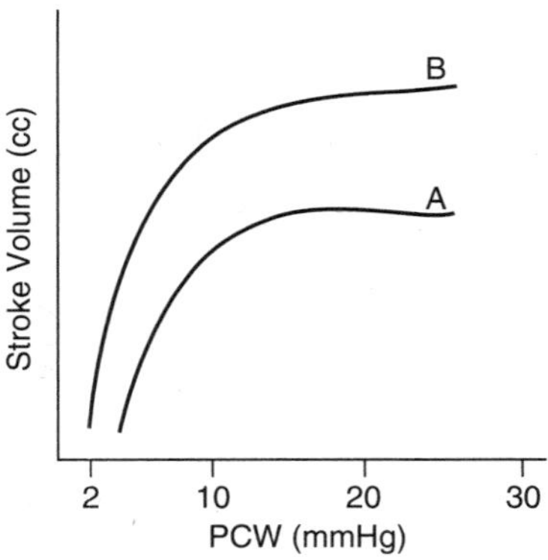

Figure 6-13 Two cardiac function curves from one patient are demonstrated. The change from **A** to **B** indicates enhanced cardiac performance, which could be caused by an increase in contractility, an increase in compliance, a reduction in afterload, the development of hypertrophy, or a combination of these elements.

EXAMPLES OF THE INTEGRATION OF SYSTOLIC MECHANICS IN ASSESSMENT OF LEFT VENTRICULAR SYSTOLIC FUNCTION

Example 1: Aortic Regurgitation

Acute Aortic Regurgitation

In acute aortic regurgitation (as might occur in staphylococcal destruction of an aortic leaflet), there is an abrupt volume overload on the left ventricle as it becomes filled both from the left atrium and from aortic regurgitation during diastole. The results of the acute aortic regurgitation are to increase left ventricular filling pressure and to decrease effective forward stroke volume. This results in congestive heart failure (CHF) because the increased filling pressure causes pulmonary congestion and the reduced effective forward stroke volume leads to reduced tissue perfusion. Acutely, pulse pressure is not greatly widened because high ventricular filling pressure maintains aortic diastolic pressure and eccentric cardiac hypertrophy has not yet had time to augment the increase in total stroke volume.

As shown in Table 6-3, an examination of systolic mechanics at this point shows that contractile function and afterload remain normal. Preload is increased greatly as the increased left ventricular filling pressure increases sarcomere stretch. Increased preload is a compensatory mechanism that helps increase total left ventricular stroke volume, a portion of which helps compensate for the decrease in forward stroke volume. However, this compensatory mechanism is not adequate to fully restore normal forward cardiac output.

Chronic Compensated Aortic Regurgitation

Whereas most patients subjected to the above events will require immediate aortic valve replacement, an occasional patient either will not require it because CHF has not occurred or the patient is deemed not to be a surgical candidate. Such a patient may then adapt to his or her chronic aortic regurgitation and become chronically compensated. As shown in Table 6-3, eccentric cardiac hypertrophy now has occurred, which increases left ventricular end-diastolic volume. Preload is still increased, but because total myocardial volume also has increased, left ventricular filling pressure can be relatively less. Contractility is still normal. Increased left ventricular volume also increases left ventricular systolic pressure. Increased pressure combined with increased radius increases systolic wall stress (afterload), which opposes ventricular contraction, leading to increased end-systolic volume. However, the increased preload offsets this afterload mismatch, and ejection performance remains normal. During the chronic compensated phase, increased preload together with eccentric cardiac hypertrophy allow for normalization of forward stroke volume and a return toward normal filling pressure. Under these circumstances the patient should be relatively asymptomatic.

Chronic Decompensated Aortic Regurgitation

Although volume overload may be tolerated for a long period of time, eventually contractile function fails. At this point the patient enters a chronic decompensated phase. The reduction in contractility produces an increase in end-systolic volume, reducing total and forward stroke volumes and ejection fraction (Table 6-3). There is further cardiac dilatation, which increases left ventricular radius, which further increases afterload, impairing left ventricular function. Left ventricular filling pressure is re-elevated. If the left ventricular dysfunction is mild or of short duration, aortic valve replacement can lead to improvement in ventricular performance (67–69). Improved ventricular performance after correction of aortic regurgitation probably results from afterload reduction (as ventricular radius and pressure return toward normal) as well as restoration of contractility (70–72). If left

TABLE 6-3
HEMODYNAMICS AND MECHANICS IN AORTIC REGURGITATION

	Base	AAR	CCAR	CDAR
EDV (cc)	150	180	270	300
ESV (cc)	50	50	70	150
Ejection fraction	0.67	0.72	0.74	0.50
Regurgitant fraction	0	0.50	0.50	0.50
TSV (cc)	100	130	200	150
FSV (cc)	100	65	100	75
LVP mm Hg	120/10	120/50	180/20	170/40
AoP mm Hg	120/80	120/60	180/70	170/70
Preload	Normal	↑↑↑	↑↑↑	↑↑↑
Afterload	Normal	Normal	↑	↑↑
Contractility	Normal	Normal	Normal	↑
LVH	Absent	Absent	↑↑↑	↑↑↑

AAR, acute aortic regurgitation; AoP, aortic pressure; Base, baseline state; CCAR, chronic compensated aortic regurgitation; CDAR, chronic decompensated aortic regurgitation; EDV, end-diastolic volume; ESV, end-systolic volume; FSV, forward stroke volume; LVH, left ventricular hypertrophy; LVP, left ventricular pressure; TSV, total stroke volume.

ventricular dysfunction is severe or prolonged, left ventricular performance remains depressed after surgery. Table 6-4 is a partial list of systolic indexes that have proven useful in predicting outcome for this disease.

Example 2: Idiopathic Dilated Cardiomyopathy

The changes in left ventricular mechanics produced by idiopathic dilated cardiomyopathy are demonstrated in the stress–volume loops depicted in Figure 6-14. Compared with normal, the patient with idiopathic dilated cardiomyopathy has a much lower ejection fraction, a much larger left ventricle, and higher afterload (wall stress). Although single stress–volume loops do not enable the assessment of contractile function, one can infer that contractile function must be reduced severely because afterload is not elevated enough to cause this severe reduction in ejection fraction; also, preload is almost surely increased, which would act to increase ejection fraction.

This figure also demonstrates the mechanisms by which vasodilator therapy improves function in this condition. Afterload (wall stress = $p \times r/2h$) is reduced when vasodilatation reduces resistance to ejection, thereby permitting the left ventricular radius to become smaller and wall thickening to increase. Systolic blood pressure is also reduced. The decrease in pressure and radius components of the stress equation, together with increased thickening due to enhanced shortening, all act in concert to reduce afterload. Reduced afterload allows for greater ejection of blood from the left ventricle, increasing cardiac output. Because the diastolic portion of the stress–volume relationship is on the steep part of its curve, diastolic stress (and diastolic pressure) can be reduced without significantly reducing end-diastolic volume. This allows for maintenance of the gain in stroke volume produced by afterload reduction, while at the same time reducing pulmonary congestion.

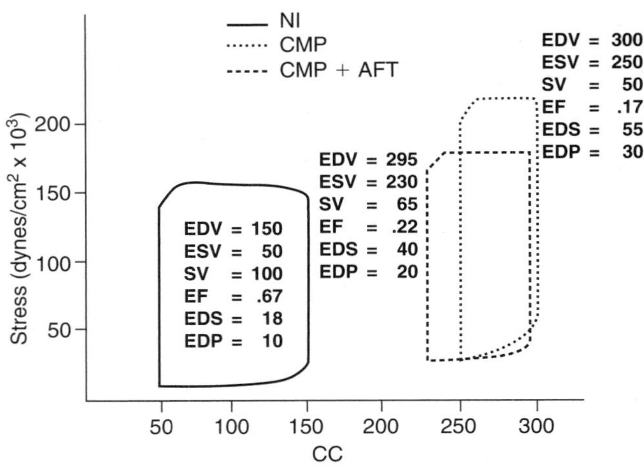

Figure 6-14 Stress volume–loops from a normal (nl) person and a patient with dilated cardiomyopathy (CMP) before and after afterload reduction therapy (CMP + AFT) are demonstrated. EDP, end-diastolic pressure; EDV, end-diastolic volume; EDS, end-diastolic stress; EF, ejection fraction; ESV, end-systolic volume; SV, stroke volume.

SUMMARY

In the complete assessment of systolic function in any given patient, preload, afterload, contractility, and myocardial mass should be evaluated. Unfortunately, this is not practical in everyday clinical practice. Contractility is a key determinant of prognosis in most cardiac diseases. However, measurements of contractile function in patients with cardiac disease are laborious and have not gained wide clinical acceptance. Because many current indexes of contractile function require load manipulation for their development, these measurements will probably continue to be limited to use as research tools. It should be noted that there has been a marked decline in the number of published papers examining contractile function since 1995. This decline may have occurred because of a general lack of acceptance of tediously derived indexes in clinical practice. Alternatively, reduced interest in indexes of contractility may stem from the fact that most cases of systolic heart failure are due either to coronary disease and myocardial infarction, or to idiopathic dilated cardiomyopathy—cases in which the reduction in contractile function is obvious and accurately predicted by ejection fraction. In the absence of an easily obtained clinical measure of contractile function, evaluation of ejection fraction often is substituted for evaluation of contractile function. In situations such as coronary disease, where loading is relatively normal, ejection fraction closely follows contractile function and is useful in the assessment of contractility and prognosis. However, in conditions such as valvular heart disease, where loading can be extremely abnormal, load must be taken into account. In such situations, use of preload-independent indexes such as end-systolic volume or dimension may be superior to ejection phase indexes in predicting outcome.

TABLE 6-4
SYSTOLIC INDEXES AS PREDICTORS OF OUTCOME IN CHRONIC AORTIC REGURGITATION

Index	Cutoff for Good Outcome	Reference
End-systolic dimension	<50 mm	26, 54
End-systolic volume	<110 cc/m^2	29, 58
Ejection fraction	>.45	54
Shortening fraction	.23–.27	26,52

Cardiology is entering an era of cell and gene therapy. It is likely that at least in the early phases, changes in cardiac function effected by insertion of a new gene or of viable myocytes or their progenitors will be modest and difficult to detect. The need to evaluate these therapies carefully is likely to once again focus interest upon accurate assessment of systolic function.

REFERENCES

1. Carabello BA, Green LH, Grossman W, et al. Hemodynamic determinants of prognosis of aortic valve replacement in critical aortic stenosis and advanced congestive heart failure. *Circulation.* 1980;62:42–8.
2. Huber D, Grimm J, Koch R, et al. Determinants of ejection performance in aortic stenosis. *Circulation.* 1981;64:126–34.
3. Starling EH. *Linacre Lecture on the Law of the Heart.* London: Longmans, Green and Co.; 1915.
4. Gordon AM, Huxley AF, Julian FJ. Tension development in highly stretched vertebrate muscle fibres. *J Physiol.* 1966;184:143–169.
5. Spotnitz HM, Sonnenblick EH, Spiro D. Relation of ultrastructure to function in the intact heart: sarcomere structure relative to pressure volume curves of intact left ventricles of dog and cat. *Circ Res.* 1966;18:49–66.
6. Gaasch WH, Battle WE, Oboler AA, et al. Left ventricular stress and compliance in man. With special reference to normalized ventricular function curves. *Circulation.* 1972;45:746–762.
7. Ross J, Jr. Afterload mismatch and preload reserve: a conceptual framework for analysis of ventricular function. *Prog Cardiovasc Dis.* 1976;18:255–264.
8. Lang RM, Borow KM, Neumann A, et al. Systemic vascular resistance: an unreliable index of left ventricular afterload. *Circulation* 1986;74:1114–1123.
9. Wolk MJ, Keefe JF, Bing OHL, et al. Estimation of V_{max} in auxotonic systoles from the rate of relative increase of isovolumic pressure: (dP/dt)/kP. *J Clin Invest.* 1971;50:1276–1285.
10. Mahler F, Ross J, Jr., O'Rourke RA, et al. Effects of changes in preload, afterload and inotropic state in ejection and isovolumic phase measures of contractility in the conscious dog. *Am J Cardiol.* 1975;35:626–634.
11. Grossman W, Haymes F, Paraskos JA, et al. Alterations in preload and myocardial mechanics in the dog and in man. *Circ Res.* 1972;31:83–94.
12. Peterson KL, Skloven D, Ludbrook P, et al. Comparison of isovolumic and ejection phase indices of myocardial performance in man. *Circulation.* 1974;49:1088–1101.
13. Kreulen TH, Bove AA, McDonough MT, et al. The evaluation of left ventricular function in man. A comparison of methods. *Circulation.* 1975;51:677–688.
14. Nemoto S, Defreitas G, Mann DL, et al. Effects of changes in left ventricular contractility on indexes of contractility in mice. *Am J Physiol Circ Physiol.* 2002;283:H2504–H2510.
15. Cohn PF, Gorlin R, Cohn LH, et al. Left ventricular ejection fraction as a prognostic guide in surgical treatment of coronary and valvular heart disease. *Am J Cardiol.* 1974;34:136–141.
16. Quinones MA, Gaasch WH, Alexander JK. Influence of acute changes in preload, afterload, contractile state and heart rate on ejection and isovolumic indices of myocardial contractility in man. *Circulation.* 1976;53:293–302.
17. Mirsky I, Tajimi T, Peterson KL. The development of the entire end-systolic pressure-volume and ejection fraction-afterload relations: a new concept of systolic myocardial stiffness. *Circulation.* 1987;76:343–356.
18. de Simone G, Devereux RB. Rationale of echocardiographic assessment of left ventricular wall stress and midwall mechanics in hypertensive heart disease. *Eur J Echocardiogr.* 2002;3: 192–198.
19. Wong CY, Spotnitz HM. Systolic and diastolic properties of the human left ventricle during valve replacement for chronic mitral regurgitation. *Am J Cardiol.* 1981;47:40–50.
20. Wisenbaugh T, Spann JF, Carabello BA. Differences in myocardial performance and load between patients with similar amounts of chronic aortic versus chronic mitral regurgitation. *J Am Coll Cardiol.* 1984;3:916–923.
21. Carabello BA, Nolan SP, McGuire LB. Assessment of preoperative left ventricular function in patients with mitral regurgitation: value of the end-systolic wall stress-end-systolic volume ratio. *Circulation.* 1981;64:1212–1217.
22. Gunther S, Grossman W. Determinants of ventricular function in pressure-overload hypertrophy in man. *Circulation.* 1979;59: 679–688.
23. Nixon JV, Murray RG, Leonard PD, et al. Effect of large variations in preload on left ventricular performance characteristics in normal subjects. *Circulation.* 1982;65:698–703.
24. Colan SD, Borow KM, Neumann A. Left ventricular end-systolic wall stress-velocity of fiber shortening relation: a load-independent index of myocardial contractility. *J Am Coll Cardiol.* 1984;4:715–724.
25. Suga H, Sagawa K, Shoukas AA. Load independence of the instantaneous pressure-volume ratio of the canine left ventricle and effects of epinephrine and heart rate on the ratio. *Circ Res.* 1973;32:314–322.
26. Henry WL, Bonow RO, Borer JS, et al. Observations on the optimum time for operative intervention for aortic regurgitation. I. Evaluation of the results of aortic valve replacement in symptomatic patients. *Circulation.* 1980;61:484–492.
27. Borow KM, Green LH, Mann T, et al. End-systolic volume as a predictor of postoperative left ventricular performance in volume overload from valvular regurgitation. *Am J Med.* 1980;68: 665–663.
28. Zile MR, Gaasch WH, Carroll JD, et al. Chronic mitral regurgitation: predictive value of preoperative echocardiographic indexes of left ventricular function and wall stress. *J Am Coll Cardiol.* 1984;3:235–242.
29. Carabello BA, Williams H, Gash AK, et al. Hemodynamic predictors of outcome in patients undergoing valve replacement. *Circulation.* 1986;74:1309–1316.
30. Carabello BA. Ratio of end-systolic to end-systolic volume: is it a useful clinical tool? [Editorial] *J Am Coll Cardiol.* 1989;14: 496–498.
31. Wisenbaugh T, Yu G, Evans J. The superiority of maximum fiber elastance over maximum stress-volume ratio as an index of contractile state. *Circulation.* 1985;72:648–653.
32. Morgan DE, Tomlinson CW, Qayumi AK, et al. Evaluation of ventricular contractility indexes in the dog with left ventricular dysfunction induced by rapid atrial pacing. *J Am Coll Cardiol.* 1989;14:489–495.
33. Daughters GT, Derby GC, Alderman EL, et al. Independence of left ventricular pressure-volume ratio from preload in man early after coronary artery bypass graft surgery. *Circulation.* 1985;71: 945–950.
34. Denenberg BS, Criner G, Jones R, et al. Cardiac function in sickle cell anemia. *Am J Cardiol.* 1983;51:1674–1678.
35. Troy AD, Chakko CS, Gash AK, et al. Left ventricular function in systemic hypertension. *J Cardiovasc Ultrasounogr.* 1983;2:251–257.
36. Ramanathan KB, Knowles J, Connor MJ, et al. Natural history of chronic mitral insufficiency: relation of peak systolic pressure/end-systolic volume ratio to morbidity and mortality. *J Am Coll Cardiol.* 1984;3:1412–1416.
37. Dehmer GJ, Lewis SE, Hillis LD, et al. Exercise-induced alterations in left ventricular volumes and the pressure-volume relationship: a sensitive indicator of left ventricular dysfunction in patients with coronary artery disease. *Circulation.* 1981;63:1008–1018.
38. Wilson MF, Sung BH, Herbst CP, et al. Evaluation of left ventricular contractility indexes for the detection of symptomatic and silent myocardial ischemia. *Am J Cardiol.* 1988;62:1176–1179.
39. Gibbons RJ, Clements IP, Zinsmeister AR, et al. Exercise response of the systolic pressure to end-systolic volume ratio in patients with coronary artery disease. *J Am Coll Cardiol.* 1987;10:33–39.
40. El-Tobgi S, Fouad FM, Kramer JR, et al. Left ventricular function in coronary artery disease. Evaluation of slope of end-systolic pressure-volume line (E_{max}) and ratio of peak systolic pressure to end-systolic volume (P/V_{es}). *J Am Coll Cardiol.* 1984;3:781–788.
41. Little WC, Cheng CP, Peterson T, et al. Response of the left ventricular end-systolic pressure-volume relation in conscious dogs to a wide range of contractile states. *Circulation.* 1988;78:736–745.
42. Kono A, Maughan WL, Sunagawa K, et al. The use of left ventricular end-ejection pressure and peak pressure in the estimation of

the end-systolic pressure-volume relationship. *Circulation.* 1984;70:1057–1065.

43. Burkhoff D, Sugiura S, Yue DT, et al. Contractility-dependent curvilinearity of end-systolic pressure-volume relations. *Am J Physiol.* 1987;252:H1218–H1227.
44. Kass DA, Beyar R, Lankford E, et al. Influence of contractile state on curvilinearity of in situ end-systolic pressure-volume relations. *Circulation.* 1989;79:167–178.
45. Carabello BA, Nakano K, Corin W, et al. Left ventricular function in experimental volume overload hypertrophy. *Am J Physiol.* 1989;256:H974–H981.
46. Corin WJ, Swindle MM, Spann JF, Jr., et al. Mechanism of decreased forward stroke volume in children and swine with ventricular septal defect and failure to thrive. *J Clin Invest.* 1988;82:544–551.
47. Suga H, Hisano R, Goto Y, et al. Normalization of end-systolic pressure volume relation and E_{max} of different sized hearts. *Jpn Circ J.* 1984;48:136–143.
48. Belcher P, Boerboom LE, Olinger GN. Standardization of end-systolic pressure-volume relation in the dog. *Am J Physiol.* 1985;249:H547–H553.
49. Berko B, Gaasch WH, Tanigawa N, et al. Disparity between ejection and end-systolic indexes of left ventricular contractility in mitral regurgitation. *Circulation.* 1987;75:1310–1319.
50. Starling MR, Walsh RA, Dell'Italia LJ, et al. The relationship of various measures of end-systole to left ventricular maximum time-varying elastance in man. *Circulation.* 1987;76: 32–43.
51. Nakano K, Sugawara M, Ishihara K, et al. Myocardial stiffness derived from end-systolic wall stress and the logarithm of the reciprocal of wall thickness: a contractility index independent of ventricular size. *Circulation.* 1990;82:1352–1361.
52. Glower DD, Spratt JA, Snow ND, et al. Linearity of the Frank-Starling relationship on the intact heart: the concept of preload recruitable stroke work. *Circulation.* 1985;71:994–1009.
53. Urabe Y, Mann DL, Kent RL, et al. Cellular and ventricular contractile dysfunction in experimental canine mitral regurgitation. *Circ Res.* 1992;70:131–147.
54. Koide M, Nagatsu M, Zile MR, et al. Premorbid determinants of left ventricular dysfunction in a novel model of gradually induced pressure overload in the adult canine. *Circulation* 1997;95:1601–1610.
55. Sutherland GR, Stewart MJ, Groundstroem KWE, et al. Color Doppler myocardial imaging: a new technique for assessment of myocardial function. *J Echocardiogr.* 1994;7:441–448.
56. Miyatake K, Yamagishi M, Tanaka N, et al. New method of evaluating left ventricular wall motion by color-coded tissue Doppler imaging: in vitro and in vivo studies. *J Am Coll Cardiol.* 1995;25:717–724.
57. Hoffman R, Altiok E, Nowak B, et al. Strain rate measurement by Doppler echocardiography allows improved assessment of myocardial viability in patients with depressed left ventricular function. *JACC.* 2002;39:443–449.
58. Yip G, Wang M, Zhang Y, et al. Left ventricular long axis function in diastolic heart failure is reduced in both diastole and systole: time for a redefinition? *Heart.* 2002;87:121–125.
59. Braunwald E, Ross J, Jr., Sonnenblick EH, eds. *Mechanisms of Contraction of the Normal and Failing Heart.* 2nd ed. Boston: Little, Brown; 1972: 77.
60. Sagawa K, Suga H, Shoukas AA, et al. End-systolic pressure/volume ratio: a new index of ventricular contractility. *Am J Cardiol.* 1977;40:748–753.
61. Carabello BA. Cardiac catheterization. In: Parmley WW, Chatterjee K, eds. *Cardiology*. Vol. 1. Physiology, pharmacology, diagnosis. Philadelphia: JB Lippincott; 1990:11.
62. Wang M, Yip GW, Wang AY, et al. Tissue Doppler imaging provides incremental prognostic value in patients with systemic hypertension and left ventricular hypertrophy. *J Hypertens.* 2005;23:183–191.
63. Lima JA, Jeremy R, Guier W, et al. Accurate systolic wall thickening by nuclear magnetic resonance imaging with tissue tagging: correlation with sonomicrometers in normal and ischemic myocardium. *J Am Coll Cardiol.* 1993;21:1741–1751.
64. Yeon SB, Reichek N, Tallant BA, et al. Validation of in vivo myocardial strain measurement by magnet resonance tagging in sonomicrometry. *J Am Coll Cardiol.* 2001;38:555–561.
65. Tei C, Lieng HL, Hodge DO, et al. New index of combined systolic and diastolic myocardial performance: a simple and reproducible measure of cardiac function—a study in normals and dilated cardiomyopathy. *J Cardiol.* 1995;26:357–366.
66. Tei C, Dujardin KS, Hodge DO, et al. Doppler index combining systolic and diastolic myocardial performance: clinical value in cardiac amyloidosis. *J Am Coll Cardiol.* 1996;28:65–66.
67. Bonow RO, Rosing DR, Maron BJ, et al. Reversal of left ventricular dysfunction after aortic valve replacement for chronic aortic regurgitation: influence of duration of preoperative left ventricular dysfunction. *Circulation.* 1984;70:570–579.
68. Carabello BA, Usher BW, Hendrix GH, et al. Predictors of outcome in patients with aortic regurgitation and left ventricular dysfunction: a change in the measuring stick. *J Am Coll Cardiol.* 1987;10:991–997.
69. Bonow RO, Dodd JT, Maron BJ, et al. Long-term serial changes in left ventricular function and reversal of ventricular dilatation after valve replacement for chronic aortic regurgitation. *Circulation.* 1988;78:1108–1120.
70. Taniguchi K, Nakano S, Kawashima Y, et al. Left ventricular ejection performance, wall stress, and contractile state in aortic regurgitation before and after aortic valve replacement. *Circulation.* 1990;82:798–807.
71. Carabello BA. Aortic regurgitation. A lesion with similarities to both aortic stenosis and mitral regurgitation [Editorial]. *Circulation.* 1990;82:1051–1053.
72. Taniguchi K, Nakano S, Hirose H, et al. Preoperative left ventricular function: minimal requirement for successful late results of valve replacement for aortic regurgitation. *J Am Coll Cardiol.* 1987;10:510–518.

7

Heart Failure with Normal Ejection Fraction

Carolyn S. P. Lam   Margaret M. Redfield

Heart failure (HF) may be defined as the inability of the heart to pump adequate blood volume relative to the metabolic needs of the body or to do so only at abnormally elevated filling pressures, with resultant congestion. Heart failure is not a single disease entity but, rather, a clinical syndrome associated with a number of cardiac abnormalities which may include impairment of valvular, systolic, diastolic, or pericardial function. The diagnosis of HF is based upon clinical signs and symptoms along with evidence of congestion on the chest radiograph. The syndrome was described and its poor prognostic implications recognized prior to the routine assessment of systolic performance by measurement of the ejection fraction (EF) (1). The most enduring diagnostic criteria established for HF, the Framingham criteria, have never included EF, and yet these criteria have served well over time and consistently identify patients with a high prevalence of cardiovascular disease and a uniformly poor prognosis associated with similar modes of death (2,3).

The predominance of systemic and pulmonary congestion in the clinical presentation of HF first directed investigators and clinicians to consider HF as a disorder of volume regulation, the so-called cardiorenal paradigm of HF (4). As contrast ventriculography, radionuclide ventriculography, and echocardiography became available, the syndrome of HF began to be equated with a reduced EF and treatment strategies focused on HF as a syndrome of contractile dysfunction. This has been referred to as the hemodynamic paradigm of HF. During this era, certain rare conditions were recognized to produce the HF syndrome despite preserved EF. However, the possibility that large numbers of patients with HF may have normal EF (HFnlEF) was never entertained.

Because numerous studies have now demonstrated that HFnlEF is very common, the reasons why it was not previously recognized are unclear. Referral bias may play a major role as methods to assess EF were first available to academic and referral centers. Such centers serve a younger and more predominantly male population, a subgroup with a lower prevalence of HFnlEF. Alternatively, it is also very possible that the prevalence of HFnlEF has increased over time, leading to its widespread recognition only as its prevalence increased. Unfortunately, the impact of referral bias and secular trends on the type of HF patients are developing (reduced versus normal EF) has never been studied, but several factors could contribute to an increased prevalence.

The percent of the population over 65 years of age has increased both due to the baby boom phenomenon and to a reduction in mortality from noncardiovascular and cardiovascular causes. Because HFnlEF (even more so than HF in general) is a disease of the elderly, the increased number of older persons and, particularly, older persons with cardiovascular disease could contribute to increases in prevalence of HFnlEF. Access to cardiologists for older persons has also increased and could contribute to increases in recognition of HFnlEF in recent years. Finally, one could also speculate that advances in the treatment of hypertension and coronary disease have modified but not prevented vascular and cardiac remodeling and dysfunction in such a manner as to preserve EF but not prevent vascular stiffening, diastolic dysfunction, or volume overload—all mechanisms postulated to lead to HFnlEF.

Whatever the reason, the fact that academic cardiologists and HF specialists had not recognized or been exposed to large numbers of patients with HFnlEF led to considerable skepticism regarding HFnlEF, despite growing epidemiological evidence of its importance. Controversy regarding the existence and prevalence of HFnlEF has largely but not completely abated. Many questions persist due to our lack of knowledge regarding the pathogenesis, natural history, and appropriate therapy for HFnlEF. For example, how HFnlEF fits into the neurohumoral paradigm of HF remains to be defined. There are few data concerning the neurohumoral profile of HFnlEF or the impact of neurohumoral antagonists on outcomes in HFnlEF. Happily, these issues are beginning to be addressed. This chapter summarizes what is currently known regarding HFnlEF, but the authors are careful to emphasize that our understanding of this syndrome is incomplete and will continue to evolve as the field advances.

NOMENCLATURE

There is controversy over proper nomenclature to use for HFnlEF. Alternative terms that have been used to divide patients with HF into two groups have included diastolic versus systolic HF, HF with preserved versus reduced systolic function, and HF with normal versus reduced EF. These three sets of terms were used interchangeably in the literature to date, but controversy over the most appropriate terminology arose as interest in the field expanded.

Diastolic Heart Failure

The term diastolic heart failure (DHF) was proposed to underscore the fundamental difference in pathophysiological mechanisms believed to cause HF in these patients, as opposed to patients with HF and reduced EF (HF↓EF), which was referred to as systolic heart failure (SHF). The term implies that HFnlEF is due to diastolic dysfunction. However, in practice there is frequently no assessment of diastolic function in patients with HFnlEF. Diastolic function is difficult to measure and there are no clear diastolic dysfunction criteria considered pathognomonic for HFnlEF. Furthermore, patients with HFnlEF often have coexistent abnormalities in systolic function, and diastolic dysfunction clearly contributes to the pathophysiology of HF↓EF. With this overlap, the term is less useful to clearly separate HF patients into two groups. The SHF/DHF distinction is easy to use and is well-recognized and supported by some studies. Although some investigators argue for a major role of diastolic dysfunction in most, if not all, patients with HFnlEF (5), others argue that the term DHF should not be applied unless or until diastolic dysfunction is proven to be the predominant mechanism in all patients with HFnlEF (6).

Heart Failure with Preserved Systolic Function

This term is also suboptimal because it is still unclear as to whether or not systolic function is indeed preserved in patients with HFnlEF. Various reports have suggested increased, unchanged, or reduced systolic function in patients with HFnlEF depending on which index is used to assess systolic function. In addition, a normal EF does not necessarily mean that myocardial contractility is normal.

Heart Failure with Normal Ejection Fraction

EF measurement makes no assumptions regarding pathophysiological mechanisms; it is clinically useful and has been the basis of inclusion for most HF clinical studies. This term has been used in the revised American College of Cardiology/American Heart Association (ACC/AHA) HF guidelines (7). The term HFnlEF will therefore be used for the purposes of this chapter. However, it should be noted that EF is a continuous variable with a normal distribution within the population, and the threshold value to define normal versus reduced EF is arbitrary. There is no clear consensus in published literature regarding an optimal cut-off value to discriminate between patients in whom systolic dysfunction is the primary mechanism responsible for the patient's HF symptoms. Indeed, as diastolic dysfunction contributes potently to symptoms and prognosis among patients with reduced EF, this terminology does not clearly distinguish the pathophysiological mechanisms involved. In support of this terminology, patients with an EF $<40\%$ and HF symptoms have been proven to derive symptomatic and survival benefit from a number of therapies, whereas benefit is unclear in those with EF $>40\%$. While consensus seems to be building toward use of an EF $\geq 50\%$ to designate HFnlEF, the proper designation of and treatment approach to patients with borderline (40% to 50%) EF adds to the complexity of the classification.

Ideally, the HF population should be divided according to pathophysiology, which, in turn, will form the basis of differential therapeutic strategies. Future nomenclature may become complicated as multiple pathophysiological mechanisms may become defined in HFnlEF. A greater understanding of the syndrome should ultimately lead to selection of terminology which reflects the underlying pathophysiological mechanisms and aids in investigating and developing therapeutic modalities.

DO PATIENTS WITH HFnlEF HAVE HEART FAILURE?

Clinical Features

Early studies compared clinical features between HF patients with normal versus reduced EF. Both Dougherty et al. (8) and Echeverria et al. (9) concluded from their respective series of HF patients that neither history, physical examination, nor chest roentgenographic findings were able to distinguish patients with normal versus reduced EF. Similarly, Aguirre et al. (10) reported that no single clinical parameter (e.g., exertional dyspnea, orthopnea, paroxysmal nocturnal dyspnea, edema, rales, jugular venous distension, S_3 or S_4 gallop) was found to discriminate between HFnlEF or HF↓EF in their series of patients with HF. Of the established clinical diagnostic criteria for HF (Framingham, Boston, or Duke criteria), none had a high sensitivity or specificity for discerning which HF patients had reduced

EF (11). More recent publications also corroborate these findings (12) and establish that decompensated HF with normal versus reduced EF are clinically indistinguishable.

Pathophysiological Features

The pathophysiological domains that characterize classic HF were studied by Kitzman et al. (13) in stable outpatients with a clinical diagnosis of HF and normal or reduced EF and age- and sex-matched healthy controls. The four key domains examined included left ventricular (LV) structure and function, exercise performance, neuroendocrine function, and quality of life (Table 7-1 and Fig. 7-1). Patients with HFnlEF were shown to have similar pathophysiological characteristics compared to patients with HF↓EF, including severely reduced exercise capacity, neuroendocrine activation, and impaired quality of life. These similar characteristics were found despite a unique LV structural and functional profile in the patients with HFnlEF, including normal LVEF, normal LV volume, and an increased LV mass to volume ratio. It must be noted that this study was performed in stable outpatients; quality of life, exercise parameters, and neurohumoral function may be more severely perturbed in more symptomatic patients studied in a hospital setting. Nonetheless, by demonstrating perturbations in these key components of the HF syndrome, the validity of the term HF in patients with HFnlEF is therefore established. This is one of the first studies to demonstrate activation of the sympathetic nervous system and the naturietic peptide system in HFnlEF. Unfortunately, characterizations of the renin-angiotensin-aldosterone system, endothelin, and cytokines in HFnlEF were not provided and remain important areas for future studies.

Epidemiologic Features

As reviewed in more detail later, several epidemiological and clinical studies have compared mortality rates in patients with HFnlEF and HF↓EF (14,15). On aggregate, the studies suggest that survival rates are nearly similar between these groups of HF patients; mortality differences, when present, are relatively minor. It should also be emphasized that compared to age-matched controls, mortality risk is clearly higher in patients with HFnlEF. As for morbidity, available comparative studies of hospital readmission rates in patients with HFnlEF versus reduced EF indicate that the readmission rates are almost identical. In a prospective study of 413 patients hospitalized for HF, Smith et al. (16) compared hospital readmission and changes in functional status in HF patients with preserved (EF $\geq$40%) versus depressed EF. After 6 months, the rates of functional decline were similar among those with preserved and depressed EF (30% versus 23%, respectively; $p = 0.14$). After adjusting for demographic and clinical covariates, there was no difference in the risk of readmission (HR 1.01; 95% CI 0.72 to 1.43; $p = 0.96$) or the odds of functional decline or death (OR 1.01; 95% CI 0.59 to 1.72; $p = 0.97$) between HF patients with preserved versus reduced EF. Thus, HFnlEF confers a considerable burden on patients with the risk of readmission, disability, and symptoms subsequent to hospital discharge, comparable to that of HF patients with reduced EF. These studies establish that patients with HFnlEF do indeed have HF, with similar implications for their quality and quantity of life as seen with HF↓EF.

Finally, it should be recognized that the diagnostic criteria for HF are somewhat nonspecific and other conditions can mimic HF clinically, particularly in elderly patients. Thus, it is likely that misdiagnosis as HF occurs in a subset of patients labeled as HFnlEF. However, the studies summarized throughout this chapter suggest that this is not common.

PATHOPHYSIOLOGY OF HFNLEF

As established in patients with systolic dysfunction, HF is a progressive syndrome characterized by complex cardiac and

TABLE 7-1

KEY PATHOPHYSIOLOGICAL DOMAINS IN HEART FAILURE WITH NORMAL OR REDUCED EJECTION FRACTION

				p Value	
Characteristic	**Controls (n = 28)**	**HF↓EF (n = 60)**	**HFnlEF (n = 59)**	**HFnlEF Versus Controls**	**HFnlEF Versus HF↓EF**
Age, mean (SD), y	68 (5)	70 (6)	70 (7)	0.34	0.83
Women, No. (%)	17 (63)	21 (35)	51 (86)	0.02	0.001
Body mass index, mean (SD)	24 (3)	26 (4)	30 (6)	0.001	0.001
LVEDV, mean (SE), mL	102 (12)	192 (10)	87 (10)	0.32	0.001
LV mass/volume ratio mean (SE)	1.49 (0.17)	1.22 (0.14)	2.12 (0.14)	0.002	0.001
Relative VO_2, mL/kg per min	19.9 (0.7)	13.1 (0.5)	14.2 (0.5)	0.001	0.12
6-minute walk, mean (SE), ft	1,802 (87)	1,356 (58)	1,430 (60)	0.001	0.28
MLHFQ total mean (SE)	—	43.8 (3.9)	24.8 (4.4)	—	0.002

SD, standard deviation; LV, left ventricular; LVEDV, left ventricular end-diastolic volume; VO_2, oxygen consumption; MLHFQ, Minnesota Living with Heart Failure Questionnaire (higher score indicates worse quality of life).
From Kitzman DW, Little WC, Brubaker PH, et al. Pathophysiological characterization of isolated diastolic heart failure in comparison to systolic heart failure. *JAMA.* 2002;288(17):2144–2150.

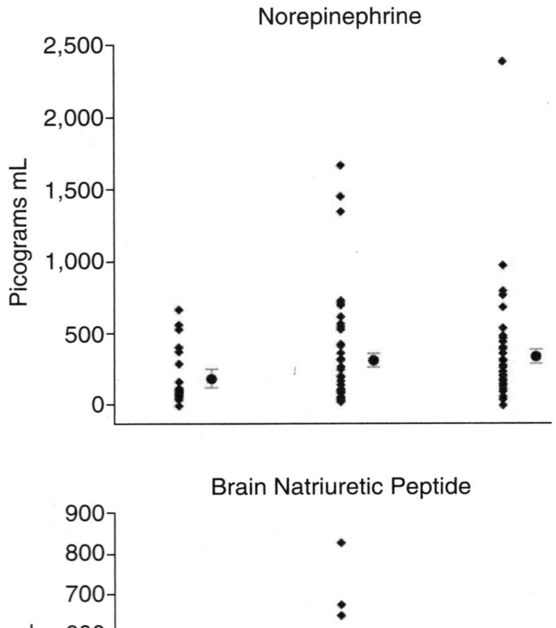

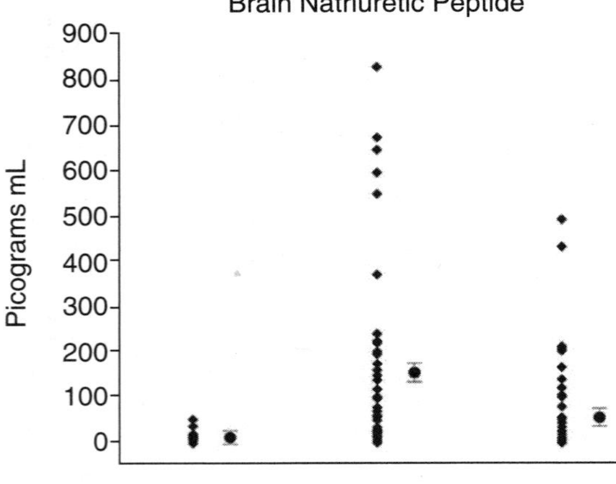

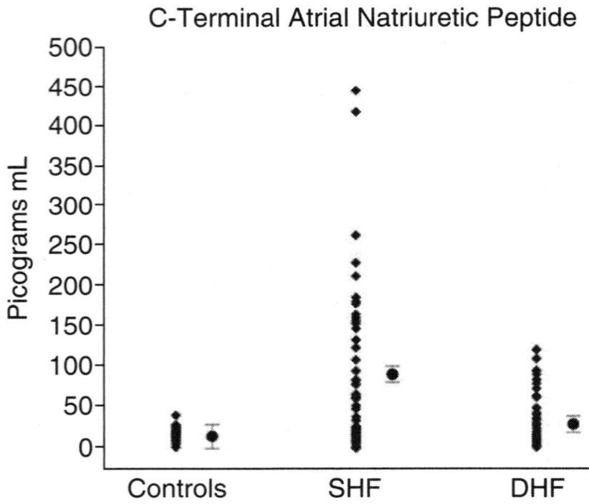

Figure 7-1 Neuroendocrine function in healthy subjects without heart failure (Controls) and in stable outpatients with HF↓EF (SHF) or HFnlEF (DHF). (From Kitzman DW, Little WC, Brubaker PH, et al. Pathophysiological characterization of isolated diastolic heart failure in comparison to systolic heart failure. *JAMA*. 2002;288(17): 2144–2150.)

systemic adaptations that vary over time. In patients with HF↓EF, a regional or global myocardial insult leads to systolic and diastolic dysfunction, LV remodeling (hypertrophy, fibrosis, and dilatation), local and systemic neurohumoral and cytokine activation, impairment of renal hemodynamic and excretory function, and vascular dysfunction. Prognostic hemodynamic subgroups are based on relative derangement in cardiac output, filling pressures, and systemic vascular resistance. Chronic elevation of left atrial pressures leads to right heart failure. Progression is modulated by comorbidities, particularly coronary and renal disease. These insights have directed development of therapeutic strategies ultimately proven in clinical trials. This process is incomplete, and genomic and proteomic paradigms for HF pathophysiology will continue to evolve.

Whether patients with HFnlEF share most pathophysiological mechanisms with HF↓EF remains to be established. The first step in this process is to understand the fundamental abnormality in ventricular function that causes (or at least accompanies) the clinical syndrome. Three theories regarding the perturbations in cardiovascular function responsible for HFnlEF have emerged. Importantly, each theory is not exclusive of the others. Multiple mechanisms may contribute in any given patient although it may be that one is predominant in some patients and others predominate in other patients. These theories are: (a) HFnlEF is due to intrinsic diastolic dysfunction (impaired relaxation and increased diastolic stiffness); (b) HFnlEF is due to increased vascular and ventricular systolic stiffness associated with enhanced sensitivity to volume and load/stress-induced diastolic dysfunction; and (c) HFnlEF is due to ventricular remodeling characterized by LV dilatation with volume-dependent elevation of filling pressures unassociated with significantly altered diastolic stiffness or impaired relaxation. Each of these theories will be discussed in turn.

HFnlEF Is Due to Intrinsic Diastolic Dysfunction

Consideration of the role of diastolic dysfunction in HFnlEF mandates clear understanding of diastolic function. Normal diastolic function allows the ventricle to fill adequately during both rest and exercise without an abnormal increase in diastolic pressures. The phases of diastole are isovolumic relaxation and the filling phase. The filling phase is divided into early rapid filling, diastasis, and atrial systole. Early rapid filling contributes 70% to 80% of LV filling in normal individuals, and this contribution diminishes with age and a variety of disease states. Early diastolic filling is driven by the left atrial (LA) to LV pressure gradient, which is dependent on a complex interplay of factors: myocardial relaxation, passive elastic properties of LV, LV elastic recoil, LV contractile state, LA pressures, ventricular interaction, pericardial constraint, elasticity of LA, pulmonary veins, and mitral orifice area. Diastasis is the period of diastole when the LA and LV pressures are usually nearly equal. It contributes less than 5% of the LV filling and its duration shortens with tachycardia. In normal subjects atrial systole contributes 15% to 25% of LV diastolic filling without raising the mean left atrial pressure. This contribution depends on the PR interval, atrial inotropic state, atrial preload, atrial afterload, autonomic tone, and heart rate (17).

Assessment of diastolic function is obtained with invasive diagnostic techniques (cardiac catheterization) or noninvasive imaging modalities (echocardiography, radionuclide angiography). Recent reviews have provided extensive analyses of the invasive and noninvasive assessment of LV diastolic function (17–21). Features of the invasive and Doppler echocardiographic assessment of diastolic function will be further discussed.

Left Ventricular Relaxation

While diastolic function is influenced by all the factors referred to above, its primary determinants are LV relaxation and LV compliance. LV relaxation is an active, energy-dependent process that begins during the ejection phase of systole and continues through isovolumic relaxation and the rapid filling phase. It is considered that the LV relaxation is under the triple control of systolic load, myofiber inactivation, and the uniformity of the distribution of load and inactivation in space and time (22–24). The time constant of relaxation, known as tau, describes the rate of decrease of LV pressure decay during isovolumic relaxation. It requires cardiac catheterization with high-fidelity manometer-tipped catheters for precise determination. The pressure data during the time from end-systole (peak – *dP/dt*) to onset of LV filling (determined from LA to LV crossover pressure or estimated as 5 mm Hg above the end-diastolic pressure) are fit to a variety of equations to calculate the time constant of isovolumic relaxation. The equations are used make different assumptions regarding the LV minimum pressure obtained. The Weiss equation assumes a zero asymptote or that the LV minimum pressure must be positive. The so-called logistic equation lets the data drive the asymptote and allows for negative LV minimum pressures as has been documented in animal studies. Another equation fits the data to a linear rather than exponential relationship by calculating the slope of the relationship between the derivative of LV pressure and LV pressure over the range of isovolumic relaxation. While the data do not fit this equation as well as the exponential relationships, this method has the advantage of being more independent of preload because the slope of the relationship does not change depending on the LA pressure. While much emphasis has been placed on the method used to derive tau, all methods have been used in clinical studies. With all methods, the larger the value for tau, the more impaired the relaxation.

While LV relaxation may become impaired in the presence of a number of cardiovascular diseases, the role of impaired relaxation in contributing to increased LA pressures at rest is unclear. However, recent data in elderly hypertensive canines (25) and in humans (5) provide evidence that impaired relaxation delays the time to LV minimum pressure well into mid- and even late-diastole and contributes to the mean LA pressures, particularly during the hypertensive episodes. With exercise, there is an increase in venous return and a decrease in the diastolic filling period due to the increase in heart rate. During exercise, the normal ventricle relaxes faster and to a lower minimal pressure, allowing an increase in diastolic filling without an increase in LA pressure, as elegantly demonstrated in conscious, chronically instrumented canines (Fig. 7-2) (26–28). This process is mediated by enhanced sympathetic tone. In HF↓EF, the acceleration of LV relaxation with exercise is absent and, therefore, the increased early diastolic filling during exercise occurs at the expense of increased LA pressures. Thus, in patients with impaired LV relaxation, exertional symptoms may occur due to an inability to augment relaxation with exercise. More recently, similar findings have been reported in patients with HFnlEF where blood pressure, tau, and filling pressures increased dramatically with exercise (Fig. 7-3) (29). LV elastic recoil results from release of the potential energy present in the shortened myocardial fibers at the end of systole and is closely related to the level of systolic function. This process has been demonstrated in both filling and nonfilling ventricles. Potentially, elastic recoil could augment the speed of LV pressure fall such that pressure decay may proceed normally even in the presence of abnormalities of myofiber inactivation. Such a situation has been postulated to occur in hypertrophic cardiomyopathy but it remains unclear as to whether elastic recoil preserves the speed of LV chamber relaxation despite myocardial diastolic dysfunction in the more common causes of HFnlEF (17).

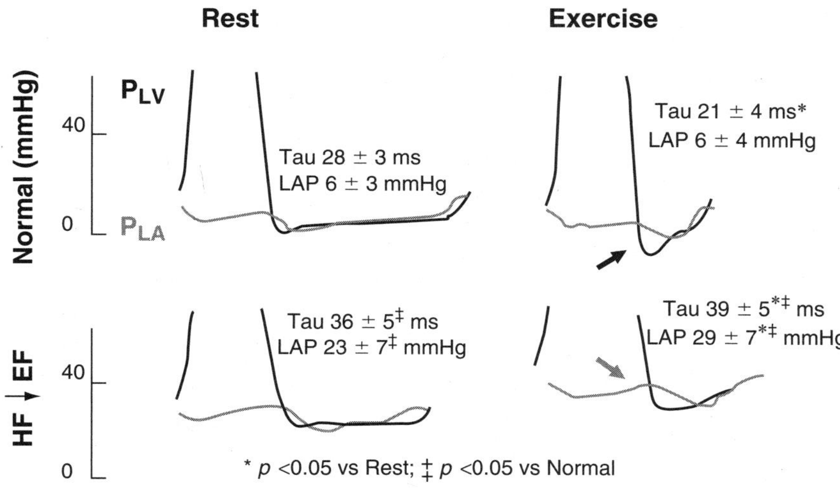

Figure 7-2 Left ventricular (P_{LV}) and left atrial (P_{LA}) pressure tracings in conscious, chronically instrumented canines before (Normal) and after (HF↓EF) induction of severe systolic dysfunction by chronic rapid right ventricular pacing. In Normals, with exercise, relaxation is enhanced with faster (decreased tau) and more complete (lower LV minimum pressure, **black arrow**) relaxation. This increases the LA to LV pressure gradient in early diastole, allowing enhanced filling without increases in P_{LA}. In contrast, after production of HF↓EF, relaxation does not improve with exercise and the LA to LV pressure gradient (and thus LV filling) can only be increased at the expense of increased P_{LA}. (Modified from Cheng CP, Noda T, Nozawa T, et al. Effect of heart failure on the mechanism of exercise-induced augmentation of mitral valve flow. *Circ Res.* 1993;72:795–806.)

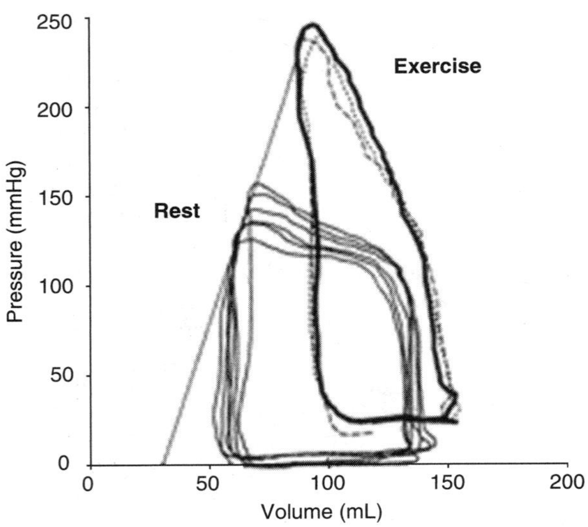

Figure 7-3 Invasive pressure volume data from a patient with HFnlEF before and during hand grip exercise, revealing a hypertensive response concordant with the high basal end-systolic elastance (Ees) and elevated diastolic pressure during stress. On average, end-systolic pressure rose to 200.5 ± 12.3 mm Hg, EDP to 32.3 ± 8.6 mm Hg, and relaxation time to 85.7 ± 23.1 milliseconds (all p <0.05 versus baseline). (Modified from Kawaguchi M, Hay I, Fetics B, Kass DA. Combined ventricular systolic and arterial stiffening in patients with heart failure and preserved ejection fraction: implications for systolic and diastolic reserve limitations. *Circulation.* 2003;107(5): 714–720.)

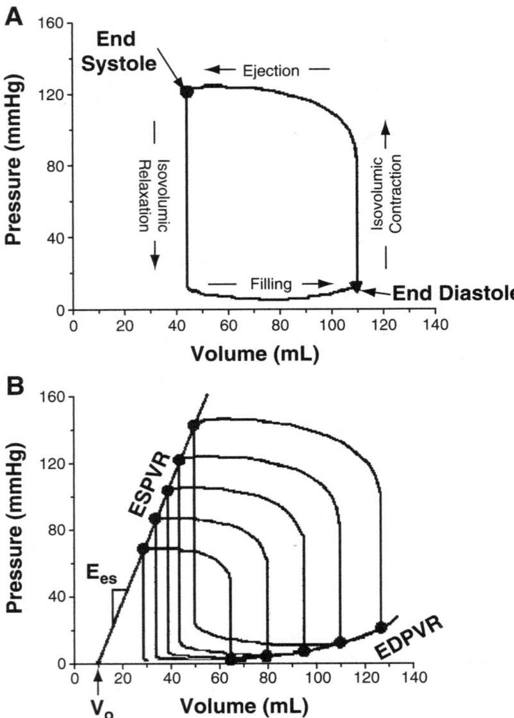

Figure 7-4 A. The four phases of the cardiac cycle are readily displayed on the pressure–volume loop, which is constructed by plotting instantaneous pressure versus volume. This loop repeats with each cardiac cycle and shows how the heart transitions from its end-diastolic state to the end-systolic state and back. **B.** With a constant contractile state and afterload resistance, a progressive reduction in ventricular filling pressure causes the loops to shift toward lower volumes at both end-systole and end-diastole. When the resulting end-systolic pressure–volume points are connected, a reasonably linear end-systolic pressure–volume relationship (ESPVR) is obtained. The linear ESPVR is characterized by a slope (Ees) and a volume axis intercept (V_o). In contrast, the diastolic pressure–volume points define a nonlinear end-diastolic pressure–volume relationship (EDPVR). (From Burkhoff D, Mirsky I, Suga H. Assessment of systolic and diastolic ventricular properties via pressure–volume analysis: a guide for clinical, translational, and basic researchers. *Am J Physiol.* (*Heart Circ Physiol.*) 2005;289(2):H501–H512.)

Left Ventricular Diastolic Stiffness

Compliance is defined as the relationship between the change in stress and the resulting strain. The inverse of compliance is stiffness or elastance. The elastance of the LV varies over the cardiac cycle (time-varying elastance), and both the end-systolic and end-diastolic elastance are defined by the relationship between pressure and volume as volume is altered (Fig. 7-4) (19). Thus, stiffness is defined by the pressure–volume relationship measured at variable preloads at end-systole (reflective of systolic performance, Ees) and end-diastole (reflective of diastolic stiffness or elastance, Ed). These relationships are altered in the presence of systolic or diastolic function. In terms of LV diastolic function, the diastolic LV stiffness is related to the rate of LV pressure change (measured at end-diastole), which occurs with a given change in LV volume. This relationship is curvilinear in the normal LV. The curvilinear nature of the normal end-diastolic pressure–volume relationship means that the normal LV becomes stiffer and more resistant to filling as the LV diastolic volume is increased.

The effective or operant compliance of the LV is defined as the change in volume and pressure during filling with a single cardiac cycle at any particular end-diastolic volume (Fig. 7-5). A ventricle will have a different operant compliance at different places on its end-diastolic pressure–volume relationship. The operant compliance is influenced not only by the intrinsic myocardial stiffness but also by continued relaxation and recoil, pericardial constraint, ventricular interaction, intrathoracic pressures, and coronary turgor. The intrinsic myocardial stiffness is related to the structure of the LV wall and the viscoelastic forces of the functioning myocardium. Evidence of decreased LV compliance has been demonstrated in patients with hypertrophic cardiomyopathy (30), hypertensive LV hypertrophy (31), acute ischemia (32), valvular disease (33), and restrictive cardiomyopathy (34) and can be inferred in any patient when filling pressures are increased in the presence of normal ventricular volume. While the slope of the curvilinear end-diastolic pressure–volume relationship increases as the compliance decreases, it is also possible to observe an upward shift of the relationship without a change in the slope of the relationship. This has been referred to as decreased distensibility by some investigators and has the same effect as altered compliance with increased pressures needed to maintain the same LV filling volume. However, the mechanisms (extrinsic forces versus intrinsic LV diastolic dysfunction) that mediate such upward shifts are less clear.

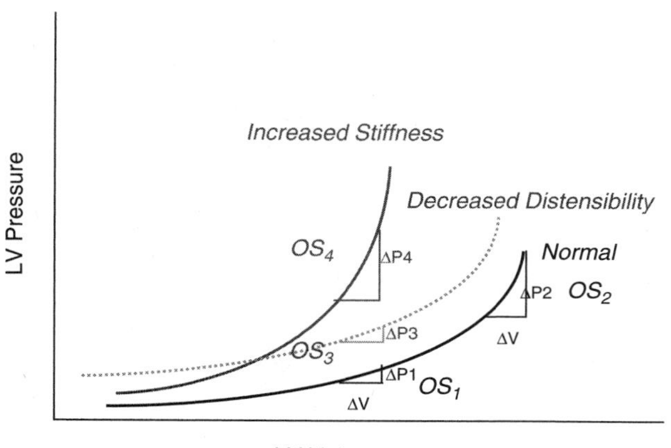

Figure 7-5 End-diastolic pressure–volume relationships showing normal diastolic stiffness, increased stiffness, and decreased distensibility. The operant stiffness (OS) can be altered by moving upward and rightward (OS_1 to OS_2) on the normal end diastolic pressure–volume relationship (EDPVR), which occurs in the absence of altered diastolic function. In contrast, if the intrinsic diastolic properties of the ventricle are altered (increased stiffness), the operant stiffness will also be increased (OS_1 to OS_4). In the presence of decreased distensibility, where the end-diastolic pressures are higher at any volume but the slope of the EDPVR is unchanged, the end-diastolic pressures will be higher than in Normals at any given volume, but the operant stiffness will not be different than in Normals.

Definition of Diastolic Dysfunction

While no standard definition for diastolic dysfunction exists, it may be described as a condition in which higher than normal LV filling pressures are needed to maintain a normal LV volume and cardiac output. It has been postulated that the natural history of diastolic dysfunction progresses through a spectrum characterized by progressive impairment of LV relaxation, which then becomes associated with progressive reduction in LV compliance and elevation in filling pressures (Fig. 7-6) (20,35). This evolution has been documented in experimental dilated cardiomyopathy using invasive assessment of LV relaxation and compliance (36) as well as in humans with the rapidly progressive infiltrative cardiomyopathy associated with amyloid deposition using noninvasive assessment of diastolic function (34,37). The natural history of diastolic dysfunction is likely highly variable in regards to the rate of progression and heavily influenced by the nature of the underlying disease state. The progression of diastolic abnormalities associated with progression to HFnlEF in patients with hypertensive heart disease or coronary disease has yet to be established in longitudinal studies with sequential assessment of diastolic function over time, and this proposed natural history remains highly plausible but as yet not definitively proven to be operative during the natural history of most or all patients who develop HFnlEF.

Evidence for Diastolic Dysfunction in HFnlEF

Several studies support the concept that intrinsic diastolic dysfunction is present and mediates elevated filling pressures in HFnlEF. Studies implicating a role for impaired relaxation and increased diastolic stiffness will be considered next.

Impaired relaxation is present in patients with HFnlEF and contributes to elevated filling pressure at rest or with exercise. When considering whether relaxation is impaired in HFnlEF, comparison to age-matched controls is important because relaxation becomes more impaired with age. If impaired relaxation contributes significantly to the pathophysiology of HFnlEF, some investigators would maintain that relaxation must be perturbed beyond what is seen in asymptomatic age-matched patients. Zile et al. characterized tau in patients with HFnlEF and reported it to be elevated (59 ± 14 milliseconds, $n = 47$) as compared to age-matched controls (35 ± 14 milliseconds, $n = 10$, $p = 0.01$) (5,38). This study also demonstrated that impaired relaxation contributed to the elevation of early (and thus, mean) diastolic pressures.

In contrast, a much smaller study did not find significant differences in tau between HFnlEF patients ($n = 10$) and age-matched controls ($n = 9$) at rest (29) but did show dramatic increases in systolic blood pressure, diastolic pressures, and tau with exercise in HFnlEF patients but not age-matched controls (Fig. 7-3). These authors speculated that while significant differences in baseline relaxation were not present in HFnlEF patients, these patients had advanced central aortic and LV *systolic* stiffening, which magnified stress-induced load and load-dependent diastolic dysfunction, resulting in elevated filling pressures with exercise. This study raises an important point, suggesting that in some HFnlEF patients, resting diastolic function may not be dramatically altered, but exercise or other stressors (hypertensive episodes, volume overload) can produce exaggerated worsening of diastolic function, resulting in stress-induced elevation of filling pressures not seen in asymptomatic age-matched controls.

The concept of differential responses to exercise in HFnlEF is supported by several earlier studies that examined the response to exercise in different ways. Sobue et al. looked at the effect of exercise on filling pressures in patients with normal EF referred to angiography for evaluation of chest pain (39). While these were not described specifically as HFnlEF patients, the findings are pertinent. In patients without coronary disease or LV hypertrophy, pulmonary capillary wedge pressure was normal at rest and at peak exercise (Table 7-2). In patients without coronary disease but with LV hypertrophy, pulmonary capillary wedge pressure was normal at rest but was elevated at peak exercise. In patients with coronary disease, pulmonary capillary wedge pressure was normal at rest but elevated at peak exercise, more so in patients with coronary disease and LV hypertrophy. These data do not define the relative contribution of impaired relaxation or compliance to the elevation of filling pressures but do demonstrate that ventricular hypertrophy and coronary disease (both common in HFnlEF) may not perturb resting filling pressures but can produce exercise-induced diastolic dysfunction and symptoms.

Cuocolo et al. demonstrated that patients with hypertension who had ventricular hypertrophy and impaired relaxation (based on Doppler evaluation) had an inability to enhance filling with exercise, resulting in a flat ejection

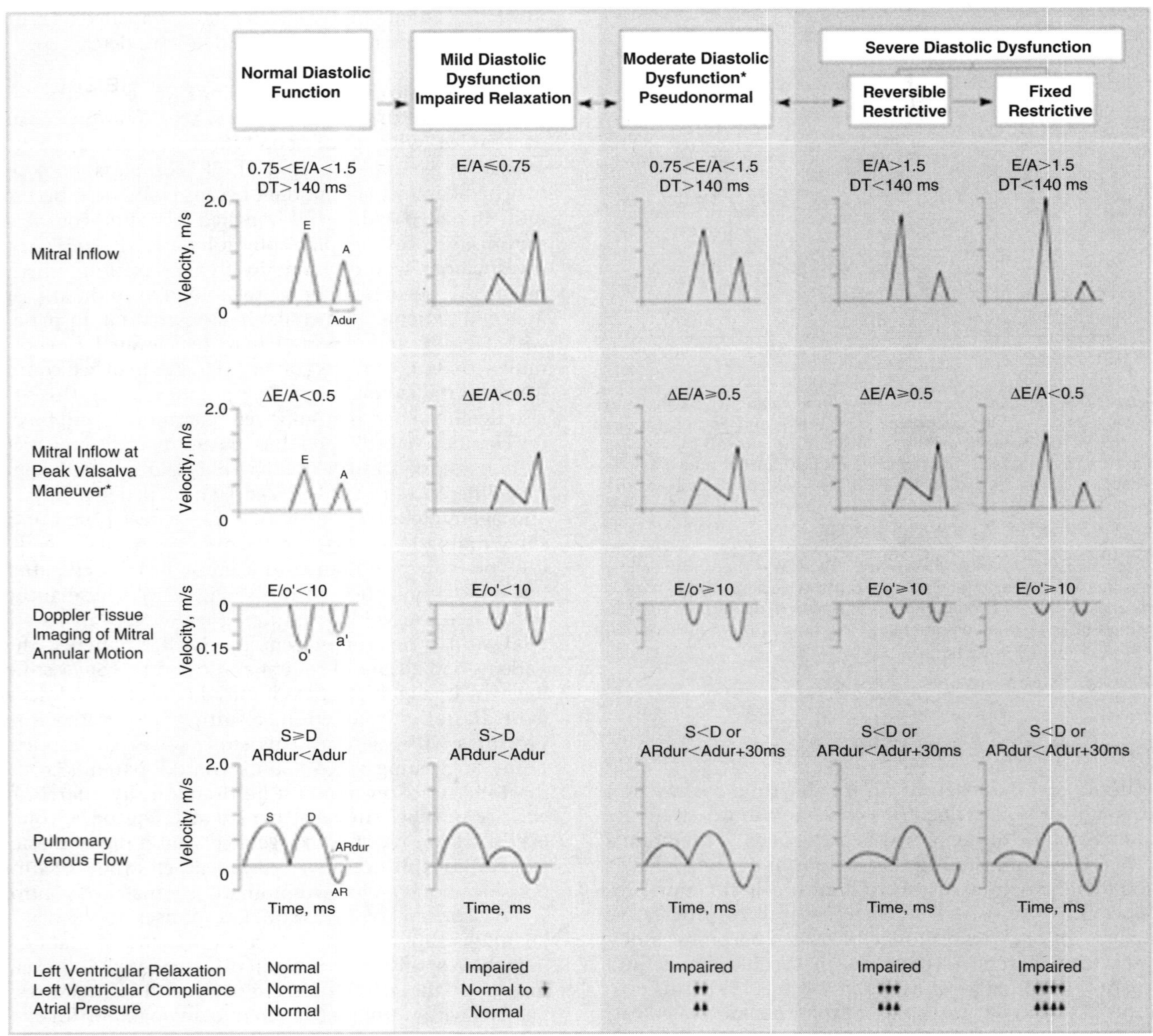

Figure 7-6 The proposed progression of diastolic function abnormalities with correlation of invasively measured diastolic properties (**text at bottom**) and the corresponding Doppler echocardiographic parameters. (From Redfield MM, Jacobsen SJ, Burnett JC, Jr., et al. Burden of systolic and diastolic ventricular dysfunction in the community: appreciating the scope of the heart failure epidemic. *JAMA.* 2003;289(2):194–202.)

fraction response to exercise and suggesting that an inability to enhance relaxation with exercise may contribute to exercise-induced symptoms (40). An elegant study by Kitzman et al. compared exercise pressures and volumes in previously treated outpatients with HFnlEF (most of whom had hypertensive heart disease) and age-matched controls. In this population, none had coronary disease (41). The HFnlEF patients had (on average) normal pulmonary capillary wedge pressures and LV volumes at rest, but with exercise developed dramatic increases in pulmonary capillary wedge pressure unassociated with increases in end-diastolic volume (Fig. 7-7). In these patients, the systolic blood pressures with exercise were not different from controls, suggesting that the exercise-induced diastolic dysfunction was not strictly load-dependent. This study suggests that the Frank-Starling mechanism is impaired in patients with HFnlEF and is consistent with the study of Cuocolo et al. However, this study did not define the relative importance of impaired relaxation versus decreased compliance in mediating the abnormal response to exercise.

Doppler echocardiography also provides supporting evidence for a role of impaired relaxation to contribute to stress-induced symptoms in HFnlEF. In patients with impaired relaxation, early filling is decreased and the contributions of diastasis flow and atrial contraction are magnified (Fig. 7-8, right panel). In these patients, the entire diastolic filling

TABLE 7-2

EFFECT OF CORONARY ARTERY DISEASE AND LEFT VENTRICULAR HYPERTROPHY ON THE EFFECT OF EXERCISE ON FILLING PRESSURES

	Patients without CAD		Patients with CAD	
	Group I (without LVH) (n = 30)	Group II (with LVH) (n = 12)	Group III (without LVH) (n = 20)	Group IV (with LVH) (n = 16)
Age (y)	53 ± 9	56 ± 10	55 ± 7	57 ± 7
1 diseased vessel	0	0	9	7
2 diseased vessels	0	0	6	5
3 diseased vessels	0	0	5	4
EF at rest (%)	74 ± 7	78 ± 9	75 ± 9	70 ± 8
LVMI (b/m^2)	105 ± 17	158 ± 32	109 ± 13	159 ± 21
HR (beats/min) rest	66 ± 11	65 ± 12	68 ± 14	66 ± 15
25 W	95 ± 10	89 ± 13	96 ± 14	95 ± 15
Peak exercise	126 ± 17	115 ± 17	113 ± 22	111 ± 17
PAWP (mm Hg) rest	6 ± 3	8 ± 2	6 ± 3	8 ± 4
25 W	9 ± 4	15 ± 6‡	16 ± 7*	22 ± 5^{*Φ}
Peak exercise	10 ± 5	18 ± 8‡	23 ± 6*	30 ± 7*†
CI (L/min/m^2) rest	2.8 ± 0.5	2.8 ± 0.5	2.7 ± 0.5	2.7 ± 0.5
25 W	4.7 / 0.8	4.8 ± 0.5	4.4 ± 0.6	4.3 ± 0.5
Peak exercise	6.8 ± 1.3	6.4 ± 1.4	5.4 ± 0.8*	5.1 ± 1.4*

$^*p < 0.01$; $^‡p < 0.05$ versus group I; $^Φp < 0.05$ versus group II; $^†p < 0.05$ versus group III. Data presented are mean value ± SD. AD, coronary artery disease; CI, cardiac index; EF, ejection fraction; HR, heart rate; LVH, left ventricular hypertrophy; LVMI, left ventricular mass index; PAWP, pulmonary artery wedge pressure; W, Watts. See text for explanation.
From Sobue T, Yokota M, Iwase M, et al. Influence of left ventricular hypertrophy on left ventricular function during dynamic exercise in the presence or absence of coronary artery disease. *J Am Coll Cardiol.* 1995;25(1):91–98.

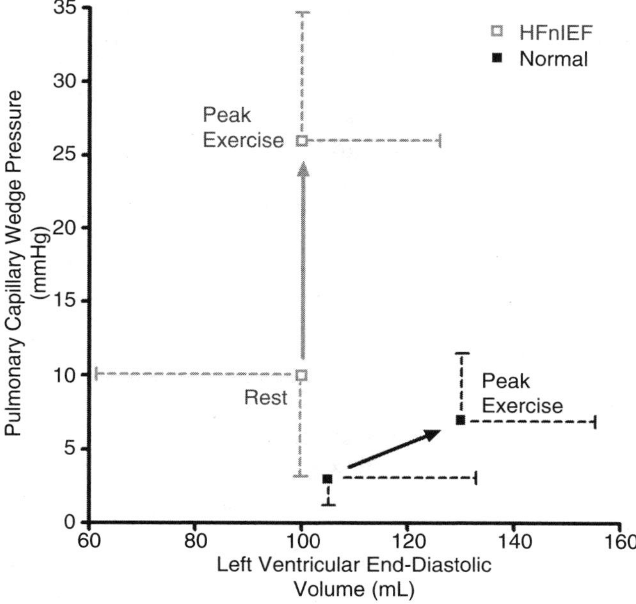

Figure 7-7 Rest and exercise pulmonary capillary wedge pressure (PCWP) and LV volume in normal subjects and patients with HFnlEF. Resting PCWP was higher in HFnlEF but the average was within the normal range. With exercise, the HFnlEF patients could not augment LV volume despite marked elevation in PCWP. In contrast, normal subjects markedly augmented LV volume during exercise without abnormal increases in PCWP. (From Kitzman DW, Higginbotham MB, Cobb FR, et al. Exercise intolerance in patients with heart failure and preserved left ventricular systolic function: failure of the Frank-Starling mechanism. *J Am Coll Cardiol.* 1991;17(5):1065–1072.)

period is needed to fill the ventricle, even at slow heart rates. During exercise, the increased venous return and shortened diastasis period will mandate the need for elevation of filling pressures to maintain filling with exercise, contributing to the elevation of filling pressures and inability to augment filling demonstrated in the studies which measured pressures and/or volumes with exercise (40,41) in HFnlEF.

Contribution of impaired relaxation to another common mode of decompensation for HFnlEF patients is also evidenced by the enhanced dependence on atrial contraction for filling. In one of the few studies that carefully examined factors contributing to decompensation in patients with HFnlEF, nearly 30% of hospitalizations for acutely decompensated HFnlEF were due to new-onset rapid atrial fibrillation (42). Exacerbation of symptoms with atrial arrhythmias is recognized and included in proposed diagnostic criteria for HFnlEF (43). The acute reduction in filling associated with loss of atrial systolic activity in atrial fibrillation, coupled with the resistance to early diastolic filling due to impaired relaxation, will again mandate acute elevation of filling pressures (44,45) and contribute to acute episodes of HFnlEF.

In contrast, in normal individuals with normal relaxation and brisk, early diastolic filling, dependence on diastasis flow and atrial filling is minimal (Fig. 7-8, left panel) and rapid atrial fibrillation is much less likely to induce acute pulmonary edema. This scenario is also supported by modeling studies which suggest that elevation of tau to levels observed in HFnlEF (60 milliseconds), while not affecting resting filling pressures, will produce dramatic increases in filling pressures with tachycardia

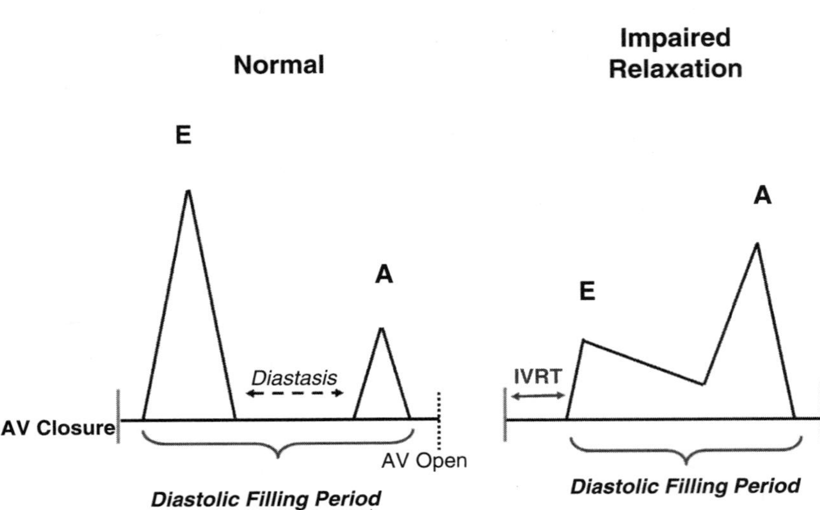

Figure 7-8 Insights into the importance of impaired relaxation in influencing atrial pressures from Doppler echocardiography. Transmitral inflow velocity profiles in normal diastolic function and in the presence of impaired relaxation are shown. In normal subjects **(left)**, the diastolic filling period is longer due to a shorter isovolumic relaxation time (IVRT). Most filling occurs in early diastole due to brisk LV relaxation, which enhances the atrial-to-LV pressure gradient in early diastole. Thus, there is little filling during diastasis and minimal contribution from atrial contraction. In the presence of markedly impaired relaxation (**right**), the diastolic filling period is shorter due to later onset of filling (longer IVRT). As the LV relaxes more slowly, the atrial-to-LV pressure gradient is smaller in early diastole and the velocity of filling is lower and filling extends into diastasis. As early diastolic filling is reduced, there is enhanced dependence on atrial contraction for filling. Tachycardia (which shortens diastasis) and loss of atrial contraction (atrial fibrillation) severely impair filling and mandate the need for elevation of left atrial pressures to restore filling and maintain cardiac output.

(46). In this experiment, compliance was held constant, suggesting that relaxation impairment alone can contribute to elevation of mean left atrial and pulmonary venous pressures with tachycardia.

There are many extracardiac and cardiac mechanisms that affect load, uniformity, and myofiber inactivation and that may mediate impaired relaxation in HF, and they have been recently reviewed in detail (47).

Increased diastolic stiffness (decreased compliance) is present in patients with HFnlEF and contributes to elevated filling pressure at rest or with exercise. Measurement of diastolic stiffness is considerably more difficult than characterization of relaxation. Ideally, LV pressure and volume are measured during acute alteration in preload to define the end-diastolic pressure–volume relationship over a range of preloads—the multiple-beat method (Figs. 7-4 and 7-5). Alternatively, pressure and volume can be measured over a single beat and the diastolic portion of the pressure–volume curve can be fit to an exponential relationship and used to estimate stiffness.

This single-beat method is subject to two important limitations. First, as previously outlined, the end-diastolic pressure–volume relationship is curvilinear, and operant stiffness measured at increased volume will yield a higher stiffness estimate than when the single beat is taken at lower volumes (see discussion of the third theory, HFnlEF Is Due to Ventricular Remodeling Characterized by LV Dilatation, later). Thus, it could be argued that increased stiffness measured by the single-beat method in HFnlEF could be due to intrinsic diastolic dysfunction or volume overload and LV dilation. This potential limitation can be addressed by carefully documenting that the volumes measured in HFnlEF are normal for age. As values for LV volume are dependent on age, sex, and the method used to measure it, this can be difficult.

The second limitation is due to the influence of impaired relaxation on the contour of the single-beat diastolic pressure–volume relationship. In the normal ventricle, relaxation is brisk and the LV minimum pressure occurs early in diastole, yielding a exponential contour to the diastolic pressure–volume relationship over a single beat. Here, only the passive stiffness of the ventricle influences the pressure–volume relationship in mid- to late-diastole, and the data fit an exponential relationship that allows calculation of a stiffness constant:

$$P = \alpha \times e^{\beta \times V}$$

where β is the stiffness constant and α is a curve-fitting constant. However, when relaxation is markedly impaired, relaxation may continue into mid- and even late-diastole under some conditions (5,25); the LV minimum pressure occurs later in diastole; and the diastolic pressure–volume relationship over the single beat is not exponential. Thus, diastolic pressures in mid- to late-diastole are influenced by relaxation as well as the passive characteristics of the ventricle. This limitation is best addressed by using preload reduction to define the end-diastolic pressure–volume relationship, avoiding measurements in other portions of diastole that may be influenced by relaxation. Alternatively, methods to correct for the affect of relaxation on diastolic pressures in the single-beat method have been used (5).

Another important limitation to both the single- and multiple-beat methods for assessment of diastolic stiffness involves the desire to express the position and contour of the exponential diastolic pressure–volume relationship in a single number. In the multiple-beat method, the end-diastolic pressure–volume data points during preload reduction are fit to one of two frequently used exponential equations.

$$EDP = \alpha \times e^{\beta \times EDV} \quad [1]$$

$$EDP = P_o + \alpha\,(e^{\beta \times EDV} - 1) \quad [2]$$

In these equations relating end-diastolic pressure (EDP) and end-diastolic volume (EDV), a curve-fitting constant (α) and a coefficient of stiffness (β) are calculated and the stiffness constant is used to characterize the stiffness of the ventricle. In the second equation, a pressure offset is also calculated (P_0) which allows for quantification of a shift in the position of the end-diastolic pressure–volume relationship with or without an accompanying change in the steepness of the relationship. However, as the pressure–volume data acquired in any experiment are not perfectly monoexponential, fitting the data to these equations can often yield very different values for α and β, even when the curves appear very similar. Both α and β convey information regarding the stiffness of the ventricle, so if β was not increased but α was, one could not conclude that stiffness was normal. Furthermore, this fact can yield considerable variability in group averages for α and β, making it difficult to detect changes.

To overcome this limitation, one can use a linear equation to characterize the pressure–volume relationship but the end-diastolic pressure–volume data do not fit a linear equation well. More recently, investigators have recommended converting the exponential pressure volume relationship to a linear one by plotting ln EDP versus EDV. This yields a linear relationship:

$$\ln EDP = \ln\alpha + \beta \times EDV$$

One can then compare the slope of this relationship (β) controlling for concomitant changes in the offset (lnα) and for the patient group in multiple linear regression analysis (19). The theoretical value of this method is considerable and deserves further study.

A final limitation to either method of characterizing stiffness with pressure–volume data is the considerable difficulty in accurately and instantaneously measuring volume along with pressure, particularly in clinical studies. While conductance catheter, echocardiography, contrast ventriculography, and radionuclide angiography have been used in clinical studies, all these methods have significant limitations when applied to a clinical population.

These difficulties have limited the characterization of ventricular diastolic stiffness in HFnlEF to only a few studies. Zile et al. used the single-beat method, measuring volumes with echocardiography and correcting for the influence of impaired relaxation on the pressure–volume contour. The patients with HFnlEF (n = 47) were relatively young and predominately male but had a firm diagnosis of HFnlEF (5,38). Compared to age-matched controls without cardiovascular disease, the stiffness coefficient was significantly higher in patients with HFnlEF (Fig. 7-9). These

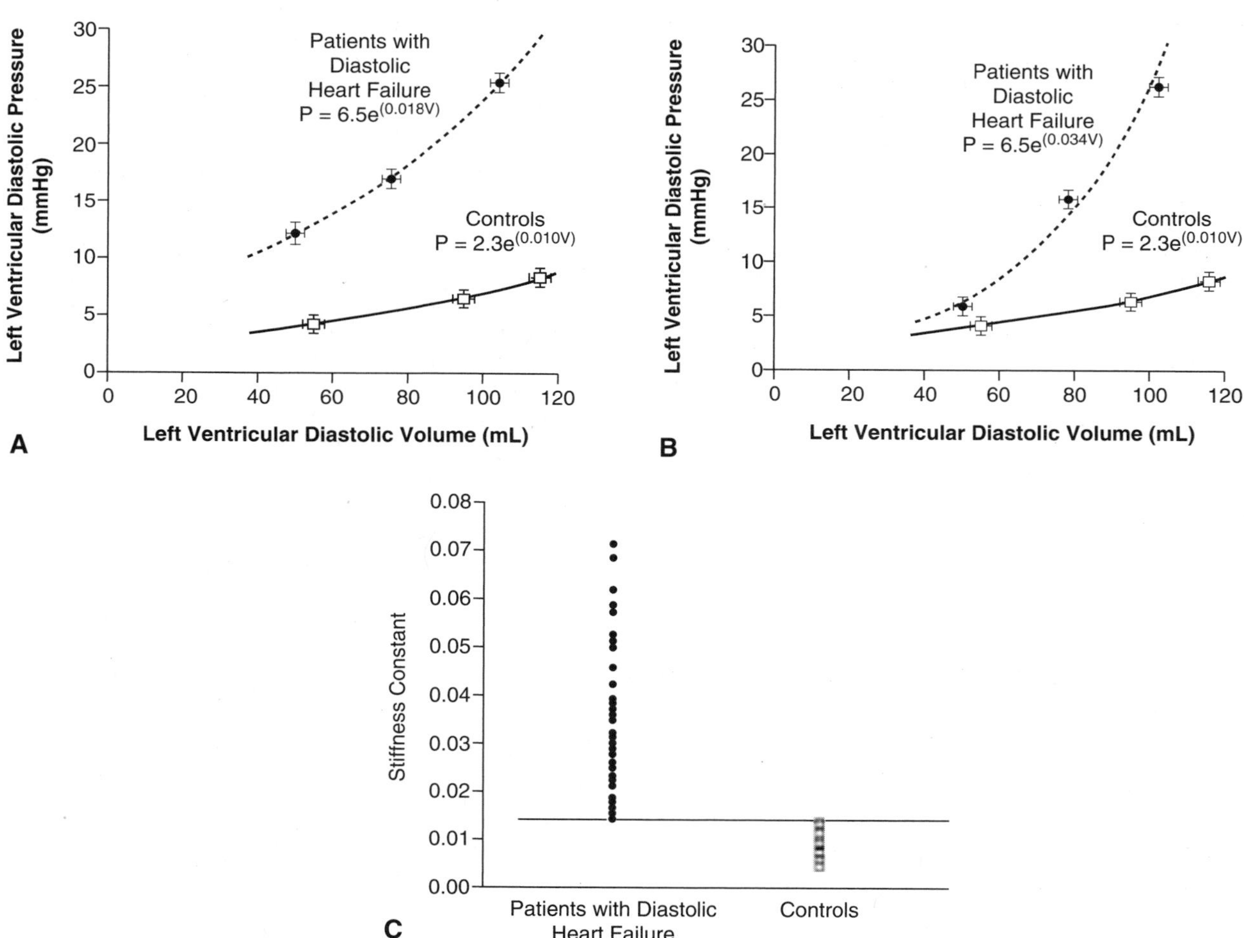

Figure 7-9 Diastolic pressure–volume relation in patients with diastolic heart failure and in controls. **A** shows measured values for the minimal left ventricular pressure and **B** shows values for the minimal left ventricular pressure, corrected for slow relaxation. The exponential value in the equation for pressure (P) is the stiffness constant. The data in both panels indicate that there was a significant increase in the passive stiffness of the left ventricle in the patients with HFnlEF (diastolic heart failure). V denotes volume, and the I-bars represent the standard error. **C** shows the individual corrected stiffness constants in patients with HFnlEF (Diastolic Heart Failure) and in Controls. The stiffness constant was increased in all the patients with HFnlEF. (From Zile MR, Baicu CF, Gaasch WH. Diastolic heart failure—abnormalities in active relaxation and passive stiffness of the left ventricle. *N Engl J Med.* 2004;350(19):1953–1959.)

investigators concluded that both impaired relaxation and increased diastolic stiffness were present in patients with HFnlEF and that these abnormalities in diastolic function were key to the pathogenesis of the syndrome.

Consistent with this concept, Liu et al. assessed diastolic stiffness invasively but fit end-diastolic pressure–volume to a linear relationship and found significant increases in diastolic stiffness in 10 patients with hypertrophy and normal EF (seven with HFnlEF) as compared to eight somewhat younger controls (48). Finally, Borbely et al. characterized chamber stiffness and, on biopsy specimens, myocardial structure, sarcomere protein composition, and myocyte stiffness in a group of 12 HFnlEF patients (five with previous cardiac transplant and all with a history of hypertension) and eight controls (six with previous cardiac transplant) (49). HFnlEF patients had increased diastolic stiffness and higher diastolic pressures at comparable indexed LV volumes consistent with increased myocardial diastolic stiffness and reduced chamber distensibility. The HFnlEF patients had more fibrosis than controls and the degree of fibrosis did correlate with LV diastolic pressures. This study showed increased passive diastolic myocyte stiffness that was unassociated with apparent changes in sarcomeric protein composition, although isoform switches in titin were not investigated. These investigators concluded that both the increased fibrosis and increased passive myocyte stiffness contribute to the increased chamber stiffness observed in vivo, with extracellular matrix contributing more as filling pressures (and presumably sarcomere length) increase. The potential contribution of collagen modification by cross-linking related to the presence of advanced glycation end-products (AGE) was not explored and could contribute to an imperfect correlation between collagen content and chamber stiffness. While this study supports a role for diastolic stiffness in HFnlEF, the special nature of the patient population must be recognized.

In contrast, Kawaguchi et al. used the conductance catheter and an inferior vena cava balloon to measure the pressure–volume relationship with the multiple-beat method during preload reduction in 10 HFnlEF patients and nine healthy, age-matched controls without hypertension or symptoms of HF (29). These patients were studied at a referral center and, while they were predominantly female, their mean age was 60 years—a value much lower than the mean age observed in most population-based studies of HFnlEF. In this study, assessment of the stiffness coefficient (β) by the single-beat method showed increased stiffness, and an increase in P_0, indicating an increased slope and an upward shift in the diastolic pressure–volume relationship (Fig. 7-10). However, when the multiple-beat method was used, there was still an upward shift in the position of the curve but the diastolic stiffness coefficient was not different in controls and HFnlEF patients. The HFnlEF patients had increased vascular stiffness (Ea), markedly increased ventricular systolic stiffness (Ees), and an exaggerated systolic pressure response to exercise. These investigators concluded that HFnlEF is not solely due to resting diastolic dysfunction but that vascular and ventricular systolic stiffening could limit cardiovascular reserve and exacerbate diastolic dysfunction during exercise, thus contributing to the pathophysiology of HFnlEF. That diastolic stiffness was not increased in the HFnlEF patients is somewhat surprising when taking the concept of time varying elastance into consideration. This concept suggests that if systolic stiffness is increased, diastolic stiffness will be as well, a concept previously confirmed in clinical studies showing concomitant age-related increases in arterial, ventricular systolic, and ventricular diastolic stiffness (50). The large variability in β observed in HFnlEF (range $\approx$0.01 to 0.05 mm Hg/mL) may be related to the limitations in calculating β discussed above previously, and this variability may prevent demonstration of differences in β in small groups. The values for α were not reported.

While most discussion has centered on ventricular compliance in HFnlEF, atrial compliance is a potentially important mediator of mean atrial and, thus, mean pulmonary venous pressures. This, in turn, can contribute to pulmonary congestion. It is important to remember that it is mean left atrial pressures, not simply ventricular end-diastolic pressures, that mediate symptoms of HF (44,45). Thus, early- and mid-diastolic as well as end-diastolic pressures in the ventricular and systolic atrial pressures (atrial V wave) are important contributors to mean left atrial pressures, namely, the resistance to filling that the pulmonary venous system faces. Indeed, an often-forgotten hemodynamic hallmark of restrictive cardiomyopathy is the presence of large V waves in the atrial wave pressure waveform in the absence of mitral regurgitation. This atrial systolic pressure wave can exceed 50 mm Hg and reflects reduced atrial compliance with increases in atrial pressures during the ventricular systolic/atrial diastolic phase of atrial filling. The Doppler correlate of this is the reduction in systolic forward flow in the pulmonary veins seen in advanced diastolic dysfunction.

Thus, although studies are few there is evidence that impaired relaxation and increased diastolic stiffness are present at rest and contribute to the pathophysiology of HFnlEF. Furthermore, even if resting diastolic dysfunction is not markedly perturbed, exercise or hypertensive episodes may lead to exaggerated impairment in relaxation or stiffness in other patients with HFnlEF. Those mechanisms that might contribute to increased LV diastolic stiffness include factors which influence ventricular interaction and extrinsic forces, the extracellular cardiac matrix, the myocyte, and the myofibrils themselves. These postulated mechanisms have been reviewed recently (47).

HfnlEF Is Due to Increased Vascular and Ventricular Systolic Stiffness Associated with Enhanced Sensitivity to Volume and Load/Stress-Induced Diastolic Dysfunction

Previous studies using a variety of indexes have established that large-artery stiffness increases with age (51–53), is higher in women (51,54–56), and increases with age even in the absence of vascular disease or risk factors (51,52,57). Arterial elastance (Ea) is a valuable means to index net ventricular afterload, which combines mean (systemic vascular resistance) and oscillatory (large-artery stiffness) components of the arterial load (58). Consistent with age-associated increases in other measures of large-artery stiff-

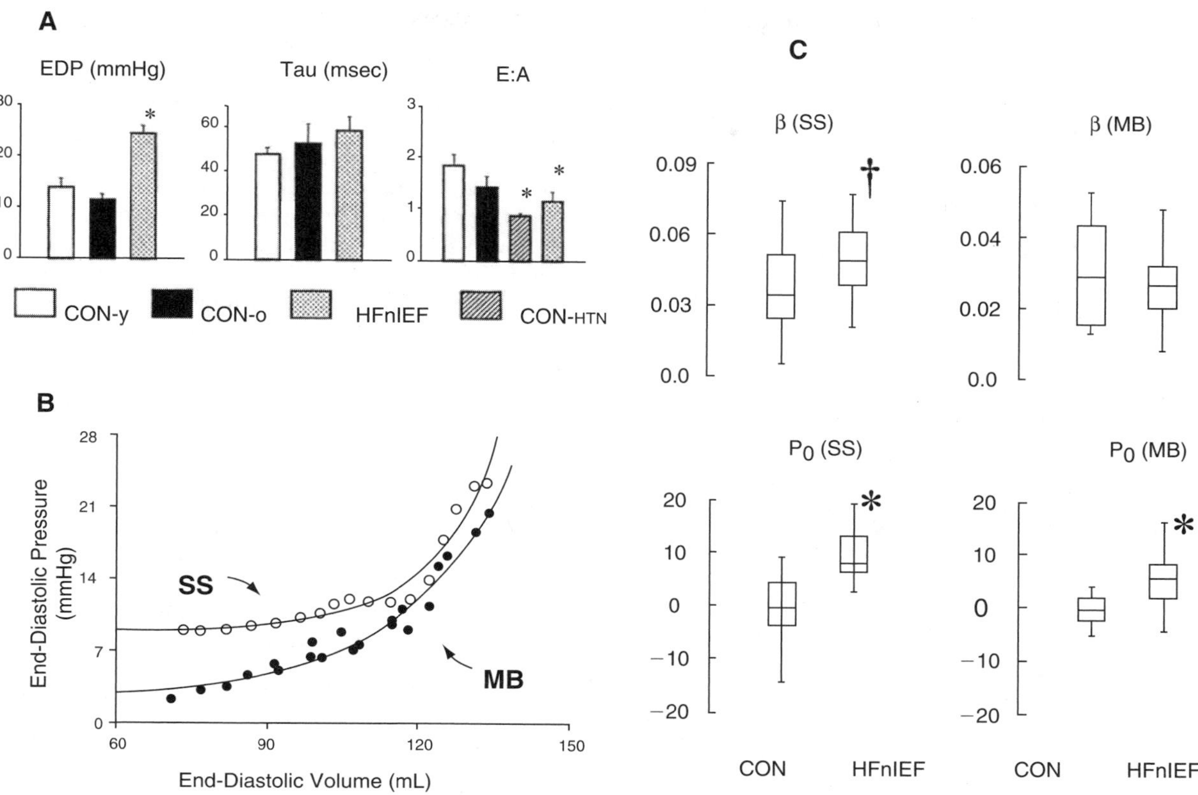

Figure 7-10 A study comparing ventricular function in young healthy persons (CON-y), older non-hypertensive persons (CON-o), patients with HFnlEF, and older hypertensive persons without HF (CON-HTN). **A.** Mean group data for end-diastolic pressure (EDP), relaxation time constant (Tau), and early/late filling ratio (E:A). **B.** Example of diastolic pressure volume data and fits from resting steady-state beat (SS) and multibeat analysis after inferior vena cava obstruction (MB). Steady-state data were typically shifted upward and were more abruptly nonlinear due to pressure elevation in the early filling phase. **C.** Summary data for end-diastolic pressure–volume relation exponential fits from steady-state and multibeat analyses. The stiffness coefficient and the pressure intercept were both elevated in SS analysis, while only the pressure intercept was elevated in MB analysis. Data for all normotensive controls were very similar and were therefore combined (CON). (From Kawaguchi M, Hay I, Fetics B, Kass DA. Combined ventricular systolic and arterial stiffening in patients with heart failure and preserved ejection fraction: implications for systolic and diastolic reserve limitations. *Circulation* 2003;107(5):714–720.) **A.** $^{*}p < 0.001$ versus young (CON-y) and age-matched (CON-o) normotensive controls. **C.** $^{*}p < 0.001$; $^{\dagger}p < 0.02$.

ness, age-related changes in Ea have also been demonstrated (50). Multiple mechanisms have been proposed to explain age-dependent vascular stiffening, including alterations in endothelial function, structural protein composition, collagen cross-linking, geometric changes, and neurohumoral signaling (59). The cause of gender differences in vascular stiffening is unclear, although most studies indicate that this is not simply a matter of differences in body size and vasculature length (51,55). Hearts coupled to a stiffer vascular system are subjected to higher systolic stresses as well as wider pulse pressures that can adversely influence the regulation of coronary flow (50,51,60,61) and contribute to microvasculature and end-organ damage (51). In order to maintain optimal interaction with the arterial system, the LV itself must develop greater systolic stiffness (50,62–64).

Importantly, age-associated increases in Ea were associated with increased systolic (Ees) and diastolic LV stiffness (Ed) in a prior invasive study which measured Ees and Ed with invasive pressure volume analysis in individuals of varying age (50) (Fig. 7-11). In this study, gender differences were not explored. However, a population-based study where Ea, Ees, and Ed were measured noninvasively demonstrated age-associated increases in Ea, Ees, and Ed and showed that these indexes were all higher in women than in men, regardless of age (65).

The chronic changes in LV systolic (and potentially diastolic) stiffness that couple with changes in vascular stiffness may represent cardiovascular adaptations to maintain optimal ventricular–vascular matching and, thus, optimal cardiac performance. Whether this is mediated by increases in inotropic state or by structural remodeling such as hypertrophy, remodeling (smaller LV cavity dimensions), or fibrosis (66) is unclear, but altered chamber geometry with age likely plays a role. While concentric hypertrophy or concentric remodeling in response to hypertension or the increases in large-artery stiffness may promote smaller (and stiffer) ventricles in elderly persons,

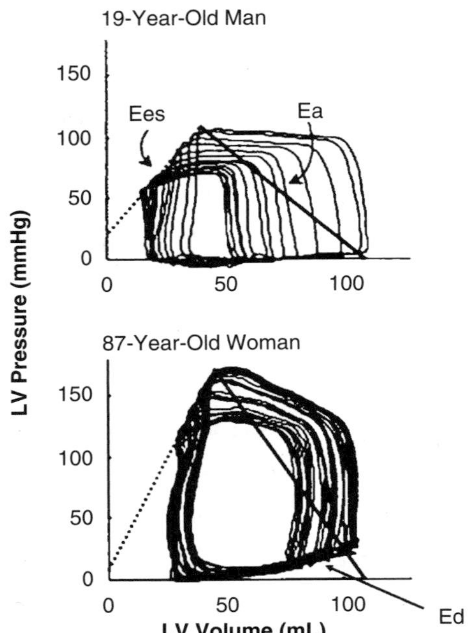

Figure 7-11 Pressure–volume curves obtained with a conductance catheter during acute reduction in preload. An example from a young (**top**) man and an elderly (**bottom**) woman are shown. End-systolic (Ees), end-diastolic (Ed), and effective arterial (Ea) elastances are elevated in the elderly woman, indicating cardiovascular stiffening. Grouped data from 57 adults confirm that all three parameters were related to age in otherwise healthy individuals. (From Chen C-H, Nakayama M, Nevo E, et al. Coupled systolic-ventricular and vascular stiffening with age: implications for pressure regulation and cardiac reserve in the elderly. *J Am Coll Cardiol.* 1998;32(5):1221–1227.)

the possibility that age-related decreases in LV volume are related to inactivity has been suggested (67).

While vascular–ventricular coupling helps to maintain stroke volume and mechanical efficiency, increases in Ees may have adverse effects. Increases in Ees result in increased sensitivity of systolic pressure to changes in volume (50). Thus, volume overload in such individuals could be associated with greater increases in systolic blood pressure and with greater increases in diastolic LV pressures. Together, increases in arterial and systolic stiffness promote load-induced impairment in LV relaxation, as previously outlined (29). Thus, age-related vascular–ventricular stiffening could contribute to increases in LV systolic blood pressure, tau, and LV diastolic pressures with exercise and could predispose to HFnlEF. As previously discussed, the recent study by Kawaguchi et al. in HFnlEF patients and age-matched controls demonstrated increased arterial and LV systolic stiffness and exaggerated increases in tau and LV diastolic pressures with exercise in HFnlEF patients as compared to normals (Fig. 7-3). While this study suggested that increases in diastolic stiffness need not be present in HFnlEF patients with increased arterial and LV systolic stiffness, it is reasonable to expect that such increases may be present in some or many patients.

The role of vascular and ventricular systolic stiffening in mediating symptoms in large numbers of HFnlEF patients has not been defined but is certainly a plausible explanation for many of the features of HFnlEF. Such age- and cardiovascular disease-associated changes in arterial and ventricular properties also are consistent with the epidemiology of HFnlEF where dramatic increases in the prevalence of HFnlEF occur with age and particularly in women (Fig. 7-12) (68). As previously discussed at length, these

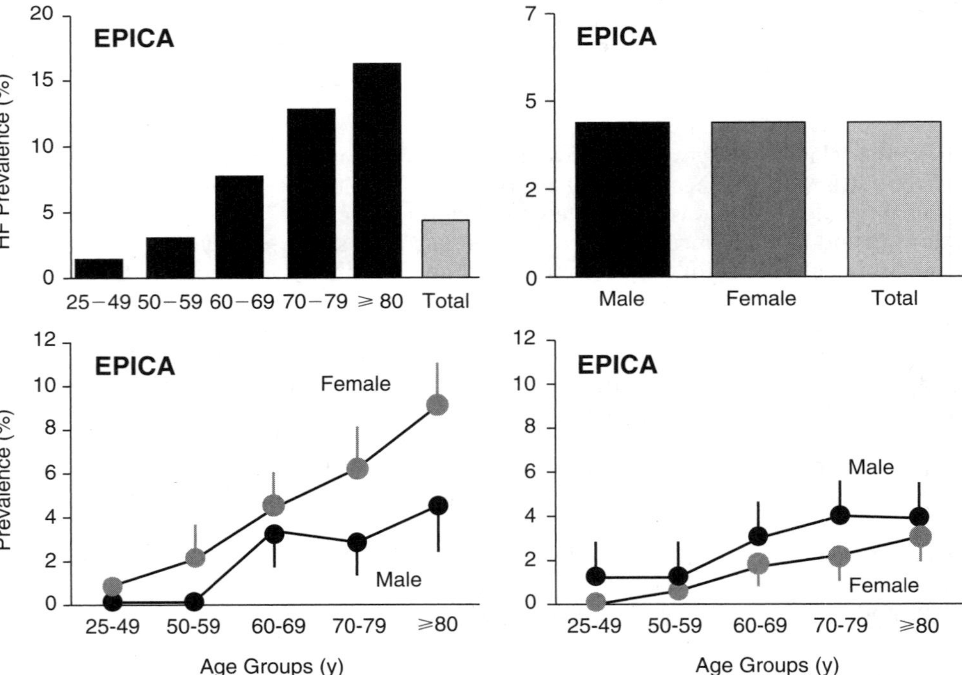

Figure 7-12 Data from a large epidemiology study in Portugal demonstrate the well-established increase in clinical HF prevalence with age (**top left**). In this study, the prevalence of HF was similar in men and women (**top right**). HFnlEF prevalence (**bottom left**) increased much more sharply with age than did the prevalence of HF↓EF (**bottom right**) and this was especially apparent in women. (From Ceia F, Fonseca C, Mota T, et al. Prevalence of chronic heart failure in Southwestern Europe: the EPICA study. *Eur J Heart Fail.* 2002;4(4):531–539.)

mechanisms do not exclude concomitant changes in resting diastolic function, either impaired relaxation or increased diastolic stiffness in some or in many persons with HFnlEF. These mechanisms do, however, provide a paradigm for understanding exercise- or other stress-induced symptoms in patients in whom resting diastolic function does not seem markedly perturbed.

HFnlEF Is Due to Ventricular Remodeling Characterized by LV Dilation with Volume-Dependent Elevation of Filling Pressures Unassociated with Significantly Altered Diastolic Stiffness or Impaired Relaxation

It has been assumed that patients with HFnlEF have normal or reduced LV volumes. This assumption is based on many studies which have reported, *on average*, normal LV cavity dimensions or volumes in patients with HFnlEF (9,13,69–77). In these types of studies where only grouped data are presented as a mean, the standard deviation of the dimension or volume measurements is wide and the potential for subgroups of patients to have enlarged, normal, and reduced cavity dimensions is almost certain.

A recent study of patients with HFnlEF studied at a tertiary referral center characterized LV geometry with three-dimensional echocardiography, estimated LV end-diastolic pressure with Doppler, and performed a noninvasive estimate of arterial and LV systolic elastance (78). The study included 99 controls without cardiovascular disease (mean age 46 ± 2 years); 11 patients with HFnlEF due to hypertrophic cardiomyopathy (n = 6), amyloid heart disease (n = 2), or restrictive cardiomyopathy (n = 3) (mean age 57 ± 20 years); and 35 patients with HFnlEF and a history of hypertension (mean age 72 ± 11 years). Patients were stratified according to the presence or absence of systemic hypertension and the findings were interpreted within the conceptual framework of pressure–volume analysis.

This study reported that most patients with hypertrophic or restrictive cardiomyopathy had normal to reduced blood pressure and normal to reduced diastolic LV volumes but increased estimated diastolic pressures (Fig. 7-13A). These patients were felt to have HFnlEF primarily due to intrinsic increase in diastolic stiffness. While other studies of hypertrophic cardiomyopathy patients report increased Ees (30), average Ees was not increased in this group. In the group with hypertension and HFnlEF, a subgroup of hypertensive HFnlEF patients had increased systolic and vascular stiffness (estimated noninvasively) (refer to the second theory, previously discussed). These patients were older, all female, and were smaller-sized with smaller ventricles. This group was considered to have combined vascular and ventricular systolic and diastolic stiffening as the etiology of their HFnlEF (Fig. 7-13B). The rest of the hypertensive HFnlEF group had normal average systolic and vascular stiffness, were younger, more obese, and had larger ventricles (on average). These investigators postulated that there was more volume expansion in such patients and that the predominant factor separating them from patients with normal volumes and no HFnlEF was increased volume (Fig. 7-13C). In support of this concept, they measured plasma volume in controls and hypertensive HFnlEF and found that, on aver-

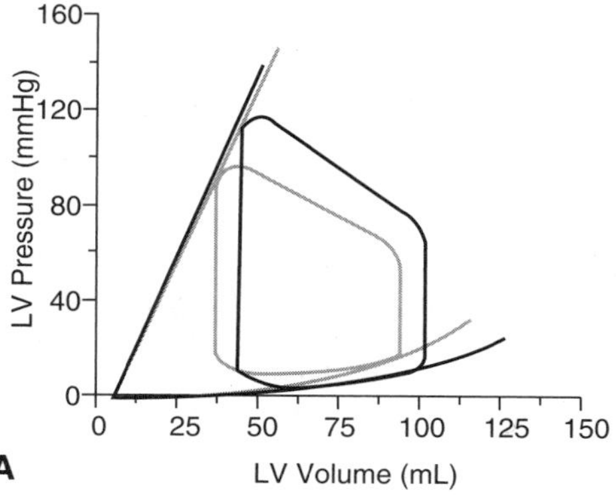

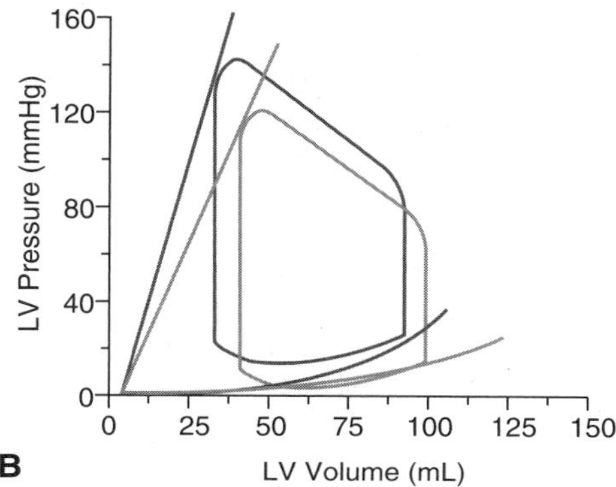

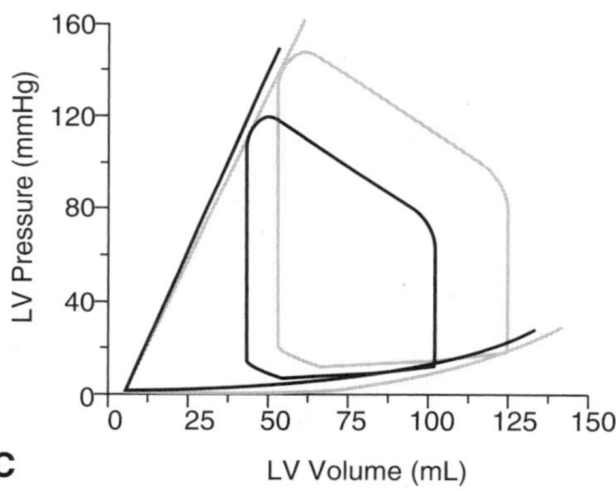

Figure 7-13 Suggested heterogeneity in the pathophysiology of HFnlEF. Ventricular systolic and diastolic properties associated with HFnlEF. Normal conditions shown in **gray**; various combinations of end-systolic pressure–volume relationship (ESPVR) and end-diastolic pressure–volume relationship (EDPVR) associated with heart failure shown in colors as detailed here. **(A)** Classic paradigm of diastolic heart failure with normal ESPVR and decreased diastolic capacitance (upward-/leftward-shifted EDPVR) accompanied by normal or low blood pressure (**black**). **(B)** Elevated ESPVR and upward-/leftward-shifted EDPVR (**black**). **(C)** Normal (or near normal) ESPVR and normal or even rightward shifted EDPVR (**black**). In the latter two cases, note that blood pressure is elevated, as is the case in patients with heart failure with a normal ejection fraction (HFnlEF) who have longstanding hypertension. (From Maurer MS, King DL, El-khoury Rumbarger L, et al. Left heart failure with a normal ejection fraction: indentification of different Pathophysiologic mechanisms. *J Card Fail.* 2005;11(3):177–187.

age, plasma volume was higher in the HFnlEF group. However, when plasma volume was indexed to body weight, this difference between normal controls and HFnlEF was minimal (42.0 versus 40.4 mL/kg, a 4% difference).

The potential for a subgroup of HFnlEF patients to have LV dilation has been previously reported (42). In persons without cardiovascular disease, ventricular volumes vary with body size, sex, and, to a lesser degree, age. Thus, selection of appropriate controls is important; here, the volume differences observed in the HFnlEF patients were more significant when controlling for these factors. While ventricular dilation and volume expansion are possible in a subgroup of patients with hypertension and HFnlEF, it is unlikely that diastolic function is completely normal in one subgroup and abnormal in a second. More likely, diastolic dysfunction plays a major role in some patients and less so in others, but there is likely a spectrum of diastolic dysfunction (even in those with HFnlEF and increased LV volumes).

It is also important to point out limitations in interpreting ventricular function according to the categories outlined in Figure 7-13. The bottom panel (Fig. 7-13C) implies that changes in systolic pressure mandate an inciting or accompanying change in volume. Such is not always the case. This model ignores the afterload enhancement of ventricular performance which results in a leftward and upward shift of Ees with or without an increase in its slope, such that systolic pressures are greater without increased end-diastolic volumes. Afterload enhancement of ventricular performance has been demonstrated in numerous animal studies (62–64,79–83). Further evidence of afterload enhancement of systolic performance comes from a study in patients with HFnlEF who were studied during acute hypertensive pulmonary edema (BP = 200/100 mm Hg) and after therapy (BP = 139/64 mm Hg). EF and end-diastolic volumes were essentially the same during these episodes (69), a phenomenon that would be impossible to predict using the construct outlined in the bottom panel of Figure 7-13C. Similarly, such a depiction does not recognize the ability of hypertrophy to normalize wall stress and maintain normal volumes and EFs.

Without recognition of afterload enhancement of ventricular performance and the effect of hypertrophy, all patients with elevated blood pressures would have reduced EF or markedly dilated ventricles. Indeed, this is not the case as normotensives (BP = 119/75 mm Hg), borderline hypertensives (BP =139/83 mm Hg), and subjects with sustained hypertension (BP = 157/99 mm Hg) in the Framingham study had identical LV dimensions (indexed to body surface area, BSA) and identical fractional shortening. This is presumably due to the development of hypertrophy, which works to normalize wall stress and prevent ventricular dilation and/or to afterload enhancement of systolic performance. Nonetheless, the concepts involved in Figure 7-13 are valuable in understanding possible mechanisms involved in the pathogenesis of HFnlEF. The true pathophysiology of the syndrome is likely heterogenous.

Systolic Function in HFnlEF

Although by definition EF is normal in patients with HFnlEF, studies have reported that other indexes of contractility are reduced in patients with preclinical diastolic dysfunction or HFnlEF despite normal EF. Studies using Doppler tissue imaging or M-mode to measure the velocity of longitudinal and short-axis fiber shortening in patients with Doppler evidence of diastolic dysfunction or HFnlEF showed that the velocity of longitudinal and short-axis myocardial shortening was reduced in patients with Doppler evidence of diastolic dysfunction and in patients with HFnlEF (84–86). However, these are indexes of the rate of contraction and may have little relevance to the extent of contraction. Other studies have reported that stress-corrected midwall shortening is reduced in some subjects with hypertension and LV hypertrophy despite normal EF (87–89). These data indicate that contractile function may decrease during the progression from preclinical diastolic dysfunction to HFnlEF and contribute to the pathogenesis of HFnlEF.

In contrast, Kawaguchi et al. measured LV Ees in patients with HFnlEF and found that Ees was increased as compared to young and old normotensive controls (29). Traditionally, Ees has been considered a load-independent index of contractility. However, structural factors may influence systolic stiffness in addition to contractility, and chronic increases in Ees observed in subjects with or at risk for cardiovascular diseases may be more reflective of structural alterations than altered inotropic state. Even if subtle changes in systolic performance do exist, their role in contributing to the pathogenesis of HFnlEF remains unclear. More importantly, whether patients with HFnlEF evolve to HF↓EF remains a frequently postulated but unproven theory.

CLINICAL PROFILE OF HFnlEF

Demographic Features and Comorbid Conditions

Clinical studies of patients with HFnlEF are summarized in Table 7-3, according to mode of presentation (acute pulmonary edema, hospitalization for HF decompensation, chronic syndrome, or mixed presentation to a referral laboratory). As shown in Table 7-3, patients with HFnlEF are often older women with a history of hypertension. The prevalence of coronary artery disease varies widely depending on the study setting. Although not reported in all studies, obesity was seen in 46% to 70% of patients, diabetes in up to 83%, and atrial fibrillation in up to 76% of cases. The prevalence of renal disease varied substantially, from 0% to 100%. The reported medications at diagnosis in patients with HFnlEF included diuretics, digoxin, anglotensin-converting enzyme (ACE) inhibitors, beta-blockers, calcium-channel blockers, and various other vasodilators, antihypertensive, and antiarrhythmic drugs. Those demographic features and comorbid conditions, which are highly prevalent in HFnlEF, will be discussed in more detail.

Aging

Although cardiovascular disease may contribute to diastolic dysfunction in older people, studies have also suggested that diastolic function deteriorates with normal

TABLE 7-3
CLINICAL STUDIES OF PATIENTS WITH HFnlEF ACCORDING TO TYPE OF PRESENTATION

				Comorbidities					
Clinical Study (Reference)	**Study Design/ Setting**	**Age**	**Female (%)**	**Obesity (%)**	**HTN (%)**	**CAD (%)**	**DM (%)**	**A-Fib (%)**	**Renal Disease (%)**
Patients presenting with acute pulmonary edema									
(139)	CS, Hsp	58	–	–	–	100	83	–	–
(171)	CS, Hsp	80	75	–	–	100	–	75	–
(172)	C, Hsp	63	31	–	–	100	–	–	–
(173)	C, Hsp	73*	60*	–	65	52	–	–	–
(174)	C, Hsp	76*	60*	–	70*	100	39*	–	–
(105)	C, Hsp	67	56	–	–	74	–	–	–
Patients hospitalized for HF decompensation									
(175)	C, Hsp	77	89	–	–	–	–	–	–
(176)	CS	68	–	–	29*	41*	–	–	–
(177)	C, Hsp	80	82	–	73	32	32	54	Excluded
(70)	C, Hsp	60	57	70	64	13	–	–	26
(178)	C, Hsp	66*	39*	–	58	–	–	76	–
(179)	C, Hsp, G	82	0	–	60	65	15	–	–
(71)	CS, Hsp	65	58	–	100	28	–	–	–
(180)	C, Hsp	76	51	–	54	31	–	42	–
(181)	C, Hsp, G	78	75	–	98	37	56	23	33
(182)	C, Hsp	81	71	–	75	58	29	–	CR = 1.6
(140)	C, Hsp	76	75	–	64	45	23	24	26
(16)	C, Hsp	73	63	–	80	24	48	39	36
(141)	C, Hsp	73	71	–	73	34	33	30	19
(72)	C, Hsp	69	51	–	66	34	30	30	11
(12)	C, Hsp	59	56	62	78	22	40	19	15
(73)	CS, Hsp	72	73	46	78	43	46	23	Dialysis 4.5%
Patients presenting with chronic stable HF									
(74)	CS, HTN	65	22	–	100	0	44	–	100
(103)	CT	56	44	–	45	67	18	–	–
(147)	CS, RL	55	79	–	83	4	30	4	11
(157)	C, CT	60	0	–	53	27	23	–	–
(183)	C, PHC	72*	62*	–	–	–	–	–	–
(184)									
(75)	C, E, G	79*	52*	–	56*	43*	40*	14*	CR=1.2*
(161)	C, HF clinic	69	50	–	40	31	21	36	–
(185)	C, G	83	77	–	70	75	–	30	–
(160)	CT	67	41		–	–	29	–	GFR = 62mL/min/m^2
(186)	C, PHC	72	72	–	83	46	35	30	22
(158)	CS, E	67*	64*	50	83	–	–	–	–
Patients with mixed presentation referred to a specialized laboratory									
(9)	C, RL	51	55	–	65	5	–	–	–
(76)	C, RL	63	53	–	65	53	35	–	18
(77)	CS	73*	76*	–	100	Excluded	Excluded	10	Excluded
(10)	C, RL	73	65	–	67	27	–	6	–
(187)	C, RL	64	2*	–	–	–	–	–	–
(188)	CS, RL	63	0	–	56	41	–	–	–
(41)	CS, RL	65	57	–	57	Excluded	–	–	–
(42)	CS, E	79	76	–	72	13	18	29	5

*For entire group of study patients. C, comparative; CS, case series; CT, clinical trial; E, epidemiology study; G, geriatric population; HTN, hypertensive population; PHC, primary health care; RL, referral lab.

aging (90). The LV early diastolic filling rate progressively slows after the age of 20 years (91–93). Recent studies using more load-independent indexes of LV relaxation have found that the speed of LV relaxation declines with age in men and women, even in the absence of cardiovascular disease (65). Structural cardiac changes with aging (increased cardiomyocyte size, increased apoptosis with decreased myocyte number, altered growth factor regulation, focal collagen deposition) are putative mechanisms for a reduced early diastolic filling rate. Functional changes at the cellular level involving excitation–contraction coupling and calcium-handling proteins that affect relaxation have also been demonstrated (60,66,94).

Fewer studies have examined potential changes in diastolic stiffness with aging. As previously noted, two studies have reported age-associated increases in LV systolic and diastolic stiffness with aging (50,65). These studies suggest that persons most at risk for HFnlEF, namely, the elderly, have alterations in ventricular function which predispose them to HFnlEF. Whether diastolic dysfunction is an inevitable consequence of aging is unclear. In a study of 12 healthy, sedentary seniors (mean age 70 years) and 12 age-matched Masters athletes undergoing cardiac catheterization, Arbab-Zadeh et al. demonstrated that although LV diastolic stiffness was substantially increased in sedentary seniors compared to young control subjects, such changes were not seen in senior Masters athletes. The authors concluded that prolonged, sustained endurance training may preserve LV compliance with aging and help to prevent HF in the elderly (67).

A final important consideration in normal cardiac aging is the change in LV afterload and vascular–ventricular load matching. As previously discussed, vascular stiffness increases with age and is coupled to increases in systolic and diastolic LV stiffness. This results in enhanced volume sensitivity and increases in load-dependent diastolic dysfunction. Increases in vascular stiffness have been shown to be related to effort intolerance in patients with HFnlEF (95). LV arterial–ventricular load mismatching in older persons during exercise may be a mechanism for the deficit in acute LV reserve that accompanies advancing age (96).

Gender

As previously outlined, female gender, along with age, is a potent risk factor for HFnlEF. Indeed, there appears to be important age–gender interactions such that the prevalence of HFnlEF increases more sharply with age in women than does the prevalence of HF↓EF (Fig. 7-12) (68). The reasons for the female predominance in HFnlEF are not entirely clear. One population-based study showed no gender difference and no evidence of age–gender interaction in load-independent indexes of LV relaxation (65), but found that women had higher LV systolic and diastolic stiffness than men. In this study, LV systolic stiffness increased more sharply with age in women than men, and indexes of arterial stiffness were also higher in women and increased more sharply with age in women than in men, even after adjusting for body size. Kelly et al. used invasive indexes and also found that LV systolic and diastolic stiffness and arterial stiffness were higher in women (97). Previous studies using a variety of indexes have established that large-artery stiffness is higher in women (51,54–56).

Thus, these studies provide some evidence that arterial and LV systolic and diastolic stiffness are increased with women and that age-related increases in cardiovascular stiffening may be accentuated in women. Whether these changes are related to differences in chamber and vascular size, hormonal influences, or other differences in risk factors in women are not clear, but increased cardiovascular stiffening with age in women may provide some explanation of the unique epidemiology of HFnlEF, where women are disproportionately afflicted.

Hypertension

Hypertension is the most commonly associated cardiac condition in patients with HFnlEF (Table 7-3). Chronically increased blood pressure load is an important stimulus for cardiac structural remodeling and functional changes. As previously reviewed in detail, the resultant hypertensive heart disease is characterized by LV hypertrophy (LVH), increasing vascular and ventricular systolic stiffness, impaired relaxation, and increased diastolic stiffness—all factors linked to the pathogenesis of HFnlEF (98). As previously discussed (Table 7-2), patients with hypertensive heart disease may be more sensitive to ischemia, and hypertensive and ischemic heart disease are often present in combination in patients with HFnlEF.

Coronary Artery Disease

The reported prevalence of coronary artery disease (CAD) or myocardial ischemia in patients with HFnlEF ranges widely (Table 7-3). Inconsistent diagnostic criteria for coronary disease may contribute to this variability. The relationship between CAD, ischemia, and HFnlEF has been nicely reviewed by Choudhury et al. (99), who emphasized the mechanisms whereby acute myocardial ischemia and chronic CAD can induce both impaired relaxation as well as increased diastolic stiffness. While diastolic dysfunction has been observed during coronary angioplasty (100), during acute myocardial infarction (101), and during exercise testing (102), the role of CAD and ischemia in patients with acute or chronic HFnlEF remains speculative. Indeed, in the Coronary Artery Surgery Study (CASS) registry, the severity of coronary disease was similar in those subjects with normal EF with or without a history of HF (103), and revascularization did not improve mortality. While LV diastolic function has been shown to improve after coronary revascularization (104), flash pulmonary edema was reported to recur in patients with CAD and HFnlEF despite revascularization (105). More studies evaluating the role of ischemia in the syndrome of HFnlEF are needed.

Atrial Fibrillation

As previously outlined, atrial contraction plays an important role in ventricular filling in the presence of impaired LV relaxation (Fig. 7-8 and accompanying text above). Indeed, atrial fibrillation has been reported in 23% to 76% of acutely decompensated HFnlEF patients and 4% to 36% of patients with the chronic syndrome (Table 7-3).

Although atrial fibrillation may cause decompensated HF in patients with diastolic dysfunction, diastolic dysfunction may also be a risk factor for atrial fibrillation by way of increased atrial pressures and atrial dilation. This issue was addressed in a study by Tsang et al. of 840 older patients with no history of atrial arrhythmia (106). Eighty patients (9.5%) developed atrial fibrillation over a mean follow-up of 4.1 years. The presence and severity of diastolic dysfunction were independently predictive of first documented atrial fibrillation in this cohort of elderly patients. Thus, diastolic dysfunction, atrial fibrillation, and HFnlEF are common and related conditions that likely share common pathogenic mechanisms in the elderly.

Obesity

Obesity has been associated with an increased risk for HF in several studies (107,108). Patients with HFnlEF are more often obese than are patients with HF↓EF (14,15), and the presence of preclinical diastolic dysfunction is increased in obese persons (109). There are several plausible mechanisms for an association between obesity and diastolic dysfunction or HFnlEF. Increased body mass index (BMI) is a risk factor for hypertension, diabetes mellitus, CAD, and atrial fibrillation, all of which are associated with HFnlEF. While an obesity cardiomyopathy has been described (110), it remains unclear whether obesity alone can produce HFnlEF. Several studies have used Doppler echocardiography to compare LV filling in obese and lean persons (111–118) and demonstrated that LV filling was impaired in patients with various degrees of obesity relative to lean subjects. A more recent study (119) using less load-dependent measures on tissue Doppler imaging also reported an association between diastolic dysfunction and obesity, as evidenced by reduced mitral annular velocity (E′) and elevated filling pressures, approximated by the mitral E/E′ ratio. In this study, E′ correlated with fasting insulin levels and reduced exercise capacity. BMI was independently related to average E′, even after adjustment for age, mean arterial pressure, LV mass index, and insulin level ($p < 0.001$). In an early study by Alexander (120) of 40 moderately to severely obese subjects, pulmonary hypertension was found at rest and with exercise in 25%, while an additional 50% had pulmonary hypertension with exercise. Increased pulmonary artery pressure was associated with raised cardiac output, stroke volume, and pulmonary capillary wedge pressure, implying that pulmonary vascular congestion was attributable to elevated LV diastolic pressures. Exercise-induced increased cardiac output associated with increased LV filling pressure in obese patients has also been reported by Backman et al. (121) and Kaltman and Goldring (122). Thus, a link between elevated filling pressures and obesity seems plausible although it remains unclear whether this is mediated by load, extrinsic factors, or intrinsic diastolic dysfunction.

Diabetes Mellitus

LV diastolic dysfunction may be the first stage of diabetic cardiomyopathy (123,124). Zabalgoitia et al. found that of 86 patients with diabetes, over 40% had diastolic dysfunction on Doppler echocardiography (125). These findings are noteworthy because the patients were young, normotensive, and under excellent diabetic control. Two large epidemiology studies found that patients with diabetes had a higher prevalence of preclinical diastolic dysfunction than did nondiabetics (109,126). Other studies have shown an association between impaired LV relaxation and glycosylated hemoglobin (HbA1c) concentrations (126,127). Most studies show that the prevalence of diabetes is similar in HFnlEF and HF↓EF, indicating that it is likely a risk factor for both forms of HF.

The morphological changes in the diabetic heart include myocyte hypertrophy, increased matrix collagen, interstitial fibrosis, and intramyocardial microangiopathy (128). These changes are probably consequences of altered myocardial glucose and fatty acid metabolism due to diabetes, as was recently reviewed (129).

An important mechanism whereby diabetes (and aging) may predispose to HFnlEF involves the role of chronic hyperglycemia and formation of AGE. Several excellent reviews on the biochemistry and potential clinical importance of AGE have recently been published (130–133). Nonenzymatic glycosylation of proteins results in formation of a Schiff base which is then modified to a more stable compound, the Amadori product. Over time, glycated proteins undergo further modification to yield the cross-linked proteins known as AGE. By cross-linking collagen molecules, AGE may increase the tensile strength of the collagen and may also make it less susceptible to degradation by matrix metalloproteases. Thus, AGE could enhance both the content and stiffness of aortic and LV collagen, contributing to increased stiffness in both tissues. There are also receptors for AGE (RAGE), which may mediate effects on intracellular second messengers and cytokines including NF-κB, tumor necrosis factor, and tissue growth factor β.

Numerous studies have reported increases in AGE tissue content in diabetes and in senescence. At what point in the aging process AGE accumulation becomes a clinically significant mediator of cardiovascular stiffening in nondiabetics remains undefined. Study of AGE in human disease is somewhat difficult as there are so many forms of AGE and standardized assay systems are lacking. Preclinical animal studies suggest the potential for dramatic effects with AGE cross-link breakers such as ALT-711. In diabetic models, marked improvement in renal damage, aortic stiffness, LV mass, and LV AGE content have been reported. In aged normoglycemic dogs, Asif et al. reported a 40% reduction in LV diastolic stiffness with 1 month of ALT-711 therapy (134). Vaitkevicius et al. reported a similarly dramatic reduction (25%) in aortic pulse wave velocity and carotid arterial augmentation index (40% reduction) after 3 weeks of therapy with ALT-711 in older rhesus monkeys (135). In the limited clinical studies to date, the effects of ALT-711 have been somewhat less dramatic than observed in animal studies. In a multicenter trial in patients with evidence of increased aortic stiffness, 8 weeks of ALT-711 therapy produced an 8% reduction in pulse wave velocity, a 7% reduction in pulse pressure, and a 15% increase in total arterial compliance (136). In two trials in patients with hypertension, no significant effect of several different doses of ALT-711 given for 6 months on systolic blood pressure or pulse pressure was seen. However, post hoc analysis in those patients with 24-hour ambulatory blood pressure monitoring did demonstrate an effect on systolic blood pressure in several dose groups (130).

A study by Little et al. was the first to test the efficacy of ALT-711 in HFnlEF (137). This was an open-label study treating 23 patients with HFnlEF for 16 weeks. Mean age of the patients was 71 years, 20% were diabetic, and all had a history of hypertension. Statistically significant improvement in symptoms (Minnesota Living with Heart Failure Questionnaire Score and New York Heart Association class) were seen but were unassociated with increases or trends toward increases in maximal exercise tolerance, raising concern over the role of the placebo effect in mediating the symptomatic response. Left ventricular mass decreased and there were trends toward improvements in some measures of aortic stiffness, although neither systolic blood pressure nor pulse pressure was changed. Doppler indexes of diastolic function were evaluated and the early diastolic mitral annular velocity increased, suggesting an improvement in the speed of LV relaxation. Whether ALT-711 will influence harder endpoints (HF hospitalizations or mortality or exercise tolerance) in HFnlEF remains to be defined.

Rare Causes of HFnlEF

Hypertrophic cardiomyopathy and infiltrative cardiomyopathies such as amyloidosis, valvular disease, and constrictive pericarditis should always be considered in young patients with HFnlEF or patients with other suggestive features. However, these diseases account for a minority of patients with HFnlEF. Idiopathic restrictive cardiomyopathy in young persons without the factors previously discussed may represent a distinct group, particularly if a family history is present. However, the clinical presentation and the echocardiographic appearance in older persons with HFnlEF may be identical to those of patients previously labeled as restrictive cardiomyopathy.

Clinical Factors Associated with Acute Decompensation in HFnlEF

Factors at clinical presentation associated with acute decompensation versus the chronic syndrome of HFnlEF were systematically examined in a few studies. Klapholz et al. (73) conducted a prospective study of 619 patients hospitalized for HFnlEF and found that severe hypertension (SBP >200 mm Hg) was the most commonly identified precipitant for symptomatic deterioration (prevalence: 13%). Other precipitating factors, in descending order of frequency, included noncompliance to medication, severe valvular regurgitation, acute coronary syndrome, renal insufficiency, supraventricular arrhythmias, severe chronic obstructive pulmonary disease (COPD)/asthma, pneumonia, severe valvular stenosis, and sepsis. Factors precipitating hospitalization were not identifiable in 47% of patients, while two or more precipitating factors were present in 19% of patients.

Chen et al. (42) retrospectively examined the factors present at diagnosis in their series of patients from Olmsted County, Minnesota, with new diagnoses of HFnlEF. These factors included uncontrolled hypertension (SBP >160 mm Hg or DBP >90 mm Hg) in 55%, atrial fibrillation or flutter in 29%, infection in 27%, ischemia in 18%, and renal insufficiency in 5% of patients. Finally, Kramer et al. (105) studied 46 patients (27 with EF >40%) with an initial presentation of flash pulmonary edema and followed them for up to 3 years, during which flash pulmonary edema recurred in half of the patients. The recurrence of flash pulmonary edema was similar in patients with normal or reduced EF, in those with or without CAD, and regardless of whether or not patients with CAD were revascularized. The acute decompensation occurred in association with marked systolic hypertension at presentation (mean SBP = 185 mm Hg). It therefore appears that uncontrolled hypertension and supraventricular arrhythmias are very common factors associated with acute decompensation. In contrast, patients with chronic, stable HF are likely to have fewer reversible features.

Symptoms and Signs

As previously addressed, clinical signs and symptoms in HFnlEF are indistinguishable from those observed in HF↓EF. Indeed, in a careful *prospective* study of consecutive patients hospitalized with HF, none of the clinical parameters was found to differentiate reliably between patients with normal and reduced EF (12). In the case of the chronic, stable outpatients, other studies have compared physical findings with invasive hemodynamic measurements and shown that physical examination is a relatively insensitive method for detecting raised filling pressures in patients with chronic HF (138). In summary, HF with normal versus reduced EF appears to be indistinguishable at the bedside and assessment of cardiac function is necessary to tell the two apart.

Findings on Chest X-Ray

Cardiomegaly, pulmonary venous congestion, and pleural effusions have all been reported in series of patients with HFnlEF (12,70,71,139–141). While some studies report a slightly higher prevalence of cardiomegaly in patients with HF↓EF as compared to HFnlEF, this feature did not reliably distinguish between the two conditions.

Findings on Doppler Echocardiography

LV size in HFnlEF

The prevalence of normal or reduced versus increased LV cavity dimensions in patients with HFnlEF was previously discussed. As was emphasized, most studies report that (on average) LV cavity size is normal in HFnlEF but a substantial subset may have LV dilatation.

LV Hypertrophy in Patients with HFnlEF

While HFnlEF has been thought to occur primarily in patients with LV hypertrophy, studies that have carefully quantified LV mass report that echocardiographic criteria for LV hypertrophy are met in less than 50% of patients (5,13,29,42). Patients with HFnlEF have (on average) increased relative wall thickness and increased mass to volume ratios (13,78) but these findings often occur in the setting of normal LV mass. Thus, despite traditional teaching, LV hypertrophy is not invariably present in HFnlEF.

Doppler Echocardiographic Assessment of Diastolic Function and Filling Pressures in Patients with HFnlEF

The Doppler assessment of diastolic function is complex. Early studies focused on the transmitral flow velocity profile. Decreases in the ratio of early to late diastolic filling (E/A), increases in the deceleration time (DT) of the early diastolic filling velocity profile, or increases in the isovolumic relaxation time (IVRT) indicate impaired relaxation. However, in the presence of impaired relaxation, increases in filling pressure modify the transmitral gradient and the mitral inflow pattern in a progressive manner (Fig. 7-6). Thus, while several studies report average values for the E/A, DT, or IVRT in patients with HFnlEF studied at various times during their presentation, these studies provide little insight into diastolic function or filling pressures. Only a few studies have utilized more advanced Doppler methods to categorize patients as currently recommended to reflect diastolic function and filling pressures (20,109) (Fig. 7-6).

Chen et al. reported that patients studied at various times during their presentation (acutely decompensated, after initial treatment of an acute decompensation episode, or as stable outpatients) were characterized by a spectrum of filling patterns (42), including abnormal relaxation, psuedonormal, and restrictive patterns. Such a spectrum has also been reported in patients with HF↓EF and reflects the potent effect of filling pressures and their interaction with underlying diastolic dysfunction on the Doppler patterns. Thus, depending on their level of compensation and their filling pressures, patients with HFnlEF may display any of the filling patterns outlined in Figure 7-6.

Other Doppler Echo Findings in HFnlEF

Regional wall motion abnormalities, left atrial dilation, right ventricular dilation, and pulmonary hypertension have also been reported at echo in patients with HFnlEF (42). The prevalence of pulmonary hypertension was 46.5% to 57% in two different studies (70,73).

EPIDEMIOLOGY OF HFNLEF

Existing clinical studies suggest that the frequency of HFnlEF among patients with HF ranges from 13% to 74%, and several reasons account for this apparent variability in the relative prevalence of HFnlEF (142). Clinical studies have been performed in diverse practice settings using a variety of methods of case ascertainment. The prevalence of HF and the frequency of HFnlEF among patients with HF vary dramatically according to age and sex, and existing studies have examined groups of varying age, gender, and ethnicity distributions—a factor that will influence estimates of the frequency of HFnlEF among patients with HF. Studies also differ in their criteria for diagnosing HF and HFnlEF. Selection biases are introduced when study patients are obtained from particular specialized laboratories within a medical facility.

Epidemiological studies have defined the prevalence or relative (to HF↓EF) prevalence of HFnlEF in a variety of populations, as was recently reviewed in detail (14,15). The review of Owan et al. also addresses the epidemiology of preclinical diastolic dysfunction (which is assumed to progress to HFnlEF), a concept supported by data from the Cardiovascular Health Study where the presence of diastolic dysfunction was predictive of future HF (143). Published epidemiological studies defining the relative prevalence of HFnlEF among patients with HF and the population prevalence of HFnlEF are summarized in Table 7-4. Although these population-based studies are not influenced by many of the referral biases inherent in the clinical studies, several limitations should be considered. As with clinical studies, epidemiological studies can be influenced by the definitions of HF and normal EF used, the imaging modality employed to assess EF, whether incident or prevalent HF is studied, whether patients with HF diagnosed in the outpatient setting are included, and, in prospective studies, by the participation rate, age, and ethnic composition of the target population. While all major epidemiological studies utilized echocardiography to assess systolic function, the specific techniques vary widely. Despite the limitations mentioned previously and the variable study design and size, estimates of the prevalence of HFnlEF among patients with clinically overt HF in epidemiological studies are more consistent than those reported in clinical studies; they range from 40% to 71% with a mean of 54%.

Of the nine cross-sectional epidemiological studies reviewed, all of them reported on the prevalence of HF and the percentage of HF cases with normal EF, thus allowing an estimation of the prevalence of HFnlEF in the population. These studies provide only estimates of the population prevalence of HFnlEF and need to be viewed within the context of the variability and limitations previously outlined. Thus, based on existing population-based epidemiological studies of HFnlEF, the prevalence of HFnlEF within the population varies from 1.14% to 5.5%, depending on the age of the population and the variables affecting the study. When younger segments of the population are included in the base population, lower estimates of prevalence are yielded, with the prevalence varying from 1.14% to 2.95% for population studies which included persons >25 or >40 to 45 years of age, respectively. For studies confined to a more elderly segment of the population (aged 65 or older), the prevalence of HFnlEF in the population varies from 3.1% to 5.5%. Importantly, the prevalence of HFnlEF among patients with HF may vary by age and sex, and only one study has had sufficient numbers of subjects to estimate the age- and sex-specific prevalence of HFnlEF in the population (68). Age- and sex-specific estimates of the prevalence of HF, HFnlEF, and HF↓EF from this study are presented in Fig. 7-12. This study highlights

TABLE 7-4

PREVALENCE OF HFnlEF AMONG PATIENTS WITH HEART FAILURE AND POPULATION PREVALENCE OF HFnlEF IN EPIDEMIOLOGIC STUDIES USING ECHOCARDIOGRAPHIC IMAGING

Reference	Study Design/ Setting	No. of Subjects (age)	CHF Criteria	Definition of Normal Systolic function	Population Prevalence of HF	% HF with HFnlEF	Population Prevalence of HFnlEF
(189)	A/Massachusetts (FHS)	73 (NR)	Framingham	EF ≥50%	NR	51%	NR
(190)	A/Hong Kong	(all ages)	Clinical Diagnosis	EF >45%	NR	66%	NR
(191)	A/Olmsted County, MN	216 (all ages)	Framingham	EF ≥50%	NR	43%	NR
(109)	B/Olmsted County, MN	2,042 (>45 y)	Framingham	EF >50%	2.60%	44%	1.14%
(68)	B/Portugal (EPICA study)	5,434 (>25 y)	ESC guidelines	EF ≥45% or FS >28%	4.36%	40%	1.70%
(75)	B/U.S. multicenter (CHS)	4,242 (>65 y)	Self-report with review	Qualitative "Normal function"	8.8%	55%	4.84%
(192)	B/Asturias, Spain	391 (>40 y)	Framingham	EF >50%	5.0%	59%	2.95%
(193)	B/Vasteras, Sweden	433 (75 y)	Clinical diagnosis	EF >43% or WMI <1.7	6.7%	46%	3.1%
(194)	B/Native Americans (SHS)	3,638 (45–74 y)	Framingham	EF >54%	3.0%	52%	1.6%
(195)	B/Rotterdam, The Netherlands	5,540 (>55 y)	Clinical score	FS >25%	3.9%	71%	2.8%
(196)	B/Poole, UK	817 (70–84 y)	Self-report	Qualitative "Normal function"	8.1%	68%	5.5%
(197)	B/Helsinki, Sweden	501 (75–86 y)	Clinical criteria, CXR	FS ≥0.25	8.2%	51%	4.2%

FHS, Framingham Heart Study; EPICA; Epidemiology of Heart Failure and Learning; CHS, Cardiovascular Health Study; SHS, Strong Heart Study; EF, ejection fraction; FS, fractional shortening; CXR, chest radiograph; NR, not reported; WMI, wall motion index; UK, United Kingdom. Population-based studies assessing the prevalence of HFnlEF among patients with HF have varied in design. Study type A: all patients with incident or prevalent HF from a defined population over a specified time period are studied prospectively or retrospectively, and the relative frequency of preserved (HFnlEF) versus reduced (HF↓EF) ejection fraction is defined. The true population prevalence of HF and HFnlEF cannot be estimated. Study B: a large, cross-sectional sample of a segment of a population (usually a specific age range) undergoes assessment for the past or current presence of HF and echocardiography. The relative frequency of preserved versus reduced ejection fraction among those with HF is defined. In this type of study, both the prevalence of HFnlEF among patients with HF and the population prevalence of HFnlEF can be estimated. However, in this type of study one cannot exclude the possibility that changes in ejection fraction have occurred between the time of HF onset and the time of the study. Thus, this type of study defines the fraction of the HF population that has preserved ejection fraction at variable times since the onset of HF.
From Owan T, Redfield M. Epidemiology of diastolic heart failure. *Prog Cardiovasc Dis.* 2005;47(5):320–332.

the age- and sex-specific variation in the prevalence of HFnlEF.

NATURAL HISTORY OF HFnlEF

Mortality

In hospitalized patients, mortality rates for HFnlEF are lower than for HF↓EF in most studies, although the differences in mortality are highly variable and, in general, not substantial, particularly in more elderly cohorts. Of the four population-based studies, three suggest that the mortality for HFnlEF is similar to that of HF↓EF. These three studies were limited by relatively small numbers of subjects with HF. In the fourth study, the Cardiovascular Health Study (144), a much larger number of HF patients were studied. In this study, mortality was higher for HF↓EF. However, in this study of free-living persons aged 65 or older, the prevalence of HFnlEF was higher than that of HF↓EF. Thus, more deaths occurred in those with HFnlEF and the population-attributable risk for death was greatest for HFnlEF. Finally, differences in etiology of HF may explain the mortality differences seen in the study by Anorow et al., which reported only on patients with HF and coronary artery disease, excluding 81 patients with HF who did not have coronary artery disease (145).

It should be emphasized that compared to age-matched controls, mortality risk is clearly higher in patients with HFnlEF (103,146,147). Also, most studies assessed the association between HF and all-cause mortality and did not assess the cause of death. A post hoc analysis from the Digitalis Investigation Group (DIG) study (148) suggested that the cause of death was somewhat different in patients with HFnlEF compared to patients with reduced EF. While worsening HF and arrhythmias were the leading causes of death in all HF patients (regardless of EF), deaths due to noncardiovascular causes were more frequent in patients with normal EF, consistent with their older age. These data need to be confirmed in more-contemporary and better-characterized cohorts but suggest that treatment strategies for HFnlEF and clinical trials testing such strategies will need to account for the considerable noncardiovascular morbidity and mortality in these patients.

Morbidity

There are only few comparative studies of hospital readmission rates in HF patients with normal versus reduced EF (Table 7-5). Most studies report similar readmission rates for HFnlEF as compared to HF↓EF. The study by Smith et al. (16) also importantly looked at functional decline after dismissal for HF and showed that this was equivalent in HF patients with normal and reduced EF. Above all, it remains clear that HF (regardless of EF) carries significant morbidity and often necessitates frequent hospital admissions and health care expenditure.

MAKING THE DIAGNOSIS OF HFnlEF

Before making a diagnosis of HFnlEF in a patient suspected to have the condition, it is important to make a diagnosis of HF itself. Since HF is a clinical syndrome, its diagnosis is a clinical one, based on the presence of characteristic symptoms and signs. Unfortunately, each of these symptoms and signs, although characteristic of the syndrome, are nonspecific. For example, several noncardiac conditions such as pulmonary disease, obesity, anemia, and even pregnancy can present with similar symptoms of breathlessness, reduced effort tolerance, and edema. Although the diagnosis of HF is supported by results of appropriate investigations, no single investigation can confirm or refute the clinical diagnosis.

Diagnostic Criteria for HFnlEF

Two different criteria for HFnlEF diagnosis have been suggested if the clinical syndrome is to be attributed to diastolic dysfunction. Neither has been formally adopted in the United States and there are limitations to both.

European Study Group on Diastolic Heart Failure

The European Society of Cardiology (ESC) Study Group on Diastolic Heart Failure (149) proposes that a diagnosis of "primary diastolic HF" requires three obligatory conditions to be simultaneously satisfied.

1. The presence of signs and symptoms of congestive heart failure.
2. The presence of normal or only mildly abnormal LV systolic function.
3. Invasive or Doppler echocardiographic evidence of abnormal LV relaxation, filling, diastolic distensibility, or stiffness.

Criteria Proposed by Vasan and Levy

The second set of criteria, proposed by Vasan and Levy (43), defines different levels of diagnostic certainty enabling a classification of definite, probable, or possible diastolic HF. A diagnosis of definite "diastolic HF" requires the triad of:

1. Definitive evidence of congestive HF.
2. Objective evidence of normal LV systolic function (ejection fraction ≥50%) in proximity to the HF event (within 72 hours of presentation with symptoms).
3. Objective evidence of diastolic dysfunction as established on cardiac catheterization.

These criteria may lack sufficient sensitivity (42) because they mandate demonstration of diastolic abnormalities, an aspect not uniformly performed or available to all clinicians. Furthermore, diastolic abnormalities are frequently present in patients without HF. The need to document abnormal diastolic function in patients with HFnlEF has been challenged (38) because such abnormalities were uniformly present in a study of patients with the clinical syndrome of HFnlEF. Furthermore, the optimal cut-off point for normal EF is unclear. EF is a continuous variable with normal distribution within the population; hence, any arbitrarily set partition value will include false-positive and false-negative findings. A higher cut-off for normal EF at >50% will be more likely to include patients with truly normal systolic function. A lower cut-off for abnormal EF at 35% to 40% would similarly include more patients with clearly abnormal systolic function and would be clinically useful since most HF treatment trials have used this as an inclusion criterion. This, however, leaves a gray zone at 40% to 49%, and better guidelines are needed to address this group.

Finally, the stipulation that patients must have EF measured within 72 hours of presentation is likely unnecessary, as was demonstrated in the study by Gandhi et al. (69) where only 4 of 29 patients with EF ≥45% 3 to 5 days after pulmonary edema had an EF <40% at the time of pulmonary edema. Thus, many have advocated the use of the term HFnlEF when clinical evidence of HF exists in the absence of valvular disease or significant reduction in EF. Whether all such patients have diastolic dysfunction remains unclear, as is previously discussed in detail.

Diagnostic Tools to Assist in the Diagnosis of HFnlEF

Brain Natriuretic Peptide (BNP) and N-terminal ProBNP

A number of small clinical studies have suggested that brain natriuretic peptide (BNP) testing has value in the diagnosis of HFnlEF (150–153). The only large study probing the utility of BNP in diagnosis of HFnlEF is a post hoc analysis of data from the Breathing Not Properly Trial (154). Of those patients thought to have HF (n = 744), 452 had an echocardiogram within 30 days of presentation; of these, 165 had preserved EF. The median BNP of the patients with HFnlEF was 413 pg/mL compared to 34 pg/mL in controls and 821 pg/mL in patients with HF↓EF. While these data might suggest that BNP lev-

TABLE 7-5
PROGNOSIS IN PATIENTS WITH HEART FAILURE AND NORMAL VERSUS REDUCED EJECTION FRACTION

Reference	Study Design/Setting	No. of Patients (% HFnlEF)	Mean Age (y) of Patients with HFnlEF	Mortality HFnlEF Versus HF↓EF*	Morbidity HFnlEF Versus HF↓EF
Hospital-Based Studies					
(172)	Retrospective/Referral hospital	39 (41%)	63	9-month mortality 25% versus 30% (NS)	9-month readmission 50% versus 48% (NS)
(187)	Retrospective/Referral hospital	91 (48%)	64#	Median survival 26 versus 11 months (p = 0.01)	
(157)	Retrospective/Multicenter	623 (13%)	60	Annual mortality rate 8% versus 19% (p = 0.0001)	
(198)	Prospective/Referral hospital	78 (28%)	60	1-year mortality 22% versus 24%; 2-year mortality 26% versus 46% (p = 0.04)	
(179)	Retrospective/Referral hospital	94 (43%)	82	1-year mortality ≈24% versus ≈24%; 2-year mortality ≈30% versus ≈42% (NS)	
(141)	Retrospective/Referral hospital	192 (46%)	73	27-month mortality 35% versus 35% (NS)	6-month readmission 41% versus 55% (NS)
(182)	Prospective/Referral hospital	501 (34%)	81	1-year mortality 28% versus 38% (p = 0.045)	3-month readmission 29% versus 42% (p = 0.011)
(199)	Retrospective/Multicenter	1,291 (24%)	75#	6-month mortality 17% versus 23% (p = 0.04)	
(16)	Prospective/Referral hospital	413 (48%)	73	6-month mortality 13% versus 21% (p = 0.02)	6-month readmission 46% versus 46% (NS) Rate of functional decline 30% versus 23% (NS)
(200)	Retrospective/VA medical center	448 (27%)	69	1-year survival 82% versus 70%; 3-year survival 56% versus 45% (p = 0.02)	6-month rehospitalization 30% versus 35%; 12-month hospitalization 37% versus 43% (NS)
Outpatient/Community-Based Studies					
(145)	Prospective/Long-term healthcare facility	166 (40%)	84	1-year mortality 22% versus 47%; 2-year mortality 38% versus 71% (p = 0.001)	
(197)	Prospective/Population-based	41 (51%)	80#	4-year mortality 43% versus 54% (NS)	
(191)	Prospective/Population-based	137 (43%)	78	1-year mortality 24% versus 24%; 3-year mortality 42% versus 42% (NS)	Hospitalization rate 1 time: 51% versus 41%; ≥2 times: 25% versus 49% (p <0.05)
(161)	Prospective/Heart failure clinic	566 (21%)	69	1-year mortality 12% versus 17%; 3-year mortality 42% versus 38% (NS)	
(189)	Prospective/Population-based nested case control	73 (51%)	72	Annual mortality 9% versus 19%; 5-year mortality 32% versus 64% (unadjusted: p = 0.023; adjusted for age and gender: p = 0.13)	
(144)	Prospective/Population-based	269 (63%)	75	Deaths per 1,000 person-years: 87 versus 154* (p = 0.007)	
(201)	Retrospective/Outpatient community-based	338 (44%)	69	22-month mortality 8% versus 12% (NS)	Cardiovascular hospitalization 27% versus 35% (NS)

*Data for HFnlEF given first.
#, All patients.

els are lower in HFnlEF, the severity of HF symptoms was milder in patients with HFnlEF. When the patients with HFnlEF were compared to patients without HF (n = 770), a BNP value of 100 pg/mL had sensitivity of 86%, a negative predictive value of 96%, and a diagnostic accuracy of 75% for diagnosing HFnlEF. There was a considerable overlap between the BNP levels in non-HF and HFnlEF, particularly in elderly women. Normal plasma BNP concentration is known to be affected by age and gender, and values increase with age and in females (155). As patients with HFnlEF are older and more often female than patients with HF↓EF, the standard partition value of 100 pg/mL suggested for the diagnosis of HF may not be appropriate in HFnlEF because normal elderly women often have BNP values >100 pg/mL. Lainchbury et al. studied N-terminal proBNP and found that values were somewhat lower in HFnlEF versus HF↓EF patients (156). Given the difficulty some clinicians have in feeling confident in the diagnosis of HFnlEF, available studies suggest BNP may be helpful but further studies are needed to establish predictive characteristics and appropriate partition values.

Cardiopulmonary Testing

Cardiopulmonary exercise testing (CPET) is useful in the evaluation of exercise intolerance and exertional dyspnea. Despite the wide application of CPET in the assessment of functional impairment and prognosis in HF↓EF, less data are available in HFnlEF. Cohn et al. (157) showed that exercise tolerance was low in patients with HFnlEF and only slightly better than in HF↓EF (peak oxygen consumption: 15.5 versus 14.6 mL/kg per minute; $p = 0.04$). Kitzman et al. (13) compared exercise performance measures in older patients with HFnlEF with those of HF↓EF patients and age-matched healthy volunteers. Peak workload, exercise time, and oxygen consumption were markedly reduced in the patients with HF (regardless of EF) compared with healthy controls. Ventilatory anaerobic threshold and peak lactate level were also markedly abnormal in both HF groups compared with controls, and no significant differences between the two types of HF were observed.

CPET may therefore be valuable in the diagnosis of HFnlEF by identifying the precise mechanism of exercise limitation in a symptomatic patient. In particular, it may help to distinguish cardiac from pulmonary or noncardiopulmonary causes of dyspnea.This clinical application was demonstrated in a study by MacFadyen et al. (158) of 67 breathless patients in the community of Arbroath, Scotland. Evaluation for the cause of breathlessness included CPET, clinical examination, rest ECG, chest radiograph, spirometry, and echocardiography. The diagnosis of HFnlEF was ultimately made in 12 (18%) patients, and the diagnosis was successfully distinguished from HF↓EF, valvular heart disease, symptomatic myocardial ischemia, pulmonary disease, and patients with noncardiopulmonary causes for breathlessness. An important caveat is the effect of age and gender on expected results on CPET. Aging causes mild to moderate declines in ventilatory capacity as a result of decreased lung elastic recoil [the average forced expiratory volume in 1 second (FEV1) of a 70-year-old person is 70% of that of an average 25-year-old person]. This is typically balanced with a fall in demand (i.e., decreased peak VO_2) due to reasons that are not fully appreciated. In normal subjects, average peak VO_2 is 20% to 30% higher in men than in women; higher percent body fat in women is postulated to be the major factor contributing to this difference. These factors must be borne in mind when interpreting CPET results.

Doppler Echocardiographic Assessment of Diastolic Function in HFnlEF

Doppler echocardiography can aid in the diagnosis of diastolic dysfunction and the assessment of filling pressures in patients with suspected HF. Despite publication of consensus papers, reviews, and numerous clinical studies, widespread routine assessment of diastolic function is not yet a clinical reality. Proper performance of the examination can be technically demanding and interpretation of Doppler indexes requires a firm understanding of the concomitant influence of loading conditions and diastolic function on these indexes.

The utility of these parameters will vary depending on the clinical scenario. An elderly patient complaining of exertional dyspnea may well have an impaired relaxation pattern at rest and this finding may support a role for diastolic dysfunction in the generation of exertional symptoms. However, although HF is more prevalent in patients with Doppler evidence of diastolic dysfunction than in those without it, diastolic dysfunction is present in nearly 25% of the adult population by Doppler examination, most of whom do not have HF (109). When present, Doppler profiles consistent with elevated filling pressures (a pseudonormal or restrictive pattern, Fig. 7-6) support a diagnosis of HFnlEF in patients with resting dyspnea or symptoms with minimal activity. Whether such patients have a restrictive or pseudonormal pattern will depend, in part, on the severity of relaxation impairment as well as on the degree of left atrial pressure elevation. On the other hand, when an impaired relaxation pattern is present in a patient with resting or severe symptoms, an alternative diagnosis should be considered because this pattern implies normal or only mildly elevated filling pressures and would be inconsistent with the severity of symptoms.

In summary, assessment of diastolic function with Doppler echocardiography can be useful in the assessment of patients with suspected HFnlEF. There is no single pattern pathognomonic of HFnlEF and the diagnosis of HFnlEF remains a clinical one.

THERAPY OF HFnlEF

In general, the management of HFnlEF has two objectives. The first is to treat the presenting syndrome of HF (relieve venous congestion and eliminate precipitating factors). The second is to reverse the factors responsible for diastolic dysfunction or other perturbations which lead to HFnlEF. Both nonpharmacologic and pharmacologic strategies may be employed to achieve these aims. Present treatment strategies for HFnlEF are largely based on assumptions regarding its pathophysiological mechanisms and extrapolations from proven strategies used in HF with reduced EF.

Nonpharmacologic Therapy

General measures that may be employed in the management of patients with chronic HFnlEF are not different from those pursued in patients with HF↓EF; they include daily monitoring of weight, attention to diet and lifestyle, patient education, and close medical follow-up. In patients with HFnlEF, aggressive control of hypertension, tachycardia, and other potential precipitants for HF decompensation should be emphasized. The role of exercise training in patients with HFnlEF has also been explored (159). Although there are no adequate clinical trials with appropriate outcome endpoints such as increased longevity, decreased symptoms, or improved quality of life (QOL) to definitively prove the benefits of exercise training in patients with HFnlEF, several clinical and experimental studies suggest that exercise training would be beneficial for such patients.

Diastolic dysfunction is usually the consequence of aging, hypertrophy, ischemia, or some combination of these factors. Exercise training has been shown to favorably influence all of these effects. Endurance-type exercise training has improved indexes of diastolic function in elderly and younger humans and in rats with LVH. Thus, exercise training may be beneficial in clinically significant, symptomatic diastolic dysfunction. Such clinical benefit remains unproved, however. This issue is confounded by the fact that many patients with diastolic dysfunction have mildly to severely limited exercise tolerance that may impair their ability to achieve conditioning. Until definitive clinical trials are performed, a reasonable policy is to recommend endurance-type exercise training, initially with careful supervision and with the caveat that training intensity is monitored to avoid excessive dyspnea or pulmonary congestion. The safety of resistance training in such patients has not been studied.

Pharmacologic Therapy

In contrast to the treatment of HF↓EF, data to guide the pharmacologic therapy of patients with HFnlEF are lacking. Limited available data from clinical studies and randomized controlled clinical trials are reviewed here, followed by a summary of the ACC/AHA practice guideline recommendations.

Clinical Studies

Several clinical studies reported on medication usage in patients with HFnlEF but only few reported on outcomes in relation to type of drugs used. Chen et al. (42) found that survival was better in patients hospitalized with HFnlEF who were discharged on ACE inhibitors or beta-blockers. In the DIG trial, univariate predictors of mortality in patients with HFnlEF included use of vasodilators and diuretics (160). McAlister et al. (161) followed outpatients in a specialized HF clinic and found that beta-blockers were associated with a reduced mortality risk in the overall group, while metolazone, thiazides, and loop diuretics were associated with increased mortality risk. Restricting their analysis to patients with normal EF, however, none of the medications was significantly associated with a survival benefit or mortality excess.

Controlled studies have been performed with various standard HF drugs in patients with HFnlEF. The drugs used have included ACE inhibitors (162,163), angiotensin-receptor antagonists (164), beta-blockers (165,166), and calcium-channel-blockers (167,168). These trials have, however, been small or have produced inconclusive results.

Randomized, Controlled Clinical Trials

To date, only two randomized, placebo-controlled, multicenter drug trials in patients with HFnlEF have been completed and published. The first is the Digoxin Investigation Group (DIG) Trial (169) that included a small subgroup of patients with HFnlEF. In that trial, digoxin did not alter mortality but did reduce HF hospitalizations. The second trial is the Candesartan in Heart Failure: Assessment of Reduction in Morbidity and Mortality (CHARM)-Preserved Trial (170), where HF patients with EF >40% were randomized to candesartan or placebo in addition to standard therapy. Cardiovascular death did not differ between groups but fewer patients in the candesartan group than in the placebo group were hospitalized for HF.

Ongoing clinical trials in HFnlEF will test the efficacy of irbesartan (I-Preserve Trial), perindopril (PEP-CHF Trial), nebivolol (SENIORS Study), combinations of diuretics, ramipril, and irbesartan (Hong Kong Diastolic Heart Failure Study), aldosterone antagonists (TOPCAT Trial), and nesiritide (Use of Nesiritde in the Management of Acute Diastolic Heart Failure Trial). Until these trials are completed, however, clinicians need to expand their understanding of this syndrome and its pathophysiology and natural history, and remain open to the possibility that the therapeutic approach to HFnlEF may well evolve into one quite different from that of HF↓EF.

Clinical Practice Guidelines.

Table 7-6 (7) summarizes the ACC/AHA 2005 recommendations for treatment of patients with HFnlEF. The committee summarized the following principles of treatment of these patients:

> In the absence of controlled clinical trials, the management of these patients with HF and preserved LVEF is based on the control of physiological factors (blood pressure, heart rate, blood volume, and myocardial ischemia) that are known to exert important effects on ventricular relaxation. Likewise, diseases that are known to cause HF with normal LVEF should be treated, such as coronary artery disease, hypertensive heart disease, or aortic stenosis. Clinically, it seems reasonable to target symptom reduction, principally by reducing cardiac filling pressures at rest and during exertion.

It is important to note that in contrast to HF↓EF, adding ACE inhibitors, beta-blockers, or aldosterone inhibition in patients with adequate blood pressure control is not strongly endorsed but potential benefit is recognized

TABLE 7-6

RECOMMENDATIONS FOR TREATMENT OF PATIENTS WITH HEART FAILURE AND NORMAL LEFT VENTRICULAR EJECTION FRACTION

Recommendation	Class	Level of Evidence
Physicians should control systolic and diastolic hypertension, in accordance with published guidelines.	I	A
Physicians should control ventricular rate in patients with atrial fibrillation.	I	C
Physicians should use diuretics to control pulmonary congestion and peripheral edema.	I	C
Coronary revascularization is reasonable in patients with coronary artery disease in whom symptomatic or demonstrable myocardial ischemia is judged to be having an adverse effect on cardiac function.	IIa	C
Restoration and maintenance of sinus rhythm in patients with atrial fibrillation might be useful to improve symptoms.	IIa	C
The use of beta-adrenergic blocking agents, angiotensin-converting enzyme inhibitors, angiotensin II receptor blockers, or calcium antagonists in patients with controlled hypertension might be effective to minimize symptoms of heart failure.	IIb	C
The use of digitalis to minimize symptoms of heart failure is not well-established.	IIb	C

Recommendations are classified in the ACC/AHA format as follows: Class I, Conditions for which there is evidence and/or general agreement that a given procedure or treatment is beneficial, useful, and effective; Class II, Conditions for which there is conflicting evidence and/or a divergence of opinion about the usefulness/efficacy of a procedure or treatment, where Class IIa is used when the weight of evidence/opinion is in favor of usefulness/efficacy and Class IIb is used when the usefulness/efficacy is less well established by evidence/opinion; and Class III, Conditions for which there is evidence and/or general agreement that a procedure/treatment is not useful/effective and in some cases may be harmful. Levels of evidence are expressed in the ACC/AHA format as follows: A, Data derived from multiple randomized clinical trials or meta-analyses; B, Data derived from a single randomized trial, or nonrandomized studies; C, Only consensus opinion of experts, case studies, or standard-of-care.
From Hunt S, Abraham W, Chin M, Feldman A, et al. ACC/AHA 2005 guideline update for the diagnosis and management of chronic heart failure in the adult: a report of the American College of Cardiology/American Heart Association Task Force on practice guidelines (Writing Committee to Update the 2001 Guidelines for the Evaluation and Management of Heart Failure). American College of Cardiology. http://acc.org/clinical/guidelines/failure/index.pdf. Accessed 8/16/2005.

(Class IIb). Furthermore, the preferential use of these agents as first-line therapy for hypertension is not endorsed, although these agents are often needed to control blood pressure in elderly patients when initial therapy with diuretics does not achieve adequate blood pressure. While heart rate control for patients with atrial fibrillation is strongly endorsed (Class I), rhythm control in such patients is less strongly endorsed (Class IIb) despite the theoretical benefit of such a strategy to preserve atrial contribution to filling as outlined above.

REFERENCES

1. McKee PA, Castelli WP, McNamara PM, et al. The natural history of congestive heart failure: the Framingham study. *New Engl J Med.* 1971;285:1441–1446.
2. Levy D, Kenchaiah S, Larson MG, et al. Long-term trends in the incidence of and survival with heart failure. *N Engl J Med.* 2002;347(18):1397–1402.
3. Ho KKK, Anderson KM, Kannel WB, et al. Survival after the onset of congestive heart failure in Framingham Heart Study subjects. *Circulation.* 1993;88:107–115.
4. Mann DL. Mechanisms and models in heart failure, a combinatorial approach. *Circulation.* 1999;100:999–1008.
5. Zile MR, Baicu CF, Gaasch WH. Diastolic heart failure—abnormalities in active relaxation and passive stiffness of the left ventricle. *N Engl J Med.* 2004;350(19):1953–1959.
6. Burkhoff D, Maurer M, Packer M. Heart failure with a normal ejection fraction: is it really a disorder of diastolic function? *Circulation.* 2003;107(5):656–658.
7. Hunt S, Abraham W, Chin M, et al. ACC/AHA 2005 guideline update for the diagnosis and management of chronic heart failure in the adult: a report of the American College of Cardiology/American Heart Association Task Force on practice guidelines (Writing Committee to Update the 2001 Guidelines for the Evaluation and Management of Heart Failure). American College of Cardiology. http://acc.org/clinical/guidelines/failure/index.pdf, accessed 8/16/2005.
8. Dougherty AH, Naccarelli GV, Gray EL, et al. Congestive heart failure withnormal systolic function. *Am J Cardiol.* 1984;54:778–782.
9. Echeverria HH, Bilsker MS, Myerburg RJ, et al. Congestive heart failure: echocardiographic insights. *Am J Med.* 1983;75(5):750–755.
10. Aguirre FV, Pearson AC, Lewen MK, et al. Usefulness of Doppler echocardiography in the diagnosis of congestive heart failure. *Am J Cardiol.* 1989;63(15):1098–1102.
11. Marantz PR, Tobin JN, Wassertheil-Smoller S, et al. The relationship between left ventricular systolic function and congestive heart failure diagnosed by clinical criteria. *Circulation.*1988;77(3):607–612.
12. Thomas JT, Kelly RF, Thomas SJ, et al. Utility of history, physical examination, electrocardiogram, and chest radiograph for differentiating normal from decreased systolic function in patients with heart failure. *Am J Med.* 2002;112(6):437–445.
13. Kitzman DW, Little WC, Brubaker PH, et al. Pathophysiological characterization of isolated diastolic heart failure in comparison to systolic heart failure. *JAMA.* 2002;288(17):2144–2150.
14. Owan T, Redfield M. Epidemiology of diastolic heart failure. *Prog Cardiovasc Dis.* 2005;47(5):320–332.
15. Hogg K, Swedberg K, McMurray J. Heart failure with preserved left ventricular systolic function; epidemiology, clinical characteristics, and prognosis. *J Am Coll Cardiol.* 2004;43(3):317–327.
16. Smith GL, Masoudi FA, Vaccarino V, et al. Outcomes in heart failure patients with preserved ejection fraction: mortality, readmission, and functional decline. *J Am Coll Cardiol.* 2003;41(9):1510–1518.
17. Maniu CV, Redfield MM. Diastolic dysfunction: insights into pathophysiology and pharmacotherapy. *Expert Opin Pharmacother.* 2001;2(6):1–12.
18. Maurer MS, Spevack D, Burkhoff D, et al. Diastolic dysfunction: can it be diagnosed by Doppler echocardiography? *J Am Coll Cardiol.* 2004;44(8):1543–1549.
19. Burkhoff D, Mirsky I, Suga H. Assessment of systolic and diastolic ventricular properties via pressure–volume analysis: a guide

for clinical, translational, and basic researchers. *Am J Physiol.* (*Heart Circ Physiol.*) 2005;289(2):H501–H512.
20. Nishimura RA, Tajik AJ. Evaluation of diastolic filling of left ventricle in health and disease: Doppler echocardiography is the clinician's Rosetta Stone. *J Am Coll Cardiol.* 1997;30(1):8–18.
21. Kass DA, Maughan WL. From 'Emax' to pressure–volume relations: a broader view. *Circulation.* 1988;77(6):1203–1212.
22. Brutsaert DL, Rademakers FE, Sys SU. Triple control of relaxation: implications in cardiac disease. *Circulation.* 1984;69:190–196.
23. Brutsaert DL, Sys SU. Relaxation and diastole of the heart. *Physiol Rev.* 1989;69(4):1228–1315.
24. Brutsaert DL, Sys SU. Diastolic dysfunction in heart failure. *J Card Fail.* 1997;3:225–242.
25. Munagala VK, Hart CY, Burnett JC, Jr., et al. Ventricular structure and function in aged dogs with renal hypertension: a model of experimental diastolic heart failure. *Circulation.* 2005;111(9): 1128–1135.
26. Cheng C-P, Freeman G, Santamore W, et al. Effect on loading conditions, contractile state, and heart rate on early diastolic left ventricular filling in conscious dogs. *Circ Res.* 1990;66:814–823.
27. Cheng CP, Noda T, Nozawa T, et al. Effect of heart failure on the mechanism of exercise-induced augmentation of mitral valve flow. *Circ Res.* 1993;72:795–806.
28. Cheng CP, Igarashi Y, Little WC. Mechanism of augmented rate of left ventricular filling during exercise. *Circ Res.* 1992;70(1):9–19.
29. Kawaguchi M, Hay I, Fetics B, et al. Combined ventricular systolic and arterial stiffening in patients with heart failure and preserved ejection fraction: implications for systolic and diastolic reserve limitations. *Circulation.* 2003;107(5):714–720.
30. Pak PH, Maughan WL, Baughman KL, et al. Marked discordance between dynamic and passive diastolic pressure–volume relations in idiopathic hypertrophic cardiomyopathy. *Circulation* 1996;94:52–60.
31. Yamakoda T, Nakano T. Left ventricular systolic and diastolic function in the huypertrophied ventricle. *Jpn Circ J.* 1990;54: 554–562.
32. De Bruyne B, Bronzwaer JCF, Heyndrickx GR, et al. Comparative effects of ischemia and hypoxemia on left ventricular systolic and diastolic function in man. *Circulation.* 1993;88:461–471.
33. Villari B, Vassalli G, Monrad SE, et al. Normalization of diastolic dysfunction in aortic stenosis late after valve replacement. *Circulation* 1995;91:2353–2358.
34. Klein AL, Hatle LK, Taliercio CP, et al. Prognositc significance of Doppler measures of diastolic function in cardiac amyloidosis. A Doppler echocardiography study. *Circulation.* 1991;83:808–816.
35. Appleton CP, Hatle LK. The natural history of left ventricular filling abnormalities: Assessment by two-dimensional and Doppler echocardiography. *Echocardiography.* 1992;9:437–457.
36. Ohno M, Cheng CP, Little WC. Mechanisms of altered patterns of left ventricular filling during the development of congestive heart failure. *Circulation.* 1994;89:2241–2250.
37. Klein AL, Burstow DJ, Tajik AJ, et al. Effects of age on left ventricular dimensions and filling dynamics in 117 normal persons. *Mayo Clinic Proc.* 1994;69:212–214.
38. Zile MR, Gaasch WH, Carroll JD, et al. Heart failure with a normal ejection fraction: is measurement of diastolic function necessary to make the diagnosis of diastolic heart failure? *Circulation* 2001;104(7):779–782.
39. Sobue T, Yokota M, Iwase M, et al. Influence of left ventricular hypertrophy on left ventricular function during dynamic exercise in the presence or absence of coronary artery disease. *J Am Coll Cardiol.* 1995;25(1):91–98.
40. Cuocolo A, Sax FL, Brush JE, et al. Left ventricular hypertrophy and impaired diastolic filling in essential hypertension. Diastolic mechanisms for systolic dysfunction during exercise. *Circulation.* 1990;81:978–986.
41. Kitzman D.W, Higginbotham MB, Cobb FR, et al. Exercise intolerance in patients with heart failure and preserved left ventricular systolic function: failure of the Frank-Starling mechanism. *J Am Coll Cardiol.* 1991;17(5):1065–1072.
42. Chen HH, Lainchbury JG, Senni M, et al. Diastolic heart failure in the community: clinical profile, natural history, therapy, and impact of proposed diagnostic criteria. *J Card Fail.* 2002;8(5): 279–287.
43. Vasan RS, Levy D. Defining diastolic heart failure: a call for standardized diagnostic criteria. *Circulation* 2000;101(17):2118–2121.
44. Braunwald E, Frahm CJ. Studies on Starling's law of the heart. IV. Observations on the hemodynamic functions of the left atrium in man. *Circulation.* 1961;24:633–642.
45. Little WC. Enhanced load dependence of relaxation in heart failure. *Circulation.* 1992;85(6):2326–2328.
46. Hay I, Rich J, Ferber P, et al. Role of impaired myocardial relaxation in the production of elevated left ventricular filling pressure. *Am J Physiol.* (*Heart Circ Physiol.*) 2005;288(3):H1203–H1208.
47. Kass DA, Bronzwaer JG, Paulus WJ. What mechanisms underlie diastolic dysfunction in heart failure? *Circ Res.* 2004;94(12): 1533–1542.
48. Liu C-P, Ting C-T, Lawrence W, et al. Diminished contractile response to increased heart rate in intact human left ventricular hypertrophy: systolic versus diastolic determinants. *Circulation* 1993;88(Part 1):1893–1906.
49. Borbely A, van der Velden J, Papp Z, et al. Cardiomyocyte stiffness in diastolic heart failure. *Circulation* 2005;111(6):774–781.
50. Chen C-H, Nakayama M, Nevo E, et al. Coupled systolic-ventricular and vascular stiffening with age: implications for pressure regulation and cardiac reserve in the elderly. *J Am Coll Cardiol.* 1998;32(5):1221–1227.
51. Mitchell GF, Parise H, Benjamin EJ, et al. Changes in arterial stiffness and wave reflection with advancing age in healthy men and women: the Framingham Heart Study. *Hypertension.* 2004;43(6): 1239–1245.
52. Vaitkevicius PV, Fleg JL, Engel JH, et al. Effects of age and aerobic capacity on arterial stiffness in healthy adults. *Circulation.* 1993;88(4 Pt 1):1456–1462.
53. Kelly R, Hayward C, Avolio A, et al. Noninvasive determination of age-related changes in the human arterial pulse. *Circulation.* 1989;80(6):1652–1659.
54. Smulyan H, Asmar RG, Rudnicki A, et al. Comparative effects of aging in men and women on the properties of the arterial tree. *J Am Coll Cardiol.* 2001;37(5):1374–1380.
55. Gatzka CD, Kingwell BA, Cameron JD, et al. Gender differences in the timing of arterial wave reflection beyond differences in body height. *J Hypertens.* 2001;19(12):2197–2203.
56. Hayward CS, Kelly RP. Gender-related differences in the central arterial pressure waveform. *J Am Coll Cardiol.* 1997;30(7):1863–1871.
57. Avolio AP, Deng FQ, Li WQ, et al. Effects of aging on arterial distensibility in populations with high and low prevalence of hypertension: comparison between urban and rural communities in China. *Circulation* 1985;71(2):202–210.
58. Kelly RP, Ting C-T, Yang T-M, et al. Effective arterial elastance as index of arterial vascular load in humans. *Circulation.* 1992;86: 513–521.
59. Safar ME, Levy BI, Struijker-Boudier H. Current perspectives on arterial stiffness and pulse pressure in hypertension and cardiovascular diseases. *Circulation.* 2003;107(22):2864–2869.
60. Lakatta EG, Levy D. Arterial and cardiac aging: major shareholders in cardiovascular disease enterprises: Part I: aging arteries: a "set up" for vascular disease. *Circulation.* 2003;107(1): 139–146.
61. Kass DA. Age-related changes in venticular-arterial coupling: pathophysiologic implications. *Heart Fail Rev.* 2002;7(1):51–62.
62. Little WC, Cheng C-P. Left ventricular-arterial coupling in conscious dogs. *Am J Physiol.* (*Heart Circ Physiol.*) 1991;261(30): H70–H76.
63. Burkhoff D, de Tombe PP, Hunter WC, et al. Contractile strength and mechanical efficiency of left ventricle are enhanced by physiological afterload. *Am J Physiol.* (*Heart Circ Physiol.*) 1991;260 29:H569–H578.
64. van der Velde ET, Burkhoff D, Steendijk P, et al. Nonlinearity and load sensitivity of end-systolic pressure–volume relation of canine left ventricle in vivo. *Circulation.* 1991;83(1):315–327.
65. Redfield M, Jacobsen S, Bourlag B, et al. Age- and gender-related ventricular-vascular stiffening: a community based study. *Circulation* 2005. In press.
66. Lakatta EG, Sollott SJ. The "heartbreak" of older age. *Mol Interv.* 2002;2(7):431–446.
67. Arbab-Zadeh A, Dijk E, Prasad A, et al. Effect of aging and physical activity on left ventricular compliance. *Circulation.* 2004;110(13):1799–1805.
68. Ceia F, Fonseca C, Mota T, et al. Prevalence of chronic heart failure in Southwestern Europe: the EPICA study. *Eur J Heart Fail.* 2002;4(4):531–539.

69. Gandhi SK, Powers JC, Nomeir AM, et al. The pathogenesis of acute pulmonary edema associated with hypertension. *N Engl J Med*. 2001;344(1):17–22.
70. Ghali JK, Kadakia S, Cooper RS, et al. Bedside diagnosis of preserved versus impaired left ventricular systolic function in heart failure. *Am J Cardiol*. 1991;67(11):1002–1006.
71. Iriarte M, Murga N, Sagastagoitia D, et al. Congestive heart failure from left ventricular diastolic dysfunction in systemic hypertension. *Am J Cardiol*. 1993;71(4):308–312.
72. Tsutsui H, Tsuchihashi M, Takeshita A. Mortality and readmission of hospitalized patients with congestive heart failure and preserved versus depressed systolic function. *Am J Cardiol*. 2001;88(5):530–533.
73. Klapholz M, Maurer M, Lowe AM, et al. Hospitalization for heart failure in the presence of a normal left ventricular ejection fraction: results of the New York Heart Failure Registry. *J Am Coll Cardiol*. 2004;43(8):1432–1438.
74. Given BD, Lee TH, Stone PH, et al. Nifedipine in severely hypertensive patients with congestive heart failure and preserved ventricular systolic function. *Arch Intern Med*. 1985;145(2):281–285.
75. Kitzman DW, Gardin JM, Gottdiener JS, et al. Importance of heart failure with preserved systolic function in patients > or = 65 years of age. CHS Research Group. Cardiovascular Health Study. *Am J Cardiol*. 2001;87(4):413–419.
76. Dougherty AH, Naccarelli GV, Gray EL, et al. Congestive heart failure with normal systolic function. *Am J Cardiol*. 1984;54(7):778–782.
77. Topol EJ, Traill TA, Fortuin NJ. Hypertensive hypertrophic cardiomyopathy of the elderly. *N Engl J Med*. 1985;312(5):277–283.
78. Maurer MS, King DL, El-Khoury Rumbarger L, et al. Left heart failure with a normal ejection fraction: identification of different pathophysiologic mechanisms. *J Card Fail*. 2005;11(3):177–187.
79. Alderman EL, Glantz SA. Acute hemodynamic interventions shift the diastolic pressure–volume curve in man. *Circulation*. 1976;54(4):662–671.
80. Chen C-H, Nakayama M, Talbot M, et al. Verapamil accutely reduces ventricular-vascular stiffening and improves aerobic exercise performance in elderly individuals. *J Am Coll Cardiol*. 1999;33(6):1602–1609.
81. Freeman GL, Little WC, O'Rourke RA. The effect of vasoactive agents on the left ventricular end-systolic pressure–volume relation in closed-chest dogs. *Circulation*. 1986;74(5):1107–1113.
82. Schipper IB, Steendijk P, Klautz RJ, et al. Cardiac sympathetic denervation does not change the load dependence of the left ventricular end-systolic pressure/volume relationship in dogs. *Pflugers Arch*. 1993;425(5–6):426–433.
83. van der Linden LP, van der Velde ET, van Houwelingen HC, et al. Determinants of end-systolic pressure during different load alterations in the in situ left ventricle. *Am J Physiol*. 1994;267(5 Pt 2):H1895–H1906.
84. Yip G, Wang M, Zhang Y, et al. Left ventricular long axis function in diastolic heart failure is reduced in both diastole and systole: time for a redefinition? *Heart*. 2002;87:121–125.
85. Yu CM, Lin H, Yang H, et al. Progression of systolic abnormalities in patients with "isolated" diastolic heart failure and diastolic dysfunction. *Circulation*. 2002;105(10):1195–1201.
86. Petrie MC, Caruana L, Berry C, et al. "Diastolic heart failure" or heart failure caused by subtle left ventricular systolic dysfunction? *Heart*. 2002;87:29–31.
87. Schussheim AE, Devereux RB, de Simone G, et al. Usefulness of subnormal midwall fractional shortening in predicting left ventricular exercise dysfunction in asymptomatic patients with systemic hypertension. *Am J Cardiol*. 1997;79:1070–1074.
88. Shimizu G, Hirota Y, Kita Y, et al. Left ventricular midwall mechanics in systemic arterial hypertension. *Circulation*. 1991;83:1676–1684.
89. Aurigemma GP, Gaasch WH, McLaughlin M, et al. Reduced left ventricular systolic pump performance and depressed myocardial contractile function in patients >65 years of age with normal ejection fraction and high relative wall thickness. *Am J Cardiol*. 1995;76:702–705.
90. Weisfeldt ML. Aging of the cardiovascular system. *N Engl J Med*. 1980;303(20):1172–1174.
91. Schulman SP, Lakatta EG, Fleg JL, et al. Age-related decline in left ventricular filling at rest and exercise. *Am J Physiol*. 1992;263-(6 Pt 2):H1932–H1938.
92. Benjamin EJ, Levy D, Anderson KM, et al. Determinants of Doppler indexes of left ventricular diastolic function in normal subjects (the Framingham Heart Study). *Am J Cardiol*. 1992;70(4):508–515.
93. Swinne CJ, Shapiro EP, Lima SD, et al. Age-associated changes in left ventricular diastolic performance during isometric exercise in normal subjects. *Am J Cardiol*. 1992;69(8):823–826.
94. Lakatta EG. Do hypertension and aging have a similar effect on the myocardium? *Circulation*. 1987;75(1 Pt 2):169–177.
95. Hundley WG, Kitzman DW, Morgan TM, et al. Cardiac cycle-dependent changes in aortic area and distensibility are reduced in older patients with isolated diastolic heart failure and correlate with exercise intolerance. *J Am Coll Cardiol*. 2001;38(3):796–802.
96. Najjar SS, Schulman SP, Gerstenblith G, et al. Age and gender affect ventricular-vascular coupling during aerobic exercise. *J Am Coll Cardiol*. 2004;44(3):611–617.
97. Hayward CS, Kalnins WV, Kelly RP. Gender-related differences in left ventricular chamber function. *Cardiovasc Res*. 2001;49(2):340–350.
98. Vasan RS, Levy D. The role of hypertension in the pathogenesis of heart failure. A clinical mechanistic overview. *Arch Intern Med*. 1996;156(16):1789–1796.
99. Choudhury L, Gheorghiade M, Bonow RO. Coronary artery disease in patients with heart failure and preserved systolic function. *Am J Cardiol*. 2002;89(6):719–722.
100. Gaasch WH. Congestive heart failure in patients with normal left ventricular systolic function: a manifestation of diastolic dysfunction. *Herz*. 1991;16(1):22–32.
101. Poulsen SH, Jensen SE, Egstrup K. Longitudinal changes and prognostic implications of left ventricular diastolic function in first acute myocardial infarction. *Am Heart J*. 1999;137(5):910–918.
102. Bonow RO, Bacharach SL, Green MV, et al. Impaired left ventricular diastolic filling in patients with coronary artery disease: assessment with radionuclide angiography. *Circulation*. 1981;64(2):315–323.
103. Judge KW, Pawitan Y, Caldwell J, et al. Congestive heart failure symptoms in patients with preserved left ventricular systolic function: analysis of the CASS registry. *J Am Coll Cardiol*. 1991;18(2):377–382.
104. Gorcsan J, 3rd, Diana P, Lee J, et al. Reversible diastolic dysfunction after successful coronary artery bypass surgery. Assessment by transesophageal Doppler echocardiography. *Chest*. 1994;106(5):1364–1369.
105. Kramer K, Kirkman P, Kitzman D, et al. Flash pulmonary edema: association with hypertension and reoccurrence despite coronary revascularization. *Am Heart J*. 2000;140(3):451–455.
106. Tsang TS, Gersh BJ, Appleton CP, et al. Left ventricular diastolic dysfunction as a predictor of the first diagnosed nonvalvular atrial fibrillation in 840 elderly men and women. *J Am Coll Cardiol*. 2002;40(9):1636–1644.
107. Hubert HB, Feinleib M, McNamara PM, et al. Obesity as an independent risk factor for cardiovascular disease: a 26-year follow-up of participants in the Framingham Heart Study. *Circulation*. 1983;67(5):968–977.
108. Kenchaiah S, Evans JC, Levy D, et al. Obesity and the risk of heart failure. *N Engl J Med*. 2002;347(5):305–313.
109. Redfield MM, Jacobsen SJ, Burnett JC, Jr., et al. Burden of systolic and diastolic ventricular dysfunction in the community: appreciating the scope of the heart failure epidemic. *JAMA*. 2003;289(2):194–202.
110. Alpert MA. Obesity cardiomyopathy: pathophysiology and evolution of the clinical syndrome. *Am J Med*. 2001;321(4):225–236.
111. Lavie CJ, Amodeo C, Ventura HO, et al. Left atrial abnormalities indicating diastolic ventricular dysfunction in cardiopathy of obesity. *Chest* 1987;92(6):1042–1046.
112. Ku CS, Lin SL, Wang DJ, et al. Left ventricular filling in young normotensive obese adults. *Am J Cardiol*. 1994;73(8):613–615.
113. Chakko S, Mayor M, Allison MD, et al. Abnormal left ventricular diastolic filling in eccentric left ventricular hypertrophy of obesity. *Am J Cardiol*. 1991;68(1):95–98.
114. Grossman E, Oren S, Messerli FH. Left ventricular filling in the systemic hypertension of obesity. *Am J Cardiol*. 1991;68(1):57–60.
115. Karason K, Wallentin I, Larsson B, et al. Effects of obesity and weight loss on cardiac function and valvular performance. *Obes Res*. 1998;6(6):422–429.

116. Stoddard MF, Tseuda K, Thomas M, et al. The influence of obesity on left ventricular filling and systolic function. *Am Heart J*. 1992;124(3):694–699.
117. Wikstrand J, Pettersson P, Bjorntorp P. Body fat distribution and left ventricular morphology and function in obese females. *J Hypertens*. 1993;11(11):1259–1266.
118. Zarich SW, Kowalchuk GJ, McGuire MP, et al. Left ventricular filling abnormalities in asymptomatic morbid obesity. *Am J Cardiol*. 1991;68(4):377–381.
119. Wong CY, O'Moore-Sullivan T, Leano R, et al. Alterations of left ventricular myocardial characteristics associated with obesity. *Circulation*. 2004;110(19):3081–3087.
120. Alexander. JK. Obesity and cardiac performance. *Am J Cardiol*. 1964;14:860–865.
121. Backman L, Freyschuss U, Hallberg D, et al. Cardiovascular function in extreme obesity. *Acta Med Scand*. 1973;193(5):437–446.
122. Kaltman AJ, Goldring RM. Role of circulatory congestion in the cardiorespiratory failure of obesity. *Am J Med*. 1976;60(5):645–653.
123. Seneviratne BI. Diabetic cardiomyopathy: the preclinical phase. *BMJ*. 1977;1(6074):1444–1446.
124. Raev DC. Which left ventricular function is impaired earlier in the evolution of diabetic cardiomyopathy? An echocardiographic study of young type I diabetic patients. *Diabetes Care*. 1994;17(7):633–639.
125. Zabalgoitia M, Ismaeil MF, Anderson L, et al. Prevalence of diastolic dysfunction in normotensive, asymptomatic patients with well-controlled type 2 diabetes mellitus. *Am J Cardiol*. 2001;87(3): 320–323.
126. Liu JE, Palmieri V, Roman MJ, et al. The impact of diabetes on left ventricular filling pattern in normotensive and hypertensive adults: the Strong Heart Study. *J Am Coll Cardiol*. 2001;37(7): 1943–1949.
127. Uusitupa M, Siitonen O, Aro A, et al. Effect of correction of hyperglycemia on left ventricular function in non-insulin-dependent (type 2) diabetics. *Acta Med Scand*. 1983;213(5): 363–368.
128. Hardin NJ. The myocardial and vascular pathology of diabetic cardiomyopathy. *Coron Artery Dis*. 1996;7(2):99–108.
129. Piccini JP, Klein L, Gheorghiade M, et al. New insights into diastolic heart failure: role of diabetes mellitus. *Am J Med*. 2004;116(Suppl 5A):64S–75S.
130. Bakris GL, Bank AJ, Kass DA, et al. Advanced glycation end-product cross-link breakers: a novel approach to cardiovascular pathologies related to the aging process. *Am J Hypertens*. 2004;17(12 Pt 2):23S–30S.
131. Kass DA. Getting better without AGE: new insights into the diabetic heart. *Circ Res*. 2003;92(7):704–706.
132. Smit AJ, Lutgers HL. The clinical relevance of advanced glycation endproducts (AGE) and recent developments in pharmaceutics to reduce AGE accumulation. *Curr Med Chem*. 2004;11(20): 2767–2784.
133. Vasan S, Foiles PG, Founds HW. Therapeutic potential of AGE-inhibitors and breakers of AGE-protein crosslinks. *Expert Opin Investig Drugs*. 2001;10(11):1–11.
134. Asif M, Egan J, Vasan S, et al. An advanced glycation endproduct cross-link breaker can reverse age-related increases in myocardial stiffness. *Proc Natl Acad Sci USA*. 2000;97(6):2809–2813.
135. Vaitkevicius PV, Lane M, Spurgeon H, et al. A cross-link breaker has sustained effects on arterial and ventricular properties in older rhesus monkeys. *Proc Natl Acad Sci USA*. 2001;98(3):1171–1175.
136. Kass DA, Shapiro EP, Kawaguchi M, et al. Improved arterial compliance by a novel advanced glycation end-product crosslink breaker. *Circulation* 2001;104:1464–1470.
137. Little WC, Zile MR, Kitzman DW, et al. The effect of alagebrium chloride (ALT-711), a novel glucose cross-link breaker, in the treatment of elderly patients with diastolic heart failure. *J Card Fail*. 2005;11(3):191–195.
138. Stevenson LW, Perloff JK. The limited reliability of physical signs for estimating hemodynamics in chronic heart failure. *JAMA*. 1989;261(6):884–888.
139. Dodek A, Kassebaum DG, Bristow JD. Pulmonary edema in coronary-artery disease without cardiomegaly. Paradox of the stiff heart. *N Engl J Med*. 1972;286(25):1347–1350.
140. McDermott MM, Feinglass J, Sy J, et al. Hospitalized congestive heart failure patients with preserved versus abnormal left ventricular systolic function: clinical characteristics and drug therapy. *Am J Med*. 1995;99(6):629–635.
141. McDermott MM, Feinglass J, Lee PI, et al. Systolic function, readmission rates, and survival among consecutively hospitalized patients with congestive heart failure. *Am Heart J*. 1997;134(4): 728–736.
142. Vasan RS, Benjamin EJ, Levy D. Prevalence, clinical features and prognosis of diastolic heart failure: an epidemiologic perspective. *J Am Coll Cardiol*. 1995;26(7):1565–1574.
143. Aurigemma GP, Gottdiener JS, Shemanski L, et al. Predictive value of systolic and diastolic function for incident congestive heart failure in the elderly: the Cardiovascular Health Study. *J Am Coll Cardiol*. 2001;37(4):1042–1048.
144. Gottdiener JS, McClelland RL, Marshall R, et al. Outcome of congestive heart failure in elderly persons: influence of left ventricular systolic function. The Cardiovascular Health Study. *Ann Intern Med*. 2002;137(8):631–639.
145. Aronow WS, Ahn C, Kronzon I. Prognosis of congestive heart failure in elderly patients with normal versus abnormal left ventricular systolic function associated with coronary artery disease. *Am J Cardiol*. 1990;66(17):1257–1259.
146. Setaro JF, Soufer R, Remetz MS, et al. Long-term outcome in patients with congestive heart failure and intact systolic left ventricular performance. *Am J Cardiol*. 1992;69(14):1212–1216.
147. Brogan WC, 3rd, Hillis LD, Flores ED, et al. The natural history of isolated left ventricular diastolic dysfunction. *Am J Med*. 1992;92(6):627–630.
148. Curtis JP, Sokol SI, Wang Y, et al. The association of left ventricular ejection fraction, mortality, and cause of death in stable outpatients with heart failure. *J Am Coll Cardiol*. 2003;42(4): 736–742.
149. European Study Group on Diastolic Heart Failure. How to diagnose diastolic heart failure. *Eur Heart J*. 1998;19(7):990–1003.
150. Bettencourt P, Ferreira A, Dias P, et al. Evaluation of brain natriuretic peptide in the diagnosis of heart failure. *Cardiology*. 2000;93(1–2):19–25.
151. Lang CC, Prasad N, McAlpine HM, et al. Increased plasma levels of brain natriuretic peptide in patients with isolated diastolic dysfunction. *Am Heart J*. 1994;127(6):1635–1636.
152. Selvais PL, Donckier JE, Robert A, et al. Cardiac natriuretic peptides for diagnosis and risk stratification in heart failure: influences of left ventricular dysfunction and coronary artery disease on cardiac hormonal activation. *Eur J Clin Invest*. 1998;28(8): 636–642.
153. Villacorta H, Duarte A, Duarte NM, et al. The role of B-type natriuretic peptide in the diagnosis of congestive heart failure in patients presenting to an emergency department with dyspnea. *Arq Bras Cardiol*. 2002;79(6):564–568, 569–572.
154. Maisel AS, McCord J, Nowak RM, et al. Bedside B-Type natriuretic peptide in the emergency diagnosis of heart failure with reduced or preserved ejection fraction. Results from the Breathing Not Properly Multinational Study. *J Am Coll Cardiol*. 2003;41(11):2010–2017.
155. Redfield MM, Rodeheffer RJ, Jacobsen SJ, et al. Plasma brain natriuretic peptide concentration: impact of age and gender. *J Am Coll Cardiol*. 2002;40(5):976–982.
156. Lainchbury JG, Campbell E, Frampton CM, et al. Brain natriuretic peptide and n-terminal brain natriuretic peptide in the diagnosis of heart failure in patients with acute shortness of breath. *J Am Coll Cardiol*. 2003;42(4):728–735.
157. Cohn JN, Johnson G. Heart failure with normal ejection fraction. The V-HeFT Study. Veterans Administration Cooperative Study Group. *Circulation*. 1990;81(Suppl 2):III48–III53.
158. MacFadyen RJ, MacLeod CM, Shiels P, et al. Isolated diastolic heart failure as a cause of breathlessness in the community: the Arbroath study. *Eur J Heart Fail*. 2001;3(2):243–248.
159. Pina IL, Apstein CS, Balady GJ, et al. Exercise and heart failure: a statement from the American Heart Association Committee on exercise, rehabilitation, and prevention. *Circulation* 2003;107(8): 1210–1225.
160. Jones RC, Francis GS, Lauer MS. Predictors of mortality in patients with heart failure and preserved systolic function in the Digitalis Investigation Group Trial. *J Am Coll Cardiol*. 2004;44(5): 1025–1029.
161. McAlister FA, Teo KK, Taher M, et al. Insights into the contemporary epidemiology and outpatient management of congestive heart failure. *Am Heart J*. 1999;138(1 Pt 1):87–94.
162. Aronow WS, Kronzon I. Effect of enalapril on congestive heart failure treated with diuretics in elderly patients with prior

myocardial infarction and normal left ventricular ejection fraction. *Am J Cardiol.* 1993;71(7):602–604.

163. Lang CC, McAlpine HM, Kennedy N, et al. Effects of lisinopril on congestive heart failure in normotensive patients with diastolic dysfunction but intact systolic function. *Eur J Clin Pharmacol.* 1995;49(1–2):15–19.

164. Warner JG, Jr., Metzger DC, Kitzman DW, et al. Losartan improves exercise tolerance in patients with diastolic dysfunction and a hypertensive response to exercise. *J Am Coll Cardiol.* 1999;33(6):1567–1572.

165. Aronow WS, Ahn C, Kronzon I. Effect of propranolol versus no propranolol on total mortality plus nonfatal myocardial infarction in older patients with prior myocardial infarction, congestive heart failure, and left ventricular ejection fraction > or = 40% treated with diuretics plus angiotensin-converting enzyme inhibitors. *Am J Cardiol.* 1997;80(2):207–209.

166. Bergstrom A, Andersson B, Edner M, et al. Effect of carvedilol on diastolic function in patients with diastolic heart failure and preserved systolic function. Results of the Swedish Doppler-echocardiographic study (SWEDIC). *Eur J Heart Fail.* 2004;6(4): 453–461.

167. Setaro JF, Zaret BL, Schulman DS, et al. Usefulness of verapamil for congestive heart failure associated with abnormal left ventricular diastolic filling and normal left ventricular systolic performance. *Am J Cardiol.* 1990;66(12):981–986.

168. Nishikawa N, Masuyama T, Yamamoto K, et al. Long-term administration of amlodipine prevents decompensation to diastolic heart failure in hypertensive rats. *J Am Coll Cardiol.* 2001;38(5):1539–1545.

169. The Digitalis Investigation Group. The effect of digoxin on mortality and morbidity in patients with heart failure. *N Engl J Med.* 1997;336(8):525–533.

170. Yusuf S, Pfeffer MA, Swedberg K, et al. Effects of candesartan in patients with chronic heart failure and preserved left-ventricular ejection fraction: the CHARM-Preserved Trial. *Lancet.* 2003;362 (9386):777–781.

171. Kunis R, Greenberg H, Yeoh CB, et al. Coronary revascularization for recurrent pulmonary edema in elderly patients with ischemic heart disease and preserved ventricular function. *N Engl J Med.* 1985;313(19):1207–1210.

172. Warnowicz MA, Parker H, Cheitlin MD. Prognosis of patients with acute pulmonary edema and normal ejection fraction after acute myocardial infarction. *Circulation.* 1983;67(2):330–334.

173. Bier AJ, Eichacker PQ, Sinoway LI, et al. Acute cardiogenic pulmonary edema: clinical and noninvasive evaluation. *Angiology.* 1988;39(3 Pt 1):211–218.

174. Stone GW, Griffin B, Shah PK, et al. Prevalence of unsuspected mitral regurgitation and left ventricular diastolic dysfunction in patients with coronary artery disease and acute pulmonary edema associated with normal or depressed left ventricular systolic function. *Am J Cardiol.* 1991;67(1):37–41.

175. Badano L, Albanese M, Fresco C, et al. Prevalence of diastolic heart failure among patients admitted to the hospital with congenstive heart failure. *Eur J Heart Fail.* 2000;2(Suppl 1):72.

176. Soufer R, Wohlgelernter D, Vita NA, et al. Intact systolic left ventricular function in clinical congestive heart failure. *Am J Cardiol.* 1985;55(8):1032–1036.

177. Wong WF, Gold S, Fukuyama O, et al. Diastolic dysfunction in elderly patients with congestive heart failure. *Am J Cardiol.* 1989;63(20):1526–1528.

178. Takarada A, Kurogane H, Minamiji K, et al. Congestive heart failure in the elderly—echocardiographic insights. *Jpn Circ J.* 1992;56(6):527–534.

179. Taffet GE, Teasdale TA, Bleyer AJ, et al. Survival of elderly men with congestive heart failure. *Age Ageing.* 1992;21(1):49–55.

180. Cohen-Solal A, Desnos M, Delahaye F, et al. A national survey of heart failure in French hospitals. The Myocardiopathy and Heart Failure Working Group of the French Society of Cardiology, the National College of General Hospital Cardiologists and the French Geriatrics Society. *Eur Heart J.* 2000;21(9):763–769.

181. Peyster E, Norman J, Domanski M. Prevalence and predictors of heart failure with preserved systolic function: community hospital admissions of a racially and gender diverse elderly population. *J Card Fail.* 2004;10(1):49–54.

182. Pernenkil R, Vinson JM, Shah AS, et al. Course and prognosis in patients ≥70 years of age with congestive heart failure and normal versus abnormal left ventricular ejection fraction. *Am J Cardiol.* 1997;79(2):216–219.

183. Wheeldon NM, MacDonald TM, Flucker CJ, et al. Echocardiography in chronic heart failure in the community. *Q J Med.* 1993;86(1):17–23.

184. Madsen BK, Hansen JF, Stokholm KH, et al. Chronic congestive heart failure. Description and survival of 190 consecutive patients with a diagnosis of chronic congestive heart failure based on clinical signs and symptoms. *Eur Heart J.* 1994;15(3):303–310.

185. Aronow WS, Ahn C, Kronzon I. Normal left ventricular ejection fraction in older persons with congestive heart failure. *Chest.* 1998;113(4):867–869.

186. Diller PM, Smucker DR, David B, et al. Congestive heart failure due to diastolic or systolic dysfunction. Frequency and patient characteristics in an ambulatory setting. *Arch Fam Med.* 1999;8(5):414–420.

187. Kinney EL, Wright RJ, Jr. Survival in patients with heart failure and normal basal systolic wall motion. *Angiology.* 1989;40(12): 1025–1029.

188. Cregler LL, Georgiou D, Sosa I. Left ventricular diastolic dysfunction in patients with congestive heart failure. *J Natl Med Assoc.* 1991;83(1):49–52.

189. Vasan RS, Larson MG, Benjamin EJ, et al. Congestive heart failure in subjects with normal versus reduced left ventricular ejection fraction: prevalence and mortality in a population-based cohort. *J Am Coll Cardiol.* 1999;33(7):1948–1955.

190. Yip GW, Ho PP, Woo KS, et al. Comparison of frequencies of left ventricular systolic and diastolic heart failure in Chinese living in Hong Kong. *Am J Cardiol.* 1999;84(5):563–567.

191. Senni M, Tribouilloy CM, Rodeheffer RJ, et al. Congestive heart failure in the community: a study of all incident cases in Olmsted County, Minnesota, in 1991. *Circulation.* 1998;98(21): 2282–2289.

192. Cortina A, Reguero J, Segovia E, et al. Prevalence of heart failure in Asturias(a region in the north of Spain). *Am J Cardiol.* 2001;87(12):1417–1419.

193. Hedberg P, Lonnberg I, Jonason T, et al. Left ventricular systolic dysfunction in 75-year-old men and women; a population-based study. *Eur Heart J.* 2001;22(8):676–683.

194. Devereux RB, Roman MJ, Liu JE, et al. Congestive heart failure despite normal left ventricular systolic function in a population-based sample: the Strong Heart Study. *Am J Cardiol.* 2000;86(10): 1090–1096.

195. Mosterd A, Hoes AW, de Bruyne MC, et al. Prevalence of heart failure and left ventricular dysfunction in the general population: the Rotterdam Study. *Eur Heart J.* 1999;20(6):447–455.

196. Morgan S, Smith H, Simpson I, et al. Prevalence and clinical characteristics of left ventricular dysfunction among elderly patients in general practice setting: cross sectional survey. *BMJ.* 1999;318(7180):368–372.

197. Kupari M, Lindroos M, Iivanainen AM, et al. Congestive heart failure in old age: prevalence, mechanisms and 4-year prognosis in the Helsinki Ageing Study. *J Intern Med.* 1997;241(5):387–394.

198. Ghali JK, Kadakia S, Bhatt A, et al. Survival of heart failure patients with preserved versus impaired systolic function: the prognostic implication of blood pressure. *Am Heart J.* 1992;123(4 Pt 1): 993–997.

199. Philbin EF, Rocco TA, Jr., Lindenmuth NW, et al. Systolic versus diastolic heart failure in community practice: clinical features, outcomes, and the use of angiotensin-converting enzyme inhibitors. *Am J Med.* 2000;109(8):605–613.

200. Agoston I, Cameron CS, Yao D, et al. Comparison of outcomes of white versus black patients hospitalized with heart failure and preserved ejection fraction. *Am J Cardiol.* 2004;94(8):1003–1007.

201. Ansari M, Alexander M, Tutar A, et al. Incident cases of heart failure in a community cohort: importance and outcomes of patients with preserved systolic function. *Am Heart J.* 2003;146(1): 115–120.

8 Cellular, Molecular, and Structural Changes During Cardiac Remodeling

Richard D. Patten

Heart failure is associated with activation of neurohormonal and cytokine signaling pathways that alter the structure and function of cardiac myocytes and nonmyocyte cells. These cellular alterations culminate in the gross morphological changes in cardiac structure termed remodeling, a maladaptive process that contributes to further left ventricular dysfunction and heart failure progression. This chapter will review the cellular basis for cardiac remodeling and the mechanisms that contribute to these cellular abnormalities and, more broadly, to the pathophysiology of heart failure and its progression.

THE CLINICAL SYNDROME OF VENTRICULAR REMODELING

Left ventricular (LV) remodeling refers to alterations in ventricular mass, chamber size, and geometry that result from myocardial injury, pressure, or volume overload. The ultrastructural changes of the remodeled ventricle are the direct result of cellular alterations that include myocyte hypertrophy, myocyte apoptosis, fibroblast proliferation, and the abnormal infiltration of mononuclear inflammatory cells. This complex, progressive, and maladaptive process promotes ongoing ventricular dilatation and dysfunction contributing directly to heart failure progression.

Because ischemic heart disease is a major risk factor for the development of heart failure, much of our understanding of LV remodeling in humans has come from the study of patients following myocardial infarction (MI). In the post-MI heart, the extent of LV chamber enlargement is directly related to infarct size (1,2). In the early period (days) following a moderate to large MI, the LV cavity enlarges because of infarct expansion (i.e., elongation and thinning of the infarcted segment) (3–5). However, progressive LV dilatation often continues over months to years (1,2,6,7), resulting primarily from elongation or eccentric hypertrophy of noninfarcted wall segments (5,8). Figure 8-1 illustrates this concept, showing outlines of LV end-diastolic and end-systolic frames from a right anterior oblique ventriculogram obtained from a patient 1 week and 1 year following a large, anterior wall MI. While the two-dimensional length measurement of the infarcted, noncontractile segment remained stable over that time period, the elongation of contractile portions of the LV resulted in further LV dilatation.

LV remodeling following MI has been shown in several studies to portend a poor prognosis (9–11). White et al. reported in a series of 605 patients 1 to 2 months after MI that the strongest independent predictor of survival was LV end-systolic volume (LVESV) (12). In the angiographic substudy of the Global Utilization of Streptokinase and t-PA for Occluded Coronary Arteries (GUSTO) I Trial, LVESV of $\geq$40mL/m^{2}was independently associated with an increase in mortality among 1,300 patients treated with thrombolytic therapy for an acute transmural MI (13). More recently, Bolognese et al. reported that among acute MI patients having undergone successful reperfusion therapy with primary percutaneous coronary intervention, 30% developed significant LV dilatation over 6 months [defined as an increase in LV end-diastolic volume (EDV) of greater than 20% above baseline] (14). As shown in Figure 8-2, patients in this study who exhibited LV remodeling had a significantly greater incidence of heart failure and death compared to patients without LV remodeling. Consistent with prior studies, 6-month LVESV was identified as a significant predictor of mortality by multivariate analysis.

Parameter	3 weeks	1 year
End-distolic volume	302mL	377mL
End-systolic volume	186mL	271mL
Circumference	59.5cm	62.8cm
Contractile segment	30.5cm	33.8cm
Noncontractile segment	23.7cm	23.5cm

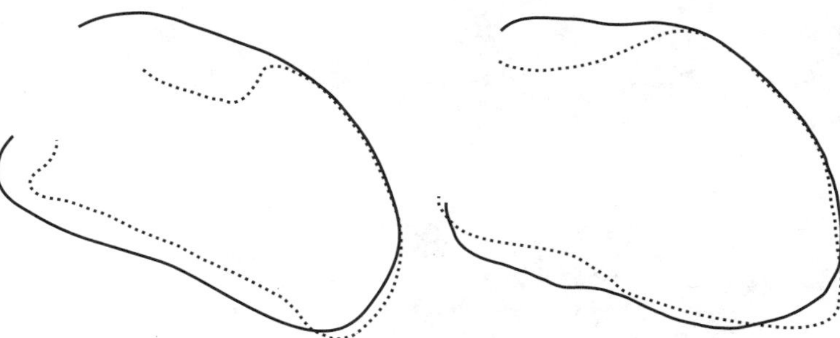

Figure 8-1 Late ventricular enlargement in a patient with anterior myocardial infarction. Marked increase in volume results from increased circumference and sphericity. The late change in circumference is due to lengthening of contractile tissue rather than further expansion of the infarcted, noncontractile segment. (Reproduced from Mitchell GF, Lamas GA, Vaughan DE, et al. Left ventricular remodeling in the year after first anterior myocardial infarction: a quantitative analysis of contractile segment lengths and ventricular shape. *J Am Coll Cardiol.* 19:1136–1144, with permission.)

Recently, two groups observed a strong association between progressive LV dilatation following MI and the incidence of sudden cardiac death and ventricular arrhythmias (15,16). These studies demonstrate that post-MI remodeling remains clinically relevant in the era of reperfusion therapy and that a direct correlation exists between remodeling and cardiac events. These data therefore support that *LV remodeling is a maladaptive process leading to the gradual decline in LV function and, hence, heart failure progression.*

Apart from the immediate post-MI setting, patients with chronic heart failure due to chronic ischemic or nonischemic etiologies also exhibit progressive LV chamber enlargement, which has been observed in placebo arms of LV remodeling substudies of clinical heart failure trials (17–21). For example, in the placebo arms of both the radionuclide and echocardiographic substudies of the Studies of Left Ventricular Dysfunction (SOLVD) trial, progressive LV dilatation and trend for increased LV mass were observed at 1 year. Thus, in addition to the post-MI setting, patients with LV systolic dysfunction with or without symptomatic heart failure exhibit progressive LV remodeling (17–19).

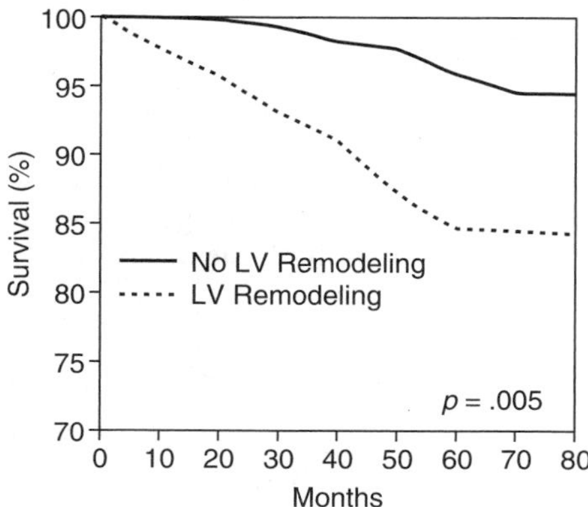

Figure 8-2 Kaplan-Meier survival curves for cardiac death in patients with and without LV remodeling at 6 months after AMI. (From Bolognese L, Neskovic AN, Parodi G, et al. Left ventricular remodeling after primary coronary angioplasty: patterns of left ventricular dilation and long-term prognostic implications. *Circulation.* 106:2351–2357, with permission.)

CELLULAR ALTERATIONS IN CARDIAC REMODELING

The clinical data previously described demonstrate that LV remodeling occurs in patients with LV systolic dysfunction and is associated with a worse prognosis. The macroscopic changes in ventricular size and shape stem from alterations in the cellular constituents of the myocardium that act in concert to bring about global LV dilatation and dysfunction and, hence, heart failure progression. This section will review the structural and biochemical alterations in cardiac myocytes and fibroblasts, and how the infiltration of inflammatory cells contributes to these pathological changes.

Cardiomyocytes

Among the cell types that exist within the myocardium, much attention (recent and remote) has focused on the cardiac myocyte. Increased myocyte size contributes importantly to the gross morphological features of ventricular enlargement. In a rat model of MI, Anversa et al. used histomorphometry to measure myocyte size distant from the infarct zone, and found that myocytes increase in length and diameter (22,23). In isolated myocytes from patients with ischemic cardiomyopathy, the Gerdes Lab (24) reported that myocyte length increased by approximately

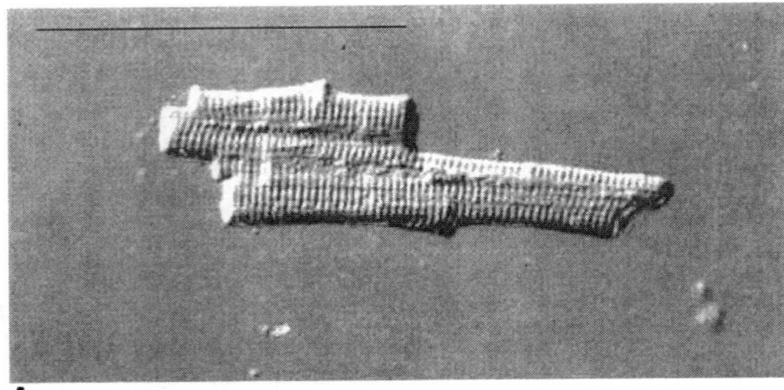

A

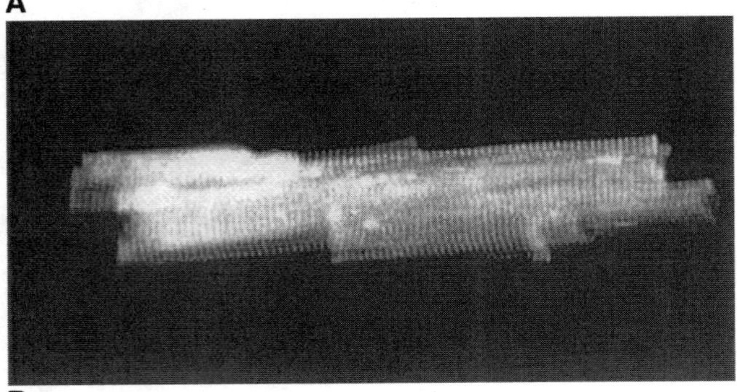

B

Figure 8-3 **(A)** Typical myocyte isolated from nonfailing human left ventricle. Bar = 100 μm. **(B)** Myocyte isolated from the LV of a patient with ischemic cardiomyopathy. (From Gerdes AM, Kellerman SE, Moore JA, et al. Structural remodeling of cardiac myocytes in patients with ischemic cardiomyopathy. *Circulation* 86:426–430, with permission.)

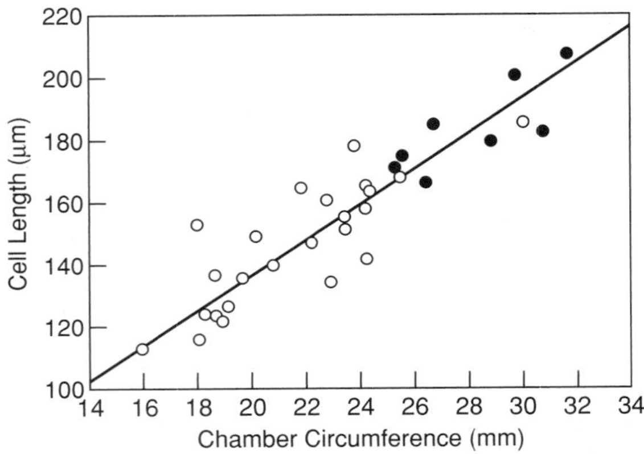

Figure 8-4 Linear regression analysis of changes in cell length and chamber circumference in aging SHHF rats. Cell length increased linearly with chamber circumference. ($r = 0.93$; $p < 0.001$; $y = 5.72x + 22.1$). (From Tamura T, Onodera T, Said S, et al. Correlation of myocyte lengthening to chamber dilation in the spontaneously hypertensive heart failure (SHHF) rat. *J Mol Cell Cardiol.* 30:2175–2181.)

40%, corresponding directly with the increase in LV chamber diameter. Figure 8-3 displays marked enlargement of isolated cardiomyocytes from cardiomyopathic human hearts (lower panel) compared with that obtained from controls (upper panel). Using the spontaneously hypertensive heart failure-prone rat model, the Gerdes Lab (25) showed further that increases in myocyte length during the transition to overt heart failure correlated directly with the degree of LV chamber dilatation (Fig. 8-4). Similarly, Anand et al. demonstrated in a rat MI model that myocyte length correlated directly with LV volume measured via passive pressure–volume curves obtained postmortem (26).

These data support that LV chamber dilatation is driven largely by myocyte enlargement, perhaps refuting the classically held notion of so-called myocyte slippage to account for LV dilatation in the failing ventricle. Myocyte slippage refers to the sliding of individual myocytes and myocyte bundles along the long axis that results from disruption of fibrillar collagen connections among these cells and bundles. The notion of myocyte slippage is based upon observations that myocyte numbers decrease across transmural segments of the LV in animal models of remodeling (27,28). Although such evidence is indirect, more recent data using scanning electron microscopy to obtain detailed structural analysis of myocytes and myocyte bundles support that myocyte slippage is likely to be a relevant phenomenon in the remodeling and dilating ventricle.

In the adult, pathological myocyte hypertrophy is characterized by the re-expression of fetal genes (i.e., genes expressed normally in ventricular myocytes during embryonic development that become quiescent soon after birth) (29). These genes include the contractile elements, β-myosin heavy chain (β-MHC), and skeletal α-actin, as well as the noncontractile protein, atrial natriuretic peptide (ANP) (29). Meggs et al. showed that increased myocyte size following experimental MI is associated with elevated expression of skeletal α-actin mRNA (30), while others have documented elevated ANP mRNA and protein within the noninfarcted myocardium (31,32). Similarly, hearts from patients with ischemic cardiomyopathy display markedly increased myocyte size (33) and elevated levels of ANP mRNA (34) in areas distant from infarction. As myocytes enlarge, they also express increasing amounts of brain natriuretic peptide (BNP) mRNA.

In addition to the pathological growth of cardiomyocytes, it has become increasingly evident over the past ten years that ongoing cardiomyocyte loss contributes to progression of ventricular remodeling and dysfunction. While there exists some controversy as to which mode of cell death, necrosis, autophagy, or apoptosis predominates among cardiomyocytes in the failing heart (35), mounting evidence supports that programmed cell death (*apoptosis*) contributes significantly to cardiomyocyte cell loss (36). Apoptosis is a tightly regulated, adenosine triphosphate (ATP)-dependent process in which intracellular proteolytic enzymes (termed caspases) are activated, causing nuclear chromatin condensation and organized disassembly of the cell. Surrounding cells or macrophages then phagocytose resulting cell fragments so that little or no classical inflammatory response occurs (37–42).

Apoptosis Signaling Pathways

Apoptosis occurs following the activation of two general pathways: (a) The extrinsic pathway that involves *agonist binding to death receptors*; and (b) the intrinsic or mitochondrial pathway, which is activated by disruption of the intracellular chemical milieu caused by accumulation of reactive oxygen species, hypoxia, and/or sudden increases in intracellular Ca^{2+} that lead to *loss of integrity of the outer mitochondrial membrane,* resulting in the cytoplasmic release of pro-apoptotic initiating factors (38,39).

Extrinsic Pathway

Apoptosis can be initiated through activation of death receptors (e.g., Fas) by death-inducing ligands (e.g., Fas ligand) that lead to the recruitment of death domain-containing adaptor proteins such as Fas-associated via death domain (FADD), and the formation of a membrane-associated, death-inducing signaling complex (DISC). FADD then recruits procaspase 8 into the complex in the form of a dimer, leading to its cleavage and activation; caspase 8 then cleaves and activates procaspase 3 to its active form, caspase 3 (Fig. 8-5) (43). Caspase 8 also activates the pro-apoptotic Bcl-2 family member, Bid (see Bcl-2 Protein Family, next page), after which the C-terminal portion of Bid (tBid) translocates to the mitochondria and inserts into the outer mitochondrial membrane, facilitating the formation of the mitochondrial permeability transition pore (MPTP). This leads to the release of cytochrome C and other pro-apoptotic factors into the cytoplasm. In this manner, the extrinsic pathway is mechanistically linked to the intrinsic or mitochondrial pathway.

Intrinsic Pathway

The intrinsic pathway of programmed cell death (38) is triggered by the accumulation of reactive oxygen species, sudden increases in intracellular calcium, or hypoxic insults (44). Following these stimuli, the outer mitochondrial membrane becomes disrupted via mechanisms that are not entirely understood, though mitochondrial localization of pro-apoptotic Bcl-2 family members leading ultimately to the formation of the MPTP appears crucial in initiating this process. Upon outer mitochondrial membrane disruption, pro-apoptotic factors are released from the intermembrane space into the cytosol. The heme-containing electron transport protein, cytochrome C, is one pro-apoptotic factor released from the intermembrane space. Once in the cytoplasm, cytochrome C binds to and induces the oligomerization of apoptosis protease activating factor (Apaf-1) that recruits procaspase 9, forming a complex known as the apoptosome. Upon recruitment to the apoptosome, procaspase 9 is cleaved and activated; caspase 9 then binds and cleaves procaspase 3, resulting in caspase 3 activation. Caspase 3 is an important terminal effector of apoptosis, cleaving substrate proteins and activating other downstream caspases within the cell (Fig. 8-5).

Bcl-2 Protein Family

The Bcl-2 family of apoptosis-related proteins is evolutionarily conserved, consisting of both pro-survival and pro-apoptotic factors (44–46). The pro-survival members of the

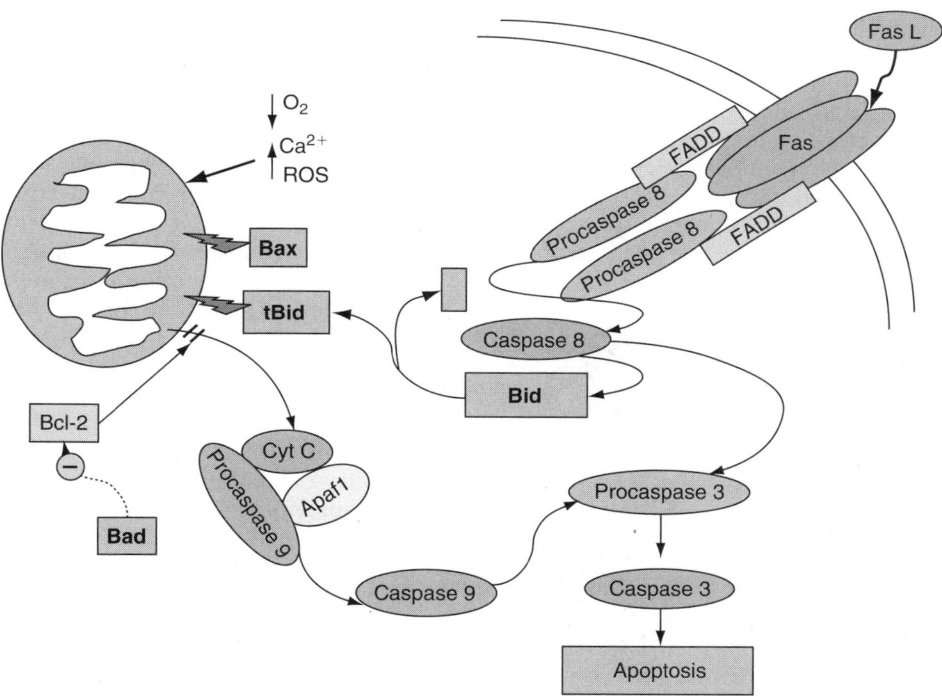

Figure 8-5 Apoptosis signaling pathways. Two major pathways converge on caspase 3, triggering apoptosis. Activation of the extrinsic pathway occurs by activation of the death receptor, Fas, by Fas ligand (Fas L). This causes cleavage and activation of procaspase 8 to caspase 8, which cleaves the pro-apoptotic protein, Bid, that contributes to mitochondrial disruption. Caspase 8 also activates caspase 3, which then cleaves target proteins and activates other downstream caspases. The intrinsic or mitochondrial pathway is activated by stimuli such as hypoxia, reactive oxygen species, or sudden increases in intracellular calcium causing disruption of the mitochondrial membrane via activation of pro-apoptotic family members such as Bax and Bid, leading to the formation of the mitochondrial permeability transition pore (MPTP). This results in cytoplasmic leakage of intermembrane contents including the pro-apoptotic factor, cytochrome C (Cyt C), that binds and activates apoptosis protease activating factor-1 (apaf-1), causing sequential activation of caspases 9 and 3. Pro-survival Bcl-2 family members, including Bcl-2 and Bcl-xl, protect the cell from apoptosis by inhibiting mitochondrial pore formation.

Bcl-2 family (Bcl-2 and Bcl-xl) inhibit apoptosis, in part, by maintaining mitochondrial membrane integrity and preventing the release of pro-apoptotic factors from the intermembrane space (e.g., cytochrome C). The anti-apoptotic Bcl-2 proteins have been shown to inhibit the pro-apoptotic members via direct protein–protein interactions. Pro-apoptotic proteins within the Bcl-2 family, such as Bad, are composed of a Bcl-2 homology (BH3) domain that induces heterodimerization with Bcl-2 and Bcl-xl, thereby blocking their anti-apoptotic effects. Other BH3 containing Bcl-2 family members such as Bid and Bax exert their pro-apoptotic effects by inducing the formation of the MPTP. Although the precise mechanisms are not clear, activation of pro-apoptotic Bid and Bax may form a protein-permeable pore in the outer mitochondrial membrane.

Role of Cardiomyocyte Apoptosis in LV Remodeling

The clinical and experimental literature is replete with evidence to support that apoptosis of cardiac myocytes contributes to remodeling (46). Elegant autopsy studies have shown that cardiomyocytes in normal hearts undergo cell death at very low rates (47–50), but the rate of apoptosis increases sharply in acutely ischemic hearts (51). Hearts from patients who died of an acute MI demonstrate a substantial increase in terminal deoxynucleotidyl transferase-mediated dUTP nick end-labeling (TUNEL)-positive cells in the infarct and peri-infarct zones (52,53). Figure 8-6 demonstrates an example of TUNEL-positive cardiomyocytes and nonmyocyte cells in the peri-infarct zone from an experimental model. Abbate et al. reported that the degree of cardiomyocyte apoptosis within the region remote from the infarct in patients who died late (>10 days) following MI correlated with greater LV remodeling. (54) These human studies provide substantial evidence that cardiomyocyte apoptosis contributes to cell death in acute myocardial injury and that the extent of apoptosis correlates with LV remodeling.

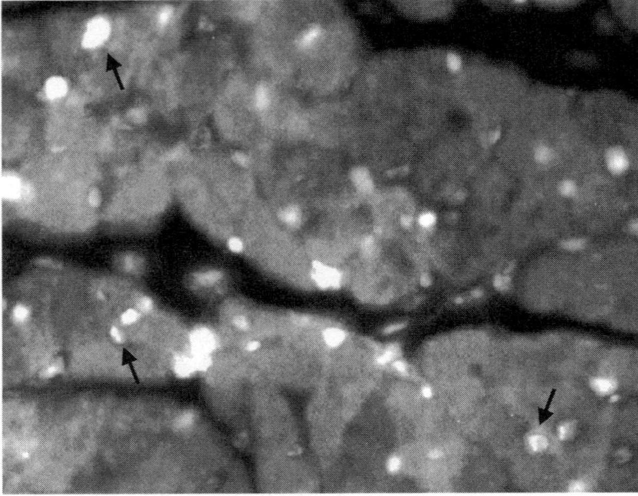

Figure 8-6 Cardiomyocyte apoptosis in the peri-infarct zone. Examples of terminal deoxynucleotidyl transferase-mediated dUTP nick end-labeling (TUNEL) staining of the peri-infarct zone in myocardial sections from mice 24 hours following permanent coronary ligation. TUNEL-positive nuclei are **bright white. Arrows** indicate examples of TUNEL-positive cardiomyocyte nuclei. Numerous TUNEL-positive nonmyocyte nuclei are also seen.

Several studies have demonstrated evidence of cardiomyocyte apoptosis in chronically failing human hearts. In cardiac biopsy samples, Saraste et al. demonstrated increased cardiomyocyte apoptosis in the myocardium of patients with dilated cardiomyopathy and heart failure. In this study, the percent of apoptotic cardiomyocytes correlated with the rapidity of heart failure progression (55). Narula et al. also reported increased TUNEL-positive cardiomyocytes in failing human myocardium and demonstrated increased levels of cytoplasmic cytochrome C and activated caspase 3 as compared to normal controls (56). These data thus support that cardiomyocyte apoptosis is present at a significantly increased rate in failing hearts and suggest that apoptotic loss of cardiac myocytes may play an important role in heart failure progression. In animal models of chronic and progressive LV dysfunction and heart failure, cardiomyocyte apoptosis occurs at an increased rate above that observed in sham or control animals. In a rat pressure overload model, Condorelli et al. demonstrated evidence of increased cardiomyocyte apoptosis following the transition from compensated hypertrophy to LV dysfunction (57). In a mouse MI model, Sam et al. noted a gradual increase in cardiomyocyte apoptosis defined both by TUNEL staining and caspase 3 activity within the noninfarcted myocardium over a span of 6 months that was associated with progressive LV dilation and heart failure (58). Both of these representative experimental studies support that progressive cardiomyocyte cell loss within the myocardium contributes to LV dilatation and progressive LV dysfunction.

Moreover, in multiple transgenic models of dilated cardiomyopathy, cardiomyocyte apoptosis is observed at an increased rate within the failing myocardium. For example, the G-protein Gq couples intracellular signaling pathways to several 7-transmembrane spanning receptors that induce cardiomyocyte hypertrophy. Overexpressing the alpha subunit of Gq (Gαq) in the heart leads to a significant rise in cardiomyocyte apoptosis, coupled with the development of compensated LV hypertrophy, followed by progressive LV dysfunction (45). Similarly, mice with a cardiac-targeted overexpression of tumor necrosis factor-alpha (TNF-α) develop increased cardiomyocyte apoptosis, significant LV dysfunction, heart failure, and premature death (59–61). These transgenic models represent a cross-section of many studies linking dilated cardiomyopathy and progressive LV dysfunction to cardiomyocyte apoptosis.

Wencker et al. (62) recently developed a transgenic mouse with cardiac-specific expression of a procaspase 8 construct that is fused to FK binding protein. This protein construct dimerizes in the presence of the pharmacologic agent, FK506. Thus, upon treatment with FK506, two procaspase 8 molecules form a dimer and their proximity leads to autocleavage and activation of caspase 8 within cardiac myocytes. These mice develop a dose-dependent increase in cardiomyocyte apoptosis, LV chamber enlargement, severe LV dysfunction, and death. One of the transgenic lines exhibited low-level caspase 8 activation that led to an apoptosis rate that was only 10-fold greater than wild type mice and was comparable to that observed in failing human hearts. These animals developed progressive LV dilation and systolic dysfunction followed by premature death, further supporting that low-level cardiomyocyte apoptosis contributes to worsening LV function and heart failure progression.

The benefit of inhibiting apoptosis has been demonstrated in several animal models of heart failure. The broad, nonspecific caspase inhibitor IDN1965 has been reported to prevent cardiomyocyte apoptosis and reduce cardiac remodeling in procaspase 8 transgenic mice previously described (62) and in female mice with cardiac-targeted overexpression of Gαq (63). In the rat MI model, Chandrashekhar et al. demonstrated that treatment of rats with a cell-permeable, broad caspase inhibitor Z-Asp 2,6-DCBMk immediately following coronary ligation reduced apoptosis in the remote myocardium at 4 weeks in association with a marked reduction of LV hypertrophy and dilatation (64). These data provide convincing support for the role of cardiomyocyte apoptosis in ventricular remodeling and heart failure progression.

Cardiac Fibroblasts

Ventricular remodeling is also characterized by changes within the interstitial compartment. Fibroblasts constitute approximately 90% of nonmyocyte cells in the myocardium and play a major role in the regulation of the extracellular matrix (65,66). Total interstitial collagen content is governed by the ongoing balance of synthesis and degradation (67), and myocardial fibroblasts produce types I and III collagen as well as fibronectin (68), the synthesis of which increases in response to myocardial injury (66). Increases in collagen deposition and collagen type I mRNA expression have been demonstrated within the noninfarcted myocardium of human hearts following MI (69) and in hearts from patients with chronic ischemic cardiomyopathy (33,70). Moreover, within the myocardium of patients with heart failure due to pressure overload (aortic stenosis), Hein et al. recently observed a marked increase in fibronectin; the greatest amount of fibrosis was evident in patients with heart failure and severe LV dysfunction (LVEF <30%) (Fig. 8-7) (78).

Similar findings have been observed in animal models of myocardial injury. For example, increased staining for collagen and increased collagen types I and III gene expression are well-established in the rat and mouse MI models. Fibroblasts also proliferate in response to myocardial injury. In the rat MI model, we and others observed increased nonmyocyte cell proliferation within the noninfarcted myocardium 14 days postcoronary ligation (71,72). Correspondingly, collagen content in the noninfarct zone increases and plateaus between days 7 and 14 (71), accompanied by elevations of collagen types 1 and III mRNA (73).

Upon activation, fibroblasts may also differentiate into myofibroblasts that develop phenotypic features of smooth muscle cells, expressing α-smooth muscle actin that is incorporated into contractile filaments and stress fibers. Myofibroblasts have important physiological functions in tissue injury and repair (74). Within the heart, myofibroblasts lie within the perivascular regions but, upon activation, translocate to the infarcted myocardium. In the rat MI model, myofibroblasts are evident within 3 days of injury and remain abundant through week 4, where they participate in the laying down of types I and III collagen and promote scar formation and contraction (75). Whether myofibroblasts infiltrate into regions remote from the infarct zone has not been firmly established. However, in models of cardiomyopathy induced by infusions of isoproterenol or angiotensin II (Ang II), myofibroblasts have been noted in areas of microfibrosis, presumably at sites of myocyte degeneration and loss (76). Thus, within the myocardium, contractile properties of myofibroblasts coupled with enhanced production of extracellular matrix material may contribute to increased stiffness of the left ventricle and, hence, lead to diastolic filling abnormalities.

Myofibroblasts have also been shown to stain positively for TGF-β1, angiotensin converting enzyme (ACE), and angiotensin II within the myocardium (73). Thus, myofibroblasts are also an important reservoir for components of the renin-angiotensin system and TGF-β signaling pathway.

Macrophages

As is evident from the previous discussion, alterations in myocyte and fibroblast biology in the progression of LV remodeling have been studied extensively, yet the potential role of inflammatory cells in the pathogenesis of remodeling has only recently gained recognition. Inflammatory cells play a clear role in infarct healing. After an MI, infiltration of polymorphonuclear neutrophils, macrophages, and other mononuclear cells (including mast cells) occurs rapidly within the infarct zone. However, as infarct healing is completed over several weeks, increased numbers of inflammatory cells appear within the noninfarcted myocardium. In hearts from patients with ischemic and idiopathic dilated cardiomyopathy, a fourfold increase in the number of macrophages per unit area (CD68-positive staining cells) are evident within the noninfarcted regions of the myocardium (77). Similar increases in macrophages have been observed in patients with heart failure due to aortic stenosis (78).

The infiltration of macrophages into the myocardium has also been observed in animal models of heart failure and remodeling. For example, in a rat pressure overload model, Shioi et al. (Fig. 8-8) observed a fourfold increase in interstitial macrophages following the transition to heart failure in association with greater interleukin-1β (IL-1β) and monocyte chemoattractant and activator protein 1 expression (MCAP1 or MCP-1) (79). In a rat MI model, Ono et al. (80) similarly observed increased numbers of macrophages in the noninfarct zone, many of which stained strongly for IL-1β, supporting that myocardial macrophages in this model may contribute to enhanced production of stress-activated cytokines which contribute further to abnormalities in cardiac myocytes and fibroblasts within the failing heart. The number of macrophages increased by approximately fourfold in the myocardium from Dahl salt-sensitive rats with heart failure compared to rats that did not develop heart failure. As in the rat MI model, the interstitial macrophages in this model stained positively for IL-1β, further emphasizing that macrophages are likely a significant if not predominant source of cytokines in these models (79).

Hayashidani et al. recently examined the remodeling effects of gene therapy directed against MCP-1, inhibited by a dominant negative construct expressed using replication-deficient, adenoviral-mediated gene transfer into the limb muscles of these mice. Following MI, wild type mice

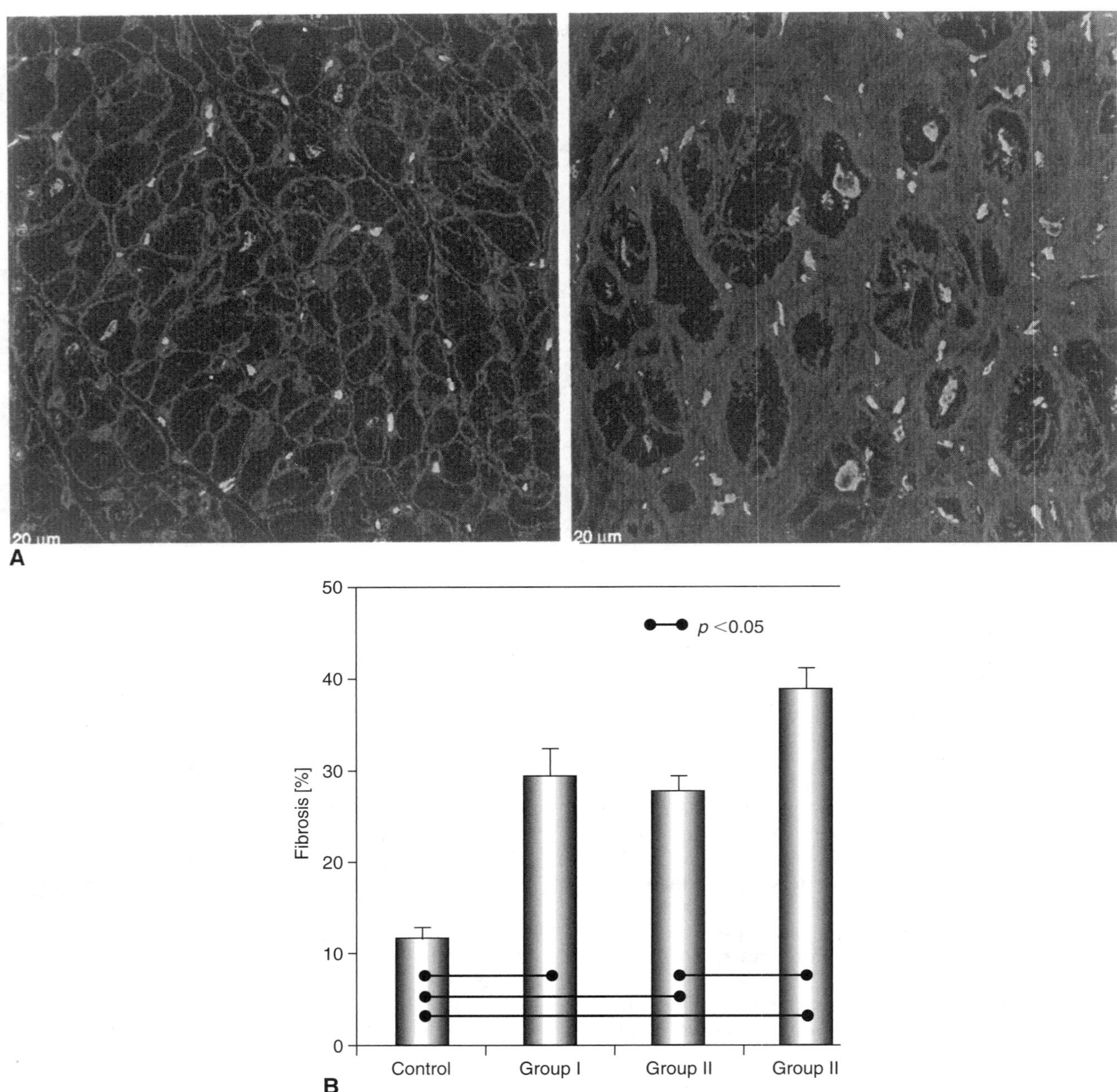

Figure 8-7 Marked fibrosis in sections from hypertrophied human hearts due to aortic stenosis. Intercellular fibronectin framework is selectively stained (nuclei are slightly brighter). **(A)** Left: Normal myocardium shows fine septa between unstained myocytes; Right: severe fibrosis with few myocytes. **(B)** Bar graphs representing area percent of myocardial fibrosis determined by fibronectin staining. Group I (preserved LVEF) and group II (LVEF ≥30% <50%) demonstrate increased fibronectin staining. Most severe fibrosis is seen in group 3 (LVEFs <30%). (From Hein S, Arnon E, Kostin S, et al. Progression from compensated hypertrophy to failure in the pressure-overloaded human heart: structural deterioration and compensatory mechanisms. *Circulation.* 107:984–991, with permission.)

exhibited potent induction of MCP-1 gene expression within the infarct and noninfarct zones that waned over the ensuing 4 weeks. Mice expressing the dominant negative MCP-1 developed less infiltration of macrophages within the noninfarct zone associated with diminished expression of both TNF-α and TGF-β1, coinciding with reduced fibrosis and myocyte hypertrophy (Fig. 8-9) (81). These findings therefore support that inhibiting mononuclear cell infiltration within the noninfarct zone limits cytokine gene expression and cardiac remodeling.

Mast Cells

Similar to macrophages, the role of mast cells in LV remodeling is not completely understood but these mononuclear inflammatory cells have recently been shown to contribute

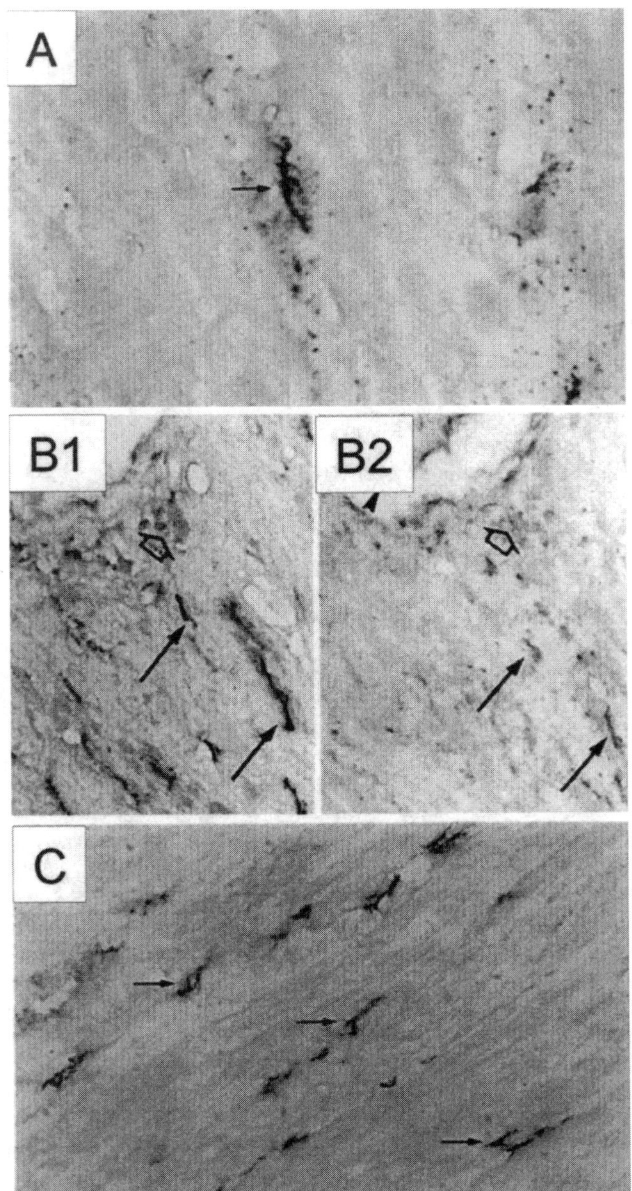

Figure 8-8 **(A)** In 11-week-old DS rats with heart failure, interstitial cells (**arrow**) stained positive for IL-1β. Original magnification 800×. **(B)** Serial sections of heart tissue stained with antibodies to macrophages **(B1)** or to IL-1β **(B2)** are shown. The interstitial cells (**arrows**) and perivascular cells (**open arrows**) positive for IL-1β were predominantly macrophages. Original magnification 220×. **(C)** The number of macrophages was increased in the hearts of DS rats with heart failure. Original magnification 220×. (From Shioi T, Matsumori A, Kihara Y, et al. Increased expression of interleukin-1β and monocyte chemotactic and activating factor/monocyte chemoattractant protein-1 in the hypertrophied and failing heart with pressure overload. *Circ Res.* 81:664–671, with permission.)

to extracellular matrix and myocyte remodeling in the failing heart. Patella et al. (82) demonstrated in samples from human dilated cardiomyopathic hearts a fourfold increase in mast cell density compared with normal control samples. Moreover, Petrovic et al. observed a twofold increase in mast cell density in human dilated cardiomyopathy, while a greater number of mast cells was observed in myocarditis (83). These studies in human tissue support that mast cells are recruited to the myocardium in response to chronic myocardial injury.

In the rat MI model, mast cells increase markedly in the infarct zone in the first day to weeks following coronary ligation, and in the noninfarct zone by day 35 (84). Mast cells are also increased in nonischemic models of dilated cardiomyopathy such as pressure overload models in rodents (85) and in the dog models of pacing-induced heart failure and mitral regurgitation (86–88). In the study by Stewart et al. (88), increased mast cell density correlated positively with matrix metalloproteinase 2 (MMP2) activity, suggesting that cardiac mast cells regulate extracellular matrix remodeling. A similar relationship between MMP activity and myocardial mast cell content was evident in the aorto-caval fistula model of volume overload in the rat (89). Moreover, in mast cell-deficient mice and in mice treated with the mast cell stabilizer, tranilast, pressure overload-induced LV hypertrophy and myocardial fibrosis were diminished in association with improved LV systolic function (85).

While the precise mechanism by which mast cells exert their remodeling effects in these heart failure models has not been completely characterized, mast cells are known to secrete a variety of factors that contribute to hypertrophy of myocytes and extracellular matrix deposition. Mast cells are the most abundant source of the serine protease, chymase, within the myocardium. Similar to ACE, chymase catalyzes the conversion of angiotensin I (Ang I) to Ang II and activates the pro-form of TGF-β1 in the failing heart (90). Thus, release of chymase by cardiac mast cells contributes to increased local levels of Ang II and TGF-β1, which activate growth responses in both cardiac myocytes and fibroblasts (see Non-ACE-Mediated Ang II-Forming pathways, next page). Cardiac mast cells also secrete tryptase and stromelysin (also known as MMP-3), which are proteases that activate other matrix metalloproteinases within the interstitium, thereby further influencing extracellular matrix composition (91).

The cellular events that initiate and propagate cardiac remodeling include cardiomyocyte hypertrophy and apoptosis, coupled with activation of fibroblasts and the abnormal accumulation of extracellular matrix material. Moreover, infiltration of inflammatory cells contributes importantly to these pathological changes in both myocytes and fibroblasts. A review of the key hormonal mechanisms known to induce these cellular abnormalities will follow next.

NEUROHORMONAL MECHANISMS CONTRIBUTING TO CARDIAC REMODELING

Renin-Angiotensin-Aldosterone System

Substantial experimental data now exist supporting a pivotal role for the renin-angiotensin-aldosterone system (RAAS) in mediating cellular changes in the remodeling and failing ventricle. The renin-angiotensin system (RAS) consists of both circulating and local tissue compartments, the activation of which leads to the formation of Ang II, the primary hormonal mediator of the RAS. Ang II signals through 7-transmembrane-spanning, G-protein-coupled receptors, causing vasoconstriction, fluid retention, and heightened

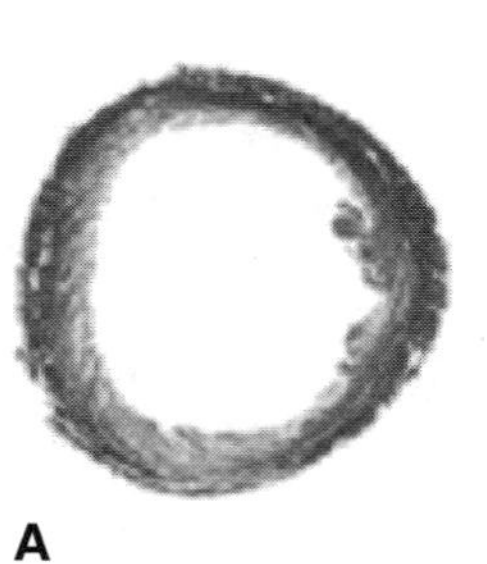

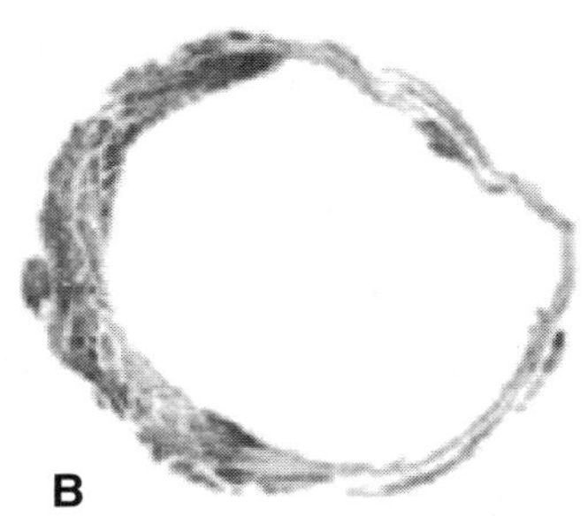

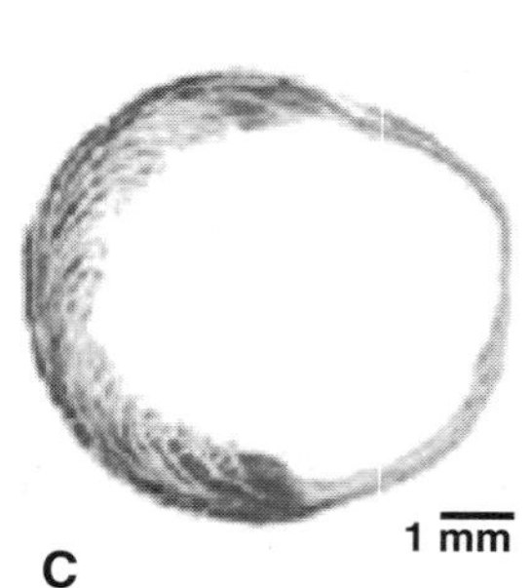

Figure 8-9 Gene therapy targeting MCP-1 reduces LV remodeling following coronary ligation in mice. Low-power **(A–C)** photomicrographs of Masson-trichrome-stained LV cross-sections obtained from sham **(A)**, MI **(B)**, and MI+DN−MCP−1 **(C)** mice 28 days after operation. (Reproduced from Hayashidani S, Tsutsui H, Shiomi T, et al. Anti-monocyte chemoattractant protein-1 gene therapy attenuates left ventricular remodeling and failure after experimental myocardial infarction. *Circulation.* 108:2134–2140, with permission.)

sympathetic outflow. The type 1 Ang II (AT_1) receptor mediates many of the known cardiovascular effects of Ang II. AT_1 receptor activation also induces the cell growth-promoting effects of Ang II. Other known Ang II receptors include the type 2 (AT_2) and type 4 (AT_4) receptors. The latter has been identified on endothelial cells and may promote the release of procoagulant substances such as plasminogen activator inhibitor-1 (92). The precise role of the AT_2 receptor remains controversial (93) but several studies suggest that AT_2 receptor activation may counter the effects of AT_1 receptor activation (reviewed later).

Role of Tissue Angiotensin-Converting Enzyme

Although circulating Ang II contributes importantly to the adverse cardiovascular effects of RAS activation, further exploration of RAS components elucidated the presence of an active RAS at the local tissue level. Several lines of evidence support that tissue ACE contributes significantly to the cellular responses taking place in the remodeling ventricle, and inhibition of tissue ACE may be important to the antiremodeling effects of ACE inhibitors. Following MI in the rat, local cardiac ACE activity and ACE mRNA levels have been shown to increase twofold in the noninfarct zone (94). Ruzicka et al. reported that prevention of LV hypertrophy in a rat volume overload model was dependent on inhibition of local (myocardial) ACE (95), and in a rat MI model, Wollert et al. found that more potent inhibition of tissue ACE activity was associated with improved survival and greater reduction in both LV mass and ventricular ANP gene expression (32). These studies support that activation of tissue ACE plays an important role in remodeling in these animal models.

Non-ACE-Mediated Ang II-Forming Pathways

In addition to ACE, other myocardial proteases have been identified that convert Ang I to Ang II [reviewed in (90)]. For example, chymase is a serine protease released by cardiac mast cells. In landmark studies by Urata et al., chymase was shown to contribute to cardiac Ang II generation in cardiac membrane preparations from failing human hearts (96,97). Thus, ACE inhibitors may not completely suppress Ang II formation. As mast cells are the primary source for chymase in the myocardium, it makes sense that mast cell infiltration into the failing heart will lead to further increases in Ang II production in an ACE-independent manner.

Role of the AT_1 Receptor in Remodeling

Locally formed Ang II exerts its cellular effects in a paracrine and autocrine fashion. Groundbreaking work by Sadoshima and Izumo demonstrated the presence of Ang II within myocyte secretory granules 30 minutes following mechanical stretch (98,99). These investigators demonstrated further that an AT_1 receptor antagonist largely blocked the increase in myocyte protein synthesis following mechanical stretch. In addition, Ang II stimulates collagen production and proliferation of cardiac fibroblasts in vitro via activation of the AT_1 receptor (99). To explore the effects of Ang II in vivo, Schunkert et al. infused Ang II into isolated rat heart preparations and observed markedly increased protein synthesis that was blocked by an AT_1 receptor antagonist (100). These experimental observations support that Ang II stimulates myocyte and fibroblast growth via AT_1 receptor activation in vitro and in vivo independent of effects on load, placing further emphasis on the role of Ang II as a growth factor.

Much work in animal models also supports the critical role of the AT_1 receptor subtype in mediating the adverse cellular effects of Ang II. We demonstrated in a mouse MI model that AT_1 receptor blockade limits the degree of myocardial hypertrophy and prevents the rise in ANP, collagen type I gene expression, and interstitial collagen content in the noninfarct zone (Fig. 8-10) (101). We and others have demonstrated in the rat MI model that AT_1 receptor blockade also limits LV hypertrophy and increased interstitial collagen (102–104). Blockade of the AT_1 receptor inhibits its activation by Ang II and leads to the unopposed stimulation of the AT_2 receptor subtype, an effect that may account for some of the observed benefits of AT_1 blockade in the rat heart following MI (102,105).

Role of the AT_2 Receptor

The precise role for AT_2 receptor activation in ventricular remodeling remains controversial (93). In rats treated with AT_1 receptor antagonists following MI, the observed reductions in LV end-diastolic volume, LV end-systolic volume,

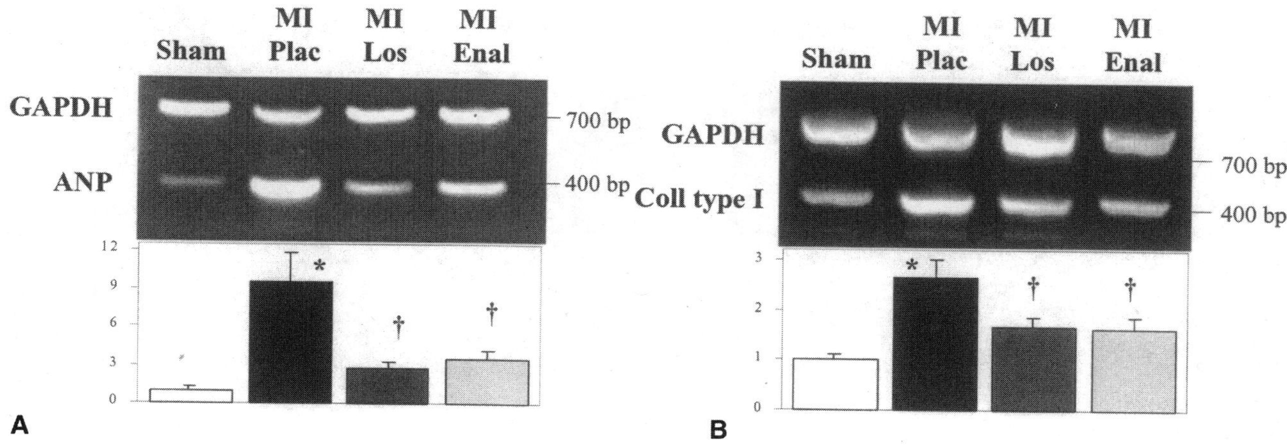

Figure 8-10 Gene expression measured within the noninfarct zone 6 weeks following MI in mice. **(A)** Ethidium bromide stained, agarose gel in which the levels of atrial natriuretic peptide (ANP) and glyceraldehyde-3-phosphate dehydrogenase (GAPDH) mRNA were measured via multiplex rtPCR. Within the ventricular myocardium, ANP expression is specific to cardiac myocytes and indicates a conversion to the hypertrophic phenotype. The bar graph below the gel image displays the mean ± SEM for the respective groups. The placebo MI group demonstrates increased ANP gene expression compared to shams, which is significantly inhibited by either the AT_1 receptor antagonist, losartan (Los) or the ACE inhibitor, enalapril (Enal). **(B)** Similar to that described for **(A)** except this ethidium bromide gel represents expression of collagen type 1 mRNA in the noninfarct zone 6 weeks following MI in mice. Both losartan and enalapril reduced collagen type 1 mRNA, supporting a role of activation of the RAS in the myocyte and fibroblast responses to myocardial injury and remodeling. (From Patten RD, Aronovitz MJ, Einstein M, et al. Effects of angiotensin II receptor blockade versus angiotensin-converting-enzyme inhibition on ventricular remodelling following myocardial infarction in the mouse. *Clin Sci. (London)* 104:109–118.) Bp, base pairs; Plac, placebo. ($p < 0.01$ versus shams; $^{\dagger}p < 0.01$ versus placebo.)

and myocyte cross-sectional area were completely reversed by simultaneous administration of an AT_2 receptor antagonist (102). This important study by Liu et al. suggested that unopposed AT_2 receptor activation might contribute to the antiremodeling effects of AT_1 blockade in this model. The advent of transgenic mice that overexpress the AT_2 receptor and mice harboring a targeted deletion of the AT_2 receptor gene have allowed the careful evaluation of its role in cardiac function and remodeling.

For example, Ichihara et al. demonstrated that mice lacking the AT_2 receptor exhibited twice the rate of cardiac rupture 1 week following coronary ligation compared to wild types, associated with reduced expression of genes encoding the extracellular matrix components, collagen type I, type III, and fibronectin in the AT_2-deficient mice (106). Adachi et al. showed further that, compared to wild types, a greater percentage of AT_2-deficient mice developed heart failure following MI (107), while Oishi et al. observed greater LV hypertrophy and dilatation coupled with an increase in mortality in AT_2 receptor knockout mice following MI (108). Taken together, these data suggest that AT_2 receptor activation plays a protective role in the post-MI heart. In a pressure overload model, AT_2 receptor knockout mice developed *less* LV hypertrophy with preservation of LV systolic function (109), supporting a growth-promoting effect of AT_2 receptor activation and emphasizing that the role of AT_2 receptor activation in cardiac remodeling may be species- or strain-specific and may depend on the stimulus for cardiac hypertrophy (110).

Role of Aldosterone in Ventricular Remodeling

The steroid hormone, aldosterone, is yet another component of the RAAS that contributes to the development of adverse ventricular remodeling in patients with LV systolic dysfunction, independent of Ang II-mediated effects. Aldosterone secretion is partially under the control of Ang II via activation of the AT_1 receptor. However, many other factors influence the secretion of aldosterone, including serum sodium and potassium concentrations, adrenocorticotropic hormone, atrial natriuretic peptide, and endothelin. (111) Aldosterone induces its cellular effects via the ligand-activated transcription factor (the mineralocorticoid receptor) which, upon stimulation, enters the nucleus and turns on the transcription of specific target genes. Mineralocorticoid receptors are present in the heart (112) and aldosterone is produced within the myocardium in experimental heart failure models, and in the myocardium of patients with hypertension or heart failure (113,114).

Aldosterone has been primarily implicated in the fibroblast responses within the myocardium that accompany remodeling of the left ventricle. In vitro, aldosterone induces an increase in collagen synthesis by cardiac fibroblasts (115). In a rat model of renovascular hypertension, Brilla et al. (116) reported that the aldosterone antagonist, spironolactone, prevented the increase in interstitial collagen within the myocardium. In a rat MI model, Silvestre et al. (117) further demonstrated that spironolactone limited the increase in interstitial collagen content within the noninfarcted myocardium (Fig. 8-11).

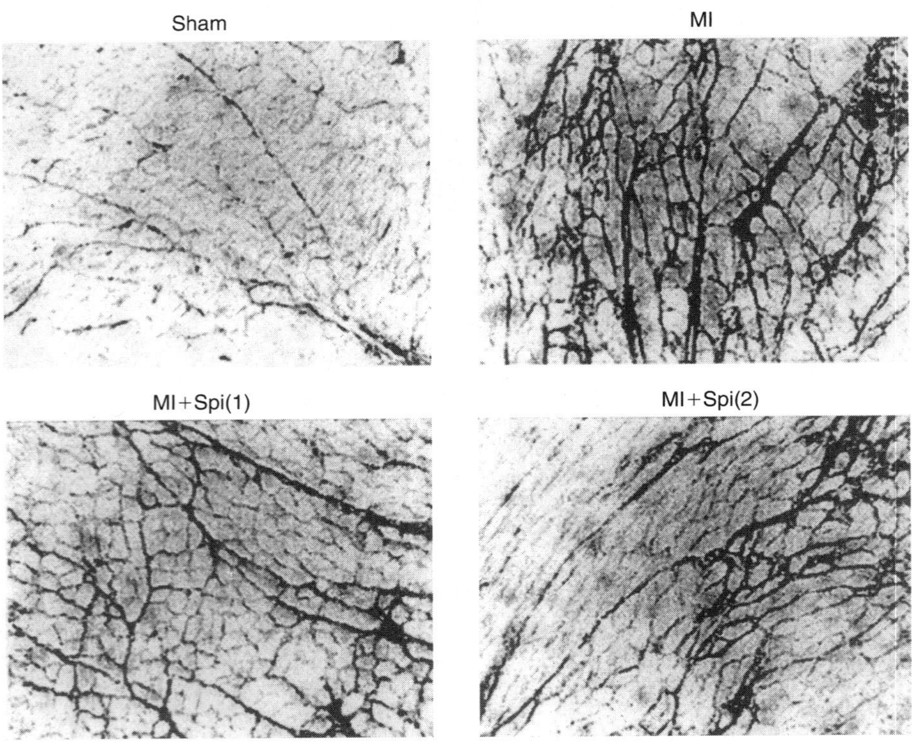

Figure 8-11 Histological images of myocardial sections stained with the collagen-specific dye, Sirius red. In this photomicrograph, collagen appears **black** and myocytes **white**. Shown are noninfarct zone sections from rats 25 days post-MI. Untreated rats (MI) demonstrate a significant increase in noninfarct zone collagen content compared to shams. Treatment with the aldosterone antagonist, spironolactone, at low [20 mg/kg/day-MI+Spi (1)] and high doses [80 mg/kg/day-MI+Spi (2)] resulted in significant decreases in interstitial collagen content as shown. (Reproduced from Silvestre JS, Heymes C, Oubenaissa A, et al. Activation of cardiac aldosterone production in rat myocardial infarction: effect of angiotensin II receptor blockade and role in cardiac fibrosis. *Circulation.* 99:2694–2701, with permission.)

Furthermore, in the dog microembolization model of heart failure, eplerenone (a novel mineralocorticoid receptor antagonist) prevented the increase in LV end-diastolic and end-systolic volumes and the decrease in fractional shortening observed in placebo-treated dogs (118). Surprisingly, eplerenone reduced cardiomyocyte hypertrophy as assessed by myocyte cross-sectional area measurements, along with the expected reduction in extracellular matrix accumulation. Taken together, these experimental studies support a pivotal role for aldosterone in the pathophysiology of ventricular remodeling following myocardial injury or pressure overload.

Sympathetic Nervous System

While sympathetic nervous system (SNS) activation was classically thought to provide a critical compensatory role in the maintenance of contractility in the failing heart, the link between sympathetic activation and mortality (119) led to the hypothesis that activation of the SNS may contribute to the progression of both LV dilation and dysfunction in patients with heart failure. Activity of the SNS is governed, in part, through the central regulation of SNS outflow, and locally via catecholamine-induced activation of G-protein-coupled receptors. Exposure of cultured cardiomyocytes to catecholamines such as norepinephrine leads to hypertrophy (120), and chronic infusions of sympathetic agonists in vivo leads to the development of a dilated cardiomyopathy characterized by myocyte hypertrophy, apoptosis, and increased fibrosis (121–124). In dog models of direct myocardial injury (125) or microembolization-induced LV dysfunction, beta-blockers limit the extent of both LV chamber dilation and myocardial hypertrophy associated with a reduction in cardiomyocyte apoptosis (126,127). Hence, heightened sympathetic activation and/or increases in circulating catecholamines promote LV remodeling and heart failure, and blockade of β-adrenergic receptors mitigates LV remodeling induced by myocardial injury.

Manipulation of adrenergic signaling using transgenic mouse models has also shed additional light on the role of adrenergic receptors in cardiac remodeling (128). For example, mice that overexpress the β2-adrenergic receptor within the heart develop gradual and progressive LV dilation and systolic dysfunction associated with myocyte hypertrophy and interstitial fibrosis (129). Moreover, using myocytes from β2-adrenergic receptor knockout mice and β1-β2-adrenergic receptor double-knockout mice, Zhou et al. elegantly demonstrated that unopposed stimulation of the β1-adrenergic receptor contributes specifically to increased cardiac myocyte apoptosis (130). Furthermore, increasing central sympathetic outflow via knocking out α2-adrenergic receptor subtypes (A and C) in mice results in the development of cardiac dilation and heart failure (131). Taken together, these experimental studies support the general conclusion that overactivation of the SNS induces cellular and structural abnormalities leading to pathological cardiac remodeling.

Endothelin System

Heart failure is associated with elevated plasma levels of endothelin-1, secreted primarily by endothelial cells. Like Ang II, endothelin-1 is a potent vasoconstrictor and the degree of endothelin-1 elevation is closely linked to the severity of heart failure (132). The main biological effects of endothelin-1 are mediated through receptor subtypes denoted ET-A and ET-B, both of which are 7-transmembrane-domain, G-protein-coupled receptors. In the failing heart, the expression of the ET-A receptor-density is increased. ET-1 stimulates cardiac hypertrophy in vitro (133) and additional data support that ET-1 may be critical to Ang II-induced cardiomyocyte hypertrophy through a paracrine mechanism (134). While ET-A blockade has been shown to prevent cardiac remodeling in the rat MI model (135), prevention of remodeling has been inconsistent among studies (136). Accordingly, given recent clinical trials demonstrating a lack of benefit of ET receptor antagonists on remodeling and clinical outcomes in patients with heart failure, it is unlikely that this hormone will receive further attention as a therapeutic target in cardiac remodeling (137,138).

Stress-Activated Cytokines in LV Remodeling

In addition to the classic neurohormonal systems previously described, stress-activated cytokines also contribute to the structural and cellular abnormalities within the remodeling and failing heart. This section will explore the roles of TGF-β, TNF-α, IL-6, and IL-1β, all of which have been shown to increase in failing hearts and contribute to remodeling.

Transforming Growth Factor-β

The relevant TGF-β isoform within the heart is TGF-β1. TGF-β1 induces its intracellular effects by activating receptor serine-threonine kinases (denoted T-βR1 and T-βR2) that are expressed in myocytes and nonmyocyte cells. TGF-β signals through the phosphorylation of small mother against decapentaplegic (Smad) proteins, leading ultimately to their nuclear translocation and transcription of target genes, many of which include components of the extracellular matrix (139). Increased levels of TGF-β1 are present in the myocardium of patients with heart failure due to either idiopathic dilated cardiomyopathy or hypertrophic cardiomyopathy. In animal models of pressure overload-induced hypertrophy, TGF-β1 expression rises in concert with the transition to heart failure (139). TGF-β1 stimulates fibroblast proliferation and promotes the phenotypic conversion of fibroblasts to contractile myofibroblasts. In vivo and in vitro studies revealed that TGF-β1 increases the transcription of procollagen 1 and fibronectin genes while also stabilizing their mRNA. Moreover, TGF-β1 decreases the activity and expression of matrix metalloproteinases—enzymes that degrade collagen and other extracellular matrix components within the interstitial space (140). Thus, TGF-β1 signaling pathway activation induces extracellular matrix material accumulation both by effecting an increase in production and inhibition of degradation. In support of this notion, Seeland et al. demonstrated that transgenic mice with cardiac-specific overexpression of TGF-β1 develop increased myocardial fibrosis that is associated with inhibition of matrix metalloproteinase activity (141). Accordingly, heterozygote TGF-β1 *knockout* mice develop *less* fibrosis of the heart associated with aging (139). In addition, treatment of rats with neutralizing antibodies to TGF-β1 prevents myocardial fibrosis and LV dysfunction that develop in response to pressure overload (142). These data therefore support a clear role for TGF-β1 in the development of myocardial fibrosis in remodeling.

Evidence also supports a role for TGF-β1 in cardiomyocyte hypertrophy. When added to neonatal rat cardiomyocytes in culture, TGF-β1 induces the expression of the fetal gene program. Accordingly, mice that overexpress TGF-β1 develop significant cardiomyocyte hypertrophy (141). Moreover, while sub-pressor doses of Ang II lead to ventricular hypertrophy in wild type mice, TGF-β1 knockout mice develop no ventricular hypertrophy in response to Ang II, supporting that the cardiomyocyte growth effects of Ang II are mediated, in part, through TFG-β signaling. (143). Thus, TGF-β contributes importantly to the pathogenesis of LV remodeling by activating fibroblasts and contributing to pathological cardiomyocyte growth.

Tumor Necrosis Factor-α

TNF-α is a potent, proinflammatory cytokine whose myocardial expression increases in concert with heart failure progression. TNF-α exists in the form of a trimer and binds its cognate receptors on the cell surface [denoted TNF receptors (TNFRs) 1 and 2]. TNFRs 1 and 2 belong to the CD45 family of cytokine receptors and exist as homotrimers. Upon stimulation by TNF-α, TNFRs activate signaling pathways (144) that lead to the activation and nuclear translocation of NFκB and AP1 transcription factors, both of which initiate the transcription of other proinflammatory cytokines, thereby creating a positive feedback loop (145). TNF-α is not constitutively expressed in the heart but its expression is rapidly activated in response to myocardial injury; this may be protective in the myocardium in the early period of the stress response (such as immediately following an MI) (146). For example, pretreating rats with TNF-α reduces the degree of myocardial injury in response to ischemia-reperfusion and in cultured cardiomyocytes, TNF-reduces apoptosis in response to hypoxia (147). However, during prolonged or sustained TNF-α expression such as that observed in the failing human myocardium, deleterious effects ensue. In vitro, TNF-α causes depression of myocyte contractility and induces cardiomyocyte hypertrophy and cardiomyocyte apoptosis (144). In vivo, overexpression of TNF-α within the heart contributes to cardiomyocyte apoptosis (61) that coincides with the development of progressive LV dilatation and dysfunction. TNF-α induces alterations of the extracellular matrix that contribute to LV dilatation. As opposed to TGF-β stimulating the heightened production of extracellular matrix material (ECM), TNF-α counters these responses. Administration of physiologically relevant concentrations of TNF-α to wild type rats for 15 days leads to significant LV dilatation and contractile dysfunction associated with the marked loss of fibrillar collagen weaves that maintain normal myocyte and myocyte bundle connections (Fig. 8-12) (148). Similarly, young (4-week-old) transgenic mice with cardiac-targeted overexpression of TNF-α develop a marked increase in MMP activity associated with a reduction in tissue inhibitor of metalloproteinase-1 (TIMP-1) protein within the myocardium, further contributing to dissolution of the extracellular matrix (146). The reduction in fibrillar

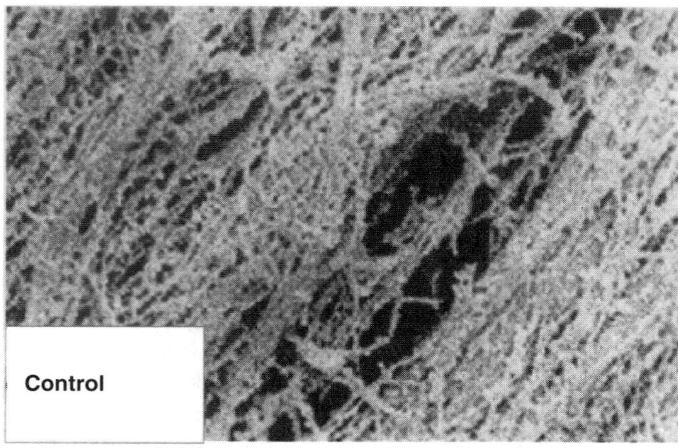

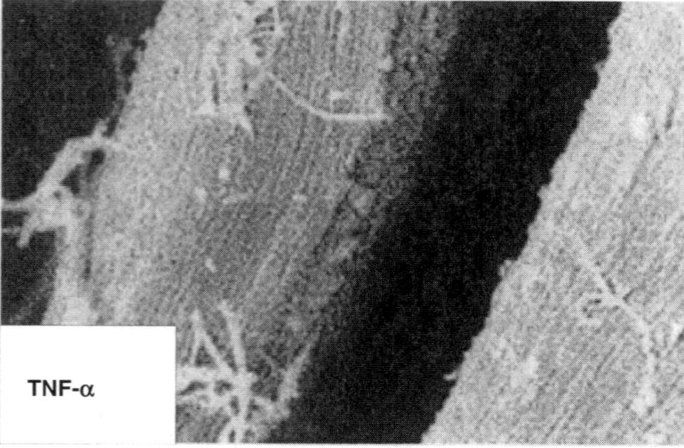

Figure 8-12 Scanning electron micrographs of LV myocardial sections taken from vehicle-treated rats (Control) and from TNF-α-treated rats (7500×). The fine weave of extracellular matrix material among myocytes in the control animals is largely absent in rats treated with TNF-α. (Reproduced from Bozkurt B, Kribbs SB, Clubb FJ, Jr., et al. Pathophysiologically relevant concentrations of tumor necrosis factor-α promote progressive left ventricular dysfunction and remodeling in rats. *Circulation.* 97:1382–1391, with permission.)

connections between myocytes and myocyte bundles may contribute to myocyte slippage and, hence, LV dilatation. Long-term exposure to elevated levels of TNF-α results in increased interstitial fibrosis related, in part, to increased TGF-β1 expression and a shift from ECM dissolution to enhanced production. These data therefore support that TNF-α contributes to the cellular alterations that drive pathological cardiac remodeling, including cardiomyocyte hypertrophy, apoptosis, and changes in the composition of the extracellular matrix.

Interleukin-6

Similar to TNF-α, circulating levels of IL-6 are elevated in patients with heart failure and the degree of elevation is related to heart failure severity and prognosis (149). IL-6 signals through its own receptor (IL-6R), which, upon ligand binding, associates with the gp130 cytokine receptor, forming a membrane complex that activates downstream signaling pathways. The myocardial source for IL-6 production is likely a combination of myocytes, fibroblasts, and mononuclear inflammatory cells (140). Similar to other cytokines, IL-6 expression increases markedly in the infarct zone postcoronary ligation. In the chronic phase post-MI, elevated IL-6 expression within the remote myocardium has been observed in both postmortem human samples (150) and rat MI models (140). Similar to TNF-α, IL-6 stimulation of fibroblasts *decreases* collagen synthesis and increases MMP activity, thereby contributing to dissolution of extracellular matrix (140). Transgenic mice expressing both IL-6 and the IL-6R within cardiac myocytes develop significant LV hypertrophy that results from continuous activation of the gp130 receptor. Moreover, in vitro, cultured neonatal rat cardiomyocytes increase in size when the combination of IL-6 and its receptor are added to the media (151). Other cytokines within the IL-6 family, including cardiotropin 1 and leukemia inhibitor factor, induce cardiomyocyte hypertrophy in vitro and in vivo (152–154). During the evolution of cardiac remodeling, therefore, IL-6 contributes to alterations in the extracellular matrix and possibly to cardiomyocyte hypertrophy.

Interleukin-1β

IL-1β expression is elevated in the myocardium of failing hearts and is present at high circulating levels in patients with heart failure. The primary sources of IL-1β within the myocardium are macrophages and cardiac fibroblasts (140,155). Similar to TNF-α and IL-6, IL-1β suppresses fibroblast-mediated production of collagen and inhibits fibroblast proliferation (156,157). IL-1β also increases the expression and activity of MMPs which cause destruction of the fibrillar collagen network that maintains proper myocyte connections and contact. In a manner distinct from TNF-α and IL-6, IL-1β potently induces the expression of inducible nitric oxide synthase. Moreover, IL-1β causes hypertrophy within cardiac myocytes but inhibits the expression of the fetal genes, β-MHC and skeletal α-actin. Thus, IL-1β alters the growth phenotype and genotype of cardiac myocytes (156,157) while also disrupting the composition of the extracellular matrix.

Cross-Talk Between Cytokine and Neurohormonal Pathways

These cytokine signaling pathways contribute significantly to the development of myocyte and extracellular matrix changes within the failing heart. Recent evidence also suggests that these pathways augment and/or sustain local neurohormonal activation, which in turn promotes the enhanced expression of these same cytokines consistent with a positive feedback mechanism (158). Gurantz et al. demonstrated that TNF-α increases the expression of the AT_1 receptor in cardiac fibroblasts by a mechanism dependent on NF-κB, thereby enhancing Ang II effects on cells via an increase in AT_1 receptor density (159). Moreover, Peng et al. showed that Ang II-mediated increase in cardiac fibroblast protein synthesis and inhibition of MMP2 activity was potentiated by pretreatment with TNF-α. A subsequent study by Gurantz et al. (160) demonstrated that both TNF-α and IL-1β increase AT_1 receptor expression, the effects of which were additive. Ang II itself activates NF-κB via the AT_1 receptor and therefore increases the transcription of proinflammatory cytokines (161). In adult cardiac myocytes, Ang II stimulates the expression of TNF-α at the mRNA and protein levels in a fashion that requires NF-κB (158). Moreover, transgenic mice with cardiac-targeted overexpression of TNF-α demonstrate significantly increased levels of both ACE and Ang II (162). These studies thus support the presence of cross-talk between the RAAS and cytokine signaling pathways in the form of a positive feedback loop that potentiates the detrimental impact of both pathways on the cellular events taking place within the remodeling ventricle.

TNF-α also enhances sympathetic activation. Infusion of physiological amounts of TNF-α into wild type rats increases central sympathetic outflow (163). Moreover, isoproterenol infusion in wild type rats and mice induces the expression of TNF-α, IL-1β, and IL-6 (164,165). These are but a few examples of the evidence supporting that the SNS positively regulates cytokine gene expression, while cytokines potentiate the effects of the catecholamines on the myocardium.

Nitric Oxide Synthases

While the contributions of neurohormonal and cytokine signaling pathways to ventricular remodeling are well-established, cytokine-mediated increases in inducible nitric oxide synthase may be an important downstream event that contributes importantly to remodeling (166,167). There are three known members of the nitric oxide synthase (NOS) family [reviewed in (166)]: neuronal NOS (nNOS or NOS I), inducible NOS (iNOS or NOS II), and endothelial or constitutive NOS (eNOS or NOS III). Cardiac myocytes constitutively express eNOS (168). eNOS-dependent NO production is regulated by the binding of calmodulin that is catalyzed by increased intracellular calcium and results in relatively low levels of NO production, which may actually confer protection from cardiac hypertrophy and remodeling (169,170). In contrast, iNOS has a high affinity for calmodulin at low calcium concentrations and, thus, its activity is independent of intracellular calcium. As a result, iNOS-dependent NO production is regulated primarily by alterations in iNOS protein abundance. Recent studies have shown that iNOS is either undetectable or detected at only low levels in healthy human hearts but it is expressed at high levels in the myocardium of failing hearts (171–173).

The precise role of iNOS in the pathophysiology of heart failure progression and in cardiomyocyte apoptosis remains controversial. In vitro experiments have shown that NO may be bifunctional, with opposing dose-dependent effects on contractility and apoptosis in cardiomyocytes (174). Vila-Petroff et al. showed that NO at low concentrations increased adult rat cardiomyocyte contraction via an increase in adenylate cyclase activity and cyclic adenosine monophosphate (cAMP). Low levels of NO have also been shown to induce a positive inotropic effect in isolated feline papillary muscle (175). High levels of NO inhibit cardiomyocyte shortening velocity in part by activation of guanylate cyclase and increased cyclic GMP (176–179). In a similar fashion, high levels of NO blunt β-adrenergic responsiveness. A similar dual functionality has been noted in cardiomyocyte apoptosis, whereby NO may protect cells from apoptotic cell death at *low* concentrations and induce apoptosis at *high* concentrations (174). Pinsky et al. demonstrated that the NO donor, S-nitroso-N-acetylpenicillamine (SNAP), induced apoptosis in adult rat ventricular myocytes in a dose-dependent fashion. In neonatal cardiomyocytes, the combination of TNF-α, IL-6, and interferon-γ stimulated a marked increase in iNOS expression associated with apoptosis (180). Arstall et al. further demonstrated that cytokine-induced apoptosis in rat cardiomyocytes could be blocked by the iNOS specific inhibitor 2-amino-5,6-dihydro-6-methyl-4H-1,3-thiazine (AMT) (181). Thus, these in vitro data support the notion that high levels of NO (as might be generated by iNOS) increase cardiomyocyte apoptosis and decrease cardiomyocyte contractile force. In this manner, increased iNOS expression within cardiomyocytes may contribute to the pathogenesis of LV remodeling and heart failure.

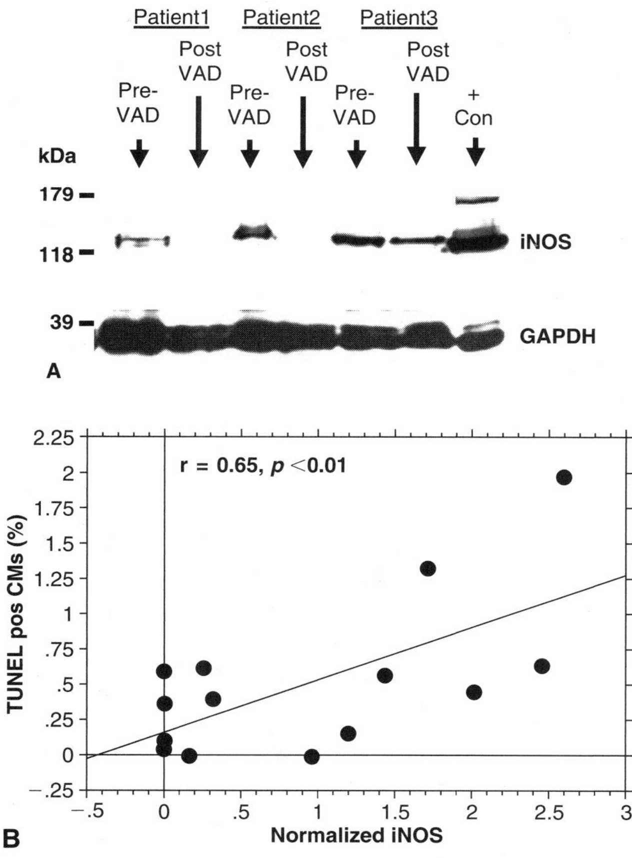

Figure 8-13 **(A)** iNOS Western blot from 3 patients with matched pre-and post-VAD myocardial samples. All three examples demonstrate a notable decrease in iNOS within-the myocardium following VAD support. The corresponding Western blot for the control protein, GAPDH, perfomed on the same membrane is shown in the lower panel. **(B)** Regression plot of percent TUNEL positive cardiomyocytes (CM) versus normalized iNOS levels (iNOS/GAPDH) in which a significant correlation was observed ($r = 0.66$; $p < 0.01$). (Reprinted from Patten RD, DeNofrio D, El-Zaru M, et al. Ventricular assist device therapy normalizes inducible nitric oxide synthase expression and reduces cardiomyocyte apoptosis in the failing human heart. *J Am Coll Cardiol.* 45:1419–1424, with permission.)

Evidence from in vivo studies also supports a detrimental effect of iNOS in the failing heart. Cardiac-specific overexpression of iNOS in transgenic mice leads to cardiac fibrosis, dilatation, and premature death (182), although another group of investigators reported no demonstrable phenotype accompanying iNOS overexpression in the mouse heart (183). Sam et al. demonstrated that 6 months after an MI the extent of LV dysfunction and myocardial apoptosis was diminished in iNOS knockout mice, supporting a detrimental role of iNOS in this chronic heart failure model (184). These data suggest that iNOS may play an important role in ventricular remodeling and cardiomyocyte apoptosis in the chronic phase of remodeling. In support of this possibility, we demonstrated that the normalization of iNOS expression in end-stage failing hearts occurs following ventricular assist device (VAD) support (Fig. 8-13). Moreover, we demonstrated that iNOS abundance correlated directly with the percent of TUNEL-positive cardiomyocytes, supporting a potential causal association between iNOS and cardiomyocyte apoptosis (173).

SUMMARY

Cardiac remodeling represents the culmination of complex interactions between neurohormonal and stress-activated cytokine signaling pathways (Fig. 8-14). These neurohormonal and cytokine signaling pathways feed back positively on one another and act in concert to initiate and propagate the cellular changes taking place within the remodeling ventricle. These include the influx of mononuclear inflammatory cells and the proliferation of fibroblasts, some of which may differentiate into contractile myofibroblasts. These pathways also stimulate myocyte hypertrophy and increase the rate at which myocytes undergo apoptotic cell death. This constellation of cellular changes ultimately leads to gross morphological features of LV dilatation, progressive LV dysfunction, and worsening heart failure. In this manner, these complex series of signaling events that lead to cardiac remodeling may very well represent the central pathophysiological mechanisms underlying heart failure progression in humans.

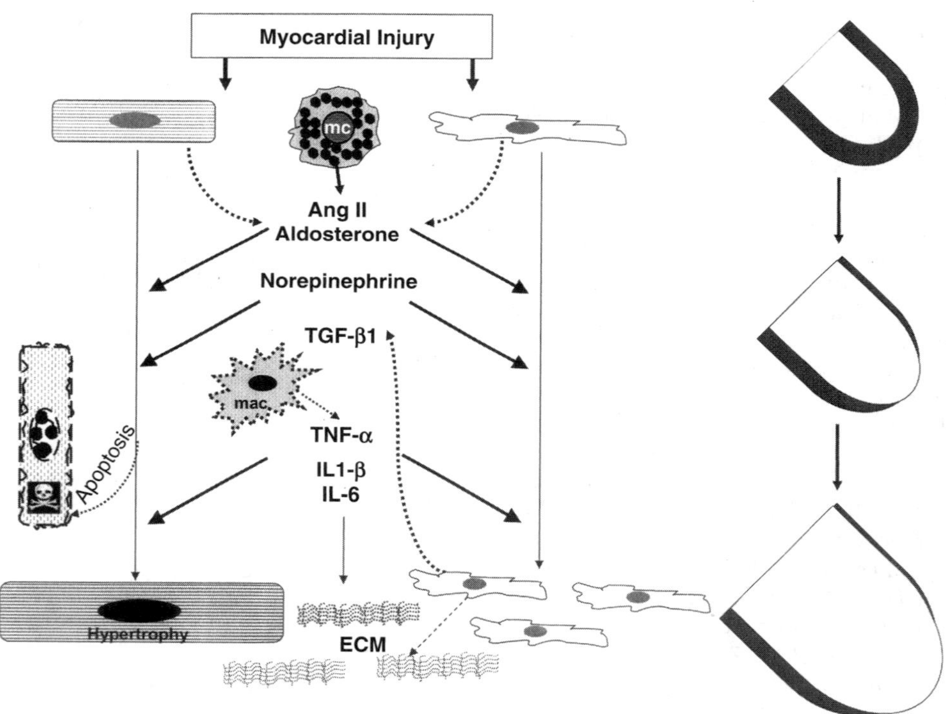

Figure 8-14 Molecular and cellular events contributing to cardiac remodeling. This figure summarizes the main points presented in this chapter. LV remodeling (depicted on the **right** by silhouettes showing progressive LV enlargement) results from pathological cellular and biochemical events that include cardiomyocyte hypertrophy and apoptosis (depicted by **skull and crossbones**), fibroblast proliferation, differentiation into myofibroblasts, and the abnormal accumulation of extracellular matrix material (ECM). Changes in these cells are driven, in part, by activation of the renin-angiotensin-aldosterone (Ang II and aldosterone) and sympathetic nervous systems (norepinephrine). The detrimental effects of these neurohormonal pathways are exacerbated further by cytokines, which further potentiate the effects of neurohormonal activation, creating a positive feedback loop and vicious cycle. Mast cells (mc) infiltrate the myocardium and contribute to the formation of Ang II via chymase release and to the activation of matrix metalloproteinases through the release of other proteases. Macrophages (mac) are also increased in the remodeling heart and are an important reservoir for cytokines (IL-1β) and inducible nitric oxide synthase within the myocardium. TGF-β1, transforming growth factor beta; TNF-α, tumor necrosis factor-alpha; IL-1β, interleukin-1-beta; IL-6, interleukin-6.

REFERENCES

1. Chareonthaitawee P, Christian TF, Hirose K, et al. Relation of initial infarct size to extent of left ventricular remodeling in the year after acute myocardial infarction. *J Am Coll Cardiol.* 25:567–573.
2. van Gilst WH, Kingma JH, Peels KH, et al., on behalf of the CATS investigators. Which patients benefit from early angiotensin-converting enzyme inhibition after myocardial infarction? Results of one-year serial echocardiographic follow-up from the Captopril and Thrombolysis Study (CATS). *J Am Coll Card.* 28:114–121.
3. Schulman SP, Weiss JL, Becker LC, et al. Effect of early enalapril therapy on left ventricular function and structure in acute myocardial infarction. *Am J Cardiol.* 76:764–770.
4. Erlebacher JA, Weiss JL, Eaton LW, et al. Late effects of acute infarct dilation on heart size: a two dimensional echocardiographic study. *Am J Cardiol.* 49:1120–1126.
5. McKay RG, Pfeffer MA, Pasternak RC, et al. Left ventricular remodeling after myocardial infarction: a corollary to infarct expansion. *Circulation.* 74:693–702.
6. Rumberger JA, Behrenbeck T, Breen JR, et al. Nonparallel changes in global left ventricular chamber volume and muscle mass during the first year after transmural myocardial infarction in humans. *J Am Coll Cardiol.* 21:673–682.
7. Jeremy RW, Allman KC, Bautovitch G, et al. Patterns of left ventricular dilation during the six months after myocardial infarction. *J Am Coll Cardiol.* 13:304–310.
8. Mitchell GF, Lamas GA, Vaughan DE, et al. Left ventricular remodeling in the year after first anterior myocardial infarction: a quantitative analysis of contractile segment lengths and ventricular shape. *J Am Coll Cardiol.* 19:1136–1144.
9. Patten RD, Udelson JE, Konstam MA. Ventricular remodeling and its prevention in the treatment of heart failure. *Curr Opinion Cardiol.* 13:162–167.
10. Pfeffer MA, Pfeffer JM. Ventricular enlargement and reduced survival after myocardial infarction. *Circulation.* 75:IV93–IV97.
11. Pfeffer MA, Braunwald E. Ventricular remodeling after myocardial infarction, experimental observations and clinical implications. *Circulation.* 81:1161–1172.
12. White HD, Norris RM, Brown MA, et al. Left ventricular end-systolic volume as the major determinant of survival after recovery from myocardial infarction. *Circulation.* 76:44–51.
13. Migrino RQ, Young JB, Ellis SG, et al., for the Global Utilization of Streptokinase and t-PA for Occluded Coronary Arteries (GUSTO)-I Angiographic Investigators. End-systolic volume index at 90 to 180 minutes into reperfusion therapy for acute myocardial infarction is a strong predictor of early and late mortality. *Circulation.* 96:116–121.
14. Bolognese L, Neskovic AN, Parodi G, et al. Left ventricular remodeling after primary coronary angioplasty: patterns of left ventricular dilation and long-term prognostic implications. *Circulation.* 106:2351–2357.
15. Gaudron P, Kugler I, Hu K, et al. Time course of cardiac structural, functional and electrical changes in asymptomatic patients after myocardial infarction: their inter-relation and prognostic impact. *J Am Coll Card.* 38:33–40.
16. St. John Sutton M, Lee D, Rouleau JL, et al. Left ventricular remodeling and ventricular arrhythmias after myocardial infarction. *Circulation.* 107:2577–2582.
17. Konstam MA, Rousseau MF, Kronenberg MW, et al., for the SOLVD Investigators. Effects of the angiotensin converting enzyme inhibitor, enalapril, on the long-term progression of left ventricular dysfunction in patients with heart failure. *Circulation.* 86:431–438.
18. Konstam MA, Kronenberg MW, Rousseau MF, et al., for the SOLVD Investigators. Effects of the angiotensin converting enzyme inhibitor, enalapril, on the long-term progression of left ventricular dilatation in patients with asymptomatic systolic dysfunction. *Circulation.* 88:2277–2283.
19. Greenberg B, Quinones MA, Koilpillai C, et al. Effects of long-term enalapril therapy on cardiac structure and function in patients with left ventricular dysfunction: results of the SOLVD echocardiography substudy. *Circulation.* 91:2573–2581.
20. Doughty M, Robert N, Whalley B, et al. Left ventricular remodeling with carvedilol in patients with congestive heart failure due to ischemic heart disease. *J Am Coll Cardiol.* 29:1060–1066.
21. Rousseau MF, Konstam MA, Benedict CR, et al. Progression of left ventricular dysfunction secondary to coronary artery disease, sustained neurohormonal activation and effects of ibopamine therapy during long-term therapy with angiotensin-converting enzyme inhibitor. *Am J Cardiol.* 73:488–493.
22. Anversa P, Loud AV, Levicky V, et al. Left ventricular failure induced by myocardial infarction. I. Myocyte hypertrophy. *Am J Physiol.* 248:H876–H882.
23. Anversa P, Olivetti G, Meggs LG, et al. Cardiac anatomy and ventricular loading after myocardial infarction. *Circulation* 87:VII22–VII27.
24. Gerdes AM, Kellerman SE, Moore JA, et al. Structural remodeling of cardiac myocytes in patients with ischemic cardiomyopathy. *Circulation.* 86:426–430.
25. Tamura T, Onodera T, Said S, et al. Correlation of myocyte lengthening to chamber dilation in the spontaneously hypertensive heart failure (SHHF) rat. *J Mol Cell Cardiol.* 30:2175–2181.
26. Anand IS, Liu D, Chugh SS, et al. Isolated myocyte contractile function is normal in postinfarct remodeled rat heart with systolic dysfunction. *Circulation.* 96:3974–3984.
27. Olivetti G, Capasso JM, Sonnenblick EH, et al. Side-to-side slippage of myocytes participates in ventricular wall remodeling acutely after myocardial infarction in rats. *Circ Res.* 67:23–34.
28. Lai T, Fallon JT, Liu J, et al. Reversibility and pathohistological basis of left ventricular remodeling in hibernating myocardium. *Cardiovasc Pathol.* 9:323–335.
29. Chien KR, Knowlton KU, Zhu H, et al. Regulation of cardiac gene expression during myocardial growth and hypertrophy: molecular studies of an adaptive physiologic response. *FASEB J.* 5:3037–3046.
30. Meggs LG, Tillotson J, Huang H, et al. Noncoordinate regulation of alpha-1 adrenoreceptor coupling and reexpression of alpha skeletal actin in myocardial infarction-induced left ventricular failure in rats. *J Clin Invest.* 86:1451–1458.
31. Michel JB, Lattio AL, Salzmann JL, et al. Hormonal and cardiac effects of converting enzyme inhibition in rat myocardial infarction. *Circ Res.* 62:641–650.
32. Wollert KC, Struder R, von Bülow B, et al. Survival after myocardial infarction in the rat: role of tissue angiotensin-converting enzyme inhibition. *Circulation.* 90:2457–2467.
33. Beltrami CA, Finato N. Rocco M, et al. Structural basis of end stage heart failure in ischemic cardiomyopathy in humans. *Circulation.* 89:151–163.
34. Feldman AM, Ray PE, Silan CM, et al. Selective gene expression in failing human heart: quantification of steady-state levels of messenger RNA in endomyocardial biopsies using the-polymerase chain reaction. *Circulation.* 83:1866–1872.
35. Kostin S, Pool L, Elsasser A, et al. Myocytes die by multiple mechanisms in failing human hearts. *Circ Res.* 92:715–724.
36. Kang PM, Izumo S. Apoptosis and heart failure: a critical review of the literature. *Circ Res.* 86:1107–1113.
37. Orike N, Middleton G, Borthwick E, et al. Role of PI 3-kinase, Akt and Bcl-2-related proteins in sustaining the survival of neurotrophic factor-independent adult sympathetic neurons. *J Cell Biol.* 154:995–1006.
38. Hare JM. Oxidative stress and apoptosis in heart failure progression. *Circ Res.* 89:198–200.
39. Green DR, Reed JC. Mitochondria and apoptosis. *Science.* 281:1309–1312.
40. Ashkenazi A, Dixit VM. Death receptors: signaling and modulation. *Science.* 281:1305–1308.
41. Thornberry NA, Lazebnik Y. Caspases: enemies within. *Science.* 281:1312–1316.
42. Reed JC, Paternostro G. Postmitochondrial regulation of apoptosis during heart failure. *Proc Natl Acad Sci USA.* 96:7614–7616.
43. Foo RS-Y, Mani K, Kitsis RN. Death begets failure in the heart. *J Clin Invest.* 115:565–571.
44. Crow MT, Mani K, Nam Y-J, et al. The mitochondrial death pathway and cardiac myocyte apoptosis. *Circ Res.* 95:957–970.
45. Adams JM, Cory S. The Bcl-2 protein family: arbiters of cell survival. *Science.* 281:1322–1326.
46. Mani K, Kitsis RN. Myocyte apoptosis: programming ventricular remodeling. *J Am Coll Cardiol.* 41:761–764.
47. Nadal-Ginard B, Kajstura J, Leri A, et al. Myocyte death, growth, and regeneration in cardiac hypertrophy and failure. *Circ Res.*92:139–150.

48. Anversa P, Nadal-Ginard B. Myocyte renewal and ventricular remodelling. *Nature.* 415:240–243.
49. Camper-Kirby D, Welch S, Walker A, et al. Myocardial Akt activation and gender: increased nuclear activity in females versus males. *Circ Res.* 88:1020–1027.
50. Olivetti G, Giordano G, Corradi D, et al. Gender differences and aging: effects on the human heart. *J Am Coll Cardiol.* 26:1068–1079.
51. Olivetti G, Abbi R, Quaini F, et al. Apoptosis in the failing human heart. *N Engl J Med.* 336:1131–1141.
52. Saraste A, Pulkki K, Kallajoki M, et al. Apoptosis in human acute myocardial infarction. *Circulation.* 95:320–323.
53. Olivetti G, Quaini F, Sala R, et al. Acute myocardial infarction in humans is associated with activation of programmed myocyte cell death in the surviving portion of the heart. *J Mol Cell Cardiol.* 28:2005–2016.
54. Abbate A, Biondi-Zoccai GGL, Bussani R, et al. Increased myocardial apoptosis in patients with unfavorable left ventricular remodeling and early symptomatic post-infarction heart failure. *J Am Coll Cardiol.* 41:753–760.
55. Saraste A, Pulkki K, Kallajoki M, et al. Cardiomyocyte apoptosis and progression of heart failure to transplantation. *Eur J Clin Invest.* 29:380–386.
56. Narula J, Pandey P, Arbustini E, et al. Apoptosis in heart failure: release of cytochrome C from mitochondria and activation of caspase-3 in human cardiomyopathy. *Proc Natl Acad Sci USA.* 96:8144–8149.
57. Condorelli G, Morisco C, Stassi G, et al. Increased cardiomyocyte apoptosis and changes in proapoptotic and antiapoptotic genes bax and bcl-2 during left ventricular adaptations to chronic pressure overload in the rat. *Circulation.* 99:3071–3078.
58. Sam F, Sawyer DB, Chang DL, et al. Progressive left ventricular remodeling and apoptosis late after myocardial infarction in mouse heart. *Am J Physiol.* (*Heart Circ Physiol.*) 279:H422–H428.
59. Kubota T, McTiernan CF, Frye CS, et al. Dilated cardiomyopathy in transgenic mice with cardiac-specific overexpression of tumor necrosis factor-α. *Circ Res.* 81:627–635.
60. Kadokami T, McTiernan CF, Kubota T, et al. Sex-related survival differences in murine cardiomyopathy are associated with differences in TNF-receptor expression. *J Clin Invest.* 106:589–597.
61. Engel D, Peshock R, Armstong RC, et al. Cardiac myocyte apoptosis provokes adverse cardiac remodeling in transgenic mice with targeted TNF overexpression. *Am J Physiol.* (*Heart Circ Physiol.*) 287:H1303–H1311.
62. Wencker D, Chandra M, Nguyen K, et al. A mechanistic role for cardiac myocyte apoptosis in heart failure. *J Clin Invest.* 111: 1497–1504.
63. Hayakawa Y, Chandra M, Miao W, et al. Inhibition of cardiac myocyte apoptosis improves cardiac function and abolishes mortality in the peripartum cardiomyopathy of Gαq transgenic mice. *Circulation.* 108:3036–3041.
64. Chandrashekhar Y, Sen S, Anway R, et al. Long-term caspase inhibition ameliorates apoptosis, reduces myocardial troponin-I cleavage, protects left ventricular function, and attenuates remodeling in rats with myocardial infarction. *J Am Coll Cardiol.* 43:295–301.
65. Brown RD, Ambler SK, Mitchell MD, et al. The cardiac fibroblast: therapeutic target in myocardial remodeling and failure. *Annual Rev Pharmacol Toxicol.* 45:657–687.
66. Booz GW, Baker KM. Molecular signalling mechanisms controlling growth and function of cardiac fibroblasts. *Cardiovasc Res.* 30:537–543.
67. Weber KT. Cardiac interstitium in health and disease: the fibrillar collagen network. *J Am Coll Cardiol.* 13:1637–1652.
68. Eghbali M, Blumenfeld OO, Seifter S, et al. Localization of types I, III, and IV collagen mRNA's in the rat heart cells by in situ hybridization. *J Mol Cell Cardiol.* 21:103–113.
69. Volders PGA, Willems IEMG, Cleutjens JPM, et al. Interstitial collagen is increased in the noninfarcted human myocardium after myocardial infarction. *J Mol Cell Cardiol.* 25:1317–1323.
70. Bishop JE, Greenbaum R, Gibson DG, et al. Enhanced deposition of predominantly type I collagen in myocardial disease. *J Mol Cell Cardiol.* 22:1157–1165.
71. van Krimpen C, Smits JFM, Cleutjens JPM, et al. DNA synthesis in the noninfarcted cardiac interstitium after left coronary artery ligation in the rat: effects of captopril. *J Mol Cell Cardiol.* 23:1245–1253.
72. Taylor K, Patten RD, Smith JJ, et al. Divergent effects of angiotensin converting enzyme inhibition and angiotensin II receptor antagonism on myocardial cellular proliferation and collagen deposition after myocardial infarction in rats. *J Cardiovasc Pharmacol.* 31:654–660.
73. Sun Y, Weber KT. Angiotensin II receptor binding following myocardial infarction in the rat. *Cardiovasc Res.* 28:1623–1628.
74. Powell DW, Mifflin RC, Valentich JD, et al. Myofibroblasts. I. Paracrine cells important in health and disease. *Am J Physiol Cell Physiol.* 277:C1–C19.
75. Sun Y, Weber KT. Angiotensin converting enzyme and myofibroblasts during tissue repair in the rat heart. *J Mol Cell Cardiol.* 28:851–858.
76. Sun Y, Cleutjens JP, Diaz-Arias AA, et al. Cardiac angiotensin converting enzyme and myocardial fibrosis in the rat. *Cardiovasc Res.* 28:1423–1432.
77. Azzawi M, Kan SW, Hillier V, et al. The distribution of cardiac macrophages in myocardial ischaemia and cardiomyopathy. *Histopathology.* 46:314–319.
78. Hein S, Arnon E, Kostin S, et al. Progression from compensated hypertrophy to failure in the pressure-overloaded human heart: structural deterioration and compensatory mechanisms. *Circulation.* 107:984–991.
79. Shioi T, Matsumori A, Kihara Y, et al. Increased expression of interleukin-1ß and monocyte chemotactic and activating factor/monocyte chemoattractant protein-1 in the hypertrophied and failing heart with pressure overload. *Circ Res.* 81:664–671.
80. Ono K, Matsumori A, Shioi T, et al. Cytokine gene expression after myocardial infarction in rat hearts possible implication in left ventricular remodeling. *Circulation.* 98:149–156.
81. Hayashidani S, Tsutsui H, Shiomi T, et al. Anti-monocyte chemoattractant protein-1 gene therapy attenuates left ventricular remodeling and failure after experimental myocardial infarction. *Circulation.* 108:2134–2140.
82. Patella V, Crescenzo GD, Lamparter-Schummert B, et al. Increased cardiac mast cell density and mediator release in patients with dilated cardiomyopathy. *Inflammation Res.* 46:31–32.
83. Petrovic D, Zorc M, Zorc-Pleskovic R, et al. Morphometrical and stereological analysis of myocardial mast cells in myocarditis and dilated cardiomyopathy. *Folia Biol (Praha).* 45:63–66.
84. Engels W, Reiters PH, Daemen MJ, et al. Transmural changes in mast cell density in rat heart after infarct induction in vivo. *J Pathol.* 177:423–429.
85. Hara M, Ono K, Hwang M-W, et al. Evidence for a role of mast cells in the evolution to congestive heart failure. *J Exp Med.* 195:375–381.
86. Matsumoto T, Wada A, Tsutamoto T, et al. Inhibition prevents cardiac fibrosis and improves diastolic dysfunction in the progression of heart failure. *Circulation.* 107:2555–2558.
87. Su X, Wei C-C, Machida N, et al. Differential expression of angiotensin-converting enzyme and chymase in dogs with chronic mitral regurgitation. *J Mol Cell Cardiol.* 31:1033–1045.
88. Stewart J, James A, Wei C-C, et al. Cardiac mast cell- and chymase-mediated matrix metalloproteinase activity and left ventricular remodeling in mitral regurgitation in the dog. *J Mol Cell Cardiol.* 35:311–319.
89. Brower GL, Chancey AL, Thanigaraj S, et al. Cause and effect relationship between myocardial mast cell number and matrix metalloproteinase activity. *Am J Physiol.* (*Heart Circ Physiol.*) 283: H518–H525.
90. Dell'Italia LJ, Husain A. Dissecting the role of chymase in angiotensin II formation and heart and blood vessel diseases. *Curr Opin Cardiol.* 17:374–379.
91. Spinale FG, Coker ML, Bond BR, et al. Myocardial matrix degradation and metalloproteinase activation in the failing heart: a potential therapeutic target. *Cardiovasc Res.* 46:225–238.
92. Kerins DM, Hao Q, Vaughan DE. Angiotensin induction of PAI-1 expression in endothelial cells is mediated by the hexapeptide angiotensin IV. *J Clin Invest.* 96:2515–2520.
93. Opie LH, Sack MN. Enhanced angiotensin II activity in heart failure: reevaluation of the counterregulatory hypothesis of receptor subtypes. *Circ Res.* 88:654–658.
94. Hirsch AT, Talsness CE, Schunkert H, et al. Tissue-specific activation of cardiac angiotensin converting enzyme in experimental heart failure. *Circ Res.* 69:475–482.

95. Ruzicka M, Skarda V, Leenen FHH. Effects of ACE inhibitors on circulating versus cardiac angiotensin II in volume overload-induced cardiac hypertrophy in rats. *Circulation.* 92:3568–3573.
96. Urata H, Healy B, Stewart RW, et al. Angiotensin II-forming pathways in normal and failing human hearts. *Circ Res.* 66:883–890.
97. Urata H, Boehm KD, Philip A, et al. Cellular localization and regional distribution of an angiotensin II-forming chymase in the human heart. *J Clin Invest.* 91:1269–1281.
98. Sadoshima J, Xu Y, Slayter HS, et al. Autocrine release of angiotensin II mediates stretch-induced hypertrophy of cardiac myocytes. *Cell.* 75:977–984.
99. Sadoshima J, Izumo S. Molecular characterization of angiotensin II-induced hypertrophy of cardiac myocytes and hyperplasia of cardiac fibroblasts: critical role of the AT_1 receptor subtype. *Circ Res.* 73:413–423.
100. Schunkert H, Sadoshima J-I, Cornelius T, et al. Angiotensin II-induced growth responses in isolated adult rat hearts: evidence for load-independent induction of cardiac protein synthesis by angiotensin II. *Circ Res.* 76:489–497.
101. Patten RD, Aronovitz MJ, Einstein M, et al. Effects of angiotensin II receptor blockade versus angiotensin-converting-enzyme inhibition on ventricular remodelling following myocardial infarction in the mouse. *Clin Sci (London).* 104:109–118.
102. Liu Y-H, Yang Y-P, Sharov VG, et al. Effects of angiotensin-converting enzyme inhibitors and angiotensin II type 1 receptor antagonists in rats with heart failure: role of kinins and angiotensin II type 2 receptors. *J Clin Invest.* 99:1926–1935.
103. Smits JFM, van Krimpen C, Schoemaker RG, et al. Angiotensin II receptor blockade after myocardial infarction in rats: effects on hemodynamics, myocardial DNA synthesis, and interstitial collagen content. *J Cardiovasc Pharm.* 20:772–778.
104. Schieffer B, Wirger A, Meybrunn M, et al. Comparative effects of chronic angiotensin-converting enzyme inhibition and angiotensin II type 1 receptor blockade on cardiac remodeling after myocardial infarction in the rat. *Circulation.* 89:2273–2282.
105. Wollert KC, Studer R, Doerfer K, et al. Differential effects of kinins on cardiomyocyte hypertrophy and interstitial collagen matrix in the surviving myocardium after myocardial infarction in the rat. *Circulation.* 95:1910–1917.
106. Ichihara S, Senbonmatsu T, Price E, Jr., et al. Targeted deletion of angiotensin II type 2 receptor caused cardiac rupture after acute myocardial infarction. *Circulation.* 106:2244–2249.
107. Adachi Y, Saito Y, Kishimoto I, et al. Angiotensin II type 2 receptor deficiency exacerbates heart failure and reduces survival after acute myocardial infarction in mice. *Circulation.* 107:2406–2408.
108. Oishi Y, Ozono R, Yano Y, et al. Cardioprotective role of AT_2 receptor in postinfarction left ventricular remodeling. *Hypertension.* 41:814–818.
109. Senbonmatsu T, Ichihara S, Price E, Jr., et al. Evidence for angiotensin II type 2 receptor-mediated cardiac myocyte enlargement during in vivo pressure overload. *J Clin Invest.* 106:R25–R29.
110. Inagami T, Senbonmatsu T. Dual effects of angiotensin II type 2 receptor on cardiovascular hypertrophy. *Trends Cardiovasc Med.* 11:324–328.
111. Mulrow PJ. Angiotensin II and aldosterone regulation. *Regul Pept.* 80:27–32.
112. Lombes M, Oblin ME, Gasc JM, et al. Immunohistochemical and biochemical evidence for a cardiovascular mineralocorticoid receptor. *Circ Res.* 71:503–510.
113. Mizuno Y, Yoshimura M, Yasue H, et al. Aldosterone production is activated in failing ventricle in humans. *Circulation.* 103:72–77.
114. Yamamoto N, Yasue H, Mizuno Y, et al. Aldosterone is produced from ventricles in patients with essential hypertension. *Hypertension.* 39:958–962.
115. Brilla CG, Zhou G, Matsubara L, et al. Collagen metabolism in cultured adult rat cardiac fibroblasts: response to angiotensin II and aldosterone. *J Mol Cell Cardiol.* 26:809–820.
116. Brilla CG, Pick R, Tan LB, et al. Remodeling of the rat right and left ventricles in experimental hypertension. *Circ Res.* 67: 1355–1364.
117. Silvestre JS, Heymes C, Oubenaissa A, et al. Activation of cardiac aldosterone production in rat myocardial infarction: effect of angiotensin II receptor blockade and role in cardiac fibrosis. *Circulation.* 99:2694–2701.
118. Suzuki G, Morita H, Mishima T, et al. Effects of long-term monotherapy with eplerenone, a novel aldosterone blocker, on progression of left ventricular dysfunction and remodeling in dogs with heart failure. *Circulation.* 106:2967–2972.
119. Francis GS, Benedict C, Johnstone DE, et al. Comparison of neuroendocrine activation in patients with left ventricular dysfunction with and without congestive heart failure. A substudy of the Studies of Left Ventricular Dysfunction (SOLVD). *Circulation.* 82:1724–1729.
120. Yamazaki T, Komuro I, Zou Y, et al. Norepinephrine induces the RAF-1 kinase/mitogen-activated protein kinase cascade through both α1- and ß-adrenoceptors. *Circulation.* 95:1260–1268.
121. Tomita H, Nazmy M, Kajimoto K, et al. Inducible cAMP early repressor (ICER) is a negative-feedback regulator of cardiac hypertrophy and an important mediator of cardiac myocyte apoptosis in response to β-adrenergic receptor stimulation. *Circ Res.* 93:12–22.
122. Dorn GW, Jr. Adrenergic pathways and left ventricular remodeling. *J Card Fail.* 8S370–S373.
123. Grimm D, Elsner D, Schunkert H, et al. Development of heart failure following isoproterenol administration in the rat: role of the renin-angiotensin system. *Cardiovasc Res.* 37:91–100.
124. Zhou Z, Liao Y-H, Wei Y, et al. Cardiac remodeling after long-term stimulation by antibodies against the [alpha]1-adrenergic receptor in rats. *Clin Immunol.* 114:164–173.
125. McDonald KM, Rector T, Carlyle PF, et al. Angiotensin-converting enzyme inhibition and beta-adrenoceptor blockade regress established ventricular remodeling in a canine model of discrete myocardial damage. *J Am Coll Cardiol.* 24:1762–1768.
126. Morita H, Suzuki G, Mishima T, et al. Effects of long-term monotherapy with metoprolol CR/XL on the progression of left ventricular dysfunction and remodeling in dogs with chronic heart failure. *Cardiovasc Drugs Ther.* 16:443–449.
127. Sabbah HN, Sharov VG, Gupta RC, et al. Chronic therapy with metoprolol attenuates cardiomyocyte apoptosis in dogs with heart failure. *J Am Coll Cardiol.* 36:1698–1705.
128. Xiang Y, Kobilka BK. Myocyte adrenoceptor signaling pathways. *Science.* 300:1530–1532.
129. Gao X-M, Agrotis A, Autelitano DJ, et al. Sex hormones and cardiomyopathic phenotype induced by cardiac β2-adrenergic receptor overexpression. *Endocrinology.* 144:4097–4105.
130. Zhu W-Z, Wang S-Q, Chakir K, et al. Linkage of β1-adrenergic stimulation to apoptotic heart cell death through protein kinase A-independent activation of Ca^{2+}/calmodulin kinase II. *J Clin Invest.* 111:617–625.
131. Hein L, Altman JD, Kobilka BK. Two functionally distinct α2-adrenergic receptors regulate sympathetic neurotransmission. *Nature.* 402:181–184.
132. Luscher TF, Barton M. Endothelins and endothelin receptor antagonists: therapeutic considerations for a novel class of cardiovascular drugs. *Circulation.* 102:2434–2440.
133. Choukroun G, Hajjar R, Kyriakis JM, et al. Role of the stress-activated protein kinases in endothelin-induced cardiomyocyte hypertrophy. *J Clin Invest.* 102:1311–1320.
134. Gray MO, Long CS, Kalinyak JE, et al. Angiotensin II stimulates cardiac myocyte hypertrophy via paracrine release of TGF-β1 and endothelin-1 from fibroblasts. *Cardiovasc Res.* 40:352–363.
135. Sakai S, Miyauchi T, Kobayashi M, et al. Inhibition of myocardial endothelin pathway improves long-term survival in heart failure. *Nature.* 384:353–355.
136. Oie E, Yndestad A, Robins SP, et al. Early intervention with a potent endothelin-A/endothelin-B receptor antagonist aggravates left ventricular remodeling after myocardial infarction in rats. *Basic Res Cardiol.* 97:239–247.
137. Anand PI, McMurray PJ, Cohn PJN, et al. Long-term effects of darusentan on left-ventricular remodelling and clinical outcomes in the EndothelinA Receptor Antagonist Trial in Heart Failure (EARTH): randomised, double-blind, placebo-controlled trial. *Lancet.* 364:347–354.
138. Rich S, McLaughlin VV. Endothelin receptor blockers in cardiovascular disease. *Circulation* 108:2184–2190.
139. Rosenkranz S. TGF-β1 and angiotensin networking in cardiac remodeling. *Cardiovasc Res.* 63:423–432.
140. Siwik DA, Colucci WS. Regulation of matrix metalloproteinases by cytokines and reactive oxygen/nitrogen species in the myocardium. *Heart Fail Rev.* 9:43–51.

141. Seeland U, Haeuseler C, Hinrichs R, et al. Myocardial fibrosis in transforming growth factor-1 (TGF-1) transgenic mice is associated with inhibition of interstitial collagenase. *Eur J Clin Invest.* 32:295–303.
142. Kuwahara F, Kai H, Tokuda K, et al. Transforming growth factor-β function blocking prevents myocardial fibrosis and diastolic dysfunction in pressure-overloaded rats. *Circulation.* 106:130–135.
143. Schultz JEJ, Witt SA, Glascock BJ, et al. TGF-β1 mediates the hypertrophic cardiomyocyte growth induced by angiotensin II. *J Clin Invest.* 109:787–796.
144. Condorelli G, Morisco C, Latronico MVG, et al. TNF-α signal transduction in rat neonatal cardiac myocytes: definition of pathways generating from the TNF–α receptor. *FASEB J.* 16:1732–1737.
145. Baud V, Karin M. Signal transduction by tumor necrosis factor and its relatives. *Trends Cell Biol.* 11:372–377.
146. Mann DL. Stress-activated cytokines and the heart: from adaptation to maladaptation. *Annual Rev Physiol.* 65:81–101.
147. Nakano M, Knowlton AA, Dibbs Z, et al. Tumor necrosis factor-α confers resistance to hypoxic injury in the adult mammalian cardiac myocyte. *Circulation.* 97:1392–1400.
148. Bozkurt B, Kribbs SB, Clubb FJ, Jr., et al. Pathophysiologically relevant concentrations of tumor necrosis factor-α promote progressive left ventricular dysfunction and remodeling in rats. *Circulation.* 97:1382–1391.
149. Tsutamoto MD T, Hisanaga MD T, Wada MD A, et al. Interleukin-6 spillover in the peripheral circulation increases with the severity of heart failure, and the high plasma level of interleukin-6 is an important prognostic predictor in patients with congestive heart failure. *J Am Coll Cardiol.* 31:391–398.
150. Kanda T, Takahashi T. Interleukin-6 and cardiovascular diseases. *Jpn Heart J.* 45:183–193.
151. Hirota H, Yoshida K, Kishimoto T, et al. Continuous activation of gp130, a signal-transducing receptor component for interleukin 6-related cytokines, causes myocardial hypertrophy in mice. *PNAS.* 92:4862–4866.
152. Nicol RL, Frey N, Pearson G, et al. Activated MEK5 induces serial assembly of sarcomeres and eccentric cardiac hypertrophy. *EMBO J.* 20:2757–2767.
153. Kato T, Sano M, Miyoshi S, et al. Calmodulin kinases II and IV and calcineurin are involved in leukemia inhibitory factor-induced cardiac hypertrophy in rats. *Circ Res.* 87:937–945.
154. Wollert KC, Taga T, Saito M, et al. Cardiotrophin-1 activates a distinct form of cardiac muscle cell hypertrophy. *J Biol Chem.* 271:9535–9545.
155. Long CS. The role of interleukin-1 in the failing heart. *Heart Fail Rev.* 6:81–94.
156. Patten M, Hartogensis WE, Long CS. Interleukin-1β is a negative transcriptional regulator of α1-adrenergic induced gene expression in cultured cardiac myocytes. *J Biol Chem.* 271:21134–21141.
157. Palmer JN, Hartogensis WE, Patten M, et al. Interleukin-1β induces cardiac myocyte growth but inhibits cardiac fibroblast proliferation in culture. *J Clin Invest.* 95:2555–2564.
158. Sekiguchi K, Li X, Coker M, et al. Cross-regulation between the renin-angiotensin system and inflammatory mediators in cardiac hypertrophy and failure. *Cardiovasc Res.* 63:433–442.
159. Gurantz D, Cowling RT, Villarreal FJ, et al. Tumor necrosis factor-α upregulates angiotensin II type 1 receptors on cardiac fibroblasts. *Circ Res.* 85:272–279.
160. Gurantz D, Cowling RT, Varki N, et al. IL-1β and TNF-α upregulate angiotensin II type 1 (AT_1) receptors on cardiac fibroblasts and are associated with increased AT_1 density in the post-MI heart. *J Mol Cell Cardiol.* 38:505–515.
161. Cowling RT, Gurantz D, Peng J, et al. Transcription factor NF-κB is necessary for up-regulation of type 1 angiotensin II receptor mRNA in rat cardiac fibroblasts treated with tumor necrosis factor-alpha or interleukin-1beta. *J Biol Chem.* 277:5719–5724.
162. Flesch M, Hoper A, Dell'Italia L, et al. Activation and functional significance of the renin-angiotensin system in mice with cardiac restricted overexpression of tumor necrosis factor. *Circulation* 108:598–604.
163. Zhang Z-H, Wei S-G, Francis J, et al. Cardiovascular and renal sympathetic activation by blood-borne TNF-alpha in rat: the role of central prostaglandins. *Am J Physiol. (Regul Integr Comp Physiol.)* 284: R916–R927.
164. Jaffre F, Callebert J, Sarre A, et al. Involvement of the serotonin 5-HT2B receptor in cardiac hypertrophy linked to sympathetic stimulation: control of interleukin-6, interleukin-1β, and tumor necrosis factor-α cytokine production by ventricular fibroblasts. *Circulation.* 110:969–974.
165. Murray DR, Prabhu SD, Chandrasekar B. Chronic β-adrenergic stimulation induces myocardial proinflammatory cytokine expression. *Circulation.* 101:2338–2341.
166. Balligand JL, Cannon PJ. Nitric oxide synthases and cardiac muscle. Autocrine and paracrine influences. *Arterioscler Thromb Vasc Biol.* 17:1846–1858.
167. Sawyer DB, Colucci WS. Nitric oxide in the failing myocardium. *Cardiol Clin.* 16:657–664, viii.
168. Feron O, Belhassen L, Kobzik L, et al. Endothelial nitric oxide synthase targeting to caveolae. Specific interactions with caveolin isoforms in cardiac myocytes and endothelial cells. *J Biol Chem.* 271:22810–22814.
169. Prabhu SD. Nitric oxide protects against pathological ventricular remodeling: reconsideration of the role of NO in the failing heart. *Circ Res.* 94:1155–1157.
170. Janssens S, Pokreisz P, Schoonjans L, et al. Cardiomyocyte-specific overexpression of nitric oxide synthase 3 improves left ventricular performance and reduces compensatory hypertrophy after myocardial infarction. *Circ Res.* 94:1256–1262.
171. Fukuchi M, Hussain SN, Giaid A. Heterogeneous expression and activity of endothelial and inducible nitric oxide synthases in end-stage human heart failure: their relation to lesion site and beta-adrenergic receptor therapy. *Circulation.* 98:132–139.
172. Haywood GA, Tsao PS, von der Leyen HE, et al. Expression of inducible nitric oxide synthase in human heart failure. *Circulation.* 93:1087–1094.
173. Patten RD, DeNofrio D, El-Zaru M, et al. Ventricular assist device therapy normalizes inducible nitric oxide synthase expression and reduces cardiomyocyte apoptosis in the failing human heart. *J Am Coll Cardiol.* 45:1419–1424.
174. Kim YM, Bombeck CA, Billiar TR. Nitric oxide as a bifunctional regulator of apoptosis. *Circ Res.* 84:253–256.
175. Vila-Petroff MG, Younes A, Egan J, et al. Activation of distinct cAMP-dependent and cGMP-dependent pathways by nitric oxide in cardiac myocytes. *Circ Res.* 84:1020–1031.
176. Mohan P, Brutsaert DL, Paulus WJ, et al. Myocardial contractile response to nitric oxide and cGMP. *Circulation.* 93:1223–1229.
177. Kinugawa KI, Kohmoto O, Yao A, et al. Cardiac inducible nitric oxide synthase negatively modulates myocardial function in cultured rat myocytes. *Am J Physiol.* 272:H35–H47.
178. Yasuda S, Lew WY. Lipopolysaccharide depresses cardiac contractility and beta-adrenergic contractile response by decreasing myofilament response to Ca^{2+} in cardiac myocytes. *Circ Res.* 81:1011–1020.
179. Joe EK, Schussheim AE, Longrois D, et al. Regulation of cardiac myocyte contractile function by inducible nitric oxide synthase (iNOS): mechanisms of contractile depression by nitric oxide. *J Mol Cell Cardiol.* 30:303–315.
180. Pinsky DJ, Aji W, Szabolcs M, et al. Nitric oxide triggers programmed cell death (apoptosis) of adult rat ventricular myocytes in culture. *Am J Physiol.* 277: H1189–H1199.
181. Arstall MA, Sawyer DB, Fukazawa R, et al. Cytokine-mediated apoptosis in cardiac myocytes: the role of inducible nitric oxide synthase induction and peroxynitrite generation. *Circ Res.* 85:829–840.
182. Mungrue IN, Gros R, You X, et al. Cardiomyocyte overexpression of iNOS in mice results in peroxynitrite generation, heart block, and sudden death. *J Clin Invest.* 109:735–743.
183. Heger J, Godecke A, Flogel U, et al. Cardiac-specific overexpression of inducible nitric oxide synthase does not result in severe cardiac dysfunction. *Circ Res.* 90:93–99.
184. Sam F, Sawyer DB, Xie Z, et al. Mice lacking inducible nitric oxide synthase have improved left ventricular contractile function and reduced apoptotic cell death late after myocardial infarction. *Circ Res.* 89:351–356.

Remodeling of the Cardiac Interstitium in Heart Failure

9

Karl T. Weber *Yao Sun* *Syamal K. Bhattacharya* *Robert A. Ahokas*
Ivan C. Gerling

Chronic cardiac failure (CCF) is a major health problem. Of the more than 4 million Americans already diagnosed with CCF, the great majority have atherosclerotic coronary artery disease with previous myocardial infarction (MI) (1,2). CCF appears over the course of several years in patients who develop progressive post-MI left ventricular dilatation in association with depressed resting ejection fraction (3–6). In others, ventricular enlargement post-MI appears early and is nonprogressive with preserved systolic performance. However, diastolic dysfunction may be evident during physical activity.

Ventricular diastolic and/or systolic dysfunction is related to a deterioration of previously normokinetic segments (i.e., sites remote to MI). Although loss of cardiac myocytes at and remote to the site of previous infarction(s) is believed to contribute to ventricular systolic dysfunction that appears in ischemic cardiomyopathy (ICM), despite hypertrophy of viable myocytes (7,8), an additional loss of myocytes through programmed cell death, or apoptosis, has recently been called into question (9–12). Abnormalities of viable myocyte contraction and relaxation have long been considered an additional cause of diastolic and systolic dysfunction in ICM (13,14). In addition to myocyte loss and faulty myocyte mechanics, a broader paradigm has recently emerged for the development of cardiac failure, one involving structural remodeling of noninfarcted myocardium by fibrous tissue (15–17).

Cardiac myocytes are highly specialized and highly differentiated parenchymal cells that impart cardiac tissue with unique morphological and functional features. Given their size, myocytes occupy 70% of the myocardium's structural space. On the other hand, myocytes represent all but one-third of all cells found in the myocardium; the remaining two-thirds are nonmyocyte cells, such as fibroblasts. Fibroblasts are undifferentiated and have a pluripotent portfolio of responses, including marked phenotypic diversity and metabolic activity. They contribute to ICM by accounting for a progressive accumulation of fibrous tissue remote to MI, which can be independent of myocyte loss.

In the failing human heart with ICM, an infarct scar(s) is a common feature. Such replacement fibrosis rebuilds myocardium, restores structural integrity at sites of myocyte loss, and resists tissue deformation. Connective tissue also appears remote to previous infarction, where it presents as an interstitial fibrosis and microscopic scars. Not unlike other organs, where interstitial fibrosis represents a final common pathway to organ failure (18), it is this adverse accumulation of matrix in viable myocardium that is considered the *major component to the adverse structural remodeling found in the explanted, failing human heart with ICM* (16). The interstitial compartment in ICM is anything but acellular and inert. Herein we review the structural remodeling of the cardiac interstitium seen in ICM, together with molecular and cellular responses associated with such remodeling.

NORMAL CARDIAC INTERSTITIUM

The extracellular space has multiple functions that make it an essential component of the myocardium. Its fibrillar collagen network, for example, serves to maintain tissue architecture and myocyte alignment throughout the cardiac cycle. It facilitates the transmission of myocyte-generated force to ventricular chambers (19). Additionally, the energy imparted to coiled collagen fibers during myocyte contraction contributes to myocyte relengthening during relaxation and active early ventricular filling (20). Of equal importance, the interstitium contains tissue fluid through which oxygen, ions, and macromolecules reach myocytes and by which various metabolic end-products exit via venous and lymphatic capillaries. The normal cardiac interstitium is integral to myocyte contraction and nutrition and has been reviewed elsewhere (21).

Fibrillar Collagens

Type I and III fibrillar collagens are the major structural proteins of the extracellular matrix (22). They normally occupy 4% of its structural space (23). Type I collagen predominates and has the tensile strength of steel (24). Type III collagen is far less abundant but is more distensible. The fibrillar collagen network of the ventricles is a structural continuum with its exteriorized portion found in chordae tendineae and valve leaflets (25). The network is segregated into various components termed epimysium, perimysium, and endomysium (19,25–29). Self-aggregating macromolecules and cytokines are bound to matrix, creating a dynamic microenvironment integral to maintaining *tissue homeostasis*, which is defined as a state of equilibrium between different yet interdependent elements and which reflects a tissue's capacity for self-regulation and determination of its cellular composition and structure.

Cellular Composition

Fibroblasts and macrophages are present in the interstitial space (23). Cardiac fibroblasts contain messenger RNAs responsible for type I and III collagen gene expression and normal collagen synthesis (30,31). Fibroblasts are also responsible for the synthesis of collagenase and gelatinases, proteolytic enzymes present in the myocardium in latent form (25,32). When activated, these matrix metalloproteinases serve to degrade collagen and to maintain steady-state collagen concentration relative to collagen synthesis. Pluripotent fibroblast-like cells with considerable phenotypic and functional diversity appear under pathological conditions and are responsible for collagen turnover (*vide infra*).

CARDIAC INTERSTITIUM IN THE INFARCTED HEART

Fibrosis

Macroscopic scarring of the infarcted myocardium is an expected finding in ICM. Remote to infarct scar(s), microscopic findings include a diffuse perivascular fibrosis of intramural arteries and arterioles; an interstitial fibrosis; foci of microscopic scarring; and a diffuse atrophy of cardiac myocytes (33). In the explanted failing human heart of ischemic origins, multiple foci of microscopic scarring, in combination with interstitial fibrosis, are found in both right and left ventricular myocardium (16). Such remodeling accounts for over two-thirds of all fibrous tissue present, while the infarct scar(s) comprises remaining fibrous tissue. Pathological remodeling of the interstitium in ICM begins with myocyte loss following MI. Its evolution is controlled by events occurring in noninfarcted myocardium involving infarcted and noninfarcted ventricles. This accumulation of extracellular matrix draws attention to tissue repair following myocardial MI.

Fibrogenesis

Repair, a property common to all vascularized tissues, is initiated by inflammatory cells that invade the site of tissue injury. Activated macrophages generate peptides integral to the initiation of repair. Fibroblasts are attracted to the site of infarction and aggregate with macrophages that border on the site of necrotic myocytes and subsequently convert to myofibroblasts (myoFb), as discussed later. Through a complex series of molecular events that include expression of immediate early-response genes and activation of multiple second-messenger systems (which act synergistically to induce mitosis), myoFb proliferate and lay down fibrillar collagen that replaces lost myocytes (34–37). Cells involved in repair are bathed by tissue fluid whose composition regulates their phenotype and behavior. A diverse array of soluble regulatory signals, whose biological properties are expressed via receptor–ligand binding, gain access to tissue fluid from necrotic myocytes, leukocytes, macrophages, and myoFb. Provided the degree of parenchymal damage is minor, regulatory signals are confined to the site of necrosis. A large, transmural MI, on the other hand, yields a large signal at the site of injury that is widely dispersed within tissue fluid of the common interstitial space of both ventricles to elicit a fibrogenic response in the noninfarcted portion of infarcted and noninfarcted ventricles (17,38–40). Signals involved in repair following MI are generally confined to the heart. When they are not, a systemic response (e.g., fever, leukocytosis) appears.

Collagen Turnover

Collagen turnover has been studied in the rat heart both at the site of MI and at remote sites following ligation of the left coronary artery (41,42). At the infarct site and during the early phase of repair, collagen degradation exceeds its synthesis. Matrix metalloproteinases (MMPs) reside in the myocardium in latent form. When activated, MMP-1 (or interstitial collagenase) degrades fibrillar collagen into one-quarter and three-quarter fragments; gelatinases (MMP-2 and MMP-9) degrade these smaller fragments. An increase in collagenase activity (Fig. 9-1, left panel) appears at the infarct site on day 2, peaks by day 7, and declines thereafter, together with increased gelatinase activity (not shown) (41). An increase in collagenase (MMP-1) mRNA expression in the infarcted ventricle does not appear until later during week 1, when it replaces the latent pool that is being consumed. Tissue inhibitors of matrix metalloproteins (TIMP) neutralize collagenolytic activity. Transcription of TIMP mRNA at the infarct site peaks on day 2 and declines slowly over the course of 14 days (Fig. 9-1, right panel). Fibroblast-like cells, not inflammatory or endothelial cells, are responsible for the transcription of MMP-1 and TIMP

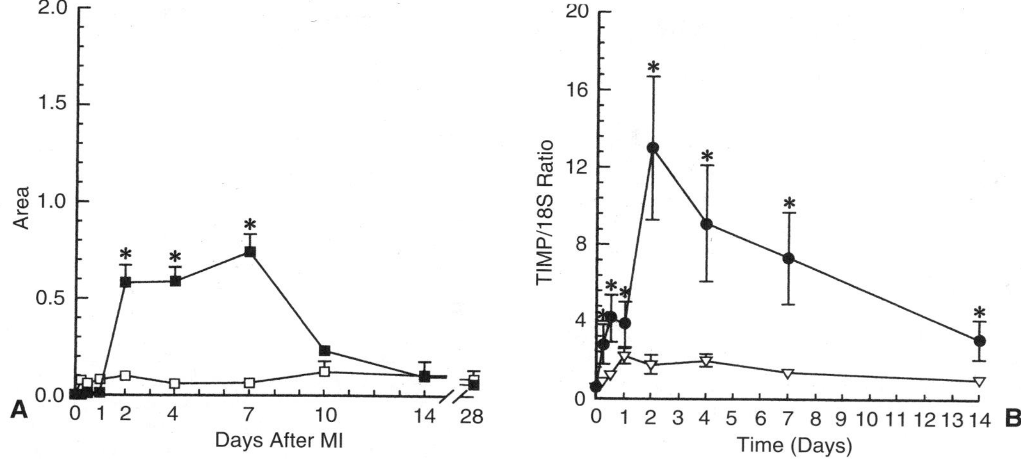

Figure 9-1 A. Scanned lytic areas of the infarcted (solid symbols) and sham-operated rat left ventricle (open symbols). Zymographic data presented for matrix metalloproteinase 1 on days following myocardial infarction. Values are means ±SD; *p <0.05 versus sham-operated animals. **B.** TIMP and 18S mRNA hybridization after Northern blotting for infarcted (solid symbols) and sham-operated animals (open symbols) rat left ventricle. Values are expressed as the TIMP/18S ratio as means ±SD; *p <0.05 versus sham-operated animals. (Adapted from Cleutjens JPM, Kandala JC, et al. Regulation of collagen degradation in the rat myocardium after infarction. *J Mol Cell Cardiol.* 1995;27:1281–1292, with permission.)

mRNAs (41). Such events pertaining to collagen degradation are not seen remote to the MI.

A fibrogenic component of healing, including an initial expression of fibronectin mRNA (43), accompanies early collagen degradation. Type III procollagen mRNA at the infarct site is increased on day 2 post-MI, reaches a peak by day 21, and declines thereafter (42). Type I procollagen mRNA is increased on day 4 at the site of infarction and remains elevated at week 4 (Fig. 9-2, left panel) and even as late as day 90 (42), suggesting collagen synthesis is an ongoing process and is in keeping with a persistence of an active myoFb phenotype at this site (44,45). A rise in procollagen mRNA is also seen remote to the infarct in the rat model with large, transmural anterior MI (42,46). Procollagen I and III mRNA are increased in the right ventricle and interventricular septum on day 4 and 7, respectively (42). In the septum, closest to the infarct, type I procollagen mRNA remains elevated until day 28 (Fig. 9-2, middle panel) while in the right ventricle only until day 7 (Fig. 9-2, right panel). These responses, involving myoFb at the infarct and fibroblasts at remote sites (*vide infra*) (42,45), are associated with increased expression of transforming growth factor-β_1 (TGF-β_1) mRNA and its receptors (*vide infra*) (46).

Collagen fibers are first evident at the infarct site on day 7, while an organized assembly of fibers in the form of scar tissue is present by day 14 and continues to accumulate for many weeks (40,47). Hydroxyproline concentration at the site of scarring increases progressively from week 1 to 6, as does collagen cross-linking (48–50). A thinning of infarct scar is evident by week 8. Remote to the infarct, including viable left ventricle, interventricular septum, and right

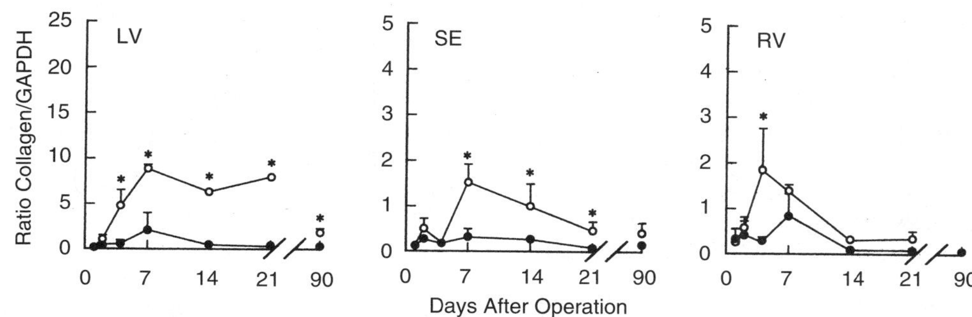

Figure 9-2 Densitometric scanning of type I procollagen versus GAPDH of the autoradiograms after Northern blotting of infarcted left ventricle (LV) and noninfarcted interventricular septum (SE) and right ventricle (RV). Infarcted (open symbols) and sham-operated animals (solid symbols). Values are means ±SD; *p <0.05. (Adapted from Cleutjens JPM, Verluyten MJA, Smits JFM, et al. Collagen remodeling after myocardial infarction in the rat heart. *Am J Pathol.* 1995;147:325–338, with permission.)

ventricle, fibrillar collagen appears by day 14 and this interstitial fibrosis continues to accumulate for weeks (16,17,38,39,50,51).

CELLULAR ASPECTS OF INTERSTITIAL REMODELING

Inflammatory Cells

Repair begins with the formation of a fibrin-fibronectin meshwork and an invasion of injured tissue by inflammatory cells, such as neutrophils and $CD4^+$ lymphocytes that secrete γ-interferon. This serves to activate macrophages (MP) that have invaded the meshwork from the circulation and local sites. Once activated, MP express the gene encoding for inducible nitric oxide synthase and produce nitric oxide, which governs their survival via apoptosis (52–54). Activated MP likewise express inducible cyclo-oxygenase that leads to their production of prostaglandins. MP have additional functional activity that includes their ability to generate AngII *de novo* (55,56). In an autocrine manner, AngII stimulates expression of TGF-β_1 that favors the recruitment of pluripotent interstitial fibroblasts and their likely conversion to the myoFb phenotype on day 4 following injury; myoFb proliferation follows. TGF-β_1 also serves to suppress the inflammatory cell response. An ACE inhibitor (ACEI) or AT_1 receptor antagonist (AT_1 Ra), introduced at the time of repair or within the first 48 hours, interferes with the ultimate appearance of fibrous tissue by abrogating this first phase of AngII generation and its important functions in cell-cell signaling and TGF-β_1 formation.

Myofibroblasts

MyoFb are central to the fibrogenic component of repair. They appear at sites of injury within days of cardiac myocyte necrosis (40,57–59) and are responsible for increased expression of genes encoding for fibrillar type I and III procollagens and their synthesis (40,60,61). Progenitor cells remain to be fully elucidated. Interstitial fibroblasts are likely candidates, not vascular smooth muscle cells or cardiac myocytes (62,63). Fibroblasts have an extensive clonal heterogeneity. MyoFb, phenotypically transformed fibroblast-like cells, have marked functional diversity (62,64) that includes their synthesis of structural proteins and expression of receptors for AngII and TGF-β_1. MyoFb also express α-SMA, and these microfilaments endow these cells with contractile behavior. MyoFb are normal residents of heart valve leaflets (45,57,58,65), and leaflet contraction, induced by AngII, is shown in Figure 9-3. MyoFb contraction governs matrix remodeling, including scar thinning (66). The contractile behavior of fibrous tissue is related not only to myoFb having α-SMA, but to their cell–cell and cell–matrix connections. Scar tissue contraction in response to AngII has been demonstrated (67). The contractile nature of fibrous tissue can therefore influence diastolic properties of the infarcted ventricle. The importance of fibrous tissue contraction to ventricular dysfunction seen in ICM remains to be systematically examined.

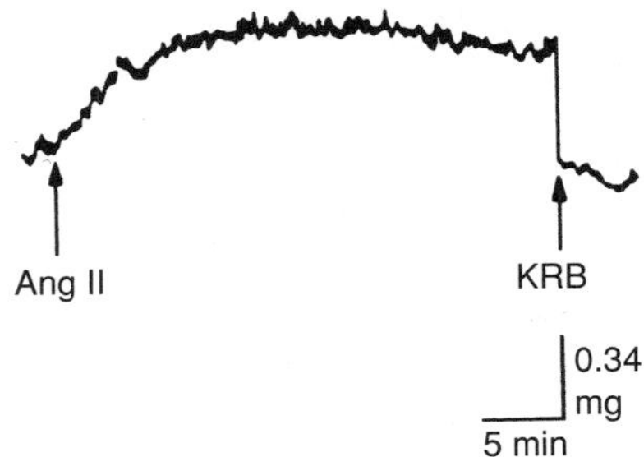

Figure 9-3 Mechanical activity of the anterior rat tricuspid valve leaflet stimulated by 10^{-5}M angiotensin II (AngII). Initial baseline was regained after return to Krebs-Ringer bicarbonate buffer (KRB). Contraction reaches a plateau 3 minutes after stimulation and is maintained for ~20 minutes. (Adapted from Filip DA, Radu A, Simionescu M. Interstitial cells of the heart valves possess characteristics similar to smooth muscle cells. *Circ Res.* 1986;59:310–320, with permission.)

Signals that determine the appearance of the myoFb phenotype are not entirely certain. TGF-β_1 is contributory. Administration of TGF-β_1 via a chamber implanted subcutaneously in rats leads to the appearance of myoFb within granulation tissue that forms around the chamber. This was not the case when the chamber contained platelet-derived growth factor or tumor necrosis factor-α (68). Cultured adult rat skin fibroblasts undergo a phenotype switch and express α-SMA when incubated with TGF-β_1 (68). The appearance of TGF-β_1 at sites of MI is likely related to necrotic myocytes (69,70), activated macrophages (71), and myoFb themselves (72).

The fibrillar fibrin-fibronectin scaffolding that forms soon after tissue injury is the precursor to granulation tissue formation and the attachment of myoFb via a fibronexus (73). MyoFb subsequently elaborate type III and then type I collagens, the major fibrillar collagens that constitute fibrous tissue (74–76). At pathological sites of tissue repair in the heart, including the site of MI, myoFb express type I and III collagen transcripts (40,42). They elaborate and metabolize substances that regulate their turnover of collagen and govern fibrous tissue contraction in an autocrine manner (*vide infra*).

A subpopulation of these myoFb are reduced in number at the infarct site via apoptosis (40,57,77). Many, however, persist long after scar tissue formation (44). This contrasts to injured skin, where they completely disappear following repair (78,79). Persistent myoFb in the kidney with experimental glomerulonephritis is associated with a progressive interstitial fibrosis (72). Persistent, active myoFb could contribute to ongoing fibrosis in ICM; this remains to be determined. Irrespective of the location or nature of the inciting stimulus to connective tissue formation in the heart, myoFb are the dominant cell involved in matrix formation at sites of injury (45).

MEDIATORS OF INTERSTITIAL REMODELING

Transforming Growth Factor-β_1

The heart's healing paradigm is still under investigation. However, it likely does not differ from other organs.

Regulatory peptides, or cytokines such as TGF-β_1, contribute to fibrogenesis. TGF-β_1 has numerous actions on the extracellular matrix (80), which include fibroblast chemotaxis, phenotype transformation and replication, and ultimately scar tissue formation (68,81). TGF-β_1 mRNA is expressed in infarcted myocardium soon after coronary artery ligation (69,70) or catecholamine-induced necrosis (82). Low-density ACE, AngII and TGF-β_1 receptor binding, and mRNA expression for type I collagen and TGF-β_1 are found in the normal heart. At sites of MI and fibrosis remote to it (including endocardial fibrosis of intraventricular septum), interstitial fibrosis of noninfarcted myocardium and fibrosis of visceral pericardium markedly increased binding of ACE, AngII and TGF-β_1 receptors is seen and colocalized with increased type I collagen and TGF-β_1 mRNA expression (83). TGF-β_1 concentration is increased at each of these sites. TGF-β_1 and type I collagen gene expression at each of these sites are attenuated in rats receiving losartan and suggest that locally generated AngII via AT_1 receptor binding governs TGF-β_1 expression and synthesis at the site of MI and at remote sites in the rat heart.

TGF-β_1 increases transcription of both type I collagen and TIMP by cultured human cardiac fibroblasts (84). AngII augments TGF-β_1 gene expression via AT_1 receptor binding in cultured neonatal or adult rat cardiac fibroblasts and myoFb (85,86), while endogenous elevations in circulating AngII are associated with upregulation of TGF-β_1 gene in the adult rat heart (87). Macrophages, clustered at sites of tissue injury (88), are a likely source of TGF-β_1 (71) and, therefore, are important to the appearance of the myoFb (68) and suppression of further inflammatory cell responses (89). A subsequent elaboration of TGF-β_1 by myoFb is integral to fibrogenesis, while persistence of myoFb elaborating TGF-β_1 leads to progressive fibrosis (72). AngII appears to play a central role in the expression of TGF-β_1 by activated macrophages and myoFb. An AT_1 Ra prevents these responses (90).

Local Angiotensin II

The role of AngII in the fibrogenic phase of tissue repair has been examined in various organs following diverse forms of injury (18). The involvement of this peptide in tissue repair includes its local production at functionally relevant concentrations and the presence of AngII receptors on myoFb responsible for collagen turnover.

Components requisite to the generation of AngII in infarcted rat hearts have been examined. Localization and density of ACE binding in the normal and injured heart (Fig. 9-4) have been addressed using quantitative in vitro autoradiography and an iodinated derivative of lisinopril (^{125}I-351A) (40,45,91–95). In the normal heart, low-density ACE binding is found throughout ventricular myocardium and atria. High-density binding is present at sites of high collagen turnover, including heart valve leaflets and the adventitia of intramyocardial coronary arteries and great vessels (95–98). High-density ACE binding is likewise found in subcutaneous skin with its metabolically active fibroblasts, but not in skeletal muscle tendon with its quiescent fibroblasts (95). Immunolabeling with a monoclonal

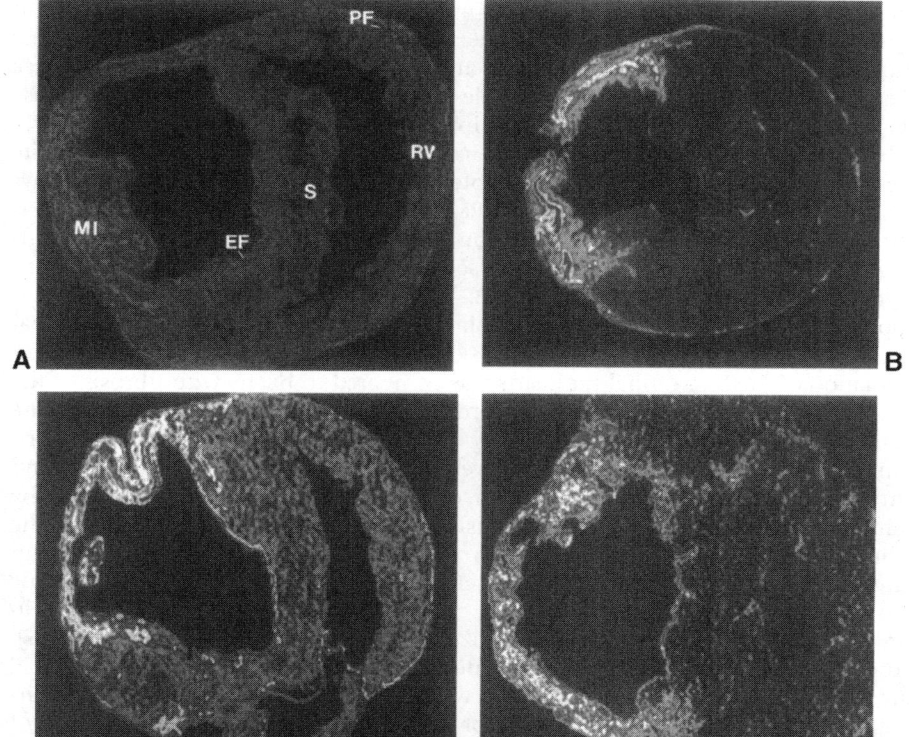

Figure 9-4 Expression of ACE, AngII receptors, type I collagen mRNA, and TGF-β_1 mRNA in the infarcted rat heart 4 weeks following coronary artery ligation. By in vitro autoradiography, high-density receptor binding of ACE (**A**) and AngII (**B**) is seen at sites of fibrosis including myocardial infarction (MI), endocardium (EF), and pericardium (PF). By in situ hybridization, high-density binding of type I collagen mRNA (**C**) and TGF-β_1 mRNA (**D**) is observed at these sites of fibrosis and are colocalized with high-density ACE and AngII receptor binding. Also involved are the interventricular septum (S) and right ventricle (RV).

ACE antibody (99) identified cells expressing this membrane-bound ectoenzyme: endothelial cells, located on the surface of each valve leaflet; myoFb-like cells residing within leaflet matrix where they are responsible for collagen turnover; and fibroblasts of the adventitia of intramural coronary arteries and great vessels. Autoradiography and immunolabeling demonstrated ACE binding in cultured intact myoFb-like cells and their cell membranes (100), where reverse transcriptase-polymerase chain reaction (RT-PCR) demonstrated the presence of ACE mRNA. Substrate utilization of membrane-bound ACE in these cells includes AngI and, in its dual capacity as a kininase II, other chemical mediators of inflammation such as BK and substance P. Thus, myoFb-like cells of valve leaflets have the potential to regulate local concentrations of AngII and other mediators of tissue repair, such as TGF-β_1, in valve leaflets. The importance of the TGF-β family of peptides in fetal heart development, including endocardial cushion formation and heart valve induction, has been identified (101,102). A role for AngII generated by these cells in contributing to this process needs to be considered.

High-affinity receptors are integral to the biological activity of ACE-related peptides. The presence of high-density AngII receptor binding in heart valves was demonstrated by autoradiography using ^{125}I[Sar^1, Ile^8]AngII (95). Competitive binding with either an AT_1 or AT_2 receptor antagonist, losartan and PD123177, respectively, provided identification of AT_1 receptors as the dominant subtype. Low-density AT_1 receptor binding is present throughout the rat myocardium, while high-density binding is present in heart valve leaflets (95). Western immunoblotting, as well as binding assay, confirmed these findings in myoFb cell membranes (100). Heart valves and myoFb cell membranes likewise contain BK receptors, as seen by ^{125}I[Tyr^8]BK autoradiographic binding and binding assay (95,100).

Cellular responses to AngII receptor–ligand binding has been examined in serum-deprived, cultured myoFb-like cells obtained from adult rat heart valve leaflets. By in situ hybridization, these cells express the transcript for type I collagen, and incubation of cultured cells with AngII in pathophysiological concentrations enhances type I collagen synthesis via AT_1 receptor binding (100,103,104). Immunohistochemistry (100,105) and electron microscopy (65,106) have shown that these cells contain α-SMA microfilaments. Like vascular smooth muscle cells these microfilaments confer contractile behavior to myoFb in response to various substances that include AngII (65,106).

A biological role for ACE in the local regulation of AngII at normal tissue sites, where collagen turnover is high, is therefore suggested. These findings led to additional autoradiographic and morphological studies in the rat using several different models of experimental injury involving the heart and related structures or systemic organs.

High-density autoradiographic ACE binding was found at the site of MI at week 1 and increased progressively over the course of 8 weeks (Fig. 9-4), in parallel with morphological evidence of fibrillar collagen accumulation found in serial heart sections (40). ACE activity, as measured by substrate conversion, is increased in aneurysmal tissue of the infarcted left ventricle (LV) as contrasted to atrial tissue (107). Additionally, a significant correlation was found between ACE activity and the extent of MI (107), as is also the case for ACE mRNA expression and activity at sites remote to the MI (108). The rat is pronate, which may sustain renal perfusion more effectively than man when in an upright posture. Accordingly, the circulating renin-angiotensin-aldosterone system (RAAS) is not activated in the rat despite extensive MI (108–112).

Monoclonal or polyclonal ACE antibodies were used to identify ACE-labeled cells at sites of healing (40,42,113). Following cardiac myocyte necrosis, these cells include macrophages, α-SMA-positive myoFb, and endothelial cells of the neovasculature. High-density ACE binding is also found at sites of fibrosis remote to MI (Fig. 9-4). This includes endocardial fibrosis of the interventricular septum; interstitial fibrosis of the right ventricle; the fibrosed pericardium that follows pericardiotomy (with or without MI); and the foreign-body fibrosis that surrounds the silk ligature placed around the left coronary artery as part of a sham operation. The anatomic coincidence between high-density ACE binding and fibrosis has been observed in other injured organs of the rat, including the infarcted kidney and incised skin sutured with silk ligature (93). Immunolabeling demonstrated myoFb-containing α-SMA as cells expressing ACE at each of these noninfarcted-related sites. High-density ACE binding is also observed at sites of isoproterenol-induced myocyte necrosis (114,115). At each of these sites of repair, in situ hybridization and immunolabeling demonstrated myoFb as expressing genes encoding for type I and III collagens (40,42).

In vitro quantitative autoradiography was used to address AngII receptor binding in the infarcted rat heart with receptor subtype determined by displacement with an AT_1 (losartan) or AT_2 (PD 123177) receptor antagonist (105,116–118). Marked AT_1 receptor binding density is present at the site of MI, as well as endocardial and pericardial fibrosis (Fig. 9-4), while AT_2 receptor binding is low at each of these sites. Cells expressing AT_1 receptors at these sites of injury are α-SMA-positive myoFb (119). These autoradiographic findings are consistent with the increase in gene transcription and protein expression of the AT_1 receptor found in homogenized tissue taken from the site of MI and remote sites using RT-PCR and binding assays (120,121). AT_1 Ra abrogates the fibrotic response, which is not the case for AT_2 Ra. Increased expression of AngII receptors likewise appears at sites of injury in other organs such as skin (122–124).

Using an isolated, crystalloid perfused organ preparation, the conversion of AngI to AngII by epicardium of normal rat hearts was compared to hearts with fibrosis of the visceral pericardium following pericardiotomy alone (without MI) (125). ACE activity of the fibrosed pericardium was several-fold higher than the normal heart and this generation of AngII was completely abrogated by ACEI. High-density ACE binding is likewise present in the perivascular fibrosis and microscopic scars that appear in the right and left atria and ventricles with the chronic administration of AngII or aldosterone (ALDO) (in uninephrectomized rats on a high-sodium diet) (91,126). These latter models, addressed later, demonstrate that ACE binding density within fibrous tissue is independent of circulating AngII or ALDO, in contrast to endothelial ACE of the pulmonary artery, which is subject to negative feedback regulation by circulating AngII (127).

The anatomic coincidence between the expression of ACE and AT_1 receptors with normal and pathological expressions of active collagen formation is apparent. High-density ACE and AngII receptor binding are markers of high collagen turnover, as defined by quantitative in situ hybridization as high-density, type I collagen expression. Alpha-SMA-containing, fibroblast-like cells, normally found within valve leaflets and vascular adventitia, and pathological sites of fibrous tissue formation express genes encoding for ACE, AT_1 receptors, and fibrillar collagens. MyoFb could therefore be considered a "metabolic entity" regulating their own collagen turnover (128).

ACE binding density correlates with the presence of myoFb. The disappearance of ACE-positive cells or a reduction in their absolute number reduces ACE binding density at sites of fibrosis, as is the case with some sarcoid granulomas (129). Both ACE and AngII receptor binding densities in the infarcted rat heart remain high for months post-MI (40,116), as does ACE activity (108). Each is in keeping with the persistence of myoFb at the infarct site (44).

Granulation tissue and its diverse cell populations, in particular, generate peptides integral to tissue repair via receptor–ligand binding. ACE, for example, regulates local concentrations of AngII. At the infarct site the concentration of AngII is increased several-fold above that found in viable myocardium (110). *De novo* Ang peptide generation requires expression of several requisite components: angiotensinogen (Ao), the precursor to all Ang peptides; a protease that cleaves amino acids to form AngI; and ACE that hydrolyzes the decapeptide AngI to AngII, an octapeptide. An independent pathway of AngII generation involving a chymase has been suggested; however, increased expression of its transcript is infrequently found in the failing human heart (130).

Ao mRNA expression in the adult rat heart and aorta is localized to fibroblasts and brown adipocytes (131,132). RT-PCR amplification identified Ao mRNA expression in the adult human heart (133). This transcript and that of renin are localized within both neonatal fibroblasts and cardiac myocytes (134), with AngI and AngII peptides detected in culture media (135). The presence of renin mRNA, however, in normal adult heart tissue is controversial and, therefore, the source of cardiac renin has been called into question (136). This aspartyl protease is taken up from the circulation and is of renal origin in normal heart (137–139); it rapidly disappears from the heart following nephrectomy (140). The presence of other aspartyl (e.g., cathepsin D) or serine (e.g., cathepsin G) proteases eliminates any absolute dependence on renin as a rate-dependent protease (55,141). This is the case for cultured myoFb that express cathepsin D and elaborate AngI despite the fact that renin mRNA or renin activity has not been detected (103,142). Several recent studies, however, have reported renin mRNA expression in the adult rat heart (143–145). The validity of a renin-angiotensin system in local AngII generation awaits further investigation.

Circulating Angiotensin II

Given connective tissue-promoting properties of AngII-generated *de novo* within injured cardiac tissue, it follows that chronic, inappropriate (relative to dietary sodium intake and intravascular volume) elevations in circulating AngII would amplify these effects throughout the heart and systemic organs (15). Endogenous elevations in circulating AngII are seen when renal perfusion is seriously compromised, such as occurs with advanced cardiac failure (146,147), with suprarenal abdominal aortic banding, or with discrete renal artery stenosis (148–150). Cardiac fibrosis seen under these circumstances need not be accompanied by cardiac myocyte (and ventricular) hypertrophy.

A hypertrophic growth of cardiac myocytes occurs when the hemodynamic workload of one or both ventricles is raised or when plasma concentrations of circulating trophic hormones of the pituitary-thyroid axis are increased (Fig. 9-5). Myocardial fibrosis, defined as increased collagen concentration, is not observed under these circumstances. Hypertrophy without fibrosis appears with banding the abdominal aorta below the renal arteries and where the RAAS is not activated (151). In animals with chronic volume overload secondary to anemia (152), arteriovenous fistula (153,154), exercise training (155), or chronic elevations in either circulating growth or thyroid hormones (156,157), ventricular hypertrophy alone appears without fibrosis. In each model of volume overload, an activation of the RAAS does not occur unless renal perfusion is seriously impaired.

In other experimental conditions, ventricular hypertrophy is associated with fibrosis (Fig. 9-5). Under these circumstances, a pressure or volume overload on one or both ventricles is associated with either an elevation in plasma renin activity (i.e., secondary hyperaldosteronism) or a

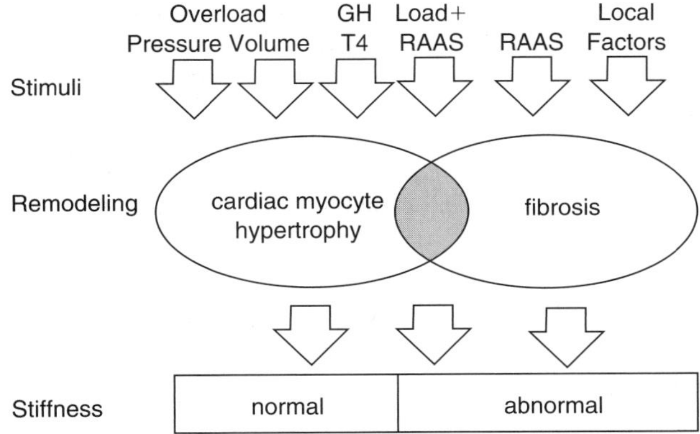

Figure 9-5 A schematic representation of various stimuli that lead to cardiac myocyte growth alone, expressed as ventricular hypertrophy, hypertrophy with myocardial fibrosis (shaded area of overlap), or fibrosis alone. With hypertrophy alone, myocardial stiffness remains normal, while fibrosis alters the stiffness of the hypertrophied or nonhypertrophied ventricle. Hypertrophy accompanies increased myocyte loading, expressed as a ventricular pressure or volume overload (load), and elevations in circulating thyroxine (T4) or growth hormone (GH). RAAS, circulating renin-angiotensin-aldosterone system activation. Local factors include *de novo* generation of angiotensin II and transforming growth factor-β_1. (Adapted from Weber KT, Brilla CG, Campbell SE, et al. Pathologic hypertrophy with fibrosis: the structural basis for myocardial failure. *Blood Press.* 1992;1:75–85, with permission.)

primary mineralocorticoid excess state, such as that which accompanies chronic mineralocorticoid administration, either ALDO or deoxycorticosterone acetate (DOCA). Myocardial fibrosis will be progressive over time under these conditions, provided such hormonal stimuli are sustained (158,159). Initially, the rise in collagen concentration creates an abnormal elevation in diastolic stiffness (160,161), while systolic function is preserved. A continued accumulation of fibrillar collagen eventuates in combined diastolic and systolic ventricular dysfunction (159).

Following surgical induction of unilateral renal ischemia, a rise in plasma renin activity, AngII, and ALDO follow, associated with the appearance of arterial hypertension (160). Left ventricular hypertrophy (LVH) is accompanied by a rise in collagen volume fraction in this model of secondary hyperaldosteronism. The fibrous tissue response begins with increased expression of type I and III collagens and presents morphologically as a perivascular fibrosis of intramyocardial coronary arteries and arterioles that extends from the perivascular space into neighboring interstitium (162). Myocardial diastolic stiffness is increased in response to this structural remodeling (150,160). Microscopic scarring following myocyte necrosis is also evident in renovascular hypertension. Its pathophysiological basis is discussed below.

A role of AngII in promoting fibrosis is evidenced by studies in which circulating AngII is chronically increased from either endogenous or exogenous sources. In experimental models associated with renal ischemia, circulating AngII is increased. Such models are associated with increased mRNA expression of renal renin, increased plasma renin activity and circulating AngII, and downregulation of AngII receptors (148–150). In keeping with a role for circulating AngII in promoting fibrogenesis, collagen synthesis is increased in tricuspid and mitral valve leaflets, which are sites of high-density AngII receptor binding. Fibrosis appears in the normotensive, nonhypertrophied right and left atria, right ventricle, and the hypertensive, hypertrophied left ventricle and is preceded by increased mRNA expression for types I and III collagens in these models of renovascular hypertension (150,160–164). Arterioles of systemic organs likewise undergo a structural remodeling that includes medial thickening and perivascular fibrosis (165–167). Myocardial fibrosis in rats with unilateral (168–170) or bilateral renal ischemia (171,172) is prevented by ACEI or AT_1 Ra. Hence, it would seem clear that elevations in circulating AngII are associated with fibrosis and this peptide does not promote biventricular or atrial hypertrophy, as is the case for elevations in circulating growth hormone or thyroxin.

Chronic infusion of AngII, using pressor or nonpressor doses of AngII, has been used to raise circulating effector hormone levels to that found in advanced heart failure. This leads to fibrosis of atria and ventricles, increased adventitial collagen of the normotensive pulmonary artery and hypertensive aorta, and systemic organs (91,126,173). Fibrosis is preceded by increased mRNA expression of fibronectin on day 3 and subsequently types I and III collagens and TGF-β_1, each of which is related to proliferating fibroblast-like cells (not myocytes) located at sites of subsequent fibrosis in each ventricle (174,175). Losartan, given in doses that either did or did not prevent arterial hypertension, abrogated these responses. This was not the case for prazosin or hydralazine, which prevented hypertension. These findings further emphasize that hemodynamic factors are not involved in promoting cardiac fibrosis (174,175). Potential mechanisms involved in the fibrogenic response associated with chronic elevations in AngII have been reviewed elsewhere (176).

In genetically modified mice, devoid of AT_{1A} receptors, aortic banding was used to further address the role of AngII in promoting LVH (177,178). Hypertrophy appeared in response to pressure overload created by the banding procedure and further suggested AT_{1A} receptor-mediated signaling by AngII was not a requisite to cardiac myocyte growth. Perivascular fibrosis, however, was evident, involving intramural coronary arteries of the left ventricle (right ventricle not examined) (178). This latter observation leaves open the question of whether this fibrous tissue response would be mediated by AT_2 receptors. AT_2 receptors, however, are thought to inhibit cell growth and collagen metabolism (179–181). Alternatively, an upregulation of other growth promoters, such as mineralocorticoids and/or endothelins, could be contributory.

Circulating Aldosterone

Renin-dependent elevations in AngII are associated with elevations in circulating ALDO (secondary hyperaldosteronism). To address a role for ALDO in contributing to cardiac fibrosis, chronic administration of D-aldosterone is given to uninephrectomized animals receiving a diet supplemented with sodium; this is referred to as aldosterone/salt treatment (ALDOST). This model of suppressed plasma renin activity and plasma AngII is associated with arterial hypertension, left ventricular pressure overload, LVH, and fibrosis of right and left ventricles (150,167). The fibrous tissue response in this model of primary hyperaldosteronism presents as a perivascular/interstitial fibrosis and as microscopic scarring, or a reparative fibrosis. Unlike AngII, where fibrosis appears within 2 weeks, reactive and reparative fibrosis in this model of mineralocorticoid excess begins to appear after 4 or more weeks of ALDO administration. In uninephrectomized rats that were maintained on a high-sodium diet without an exogenous source of ALDO, LVH accompanied the expansion in intravascular volume without the appearance myocardial fibrosis (150). The administration of ALDO to animals maintained on a low-sodium diet was not associated with arterial hypertension, LVH, or myocardial fibrosis, despite an increase in plasma AngII (renin-dependent) and a marked increase in ALDO (renin-dependent and exogenous source). Thus, the abnormal fibrous tissue response is most closely related to an inappropriate rise in plasma mineralocorticoid in association with enhanced dietary sodium intake.

LVH with fibrosis is also seen with the primary mineralocorticoid excess state that accompanies the chronic administration of DOCA in uninephrectomized rats maintained on a high-sodium diet (182). In this model, plasma renin activity, AngII, and ALDO are each suppressed. Nonetheless, fibrosis appears in both ventricles, but again requires 4 or more weeks of DOCA administration. A mineralocorticoid excess state itself, which includes sodium loading together with the chronic administration of either ALDO or DOCA, is the essential link to the fibrous tissue response. Selye (166) has previously noted that chronic DOCA administration was associated with perivascular and interstitial fibrosis of systemic organs. The heart therefore is not unique in its response. In autopsy-proven cases of adrenal adenoma, a similar fibrous tissue response is present in the human myocardium, pancreas, and adrenal glands (183).

In each of the aforementioned models that simulate advanced symptomatic heart failure or acquired arterial hypertension, where elevated plasma mineralocorticoid was inappropriate for the level of sodium intake and excretion, the abnormal fibrous tissue response was not only found in the hypertensive, hypertrophied left ventricle, but also the normotensive, nonhypertrophied right ventricle (150). This finding again underscores that factors which regulate myocyte growth and fibrosis are independent of one another (Fig. 9-5). At the same time, it is clear that myocyte growth and ventricular hypertrophy occur in association with ventricular systolic pressure overload, not elevations in these effector hormones of the RAAS. Accordingly, right ventricular hypertrophy (RVH) was not observed in any of these models of arterial hypertension (150). The presence of fibrosis in each ventricle, despite inherent differences in loading and the presence or absence of hypertrophy, is in keeping with the importance of a circulating substance in promoting the disproportionate accumulation of fibrillar collagen.

Robert et al. (184,185) have found that the biventricular fibrosis that accompanies chronic ALDO administration is preceded by increased expression of type I and III collagens in both the right and left ventricles. However, ventricular hypertrophy, expressed by weight or increased expression of atrial natriuretic peptide (ANP), is related to arterial hypertension. Young et al. (186,187) have confirmed the association between cardiac fibrosis and either ALDO or DOCA, together with enhanced dietary sodium. Moreover, Young's findings underscore the importance of circulating ALDO and its interaction with the heart as target tissue. By combining systemic ALDO administration with an intracerebroventricular infusion of a mineralocorticoid receptor antagonist, these investigators found it possible to prevent arterial hypertension, but not cardiac fibrosis. Alternatively, a central infusion of ALDO produces hypertension without fibrosis (188). Hence, it is apparent that the mineralocorticoid must interact directly with cardiac tissue, a now recognized site of mineralocorticoid (MC) receptors and its population of fibroblasts specifically (189–192).

Slight et al. (193–195) addressed the presence a guardian enzyme, 11β-hydroxysteroid dehydrogenase (11ß-HSD), that metabolizes more plentiful glucocorticoids into inactive metabolites. In doing so, 11ß-HSD preserves the specificity of promiscuous MC receptors having equal affinity for glucocorticoids and mineralocorticoids. 11ß-HSD activity was found in human cardiac tissue and cultured cardiac fibroblasts. Thus, circulating mineralocorticoid excess, represented by either plasma ALDO or DOC, relative to dietary sodium intake and elimination is responsible for the reactive fibrous tissue response seen in the myocardium and systemic organs and is independent of hemodynamic factors.

A systemic response involving a circulating factor is considered integral to the proinflammatory vascular phenotype that accompanies ALDOST. Several other lines of evidence support this view. First, cotreatment with spironolactone (Spi), an aldosterone receptor antagonist, prevents the appearance of these lesions. This is the case for either a large or a small dose of Spi, which, respectively, does or does not prevent arterial hypertension. This contrasts to nonspecific vasodilator agents, which provide a comparable attenuation in arterial pressure but do not prevent vascular remodeling. Second, pharmacological interference with the inflammatory cell response prevents these lesions without attenuating arterial pressure. This includes mycophenolate mofetil, peroxisome proliferator-activated receptor-alpha or gamma and 3-hydroxy-3-methylglutaryl coenzyme A reductase (reviewed in 196). Third, when ALDOST is combined with an intracerebroventricular infusion of a mineralocorticoid receptor antagonist, arterial pressure fails to rise while vascular lesions still appear. Finally, coronary lesions are not found in a transgenic mouse having a cardioselective overexpression of aldosterone synthase, a terminal enzyme in aldosterone biosynthesis, with increased levels of aldosterone in cardiac tissue.

Thus, a systemic response involving a circulating "factor" accounts for the appearance of the proinflammatory vascular phenotype in aldosteronism. The nature of this "factor" remains to be identified. Because there is no injury to the heart or systemic organs prior to initiating ALDOST, a circulating self-antigen and antibody response to said antigen is considered unlikely. Elevations in arterial pressure govern the hypertrophic growth of cardiomyocytes but are not responsible for the vascular remodeling found in aldosteronism.

A Role for Oxi/Nitrosative Stress

Immunohistochemical evidence of reactive oxygen and nitrogen intermediates and an activation of nicotinamide adenine dinucleotide phosphate (NADPH) oxidase, integral to superoxide formation, is found in vascular tissue in rats receiving an infusion of AngII or ALDOST. This includes invading inflammatory cells and the endothelium of the affected vasculature (197–199). Markers of oxi/nitrosative stress are also present in blood, suggesting a widespread, systemic response (199,200). In the right and left heart and mesenteric circulation there is immunohistochemical evidence of NFκB activation, a redox-sensitive transcription factor that regulates the expression of such proinflammatory genes as intercellular adhesion molecule (ICAM)-1, monocyte chemoattractant protein (MCP)-1, and tumor necrosis factor (TNF)-α. Cotreatment with an antioxidant (either N-acetylcysteine or pyrrolidine dithiocarbamate) or with spironolactone prevents NFκB activation and the upregulated mRNA expression for ICAM-1, MCP-1, and TNF-α, as well as the appearance of these vascular lesions that accompany ALDOST (197,198,201).

Thus, during AngII infusion or with ALDOST, evidence of oxi/nitrosative stress is present in blood plasma and the endothelium and invading inflammatory cells of the affected vasculature. In the next section, what accounts for this altered redox state will be addressed.

An Immunostimulatory State and Altered Ca^{2+} and Mg^{2+} Homeostasis

Lymphocyte cytosolic-free $[Mg^{2+}]_i$ is reduced in patients with primary aldosteronism (202). Reduced $[Mg^{2+}]_i$, the biologically active component of this intracellular cation, could lead to Ca^{2+} loading of cells, a well-known stimulus to the induction of oxi/nitrosative stress, especially within mitochondria. $[Ca^{2+}]_i$ and $[Mg^{2+}]_i$ in peripheral blood mononuclear cells (PBMC, lymphocytes and monocytes) were monitored during preclinical and clinical stages of ALDOST. An early and persistent decline in $[Mg^{2+}]_i$ is accompanied by a rise in $[Ca^{2+}]_i$ and increased H_2O_2 production by these cells. H_2O_2 serves as an intracellular messenger involved in signal transduction (203). Spironolactone cotreatment prevents these responses, as does a Ca^{2+} channel blocker and an antioxidant (200,201).

Evidence that the transcriptome of PBMC is activated during week 1 was found by gene chip array. This includes upregulated expression of genes representing antioxidant defenses, proinflammatory behavior (e.g., adhesion molecules, CC and CXC chemokines, interleukin-1β) and lymphocyte activation. Considered an immunostimulatory state, PBMC activation precedes the invasion of the coronary circulation by several weeks. Given the absence of previous cardiac injury, these vascular lesions appear to be a consequence of autoactivation of circulating immune cells. In this connection, there is evidence of B lymphocyte activation and expression of MHC Class II and downregulated expression of RT-6.2, an autoantigen lost upon cell activation (200). This proinflammatory PBMC phenotype persists throughout the weeks of ALDOST and is prevented by cotreatment with spironolactone (200). Cotreatment with amlodipine, an L-type Ca^{2+} channel blocker, prevents Ca^{2+} loading of PBMC, the increased production of H_2O_2 by these cells, and attenuates vasculature invasion (201).

What accounts for the iterations in PBMC $[Ca^{2+}]_i$ and $[Mg^{2+}]_i$ and the induction of oxi/nitrosative stress? Is this an Na^+-dependent, direct effect of ALDO on lymphocytes and monocytes (202)? Alternatively, and given the time-dependent response seen in animal studies, could this be an indirect effect of ALDOST on these cells?

In his original series of 18 patients with primary aldosteronism reported in 1963 (204,205), Conn identified hypomagnesemia as one of its prominent metabolic features. Horton and Biglieri (206) found hypermagnesuria to accompany primary aldosteronism, which is normalized by spironolactone or adrenal surgery. Others have reported on the hypercalciuria that accompanies primary aldosteronism or treatment with a mineralocorticoid and which is accentuated by increased dietary Na^+ (207–209).

Based on this information, metabolic studies were undertaken in rats with ALDOST. Given the presence of high-density aldosterone receptor binding in both kidneys and colon, urinary and fecal Ca^{2+} and Mg^{2+} excretion were monitored. In response to ALDOST a marked increase in excretion of these divalent cations was found at weeks 1 to 6. This includes microgram quantities of Mg^{2+} and Ca^{2+} found in urine and a thousand-fold greater levels (or milligrams) of these cations in feces. These losses were accompanied by a fall in both plasma-ionized $[Ca^{2+}]_o$ and $[Mg^{2+}]_o$, each of which is an important determinant of the parathyroid glands' secretion of such calcitropic hormones as parathyroid hormone (PTH) and endothelin (ET)-1. Spironolactone cotreatment prevents urinary and fecal losses of Ca^{2+} and Mg^{2+} and thereby the fall in plasma $[Ca^{2+}]_o$ and $[Mg^{2+}]_o$.

Hyperparathyroidism and the Ca^{2+} Paradox

Plasma PTH levels are increased as early as week 1 of ALDOST and remain so over ensuing weeks. In an attempt to restore extracellular Ca^{2+} and Mg^{2+} homeostasis, PTH promotes bone resorption (Fig. 9-6). Bone loss with a reduction in bone mineral density of the tibia and femur appears at weeks 4 to 6 of ALDOST and is accompanied by a reduction in bone strength (210,211). PTH-driven formation of $1,25(OH)_2D_3$ by the kidneys serves to promote Ca^{2+} absorption from the gut and kidneys. However, and as shown in Fig. 9-6, hyperparathyroidism leads to a Ca^{2+} loading of cells and a Ca^{2+}-mediated alteration in cell redox state with generation of reactive oxygen and nitrogen species within mitochondria and the cytosol.

Intracellular Ca^{2+} loading and induction of oxi/nitrosative stress involves diverse cells and tissues: lymphocytes and monocytes, platelets, endothelial and vascular smooth muscle cells, and cardiac and skeletal muscle (211–213). This Ca^{2+} overload of myocyte and nonmyocyte cells in the presence of heightened urinary and fecal losses of Ca^{2+} and reduced plasma-ionized $[Ca^{2+}]_o$ is termed a Ca^{2+} paradox. A Ca^{2+} loading of cells leads to their activation and accounts for a structural remodeling of vascular tissue and an electrical remodeling of cardiomyocytes and skeletal muscle. Such remodeling can lead to adverse cardiovascular events such as thrombosis with myocardial infarction or stroke; hypertension (HPT) due to abnormal vasomotor reactivity of media,

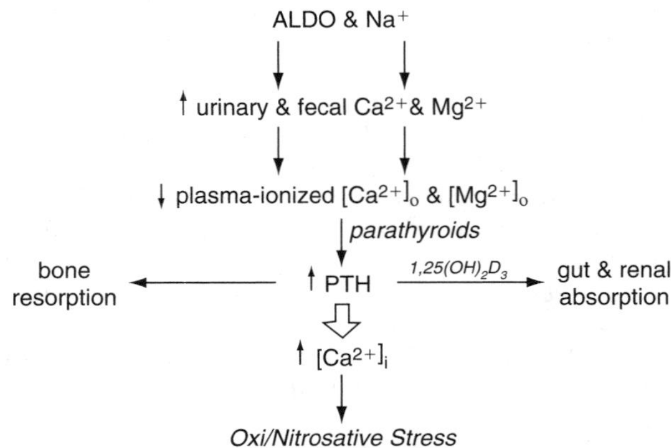

Figure 9-6 Aldosterone is accompanied by increased excretion of Ca^{2+} and Mg^{2+} in both urine and feces. A subsequent fall in plasma-ionized levels of these cations stimulates the parathyroid glands to release parathyroid hormone (PTH). The resultant hyperparathyroidism leads to intracellular Ca^{2+} loading and induction of oxi/nitrosative stress and cell activation.

dysfunction of the endothelium, and adventitial fibrosis; a heightened propensity for ventricular arrhythmias; and skeletal muscle atrophy. Insulin resistance accompanies HPT and may be fostered by reduced intracellular Mg^{2+} and Ca^{2+} loading of target cells.

Parathyroidectomy, performed prior to administering ALDOST, prevents or attenuates Ca^{2+} loading of PBMC, cardiac tissue, and skeletal muscle; the heightened production of H_2O_2 by PBMC and the fall in plasma α_1-antiproteinase activity, an inverse correlate of oxi/nitrosative stress; and the appearance of vascular lesions. The role of calcitropic hormones elaborated by the parathyroid glands, including PTH and ET-1, remain to be identified. ET receptor blockade prevents the appearance of oxi/nitrosative stress in vascular tissue and blood during deoxycorticosterone/salt treatment (DOCST) (198,199,214).

Thus, the parathyroid glands and their calcitropic hormones promote a Ca^{2+} loading of PBMC and other tissues and lead to the resultant alteration in their redox state. Reactive oxygen and nitrogen intermediates function as intracellular messengers to activate downstream signaling molecules to alter cell behavior and survival. They account for PBMC activation and the immunostimulatory state that eventuates in the proinflammatory vascular phenotype involving the coronary and systemic circulations. Hyperparathyroidism is held responsible for the systemic nature of the response and suggests activated immune cells are the circulating "factor" responsible for vascular remodeling in aldosteronism.

FUNCTIONAL CONSEQUENCES OF INTERSTITIAL REMODELING

Fibrillar collagen is the anatomic counterpart of theoretical elastic elements, which, together with a contractile element (myocytes), are invoked to explain basic principles of cardiac muscle mechanics. The alignment of collagen fibers with respect to cardiac myocytes determines whether they are considered in-parallel or in-series elastic elements. Both active (systolic) and passive (diastolic) tissue stiffness will be influenced by the amount and alignment of collagen fibers relative to myocytes; the configuration of collagen fibers; the ratio of type I/III collagens; and the degree of collagen cross-linking. These issues have been addressed elsewhere (215).

Diastolic Dysfunction

Postmortem studies of diseased hearts with known diastolic dysfunction have identified abnormal collagen accumulation, as have endomyocardial biopsy tissues (216–219). Fibrillar type I collagen with its tensile strength of steel is a recognized, important determinant of tissue stiffness. This has been systemically demonstrated in experimental models associated with or without fibrous tissue accumulation in association with or without myocyte hypertrophy. In rats with MI following coronary artery ligation, stiffness of noninfarcted papillary muscle rises in association with hydroxyproline content (51). Papillary muscle passive stiffness likewise is increased when its hydroxyproline concentration rises in association with the appearance of cardiac fibrosis in rats with genetic hypertension (220).

Prevention of tissue fibrosis by captopril abrogated this response in papillary muscle stiffness. When introduced after fibrosis was established, short-term captopril treatment was unable to regress fibrosis or to restore normal tissue stiffness (51,221). Longer-term lisinopril treatment of 14-week-old hypertensive rats, having established cardiac fibrosis and hypertrophy, was able to regress excess connective tissue and normalize ventricular stiffness. This was the case for a small dose of the ACE inhibitor that did not normalize arterial pressure or regress LVH and a larger dose that achieved these endpoints (151). This further underscores the importance of collagen on tissue stiffness. In senescent spontaneously hypertensive rats (SHRs) with more advanced fibrosis, long-term lisinopril treatment was able to partially regress fibrosis and improve diastolic stiffness through activation of latent myocardial collagenase (222). A further discussion of the impact of fibrous tissue on diastolic function can be found elsewhere (223–225).

Matrix accumulation in diseased hearts is dependent upon collagen-producing myoFb having α-smooth muscle actin microfilaments. Together with cell–cell connections and cell–matrix connections, these cells impart fibrous tissue with contractile behavior that resembles vascular smooth muscle cells. Agents that promote smooth muscle contraction induce a similar response in fibrous tissue. Figure 9-3 demonstrates AngII-induced contraction of valve leaflet tissue. The same has been found for infarct scar tissue (44) and subcutaneous pouch tissue (226). This dynamic nature of fibrous tissue may explain acute responses to infusion of AngII or ACE inhibitor. In the normal rat left ventricle, intracoronary administration of AngII does not raise end-diastolic pressure (149). In the hypertrophied left ventricle that accompanies suprarenal aortic banding, on the other hand, and where cardiac fibrosis coincident with high-density AngII receptor binding and myoFb at these sites are expected (*vide supra*), AngII is associated with an acute rise in filling pressure that can be prevented by losartan (149). This response in diastolic distensibility could therefore be interpreted as fibrous tissue contraction. AngII-induced alterations in abnormal cardiac myocyte calcium handling cannot be discounted.

In human hypertensive heart disease, where end-diastolic pressure is elevated and myocardial fibrosis is expected (216,217), left coronary artery infusion of enalapril leads to an acute fall in filling pressure (227). Similarly, an intracoronary infusion of enalaprilat leads to an acute reduction in left ventricular end-diastolic pressure and improvement in diastolic distensibility in patients with LVH and significant aortic valvular stenosis (228), where myocardial fibrosis is a well-recognized accompaniment (219,229,230). An acute reduction in end-diastolic pressure and diastolic wall stress accompanies intravenous benazeprilat in patients with coronary artery disease and previous transmural MI (231).

These responses to ACE inhibitor, where systemic effects were negligible, suggest an acute improvement in diastolic dysfunction that may be related to relaxation of fibrous tissue tonicity and the tension it exerts within diseased myocardium.

Systolic Dysfunction

Failure of the heart as a muscular pump can have diverse pathophysiological origins. An adverse accumulation of extracellular matrix is one. Myocardial contractility, defined by the slope of the developed stress–length relation observed in the isovolumetrically beating ventricle or its equivalent (end-systolic stress–strain relation) in the ejecting ventricle, is depressed when tissue collagen concentration rises fourfold or more (232,233). Papillary muscle-developed isometric stress and maximum rate of stress development are reduced in association with the appearance of interstitial fibrosis in the infarcted rat heart or in rats with genetic hypertension (51,220,221). Decompensated heart failure in these hypertensive rats, manifested by tachypnea and pleural and pericardial effusions, is coincident with a marked upregulation of genes encoding for matrix components (fibronectin, type I and III collagens) and the fibrogenic cytokine TGF-β (234). Fibrous tissue that envelopes myocytes further serves to hinder myocyte stretch and force development, and this would lead to a reduction in myocyte cross-sectional area, or atrophy, that further impairs contractile function (161,221).

CARDIOPROTECTIVE INTERVENTIONS

Prevention trials are designed to attenuate or completely prevent the appearance of fibrosis. Various pharmacological interventions have been used with this objective in mind. Such strategies contrast to treatment trials, where fibrosis is established and an intervention is introduced to determine whether it will regress and perhaps normalize tissue structure by removing fibrosis.

ACE inhibitors have proven an effective management strategy in patients with ischemic cardiomyopathy (ICM) and chronic heart failure. This includes patients with and without an activation of the circulating RAAS and who accordingly were symptomatic or asymptomatic, respectively, despite comparable reductions in ejection fraction of 35% or less (1,2). Efficacy of ACEI intervention on the progressive nature of ICM is likely multifactorial. Herein, evidence is reviewed and the perspective raised as to a favorable outcome related to prevented adverse structural remodeling of the interstitium, or extracellular matrix.

Directed at Local Angiotensin II

Evidence supporting a contribution of locally produced AngII in regulating myoFb collagen synthesis is obtained using pharmacological probes that interfere with local AngII generation (i.e., ACEI) or occupancy of its AT_1 receptor when the circulating RAAS has not been activated. Collagen formation in the heart and vasculature is rapid soon after birth. In 4-week-old rats treated with enalapril for 6 weeks, collagen formation in both the right and left ventricles, aorta, and superior mesenteric artery is retarded compared to untreated, normal 10-week-old controls (235). In 4-week-old SHRs, a small dose of quinapril, which did not prevent the ultimate appearance of hypertension, prevents the expected rise in aortic collagen volume fraction compared to untreated 30-week-old SHRs (236). Each of these studies implicates local AngII in regulating collagen formation in the heart and vasculature.

Captopril and enalapril, begun at or close to the onset of MI, have each reduced infarct size, expansion, and thinning, and have attenuated a rise in hydroxyproline concentration at the infarct site in dogs with coronary artery occlusion (237–239). The potential contribution of reduced bradykinin degradation to tissue repair (and which would accompany ACEI) is under investigation. Several studies suggest BK is released post-MI (240–242). A BK_2 receptor antagonist (Hoe140 or icatibant) accentuates collagen accumulation remote to the MI site (243).

Losartan, begun on day 1 after coronary artery ligation and in a dose that reduced AT_1 receptor binding by 50%, reduces infarct scar area (244). Moreover, the expected rise in tissue AngII concentration found at the infarct site 3 weeks postcoronary artery ligation is markedly attenuated by either delapril or TCV-116, an AT_1 Ra, introduced on postoperative day 1 (110). These findings raise the prospect that the number of myoFb or their AngII-generating activity per cell at sites of repair may be influenced by AngII. Other studies (120,245) have not found an AT_1 Ra, introduced at or soon after coronary artery ligation, to influence fibrosis post-MI. An explanation for these divergent findings is presently unclear.

Fibrous tissue formation at sites remote to MI has also been examined in response to these pharmacological interventions. Perindopril, given 1 week after MI, attenuates the endomyocardial fibrosis that appears in the non-necrotic segment of the rat left ventricle (109). Captopril, commenced at the time of coronary artery ligation, prevents the expected fibrosis of noninfarcted left and right ventricles (38,246) and proliferation of fibroblasts and endothelial cells that appears at remote sites 1 and 2 weeks following MI (38). Under these circumstances, captopril prevents the rise in LV end-diastolic pressure that appears in untreated or propranolol-treated rats; captopril also reduces inducibility of ventricular arrhythmias in this model (246). When initiated 3 weeks post-MI, well after the tissue repair process has developed, captopril does not prevent fibrosis remote to the infarct site or the rise in ventricular stiffness (51). Losartan prevents fibrosis at remote sites (39,244,247) but not the cellular proliferation that appears (39). Other investigators did not find an inhibition of types I and III collagen mRNA expression at remote sites (46,248) and have suggested posttranslational modification in collagen turnover to explain why fibrosis fails to appear at remote sites (248).

ACEI and/or AT_1 Ra prevent the appearance of fibrosis in diverse organs with experimentally induced or naturally occurring tissue injury and where circulating RAAS is not activated. These include pericardial fibrosis post-pericardiotomy (105); tubulointerstitial fibrosis associated with unilateral urethral obstruction (90,249–254), toxic nephropathy (255–257), remnant kidney (258–261), or renal injury following irradiation (262); cardiovascular and glomerulosclerosis that appear in stroke-prone SHRs (263–266); interstitial pulmonary fibrosis that follows irradiation (267–269) or monocrotaline administration (270); and subcutaneous fibrous tissue pouch model (271). A more detailed review of

AngII and tissue repair involving systemic organs can be found elsewhere (18).

Attenuation of fibrous tissue formation by ACEI and by AT_1 Ra, in particular, in diverse organs with various forms of injury supports the importance of local AngII in promoting fibrosis. Further evidence that this peptide influences collagen turnover has been obtained in cultured adult rat cardiac fibroblasts and myoFb. In serum-deprived cells, incubation with AngII in pathophysiologic concentrations increases type I collagen mRNA expression and synthesis and reduces collagenolytic activity of culture medium (142,272–274). The importance of AngII-induced expression of TGF-β_1 in contributing to this fibrogenic response has been suggested (18,35,86,275).

Directed at Circulating Hormones

Based on the importance of circulating hormones and ventricular workload in regulating myocyte growth and reactive myocardial fibrosis, various pharmacological probes have been used to determine if either or both of these responses could be prevented. Agents were administered either before or at the time of model induction and continued thereafter. Captopril prevented arterial hypertension, LVH, and fibrosis in rats with unilateral renal ischemia (168). Spironolactone, an ALDO receptor antagonist, was used to address the importance of this steroid hormone in contributing to cardiac fibrosis. A small, nonantihypertensive dose of spironolactone was compared to a larger dose with antihypertensive effects. Each dose was able to prevent fibrosis irrespective of the presence of arterial hypertension and LVH.

The absence of ventricular pressure or volume overload and the development of hypertrophy does not preclude the appearance of myocardial fibrosis. The increased collagen volume fraction that was found in the normotensive, nonhypertrophied right ventricle in the aforementioned models of primary or secondary hyperaldosteronism or chronic DOCA administration underscores this point (Fig. 9-2). This is further emphasized by the absence of right ventricular fibrosis in the arterial hypertension that is not associated with an elevation in plasma renin activity or circulating ALDO, such as that seen with infrarenal aorta banding. These in vivo findings therefore provide additional confirmation as to the importance of circulating hormones of the RAAS in mediating the disproportionate fibrous tissue response.

Microscopic scars replace necrotic cardiac myocytes that have been lost from the myocardium. These scars are morphologically distinct from the perivascular/interstitial fibrosis previously considered and are found in both ventricles in states of primary or secondary mineralocorticoid excess. Their presence in the right ventricle indicates that they have no relationship to the hypertrophic process or to hemodynamic overload. This perspective is confirmed by previous studies (276) that examined cardiac myocyte necrosis in response to endogenous or exogenous elevations in plasma AngII. Necrosis occurred on day 1 following elevation in endogenous circulating AngII induced by unilateral renal ischemia. Necrosis was also seen on day 1 when plasma AngII was increased by the administration of a suppressor dose of AngII. The necrosis of myocytes, detected by antimyosin antibody labeling, could be prevented by captopril in renovascular hypertension. Necrosis, on the other hand, was not observed with infrarenal aorta banding.

In addition to the early cytotoxicity that accompanies elevations in plasma AngII, another factor is involved in the appearance of microscopic scarring that accompanies 4 weeks or more of mineralocorticoid excess. Here, myocyte necrosis is related to enhanced urinary potassium excretion and myocardial potassium depletion that accompany chronic elevations in plasma ALDO or DOCA (277,278).

Replacement fibrosis in rats administered ALDO for 8 weeks could be prevented by spironolactone (279). Amiloride, a potassium-sparing diuretic devoid of ALDO receptor antagonistic properties, prevents scarring in rats with primary hyperaldosteronism (280). Unlike spironolactone, however, amiloride did not prevent the reactive perivascular/interstitial fibrosis that also appears in these hearts. These findings broaden our understanding of the multifactorial nature of myocardial fibrosis, which includes a reactive component, associated with mineralocorticoid excess, and a reparative (replacement) component that follows myocyte necrosis due to cytotoxicity of elevated plasma AngII and reduced stores of intracellular potassium. The preceding results of the prevention trials using either ACE inhibition or ALDO receptor antagonism indicate that it is possible to prevent the reactive and replacement fibrosis that appears in the myocardium associated with unilateral renal ischemia or hyperaldosteronism. These cardioprotective properties suggest these agents would be useful in preventing fibrosis and ventricular dysfunction in patients with heart failure or arterial hypertension.

SUMMARY

The cardiac interstitium, often referred to as an extracellular space, normally includes a fibrillar collagen network; a population of pluripotent, undifferentiated fibroblasts; and both soluble and matrix-bound signals that regulate cell growth and behavior. An adverse accumulation of fibrillar collagen occurs within the interstitium and contributes to the appearance and progressive nature of heart failure in ICM. Such fibrosis remote to an infarct is considered the major component to the adverse structural remodeling of the failing human heart with ICM.

Tissue repair, a fundamental property of vascularized tissues, takes place within the interstitium following MI. It is driven by cell–cell signaling between invading macrophages and fibroblasts, whose differentiation and replication result in a population of phenotypically transformed fibroblasts termed myofibroblasts (the cells of fibrogenesis). They possess a diverse portfolio of activities: their expression of α-smooth muscle actin confers fibrous tissue with contractile behavior that contributes to scar tissue thinning and stiffness; their expression of components requisite to Ang peptide generation leads to *de novo* generation of AngII, whose autocrine properties include induction of the fibrogenic cytokine TGF-β; and their persistence and sustained collagen turnover at sites of repair leads to a progressive remodeling of the interstitium with adverse matrix accumulation at and remote to the MI.

The growth and behavior of fibroblasts and fibroblast-like cells are not regulated by hemodynamic factors. Instead, locally produced AngII at sites of repair and inappropriate (relative to intravascular volume and dietary sodium intake), chronic activation of the circulating RAAS with elevations in plasma AngII and ALDO contribute to matrix accumulation in ICM. Pharmacological interventions aimed at preventing cardiac fibrosis at sites remote to MI have therefore focused on this peptide and steroid. They have included ACEI and corresponding receptor antagonists. Such cardioprotective strategies have proven effective in attenuating fibrous tissue formation in the infarcted rat heart when initiated soon after myocardial infarction.

Congestive heart failure (CHF) is a clinical syndrome that features signs and symptoms that arise from Na^+ and water retention. Additionally, the neurohormonal activation of CHF gives rise to a systemic illness that features an altered redox state in multiple cells, tissues, and blood; elevations in circulating chemokines with cytokines and activated lymphocytes and monocytes; and a wasting of tissues that includes bone. As a result of this neuroendocrine–immune interface gone awry, CHF represents a proinflammatory phenotype that includes the structure of the cardiac interstitium. Based on experimental studies in rats and patients with primary aldosteronism, it is likely that hyperparathyroidism complicates the secondary aldosteronism of CHF. The attendant Ca^{2+} loading of diverse cells, mediated by calcitropic hormones, can lead to cardiac fibrosis.

REFERENCES

1. The SOLVD Investigators. Effect of enalapril on survival in patients with reduced left ventricular ejection fractions and congestive heart failure. *N Engl J Med.* 1991;325:293–302.
2. The SOLVD Investigators. Effect of enalapril on mortality and the development of heart failure in asymptomatic patients with reduced left ventricular ejection fractions. *N Engl J Med.* 1992;327:685–691.
3. Konstam MA, Rousseau MF, Kronenberg MW, et al. Effects of the angiotensin converting enzyme inhibitor enalapril on the long-term progression of left ventricular dysfunction in patients with heart failure. SOLVD Investigators. *Circulation.* 1992;86:431–438.
4. Gaudron P, Eilles C, Kugler I, et al. Progressive left ventricular dysfunction and remodeling after myocardial infarction. Potential mechanisms and early predictors. *Circulation.* 1993;87:755–763.
5. St. John Sutton M, Pfeffer MA, Plappert T, et al. Quantitative two-dimensional echocardiographic measurements are major predictors of adverse cardiovascular events after acute myocardial infarction. The protective effects of captopril. *Circulation.* 1994;89:68–75.
6. St. John Sutton M, Pfeffer MA, Moye L, et al. Cardiovascular death and left ventricular remodeling two years after myocardial infarction. Baseline predictors and impact of long-term use of captopril: information from the Survival and Ventricular Enlargement (SAVE) trial. *Circulation.* 1997;96:3294–3299.
7. Anversa P, Loud AV, Levicky V, et al. Left ventricular failure induced by myocardial infarction. I. Myocyte hypertrophy. *Am J Physiol.* 1985;248:H876–H882.
8. Anversa P, Kajstura J, Cheng W, et al. Insulin-like growth factor-1 and myocyte growth: the danger of a dogma. Part II. Induced myocardial growth: pathologic hypertrophy. *Cardiovasc Res.* 1996;32:484–495.
9. Anversa P, Kajstura J, Olivetti G. Myocyte death in heart failure. *Curr Opin Cardiol.* 1996;11:245–251.
10. Itoh G, Tamura J, Suzuki M, et al. DNA fragmentation of human infarcted myocardial cells demonstrated by the nick end labeling method and DNA agarose gel electrophoresis. *Am J Pathol.* 1995;146:1325–1331.
11. Bardales RH, Hailey LS, Xie SS, et al. In situ apoptosis assay for the detection of early acute myocardial infarction. *Am J Pathol.* 1996;149:821–829.
12. Saraste A, Pulkki K, Kallajoki M, et al. Apoptosis in human acute myocardial infarction. *Circulation.* 1997;95:320–323.
13. Cooper G, IV. Basic determinants of myocardial hypertrophy: a review of molecular mechanisms. *Annu Rev Med.* 1997;48:13–23.
14. Katz AM. Biochemical "defect" in the hypertrophied and failing heart. Deleterious or compensatory? *Circulation.* 1973;47: 1076–1079.
15. Weber KT. Extracellular matrix remodeling in heart failure. A role for de novo angiotensin II generation. *Circulation.* 1997;96: 4065–4082.
16. Beltrami CA, Finato N, Rocco M, et al. Structural basis of end-stage failure in ischemic cardiomyopathy in humans. *Circulation.* 1994;89:151–163.
17. Volders PGA, Willems IEMG, Cleutjens JPM, et al. Interstitial collagen is increased in the non-infarcted human myocardium after myocardial infarction. *J Mol Cell Cardiol.* 1993;25:1317–1323.
18. Weber KT. Fibrosis, a common pathway to organ failure: angiotensin II and tissue repair. *Semin Nephrol.* 1997;17:467–491.
19. Caulfield JB. Alterations in cardiac collagen with hypertrophy. In: Tarazi RC, Dunbar JB, eds. *Cardiac Hypertrophy in Hypertension.* New York: Raven Press; 1983: 49–57. (Katz AM, ed. Perspectives in cardiovascular research series).
20. Factor SM, Robinson TF. Comparative connective tissue structure-function relationships in biologic pumps. *Lab Invest.* 1988;58:150–156.
21. Weber KT. Cardiac interstitium: extracellular space of the myocardium. In: Fozzard HA, Haber E, Jennings RB, et al, eds. *The Heart and Cardiovascular System.* 2nd ed. New York: Raven Press; 1991:1465–1480.
22. Weber KT, Janicki JS, Pick R, et al. Collagen in the hypertrophied, pressure-overloaded myocardium. *Circulation.* 1987;75(Suppl I): I-40–I-47.
23. Frank JS, Langer GA. The myocardial interstitium: its structure and its role in ionic exchange. *J Cell Biol.* 1974;60:586–601.
24. Burton AC. Relation of structure to function of the tissues of the wall of blood vessels. *Physiol Rev.* 1954;34:619–642.
25. Robinson TF, Geraci MA, Sonnenblick EH, et al. Coiled perimysial fibers of papillary muscle in rat heart: morphology, distribution, and changes in configuration. *Circ Res.* 1988;63:577–592.
26. Caulfield JB, Borg TK. The collagen network of the heart. *Lab Invest.* 1979;40:364–372.
27. Abrahams C, Janicki JS, Weber KT. Myocardial hypertrophy in *Macaca fascicularis*: structural remodeling of the collagen matrix. *Lab Invest.* 1987;56:676–683.
28. Robinson TF, Cohen-Gould L, Factor SM, et al. Structure and function of connective tissue in cardiac muscle: collagen types I and III in endomysial struts and pericellular fibers. *Scanning Microsc.* 1988;2:1005–1015.
29. Robinson TF, Cohen-Gould L, Factor SM. The skeletal framework of mammalian heart muscle: arrangement of inter- and pericellular connective tissue structures. *Lab Invest.* 1983;49:482–498.
30. Eghbali M, Czaja MJ, Zeyel M, et al. Collagen chain mRNAs in isolated heart cells from young and adult rats. *J Mol Cell Cardiol.* 1988;20:267–276.
31. Eghbali M, Blumenfeld OO, Seifter S, et al. Localization of types I, III, and IV collagen mRNAs in rat heart cells by *in situ* hybridization. *J Mol Cell Cardiol.* 1989;21:103–113.
32. Chakraborty A, Eghbali M. Collagenase activity in the normal rat myocardium: an immunohistochemical method. *Histochemistry* 1989;92:391–396.
33. Cotran RS, Kumar V, Robbins SL, eds. *Robbins' Pathologic Basis of Disease.* 4th ed. Philadelphia: WB Saunders; 1989: 1519.
34. Booz GW, Baker KM. Molecular signalling mechanisms controlling growth and function of cardiac fibroblasts. *Cardiovasc Res.* 1995;30:537–543.
35. Sharma HS, van Heugten HAA, Goedbloed MA, et al. Angiotensin II induced expression of transcription factors pre-

cedes increase in transforming growth factor-β1 mRNA in neonatal cardiac fibroblasts. *Biochem Biophys Res Commun.* 1994;205:105–112.

36. Puri PL, Avantaggiati ML, Burgio VL, et al. Reactive oxygen intermediates angiotensin II-induced c-Jun•c-Fos heterodimer DNA binding activity and proliferative hypertrophic responses in myogenic cells. *J Biol Chem.* 1995;270:22129–22134.
37. Crabos M, Roth M, Hahn AWA, et al. Characterization of angiotensin II receptors in cultured adult rat cardiac fibroblasts. *J Clin Invest.* 1994;93:2372–2378.
38. van Krimpen C, Smits JFM, Cleutjens JPM, et al. DNA synthesis in the non-infarcted cardiac interstitium after left coronary artery ligation in the rat heart: effects of captopril. *J Mol Cell Cardiol.* 1991;23:1245–1253.
39. Smits JFM, van Krimpen C, Schoemaker RG, et al. Angiotensin II receptor blockade after myocardial infarction in rats: effects on hemodynamics, myocardial DNA synthesis, and interstitial collagen content. *J Cardiovasc Pharmacol.* 1992;20:772–778.
40. Sun Y, Cleutjens JPM, Diaz-Arias AA, et al. Cardiac angiotensin converting enzyme and myocardial fibrosis in the rat. *Cardiovasc Res.* 1994;28:1423–1432.
41. Cleutjens JPM, Kandala JC, et al. Regulation of collagen degradation in the rat myocardium after infarction. *J Mol Cell Cardiol.* 1995;27:1281–1292.
42. Cleutjens JPM, Verluyten MJA, Smits JFM, et al. Collagen remodeling after myocardial infarction in the rat heart. *Am J Pathol.* 1995;147:325–338.
43. Knowlton AA, Connelly CM, Romo GM, et al. Rapid expression of fibronectin in the rabbit heart after myocardial infarction with and without reperfusion. *J Clin Invest.* 1992;89:1060–1068.
44. Willems IEMG, Havenith MG, De Mey JGR, et al. The α-smooth muscle actin-positive cells in healing human myocardial scars. *Am J Pathol.* 1994;145:868–875.
45. Sun Y, Weber KT. Angiotensin converting enzyme and myofibroblasts during tissue repair in the rat heart. *J Mol Cell Cardiol.* 1996;28:851–858.
46. Hanatani A, Yoshiyama M, Kim S, et al. Inhibition by angiotensin II type 1 receptor antagonist of cardiac phenotypic modulation after myocardial infarction. *J Mol Cell Cardiol.* 1995;27:1905–1914.
47. Whittaker P. Unravelling the mysteries of collagen and cicatrix after myocardial infarction. *Cardiovasc Res.* 1996;31:19–27.
48. Jugdutt BI, Amy RWM. Healing after myocardial infarction in the dog: changes in infarct hydroxyproline and topography. *J Am Coll Cardiol.* 1986;7:91–102.
49. McCormick RJ, Musch TI, Bergman BC, et al. Regional differences in LV collagen accumulation and mature cross-linking after myocardial infarction in rats. *Am J Physiol.* 1994;266: H354–H359.
50. Pelouch V, Dixon IMC, Sethi R, et al. Alteration of collagenous protein profile in congestive heart failure secondary to myocardial infarction. *Mol Cell Biochem.* 1993;129:121–131.
51. Litwin SE, Litwin CM, Raya TE, et al. Contractility and stiffness of noninfarcted myocardium after coronary ligation in rats. Effects of chronic angiotensin converting enzyme inhibition. *Circulation.* 1991;83:1028–1037.
52. Vane JR, Mitchell JA, Appleton I, et al. Inducible isoforms of cyclooxygenase and nitric-oxide synthase in inflammation. *Proc Natl Acad Sci USA.* 1994;91:2046–2050.
53. Stuehr DJ, Nathan CF. Nitric oxide. A macrophage product responsible for cytostasis and respiratory inhibition in tumor target cells. *J Exp Med.* 1989;169:1543–1555.
54. Albina JE, Cui S, Mateo RB, et al. Nitric oxide-mediated apoptosis in murine peritoneal macrophages. *J Immunol.* 1993;150: 5080–5085.
55. Klickstein LB, Kaempfer CE, Wintroub BU. The granulocyte-angiotensin system. Angiotensin I-converting activity of cathepsin G. *J Biol Chem.* 1982;257:15042–15046.
56. Silverstein E, Friedland J, Vuletin JC. Marked elevation of serum angiotension-converting enzyme and hepatic fibrosis containing long-spacing collagen fibrils in type 2 acute neuronopathic Gaucher's disease. *Am J Clin Pathol.* 1978;69:467–471.
57. Vracko R, Thorning D. Contractile cells in rat myocardial scar tissue. *Lab Invest.* 1991;65:214–227.
58. Campbell SE, Janicki JS, Weber KT. Temporal differences in fibroblast proliferation and phenotype expression in response to chronic administration of angiotensin II or aldosterone. *J Mol Cell Cardiol.* 1995;27:1545–1560.
59. Leslie KO, Taatjes DJ, Schwarz J, et al. Cardiac myofibroblasts express alpha smooth muscle actin during right ventricular pressure overload in the rabbit. *Am J Pathol.* 1991;139:207–216.
60. Bishop JE, Rhodes S, Laurent GJ, et al. Increased collagen synthesis and decreased collagen degradation in right ventricular hypertrophy induced by pressure overload. *Cardiovasc Res.* 1994;28:1581–1585.
61. Majno G. The story of the myofibroblasts. *Am J Surg Pathol.* 1979;3:535–542.
62. Sappino AP, Schürch W, Gabbiani G. Differentiation repertoire of fibroblastic cells: expression of cytoskeletal proteins as marker of phenotypic modulations. *Lab Invest.* 1990;63:144–161.
63. Skalli O, Schürch W, Seemayer T, et al. Myofibroblasts from diverse pathologic settings are heterogeneous in their content of actin isoforms and intermediate filament proteins. *Lab Invest.* 1989;60:275–285.
64. McCulloch CAG, Bordin S. Role of fibroblast subpopulations in periodontal physiology and pathology. *J Periodont Res.* 1991;26:144–154.
65. Filip DA, Radu A, Simionescu M. Interstitial cells of the heart valves possess characteristics similar to smooth muscle cells. *Circ Res.* 1986;59:310–320.
66. Gabbiani G, Hirschel BJ, Ryan GB, et al. Granulation tissue as a contractile organ. A study of structure and function. *J Exp Med.* 1972;135:719–734.
67. De Mey JGR, Fazzi GE. A smooth muscle-like component in rat myocardial infarcts [abstract]. *Hypertension.* 1996;28:696.
68. Desmouliére A, Geinoz A, Gabbiani F, et al. Transforming growth factor-β1 induces α-smooth muscle actin expression in granulation tissue myofibroblasts and in quiescent and growing cultured fibroblasts. *J Cell Biol.* 1993;122:103–111.
69. Thompson NL, Bazoberry F, Speir EH, et al. Transforming growth factor beta-1 in acute myocardial infarction in rats. *Growth Factors.* 1988;1:91–99.
70. Casscells W, Bazoberry F, Speir E, et al. Transforming growth factor-β1 in normal heart and in myocardial infarction. *Ann NY Acad Sci.* 1990;593:148–160.
71. Riches DWH. Macrophage involvement in wound repair, remodeling, and fibrosis. In: Clark RAF, ed. *The Molecular and Cellular Biology of Wound Repair.* 2nd ed. New York: Plenum Press; 1996: 95–141.
72. Zhang G, Moorhead PJ, el Nahas AM. Myofibroblasts and the progression of experimental glomerulonephritis. *Exp Nephrol.* 1995;3:308–318.
73. Singer II, Kawka DW, Kazazis DM, et al. In vivo co-distribution of fibronectin and actin fibers in granulation tissue: immunofluorescence and electron microscope studies of the fibronexus at the myofibroblast surface. *J Cell Biol.* 1984;98:2091–2106.
74. Bishop J, Greenbaum J, Gibson D, et al. Enhanced deposition of predominantly type I collagen in myocardial disease. *J Mol Cell Cardiol.* 1990;22:1157–1165.
75. Mukherjee D, Sen S. Collagen phenotypes during development and regression of myocardial hypertrophy in spontaneously hypertensive rats. *Circ Res.* 1990;67:1474–1480.
76. Weber KT, Janicki JS, Shroff SG, et al. Collagen remodeling of the pressure-overloaded, hypertrophied nonhuman primate myocardium. *Circ Res.* 1988;62:757–765.
77. Ohsato K, Shimizu M, Sugihara N, et al. Histopathological factors related to diastolic function in myocardial hypertrophy. *Jpn Circ J.* 1992;56:325–333.
78. Darby I, Skalli O, Gabbiani G. α-smooth muscle actin is transiently expressed by myofibroblasts during experimental wound healing. *Lab Invest.* 1990;63:21–29.
79. Desmouliére A, Redard M, Darby I, et al. Apoptosis mediates the decrease in cellularity during the transition between granulation tissue and scar. *Am J Pathol.* 1995;146:56–66.
80. Border WA, Ruoslahti E. Transforming growth factor-β in disease: the dark side of tissue repair. *J Clin Invest.* 1992;90:1–7.
81. Lawrence WT, Diegelmann RF. Growth factors in wound healing. *Clin Dermatol.* 1994;12:157–169.
82. Omura T, Kim S, Takeuchi K, et al. Transforming growth factor β_1 and extracellular matrix gene expression in isoprenaline induced cardiac hypertrophy: effects of inhibition of the renin-angiotensin system. *Cardiovasc Res.* 1994;28:1835–1842.

83. Sun Y, Zhang JQ, Zhang J, et al. Angiotensin II, transforming growth factor-β_1 and repair in the infarcted heart. *J Mol Cell Cardiol*. 1998;30:1559–1569.
84. Chua CC, Chua BHL, Zhao ZY, et al. Effect of growth factors on collagen metabolism in cultured human heart fibroblasts. *Connect Tissue Res*. 1991;26:271–281.
85. Sadoshima J, Izumo S. Molecular characterization of angiotensin II-induced hypertrophy of cardiac myocytes and hyperplasia of cardiac fibroblasts. Critical role of the AT_1 receptor subtype. *Circ Res*. 1993;73:413–423.
86. Campbell SE, Katwa LC. Angiotensin II stimulated expression of transforming growth factor-β_1 in cardiac fibroblasts and myofibroblasts. *J Mol Cell Cardiol*. 1997;29:1947–1958.
87. Everett AD, Tufro-McReddie A, Fisher A, et al. Angiotensin receptor regulates cardiac hypertrophy and transforming growth factor-β1 expression. *Hypertension*. 1994;23:587–592.
88. Hinglais N, Heudes D, Nicoletti A, et al. Colocalization of myocardial fibrosis and inflammatory cells in rats. *Lab Invest*. 1994;70:286–294.
89. Wardle N. Glomerulosclerosis: the final pathway is clarified, but can we deal with the triggers? *Nephron*. 1996;73:1–7.
90. Pimentel JL, Jr., Martinez-Maldonado M, Wilcox JN, et al. Regulation of renin-angiotensin system in unilateral ureteral obstruction. *Kidney Int*. 1993;44:390–400.
91. Sun Y, Ratajska A, Zhou G, et al. Angiotensin converting enzyme and myocardial fibrosis in the rat receiving angiotensin II or aldosterone. *J Lab Clin Med*. 1993;122:395–403.
92. Sun Y, Weber KT. Angiotensin II and aldosterone receptor binding in rat heart and kidney: response to chronic angiotensin II or aldosterone administration. *J Lab Clin Med*. 1993;122:404–411.
93. Sun Y, Ratajska A, Weber KT. Inhibition of angiotensin-converting enzyme and attenuation of myocardial fibrosis by lisinopril in rats receiving angiotensin II. *J Lab Clin Med*. 1995;126:95–101.
94. Sun Y, Ratajska A, Weber KT. Bradykinin receptor and tissue ACE binding in myocardial fibrosis: response to chronic angiotensin II or aldosterone administration in rats. *J Mol Cell Cardiol*. 1995;27:813–822.
95. Sun Y, Diaz-Arias AA, Weber KT. Angiotensin-converting enzyme, bradykinin and angiotensin II receptor binding in rat skin, tendon and heart valves: an in vitro quantitative autoradiographic study. *J Lab Clin Med*. 1994;123:372–377.
96. Allen AM, Yamada H, Mendelsohn FAO. In vitro autoradiographic localization of binding to angiotensin receptors in the rat heart. *Int J Cardiol*. 1990;28:25–33.
97. Yamada H, Fabris B, Allen AM, et al. Localization of angiotensin converting enzyme in rat heart. *Circ Res*. 1991;68:141–149.
98. Pinto JE, Viglione P, Saavedra JM. Autoradiographic localization and quantification of rat heart angiotensin converting enzyme. *Am J Hypertens*. 1991;4:321–326.
99. Danilov SM, Faerman AI, Printseva OY, et al. Immunohistochemical study of angiotensin-converting enzyme in human tissues using monoclonal antibodies. *Histochemistry*. 1987;87:487–490.
100. Katwa LC, Ratajska A, Cleutjens JPM, et al. Angiotensin converting enzyme and kininase-II-like activities in cultured valvular interstitial cells of the rat heart. *Cardiovasc Res*. 1995;29:57–64.
101. Nakajima Y, Miyazono K, Kato M, et al. Extracellular fibrillar structure of latent TGFβ binding protein-1: role in TGFβ-dependent endothelial-mesenchymal transformation during endocardial cushion tissue formation in mouse embryonic heart. *J Cell Biol*. 1997;136:193–204.
102. Potts JD, Vincent EB, Runyan RB, et al. Sense and antisense TGFβ3 mRNA levels correlate with cardiac valve induction. *Dev Dyn*. 1992;193:340–345.
103. Katwa LC, Tyagi SC, Campbell SE, et al. Valvular interstitial cells express angiotensinogen, cathepsin D, and generate angiotensin peptides. *Int J Biochem Cell Biol*. 1996;28:807–821.
104. Weber KT, Sun Y, Katwa LC. Myofibroblasts and local angiotensin II in rat cardiac tissue repair. *Int J Biochem Cell Biol*. 1997;29:31–42.
105. Sun Y, Weber KT. Angiotensin II receptor binding following myocardial infarction in the rat. *Cardiovasc Res*. 1994;28:1623–1628.
106. Sims DE. The pericyte—a review. *Tissue Cell*. 1986;18:153–174.
107. Hokimoto S, Yasue H, Fujimoto K, et al. Increased angiotensin converting enzyme activity in left ventricular aneurysm of patients after myocardial infarction. *Cardiovasc Res*. 1995;29:664–669.
108. Hirsch AT, Talsness CE, Schunkert H, et al. Tissue-specific activation of cardiac angiotensin converting enzyme in experimental heart failure. *Circ Res*. 1991;69:475–482.
109. Michel J-B, Lattion A-L, Salzmann J-L, et al. Hormonal and cardiac effects of converting enzyme inhibition in rat myocardial infarction. *Circ Res*. 1988;62:641–650.
110. Yamagishi H, Kim S, Nishikimi T, et al. Contribution of cardiac renin-angiotensin system to ventricular remodeling in myocardial-infarcted rats. *J Mol Cell Cardiol*. 1993;25:1369–1380.
111. Pinto YM, de Smet BG, van Gilst WH, et al. Selective and time related activation of the cardiac renin-angiotensin system after experimental heart failure: relation to ventricular function and morphology. *Cardiovasc Res*. 1993;27:1933–1938.
112. Hodsman GP, Kohzuki M, Howes LG, et al. Neurohumoral responses to chronic myocardial infarction in rats. *Circulation*. 1988;78:376–381.
113. Falkenhahn M, Franke F, Bohle RM, et al. Cellular distribution of angiotensin-converting enzyme after myocardial infarction. *Hypertension*. 1995;25:219–226.
114. Benjamin IJ, Jalil JE, Tan LB, et al. Isoproterenol-induced myocardial fibrosis in relation to myocyte necrosis. *Circ Res*. 1989;65:657–670.
115. Sun Y, Weber KT. Angiotensin-converting enzyme and wound healing in diverse tissues of the rat. *J Lab Clin Med*. 1996;127:94–101.
116. Lefroy DC, Wharton J, Crake T, et al. Regional changes in angiotensin II receptor density after experimental myocardial infarction. *J Mol Cell Cardiol*. 1996;28:429–440.
117. Sechi LA, Griffin CA, Grady EF, et al. Characterization of angiotensin II receptor subtypes in rat heart. *Circ Res*. 1992;71:1482–1489.
118. Regitz-Zagrosek V, Friedel N, Heymann A, et al. Regulation, chamber localization, and subtype distribution of angiotensin II receptors in human hearts. *Circulation*. 1995;91:1461–1471.
119. Sun Y, Weber KT. Cells expressing angiotensin II receptors in fibrous tissue of rat heart. *Cardiovasc Res*. 1996;31:518–525.
120. Nio Y, Matsubara H, Murasawa S, et al. Regulation of gene transcription of angiotensin II receptor subtypes in myocardial infarction. *J Clin Invest*. 1995;95:46–54.
121. Makino N, Hata T, Sugano M, et al. Regression of hypertrophy after myocardial infarction is produced by the chronic blockade of angiotensin type I receptor in rats. *J Mol Cell Cardiol*. 1996;28:507–517.
122. Kimura B, Sumners C, Phillips MI. Changes in skin angiotensin II receptors in rats during wound healing. *Biochem Biophys Res Commun*. 1992;187:1083–1090.
123. Phillips MI, Kimura B, Gyurko R. Angiotensin receptor stimulation of transforming growth factor-β in rat skin and wound healing. In: Saavedra JM, Pieter BMWM, eds. *Angiotensin Receptors*. New York: Plenum Press; 1994: 377–396.
124. Viswanathan M, Saavedra JM. Expression of angiotensin II AT2 receptors in the rat skin during experimental wound healing. *Peptides*. 1992;13:783–786.
125. Ou R, Sun Y, Ganjam VK, Weber KT. In situ production of angiotensin II by fibrosed rat pericardium. *J Mol Cell Cardiol*. 1996;28:1319–1327.
126. Sun Y, Ramires FJA, Weber KT. Fibrosis of atria and great vessels in response to angiotensin II or aldosterone infusion. *Cardiovasc Res*. 1997;35:138–147.
127. Schunkert H, Ingelfinger JR, Hirsch AT, et al. Feedback regulation of angiotensin converting enzyme activity and mRNA levels by angiotensin II. *Circ Res*. 1993;72:312–318.
128. Weber KT, Sun Y, Katwa LC, et al. Connective tissue: a metabolic entity? *J Mol Cell Cardiol*. 1995;27:107–120.
129. Allen RKA, Chai SY, Dunbar MS, et al. In vitro autoradiographic localization of angiotensin-converting enzyme in sarcoid lymph nodes. *Chest*. 1986;90:315–320.
130. Studer R, Reinecke H, Müller B, et al. Increased angiotensin-I converting enzyme gene expression in the failing human heart. Quantification by competitive RNA polymerase chain reaction. *J Clin Invest*. 1994;94:301–310.
131. Campbell DJ, Habener JF. Cellular localization of angiotensinogen gene expression in brown adipose tissue and mesentery:

quantification of messenger ribonucleic acid abundance using hybridization in situ. *Endocrinology.* 1987;121:1616–1626.
132. Cassis LA, Lynch KR, Peach MJ. Localization of angiotensinogen messenger RNA in rat aorta. *Circ Res.* 1988;62:1259–1262.
133. Sawa H, Tokuchi F, Mochizuki N, et al. Expression of the angiotensinogen gene and localization of its protein in the human heart. *Circulation.* 1992;86:138–146.
134. Dostal DE, Rothblum KN, Chernin MI, et al. Intracardiac detection of angiotensinogen and renin: a localized renin-angiotensin system in neonatal rat heart. *Am J Physiol.* 1992;263:C838–C850.
135. Dostal DE, Rothblum KN, Conrad KM, et al. Detection of angiotensin I and II in cultured rat cardiac myocytes and fibroblasts. *Am J Physiol.* 1992;263:C851–C863.
136. von Lutterotti N, Catanzaro DF, Sealey JE, et al. Renin is not synthesized by cardiac and extrarenal vascular tissues. A review of experimental evidence. *Circulation.* 1994;89:458–470.
137. Danser AHJ, Koning MMG, Admiraal PJJ, et al. Production of angiotensins I and II at tissue sites in intact pigs. *Am J Physiol.* 1992;263:H429–H437.
138. Danser AHJ, Koning MMG, Admiraal PJJ, et al. Metabolism of angiotensin I by different tissues in the intact animal. *Am J Physiol.* 1992;263:H418–H428.
139. Danser AHJ, van Katz JP, Admiraal PJJ, et al. Cardiac renin and angiotensins: uptake from plasma versus in situ synthesis. *Hypertension* 1994;24:37–48.
140. Campbell DJ, Kladis A, Duncan AM. Nephrectomy, converting enzyme inhibition, and angiotensin peptides. *Hypertension.* 1993;22:513–522.
141. Wintroub BU, Klickstein LB, Dzau VJ, et al. Granulocyte-angiotensin system. Identification of angiotensinogen as the plasma protein substrate of leukocyte cathepsin G. *Biochemistry.* 1984;23:227–232.
142. Katwa LC, Campbell SE, Tyagi SC, et al. Cultured myofibroblasts generate angiotensin peptides de novo. *J Mol Cell Cardiol.* 1997;29:1375–1386.
143. Passier RCJJ, Smits JFM, Verluyten MJA, et al. Activation of angiotensin-converting enzyme expression in infarct zone following myocardial infarction. *Am J Physiol.* 1995;269: H1268–H1276.
144. Iwai N, Inagami T, Ohmichi N, et al. Renin is expressed in rat macrophage/monocyte cells. *Hypertension.* 1996;27:399–403.
145. Zhang X, Dostal DE, Reiss K, et al. Identification and activation of autocrine renin-angiotensin system in adult ventricular myocytes. *Am J Physiol.* 1995;269:H1791–H1802.
146. Francis GS, Benedict C, Johnstone DE, et al. Comparison of neuroendocrine activation in patients with left ventricular dysfunction with and without congestive heart failure: a substudy of the Studies of Left Ventricular Dysfunction (SOLVD). *Circulation* 1990;82:1724–1729.
147. Swedberg K, Eneroth P, Kjekshus J, et al. Hormones regulating cardiovascular function in patients with severe congestive heart failure and their relation to mortality. CONSENSUS Trial Study Group. *Circulation.* 1990;82:1730–1736.
148. Tufro-McReddie A, Chevalier RL, Everett AD, et al. Decreased perfusion pressure modulates renin and ANG II type 1 receptor gene expression in the rat kidney. *Am J Physiol.* 1993;264:R696–R702.
149. Lopez JJ, Lorell BH, Ingelfinger JR, et al. Distribution and function of cardiac angiotensin AT_1- and AT_2-receptor subtypes in hypertrophied rat hearts. *Am J Physiol.* 1994;267:H844–H852.
150. Brilla CG, Pick R, Tan LB, et al. Remodeling of the rat right and left ventricle in experimental hypertension. *Circ Res.* 1990;67: 1355–1364.
151. Brilla CG, Janicki JS, Weber KT. Impaired diastolic function and coronary reserve in genetic hypertension: role of interstitial fibrosis and medial thickening of intramyocardial coronary arteries. *Circ Res.* 1991;69:107–115.
152. Bartosova D, Chvapil M, Korecky B, et al. The growth of the muscular and collagenous parts of the rat heart in various forms of cardiomegaly. *J Physiol.* 1969;200:285–295.
153. Michel JB, Salzmann JL, Ossondo Nlom M, et al. Morphometric analysis of collagen network and plasma perfused capillary bed in the myocardium of rats during evolution of cardiac hypertrophy. *Basic Res Cardiol.* 1986;81:142–154.
154. Weber KT, Brilla CG. Pathological hypertrophy and cardiac interstitium: fibrosis and renin-angiotensin-aldosterone system. *Circulation.* 1991;83:1849–1865.
155. Tomanek RJ, Taunton CA, Liskop KS. Relationship between age, chronic exercise, and connective tissue of the heart. *J Gerontol.* 1972;27:33–38.
156. Gilbert PL, Siegel RJ, Melmed S, et al. Cardiac morphology in rats with growth hormone-producing tumours. *J Mol Cell Cardiol.* 1985;17:805–811.
157. Bonnin CM, Sparrow MP, Taylor RR. Increased protein synthesis and degradation in the dog heart during thyroxine administration. *J Mol Cell Cardiol.* 1983;15:245–250.
158. Silver MA, Pick R, Brilla CG, et al. Reactive and reparative fibrosis in the hypertrophied rat left ventricle: two experimental models of myocardial fibrosis. *Cardiovasc Res.* 1990;24: 741–747.
159. Weber KT, Janicki JS, Pick R, et al. Myocardial fibrosis and pathologic hypertrophy in the rat with renovascular hypertension. *Am J Cardiol.* 1990;65:1G–7G.
160. Doering CW, Jalil JE, Janicki JS, et al. Collagen network remodeling and diastolic stiffness of the rat left ventricle with pressure overload hypertrophy. *Cardiovasc Res.* 1988;22:686–695.
161. Jalil JE, Doering CW, Janicki JS, et al. Fibrillar collagen and myocardial stiffness in the intact hypertrophied rat left ventricle. *Circ Res.* 1989;64:1041–1050.
162. Chapman D, Weber KT, Eghbali M. Regulation of fibrillar collagen types I and III and basement membrane type IV collagen gene expression in pressure overloaded rat myocardium. *Circ Res.* 1990;67:787–794.
163. Averill DB, Ferrario CM, Tarazi RC, et al. Cardiac performance in rats with renal hypertension. *Circ Res.* 1976;38:280–288.
164. Willems IEMG, Havenith MG, Smits JFM, et al. Structural alterations in heart valves during left ventricular pressure overload in the rat. *Lab Invest.* 1994;71:127–133.
165. Goldblatt H. Experimental hypertension induced by renal ischemia (Harvey Lecture). *Bull NY Acad Med.* 1938;14:523–553.
166. Selye H. The general adaptation syndrome and the diseases of adaptation. *J Clin Endocrinol.* 1946;6:117–230.
167. Hall CE, Hall O. Hypertension and hypersalimentation. I. Aldosterone hypertension. *Lab Invest.* 1965;14:285–294.
168. Jalil JE, Janicki JS, Pick R, et al. Coronary vascular remodeling and myocardial fibrosis in the rat with renovascular hypertension: response to captopril. *Am J Hypertens.* 1991;4:51–55.
169. Nicoletti A, Mandet C, Challah M, et al. Mediators of perivascular inflammation in the left ventricle of renovascular hypertensive rats. *Cardiovasc Res.* 1996;31:585–595.
170. Nicoletti A, Heudes D, Hinglais N, et al. Left ventricular fibrosis in renovascular hypertensive rats. Effect of losartan and spironolactone. *Hypertension.* 1995;26:101–111.
171. Regan CP, Anderson PG, Bishop SP, et al. Captopril prevents vascular and fibrotic changes but not cardiac hypertrophy in aortic-banded rats. *Am J Physiol.* 1996;271:H906–H913.
172. Linz W, Schaper J, Wiemer G, et al. Ramipril prevents left ventricular hypertrophy with myocardial fibrosis without blood pressure reduction: a one year study in rats. *Br J Pharmacol.* 1992;107:970–975.
173. Johnson RJ, Alpers CE, Yoshimura A, et al. Renal injury from angiotensin II-mediated hypertension. *Hypertension.* 1992;19: 464–474.
174. Crawford DC, Chobanian AV, Brecher P. Angiotensin II induces fibronectin expression associated with cardiac fibrosis in the rat. *Circ Res.* 1994;74:727–739.
175. Kim S, Ohta K, Hamaguchi A, et al. Angiotensin II induces cardiac phenotypic modulation and remodeling in vivo in rats. *Hypertension.* 1995;25:1252–1259.
176. Weber KT, Sun Y, Guarda E. Nonclassic actions of angiotensin II and aldosterone in nonclassic target tissue (the heart): relevance to hypertensive heart disease. In: Laragh JH, Brenner BM, eds. *Hypertension: Pathophysiology, Diagnosis, and Management.* 2nd ed. New York: Raven Press; 1995: 2203–2223.
177. Hamawaki M, Coffman TM, Lashus A, et al. Pressure-overload hypertrophy is unabated in mice devoid of AT_{1A} receptors. *Am J Physiol.* 1998;274:H868–H873.
178. Harada K, Komuro I, Shiojima I, et al. Pressure overload induced cardiac hypertrophy in angiotensin II type 1A receptor knockout mice. *Circulation.* 1998;97:1952–1959.
179. Ohkubo N, Matsubara H, Nozawa Y, et al. Angiotensin type 2 receptors are reexpressed by cardiac fibroblasts from failing myopathic hamster hearts and inhibit cell growth and fibrillar collagen metabolism. *Circulation* 1997;96:3954–3962.

180. Nakajima M, Hutchinson HG, Fuginaga M, et al. The angiotensin II type 2 (AT2) antagonizes the growth effects of the AT1 receptor: gain-of-function study using gene transfer. *Proc Natl Acad Sci USA*. 1995;92:10663–10667.
181. Stoll M, Steckelings UM, Paul M, et al. The angiotensin AT2-receptor mediates inhibition of cell proliferation in coronary endothelial cells. *J Clin Invest*. 1995;95:651–657.
182. Brilla CG, Weber KT. Mineralocorticoid excess, dietary sodium and myocardial fibrosis. *J Lab Clin Med*. 1992;120:893–901.
183. Campbell SE, Diaz-Arias AA, Weber KT. Fibrosis of the human heart and systemic organs in adrenal adenoma. *Blood Press*. 1992;1:149–156.
184. Robert V, Van Thiem N, Cheav SL, et al. Increased cardiac types I and III collagen mRNAs in aldosterone-salt hypertension. *Hypertension*. 1994;24:30–36.
185. Robert V, Silvestre JS, Charlemagne D, et al. Biological determinants of aldosterone-induced cardiac fibrosis in rats. *Hypertension*. 1995;26:971–978.
186. Young M, Fullerton M, Dilley R, et al. Mineralocorticoids, hypertension, and cardiac fibrosis. *J Clin Invest*. 1994;93:2578–2583.
187. Young M, Head G, Funder J. Determinants of cardiac fibrosis in experimental hypermineralocorticoid states. *Am J Physiol*. 1995;269:E657–E662.
188. Gómez-Sánchez EP. Mineralocorticoid modulation of central control of blood pressure. *Steroids*. 1995;60:69–72.
189. Lombes M, Oblin M-E, Gasc J-M, et al. Immunohistochemical and biochemical evidence for a cardiovascular mineralocorticoid receptor. *Circ Res*. 1992;71:503–510.
190. Lombès M, Alfaidy N, Eugene E, et al. Prerequisite for cardiac aldosterone action. Mineralocorticoid receptor and 11β-hydroxysteroid dehydrogenase in the human heart. *Circulation*. 1995;92:175–182.
191. Pearce P, Funder JW. High affinity aldosterone binding sites (type I receptors) in rat heart. *Clin Exp Pharmacol Physiol*. 1987;14:859–866.
192. Meyer WJ, III, Nichols NR. Mineralocorticoid binding in cultured smooth muscle cells and fibroblasts from rat aorta. *J Steroid Biochem*. 1981;14:1157–1168.
193. Slight S, Ganjam VK, Nonneman DJ, et al. Glucocorticoid metabolism in the cardiac interstitium: 11β-hydroxysteroid dehydrogenase activity in cardiac fibroblasts. *J Lab Clin Med*. 1993;122:180–187.
194. Slight S, Ganjam VK, Weber KT. Species diversity of 11β-hydroxysteroid dehydrogenase in the cardiovascular system. *J Lab Clin Med*. 1994;124:821–826.
195. Slight SH, Ganjam VK, Gómez-Sánchez CE, et al. High affinity NAD^+-dependent 11β-hydroxysteroid dehydrogenase in the human heart. *J Mol Cell Cardiol*. 1996;28:781–787.
196. Weber KT. Aldosterone in congestive heart failure. *N Engl J Med*. 2001;345:1689–1697.
197. Sun Y, Zhang J, Lu L, et al. Aldosterone-induced inflammation in the rat heart. Role of oxidative stress. *Am J Pathol*. 2002;161:1773–1781.
198. Virdis A, Neves MF, Amiri F, et al. Spironolactone improves angiotensin-induced vascular changes and oxidative stress. *Hypertension*. 2002;40:504–510.
199. Pu Q, Neves MF, Virdis A, et al. Endothelin antagonism on aldosterone-induced oxidative stress and vascular remodeling. *Hypertension*. 2003;42:49–55.
200. Ahokas RA, Warrington KJ, Gerling IC, et al. Aldosteronism and peripheral blood mononuclear cell activation. A neuroendocrine-immune interface. *Circ Res*. 2003;93:E124–E135.
201. Ahokas RA, Sun Y, Bhattacharya SK, et al. Aldosteronism and a proinflammatory vascular phenotype. Role of Mg^{2+}, Ca^{2+} and H_2O_2 in peripheral blood mononuclear cells. *Circulation* 2005;111:51–57.
202. Delva P, Pastori C, Degan M, et al. Intralymphocyte free magnesium in patients with primary aldosteronism: aldosterone and lymphocyte magnesium homeostasis. *Hypertension* 2000;35:113–117.
203. Reth M. Hydrogen peroxide as second messenger in lymphocyte activation. *Nat Immunol*. 2002;3:1129–1134.
204. Conn JW. Aldosteronism in man. Some clinical and climatological aspects. Part I. *JAMA*. 1963;183:775–781.
205. Conn JW. Aldosteronism in man. Some clinical and climatological aspects. Part II. *JAMA*. 1963;183:871–878.
206. Horton R, Biglieri EG. Effect of aldosterone on the metabolism of magnesium. *J Clin Endocrinol Metab*. 1962;22:1187–1192.
207. Rastegar A, Agus Z, Connor TB, et al. Renal handling of calcium and phosphate during mineralocorticoid "escape" in man. *Kidney Int*. 1972;2:279–286.
208. Gehr MK, Goldberg M. Hypercalciuria of mineralocorticoid escape: clearance and micropuncture studies in the rat. *Am J Physiol*. 1986;251(5 Pt 2):F879–F888.
209. Cappuccio FP, Markandu ND, MacGregor GA. Renal handling of calcium and phosphate during mineralocorticoid administration in normal subjects. *Nephron*. 1988;48:280–283.
210. Chhokar VS, Sun Y, Bhattacharya SK, et al. Loss of bone minerals and strength in rats with aldosteronism. *Am J Physiol Heart Circ Physiol*. 2004;287:H2023–H2026.
211. Chhokar VS, Sun Y, Bhattacharya SK, et al. Hyperparathyroidism and the calcium paradox of aldosteronism. *Circulation*. 2005;111:871–878.
212. Haller H, Thiede M, Lenz T, et al. Intracellular free calcium and ionized plasma calcium during mineralocorticoid-induced blood pressure increase in man. *J Hypertens Suppl*. 1985;3(Suppl 3):S41–S43.
213. Vidal A, Sun Y, Bhattacharya SK, et al. The calcium paradox of aldosteronism and the role of the parathyroid glands. *Am J Physiol Heart Circ Physiol*. 2006;290:H286–H294.
214. Ammarguellat FZ, Gannon PO, Amiri F, et al. Fibrosis, matrix metalloproteinases, and inflammation in the heart of DOCA-salt hypertensive rats: role of ET_A receptors. *Hypertension*. 2002;39(Part 2):679–684.
215. Weber KT, Janicki JS, Shroff SG, et al. Collagen compartment remodeling in the pressure overloaded left ventricle. *J Appl Cardiol*. 1988;3:37–46.
216. Pearlman ES, Weber KT, Janicki JS, et al. Muscle fiber orientation and connective tissue content in the hypertrophied human heart. *Lab Invest*. 1982;46:158–164.
217. Huysman JAN, Vliegen HW, Van der Laarse A, et al. Changes in nonmyocyte tissue composition associated with pressure overload of hypertrophic human hearts. *Pathol Res Pract*. 1989;184:577–581.
218. Hess OM, Schneider J, Koch R, et al. Diastolic function and myocardial structure in patients with myocardial hypertrophy. Special reference to normalized viscoelastic data. *Circulation*. 1981;63:360–371.
219. Villari B, Campbell SE, Hess OM, et al. Influence of collagen network on left ventricular systolic and diastolic function in aortic valve disease. *J Am Coll Cardiol*. 1993;22:1477–1484.
220. Conrad CH, Brooks WW, Hayes JA, et al. Myocardial fibrosis and stiffness with hypertrophy and heart failure in the spontaneously hypertensive rat. *Circulation*. 1995;91:161–170.
221. Brooks WW, Bing OHL, Robinson KG, et al. Effect of angiotensin-converting enzyme inhibition on myocardial fibrosis and function in hypertrophied and failing myocardium from the spontaneously hypertensive rat. *Circulation*. 1997;96:4002–4010.
222. Brilla CG, Matsubara L, Weber KT. Advanced hypertensive heart disease in spontaneously hypertensive rats: lisinopril-mediated regression of myocardial fibrosis. *Hypertension*. 1996;28:269–275.
223. Weber KT. Cardiac interstitium in health and disease: the fibrillar collagen network. *J Am Coll Cardiol*. 1989;13:1637–1652.
224. Weber KT, Brilla CG, Janicki JS. Myocardial fibrosis: functional significance and regulatory factors. *Cardiovasc Res*. 1993;27:341–348.
225. Weber KT. Cardiac interstitium. In: Poole-Wilson PA, Colucci WS, Massie BM, Chatterjee K, Coats AJS, eds. *Heart Failure: Scientific Principles and Clinical Practice*. New York: Churchill Livingstone; 1997: 13–31.
226. Gabbiani G, Ryan GB, Majno G. Presence of modified fibroblasts in granulation tissue and their possible role in wound contraction. *Experientia*. 1971;27:549–550.
227. Haber HL, Powers ER, Gimple LW, et al. Intracoronary angiotensin-converting enzyme inhibition improves diastolic function in patients with hypertensive left ventricular hypertrophy. *Circulation*. 1994;89:2616–2625.
228. Friedrich SP, Lorell BH, Rousseau MF, et al. Intracardiac angiotensin-converting enzyme inhibition improves diastolic function in patients with left ventricular hypertrophy due to aortic stenosis. *Circulation*. 1994;90:2761–2771.

229. Krayenbuehl HP, Hess OM, Schneider J, et al. Physiologic or pathologic hypertrophy. *Eur Heart J*. 1983;4:29–34.
230. Hess OM, Ritter M, Schneider J, et al. Diastolic stiffness and myocardial structure in aortic valve disease before and after valve replacement. *Circulation*. 1984;69:855–865.
231. Rousseau MF, Gurné O, van Eyll C, et al. Effects of benazeprilat on left ventricular systolic and diastolic function and neurohormonal status in patients with ischemic heart disease. *Circulation* 1990;81(Suppl III):III123–III129.
232. Jalil JE, Doering CW, Janicki JS, et al. Structural vs. contractile protein remodeling and myocardial stiffness in hypertrophied rat left ventricle. *J Mol Cell Cardiol*. 1988;20:1179–1187.
233. Carroll EP, Janicki JS, Pick R, et al. Myocardial stiffness and reparative fibrosis following coronary embolization in the rat. *Cardiovasc Res*. 1989;23:655–661.
234. Boluyt MO, O'Neill L, Meredith AL, et al. Alterations in cardiac gene expression during the transition from stable hypertrophy to heart failure. Marked upregulation of genes encoding extracellular matrix components. *Circ Res*. 1994;75:23–32.
235. Keeley FW, Elmoselhi A, Leenen FHH. Enalapril suppresses normal accumulation of elastin and collagen in cardiovascular tissues of growing rats. *Am J Physiol*. 1992;262:H1013–H1021.
236. Albaladejo P, Bouaziz H, Duriez M, et al. Angiotensin converting enzyme inhibition prevents the increase in aortic collagen in rats. *Hypertension*. 1994;23:74–82.
237. Jugdutt BI, Khan MI, Jugdutt SJ, et al. Effect of enalapril on ventricular remodeling and function during healing after anterior myocardial infarction in the dog. *Circulation*. 1995;91:802–812.
238. Jugdutt BI, Schwarz-Michorowski BL, Khan MI. Effect of long-term captopril therapy on left ventricular remodeling and function during healing of canine myocardial infarction. *J Am Coll Cardiol*. 1992;19:713–721.
239. Jugdutt BI. Effect of captopril and enalapril on left ventricular geometry, function and collagen during healing after anterior and inferior myocardial infarction in a dog model. *J Am Coll Cardiol*. 1995;25:1718–1725.
240. Hashimoto K, Hirose M, Furukawa K, et al. Changes in hemodynamics and bradykinin concentration in coronary sinus blood in experimental coronary artery occlusion. *Jpn Heart J*. 1977;18:679–689.
241. Needleman P, Marshall GR, Sobel BE. Hormone interactions in the isolated rabbit heart. Synthesis and coronary vasomotor effects of prostaglandins, angiotensin, and bradykinin. *Circ Res*. 1975;37:802–808.
242. Noda K, Sasaguri M, Ideishi M, et al. Role of locally formed angiotensin II and bradykinin in the reduction of myocardial infarct size in dogs. *Cardiovasc Res*. 1993;27:334–340.
243. Wollert KC, Studer R, Doerfer K, et al. Differential effects of kinins on cardiomyocyte hypertrophy and interstitial collagen matrix in the surviving myocardium after myocardial infarction in the rat. *Circulation*. 1997;95:1910–1917.
244. Frimm CdC, Sun Y, Weber KT. Angiotensin II receptor blockade and myocardial fibrosis of the infarcted rat heart. *J Lab Clin Med*. 1997;129:439–446.
245. Makino N, Matsui H, Masutomo K, et al. Effect of angiotensin converting enzyme inhibitor on regression in cardiac hypertrophy. *Mol Cell Biochem*. 1993;119:23–28.
246. Bélichard P, Savard P, Cardinal R, et al. Markedly different effects on ventricular remodeling result in a decrease in inducibility of ventricular arrhythmias. *J Am Coll Cardiol*. 1994;23:505–513.
247. Schieffer B, Wirger A, Meybrunn M, et al. Comparative effects of chronic angiotensin-converting enzyme inhibition and angiotensin II type 1 receptor blockade on cardiac remodeling after myocardial infarction in the rat. *Circulation*. 1994;89:2273–2282.
248. Dixon IMC, Ju H, Jassal DS, et al. Effect of ramipril and losartan on collagen expression in right and left heart after myocardial infarction. *Mol Cell Biochem*. 1996;165:31–45.
249. Pimentel JL, Jr., Sundell CL, Wang S, et al. Role of angiotensin II in the expression and regulation of transforming growth factor-β in obstructive nephropathy. *Kidney Int*. 1995;48:1233–1246.
250. Morrissey JJ, Ishidoya S, McCracken R, et al. The effect of ACE inhibitors on the expression of matrix genes and the role of p53 and p21 (WAF1) in experimental renal fibrosis. *Kidney Int*. 1996;49(Suppl 54):S83–S87.
251. Ishidoya S, Morrissey J, McCracken R, et al. Angiotensin II receptor antagonist ameliorates renal tubulointerstitial fibrosis caused by unilateral ureteral obstruction. *Kidney Int*. 1995;47:1285–1294.
252. Kaneto H, Morrissey J, McCracken R, et al. Enalapril reduces collagen type IV synthesis and expansion of the interstitium in the obstructed rat kidney. *Kidney Int*. 1994;45:1637–1647.
253. Ishidoya S, Morrissey J, McCracken R, et al. Delayed treatment with enalapril halts tubulointerstitial fibrosis in rats with obstructive nephropathy. *Kidney Int*. 1996;49:1110–1119.
254. Yanagisawa H, Morrissey J, Morrison AR, et al. Eicosanoid production by isolated glomeruli of rats with unilateral ureteral obstruction. *Kidney Int*. 1990;37:1528–1535.
255. Diamond JR, Anderson S. Irreversible tubulointerstitial damage associated with chronic aminonucleoside nephrosis. *Am J Pathol*. 1990;137:1323–1332.
256. Lafayette RA, Mayer G, Meyer TW. The effects of blood pressure reduction on cyclosporine nephrotoxicity in the rat. *J Am Soc Nephrol*. 1993;3:1892–1899.
257. Cohen EP, Moulder JE, Fish BL, et al. Prophylaxis of experimental bone marrow transplant nephropathy. *J Lab Clin Med*. 1994;124:371–380.
258. Tanaka R, Sugihara K, Tatematsu A, et al. Internephron heterogeneity of growth factors and sclerosis—modulation of platelet-derived growth factor by angiotensin II. *Kidney Int*. 1995;47:131–139.
259. Ikoma M, Kawamura T, Kakinuma Y, et al. Cause of variable therapeutic efficiency of angiotensin converting enzyme inhibitor on glomerular lesions. *Kidney Int*. 1991;40:195–202.
260. Shibouta Y, Chatani F, Ishimura Y, et al. TCV-116 inhibits renal interstitial and glomerular injury in glomerulosclerotic rats. *Kidney Int*. 1996;49(Suppl 55):S115–S118.
261. Anderson S, Rennke HG, Brenner BM. Therapeutic advantage of converting enzyme inhibitors in arresting progressive renal disease associated with systemic hypertension in the rat. *J Clin Invest*. 1986;77:1993–2000.
262. Juncos LI, Carrasco Dueñas S, Cornejo JC, et al. Long-term enalapril and hydrochlorothiazide in radiation nephritis. *Nephron*. 1993;64:249–255.
263. Nakamura T, Honma H, Ikeda Y, et al. Renal protective effects of angiotensin II receptor I antagonist CV-11974 in spontaneously hypertensive stroke-prone rats (SHR-sp). *Blood Press*. 1994;3(Suppl 5):61–66.
264. Nakamura T, Obata J, Kuroyanagi R, et al. Involvement of angiotensin II in glomerulosclerosis of stroke-prone spontaneously hypertensive rats. *Kidney Int*. 1996;49(Suppl 55):S109–S112.
265. Kim S, Ohta K, Hamaguchi A, et al. Contribution of renal angiotensin II type I receptor to gene expressions in hypertension-induced renal injury. *Kidney Int*. 1994;46:1346–1358.
266. Kim S, Ohta K, Hamaguchi A, et al. Angiotensin II type I receptor antagonist inhibits the gene expression of transforming growth factor-β 1 and extracellular matrix in cardiac and vascular tissues of hypertensive rats. *J Pharmacol Exp Ther*. 1995;273:509–515.
267. Ward WF, Molteni A, Ts'ao C. Radiation-induced endothelial dysfunction and fibrosis in rat lung: modification by the angiotensin converting enzyme inhibitor CL242817. *Radiat Res*. 1989;117:342–350.
268. Ward WF, Molteni A, Ts'ao C, et al. Radiation pneumotoxicity in rats: modification by inhibitors of angiotensin converting enzyme. *Int J Radiat Oncol Biol Phys*. 1992;22:623–625.
269. Ward WF, Molteni A, Ts'ao C-H, et al. Captopril reduces collagen and mast cell accumulation in irradiated rat lung. *Int J Radiat Oncol Biol Phys*. 1990;19:1405–1409.
270. Molteni A, Ward WF, Ts'ao C, et al. Monocrotaline-induced pulmonary fibrosis in rats: amelioration by captopril and penicillamine. *Proc Soc Exp Biol Med*. 1985;180:112–120.
271. Sun Y, Ramires FJA, Zhou G, et al. Fibrous tissue and angiotensin II. *J Mol Cell Cardiol*. 1997;29:2001–2012.
272. Villarreal FJ, Kim NN, Ungab GD, et al. Identification of functional angiotensin II receptors on rat cardiac fibroblasts. *Circulation* 1993;88:2849–2861.
273. Brilla CG, Zhou G, Matsubara L, et al. Collagen metabolism in cultured adult rat cardiac fibroblasts: response to angiotensin II and aldosterone. *J Mol Cell Cardiol*. 1994;26:809–820.

274. Zhou G, Kandala JC, Tyagi SC, et al. Effects of angiotensin II and aldosterone on collagen gene expression and protein turnover in cardiac fibroblasts. *Mol Cell Biochem*. 1996;154:171–178.
275. Lee AA, Dillmann WH, McCulloch AD, et al. Angiotensin II stimulates the autocrine production of transforming growth factor-β 1 in adult rat cardiac fibroblasts. *J Mol Cell Cardiol*. 1995;27:2347–2357.
276. Tan LB, Jalil JE, Pick R, et al. Cardiac myocyte necrosis induced by angiotensin II. *Circ Res*. 1991;69:1185–1195.
277. Darrow DC, Miller HC. The production of cardiac lesions by repeated injections of desoxycorticosterone acetate. *J Clin Invest*. 1942;21:601–611.
278. Potts JL, Dalakos TG, Streeten DHP, et al. Cardiomyopathy in an adult with Bartter's syndrome: hemodynamic, angiographic, and metabolic studies. *Am J Cardiol*. 1977;40:995–999.
279. Brilla CG, Weber KT. Reactive and reparative myocardial fibrosis in arterial hypertension in the rat. *Cardiovasc Res*. 1992;26:671–677.
280. Campbell SE, Janicki JS, Matsubara BB, et al. Myocardial fibrosis in the rat with mineralocorticoid excess: prevention of scarring by amiloride. *Am J Hypertens*. 1993;6:487–495.
281. Weber KT, Brilla CG, Campbell SE, et al. Pathologic hypertrophy with fibrosis: the structural basis for myocardial failure. *Blood. Press*. 1992;1:75–85.

The Renin-Angiotensin System

10

Barry H. Greenberg

Our understanding of the important role of the renin-angiotensin system (RAS) in maintaining circulatory homeostasis and in the pathogenesis of cardiovascular disease has evolved considerably since the late 1890s, when Tigerstedt first observed that aqueous extracts of the kidneys could produce a prolonged increase in blood pressure in an experimental animal model (1). In particular, involvement of the RAS in conditions that lead to the development of heart failure such as hypertension, myocardial infarction (MI), and especially cardiac remodeling, has been well-established for many years now. Moreover, we have come to recognize that the extent, pathways, actions, and interactions ascribed to the RAS are much more varied, far-reaching, and complex than was previously imagined. In this chapter, a description of the RAS and its role in heart failure will be presented. New and emerging pathways and evidence that relates the RAS to the pathogenesis of heart failure will be emphasized. The use of drugs that block RAS activation as a strategy for treating heart failure patients will be discussed briefly and then only in the service of providing evidence that the RAS is involved. Since targeting the RAS has become a cornerstone of heart failure therapy treatment, options will be presented in detail in another chapter of this text.

DESCRIPTION OF THE RENIN-ANGIOTENSIN SYSTEM

As shown in Figure 10-1, initial descriptions of the RAS depicted a cascade of events in which angiotensinogen is released from the liver into the circulation where it is acted upon by renin (generated and released from the juxtaglomerular apparatus of the kidneys) to form the physiologically inactive decapeptide angiotensin I (Ang I). Further degradation of this peptide by angiotensin-converting enzyme (ACE) occurs on the endothelial surface of blood vessels, particularly in the lungs, and results in the formation of Ang II, the main effector molecule of the RAS. Ang II is then distributed in the bloodstream throughout the body where it initiates a wide variety of physiological and pathophysiological effects, most of which are mediated through interactions with its type I (AT_1) receptor. Effects of Ang II include arterial vasoconstriction, stimulation of thirst, salt and water retention by the kidney, release of antidiuretic hormone from the posterior pituitary, augmentation of norepinephrine release from sympathetic nerve endings (and inhibition of its reuptake), and remodeling of the heart and blood vessels.

While the circulatory RAS clearly plays an important role in cardiovascular homeostasis, it fails to account for many of the pathophysiological changes that have been ascribed to Ang II during the development and progression of heart failure. For instance, little if any evidence of activation of the circulatory RAS can be detected post-MI once the acute phase is passed (2–4). During this quiescent period wherein both plasma renin activity and angiotensin levels are within the normal range, progressive changes in cardiac structure and function that result in the development of heart failure are known to occur. In support of a role of the RAS in this process is a substantial body of evidence from studies done in both experimental animal models and in human patients demonstrating that blocking the generation of Ang II or its interaction with the AT_1 receptor can greatly ameliorate the remodeling process (4–8).

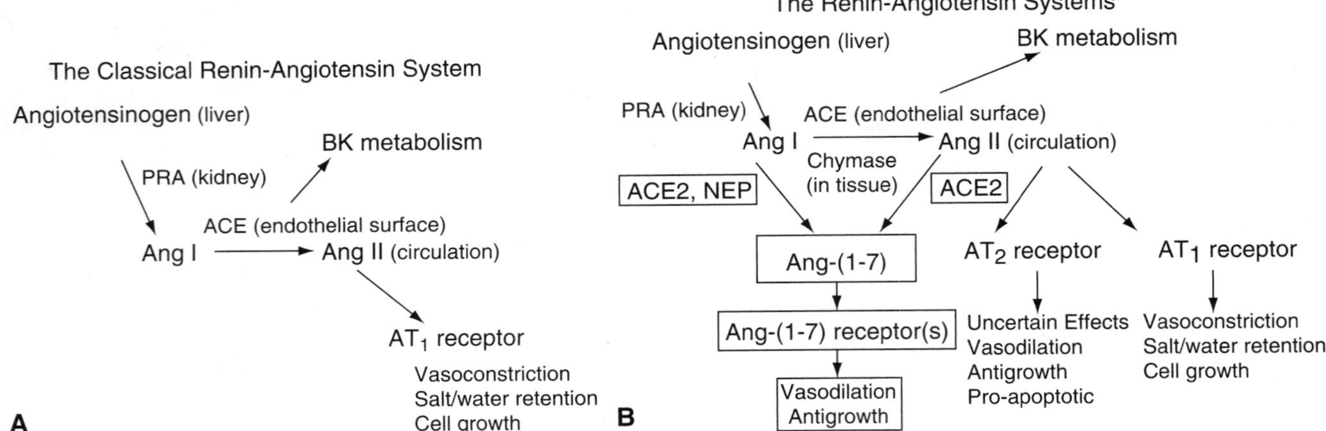

Figure 10-1 Expanding pathways of the renin-angiotensin system (RAS). **(A)** depicts the classical RAS, while in **(B)** an expanded version of this system is shown. As discussed in the text, there is information that the tissue-based RAS, the AT_2 receptor, and an alternative pathway involving ACE2 all play important roles in regulating cardiac structure and function.

Discovery that the genes for virtually all components of the RAS are expressed in the heart resulted in the recognition of a tissue-based cardiac RAS (9–14). In addition, alternative enzymatic pathways for converting Ang I to Ang II that do not require ACE have been identified. The pathway that has been best-described involves chymase, an enzyme derived from mast cells in the heart (15). There is evidence that the alternative chymase pathway, rather than the one involving ACE, is responsible for the generation of most of the Ang II that is found in human cardiac tissue. The only component of the RAS that may not be generated in sufficient amounts in the heart is renin activity. However, renin from the kidneys can be transported in the bloodstream to the heart, where it is extracted from the coronary circulation (16) and is able to act on locally generated angiotensinogen. The cardiac RAS system is regulated independently of the circulatory system and it functions in an autocrine/paracrine manner to influence cardiac structure and function (10,13,17). In the post-MI setting, substantial upregulation of the cardiac RAS is associated with increases in local concentrations of Ang II (12,18,19). The importance of the cardiac RAS in remodeling is suggested by the close correlation between the extent of structural changes in the heart and cardiac RAS activation (18,19) and by evidence that Ang II levels in the interstitial fluid of the heart are much higher than plasma levels (20).

The use of cardiac-specific transgenic approaches has helped confirm the critical role of the cardiac RAS in the remodeling process (21–23). Transgenic mice overexpressing angiotensinogen in cardiomyocytes have been shown to develop cardiac hypertrophy without fibrosis, despite the presence of normal blood pressure. This effect could be inhibited by administration of either an ACE inhibitor or an angiotensin receptor blocker (ARB) (23). Cardiac-specific overexpression of the AT_1 receptor results in significant remodeling that is characterized by cardiac hypertrophy and fibrosis (21). Since most effects of Ang II in promoting cardiac remodeling are mediated through its AT_1 receptor, the role of the RAS in post-MI cardiac remodeling has been studied in knockout mice that are null for the AT_1 receptor. As shown in Figure 10-2, when these mice undergo coronary artery ligation to induce a large MI they develop significantly less left ventricular (LV) dilatation, less fibrosis in noninfarcted segments of myocardium, and better LV systolic function over time than do wild type controls, despite the fact that infarct sizes in the study groups were equal (22). Moreover, post-MI survival is significantly improved in AT_1 knockout mice compared to wild type controls.

EFFECTS OF ANGIOTENSIN II

As previously noted, the AT_1 receptor mediates most known effects of the RAS. The mammalian AT_1 receptor is a 359-amino-acid protein that has a typical 7-transmembrane domain structure that is similar to other guanine nucleotide regulatory-protein coupled receptors (24–26). It has been identified on numerous cell types in tissue throughout the body, including the adrenal gland, heart, kidney, blood vessels, and brain (25,25–28). In the heart, AT_1 receptors are present on cardiac myocytes, fibroblasts, mast cells, and vascular cells (29,30). The AT_1 receptor is coupled via heterotrimeric G-proteins to the phospholipase C signal transduction pathway, as evidenced by intracellular calcium mobilization and inositol triphosphate production upon receptor activation (24,31). It has also been linked to transactivation of the epidermal growth factor and other receptor tyrosine kinases and activation of protein kinase C, MAP kinases such as ERK, the JAK/STAT signaling pathway, c-src, and PYK2 kinase (32–43). Another important effect of Ang II is activation of the NAD(P)H oxidase, a major source of reactive oxygen species (ROS) production by vascular cells (44).

It is not surprising (given the potential for both local and systemic generation of Ang II, the presence of relevant receptors on numerous cell types throughout the body, and the widely varied signaling pathways that are activated

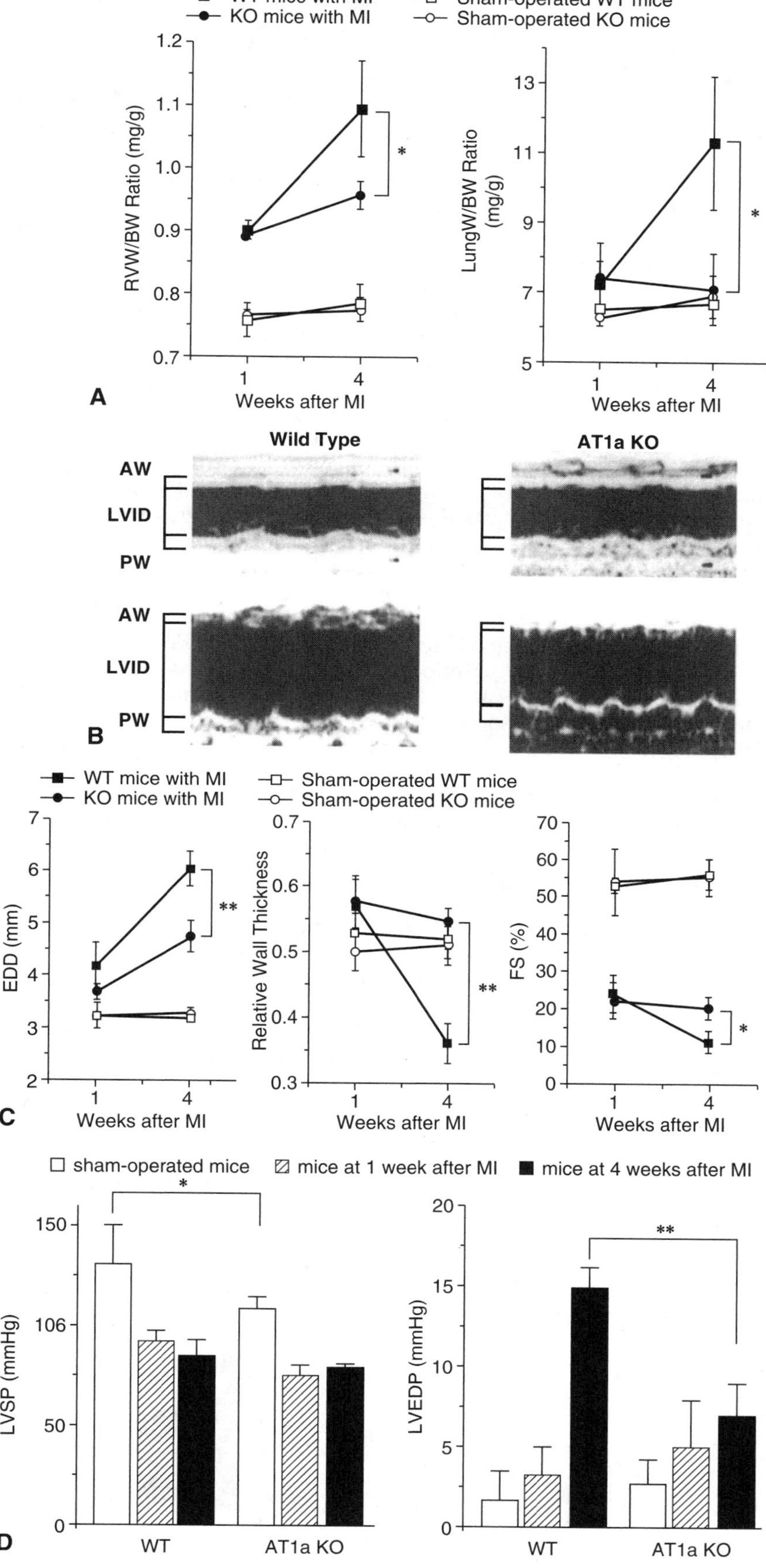

Figure 10-2 Effects of AT_1 ablation on post-MI cardiac remodeling. Depicted are echocardiographic and hemodynamic results from AT_1 receptor knockout (KO) mice compared to wild type (WT) mice at 1 and 4 weeks post-MI. RVW/BW ratio, right ventricular to body weight ratio; LVID, left ventricular internal dimension; AW, anterior wall; PW, posterior wall. Data expressed as mean ± SEM of 5 to 15 mice per group. $^{*}p < 0.05$; $^{**}p$ 0.01. (From Harada K, Sugaya T, Murakami K, et al. Angiotensin II type 1A receptor knockout mice display less left ventricular remodeling and improved survival after myocardial infarction. *Circulation.* 1999;100 (20):2093–2099, with permission.)

via the AT_1 receptor) that Ang II has substantial effects on the structure and function of numerous organs and organ systems throughout the body. In considering the pathophysiology of heart failure, the effects of Ang II on kidneys, blood vessels, and the heart itself are of greatest interest. Ang II has been associated with many of the conditions that can result in cardiac damage and dysfunction, including hypertension, atherosclerosis, coronary thrombosis, and valvular disease. In the kidney, Ang II promotes the retention of salt and water by both direct effects on the nephron as well as by stimulating the production and release of aldosterone from the adrenal glands. In blood vessels, Ang II has been shown to be a potent vasoconstrictor agent. The renal and vascular effects of Ang II are most important when there is already evidence of cardiac dysfunction. In this setting, salt and water retention predispose to both pulmonary and systemic congestion, while peripheral vasoconstriction reduces delivery of oxygen and nutrients to tissue throughout the body. Moreover, both the salt/water and vascular effects increase load on the heart. While this increase in load may have some favorable short-term benefits (e.g., increasing stroke volume by increasing stretch on cardiac myocytes), these effects are limited and are more than offset by long-term adverse consequences, most notably effects on cardiac remodeling.

In addition to the indirect effects of the RAS on cardiac remodeling that are mediated by increases in load, it is now recognized that Ang II has direct effects on cells in the heart that promote growth and organ remodeling. Despite the fact that cardiac myocytes have been reported to contain a relatively low density of AT_1 receptors (45,46), Ang II (the main effector molecule of the RAS) has been shown to induce cardiac myocyte hypertrophy (30,47–49). A possible explanation for this paradox is that Ang II stimulation of other cells that are more richly endowed with AT_1 receptors (e.g., cardiac fibroblasts) leads to the generation of numerous secondary growth factors, including interleukin-6 (IL-6), leukemia inhibitory factor-1 (LIF-1), transforming growth factor-beta (TGF-β), and endothelin-1 (ET-1), all of which have been postulated to play a role in promoting cardiac remodeling (46,50–59). Evidence that Ang II induces hypertrophy of cardiac myocytes only when these cells are co-cultured with cardiac fibroblasts, or when conditioned media from fibroblasts stimulated by Ang II is added to myocyte culture, supports the notion that production of growth factors from fibroblasts is a critical component of the remodeling process (46,51) and that Ang II-mediated cardiac myocyte hypertrophy may not be a direct effect of the peptide. Thus, whether or not Ang II directly causes cardiac myocyte hypertrophy or whether this effect is mediated through the release of secondary growth factors from other cells in the heart is open to question.

Ang II stimulates numerous cardiac fibroblast functions that are involved in remodeling. These include replication, migration, and production of extracellular matrix (ECM) proteins and secondary growth factors. Most of these effects are mediated through the AT_1 receptor (31,60–64), which is considerably more abundant on cardiac fibroblasts than on cardiac myocytes (45). Furthermore, in pathological settings in which cardiac remodeling occurs (e.g., following an MI), the density of the AT_1 receptor on cardiac fibroblasts is increased (65–68). As shown in Figure 10-3, the proinflammatory cytokines, tumor necrosis factor-alpha (TNF-α), and interleukin-1beta (IL-1β) have been shown to be potent inducers of AT_1 receptor upregulation in cultured cardiac fibroblasts, whereas other growth factors known to be present in the remodeling heart either fail to increase or actually decrease AT_1 receptor expression (69). Proinflammatory cytokine-mediated AT_1 receptor upregulation involves activation of the transcription factor nuclear factor-kappa B (NF-κB) since it can be selectively blocked by interfering with NF-κB dissociation from IκB, a regulatory protein that restricts nuclear translocation which is essential to activate gene expression (70).

In the post-MI heart there are both temporal and spatial associations between increases in AT_1 receptor density and the appearance of these proinflammatory cytokines that are consistent with the possibility that the relationship may be causal in nature (71). In addition, receptor upregulation induced by TNF-α and IL-1β appear to be additive. Although the significance of increased AT_1 receptor density on cardiac fibroblasts during remodeling is uncertain, there is evidence that proinflammatory cytokine-induced AT_1 upregulation enhances Ang II-stimulated proline incorporation (depicted in Figure 10-4) and production of

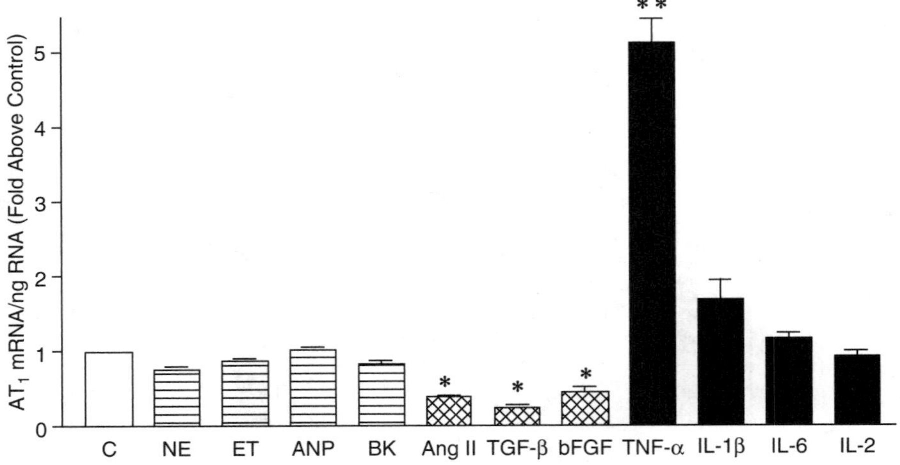

Figure 10-3 AT_1 receptor expression in cultured neonatal rat cardiac fibroblasts is increased by proinflammatory cytokines but not by other agents that have been identified in the remodeling heart. $^{*}p < 0.02$; $^{**}p < 0.01$; $^{***}p < 0.04$. (From Gurantz D, Cowling RT, Villarreal FJ, et al. Tumor necrosis factor-alpha upregulates angiotensin II type 1 receptors on cardiac fibroblasts. *Circ Res.* 1999;85(3):272–279, with permission.)

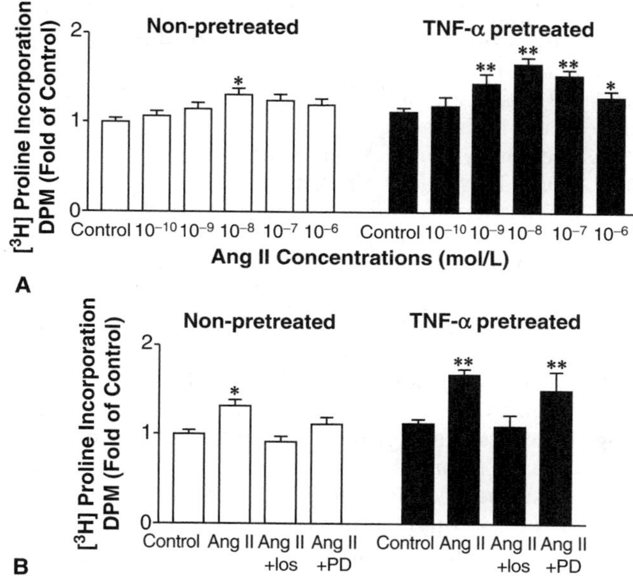

Figure 10-4 **(A)** Ang II-stimulated [(3)H]proline incorporation is enhanced by TNF-α pretreatment. In nonpretreated fibroblasts (**open bars**), Ang II-stimulated [(3)H]proline incorporation throughout a concentration range of 10^{-10} to 10^{-6} mol/L. Pretreatment of the cells with TNF-α (10 ng/mL) for 48 hours, however, enhanced the profile of [(3)H]proline incorporation by Ang II (**filled bars**). **(B)** Effect of losartan and PD123319 (both at 10–(6) mol/L) on [(3)H]proline incorporation by Ang II (10^{-8} mol/L). Losartan (Los), the AT_1 receptor antagonist, but not PD123319 (PD), the AT_2 receptor antagonist, blocked the Ang II effects in both nonpretreated (**open bars**) and TNF-α-pretreated (filled bars) cells. Data are presented as mean ± SEM fold of control.
For **(A)** and **(B)**, $^{*}p < 0.05$, $^{**}p < 0.01$, n = 7 to 8). (From Peng J, Gurantz D, Tran V, et al. Tumor necrosis factor-alpha-induced AT1 receptor upregulation enhances angiotensin II-mediated cardiac fibroblast responses that favor fibrosis. *Circ Res.* 2002;91(12):1119–1126, with permission.)

TIMP-1 (72). These findings strongly suggest that upregulation of the AT_1 receptor contributes to the remodeling process by increasing the responsiveness of cardiac fibroblasts to the profibrotic effects of Ang II (69,72).

As previously noted, most Ang II effects are mediated by the AT_1 receptor. It is now recognized, however, that Ang II can also bind to its type 2 (AT_2) receptor with effects that may have important consequences in the cardiovascular system (Fig. 10-1B). Although both receptor subtypes are 7-transmembrane domain G-protein-coupled receptors of the class A rhodopsin-like family, there is only ~30% sequence homology between them (73,74). Both the AT_1 and the AT_2 receptors have affinities for Ang II that are in the nanomolar range. The AT_2 receptor is highly expressed in developing fetuses (27,75). After birth, its expression declines rapidly and in the adult it is expressed in very low abundance in the cardiovascular system. Under pathological, conditions, however, expression levels may increase substantially (76–78). Signaling pathways associated with the AT_2 receptor include activation of protein phosphatases (with resultant protein dephosphorylation), activation of phospholipase A_2, regulation of the bradykinin-NO-cyclic guanosine monophosphate (cGMP) system, and sphingolipid-derived ceramide formation (79–82). Activation of the AT_2 receptor has been associated with an increased rate of cell apoptosis (83).

The role of the AT_2 receptor in cardiovascular homeostasis and, particularly, in remodeling of the heart has not yet been fully delineated. Consistent with evidence indicating an association between the AT_2 receptor and protein phosphatase activity, initial reports of the effects of AT_2 receptor activation suggested that it mediated antigrowth effects that opposed those of the AT_1 receptor in cardiac myocytes and fibroblasts (84–87). However, some experiments in mice that were null for the AT_2 receptor gene have provided conflicting results in regard to its impact on the remodeling process. For instance, Ichihara et al. found that the chronic loss of the AT_2 receptor abolished the development of LV hypertrophy and cardiac fibrosis in chronic Ang II-induced hypertension, suggesting the necessity of this receptor subtype for the development of these pathological structural changes (88). Of interest is the observation that transgenic mice with ventricular-specific increases in AT_2 receptor density develop a phenotype of dilated cardiomyopathy characterized by ventricular dilatation, wall thinning, increased fibrosis, and depressed contractile function (89). Although the mechanism for these abnormalities in ventricular structure and function are uncertain, increased apoptosis within the ventricular myocardium may be involved. In support of this possibility was the observation that the severity of the phenotype and extent of apoptosis were directly related to the level of expression of AT_2 receptor gene expression (83). Furthermore, the transgenic animals with cardiac-specific AT_2 receptor overexpression also demonstrated evidence of increased levels of activation of PKC-α and -β, both of which have been implicated in cardiac remodeling and the development of heart failure.

Complicating this picture is evidence that the AT_2 receptor might influence the response to Ang II through formation of structural heterodimers with the AT_1 receptor. In this case the interposition of the AT_2 molecule into the usual AT_1 homodimer has been shown to inhibit AT_1 receptor signaling. Thus, AT_2 molecules could serve a dominant-negative function and antagonize the AT_1 receptor (84). Since both of these Ang receptor subtypes are co-expressed in many tissues, the precise effects of Ang II signaling might well be related to the relative abundance of the two receptor subtypes. Thus, in settings where the AT_2 receptor is downregulated, the ratio between the receptors would result in a lower likelihood of heterodimerization, an effect that would tend to favor an enhanced response of the AT_1 receptor to Ang II. Conversely, situations that result in an increase in the ratio of AT_2 to AT_1 would be expected to decrease AT_1-mediated effects of Ang II.

A role for the AT_2 receptor in the development of cardiac hypertrophy in humans was suggested by the results of a recent study evaluating the association between a common intronic polymorphism of the AT_2 gene (-1332 G/A) and the presence of LV hypertrophy in hypertensive patients (90). The AT_2 gene consists of 3 exons and 2 introns, with the entire reading frame for the AT_2 receptor located on exon 3. The polymorphism site is located just downstream from exon 2 in a region that is important for transcriptional activity. Individuals with the G allele lack exon 2 of the AT_2 gene; this leads to less-effective transcription. The fact that there was an association between the G allele and LV hypertrophy (despite the fact that patients had been treated for their hypertension) is consistent with the possibility that the AT_2 receptor may mediate antihypertrophic effects in this setting. Clearly, the role of the AT_2 receptor in cardiac remodeling and heart failure will require further study in order to determine its importance.

THE ANGIOTENSIN-CONVERTING ENZYME -2 PATHWAY

Recently, an alternative pathway of the RAS involving a homolog of ACE, termed ACE2, has been described (91,92) and there is emerging evidence that it may play an important role in the cardiovascular system (93). Human ACE2 cDNA predicts an 805-amino-acid protein that has a 42% homology with the N-terminal catalytic domain of ACE (91). Although first identified in the heart, kidney, and testes (91,94), the distribution of ACE2 now appears to be considerably more widespread than was originally believed (92).

As shown in Figure 10-1B, ACE2 functions as a carboxypeptidase that cleaves the terminal amino acid from either the decapeptide Ang I to form Ang-(1–9) or the octapeptide Ang II to form Ang-(1–7). The catalytic activity of ACE2 for Ang II is substantially greater than for Ang I, suggesting that its primary role may be in the conversion of Ang II to Ang-(1–7) (95). Unlike ACE activity, ACE2 is neither able to convert Ang I to Ang II nor break down bradykinin (91,95). Of particular importance is the fact that the activity of ACE2 is not affected by ACE inhibitors (91,94). ACE2 has also been found to be a functional receptor for the severe acute respiratory syndrome coronavirus (SARS-CoV) (96) and there is evidence that the Spike protein of the virus reduces ACE2 expression, an effect that has been postulated to be related to the virulence of the pneumonia caused by this agent.

There is evidence that ACE2 is involved in the regulation of blood pressure and that it might protect against elevations in arterial pressure. In three different rat models of hypertension the ACE2 gene maps to a quantitative trait locus (QTL) on the X chromosome, and in all three of these strains of rat ACE2 levels are reduced (97). ACE2 has also been implicated in regulating cardiac function. Knockout mice null for the ACE2 gene mice develop LV dilatation in association with severe cardiac contractile abnormalities (97). These abnormalities are both gender- and time-dependent since they are more severe in males and they progress with age. The fact that ablation of ACE expression can prevent cardiac dysfunction in ACE2-null mice suggests that the balance between ACE and ACE2 may play a critical role in regulating cardiac function (97). This situation may be analogous to what is seen in the lung, where a reduction in ACE2 activity has been associated with worsening acute lung injury and this effect can be attenuated by blocking the RAS (98).

Although the mechanisms and pathways through which ACE2 may exert beneficial effects on the cardiovascular (CV) system have not yet been defined, regulation of Ang II levels seems likely to be involved. Increases in ACE2 activity would be expected to reduce Ang II levels by both decreasing its degradation and also by reducing availability of Ang I, its immediate precursor. An additional mechanism might be through the production of Ang-(1–7), a peptide that has the property of being able to inhibit the C-terminal active site of ACE (99) and thus prevent conversion of Ang I to Ang II.

As previously noted, Ang II is the preferred substrate for ACE2 (95). This reaction results in the formation of Ang-(1–7). This heptapeptide can be generated from either Ang II (by ACE2 activity) or from Ang I (in a single step via neutral endopeptidase activity or in two steps via successive ACE2 and ACE activity). Ang-(1–7) is believed to have beneficial effects on cardiac structure and function by virtue of its ability to inhibit the pressor, proliferative, and cell growth-promoting effects of Ang II (100,101). In vascular smooth muscle cells (VSMCs) Ang-(1–7) inhibits Ang II-mediated cell growth, and infusion of Ang-(1–7) after vascular injury inhibits neointimal growth through a mechanism independent of effects on heart rate or blood pressure (102). Ang-(1–7) has been shown to significantly attenuate protein synthesis (103). In cultured neonatal rat cardiac myocytes this peptide has also been shown to have antigrowth effects. Iwata et al. found that exposure of adult rat cardiac fibroblasts to nanomolar concentrations of Ang-(1–7) had inhibitory effects on collagen synthesis as well as the expression of the secondary growth factors ET-1 and LIF (Fig. 10-5) (104). Moreover, Ang II-mediated increases in expression of these growth factors were attenuated by Ang-(1–7). Conditioned media from cardiac fibroblasts promotes cardiac myocyte hypertrophy and this effect is increased when the fibroblasts are exposed to Ang II, indicating enhanced release of secondary growth factors from these cells. However, as depicted in Figure 10-6, when fibroblasts are pretreated with Ang-(1–7), growth induced by conditioned media is significantly reduced, suggesting that growth factor production and/or release has been suppressed by the heptapeptide (104). These findings may explain results from the rat coronary ligation model of MI where Ang-(1–7) administration helped preserve cardiac function and limit increases in cardiac myocyte diameter (105). In this same experimental model the administration of an angiotensin receptor blocker (ARB) increases cardiac ACE2 gene expression and circulating Ang-(1–7) levels, both of which may contribute to the inhibition in post-MI cardiac hypertrophy that is seen (106).

The signaling pathways through which Ang-(1–7) affects cell structure and function have not yet been clearly defined. Although Ang-(1–7) could conceivably interfere with Ang II signaling through the AT_1 receptor by competing for receptor binding sites or by inducing AT_1 receptor internalization (107), the concentrations required for these effects are substantially higher than are required for the effects on cell functions; this makes it unlikely that interference with Ang II binding is the major pathway involved. In cultured rat aortic VSMCs the antiproliferative effects of Ang-(1–7) involve release of prostacyclin and prostacyclin-mediated production of cyclic adenosine monophosphate (cAMP), activation of cAMP-dependent protein kinase, and attenuation of ERK1 and ERK2 phosphorylation (108). Ang-(1–7) has also been shown to inhibit Ang II effects by stimulating production of nitric oxide and vasodilatory prostaglandins (99,108–110). Another mechanism through

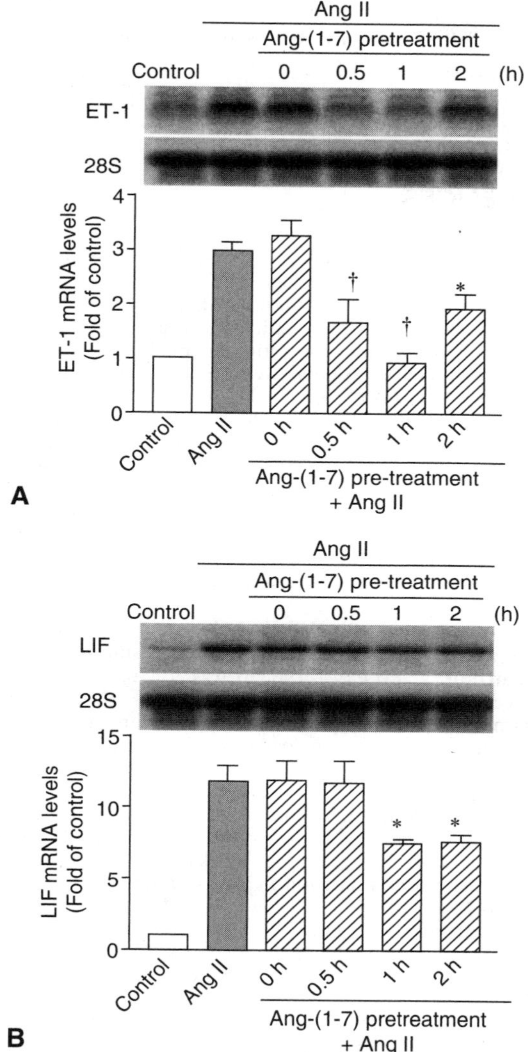

Figure 10-5 Effects of pretreatment with Ang-(1–7) on Ang II-induced increase in ET-1 and LIF mRNA expression in adult rat cardiac fibroblasts (ARCFs). ARCFs were pretreated with Ang-(1–7) (10^{-7} M) for the indicated periods and then stimulated with Ang II (10^{-7} M) for 30 minutes (ET-1) or 1 hour (LIF). Representative Northern blots are depicted above the composite data on time-dependent effects of pretreatment with Ang-(1–7) on Ang II-induced increase in mRNA expression of ET-1. **(A)**, $n = 4$ and LIF; **(B)**, $n = 3$. Data are means ± SE. $^{*}p < 0.05$; $^{\dagger}p < 0.01$ versus Ang II stimulation alone (Dunnett's post hoc test). (Adapted from Iwata M, Cowling RT, Gurantz D, et al. Angiotensin-(1–7) binds to specific receptors on cardiac fibroblasts to initiate antifibrotic and antitrophic effects. *Am J Physiol.* [*Heart Circ Physiol.*] 2005;289[6]:H2356–H2363, with permission.)

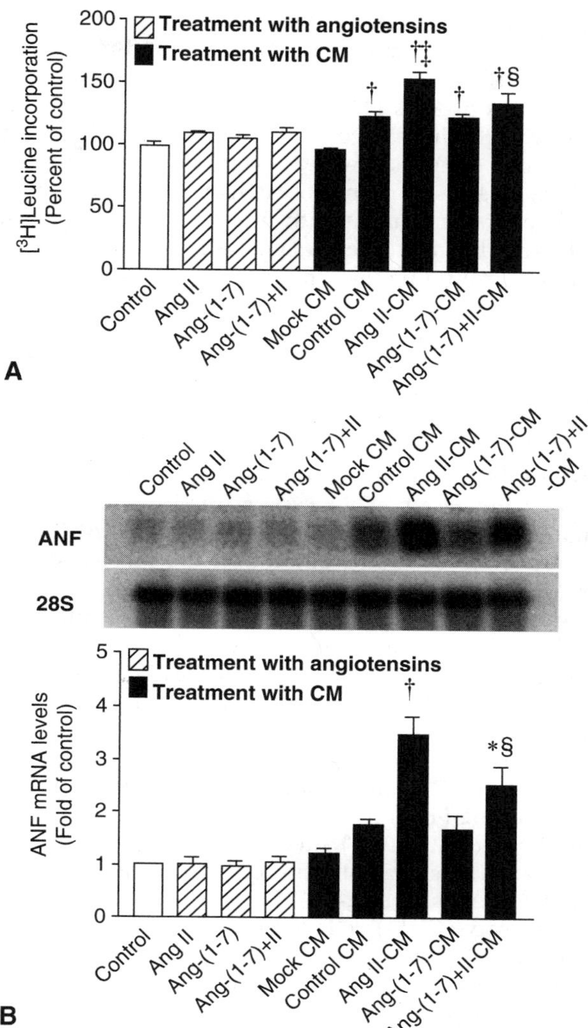

Figure 10-6 Effects of angiotensins and conditioned media (CM) from adult rat cardiac fibroblasts (ARCFs) treated with angiotensins on [(3)H]leucine incorporation and atrial natriuretic factor (ANF) mRNA expression in cardiomyocytes. Cardiomyocytes were stimulated for 24 hours with Ang II (10^{-7} M), Ang-(1–7) (10^{-7} M), or both after 1-hour pretreatment with Ang-(1–7) [10^{-7} M; Ang-(1–7)+II] or CM from ARCFs in the presence of [Sar(1),Thr(8)]-Ang II (10^{-6} M) to assess [(3)H]leucine incorporation and rat ANF mRNA expression. **(A)** Effects of angiotensins and CM on [(3)H]leucine incorporation in cardiomyocytes. **(B)** Effects of angiotensins and CM on ANF mRNA expression in cardiomyocytes. Representative Northern blots of ANF mRNA and 28S rRNA are depicted above the composite data.
Ang II-CM, CM from Ang II-treated ARCFs; Ang-(1–7)-CM, CM from Ang-(1–7)-treated ARCFs; Ang-(1–7)+II-CM, CM from ARCFs treated with both angiotensins after 1-hour pretreatment with Ang-(1–7). Data are means ± SE. **(A)** $n = 4$; **(B)** $n = 3$ or 4). $^{*}p < 0.01$; $^{\dagger}p < 0.001$ versus mock CM; $\ddagger p < 0.001$ versus control CM; $^{\S}p < 0.05$ versus Ang II-CM (Bonferroni's post hoc test). (From Iwata M, Cowling RT, Gurantz D, et al. Angiotensin-(1–7) binds to specific receptors on cardiac fibroblasts to initiate antifibrotic and antitrophic effects. *Am J Physiol.* [*Heart Circ Physiol.*] 2005; 289[6]:H2356–H2363, with permission.)

which Ang-(1–7) might counter Ang II effects is its ability to inhibit ACE activity (99), thereby reducing production of Ang II. Inhibition of ACE would have the added benefit of blocking the breakdown of antigrowth factors such as bradykinin (BK).

Ang-(1–7) can be generated locally in the myocardium of various species (20,111). It is formed from Ang I or Ang II in the interstitium of the canine LV, and the concentration of Ang-(1–7) immunoreactivity is increased in the rat heart following induction of a large MI due to coronary artery ligation (112). In the failing human heart, Ang-(1–7)-forming activity related to both neutral endopeptidase (NEP) and ACE2 is increased (113). In this setting, NEP has a preference for Ang I while ACE2 appears to have substrate preference for Ang II (113).

Evidence that the major pathway for the generation of Ang-(1–7) in the human heart depends on the availability of Ang II as a substrate suggests the importance of ACE2 in this process (113). Neither localization within the myocardium nor the cell type involved in the generation of Ang-(1–7) is known with certainty. In the post-MI rat heart, Ang-(1–7) immunoreactivity is associated with cardiac myocytes but not with interstitial cells or blood vessels, and the most intense signal is noted at 4 weeks in the zone surrounding the replacement scar. Although the increase in Ang-(1–7) in the post-MI heart suggests that ACE2 is likely to be increased in this setting (93) in a manner analogous to what has been reported with ACE (18, 114), whether or not this actually occurs is uncertain. In one report neither ACE nor ACE2 mRNA levels were increased in noninfarcted segments of LV in rats 4 weeks post-MI (106), whereas in another study there was evidence of increased ACE2 expression in both rat and human hearts post-MI (115). Expression of ACE2 has been reported to be upregulated in the failing human heart (116).

The effects of Ang-(1–7) on cells appear to be mediated through an interaction with a distinct receptor that is encoded by the *Mas* proto-oncogene (117). This is a 7-transmembrane domain receptor that contains features characteristic of class I G-protein-coupled receptors. Studies done in *Mas*-null mice demonstrated that the absence of this G-protein-coupled receptor abolishes the binding of Ang-(1–7) to kidney cells as well as the antidiuretic effects of Ang-(1–7) after administration of an acute water load. The aortas of *Mas*-deficient mice also fail to relax in response to Ang-(1–7). Transfection of Chinese hamster ovary (CHO) cells with the *Mas* proto-ocogene increased arachidonic acid release. When cardiac myocytes were transfected with antisense oligonucleotide to the *Mas* receptor, Ang-(1–7)-induced MAP kinase activation was blocked (103). There is also evidence that the *Mas* receptor can hetero-oligomerize with the AT_1 receptor in a manner similar to what has been described for the AT_2 receptor (118). As in the case of the AT_2 receptor, this interaction would have the effect of inhibiting some of the actions of Ang II on cells.

CONCLUSIONS

While it is clear that the RAS plays a major role in the development and progression of heart failure, the exact mechanisms involved have not yet been fully delineated. The concept that circulating Ang II was the only (or even the major) effector molecule of this system has long been disproved, first with evidence that this peptide could be produced locally within the heart and, more recently, by reports indicating that other angiotensin peptides such as Ang-(1–7) could influence cardiac structure and function. The presence of receptors in addition to the AT_1 receptor has added a degree of complexity to the system. Whether the AT_2 receptor mediates effects that are harmful or beneficial is uncertain and may be dependent on the context in which activation occurs. Discovery of the alternative pathway involving ACE2 has also opened new possibilities that need to be explored. In addition to affirming the importance of the RAS in heart failure, what can be said with certainty at this time is that the final word regarding the workings of this system has not yet been spoken.

REFERENCES

1. Tigerstedt R, Bergman PG. Niere und Kreislauf. *Scandinav Arch J Physiol.* 1898, 8:223.
2. Francis GS, Benedict C, Johnstone DE, et al. Comparison of neuroendocrine activation in patients with left ventricular dysfunction with and without congestive heart failure. A substudy of the Studies of Left Ventricular Dysfunction (SOLVD). *Circulation.* 1990;82(5):1724–1729.
3. Hodsman GP, Kohzuki M, Howes LG, et al. Neurohumoral responses to chronic myocardial infarction in rats. *Circulation.* 1988;78(2):376–381.
4. Michel JB, Lattion AL, Salzmann JL, et al. Hormonal and cardiac effects of converting enzyme inhibition in rat myocardial infarction. *Circ Res.* 1988;62(4):641–650.
5. Pfeffer JM, Pfeffer MA, Braunwald E. Influence of chronic captopril therapy on the infarcted left ventricle of the rat. *Circ Res.* 1985;57(1):84–95.
6. Pfeffer MA, Lamas GA, Vaughan DE, et al. Effect of captopril on progressive ventricular dilatation after anterior myocardial infarction. *N Engl J Med.* 1988;319(2):80–86.
7. Greenberg B, Quinones MA, Koilpillai C, et al. Effects of long-term enalapril therapy on cardiac structure and function in patients with left ventricular dysfunction. Results of the SOLVD echocardiography substudy. *Circulation.* 1995;91(10): 2573–2581.
8. Schieffer B, Wirger A, Meybrunn M, et al. Comparative effects of chronic angiotensin-converting enzyme-inhibition and angiotensin-II type-1 receptor blockade on cardiac remodeling after myocardial infarction in the rat. *Circulation.* 1994; 89(5): 2273–2282.
9. Paul M, Wagner J, Dzau VJ. Gene expression of the renin-angiotensin system in human tissues. Quantitative analysis by the polymerase chain reaction. *J Clin Invest.* 1993;91(5): 2058–2064.
10. Zhang X, Dostal DE, Reiss K, et al. Identification and activation of autocrine renin-angiotensin system in adult ventricular myocytes. *Am J Physiol.* 1995;269(5 Pt 2):H1791–H1802.
11. Katwa LC, Ratajska A, Cleutjens JP, et al. Angiotensin converting enzyme and kinase-II-like activities in cultured valvular interstitial cells of the rat heart. *Cardiovasc Res.* 1995;29(1):57–64.
12. Lindpaintner K, Lu W, Neidermajer N, et al. Selective activation of cardiac angiotensinogen gene expression in post-infarction ventricular remodeling in the rat. *J. Mol Cell Cardiol.* 1993;25(2): 133–143.
13. Dostal DE, Rothblum KN, Chernin MI, et al. Intracardiac detection of angiotensinogen and renin: a localized renin-angiotensin system in neonatal rat heart. *Am J Physiol.* 1992;263(4 Pt 1):C838–C850.
14. Endo-Mochizuki Y, Mochizuki N, Sawa H, et al. Expression of renin and angiotensin-converting enzyme in human hearts. *Heart Vessels.* 1995;10(6):285–293.
15. Urata H, Boehm KD, Philip A, et al. Cellular localization and regional distribution of an angiotensin II-forming chymase in the heart. *J Clin Invest.* 1993;91(4):1269–1281.
16. Muller DN, Fischli W, Clozel JP, et al. Local angiotensin II generation in the rat heart: role of renin uptake. *Circ Res.* 1998;82(1):13–20.
17. De Mello WC, Danser AH. Angiotensin II and the heart: on the intracrine renin-angiotensin system. *Hypertension.* 2000;35(6): 1183–1188.
18. Hirsch AT, Talsness CE, Schunkert H, et al. Tissue-specific activation of cardiac angiotensin converting enzyme in experimental heart failure. *Circ Res.* 1991;69(2):475–482.
19. Serneri GG, Boddi M, Cecioni I, et al. Cardiac angiotensin II formation in the clinical course of heart failure and its relationship with left ventricular function. *Circ Res.* 2001;88(9):961–968.

20. Wei CC, Ferrario CM, Brosnihan KB, et al. Angiotensin peptides modulate bradykinin levels in the interstitium of the dog heart in vivo. *J Pharmacol Exp Ther*. 2002;300(1):324–329.
21. Paradis P, Dali-Youcef N, Paradis FW, et al. Overexpression of angiotensin II type I receptor in cardiomyocytes induces cardiac hypertrophy and remodeling. *Proc Natl Acad Sci USA*. 2000;97(2):931–936.
22. Harada K, Sugaya T, Murakami K, et al. Angiotensin II type 1A receptor knockout mice display less left ventricular remodeling and improved survival after myocardial infarction. *Circulation*. 1999;100(20):2093–2099.
23. Mazzolai L, Nussberger J, Aubert JF, et al. Blood pressure-independent cardiac hypertrophy induced by locally activated renin-angiotensin system. *Hypertension*. 1998;31(6):1324–1330.
24. Sandberg K. Structural analysis and regulation of angiotensin II receptors. *Trends Endcrinol Metab*. 1994;5:28–35.
25. Murphy TJ, Alexander RW, Griendling KK, et al. Isolation of a cDNA encoding the vascular type-1 angiotensin II receptor. *Nature*. 1991;351(6323):233–236.
26. Inagami T, Guo DF, Kitami Y. Molecular biology of angiotensin II receptors: an overview. *J Hypertens*. 1994;12(10)(Suppl): S83–S94.
27. Sechi LA, Griffin CA, Grady EF, et al. Characterization of angiotensin II receptor subtypes in rat heart. *Circ Res*. 1992;71(6):1482–1489.
28. Shanmugam S, Monnot C, Corvol P, et al. Distribution of type 1 angiotensin II receptor subtype messenger RNAs in the rat fetus. *Hypertension*. 1994;23(1):137–141.
29. Everett AD, Heller F, Fisher A. AT1 receptor gene regulation in cardiac myocytes and fibroblasts. *J Mol Cell Cardiol*. 1996;28(8):1727–1736.
30. Sadoshima J, Izumo S. Molecular characterization of angiotensin II-induced hypertrophy of cardiac myocytes and hyperplasia of cardiac fibroblasts. Critical role of the AT1 receptor subtype. *Circ Res*. 1993;73(3):413–423.
31. Sadoshima J, Izumo S. Signal transduction pathways of angiotensin II-induced c-fos gene expression in cardiac myocytes in vitro. Roles of phospholipid-derived second messengers. *Circ Res*. 1993;73(3):424–438.
32. Kalra D, Sivasubramanian N, Mann DL. Angiotensin II induces tumor necrosis factor biosynthesis in the adult mammalian heart through a protein kinase C-dependent pathway. *Circulation*. 2002;105(18):2198–2205.
33. Murasawa S, Mori Y, Nozawa Y, et al. Angiotensin II type 1 receptor-induced extracellular signal-regulated protein kinase activation is mediated by Ca2+/calmodulin-dependent transactivation of epidermal growth factor receptor. *Circ Res*. 1998;82(12): 1338–1348.
34. Bhat GJ, Baker KM. Angiotensin II stimulates rapid serine phosphorylation of transcription factor Stat3. *Mol Cell Biochem*. 1997;170(1–2):171–176.
35. Wang D, Yu X, Cohen RA, et al. Distinct effects of N-acetylcysteine and nitric oxide on angiotensin II-induced epidermal growth factor receptor phosphorylation and intracellular Ca(2+) levels. *J Biol Chem*. 2000;275(16):12223–12230.
36. Bhat GJ, Thekkumkara TJ, Thomas WG, et al. Activation of the STAT pathway by angiotensin II in T3CHO/AT1A cells. Cross-talk between angiotensin II and interleukin-6 nuclear signaling. *J Biol Chem*. 1995;270(32):19059–19065.
37. Fischer TA, Singh K, O'Hara DS, et al. Role of AT1 and AT2 receptors in regulation of MAPKs and MKP-1 by ANG II in adult cardiac myocytes. *Am J Physiol*. 1998;275(3 Pt 2):H906–H916.
38. Paxton WG, Marrero MB, Klein JD, et al. The angiotensin II AT1 receptor is tyrosine and serine phosphorylated and can serve as a substrate for the src family of tyrosine kinases. *Biochem Biophys Res Commun*. 1994;200(1):260–267.
39. Seta K, Nanamori M, Modrall JG, et al. AT1 receptor mutant lacking heterotrimeric G protein coupling activates the Src-Ras-ERK pathway without nuclear translocation of ERKs. *J Biol Chem*. 2002;277(11):9268–9277.
40. Booz GW, Baker KM. Protein kinase C in angiotensin II signalling in neonatal rat cardiac fibroblasts. Role in the mitogenic response. *Ann NY Acad Sci*. 1995;752:158–167.
41. Pan J, Fukuda K, Kodama H, et al. Role of angiotensin II in activation of the JAK/STAT pathway induced by acute pressure overload in the rat heart. *Circ Res*. 1997;81(4):611–617.
42. Wang HD, Xu S, Johns DG, et al. Role of NADPH oxidase in the vascular hypertrophic and oxidative stress response to angiotensin II in mice. *Circ Res*. 2001;88(9):947–953.
43. Eguchi S, Iwasaki H, Inagami T, et al. Involvement of PYK2 in angiotensin II signaling of vascular smooth muscle cells. *Hypertension*. 1999;33(1 Pt 2):201–206.
44. Harrison DG, Cai H, Landmesser U, et al. Interactions of angiotensin II with NAD(P)H oxidase, oxidant stress and cardiovascular disease. *J Renin Angiotensin Aldosterone Syst*. 2003;4(2): 51–61.
45. Villarreal FJ, Kim NN, Ungab GD, et al. Identification of functional angiotensin II receptors on rat cardiac fibroblasts. *Circulation*. 1993;88(6):2849–2861.
46. Gray MO, Long CS, Kalinyak JE, et al. Angiotensin II stimulates cardiac myocyte hypertrophy via paracrine release of TGF-beta 1 and endothelin-1 from fibroblasts. *Cardiovasc Res*. 1998;40(2): 352–363.
47. Aikawa R, Komuro I, Nagai R, et al. Rho plays an important role in angiotensin II-induced hypertrophic responses in cardiac myocytes. *Mol Cell Biochem*. 2000;212(1–2):177–182.
48. Hunton DL, Lucchesi PA, Pang Y, et al. Capacitative calcium entry contributes to nuclear factor of activated T-cells nuclear translocation and hypertrophy in cardiomyocytes. *J Bioll Chem*. 2002;277(16):14266–14273.
49. Aceto JF, Baker KM. [Sar1]angiotensin II receptor-mediated stimulation of protein synthesis in chick heart cells. *Am J Physiol*. 1990;258(3 Pt 2):H806–H813.
50. Campbell SE, Katwa LC. Angiotensin II-stimulated expression of transforming growth factor-beta1 in cardiac fibroblasts and myofibroblasts. *J Mol Cell Cardiol*. 1997;29(7):1947–1958.
51. Harada M, Itoh H, Nakagawa O, et al. Significance of ventricular myocytes and nonmyocytes interaction during cardiocyte hypertrophy: evidence for endothelin-1 as a paracrine hypertrophic factor from cardiac nonmyocytes. *Circulation*. 1997;96(10): 3737–3744.
52. Fujisaki H, Ito H, Hirata Y, et al. Natriuretic peptides inhibit angiotensin II-induced proliferation of rat cardiac fibroblasts by blocking endothelin-1 gene expression. *J Clin Invest*. 1995; 96(2):1059–1065.
53. Sano M, Fukuda K, Sato T, et al. ERK and p38 MAPK, but not NF-kappaB, are critically involved in reactive oxygen species-mediated induction of IL-6 by angiotensin II in cardiac fibroblasts. *Circ Res*. 2001;89(8):661–669.
54. Sano M, Fukuda K, Kodama H, et al. Interleukin-6 family of cytokines mediate angiotensin II-induced cardiac hypertrophy in rodent cardiomyocytes. *J Biol Chem*. 2000;275(38): 29717–29723.
55. Piacentini L, Gray M, Honbo NY, et al. Endothelin-1 stimulates cardiac fibroblast proliferation through activation of protein kinase C. *J Mol Cell Cardiol*. 2000;32(4):565–576.
56. Wang F, Trial J, Diwan A, et al. Regulation of cardiac fibroblast cellular function by leukemia inhibitory factor. *J Mol Cell Cardiol*. 2002;34(10):1309–1316.
57. Yue TL, Gu JL, Wang C, et al. Extracellular signal-regulated kinase plays an essential role in hypertrophic agonists, endothelin-1 and phenylephrine-induced cardiomyocyte hypertrophy. *J Biol Chem*. 2000;275(48):37895–37901.
58. Kodama H, Fukuda K, Pan J, et al. Leukemia inhibitory factor, a potent cardiac hypertrophic cytokine, activates the JAK/STAT pathway in rat cardiomyocytes. *Circ Res*. 1997;81(5): 656–663.
59. Murata M, Fukuda K, Ishida H, et al. Leukemia inhibitory factor, a potent cardiac hypertrophic cytokine, enhances L-type Ca2+ current and [Ca2+]i transient in cardiomyocytes. *J Mol Cell Cardiol*. 1999;31(1):237–245.
60. Kim NN, Villarreal FJ, Printz MP, et al. Trophic effects of angiotensin II on neonatal rat cardiac myocytes are mediated by cardiac fibroblasts. *Am J Physiol*. 1995;269(3 Pt 1):E426–E437.
61. Crawford DC, Chobanian AV, Brecher P. Angiotensin II induces fibronectin expression associated with cardiac fibrosis in the rat. *Circ Res*. 1994;74(4):727–739.
62. Brilla CG, Zhou G, Matsubara L, et al. Collagen metabolism in cultured adult rat cardiac fibroblasts: response to angiotensin II and aldosterone. *J Mol Cell Cardiol*. 1994;26(7):809–820.
63. Sun Y, Ramires FJ, Zhou G, et al. Fibrous tissue and angiotensin II. *J Mol Cell Cardiol*. 1997;29(8):2001–2012.

64. Schorb W, Booz GW, Dostal DE, et al. Angiotensin II is mitogenic in neonatal rat cardiac fibroblasts. *Circ Res.* 1993;72(6):1245–1254.
65. Nio Y, Matsubara H, Murasawa S, et al. Regulation of gene transcription of angiotensin II receptor subtypes in myocardial infarction. *J Clin Invest.* 1995;95(1):46–54.
66. Sun Y, Cleutjens JP, Diaz-Arias AA, et al. Cardiac angiotensin converting enzyme and myocardial fibrosis in the rat. *Cardiovasc Res.* 1994;28(9):1423–1432.
67. Lefroy DC, Wharton J, Crake T, et al. Regional changes in angiotensin II receptor density after experimental myocardial infarction. *J Mol Cell Cardiol.* 1996;28(2):429–440.
68. Sun Y, Weber KT. Angiotensin II receptor binding following myocardial infarction in the rat. *Cardiovasc Res.* 1994;28(11):1623–1628.
69. Gurantz D, Cowling RT, Villarreal FJ, et al. Tumor necrosis factor-alpha upregulates angiotensin II type 1 receptors on cardiac fibroblasts. *Circ Res.* 1999;85(3):272–279.
70. Cowling RT, Gurantz D, Peng J, et al. Transcription factor NF-kappa B is necessary for up-regulation of type 1 angiotensin II receptor mRNA in rat cardiac fibroblasts treated with tumor necrosis factor-alpha or interleukin-1 beta. *J Biol Chem.* 2002;277(8):5719–5724.
71. Gurantz D, Cowling RT, Varki N, et al. IL-1B and TNF-a upregulate angiotensin II type 1 (AT1) receptors on cardiac fibroblasts and are associated with increased AT1 density in the post-MI heart. *J Mol Cell Cardiol.* In press.
72. Peng J, Gurantz D, Tran V, et al. Tumor necrosis factor-alpha-induced AT1 receptor upregulation enhances angiotensin II-mediated cardiac fibroblast responses that favor fibrosis. *Circ Res.* 2002;91(12):1119–1126.
73. Kambayashi Y, Bardhan S, Takahashi K, et al. Molecular cloning of a novel angiotensin II receptor isoform involved in phosphotyrosine phosphatase inhibition. *J Biol Chem.* 1993;268(33):24543–24546.
74. Mukoyama M, Nakajima M, Horiuchi M, et al. Expression cloning of type 2 angiotensin II receptor reveals a unique class of seven-transmembrane receptors. *J Biol Chem.* 1993;268(33):24539–24542.
75. Shanmugam S, Lenkei ZG, Gasc JM, et al. Ontogeny of angiotensin II type 2 (AT2) receptor mRNA in the rat. *Kidney Int.* 1995;47(4):1095–1100.
76. Lopez JJ, Lorell BH, Ingelfinger JR, et al. Distribution and function of cardiac angiotensin AT1- and AT2-receptor subtypes in hypertrophied rat hearts. *Am J Physiol.* 1994;267(2 Pt 2):H844–H852.
77. Asano K, Dutcher DL, Port JD, et al. Selective downregulation of the angiotensin II AT1-receptor subtype in failing human ventricular myocardium. *Circulation.* 1997;95(5):1193–1200.
78. Wharton J, Morgan K, Rutherford RA, et al. Differential distribution of angiotensin AT2 receptors in the normal and failing human heart. *J Pharmacol Exp Ther.* 1998;284(1):323–336.
79. Booz GW. Cardiac angiotensin AT2 receptor: what exactly does it do? *Hypertension.* 2004;43(6):1162–1163.
80. Nouet S, Nahmias C. Signal transduction from the angiotensin II AT2 receptor. *Trends Endocrinol Metab.* 2000;11(1):1–6.
81. Siragy HM, Carey RM. The subtype 2 (AT2) angiotensin receptor mediates renal production of nitric oxide in conscious rats. *J Clin Invest.* 1997;100(2):264–269.
82. Horiuchi M, Hayashida W, Kambe T, et al. Angiotensin type 2 receptor dephosphorylates Bcl-2 by activating mitogen-activated protein kinase phosphatase-1 and induces apoptosis. *J Biol Chem.* 1997;272(30):19022–19026.
83. Yamada T, Horiuchi M, Dzau VJ. Angiotensin II type 2 receptor mediates programmed cell death. *Proc Natl Acad Sci USA.* 1996;93(1):156–160.
84. AbdAlla S, Lother H, Abdel-tawab AM, et al. The angiotensin II AT2 receptor is an AT1 receptor antagonist. *J Biol Chem.* 2001;276(43):39721–39726.
85. Masaki H, Kurihara T, Yamaki A, et al. Cardiac-specific overexpression of angiotensin II AT2 receptor causes attenuated response to AT1 receptor-mediated pressor and chronotropic effects. *J Clin Invest.* 1998;101(3):527–535.
86. Stoll M, Steckelings UM, Paul M, et al. The angiotensin AT2-receptor mediates inhibition of cell proliferation in coronary endothelial cells. *J Clin Invest.* 1995;95(2):651–657.
87. Booz GW, Baker KM. Role of type 1 and type 2 angiotensin receptors in angiotensin II-induced cardiomyocyte hypertrophy. *Hypertension.* 1996;28(4):635–640.
88. Ichihara S, Senbonmatsu T, Price E Jr., et al. Angiotensin II type 2 receptor is essential for left ventricular hypertrophy and cardiac fibrosis in chronic angiotensin II-induced hypertension. *Circulation.* 2001;104(3):346–351.
89. Yan X, Price RL, Nakayama M, et al. Ventricular-specific expression of angiotensin II type 2 receptors causes dilated cardiomyopathy and heart failure in transgenic mice. *Am J Physiol.* (*Heart Circ Physiol.*) 2003;285(5):H2179–H2187.
90. Alfakih K, Maqbool A, Sivananthan M, et al. Left ventricle mass index and the common, functional, X-linked angiotensin II type-2 receptor gene polymorphism (-1332 G/A) in patients with systemic hypertension. *Hypertension.* 2004;43(6):1189–1194.
91. Donoghue M, Hsieh F, Baronas E, et al. A novel angiotensin-converting enzyme-related carboxypeptidase (ACE2) converts angiotensin I to angiotensin 1–9. *Circ Res.* 2000;87(5):E1–E9.
92. Harmer D, Gilbert M, Borman R, et al. Quantitative mRNA expression profiling of ACE 2, a novel homologue of angiotensin converting enzyme. *FEBS Lett.* 2002;532(1–2):107–110.
93. Burrell LM, Johnston CI, Tikellis C, et al. ACE2, a new regulator of the renin-angiotensin system. *Trends Endocrinol Metab.* 2004;15(4):166–169.
94. Tipnis SR, Hooper NM, Hyde R, et al. A human homolog of angiotensin-converting enzyme—Cloning and functional expression as a captopril-insensitive carboxypeptidase. *J Biol Chem.* 2000;275(43):33238–33243.
95. Vickers C, Hales P, Kaushik V, et al. Hydrolysis of biological peptides by human angiotensin-converting enzyme-related carboxypeptidase. *J Biol Chem.* 2002;277(17):14838–14843.
96. Li W, Moore MJ, Vasilieva N, et al. Angiotensin-converting enzyme 2 is a functional receptor for the SARS coronavirus. *Nature.* 2003;426(6965):450–454.
97. Crackower MA, Sarao R, Oudit GY, et al. Angiotensin-converting enzyme 2 is an essential regulator of heart function. *Nature* 2002;417(6891):822–828.
98. Imai Y, Kuba K, Rao S, et al. Angiotensin-converting enzyme 2 protects from severe acute lung failure. *Nature.* 2005;436(7047):112–116.
99. Li P, Chappell MC, Ferrario CM, et al. Angiotensin-(1–7) augments bradykinin-induced vasodilation by competing with ACE and releasing nitric oxide. *Hypertension.* 1997;29(1 Pt 2):394–400.
100. Freeman EJ, Chisolm GM, Ferrario CM, et al. Angiotensin-(1–7) inhibits vascular smooth muscle cell growth. *Hypertension.* 1996;28(1):104–108.
101. Zhu Z, Zhong J, Zhu S, et al. Angiotensin-(1–7) inhibits angiotensin II-induced signal transduction. *J Cardiovasc Pharmacol.* 2002;40(5):693–700.
102. Strawn WB, Ferrario CM, Tallant EA. Angiotensin-(1–7) reduces smooth muscle growth after vascular injury. *Hypertension.* 1999;33(1 Pt 2):207–211.
103. Tallant EA, Ferrario CM, Gallagher PE. Angiotensin-(1–7) inhibits growth of cardiac myocytes through activation of the mas receptor. *Am J Physiol.* (*Heart Circ Physiol.*) 2005;289(4):H1560–H1566.
104. Iwata M, Cowling RT, Gurantz D, et al. Angiotensin-(1–7) binds to specific receptors on cardiac fibroblasts to initiate antifibrotic and antitrophic effects. *Am J Physiol.* (*Heart Circ Physiol.*) 2005;289(6):H2356–H2363.
105. Loot AE, Roks AJ, Henning RH, et al. Angiotensin-(1–7) attenuates the development of heart failure after myocardial infarction in rats. *Circulation.* 2002;105(13):1548–1550.
106. Ishiyama Y, Gallagher PE, Averill DB, et al. Upregulation of angiotensin-converting enzyme 2 after myocardial infarction by blockade of angiotensin II receptors. *Hypertension.* 2004;43(5):970–976.
107. Clark MA, Diz DI, Tallant EA. Angiotensin-(1–7) downregulates the angiotensin II type 1 receptor in vascular smooth muscle cells. *Hypertension.* 2001;37(4):1141–1146.
108. Tallant EA, Clark MA. Molecular mechanisms of inhibition of vascular growth by angiotensin-(1–7). *Hypertension.* 2003;42(4):574–579.

109. Brosnihan KB, Li P, Ferrario CM. Angiotensin-(1–7) dilates canine coronary arteries through kinins and nitric oxide. *Hypertension*. 1996;27(3 Pt 2):523–528.
110. Muthalif MM, Benter IF, Uddin MR, et al. Signal transduction mechanisms involved in angiotensin-(1–7)-stimulated arachidonic acid release and prostanoid synthesis in rabbit aortic smooth muscle cells. *J Pharmacol Exp Ther*. 1998;284(1): 388–398.
111. Zisman LS, Meixell GE, Bristow MR, et al. Angiotensin-(1–7) formation in the intact human heart: in vivo dependence on angiotensin II as substrate. *Circulation* 2003;108(14):1679–1681.
112. Averill DB, Ishiyama Y, Chappell MC, et al. Cardiac angiotensin-(1–7) in ischemic cardiomyopathy. *Circulation*. 2003;108(17): 2141–2146.
113. Zisman LS, Keller RS, Weaver B, et al. Increased angiotensin-(1–7)-forming activity in failing human heart ventricles: evidence for upregulation of the angiotensin-converting enzyme Homologue ACE2. *Circulation*. 2003;108(14):1707–1712.
114. Duncan AM, Burrell LM, Kladis A, et al. Effects of angiotensin-converting enzyme inhibition on angiotensin and bradykinin peptides in rats with myocardial infarction. *J Cardiovasc Pharmacol*. 1996;28(6):746–754.
115. Burrell LM, Risvanis J, Kubota E, et al. Myocardial infarction increases ACE2 expression in rat and humans. *Eur Heart J*. 2005;26(4):369–375.
116. Goulter AB, Goddard MJ, Allen JC, et al. ACE2 gene expression is up-regulated in the human failing heart. *BMC Med*. 2004; 2:19.
117. Santos RAS, Silva ACSE, Maric C, et al. Angiotensin-(1–7) is an endogenous ligand for the G protein-coupled receptor Mas. *Proc Natl Acad Sci USA*. 2003;100(14):8258–8263.
118. Kostenis E, Milligan G, Christopoulos A, et al. G-protein-coupled receptor Mas is a physiological antagonist of the angiotensin II type 1 receptor. *Circulation*. 2005;111(14): 1806–1813.

Sympathetic Nervous System in Heart Failure

G. Michael Felker Wilson S. Colucci Howard A. Rockman

The sympathetic nervous system (SNS) plays a central role in cardiovascular physiology by releasing endogenous neurohormones that primarily act on a family of cellular receptors known as 7-transmembrane or heptahelical receptors. Activation of these heptahelical receptors transduces extracellular signals across the cell surface to mediate numerous cellular processes. In the event of an acute decrease in myocardial performance, increased SNS activity serves as a critical compensatory mechanism that supports the cardiovascular system. This is accomplished through a variety of physiology changes, including increasing heart rate, myocardial contractility, and venous return, all of which help to restore and maintain cardiac output. Adequate blood pressure to preserve organ perfusion is further supported by systemic arterial constriction, and intravascular volume is expanded through increased renal retention of sodium and water. While adaptive in the short term, these have deleterious effects on the cardiovascular system when maintained chronically. Vasoconstriction, salt and water retention, increased heart rate, and increased contractility lead to increases in myocardial wall stresses, oxygen consumption, and energetic requirements. Chronically elevated levels of SNS activity may also cause arrhythmias, desensitization of the postsynaptic β-adrenergic receptor pathway, and activation of other neurohumoral systems (e.g., the renin-angiotensin system), which may themselves exert adverse effects. Finally, prolonged exposure to norepinephrine (NE) may contribute to disease progression by acting directly on the biology of the myocardium to modify cellular phenotype and cause myocyte death (1). The balance between the compensatory and the maladaptive effects of SNS activation is central to the understanding of heart failure pathophysiology.

REGULATION OF SYMPATHETIC NERVOUS SYSTEM IN HEART FAILURE

Sympathetic activity, as measured by an increase in circulating plasma NE, is increased in patients with heart failure and is related to both disease severity and prognosis (Fig. 11-1) (2). In addition to elevations in plasma NE, SNS activation in heart failure is demonstrated by increases in the urinary excretion of catecholamines and electrical activity in skeletal muscle (2–6). Of note, plasma NE is elevated even in patients with mild or asymptomatic heart failure in whom there is little or no increase in circulating renin levels (7). While plasma NE levels reflect overall systemic activity, they do not address the level of cardiac sympathetic activity. Direct measurements of cardiac sympathetic nerve activity are not feasible in patients. However, the aorta-to-coronary-sinus gradient of plasma NE is increased in patients with heart failure (8), indicating an increase in the net release of NE from the heart.

Studies using tracer quantities of ^{3}H-NE to measure NE turnover kinetics across the heart have provided additional important information about cardiac sympathetic activity. These techniques have demonstrated that NE spillover is increased in the heart of patients with more severe heart failure (Fig. 11-2) (9,10). Cardiac spillover of NE is increased even in patients with mild symptoms of heart failure, at a time when there is no increase in total body or renal NE spillover (11), indicating that with early heart failure there is selective activation of cardiac sympathetic nerves.

An increase in cardiac spillover may reflect an increase in NE release, a decrease in reuptake, or both (10). In one study (12), cardiac NE spillover and dihydroxyphenylalanine (DOPA) production were increased eightfold and

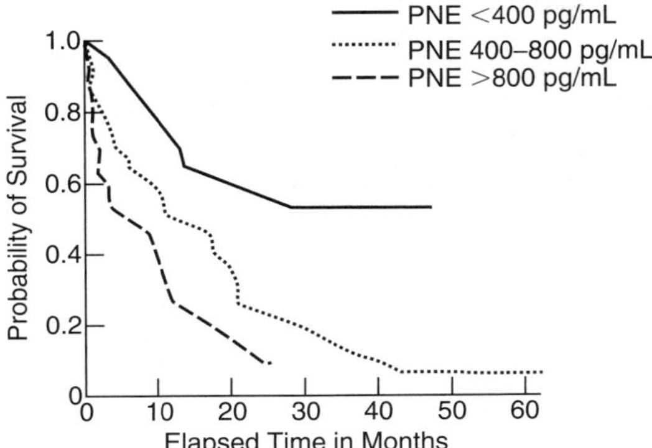

Figure 11-1 Plasma norepinephrine levels in patients with heart failure. Patients with the most elevated levels had the worst prognosis. (From Cohn JN, Levine TB, Olivari MT, et al. Plasma norepinephrine as a guide to prognosis in patients with chronic congestive heart failure. *N Engl J Med.* 1984;311:819–820, with permission.)

twofold, respectively, in patients with heart failure, whereas cardiac extraction of NE was unchanged. The outward flux of dihydroxylphenylglycol (DHPG), which reflects neuronal reuptake and intraneuronal metabolism of NE, was similar in normal subjects and patients with heart failure and was reduced to a comparable degree by desipramine, which blocks neuronal reuptake, suggesting that their NE reuptake was not impaired. However, another study found a modest reduction in neuronal reuptake (13), leading to the conclusion that although increased NE release is the major mechanism of NE spillover, reduced reuptake may contribute, particularly in patients with more severe heart failure (10). The mechanism responsible for increased neuronal release of NE in heart failure is not certain but, as discussed below, may involve reflex mechanisms and/or presynaptic facilitation of NE release.

Blunted Baroreceptor Function in Heart Failure

Baroreceptor function is abnormal in both experimental animals and humans with heart failure (14,15). Increases in mean arterial or pulse pressure, or increased atrial or ventricular filling pressures and distention, or both, normally cause activation of cardiopulmonary and arterial baroreceptors, which inhibit SNS outflow from cardiovascular centers and cause a reciprocal increase in parasympathetic activity. Baroreceptor sensitivity is blunted in animal models and patients with heart failure, as evidenced by the observation that the reflex sympathetic response to reductions in arterial pressure (e.g., caused by nitroprusside infusion, head-up tilt, or lower-body negative pressure) is decreased (14–19). Conversely, the reflex withdrawal of sympathetic tone that normally follows the infusion of a vasopressor (e.g., phenylephrine) is attenuated.

Baroreceptor sensitivity can be quantified by measuring the relative changes in heart rate (R-R interval) and arterial pressure during the infusion of phenylephrine, which in normal persons causes an approximately 10-millisecond increase in the R-R interval for each 1 mm Hg rise in arterial pressure. In patients with severe heart failure, this slope is markedly reduced to the range of 2 ms/mm Hg (Fig. 11-3). Cardiac transplantation causes normalization of baroreceptor function with a return of the slope to the normal range (20), suggesting that baroreceptor dysfunction is not a primary abnormality but, rather, is secondary to cardiac dysfunction. An important consequence of reduced baroreceptor sensitivity may be that SNS efferent activity is inappropriately elevated relative to the level of cardiovascular performance.

The cellular basis for baroreceptor dysfunction is not known but may involve a number of factors such as mechanical alterations in the environment of the baroreceptor (e.g., vessel wall, myocardium), a resetting of baroreceptor reflex pathways (perhaps at the brainstem level), or alterations in the biochemical function of the baroreceptor, such as altered Na^+,K^+-ATPase activity (15). In animals, perfusion of isolated baroreceptors with digitalis or low K^+ to inhibit Na^+,K^+-ATPase partially corrects abnormal baroreceptor sensitivity (16), suggesting that increased Na^+,K^+-ATPase activity may contribute to reduced baroreceptor sensitivity in heart failure. Likewise, in patients with heart failure the acute intravenous administration of a digitalis glycoside normalizes baroreceptor sensitivity, as reflected by decreases in both forearm vascular

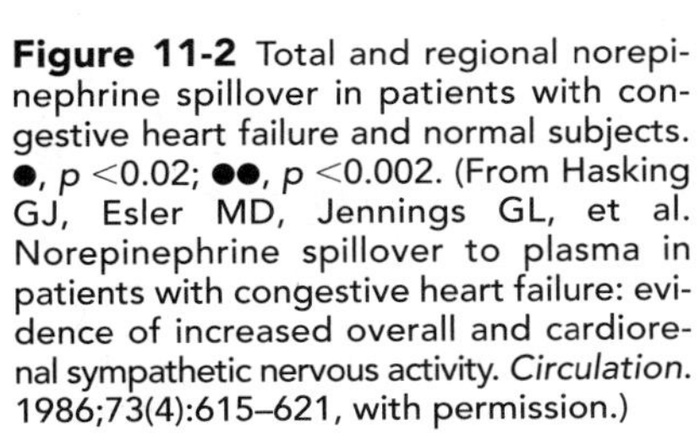

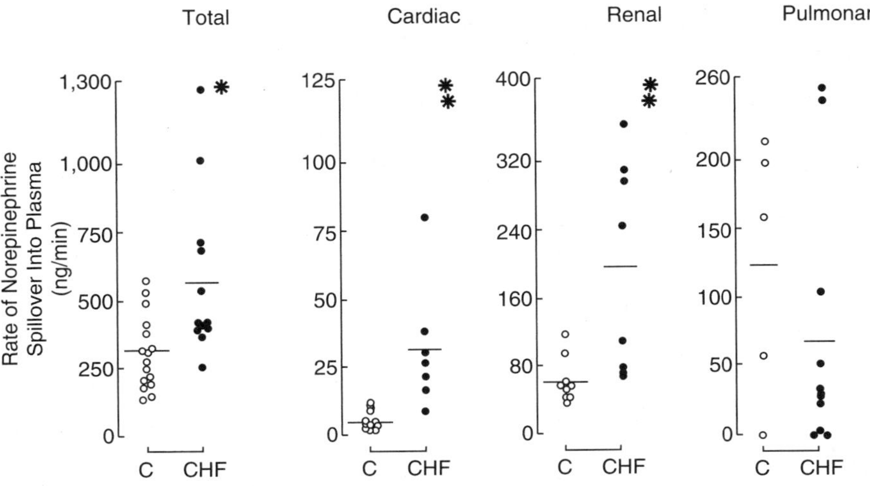

Figure 11-2 Total and regional norepinephrine spillover in patients with congestive heart failure and normal subjects. ●, $p < 0.02$; ●●, $p < 0.002$. (From Hasking GJ, Esler MD, Jennings GL, et al. Norepinephrine spillover to plasma in patients with congestive heart failure: evidence of increased overall and cardiorenal sympathetic nervous activity. *Circulation.* 1986;73(4):615–621, with permission.)

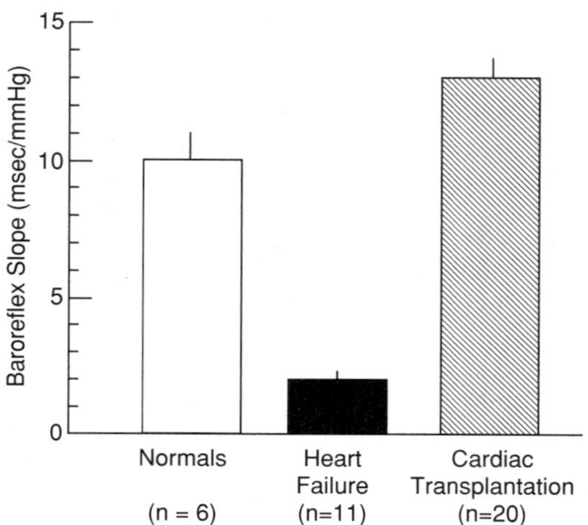

Figure 11-3 Arterial baroreflex slopes in normal persons, patients with congestive heart failure, and patients after cardiac transplantation. The arterial baroreflex slope is determined as the increase in R-R interval (milliseconds) per increase in arterial blood pressure (mm Hg) during administration of a vasoconstrictor such as phenylephrine. The baroreflex slope is typically reduced in patients with congestive heart failure, reflecting reduced sensitivity of arterial baroreceptors. After cardiac transplantation, baroreceptor sensitivity is restored to normal, indicating that reduced baroreceptor sensitivity in heart failure is reversible. (From Hirsch AT, Dzau VJ, Creager MA. Baroreceptor function in congestive heart failure: effect on neurohumoral activation and regional vascular resistance. *Circulation.* 1987;75(5 Pt 2):IV36–IV48, with permission.)

resistance and sympathetic nerve activity to skeletal muscle (21).

Most studies of reflex regulation in heart failure have focused on arterial baroreceptor function. It has been observed that cardiac NE spillover is increased in proportion to right heart pressures in patients with heart failure (22), leading to the suggestion that increased pulmonary pressures might be a stimulus for increased SNS activity. However, in contrast to arterial baroreceptors, the responsiveness of low-pressure cardiac receptors appears to be relatively preserved in patients with heart failure and would be anticipated to mediate a decrease rather than an increase in sympathetic activity in response to increased filling pressures (23).

Potentiation of Peripheral Norepinephrine Release

Norepinephrine is stored in vesicles in sympathetic nerve endings, where exocytotic release is triggered by a membrane depolarization-induced increase in the intracellular calcium concentration. The amount of NE released in response to a nerve impulse can be modulated by a variety of hormones and substances that act on specific receptors located on the nerve ending (Table 11-1) (24). By this mechanism, stimulation of presynaptic α2-adrenergic receptors decreases NE release, whereas stimulation of β2-adrenergic or angiotensin (25) receptors increases NE release. In humans it can be shown that the nonselective α-adrenergic antagonist phentolamine, which inhibits presynaptic α2-adrenergic receptors, increases NE release in the forearm (26) and heart (27). Conversely, stimulation of β2-adrenergic receptors increases NE spillover from the heart (28).

TABLE 11-1 PRESYNAPTIC RECEPTORS THAT MAY MODULATE THE RELEASE OF NOREPINEPHRINE

Inhibit Norepinephrine Release	Stimulate Norepinephrine Release
α_2-adrenergic	β_2-adrenergic
Dopamine	Angiotensin
Muscarinic	
Opiate	
Prostaglandin	
Adenosine	
Serotonin	
Histamine	

Given the increased levels of angiotensin and NE in heart failure, these observations could have important pathophysiological and therapeutic implications. Converting enzyme inhibitors and angiotensin receptor-blockers may reduce NE release by reducing the availability of angiotensin at presynaptic nerve endings. Conversely, increased NE availability at the nerve ending may facilitate additional NE release. Likewise, there may be release of epinephrine from extraneuronal sources in the hearts of patient with heart failure (29), which may in turn facilitate NE release via stimulation of presynaptic β2-adrenergic receptors.

Neuronal Norepinephrine Stores

Adrenergic nerves take up tyrosine, which is acted on by a series of enzymes (tyrosine hydroxylase, amino acid decarboxylase, and dopamine β-hydroxylase) to yield NE (30). Most of the NE released from the nerve ending is taken up by neuronal and, to a lesser extent, extraneuronal tissues (e.g., endothelial cells, vascular smooth muscle cells). The NE taken up by neurons may be recycled into vesicles for future release or converted to metabolites that are released into the circulation. The NE taken up by extraneuronal cells is likewise converted to metabolites that are released to the interstitial space and may be recovered in the plasma. As discussed previously, a decrease in the reuptake of NE by sympathetic neurons may contribute to increased NE spillover in patients with heart failure (10). Early work in patients with heart failure and in animal models found that the tissue concentration of NE was decreased in myocardium (3,30). Likewise, the release of myocardial NE stores by tyrosine was decreased in patients with heart failure. This depletion of cardiac NE may reflect a defect in NE biosynthesis (30) or a decrease in the neuronal reuptake of NE (13).

POSTSYNAPTIC REGULATION OF THE ADRENERGIC RESPONSE

β-adrenergic responsiveness is reduced in patients with heart failure, a phenomenon known as desensitization. In vitro,

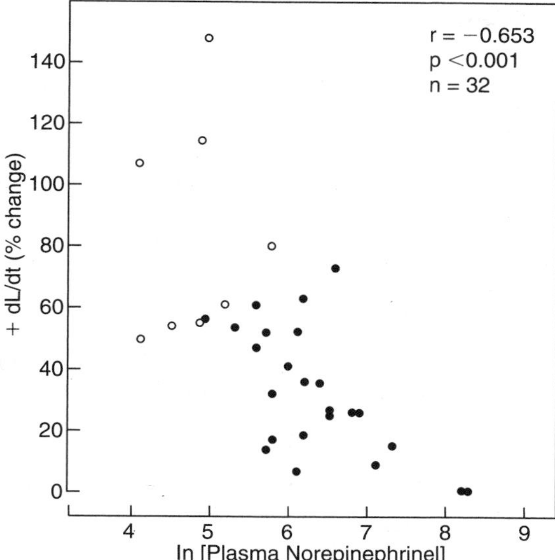

Figure 11-4 The positive inotropic response to an intracoronary infusion of dobutamine, 25 μg/min, in patients with congestive heart failure (**solid circles**) and persons without congestive heart failure (**open circles**).The magnitude of positive inotropic response to β-adrenergic receptor stimulation with intracoronary dobutamine is inversely related to the resting plasma NE concentration at the time of study, suggesting that decreased β-adrenergic responsiveness of the heart in patients with heart failure is caused, at least in part, by tonic elevation of sympathetic tone. (From Colucci WS, Denniss AR, Leatherman GF, et al. Intracoronary infusion of dobutamine to patients with and without severe congestive heart failure. Dose-response relationships, correlation with circulating catecholamines, and effect of phosphodiesterase inhibition. *J Clin Invest.* 1988;81(4):1103–1110.)

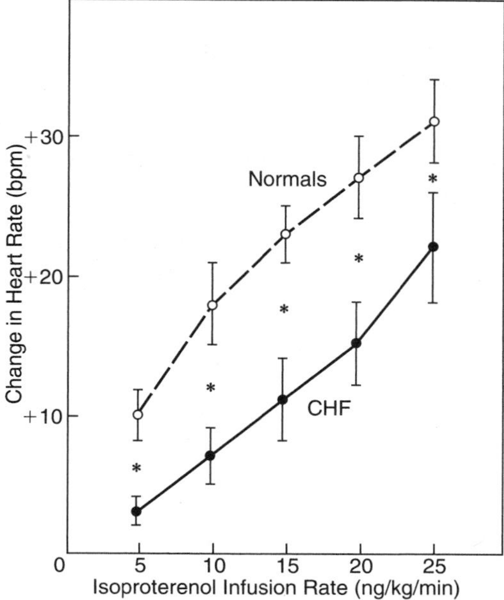

Figure 11-5 Dose-response relationship for isoproterenol-stimulated heart rate increase in normal persons (**dashed line**) and patients with severe congestive heart failure (**solid line**). (From Colucci WS, Ribeiro JP, Rocco MB, et al. Impaired chronotropic response to exercise in patients with congestive heart failure. Role of postsynaptic beta-adrenergic desensitization. *Circulation* 1989;80(2):314–323, with permission.)

myocardium obtained from patients with end-stage heart failure at the time of transplantation exhibits a normal contractile response to calcium but a markedly attenuated response to β-adrenergic agonists (31). In situ, the positive inotropic response to intracoronary infusion of a β-adrenergic agonist (dobutamine) is markedly depressed (Fig. 11-4) (32), as is the chronotropic response to a β-adrenergic agonist (isoproterenol) or exercise (Fig. 11-5) (33). Because heart rate is the predominant determinant of the increase in cardiac output that occurs with exercise, this may be a major way in which β-adrenergic receptor pathway dysfunction impacts the physiology of a patient with heart failure. The degree of attenuation of the inotropic and chronotropic response to β-adrenergic stimulation is inversely related to plasma NE (32,33). In contrast, the isovolumic relaxation response to β-adrenergic receptor stimulation is preserved, even in patients with end-stage heart failure (34). Several mechanisms may contribute to reduced β-adrenergic responsiveness in heart failure (Table 11-2). In the following, we summarize the body of animal and human studies that contribute to the current understanding of regulation of β-adrenergic responsiveness at the receptor level.

BIOLOGY OF HEPTAHELICAL RECEPTORS

Adrenergic receptors belong to the large superfamily of receptors known as 7-transmembrane or heptahelical receptors. Two classes of adrenergic receptors (ARs), α and β, have been described and, even though they both respond to norepinephrine and epinephrine, the cellular responses they mediate differ significantly. There are three known subtypes of βARs (β_1, β_2, and β_3), all of which are expressed in the heart (35) wherein, despite the existence of species-related differences (36), β_1ARs are the most abundant.

Activation of all types of adrenergic receptors results in G-protein-mediated generation of second messengers and/or activation of ion channels; therefore, these receptors are commonly referred to as G-protein-coupled receptors (GPCRs). By inducing conformational changes in the receptor, agonist stimulation allows interaction with the cognate heterotrimeric G-proteins, promoting dissociation

TABLE 11-2
POTENTIAL MECHANISMS FOR DECREASED β-ADRENERGIC RESPONSIVENESS IN FAILING HUMAN MYOCARDIUM

Downregulation of β_1-adrenergic receptors
Uncoupling of β_1-adrenergic receptors
Uncoupling of β_2-adrenergic receptors
Upregulation of β-adrenergic receptor kinase (βARK)
Increased activity of G_i
Decreased activity of adenylyl cyclase
Increased nitric oxide

Modified from Bristow MR, Hershberger RE, Port JD, et al. Beta-adrenergic pathways in nonfailing and failing human ventricular myocardium. *Circulation.* 1990;82(Suppl 2):I12–I25, with permission.

of G-proteins into G_α and $G_{\beta\gamma}$ subunits and activation. Both G_α subunits and $G_{\beta\gamma}$ dimers amplify and propagate signals intracellularly by activating one or more effector molecules, which in turn activate different signaling pathways by generating second messengers (Fig. 11-6). All known βAR subtypes couple to G_s and activate adenylyl cyclase, resulting in elevated cyclic adenosine monophosphate (cAMP) levels and subsequent activation of protein kinase (PKA) (37). PKA activation is a critical step in the mediation of contractility through phosphorylation of L-type calcium channels and regulation of calcium influx and reuptake (36). In addition to G_s, β_2ARs have been shown to couple to G_i both in vitro (38), and in the heart (36,39–41).

Given the biological relevance of these receptors, it is not surprising that they have evolutionarily developed a highly regulated mechanism to turn off the signal (42). Rapid waning of receptor responsiveness to agonist stimulation (within seconds or minutes) is dependent on receptor phosphorylation, and results in uncoupling of the receptor from its signal-transducing G-protein. A slow mechanism for receptor desensitization (hours or days) is receptor downregulation (42). In this case a decrease in receptor synthesis, a destabilization of receptor messenger RNA, or an increase in receptor degradation leads to the net loss of cell surface receptors (43,44).

The processes of desensitization and downregulation are initiated by a phosphorylation signal that determines the uncoupling of the receptor from its signal-transducing G-protein and enhances the affinity of the receptor for cytosolic proteins known as the β-arrestins (42). Once bound to the receptor, β-arrestins not only interdict further G-protein coupling and target the activated receptor for endocytosis (45), but also act as a scaffold for the assembly of complex signaling cascades, like the mitogen-activated protein kinase (MAPK) pathway (46–48). Once internalized, receptors are targeted to specialized intracellular compartments, where they can be dephosphorylated and recycled to the plasma membrane (early endosomes) or sent down a degradation pathway (late endosomes) (42,49). Interestingly, accumulating evidence suggests that the process of βAR internalization per se may be pathological because the activation of signals arising from internalizing receptors can directly activate maladaptive signaling pathways (50,51). Therefore, strategies that prevent this redistribution may exert a beneficial effect in the failing cardiomyocytes (49,51).

βAR phosphorylation can be mediated by second messenger kinases (for example, protein kinase A or protein kinase C), in a process known as heterologous desensitization or non-agonist-specific desensitization, or by G-protein-coupled receptors kinases (GRKs) (42). The β-adrenergic receptor kinase (βARK1), now commonly known as GRK2, is the most abundant GRK expressed in the heart (52,53). An important binding partner for GRK2 is the multifunctional enzyme phosphoinositide 3-kinase (PI3K). Binding of cytosolic GRK2 to liberated $G_{\beta\gamma}$ subunits of the heterotrimeric G-protein facilitates its translocation to the plasma membrane where it then phosphorylates the agonist-bound receptor (Fig. 11-7) (54). Following agonist stimulation and release of $G_{\beta\gamma}$ subunits, PI3K is recruited to activated βARs by GRK2, where it catalyzes the generation D-3 phosphoinositides that are required for receptor endocytosis (Fig. 11-7) (55,56).

βARs renew their ability to respond to ligands through a process of *resensitization*, that has been shown to require internalization into intracellular compartments where the acidic environment allows for dephosphorylation of the receptor (54,57). Indeed, it has been recently suggested that a continuous equilibrium between internalization and recycling of βARs to the sarcolemma exists in vivo under physiological conditions, and this plasma membrane–endosome bidirectional trafficking of βARs may be responsible for the resensitization of receptors after prolonged catecholamine exposure (58). Molecular interventions that promote a rapid cycle of receptor dephosphorylation and recycling to the plasma membrane might also represent novel possible therapeutic strategies to normalize βAR function.

NEW PARADIGMS FOR HEPTAHELICAL RECEPTOR SIGNALING AND TRAFFICKING

Phosphoinositide 3-Kinase: Lipid and Protein Kinase Activity

Agonist binding to βARs leads to its phosphorylation primarily by the cytosolic enzyme GRK2. Following

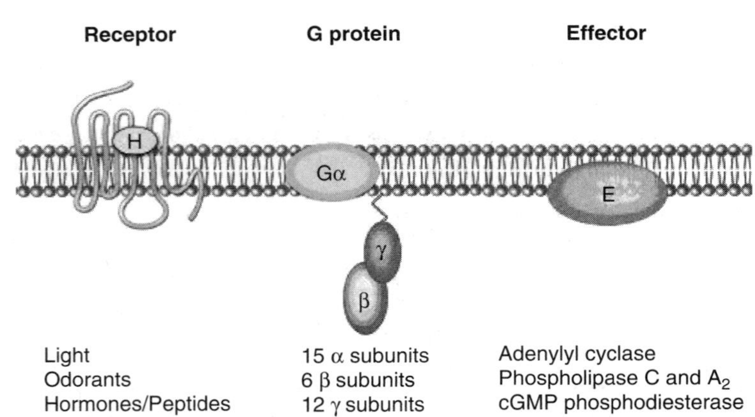

Figure 11-6 Summary of G-protein-coupled receptor signaling. The basic unit of G-protein-coupled receptor signaling comprises a 7-transmembrane-spanning receptor, a heterotrimeric G-protein, and an effector molecule such as an enzyme or ion channel. (Adapted from Rockman HA, Koch WJ, Lefkowitz RJ. Seven-transmembrane-spanning receptors and heart function. *Nature*. 2002;415(6868): 206–212, with permission.)

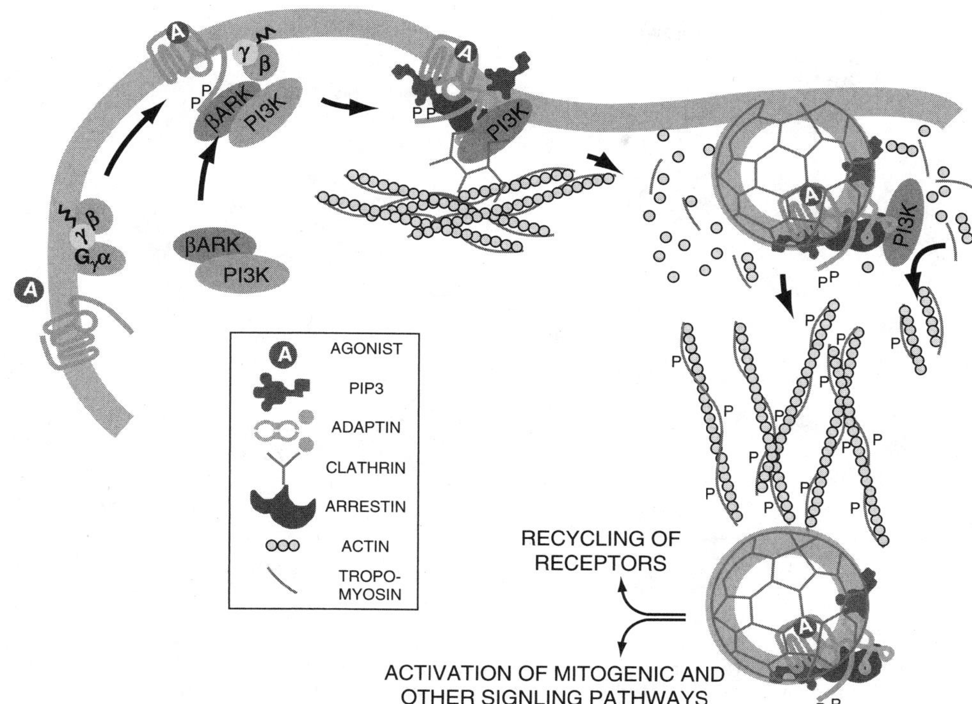

Figure 11-7 Mechanisms of regulation of β-adrenergic receptor signaling. βARK1 forms a cytosolic complex with PI3K. Following agonist binding to βARs, heterotrimeric G-proteins dissociate into G_α and $G_{\beta\gamma}$ subunits. The release of $G_{\beta\gamma}$ subunits activates and translocates βARK1, along with PI3K, to the agonist-occupied receptor complex. At the plasma membrane, PI3K generates D-3 phosphoinositides that regulate receptor internalization through the recruitment of essential adaptor proteins. Following internalization, receptors can be dephosphorylated (resensitized) and recycled to the plasma membrane or sent to the degradation pathway.
This is a schematic diagram showing the role of lipid and protein kinase activity of PI3K in regulating βAR endocytosis. Agonist binding to βARs leads to the dissociation of heterotrimeric G-proteins into Gα and Gβγ subunits. The release of Gβγ subunits activates GRK2 (βARK1) and facilitates its translocation to the agonist-occupied receptor. βARK1 interacts with PI3K and mediates translocation of PI3K to the receptor complex. βARK1 phosphorylates the receptor, leading to β-arrestin recruitment while the lipid kinase activity of PI3K generates D-3 phosphoinositides, allowing for efficient recruitment of AP-2 adaptor protein to the receptor complex. AP-2 recruitment to the receptor complex targets the receptor complex to clathrin-coated pits. The protein kinase activity of PI3K phosphorylates the nonmuscle tropomyosin at the receptor complex, allowing for stronger head-to-tail interactions between tropomyosin molecules and resulting in changes in actin bundling that are known to be critical for endocytosis. (Adapted from Naga Prasad SV, Jayatilleke A, Rockman HA. Protein kinase activity of phosphoinositide 3-kinase regulates regulates beta2-adrenergic receptor endocytosis. *Nature Cell Biol.* 20057:785–787.)

phosphorylation, receptors are bound by β-arrestin, resulting in targeting of the β-arrestin/receptor complex to clathrin-coated pits for internalization. Internalization involves the recruitment of the AP-2 adaptor protein to the receptor complex, a process that is regulated by the generation of phospholipids by the multifunctional enzyme PI3K (Fig. 11-7). Recently, it has been found that the cellular trafficking of βARs after agonist stimulation requires both lipid and protein kinase activity of PI3K (59). Using a variety of PI3K mutants with either protein or lipid phosphorylation activity, it was found that the substrate for PI3K is the cytoskeletal protein, nonmuscle tropomyosin (Fig. 11-7) (59). Tropomyosin is a dimeric, α-helical coiled protein with adjacent molecules interacting head-to-tail and belongs to a family of widely distributed actin filament binding proteins that is classified into muscle and nonmuscle isoforms. Nonmuscle tropomyosin isoform interacts with actin and regulates actin filament stability, vesicular trafficking, motility, and cell structure. It is postulated that phosphorylated tropomyosin stabilizes actin filaments and allows for proper actin cytoskeletal remodeling necessary to support βAR internalization (Fig. 11-7) (59).

G-Protein-Independent Signaling: Role of the β-Arrestins

Recently, it has been appreciated that heptahelical receptors regulate intracellular signaling pathways independent of their ability to couple and activate G-proteins. The primary architects of this process are the β-arrestins, which are multifunctional endocytic adaptors and signal transducers. By binding to a growing list of endocytic and signaling proteins, β-arrestins mediate a variety of receptor signaling and cellular regulatory processes (48,50) (Fig. 11-8). The traditional concept has been that receptor stimulation leads to the intracellular accumulation of second messengers such as cAMP, leading to activation of downstream signaling pathways (Fig. 11-8A).

Currently, a new paradigm is evolving where the initiation of signaling pathways requires the formation and activation of multicomponent signaling complexes that primarily involve the agonist-dependent receptor recruitment of β-arrestin (Fig. 11-8B). G-protein-mediated activation is rapid, transient, and leads to the nuclear translocation of molecules that regulate transcription and cellular proliferation. In contrast, β-arrestin-mediated signaling is associated with being slower in onset, persistent, the formation of

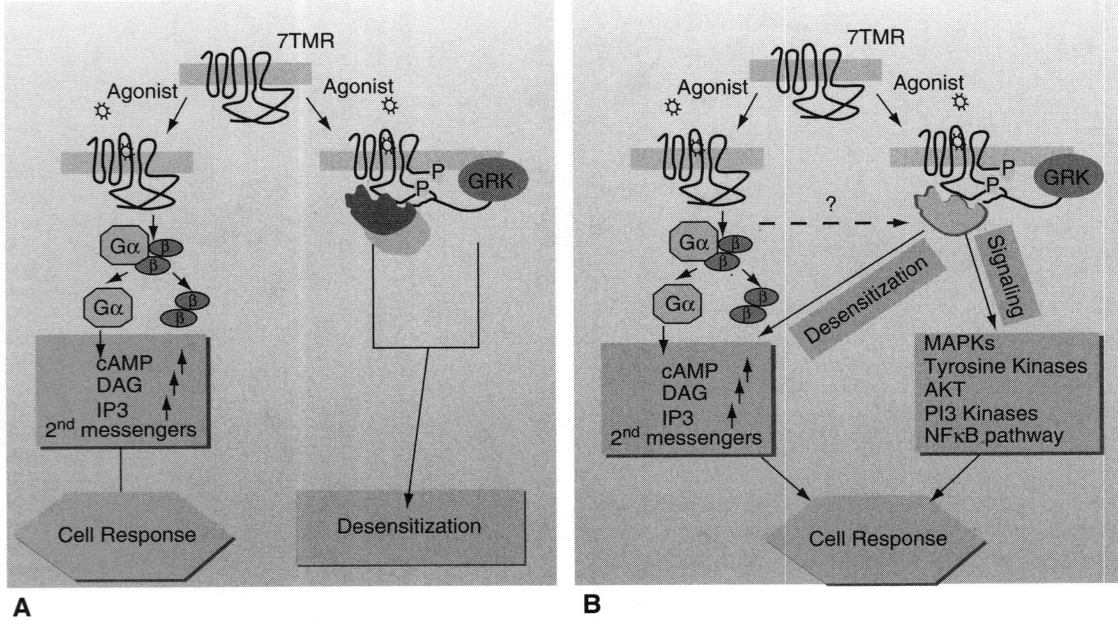

Figure 11-8 Signal transduction by seven transmembrane receptors. **(A)** Classical paradigm. The active form of the receptor (R*) stimulates heterotrimeric G-proteins and is rapidly phosphorylated by G-protein-coupled receptor kinases (GRKs), which leads to β-arrestin recruitment. The receptor is thereby desensitized and the signaling is stalled. **(B)** New paradigm. β-arrestins not only mediate desensitization of G-protein signaling but also act as signal transducers themselves. (From Lefkowitz RJ, Shenoy SK. Transduction of receptor signals by beta-arrestins. *Science.* 2005;308(5721):512–517.)

cytosolic endocytic vesicles, and little modulation of transcriptional activity (60).

Receptor Dimerization

In addition to the signals arising from single βARs, a rapidly growing field of research is elucidating the role of possible protein–protein interactions among receptors (61,62). Against the traditional paradigm for signaling of GPCRs as single units (monomers), a large body of evidence now indicates that GPCRs exist as homodimers and heterodimers (63,64). Interestingly, heterodimers between GPCRs often present properties that differ from homogeneous populations of receptors, thereby generating previously unrealized diversity of function. Interactions between same family members of adrenergic receptors can occur, as well as oligomerization with receptors from different GPCR families (62,65). Interfamily interactions between endogenous βARs and angiotensin II receptors (AT_1Rs) were recently demonstrated to take place in cardiomyocytes (Fig. 11-9) (62). An important consequence of this interaction was that blockade of one of the two receptors in the complex was sufficient to inhibit signaling and trafficking of both receptors (62). Thus, treatment of myocytes with a β-blocker completely inhibited angiotensin/Gq coupling and contractility, and treatment of mice with a selective angiotensin receptor-blocker reduced heart rate response to β-agonist stimulation (Fig. 11-9) (62,65). The accumulating data regarding homodimerization or heterodimerization of adrenergic receptors suggest a much more complex role for each receptor in regulating cardiomyocyte contractility, particularly under conditions of heart failure.

β-Adrenergic Receptor Signaling in the Normal Heart

Targeted gene disruption and transgenic overexpression techniques in mice have clarified the roles of specific βAR subtypes in the cardiovascular system. Studies in β_1AR knockout mice have demonstrated that this receptor is critical for proper mouse development in utero, since almost 70% of β_1 knockout mice die before reaching the later stage of embryos (66). While βARs generally do not regulate resting heart rate, blood pressure, or metabolic rate (66,67), they play a cardinal role in mediating the cardiovascular response to sympathetic stimulation. The positive chronotropic and inotropic response of the heart to catecholamine stimulation is mediated almost exclusively by β_1ARs (66–68). Coupling of β_2ARs to cardiac contractility is less-defined and species-related, showing a positive effect in human hearts (69) while not affecting contractility in the mouse (66,67,70). In contrast, β_2ARs mainly affect vascular tone, with no effects on prenatal development or basal and ISO-stimulated chronotropic response (71).

β-Adrenergic Receptor Signaling in the Failing Heart

The chronic increase in circulating catecholamine levels is largely responsible for the extensive abnormalities of the βAR system in failing cardiomyocytes, including marked impairment in the ability of both β_1ARs and β_2ARs to couple to their respective G-proteins and selective downregulation of β_1ARs (72).

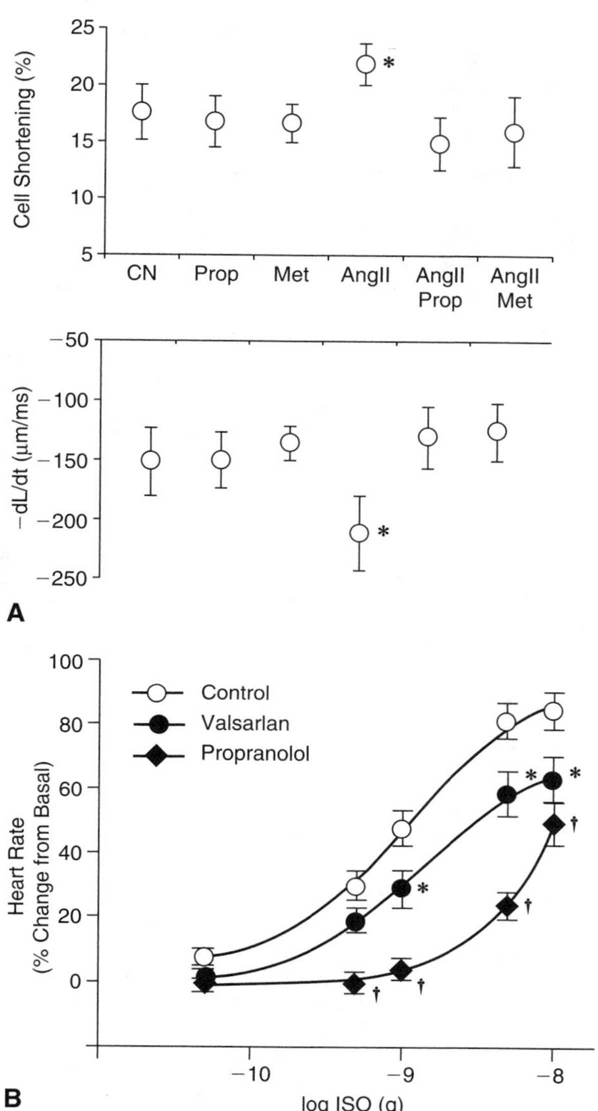

Figure 11-9 βAR-AT$_1$R heterodimerization in cardiomyocytes. **(A)** Summary data of percent cellular shortening (%CS) and rate of cell shortening (*−dL/dt*) in cardiomyocytes at baseline and following stimulation with the different agents. Co-administration of the βblockers propranolol or metoprolol together with Ang II abolishes the Ang II-mediated myocyte contractility. **(B)** In vivo assessment of change of intact, vagotomized, wild type mice in heart rate in response to increasing doses of the β-agonist isoproterenol ISO (O) following acute administration of 250 μg valsartan (●) or 1 μg propranolol (◆). Increasing doses of ISO yielded a marked elevation in heart rate. Pretreatment with a single dose of propranolol resulted in a marked shift of the ISO response curve to the right, as expected from a classical competitive β-antagonist. In contrast, a single dose of valsartan resulted in a significant 25% reduction in the maximal heart rate, without a rightward shift, indicating that valsartan-mediated attenuation of the ISO response is not through competitive antagonism of the βAR. (Adapted from Barki-Harrington L, Luttrell LM, Rockman HA. Dual inhibition of beta-adrenergic and angiotensin II receptors by a single antagonist: a functional role for receptor-receptor interaction in vivo. *Circulation.* 2003;108(13):1611–1618, with permission.)

Excessive agonist stimulation of β$_1$ARs is known to cause deleterious effects on cardiomyocytes (73). Indeed, overexpression of β$_1$ARs in transgenic mice was shown to cause hypertrophy and interstitial fibrosis in young animals, which proceeded to cardiac dysfunction as the animals aged (74,75). Hemodynamic studies in these mice showed that although maximal contractility and rate of isovolumic relaxation were initially increased in young animals, systolic and diastolic functions were already impaired and progressed to a steady decline of left ventricular contractility and relaxation (76,77). Studies in transgenic animals overexpressing G$_s$ confirm that increased signaling in the βAR/G$_s$/adenylyl cyclase pathway initially leads to increased cardiac function but is detrimental to the heart in the long run (78). While overstimulation of β$_1$AR signaling in the healthy myocardium is clearly deleterious, it remains controversial whether restoration of normal β$_1$AR coupling under conditions of heart failure is advantageous or detrimental (42,79).

Downregulation and desensitization of β$_1$ARs in failing human cardiomyocytes (72,80) are attributed, at least in part, to a significant increase in the levels of βARK1 (81). While the classical paradigm has been that βAR downregulation is beneficial because it protects cardiomyocytes against catecholamine damage, a large body of data now indicates that pathological signaling pathways arise from internalizing receptors (42,48,50). Indeed, preventing the internalization and chronic downregulation of βARs under conditions of high catecholamines or elevated hemodynamic stress restores normal βAR-G-protein coupling and consistently has demonstrated improved long-term cardiac function and survival in a variety of species and animal models (42,49,82–85). These studies suggest that abnormalities in βAR signaling might indeed promote cardiomyocyte dysfunction.

As opposed to a specific, marked downregulation of β$_1$ARs, there is no significant change in the levels of β$_2$ARs in the failing heart (72). The result is a change in the ratio of β$_1$/β$_2$ARs, suggesting a possible role for β$_2$ARs under conditions where β$_1$AR signaling is suppressed. Several studies have addressed the issue of whether β$_2$ARs are advantageous or deleterious during cardiac hypertrophy and failure (75,86,87). Coupling of β$_2$AR to G$_i$ is likely to play an important role in failing cardiomyocytes, since β$_2$AR/G$_i$ coupling may act to activate a protective anti-apoptotic pathway during hyperactivation of β$_1$ARs by excess of catecholamines (88).

Reversal of Cardiac Failure through Targeted Inhibition of GRK2-Associated PI3K Activity

As discussed earlier, recent studies have shown that GRK2 and PI3K interact in the cytosol of cardiac cells to form a complex that is recruited to the plasma membrane at the site of activated receptors in response to agonist stimulation (55). At the plasma membrane, PI3K activity is required for agonist-stimulated receptor endocytosis (51,55). Recent studies have shown that established βAR abnormalities under conditions of heart failure can be rapidly reversed by a gene therapy approach that targets the GRK2/PI3K complex (49), to result in not only

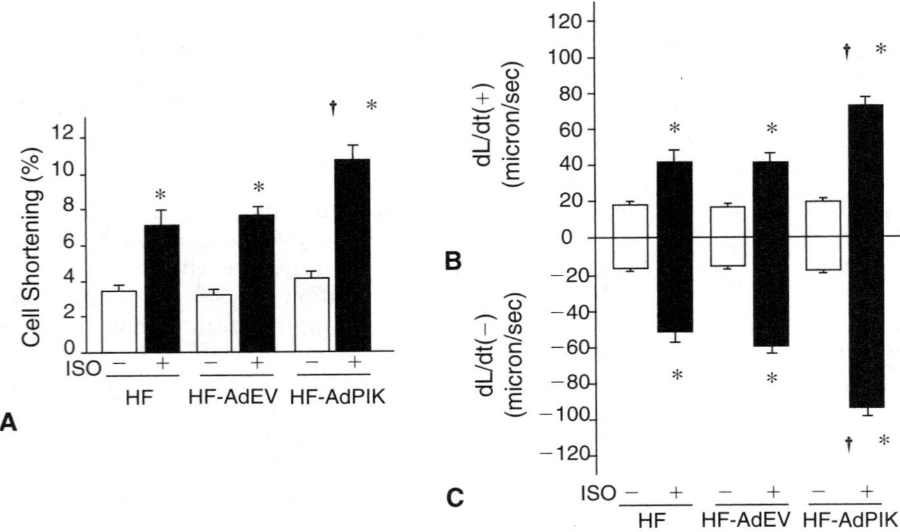

Figure 11-10 Competitive displacement of PI3K from βARK1 reverses contractile dysfunction of failing cardiac myocytes. Summary data of **(A)** percent cell shortening, **(B)** velocity of cell shortening ($-dL/dt_{max}$), and **(C)** velocity of cell relaxation ($+dL/dt_{max}$) in failing porcine cardiomyocytes under basal conditions (**white bars**) and upon isoproterenol (ISO) 1μM (**black bars**) following treatment with the adenoviral backbone (HF-AdEV), adenovirus coding for PIK (HF-AdPIK), or no treatment (HF). (Adapted from Perrino C, Naga Prasad SV, Schroder JN, et al. Restoration of beta-adrenergic receptor signaling and contractile function in heart failure by disruption of the betaARK1/phosphoinositide 3-kinase complex. *Circulation.* 2005;111(20): 2579–2587, with permission.)
$^*p < 0.01$ for all ISO versus basal; $^\dagger p < 0.05$ AdPIK ISO versus HF ISO and AdEV ISO.

improved contractility parameters of failing cardiomyocytes (Fig. 11-10) (49) but also improved cardiac function and survival (84).

Thus, abnormalities of βAR signaling are hallmarks of cardiomyocyte failure. Moreover, recent data suggest that chronic βAR dysfunction promotes deterioration of cardiomyocyte function. Indeed, preservation of βAR signaling through a variety of different strategies, including GRK2 inhibition (42,83,85), or preventing targeting of PI3K to activated βARs, consistently ameliorates cardiac dysfunction and survival in experimental heart failure (49,82,84,85). These studies also highlight novel therapeutic opportunities to reverse established βAR abnormalities in failing cardiomyocytes.

ADVERSE EFFECTS OF ADRENERGIC STIMULATION

Increased SNS activity may exert adverse effects on the structure and function of the myocardium, both indirectly and directly. Increased arterial and venous tone, and salt and water retention by the kidneys, result in increases in myocardial wall stresses. Increased SNS activity may activate other neurohumoral systems, such as the renin-angiotensin system, that themselves exert potent effects on vascular tone and salt and water retention. In addition to these indirect effects, NE may also directly affect the biology of the myocardium by mediating a process referred to as remodeling (Fig. 11-11).

Myocardial remodeling refers to the process of progressive deterioration in the structure and function of the ventricle over time, typically in response to an initial insult such as myocardial infarction (89). Myocardial remodeling involves hypertrophy and apoptosis of myocytes, regression to a fetal phenotype, and changes in the nature of the extracellular matrix. It appears that NE can contribute to many of these changes by direct stimulation of adrenergic receptors on cardiac myocytes and fibroblasts. In addition, several other factors not considered here (including endothelin, inflammatory cytokines, peptide growth factors, nitric oxide, reactive oxygen species) are produced within the myocardium and may be involved in myocardial remodeling (1).

Myocyte Hypertrophy and Fetal Phenotype

A central feature in myocardial remodeling is an increase in myocardial mass through hypertrophy of individual myocytes. In vitro experiments with cardiac myocytes cultured from neonatal rat heart have demonstrated that NE stimulates myocyte growth via increased protein synthesis (90,91). This pathological hypertrophic remodeling is mediated primarily by stimulation of Gq-coupled heptahelical receptors, both in vitro in isolated myocytes and in vivo in the intact organism (61,92,93). The hypertrophic effect of NE is associated with the re-expression of fetal genes such as atrial natriuretic peptide, α-skeletal actin, and β-myosin heavy chain and the reciprocal downregulation of several adult genes that are important in excitation–contraction coupling such as the sarcoplasmic reticulum Ca^{2+}-ATPase (SERCA2) (91).

Myocyte Apoptosis

The death of cardiac myocytes by apoptosis, or programmed cell death, may contribute to pathological remodeling (94). Apoptosis is a highly regulated sequence of energy-dependent molecular and biochemical events that are guided by a genetic program. Although it was thought that apoptosis did not occur in terminally differentiated cardiac myocytes, it has now been shown that apoptosis is present in the myocardium of patients with end-stage dilated cardiomyopathy (95,96). Although the relevance of these observations is not yet clear, they have led to the thesis that continuing loss of viable myocytes contributes to progressive myocardial failure.

High levels of NE are toxic to cardiac myocytes (97). Several mechanisms have been suggested, including

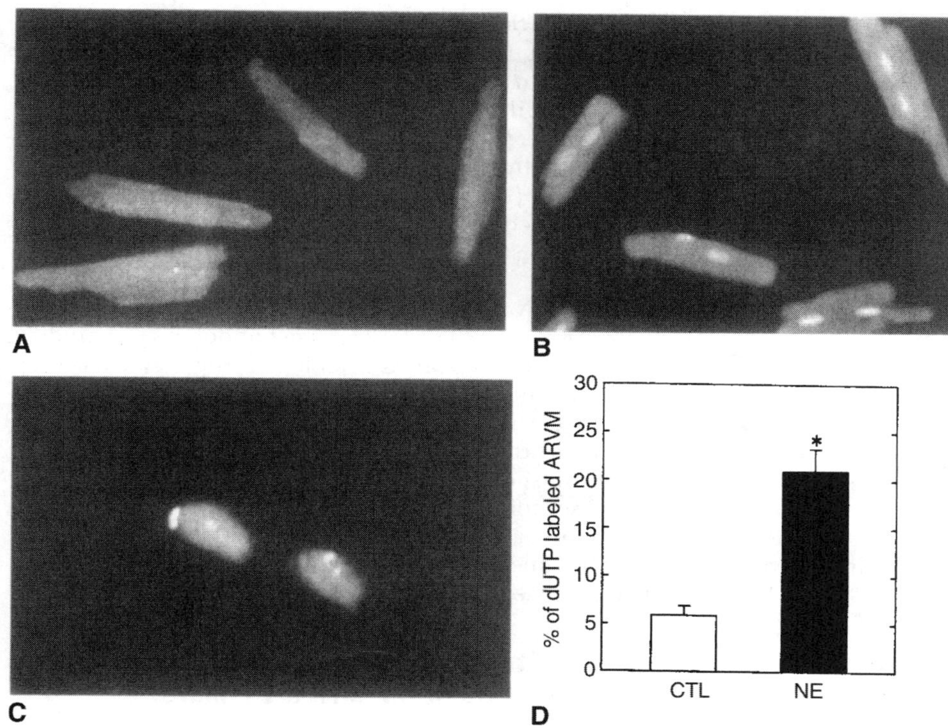

Figure 11-11 Effect of norepinephrine on apoptosis in cultured cardiac myocytes obtained from adult rats. The cells were exposed to norepinephrine for 24 hours, and apoptosis was assessed by terminal deoxynucleotidyl transferase mediated nick end-labeling (TUNEL) staining to detect double-stranded DNA breaks. **(A)** Control myocytes. **(B)** Myocytes exposed to DNase to serve as a positive control. **(C)** Myocytes exposed to norepinephrine for 24 hours. **(D)** The mean percentage of TUNEL-positive cells in control and norepinephrine-treated cultures. (Adapted from Communal C, Singh K, Pimentel DR, et al. Norepinephrine stimulates apoptosis in adult rat ventricular myocytes by activation of the beta-adrenergic pathway. *Circulation.* 1998;98(13):1329–1334.)
*$p < 0.01$ versus control.

hypoxia, increased sarcolemmal permeability, calcium overload, elevation of cAMP, activation of α- or β-adrenergic receptors, and the formation of oxidative catecholamine metabolites (98,99). A direct toxic effect mediated by receptor activation was suggested by Mann et al. (100), who demonstrated that exposure to NE was toxic to adult cardiac myocytes in vitro and that the toxic effect was completely blocked by a β-adrenergic antagonist. Several studies now suggest that the toxic effect of β-adrenergic receptor stimulation is mediated, at least in part, by apoptosis. In cardiac myocytes cultured from adult rat hearts, Communal et al. (101) showed that exposure to NE for 24 hours stimulated the frequency of apoptosis (Fig. 11-12). In these cells, NE-stimulated apoptosis was

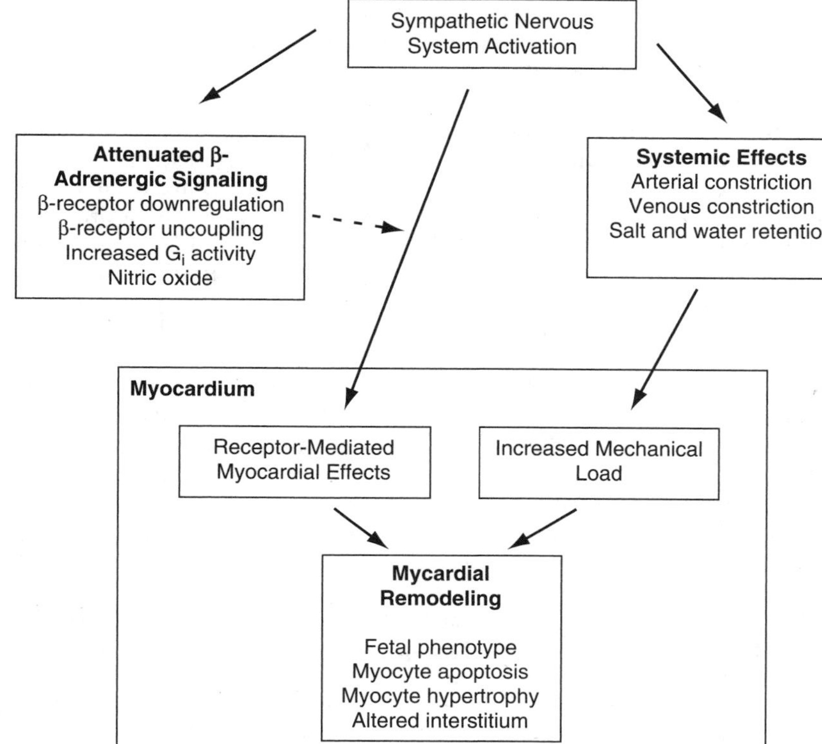

Figure 11-12 Schematic illustrating the relationship between sympathetic nervous system activation and myocardial remodeling. Norepinephrine acts directly on adrenergic receptors in the myocardium and indirectly through systemic effects on vascular tone and volume to promote myocardial remodeling. Increased sympathetic activity also leads to reduced β-adrenergic responsiveness, which may impair myocardial function but may also help to protect the myocardium from the direct effects of sympathetic activation.

inhibited by the β-adrenergic antagonist propranolol, mimicked by isoproterenol and forskolin, and abolished by the PKA inhibitor H-89. Consistent with these in vitro experiments, it has been shown that transgenic mice over-expressing the Gs_{α} subunit in the myocardium develop a dilated cardiomyopathy which is associated with apoptosis (102).

Extracellular Matrix

Relatively little is known about the effects of NE on the extracellular matrix. However, in cardiac myocytes from the neonatal rat heart, NE stimulates the expression of transforming growth factor-β (TGF-β), an important regulator of extracellular matrix proteins (103). In neonatal rat cardiac fibroblasts, NE stimulates proliferation, as indicated by increased DNA synthesis and increased protein synthesis (104). Likewise, in rats, the chronic infusion of isoproterenol causes interstitial fibrosis and increased levels of fibronectin and TGF-β (105).

CLINICAL ASPECTS OF SYMPATHETIC NERVOUS SYSTEM ACTIVATION IN HUMAN HEART FAILURE

Clinical Assessment of Sympathetic Nervous System Activity

Given the critical role of the SNS in the pathogenesis of heart failure, the possibility of clinical assessment of SNS activity in vivo remains a subject of substantial interest. Assessment of SNS activity may be useful in establishing prognosis, in targeting therapies, in monitoring response to therapy, or as a surrogate endpoint in the evaluation of new heart failure treatments. Elevated levels of plasma NE have been shown to be powerful predictors of adverse outcomes (2). As previously noted, however, levels of NE in the venous circulation reflect primarily systemic rather than cardiac sympathetic activation, and measurement of norepinephrine is technically burdensome, limiting its clinical usefulness. Likewise, radiotracer methods and direct recording of sympathetic motor activity are unsuited for clinical use. Several methods of evaluating autonomic balance in vivo for clinical use do, however exist, as discussed later.

Heart rate variability has been suggested as a physiological correlate of autonomic tone (106). A variety of studies have demonstrated that diminished variability in heart rate over time is a sign of sympathetic overactivity (or, alternatively, parasympathetic withdrawal). Lower heart rate variability is associated with a higher rate of adverse events in a variety of populations with heart failure (107–109). Although heart rate variability has traditionally been laborious to measure accurately, the proliferation of implantable cardiac defibrillators and biventricular pacemakers in patients with chronic heart failure has resulted in ready access to detailed data on heart rate variability in an ever-increasing proportion of the heart failure population (110). Validated algorithms for incorporating these data into clinical care remain undeveloped, but potentially such "heart rate variability footprints" could be used to quantify changes in prognosis as well as response to therapy. Many treatments that have been demonstrated to be efficacious (including statins, exercise training, and cardiac resynchronization therapy) have been shown to decrease SNS activation in patients with heart failure (111–115).

Alternatively, SNS activity in the heart may be estimated with iodine-123 (I-123) metaiodobenzylguanidine (MIBG) scanning. MIBG is an NE analog that is taken up by myocardial cells in proportion to cardiac sympathetic activity (116). The relative activity of heart versus mediastinum (heart/mediastinum ratio) can be calculated and a MIBG washout rate calculated using delayed imaging. MIBG scanning has been demonstrated to have prognostic value in heart failure patients in a variety of studies and may be superior to heart rate variability measurements or plasma norepinephrine levels (116–119).

Clinical Studies of Sympathetic Nervous System Modulation in Heart Failure

In addition to the body of basic, animal, and human research previously described, several lines of clinical evidence attest to the importance of SNS activation in patients with heart failure. Circulating levels of NE are elevated in chronic heart failure in relation to disease severity, and have been shown to be a marker of poor prognosis (2). Additionally, β-adrenergic-blockers have become a mainstay of the medical management of chronic heart failure. Although once thought to be contraindicated in patients with heart failure due to their acute negative inotropic effects, the unequivocal long-term benefits of these agents in heart failure attest to the adverse consequences of chronic SNS activation (120–122).

Notably, however, not all sympathetic antagonism appears to be beneficial in heart failure. Despite the salutary effects of β-adrenergic blockade, agents targeting central sympathetic outflow (moxonidine) have been shown to increase mortality in heart failure, despite a dramatic decrease in measurable SNS activation (123). Data from the Beta-blocker Evaluation of Survival Trial (BEST) on bucindolol (a β-adrenergic-blocker with sympatholytic properties) have suggested that patients with the greatest acute decrease in circulating norepinephrine levels with treatment have increased mortality, a finding that may explain the negative results of the overall trial (124,125). Such studies suggest that some minimal level of adrenergic support may be required in human heart failure and that the most effective therapies may be those that modulate rather than remove adrenergic support from the heart.

Apical Ballooning Syndrome: A Case Study in Sympathetic Nervous System Overactivity

In addition to the role of SNS activation in the general heart failure population, data have emerged on a specific acute

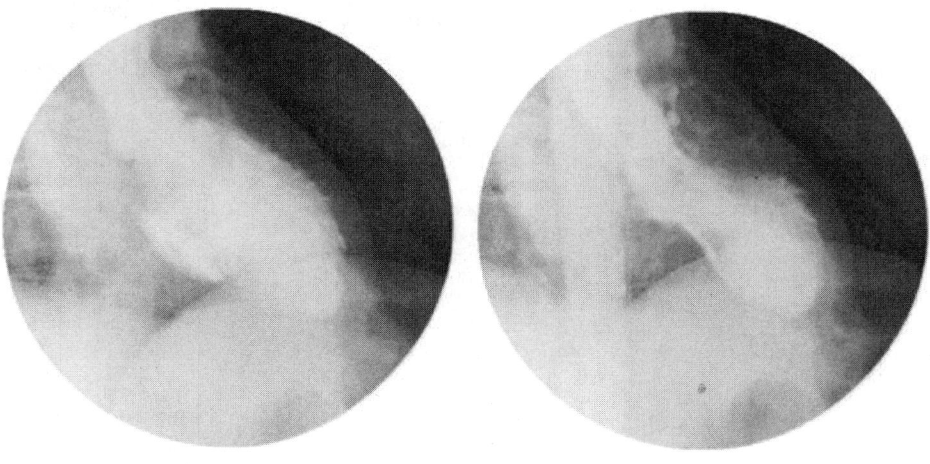

Figure 11-13 Left ventriculogram in diastole and systole in patient with apical ballooning syndrome in the setting of acute emotional stress. (Images courtesy of Ilan Wittstein, M.D., The Johns Hopkins Hospital, Baltimore, MD.)

cardiomyopathy syndrome that appears to be directly related to acute increases in SNS activation. This syndrome was originally described in Japan as apical ballooning syndrome or "tako-tsubo-like cardiomyopathy," due to the characteristic appearance of the left ventriculogram that resembles a trap used for catching octopus (126,127). Clinically, this syndrome is characterized by the acute onset of severe systolic dysfunction and acute heart failure, with a characteristic systolic apical ballooning due to dyskinesis of the ventricular apex (Fig. 11-13). This syndrome appears to be much more common in women and is often mistaken for acute myocardial infarction. Notably, an association with acute emotional stressors has been identified in this syndrome (126,127). Recently, careful study has implicated dramatic increase in circulating catecholamine levels in patients with this syndrome, several times higher than a control group of patients with acute myocardial infarction (128). Ongoing research into the pathophysiology of this disorder may shed light on both this clinical syndrome and the role of the SNS in heart failure generally.

REFERENCES

1. Colucci WS. Molecular and cellular mechanisms of myocardial failure. *Am J Cardiol.* 1997;80(11A):15L–25L.
2. Cohn JN, Levine TB, Olivari MT, et al. Plasma norepinephrine as a guide to prognosis in patients with chronic congestive heart failure. *N Engl J Med.* 1984;311:819–823.
3. Chidsey CA, Braunwald E. Sympathetic activity and neurotransmitter depletion in congestive heart failure. *Pharmacol Rev.* 1966;18(1):685–700.
4. Thomas JA, Marks BH. Plasma norepinephrine in congestive heart failure. *Am J Cardiol.* 1978;41(2):233–243.
5. Levine TB, Francis GS, Goldsmith SR, et al. Activity of the sympathetic nervous system and renin-angiotensin system assessed by plasma hormone levels and their relation to hemodynamic abnormalities in congestive heart failure. *Am J Cardiol.* 1982;49(7):1659–1666.
6. Leimbach WN, Jr., Wallin BG, Victor RG, et al. Direct evidence from intraneural recordings for increased central sympathetic outflow in patients with heart failure. *Circulation.* 1986;73-(5):913–919.
7. Francis GS, Benedict C, Johnstone DE, et al. Comparison of neuroendocrine activation in patients with left ventricular dysfunction with and without congestive heart failure. A substudy of the Studies of Left Ventricular Dysfunction (SOLVD). *Circulation.* 1990;82(5):1724–1729.
8. Swedberg K, Viquerat C, Rouleau JL, et al. Comparison of myocardial catecholamine balance in chronic congestive heart failure and in angina pectoris without failure. *Am J Cardiol.* 1984;54(7):783–786.
9. Hasking GJ, Esler MD, Jennings GL, et al. Norepinephrine spillover to plasma in patients with congestive heart failure: evidence of increased overall and cardiorenal sympathetic nervous activity. *Circulation* 1986;73(4):615–621.
10. Esler M, Kaye D, Lambert G, et al. Adrenergic nervous system in heart failure. *Am J Cardiol.* 1997;80(11A):7L–14L.
11. Rundqvist B, Elam M, Bergmann-Sverrisdottir Y, et al. Increased cardiac adrenergic drive precedes generalized sympathetic activation in human heart failure. *Circulation.* 1997;95(1):169–175.
12. Meredith IT, Eisenhofer G, Lambert GW, Dewar EM, Jennings GL, Esler MD. Cardiac sympathetic nervous activity in congestive heart failure. Evidence for increased neuronal norepinephrine release and preserved neuronal uptake. *Circulation.* 1993;88(1): 136–145.
13. Eisenhofer G, Friberg P, Rundqvist B, et al. Cardiac sympathetic nerve function in congestive heart failure. *Circulation.* 1996;93-(9):1667–1676.
14. Hirsch AT, Dzau VJ, Creager MA. Baroreceptor function in congestive heart failure: effect on neurohumoral activation and regional vascular resistance. *Circulation.* 1987;75(5 Pt 2):IV36–IV48.
15. Rea RF, Berg WJ. Abnormal baroreflex mechanisms in congestive heart failure. Recent insights. *Circulation.* 1990;81(6):2026–2027.
16. Wang W, Chen JS, Zucker IH. Carotid sinus baroreceptor sensitivity in experimental heart failure. *Circulation.* 1990;81(6): 1959–1966.
17. Olivari MT, Levine TB, Cohn JN. Abnormal neurohumoral response to nitroprusside infusion in congestive heart failure. *J Am Coll Cardiol.* 1983;2(3):411–417.
18. Levine TB, Francis GS, Goldsmith SR, et al. The neurohumoral and hemodynamic response to orthostatic tilt in patients with congestive heart failure. *Circulation.* 1983;67(5):1070–1075.
19. Kubo SH, Cody RJ. Circulatory autoregulation in chronic congestive heart failure: responses to head-up tilt in 41 patients. *Am J Cardiol.* 1983;52(5):512–518.
20. Ellenbogen KA, Mohanty PK, Szentpetery S, et al. Arterial baroreflex abnormalities in heart failure. Reversal after orthotopic cardiac transplantation. *Circulation.* 1989;79(1):51–58.
21. Ferguson DW, Abboud FM, Mark AL. Selective impairment of baroreflex-mediated vasoconstrictor responses in patients with ventricular dysfunction. *Circulation.* 1984;69(3):451–460.
22. Kaye DM, Lambert GW, Lefkovits J, et al. Neurochemical evidence of cardiac sympathetic activation and increased central nervous system norepinephrine turnover in severe congestive heart failure. *J Am Coll Cardiol.* 1994;23(3):570–578.

23. Creager MA, Hirsch AT, Dzau VJ, et al. Baroreflex regulation of regional blood flow in congestive heart failure. *Am J Physiol.* 1990;258(5 Pt 2):H1409–H1414.
24. Langer SZ. Presynaptic regulation of the release of catecholamines. *Pharmacol Rev.* 1980;32(4):337–362.
25. Isaacson JS, Reid IA. Importance of endogenous angiotensin II in the cardiovascular responses to sympathetic stimulation in conscious rabbits. *Circ Res.* 1990;66(3):662–671.
26. Kubo SH, Rector TS, Heifetz SM, et al. Alpha 2-receptor-mediated vasoconstriction in patients with congestive heart failure. *Circulation.* 1989;80(6):1660–1667.
27. Parker JD, Newton GE, Landzberg JS, et al. Functional significance of presynaptic alpha-adrenergic receptors in failing and nonfailing human left ventricle. *Circulation.* 1995;92(7): 1793–1800.
28. Newton GE, Parker JD. Acute effects of beta 1-selective and nonselective beta-adrenergic receptor blockade on cardiac sympathetic activity in congestive heart failure. *Circulation.* 1996;94(3):353–358.
29. Kaye DM, Lefkovits J, Cox H, et al. Regional epinephrine kinetics in human heart failure: evidence for extra-adrenal, nonneural release. *Am J Physiol.* 1995;269(1 Pt 2):H182–H188.
30. Daly PA, Sole MJ. Myocardial catecholamines and the pathophysiology of heart failure. *Circulation.* 1990;82(Suppl 2):I35–I43.
31. Bristow MR, Hershberger RE, Port JD, et al. Beta-adrenergic pathways in nonfailing and failing human ventricular myocardium. *Circulation.* 1990;82(Suppl 2):I12–I25.
32. Colucci WS, Denniss AR, Leatherman GF, et al. Intracoronary infusion of dobutamine to patients with and without severe congestive heart failure. Dose-response relationships, correlation with circulating catecholamines, and effect of phosphodiesterase inhibition. *J Clin Invest.* 1988;81(4):1103–1110.
33. Colucci WS, Ribeiro JP, Rocco MB, et al. Impaired chronotropic response to exercise in patients with congestive heart failure. Role of postsynaptic beta-adrenergic desensitization. *Circulation.* 1989;80(2):314–323.
34. Parker JD, Landzberg JS, Bittl JA, et al. Effects of beta-adrenergic stimulation with dobutamine on isovolumic relaxation in the normal and failing human left ventricle. *Circulation.* 1991;84(3): 1040–1048.
35. Brodde OE, Michel MC. Adrenergic and muscarinic receptors in the human heart. *Pharmacol Rev.* 1999;51(4):651–690.
36. Xiao RP, Cheng H, Zhou YY, et al. Recent advances in cardiac beta(2)-adrenergic signal transduction. *Circ Res.* 1999;85(11): 1092–1100.
37. Brodde OE, Michel MC, Zerkowski HR. Signal transduction mechanisms controlling cardiac contractility and their alterations in chronic heart failure. *Cardiovasc Res.* 1995;30(4): 570–584.
38. Abramson SN, Martin MW, Hughes AR, et al. Interaction of beta-adrenergic receptors with the inhibitory guanine nucleotide-binding protein of adenylate cyclase in membranes prepared from cyc-S49 lymphoma cells. *Biochem Biophys Res Commun.* 1988;37(22):4289–4297.
39. Xiao RP, Ji X, Lakatta EG. Functional coupling of the beta 2-adrenoceptor to a pertussis toxin-sensitive G-protein in cardiac myocytes. *Mol Pharmacol.* 1995;47(2):322–329.
40. Communal C, Singh K, Sawyer DB, et al. Opposing effects of beta(1)- and beta(2)-adrenergic receptors on cardiac myocyte apoptosis: role of a pertussis toxin-sensitive G-protein. *Circulation.* 1999;100(22):2210–2212.
41. Kilts JD, Gerhardt MA, Richardson MD, et al. Beta(2)-adrenergic and several other G-protein-coupled receptors in human atrial membranes activate both G(s) and G(i). *Circ Res.* 2000;87(8): 705–709.
42. Rockman HA, Koch WJ, Lefkowitz RJ. Seven-transmembrane-spanning receptors and heart function. *Nature.* 2002;415(6868): 206–212.
43. Lefkowitz RJ. G-protein-coupled receptors. III. New roles for receptor kinases and beta-arrestins in receptor signaling and desensitization. *J Biol Chem.* 1998;273(30):18677–18680.
44. Pitcher JA, Freedman NJ, Lefkowitz RJ. G-protein-coupled receptor kinases. *Annu Rev Biochem.* 1998;67:653–692.
45. Laporte SA, Oakley RH, Holt JA, et al. The interaction of beta-arrestin with the AP-2 adaptor is required for the clustering of beta 2-adrenergic receptor into clathrin-coated pits. *J Biol Chem.* 2000;275(30):23120–23126.
46. DeFea KA, Zalevsky J, Thoma MS, et al. Beta-arrestin-dependent endocytosis of proteinase-activated receptor 2 is required for intracellular targeting of activated ERK1/2. *J Cell Biol.* 2000;148(6):1267–1281.
47. Luttrell LM, Ferguson SS, Daaka Y, et al. Beta-arrestin-dependent formation of beta2 adrenergic receptor-Src protein kinase complexes. *Science.* 1999;283(5402):655–661.
48. Lefkowitz RJ, Shenoy SK. Transduction of receptor signals by beta-arrestins. *Science* 2005;308(5721):512–517.
49. Perrino C, Naga Prasad SV, Schroder JN, et al. Restoration of beta-adrenergic receptor signaling and contractile function in heart failure by disruption of the betaARK1/phosphoinositide 3-kinase complex. *Circulation.* 2005;111(20):2579–2587.
50. Lefkowitz RJ, Whalen EJ. Beta-arrestins: traffic cops of cell signaling. *Curr Opin Cell Biol.* 2004;16(2):162–168.
51. Prasad SV, Perrino C, Rockman HA. Role of phosphoinositide 3-kinase in cardiac function and heart failure. *Trends Cardiovasc Med.* 2003;13(5):206–212.
52. Inglese J, Freedman NJ, Koch WJ, et al. Structure and mechanism of the G-protein-coupled receptor kinases. *J Biol Chem.* 1993;268(32):23735–23738.
53. Iaccarino G, Tomhave ED, Lefkowitz RJ, et al. Reciprocal in vivo regulation of myocardial G-protein-coupled receptor kinase expression by beta-adrenergic receptor stimulation and blockade. *Circulation.* 1998;98(17):1783–1789.
54. Perry SJ, Lefkowitz RJ. Arresting developments in heptahelical receptor signaling and regulation. *Trends Cell Biol.* 2002;12(3): 130–138.
55. Naga Prasad SV, Barak LS, Rapacciuolo A, et al. Agonist-dependent recruitment of phosphoinositide 3-kinase to the membrane by beta-adrenergic receptor kinase 1. A role in receptor sequestration. *J Biol Chem.* 2001;276(22):18953–18959.
56. Prasad SV, Laporte SA, Chamberlain D, et al. Phosphoinositide 3-kinase regulates beta2-adrenergic receptor endocytosis by AP-2 recruitment to the receptor/beta-arrestin complex. *J Cell Biol.* 2002;158(3):563–575.
57. Krueger KM, Daaka Y, Pitcher JA, et al. The role of sequestration in G-protein-coupled receptor resensitization. Regulation of beta2-adrenergic receptor dephosphorylation by vesicular acidification. *J Biol Chem.* 1997;272(1):5–8.
58. Odley A, Hahn HS, Lynch RA, et al. Regulation of cardiac contractility by Rab4-modulated beta2-adrenergic receptor recycling. *Proc Natl Acad Sci USA.* 2004;101(18):7082–7087.
59. Naga Prasad SV, Jayatilleke A, Rockman HA. Protein kinase activity of phosphoinositide 3-kinase regulates regulates beta2-adrenergic receptor endocytosis. *Nature Cell Biol.* 2005, 785–796.
60. Ahn S, Shenoy SK, Wei H, et al. Differential kinetic and spatial patterns of beta-arrestin and G-protein-mediated ERK activation by the angiotensin II receptor. *J Biol Chem.* 2004;279(34): 35518–35525.
61. Barki-Harrington L, Perrino C, Rockman HA. Network integration of the adrenergic system in cardiac hypertrophy. *Cardiovasc Res.* 2004;63(3):391–402.
62. Barki-Harrington L, Luttrell LM, Rockman HA. Dual inhibition of beta-adrenergic and angiotensin II receptors by a single antagonist: a functional role for receptor-receptor interaction in vivo. *Circulation.* 2003;108(13):1611–1618.
63. George SR, O'Dowd BF, Lee SP. G-protein-coupled receptor oligomerization and its potential for drug discovery. *Nat Rev Drug Discov.* 2002;1(10):808–820.
64. Bulenger S, Marullo S, Bouvier M. Emerging role of homo- and heterodimerization in G-protein-coupled receptor biosynthesis and maturation. *Trends Pharmacol Sci.* 2005;26(3):131–137.
65. Jordan BA, Trapaidze N, Gomes I, et al. Oligomerization of opioid receptors with beta 2-adrenergic receptors: a role in trafficking and mitogen-activated protein kinase activation. *Proc Natl Acad Sci USA.* 2001;98(1):343–348.
66. Rohrer DK, Desai KH, Jasper JR, et al. Targeted disruption of the mouse beta1-adrenergic receptor gene: developmental and cardiovascular effects. *Proc Natl Acad Sci USA.* 1996;93(14): 7375–7380.
67. Rohrer DK, Schauble EH, Desai KH, et al. Alterations in dynamic heart rate control in the beta 1-adrenergic receptor knockout mouse. *Am J Physiol.* 1998;274(4 Pt 2):H1184–H1193.

68. Brodde OE. Beta 1- and beta 2-adrenoceptors in the human heart: properties, function, and alterations in chronic heart failure. *Pharmacol Rev.* 1991;43(2):203–242.
69. Brodde OE. Beta 1- and beta 2-adrenoceptors in the human heart: properties, function, and alterations in chronic heart failure. *Pharmacol Rev.* 1991;43(2):203–242.
70. Rohrer DK, Chruscinski A, Schauble EH, et al. Cardiovascular and metabolic alterations in mice lacking both beta1- and beta2-adrenergic receptors. *J Biol Chem.* 1999;274(24):16701–16708.
71. Chruscinski AJ, Rohrer DK, Schauble E, et al. Targeted disruption of the beta2 adrenergic receptor gene. *J Biol Chem.* 1999;274(24):16694–16700.
72. Bristow MR. Why does the myocardium fail? Insights from basic science. *Lancet.* 1998;352 (Suppl 1):SI8–S14.
73. Colucci WS, Sawyer DB, Singh K, et al. Adrenergic overload and apoptosis in heart failure: implications for therapy. *J Card Fail.* 2000;6(2 Suppl 1):1–7.
74. Bisognano JD, Weinberger HD, Bohlmeyer TJ et al. Myocardial-directed overexpression of the human beta(1)-adrenergic receptor in transgenic mice. *J. Mol Cell Cardiol.* 2000;32(5):817–830.
75. Engelhardt S, Hein L, Wiesmann F, et al. Progressive hypertrophy and heart failure in beta1-adrenergic receptor transgenic mice. *Proc Natl Acad Sci USA.* 1999;96(12):7059–7064.
76. Engelhardt S, Grimmer Y, Fan GH, et al. Constitutive activity of the human beta(1)-adrenergic receptor in beta(1)-receptor transgenic mice. *Mol Pharmacol.* 2001;60(4):712–717.
77. Engelhardt S, Boknik P, Keller U, et al. Early impairment of calcium handling and altered expression of junctin in hearts of mice overexpressing the beta1-adrenergic receptor. *Faseb J.* 2001;15(14):2718–2720.
78. Iwase M, Bishop SP, Uechi M, et al. Adverse effects of chronic endogenous sympathetic drive induced by cardiac GS alpha overexpression. *Circ Res.* 1996;78(4):517–524.
79. Frey N, Katus HA, Olson EN, et al. Hypertrophy of the heart: a new therapeutic target? *Circulation.* 2004;109(13):1580–1589.
80. Bristow MR, Minobe WA, Raynolds MV, et al. Reduced beta 1 receptor messenger RNA abundance in the failing human heart. *J Clin Invest.* 1993;92(6):2737–2745.
81. Ungerer M, Bohm M, Elce JS, et al. Altered expression of beta-adrenergic receptor kinase and beta 1-adrenergic receptors in the failing human heart. *Circulation.* 1993;87(2):454–463.
82. Nienaber JJ, Tachibana H, Naga Prasad SV, et al. Inhibition of receptor-localized PI3K preserves cardiac beta-adrenergic receptor function and ameliorates pressure overload heart failure. *J Clin Invest.* 2003;112(7):1067–1079.
83. Harding VB, Jones LR, Lefkowitz RJ, et al. Cardiac beta ARK1 inhibition prolongs survival and augments beta blocker therapy in a mouse model of severe heart failure. *Proc Natl Acad Sci USA.* 2001;98(10):5809–5814.
84. Perrino C, Naga Prasad SV, Patel M, et al. Targeted inhibition of beta-adrenergic receptor kinase-1-associated phosphoinositide-3 kinase activity preserves beta-adrenergic receptor signaling and prolongs survival in heart failure induced by calsequestrin overexpression. *J Am Coll Cardiol.* 2005;45(11):1862–1870.
85. Rockman HA, Chien KR, Choi DJ, Iaccarino et al. Expression of a beta-adrenergic receptor kinase 1 inhibitor prevents the development of myocardial failure in gene-targeted mice. *Proc Natl Acad Sci USA.* 1998;95(12):7000–7005.
86. Milano CA, Dolber PC, Rockman HA, et al. Myocardial expression of a constitutively active alpha 1B-adrenergic receptor in transgenic mice induces cardiac hypertrophy. *Proc Natl Acad Sci USA.* 1994;91(21):10109–10113.
87. Liggett SB, Tepe NM, Lorenz JN, et al. Early and delayed consequences of beta(2)-adrenergic receptor overexpression in mouse hearts: critical role for expression level. *Circulation.* 2000;101(14):1707–1714.
88. Xiang Y, Rybin VO, Steinberg SF, et al. Caveolar localization dictates physiologic signaling of beta 2-adrenoceptors in neonatal cardiac myocytes. *J Biol Chem.* 2002;277(37):34280–34286.
89. Cohn JN. Structural basis for heart failure. Ventricular remodeling and its pharmacological inhibition. *Circulation* 1995;91(10):2504–2507.
90. Simpson P. Norepinephrine-stimulated hypertrophy of cultured rat myocardial cells is an alpha 1 adrenergic response. *J Clin Invest.* 1983;72(2):732–738.
91. Knowlton KU, Michel MC, Itani M, et al. The alpha 1A-adrenergic receptor subtype mediates biochemical, molecular, and morphologic features of cultured myocardial cell hypertrophy. *J Biol Chem.* 1993;268(21):15374–15380.
92. Akhter MW, Luttrell DK, Rockman HA, et al. Transgenic mice with deficient myocardial signaling through the guanine nucleotide binding protein Gq are resistant to pressure overload hypertrophy. *Science.* 1998;280:574–577.
93. Dorn GW, Force T. Protein kinase cascades in the regulation of cardiac hypertrophy. *J Clin Invest.* 2005;115(3):527–537.
94. Colucci WS. Apoptosis in the heart. *N Engl J Med.* 1996;335(16):1224–1226.
95. Narula J, Haider N, Virmani R, et al. Apoptosis in myocytes in end-stage heart failure. *N Engl J Med.* 1996;335(16):1182–1189.
96. Olivetti G, Abbi R, Quaini F, et al. Apoptosis in the failing human heart. *N Engl J Med.* 1997;336(16):1131–1141.
97. Rona G. Catecholamine cardiotoxicity. *J. Mol Cell Cardiol.* 1985;17(4):291–306.
98. Opie LH, Walpoth B, Barsacchi R. Calcium and catecholamines: relevance to cardiomyopathies and significance in therapeutic strategies. *J.Mol Cell Cardiol.* 1985;17 (Suppl 2):21–34.
99. Singal PK, Kapur N, Dhillon KS, et al. Role of free radicals in catecholamine-induced cardiomyopathy. *Can J Physiol Pharmacol.* 1982;60(11):1390–1397.
100. Mann DL, Kent RL, Parsons B, et al. Adrenergic effects on the biology of the adult mammalian cardiocyte. *Circulation.* 1992;85(2):790–804.
101. Communal C, Singh K, Pimentel DR, et al. Norepinephrine stimulates apoptosis in adult rat ventricular myocytes by activation of the beta-adrenergic pathway. *Circulation.* 1998;98(13):1329–1334.
102. Iwase M, Uechi M, Vatner DE, et al. Cardiomyopathy induced by cardiac Gs alpha overexpression. *Am J Physiol.* 1997;272(1 Pt 2):H585–H589.
103. Takahashi N, Calderone A, Izzo NJ, Jr., et al. Hypertrophic stimuli induce transforming growth factor-beta 1 expression in rat ventricular myocytes. *J Clin Invest.* 1994;94(4):1470–1476.
104. Calderone A, Takahashi N, Izzo NJ, Jr., et al. Pressure- and volume-induced left ventricular hypertrophies are associated with distinct myocyte phenotypes and differential induction of peptide growth factor mRNAs. *Circulation.* 1995;92(9):2385–2390.
105. Boluyt MO, Long X, Eschenhagen T, et al. Isoproterenol infusion induces alterations in expression of hypertrophy-associated genes in rat heart. *Am J Physiol.* 1995;269(2 Pt 2):H638-H647.
106. Task Force of the European Society of Cardiology and the North American Society of Pacing and Electrophysiology. Heart rate variability: standards of measurement, physiological interpretation and clinical use. *Circulation.* 1996;93(5):1043–1065.
107. Aronson D, Mittleman MA, Burger AJ. Measures of heart period variability as predictors of mortality in hospitalized patients with decompensated congestive heart failure. *Am J Cardiol.* 2004;93(1):59–63.
108. Nolan J, Batin PD, Andrews R, et al. Prospective study of heart rate variability and mortality in chronic heart failure: results of the United Kingdom heart failure evaluation and assessment of risk trial (UK-heart). *Circulation.* 1998;98(15):1510–1516.
109. Fauchier L, Babuty D, Cosnay P, et al. Heart rate variability in idiopathic dilated cardiomyopathy: characteristics and prognostic value. *J Am Coll Cardiol.* 1997;30(4):1009–1014.
110. Adamson PB, Smith AL, Abraham WT, et al. Continuous autonomic assessment in patients with symptomatic heart failure: prognostic value of heart rate variability measured by an implanted cardiac resynchronization device. *Circulation.* 2004;110(16):2389–2394.
111. Hamdan MH, Zagrodzky JD, Joglar JA, et al. Biventricular pacing decreases sympathetic activity compared with right ventricular pacing in patients with depressed ejection fraction. *Circulation.* 2000;102(9):1027–1032.
112. Pliquett RU, Cornish KG, Zucker IH. Statin therapy restores sympathovagal balance in experimental heart failure. *J Appl Physiol.* 2003;95(2):700–704.

113. Adamson PB, Kleckner KJ, VanHout WL, et al. Cardiac resynchronization therapy improves heart rate variability in patients with symptomatic heart failure. *Circulation.* 2003;108(3):266–269.
114. Roveda F, Middlekauff HR, Rondon MU, et al. The effects of exercise training on sympathetic neural activation in advanced heart failure: a randomized controlled trial. *J Am Coll Cardiol.* 2003;42(5):854–860.
115. Grassi G, Vincenti A, Brambilla R, et al. Sustained sympathoinhibitory effects of cardiac resynchronization therapy in severe heart failure. *Hypertension.* 2004;44(5):727–731.
116. Henderson EB, Kahn JK, Corbett JR, et al. Abnormal I-123 metaiodobenzylguanidine myocardial washout and distribution may reflect myocardial adrenergic derangement in patients with congestive cardiomyopathy. *Circulation.* 1988;78(5 Pt 1): 1192–1199.
117. Cohen-Solal A, Esanu Y, Logeart D, et al. Cardiac metaiodobenzylguanidine uptake in patients with moderate chronic heart failure: relationship with peak oxygen uptake and prognosis. *J Am Coll Cardiol.* 1999;33(3):759–766.
118. Somsen GA, Szabo BM, van Veldhuisen DJ, et al. Comparison between iodine 123 metaiodobenzylguanidine scintigraphy and heart rate variability for the assessment of cardiac sympathetic activity in mild to moderate heart failure. *Am Heart J.* 1997; 134(3):456–458.
119. Yamada T, Shimonagata T, Fukunami M, et al. Comparison of the prognostic value of cardiac iodine-123 metaiodobenzylguanidine imaging and heart rate variability in patients with chronic heart failure: a prospective study. *J Am Coll Cardiol.* 2003;41(2):231–238.
120. Packer M, Coats AJS, Fowler MB, et al. Effect of carvedilol on survival in severe chronic heart failure. *N Engl J Med.* 2001;344(22): 1651–1658.
121. Poole-Wilson PA, Swedberg K, Cleland JGF, et al. Comparison of carvedilol and metoprolol on clinical outcomes in patients with chronic heart failure in the Carvedilol Or Metoprolol, European Trial (COMET): randomised controlled trial. *Lancet.* 2003;362-(9377):7–13.
122. MERIT-HF Study Group. Effect of metoprolol CR/XL in chronic heart failure: Metoprolol CR/XL Randomised Intervention Trial in Congestive Heart Failure (MERIT-HF). *Lancet.* 1999;353: 2001–2007.
123. Cohn JN, Pfeffer MA, Rouleau J, et al. Adverse mortality effect of central sympathetic inhibition with sustained-release moxonidine in patients with heart failure (MOXCON). *Eur J Heart Fail.* 2003;5(5):659–667.
124. Bristow MR, Krause-Steinrauf H, Nuzzo R, et al. Effect of baseline or changes in adrenergic activity on clinical outcomes in the Beta-Blocker Evaluation of Survival Trial. *Circulation.* 2004;110(11): 1437–1442.
125. The Beta-Blocker Evaluation of Survival Trial Investigators. A trial of the beta-blocker bucindolol in patients with advanced heart failure. *N Engl J Med.* 2001;344:1659–1667.
126. Abe Y, Kondo M, Matsuoka R, et al. Assessment of clinical features in transient left ventricular apical ballooning. *J Am Coll Cardiol.* 2003;41(5):737–742.
127. Tsuchihashi K, Ueshima K, Uchida T, et al. Transient left ventricular apical ballooning without coronary artery stenosis: a novel heart syndrome mimicking acute myocardial infarction. Angina Pectoris-Myocardial Infarction Investigations in Japan. *J Am Coll Cardiol.* 2001;38(1):11–18.
128. Wittstein IS, Thiemann DR, Lima JA, et al. Neurohumoral features of myocardial stunning due to sudden emotional stress. *N Engl J Med.* 2005;352(6):539–548.

Other Neurohormonal Systems

12

Steven Goldsmith   Bradley A. Bart

Interference with the maladaptive consequences of imbalances in activity of the renin-angiotensin-aldosterone system (RAAS) and the adrenergic nervous system forms the bedrock of current therapy for left ventricular systolic dysfunction (LVSD) and the heart failure (HF) syndrome that frequently follows. Detailed discussion of the proof of this assertion, as well as an exploration of the potential mechanisms involved, are found elsewhere in this text. However, it is clear that the benefit of angiotensin-converting enzyme inhibitors (ACEIs), angiotensin receptor blockers, aldosterone antagonists, and beta-adrenergic blockers cannot be attributed primarily to direct effects on ventricular loading conditions or to a direct effect to improve myocardial function. Indeed, while such treatments stabilize and improve myocardial structure and function over time, they may have little or no acute beneficial effect; beta-blockers might even have adverse acute effects on such measures. These observations have forced us to search more deeply into the nature of the fundamental processes affecting progressive structural and functional abnormalities governing LV dysfunction (LVD) and HF. They have also made it considerably more difficult to design and conduct therapeutic trials, since clearly it is not always appropriate to use traditional functional measures as surrogates for assessing long-term effectiveness. In the case of certain vasodilators and inotropes, reliance on the response of traditional hemodynamic measurements as a guide to the design of long-term, placebo-controlled trials led to the unhappy result of achieving worse outcomes on active therapy.

We have therefore had to focus more closely on the impact of a potential new treatment, not just on ventricular function and loading conditions but also on the deeper biological processes suspected to be involved in HF (1). Unfortunately, these are not yet fully characterized. However, since treatments directed at neurohormonal imbalance have been our most successful efforts to date, it is logical to extrapolate from this success to other candidate pathogens within the neurohormonal milieu of HF. In general, most theoretically maladaptive elements of this milieu act on cell-surface receptors which are coupled to related intracellular signaling processes implicated in progressive structural and functional abnormalities. Hence, it is logical, based on the beneficial response to interfering with the receptors (or activity) of the RAAS and adrenergic nervous system, to extrapolate to interfering with the elements of other systems which may cause similar downstream effects over time. The two candidate substances most-studied to date are arginine vasopressin (AVP) and endothelin. Alternatively, since at least one system, involving the natriuretic peptide family, is most likely a beneficial counterresponse to LVD, vasoconstriction, and fluid retention, it has also been suggested that further increasing the level or effect of such peptides would be of benefit. We must stress that as of this writing there are not yet any approved agents for treating LVD or clinical HF based on antagonism of either AVP or endothelin, or on an attempt to chronically enhance natriuretic peptide activity. In fact, despite great theoretical promise and considerable effort, data regarding endothelin antagonism and natriuretic peptide enhancement are thus far disappointing and it is still too early to conclude anything definitive about AVP antagonists. Nonetheless, preliminary data with the latter approach are promising, and Phase III trials are under way. Because of both the clinical and pathophysiological importance of the attempt to further exploit neurohormonal imbalance as a target for drug development in HF, this chapter will attempt not only to summarize the rationale for and current status of each of these three newer treatment strategies, but also to place the results to date in the overall context of HF therapy with an attempt to explicate the lessons learned thus far.

VASOPRESSIN ANTAGONISM

Rationale

The case for antagonizing the effects of AVP in HF rests on the possible contributions of AVP to both load-related and load-independent processes known to be important in progressive LVD (Fig. 12-1) (2). AVP is a nonapeptide made in the hypothalamus and stored in the posterior pituitary gland. Its secretion is primarily regulated by serum osmolality but is also influenced by numerous hemodynamic and neurohormonal stimuli (3). AVP signals through at least three receptor subtypes: the V1a, V2 and V1b, or V3 receptors (4). These receptors are structurally dissimilar, are coupled to different intracellular processes, and are linked to very different end-organ responses. Briefly, the V1a receptor is G-protein-coupled, increases intracellular calcium via the IP3 pathway, causes vasoconstriction in smooth muscle, and has both a positively inotropic and mitogenic effect in myocardial cells (5,6). The V2 receptor is also G-protein-coupled but acts via increasing cyclic adenosine monophosphate (cAMP) to alter the expression of aquaporin channels in the renal collecting duct (7). The result is water retention (hence the other name for AVP, ADH—the antidiuretic hormone). V2 receptors also cause endothelium-dependent vasodilation but probably not at physiologic hormone levels, although this has only been investigated in normal humans (8). The V1b or V3 receptor is much less well-characterized, resides in the midbrain or hypothalamus, and is thought be involved in regulating cortisol secretion.

From the standpoint of LV dysfunction and HF, the V1a and V2 receptors are of the most importance. Given our current understanding of the pathophysiology of these syndromes, excessive AVP-mediated effects at either or both of these receptors could be maladaptive. Too much V1a signaling could contribute to increased systemic resistance, increased venous tone, and increased afterload and preload, thereby aggravating myocardial dysfunction and structural remodeling. Direct myocardial V1a effects could promote ventricular remodeling and hypertrophy independent of any load-related stimuli. An effective V1a antagonist might therefore be expected to be beneficial, both indirectly (via afterload and preload reduction) and directly (via interruption of adverse myocardial stimulation). Such effects would be analogous to those expected from interfering with excessive angiotensin II stimulation on the vasculature and myocardium.

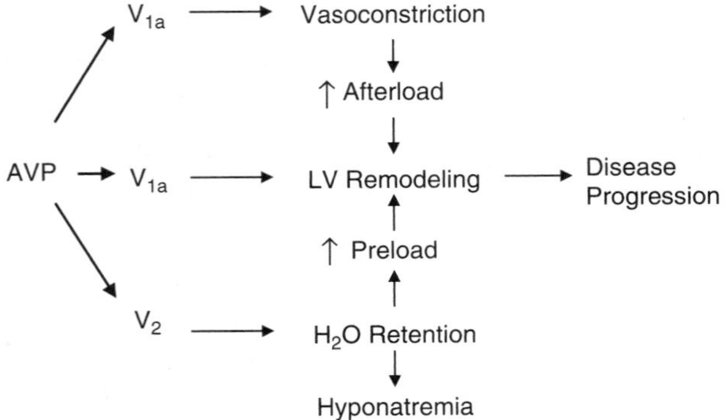

Figure 12-1 Proposed pathophysiological effects of arginine vasopressin (AVP) in congestive heart failure. By interacting with both V1a and V2 receptors, inappropriately increased AVP levels could adversely influence the progression of left ventricular dysfunction and remodeling in multiple ways. See the text for details.

Excessive V2 stimulation could lead to volume expansion and an increase in both ventricular preload and afterload, again contributing to adverse LV remodeling and eventual contractile dysfunction. Hyponatremia is another possible result of excessive and inappropriate AVP secretion. Hyponatremia is emerging as one of the most powerful predictors of poor outcome in congestive heart failure (CHF), even in this era of modern therapeutics (9). While long-assumed to be just a marker for disease severity, this assumption is now under vigorous challenge, with a number of possible reasons being advanced for a possible bidirectional relationship between progressive CHF and a fall in serum sodium. Some of these hypotheses include possible underuse of ACEIs and diuretics because of fear of further lowering sodium; adverse effects of low sodium on quality of life and neurological function; and direct, adverse effects of low sodium on myocardial cell structure and function. If any or all of these prove true, chronically excessive V2 signaling could play a role in LVD and CHF well beyond the more obvious one of contributing to volume expansion. In this regard a most interesting recent clinical study demonstrated better outcomes in a group of patients with advanced HF as a function of directly increasing serum sodium, despite the challenging difficulties inherent in the use of hypertonic saline to achieve this goal (10).

Another related issue for considering a beneficial effect of interference with V2 signaling (if it is, in fact, excessive) would be the possibility of reducing dependence on loop diuretics as our primary means of maintaining volume homeostasis in CHF. Loop diuretics do effectively remove salt and water acutely, but their actual efficacy in either short- or long-term use has never been established. Their beneficial effects are rapidly attenuated, however, and there are a number of adverse results of their use which may either limit their effectiveness or, worse, actually contribute to disease progression and its consequences (11). These include electrolyte depletion, the myocardial and renal consequences of such depletion (particularly magnesium depletion and its effect on myocardial, vascular, and renal calcium overload), and direct stimulation of the very neurohormonal systems being targeted by other therapeutic agents. If volume control could be achieved, at least in part, without these effects, a safer and more effective diuresis could theoretically be the result.

The foregoing discussion makes it abundantly clear that there are many reasons to target AVP as a contributor to LVD and progressive CHF. The remaining part of the rationale rests on demonstrating excessive AVP signaling in the presence of these conditions. This demonstration must be based not just on hormone levels but also on proof that interfering with AVP signaling has a meaningful and positive biological effect. Unfortunately, that is not always evident from acute experience and, in the absence of universally accepted surrogates, all acute experiences must be interpreted with caution. Nonetheless, there is abundant evidence from animal models for both excessive V1a and V2 signaling, some evidence (albeit scant) for excessive V1a signaling in human HF, and quite a bit of evidence for excessive, or at least demonstrable, V2 signaling in human HF.

Preclinical Studies

A possible role for AVP in the pathophysiology of HF has been explored in several animal models (12–20). In general, the results of these studies indicate the presence of significant V1a- and V2-mediated signaling. Most studies have focused on acute responses but several have looked at the impact of AVP antagonism over time.

Studies have been conducted with selective V1a antagonists in three separate models: adriamycin toxicity (13), tricuspid avulsion/pulmonary artery banding (12), and rapid ventricular pacing (14). All yielded positive results, using decreased systemic vascular resistance and/or improved cardiac output as the measure of V1a signaling. The combination of V1a antagonism and angiotensin II blockade produced greater improvement in myocyte function in an in vitro experiment than did either agent alone (15), but in vivo studies with pure V1a antagonism and other neurohormonal blockers have not been reported. There have been no studies reported with chronic administration of a V1a antagonist.

V2 antagonism has been studied in both the rapid ventricular pacing model (dogs) (14) and the post-myocardial infarction (MI) model (rats) (16). In each acute study, the administration of a selective V2 antagonist yielded a brisk diuresis (largely purely free water) and/or a decrease in cardiac filling pressure, depending on what was measured. A longer-term experience using a V2 antagonist in rats yielded a sustained response analogous to a clinical benefit (17).

Studies with combined V1a/V2 antagonism have also been performed. One acute study demonstrated apparent hemodynamic synergism with the administration of both a V1a and a V2 antagonist to dogs with pacing-induced failure (14). The V1a antagonist produced primarily an improvement in cardiac output with a fall in systemic resistance, while the V2 antagonist largely affected filling pressure. The combination, however, yielded greater and more sustained effects on each measure than did either alone. When an antagonist with both V1a and V2 antagonizing properties was administered in the same model, hemodynamic and renal responses were seen which were comparable to those observed with the administration of the individual agents (19). This agent (conivaptan, Astellas Pharma) has also been administered to rats with post-MI LVD, both alone and in combination with an ACEI (20). That study focused on the impact of treatment on left and right ventricular remodeling. No hemodynamics beyond blood pressure were measured. At 1 week there was evidence of V1a signaling since blood pressure fell with conivaptan alone. Conivaptan alone did not exert major effects on either RV or LV mass, but the combination of conivaptan and captopril yielded greater effects on RV mass beyond that seen with captopril alone. There was a trend for a greater effect on the LV response.

The mechanism of the results is not clear but could involve interruption primarily of V2-mediated signaling, causing a reduction in preload, pulmonary venous pressure, and thus right ventricular remodeling. A role for the V1a moiety on venous tone, the pulmonary vasculature, or the LV could not be excluded, however. Perhaps the major importance of this study is the demonstration that AVP-mediated signaling is possible, and even more likely, in the presence of other clinically used neurohormonal antagonists. This is obviously relevant to the clinical situation and could be predicted by experimental work in models other than LVD or CHF which clearly established greater potency of AVP-mediated effects, especially V1a effects, in the presence of diminished activity of the RAAS and/or adrenergic nervous system (21,22).

Taken together, the preclinical results establish the presence of tonic V1a- and V2-mediated signaling in several animal models of ventricular dysfunction and HF, which can be interrupted by effective nonpeptide and peptide antagonists to AVP. However, only very limited information is available with chronic administration of any antagonist. What has been reported does suggest that it is possible to produce clinically relevant, sustained interference with either V2-mediated signaling alone or with both V1a and V2 signaling using a combined antagonist in association with interruption of the RAAS.

Clinical Studies

It has been known for some time that plasma AVP levels are elevated, or at least incompletely suppressed for the prevailing osmolality, in patients with chronic or acutely decompensated CHF (Fig. 12-2) (23–26). As with other measured neurohormones, AVP levels are correlated to poor outcome in this syndrome (27). AVP, similar to

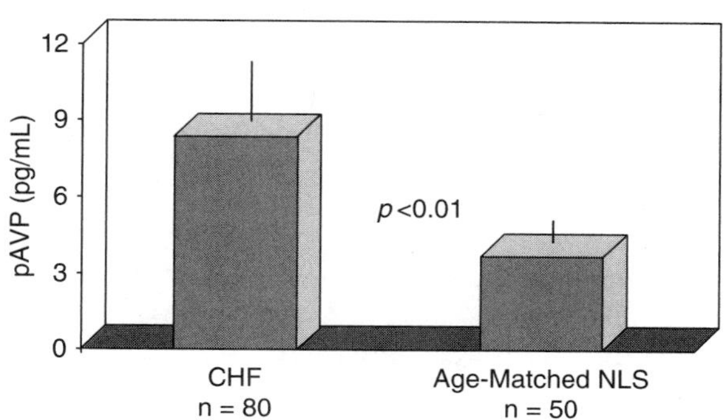

Figure 12-2 Plasma arginine vasopressin (AVP) levels from 80 patients with chronic congestive heart failure (CHF) and 50 age-matched control subjects. Plasma levels were collected on subjects between 1980 and 1985, prior to the widespread use of angiotensin-converting enzyme inhibitors (ACEIs).

plasma norepinephrine and atrial natriuretic peptide, is elevated early in the disease, including in patients with asymptomatic LVD (28). The reason for the increase in AVP secretion has thus far escaped clear delineation but must involve nonosmotic inputs (either hemodynamic or neurohormonal), since the osmotic regulation of the hormone is intact but shifted to higher plasma levels, with incomplete suppression in many patients despite very low serum sodium (29). The demonstration of either increased AVP levels or an association between plasma AVP and outcome in HF does not prove any pathophysiological contribution of AVP in HF, although such a relationship has been demonstrated with other neurohormones that have intracellular signaling pathways similar to AVP, such as norepinephrine, angiotensin II, and aldosterone. To do so, of course, requires proof that interfering with the secretion or effects of AVP produces chronic benefit in the syndrome of HF. Such data are not yet available for AVP but there are several acute and modestly prolonged experiences with AVP antagonists to consider.

To date, human studies attempting to establish a role for AVP in the pathophysiology of HF at the plasma levels seen in the syndrome have included the infusion of exogenous vasopressin to determine its hemodynamic effects in patients with chronic HF; single-dose administration of a peptide antagonist to the V1a receptor in patients with HF and hypertension; administration of a V2 antagonist for up to 60 days in patients with chronic HF; and the acute administration of a mixed antagonist, also to patients with chronic HF.

Goldsmith et al. infused exogenous AVP into 11 patients with advanced, but stable, HF due to either ischemic or primary dilated cardiomyopathy (30). The result (Fig. 12-3) was a decline in stroke volume, an increase in systemic vascular resistance, and a rise in filling pressures at moderately increased plasma AVP levels. These findings suggested that modest increases in plasma AVP could produce adverse hemodynamic effects in chronic HF, presumably via the V1a receptor.

Two single-dose studies using a selective V1a antagonist to AVP were reported at about the time of the infusion studies conducted by Goldsmith et al. Both studies found that if plasma AVP was increased, a fall in systemic vascular resistance and an increase in cardiac output occurred (Fig. 12-4) (31,32). These results thus complemented those by Goldsmith et al. and confirmed that hemodynamically important V1a-mediated signaling could be demonstrated under basal conditions in CHF if plasma AVP levels were increased.

A relevant, related study with the same compound in patients with severe hypertension demonstrated a fall in arterial pressure, even if plasma AVP levels were normal (33). This was an important observation since it established clinically relevant V1a signaling in humans with hypertension under basal conditions, and that (at least in this patient population) one could not necessarily predict a hemodynamic response to a V1a antagonist by measuring plasma AVP levels. No chronic experience in either HF or hypertension has been reported with selective V1a antagonism.

Selective V2 antagonism produces both an acute and sustained diuresis in patients with chronic CHF, which is largely an aquaresis since the major effect of these compounds is to increase free water clearance. One of these agents, tolvaptan (Otsuka Pharma), has now been given for 30 and 60 days to patients with CHF of mixed etiologies (34) and to those with acute decompensated heart failure (ADHF) due to LVD, respectively (35). The latter experience was placebo-controlled. Both studies confirmed sustained weight loss and a rise in serum sodium in those patients with hyponatremia (Figs. 12-5, 12-6). The drug was well-tolerated with only thirst as a common side effect. Neither study was powered for clinical endpoints as such, but the study in ADHF patients did include "worsening HF" as one measure, and it was unaffected. An intriguing post hoc analysis did demonstrate improved outcomes, including an unexpectedly large effect on mortality, in those patients with renal insufficiency or severe congestive symptoms. These results, taken together, demonstrate that one can produce a sustained interruption of V2 signaling in patients with chronic CHF using an appropriate agent.

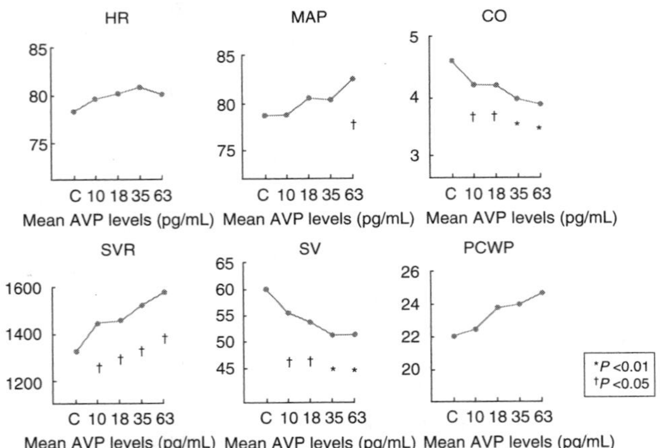

Figure 12-3 Hemodynamic effects of infusing exogenous AVP in patients with chronic CHF. Results were obtained via Swan-Ganz catheter in clinically stable patients. Goldsmith S, Francis GS, Cowley AW, et al. Hemodynamic effects of infused arginine vasopressin in congestive heart failure. *J Am Coll Cardiol.* 1986;8: 779–783.
HR, heart rate; MAP, mean arterial pressure; SVR, systemic vascular resistance; CO, cardiac output; SV, stroke volume; PCWP, pulmonary capillary wedge pressure.

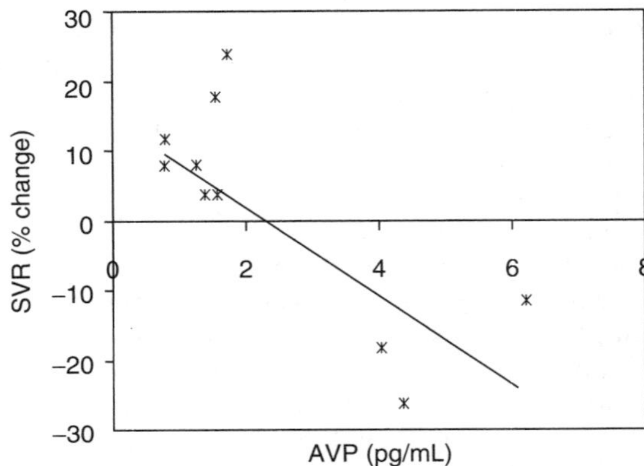

Figure 12-4 Effect of single-dose administration of a V1a antagonist on systemic vascular resistance (SVR) in patients with chronic, stable CHF.

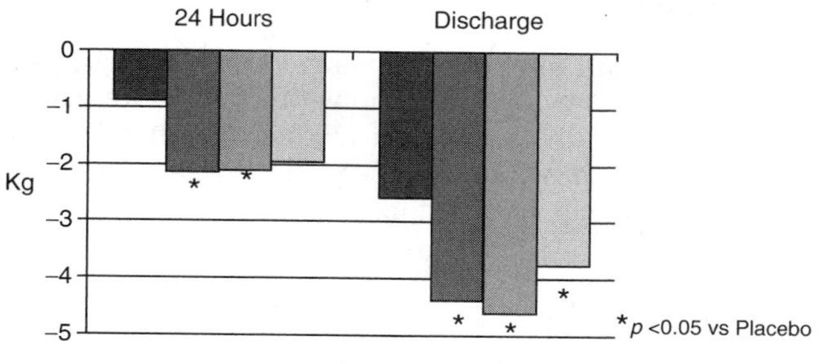

Figure 12-5 Effect of the V2 antagonist tolvaptan compared to standard care on body weight during hospitalization for acute decompensated heart failure.

Only one experience has been published with a mixed V1a/V2 antagonist in patients with chronic CHF. This study, measuring the effect of various doses of conivaptan against placebo in patients with advanced but stable HF, demonstrated an acute fall in cardiac filling pressure and a brisk aquaresis, but no effect on systemic vascular resistance or stroke volume (36). Plasma AVP levels were low in this population of patients. The most likely explanation for these findings is an interruption primarily of V2-mediated signaling, but venodilating effects from the V1a-blocking moiety or a balanced effect of the agent on preload and afterload leaving stroke volume unchanged are not excluded. No chronic experience with this agent is available, although it has been given to many patients with hyponatremia, many of whom have CHF. These results suggest safety and a sustained effect on serum sodium for a period up to several days.

Implications of Current Data and Future Development Plans

As of this writing, no selective V1a antagonist is under active development for LVD or CHF. The selective V2 antagonist tolvaptan is currently being investigated for short-term use against furosemide in chronic, stable CHF, with the endpoints being renal function and plasma neurohormones. Tolvaptan is also being investigated against placebo in a 12-month study in chronic CHF with ventricular remodeling as the endpoint. Finally, this agent is being evaluated against placebo for its effect on mortality in a large population of patients with LVD, presenting with ADHF. Preliminary experience with the similar compound lixivaptan has been reported (37) and this agent may be slated for additional study, as well.

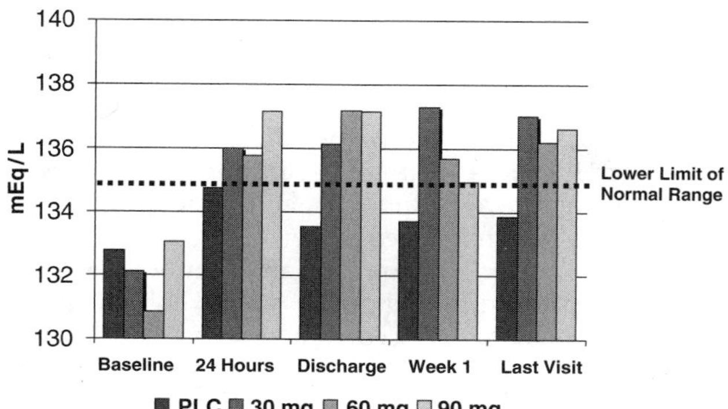

Figure 12-6 Effect of 60 days administration of the V2 antagonist tolvaptan on serum sodium in patients presenting initially with acute decompensated heart failure.

The combined antagonist conivaptan has been studied in a Phase II pilot for acute decompensated HF; results are not yet available. A New Drug Application (NDA) has been submitted to the U.S. Food and Drug Administration (FDA) for approval of this agent specifically for hyponatremia. Due to interactions with the cytochrome P450 system, however, this agent will be used only in an intravenous form (if approved), limiting its potential use to acute or intermittent administration. As of this writing, to our knowledge no other mixed antagonist is being studied in CHF.

The case for interfering with AVP signaling is certainly strong based on our current pathophysiological concept of LV dysfunction and HF. There does seem to be active signaling at both the V1a and V2 receptors in the clinical syndrome, although at this point the evidence is stronger regarding the V2 receptor. However, it should be noted that there is much less information actually available with V1a or mixed antagonists, and that while both the preclinical and early clinical studies would predict a positive response to such agents, it may depend more on the nature of concomitant therapy or the prevailing plasma AVP level than does the V2 signaling. In any event, if one considers the possible utility of vasopressin antagonism in CHF, several important points should be borne in mind.

A pure V1a antagonist would have the expected hemodynamic and myocardial effects but could, if AVP levels rose in response to competitive displacement of hormone from V1a receptors, lead to unwanted water retention. An increase in ventricular preload might therefore offset any gains from lower afterload or direct benefits to the myocardium. A pure V2 antagonist may well lead to sustained water diuresis but, as AVP levels rise in response to increased plasma osmolality and/or competitive displacement of hormone from V2 receptors, undesirable V1a stimulation could occur. For these reasons, it might be most useful to employ agents that block both receptor sites, although the impact of the V1a antagonizing moiety might not be readily apparent in shorter-term studies and the utility of V2 receptor antagonism in patients not already volume-expanded might well be questionable. Since it may be possible to adjust the relative degree of receptor antagonism in newer compounds, the use of a particular agent might be tailored to particular clinical settings. For acutely ill or chronically congested patients, a major component of V2 antagonism would be desirable, while for prophylactic use in patients with LVD but without a great deal of volume expansion, an agent with primarily V1a activity might be best.

The settings in which these agents might be used also deserve consideration. Chronic, stable LVD with or without mild CHF now carries a very favorable prognosis (38). The success of current therapies renders it challenging from a statistical point of view to demonstrate the effectiveness of newer treatment. On the other hand, episodes of ADHF and the presence of persistent congestion identify a high-risk population (39) in which it may be easier to demonstrate effectiveness of newer treatment. Effective V2 antagonism, especially if combined (for the reason previously discussed) with V1a antagonism, could be very useful in these patients since the most obvious and direct effect of these agents is volume removal. Given the limitations and toxicity of diuresis produced only by loop diuretics, adjunctive or replacement diuretic therapy with a V2 antagonist could provide more effective (and actually safer) long-term volume control.

Finally, hyponatremia is, as previously noted, a marker for very poor outcome in CHF. Agents such as V2 antagonists that rapidly and safely correct hyponatremia conceivably could lead directly to improved outcomes in this group of patients if the association is causative in any way. Since V2 antagonists have been shown to correct and maintain sodium homeostasis over a period of weeks in patients with CHF and hyponatremia, longer-term study of V2 or mixed antagonists specifically in this patient group seems warranted.

ADDITIONAL NEUROHORMONAL TARGETS IN HEART FAILURE: ENDOTHELIN AND NEUTRAL ENDOPEPTIDASE

As discussed in the introduction to this chapter, a number of additional neurohormonal targets for the treatment of HF have been suggested, based on the success of agents which interfere with the adrenergic nervous system and the RAAS. This section of the chapter will review the rationale and experience for targeting endothelin and neutral endopeptidase.

Description of Endothelin

Endothelin is a potent vasoconstrictor peptide that was first isolated in 1988 (40). It is synthesized as a pre-prohormone (big endothelin-1) that is converted to proendothelin and later to four isoforms (endothelins 1–4) (41). Endothelin-1 is the predominant isoform in the vasculature and is felt to play a role in cardiovascular disease. The other endothelin isoforms are less well-understood and will not be discussed in this chapter.

Endothelin-1 synthesis is stimulated by hypoxia, ischemia, neurohormones (norepinephrine, angiotensin II, arginine vasopressin), and inflammatory cytokines (42–44). It is formed in endothelial cells and is released toward the vascular smooth muscle consistent with a paracrine role, but it is also produced by smooth muscle cells and cardiac myocytes (41). Endothelins are cleared largely by the lungs, liver, and kidneys (45).

Endothelin Receptors

There are two major receptors to endothelin (A and B) expressed on several cells in the cardiovascular system, including endothelial cells, vascular smooth muscle cells, cardiac myocytes, and fibroblasts (41,46). Endothelin-A receptors are found on vascular smooth muscle cells and cardiac myocytes and, when stimulated, result in vasoconstriction, smooth muscle cell proliferation, fibroblast proliferation, and myocyte hypertrophy (47,48). Endothelin-B receptors are mainly located on vascular endothelial cells; stimulation of these receptors leads to increased production of nitric oxide, resulting in vasodilation (49).

Endothelin in Heart Failure

Tissue and plasma levels of endothelin-1 and its precursor (big endothelin-1) are elevated in patients with HF (50–55). These increases are probably due to increased endothelin synthesis primarily in the pulmonary vascular bed (56) and the myocardium (57). The vascular distention seen in HF (especially in the pulmonary vascular bed) may be a stimulus for increased endothelin-1 production (58). This idea is supported by the observation that endothelin concentrations decrease significantly when the pulmonary hypertension associated with acute pulmonary edema is effectively treated with continuous positive airway pressure (59) or short-term vasodilator therapy (60). Another potential contributor to the increased endothelin-1 concentrations observed in HF is the downregulation of endothelin-B receptors, which has been observed in the lung tissue of animals with experimental HF (61,62). Endothelin-B receptors are felt to play a role in the clearance of endothelin-1. Pulmonary vascular tone in HF may be largely mediated by endothelin-A receptors since HF patients treated with endothelin antagonists experience decreases in pulmonary vascular resistance, whereas no such change is seen when the same agent is given to normal subjects (63,64). Increased levels of endothelin-1 and its precursor (big endothelin-1) are associated with increased angiotensin II levels, more advanced HF symptoms, worse hemodynamics, lower LV ejection fractions, and decreased survival (42,52,55,58,65–74).

Animal Studies of Endothelin Antagonists in Heart Failure

Endothelin antagonists have been developed for a number of cardiovascular conditions. They can generally be classified according to the type of endothelin receptor that the agent inhibits: endothelin-A receptor antagonists, endothelin-B receptor antagonists, and drugs that inhibit interaction of endothelin at both the A and B receptors. Both endothelin-A receptor antagonists and mixed type A/B receptor antagonists have beneficial effects in animal models of HF. Endothelin-A receptor antagonists prevent remodeling, improve LV function, and prolong survival in rats (75–77). They have been shown to attenuate the deterioration of cardiac performance and hemodynamics in dogs with a pacing-induced model of HF (78). The mixed endothelin antagonists bosentan and tezosentan improve LV function, reduce remodeling, and increase survival in dog and rat models of post-infarction HF (79–82).

Given the potential theoretical benefits of increased endothelin signaling at the B receptor, antagonizing this receptor has not been pursued as a target for therapy.

Increased signaling at this receptor could, however, theoretically contribute to any benefit of pure endothelin-A antagonism, assuming endothelin levels increase following the administration of a selective antagonist.

Not all the preclinical experiences with selective and nonselective antagonists have been positive. Early therapy after onset of infarction in an animal model impaired scar healing and was associated with LV dilation (83). In another model, dogs with pacing-induced HF developed neurohormonal activation and increased fluid retention after treatment with an endothelin-A antagonist (84). A problem in many of these preclinical studies is the administration of endothelin antagonists without additional neurohormonal blockade. The lack of neurohormanal blockade could mitigate any potential benefit of these agents if it were overwhelmed by vasoconstriction, volume retention, and myocardial stimulation as a result of activation of the other systems. This is a generic problem in testing any new, neurohormonally active agent and suggests the need for such experiments to more closely mimic human LV dysfunction and HF, wherein the potential benefit of additional therapy must be demonstrated against a background of treatment with agents interfering with the renin-angiotensin-aldosterone and adrenergic nervous systems.

Endothelin Antagonists in Human Heart Failure

The rationale and body of experimental evidence supporting the use of endothelial receptor antagonists in the treatment of patients with HF is compelling: concentrations of endothelin and its precursors are increased in HF and are independently associated with more advanced HF symptoms and poor prognosis; infusion of endothelin into patients with LV dysfunction increases mean arterial pressure and systemic vascular resistance and decreases cardiac index (85); effective treatment of HF decreases endothelin concentrations (68,86–88); and preclinical data demonstrate beneficial hemodynamic effects with both endothelin-A and mixed A/B endothelin antagonists. Unfortunately, to date no study has clearly demonstrated the benefit of such antagonists in reducing symptoms or improving outcomes in patients with acute or chronic HF.

The acute administration of both endothelin-A and mixed A/B receptor antagonists can improve cardiac index and decrease pulmonary artery pressure, pulmonary vascular resistance, and pulmonary capillary wedge pressure (53,89–101). However, not all of these agents have been effective. The Randomized Intravenous Tezosentan Study (RITZ) program has studied the effectiveness of tezosentan (a mixed endothelin A/B receptor antagonist) administered acutely in a variety of clinical settings. RITZ 1 studied 669 patients hospitalized for decompensated HF requiring parenteral therapy. The control group received usual care for HF plus placebo, and the intervention group received standard therapy plus 25 mg of tezosentan per hour intravenously for 1 hour followed by a titration to 50 mg per hour intravenously for 24 to 72 hours. The primary endpoint was patient assessment of dyspnea at 24 hours. There were no significant differences between the two treatment groups. However, patients receiving higher doses of tezosentan experienced more hypotension, dizziness, and renal failure, suggesting that this dose might have been excessive (102). More recently, this trial was repeated in 130 patients with ADHF using lower doses of tezosentan. The primary endpoint of cardiac index at 24 hours was significantly improved in the tezosentan group compared to placebo, suggesting that lower doses are effective and better-tolerated (103).

Value of Endothelin Receptor Inhibition with Tezosentan in Acute Heart Failure Study (VERITAS), the largest clinical trial of an endothelin receptor antagonist for ADHF, enrolled 1,435 patients and randomized them to receive placebo or tazosentan. The dose of tazosentan was 5 mg per hour for 30 minutes followed by 1 mg per hour for up to 72 hours (considerably less than that used in RITZ 1). Patients treated with tezosentan experienced significant reductions in pulmonary artery pressure and pulmonary capillary wedge pressure, as well as an increase in cardiac index. Despite these significant improvements in hemodynamics, use of tazosentan did not improve the primary endpoints of dyspnea at 24 hours or worsening HF or death at 7 days (104).

Chronic treatment with endothelin receptor antagonists has been evaluated in a number of clinical trials. The Endothelin Antagonist Bosentan for Lowering cardiac Events (ENABLE) trials were two Phase III trials conducted in Europe and Australia (ENABLE 1) and in the United States and Canada (ENABLE 2) (105). In these trials, 1,613 patients with advanced HF and an ejection fraction less than 35% were randomized to receive either bosentan (a mixed endothelin A/B receptor antagonist) 125 mg twice daily, or placebo. The primary endpoints were clinical status, all-cause mortality, and HF-related hospitalizations after 9 months of treatment. There were no significant differences between the two treatment groups in the primary endpoint of clinical status and there was an early worsening of HF leading to a greater rate of hospitalization in patients randomized to bosentan during the first 1 to 2 months. This was manifested by a higher incidence of weight gain, increased edema, and lower hemoglobin concentration (105).

Resource utilization Among Congestive Heart Failure Study (REACH) was another trial examining the effect of chronic bosentan therapy in 370 patients with advanced HF and an ejection fraction less than 35%. Patients were randomized to be treated either with placebo or bosentan for 6 months. The primary endpoint was change in clinical status from baseline (106). The trial was stopped prematurely due to elevations in liver transaminases. At the time the study was stopped, there were no significant differences in outcomes between the two treatment groups. However, a post hoc analysis of 174 patients who completed the 6-month follow-up demonstrated significant clinical improvement and a decreased probability of worsening clinical status among patients treated with bosentan ($p = 0.045$). These data suggest a biphasic response to bosentan, with early worsening and late improvement in symptoms.

Enrasentan Cooperative Randomized Evaluation (ENCOR) studied the use of enrasentan, a mixed endothelin A/B receptor antagonist, in 419 patients with stable New York Heart Association (NYHA) Class II and III HF and LV ejection fractions less than or equal to 35%. There was no significant improvement in the primary endpoint of clinical HF score after 9 months associated with the use of enrasentan, and there was a trend for increased adverse events and increased hospitalizations in the active treatment arm compared to placebo (107).

On theoretical grounds, it has been argued that selective endothelin-A antagonism might be preferable to mixed antagonism, since the endothelin-B receptor may subserve useful functions in HF. Less experience is available with this approach but, unfortunately, what is available is also disappointing. The Endothelin-A Receptor Antagonist Trial in Heart Failure (EARTH) studied LV remodeling (a very potent surrogate endpoint for benefit in chronic HF) in 642 patients with stable Class II to IV HF and LV ejection fractions less than 35% after 6 months of treatment with the selective endothelin-A receptor antagonist, darusentan. There was no change in the primary endpoint of LV end-systolic volume as assessed by magnetic resonance imaging (MRI) at the 6-month endpoint (108). Thus far in clinical studies, there is a nearly perfect parallel between effects on remodeling and effects on survival; therefore, the negative results in this trial are not encouraging for future development of this or other similar agents.

Endothelin remains an attractive therapeutic target for the management of HF. The explanation for the failure of the therapeutic trials remains elusive but, given the remarkable consistency of the findings, it is unlikely that the reason lies with the specific agents tested. They are hemodynamically effective but, in the case of this approach, there must be activation of other poorly understood systems which offsets any purely load-related effects or any directly beneficial myocardial effects of antagonizing the endothelin-A receptor. Or, in some poorly understood way, perhaps endothelin has some beneficial adaptive function in chronic HF. Whatever the explanation, these results are not consistent with those from the results from the trials with agents interfering with the renin-angiotensin-aldosterone and adrenergic nervous systems, in which, presumably, a mix of load-related and non-load-related effects of the agents tested actually does influence the course of the disease. We may never know the explanation for the failure of endothelin antagonism but, given the data, it is unlikely that the pharmaceutical industry will vigorously pursue further research based on this approach. However, a related effort based on inhibiting endothelin-converting enzyme is being developed (109); clinical trials are ongoing.

Neutral Endopeptidase Inhibition

Neutral endopeptidase (NEP) is an endothelial cell surface enzyme that catalyzes the degradation of bradykinin and the natriuretic peptides ANP, BNP, and CNP. Natriuretic peptides are produced by the myocardium and endothelium and have salutary effects on hemodynamics, vascular and myocardial remodeling, renal perfusion, and sodium excretion (please refer to the chapter on natriuretic peptides). Bradykinin is a potent vasodilator, plays a role in the regulation of coronary vascular tone, and may mediate some of the beneficial effects associated with the use of ACEIs (110,111). Therefore, NEP inhibitors may be beneficial in HF due to increased circulating levels of the aforementioned endogenous vasoactive peptides.

Similar to ACE, NEP is found in a wide variety of tissues, including the vascular endothelium, smooth muscle cells, cardiac myocytes and fibroblasts, renal tubular cells, and the brain. It acts on many substrates in addition to natriuretic peptides and bradykinin, including angiotensin I, angiotensin II, substance P, adrenomedullin, endothelin, and enkephalins (111). NEP inhibitors have beneficial effects on hemodynamics, renal function, and survival in some animal models of HF (112–115).

Due to NEP's role in regulating vasodilator and vasoconstrictor substances, NEP inhibition can result in variable affects on blood pressure depending on the degree to which the degradation of vasodilator or vasoconstrictor substances is diminished (116). Indeed, increased levels of endothelin have been detected in healthy volunteers treated with NEP inhibitors, and intra-arterial infusions of an NEP inhibitor results in increased vascular resistance in the forearm of human subjects—a response that is prevented by an endothelin antagonist (117,118).

The combination of ACE and NEP inhibition may be particularly helpful for HF because an increase in natriuretic peptide levels caused by NEP inhibition could lead to improved blood pressure control (the combination of ACEIs and diuretics decreases blood pressure), enhanced vasodilation, and reductions in sympathetic activity, smooth muscle cell proliferation, and cardiac fibrosis (111). Moreover, the degradation of bradykinin is catalyzed by both ACE and NEP. When the actions of ACE are inhibited, NEP is the major pathway for bradykinin degradation. The combination of ACE and NEP inhibition leads to striking increases in bradykinin levels that could account for significant improvements in blood pressure, but might also explain the increased incidence of angioedema observed in some studies (111).

Initial studies in patients with HF demonstrated that the use of vasopeptidase inhibitors (the combination of an ACEI and an NEP inhibitor) was associated with improved hemodynamics, a decrease in death or hospitalization from HF, increases in ANP levels, decreases in plasma norepinephrine levels, and improvements in exercise tolerance (119–121). The promising results of the early trials using vasopeptidase inhibitors, however, were not borne out in a large mortality trial. The Omapatrilat Versus Enalapril Randomized Trial of Utility in Reducing Events (OVERTURE) was a double-blind, randomized trial comparing omapatrilat 40 mg once daily to the ACE inhibitor enalapril 10 mg twice daily in 5,770 patients with NYHA Class II to IV HF (122). After a mean follow-up of 14.5 months, there was no significant difference in the primary endpoint of the combined risk of death or hospitalization for HF requiring intravenous treatment. Patients treated with omapatrilat had a 9% lower risk of cardiovascular death or hospitalization and a 6% lower risk of death compared to the enalapril group. The incidence of angioedema was low in both treatment groups (0.8% and 0.5%, respectively, NS). This low incidence of angioedema was probably due to the fact that all patients were required to be on ACEIs prior to enrollment in the study, effectively selecting patients who were less likely to develop angioedema. In a large population of hypertensive patients, omapatrilat was associated with an increased incidence of angioedema compared to treatment with an ACEI (2.17% and 0.68%, respectively) (123). Episodes of angioedema associated with omapatrilat tended to be more severe and occurred early after the initial dose. For this reason, omapatrilat is currently not available in the United States.

Therefore, similar to endothelin antagonism, NEP inhibition's solid rationale, strong preclinical data, and early therapeutic success have not yet been converted to clinical benefit in HF. Unlike the endothelin story, however, there is really only one negative experience to date with NEP inhibitions in HF; the agent is unquestionably effective in treating hypertension, although (as noted) limited by a possible increase in the incidence or severity of angioedema. Questions remain regarding the adequacy of the inhibition of the enzyme with omapatrilat in a population characterized by very high BNP levels, for example. Other agents with varying potency of enzyme inhibition are available and may see further study. Also, given the likelihood that side effects might ultimately limit the use of this class of agents, it is possible that increasing the putative benefits of the natriuretic peptide system might be better accomplished by administering pharmacologic doses of the peptides themselves. Preliminary work is under way based on subcutaneous administration of at least one peptide (BNP) since peptides are not effective via the oral route.

SUMMARY

The progression from LV dysfunction to HF is clearly a complicated process. Naturally, prevention and treatment of HF are therefore challenging. One cannot overlook cardiac loading conditions and LV function, yet how one goes about altering these factors makes a difference. Simply producing a diuresis or causing vasorelaxation is insufficient in altering the natural history of the syndrome. The likely reason is the effect of such treatment on intermediaries which connect to the basic molecular and cellular pathology of HF. It is clearly not desirable to increase adrenergic signaling or the activity of the RAAS. Inhibiting these systems (assuming adequate control of volume and pressure) to date has produced the best outcomes in HF. By extension, inhibiting other neurohormonal systems that share intracellular signaling pathways should be desirable, as would be the potentiation of other systems such as those involving the natriuretic peptides, which counteract the maladaptive effects of excessive adrenergic signaling and activation of the RAAS.

Whether this can be accomplished with the three candidate approaches discussed in this chapter—AVP antagonism, endothelin antagonism, and the potentiation of natriuretic peptide signaling via endopeptidase inhibition—is not yet clear. Strong theoretical rationales and preclinical data are present for each. It is simply too early to conclude anything about AVP antagonism since no long-term clinical trials are yet completed, although preliminary results are encouraging. Only one study of endopeptidase inhibition has been completed and, although there were trends toward benefit, they were not statistically significant; it is possible that the dose or formulation was inadequate. While further exploration of the value of potentiating the natriuretic peptide systems may not be forthcoming using this approach, the more direct method of injecting or infusing these compounds is only in its earliest stages of development.

With endothelin antagonism, the prognosis is much poorer since a number of trials in both acute and chronic HF are complete. None show benefit and there are trends toward adverse effects in some. The reasons are unclear and likely involve the induction of unexpected genomic or other cellular effects which arise in the presence of such antagonists. It is, however, a cautionary tale both in terms of the completeness of our model of HF and of the predictive value of even the best theoretical rationales and preclinical data for outcomes assessment in HF. We do not yet completely understand the biology of this disease; until we do, future development of therapy whether based on neurohormonal imbalance or more direct approaches to loading conditions and ventricular performance must be guided by the effect of such treatments on clinical outcomes. Surrogate measures such as ventricular remodeling and biomarkers can aid us in this process but probably are not yet ready to substitute for clinical effects. It will be most interesting to revisit these issues after the studies with the AVP antagonists are completed, since they will, at minimum, provide a wealth of data regarding these surrogate markers and outcomes in HF in the face of additional neurohormonal inhibition.

REFERENCES

1. Goldsmith SR. Therapeutics in congestive heart failure: from hemodynamics to neurohormones. In: *Cardiac Remodeling and Failure*. Boston: Kluwer Academic Publishers; 2003:17–34.
2. Goldsmith SR. Vasopressin: a therapeutic target in congestive heart failure? *J Card Fail*. 1999;5:347–356.
3. Goldsmith SR. Baroreflex control of vasopressin secretion in normal humans. In: Cowley AW, Liard J-F, Ausiello DA, eds. *Vasopressin: Cellular and Integrative Functions*. New York: Raven Press; 1988: 389–397.
4. Jard S. Mechanisms of action of vasopressin and vasopressin antagonists. *Kidney Int Suppl*. 1988;26:S38–S42.
5. Xu YJ, Gopalakrishnan V. Vasopressin increases cytosolic free [Ca2+] in the neonatal rat cardiomyocyte. Evidence for V1 subtype receptors. *Circ Res*. 1991;69:239–245.
6. Nakamura Y, Haneda T, Osaki J, et al. Hypertrophic growth of cultured neonatal rat heart cells mediated by vasopressin V(1A) receptor. *Eur J Pharmacol*. 2000;391:39–48.
7. Verbalis JG. Vasopressin V2 receptor antagonists. *J Mol Endocrinol*. 2002;29:1–9.
8. Hirsch AT, Dzau VJ, Majzoub JA, et al. Vasopressin-mediated forearm vasodilation in normal humans. Evidence for a vascular vasopressin V2 receptor. *J Clin Invest*. 1989;84:418–426.
9. Liviu Klein, Gattis WA. Prognostic value of hyponatremia in hospitalized patients with worsening heart failure: insights from the Outcomes of a Prospective Trial of Intravenous Milrinone for Exacerbations of Chronic Heart Failure (OPTIME-CHF) [abstract]. *J Card Fail*. 2004.
10. Licata G, Di Pasquale P, Parrinello G, et al. Effects of high-dose furosemide and small-volume hypertonic saline solution infusion in comparison with a high dose of furosemide as bolus in refractory congestive heart failure: long-term effects. *Am Heart J*. 2003;145:459–466.
11. Weber KT. Furosemide in the long-term management of heart failure: the good, the bad, and the uncertain. *J Am Coll Cardiol*. 2004;44:1308–1310.
12. Stone CK, Imai N, Thomas A, et al. Hemodynamic effects of vasopressin inhibition in congestive heart failure. *Clin Res*. 1986;34:632A-0.

13. Arnolda L, McGrath BP, Cocks M, et al. Vasoconstrictor role for vasopressin in experimental heart failure in the rabbit. *J Clin Invest.* 1986;78:674–679.
14. Naitoh M, Suzuki H, Murakami M, et al. Effects of oral AVP receptor antagonists OPC-21268 and OPC-31260 on congestive heart failure in conscious dogs. *Am J Physiol.* 1994;267: H2245–H2254.
15. Clair MJ, King MK, Goldberg AT, et al. Selective vasopressin, angiotensin II, or dual receptor blockade with developing congestive heart failure. *J Pharmacol Exp Ther.* 2000;293:852–860.
16. Burrell LM, Phillips PA, Rolls KA, et al. Vascular responses to vasopressin antagonists in man and rat. *Clin Sci.* (Lond) 1994; 87:389–395.
17. Wang YX, Franco R, Gavras I, et al. Effects of chronic administration of a vasopressin antagonist with combined antivasopressor and antiantidiuretic activities in rats with left ventricular dysfunction. *J Lab Clin Med.* 1991;117:313–318.
18. Nishikimi T, Kawano Y, Saito Y, et al. Effect of long-term treatment with selective vasopressin V1 and V2 receptor antagonist on the development of heart failure in rats. *J Cardiovasc Pharmacol.* 1996;27:275–282.
19. Yatsu T, Tomura Y, Tahara A, et al. Cardiovascular and renal effects of conivaptan hydrochloride (YM087), a vasopressin V1A and V2 receptor antagonist, in dogs with pacing-induced congestive heart failure. *Eur J Pharmacol.* 1999;376:239–246.
20. Naitoh M, Risvanis J, Balding LC, et al. Neurohormonal antagonism in heart failure; beneficial effects of vasopressin V(1a) and V(2) receptor blockade and ACE inhibition. *Cardiovasc Res.* 2002;54:51–57.
21. Share L. Interrelations between vasopressin and the renin-angiotensin system. *Fed Proc.* 1979;38:2267–2271.
22. Cowley AW, Jr., Liard JF. Vasopressin and arterial pressure regulation. Special lecture. *Hypertension.* 1988;11(2 Pt 2):125–132.
23. Yamane Y. Plasma ADH level in patients with chronic congestive heart failure. *Japn Circ J.* 1968;32:745–759.
24. Szatalowicz VL, Arnold PE, Chaimovitz C, et al. Radioimmunoassay of plasma arginine vasopressin in hyponatremic patients with congestive heart failure. *N Engl J Med.* 1981;305:263–266.
25. Goldsmith SR, Francis GS, Cowley AW, et al. Increased plasma arginine vasopressin levels in patients with congestive heart failure. *J Am Coll Cardiol.* 1983;1 (6):1385–1390.
26. Prebiscz J, Seasley J, Laragh J, et al. Platelet and plasma vasopressin in essential hypertension and congestive heart failure. *Hypertension.* 1983; (5 Suppl I) I:129–132.
27. Rouleau JL, Packer M, Moye L, et al. Prognostic value of neurohumoral activation in patients with an acute myocardial infarction: effect of captopril. *J Am Coll Cardiol.* 1994;24:583–591.
28. Francis GS, Benedict C, Johnstone DE, et al. Comparison of neuroendocrine activation in patients with left ventricular dysfunction with and without congestive heart failure. A substudy of the Studies of Left Ventricular Dysfunction (SOLVD). *Circulation.* 1990;82:1724–1729.
29. Goldsmith SR, Cowley AW, Francis GS, et al. Arginine vasopressin and the renal response to water loading in congestive heart failure. *Am J Cardiol.* 1986;58:295–299.
30. Goldsmith SR, Francis GS, Cowley AW, et al. Hemodynamic effects of infused arginine vasopressin in congestive heart failure. *J Am Coll Cardiol.* 1986;8:779–783.
31. Creager MA, Faxon DP, Cutler SS, et al. Contribution of vasopressin to vasoconstriction in patients with congestive heart failure: comparison with the renin-angiotensin system and the sympathetic nervous system. *J Am Coll Cardiol.* 1986;7:758–765.
32. Nicod P, Waeber B, Bussien JP, et al. Acute hemodynamic effects of a vascular antagonist of vasopressin in patients with congestive heart failure. *Am J Cardiol.* 1985;55:1043–1047.
33. Ribiero A, Mulinasi R, Gavras I, et al. Sequential elimination of pressor mechanisms in severe hypertension in humans. *Hypertension.* 1986; (8 Suppl I) I:169–173.
34. Gheorghiade M, Niazi I, Ouyang J, et al. Vasopressin V2-receptor blockade with tolvaptan in patients with chronic heart failure: results from a double-blind, randomized trial. *Circulation* 2003;107:2690–2696.
35. Gheorghiade M, Gattis WA, O'Connor CM, et al. Effects of tolvaptan, a vasopressin antagonist, in patients hospitalized with worsening heart failure: a randomized controlled trial (ACTIV). *JAMA.* 2004;291:1963–1971.
36. Udelson JE, Smith WB, Hendrix GH, et al. Acute hemodynamic effects of conivaptan, a dual V(1A) and V(2) vasopressin receptor antagonist, in patients with advanced heart failure. *Circulation.* 2001;104:2417–2423.
37. Wong F, Blei AT, Blendis LM, et al. A vasopressin receptor antagonist (VPA-985) improves serum sodium concentration in patients with hyponatremia: a multicenter, randomized, placebo-controlled trial. *Hepatology.* 2003;37:182–191.
38. Fonarow GC. The Acute Decompensated Heart Failure National Registry (ADHERE): opportunities to improve care of patients hospitalized with acute decompensated heart failure. *Rev Cardiovasc Med.* 2003;(4 Suppl 7):S21–S30.
39. Yanagisawa M, Kurihara H, Kimura S, et al. A novel potent vasoconstrictor peptide produced by vascular endothelial cells. *Nature* 1988;332:411–415.
40. Rich S, McLaughlin VV. Endothelin receptor blockers in cardiovascular disease. *Circulation.* 2003;108:2184–2190.
41. McMurray JJ, Ray SG, Abdullah I, et al. Plasma endothelin in chronic heart failure. *Circulation.* 1992;85:1374–1379.
42. Clavell AL, Mattingly MT, Stevens TL, et al. Angiotensin converting enzyme inhibition modulates endogenous endothelin in chronic canine thoracic inferior vena caval constriction. *J Clin Invest.* 1996;97:1286–1292.
43. Noll G, Wenzel RR, Luscher TF. Endothelin and endothelin antagonists: potential role in cardiovascular and renal disease. *Mol Cell Biochem.* 1996;157:259–267.
44. Fukuroda T, Fujikawa T, Ozaki S, et al. Clearance of circulating endothelin-1 by ETB receptors in rats. *Biochem Biophys Res Commun.* 1994;199:1461–1465.
45. Colucci WS. Myocardial endothelin. Does it play a role in myocardial failure? *Circulation.* 1996;93:1069–1072.
46. Choukroun G, Hajjar R, Kyriakis JM, et al. Role of the stress-activated protein kinases in endothelin-induced cardiomyocyte hypertrophy. *J Clin Invest.* 1998;102:1311–1320.
47. Inada T, Fujiwara H, Hasegawa K, et al. Upregulated expression of cardiac endothelin-1 participates in myocardial cell growth in Bio14.6 Syrian cardiomyopathic hamsters. *J Am Coll Cardiol.* 1999;33:565–571.
48. de Nucci G, Thomas R, D'Orleans-Juste P, et al. Pressor effects of circulating endothelin are limited by its removal in the pulmonary circulation and by the release of prostacyclin and endothelium-derived relaxing factor. *Proc Natl Acad Sci USA.* 1988;85:9797–9800.
49. Zolk O, Quattek J, Sitzler G, et al. Expression of endothelin-1, endothelin-converting enzyme, and endothelin receptors in chronic heart failure. *Circulation.* 1999;99:2118–2123.
50. Fukuchi M, Giaid A. Expression of endothelin-1 and endothelin-converting enzyme-1 mRNAs and proteins in failing human hearts. *J Cardiovasc Pharmacol.* 1998;31(Suppl 1):S421–S423.
51. Genth-Zotz S, Zotz RJ, Cobaugh M, et al. Changes of neurohumoral parameters and endothelin-1 in response to exercise in patients with mild to moderate congestive heart failure. *Int J Cardiol.* 1998;66:137–142.
52. Kiowski W, Sutsch G, Hunziker P, et al. Evidence for endothelin-1-mediated vasoconstriction in severe chronic heart failure. *Lancet* 1995;346:732–736.
53. Good JM, Nihoyannopoulos P, Ghatei MA, et al. Elevated plasma endothelin concentrations in heart failure; an effect of angiotensin II? *Eur Heart J.* 1994;15:1634–1640.
54. Pacher R, Stanek B, Hulsmann M, et al. Prognostic impact of big endothelin-1 plasma concentrations compared with invasive hemodynamic evaluation in severe heart failure. *J Am Coll Cardiol.* 1996;27:633–641.
55. Tsutamoto T, Wada A, Maeda Y, et al. Relation between endothelin-1 spillover in the lungs and pulmonary vascular resistance in patients with chronic heart failure. *J Am Coll Cardiol.* 1994;23: 1427–1433.
56. Sakai S, Miyauchi T, Sakurai T, et al. Endogenous endothelin-1 participates in the maintenance of cardiac function in rats with congestive heart failure. Marked increase in endothelin-1 production in the failing heart. *Circulation.* 1996;93:1214–1222.
57. Cody RJ, Haas GJ, Binkley PF, et al. Plasma endothelin correlates with the extent of pulmonary hypertension in patients with chronic congestive heart failure. *Circulation.* 1992;85: 504–509.

58. Takeda S, Takano T, Ogawa R. The effect of nasal continuous positive airway pressure on plasma endothelin-1 concentrations in patients with severe cardiogenic pulmonary edema. *Anesth Analg.* 1997;84:1091–1096.
59. Stangl K, Dschietzig T, Richter C, et al. Pulmonary release and coronary and peripheral consumption of big endothelin and endothelin-1 in severe heart failure: acute effects of vasodilator therapy. *Circulation.* 2000;102:1132–1138.
60. Dupuis J, Rouleau JL, Cernacek P. Reduced pulmonary clearance of endothelin-1 contributes to the increase of circulating levels in heart failure secondary to myocardial infarction. *Circulation.* 1998;98:1684–1687.
61. Kobayshi T, Miyauchi T, Sakai S, et al. Down-regulation of ET(B) receptor, but not ET(A) receptor, in congestive lung secondary to heart failure. Are marked increases in circulating endothelin-1 partly attributable to decreases in lung ET(B) receptor-mediated clearance of endothelin-1? *Life Sci.* 1998; 62:185–193.
62. Ooi H, Colucci WS, Givertz MM. Endothelin mediates increased pulmonary vascular tone in patients with heart failure: demonstration by direct intrapulmonary infusion of sitaxsentan. *Circulation.* 2002;106:1618–1621.
63. Fleisch M, Sutsch G, Yan XW, et al. Systemic, pulmonary, and renal hemodynamic effects of endothelin ET(A/B)-receptor blockade in patients with maintained left ventricular function. *J Cardiovasc Pharmacol.* 2000;36:302–309.
64. Rodeheffer RJ, Lerman A, Heublein DM, et al. Increased plasma concentrations of endothelin in congestive heart failure in humans. *Mayo Clin Proc.* 1992;67:719–724.
65. Pacher R, Stanek B, Hulsmann M, et al. Prognostic impact of big endothelin-1 plasma concentrations compared with invasive hemodynamic evaluation in severe heart failure. *J Am Coll Cardiol.* 1996;27:633–641.
66. Wei CM, Lerman A, Rodeheffer RJ, et al. Endothelin in human congestive heart failure. *Circulation.* 1994;89:1580–1586.
67. Tsutamoto T, Hisanaga T, Fukai D, et al. Prognostic value of plasma soluble intercellular adhesion molecule-1 and endothelin-1 concentration in patients with chronic congestive heart failure. *Am J Cardiol.* 1995;76:803–808.
68. Krum H, Goldsmith R, Wilshire-Clement M, et al. Role of endothelin in the exercise intolerance of chronic heart failure. *Am J Cardiol.* 1995;75:1282–1283.
69. Omland T, Lie RT, Aakvaag A, et al. Plasma endothelin determination as a prognostic indicator of 1-year mortality after acute myocardial infarction. *Circulation.* 1994;89:1573–1579.
70. Pousset F, Isnard R, Lechat P, et al. Prognostic value of plasma endothelin-1 in patients with chronic heart failure. *Eur Heart J.* 1997;18:254–258.
71. Hulsmann M, Stanek B, Frey B, et al. Value of cardiopulmonary exercise testing and big endothelin plasma levels to predict short-term prognosis of patients with chronic heart failure. *J Am Coll Cardiol.* 1998;32:1695–1700.
72. Frey B, Pacher R, Locker G, et al. Prognostic value of hemodynamic vs big endothelin measurements during long-term IV therapy in advanced heart failure patients. *Chest.* 2000;117: 1713–1719.
73. Stanek B, Frey B, Hulsmann M, et al. Validation of big endothelin plasma levels compared with established neurohumoral markers in patients with severe chronic heart failure. *Transplant Proc.* 1997;29:595–596.
74. Sakai S, Miyauchi T, Kobayashi M, et al. Inhibition of myocardial endothelin pathway improves long-term survival in heart failure. *Nature.* 1996;384:353–355.
75. Spinale FG, Walker JD, Mukherjee R, et al. Concomitant endothelin receptor subtype-A blockade during the progression of pacing-induced congestive heart failure in rabbits. Beneficial effects on left ventricular and myocyte function. *Circulation* 1997;95:1918–1929.
76. Borgeson DD, Grantham JA, Williamson EE, et al. Chronic oral endothelin type A receptor antagonism in experimental heart failure. *Hypertension.* 1998;31:766–770.
77. Moe GW, Albernaz A, Naik GO, et al. Beneficial effects of long-term selective endothelin type A receptor blockade in canine experimental heart failure. *Cardiovasc Res.* 1998;39:571–579.
78. Fraccarollo D, Hu K, Galuppo P, et al. Chronic endothelin receptor blockade attenuates progressive ventricular dilation and improves cardiac function in rats with myocardial infarction: possible involvement of myocardial endothelin system in ventricular remodeling. *Circulation.* 1997;96:3963–3973.
79. Mishima T, Tanimura M, Suzuki G, et al. Effects of long-term therapy with bosentan on the progression of left ventricular dysfunction and remodeling in dogs with heart failure. *J Am Coll Cardiol.* 2000;35:222–229.
80. Clozel M, Qiu C, Qiu CS, et al. Short-term endothelin receptor blockade with tezosentan has both immediate and long-term beneficial effects in rats with myocardial infarction. *J Am Coll Cardiol.* 2002;39:142–147.
81. Mulder P, Richard V, Derumeaux G, et al. Role of endogenous endothelin in chronic heart failure: effect of long-term treatment with an endothelin antagonist on survival, hemodynamics, and cardiac remodeling. *Circulation.* 1997;96:1976–1982.
82. Nguyen QT, Cernacek P, Calderoni A, et al. Endothelin A receptor blockade causes adverse left ventricular remodeling but improves pulmonary artery pressure after infarction in the rat. *Circulation.* 1998;98:2323–2330.
83. Schirger JA, Chen HH, Jougasaki M, et al. Endothelin A receptor antagonism in experimental congestive heart failure results in augmentation of the renin-angiotensin system and sustained sodium retention. *Circulation.* 2004;109:249–254.
84. Cowburn PJ, Cleland JG, McArthur JD, et al. Pulmonary and systemic responses to exogenous endothelin-1 in patients with left ventricular dysfunction. *J Cardiovasc Pharmacol.* 1998;31(Suppl 1): S290–S293.
85. Krum H, Gu A, Wilshire-Clement M, et al. Changes in plasma endothelin-1 levels reflect clinical response to beta-blockade in chronic heart failure. *Am Heart J.* 1996;131:337–341.
86. Galatius-Jensen S, Wroblewski H, Emmeluth C, et al. Plasma endothelin in congestive heart failure: effect of the ACE inhibitor, fosinopril. *Cardiovasc Res.* 1996;32:1148–1154.
87. Davidson NC, Coutie WJ, Webb DJ, et al. Hormonal and renal differences between low dose and high dose angiotensin converting enzyme inhibitor treatment in patients with chronic heart failure. *Heart.* 1996;75:576–581.
88. Sutsch G, Kiowski W, Yan XW, et al. Short-term oral endothelin-receptor antagonist therapy in conventionally treated patients with symptomatic severe chronic heart failure. *Circulation.* 1998;98:2262–2268.
89. Sutsch G, Bertel O, Kiowski W. Acute and short-term effects of the nonpeptide endothelin-1 receptor antagonist bosentan in humans. *Cardiovasc Drugs Ther.* 1997;10:717–725.
90. Torre-Amione G, Young JB, Durand J, et al. Hemodynamic effects of tezosentan, an intravenous dual endothelin receptor antagonist, in patients with class III to IV congestive heart failure. *Circulation.* 2001;103:973–980.
91. Torre-Amione G, Young JB, Colucci WS, et al. Hemodynamic and clinical effects of tezosentan, an intravenous dual endothelin receptor antagonist, in patients hospitalized for acute decompensated heart failure. *J Am Coll Cardiol.* 2003;42: 140–147.
92. Cotter G, Kiowski W, Kaluski E, et al. Tezosentan (an intravenous endothelin receptor A/B antagonist) reduces peripheral resistance and increases cardiac power therefore preventing a steep decrease in blood pressure in patients with congestive heart failure. *Eur J Heart Fail.* 2001;3:457–461.
93. Schalcher C, Cotter G, Reisin L, et al. The dual endothelin receptor antagonist tezosentan acutely improves hemodynamic parameters in patients with advanced heart failure. *Am Heart J.* 2001;142:340–349.
94. Louis A, Cleland JG, Crabbe S, et al. Clinical trials update: CAPRICORN, COPERNICUS, MIRACLE, STAF, RITZ-2, RECOVER and RENAISSANCE and cachexia and cholesterol in heart failure. Highlights of the Scientific Sessions of the American College of Cardiology, 2001. *Eur J Heart Fail.* 2001;3:381–387.
95. Torre-Amione G, Durand JB, Nagueh S, et al. A pilot safety trial of prolonged (48 h) infusion of the dual endothelin-receptor antagonist tezosentan in patients with advanced heart failure. *Chest* 2001;120:460–466.
96. Luscher TF, Enseleit F, Pacher R, et al. Hemodynamic and neurohumoral effects of selective endothelin A (ET(A)) receptor blockade in chronic heart failure: the Heart Failure ET(A) Receptor Blockade Trial (HEAT). *Circulation.* 2002;106:2666–2672.

97. Philipp S, Monti J, Pagel I, et al. Treatment with darusentan over 21 days improved cGMP generation in patients with chronic heart failure. *Clin Sci.* (Lond) 2002;103(Suppl 48):249S–53S.
98. Givertz MM, Colucci WS, LeJemtel TH, et al. Acute endothelin A receptor blockade causes selective pulmonary vasodilation in patients with chronic heart failure. *Circulation.* 2000;101: 2922–2927.
99. Cowburn PJ, Cleland JG, McArthur JD, et al. Short-term haemodynamic effects of BQ-123, a selective endothelin ET(A)-receptor antagonist, in chronic heart failure. *Lancet.* 1998;352: 201–202.
100. Wenzel RR, Fleisch M, Shaw S, et al. Hemodynamic and coronary effects of the endothelin antagonist bosentan in patients with coronary artery disease. *Circulation.* 1998;98:2235–2240.
101. Coletta AP, Cleland JG. Clinical trials update: highlights of the scientific sessions of the XXIII Congress of the European Society of Cardiology: WARIS II, ESCAMI, PAFAC, RITZ-1 and TIME. *Eur J Heart Fail.* 2001;3:747–750.
102. Cotter G, Kaluski E, Stangl K, et al. The hemodynamic and neurohormonal effects of low doses of tezosentan (an endothelin A/B receptor antagonist) in patients with acute heart failure. *Eur J Heart Fail.* 2004;6:601–609.
103. McMurray JJ. Results from late breaking clinical trials sessions at the American College of Cardiology 54th Annual Scientific Session [abstract]. *J Am Coll Cardiol.* 2005;45.
104. Kalra PR, Moon JC, Coats AJ. Do results of the ENABLE (Endothelin Antagonist Bosentan for Lowering Cardiac Events in Heart Failure) study spell the end for non-selective endothelin antagonism in heart failure? *Int J Cardiol.* 2002;85:195–197.
105. Packer M, McMurray J, Massie BM, et al. Clinical effects of endothelin receptor antagonism with bosentan in patients with severe chronic heart failure: results of a pilot study. *J Card Fail.* 2005;11:12–20.
106. Cosenzi A. Enrasentan, an antagonist of endothelin receptors. *Cardiovasc Drug Rev.* 2003;21:1–16.
107. Anand I, McMurray J, Cohn JN, et al. Long-term effects of darusentan on left-ventricular remodelling and clinical outcomes in the EndothelinA Receptor Antagonist Trial in Heart Failure (EARTH): randomised, double-blind, placebo-controlled trial. *Lancet.* 2004;364:347–354.
108. Dickstein K, De Voogd HJ, Miric MP, et al. Effect of single doses of SLV306, an inhibitor of both neutral endopeptidase and endothelin-converting enzyme, on pulmonary pressures in congestive heart failure. *Am J Cardiol.* 2004;94:237–239.
109. Tschope C, Gohlke P, Zhu YZ, et al. Antihypertensive and cardioprotective effects after angiotensin-converting enzyme inhibition: role of kinins. *J Card Fail.* 1997;3:133–148.
110. Campbell DJ. Vasopeptidase inhibition: a double-edged sword? *Hypertension.* 2003;41:383–389.
111. Rademaker MT, Charles CJ, Espiner EA, et al. Neutral endopeptidase inhibition: augmented atrial and brain natriuretic peptide, haemodynamic and natriuretic responses in ovine heart failure. *Clin Sci.* (Lond) 1996;91:283–291.
112. Seymour AA, Asaad MM, Lanoce VM, et al. Inhibition of neutral endopeptidase 3.4.24.11 in conscious dogs with pacing induced heart failure. *Cardiovasc Res.* 1993;27:1015–1023.
113. Trippodo NC, Fox M, Monticello TM, et al. Vasopeptidase inhibition with omapatrilat improves cardiac geometry and survival in cardiomyopathic hamsters more than does ACE inhibition with captopril. *J Cardiovasc Pharmacol.* 1999;34:782–790.
114. Chen HH, Lainchbury JG, Matsuda Y, et al. Endogenous natriuretic peptides participate in renal and humoral actions of acute vasopeptidase inhibition in experimental mild heart failure. *Hypertension.* 2001;38:187–191.
115. Corti R, Burnett JC, Jr., Rouleau JL, et al. Vasopeptidase inhibitors: a new therapeutic concept in cardiovascular disease? *Circulation.* 2001;104:1856–1862.
116. Ando S, Rahman MA, Butler GC, et al. Comparison of candoxatril and atrial natriuretic factor in healthy men. Effects on hemodynamics, sympathetic activity, heart rate variability, and endothelin. *Hypertension.* 1995;26:1160–1166.
117. Ferro CJ, Spratt JC, Haynes WG, et al. Inhibition of neutral endopeptidase causes vasoconstriction of human resistance vessels in vivo. *Circulation.* 1998;97:2323–2330.
118. McClean DR, Ikram H, Garlick AH, et al. The clinical, cardiac, renal, arterial and neurohormonal effects of omapatrilat, a vasopeptidase inhibitor, in patients with chronic heart failure. *J Am Coll Cardiol.* 2000;36:479–486.
119. Ikram H, Chan W, Espiner EA, et al. Haemodynamic and hormone responses to acute and chronic furosemide therapy in congestive heart failure. *Clin Sci.* (Lond) 1980;59(6):443–449.
120. Rouleau JL, Pfeffer MA, Stewart DJ, et al. Comparison of vasopeptidase inhibitor, omapatrilat, and lisinopril on exercise tolerance and morbidity in patients with heart failure: IMPRESS randomised trial. *Lancet.* 2000;356:615–620.
121. Packer M, Califf RM, Konstam MA, et al. Comparison of omapatrilat and enalapril in patients with chronic heart failure: the Omapatrilat Versus Enalapril Randomized Trial of Utility in Reducing Events (OVERTURE). *Circulation.* 2002;106:920–926.
122. Armstrong PW, Lorell BH, Nissen S, et al. Omapatrilat. *Circulation.* 2002;106:e9011–e9012.
123. Armstrong PW, Lorell BH, Nissen S, Borer J. Candesartan. [News] *Circulation.* 2002;106(6):e9011–9012.

Cytokines as Mediators of Disease Progression in the Failing Heart

13

Douglas L. Mann

Since the original description of inflammatory cytokines in patients with heart failure in 1990 (1), there has been a growing interest in the role that these molecules play in regulating cardiac structure and function, particularly with regard to their potential role in disease progression in heart failure. The growing appreciation of the pathophysiological consequences of sustained expression of proinflammatory mediators in preclinical and clinical heart failure models culminated in a series of multicenter clinical trials that utilized targeted approaches to neutralize tumor necrosis factor (TNF) in patients with moderate to advanced heart failure. However, these targeted approaches appear to have resulted in worsening heart failure (2), thereby raising a number of important questions about what role, if any, proinflammatory cytokines play in the pathogenesis of heart failure. To this end, in the present review we will summarize the tremendous growth of knowledge that has taken place in this field since 1990, with an emphasis on discussing the adaptive and maladaptive effects of cytokine signaling in the heart, as well as discuss what we have learned from the negative clinical trials that have used targeted anticytokine approaches in heart failure.

THE BIOLOGY OF PROINFLAMMATORY (STRESS-ACTIVATED) CYTOKINES AND THEIR RECEPTORS

The term cytokine is applied to a group of relatively low–molecular-weight protein molecules (generally 15 to 30 Kda) that are secreted by cells in response to a variety of different inducing stimuli. Although cytokines are similar to polypetide hormones in many respects, cytokines can be produced by a variety of different cell types in a number of different tissues, as opposed to being produced by a specific cell type in a specific organ, as is the case for polypeptide hormones. Whereas proinflammatory cytokines have traditionally been thought to be produced by the immune system, one of the more recent intriguing observations is that virtually all nucleated cell types within the myocardium, including cardiac myocytes themselves, are capable of synthesizing a portfolio of proinflammatory cytokines in response to various forms of cardiac injury (Table 13-1). Thus, from a conceptual standpoint, these molecules should be envisioned as proteins that are produced locally within the myocardium by cardiocytes (i.e., cells that reside within the myocardium), in response to one or more different forms of environmental stress. An important corollary of this statement is that the expression of these stress-activated cytokines can occur in the complete absence of activation of the immune system. The biological properties of several important proinflammatory cytokines, including TNF, members of the interleukin-1 (IL-1) family as well as the interleukin-6 (IL-6) family of cytokines, have been reviewed recently and will not be discussed further herein (3).

ADAPTIVE EFFECTS OF PROINFLAMMATORY CYTOKINE SIGNALING IN THE HEART

Although the exact role proinflammatory cytokines play in the heart is not known with certainty, two important themes have emerged from recent studies of proinflammatory

TABLE 13-1
CARDIAC PATHOPHYSIOLOGICAL CONDITIONS ASSOCIATED WITH ACTIVATION OF INFLAMMATORY MEDIATORS

Acute viral myocarditis
Cardiac allograft rejection
Myocardial infarction
Unstable angina
Myocardial reperfusion injury
Hypertrophic cardiomyopathy*
Heart failure*
Cardiopulmonary bypass*
Magnesium deficiency*
Pressure overload*

*Indicates conditions not traditionally associated with immunologically mediated inflammation.

cytokine gene regulation in the heart. One consistent theme is that proinflammatory cytokines are not expressed constitutively in the heart (4,5). The second theme is that these molecules are consistently and rapidly expressed in response to a variety of different forms of myocardial injury (Table 13-1). The observation that proinflammatory cytokine gene expression is not coupled to a specific form of cardiac injury, but is instead observed in *all* forms of cardiac injury, suggests that these molecules constitute part of an intrinsic or innate stress response system in the heart. Thus, analogous to the role that proinflammatory cytokines play as effector molecules in the innate immune system, which is intended to act as an early warning system that allows the host to rapidly discriminate self from nonself (6), the expression of proinflammatory cytokines in the heart may permit the myocardium to rapidly respond to tissue injury as part of an early warning system that coordinates and integrates a panoply of homeostatic responses within the heart following tissue injury.

As will be discussed later, there is a now growing body of evidence that supports the point of view that short-term expression of proinflammatory cytokines is beneficial in the heart. However, it bears emphasizing that the family of proinflammatory molecules that comprise this innate stress response system are phylogenetically ancient, and are thus likely evolved in organisms with relatively short life spans (weeks to months). Thus, activation of the innate stress response system was never intended to provide long-term adaptive responses to the host organism. As will be discussed toward the end of this review, sustained and/or dysregulated expression of proinflammatory cytokines is sufficient to produce tissue injury and provoke overt cardiac decompensation.

The first line of evidence in support of a beneficial role for cytokines in the heart is implicit in phylogenetic studies of so-called primitive cytokines, such as TNF and IL-1. TNF and IL-1-like activity has been identified in both protostome vertebrates (annelids) and deuterostome invertebrates (echinoderms) (7,8), suggesting that these molecules came into existence during the onset of the Cambrian period, before the split of the major animal phyla into vertebrate and invertebrate species. The evolutionary development of cytokines was probably necessary for the development of large, multicellular organisms that required intercellular messengers such as cytokines to coordinate complex biological cellular responses. The observation that primitive cytokines such as TNF and IL-1 have been conserved by nature throughout the animal kingdom for nearly 600,000 million years, coupled with the observation that these same cytokines are expressed in virtually all forms of cardiac injury (Table 13-2), suggests that these molecules may in some way confer a survival benefit in the host organism. Nonetheless, this argument is based on teleological evidence and must therefore be regarded as indirect proof in support of the point of view that cytokines confer beneficial responses in the heart.

The second line of evidence in support of a beneficial role for proinflammatory cytokines in the heart comes from a series of gain of function studies that have shown that proinflammatory cytokines confer cytoprotective responses in the heart. The first study to demonstrate the potential beneficial effects of cytokines showed that pretreating rats with TNF protected the heart from ischemic reperfusion injury ex vivo (9). Following ischemia reperfusion injury the hearts from TNF-pretreated animals had a threefold reduction in the amount of lactate dehydrogenase release (9), and showed an increase in the percent of recovery of developed left ventricular pressure when compared to control hearts (10). IL-1 has also been shown to protect rat hearts against ischemia reperfusion injury in vitro (11). Subsequent in vitro studies have demonstrated that physiological levels of TNF are sufficient to protect cardiac myocytes against either hypoxic or ischemic injury, respectively (12). Moreover, the cytoprotective effects of TNF could be mimicked by stimulating either the type 1 (p55, TNFR1) or the type 2 (p75, TNFR2) receptor, suggesting that the cytoprotective effects of TNF are mediated by activation of TNFR1 or TNFR2.

Although these studies did not clearly identify the mechanism for these findings, proinflammatory cytokines are known to upregulate the expression of at least two sets of protective proteins in the heart: the free radical scavenger manganese-superoxide dismutase (MnSOD) (9,13) and the cytoprotective heat shock proteins (HSPs) (14,15). Relevant to this discussion is the finding that TNF-induced MnSOD induction is very rapid (<1 hour) and requires very low levels of TNF (0.1 ng/mL^{-1}), consistent with the proposed homeostatic role for these proteins (13). Given

TABLE 13-2
DELETERIOUS EFFECTS OF INFLAMMATORY MEDIATORS IN HEART FAILURE

Left ventricular dysfunction
Pulmonary edema in humans
Cardiomyopathy in humans
Reduced skeletal muscle blood flow
Endothelial dysfunction
Anorexia and cachexia
Receptor uncoupling from adenylate cyclase experimentally
Activation of the fetal gene program experimentally
Cardiac myocyte apoptosis experimentally

that contracting myocardial cells are continually susceptible to oxygen-derived free radicals, TNF and IL-1 may play important roles in protecting the heart against oxidative stress, particularly during ischemia and reperfusion injury. TNF has also been shown recently to upregulate the expression of heat shock protein 72 (HSP 72) (14), a protein that is thought to protect the heart against ischemia reperfusion injury (16,17).

Finally, proinflammatory cytokines such as TNF and IL-1β have been shown to activate the transcription factor nuclear factor-kappa B (NF-κB), which has been shown to be cytoprotective under certain circumstances, presumably through upregulation of one or more cytoprotective genes, including MnSOD, the cellular inhibitors of apoptosis 1 and 2 (c-IAP1 and cIAP2), and the members of the Bcl-2 family, including Bcl-2, Bcl-1 and Bcl-xL (18–22).

Similar findings have been obtained in gain of function studies for the so-called IL-6 family of cytokines, that include interleukin-6 (IL-6), leukemia inhibitory factor (LIF), cardiotrophin-1 (CT-1), ciliary neurotrophic factor (CNTF), interleukin-11 (IL-11), and oncostatin M (OSM). This family of cytokines triggers downstream signaling pathways in multiple cell types, including cardiac myocytes, either through the homodimerization of the gp130 receptor or through the heterodimerization of gp130 with a related transmembrane receptor. Studies with CT-1 have shown that CT-1 blunts serum deprivation-induced apoptosis in isolated neonatal cardiac myocytes through a pathway that was dependent on activation of the mitogen-activated protein kinase (MAPK). In these studies, transfection of an MAP kinase kinase 1 (MEK1)–dominant negative-mutant cDNA into myocardial cells or treatment with a MEK-specific inhibitor (PD098059) blocked the antiapoptotic effects of CT-1, indicating a requirement of the MAP kinase pathway for the survival effect of CT-1. Similarly, studies have shown that LIF confers cytoprotective responses in isolated myocytes, as well as in intact myocardial tissue (10,23). However, the mechanisms for LIF-mediated cytoprotective effects appear to be more complex than those reported for CT-1. Although studies in isolated neonatal myocytes suggest an important role for the Janus kinase (JAK) and the signal transducer and activator of transcription (STAT)-mediated signaling pathways (23), more recent studies in adult myocytes suggest that the cytoprotective effects of LIF are mediated through activation of the MAPK pathway, consistent with what has been reported for CT-1. One explanation for these apparent differences in the cytoprotective mechanisms for LIF is that there may be functionally significant cross-talk between the MAPK and the JAK/STAT pathways, as has been suggested recently (23). Thus, the cytoprotective signaling pathways that are downstream from gp130-mediated signaling may involve both JAK/STAT- and MAPK-mediated signaling pathways.

The third, and perhaps most striking line of evidence in support of a beneficial role for proinflammatory cytokines in the heart comes from a series of loss of function studies in mice deficient in proinflammatory cytokine receptor-mediated signaling. Mice with targeted disruption of gp130 have been developed recently (24). Mice homozygous for the gp130 knockout (gp130$^{-/-}$) died between 12.5 days postcoitum and term. The ventricular myocardium in these mice developed normally until 14.5 days postcoitum; however, beyond 16.5 days postcoitum the gp130$^{-/-}$ mice demonstrated a markedly hypoplastic ventricle, with an abnormally thin ventricular wall that had a minimum thickness of one cell. Studies employing mice that harbor a ventricular restricted knockout of the gp130 cytokine receptor via Cre- LoxP-mediated recombination showed that these mice have normal embryonic viability and no evidence of cardiac morphological abnormalities that were observed in the gp130 knockout (gp130$^{-/-}$) (25). Moreover, these mice had normal cardiac structure (Fig. 13-1B) and function under basal conditions. Thus, the most likely explanation for the findings in the gp130$^{-/-}$ mice is that the cardiac developmental defects and embryonic lethality in these mice were the result of hematopoietic abnormalities and associated oxygen deprivation, as opposed to a primary gp130-mediated defect in myocytes. Interestingly, mice harboring the ventricular restricted knockout of the gp130 cytokine receptor demonstrated a critical role for a gp130-dependent myocyte survival pathway following aortic banding (25). That is, following hemodynamic overloading by transaortic constriction, these mice displayed a decrease in survival (Fig. 13-1A), ventriclar enlargement involving both the right and left ventricular chambers (Fig. 13-1B), and a striking increase in the prevalence of cardiac myocyte apoptosis when compared to control mice that exhibited normal compensatory cardiac hypertrophy (25). These studies suggest that the gp130 pathway is an essential stress-activated myocyte survival pathway.

More recently, studies in mice that are doubly deficient for the type 1 and type 2 TNF receptors (TNFR1$^{-/-}$/TNFR2$^{-/-}$) have been shown to have an increase in infarct size in response to ischemic injury (26). However, unlike gp130 mice, TNFR1$^{-/-}$/TNFR2$^{-/-}$ mice displayed a normal cardiac phenotype under nonstressed conditions. However, following acute coronary artery ligation there was a striking increase in infarct size in TNFR1$^{-/-}$/TNFR2$^{-/-}$ mice (Fig. 13-2A) compared to littermate controls (Fig. 13-2B). As shown by the group data summarized in Figure 13-2C, infarct size was the same in wild-type, TNFR1$^{-/-}$/TNFR2$^{-/-}$ mice; however, infarct size was 40% greater in the TNFR1$^{-/-}$/ TNFR2$^{-/-}$ mice. Interestingly, the increase in infarct size in the TNFR1$^{-/-}$ /TNFR2$^{-/-}$ mice was shown to be secondary to accelerated apoptosis in the TNFR1$^{-/-}$/TNFR2$^{-/-}$ mice, as opposed to increased myocyte necrosis. Although this study did not identify the biological mechanisms that were responsible for the cytoprotective effects of TNF, the observation that deletion of both TNFR1 and TNFR2 was necessary to provoke increased tissue injury suggested that TNFR1 and TNFR2 activated redundant cytoprotective signaling pathways in the heart. Although the complete portfolio of cytoprotective signaling pathways that are common to both TNFR1 and TNFR2 is not known, it is interesting to note that NF-κB activation is common to both TNF receptors (27).

As previously noted, NF-κB activation has been shown to be cytoprotective in certain settings. Thus, taken together, the gain of function and loss of function studies for gp130- and TNF-mediated signaling described in this section suggest that proinflammatory cytokines may play an important role in the orchestration and timing of the myocardial stress response, by providing early antiapop-

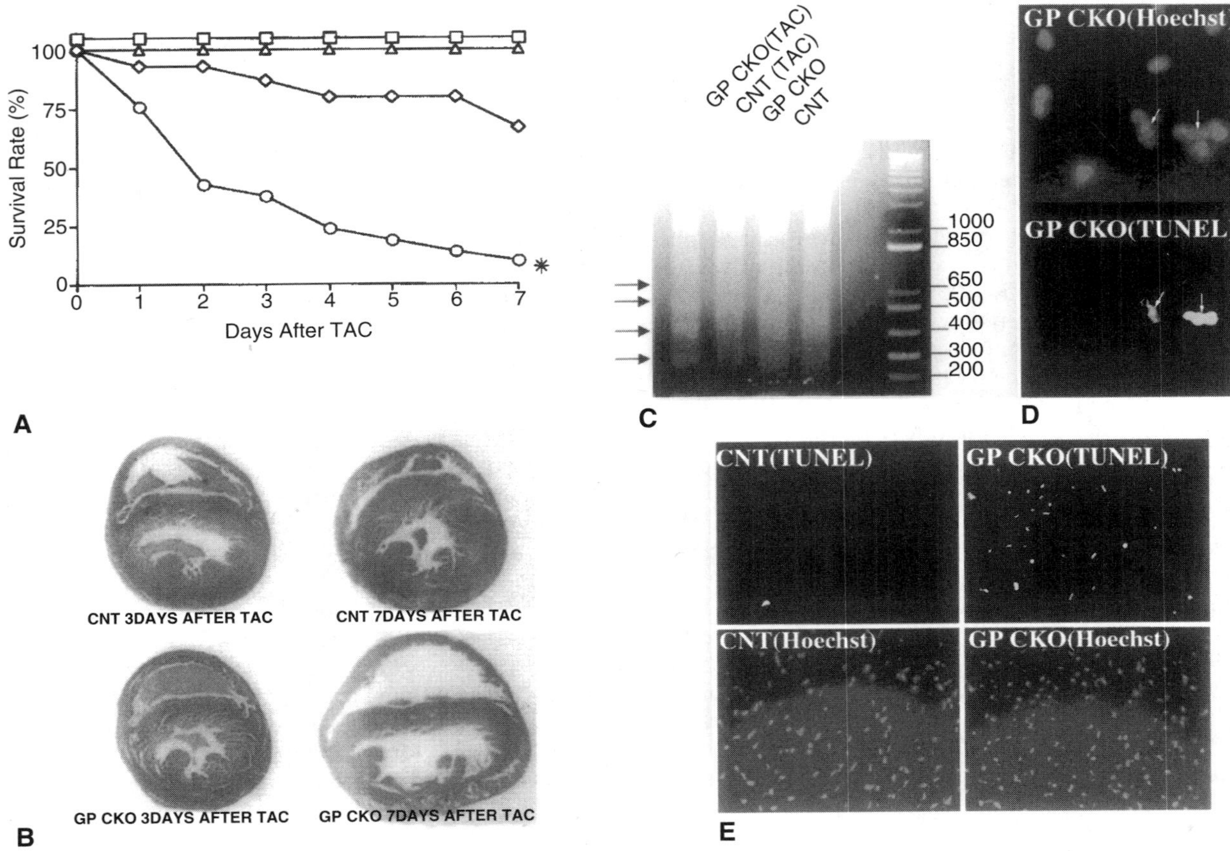

Figure 13-1 Effect of hemodynamic overload in mice with a ventricular restricted knockout of the gp130 signaling pathway. **(A)** Analysis of survival of gp130 conditional knockout mice after transaortic constriction (TAC). Control mice (CNT) mice were subjected to a sham operation (squares) or transaortic constriction (diamonds). Mice with conditional ventricular restricted knockout of the gp130 signaling pathway (CKO) were subjected to a sham operation (triangles) or transaortic constriction (circles). Differences in survival rates between the CNT and gp130 conditional knockout mice after TAC were significant by the Peto-Peto-Wilcoxon test (* = $p < 0.001$). **(B)** Pathological analysis of the gp130 conditional knockout mice hearts. Histological sections of hearts from 3 days and 7 days after transaortic constriction were found in wild-type and gp130 conditional knockout mice. Histological examination of the hearts demonstrated ventriclar enlargement involving both the right and left ventricular chambers in the gp130 conditional knockout mice. **(C)** A DNA laddering assay (TUNEL) revealed evidence of increased apoptosis in the gp130 conditional knockout mice after **(D)** low-power (100×) and **(E)** high-power (1,000×) images showing DNA labeling visualized by fluoresence (green) and counterstained with Hoechst dye (blue). In agreement with the DNA laddering assay, there was significant increase in apoptotic cells in the hearts from the gp130 conditional knockout mice after transaortic constriction, with apoptotic indices of 34% ± 11% in gp130 conditional knockout mice after transaortic constriction versus 3% ± 0.5% in control mice following transaortic constriction ($p < 0.05$). (Modified from Hirota H, Chen J, Betz UA, et al. Loss of a gp130 cardiac muscle cell survival pathway is a critical event in the onset of heart failure during biomechanical stress. *Cell*. 1999;97:189–198, with permission.)

totic cytoprotective signals that are responsible for delimiting tissue injury, as well as providing delayed signals that facilitate tissue repair and/or tissue remodeling once myocardial tissue damage has supervened. In keeping with this latter point of view, previous studies have shown that CT-1, LIF, and TNF are all sufficient to provoke modest hypertrophic growth response in cardiac myocytes (28) and that TNF is sufficient to lead to degradation and remodeling of the extracellular matrix in the heart (29).

MALADAPTIVE EFFECTS OF CYTOKINE SIGNALING IN THE HEART

The interest in understanding the role of inflammatory mediators in a variety of cardiac disease states, including heart failure, arises from the observation that many aspects of the syndrome of heart failure can be explained by the known biological effects of proinflammatory cytokines (Table 13-2). When expressed at sufficiently high concen-

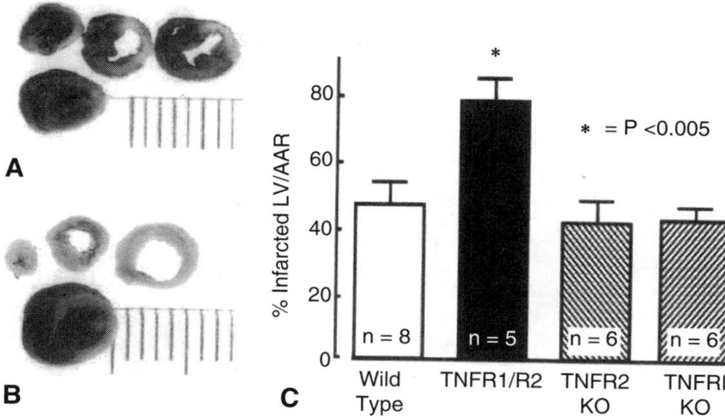

Figure 13-2 Effect of acute coronary artery ligation in TNFR1/TNFR2 knockout mice. The triphenyltetrazolium chloride (TTC) staining deficit, a marker of infarct size, was significantly greater in mice lacking both TNF receptors **(B)** when compared to littermate control mice **(A)**. The results of group data show that the TTC staining deficit was similar in wild-type mice and mice lacking either the type 1 or type 2 TNF receptors; however, there was a 40% increase in infarct size in the mice lacking both TNF receptors **(C)**. TNFR1/TNFR2 KO, TNFR1/TNFR2 knockout mice; TNFR1 KO, TNFR1 knockout mice; TNFR2 KO, TNFR2 knockout mice). (Modified from Kurrelmeyer K, Michael L, Baumgarten G, et al. Endogenous myocardial tumor necrosis factor protects the adult cardiac myocyte against ischemic-induced apoptosis in a murine model of acute myocardial infarction. *Proc Natl Acad Sci USA.* 2000;290:5456–5461.)

trations, such as those that are observed in heart failure, cytokines are sufficient to mimic some aspects of the so-called heart failure phenotype, including (but not limited to) progressive left ventricular (LV) dysfunction, pulmonary edema, LV remodeling, fetal gene expression, and cardiomyopathy (29–31). Thus, the cytokine hypothesis (32) for heart failure holds that heart failure progresses, at least in part, as a result of the toxic effects exerted by endogenous cytokine cascades on the heart and the peripheral circulation. It should be emphasized that the cytokine hypothesis does not imply that cytokines cause heart failure per se but, rather, that the overexpression of cytokine cascades contributes to disease progression of heart failure. Thus, the elaboration of cytokines, much like the elaboration of neurohormones, may represent a biological mechanism that is responsible for worsening heart failure. Although the deleterious effects of cytokines on myocardial function have received the most attention thus far, cytokines may also produce deleterious effects on LV structure (remodeling) and endothelial function. Accordingly, in the following section, the studies that form the scientific basis for studying the role of proinflammatory mediators in the failing heart will be discussed.

Effects of Cytokines on Left Ventricular Function

The negative inotropic effects of TNF have been observed in studies in which rats were infused with pathophysiologically levels of TNF, as well as in transgenic mice with targeted overexpression of TNF (29,33,34). Franco et al. used cinemagnetic resonance imaging to demonstrate that there was a significant increase in LV volume and a significant decrease in LV ejection fraction over time in transgenic mice with targeted overexpression of TNF (33). Importantly, these effects were shown to be dependent upon gene dosage. That is, when the line of transgenic mice with high TNF expression (lineage 1) was compared to a transgenic line with lower myocardial TNF expression (lineage 2), there was a significantly greater increase in LV volume (Fig. 13-3A) and a significantly greater decrease in LV ejection fraction (Fig. 13-3B) in the transgenic mouse lines with higher TNF expression (33).

In studies from our laboratory, we measured LV function in line of transgenic mice with targeted overexpression of TNF (34) using Millar catheters. The animals were paced from the atrium to a heart rate at which *dP/dt* was maximal, as defined by examination of the force–frequency curves for each animal, and peak positive and negative *dP/dt* were assessed for TNF transgenic mice and littermate controls. As shown in Figure 13-3C, there was significant decrease in peak +*dP/dt* and peak –*dP/dt* in the TNF transgenic mice, consistent with the findings reported by Franco et al. (33). Experimental studies in rats have shown that circulating concentrations of TNF that overlap those observed in patients with heart failure are sufficient to produce persistent negative inotropic effects that are detectable at the level of the cardiac myocyte; moreover, the negative inotropic effects of TNF were completely reversible when the TNF infusion was stopped (29). Subsequent studies in transgenic mice with targeted overexpression of TNF in the cardiac compartment have shown that forced overexpression of TNF results in depressed LV ejection performance and that the depressed LV ejection performance was dependent on TNF gene dosage (31,33).

With respect to the potential mechanisms for the deleterious effects of TNF on LV function, the literature suggests that TNF modulates myocardial function through at least two different pathways: an immediate pathway that is manifest within minutes and is mediated by activation of the neutral sphingomyelinase pathway (35) and a delayed pathway that requires hours to days to develop and is mediated by nitric oxide (36,37). Recently, it has been suggested that TNF and IL-1 may produce negative inotropic effects *indirectly* through activation and/or release of IL-18, which is a recently described member of the IL-1 family of cytokines (38). Relevant to the present discussion is the observation that specific blockade of IL-18 using neutralizing IL-18 binding protein leads to an improvement in myocardial contractility in atrial tissue that was subjected ischemia reperfusion injury (39). Although the signaling pathways that are responsible for the IL-18-induced negative inotropic effects have not been delineated thus far, it is likely that they will overlap those for IL-1, given that the IL-18 receptor complex utilizes components of the IL-1 signaling chain, including IL-1R-activating kinase (IRAK) and TNFR-associated factor-6 (TRAF-6) (38). IL-6 has been shown to decrease cardiac contractility via a nitric oxide (NO)-dependent pathway that is secondary to IL-6-induced phosphorylation of signal transducer and activator of transcription 3 (STAT3). In this study, IL-6 enhanced

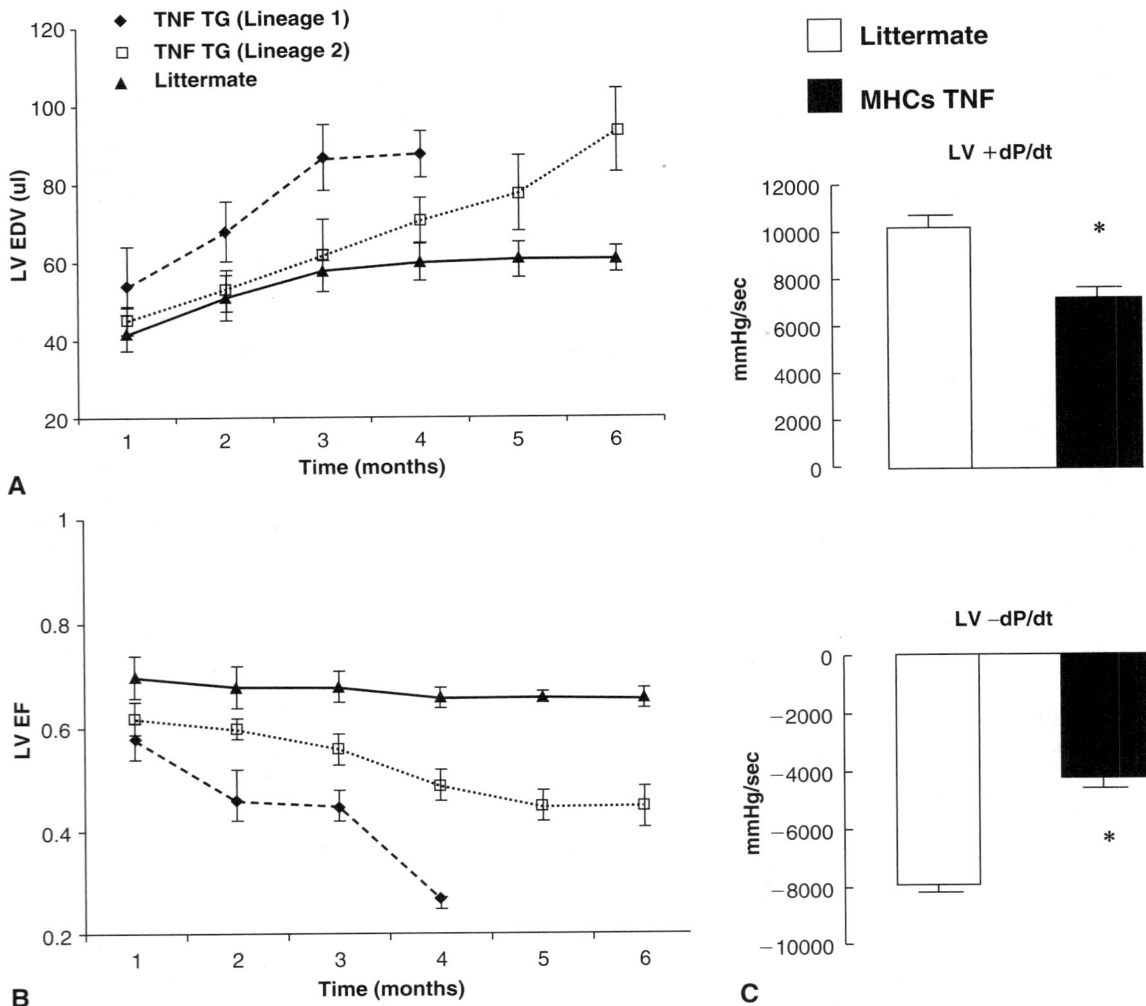

Figure 13-3 Effect of TNF on left ventricular function. LV volume and LV ejection fraction were serially examined by magnetic resonance imaging in two lines of transgenic mice (TNF TG) with high (lineage 1) and low (lineage 2) levels of myocardial TNF expression in comparison to age-matched, littermate control mice (33). **(A)** Serial changes in LV volume in transgenic mice and littermate control mice. **(B)** Serial changes in LV ejection fraction in transgenic mice and littemate control mice. **(C)** LV contractility in mice with targeted overexpression of TNF (MHCsTNF). (From Sivasubramanian N, Coker ML, Kurrelmeyer K, et al. Left ventricular remodeling in transgenic mice with cardiac restricted overexpression of tumor necrosis factor. *Circulation.* 2001;2001:826–831.) For these studies the animals were paced via the atrium to a heart rate at which positive *dP/dt* was maximal, as defined by examination of the force–frequency curves for each animal, and peak positive and negative *dP/dt* were assessed for MHCs TNF mice and littermate controls. (**A** and **B** were reproduced from Franco F, Thomas GD, Giroir BP, et al. Magnetic resonance imaging and invasive evaluation of development of heart failure in transgenic mice with myocardial expression of tumor necrosis factor-alpha. *Circulation.* 1999;99:448–454, and the American Heart Association, with permission.)

de novo synthesis of inducible nitric-oxide synthase (iNOS) protein, increased NO production, and decreased rat cardiac myocyte contractility after 2 hours of incubation. The effects of IL-6 on iNOS production and myocyte contractility were blocked by genistein at concentrations that were sufficient to block IL-6-induced activation of STAT3. Taken together, these observations suggest that IL-6 is sufficient to produce negative inotropic effects through STAT3-mediated activation of iNOS (40).

Effects of Proinflammatory Cytokines on Left Ventricular Remodeling

The term left ventricular remodeling has been used to describe the multitude of changes that occur in cardiac shape, size, and composition in response to myocardial injury. As shown in Table 13-3, inflammatory mediators have a number of important effects that may play an important role in the process of LV remodeling, including myocyte hypertro-

TABLE 13-3

EFFECTS OF INFLAMMATORY MEDIATORS ON LEFT VENTRICULAR REMODELING

Alterations in the biology of the myocyte
Myocyte hypertrophy
Contractile abnormalities
Fetal gene expression
Alteration in the extracellular matrix
MMP activation
Degradation of the matrix
Fibrosis
Progressive myocyte loss
Necrosis
Apoptosis

phy (28), alterations in fetal gene expression (30,31), as well as progressive myocyte loss through apoptosis (41).

In addition to these effects, there are several lines of evidence that suggest that TNF may promote LV remodeling through alterations in the extracellular matrix. First, when concentrations of TNF that overlap those observed in patients with heart failure are infused continuously in rats, there is a time-dependent change in LV dimension that is accompanied by progressive degradation of the extracelluar matrix. Moreover, similar findings have been reported following a single infusion of TNF in dogs (42). Second, recent studies in transgenic mice with targeted overexpression of TNF have shown that these mice develop progressive LV dilation. For example, Kubota et al. showed that a transgenic mouse line that overexpressed TNF in the cardiac compartment developed progressive LV dilatation over a 24-week period of observation (31). Similar findings have also been reported by Bryant et al. (43) and Sivasubramanian et al. (34), who observed identical findings with respect to LV dysfunction and LV dilation in transgenic mice with targeted overexpression of TNF in the heart. With respect to the mechanisms that are involved in TNF-induced LV dilation, it has been suggested that TNF-induced activation of matrix metalloproteinases (MMPs) is responsible for this effect (34,44).

As shown in Figures 13-4 and 13-5, respectively, there was progressive loss of fibrillar collagen and increased

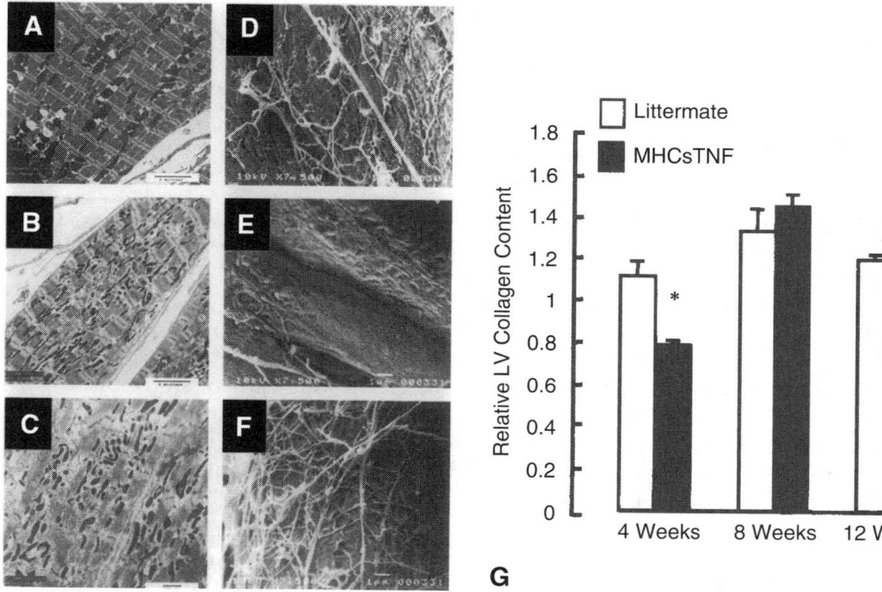

Figure 13-4 Effects of sustained proinflammatory cytokine expression on myocardial ultrastructure and collagen content. **A–C** show representative transmission electron micrographs in littermate controls **(A)** and the TNF transgenic mice at 4 weeks **(B)** and 8 weeks of age **(C)**. The transmission electron micrographs from the littermate control mice at 4 weeks **(A)** revealed a characteristic linear array of sarcomere and myofibril. In contrast, the myofibril in the 4-week-old TNF transgenic mice were less organized, with loss of sarcomeric registration observed in many of the sections **(B)**. The ultrastructural abnormalities in the TNF transgenic mice were further exaggerated in the 12-week-old TNF transgenic mice, which showed a significant loss of sarcomere registration and myofibril disarray **(C)**. **D–F** show representative scanning electron micrographs in littermate controls **(D)** and the TNF transgenic mice at 4 weeks **(E)** and 8 weeks of age **(F)**. **E** shows that there was a significant loss of fibrillar collagen in the TNF transgenic mice at 4 weeks of age when compared to age-matched, littermate controls **(D)**. However, as the TNF transgenic mice aged (12 weeks), there was an obvious increase in myocardial fibrillar collagen content. **G** illustrates the myocardial collagen content as determined by picrosirius red staining. There was a loss of myocardial collagen content at 4 weeks of age in the TNF transgenic mice, which was later followed by a progressive increase in myocardial collagen content at 8 and 12 weeks of age. (Reproduced from Sivasubramanian N, Coker ML, Kurrelmeyer K, et al. Left ventricular remodeling in transgenic mice with cardiac restricted overexpression of tumor necrosis factor. *Circulation*. 2001;2001: 826–831, and the American Heart Association, with permission.)

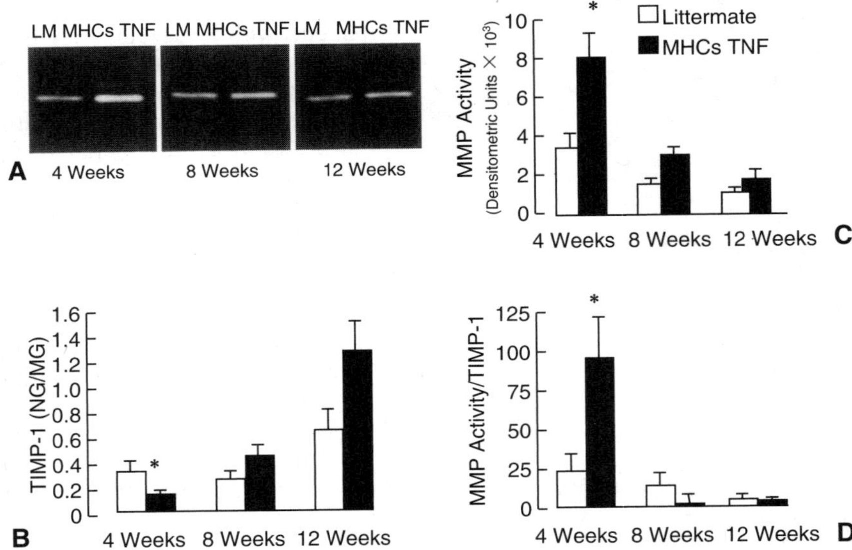

Figure 13-5 Effects of sustained proinflammatory cytokine expression on MMP activity and TIMP levels. **A** shows a zymogram of total MMP activity in the TNF transgenic mice (TNF-TG) and littermate (LM) control mice at 4, 8, and 12 weeks of age, whereas **B** summarizes the results of group data for total MMP zymographic activity. MMP activity was significantly ($p < 0.001$) greater in the TNF transgenic mice at 4 weeks of age; however, MMP activity was no different from littermate control mice at 8 and 12 weeks of age. **C** depicts the time-dependent changes in TIMP levels at 4, 8, and 12 weeks in the TNF transgenic and littermate control mice. At 4 weeks of age, TIMP-1 levels were significantly less in the TNF transgenic mice at 4 weeks of age; however, TIMP-1 levels increased progressively in the TNF transgenic mice from 8 to 12 weeks of age. **D** depicts the time-dependent changes in the ratio of MMP activity/TIMP levels in the TNF transgenic and littermate control mice. As shown, at 4 weeks of age the ratio of MMP activity/TIMP-1 levels was significantly greater in the TNF transgenic mice, thus favoring collagen degradation (Fig. 13-4D); however, the ratio of MMP activity/TIMP-1 decreased progressively from 8 to 12 weeks of age, thus favoring collagen accumulation (Fig. 13-4D). (Reproduced from Sivasubramanian N, Coker ML, Kurrelmeyer K, et al. Left ventricular remodeling in transgenic mice with cardiac restricted overexpression of tumor necrosis factor. *Circulation.* 2001;2001:826–831, and the American Heart Association, with permission.)

MMP activation in the hearts of the transgenic mice overexpressing TNF in the cardiac compartment. The dissolution of the fibrillar collagen weave that surrounds the individual cardiac myocytes and links the myocytes together would be expected to allow for rearrangement (slippage) of myofibrillar bundles within the ventricular wall (45). However, Figure 13-5 shows that long-term stimulation (i.e., 8 to 12 weeks) with TNF resulted in an increase in fibrillar collagen content that was accompanied by decreased MMP activity (Fig. 13-5) and increased expression of the tissue inhibitors of matrix metalloproteinases (TIMPs) (Fig. 13-5).

Taken together, these observations suggest that sustained myocardial inflammation provokes time-dependent changes in the balance between MMP activity and TIMP activity (i.e., during the early stages of inflammation there is an increase in the ratio of MMP activity to TIMP levels that fosters LV dilation). However, with chronic inflammatory signaling there is a time-dependent increase in TIMP levels, with a resultant decrease in the ratio of MMP activity to TIMP activity and a subsequent increase in myocardial fibrillar collagen content. Although the molecular mechanisms that are responsible for the transition between excessive degradation and excessive synthesis of the extracellular matrix are not known, studies in experimental models of chronic injury/inflammation in an array of different organs, including liver, lung, and kidney, wherein an initial increase in MMP expression is superseded by increased TIMP expression and increased expression of a number of fibrogenic cytokines, most notably TGF-β (46,47). Thus, excessive activation of proinflammatory cytokines may contribute to LV remodeling through a variety of different mechanisms that involve both the myocyte and nonmyocyte components of the myocardium.

INTERACTIONS BETWEEN THE RENIN ANGIOTENSIN SYSTEM AND PROINFLAMMATORY CYTOKINES IN ADVERSE CARDIAC REMODELING

Although neurohormonal and cytokine systems have been regarded as functionally distinct biological systems, recent studies suggest that these two systems can crossregulate each other, with the result that neurohormonal and cytokine systems may participate in positive feed-forward loops that contribute to adverse cardiac remodeling.

Angiotensin II was traditionally viewed as a circulating neurohormone that stimulated the constriction of vascular smooth muscle cells; aldosterone release from the adrenal gland; sodium reabsorption in the renal tubule, and/or growth of cardiac myocytes or fibroblasts (48). However, it is becoming increasingly apparent that angiotensin II provokes inflammatory responses in a variety of different cell and tissue types.

For example, angiotensin II activates the redox-sensitive transcription factor NF-κB (49) that is critical for initiating the coordinated expression of classical components of the myocardial inflammatory response, including increased expression of proinflammatory cytokines, nitric oxide, chemokines, and cell adhesion molecules (50,51). Pathophysiologically relevant concentrations of angiotensin II are sufficient to provoke TNF mRNA and protein synthesis in the adult heart through a NF-κB-dependent pathway (52). Figure 13-6 shows that treatment with angiotensin II resulted in a rapid increase in TNF mRNA (Fig. 13-6A) and protein synthesis (Fig. 13-6B) in isolated buffer perfused hearts. Stimulation of isolated adult cardiac myocytes with angiotensin II resulted in a threefold increase in TNF protein biosynthesis within 1 hour, and a 15-fold increase in TNF protein biosynthesis within 24 hours, suggesting that the increase in TNF biosynthesis in the intact heart was mediated, at least in part, at the level of the cardiac myocyte.

The effects of angiotensin II on TNF mRNA and protein synthesis were mediated exclusively through the angiotensin type 1 receptor, insofar as pretreatment with the angiotensin type 1 receptor antagonist losartan completely abolished the effects of angiotensin II on TNF biosynthesis. Conversely, pretreatment with the angiotensin type 2 receptor antagonist PD123319 had no effect on angiotensin II-induced TNF biosynthesis (Fig. 13-6B). This study further showed that the effects of angiotensin II on TNF myocardial biosynthesis were dependent upon protein kinase C (PKC)-mediated activation of NF-κB (52).

There is also increasing evidence that inflammatory mediators are capable of upregulating various components of the renin angiotensin system in a variety of mammalian tissues, including the heart. As one recent example, studies using transgenic mice with cardiac restricted overexpression of TNF have shown that targeted overexpression of TNF leads to an increase in angiotensin II peptide levels in the heart (53). This study serially examined several components of the renin angiotensin system, including angiotensinogen, renin, angiotensin converting enzyme (ACE), and angiotensin I and II peptide levels in a transgenic mouse line with cardiac restricted overexpression of TNF (MHCsTNF). There was a significant increase in ACE mRNA levels (Figs. 13-7AB) and ACE activity (Fig. 13-7C), as well as increased angiotensin II peptide levels (Fig. 13-7D) in the hearts of the MHCsTNF mice relative to littermate controls.

Significantly, the expression of renin and angiotensinogen was not increased in MHCsTNF mice compared with littermate controls. Thus, this study suggested that the increased levels of angiotensin II peptide levels in the MHCsTNF mice was principally the result of increased ACE activity, as opposed to increased activation of the more proximal components of the renin-angiotensin system, namely, renin and angiotensinogen. This study also showed that the activation of the renin-angiotensin system

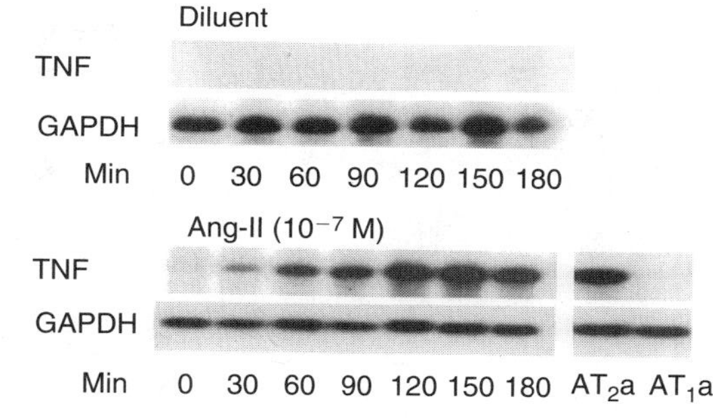

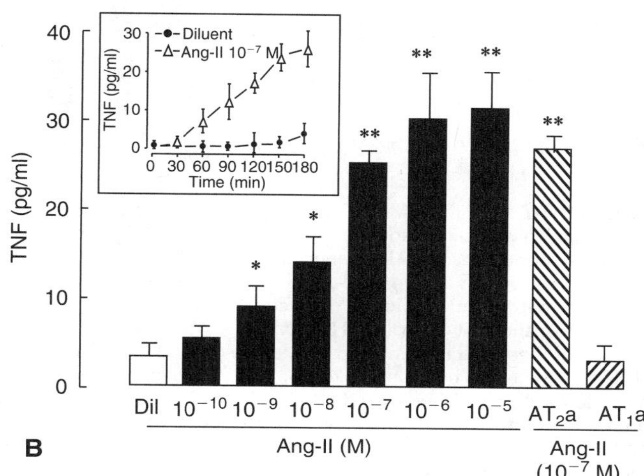

Figure 13-6 Angiotensin II-induced myocardial TNF biosynthesis in the adult heart. **(A)** TNF mRNA expression (RNase protection assay) was assessed ex vivo in diluent and angiotensin II (10^{-7} M) treated (0 to 180 minutes) buffer perfused Langendorf hearts, in the presence or absence of 10^{-6} M PD123319, an AT_2 receptor antagonist (AT_2a) or 10^{-6} M losartan, an AT_1 receptor antagonist (AT_1a). **(B)** Myocardial TNF protein production was assessed in the superfusates of the angiotensin II-treated hearts using enzyme-linked immunosorbent assay (ELISA), in the presence or absence of PD123319 (10^{-6} M) or losartan (10^{-6} M) pretreatment. The main panel **B** shows the dose-dependent effects of angiotensin II (10^{-10} M to 10^{-5} M), whereas the inset shows the time course (0 to 180 minutes) for TNF protein synthesis following stimulation with either diluent (solid circles) or 10^{-7} M Ang-II (open triangles). AT_{1a}, AT_1 receptor antagonist (losartan); AT_{2a}, AT_2 receptor antagonist (PD123319); *, $p < 0.05$ and **, $p < 0.01$ compared to diluent treated hearts. (Reproduced from Kalra D, Sivasubramanian N, Mann DL. Angiotensin II induces tumor necrosis factor biosynthesis in the adult mammalian heart through a protein kinase C-dependent pathway. *Circulation*. 2002;105:2198–2205, and the American Heart Association, with permission.)

was functionally significant in the TNF transgenic mice. That is, treatment of the MHCsTNF mice from 4 to 8 weeks of age with losartan significantly attenuated cardiac hypertrophy, myocardial fibrosis, and cardiac myocyte apoptosis in the MHCsTNF mice (53). Taken together, these observations suggest that interactions between the renin-angiotensin system and inflammatory mediators may contribute to adverse cardiac remodeling in the adult mammalian heart. Although speculative, one potential reason for the so-called phenomenon of neurohormonal escape (54), in which there is progressive cardiac remodeling despite pharmacological blockade of renin-angiotensin

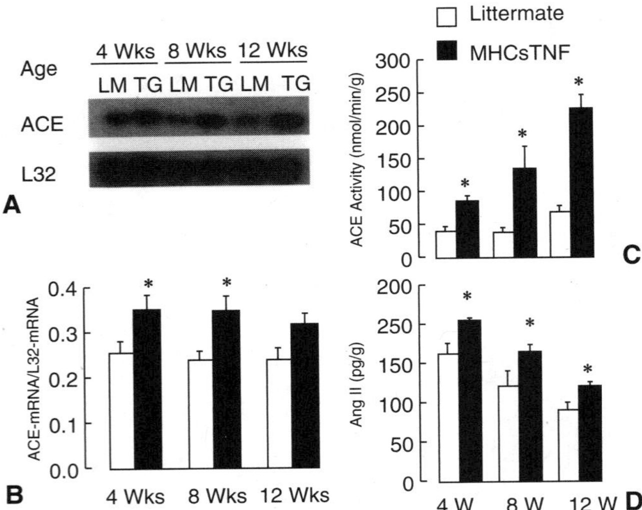

Figure 13-7 ACE mRNA, ACE activity, and angiotensin II peptide levels in mice with targeted overexpression of TNF (MHCsTNF) and littermate control mice. **(A)** Ribonuclease protection assay for ACE mRNA in the hearts of the 4-, 8-, and 12-week-old MHCsTNF (TG) and littermate control mice (LM) mice. **(B)** Group data in hearts from 4-, 8-, and 12-week-old MHCsTNF (n = 7 hearts/time) and 4-, 8-, and 12-week-old littermate control mice (n = 7 hearts/time). **(C)** ACE activity in the hearts from 4-, 8-, and 12-week-old MHCsTNF and the 4-, 8-, and 12-week-old littermate control mice. **(D)** Group data for angiotensin II peptide levels in the hearts of the MHCsTNF and littermate control mice at 4, 8, and 12 weeks of age. LM, littermate control; TG, transgenic; *, $p < 0.05$ versus age-matched control group by Tukey's test. (Reproduced from Flesch M, Hoper A, Dell'Italia L, et al. Activation and functional significance of the renin-angiotensin system in mice with cardiac restricted overexpression of tumor necrosis factor. *Circulation.* 2003;108:598–604, and the American Heart Association, with permission.)

system, may relate to the redundancy that exists between crossregulated biological systems, such as the renin angiotensin systems and proinflammatory cytokines.

CLINICAL RATIONALE FOR STUDYING INFLAMMATORY MEDIATORS IN HEART FAILURE

As previously noted, the interest in understanding the role of inflammatory mediators in heart failure arises from the observation that many aspects of the syndrome of heart failure can be explained by the known biological effects of proinflammatory cytokines (Table 13-2). A second rationale for studying inflammatory mediators in heart failure is that the pattern of expression of cytokines is very similar to that observed with the classical neurohormones (e.g., angiotensin II and norepineprhine) that are believed to play an important role in disease progression in heart failure (reviewed in [55]). That is, proinflammatory cytokines, including TNF, IL-1β, and IL-6, are expressed in direct relation to worsening New York Heart Association (NYHA) functional classification. Moreover, the observation that a variety of redundant inflammatory mediators are activated in heart failure also has potential therapeutic implications for the types of anti-inflammatory strategies that should be employed in clinical trials.

Insofar as proinflammatory cytokines were initially identified in patients with cardiac cachexia (1), there is a common misperception that these molecules are elaborated only in patients with end-stage heart failure. However, as is consistently reported in a number of studies (56–59), there is a progressive increase in proinflammatory cytokines levels in direct relation to deteriorating NYHA functional class. Indeed, proinflammatory cytokines are activated earlier in heart failure (i.e, NYHA class I and II) than are the classical neurohormones, which tend to be activated in the latter stages of heart failure (i.e., NYHA class III–IV) (60,61). Another clinical similarity between both inflammatory mediators and classical neurohormones is that circulating levels of both families of molecules have prognostic importance in the setting of heart failure (62). As shown in Figure 13-8A, data from the multicenter Vesnarinone trial (VEST) showed that there was a significant overall difference in survival as a function of increasing TNF levels, with the worst survival in patients with TNF levels >75th percentile (59). Similar findings were observed with respect to the Kaplan-Meier analysis of circulating levels of IL-6 (Fig. 13-8B). This analysis further showed that levels of soluble TNF receptor type 1 (sTNFR1) and soluble TNF receptor type 2 (sTNFR2) were highly predictive of adverse outcomes, consistent with prior reports (Figs. 13-8C–D) (63,64). Indeed, a univariate Cox analysis of the VEST cytokine database showed that TNF, IL-6, sTNFR1, and sTNFR2 were significant univariate predictors of mortality. Moreover, when the cytokine and/or cytokine receptor were separately entered into a multivariate Cox proportional hazards model that included age, gender, etiology of heart failure, NYHA class, ejection fraction, and serum sodium, TNF, IL-6, sTNFR1, and sTNFR2 remained significant independent predictors of mortality, along with NYHA class and ejection fraction.

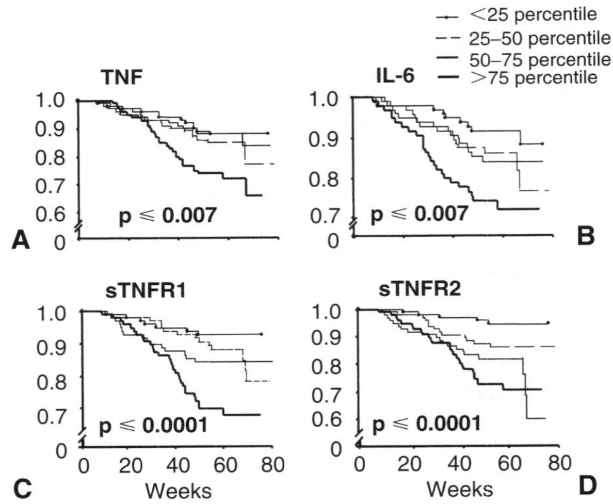

Figure 13-8 Kaplan-Meier survival analysis of inflammatory mediators in the VEST trial. The circulating levels of **(A)** TNF (6A), **(B)** IL-6 (6B), **(C)** sTNFR1 (6C), **(D)** and sTNFR2 (6D) were examined in relation to patient survival during follow-up (mean duration = 55 weeks; maximum duration = 78 weeks). For this analysis, the circulating levels of cytokines and cytokine receptors were arbitrarily divided into quartiles. (Reproduced with permission from Deswal et al [59] and the American Heart Association.)

The striking negative prognostic significance of elevated levels of circulating soluble TNF receptors in heart failure merits further discussion. Previous studies have shown that both the type 1 (TNFR1; p55) and the type 2 (TNFR2; p75) TNF receptors are proteolytically cleaved (shed) from cell membranes. These shed TNF receptors remain in the periphery as circulating soluble receptors that retain the ability to bind ligand, as well as the ability to inhibit TNF cytotoxicity by preventing TNF from binding to its cognate receptors on cell surface membranes. While the exact biological role for these soluble TNF receptors in vivo is not known with certainty, it has been suggested that they may serve as biological buffers that are capable of rapidly binding to and neutralizing the acute cytotoxic effects of TNF following release of TNF into the circulation. However, soluble TNF receptors are also capable of stabilizing TNF in the periphery, and may thus act as circulating TNF reservoirs (65). Importantly, TNF is not tightly bound to the circulating TNF receptors and thus retains full bioactivity (66). Whether the potential reservoir function of soluble TNF receptors explains the negative prognostic significance of the soluble TNF receptors, or whether the soluble TNF receptors are simply indirect markers of the degree of immune activation, remains unknown. However, given the worsening heart failure that has been observed in the clinical trials that have utilized recombinant human TNF receptors (see later), the reservoir function of circulating TNF receptors may prove to have mechanistic, as well as prognostic significance in heart failure.

A third rationale for studying the role of proinflammatory mediators in the setting of heart failure stems from the growing evidence that there are critical interactions between inflammatory mediators and the mediators of the classical neurohormonal systems. Indeed, over the past two decades our perception of the role of angiotensin II in the cardiovascular system has changed dramatically. Whereas angiotensin II was traditionally viewed as a circulating neurohormone that stimulated the constriction of vascular smooth muscle cells, aldosterone release from the adrenal gland, sodium reabsorption in the renal tubule, and/or the growth of cardiac myocytes or fibroblasts (48), it is becoming increasingly apparent that angiotensin II provokes inflammatory responses in a variety of different tissues and cell and tissue types. Moreover, clinical studies that have examined long-term administration of ACE inhibitors or angiotensin receptor blockers have shown that although ACE inhibitors have mixed results in terms of inhibiting proinflammatory cytokines (67,68), angiotensin type 1 receptor antagonists have consistently led to significant decreases in circulating levels of inflammatory mediators (TNF), and/or cell adhesion molecules (intercellular adhesion molecule-1 and vascular adhesion molecule-1) in patients with heart failure (68,69). Similarly, findings have recently been reported for the use of β-adrenergic blocking agents in experimental and clinical heart failure studies. That is, β-adrenergic blockade with a β_1-selective adrenergic antagonist has been shown to prevent the expression of proinflammatory mediators in an experimental model of post-infarct LV remodeling (70).

In a subset analysis of the Metoprolol CR/XL Randomized Intervention Trial in Congestive Heart Failure (MERIT-HF) (71), treatment with metoprolol did not lead to a decrease in the level of proinflammatory mediators (72), whereas in a different study the use of a nonselective β_1- and B_{a2}-adrenergic antagonist with ancillary antioxidant properties (carvedilol) resulted in a significant reduction in the transcardiac production of TNF in a small number of patients (73). Whether the differences in these two studies relates to the differences in selective versus nonselective β-adrenergic blockade, differences in ancillary properties between metoprolol and carvedilol, differences in the degree of ACE inhibition in the two studies, or a sample bias remains unclear. Nonetheless, the aggregate data suggest that there are important interactions between the renin angiotensin/adrenergic systems and proinflammatory cytokines. Moreover, there is increasing evidence that many of the conventional therapies for heart failure may work, at least in part, through modulation of proinflammatory cytokines.

INFLAMMATORY MEDIATORS AS THERAPEUTIC TARGETS IN HEART FAILURE

The rationale for employing anti-inflammatory strategies in patients with heart failure is threefold. First, as previsouly noted, the excessive elaboration of proinflammatory cytokines appears to mimic many aspects of the heart failure phenotype. Second, many of the deleterious effects of inflammatory mediators are potentially reversible once inflammation subsides. Third, heart failure remains an ineluctably progressive disease process despite optimal therapy with ACE inhibitors and β-blockers. As shown in Figure 13-9, the biological effects of proinflammatory mediators can be antagonized through transcriptional or translational approaches, or by so-called biological response modifiers that bind and/or neutralize soluble mediators (e.g., TNF or IL-1β). In addition, there are several novel immunomodulatory strategies that alter the levels of inflammatory mediators through multiple mechanisms.

Transcriptional Suppression of Proinflammatory Cytokines

Experimental studies have shown that agents that raise cyclic adenosine monophosphate (cAMP) levels, such as pentoxifylline, dobutamine, and milrinone, prevent TNF mRNA accumulation, largely by blocking the transcriptional activation of TNF (74–77). Although a short-term infusion of dobutamine infusion suppresses TNF production (78), Deng et al. reported administration of dobutamine increased IL-6 levels in patients with NYHA class III–IV heart failure (79). Thus, it is unclear at the time of this writing whether dobutamine has pro- or anti-inflammatory effects in the setting of heart failure.

More encouraging results with respect to modulating levels of inflammatory mediators through alterations in intracellular cAMP levels have been reported recently by Wagner et al. (80) and Sliwa et al. (81). Wagner et al. showed that adenosine was sufficient to block lipolysaccharide-induced TNF production in cultured neonatal and adult rat myocytes, as well as in slices of human myocardium obtained from explanted failing human hearts. The effect of adenosine could be mimicked by PD-125944, a selective A_2 receptor agonist (which is known to increase cAMP levels), or forskolin, and

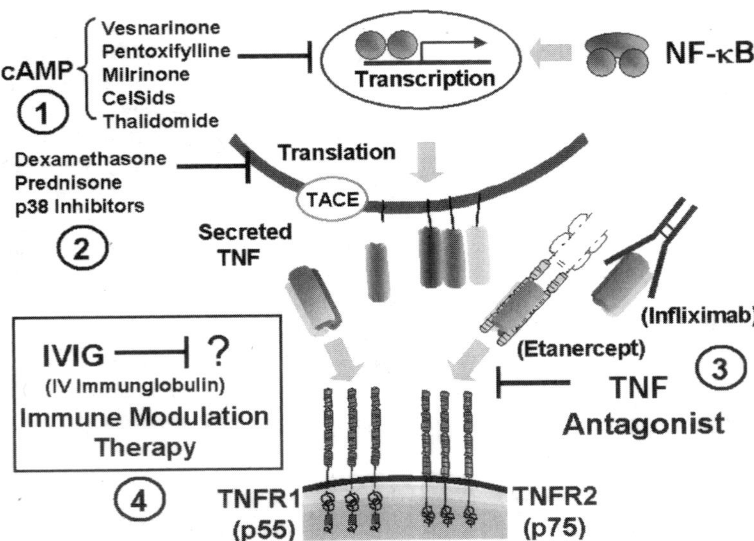

Figure 13-9 Therapeutic strategies for antagonizing proinflammatory mediators. TNF gene transcription is mediated, in part, by activation of NF-κB. Agents that increase intracellular levels of cAMP **(1)**, such as vesnarinone, penoxifylline, milrinone, thalidomide and thalidomide analogs (e.g., CelSids), decrease the level of inflammatory mediators through transcriptional blockade of inflammatory gene expression. Agents such as dexamethasone and prednisone and some p38 inhibitors suppress inflammation by blocking the translation of inflammatory mediators **(2)**. Secreted TNF can be neutralized **(3)** by soluble TNF antagonists (etanercept) or by neutralizing antibodies (infliximab) that prevent TNF from binding to its cognate type 1 (p55) and type 2 (p75) TNF receptors. In addition to these targeted approaches, immodulatory strategies have been employed **(4)** using intravenous immunoglobulin (IVIg) and immune modulation therapy using irradiated whole blood. (Reproduced from Mann DL. Inflammatory mediators and the failing heart: past, present, and the foreseeable future. *Circ Res.* 2002;91:988–98, and the American Heart Association, with permission.)

antagonized by DPMX, an A_2-selective antagonist. However, adenosine was only able to block TNF production if given before lipopolysaccharide challenge. Adenosine has also been shown to suppress intramyocardial TNF levels in an ex vivo model of ischemia reperfusion in the rat, as well as improve post-ischemic myocardial function (82).

Sliwa et al. studied the effects of pentoxifylline in patients with dilated cardiomyopathy and NYHA class II–III heart failure. A total of 14 patients received pentoxifylline at a dose of 400 mg 3 times daily and an equal number received placebo. Four patients died as a result of progressive pump dysfunction during the 6-month study period, all in the placebo group. At the end of 6 months there was an improvement in functional class in the pentoxifylline group, whereas there was functional deterioration in the placebo group. At 6 months there was a significant increase in the ejection fraction (from 22.3 ± 9.0 [S.D.] to 38.7 ± 15.0 [S.D.]) in the pentoxifylline group, whereas there was no significant change in the placebo group. There was, however, no change in the LV end-diastolic dimension in either group. An important observation was that TNF levels fell significantly ($p < 0.002$) from 6.5 ± pg/mL to 2.1 ± 1.0 pg/mL in the pentoxifylline group, whereas there was no significant change in the TNF levels in the placebo group.

In a subsequent study in patients with more advanced heart failure (NYHA class IV), pentoxifylline (400 mg 3 times daily) was shown to reduce TNF and Fas/Apo-1 concentrations, and improve ejection fraction at 1 month ($p < 0.05$) when compared with baseline and with patients receiving placebo. Significantly, these effects were not observed in the placebo-treated group (83). Similar findings with respect to pentoxifylline were observed in patients with ischemic and postpartum cardiomyopathies (84,85). Taken together, these data suggest that pentoxifylline may be a useful adjunct to conventional therapy in patients with severe heart failure. Thus, it appears that modulation of TNF levels via agents that alter intracellular cAMP levels, thus blocking transcriptional activation of TNF, may be a useful strategy for altering cytokine levels in heart failure.

Thalidomide (αN-pthalimidoglutarimide) is another class of drug that may be useful in suppressing TNF production. Thalidomide selectively inhibits TNF production in monocytes, (86) but has no effect on the production of IL-1β, IL-6, or granulocyte/macrophage colony-stimulating factor (GM-CSF). Thalidomide appears to reduce TNF levels by enhancing mRNA degradation (87). Since the teratogenic and sedative properties of thalidomide may limit its clinical utility, thalidomide analogs that have more potent TNF-lowering properties, and at the same time appear to be nonteratogenic, are being developed. A provisional report from an open-label study of a small number of patients showed that treatment with thalidomide led to a significant improvement in 6-minute walk distance and a trend toward a significant improvement in the quality of life and LV ejection performance (88). A similar, small open-label study in nine patients showed that 200 mg thalidomide daily for 6 weeks, in patients who were receiving optimal medical therapy, led to an increase in ejection fraction (from 26% ± 9% to 34% ± 10%) and a fall in baseline elevated levels of TNF (89). The effects of thalidomide are currently being tested in a larger, ongoing clinical trial in Europe.

Translational Suppression of Proinflammatory Cytokines

Dexamethasone, which is thought to primarily suppress TNF biosynthesis at the translational level, may also block TNF biosynthesis at the transcriptional level (90). One of the earliest studies to use this type of approach was performed by Parrillo et al. (91), who randomized 102 patients to treatment with prednisone (60 mg per day) or placebo. Following 3 months of therapy, they observed an increase in ejection fraction of >5% in 53% of the patients receiving prednisone, whereas only 27% of the controls had a significant improvement in ejection fraction ($p = 0.005$). Overall, the mean ejection fraction increased 4.3% ± 1.5% in the prednisone group, as compared with 2.1% ± 0.8% in the control group ($p = 0.054$). The patients were then categorized prospectively in two separately randomized subgroups. So-called reactive patients had fibroblastic or lymphocytic infiltration or immunoglobulin deposition on endomyocardial biopsy, a positive gallium scan, or an elevated erythrocyte sedimentation rate, and nonreactive patients had none of these features. At 3 months, 67% of the reactive patients who received prednisone had improvement in LV function, as compared with 28% of the reactive controls ($p = 0.004$). In contrast, nonreactive patients did not improve significantly with prednisone ($p = 0.51$). Although specific cytokine levels were not measured in this study, their data suggest that patients with idiopathic dilated cardiomyopathy may have some improvement when given a high dose of prednisone daily.

Targeted Anticytokine Approaches Using Biological Response Modifiers

Two different targeted approaches have been taken to selectively antagonize proinflammatory cytokines in heart failure patients. In the first approach, investigators have used recombinant human TNF receptors that act as decoys to bind TNF, thereby preventing TNF from binding to TNF receptors on cell surface membranes of target cells. The second approach is to use monoclonal antibodies to bind to and neutralize circulating cytokines.

Soluble TNF Receptors

Etanercept (Enbrel) is a genetically engineered, dimerized, fusion protein composed of two TNF p75 receptors and an IgG_1:Fc portion. Based on early, preclinical studies which showed that etanercept was sufficient to reverse the deleterious, negative inotropic effects of TNF in vitro (92) and in vivo (29), a series of phase I clinical studies were performed on patients with moderate to advanced heart failure. These early, short-term studies of small numbers of patients showed improvements in quality of life, 6-minute walk distance, and LV ejection performance following treatment with etanercept for up to 3 months (93,94). Following this, two multicenter clinical trials were initiated using etanercept in patients with NYHA class II–IV heart failure. The trial in North America, entitled Randomized Etanercept North AmerIcan Strategy to Study AntagoNism of CytokinEs (RENAISSANCE; n = 900), and the trial in Europe and Australia, entitled Research into Etanercept Cytokine Antagonism in Ventricular Dysfunction (RECOVER; n = 900), were both quality-of-life trials that used a clinical composite as the primary endpoint. The clinical composite score classifies patients as better, worse, or the same after a clinical intervention, based on the patient and the physician's assessment at the end of the study (95).

Both trials had parallel study designs, but differed in the doses of etanercept that were used in the two studies. RENAISSANCE employed doses of 25 mg biw and 25 mg tiw, whereas RECOVER employed doses of 25 mg qw and 25 mg biw. A third trial, which utilized the pooled data from the RENAISSANCE (biw and tiw dosing) and RECOVER (biw dosing only), termed Randomized Etanercept World-wide EvALuation (RENEWAL; n = 1,500), had a primary endpoint of all-cause mortality and hospitalization for heart failure. Based upon prespecified guidelines set forth in the charter of the trials, the trials were stopped prematurely because it was deemed unlikely that they would show benefit on the primary endpoints of the trials if the two trials were allowed to go to completion (96). Analysis of the data showed no benefit for etanercept on the clinical composite endpoint in RENAISSANCE and RECOVER (Fig. 13-10), and no benefit for etanercept on all-cause mortality and heart failure hospitalization in RENEWAL (Fig. 13-11) (96). In a post hoc analysis of hazard ratios for death or worsening heart failure, patients taking the biw dose of etanercept appeared to fare slightly better than patients taking the qw dose of etanercept in RECOVER, with hazard ratios for death or heart failure hospitalization of 0.87 and 1.01, respectively. In contrast, RENAISSANCE patients receiving biw etanercept experienced a 1.21 risk of death or heart failure hospitalization compared with placebo, while patients receiving the tiw dose had a slightly worse hazard ratio of 1.23.

These disparities in trial findings are likely related to the different length of follow-up in the two trials. Patients in RECOVER received etanercept for a median time of 5.7 months, whereas patients in RENAISSANCE received etancercept for 12.7 months. It it significant that these studies were stopped prematurely; had they been allowed to continued to completion, the hazard ratios may have been worse. On the basis of these findings, the prescribing information for etanercept has been updated and now suggests that physicians exercise caution in the use of etanercept in patients with heart failure.

Monoclonal Antibodies

A second targeted approach that has been tried in clinical heart failure trials is to use monoclonal antibodies directed against a particular cytokine. Infliximab (Remicade) is a chimeric monoclonal antibody consisting of a genetically engineered murine Fab fragment (that binds human TNF) fused to a human Fc portion of human IgG_1. Although infliximab had been shown to be effective in effective in Crohn disease and rheumatoid arthritis, there were no preclinical or early phase I clinical studies to support the use of this specific agent in heart failure. The Anti-TNF Therapy Against Congestive Heart failure (ATTACH) was a phase II study of 150 patients with moderate to advanced heart failure. The primary endpoint of the ATTACH trial was the clinical composite score previously described (95). In this study, patients with NYHA class III and IV heart failure were treated with a single intravenous infusion of infliximab (5 mg and 10 mg) or placebo at 0, 2, and 6 weeks and were followed for up to 28 weeks. Treatment with inflixmab did not result in a significant improvement in inflammatory mediators. However, as shown in Figure 13-12, at 28 weeks there was a dose-related increase in death and heart failure hospitalizations with infliximab when compared to placebo at 14 weeks (21% increase) and at 28 weeks (26% increase). By 38 weeks of follow-up, nine infliximab patients had died (two in the 5 mg per kg group and seven in the 10 mg per kg group) compared

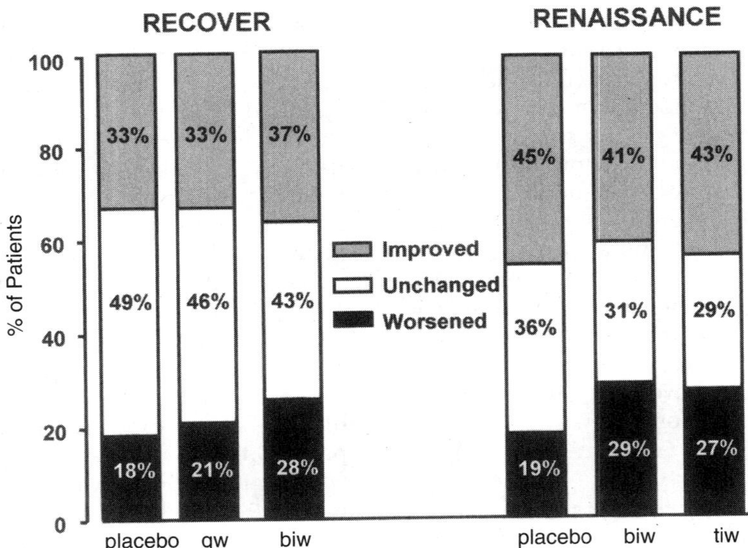

Figure 13-10 Analysis of the clinical status composite score for the RECOVER and RENAISSANCE trials in the placebo and etanercept groups (number of patients who had completed planned 24 weeks of treatment by the time these trials were stopped). (Reproduced from Mann DL, McMurray JJV, Packer M, et al. Targeted anti-cytokine therapy in patients with chronic heart failure: results of the Randomized EtaNcercept Worldwide evALuation (RENEWAL). *Circulation.* 2004;109:1594–1602, and the American Heart Association, with permission.)

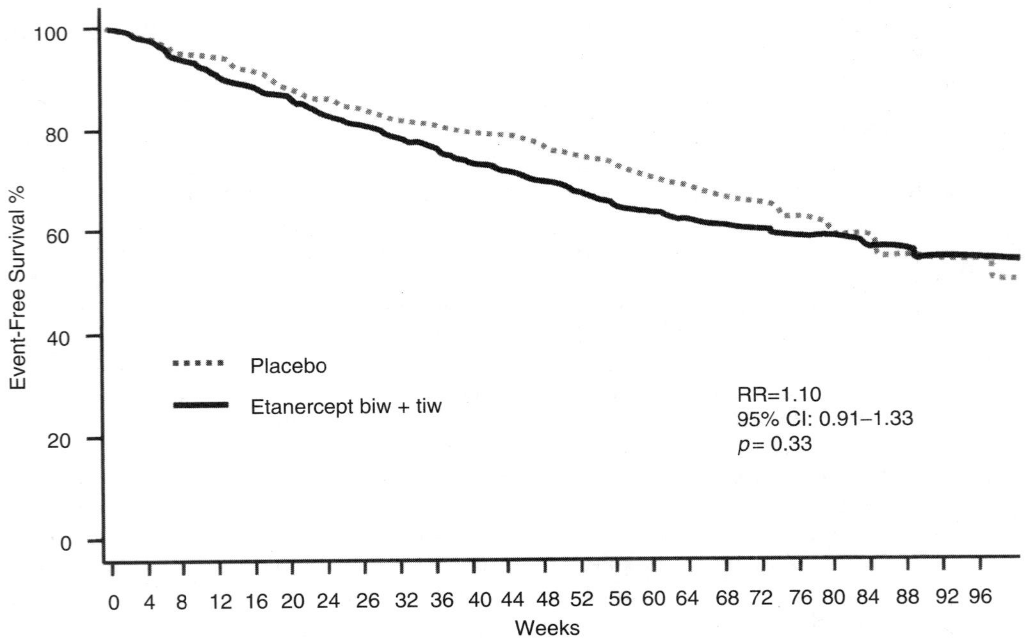

Figure 13-11 Kaplan-Meier analysis of the time to death or heart failure hospitalizations in the placebo and etanercept group (biw and tiw) in the RENEWAL analysis. (Reproduced from Mann DL, McMurray JJV, Packer M, et al. Targeted anti-cytokine therapy in patients with chronic heart failure: results of the Randomized EtaNcercept Worldwide evALuation [RENEWAL]. *Circulation.* 2004;109:1594–602, and the American Heart Association, with permission.)

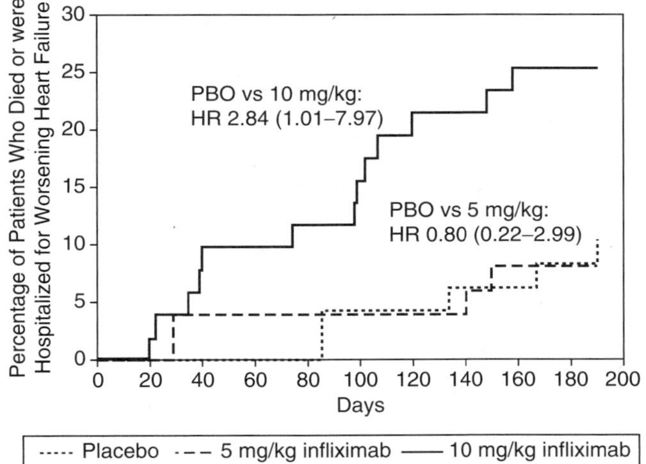

Figure 13-12 Kaplan-Meier analysis of the time to death and heart failure hospitalization in the placebo (dotted line) and infliximab [5 mg/kg (dashed line) and 10 mg/kg (solid line)] in the ATTACH trial. (Reproduced from Chung ES, Packer M, Lo KH, et al. Randomized, double-blind, placebo-controlled, pilot trial of infliximab, a chimeric monoclonal antibody to tumor necrosis factor-α, in patients with moderate-to-severe heart failure: results of the Anti-TNF Therapy Against Congestive Heart failure [ATTACH] trial. *Circulation*. 2003;107:3133–3140, with permission.)

with just one death in the placebo group (97). On the basis of these findings, the prescribing information for infliximab in rheumatoid arthritis and Crohn disease now cautions against its use for patients with heart failure.

Why Have Targeted Anti-TNF Therapies Failed in Heart Failure Trials?

Given the wealth of preclinical data and early clinical studies that suggested a role for TNF antagonism in heart failure, the negative results of the clinical trials have been discouraging. Nevertheless, analysis of the aggregate clinical trial data permits some insight into the potential reasons for why these studies have had negative results. It is important to recognize that neither the trials with etanercept nor the trial with infliximab was neutral (i.e., no effect); in both trials there was evidence for dose- and time-dependent worsening of heart failure and/or worsening outcomes. This, in turn, suggests that the biological agents used in the trials either had intrinsic effects themselves or, alternatively, that TNF antagonism has untoward effects in the setting of heart failure. With respect to the first explanation, it is significant that infliximab exerts its effects, at least in part, by fixing complement in cells that express TNF on the membrane. As shown in Figure 13-13A, infliximab is directly cytotoxic to cells expressing TNF on the membrane. Although this type of biological action is beneficial in eliminating activated T cells that have invaded the gastrointestinal mucosa of patients with Crohn disease, it is likely to be overtly deleterious in the setting of heart failure, wherein failing myocytes express TNF on their cell membranes (98).

A second line of evidence in support of the cytotoxic actions of infliximab comes from an analysis of the cytokine levels in the ATTACH trial. There was a 20-fold increase in the level of immunoreactive TNF in the ATTACH trial following treatment with infliximab. Given that TNF is released in response to tissue injury, the rise in TNF levels in the ATTACH is consistent with infliximab-mediated complement fixation leading to myocarditis, progressive myocyte cell loss, and worsening heart failure (99). The observation that heart failure developed at 28 weeks in the ATTACH trial, which was 22 weeks after the last dose of infliximab was given and 14 weeks after the circulating levels of infliximab became subtherapeutic, is consistent with this point of view. A second potential explanation for the increase in TNF levels in the ATTACH trial may have been because of a so-called TNF rebound effect (100) following cessation of therapy with infliximab. However, it should be emphasized that precise mechanistic explanations for the untoward outcomes in the ATTACH trial are not known.

Cytokine binding proteins such as etanercept also have intrinsic biological activity and, in certain settings, can act as agonists for the cytokine they bind (101). As a case in point, in human studies etanercept acts as a carrier protein that stabilizes TNF and results in the accumulation of high concentrations of immunoreactive TNF in the peripheral circulation (Fig. 13-13B) (102). As shown in Figure 13-13C, TNF complexed to etanercept does not remain tightly bound but, rather, dissociates with an extremely fast off-rate (620 milliseconds) (66). The increase in the levels of TNF bound to etanercept and the rapid off-rates of TNF from etanercept can lead to an increase in the duration of TNF bioactivity, as shown in Figure 13-13D.

In summary, Figures 13B–D show that etanercept can, in certain settings, act as a stimulating antagonist (101). The aforementioned biological effects of etanercept might not be problematic in rheumatoid arthritis, wherein TNF is encapsulated within a joint space and peripheral circulating TNF levels are relatively low (compared to heart failure) or are nonexistent (103). However, an increase in the circulating levels of biologically active TNF in a patient with heart failure might be expected to produce worsening heart failure, for all of the reasons articulated at the outset of this review (Table 13-2).

With respect to the second explanation for worsening heart failure in the clinical trials, there is a well-established body of literature that suggests that relatively low levels of TNF are cytoprotective in the heart. As noted at the outset, physiological concentrations of TNF have been shown to protect the adult cardiac myocytes against ischemic and/or hypoxic cell injury (12,26,104). Thus, one potential explanation for the worsening heart failure observed in the anti-TNF trials, albeit speculative, is that our current attempts to antagonize TNF result in the loss of one or more of the beneficial effects of TNF. Accordingly, TNF antagonism might be expected to attenuate both the deleterious and beneficial effects of TNF. The observation that TNF antagonism provides short-term beneficial effects in heart failure patients (93,94) and yet results in worsening heart failure when used chronically is entirely consistent with this point of view.

IMMUNOMODULATORY STRATEGIES

An alternative approach to targeting specific components of the inflammatory cascade is to use approaches that

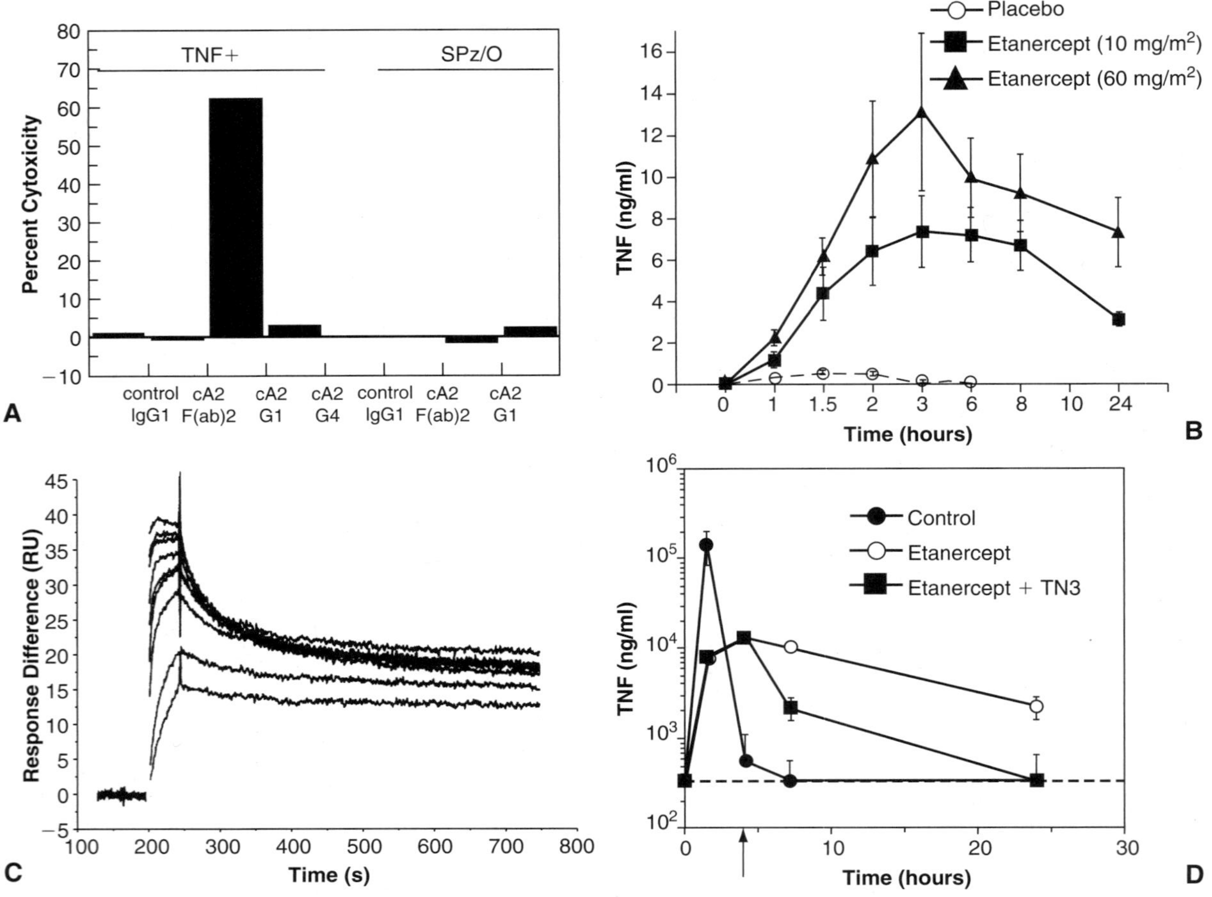

Figure 13-13 Biological properties of infliximab and etanercept. **(A)** Infliximab (cA2 G1) is cytotoxic for cells that express TNF on their cell membranes (TNF+), whereas it is not cytotoxic for cells that do not express TNF on their membranes (SPz/O). The mechanism for the cytotoxic effects of infliximab was demonstrated using F(ab)2 fragments of infliximab, which lack the Fc domain and therefore cannot fix complement. As shown, the F(ab)2 fragment of infliximab was not cytotoxic for TNF+ cells. (Reproduced from Scallon BJ, Moore MA, Trinh H, et al. Chimeric anti-TNF-alpha monoclonal antibody cA2 binds recombinant transmembrane TNF-alpha and activates immune effector functions. *Cytokine.* 1995;7:251–259, with permission.) **(B)** Etanercept increases the levels of immunoreactive TNF in the peripheral circulation of human subjects following intravenous endotoxin administration. As shown, high-dose etanercept (60 mg/m^2) increased immunoreactive TNF levels more than low-dose etanercept (10 mg/m^2). (Modified from Suffredini AF, Reda D, Banks SM, et al. Effects of recombinant dimeric TNF receptor on human inflammatory responses following intravenous endotoxin administration. *J Immunol.* 1995;155:5038–5045.) **(C)** Kinetic analysis of TNF binding to etanercept using surface plasmon resonance biosensor technology (BIAcore assay, as described in Weinberger SR, Morris TS, Pawlak M. Recent trends in protein biochip technology. *Pharmacogenomics.* 2000;1:395–416.) Etanercept was exposed to 1,000, 500, 250, 125, 62.5, 31.25, 16.63, 3.90, and 1.95 nmol/L of TNF, and the kinetics of TNF binding were determined by the decay of the light signal after peak binding to etanercept. The off-rate of TNF from etanercept was determined to be 620 milliseconds. (Reproduced from Frishman JI, Edwards CK, III, et al. Tumor necrosis factor (TNF)-alpha-induced interleukin-8 in human blood cultures discriminates neutralization by the p55 and p75 TNF soluble receptors. *J Infect Dis.* 2000;182:1722–1730, with permission.) **(D)** Etanercept increases TNF bioactivity. Animals were inoculated with bacteria and levels of TNF bioactivity measured at the indicated time points. TNF bioactivity peaked at 90 minutes after bacterial inoculation but was undetectable at later time points. Mice treated with etanercept after bacterial inoculation showed a significant reduction in the level of peak TNF bioactivity; however, as shown, TNF bioactivity was significantly prolonged by etanercept. Mice that received etanercept after bacterial inoculation followed by an anti-TNF neutralizing antibody (TN3) had a shorter duration of TNF bioactivity. The **arrow** indicates the timing of the administration of the neutralizing anti-TNF antibody. (Reproduced from Mann DL, McMurray JJV, Packer M, et al. Targeted anti-cytokine therapy in patients with chronic heart failure: results of the Randomized EtaNcercept Worldwide evALuation (RENEWAL). *Circulation.* 2004;109:1594–1602, with permission.)

result in a decrease in the systemic inflammatory response. Thus far, three different approaches have been employed in heart failure studies: intravenous immunoglobulin, immune modulation therapy, and hydroxymethylglutaryl coenzyme A reductase inhibitors (statins).

Intravenous Immuoglobulin

Therapy with intravenous immunoglobulin (IVIg) has been tried in a wide range of immune-mediated disorders, such as Kawasaki syndrome, dermatomyositis, and multiple sclerosis. Although the exact mechanism of action of IV Ig is not known, a number of different mechanisms have been proposed, including Fc receptor blockade, neutralization of autoantibodies, modulation of cytokine activity, and activation of an inhibitory Fc receptor (105). Based on an initial report that IV Ig was beneficial in acute cardiomyopathy (106), Gullestad et al. conducted a double-blind trial with IVIg for 26 weeks in 47 patients with moderate heart failure who were receiving conventional therapy for heart failure, including ACE inhibitors and β-blockers. They observed that, in comparison to placebo, IVIg induced a marked rise in plasma levels of the anti-inflammatory mediators (IL-10, and IL-1 receptor antagonist), and that these changes were accompanied by a significant increase in LV ejection performance by 10%, and a decrease in N-terminal proatrial natriuretic peptide levels (107). Thus, in this small study immunomodulatory therapy with IVIg was effective in patients with heart failure.

Immune Modulation Therapy

Immune modulation therapy uses a medical device (the VC7000 Blood Treatment System) to expose a sample of blood to a combination of physiochemical stressors ex vivo. The treated blood sample is then administered intramuscularly, along with local anesthetic, into the same patient from whom the sample was obtained. The physiochemical stresses to which the autologous blood sample is subjected are known to initiate or facilitate apoptotic cell death. The uptake of apoptotic cells by macrophages results in a downregulation of proinflammatory cytokines, including TNF, IL-1β, and IL-8, and an increase in production of the anti-inflammatory cytokines, including TGF-β and IL-10 (108,109). Recent studies have shown that immune modulation therapy leads to a decrease in the production of proinflammatory cytokines and a corresponding increase in anti-inflammatory cytokines in human subjects (110).

Given that an imbalance exists between pro- and anti-inflammatory cytokines in patients with heart failure (58), immune modulation therapy may restore this balance more toward normal. In a recent trial, 75 patients with NYHA functional class III–IV heart failure were randomized in a double-blind manner to receive either immune modulation therapy (n = 38) or placebo (n = 37). This study showed that treatment with immune modulation therapy for 6 months led to a trend toward improvement in NYHA functional classification by at least one class ($p = 0.14$), whereas there was no between-group difference in 6-minute walk test or the ejection fraction between groups (111). However, the striking finding of

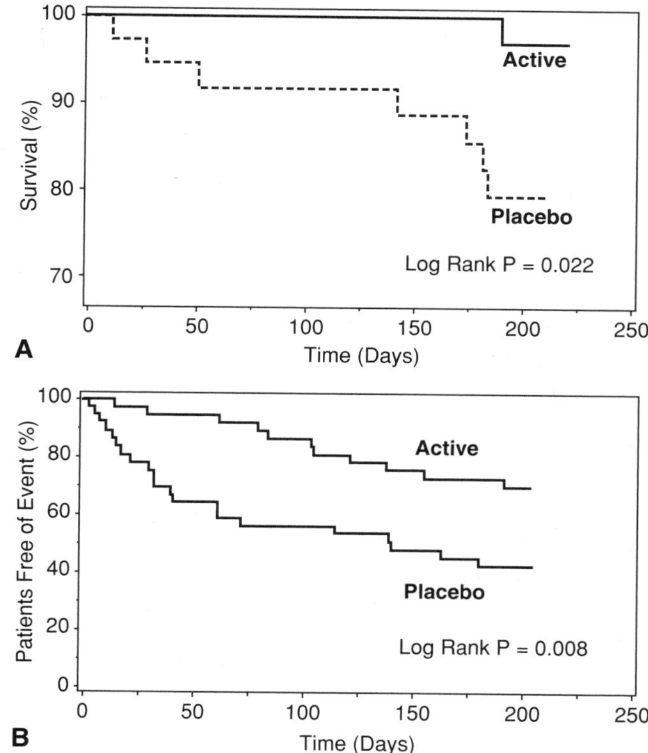

Figure 13-14 Effect of immune modulation therapy in patients with heart failure. **A** shows the Kaplan-Meier analysis of the time to death; **B** shows the Kaplan Meier analysis of hospital-free survival in the control and immune modulation therapy groups. (Reproduced from Torre-Amione G, Sestier F, Radovancevic B, et al. Effects of a novel immune modulation therapy in patients with advanced chronic heart failure: results of a randomized, controlled, phase II trial. *J Am Coll Cardiol*. 2004;44:1181–1186, with permission.)

this study was that the Kaplan-Meier survival analysis (Fig. 13-14) showed that immune modulation significantly reduced the risk of death ($p = 0.022$) and hospitalization ($p = 0.008$). Analysis of a clinical composite score demonstrated a significant between-group difference ($p = 0.006$). Based on the encouraging results of this pilot trial, a larger, pivotal trial with immune modulation therapy is being planned (111).

Hydroxymethylglutaryl Coenzyme A Reductase Inhibitors (Statins)

Large-scale clinical trials involving thousands of patients in both primary and secondary prevention of coronary artery disease (CAD) have clearly demonstrated that statin therapy will reduce cardiovascular mortality across a broad spectrum of patient subgroups. However, in addition to the pure lipid-lowering effects of hydroxymethylglutaryl coenzyme A reductase inhibitors, statins are also believed to impart immunomodulatory and/or anti-inflammatory effects. Relevant to the present discussion, several retrospective analyses have shown that treatment with statins also appears to reduce the risk of developing heart failure (112–114).

For example, Kjekshus et al. performed a retrospective analysis of patients with known CAD who were enrolled in the Scandinavian Simvastatin Survival Study (112). They found that 10.3% of the patients in that study that were randomized to receive placebo developed heart failure during follow-up, whereas heart failure developed in 8.3% of patients who received simvastatin ($p < 0.015$). Similar findings were reported by Horwich et al., who studied a cohort of 551 patients with systolic heart failure who were referred for clinical management and/or transplant evaluation (114). In this retrospective, single-center study, statin use was associated with improved survival without the necessity of urgent transplantation in both nonischemic and ischemic heart failure patients, even after adjustment for confounding variables (hazard ratio 0.41; 95% confidence interval 0.18–0.94).

Finally, in a recent prospective trial, 63 patients with symptomatic, nonischemic dilated cardiomyopathy were randomly assigned to receive simvastatin (n = 24) or placebo (n = 27). After 14 weeks, patients treated with simvastatin had a significantly lower NYHA functional class compared with patients receiving placebo, as well as a corresponding increase in LV ejection fraction. In addition, plasma concentrations of TNF, IL-6, and brain natriuretic peptide were significantly lower in the simvastatin group when compared with the placebo group, suggesting that short-term statin therapy improves cardiac function, neurohormonal imbalance, and symptoms associated with idiopathic dilated cardiomyopathy (118). At the time of this writing there are several ongoing clinical trials of statins in heart failure patients in Europe (GISSI, CORONA, and UNIVERSE), which should more definitively address the immunomodulatory role of statins in heart failure.

CONCLUSION

In the present review we have summarized experimental material which suggests that activation of cytokines within the heart following cardiac injury may have either beneficial or detrimental consequences for the host, depending on the duration and degree of cytokine exposure. Short-term expression of these stress-activated cytokines may be beneficial by upregulating the expression of families of so-called protective proteins in the heart, as well as by integrating the various components of the myocardial stress response (i.e., cardiac hypertrophy, cardiac remodeling, and cardiac repair). On the other hand, the short-term beneficial effects of stress-activated cytokines may be lost if myocardial expression of these molecules either becomes sustained and/or excessive, in which case the salutary effects of these proteins may be contravened by their known deleterious effects. Pathophysiologically relevant concentrations of these molecules appear to be able to mimic many aspects of the so-called heart failure phenotype in experimental animals, including LV dysfunction, LV dilation, activation of fetal gene expression, cardiac myocyte hypertrophy, and cardiac myocyte apoptosis (Table 13-2). The early attempts to translate this information to the bedside have not only been disappointing but have, in many instances, led to worsening heart failure.

While one interpretation of these findings is that inflammatory mediators are not viable targets in cardiac disease states such as heart failure, based on the arguments previously delineated, the countervailing point of view is that we simply have not targeted proinflammatory mediators with agents that can be used safely in the context of heart failure or, alternatively, that targeting a single component of the inflammatory cascade is not sufficient in a disease as complex as heart failure. As with all therapeutic approaches in heart failure, the only way to really answer the question of whether broader-spectrum anti-inflammatory strategies will have any added value in heart failure is through well-designed clinical trials. Strategies that use small molecules that have a broad spectrum of anti-inflammatory properties [e.g., pentoxifylline and thalidomide (or its analogs)] and immunomodulatory strategies that activate anti-inflammatory pathways (e.g., immune modulation therapy) are currently being evaluated.

ACKNOWLEDGMENTS

The author would like to thank Ms. Mary Helen Soliz for secretarial support. This work was supported, in part, by research funds from the U.S. Department of Veterans Affairs and the National Institutes of Health (P50 HL-O6H and RO1 HL58081-01, RO1 HL61543-01, HL-42250-10/10, RO1 HL73017-01).

REFERENCES

1. Levine B, Kalman J, Mayer L, et al. Elevated circulating levels of tumor necrosis factor in severe chronic heart failure. *N Engl J Med.* 1990;223:236–241.
2. Mann DL. Inflammatory mediators and the failing heart: past, present, and the foreseeable future. *Circ Res.* 2002;91:988–998.
3. Mann DL. Cytokines as mediators of disease progression in the failing heart. In: Hosenpud JD, Greenberg BH, eds. *Congestive Heart Failure.* Philadelphia: Lippincott Williams & Wilkins; 1999: 213–232.
4. Kapadia S, Lee JR, Torre-Amione G, et al. Tumor necrosis factor gene and protein expression in adult feline myocardium after endotoxin administration. *J Clin Invest.* 1995;96:1042–1052.
5. Kapadia S, Oral H, Lee J, et al. Hemodynamic regulation of tumor necrosis factor-α gene and protein expression in adult feline myocardium. *Circ Res.* 1997;81:187–195.
6. Hoffmann JA, Kafatos FC, Janeway CA, Jr., et al. Phylogenetic perspectives in innate immunity. *Science.* 1999;284:1313–1318.
7. Raftos DA, Cooper EL, Habicht GS, et al. Invertebrate cytokines: tunicate cell proliferation stimulated by an interleukin 1-like molecule. *Proc Natl Acad Sci USA.* 1991;88:9518–9522.
8. Beck G, Habicht GS. Primitive cytokines: harbingers of vertebrate defense. *Immunol Today.* 1991;12:180–183.
9. Eddy LJ, Goeddel DV, Wong GHW. Tumor necrosis factor-α pretreatment is protective in a rat model of myocardial ischemia-reperfusion injury. *Biochem Biophys Res Commun.* 1992;184:1056–1059.
10. Nelson SK, Wong GHW, McCord JM. Leukemia inhibitory factor and tumor necrosis factor induce manganese superoxide dismutase and protect rabbit hearts from reperfusion injury. *J Mol Cell Cardiol.* 1995;27:223–229.
11. Maulik N, Engelman RM, Wei ZJ, et al. Interleukin-1 alpha preconditioning reduces myocardial ischemia reperfusion injury. *Circulation.* 1993;88:387–394.
12. Nakano M, Knowlton AA, Dibbs Z, et al. Tumor necrosis factor-α confers resistance to injury induced by hypoxic injury in the adult mammalian cardiac myocyte. *Circulation.* 1998;97:1392–1400.
13. Wong GHW, Goeddel DV. Induction of manganous superoxide dismutase by tumor necrosis factor: possible protective mechanism. *Science.* 1988;242:941–944.
14. Nakano M, Knowlton AA, Yokoyama T, et al. Tumor necrosis factor-α induced expression of heat shock protein 72 in adult feline cardiac myocytes. *Am J Physiol.* 1996;270:H1231–H1239.

15. Low-Friedrich I, Weisensee D, Mitrou P, et al. Cytokines induce stress protein formation in cultured cardiac myocytes. *Basic Res Cardiol.* 1992;87:12–18.
16. Marber MS, Mestril R, Chi SH, et al. Overexpression of the rat inducible 70-kd heat stress protein in a transgenic mouse increases the resistance of the heart to ischemic injury. *J Clin Invest.* 1995;95:1446–1456.
17. Plumier JCL, Ross BM, Currie RW, et al. Transgenic mice expressing the human heat shock protein 70 have improved post-ischemic myocardial recovery. *J Clin Invest.* 1995;95:1854–1860.
18. Narula J, Pandey P, Arbustini E, et al. Apoptosis in heart failure: release of cytochrome C from mitochondria and activation of caspase-3 in human cardiomyopathy. *Proc Natl Acad Sci USA.* 1999;96:8144–8149.
19. Erl W, Hansson GK, de Martin RC. Nuclear factor-kappa B regulates induction of apoptosis and inhibitor of apoptosis protein-1 expression in vascular smooth muscle cells. *Circ Res.* 1999;84:668–677.
20. Wang CY, Mayo MW, Korneluk RC. NF-kappaB antiapoptosis: induction of TRAF1 and TRAF2 and c-IAP1 and c- IAP2 to suppress caspase-8 activation. *Science.* 1998;281:1680–1683.
21. Stehlik C, de Martin R, Binder BR, et al. Cytokine induced expression of porcine inhibitor of apoptosis protein (iap) family member is regulated by NF-kappa B. *Biochem Biophys Res Commun.* 1998;243:827–832.
22. Lee JP, Palfrey HC, Bindokas VP, et al. The role of immunophilins in mutant superoxide dismutase-1linked familial amyotrophic lateral sclerosis. *Proc Natl Acad Sci USA.* 1999;96:3251–3256.
23. Fujio Y, Kunisada K, Hirota H, et al. Signals through gp130 upregulate *bcl-x* gene expression via STAT1-binding *cis*-element in cardiac myocytes. *J Clin Invest.* 1997;99:2898–2905.
24. Yoshida K, Taga T, Saito M, et al. Targeted disruption of gp130, a common signal transducer for the interleukin 6 family of cytokines, leads to myocardial and hematological disorders. *Proc Natl Acad Sci USA.* 1996;93:407–411.
25. Hirota H, Chen J, Betz UA, et al. Loss of a gp130 cardiac muscle cell survival pathway is a critical event in the onset of heart failure during biomechanical stress. *Cell.* 1999;97:189–198.
26. Kurrelmeyer K, Michael L, Baumgarten G, et al. Endogenous myocardial tumor necrosis factor protects the adult cardiac myocyte against ischemic-induced apoptosis in a murine model of acute myocardial infarction. *Proc Natl Acad Sci USA.* 2000;290:5456–5461.
27. Rothe M, Sarma V, Dixit VM, et al. TRAF2-mediated activation of NF-kB by TNF receptor 2 and CD40. *Science* 1995;269:1424–1427.
28. Yokoyama T, Nakano M, Bednarczyk JL, et al. Tumor necrosis factor-α provokes a hypertrophic growth response in adult cardiac myocytes. *Circulation.* 1997;95:1247–1252.
29. Bozkurt B, Kribbs S, Clubb FJ, Jr., et al. Pathophysiologically relevant concentrations of tumor necrosis factor-α promote progressive left ventricular dysfunction and remodeling in rats. *Circulation.* 1998;97:1382–1391.
30. Thaik CM, Calderone A, Takahashi N, et al. Interleukin-1β modulates the growth and phenotype of neonatal rat cardiac myocytes. *J Clin Invest.* 1995;96:1093–1099.
31. Kubota T, McTiernan CF, Frye CS, et al. Dilated cardiomyopathy in transgenic mice with cardiac specific overexpression of tumor necrosis factor-alpha. *Circ Res.* 1997;81:627–635.
32. Seta Y, Shan K, Bozkurt B, et al. Basic mechanisms in heart failure: the cytokine hypothesis. *J Cardiac Fail.* 1996;2:243–249.
33. Franco F, Thomas GD, Giroir BP, et al. Magnetic resonance imaging and invasive evaluation of development of heart failure in transgenic mice with myocardial expression of tumor necrosis factor-alpha. *Circulation.* 1999;99:448–454.
34. Sivasubramanian N, Coker ML, Kurrelmeyer K, et al. Left ventricular remodeling in transgenic mice with cardiac restricted overexpression of tumor necrosis factor. *Circulation.* 2001;2001: 826–831.
35. Oral H, Dorn GW, II, Mann DL. Sphingosine mediates the immediate negative inotropic effects of tumor necrosis factor-α in the adult mammalian cardiac myocyte. *J Biol Chem.* 1997;272:4836–4842.
36. Gulick TS, Chung MK, Pieper SJ, et al. Interleukin 1 and tumor necrosis factor inhibit cardiac myocyte β-adrenergic responsiveness. *Proc Natl Acad Sci USA.* 1989;86:6753–6757.
37. Balligand JL, Ungureanu D, Kelly RA, et al. Abnormal contractile function due to induction of nitric oxide synthesis in rat cardiac myocytes follows exposure to activated macrophage-conditioned medium. *J Clin Invest.* 1993;91:2314–2319.
38. Dinarello CA. Interleukin-18. *Methods.* 1999;19:121–132.
39. Maisel AS, Koon J, Krishnaswamy P, et al. Utility of B-natriuretic peptide as a rapid, point-of-care test for screening patients undergoing echocardiography to determine left ventricular dysfunction. *Am Heart J.* 2001;141:367–74.
40. Yu X, Kennedy RH, Liu SJ. JAK2/STAT3, not ERK1/2, mediates interleukin-6-induced activation of inducible nitric-oxide synthase and decrease in contractility of adult ventricular myocytes. *J Biol Chem.* 2003;278:16304–16309.
41. Krown KA, Page MT, Nguyen C, et al. Tumor necrosis factor alpha-induced apoptosis in cardiac myocytes: involvement of the sphingolipid signaling cascade in cardiac cell death. *J Clin Invest.* 1996;98:2854–2865.
42. Pagani FD, Baker LS, Hsi C, et al. Left ventricular systolic and diastolic dysfunction after infusion of tumor necrosis factor-α in conscious dogs. *J Clin Invest.* 1992;90:389–398.
43. Bryant D, Becker L, Richardson J, et al. Cardiac failure in transgenic mice with myocardial expression of tumor necrosis factor-α (TNF). *Circulation* 1998;97:1375–1381.
44. Li YY, Feng YQ, Kadokami T, et al. Myocardial extracellular matrix remodeling in transgenic mice overexpressing tumor necrosis factor alpha can be modulated by anti- tumor necrosis factor alpha therapy. *Proc Natl Acad Sci USA.* 2000;97:12746–12751.
45. Weber KT. Cardiac intersitium in health and disease: the fibrillar collagen network. *J Am Coll Cardiol.* 1989;13(7):1637–1652.
46. Knittel T, Mehde M, Grundmann A, et al. Expression of matrix metalloproteinases and their inhibitors during hepatic tissue repair in the rat [In Process Citation]. *Histochem Cell Biol.* 2000;113:443–453.
47. Sime PJ, Marr RA, Gauldie D, et al. Transfer of tumor necrosis factor-alpha to rat lung induces severe pulmonary inflammation and patchy interstitial fibrogenesis with induction of transforming growth factor-beta1 and myofibroblasts. *Am J Pathol.* 1998;153:825–832.
48. Dostal DE, Baker KM. The cardiac renin-angiotensin system: conceptual, or a regulator of cardiac function? *Circ Res.* 1999;85:643–650.
49. Brasier AR, Jamaluddin M, Han Y, et al. Angiotensin II induces gene transcription through cell-type-dependent effects on the nuclear factor-kappaB (NF-kappaB) transcription factor. *Mol Cell Biochem.* 2000;212:155–169.
50. Hernandez-Presa M, Bustos C, Ortega M, et al. Angiotensin-converting enzyme inhibition prevents arterial nuclear factor-kB activtion, monocyte chemoattractant protein-1 expression, and macrophage infiltration in a rabbit model of early accelerated atherosclerosis. *Circulation.* 1997;95:1532–1541.
51. Luft FC. Workshop: mechanisms and cardiovascular damage in hypertension. *Hypertension.* 2001;37:594–598.
52. Kalra D, Baumgarten G, Dibbs Z, et al. Nitric oxide provokes tumor necrosis factor-alpha expression in adult feline myocardium through a cGMP-dependent pathway. *Circulation.* 2000;102:1302–1307.
53. Flesch M, Hoper A, Dell'Italia L, et al. Activation and functional significance of the renin-angiotensin system in mice with cardiac restricted overexpression of tumor necrosis factor. *Circulation.* 2003;108:598–604.
54. Francis GS, Cohn JN, Johnson G, et al. Plasma norepinephrine, plasma renin activity, and congestive heart failure. *Circulation.* 1993;87:VI40–VI48.
55. Mann DL. Mechanisms and models in heart failure: a combinatorial approach. *Circulation.* 1999;100:999–1088.
56. Torre-Amione G, Kapadia S, Benedict CR, et al. Proinflammatory cytokine levels in patients with depressed left ventricular ejection fraction: a report from the studies of left ventricular dysfunction (SOLVD). *J Am Coll Cardiol.* 1996;27:1201–1206.
57. Testa M, Yeh M, Lee P, et al. Circulating levels of cytokines and their endogenous modulators in patients with mild to severe congestive heart failure due to coronary artery disease or hypertension. *J Am Coll Cardiol.* 1996;28:964–971.
58. Aukrust P, Ueland T, Lien E, et al. Cytokine network in congestive heart failure secondary to ischemic or idiopathic dilated cardiomyopathy. *Am J Cardiol.* 1999;83:376–382.

59. Deswal A, Petersen NJ, Feldman AM, et al. Cytokines and cytokine receptors in advanced heart failure: an analysis of the cytokine database from the Vesnarinone Trial (VEST). *Circulation.* 2001;103:2055–2059.
60. Benedict CR, Weiner DH, Johnstone DE, et al. Comparative neurohormonal responses in patients with preserved and impaired left ventricular ejection fraction: results of the studies of left ventricular dysfunction (SOLVD) registry. *J Am Coll Cardiol.* 1993;22:146A–53A.
61. Benedict CR, Johnstone DE, Weiner DH, et al. Relation of neurohormonal activation to clinical variables and degree of ventricular dysfunction: a report from the registry of studies of left ventricular dysfunction. *J Am Coll Cardiol.* 1994; 23: 1410–1420.
62. Cohn JN, Levine TB, Olivari MT, et al. Plasma norepinephrine as a guide to prognosis in patients with chronic congestive heart failure. *N Engl J Med.* 1984;311:819–823.
63. Ferrari R, Bachetti T, Confortini R, et al. Tumor necrosis factor soluble receptors in patients with various degrees of congestive failure. *Circulation.* 1995;92:1479–1486.
64. Rauchhaus M, Doehner W, Francis DP, et al. Plasma cytokine parameters and mortality in patients with chronic heart failure. *Circulation.* 2000;102:3060–3067.
65. Aderka D, Engelmann H, Maor Y, et al. Stabilization of the bioactivity of tumor necrosis factor by its soluble receptors. *J Exp Med.* 1992;175:323–329.
66. Frishman JI, Edwards CK, III, Sonnenberg MG, et al. Tumor necrosis factor (TNF)-alpha-induced interleukin-8 in human blood cultures discriminates neutralization by the p55 and p75 TNF soluble receptors. *J Infect Dis.* 2000;182:1722–1730.
67. Eriksson SV, Kjekshus J, Eneroth P, et al. Neopterin, tumor necrosis factor, C-reactive and prostaglandin E2 in patients with severe congestive heart failure treated with enalapril [abstr]. *Circulation.* 2000;96:I-322.
68. Gullestad L, Aukrust P, Ueland T, et al. Effect of high- versus low-dose angiotensin converting enzyme inhibition on cytokine levels in chronic heart failure. *J Am Coll Cardiol.* 1999;34: 2061–2067.
69. Gurlek A, Kilickap M, Dincer I, et al. Effect of losartan on circulating TNFalpha levels and left ventricular systolic performance in patients with heart failure. *J Cardiovasc Risk.* 2001;8:279–282.
70. Prabhu SD, Chandrasekar B, Murray DR, et al. beta-adrenergic blockade in developing heart failure: effects on myocardial inflammatory cytokines, nitric oxide, and remodeling. *Circulation* 2000;101:2103–2109.
71. MERIT-HF Study Group. Effect of metoprolol CR/XL in chronic heart failure: Metoprolol CR/XL Randomised Intervention Trial in Congestive Heart Failure (MERIT-HF). *Lancet.* 1999;353: 2001–2007.
72. Gullestad L, Ueland T, Brunsvig A, et al. Effect of metoprolol on cytokine levels in chronic heart failure—a substudy in the Metoprolol Controlled-Release Randomised Intervention Trial in Heart Failure (MERIT-HF). *Am Heart J.* 2001;141:418–421.
73. Tsutamoto T, Wada A, Matsumoto T, et al. Relationship between tumor necrosis factor-alpha production and oxidative stress in the failing hearts of patients with dilated cardiomyopathy. *J Am Coll Cardiol.* 2001;37:2086–2092.
74. Zabel P, Schade FU, Schlaak M. Inhibition of endogenous TNF formation by pentoxifylline. *Immunbiol.* 1993;187:447–463.
75. Zabel P, Greinert U, Entzian P, et al. Effects of pentoxifylline on circulating cytokines (TNF and IL- 6) in severe pulmonary tuberculosis. In: Fiers W, Buurman WA, eds. *Tumor Necrosis Factor: Molecular and Cellular Biology and Clinical Relevance.* Basel: S. Karger; 1993: 178–181.
76. Dezube BJ, Pardee AB, Chapman B, et al. Pentoxifylline decreases tumor necrosis factor expression and serum triglycerides in people with AIDS. *J Acq Immun Defic Syndrome.* 1993;6:787–794.
77. Giroir BP, Beutler B. Effect of amrinone on tumor necrosis factor production in endotoxin shock. *Circ Shock.* 1992;36:200–207.
78. Sindhwani R, Yuen J, Hirsch H, et al. Reversal of low flow state attenuates immune activation in severe decompensated congestive heart failure [abstr]. *Circulation* 1993;88:I-255.
79. Deng MC, Erren M, Lutgen A, et al. Interleukin-6 correlates with hemodynamic impairment during dobutamine administration in chronic heart failure. *Int J Cardiol.* 1996;57:129–134.
80. Wagner DR, Combes A, McTiernan CF, et al. Adenosine inhibitis lipopolysaccharide-induced cardiac expression of tumor necrosis factor-α. *Circ Res.* 1998;82:47–56.
81. Sliwa K, Skudicky D, Candy G, et al. Randomized investigation of effects of pentoxifylline on left ventricular performance in idiopathic dilated cardiomyopathy. *Lancet* 1998;351:1091–1093.
82. Meldrum DR, Cain BS, Cleveland JC, Jr., et al. Adenosine decreases post-ischemic cardiac TNFα production: anti-inflammatory implications for preconditioning and transplantation. *Immunology* 1997;92:472–477.
83. Sliwa K, Woodiwiss A, Candy G, et al. Effects of pentoxifylline on cytokine profiles and left ventricular performance in patients with decompensated congestive heart failure secondary to idiopathic dilated cardiomyopathy. *Am J Cardiol.* 2002;90:1118–1122.
84. Sliwa K, Skudicky D, Bergemann A, et al. Peripartum cardiomyopathy: analysis of clinical outcome, left ventricular function, plasma levels of cytokines and Fas/APO-1. *J Am Coll Cardiol.* 2000;35:701–705.
85. Sliwa K, Woodiwiss A, Kone VN, et al. Therapy of ischemic cardiomyopathy with the immunomodulating agent pentoxifylline: results of a randomized study. *Circulation.* 2004;109:750–755.
86. Sampaio EP, Sarno EN, Galilly R, et al. Thalidomide selectively inhibits tumor necrosis factor α production by stimulated human monocytes. *J Exp Med.* 1991;173:699–703.
87. Moreira AL, Sampaio EP, Zmuidzinas A, et al. Thalidomide exerts its inhibitory action on tumor necrosis factor-alpha by enhancing messenger RNA degradation. *J Exp Med.* 1993;177:1675–1680.
88. Agoston I, Dibbs ZI, Wang F, et al. Preclinical and clinical assessment of the safety and potential efficacy of thalidomide in heart failure. *J Card Fail.* 2002;8:306–314.
89. Gullestad L, Semb AG, Holt E, et al. Effect of thalidomide in patients with chronic heart failure. *Am Heart J.* 2002;144:847–850.
90. Remick DG, Strieter RM, Lynch IJP, et al. In vivo dynamics of murine tumor necrosis factor-α gene expression. Kinetics of dexamethasone-induced suppression. *Lab Invest.* 1989;60: 766–771.
91. Parrillo JE, Cunnion RE, Epstein SE, et al. A prospective randomized controlled trial of prednisone for dilated cardiomyopathy. *N Engl J Med.* 1989;321:1061–1068.
92. Kapadia S, Torre-Amione G, Yokoyama T, et al. Soluble tumor necrosis factor binding proteins modulate the negative inotropic effects of TNF-α in vitro. *Am J Physiol.* 1995;37: H517–H525.
93. Deswal A, Bozkurt B, Seta Y, et al. A phase I trial of tumor necrosis factor receptor (p75) fusion protein (TNFR:Fc) in patients with advanced heart failure. *Circulation.* 1999;99: 3224–3226.
94. Bozkurt B, Torre-Amione G, Warren MS, et al. Results of targeted ant-tumor necrosis factor therapy with etanercept (ENBREL) in patients with advanced heart failure. *Circulation.* 2001;103: 1044–1047.
95. Packer M. Proposal for a new clinical end point to evaluate the efficacy of drugs and devices in the treatment of chronic heart failure. *J Card Fail.* 2001;7:176–182.
96. Mann DL, McMurray JJV, Packer M, et al. Targeted anti-cytokine therapy in patients with chronic heart failure: results of the Randomized EtaNcercept Worldwide evALuation (RENEWAL). *Circulation.* 2004;109:1594–1602.
97. Chung ES, Packer M, Lo KH, et al. Randomized, double-blind, placebo-controlled, pilot trial of infliximab, a chimeric monoclonal antibody to tumor necrosis factor-α, in patients with moderate-to-severe heart failure: results of the Anti-TNF Therapy Against Congestive Heart failure (ATTACH) trial. *Circulation.* 2003;107:3133–3140.
98. Torre-Amione G, Kapadia S, Lee J, et al. Tumor necrosis factor-α and tumor necrosis factor receptors in the failing human heart. *Circulation.* 1996;93:704–711.
99. Homeister JW, Lucchesi BR. Complement activation and inhibition in myocardial ischemia and reperfusion injury. *Ann Rev Pharmacol Toxicol.* 1994;34:17–40.
100. Clark MA, Plank LD, Connolly AB, et al. Effect of a chimeric antibody to tumor necrosis factor-alpha on cytokine and physiologic responses in patients with severe sepsis—a randomized, clinical trial. *Crit Care Med.* 1998;26:1650–1659.
101. Klein B, Brailly H. Cytokine-binding proteins: stimulating antagonists. *Immunol Today.* 1995;16:216–220.

102. Suffredini AF, Reda D, Banks SM. Effects of recombinant dimeric TNF receptor on human inflammatory responses following intravenous endotoxin administration. *J Immunol.* 1995;155:5038–5045.
103. Maury CP, Teppo AM. Cachectin/tumour necrosis factor-alpha in the circulation of patients with rheumatic disease. *Int J Tissue React.* 1989;11:189–193.
104. Lecour S, Smith RM, Woodward B, et al. Identification of a novel role for sphingolipid signaling in TNF alpha and ischemic preconditioning mediated cardioprotection. *J Mol Cell Cardiol.* 2002;34:509–518.
105. Samuelsson A, Towers TL, Ravetch JV. Anti-inflammatory activity of IVIG mediated through the inhibitory Fc receptor. *Science.* 2001;291:484–486.
106. McNamara DM, Holubkov R, Starling RC, et al. Controlled trial of intravenous immune globulin in recent-onset dilated cardiomyopathy. *Circulation.* 2001;103:2254–2259.
107. Gullestad L, Aass H, Fjeld JG, et al. Immunomodulating therapy with intravenous immunoglobulin in patients with chronic heart failure. *Circulation.* 2001;103:220–225.
108. Fadok VA, Bratton DL, Konowal A, et al. Macrophages that have ingested apoptotic cells in vitro inhibit proinflammatory cytokine production through autocrine/paracrine mechanisms involving TGF-beta, PGE2, and PAF. *J Clin Invest.* 1998;101:890–898.
109. Voll RE, Herrmann M, Roth EA, et al. Immunosuppressive effects of apoptotic cells. *Nature.* 1997;390:350–351.
110. Babaei S, Stewart DJ, Picard P, et al. Effects of VasoCare therapy on the initiation and progression of atherosclerosis. *Atherosclerosis.* 2002;162:45–53.
111. Torre-Amione G, Sestier F, Radovancevic B, et al. Effects of a novel immune modulation therapy in patients with advanced chronic heart failure: results of a randomized, controlled, phase II trial. *J Am Coll Cardiol.* 2004;44:1181–1186.
112. Kjekshus J, Pedersen TR, Olsson AG, et al. The effects of simvastatin on the incidence of heart failure in patients with coronary heart disease. *J Card Fail.* 1997;3:249–254.
113. Aronow WS, Ahn C. Frequency of congestive heart failure in older persons with prior myocardial infarction and serum low-density lipoprotein cholesterol ≥125 mg/dl treated with statins versus no lipid-lowering drug. *Am J Cardiol.* 2002;90:147–149.
114. Horwich TB, MacLellan WR, Fonarow GC. Statin therapy is associated with improved survival in ischemic and non-ischemic heart failure. *J Am Coll Cardiol.* 2004;43:642–648.
115. Kalra D, Sivasubramanian N, Mann DL. Angiotensin II induces tumor necrosis factor biosynthesis in the adult mammalian heart through a protein kinase C-dependent pathway. *Circulation.* 2002;105:2198–2205.
116. Scallon BJ, Moore MA, Trinh H, et al. Chimeric anti-TNF-alpha monoclonal antibody cA2 binds recombinant transmembrane TNF-alpha and activates immune effector functions. *Cytokine.* 1995;7:251–259.
117. Weinberger SR, Morris TS, Pawlak M. Recent trends in protein biochip technology. *Pharmacogenomics.* 2000;1:395–416.
118. Node K, Fujita M, kitakaze M, et al. Short-term statin therapy improves cardiac function and symptoms in patients with idiopathic dilated cardiomyopathy. *Circulation.* 2003;108: 839–843.

14

The Peripheral Circulation in Heart Failure

Anju Nohria   *Mark A. Creager*

The development and progression of myocardial failure are heralded by the activation of circulating neurohormonal systems that modulate both vascular tone and renal retention of salt and water. The peripheral circulation undergoes local changes in response to heart failure that are fundamental to the pathophysiology of this disease state. The fractional distribution of blood flow to the kidneys, limbs, and splanchnic beds decreases, whereas blood flow to the heart and brain is preserved (1,2). The diminished exercise capacity of limb muscles in patients with heart failure may be due in part to chronically diminished nutritive perfusion (3,4). Renal hypoperfusion and altered intrarenal hemodynamics may contribute to sodium and water retention (5,6). Previous chapters have focused on the mechanisms underlying systemic activation of the sympathetic nervous system, the renin-angiotensin system, as well as other circulatory neurohormones, such as arginine vasopressin and natriuretic peptides. In this chapter we will examine the structural and functional changes that occur in the peripheral vasculature. Specifically, this chapter will focus on local vasodilator and vasoconstrictor mechanisms that are mediated by the endothelium, by tissue production of angiotensin II, and by adrenergic and vasopressinergic receptors. The vascular effects of endogenous vasodilators, including the natriuretic peptides and adrenomedullin, will be discussed as well.

ENDOTHELIAL MECHANISMS IN HEART FAILURE

The response of large arteries and arterioles to both physiological and pharmacological stimuli is influenced by the presence of an intact endothelium. Vascular endothelial cells have been shown to synthesize endogenous vasodilators (e.g., nitric oxide and prostacyclin) as well as vasoconstrictors (e.g., endothelin and vasoconstrictor prostanoids). Regulation of endothelium-derived vasodilation and constriction may be altered in heart failure and contribute to the vasoconstricted state (Table 14-1). The data supporting this contention are reviewed next.

Nitric Oxide

Furchgott and Zawadzki initially demonstrated that relaxation of vascular rings in response to acetylcholine was dependent on an intact endothelium and was abolished by removal of the endothelium (7). This relaxation is due to the release of an endogenous substance called nitric oxide (8–10). Nitric oxide elicits vascular smooth muscle dilation by activating soluble guanylyl cyclase, thereby increasing intracellular levels of cyclic guanosine monophosphate (cGMP).

Nitric oxide is the most potent endogenous vasodilator yet identified and contributes to the regulation of basal vascular tone. Nitric oxide is synthesized by nitric oxide synthase from the amino acid, L-arginine (11,12) in response to a wide variety of stimuli (Fig. 14-1). A number of vasoconstrictors, such as norepinephrine, vasopressin, thrombin, and endothelin, interact with specific receptors on the endothelial surface to induce the release of nitric oxide, thus modulating the direct vasoconstrictor effect of these substances. Aggregating platelets also release vasoactive substances (e.g., adenosine diphosphate and serotonin) that stimulate nitric oxide production and thereby prevent further platelet aggregation. Thus, in the presence of an intact endothelium, nitric oxide counterbalances the deleterious effects

TABLE 14-1
EFFECTS OF ENDOGENOUS VASOACTIVE SUBSTANCES IN HEART FAILURE

Vasoactive Factor	Action	Alteration in Heart Failure	Stimulus for Production/Release
Nitric oxide	Mediator of endothelium-dependent vasodilation	Bioavailability is reduced	Sheer stress, exercise, arterial occlusion, acetylcholine
Prostaglandin	Vasodilation, likely counterbalancing endogenous vasoconstrictors	Increased circulating metabolites in some patients	Possibly regional hypoperfusion, angiotensin, vasopressin, norepinephrine
Endothelin-1	Vasoconstriction, autocoid modulation of vascular tone, increases contractility, vascular smooth-muscle cell proliferation	Increased production, decreased clearance	Catecholamines, angiotensin II, vasopressin
Angiotensin II	Vasoconstriction, vascular smooth muscle cell proliferation, decreased arterial compliance, may facilitate release of NE, promotes superoxide anion generation	Increased circulating levels, increased local tissue and vascular levels	Low renal perfusion pressure, increased sympathetic activity, diuretics, decreased distal tubule Na^+ load
Arginine vasopressin	Vasoconstriction (V_1 receptor), fluid retention (V_2 receptor), indirect vasodilator effects	Increased circulating levels in a subset of patients	Increased osmolality, unloading baroreceptors, angiotensin II
Atrial natriuretic peptide	Endothelium-independent vascular smooth-muscle cell relaxation, natriuresis, renin inhibition	Increased plasma levels, possibly decreased receptor number or sensitivity, increased local clearance, or receptor uncoupling	Elevated venous filling pressures, possibly endothelin-1
Brain natriuretic peptide	Vasodilation, natriuresis, renin inhibition	Increased plasma levels, possibly receptor downregulation and uncoupling	Elevated venous pressures, possibly ventricular wall tension, ischemia, and necrosis
C-type natriuretic peptide	Vasodilation	Increased plasma levels, increased endothelial production	ANP, BNP, hypoxia, inflammation
Adrenomedullin	Vasodilation (nitric oxide-dependent), natriuresis, may increase ANP and BNP, and decrease aldosterone	Increased plasma levels, increased ventricular levels	Angiotensin II, endothelin-1

NE, norepinephrine.

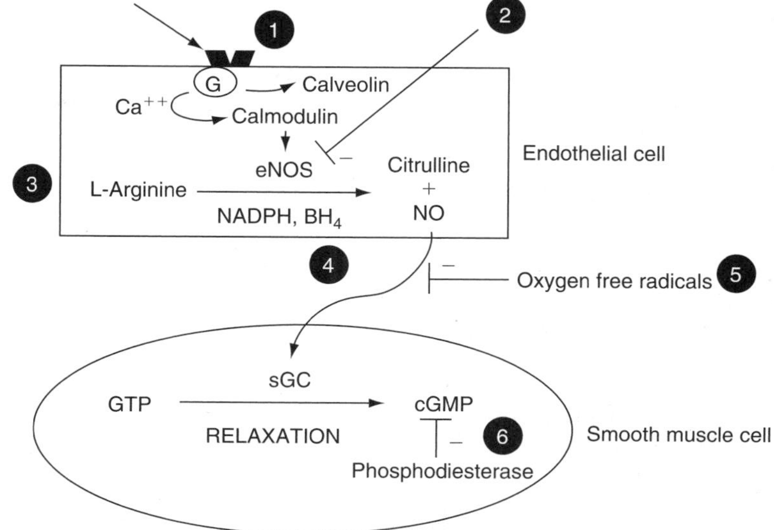

Figure 14-1 Endothelial cell production of nitric oxide (NO) and the potential mechanisms for endothelial dysfunction in heart failure. Stimulation of endothelial cells leads to an increase in intracellular calcium (Ca^{2+}), displacing calveolin from calmodulin, activating endothelial nitric oxide synthase (eNOS). eNOS synthesizes NO from L-arginine in the presence of several cofactors, including NADPH and tetrahydrobiopterin (BH_4). NO diffuses to the underlying vascular smooth muscle and causes vasodilation by activating soluble guanylate cyclase (sGC), thereby increasing intracellular cyclic guanosine monophosphate (cGMP). Heart failure reduces the bioavailability of NO by several potential mechanisms: **(1)** uncoupling of endothelial receptors from associated G-proteins needed for signal transduction; **(2)** decreasing synthesis and activity of eNOS; **(3)** reducing substrate availability for the synthesis of NO; **(4)** reducing cofactors necessary for the activity of eNOS; **(5)** degradation of NO by oxygen free radicals; and **(6)** inactivation of cGMP by increased phosphodiesterase activity.

of vasoconstrictive and thrombogenic stimuli. However, after endothelial cell injury, the predominant effects of these stimuli are mediated by their receptors on vascular smooth muscle, activation of which causes vasoconstriction (13–15). Thus, alterations in the bioavailability of nitric oxide in disease states might lead to increased vascular resistance and may be associated with changes in vascular structure and increased thrombosis.

Nitric Oxide in Heart Failure

Endothelium-dependent vasodilation is attenuated in animal models of heart failure. Vasodilator responses to acetylcholine, but not to nitroglycerin, are diminished in the peripheral and coronary arteries of dogs with pacing-induced heart failure (16,17). Moreover, inhibition of basal nitric oxide biosynthesis by the administration of L-N mono methyl arginine (L-NMMA), an inhibitor of nitric oxide synthase, results in a marked increase in mean arterial pressure in conscious healthy dogs but not in dogs with pacing-induced heart failure (18). These results suggest that basal release of nitric oxide is reduced in this model of heart failure.

A number of studies have shown that endothelium-dependent vasodilation is also abnormal in humans with heart failure. Acetylcholine-mediated coronary vasodilation is diminished in patients with idiopathic dilated cardiomyopathy (19). Several groups of investigators have also evaluated the responsiveness of the forearm circulation to endothelium-dependent and endothelium-independent vasodilators (20–22). The increase in forearm blood flow during intrabrachial artery infusion of acetylcholine and methacholine, both endothelium-dependent vasodilators, is blunted in patients with heart failure, whereas forearm vascular responsiveness to the endothelium-independent vasodilator, nitroprusside, is preserved (Fig. 14-2). Acetylcholine-induced changes in brachial artery diameter, a measure of peripheral conduit vessel dilation, are also abnormal in patients with heart failure (20). The blunted forearm blood flow response to acetylcholine is not associated with duration of symptoms or abnormal hemodynamic indexes; rather, it correlates with maximal oxygen consumption at peak exercise (23). Hence, it is not surprising that endothelial dysfunction is an early predictor of mortality in patients with heart failure (24,25).

The exact mechanism contributing to the decreased bioavailability of nitric oxide in patients with heart failure remains unclear. Decreased production of nitric oxide might contribute to endothelial dysfunction in heart failure (Fig. 14-1). Endothelial cells produce nitric oxide from L-arginine via nitric oxide synthase. It has been suggested that a reduction in the expression of cationic amino acid transporters and thus arginine transport by endothelial cells may lead to a relative deficiency of intracellular arginine, affecting nitric oxide synthesis (26). This may provide one explanation for impaired nitric oxide synthesis and for the beneficial response to acetylcholine seen after the intravenous (27) and oral administration of L-arginine in patients with heart failure (28). A decrease in the bioavailability of tetrahydrobiopterin, an essential cofactor of nitric

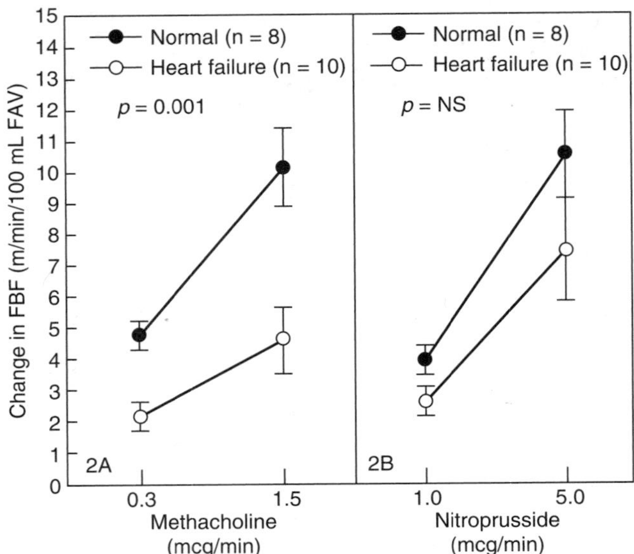

Figure 14-2 The vascular effects of intrabrachial infusion of an endothelium-dependent vasodilator (methacholine) and an endothelium-independent vasodilator (nitroprusside) in normal subjects and in patients with heart failure. The methacholine dose response was blunted in patients with heart failure **(left panel)**; in contrast, the nitroprusside dose response was not significantly decreased in heart failure patients. FBF, forearm blood flow. (Adapted from Kubo SH, Rector TS, Bank AJ, et al. Endothelium-dependent vasodilation is attenuated in patients with heart failure. *Circulation.* 1991;84:1589–1596.)

oxide synthase, may also contribute to decreased nitric oxide production since infusion of tetrahydrobiopterin improves acetylcholine mediated forearm vasodilation in patients with heart failure (29). Conversely, increased degradation of nitric oxide or its downstream effectors might also contribute to endothelial dysfunction in heart failure (Fig. 14-1). Increased oxidative stress and nitric oxide inactivation by superoxide anions have been proposed as an additional mechanisms contributing to endothelial dysfunction in heart failure.

The three enzyme systems responsible for free radical production within the vessel wall include nicotinamide adenine dinucleotide/nicotinamide adenine dinucleotide phosphate (NADH/NADPH) oxidase, xanthine oxidoreductase, and endothelial nitric oxide synthase (30). Strategies aimed at preventing superoxide anion formation, such as inhibition of NADPH oxidase by statins (31) and xanthine oxidoreductase by allopurinol (32,33), have been shown to improve the forearm blood flow response to acetylcholine in patients with heart failure. Furthermore, neutralization of the harmful effects of superoxide anions by the antioxidant vitamin C improves flow-dependent vasodilation in chronic heart failure (34). Exercise training improves endothelial function and is associated with a 100% increase in the transcript levels of genes encoding the antioxidant enzymes, copper zinc superoxide dismutase and glutathione peroxidase (35). Reduction in oxidant stress may be one mechanism to explain the improvement in endothelial function associated with exercise training in patients with heart failure (36).

Nitric oxide mediates its effects via cGMP. Increased degradation of cGMP by phosphodiestereases, in particular type 5 phosphodiesterase, might also lead to increased vasoconstriction in heart failure. Inhibition of type 5 phosphodiesterase with sildenafil has also been shown to increase flow-mediated, endothelium-dependent vasodilation in patients with heart failure (37). The relative contribution of these potential mechanisms for decreased nitric oxide bioavailability in heart failure remains unclear.

Many patients with heart failure have other coexisting diseases, such as atherosclerosis. It is well-established that endothelium-dependent vasodilation is abnormal in atherosclerotic vessels (38). Endothelial function is impaired in animals and humans with risk factors for atherosclerosis, such as hypercholesterolemia, hypertension, hyperhomocysteinemia, and diabetes, even in vessels without overt atherosclerotic lesions (39). Therefore, it is conceivable that abnormalities in endothelium-dependent vasodilation in some patients with heart failure reflect the presence of these other disease states, in addition to the effect of heart failure alone.

Prostaglandins

Endothelial cells synthesize the vasodilator prostaglandins E_2 and I_2 (PGE_2 and PGI_2) from arachidonic acid. Increased systemic levels of vasodilator prostaglandins are observed in patients with heart failure. In patients with severe left ventricular dysfunction, the prostaglandin metabolites of PGE_2 and PGI_2 are three- to tenfold higher than levels measured in normal subjects (40). The mechanisms underlying increased prostaglandin levels in heart failure are not known. Local synthesis of vasoactive prostanoids is increased by hypoperfusion of regional vascular beds (e.g., the renal and coronary circulations [41,42] and production of prostaglandins may directly be stimulated by vasoconstrictor hormones, such as angiotensin, vasopressin, and norepinephrine [43–45]). The concentration of prostanoids is not increased in all patients, but levels of these vasodilator prostaglandins correlate directly with the concentrations of angiotensin II and plasma renin activity. Thus, it appears that synthesis of prostaglandins by blood vessels counterbalances vasoconstrictor mechanisms in heart failure.

The contribution of local vasodilator prostaglandins to vascular resistance has important clinical implications. Prostaglandin-synthetase inhibition in patients with heart failure causes a decline in cardiac output and an increase in pulmonary capillary wedge pressure, particularly in those subjects with the greatest activation of circulating vasoconstrictor hormones (40). Additionally, some pharmacological agents produce their beneficial effects in part by increasing the production of endogenous vasodilator prostaglandins. The vasodilation induced by captopril, nitroglycerin, nitroprusside, and hydralazine is attenuated by pretreatment with indomethacin (46–48). In addition to its effects on angiotensin, captopril inhibits the breakdown of bradykinin by kininase II. Bradykinin may be an important contributor to the short-term vasodilatory effect of captopril (49), potentially by stimulating release of prostacyclin (50). Acetylsalicylic acid, another inhibitor of cyclooxygenase, has been found to blunt the augmentation in endothelium-dependent vasodilation induced by enalaprilat in patients with mild heart failure, highlighting the contribution of prostaglandins to the peripheral vascular effects of angiotensin-converting enzyme (ACE) inhibitors in this population (51,52).

Endothelin

The endothelium also produces potent vasoconstrictor substances. Yanagisawa et al. identified the endothelium-derived vasoconstrictor, endothelin, in 1988 (53). Endothelin, a 21-amino acid peptide hormone, is the most potent endogenous vasoconstrictor substance identified to date. Endothelin is synthesized from its messenger RNA (mRNA) in endothelial cells as a pre-propeptide and is cleaved to big endothelin by an endogenous endopeptidase. Mature endothelin is then produced by an endothelin-specific converting enzyme, which is present in the lung and in other endothelial cells (54). Many of the same stimuli that increase release of nitric oxide (including shear stress, epinephrine, thrombin, angiotensin II, arginine vasopressin, and calcium ionophore) also increase transcription of the pre-proendothelin mRNA and increase release of endothelin (53,55–58).

Three isoforms of endothelin have been identified and sequenced: endothelin-1 (ET-1), ET-2, and ET-3. The ET-1 isoform is most widely associated with cardiovascular regulation. ET-1 acts through the endothelin A (ET_A) and endothelin B (ET_B) receptor subtypes. The ET_A receptor, found on vascular smooth muscle cells, mediates vasoconstriction as well as smooth muscle cell proliferation (53,59) (Fig. 14-3). ET_B is present on both vascular smooth muscle cells and endothelial cells, where it mediates ET-1-induced vasoconstriction and vasodilation, respectively (60,61) (Fig. 14-3).

Endothelin binds to these specific receptors and activates several intracellular signal transduction systems via guanosine triphosphate (GTP)-binding proteins. Endothelin stimulates phospholipase C (PLC) and opens voltage-dependent calcium channels. Activation of PLC degrades phosphoinositide to form inositol triphosphate (IP_3) and diacylglycerol. IP_3 releases calcium from intracellular stores, and diacylglycerol sensitizes contractile proteins via protein kinase C (62–65). Endothelin may also promote vasoconstriction by upregulation of the endogenous nitric oxide synthase inhibitor, asymmetric dimethylarginine, thus reducing nitric oxide synthesis (66). Endothelin also stimulates phospholipase A_2 to produce several vasoconstrictor prostanoids (62,64). The effects of endothelin are most prominent in adjacent vascular regions and, thus, endothelin serves as an autocoid modulator of arteriolar resistance.

The vascular effects of endothelin are complex and potentially clinically important. During exogenous infusion of endothelin there is an initial, brief vasodilation followed by prolonged vasoconstriction (60,61,67–69). Infusion of exogenous endothelin into normal animals increases systemic vascular resistance and consequently reduces cardiac output via cardiac and associated peripheral vascular effects (67,68,70). Chronic exposure of vascular smooth muscle cells to endothelin has been shown to cause proliferation in vitro (71–73). Like peptide growth factors, endothelin mediates cellular growth via tyrosine kinases and mitogen-activated protein kinase pathways (74).

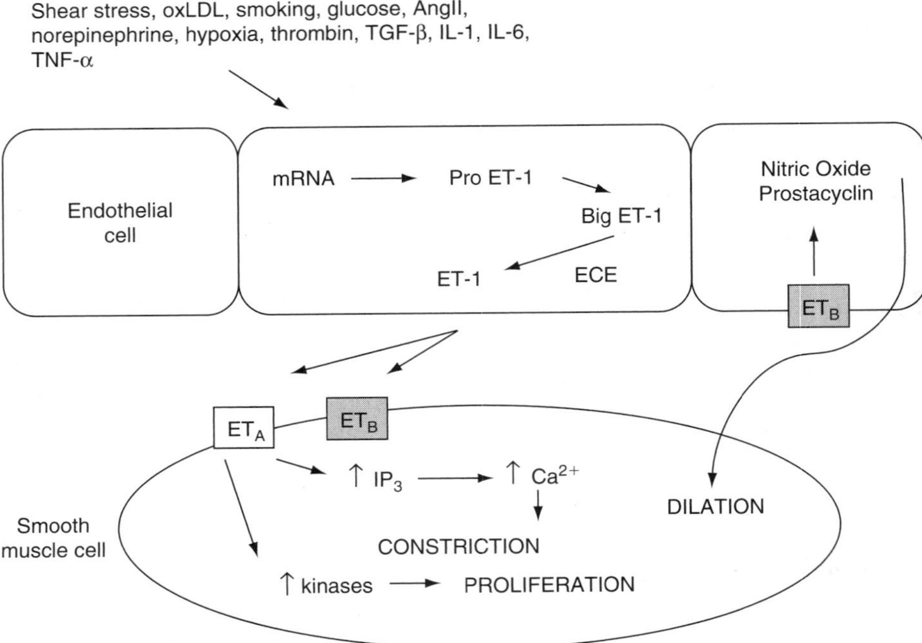

Figure 14-3 Synthesis and effects of endothelin. In response to several stimuli, endothelin (ET-1) is synthesized from its messenger RNA (mRNA) as a prepropeptide (pro ET-1) and is cleaved to big endothelin (Big ET-1) by an endogenous endopeptidase. Mature ET-1 is then produced by endothelin converting enzyme (ECE). ET-1 acts on endothelin A (ET_A) receptors on vascular smooth muscle cells to activate phospholipase C that degrades phosphoinositide to form inositol triphosphate (IP_3) and diacylglycerol. IP_3 releases calcium (Ca^{2+}) from intracellular stores to cause contraction. ET-1 also activates (ET_A) receptors to mediate cellular growth via tyrosine kinase and mitogen-activated protein kinase pathways. ET-1 also activates the endothelin B (ET_B) receptor present on vascular smooth muscle cells to mediate vasoconstriction. However, the ET_B receptor on endothelial cells promotes the release of nitric oxide (NO) and stimulates phospholipase A_2 to produce prostanoids that mediate vasodilation.

Endothelin in Heart Failure

A two- to threefold increase in plasma concentrations of endothelin has been observed in experimental heart failure induced by rapid ventricular pacing in the dog (75,76). Elevations in plasma endothelin concentration also occur in humans with stable or decompensated heart failure (76–80).

Plasma endothelin levels may be increased in heart failure by several mechanisms. Catecholamines, angiotensin II, and arginine vasopressin stimulate endothelin synthesis (53,56,81) and endothelin clearance also is decreased in heart failure. The pathophysiological significance of increased plasma endothelin levels has become more apparent with the advent of endothelin receptor antagonists. In a rat model of post-myocardial infarction heart failure, both ET_A and combined $ET_{A/B}$ receptor antagonism improved acetylcholine-mediated vasodilation and reduced superoxide anion formation (82) (Fig. 14-4). Similarly, treatment with the ET_A receptor blocker, LU135252, improved flow-mediated vasodilation in the brachial artery of humans with heart failure (83). Blockade of endogenous endothelin with a short-term infusion of the nonselective antagonist, bosentan, lowered ventricular filling pressures and systemic vascular resistance in patients with heart failure (84). However, the promise of both specific and combined endothelin receptor antagonists has not been realized in large clinical trials, suggesting that the effects and importance of the two endothelin receptors are poorly understood (85–87) (Table 14-2).

RENIN-ANGIOTENSIN SYSTEM

The role of the circulating renin-angiotensin system in the maintenance of cardiovascular homeostasis has been defined by use of specific antagonists. Antirenin antibodies (88), angiotensin II antagonists (89), and ACE inhibitors (90) have all been used in this context. Studies with these agents have demonstrated that acute hemodynamic responses correlate with pretreatment plasma renin-angiotensin system activity, and are most profound in individuals with high plasma renin activity and angiotensin II concentrations. In contrast, chronic responses to these agents are not predicted by plasma renin-angiotensin system activity. Indeed, ACE inhibition is also effective in heart failure patients with normal plasma renin activity (91,92). Therefore, circulating angiotensin II may not account wholly for angiotensin II-mediated vasoconstriction in heart failure.

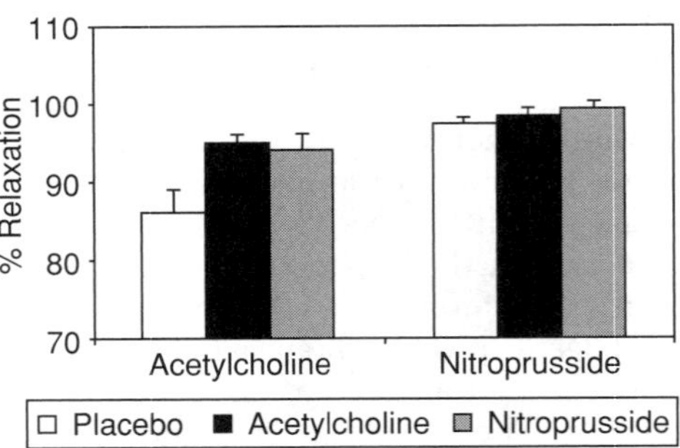

Figure 14-4 Acetylcholine (endothelium-dependent)– and nitroprusside (endothelium-independent)– induced relaxation of phenylephrine preconstricted aortic rings from rats with heart failure after myocardial infarction. Both the endothelin A specific receptor antagonist, LU135252, and the nonspecific endothelin A and B receptor antagonist, bosentan, improved acetylcholine-mediated relaxation relative to placebo. These data suggest that endothelin antagonists improve nitric oxide bioavailability in blood vessels from animal models of heart failure. (Adapted from Bauersachs J, Fraccarollo D, Galuppo P, et al. Endothelin-receptor blockade improves endothelial vasomotor dysfunction in heart failure. *Cardiovasc Res.* 2000;47:142–149.)

TABLE 14-2
SELECTED RANDOMIZED CLINICAL TRIALS OF ENDOTHELIN ANTAGONISTS IN HEART FAILURE

Study	Agent	ET-1 Receptor Selectivity	Patients	Primary Outcome	Results
RITZ-5 (87)	Tezosentan	Nonselective	Acute HF O_2 sat <90%	Δ in O_2 sat @ 1 h	NS
ENABLE (86)	Bosentan	Nonselective	Chronic HF EF <35% NYHA IIIB/IV	HF hospitalization and death @ 9 mo	NS
EARTH (85)	Darusentan	ET_A selective	Chronic HF EF <35% NYHA II-IV	Δ in LVESV @ 24 wk	NS

ET-1, endothelin; HF, heart failure; EF, ejection fraction; NYHA, New York Heart Association functional class; LVESV, left ventricular end systolic volume; NS, no significant difference between treatment and placebo

Endogenous renin-angiotensin systems have been demonstrated in tissues that are important in cardiovascular regulation (e.g., blood vessels, heart, kidney, brain, and adrenal tissues). The evidence supporting the existence and physiological role of vascular and renal renin-angiotensin systems is reviewed below. The possibility that the tissue renin-angiotensin system might contribute to local angiotensin II production has important pathophysiological and therapeutic implications.

The Vascular Renin-Angiotensin System

The presence of renin, angiotensinogen, and angiotensin II in blood vessels has been reported by a number of laboratories (93,94). The vessel wall distribution of renin has been examined by use of antirenin-specific antibody, and intense staining has been noted throughout the thickness of the aorta, large and smaller arteries, as well as arterioles, particularly in endothelial and smooth muscle cells (95). Additionally, kinetic analysis of arterial-venous angiotensin I and angiotensin II differences in humans indicates that both angiotensin I and angiotensin II are synthesized in vascular tissues (96).

The local synthesis of angiotensin II in the blood vessel wall has important physiological implications. Angiotensin II has multiple effects on the cardiovascular system, which include not only vasoconstriction, but also smooth muscle cell proliferation, myocardial hypertrophy, and altered ventricular remodeling (97). Conceptually, local increases in vascular angiotensin II can cause constriction of large arteries and resistance vessels via the angiotensin type I receptor, resulting in increased systemic vascular resistance and reduced arterial compliance. Local angiotensin II also may contribute directly to regional blood flow regulation by activating vascular receptors in specific circulations (e.g., the kidney). Angiotensin II receptors are also found on endothelial cells, and activation can result in release of both nitric oxide (98) and vasoconstrictor prostanoids (99). Angiotensin II also may alter vascular function by facilitating norepinephrine release from local noradrenergic nerve terminals (100). In addition to these mechanisms, there is data suggesting that angiotensin II activates membrane-bound NADH/NADPH-driven oxidases that promote superoxide anion generation in cultured vascular smooth muscle cells (101). Cells exposed to angiotensin II for 4 hours produce two- to sevenfold more superoxide anion than control cells. This increase can be reversed by co-incubation with an angiotensin II receptor antagonist. Angiotensin II-induced, but not norepinephrine-induced, hypertension is associated with impaired vascular response to acetylcholine (102). Treatment with the angiotensin II receptor antagonist, losartan, improves the response to acetylcholine and normalizes vascular superoxide production, implicating the angiotensin type-1 receptor as a mediator in this process. These autocoid mechanisms may affect regional vascular tone, even when circulating levels of angiotensin II are not increased.

Evidence to support the importance of local angiotensin II to arteriolar and conduit artery function is derived from experiments involving ACE inhibition or angiotensin receptor blockade. Local infusion of ACE inhibitors to humans causes limb and coronary vasodilation, indicating that local generation of angiotensin II may contribute to vascular resistance (103). Intra-arterial infusion of quinapril augments the forearm blood flow response to bradykinin. The increase in arterial flow caused by quinapril can be inhibited by L-NMMA, suggesting that this ACE inhibitor may increase vascular nitric oxide, perhaps through a bradykinin-mediated pathway (104). The compliance and diameter of large (brachial and carotid) arteries are increased by ACE inhibition, even at doses that do not reduce blood pressure (105,106). This latter observation suggests that the local vascular renin-angiotensin system activity influences distensibility of these conduit vessels.

The Renal Renin-Angiotensin System

The juxtaglomerular apparatus is capable of releasing large amounts of renin into the circulation. In patients with heart failure, low renal perfusion pressure, decreased distal tubular sodium load, increased sympathetic activity, and diuretic administration all increase systemic levels of renin and angiotensin II. The presence of a locally active renin-angiotensin system in the kidney, in sites other than the juxtaglomerular cells, has been documented using molecular biological, immunocytochemical, and biochemical techniques. Renin has been demonstrated in afferent and efferent arterioles and in the proximal tubule by antirenin antiserum staining (107,108). Cultured glomerular mesangial cells synthesize renin (93). Angiotensinogen mRNA expression in the renal cortex has been demonstrated and in situ hybridization studies have shown that angiotensinogen mRNA is expressed principally in the proximal tubule (109,110), while renin mRNA is primarily localized to the juxtaglomerular cells (110). Intrarenal ACE also has been demonstrated by the presence of ACE mRNA (111). In addition to the vasculature, ACE has been localized to the proximal tubule brush border using immunohistochemical and radioligand binding techniques (112). Because all the components are found in the proximal tubule, local synthesis of angiotensin II has been hypothesized (110). Indeed, a micropuncture study demonstrated that proximal tubular fluid angiotensin II concentration is 1,000-fold greater than in the plasma (113). Local angiotensin II production might be a major factor in regulation of basal renal hemodynamics and sodium reabsorption.

Experimental heart failure causes profound changes in the activity of the intrarenal renin-angiotensin system. In rats with chronic left ventricular dysfunction after experimental myocardial infarction, the renal angiotensinogen mRNA level increases twofold as compared with sham-operated controls (114). The magnitude of increase correlates closely with the histopathological size of the myocardial infarction, implying a relationship with the degree of ventricular dysfunction (114). The effect of heart failure on the kidney renin-angiotensin system appears to be selective for this single component of the renin-angiotensin system because renal renin and ACE activities are unchanged. Chronic ACE inhibition with enalapril normalizes renal angiotensinogen expression to that of sham-operated control rats, suggesting that angiotensin may have a positive feedback role on angiotensinogen expression in the kidney. Treatment with a single oral dose of captopril reverses renal vasoconstriction by improving renal blood flow in patients with heart failure. This is accompanied by a decrease in systemic vascular resistance, increase in cardiac output, and increase in the proportional regional blood flow to the kidney (5).

VASCULAR ADRENERGIC MECHANISMS

In patients with heart failure, sympathetic efferent activity is increased and plasma norepinephrine concentration often is elevated. The mechanisms underlying activation of the sympathetic nervous system are discussed in Chapter 11. The effect of sympathetic nervous system activation on vascular tone is a consequence of the regulation and responsiveness of the adrenergic receptor pathways.

Adrenergic Receptor Pharmacology

There are two categories of α-adrenergic receptors: α_1 and α_2 (115). Three distinct subtypes of α_1 receptors have been identified (116–120). α_{1a}, α_{1b}, and α_{1d} receptors modulate vascular smooth muscle tone (120–122). α_1 receptors activate phospholipase C to promote mobilization of calcium and sensitization of contractile proteins via protein kinase C. Both the density and coupling of α_1-adrenergic receptors in vascular smooth muscle are affected by the adrenergic hormonal milieu. The density of α_1-adrenergic receptors on vascular smooth muscle is decreased in animals chronically exposed to high catecholamine levels (123,124). In cultured rabbit aortic smooth muscle cells, norepinephrine decreases mRNA for the α_1-adrenergic receptor, decreases α_1-adrenergic receptor density, and uncouples the receptor from its intracellular second messenger pathways (125,126). In rabbit aorta, norepinephrine decreases α-adrenergic receptor sensitivity, but not receptor density (127). α_2-adrenergic receptors inhibit neural release of norepinephrine from the presynaptic nerve terminal. Postjunctional vascular α_2-adrenergic receptors mediate vasoconstriction (128). In general, α_2-adrenergic receptors inhibit adenylyl cyclase (129) but in certain instances may stimulate it, perhaps related to differential subtype activation. Three α_2-adrenergic receptor subtypes have been identified (130): α_{2A}, α_{2B} and α_{2C}. Of these, the α_{2A} and α_{2C} receptors are important in inhibiting presynaptic norepinephrine release.

Three subtypes of β-adrenergic receptors have been identified (131,132). β_1-adrenergic receptors, when activated, increase cardiac contractility and heart rate and stimulate lipolysis. β_2-adrenergic receptors are located in the heart, as well as on blood vessels and bronchi. Activation of β_2-adrenergic receptors causes vasodilation and bronchial dilation, and increases cardiac contractility and heart rate. β_2-adrenergic receptors also are present on lymphocytes and pancreatic islet cells. β_3-adrenergic receptors have been isolated and described in adipose cells, liver, muscle, and ileum and may mediate adipose tissue thermogenesis, glycogen synthesis, and ileum relaxation (131). β-adrenergic receptors are membrane-bound proteins that stimulate adenylyl cyclase via GTP-binding proteins. Adenylyl cyclase hydrolyzes adenosine triphosphate (ATP) to cyclic adenosine monophosphate (cAMP). cAMP has selective effects depending on the β-adrenergic receptor subtype. In β_1-adrenergic receptor cell types, an inotropic effect occurs when cAMP binds to protein kinase C, ultimately resulting in an increase in intracellular calcium. In vascular smooth muscle, the increase in cAMP consequent to stimulation of β_2-adrenergic receptors causes vasodilation. This results from the sequestration of intracellular calcium by the sarcoplasmic reticulum, hyperpolarization of the cell due to increased potassium permeability, effects on the myosin light chain, or activation of the electrogenic sodium pump (133).

Both the density and coupling of β-adrenergic receptors can be regulated. Norepinephrine or isoproterenol desensitizes β-adrenergic receptors in cultured tissue, such as rat myocardium and human fibroblasts (134–136). In vivo, chronic administration of norepinephrine uncouples the β-adrenoceptor from its second messengers (137). The regulation of β-adrenergic receptors may be specific for each subtype and dependent on the level of specific agonists (137–141).

Vascular Adrenergic Receptor Function in Heart Failure

Vascular α-adrenergic responsiveness has been studied in experimental models and in humans with heart failure. Studies performed in dogs with heart failure caused by rapid ventricular pacing have yielded different findings. Wilson et al. found no difference in hindlimb vascular responsiveness to intra-arterial norepinephrine between healthy dogs and those with heart failure (142). In contrast, Forster et al. reported that the responses to the α-adrenergic agonists norepinephrine and phenylephrine were increased in the isolated pedal artery of dogs following the development of heart failure, and suggested that the increased responsiveness to these agonists was due to increased responsiveness of the α_1-adrenergic pathway (143). Yet others have reported that the response to phenylephrine is decreased in rats with heart failure induced by coronary ligation compared to sham-operated animals, suggesting downregulation of postsynaptic α_1 adrenoreceptors in heart failure (144). In humans, intra-arterial infusion of phenylephrine, a relatively selective α_1-adrenergic receptor agonist, causes a dose-related increase in forearm vascular resistance that is similar in normal subjects and patients with heart failure (145,146) (Fig. 14-5). Thus, altered α_1-adrenergic vascular responsiveness is not apparent in humans with congestive heart failure.

As previously mentioned, the α_{2A} and α_{2C} adrenoreceptors are important for central and peripheral nervous system inhibition of norepinephrine release from presynaptic nerve terminals. Genetic polymorphisms of these receptors, specifically in-frame deletion of the α_{2C}-adrenoreceptor subtype (alpha2CDel322–325), increases total body norepinephrine spillover (147) and increases the risk of developing congestive heart failure (148). Heart failure patients with this dysfunctional variant of the α_{2C} adrenoceptor have a worse clinical status and decreased cardiac function as determined by invasive catheterization and echocardiography (149). In addition to these genetic polymorphisms that may predispose individuals to the development of heart failure, there is evidence supporting the downregulation of presynaptic α_2-adrenergic receptor activity in humans with heart failure. Intra-arterial infusion of the α_2 agonist, clonidine, decreases norepinephrine spillover in healthy humans but not in patients with heart failure (150). Contrary to animal data that suggest downregulation of postjunctional vascular α_2-adrenergic receptors (151), human studies do not support decreased α_2-adrenergic vascular responsiveness in heart failure. Intra-arterial infusion of the α_2 agonist, clonidine, or the α_2 antagonist, yohimbine, does not alter forearm vascular resistance in patients with heart failure compared to healthy subjects (145,152). Thus, altered α_2-adrenergic vascular responsiveness is not apparent in humans with congestive heart failure.

Changes in ventricular β-adrenoceptor number and sensitivity in animal models of patients with heart failure have been studied extensively and are reviewed in Chapters 11 and 28 (137,139,153–155). Little information is available regarding peripheral vascular β-adrenergic receptors in heart failure. Marzo et al. reported that β_2-adrenergic receptor density is reduced in the hindlimb vessels of dogs with heart failure induced by rapid ventricular pacing (156). Yet, isoproterenol-induced hindlimb vasodilation was similar in the control dogs and the dogs with heart failure. Creager et al. examined β-adrenoceptor–mediated vasodilator function in the forearm resistance vessels of patients with congestive heart failure and normal subjects (157). Intra-arterial isoproterenol adminis-tration to normal subjects and patients with heart failure in- creased forearm blood flow and decreased forearm vascular resistance comparably in each group (Fig. 14-6). Thus, studies in one animal model of heart failure and in humans indicate that peripheral β_2-adrenoceptor–mediated vasodilation is not downregulated. However, like the α_2-adrenergic receptor, the β-adrenoceptor exhibits significant genetic heterogeneity in the population. In particular, carriers of the Ile164 polymorphism of the β_2 receptor have a significantly reduced survival compared to heart failure patients with the wild-type receptor (158). In addition to blunted cardiac responsiveness (159), humans with the Ile164 β_2-receptor genotype have altered vascular responsiveness to the β agonist, isoproterenol. The dose of isoproterenol required to achieve 50% venodilation is significantly higher in healthy individuals with the Ile164 allele than those without this genetic polymorphism (160). Therefore, it is possible that in addition to con-

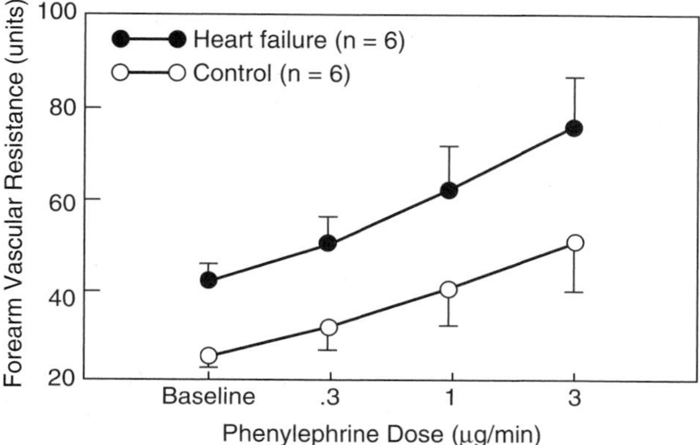

Figure 14-5 The effect of intra-arterial phenylephrine on forearm vascular resistance in normal subjects and patients with congestive heart failure. There was no significant difference in the dose–response curves to the α_1-adrenoceptor agonist between the two groups. (Adapted from Creager MA, Hirsch AT, Dzau VJ, et al. Baroreflex regulation of regional blood flow in congestive heart failure. *Am J Physiol.* 1990;258:H1409–1414.)

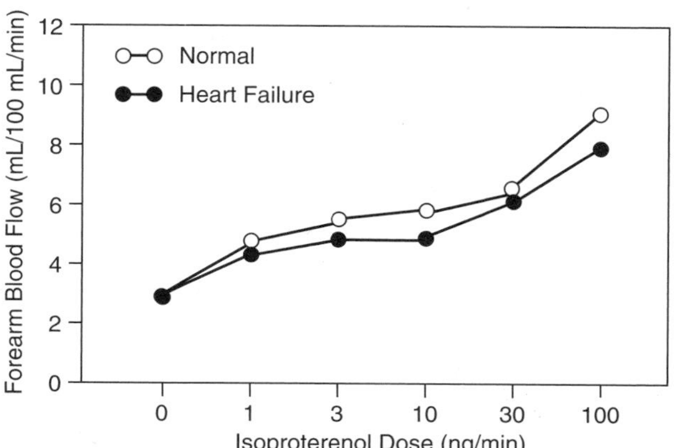

Figure 14-6 The effect of intra-arterial isoproterenol on forearm blood flow in normal subjects and patients with congestive heart failure. There was no significant difference in the dose–response curves to the β-adrenoceptor agonist between the two groups. (Adapted from Creager MA, Quigg RJ, Ren CJ, et al. Limb vascular responsiveness to beta-adrenergic receptor stimulation in patients with congestive heart failure. *Circulation.* 1991;83:1873–1879.)

tributing to contractile dysfunction, the β_2 receptor Ile164 polymorphism may make the peripheral vasculature more prone to vasoconstriction and contribute to the poor prognosis seen in carriers of this mutation.

VASOPRESSIN

Arginine vasopressin is a potent nonapeptide with dual vasopressor and antidiuretic properties. This peptide is synthesized by the hypothalamic magnocellular neurons of the supraoptic and paraventricular nuclei and is released into the circulation by axonal terminals of the posterior pituitary gland. Vasopressin release is modulated in animals and humans by both osmotic and nonosmotic stimuli. Increases in plasma osmolality are sensed by hypothalamic osmoreceptors, and vasopressin is secreted into the circulation. Nonosmotic stimuli that increase vasopressin release include unloading of the cardiopulmonary and arterial baroreceptors, activation of chemoreceptors, and elevated concentration of angiotensin II.

The effects of vasopressin are mediated by V_1 and V_2 receptors. Activation of the V_1 receptor causes vasoconstriction via GTP-binding proteins that activate phospholipase C and produce inositol triphosphate and diacylglycerol. Subsequently, intracellular calcium levels increase. Vasopressin also activates a vascular V_2 receptor and causes direct vasodilation of skeletal muscle (161–163). In addition, vasopressin affects vascular tone indirectly. It sensitizes baroreceptors and causes vasodilation by withdrawing sympathetic activity. Moreover, vasopressin may mediate vasodilation by increasing the synthesis and release of nitric oxide and vasodilator prostaglandins (44,164). Thus, the peripheral vascular effects of vasopressin are complex and include both vasoconstriction and vasodilation.

The renal hydro-osmotic effects of vasopressin are mediated by the V_2 receptor present on the basolateral membrane of principal cells in the collecting duct. Activation of the V_2 receptor leads to translocation of aquaporin-2 water channels from cytoplasmic vescicles to the apical surface of the collecting duct. These channels then allow water molecules to traverse the apical membrane in response to the osmotic gradient generated by the urinary countercurrent mechanism (165).

Vasopressin in Heart Failure

The vasoactive effects of vasopressin may be pertinent to the pathophysiology of heart failure. The availability of pharmacological probes that specifically block vasopressin receptors has permitted investigation of the pressor action of this peptide in pathophysiological states. In dogs with low-output failure caused by tricuspid valve occlusion and pulmonary artery constriction, Stone et al. found that a vasopressin (V_1) receptor antagonist decreased systemic vascular resistance and increased peripheral blood flow (166). In the rat aortocaval fistula model of heart failure, chronic therapy with a V_2-receptor antagonist significantly reduced ventricular filling pressures, while chronic treatment with a V_1-receptor antagonist had no hemodynamic effect (167). High plasma vasopressin concentrations have been demonstrated in some patients with heart failure (168–172). Creager et al. have evaluated the role of endogenous vasopressin in clinical heart failure (171). Administration of a V_1-receptor antagonist caused a decrease in systemic vascular resistance and increase in cardiac output only in those subjects with the highest vasopressin concentrations. Nicod et al. evaluated the role of vasopressin blockade in an additional ten patients with heart failure, similarly demonstrating that V_1-receptor blockade was effective only in the single subject with an elevated baseline plasma vasopressin level (173). In a larger study of 142 patients with symptomatic heart failure, Udelson et al. demonstrated that the combined V_1/ V_2 receptor antagonist, conivaptan, increased urine output and lowered cardiac filling pressures in a dose-dependent fashion without significantly altering systemic vascular resistance or cardiac output (174). Thus, the relative contribution of vascular V_1 and V_2 receptors and the role of vasopressin in modulating vascular tone in heart failure remain unclear.

The aquaretic effects of V_2-receptor antagonists have been evaluated in patients with heart failure. The synthesis and apical translocation of aquaporin-2 water channels is increased in rats with heart failure (165). Treatment of heart failure patients with a V_2-receptor antagonist increased urinary free water excretion and decreased urinary aquaporin-2 excretion, consistent with the notion that vasopressin exerts it antidiuretic effects via the aquaporin-2 water channel (175). The V_2-receptor antagonist, tolvaptan, also increased urine output and decreased body weight, consistent with the water-retentive properties of vasopressin in humans with heart failure (176,177).

NATRIURETIC PEPTIDES

Atrial natriuretic peptide (ANP), brain natriuretic peptide (BNP), and C-type natriuretic peptide (CNP) constitute a family of vasoactive peptides that has important effects on cardiovascular and renal function. In the normal heart, ANP is produced chiefly by atrial myocytes (178), whereas BNP originates from both ventricular and atrial tissue (179). CNP is produced in endothelial cells (180,181) (Fig 14-7). ANP is a 28-amino acid peptide that has vasoactive, natriuretic, and renin-inhibiting activities. BNP, a 32-amino acid peptide, has structural similarities to ANP, including a 17-amino acid ring formed by a disulfide bond, and shares the same biological functions. Both peptides act via the guanylyl cyclase-linked natriuretic peptide A receptor (NPR-A), which has a higher affinity for ANP (Fig. 14-7). CNP carries the same ring structure as ANP and BNP, but lacks a COOH amino acid extension from the ring, and appears not to have natriuretic effects (180). CNP activates the guanylyl cyclase-linked natriuretic peptide B receptor (NPR-B) (Fig. 14-7). ANP and BNP also bind NPR-B, but with lower affinity. Natriuretic peptides are degraded intracellularly via a common receptor, the natriuretic peptide C receptor (NPR-C) (182). Neutral endopeptidase, an enzyme with wide tissue distribution, inactivates all of the natriuretic peptides with a relative affinity for CNP greater than for ANP and BNP. All three peptides are increased in heart failure, but appear to be differentially regulated (6,179,183–185).

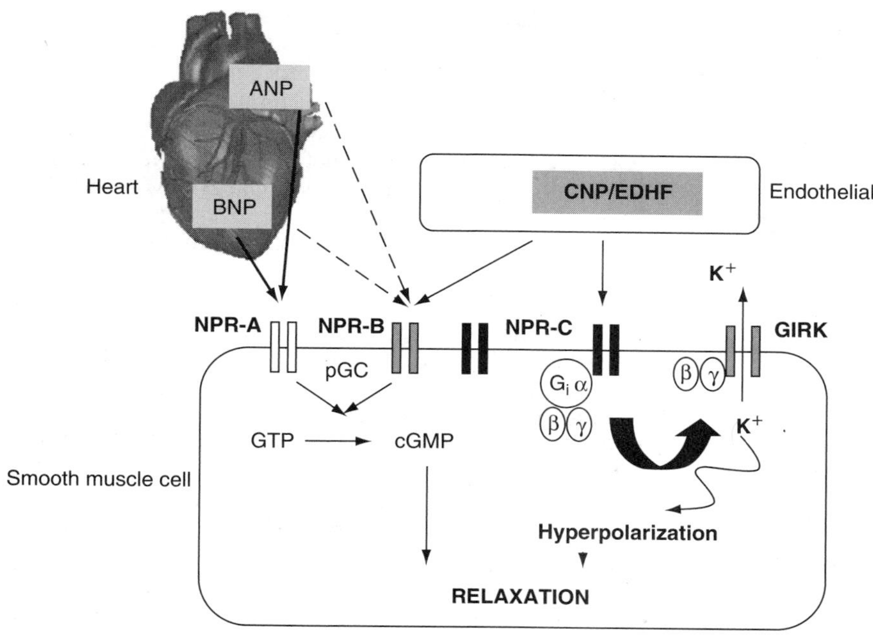

Figure 14-7 The natriuretic peptide system. Atrial natriuretic peptide (ANP) and brain natriuretic peptide (BNP) are released predominantly from the atria and ventricles, respectively, in response to increased wall stress. They act via the natriuretic peptide A (NPR-A) receptor on vascular smooth muscle cells to activate particulate guanylate cyclase (pGC) to increase intracellular cyclic guanosine monophosphate (cGMP), thereby promoting vasodilation. C-type natriuretic peptide (CNP) is released by endothelial cells and acts via natriuretic peptide receptor B (NPR-B) to activate pGC and increase cGMP. It also promotes vasodilation by activating the natriuretic peptide clearance receptor (NPR-C) and inducing hyperpolarization of the smooth muscle cell via a pertussis-toxin sensitive G protein (G_i) pathway.

Atrial Natriuretic Peptide

The natriuretic peptide A receptor has been localized in vascular smooth muscle, endothelial cells, cardiac myocytes, platelets, the adrenal glomerulosa, and renal epithelial and glomerular sites. Activation of particulate guanylyl cyclase via NPR-A increases the intracellular second messenger, cGMP (186,187). Through this receptor pathway, ANP is a potent inhibitor of vascular smooth muscle contraction, and the effect is not dependent on the presence of normal endothelium (186). Regional vascular beds have heterogeneous responses to ANP. Aortic and renal vascular strips are more sensitive to ANP than coronary, mesenteric, femoral, and carotid vessels (188,189).

Plasma ANP levels are increased in patients with heart failure and correlate with atrial filling pressures and disease severity (6,179,183,190,191). It is possible that high circulating levels of ANP reduce receptor number or sensitivity in vascular smooth muscle. The vascular and renal responses to ANP are attenuated in both animal models and in patients with heart failure. The vasodepressor response to infusion of ANP is markedly blunted in rats with heart failure due to myocardial infarction (192). Cody et al. have demonstrated that the hemodynamic effects of exogenous ANP are decreased in patients with heart failure (193). The forearm vascular responses to intrabrachial arterial ANP infusion in heart failure patients and normal subjects were examined by Hirooka et al. (194). ANP caused comparable increases in local venous plasma ANP and cGMP concentrations in heart failure patients and healthy subjects; however, the direct vasodilator effect of ANP was markedly blunted in the heart failure patients. In contrast, the forearm vasodilator responses to the intra-arterial infusion of nitroglycerin, which causes vasodilation by activating soluble guanylyl cyclase, were similar in healthy subjects and heart failure patients. The mechanisms underlying altered vascular responsiveness to ANP in heart failure are not known but might be due to changes in vascular smooth muscle ANP receptor density, uncoupling of intracellular signal transduction pathways, or increased local clearance of active ANP.

Brain Natriuretic Peptide

Brain natriuretic peptide shares substantial structural homology with ANP. In contrast, the sites and modulators of synthesis, clearance mechanisms, and receptor affinity in tissues are different. Like ANP, BNP exhibits vasodilatory, renin-inhibiting, natriuretic, and growth-suppressing actions through its activation of particulate guanylyl cyclase via the natriuretic peptide A receptor. In addition to elevated venous pressures, stimuli for BNP release include ventricular wall stress and myocardial ischemia or necrosis (195,196). Plasma levels of BNP are elevated and predict outcomes in patients with heart failure (197). In humans with acute heart failure, exogenous BNP results in enhanced natriuresis, diuresis, renin/aldosterone inhibition, vasodilation, and preload reduction (198) (Fig. 14-8). Similarly, in larger studies of humans with chronic heart failure, infusion of intravenous nesiritide reduced systemic vascular resistance and increased cardiac output in a dose-dependent manner (199,200).

C-Type Natriuretic Peptide

CNP is a vasodilator produced by the vascular endothelium. It shares structural and physiological properties with ANP and BNP, but little is known about its pathophysiological role in chronic heart failure. Since CNP binds selectively to NPR-B, it is assumed that the vasodilatory effects of CNP are mediated via this receptor (201). While NPR-B antagonism does not inhibit acetylcholine-mediated vasodilation of canine coronary arteries, inhibition of nitric oxide and NPR-B results in greater vasoconstriction than inhibition of nitric oxide alone (202). This cross-talk between these two pathways indicates that the activity of CNP and nitric oxide is closely linked, and CNP may serve

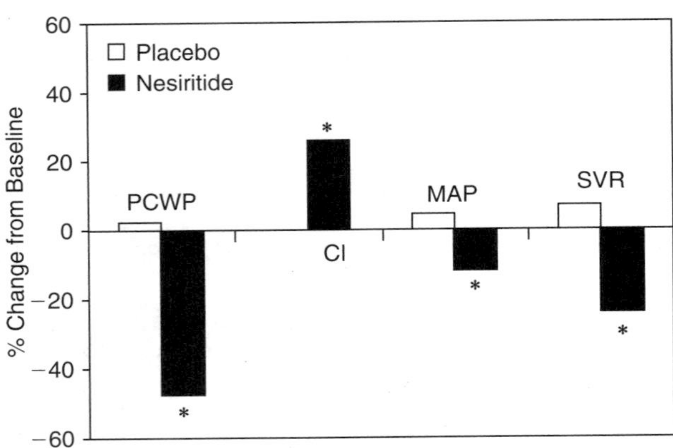

Figure 14-8 Effects of placebo and human BNP on pulmonary capillary wedge pressure (PCWP), cardiac index (CI), mean arterial pressure (MAP), and systemic vascular resistance (SVR) in 19 patients with severe congestive heart failure. BNP resulted in significant vasodilation accompanied by a decline in cardiac filling pressures and increase in cardiac output. *$p < 0.01$ versus placebo. (Adapted from Marcus LS, Hart D, Packer M, et al. Hemodynamic and renal excretory effects of human brain natriuretic peptide infusion in patients with congestive heart failure. A double-blind, placebo-controlled, randomized crossover trial. *Circulation*. 1996;94:3184–3189.)

a compensatory function in disease states associated with decreased nitric oxide bioavailability.

There is increasing evidence that activation of the clearance receptor (NPR-C) by CNP can also elicit vascular effects via a pertussis toxin-sensitive G_i pathway (203). CNP may cause vasodilation of resistance and conduit vessels by hyperpolarization of the underlying smooth muscle (Fig. 14-7). It has been shown that acetylcholine directly stimulates the release of CNP from the vascular endothelium of rat mesenteric arteries and results in vasodilation via NPR-C-mediated coupling of G_i with inwardly rectifying potassium channels present in the smooth muscle (204). Furthermore, removal of the endothelium in canine coronary artery rings does not inhibit the vasodilatory effects of exogenous CNP, supporting its role as a hyperpolarizing factor (202). Therefore, it appears that CNP acts via both NPR-B and particulate cGMP and NPR-C and G_i to promote vasodilation. Furthermore, it has been suggested that CNP is an endogenous inhibitor of ACE in the vasculature and thus may promote vasodilation by inhibiting the synthesis of angiotensin II (205). Plasma CNP levels are increased in patients with heart failure (206); however, the clinical significance of this peptide in heart failure remains unclear.

ADRENOMEDULLIN

Adrenomedullin (ADM) is an endogenous vasodilator and natriuretic 52-amino acid peptide first isolated in 1993 from human pheochromocytoma tissue (207). Subsequently, it has been found in a variety of tissues, including adrenal medulla, brain, kidney, gastrointestinal tract, lung, heart, aorta, vascular smooth muscle cells, and endothelial cells. Adrenomedullin belongs to the calcitonin superfamily of regulatory peptides and exerts its effects via two receptors: AM_1 and AM_2. These receptors are heterodimers composed of the calcitonin-like receptor (CLR) and receptor activity-modifying proteins (RAMP) 2 and 3 (208). RAMP 2 and 3 serve as accessory proteins that transport CLR to the cell surface to form functional AM_1 (CLR/RAMP2) and AM_2 (CLR/RAMP3) receptors that mediate the effects of adrenomedullin via increased intracellular cAMP production (209,210). Early animal data suggest that adrenomedullin has multiple biological effects, including inhibition of aldosterone secretion from the adrenal zona glomerulosa (211), suppression of catecholamine release from the adrenal medulla, inhibition of endothelin-1 and angiotensin II release from isolated aorta (212), and decreased vascular smooth-muscle cell proliferation (213). Cardiac myocyte expression of adrenomedullin and RAMP 2 and RAMP 3 mRNA is increased in animal models of heart failure (214). Immunostaining of ventricular tissue for adrenomedullin from canines with pacing-induced heart failure is more intense than from control dogs and is correlated with left ventricular mass (215). Similarly, Jougasaki et al. found more intense immunohistochemical staining for adrenomedullin in failing human ventricular myocardium than in normal human ventricles (216). Subsequent studies using coronary sinus and anterior interventricular vein sampling demonstrated that the failing human heart itself secretes adrenomedullin (216,217) and plasma levels correlate directly with left ventricular end-diastolic pressure, and inversely with ejection fraction and cardiac output (215).

Systemic administration of human adrenomedullin to animals with experimental heart failure decreases peripheral vascular resistance and left atrial pressure, whereas cardiac output, urine sodium excretion, creatinine clearance, and urine output increase (218). Also, adrenomedullin decreases plasma aldosterone levels and increases ANP and BNP concentrations. Intravenous infusion of adrenomedullin (0.05 μg/kg/min) in seven heart failure patients decreased arterial pressure, increased cardiac output, increased diuresis and natriuresis, and decreased aldosterone levels (219) (Fig 14-9). In humans, intrabrachial infusion of adrenomedullin caused potent and sustained vasodilation; however, this effect was attenuated in patients with heart failure compared to healthy controls (220). In a canine model of pacing-induced heart failure, adrenomedullin infusion increased nitrite production by coronary microvessels despite a decrease in endothelial nitric oxide synthase expression. This increase in nitric oxide production appeared to occur via a cAMP-dependent pathway (221). Taken together, these observations indicate that adrenomedullin is an important mediator of integrated cardiac, renal, and vascular function in heart failure and may serve an important compensatory role for microvascular nitric oxide production in heart failure.

STRUCTURAL CONTRIBUTIONS TO VASCULAR TONE

In chronic heart failure, abnormalities in vascular structure may contribute to increased vascular resistance at rest and impair the vasodilator response to exercise or hormonal stimuli. Although there is no direct histopathological

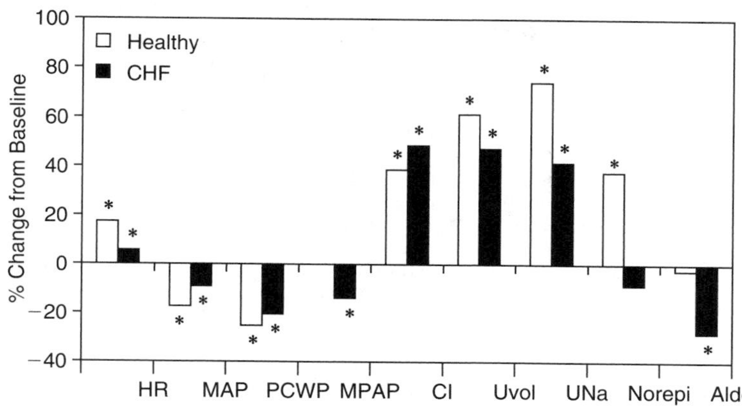

Figure 14-9 Effects of adrenomedullin infusion in patients with heart failure. 0.05 μg/kg/min of adrenomedullin was infused for 30 minutes in seven congestive heart failure (CHF) patients and seven healthy controls. Adrenomedullin significantly decreased heart rate (HR), mean arterial pressure (MAP), pulmonary capillary wedge pressure (PCWP), and mean pulmonary artery pressure (MPAP), while increasing cardiac index (CI) in patients with CHF. It also promoted diuresis (Uvol) and natriuresis (UNa) and reduced deleterious neurohormone levels (aldosterone) in patients with heart failure. $^*p < 0.05$ versus healthy controls. (Adapted from Nagaya N, Satoh T, Nishikimi T, et al. Hemodynamic, renal, and hormonal effects of adrenomedullin infusion in patients with congestive heart failure. *Circulation.* 2000;101:498–503.)

evidence of altered vascular structure in humans with heart failure, physiological evidence suggests that vascular remodeling does occur in this disease state. Structural abnormalities in resistance vessels have been suggested by experiments in which vascular tone is minimized by a maximal metabolic vasodilatory stimulus; the residual vascular resistance would then represent the structural contribution. The blunted response of peak hyperemic blood flow and exercise in many patients with heart failure has implicated a structural component. It is possible that structural alterations, caused in part by vascular wall salt and water retention, may prevent maximal vasodilation. Additionally, aldosterone escape or increased plasma aldosterone concentrations (despite adequate ACE inhibition) may lead to increased collagen synthesis and decreased vascular distensibility in patients with heart failure (222).

Structural changes in conductance vessels have been suggested by studies that measure impedance or arterial compliance. Indirect measurements of compliance usually indicate that elasticity is reduced in conduit vessels of patients with heart failure. Pulse wave velocity correlates inversely with compliance and is increased in heart failure (223). Moreover, characteristic impedance is elevated in patients with heart failure (224,225). Direct measurements of brachial artery compliance using high-resolution ultrasonography have confirmed decreased distensibility in patients with heart failure compared with healthy subjects and have shown that decreased arterial elasticity correlates with impairment in flow-mediated vasodilation in these individuals (226). The structural changes contributing to altered compliance are not known. Nonetheless, decreased distensibility will increase the load on the heart during systole and will further compromise cardiac function. These implied structural changes in conjunction with functional metabolic and neurohormonal effects are interwoven to create a complex tapestry of abnormal vascular function that contributes to both symptoms of heart failure and progression of disease.

ACKNOWLEDGMENTS

Dr. Mark A. Creager is the Simon C. Fireman Scholar in Cardiovascular Medicine at Brigham and Women's Hospital, Boston, MA.

REFERENCES

1. Leithe ME, Margorien RD, Hermiller JB, et al. Relationship between central hemodynamics and regional blood flow in normal subjects and in patients with congestive heart failure. *Circulation.* 1984;69:57–64.
2. Zelis R, Flaim SF. Alterations in vasomotor tone in congestive heart failure. *Prog Cardiovasc Dis.* 1982;24:437–459.
3. Wiener DH, Maris J, Chance B, et al. Detection of skeletal muscle hypoperfusion during exercise using phosphorus-31 nuclear magnetic resonance spectroscopy. *J Am Coll Cardiol.* 1986;7:793–799.
4. Wilson JR, Wiener DH, Fink LI, et al. Vasodilatory behavior of skeletal muscle arterioles in patients with nonedematous chronic heart failure. *Circulation.* 1986;74:775–779.
5. Creager MA, Halperin JL, Bernard DB, et al. Acute regional circulatory and renal hemodynamic effects of converting-enzyme inhibition in patients with congestive heart failure. *Circulation.* 1981;64:483–489.
6. Cody RJ, Covit AB, Schaer GL, et al. Sodium and water balance in chronic congestive heart failure. *J Clin Invest.* 1986;77:1441–1452.
7. Furchgott RF, Zawadzki JV. The obligatory role of endothelial cells in the relaxation of arterial smooth muscle by acetylcholine. *Nature.* 1980;288:373–376.
8. Ignarro LJ, Byrns RE, Buga GM, et al. Endothelium-derived relaxing factor from pulmonary artery and vein possesses pharmacologic and chemical properties identical to those of nitric oxide radical. *Circ Res.* 1987;61:866–879.
9. Palmer RM, Ferrige AG, Moncada S. Nitric oxide release accounts for the biological activity of endothelium-derived relaxing factor. *Nature.* 1987;327:524–526.
10. Myers PR, Guerra R, Jr., Harrison DG. Release of NO and EDRF from cultured bovine aortic endothelial cells. *Am J Physiol.* 1989;256:H1030–H1037.
11. Palmer RM, Ashton DS, Moncada S. Vascular endothelial cells synthesize nitric oxide from L-arginine. *Nature.* 1988;333:664–666.
12. Lamas S, Marsden PA, Li GK, et al. Endothelial nitric oxide synthase: molecular cloning and characterization of a distinct constitutive enzyme isoform. *Proc Natl Acad Sci USA.* 1992;89:6348–6352.
13. Cohen RA, Zitnay KM, Haudenschild CC, et al. Loss of selective endothelial cell vasoactive functions caused by hypercholesterolemia in pig coronary arteries. *Circ Res.* 1988;63:903–910.
14. De Mey JG, Vanhoutte PM. Heterogeneous behavior of the canine arterial and venous wall. Importance of the endothelium. *Circ Res.* 1982;51:439–447.
15. Shimokawa H, Vanhoutte PM. Impaired endothelium-dependent relaxation to aggregating platelets and related vasoactive substances in porcine coronary arteries in hypercholesterolemia and atherosclerosis. *Circ Res.* 1989;64:900–914.
16. Kaiser L, Spickard RC, Olivier NB. Heart failure depresses endothelium-dependent responses in canine femoral artery. *Am J Physiol.* 1989;256:H962–H967.

17. Wang J, Seyedi N, Xu XB, et al. Defective endothelium-mediated control of coronary circulation in conscious dogs after heart failure. *Am J Physiol.* 1994;266:H670–H680.
18. Elsner D, Muntze A, Kromer EP, et al. Systemic vasoconstriction induced by inhibition of nitric oxide synthesis is attenuated in conscious dogs with heart failure. *Cardiovasc Res.* 1991;25:438–440.
19. Treasure CB, Vita JA, Cox DA, et al. Endothelium-dependent dilation of the coronary microvasculature is impaired in dilated cardiomyopathy. *Circulation.* 1990;81:772–779.
20. Drexler H, Hayoz D, Munzel T, et al. Endothelial function in chronic congestive heart failure. *Am J Cardiol.* 1992;69:1596–1601.
21. Katz SD, Schwarz M, Yuen J, et al. Impaired acetylcholine-mediated vasodilation in patients with congestive heart failure. Role of endothelium-derived vasodilating and vasoconstricting factors. *Circulation.* 1993;88:55–61.
22. Kubo SH, Rector TS, Bank AJ, et al. Endothelium-dependent vasodilation is attenuated in patients with heart failure. *Circulation.* 1991;84:1589–1596.
23. Nakamura M, Ishikawa M, Funakoshi T, et al. Attenuated endothelium-dependent peripheral vasodilation and clinical characteristics in patients with chronic heart failure. *Am Heart J.* 1994;128:1164–1169.
24. Heitzer T, Baldus S, von Kodolitsch Y, et al. Systemic endothelial dysfunction as an early predictor of adverse outcome in heart failure. *Arterioscler Thromb Vasc Biol.* 2005;25:1174–1179.
25. Katz SD, Hryniewicz K, Hriljac I, et al. Vascular endothelial dysfunction and mortality risk in patients with chronic heart failure. *Circulation.* 2005;111:310–314.
26. Kaye DM, Ahlers BA, Autelitano DJ, et al. In vivo and in vitro evidence for impaired arginine transport in human heart failure. *Circulation.* 2000;102:2707–2712.
27. Hirooka Y, Imaizumi T, Tagawa T, et al. Effects of L-arginine on impaired acetylcholine-induced and ischemic vasodilation of the forearm in patients with heart failure. *Circulation.* 1994;90:658–668.
28. Rector TS, Bank AJ, Mullen KA, et al. Randomized, double-blind, placebo-controlled study of supplemental oral L-arginine in patients with heart failure. *Circulation.* 1996;93:2135–2141.
29. Setoguchi S, Hirooka Y, Eshima K, et al. Tetrahydrobiopterin improves impaired endothelium-dependent forearm vasodilation in patients with heart failure. *J Cardiovasc Pharmacol.* 2002;39:363–368.
30. Zalba G, Beaumont J, San Jose G, et al. Vascular oxidant stress: molecular mechanisms and pathophysiological implications. *J Physiol Biochem.* 2000;56:57–64.
31. Takayama T, Wada A, Tsutamoto T, et al. Contribution of vascular NAD(P)H oxidase to endothelial dysfunction in heart failure and the therapeutic effects of HMG-CoA reductase inhibitor. *Circ J.* 2004;68:1067–1075.
32. Doehner W, Schoene N, Rauchhaus M, et al. Effects of xanthine oxidase inhibition with allopurinol on endothelial function and peripheral blood flow in hyperuricemic patients with chronic heart failure: results from 2 placebo-controlled studies. *Circulation.* 2002;105:2619–2624.
33. Farquharson CA, Butler R, Hill A, et al. Allopurinol improves endothelial dysfunction in chronic heart failure. *Circulation.* 2002;106:221–226.
34. Hornig B, Arakawa N, Kohler C, et al. Vitamin C improves endothelial function of conduit arteries in patients with chronic heart failure. *Circulation.* 1998;97:363–368.
35. Ennezat PV, Malendowicz SL, Testa M, et al. Physical training in patients with chronic heart failure enhances the expression of genes encoding antioxidative enzymes. *J Am Coll Cardiol.* 2001;38:194–198.
36. Hornig B, Maier V, Drexler H. Physical training improves endothelial function in patients with chronic heart failure. *Circulation.* 1996;93:210–214.
37. Katz SD, Balidemaj K, Homma S, et al. Acute type 5 phosphodiesterase inhibition with sildenafil enhances flow-mediated vasodilation in patients with chronic heart failure. *J Am Coll Cardiol.* 2000;36:845–851.
38. Ludmer PL, Selwyn AP, Shook TL, et al. Paradoxical vasoconstriction induced by acetylcholine in atherosclerotic coronary arteries. *N Engl J Med.* 1986;315:1046–1051.
39. Vita JA, Treasure CB, Nabel EG, et al. Coronary vasomotor response to acetylcholine relates to risk factors for coronary artery disease. *Circulation.* 1990;81:491–497.
40. Dzau VJ, Packer M, Lilly LS, et al. Prostaglandins in severe congestive heart failure. Relation to activation of the renin-angiotensin system and hyponatremia. *N Engl J Med.* 1984;310:347–352.
41. Oliver JA, Sciacca RR, Pinto J, et al. Participation of the prostaglandins in the control of renal blood flow during acute reduction of cardiac output in the dog. *J Clin Invest.* 1981;67:229–237.
42. Friedman PL, Brown EJ, Jr., Gunther S, et al. Coronary vasoconstrictor effect of indomethacin in patients with coronary-artery disease. *N Engl J Med.* 1981;305:1171–1175.
43. Shebuski RJ, Aiken JW. Angiotensin II stimulation of renal prostaglandin synthesis elevates circulating prostacyclin in the dog. *J Cardiovasc Pharmacol.* 1980;2:667–677.
44. Zusman RM, Keiser HR. Prostaglandin biosynthesis by rabbit renomedullary interstitial cells in tissue culture. Stimulation by angiotensin II, bradykinin, and arginine vasopressin. *J Clin Invest.* 1977;60:215–223.
45. McGiff JC, Crowshaw K, Terragno NA, et al. Differential effect of noradrenaline and renal nerve stimulation on vascular resistance in the dog kidney and the release of a prostaglandin E-like substance. *Clin Sci.* 1972;42:223–233.
46. Levin RI, Jaffe EA, Weksler BB, et al. Nitroglycerin stimulates synthesis of prostacyclin by cultured human endothelial cells. *J Clin Invest.* 1981;67:762–769.
47. Morcillio E, Reid PR, Dubin N, et al. Myocardial prostaglandin E release by nitroglycerin and modification by indomethacin. *Am J Cardiol.* 1980;45:53–57.
48. Rubin LJ, Lazar JD. Influence of prostaglandin synthesis inhibitors on pulmonary vasodilatory effects of hydralazine in dogs with hypoxic pulmonary vasoconstriction. *J Clin Invest.* 1981;67:193–200.
49. Gainer JV, Morrow JD, Loveland A, et al. Effect of bradykinin-receptor blockade on the response to angiotensin-converting-enzyme inhibitor in normotensive and hypertensive subjects. *N Engl J Med.* 1998;339:1285–1292.
50. Brown NJ, Ryder D, Gainer JV, et al. Differential effects of angiotensin converting enzyme inhibitors on the vasodepressor and prostacyclin responses to bradykinin. *J Pharmacol Exp Ther.* 1996;279:703–712.
51. Nakamura M, Funakoshi T, Arakawa N, et al. Effect of angiotensin-converting enzyme inhibitors on endothelium-dependent peripheral vasodilation in patients with chronic heart failure. *J Am Coll Cardiol.* 1994;24:1321–1327.
52. Spaulding C, Charbonnier B, Cohen-Solal A, et al. Acute hemodynamic interaction of aspirin and ticlopidine with enalapril: results of a double-blind, randomized comparative trial. *Circulation.* 1998;98:757–765.
53. Yanagisawa M, Kurihara H, Kimura S, et al. A novel potent vasoconstrictor peptide produced by vascular endothelial cells. *Nature.* 1988;332:411–415.
54. Wu-Wong JR, Budzik GP, Devine EM, et al. Characterization of endothelin converting enzyme in rat lung. *Biochem Biophy Res Commun.* 1990;171:1291–1296.
55. Yanagisawa M, Masaki T. Endothelin, a novel endothelium-derived peptide. Pharmacological activities, regulation and possible roles in cardiovascular control. *Biochem Biophy Res Commun.* 1989;38:1877–1883.
56. Resink TJ, Hahn AW, Scott-Burden T, et al. Inducible endothelin mRNA expression and peptide secretion in cultured human vascular smooth muscle cells. *Biochem Biophy Res Commun.* 1990;168:1303–1310.
57. Brenner BM, Troy JL, Ballermann BJ. Endothelium-dependent vascular responses. Mediators and mechanisms. *J Clin Invest.* 1989;84:1373–1378.
58. Yoshizumi M, Kurihara H, Sugiyama T, et al. Hemodynamic shear stress stimulates endothelin production by cultured endothelial cells. *Biochem Biophy Res Commun.* 1989;161:859–864.
59. Arai H, Hori S, Aramori I, et al. Cloning and expression of a cDNA encoding an endothelin receptor. *Nature* 1990;348:730–732.
60. King AJ, Pfeffer JM, Pfeffer MA, et al. Systemic hemodynamic effects of endothelin in rats. *Am J Physiol.* 1990;258:H787–H792.

61. Otsuka A, Mikami H, Katahira K, et al. Haemodynamic effect of endothelin, a novel potent vasoconstrictor in dogs. *Clin Exp Pharmacol Physiol.* 1990;17:351–360.
62. Masaki T, Kimura S, Yanagisawa M, et al. Molecular and cellular mechanism of endothelin regulation. Implications for vascular function. *Circulation.* 1991;84:1457–1468.
63. Marsden PA, Danthuluri NR, Brenner BM, et al. Endothelin action on vascular smooth muscle involves inositol trisphosphate and calcium mobilization. *Biochem Biophy Res Commun.* 1989;158:86–93.
64. Resink TJ, Scott-Burden T, Buhler FR. Activation of phospholipase A2 by endothelin in cultured vascular smooth muscle cells. *Biochem Biophy Res Commun.* 1989;158:279–286.
65. Simonson MS, Wann S, Mene P, et al. Endothelin stimulates phospholipase C, Na+/H+ exchange, c-fos expression, and mitogenesis in rat mesangial cells. *J Clin Invest.* 1989;83:708–712.
66. Ohnishi M, Wada A, Tsutamoto T, et al. Endothelin stimulates an endogenous nitric oxide synthase inhibitor, asymmetric dimethylarginine, in experimental heart failure. *Clin Sci.* (Lond) 2002;103(Suppl)48:241S–244S.
67. Goetz KL, Wang BC, Madwed JB, et al. Cardiovascular, renal, and endocrine responses to intravenous endothelin in conscious dogs. *Am J Physiol.* 1988;255:R1064–R1068.
68. Miller WL, Redfield MM, Burnett JC, Jr. Integrated cardiac, renal, and endocrine actions of endothelin. *J Clin Invest.* 1989;83: 317–320.
69. Knuepfer MM, Han SP, Trapani AJ, et al. Regional hemodynamic and baroreflex effects of endothelin in rats. *Am J Physiol.* 1989;257:H918–H926.
70. Kramer BK, Nishida M, Kelly RA, et al. Endothelins. Myocardial actions of a new class of cytokines. *Circulation.* 1992;85:350–356.
71. Janakidevi K, Fisher MA, Del Vecchio PJ, et al. Endothelin-1 stimulates DNA synthesis and proliferation of pulmonary artery smooth muscle cells. *Am J Physiol.* 1992;263:C1295–C301.
72. Alberts GF, Peifley KA, Johns A, et al. Constitutive endothelin-1 overexpression promotes smooth muscle cell proliferation via an external autocrine loop. *J Biol Chem.* 1994;269:10112–10118.
73. Lonchampt MO, Pinelis S, Goulin J, et al. Proliferation and Na+/H+ exchange activation by endothelin in vascular smooth muscle cells. *Am J Hypertens..* 1991;4:776–779.
74. Bogoyevitch MA, Glennon PE, Andersson MB, et al. Endothelin-1 and fibroblast growth factors stimulate the mitogen-activated protein kinase signaling cascade in cardiac myocytes. The potential role of the cascade in the integration of two signaling pathways leading to myocyte hypertrophy. *J Biol Chem.* 1994;269:1110–1119.
75. Cavero PG, Miller WL, Heublein DM, et al. Endothelin in experimental congestive heart failure in the anesthetized dog. *Am J Physiol.* 1990;259:F312–F317.
76. Margulies KB, Hildebrand FL, Jr., Lerman A, et al. Increased endothelin in experimental heart failure. *Circulation.* 1990;82: 2226–2230.
77. Stewart DJ, Cernacek P, Costello KB, et al. Elevated endothelin-1 in heart failure and loss of normal response to postural change. *Circulation.* 1992;85:510–517.
78. Cody RJ, Haas GJ, Binkley PF, et al. Plasma endothelin correlates with the extent of pulmonary hypertension in patients with chronic congestive heart failure. *Circulation.* 1992;85:504–509.
79. McMurray JJ, Ray SG, Abdullah I, et al. Plasma endothelin in chronic heart failure. *Circulation.* 1992;85:1374–1379.
80. Cernacek P, Stewart DJ. Immunoreactive endothelin in human plasma: marked elevations in patients in cardiogenic shock. *Biochem Biophy Res Commun.* 1989;161:562–567.
81. Emori T, Hirata Y, Ohta K, et al. Secretory mechanism of immunoreactive endothelin in cultured bovine endothelial cells. *Biochem Biophy Res Commun.* 1989;160:93–100.
82. Bauersachs J, Fraccarollo D, Galuppo P, et al. Endothelin-receptor blockade improves endothelial vasomotor dysfunction in heart failure. *Cardiovasc Res.* 2000;47:142–149.
83. Berger R, Stanek B, Hulsmann M, et al. Effects of endothelin a receptor blockade on endothelial function in patients with chronic heart failure. *Circulation.* 2001;103:981–986.
84. Kiowski W, Sutsch G, Hunziker P, et al. Evidence for endothelin-1-mediated vasoconstriction in severe chronic heart failure. *Lancet.* 1995;346:732–736.
85. Anand I, McMurray J, Cohn JN, et al. Long-term effects of darusentan on left-ventricular remodelling and clinical outcomes in the EndothelinA Receptor Antagonist Trial in Heart Failure (EARTH): randomised, double-blind, placebo-controlled trial. *Lancet.* 2004;364:347–354.
86. Teerlink JR. Recent heart failure trials of neurohormonal modulation (OVERTURE and ENABLE): approaching the asymptote of efficacy? *J Card Fail.* 2002;8:124–127.
87. Kaluski E, Kobrin I, Zimlichman R, et al. RITZ-5: randomized intravenous TeZosentan (an endothelin-A/B antagonist) for the treatment of pulmonary edema: a prospective, multicenter, double-blind, placebo-controlled study. *J Am Coll Cardiol.* 2003;41: 204–210.
88. Dzau VJ, Kopelman RI, Barger AC, et al. Renin-specific antibody for study of cardiovascular homeostasis. *Science* 1980;207:1091–1093.
89. Pals DT, Masucci FD, Sipos F, et al. A specific competitive antagonist of the vascular action of angiotensin. II. *Circ Res.* 1971;29:664–672.
90. Ondetti MA, Rubin B, Cushman DW. Design of specific inhibitors of angiotensin-converting enzyme: new class of orally active antihypertensive agents. *Science.* 1977;196:441–444.
91. Creager MA, Faxon DP, Halperin JL, et al. Determinants of clinical response and survival in patients with congestive heart failure treated with captopril. *Am Heart J.* 1982;104:1147–1154.
92. Kubo SH, Clark M, Laragh JH, et al. Identification of normal neurohormonal activity in mild congestive heart failure and stimulating effect of upright posture and diuretics. *Am J Cardiol.* 1987;60:1322–1328.
93. Dzau VJ, Gibbons GH. Autocrine-paracrine mechanisms of vascular myocytes in systemic hypertension. *Am J Cardiol.* 1987;60: 991–1031.
94. Rosenthal JH, Pfeifle B, Michailov ML, et al. Investigations of components of the renin-angiotensin system in rat vascular tissue. *Hypertension.* 1984;6:383–390.
95. Re R, Fallon JT, Dzau V, et al. Renin synthesis by canine aortic smooth muscle cells in culture. *Life Sci.* 1982;30:99–106.
96. Admiraal PJ, Derkx FH, Danser AH, et al. Metabolism and production of angiotensin I in different vascular beds in subjects with hypertension. *Hypertension.* 1990;15:44–55.
97. Lee MA, Bohm M, Paul M, et al. Tissue renin-angiotensin systems. Their role in cardiovascular disease. *Circulation.* 1993;87: IV7–IV13.
98. Seyedi N, Xu X, Nasjletti A, et al. Coronary kinin generation mediates nitric oxide release after angiotensin receptor stimulation. *Hypertension.* 1995;26:164–170.
99. Lin L, Nasjletti A. Role of endothelium-derived prostanoid in angiotensin-induced vasoconstriction. *Hypertension.* 1991;18: 158–164.
100. Shepherd JT, Vanhoutte PM. George E. Brown memorial lecture. Local modulation of adrenergic neurotransmission. *Circulation.* 1981;64:655–666.
101. Griendling KK, Minieri CA, Ollerenshaw JD, et al. Angiotensin II stimulates NADH and NADPH oxidase activity in cultured vascular smooth muscle cells. *Circ Res.* 1994;74:1141–1148.
102. Rajagopalan S, Kurz S, Munzel T, et al. Angiotensin II-mediated hypertension in the rat increases vascular superoxide production via membrane NADH/NADPH oxidase activation. Contribution to alterations of vasomotor tone. *J Clin Invest.* 1996;97: 1916–1923.
103. Bank AJ, Kubo SH, Rector TS, et al. Local forearm vasodilation with intra-arterial administration of enalaprilat in humans. *Clin Pharmacol Ther.* 1991;50:314–321.
104. Haefeli WE, Linder L, Luscher TF. Quinaprilat induces arterial vasodilation mediated by nitric oxide in humans. *Hypertension.* 1997;30:912–917.
105. Simon AC, Levenson JA, Bouthier JD, et al. Comparison of oral MK 421 and propranolol in mild to moderate essential hypertension and their effects on arterial and venous vessels of the forearm. *Am J Cardiol.* 1984;53:781–785.
106. Dzau VJ, Safar ME. Large conduit arteries in hypertension: role of the vascular renin-angiotensin system. *Circulation.* 1988;77: 947–954.
107. Taugner R, Hackenthal E, Rix E, et al. Immunocytochemistry of the renin-angiotensin system: renin, angiotensinogen, angiotensin I, angiotensin II, and converting enzyme in the kidneys of mice, rats, and tree shrews. *Kidney Int Suppl.* 1982;12:S33–S43.

108. Taugner R, Hackenthal E, Helmchen U, et al. The intrarenal renin-angiotensin-system. An immunocytochemical study on the localization of renin, angiotensinogen, converting enzyme and the angiotensins in the kidney of mouse and rat. *Klin Wochenschr*. 1982;60:1218–1222.
109. Dzau VJ, Ellison KE, Brody T, et al. A comparative study of the distributions of renin and angiotensinogen messenger ribonucleic acids in rat and mouse tissues. *Endocrinology.* 1987;120:2334–2338.
110. Ingelfinger JR, Zuo WM, Fon EA, et al. In situ hybridization evidence for angiotensinogen mRNA in the rat proximal tubule. An hypothesis for the intrarenal renin angiotensin system. *J Clin Invest*. 1990;85:417–423.
111. Soubrier F, Alhenc-Gelas F, Hubert C, et al. Two putative active centers in human angiotensin I-converting enzyme revealed by molecular cloning. *Proc Natl Acad Sci USA*. 1988;85:9386–9390.
112. Sakaguchi K, Chai SY, Jackson B, et al. Inhibition of tissue angiotensin converting enzyme. Quantitation by autoradiography. *Hypertension.* 1988;11:230–238.
113. Seikaly MG, Arant BS, Jr., Seney FD, Jr. Endogenous angiotensin concentrations in specific intrarenal fluid compartments of the rat. *J Clin Invest*. 1990;86:1352–1357.
114. Schunkert H, Tang SS, Litwin SE, et al. Regulation of intrarenal and circulating renin-angiotensin systems in severe heart failure in the rat. *Cardiovasc Res*. 1993;27:731–735.
115. Hoffman BB, Lefkowitz RJ. Alpha-adrenergic receptor subtypes. *N Engl J Med*. 1980;302:1390–1396.
116. Cotecchia S, Schwinn DA, Randall RR, et al. Molecular cloning and expression of the cDNA for the hamster alpha 1-adrenergic receptor. *Proc Natl Acad Sci USA*. 1988;85:7159–7163.
117. Schwinn DA, Lomasney JW, Lorenz W, et al. Molecular cloning and expression of the cDNA for a novel alpha 1-adrenergic receptor subtype. *J Biol Chem*. 1990;265:8183–8189.
118. Han C, Abel PW, Minneman KP. Alpha 1-adrenoceptor subtypes linked to different mechanisms for increasing intracellular Ca2+ in smooth muscle. *Nature.* 1987;329:333–335.
119. Suzuki E, Tsujimoto G, Tamura K, et al. Two pharmacologically distinct alpha 1-adrenoceptor subtypes in the contraction of rabbit aorta: each subtype couples with a different Ca2+ signalling mechanism and plays a different physiological role. *Mol Pharmacol*. 1990;38:725–736.
120. Deng XF, Chemtob S, Varma DR. Characterization of alpha 1 D-adrenoceptor subtype in rat myocardium, aorta and other tissues. *Br J Pharmacol*. 1996;119:269–276.
121. Buckner SA, Oheim KW, Morse PA, et al. Alpha 1-adrenoceptor-induced contractility in rat aorta is mediated by the alpha 1D subtype. *Eur J Pharmacol*. 1996;297:241–248.
122. Daniel EE, Low AM, Gaspar V, et al. Unusual alpha-adrenoceptor subtype in canine saphenous vein: comparison to mesenteric vein. *Br J Pharmacol*. 1996;117:1535–1543.
123. Colucci WS, Gimbrone MA, Jr., Alexander RW. Regulation of the postsynaptic alpha-adrenergic receptor in rat mesenteric artery. Effects of chemical sympathectomy and epinephrine treatment. *Circ Res*. 1981;48:104–111.
124. Tsujimoto G, Honda K, Hoffman BB, et al. Desensitization of postjunctional alpha 1- and alpha 2-adrenergic receptor-mediated vasopressor responses in rat harboring pheochromocytoma. *Circ Res*. 1987;61:86–98.
125. Colucci WS, Alexander RW. Norepinephrine-induced alteration in the coupling of alpha 1-adrenergic receptor occupancy to calcium efflux in rabbit aortic smooth muscle cells. *Proc Natl Acad Sci USA*. 1986;83:1743–1746.
126. Izzo NJ, Jr., Seidman CE, Collins S, et al. Alpha 1-adrenergic receptor mRNA level is regulated by norepinephrine in rabbit aortic smooth muscle cells. *Proc Natl Acad Sci USA*. 1990;87: 6268–6271.
127. Lurie KG, Tsujimoto G, Hoffman BB. Desensitization of alpha-1 adrenergic receptor-mediated vascular smooth muscle contraction. *J Pharmacol Exp Ther*. 1985;234:147–152.
128. Goldberg MR, Robertson D. Evidence for the existence of vascular alpha 2-adrenergic receptors in humans. *Hypertension.* 1984;6:551–556.
129. Cotecchia S, Kobilka BK, Daniel KW, et al. Multiple second messenger pathways of alpha-adrenergic receptor subtypes expressed in eukaryotic cells. *J Biol Chem*. 1990;265:63–69.
130. Lorenz W, Lomasney JW, Collins S, et al. Expression of three alpha 2-adrenergic receptor subtypes in rat tissues: implications for alpha 2 receptor classification. *Mol Pharmacol*. 1990;38: 599–603.
131. Emorine LJ, Marullo S, Briend-Sutren MM, et al. Molecular characterization of the human beta 3-adrenergic receptor. *Science.* 1989;245:1118–1121.
132. Lefkowitz RJ, Stadel JM, Caron MG. Adenylate cyclase-coupled beta-adrenergic receptors: structure and mechanisms of activation and desensitization. *Annu Rev Biochem*. 1983;52: 159–186.
133. Bulbring E, Tomita T. Catecholamine action on smooth muscle. *Pharmacol Rev*. 1987;39:49–96.
134. Hertel C, Perkins JP. Receptor-specific mechanisms of desensitization of beta-adrenergic receptor function. *Mol Cell Endocrinol*. 1984;37:245–256.
135. Kassis S, Fishman PH. Different mechanisms of desensitization of adenylate cyclase by isoproterenol and prostaglandin E1 in human fibroblasts. Role of regulatory components in desensitization. *J Biol Chem*. 1982;257:5312–5318.
136. Strasser RH, Lefkowitz RJ. Homologous desensitization of beta-adrenergic receptor coupled adenylate cyclase. Resensitization by polyethylene glycol treatment. *J Biol Chem*. 1985;260: 4561–4564.
137. Vatner DE, Vatner SF, Nejima J, et al. Chronic norepinephrine elicits desensitization by uncoupling the beta-receptor. *J Clin Invest*. 1989;84:1741–1748.
138. Brodde OE, Daul A, Michel-Reher M, et al. Agonist-induced desensitization of beta-adrenoceptor function in humans. Subtype-selective reduction in beta 1- or beta 2-adrenoceptor-mediated physiological effects by xamoterol or procaterol. *Circulation*. 1990;81:914–921.
139. Vatner DE, Vatner SF, Fujii AM, et al. Loss of high affinity cardiac beta adrenergic receptors in dogs with heart failure. *J Clin Invest*. 1985;76:2259–2264.
140. Rothwell NJ, Stock MJ, Sudera DK. Changes in tissue blood flow and beta-receptor density of skeletal muscle in rats treated with the beta2-adrenoceptor agonist clenbuterol. *Br J Pharmacol*. 1987;90:601–607.
141. Colucci WS, Alexander RW, Williams GH, et al. Decreased lymphocyte beta-adrenergic-receptor density in patients with heart failure and tolerance to the beta-adrenergic agonist pirbuterol. *N Engl J Med*. 1981;305:185–190.
142. Wilson JR, Lanoce V, Frey MJ, et al. Arterial baroreceptor control of peripheral vascular resistance in experimental heart failure. *Am Heart J*. 1990;119:1122–1130.
143. Forster C, Carter SL, Armstrong PW. Alpha 1-adrenoceptor activity in arterial smooth muscle following congestive heart failure. *Can J Physiol Pharmacol*. 1989;67:110–115.
144. Feng Q, Sun X, Lu X, et al. Decreased responsiveness of vascular postjunctional alpha1-, alpha2-adrenoceptors and neuropeptide Y1 receptors in rats with heart failure. *Acta Physiol Scand*. 1999;166:285–291.
145. Indolfi C, Maione A, Volpe M, et al. Forearm vascular responsiveness to alpha 1- and alpha 2-adrenoceptor stimulation in patients with congestive heart failure. *Circulation*. 1994;90:17–22.
146. Creager MA, Hirsch AT, Dzau VJ, et al. Baroreflex regulation of regional blood flow in congestive heart failure. *Am J Physiol*. 1990;258:H1409–414.
147. Neumeister A, Charney DS, Belfer I, et al. Sympathoneural and adrenomedullary functional effects of alpha2C-adrenoreceptor gene polymorphism in healthy humans. *Pharmacogenet Genomics*. 2005;15:143–149.
148. Small KM, Wagoner LE, Levin AM, et al. Synergistic polymorphisms of beta1- and alpha2C-adrenergic receptors and the risk of congestive heart failure. *N Engl J Med*. 2002;347:1135–1142.
149. Brede M, Wiesmann F, Jahns R, et al. Feedback inhibition of catecholamine release by two different alpha2-adrenoceptor subtypes prevents progression of heart failure. *Circulation*. 2002;106: 2491–2496.
150. Aggarwal A, Esler MD, Socratous F, et al. Evidence for functional presynaptic alpha-2 adrenoceptors and their down-regulation in human heart failure. *J Am Coll Cardiol*. 2001;37: 1246–1251.
151. Feng QP, Bergdahl A, Lu XR, et al. Vascular alpha-2 adrenoceptor function is decreased in rats with congestive heart failure. *Cardiovasc Res*. 1996;31:577–584.

152. Kubo SH, Rector TS, Heifetz SM, et al. Alpha 2-receptor-mediated vasoconstriction in patients with congestive heart failure. *Circulation.* 1989;80:1660–1667.
153. Gilson N, el Houda Bouanani N, Corsin A, et al. Left ventricular function and beta-adrenoceptors in rabbit failing heart. *Am J Physiol.* 1990;258:H634–H641.
154. Fan TH, Liang CS, Kawashima S, et al. Alterations in cardiac beta-adrenoceptor responsiveness and adenylate cyclase system by congestive heart failure in dogs. *Eur J Pharmacol.* 1987;140:123–132.
155. Bristow MR, Hershberger RE, Port JD, et al. Beta-adrenergic pathways in nonfailing and failing human ventricular myocardium. *Circulation.* 1990;82:I12–I25.
156. Marzo KP, Frey MJ, Wilson JR, et al. Beta-adrenergic receptor-G protein-adenylate cyclase complex in experimental canine congestive heart failure produced by rapid ventricular pacing. *Circ Res.* 1991;69:1546–1556.
157. Creager MA, Quigg RJ, Ren CJ, et al. Limb vascular responsiveness to beta-adrenergic receptor stimulation in patients with congestive heart failure. *Circulation.* 1991;83:1873–1879.
158. Liggett SB, Wagoner LE, Craft LL, et al. The Ile164 beta2-adrenergic receptor polymorphism adversely affects the outcome of congestive heart failure. *J Clin Invest.* 1998;102:1534–1539.
159. Brodde OE, Buscher R, Tellkamp R, et al. Blunted cardiac responses to receptor activation in subjects with Thr164Ile beta(2)-adrenoceptors. *Circulation.* 2001;103:1048–1050.
160. Dishy V, Landau R, Sofowora GG, et al. Beta2-adrenoceptor Thr164Ile polymorphism is associated with markedly decreased vasodilator and increased vasoconstrictor sensitivity in vivo. *Pharmacogenetics.* 2004;14:517–522.
161. Walker BR. Evidence for a vasodilatory effect of vasopressin in the conscious rat. *Am J Physiol.* 1986;251:H34–H39.
162. Liard JF. Cardiovascular effects associated with antidiuretic activity of vasopressin after blockade of its vasoconstrictor action in dehydrated dogs. *Circ Res.* 1986;58:631–640.
163. Hirsch AT, Dzau VJ, Majzoub JA, et al. Vasopressin-mediated forearm vasodilation in normal humans. Evidence for a vascular vasopressin V2 receptor. *J Clin Invest.* 1989;84:418–426.
164. Katusic ZS, Shepherd JT, Vanhoutte PM. Vasopressin causes endothelium-dependent relaxations of the canine basilar artery. *Circ Res.* 1984;55:575–579.
165. Nielsen S, Chou CL, Marples D, et al. Vasopressin increases water permeability of kidney collecting duct by inducing translocation of aquaporin-CD water channels to plasma membrane. *Proc Natl Acad Sci USA.* 1995;92:1013–1017.
166. Stone CK, Liang CS, Imai N, et al. Short-term hemodynamic effects of vasopressin V1-receptor inhibition in chronic right-sided congestive heart failure. *Circulation.* 1988;78:1251–1259.
167. Nishikimi T, Kawano Y, Saito Y, et al. Effect of long-term treatment with selective vasopressin V1 and V2 receptor antagonist on the development of heart failure in rats. *J Cardiovasc Pharmacol.* 1996;27:275–282.
168. Yamane Y. Plasma ADH level in patients with chronic congestive heart failure. *Jpn Circ J.* 1968;32:745–759.
169. Riegger GA, Liebau G, Kochsiek K. Antidiuretic hormone in congestive heart failure. *Am J Med.* 1982;72:49–52.
170. Goldsmith SR, Francis GS, Cowley AW, Jr., et al. Increased plasma arginine vasopressin levels in patients with congestive heart failure. *J Am Coll Cardiol.* 1983;1:1385–1390.
171. Creager MA, Faxon DP, Cutler SS, et al. Contribution of vasopressin to vasoconstriction in patients with congestive heart failure: comparison with the renin-angiotensin system and the sympathetic nervous system. *J Am Coll Cardiol.* 1986;7:758–765.
172. Szatalowicz VL, Arnold PE, Chaimovitz C, et al. Radioimmunoassay of plasma arginine vasopressin in hyponatremic patients with congestive heart failure. *N Engl J Med.* 1981;305:263–266.
173. Nicod P, Waeber B, Bussien JP, et al. Acute hemodynamic effect of a vascular antagonist of vasopressin in patients with congestive heart failure. *Am J Cardiol.* 1985;55:1043–1047.
174. Udelson JE, Smith WB, Hendrix GH, et al. Acute hemodynamic effects of conivaptan, a dual V(1A) and V(2) vasopressin receptor antagonist, in patients with advanced heart failure. *Circulation.* 2001;104:2417–2423.
175. Martin PY, Abraham WT, Lieming X, et al. Selective V2-receptor vasopressin antagonism decreases urinary aquaporin-2 excretion in patients with chronic heart failure. *J Am Soc Nephrol.* 1999;10:2165–2170.
176. Gheorghiade M, Niazi I, Ouyang J, et al. Vasopressin V2-receptor blockade with tolvaptan in patients with chronic heart failure: results from a double-blind, randomized trial. *Circulation.* 2003;107:2690–2696.
177. Gheorghiade M, Gattis WA, O'Connor CM, et al. Effects of tolvaptan, a vasopressin antagonist, in patients hospitalized with worsening heart failure: a randomized controlled trial. *JAMA.* 2004;291:1963–1971.
178. Kangawa K, Fukuda A, Kubota I, et al. Human atrial natriuretic polypeptides (hANP): purification, structure synthesis and biological activity. *J Hypertens. Suppl.* 1984;2:S321–S323.
179. Mukoyama M, Nakao K, Hosoda K, et al. Brain natriuretic peptide as a novel cardiac hormone in humans. Evidence for an exquisite dual natriuretic peptide system, atrial natriuretic peptide and brain natriuretic peptide. *J Clin Invest.* 1991;87: 1402–1412.
180. Stingo AJ, Clavell AL, Heublein DM, et al. Presence of C-type natriuretic peptide in cultured human endothelial cells and plasma. *Am J Physiol.* 1992;263:H1318–H1321.
181. Suga S, Nakao K, Itoh H, et al. Endothelial production of C-type natriuretic peptide and its marked augmentation by transforming growth factor-beta. Possible existence of "vascular natriuretic peptide system." *J Clin Invest.* 1992;90:1145–1149.
182. Koller KJ, Lowe DG, Bennett GL, et al. Selective activation of the B natriuretic peptide receptor by C-type natriuretic peptide (CNP). *Science.* 1991;252:120–123.
183. Burnett JC, Jr., Kao PC, Hu DC, et al. Atrial natriuretic peptide elevation in congestive heart failure in the human. *Science* 1986;231:1145–1147.
184. Wei CM, Heublein DM, Perrella MA, et al. Natriuretic peptide system in human heart failure. *Circulation.* 1993;88: 1004–1009.
185. Takahashi T, Allen PD, Izumo S. Expression of A-, B-, and C-type natriuretic peptide genes in failing and developing human ventricles. Correlation with expression of the Ca(2+)-ATPase gene. *Circ Res.* 1992;71:9–17.
186. Winquist RJ, Faison EP, Waldman SA, et al. Atrial natriuretic factor elicits an endothelium-independent relaxation and activates particulate guanylate cyclase in vascular smooth muscle. *Proc Natl Acad Sci USA.* 1984;81:7661–7664.
187. Waldman SA, Rapoport RM, Murad F. Atrial natriuretic factor selectively activates particulate guanylate cyclase and elevates cyclic GMP in rat tissues. *J Biol Chem.* 1984;259: 14332–14334.
188. Garcia R, Thibault G, Gutkowska J, et al. Changes of regional blood flow induced by atrial natriuretic factor (ANF) in conscious rats. *Life Sci.* 1985;36:1687–1692.
189. Ishihara T, Aisaka K, Hattori K, et al. Vasodilatory and diuretic actions of alpha-human atrial natriuretic polypeptide (alpha-hANP). *Life Sci.* 1985;36:1205–1215.
190. Raine AE, Erne P, Burgisser E, et al. Atrial natriuretic peptide and atrial pressure in patients with congestive heart failure. *N Engl J Med.* 1986;315:533–537.
191. Creager MA, Hirsch AT, Nabel EG, et al. Responsiveness of atrial natriuretic factor to reduction in right atrial pressure in patients with chronic congestive heart failure. *J Am Coll Cardiol.* 1988;11:1191–1198.
192. Kohzuki M, Hodsman GP, Johnston CI. Attenuated response to atrial natriuretic peptide in rats with myocardial infarction. *Am J Physiol.* 1989;256:H533–H538.
193. Cody RJ, Atlas SA, Laragh JH, et al. Atrial natriuretic factor in normal subjects and heart failure patients. Plasma levels and renal, hormonal, and hemodynamic responses to peptide infusion. *J Clin Invest.* 1986;78:1362–1374.
194. Hirooka Y, Takeshita A, Imaizumi T, et al. Attenuated forearm vasodilative response to intra-arterial atrial natriuretic peptide in patients with heart failure. *Circulation.* 1990;82:147–153.
195. Nakao K, Mukoyama M, Hosoda K, et al. Biosynthesis, secretion, and receptor selectivity of human brain natriuretic peptide. *Can J Physiol Pharmacol.* 1991;69:1500–1506.
196. Hama N, Itoh H, Shirakami G, et al. Rapid ventricular induction of brain natriuretic peptide gene expression in experimental acute myocardial infarction. *Circulation.* 1995;92:1558–1564.

197. Tsutamoto T, Wada A, Maeda K, et al. Attenuation of compensation of endogenous cardiac natriuretic peptide system in chronic heart failure: prognostic role of plasma brain natriuretic peptide concentration in patients with chronic symptomatic left ventricular dysfunction. *Circulation.* 1997;96:509–516.
198. Marcus LS, Hart D, Packer M, et al. Hemodynamic and renal excretory effects of human brain natriuretic peptide infusion in patients with congestive heart failure. A double-blind, placebo-controlled, randomized crossover trial. *Circulation.* 1996;94:3184–189.
199. Colucci WS, Elkayam U, Horton DP, et al. Intravenous nesiritide, a natriuretic peptide, in the treatment of decompensated congestive heart failure. Nesiritide Study Group. *N Engl J Med.* 2000;343:246–253.
200. Publication Committee for the VMAC Investigators (Vasodilatation in the Management of Acute CHF). Intravenous nesiritide vs nitroglycerin for treatment of decompensated congestive heart failure: a randomized controlled trial. *JAMA.* 2002;287:1531–1540.
201. Wright RS, Wei CM, Kim CH, et al. C-type natriuretic peptide-mediated coronary vasodilation: role of the coronary nitric oxide and particulate guanylate cyclase systems. *J Am Coll Cardiol.* 1996;28:1031–1038.
202. Wennberg PW, Miller VM, Rabelink T, et al. Further attenuation of endothelium-dependent relaxation imparted by natriuretic peptide receptor antagonism. *Am J Physiol.* 1999;277: H1618–H1621.
203. Maack T, Suzuki M, Almeida FA, et al. Physiological role of silent receptors of atrial natriuretic factor. *Science.* 1987;238:675–678.
204. Chauhan SD, Nilsson H, Ahluwalia A, et al. Release of C-type natriuretic peptide accounts for the biological activity of endothelium-derived hyperpolarizing factor. *Proc Natl Acad Sci USA.* 2003;100:1426–1431.
205. Davidson NC, Barr CS, Struthers AD. C-type natriuretic peptide. An endogenous inhibitor of vascular angiotensin-converting enzyme activity. *Circulation.* 1996;93:1155–1159.
206. Del Ry S, Passino C, Maltinti M, et al. C-type natriuretic peptide plasma levels increase in patients with chronic heart failure as a function of clinical severity. *Eur J Heart Fail.* 2005 (May 25).
207. Kitamura K, Kangawa K, Kawamoto M, et al. Adrenomedullin: a novel hypotensive peptide isolated from human pheochromocytoma. *Biochem Biophy Res Commun.* 1993;192:553–560.
208. Kuwasako K, Cao YN, Nagoshi Y, et al. Adrenomedullin receptors: pharmacological features and possible pathophysiological roles. *Peptides.* 2004;25:2003–2012.
209. Ishizaka Y, Tanaka M, Kitamura K, et al. Adrenomedullin stimulates cyclic AMP formation in rat vascular smooth muscle cells. *Biochem Biophy Res Commun.* 1994;200:642–646.
210. Jougasaki M, Rodeheffer RJ, Redfield MM, et al. Cardiac secretion of adrenomedullin in human heart failure. *J Clin Invest.* 1996;97:2370–2376.
211. Yamaguchi T, Baba K, Doi Y, et al. Effect of adrenomedullin on aldosterone secretion by dispersed rat adrenal zona glomerulosa cells. *Life Sci.* 1995;56:379–387.
212. Tian Q, Zhao D, Tan DY, et al. Vasodilator effect of human adrenomedullin(13–52) on hypertensive rats. *Can J Physiol Pharmacol.* 1995;73:1065–1069.
213. Kano H, Kohno M, Yasunari K, et al. Adrenomedullin as a novel antiproliferative factor of vascular smooth muscle cells. *J Hypertens.* 1996;14:209–213.
214. Oie E, Vinge LE, Andersen GO, et al. RAMP2 and RAMP3 mRNA levels are increased in failing rat cardiomyocytes and associated with increased responsiveness to adrenomedullin. *J. Mol Cell Cardiol.* 2005;38:145–151.
215. Jougasaki M, Stevens TL, Borgeson DD, et al. Adrenomedullin in experimental congestive heart failure: cardiorenal activation. *Am J Physiol.* 1997;273:R1392–R1399.
216. Jougasaki M, Wei CM, McKinley LJ, et al. Elevation of circulating and ventricular adrenomedullin in human congestive heart failure. *Circulation.* 1995;92:286–289.
217. Nishikimi T, Horio T, Sasaki T, et al. Cardiac production and secretion of adrenomedullin are increased in heart failure. *Hypertension.* 1997;30:1369–1375.
218. Rademaker MT, Charles CJ, Lewis LK, et al. Beneficial hemodynamic and renal effects of adrenomedullin in an ovine model of heart failure. *Circulation.* 1997;96:1983–1990.
219. Nagaya N, Satoh T, Nishikimi T, et al. Hemodynamic, renal, and hormonal effects of adrenomedullin infusion in patients with congestive heart failure. *Circulation.* 2000;101:498–503.
220. Nakamura M, Yoshida H, Makita S, et al. Potent and long-lasting vasodilatory effects of adrenomedullin in humans. Comparisons between normal subjects and patients with chronic heart failure. *Circulation.* 1997;95:1214–1221.
221. Zhang XP, Tada H, Wang Z, et al. cAMP signal transduction, a potential compensatory pathway for coronary endothelial NO production after heart failure. *Arterioscler Thromb Vasc Biol.* 2002;22:1273–1278.
222. Duprez DA, De Buyzere ML, Rietzschel ER, et al. Inverse relationship between aldosterone and large artery compliance in chronically treated heart failure patients. *Eur Heart J.* 1998;19:1371–1376.
223. Arnold JM, Marchiori GE, Imrie JR, et al. Large artery function in patients with chronic heart failure. Studies of brachial artery diameter and hemodynamics. *Circulation.* 1991;84: 2418–2425.
224. Finkelstein SM, Cohn JN, Collins VR, et al. Vascular hemodynamic impedance in congestive heart failure. *Am J Cardiol.* 1985;55:423–427.
225. Pepine CJ, Nichols WW, Conti CR. Aortic input impedance in heart failure. *Circulation.* 1978;58:460–465.
226. Nakamura M, Sugawara S, Arakawa N, et al. Reduced vascular compliance is associated with impaired endothelium-dependent dilatation in the brachial artery of patients with congestive heart failure. *J Card Fail.* 2004;10:36–42.
227. Ontkean M, Gay R, Greenberg B. Diminished endothelium-derived relaxing factor activity in an experimental model of chronic heart failure. *Circ Res.* 1991;69:1088–1096.

The Kidney in Heart Failure

15

JoAnn Lindenfeld Robert W. Schrier

Sodium and water retention are hallmarks of heart failure (HF) and link the heart and kidney in this common medical problem. Only recently has it been recognized that renal dysfunction is an important predictor of morbidity and mortality due to HF. When renal dysfunction occurs in the setting of HF, there is a higher mortality, a more prolonged hospital stay, and a higher rate of readmission for HF (1–5). However, it remains uncertain whether renal dysfunction occurring with HF is merely a reflection of the severity of the HF or whether the renal dysfunction actually accelerates the progression of HF (6). In this chapter we review what is known about renal salt and water handling in HF and describe the clinical characteristics of the so-called cardiorenal syndrome. We then explore potential mechanisms whereby renal dysfunction may exacerbate the progression of HF and address potential therapeutic strategies to ameliorate worsening renal function in patients with HF.

RENAL SALT AND WATER HANDLING IN HEART FAILURE

A substantial body of evidence supports a unifying hypothesis of body fluid volume regulation in health and disease (7–9). While the exact nature of this volume-regulatory system remains incompletely understood, the factors involved in renal salt and water handling in HF can be broadly classified as belonging to either afferent (sensor) or efferent (effector) limbs. This integrated mechanism provides an understanding of why patients with HF have expanded total plasma and blood volumes and yet their kidneys, which are otherwise normal, continue to retain sodium and water.

AFFERENT MECHANISMS

The Concept of Adequate Arterial Filling or the Compartment Sensed

There are a number of circumstances in which there is avid renal sodium and water retention despite expanded extracellular fluid (ECF), interstitial fluid (ISF), and intravascular volumes. For example, patients with advanced HF often have increased ECF volumes, including interstitial edema, expanded total plasma, and blood volumes (7–9). In fact, the edematous disorders, including HF, cirrhosis, and pregnancy are defined by avid renal sodium and water retention despite total body salt and water excess. In these disease states, it is clear that the integrity of the kidney as the ultimate effector organ of body fluid regulation is intact. For example, renal sodium and water retention in cirrhotic patients is reversed by transplantation of the kidney from a cirrhotic patient to a subject with normal liver function (10). Moreover, the transplantation of a normal liver into the edematous cirrhotic patient or implantation of a left ventricular assist device into an edematous HF patient have both been shown to reverse renal sodium and water retention (11,12). Thus, in such edematous disorders the kidney must be responding to extrarenal signals from the afferent limb of a volume-regulatory system. The pathogenesis of these extrarenal signals, although not completely understood, is discussed next.

If afferent volume receptors sense primarily total blood volume, then the kidneys of edematous patients should increase their excretion of sodium and water as total blood volume increases. Since this does not occur in patients with severe cardiac or liver disease, there must be some body fluid compartment that remains underfilled even in the presence of expansion of total ECF and blood volume. This underfilled compartment is the afferent limb of renal sodium and water retention in patients with edematous disorders. In 1948, John Peters at Yale coined the term *effective blood volume* as a reference to just such an underfilled body fluid compartment (13). Peters postulated that a decrease in effective blood volume triggers extrarenal signals that enhance tubular sodium and water reabsorption by the otherwise normal kidney. Indeed, renal sodium and water retention can occur in patients with cardiac failure prior to any diminution in glomerular filtration rate (GFR).

Borst and De Vries (14) first suggested that cardiac output was the effective blood volume postulated by Peters and, as such, was the primary modulator of renal sodium and water excretion. However, cardiac output is unlikely the only candidate for effective blood volume because profound renal salt and water retention may occur in the presence of increased in cardiac output. Cirrhosis, pregnancy, large arteriovenous (AV) fistulas, and other causes of high-output cardiac failure such as thyrotoxicosis and beriberi are all associated with significant elevations in cardiac output and avid renal sodium and water retention with expansion of ECF volume (7–9).

Primacy of the Arterial Circulation in Volume Regulation

A unifying hypothesis for body fluid volume regulation in health and disease (7–9) has been developed from a series of investigations in experimental animals and in humans (15–25). This unifying hypothesis states that total ECF, ISF, or intravascular volumes are not primary determinants of renal sodium and water excretion. With this hypothesis, the venous component of intravascular volume is likewise excluded as the primary determinant of sodium and water excretion. However, it is acknowledged that there are experimental and clinical circumstances in which selective increases in right and left or only left atrial pressure stimulate the release of atrial natriuretic peptide (ANP) (9) and suppression of arginine vasopressin (AVP) (26), respectively, which may enhance sodium and water excretion. However, these events must be subservient to more potent determinants of body fluid volume regulation because the patient with advanced left or right ventricular dysfunction, or both, exhibits avid sodium and water retention despite markedly elevated atrial pressures.

The unifying hypothesis of body fluid volume regulation proposes that the arterial circulation is the primary body fluid compartment modulating renal sodium and water excretion (7–9). In a 70-kg man, total body water approximates 42 L, of which only 0.7 L (1.7% of total body water) resides in the arterial circulation (Table 15-1). From a teleologic viewpoint, it is attractive to propose that the primary regulation of renal sodium and water excretion, and thus body fluid volume homeostasis, is modulated by the smallest body fluid compartment, thus endowing the system with exquisite sensitivity to relatively small changes in body fluid volume, and resides in that fluid compartment responsible for the arterial perfusion of the body's vital organs and tissues.

TABLE 15-1
BODY FLUID VOLUME DISTRIBUTION

Compartment	Amount	Volumes in 70-kg Man
Total body fluid	60% of body weight	42 L
Intracellular fluid	40% of body weight	28 L
Extracellular fluid (ECF)	20% of body weight	14 L
Interstitial fluid	Two-thirds of ECF	9.4 L
Plasma fluid	One-third of ECF	4.6 L
Venous fluid	85% of plasma fluid	3.9 L
Arterial fluid	15% of plasma fluid	0.7 L

Cardiac Output and Peripheral Arterial Resistance as Determinants of Arterial Filling

The body fluid volume regulation hypothesis proposes that cardiac output and peripheral vascular resistance are the two primary determinants of overfilling or underfilling of the arterial circulation. In this context, it is proposed that all renal sodium- and water-retaining states, which occur in the absence of intrinsic renal disease, are initiated by either a decrease in cardiac output, peripheral arterial vasodilation, or both. Thus, this hypothesis accounts for sodium and water retention in both low-output and high-output cardiac failure as well as in other edematous disorders with intact kidney function.

Afferent Volume Receptors

The afferent volume receptors for such a volume regulatory system must reside in the arterial vascular tree, such as the high-pressure baroreceptors in the carotid sinus, aortic arch, left ventricle, and juxtaglomerular apparatus. As previously mentioned, the low-pressure volume receptors of the thorax (atria, right ventricle, and pulmonary vessels) must be of some importance to the volume regulatory system. However, there is considerable evidence that arterial receptors predominate over low-pressure receptors in volume control in mammals (27–35).

Low-pressure Volume Receptors

Various maneuvers that decrease central venous return, such as positive pressure breathing (36), lower extremity tourniquets (37,38), and prolonged standing (39) are associated with decreased renal sodium excretion. Conversely, maneuvers that increase thoracic venous return, such as negative pressure breathing (40) and recumbency (41), are associated with enhanced renal sodium excretion. Head-out water immersion, a technique that increases venous return to the heart, results in a significant increase in renal salt and water excretion independent of major changes in either GFR or renal hemodynamics (42). Moreover, in the dog a direct correlation between renal sodium excretion and left atrial pressure has been demonstrated (43,44), supporting a role for an atrial receptor in volume regulation. As first suggested by Gauer and Henry (40,45), physiologically important left atrial receptors have also been shown to contribute to ECF volume regulation by exerting nonosmotic control over the antidiuretic hormone AVP (26,43, 45). In addition, changes in atrial stretch and transmural pressures have been shown to determine circulating plasma concentrations of the vasoactive and natriuretic hormone ANP (46–48). Another normal response to increased left atrial pressure is a decrease in renal sympathetic tone (49). In chronic HF these atrial-renal reflexes are impaired. For example, the atrial-renal sympathetic reflex is also blunted in a dog model of HF (50). In patients with dilated cardiomyopathy and mild HF, a volume load failed to increase ANP and the natriuretic response was blunted (51).

High-Pressure Volume Receptors

Evidence for the presence of volume-sensitive receptors in the arterial circulation in humans originated from observations in subjects with traumatic AV fistulas (52). Closure of an AV fistula is associated with a decreased rate of emptying of the arterial blood into the venous circulation, as demonstrated by closure-induced increases in diastolic arterial pressure and decreases in cardiac output, and results in an immediate increase in renal sodium excretion without changes in either GFR or renal blood flow (RBF) (52). Further evidence implicating the fullness of the arterial vascular tree as a sensor in modulating renal sodium excretion can be found in denervation experiments. In these studies, pharmacologic or surgical interruption of sympathetic afferent neural pathways emanating from high-pressure areas inhibited the natriuretic response to volume expansion (15,16,53–57). Moreover, reduction of pressure or stretch at the carotid sinus has been shown to activate the sympathetic nervous system and to promote renal sodium and water retention (58,59). High-pressure baroreceptors also appear to be important factors in regulating the nonosmotic release of AVP and, thus, renal water excretion (60,61).

Located in the afferent arterioles within the kidney, the juxtaglomerular apparatus is one of the best-defined of the high-pressure receptors implicated in body fluid volume regulation. The juxtaglomerular apparatus responds to decreased stretch or increased renal sympathetic tone with enhanced renal secretion of renin (59). Thus, this baroreceptor is an important factor in the control of angiotensin II formation and aldosterone secretion and, ultimately, in renal sodium and water retention.

Other Afferent Receptors

While unloading of high-pressure volume receptors appears to play the predominant role in initiating renal salt and water retention in HF and in other edematous disorders with intact kidney function, experimental evidence suggests a possible role for various chemoreceptors found in the heart and elsewhere in the body. For example, in the heart and lungs, both vagal and sympathetic afferent nerve endings respond to a variety of exogenous and endogenous chemical substances, including capsaicin, phenyldiguanidine, bradykinin, substance P, and prostaglandins (62–64). Significantly, Zucker et al. (63) have shown that prostaglandin I_2 (PGI_2) attenuates the baroreflex control of renal nerve activity via a cardiac afferent vagal mechanism. Because substances such as bradykinin and prostaglandins may circulate at increased concentrations in HF patients (65), it is possible that altered central nervous system input from chemically sensitive cardiac or pulmonary afferents contributes to the sodium and water retention of chronic HF. However, the exact role in HF of these and other chemoreceptors remains to be defined.

EFFERENT MECHANISMS

Renal Hemodynamics

The GFR usually is normal in early or mild HF and is reduced only as cardiac performance becomes more severely impaired. Renal vascular resistance is increased with a concomitant decrease in RBF. In general, RBF decreases in proportion to the decrease in cardiac performance. Thus, the ratio of GFR to renal plasma flow, or the filtration fraction, usually is increased in patients with cardiac failure. This increased filtration fraction is a consequence of constriction of the efferent arterioles within the kidney. These changes in renal hemodynamics alter the hydrostatic and oncotic forces in the peritubular capillaries to favor increased proximal tubular reabsorption of sodium and water (Fig. 15-1). The renal hemodynamic changes seen in HF are primarily mediated by activation of various neurohormonal vasoconstrictor

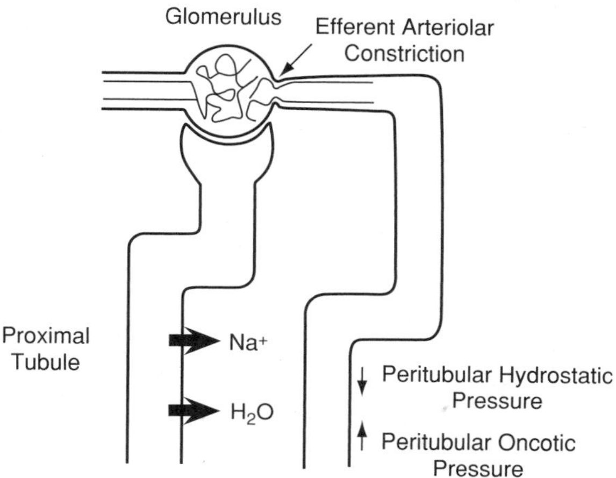

Figure 15-1 Efferent arteriolar constriction, mediated in congestive heart failure (CHF) by increased renal sympathetic nerve activity and angiotensin II concentrations, alters net postglomerular Starling forces in a direction to enhance proximal tubular sodium and water reabsorption.

systems. In addition, neurohormonal activation directly contributes to enhanced sodium and water reabsorption in both the proximal and distal nephron in HF, as discussed next.

The Neurohormonal Response to Heart Failure

Arterial underfilling secondary to a diminished cardiac output elicits a number of compensatory neurohormonal responses that act to maintain the integrity of the arterial circulation by promoting peripheral vasoconstriction as well as expansion of the ECF volume through renal sodium and water retention. The three best-described neurohor-monal vasoconstrictor systems activated in response to cardiac failure are the sympathetic nervous system, the renin-angiotensin-aldosterone system (RAAS), and the nonosmotic release of AVP. Baroreceptor activation of the sympathetic nervous system appears to be the primary integrator of the hormonal vasoconstrictor systems involved in the volume control system because the nonosmotic release of AVP involves sympathetic stimulation of the supraoptic and paraventricular nuclei in the hypothalamus (66), and activation of the RAAS involves renal adrenergic stimulation (67). Thus, in low-output cardiac failure, diminished integrity of the arterial circulation, as determined by decreased cardiac output, causes unloading of arterial baroreceptors in the carotid sinus and aortic arch. Peripheral vasodilation causes unloading of these arterial baroreceptors in the setting of high-output cardiac failure (Fig. 15-2). This baroreceptor inactivation results in diminution of the tonic inhibitory effect of afferent vagal and glossopharyngeal pathways to the central nervous system and initiates an increase in sympathetic efferent adrenergic tone with subsequent activation of the other two major vasoconstrictor hormonal systems. Various counterregulatory vasodilatory and natriuretic hormones are also activated in HF, including the natriuretic peptides (NPs) and renal prostaglandins. Table 15-2 summarizes the renal effects of some of the neurohormonal systems that are activated in HF.

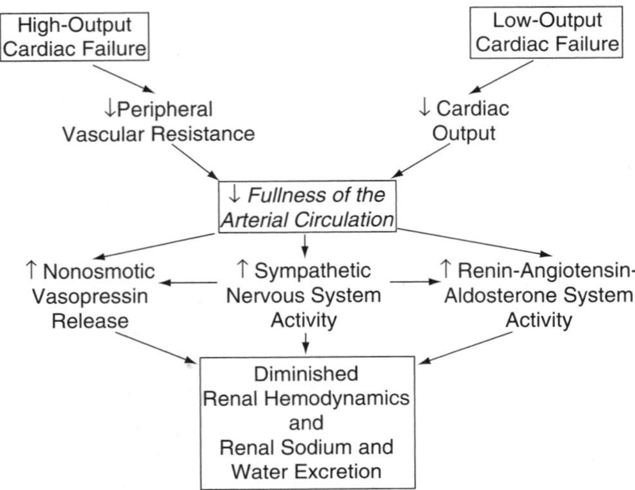

Figure 15-2 Proposed mechanism of renal sodium and water retention in high-output and low-output cardiac failure.

TABLE 15-2
RENAL EFFECTS OF NEUROHORMONAL ACTIVATION IN CONGESTIVE HEART FAILURE

Vasoconstrictor Systems

Renal nerves
- Promote afferent and efferent arteriolar constriction
- Enhance sodium reabsorption in proximal tubule
- Stimulate renal renin release

Renin-angiotensin-aldosterone system
- Angiotensin II
  - Promotes efferent greater than afferent arteriolar constriction
  - Enhances sodium reabsorption in proximal tubule
  - Stimulates adrenal aldosterone synthesis and release
  - Causes cardiac remodeling
- Aldosterone
  - Enhances sodium reabsorption and potassium secretion in collecting duct
  - Increases cardiac fibrosis

Arginine vasopressin
- Increases water reabsorption in cortical and medullary collecting duct
- Increases sodium chloride reabsorption in medullary ascending limb of the loop of Henle (in animal models)
- Increases vasoconstriction of predominantly efferent arteriole

Endothelin
- Increases renal vasoconstriction
- Unknown effect on tubular sodium handling

Vasodilator Systems

Natriuretic peptides
- Increase glomerular filtration rate
- Promote diminished sodium reabsorption in collecting duct
- Suppress plasma renin activity
- Inhibit aldosterone synthesis and release
- Possible inhibition of vasopressin release

Renal prostaglandins
- Promote renal vasodilation
- Decrease tubular sodium reabsorption in ascending limb of the loop of Henle
- Inhibit vasopressin hydro-osmotic action in collecting duct

The Sympathetic Nervous System in Heart Failure

The sympathetic nervous system is activated early in patients with HF. Evidence for this comes both from indirect and direct measurements of sympathetic nervous system activity in HF patients. Various studies have documented elevated peripheral venous plasma norepinephrine (NE) concentrations in patients with HF (68–73). Previous studies in advanced HF, using tritiated NE to determine NE kinetics, demonstrated that both increased NE secretion and decreased NE clearance contribute to the high venous plasma NE concentrations seen in these patients, suggesting that increased sympathetic activity is at least partially responsible for the elevated circulating plasma NE (70,71). A more recent investigation of NE kinetics in earlier stages of HF demonstrated that the initial increase in plasma NE in HF is solely due to increased NE secretion, providing evidence of increased sympathetic nervous activity early in the course of HF (72). Studies using peroneal nerve microneurography to directly assess sympathetic nerve activity to muscle also demonstrate increased sympathetic activity in HF patients. Using this technique, one group of investigators recorded sympathetic nerve activity to muscle while simultaneously measuring plasma NE concentrations in patients with HF (74). Sympathetic nerve activity was increased in these patients and strongly correlated with plasma NE levels (74). Finally, the SOLVD Investigators (75) have reported the presence of sympathetic activation, as determined by plasma NE concentrations, in patients with asymptomatic LV dysfunction.

A study in human HF have demonstrated the presence of selective cardiorenal sympathetic activation (70). In this study of whole-body and organ-specific NE kinetics in HF patients, cardiac and renal NE spillover rates were increased 504% and 206%, respectively, whereas the NE spillover rate from the lungs was normal. Thus, it is perhaps not surprising that the deleterious effects of chronic sympathetic activation in HF are seen primarily in the heart and kidney. The importance of increased renal sympathetic nerve activity was demonstrated in a recent study of 61 HF patients. In a model that included total body NE spillover, left ventricular ejection fraction (LVEF), GFR, RBF, cardiac index, etiology of HF, and age, renal NE spillover was the most important predictor of all-cause mortality and need for heart transplantation.

The adverse effects of systemic and cardiac adrenergic activation in chronic HF include peripheral vasoconstriction, renal sodium and water retention, direct myocardial toxicity via calcium overload or the induction of apoptosis, stimulation of tachycardia and other arrhythmias, activation of the RAAS, stimulation of nonosmotic AVP release, and downregulation of cardiac β_1-adrenergic receptors and other myocardial receptor-signal transduction abnormalities. This latter effect, which occurs in response to increased cardiac sympathetic activity, may be alternatively viewed as a protective mechanism to withdraw the heart from the effects of excessive adrenergic stimulation. Sympathetic activation, as measured by the plasma NE concentration, correlates directly with the degree of LV dysfunction in HF (68,69,76). Moreover, the plasma NE concentration correlates negatively with prognosis in HF (77). That is, high plasma NE levels are associated with poor prognosis in HF patients. This was demonstrated by Cohn et al. (77), who prospectively studied 106 patients with moderate or severe HF and found that a single resting venous plasma NE level provided a better guide to prognosis than did other commonly measured indexes of cardiac and functional performance. Recent studies confirm the predictive value of plasma NE even in patients treated with angiotensin-converting enzyme (ACE) inhibitors and β-blockers (78). Finally, β-adrenergic receptor antagonists have been demonstrated to improve LVEF and mortality and reduce hospital admissions in patients with HF (79–81). Taken together, these observations support the hypothesis that NE contributes to disease progression in chronic HF.

Effects of Increased Renal Sympathetic Activity in Heart Failure

Through renal vasoconstriction, stimulation of the RAAS, and direct effects on the proximal convoluted tubule, enhanced renal sympathetic activity may contribute to the avid sodium and water retention of HF. Indeed, intrarenal adrenergic blockade has been shown to cause a natriuresis in experimental animals and in humans with HF (82–84). Moreover, in the rat, renal nerve stimulation has been demonstrated to produce an approximate 25% reduction in sodium excretion and urine volume (85). The diminished renal sodium excretion that accompanies renal nerve stimulation may be mediated by at least two mechanisms. Studies performed in rats have demonstrated that NE-induced efferent arteriolar constriction alters peritubular hemodynamic forces in favor of increased tubular sodium reabsorption (86). As previously mentioned, the increase in filtration fraction with a normal or only slightly reduced GFR that is often seen in HF patients must be due to predominant efferent arteriolar constriction. Constriction of the efferent arterioles in HF has been confirmed by renal micropuncture studies performed in rats (87), and is at least partially mediated by increased renal sympathetic activity and by angiotensin II. Thus, efferent arteriolar constriction in HF alters the balance of hemodynamic forces in the peritubular capillaries in favor of enhanced proximal tubular sodium reabsorption.

In addition, renal nerves have been shown to exert a direct influence on sodium reabsorption in the proximal convoluted tubule (85,88). Bello-Reuss et al. (85) demonstrated this direct effect of renal nerve activation to enhance proximal tubular sodium reabsorption in whole-kidney and individual nephron studies in the rat. In these animals, renal nerve stimulation produced an increase in the tubular fluid/plasma inulin concentration ratio in the late proximal tubule, an outcome of increased fractional sodium and water reabsorption in this segment of the nephron (85). Hence, increased renal nerve activity may promote sodium retention by a mechanism independent of changes in renal hemodynamics. However, in dogs with denervated transplanted kidneys and chronic vena caval constriction, the sodium retention persists (89). Moreover, renal denervation does not prevent ascites in the dog with chronic vena caval constriction (90). Thus, renal nerves probably contribute to, but do not fully account for, the avid sodium and water retention of HF.

The Renin-Angiotensin-Aldosterone System in Heart Failure

The RAAS is also activated in HF, as assessed by plasma renin activity (PRA) (69,91,92). Renin acts on angiotensinogen to produce angiotensin I, which is then converted by ACE to angiotensin II. In HF, the resultant increased plasma concentration of angiotensin II exerts circulatory effects similar to sympathetic activation, including peripheral arterial and venous vascular constriction, renal vasoconstriction, and cardiac inotropism. Angiotensin II also acts to promote the secretion of the sodium-retaining hormone aldosterone by the adrenal cortex and in positive-feedback stimulation of the sympathetic nervous system (93). Thus, in the kidney, activation of this hormonal system promotes sodium retention via several mechanisms, as discussed later.

Activation of the RAAS is associated with hyponatremia and an unfavorable prognosis in HF (65,94). The association of PRA and hyponatremia was first described by Dzau et al. (65) in a cohort of 15 HF patients. These data demonstrated that normal or suppressed PRA is associated with a normal serum sodium level, whereas the highest PRA is associated with the lowest serum sodium concentrations (65). This association of hyponatremia with RAAS activation was later confirmed by Lee and Packer (94) in a larger group of HF patients. Moreover, these investigators demonstrated the association of this hyponatremic, hyperreninemic state with poor survival (94). The mechanisms by which activation of the RAAS might negatively impact on survival in HF are primarily mediated by increased angiotensin II levels. As previously noted, increased angiotensin II causes venous and arteriolar vasoconstriction, thus increasing ventricular preload and afterload. Angiotensin II may stimulate nonosmotic AVP release, promoting renal water retention, and increase thirst. Angiotensin II also may act as a growth factor, promoting myocardial hypertrophy and thus ventricular ischemia and remodeling, as well as vascular and glomerular hypertrophy and remodeling. Angiotensin II, via several mechanisms, augments renal sodium reabsorption.

Renal Effects of Increased Angiotensin II in Heart Failure

Angiotensin II may contribute to the sodium and water retention of HF through direct and indirect effects on proximal tubular sodium reabsorption and by stimulating the release of aldosterone from the adrenal gland. Angiotensin II causes renal efferent arteriolar vasoconstriction, resulting in decreased RBF and an increased filtration fraction. As with renal nerve stimulation, this results in increased peritubular capillary oncotic pressure and reduced peritubular capillary hydrostatic pressure, which favors the reabsorption of sodium and water in the proximal tubule (87,95). In addition, angiotensin II has been shown to have a direct effect on enhanced sodium reabsorption in the proximal tubule (96,97). This direct effect of angiotensin II on the proximal tubule has been associated with angiotensin II-mediated activation of the basolateral sodium-bicarbonate cotransporters and apical sodium-hydrogen exchanger and is inhibited by angiotensin II AT_1-receptor blockade (97). Finally, angiotensin II enhances aldosterone secretion by the adrenal gland, which promotes tubular sodium reabsorption in the distal tubule and collecting duct.

A role for RAAS activation in the sodium retention of HF is suggested by the finding that urinary sodium excretion inversely correlates with PRA and urinary aldosterone excretion in HF patients (98,99). However, the administration of an ACE inhibitor during HF does not consistently increase urinary sodium excretion, despite a consistent decrease in plasma aldosterone concentration (100). The simultaneous decrease in blood pressure due to decreased circulating concentrations of angiotensin II, however, may activate hemodynamic and neurohormonal mechanisms, which could obscure the natriuretic response to lowered angiotensin II and aldosterone concentrations.

Support for this hypothesis comes from a study performed by Hensen et al. (101). The effect of the specific aldosterone antagonist, spironolactone, on urinary sodium excretion was examined in patients with mild to moderate HF who were withdrawn from all medications prior to study. Sodium was retained in all patients throughout the period prior to aldosterone antagonism. On an average sodium intake was 97 ± 8 mmol per day, and the average sodium excretion prior to spironolactone was 78 ± 8 mmol per day. During therapy with spironolactone, all HF patients exhibited a significant increase in urinary sodium excretion to an average of 131 ± 13 mmol per day. Plasma renin activity and NE increased during the administration of spironolactone. Thus, this investigation demonstrates reversal of the sodium retention of HF with the administration of an aldosterone antagonist, despite further activation of various antinatriuretic influences, including stimulation of the renin-angiotensin and sympathetic nervous systems. These results indicate that the RAAS is an important mediator of sodium retention in HF.

The Nonosmotic Release of Vasopressin in Heart Failure

Plasma AVP is usually elevated in patients with HF and correlates in general with the clinical and hemodynamic severity of disease and with the serum sodium level (18,102–105). Plasma AVP concentrations are elevated in spite of hypo-osmality in patients with HF, and these levels fail to suppress normally to acute water loading (102,106). Taken together, these observations suggest that there is enhanced release of AVP in HF and that nonosmotic mechanisms are responsible. As already suggested, baroreceptor activation of the sympathetic nervous system likely mediates the nonosmotic release of AVP in HF patients (66).

Through its effects on vascular (V_1) and renal (V_2) receptors, AVP is a potent mediator of peripheral vasoconstriction and renal water retention, respectively. By analogy to NE and angiotensin II, it can be speculated that both of these effects may be of some pathophysiological importance in HF. Several findings support a role for AVP in the altered hemodynamics of HF. For example, small increases in plasma AVP concentrations, within the basal range seen in HF patients, increase peripheral vascular resistance and produce a corresponding decrease in cardiac output in patients with cardiac failure (105). Moreover, experimental antagonists of the V_1 vasopressin receptor have been used in patients with low-output cardiac failure (107,108). Selective antagonism of these receptors in humans is associated with peripheral vasodilation and improved cardiac function in a subset of patients with severe HF (107,108). Finally, it has been shown that a nonpeptide V_1 receptor antagonist decreases systemic vascular resistance and increases cardiac output in dogs with tachycardia-induced HF (109). These observations suggest a role for AVP in the peripheral vasoconstriction and, hence, increased afterload of HF.

Renal Effects of Increased Arginine Vasopressin in Heart Failure

Arginine vasopressin, via stimulation of its V_2 receptor, enhances water reabsorption in the distal nephron, including the cortical and medullary collecting ducts. Three lines of evidence implicate nonosmotic AVP release in the abnormal water retention of HF. First, in animal models of HF, the absence of a pituitary source of AVP is associated with normal or near-normal water excretion (30,110). This observation was first demonstrated by decreasing cardiac preload with acute thoracic vena caval constriction (30). In these animals, acute removal of the pituitary source of AVP by surgical hypophysectomy virtually abolished the defect in water excretion. Abnormal water excretion also occurs in the rat with an aortocaval fistula (110). The impairment in water excretion seen in this high-output model of cardiac failure is presumably the result of AVP release because the defect is not demonstrable in rats with central diabetes insipidus (110).

The second line of evidence supporting a role for AVP in the water retention of HF comes from studies using selective antagonists of the V_2 receptor of AVP in animals and in humans with HF (111–114). Ishikawa et al. (112) assessed the antidiuretic effect of plasma AVP in a low-output model of cardiac failure secondary to vena caval constriction in the rat. In these animals, plasma AVP concentrations were increased and a peptide antagonist of the antidiuretic effect of AVP reversed the defect in water excretion. Yared et al. (113) have also shown a reversal of water retention using a peptide antagonist to the antidiuretic effect of AVP in another model of HF, the rat coronary artery ligation model. In addition, studies in human HF of an orally available nonpeptide AVP antagonist have demonstrated reversal of the impaired urinary diluting capacity, increased solute-free water excretion, and correction of hyponatremia following drug administration (111,113,114). AVP-sensitive water channels have been shown to be upregulated in the cortex and papilla of rats with cardiac failure, an effect that was reversed with a nonpeptide V_2-receptor antagonist (115).

In a study by Bichet et al. (104), the effect of the ACE inhibitor captopril or the α_1-adrenergic-blocker prazosin to reverse the abnormality in water retention in patients with stage III and IV HF was examined. The afterload reduction and increased cardiac output with either agent were associated with improved water excretion and suppression of plasma AVP in response to an acute water load. A role of angiotensin II in modulating the effect of AVP in HF seems unlikely because captopril and prazosin had opposing effects on the renin-angiotensin system, yet their effects to improve water excretion as plasma AVP was suppressed were comparable (104). In this regard, it is important to note that in this study by Bichet et al. the average decrease in mean arterial pressure was 5 mm Hg, a decrement that is less than the 7% to 10% necessary to activate the nonosmotic release of AVP (116). Thus, these results are compatible with the suggestion that a decrease in stroke volume, in addition to a decrease in mean arterial pressure, may be a stimulus for the nonosmotic release of AVP in low-output cardiac failure. The association of improved cardiac output and water excretion during afterload reduction is compatible with an influence of ventricular receptors and/or baroreceptors sensing arterial pressure and stroke volume in modulating AVP release.

Endothelin in Heart Failure

Endothelin is a potent vasoconstrictor and its concentration is increased in patients with HF (117). A study from Teerlink et al. (118) supports a role for endothelin in the arterial vasoconstriction of experimental HF. This study demonstrated a significant decrease in blood pressure following the administration of the endothelin antagonist, bosentan, in rats with HF following coronary artery ligation. Moreover, elevated plasma endothelin concentrations have been found to be associated with a poor prognosis in patients with New York Heart Association (NYHA) Class III and IV HF (119). In the kidney, mesangial cells, endothelial cells, epithelial glomerular cells, and inner medullary collecting duct cells can synthesize endothelin (120). Despite these observations, the role of increased endothelin in the pathogenesis of the renal sodium and water retention of HF is as yet unknown. In this regard, however, endothelin (as an autocrine/paracrine hormone) may be a potent mediator of renal vasoconstriction and thus influence renal sodium and water handling.

Natriuretic Peptides in Heart Failure

The NPs, including ANP and brain or B-type natriuretic peptide (BNP), circulate at increased concentrations in patients with HF (46,47,121–125). These peptide hormones possess natriuretic; vasorelaxant; and renin-, aldosterone-, and possibly AVP- and sympatho-inhibiting properties (126–130). These attributes suggest the possibility of an important counterregulatory role for ANP and BNP in cardiac failure. These hormones are released primarily from the heart in response to increased atrial or ventricular end-diastolic pressure or to increased transmural cardiac pressure (48,99).

In a recent study of ANP kinetics, increased ANP production rather than decreased metabolic clearance was the major factor contributing to the elevated plasma ANP concentrations in HF patients (101). This finding is consistent with the observed increase in expression of both ANP and BNP mRNA in the cardiac atria and ventricles, respectively, of animals and humans with HF (131,132). The significant vasodilatory action of elevated endogenous ANP concentrations in chronic HF has been demonstrated during the infusion of a monoclonal ANP antibody in the rat (133). In this coronary artery ligation model of HF, infusion of a monoclonal antibody shown to specifically block endogenous ANP in vivo caused a significant increase in right atrial pressure, LV end-diastolic pressure, and peripheral vascular resistance. Thus, ANP appears to attenuate to some degree the systemic venous and arterial vasoconstriction of HF. In human HF, NP infusions result in decreased pulmonary arterial wedge pressure and decreased peripheral vascular resistance with an associated increase in cardiac output (99,133–135).

Renal Effects of Increased Natriuretic Peptides in Heart Failure

In normal human subjects, NPs increase GFR with no change or only a modest decrease in RBF (99,136). These changes in renal hemodynamics are likely mediated by afferent arteriolar vasodilation and constriction of the efferent arterioles, as demonstrated by micropuncture studies during ANP exposure in the rat (137,138). NP infusions appear to be associated with diminished sodium reabsorption in the proximal tubule (99,136). This effect of infused NPs may be a consequence of renal hemodynamic changes or a result of a direct tubular effect. Against this latter possibility are enzymatic and binding studies of ANP in rat glomeruli and nephrons that demonstrate that the glomerulus and distal nephron are the important sites of renal ANP action, rather than the proximal tubule (139–141). Thus, in addition to increasing GFR and filtered sodium load as a mechanism of their natriuretic effect, NPs have been proposed as specific inhibitors of sodium reabsorption in the collecting tubule.

An important functional role for endogenous ANP in the renal sodium balance of HF has been proposed by Lee et al. (142). These investigators examined sodium excretion in two models of low-output cardiac failure in the dog: acute HF produced by rapid ventricular pacing, and a thoracic inferior vena caval constriction model. In the case of acute HF produced by rapid ventricular pacing, cardiac output and arterial pressure were diminished while atrial pressures and plasma ANP concentrations were increased. Despite the arterial hypotension, sodium excretion was maintained. In addition, PRA and plasma aldosterone concentrations were not increased. In contrast, similar reductions in cardiac output and arterial pressure by thoracic inferior vena caval constriction were not associated with increased atrial pressures or plasma ANP. In these animals, PRA and plasma aldosterone were significantly increased. Moreover, avid sodium retention was observed in these animals with normal circulating, rather than elevated, ANP concentrations. Finally, dogs with thoracic inferior vena caval obstruction were administered exogenous ANP to achieve circulating levels comparable with those seen in the animals with HF secondary to ventricular pacing. The exogenous administration of ANP to such levels prevented sodium retention, renal vasoconstriction, and activation of the RAAS (142). These results suggest that the high plasma ANP (and probably BNP) concentrations observed in HF are important in attenuating the renal sodium retention.

Despite such observations supporting a natriuretic role for NPs in HF, the intravenous infusion of synthetic NPs to patients with low-output cardiac failure results in a much smaller increase in renal sodium excretion and less-significant alterations in renal hemodynamics compared with normal subjects (99,133). The mechanism of this relative resistance to the natriuretic effect of NPs in HF is uncertain. Possible mechanisms include (a) downregulation of renal natriuretic peptide receptors; (b) secretion of inactive immunoreactive natriuretic peptides; (c) enhanced renal neutral endopeptidase activity limiting the delivery of NPs to the collecting duct receptor sites; (d) hyperaldosteronism by an increased sodium reabsorption in the distal renal tubule; (e) increased intracellular phosphodiesterase activity diminishing second messenger cyclic guanosine monophosphate (cGMP) concentrations; and (f) diminished sodium delivery to the distal renal tubule site of natriuretic peptide action. This latter possibility suggests that NPs activate their collecting duct receptors normally with subsequent activation of the secondary messenger, cGMP; however, decreased distal sodium delivery to the collecting duct secondary to a decrease in GFR or increased proximal tubule sodium reabsorption occurs and is responsible for the NP resistance in HF. Support for this possibility is the finding of a linear correlation between plasma ANP and urinary cGMP excretion in HF patients (143). Moreover, a similar ANP resistance in cirrhotic patients has been reversed by increasing distal sodium delivery to the collecting duct with an infusion of mannitol (144). Finally, the best correlate of the natriuretic response to infused BNP in HF patients has been shown to be distal tubular sodium delivery (133).

These data thus support the hypothesis that the NP resistance seen in patients with HF is primarily due to decreased sodium delivery to the collecting duct site of NP action rather than a direct impairment of the NP receptor-signal transduction system involving cGMP. This decreased distal delivery mechanism may also account for the impairment in aldosterone escape seen in HF and may be mediated by neurohormonal vasoconstrictor activation. Figure 15-3 shows the various factors that are activated in HF and contribute to decreased distal sodium delivery.

In addition to ANP and BNP, other members of the NP family have been described, including urodilatin and C-type natriuretic peptide (CNP) (134). Urodilatin, a slightly extended form of ANP, is synthesized primarily in the distal nephron of the kidney. When infused exogenously, urodilatin exerts vasodilating and natriuretic effects similar to ANP and BNP. It remains to be seen whether or not urodilatin has a role in the regulation of renal sodium excretion in cardiac failure. CNP, a 22-amino-acid peptide synthesized in the endothelium, produces relaxation of vascular smooth muscle cells and thus may promote vasodilation. It may be a more potent inhibitor of myocyte growth than either ANP or BNP. Its role in renal sodium excretion is unknown. In a recent study in individuals without known cardiovascular disease the plasma n-terminal pro-BNP was shown to correlate with mortality and first cardiovascular complication better than C-reactive protein and comparable to urinary albumin/creatinine ratios (145).

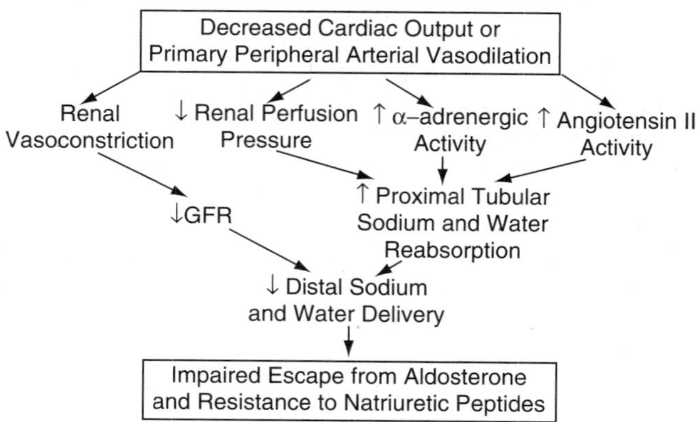

Figure 15-3 Factors that contribute to decreased distal tubular sodium and water delivery in CHF. Decreased distal sodium delivery is the postulated cause of impaired aldosterone escape and natriuretic peptide resistance in CHF.

Renal Prostaglandins in Heart Failure

In normal subjects and in intact animals, renal prostaglandins do not regulate renal sodium excretion or renal hemodynamics to any significant extent (146,147). In HF patients, prostaglandin activity is increased and has been shown to correlate with the severity of disease as assessed by the degree of hyponatremia (65). Moreover, it has been well-documented that the administration of a cyclo-oxygenase inhibitor in HF patients may result in reversible acute renal failure, an effect proposed to be due, at least in part, to inhibition of renal prostaglandins (148). An investigation in patients with moderate HF and a normal sodium intake demonstrated that the administration of acetylsalicylic acid in doses that decrease the synthesis of renal PGE_2 results in a significant reduction in urinary sodium excretion (149). These observations suggest a possible role for vasodilating prostaglandins in HF; however, their exact role in renal sodium handling in HF remains to be elucidated. Figure 15-4 shows the renal sites of action of some of the neurohormonal systems activated in HF.

THE CARDIORENAL SYNDROME

The cardiorenal syndrome describes the clinical scenario of concomitant renal and cardiac dysfunction (150,151). In patients with HF, both baseline renal dysfunction and worsening renal function (WRF) are common and both are potent predictors of mortality and rehospitalization for HF.

In outpatients with asymptomatic and symptomatic HF, mild or moderate renal dysfunction as measured by a creatinine clearance of <70 mL per minute have been associated with increased morbidity and mortality (1).

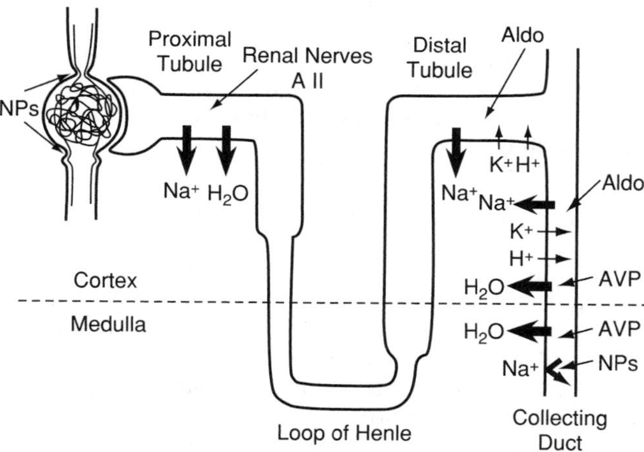

Figure 15-4 Glomerular and tubular sites of action of various neurohormonal systems that are activated in CHF. Renal nerves and angiotensin II (Ang II) influence sodium reabsorption in the proximal tubule. Aldosterone (Aldo) enhances sodium reabsorption and promotes potassium and hydrogen excretion in the cortical and medullary collecting duct. Arginine vasopressin (AVP) acts to increase water reabsorption in the cortical and medullary collecting duct. Natriuretic peptides (NPs) promote afferent arteriolar vasodilation and constriction of the efferent arterioles and inhibit sodium reabsorption in the collecting duct.

The increased risk for mortality conferred by renal dysfunction was as important as other prognostic factors such as NYHA functional classification, age, LVEF, and diabetes (1). In another study of outpatients with left ventricular dysfunction and NYHA Class III to IV symptoms, GFR was the most powerful predictor of mortality and the increased risk was largely independent of the LVEF, although an LVEF of <35% was present in all subjects (152). In both of these studies multivariate analysis demonstrated that mortality increased progressively with decreasing GFR (1,152). In a registry of over 65,000 hospital admissions for HF, abnormal renal function (as defined by a blood urea nitrogen [BUN] of ≥43 mg/dL) was determined to be the strongest predictor of hospital mortality (5).

A number of studies have demonstrated that renal dysfunction is common in patients with HF. In the large HF registry mentioned above, renal insufficiency was present in 30% (5). In the Studies of Left Ventricular Dysfunction (SOLVD), a creatinine clearance of <60 mL per minute determined by the Cockcroft-Gault formula was noted in 21% of subjects in the prevention trial and 36% in the treatment trial, despite an exclusion for a plasma creatinine of >2 mg/dL (1). In another study of 1,004 patients hospitalized for acutely decompensated HF, 35.8% had a baseline creatinine of 1.5 mg/dL or greater (153). Thus, renal dysfunction in the setting of HF is both a common and morbid problem.

In patients with acutely decompensated HF, WRF is also a common and morbid condition occurring in 27% to 28% of all patients when WRF was defined as a plasma creatinine increase of 0.3 mg/dL or greater (2,153). Smaller increases in plasma creatinine are even more common (3). WRF in patients with decompenstated HF is a potent predictor of mortality. In a prospective cohort of 412 patients hospitalized for HF, a plasma creatinine elevation of ≥0.1 mg/dL and ≥0.5 mg/dL occurred in 75% and 24% of patients, respectively (4). Mortality increased more in patients with the greater elevations in plasma creatinine, and WRF during treatment for decompensated HF was a more important predictor of mortality than was baseline plasma creatinine (4).

Only a few studies have evaluated risk factors for WRF in HF patients. In the same study of 1,004 patients admitted for decompensated HF, the factors associated with WRF were a previous history of HF or diabetes and an admission plasma creatinine ≥1.5 mg/dL (153). Hypertension (systolic BP >160 mm Hg), but not hypotension, was also associated with WRF; hypotension, however, was uncommon in this study. LVEF was not a predictor of WRF (153). In a similar study of 1,681 patients ≥65 years of age, predictors of WRF were female sex, admission systolic BP >200 mm Hg, greater bibasilar rales, a baseline creatinine of ≥1.5 mg/dL, and a heart rate of >100 beats per minute (2). Once again, LVEF was not predictive of WRF. In general, WRF occurs in the first few days of hospitalization for HF; specifically, within 7 days 81% to 90% of patients exhibited decreased renal function (2,3,153).

As many as 45% of patients who develop WRF during treatment for decompensated HF have preserved systolic function as assessed by a normal ejection fraction (EF)

(153). In addition, hypertension, rather than hypotension, is a predictor of WRF (2,153). It is perplexing how these findings of hypertension and normal LVEF can be integrated into the unifying hypothesis of body fluid regulation depicted in Figure 15-3. In this regard, several lines of evidence suggest that this unifying hypothesis is compatible with WRF, even in patients with HF and normal LVEF. In patients admitted for acutely decompensated HF, the development of WRF is not related to EF (2,153). In a recent comparison of HF patients, one group with LVEF ≥50% and the other with LVEF <50%, there were similar decreases in left ventricular stroke volume, and thus cardiac output was shown to be an initiator of arterial underfilling (154). In addition, levels of circulating NE were the same in patients with normal and abnormal LVEF, demonstrating similar levels of sympathetic activation (154).

Furthermore, patients with HF and preserved EF have a high prevalence of hypertension and/or diabetes, both of which are associated with neurohormonal activation (155). Indeed, even in young people with hypertension and no HF, plasma NE spillover is increased (156). The neurohormonal activation includes increased renal sympathetic nerve activity, which decreases renal sodium and water excretion (155). Increased activation of cardiac sympa-thetic afferents stimulated by increased filling pressure or relative ischemia may be sensed by the ventricular receptors with stimulation of the sympathetic nervous system (157,158). Patients with HF and preserved EF (i.e., diasolic dysfunction) also have increased vascular stiffness with decreased arterial compliance causing systolic hypertension (159–161). Diastolic dysfunction, which is very common in elderly patients with HF, is associated with hypertension. In these patients the ventricular receptors may initiate the afferent pathway for sympathetic stimulation with a normal EF and diastolic dysfunction. Hypertensive patients may also have nephrosclerosis and thus may be more likely to have WRF with an additional insult. In addition, intrinsic renal disease resulting from either hypertension or diabetes may exacerbate fluid retention and neurohormonal activation in these patients.

In both the prevention and treatment arms of the SOLVD studies, WRF was primarily predictive for an increase in pump failure deaths and hospitalizations for HF, with little predictive value for arrhythmic death (1). This has led to the speculation that renal dysfunction may not be only a marker for worsening HF but may also be a factor exacerbating the progression of HF (1,6,150).

THE POTENTIAL ROLE OF DIMINISHED RENAL FUNCTION IN THE PROGRESSION OF HEART FAILURE

There are a number of potential mechanisms whereby renal dysfunction may contribute to the progression of HF. These mechanisms include increased left ventricular volume; activation of the RAAS and the sympathetic nervous system as well as other neurohormonal systems; decreased erythropoietin and resultant anemia; and inflammation and increased reactive oxygen species (ROS) (6,151). Each of these mechanisms may influence myocardial remodeling with increasing left ventricular dilatation and resultant worsening mitral regurgitation, increased left ventricular wall mass, and increased myocardial fibrosis and myocyte apoptosis.

Myocardial Remodeling

Cardiac Dilatation and Increasing Mitral Regurgitation

Renal sodium retention with ECF expansion causes increased cardiac preload, resulting in cardiac dilatation. Cardiac dilatation is an important risk factor for mortality in HF. In fact, it is so closely associated with mortality and hospitalization for HF that is has been suggested as a surrogate marker for these outcomes (162). With cardiac dilatation, myocardial wall stress increases, resulting in increased myocardial oxygen demands. Ventricular dilatation may also worsen or initiate mitral regurgitation, which leads to reduced forward cardiac output and increased pulmonary pressures placing an additional strain on the right ventricle.

Early in HF, ventricular dilatation is associated with an increase in BNP, facilitating the maintenance of sodium balance and suppressing the RAAS. Potential beneficial effects of exogenous BNP include decreased cardiac preload (135), decreased cardiac fibrosis (163), and an enhanced response to the diuretic effect of furosemide (164). However, exogenous BNP does not appear to ameliorate WRF associated with treatment of acutely decompensated HF (165,166). Perhaps the failure to prevent WRF is due, at least in part, to the fact that beneficial effects of NPs may be blunted because of renal vasoconstriction and decreased renal perfusion pressure, as well as decreased sodium delivery to the distal tubule site of BNP action. Although administration of BNP may not result in improved renal function, the potential still exists for BNP given chronically to improve myocardial remodeling (167).

Increased Left Ventricular Mass Index

Increased wall stress results in an increased left ventricular mass index (LVMI) or left ventricular hypertrophy (LVH). LVH results in diastolic dysfunction, worsening wall stress, and increasing left ventricular filling pressures. Anemia, discussed later, may also exacerbate LVH, and LVH is associated with increased mortality (168).

Activation of the Renin-Angiotensin-Aldosterone System

Several factors in patients with HF and renal dysfunction may result in further activation of the RAAS. Fluid retention with cardiac dilatation and increased mitral regurgitation reduces cardiac output, resulting in diminished renal perfusion and further activation of the RAAS. Increased renin correlates with mortality in HF (169). Increased aldosterone levels may block myocardial reuptake of NE, resulting in increased sympathetic activation of the myocardium and progressive myocardial dysfunction (170).

In addition, angiotensin II stimulates the sympathetic nervous system (171). Myocardial remodeling is exacerbated by angiotensin II and aldosterone stimulates myocardial fibrosis, apoptosis, and necrosis (171,172). HF is associated with angiotensin II generation in the cerebrospinal fluid, and increased angiotensin II and decreased nitric oxide (NO) in the central nervous system have been implicated as mediators of the blunted baroreflexes described in HF. (158). Decreased baroreceptor sensitivity, by reducing the tonic inhibition of renal sympathetic nerve activity, would result in sodium retention as shown in Figure 15-5. Both angiotensin II and increased renal sympathetic activity activate proximal tubular epithelial receptors that enhance sodium absorption (85,173). Decreased sodium delivery to the distal nephron prevents escape from the sodium-retaining effects of aldosterone. Angiotensin II causes glomerular efferent arteriolar constriction resulting in enhanced sodium, an absorption due to decreased hydrostatic and increased oncotic pressure in the peritubular capillary (174). Thus, in the proximal tubule, enhanced sodium reabsorption occurs due to the direct effect of angiotensin II and α-adrenergic stimulation and also by renal vasoconstriction. Sodium reabsorption in the collecting duct is increased by aldosterone. The juxtaglomerular apparatus plays a major role in activation of the RAAS. β-adrenergic stimulation and decreased sodium chloride delivery to the macula densa (both common events in HF) stimulate the RAAS (67,175). In addition, loop diuretics, discussed later, further activate the RAAS (176).

Erythropoietin and Anemia

Anemia is common in patients with HF and is associated with an excess mortality (177). Both anemia and relative resistance to erythopoietin (EPO) may contribute to cardiac dysfunction in HF. Renal dysfunction appears to be a causative factor in the anemia of HF. (177,178). Anemia results in LVH in patients with even mild kidney disease (179). In addition, anemia causes peripheral vasodilation, and thus relative arterial underfilling, with reduced renal perfusion pressure exacerbating sodium and water retention. Since red blood cells contain antioxidants, anemia may also result in increased oxidative stress (180). EPO levels are generally increased in HF (181,182) but it has been suggested that levels are not increased adequately for the level of anemia. The causes(s) of resistance to EPO are not known but have been postulated to be due to the elevated levels of inflammatory cytokines described in HF (180,183). This, however, is not the only factor because EPO levels and hemoglobin concentration demonstrate only a mild inverse correlation in HF (181). Insensitivity to the hematopoietic effects of EPO, possibly due to inflammatory cytokines, has also been described (180,181). Erythropoietin has other important effects in addition to stimulation of hematopoiesis. Erythropoietin receptors are present in endothelial and smooth muscle cells (4,184,185) and erythropoietin reduces the production and release of proinflammatory cytokines and chemokines, and also decreases the influx of inflammatory cells into injured myocardium with a potential decrease in myocardial remodeling (186). If the resistance to EPO, as noted for the bone marrow, is present for these other beneficial anti-inflammatory and antioxidant effects, then myocardial remodeling may be adversely affected.

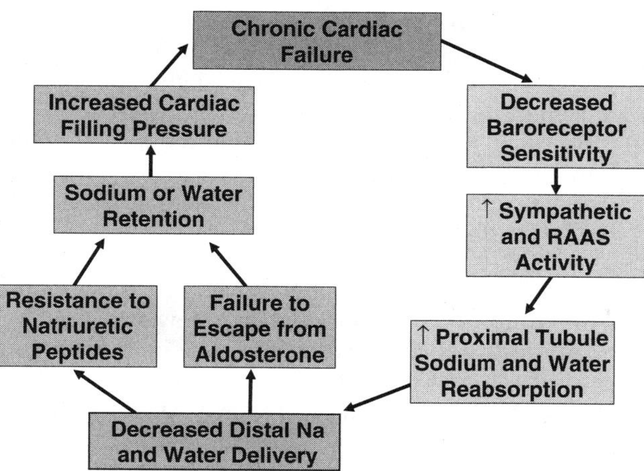

Figure 15-5 Decreased baroreceptor sensitivity in patients with chronic HF can worsen cardiac function by increasing RAAS and sympathetic activity, enhancing proximal fluid reabsorption, impairing aldosterone escape, and blunting the response to natriuretic peptides. (From Schrier RW. Role of diminished renal function in cardiovascular mortality: marker or pathogenic factor? *J Am Coll Cardiol.* 2006;47(1):1–8, with permission.)

Inflammation

Both HF and renal dysfunction are characterized by high levels of circulating proinflammatory cytokines such as tumor necrosis factor (TNF)-α and interleukin-6 (IL-6) (187,188). It is likely that the inflammation associated with both HF and renal dysfunction creates a vicious cycle of inflammation, with one amplifying the other. For example, TNF-α is increased in renal failure (189) and is also a myocardial depressant. As is the case with neurohormonal activation, overexpression of cytokines results in direct toxic effects in the heart and kidney (188,190). Furthermore, there is significant cross-talk between the classic neurohormonal and the cytokine systems (188). Angiotensin II is known to activate nuclear factor-kappa B (NF-κB), a redox-sensitive transcription factor, that is important in stimulating the myocardial inflammatory response (191). Both angiotensin II and TNF-α induce oxidative stress that results in hypertrophy in myocytes (188). Thus, the additional inflammation that results when renal dysfunction occurs with HF is likely to exacerbate myocardial remodeling.

The Role of Diuretics

Loop diuretics are clearly beneficial agents in managing the sodium and water retention that occurs in patients with HF. However, these agents have potential negative effects, as they may worsen renal function in these patients (192). Loop diuretics activate the RAAS by blocking sodium chloride transport at the macula densa (176). Indeed, in a porcine pacing model of HF, initiation of furosemide at the onset of pacing resulted in more rapidly progressive LV remodeling and elevated aldosterone levels without differences in plasma NE (193). This occurred without an early difference in preload, suggesting that activation of the RAAS was an important factor. Activation of the RAAS by loop diuretics is also an

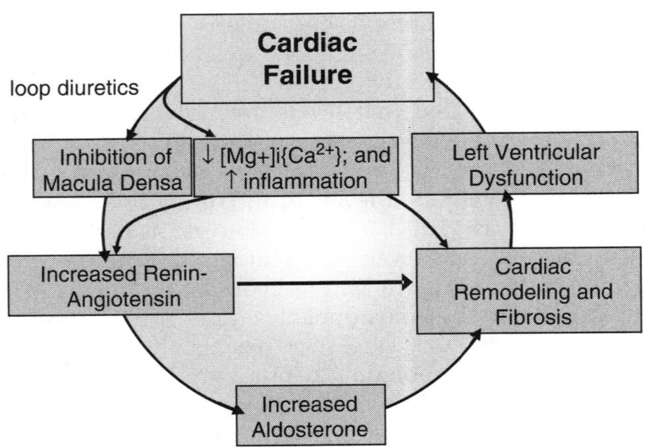

Figure 15-6 Mechanisms whereby loop diuretics may worsen HF. Based on this schema, it could be theoretically argued that loop diuretics should always be accompanied by treatment with ACE inhibitors or ARBs.

important mechanism of diuretic resistance (194). There are additional potential adverse effects of loop diuretics in HF. Loop diuretics promote urinary magnesium and calcium excretion which may lead to a reduction in cardiomyocyte cytosolic Ca^{2+} and $[Mg^{+}]$, with resultant decreased myocardial contractions (195). A decrease in intracellular $[Mg^{+}]$ may also result in activation of peripheral blood mononuclear cells to produce inflammatory cytokines that could adversely affect both myocardial and renal function and remodeling (196). Finally, thiamine deficiency may worsen cardiac function (195). Potential negative effects of loop diuretics in HF are shown in Figure 15-6.

THERAPEUTIC STRATEGIES TO PREVENT WORSENING RENAL FUNCTION IN PATIENTS WITH HEART FAILURE

Prevention of renal dysfunction in patients with HF is likely to result in fewer and shorter hospitalizations, improved symptoms, and a lower mortality. However, no clear strategies have yet been devised to prevent renal dysfunction. While diuretics clearly improve symptoms in patients with HF, there remain questions, as previously described, about their contribution to the progression of HF. Thus, when the plasma creatinine begins to increase in a patient treated for decompensated HF, the physician is in a quandary as to whether to halt diuresis and leave the patient with increased cardiac preload and cardiac dilatation and dyspnea, or continue diuresis at the expense of WRF. We summarize below what is known about the effects of current therapy on WRF in HF.

ACE Inhibitors, Adrenergic Receptor Blockers, β-Blockers, and Vasodilators

Conventional medical therapy of HF with dietary salt restriction, diuretics, and direct-acting vasodilators without neurohormonal antagonists (e.g., nitrates and hydralazine), although observed to modestly improve survival in HF (197), may be limited by the development of drug tolerance. The emergence of diuretic resistance or vasodilator tolerance in patients with chronic HF may be due in part to further activation of vasoconstrictor mechanisms induced by these therapeutic agents. In fact, sodium depletion due to dietary salt restriction and the use of diuretics may activate all three of the aforementioned major neurohormonal vasoconstrictor systems (198,199). Moreover, in HF patients, continuous vasodilator therapy with nitroglycerin results in the rapid development of drug tolerance and in weight gain occurring simultaneously with activation of the RAAS (200). The ACE inhibitor enalapril was associated with improved mortality and decreasing plasma norepinephrine compared to hydralazine and isordil, which were associated with increases in plasma norepinephrine (169). Thus, it can be postulated that diuretic- or vasodilator-induced activation of neurohormonal vasoconstrictor mechanisms attenuates the beneficial hemodynamic effects of these agents and stimulates renal sodium and water retention.

A study that examined the interaction of continuous nitroglycerin administration and ACE inhibition in normal subjects supports this hypothesis (201). This study showed that the development of nitrate tolerance and the weight gain observed with chronic nitrate therapy were prevented by the simultaneous administration of either captopril or enalapril, suggesting that the development of drug tolerance and expansion of body fluid volume seen with chronic nitrate therapy is mediated by activation of the RAAS (201). Indeed, a recent trial, using a combination of hydralazine and isordil in African-Americans with HF who were taking ACE inhibitors and β-blockers demonstrated a 44% reduction in HF mortality and a substantial reduction in hospitalizations, with marked improvements in quality of life (202). These findings demonstrate that maneuvers that inhibit or antagonize neurohormonal vasoconstrictor activation might be more beneficial than, or are of additive value to, diuretics and vasodilator therapy in HF. The proven beneficial effects of ACE inhibitors and β-adrenergic receptor blockers (ARBs) on symptoms, hemodynamics, and survival in advanced HF support the routine use of these agents in HF (79–81,203–208). However, there is the potential for ACE inhibitors and ARBs to worsen renal function by blocking the effect of angiotensin in vasoconstricting the efferent arteriole. Blockade of this effect would reduce glomerular hydrostatic pressure and thus glomerular filtration rate and perpetuate sodium retention and volume overload (209). Patients with abnormal renal function at baseline and are on loop diuretics would be most susceptible to this effect. In most circumstances, vasodilators improve cardiac output and thus improve renal blood flow. However, if arterial vasodilation is not balanced by adequate improvement in cardiac output and there is relative worsening of arterial underfilling and reduced renal perfusion pressure, tubular sodium reabsorption may be increased (104,210).

B-Type Natriuretic Peptide (Nesiritide)

While a number of studies have suggested a benefit of BNP on renal function in patients with HF, two recent publications suggest that BNP may not be of therapeutic benefit in patients with HF and renal dysfunction or WRF. In a meta-analysis of several studies using BNP in patients with HF, renal dysfunction was significantly more common in patients receiving BNP (nesiritide) compared to placebo or other forms of therapy (166). In a recent study of 15 patients with HF and WRF, Wang et al. demonstrated no benefit of nesiritide on sodium excretion or GFR (165). The reasons for the absence of benefit are uncertain, although one might postulate that systemic vasodilation with worsening arterial underfilling counteracts the potential benefits of BNP on ventricular filling pressures and neurohormonal activation.

Arginine Vasopressin Antagonists

Ongoing investigations of AVP receptor antagonists may broaden the application of such antihormonal therapy in HF. A recent trial with a vasopressin (V_2) antagonist in HF patients demonstrated weight loss accompanied by increased solute-free water excretion without changes in blood pressure, renal function, or neurohormones (114). It is important to understand, despite these promising results, that only one-third of electrolyte-free water excretion comes from the extracellular fluid; the remaining comes from the intracellular compartment. Furthermore, vasopressin agonism of the unblocked V_{1a} receptors on cardiomyocytes and vascular smooth muscle might be detrimental. There are, however, nonpeptide orally active antagonists on both V_{1a} and V_2 vasopressin receptors under investigation. Figure 15-7 outlines the potential effects of V_{1a} or V_2 agonism, which could continue worsening of myocardial dysfunction in HF patients and be amenable to V_{1a} and V_2 receptor antagonism.

Endothelin Antagonists

Studies of endothelin antagonists in HF have not demonstrated additional benefits over the combination of ACE inhibitors and β-blockers on mortality and hospitalizations, although specific effects on renal function from these studies have not yet been reported (211,212).

Ultrafiltration

The use of ultrafiltration has been suggested when loop diuretics are associated with WRF (213). There are theoretical advantages to ultrafiltration in this setting. Diuretic resistance is often present when large doses of loop diuretics are used and, as previously discussed, these may have adverse effects (194). Ultrafiltration, however, may be associated with neurohormonal activation if the rate of fluid removal (and thus the transfer of fluid from the interstitium to vascular compartment) is too aggressive (214). The fluid removed by ultrafiltration is isotonic with plasma, while the fluid removed with diuretics is hypotonic to plasma. Thus, ultrafiltration is likely to remove more sodium with fewer electrolyte disturbances than loop diuretics. Although ultrafiltration has demonstrated beneficial effects in small, nonrandomized studies, it is invasive and more expensive than diuretic therapy; a large, prospective, randomized trial is necessary to determine if ultrafiltration provides improved outcomes in HF patients with renal dysfunction on loop diuretics. The potential benefits of both loop diuretics and ultrafiltration are outlined in Figure 15-8.

SUMMARY

Renal dysfunction and WRF are both associated with increased morbidity and mortality in HF. Evidence from several studies suggests renal dysfunction may result in a more accelerated course of HF. While neurohormonal antagonism with ACE inhibitors and β-blockers improves mortality and (presumably) renal function in these patients, no other

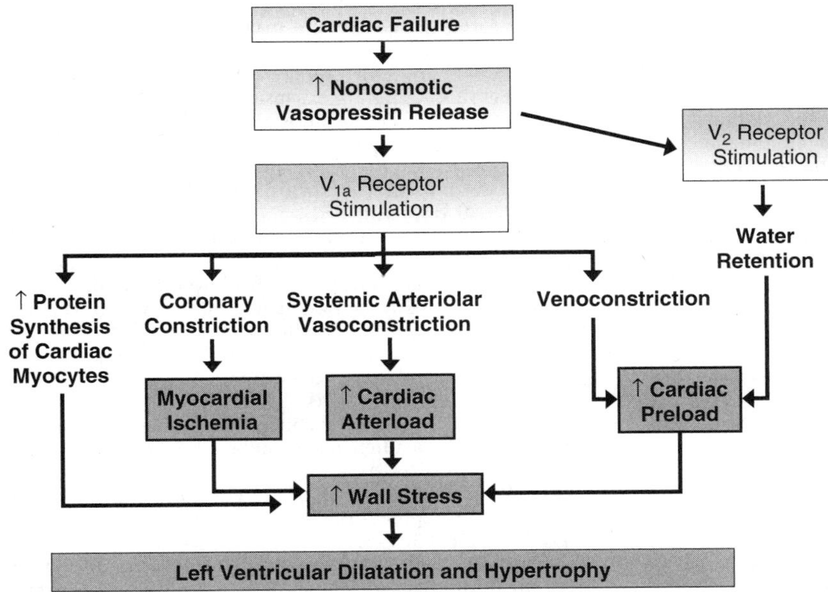

Figure 15-7 Pathways whereby vasopressin stimulation of V_2 and V_{1a} receptors can contribute to worsening HF. (From Schrier RW. Role of diminished renal function in cardiovascular mortality: marker or pathogenic factor? *J Am Coll Cardiol.* 2006;47(1):1–8, with permission.)

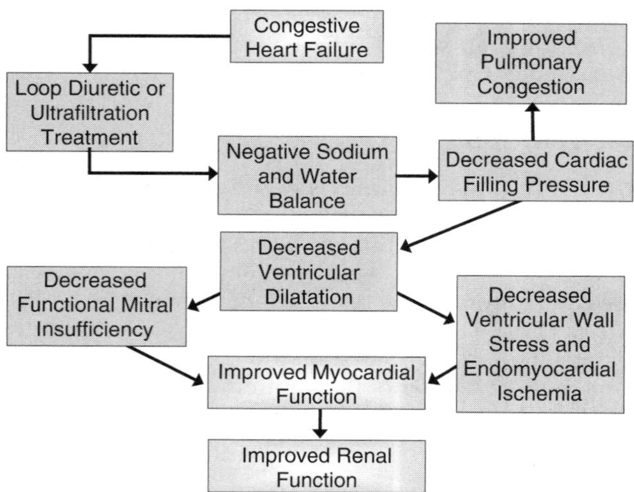

Figure 15-8 Mechanisms whereby negative sodium and water balance in HF caused by either loop diuretics or ultrafiltration may improve myocardial function. (From Schrier RW, Role of diminished renal function in cardiovascular mortality: marker or pathogenic factor? *J Am Coll Cardiol.* 2006;47(1):1–8, with permission.)

effective strategies have been devised to prevent or reverse renal dysfunction. Improved understanding of the complex relationship between cardiac and renal dysfunction is likely to provide beneficial treatment to reverse these complex cardiorenal interactions. Unfortunately, some patients with advanced HF are frequently deprived of the proven efficacy on survival of RAAS inhibition with ACE inhibitors or ARBs because of elevated plasma creatinine or WRF. Prospective randomized studies are necessary to assess whether this is a wise therapeutic decision, since persistent cardiac filling pressure, and the consequence thereof, and the deleterious cardiac effects of angiotensin and aldosterone may be pivotal pathological factors in HF mortality.

REFERENCES

1. Dries DL, Exner DV, Domanski MJ, et al. The prognostic implications of renal insufficiency in asymptomatic and symptomatic patients with left ventricular systolic dysfunction. *J Am Coll Cardiol.* 2000;35(3):681–689.
2. Krumholz HM, Chen YT, Vaccarino V, et al. Correlates and impact on outcomes of worsening renal function in patients ≥or =65 years of age with heart failure. *Am J Cardiol.* 2000;85(9): 1110–1113.
3. Gottlieb SS, Abraham W, Butler J, et al. The prognostic importance of different definitions of worsening renal function in congestive heart failure. *J Card Fail.* 2002;8(3):136–141.
4. Smith KJ, Bleyer AJ, Little WC, et al. The cardiovascular effects of erythropoietin. *Cardiovasc Res.* 2003;59(3):538–548.
5. Fonarow GC, Adams KF, Jr., Abraham WT, et al. Risk stratification for in-hospital mortality in acutely decompensated heart failure: classification and regression tree analysis. *JAMA.* 2005;293(5):572–580.
6. Schrier RW. Role of diminished renal function in cardiovascular mortality: marker or pathogenic factor? *J AM Coll Cardiol.* 2006;47(1):1–8.
7. Schrier RW. Body fluid volume regulation in health and disease: a unifying hypothesis. *Ann Intern Med.* 1990;113(2): 155–159.
8. Schrier RW. A unifying hypothesis of body fluid volume regulation. The Lilly Lecture 1992. *J R Coll Physicians Lond.* 1992;26(3): 295–306.
9. Schrier RW, Abraham WT. Hormones and hemodynamics in heart failure. *N Engl J Med.* 1999;341(8):577–585.
10. Koppel MH, Coburn JW, Mims MM, et al. Transplantation of cadaveric kidneys from patients with hepatorenal syndrome. Evidence for the functional nature of renal failure in advanced liver disease. *N Engl J Med.* 1969;280(25):1367–1371.
11. Iwatsuki S, Popovtzer MM, Corman JL, et al. Recovery from "hepatorenal syndrome" after orthotopic liver transplantation. *N Engl J Med.* 1973;289(22):1155–1159.
12. Farrar DJ, Hill JD. Recovery of major organ function in patients awaiting heart transplantation with Thoratec ventricular assist devices. Thoratec Ventricular Assist Device Principal Investigators. *J Heart Lung Transplant.* 1994;13(6):1125–1132.
13. Peters JP. The role of sodium in the production of edema. *N Engl J Med.* 1948;239:353–362.
14. Borst JG, De Vries LA. The three types of "natural" diuresis. *Lancet.* 1950;2(1):1–6.
15. Schrier RW, Humphreys MH. Factors involved in antinatriuretic effects of acute constriction of the thoracic and abdominal inferior vena cava. *Circ Res.* 1971;29(5):479–489.
16. Schrier RW, Humphreys MH, Ufferman RC. Role of cardiac output and the autonomic nervous system in the antinatriuretic response to acute constriction of the thoracic superior vena cava. *Circ Res.* 1971;29(5):490–498.
17. Schrier RW, Berl T, Anderson RJ. Osmotic and nonosmotic control of vasopressin release. *Am J Physiol.* 1979;236(4):F321–F332.
18. Szatalowicz VL, Arnold PE, Chaimovitz C, et al. Radioimmunoassay of plasma arginine vasopressin in hyponatremic patients with congestive heart failure. *N Engl J Med.* 1981;305(5):263–266.
19. Bichet D, Szatalowicz V, Chaimovitz C, et al. Role of vasopressin in abnormal water excretion in cirrhotic patients. *Ann Intern Med.* 1982;96(4):413–417.
20. Bichet DG, Van Putten VJ, Schrier RW. Potential role of increased sympathetic activity in impaired sodium and water excretion in cirrhosis. *N Engl J Med.* 1982;307(25):1552–1557.
21. Bichet DG, Groves BM, Schrier RW. Mechanisms of improvement of water and sodium excretion by immersion in decompensated cirrhotic patients. *Kidney Int.* 1983;24(6):788–794.
22. Nicholls KM, Shapiro MD, Van Putten VJ, et al. Elevated plasma norepinephrine concentrations in decompensated cirrhosis. Association with increased secretion rates, normal clearance rates, and suppressibility by central blood volume expansion. *Circ Res.* 1985;56(3):457–461.
23. Shapiro MD, Nicholls KM, Groves BM, et al. Interrelationship between cardiac output and vascular resistance as determinants of effective arterial blood volume in cirrhotic patients. *Kidney Int.* 1985;28(2):206–211.
24. Nicholls KM, Shapiro MD, Kluge R, et al. Sodium excretion in advanced cirrhosis: effect of expansion of central blood volume and suppression of plasma aldosterone. *Hepatology.* 1986;6(2): 235–238.
25. Bichet D. [Anomalies of water and sodium excretion by the kidney in decompensated cirrhosis. The theory of blood volume overload opposed to the theory of the diminution of effective circulating volume]. *Gastroenterol Clin Biol.* 1985; 9(11):829–837.
26. de Torrente A, Robertson GL, McDonald KM, et al. Mechanism of diuretic response to increased left atrial pressure in the anesthetized dog. *Kidney Int.* 1975;8(6):355–361.
27. Schrier RW, Berl T. Mechanism of the antidiuretic effect associated with interruption of parasympathetic pathways. *J Clin Invest.* 1972;51(10):2613–2620.
28. Schrier RW, Lieberman R, Ufferman RC. Mechanism of antidiuretic effect of beta adrenergic stimulation. *J Clin Invest.* 1972; 51(1):97–111.
29. Schrier RW, Berl T. Mechanism of effect of alpha adrenergic stimulation with norepinephrine on renal water excretion. *J Clin Invest.* 1973;52(2):502–511.
30. Anderson RJ, Cadnapaphornchai P, Harbottle JA, et al. Mechanism of effect of thoracic inferior vena cava constriction on renal water excretion. *J Clin Invest.* 1974;54(6): 1473–1479.

31. Berl T, Cadnapaphornchai P, Harbottle JA, et al. Mechanism of stimulation of vasopressin release during beta adrenergic stimulation with isoproterenol. *J Clin Invest.* 1974;53(3):857–867.
32. Berl T, Cadnapaphornchai P, Harbottle JA, et al. Mechanism of suppression of vasopressin during alpha-adrenergic stimulation with norepinephrine. *J Clin Invest.* 1974;53(1):219–227.
33. Goetz KL, Bond GC, Bloxham DD. Atrial receptors and renal function. *Physiol Rev.* 1975;55(2):157–205.
34. Zucker IH, Earle AM, Gilmore JP. The mechanism of adaptation of left atrial stretch receptors in dogs with chronic congestive heart failure. *J Clin Invest.* 1977;60(2):323–331.
35. Anderson RJ, Pluss RG, Berns AS, et al. Mechanism of effect of hypoxia on renal water excretion. *J Clin Invest.* 1978;62(4):769–777.
36. Murdaugh HV, Jr., Sieker HO, Manfredi F. Effect of altered intrathoracic pressure on renal hemodynamics, electrolyte excretion and water clearance. *J Clin Invest.* 1959;38(5):834–842.
37. Smith HW. Salt and water volume receptors: an exercise in physiologic apologetics. *Am J Med.* 1957;23(4):623–652.
38. Gauer OH, Henry JP. Circulatory basis of fluid volume control. *Physiol Rev.* 1963;43:423–481.
39. Epstein FH, Goodyer AV, Lawrason FD, et al. Studies of the antidiuresis of quiet standing: the importance of changes in plasma volume and glomerular filtration rate. *J Clin Invest.* 1951;30(1):63–72.
40. Gauer OH, Henry JP, Sieker HO, et al. The effect of negative pressure breathing on urine flow. *J Clin Invest.* 1954;33(2):287–296.
41. Hulet WH, Smith HW. Postural natriuresis and urine osmotic concentration in hydropenic subjects. *Am J Med.* 1961;30:8–25.
42. Epstein M, Duncan DC, Fishman LM. Characterization of the natriuresis caused in normal man by immersion in water. *Clin Sci.* 1972;43(2):275–287.
43. Gillespie DJ, Sandberg RL, Koike TI. Dual effect of left atrial receptors on excretion of sodium and water in the dog. *Am J Physiol.* 1973;225(3):706–710.
44. Reinhardt HW, Kaczmarczyk G, Eisele R, et al. Left atrial pressure and sodium balance in conscious dogs on a low sodium intake. *Pflugers Arch.* 1977;370(1):59–66.
45. Henry JP, Gauer OH, Reeves JL. Evidence of the atrial location of receptors influencing urine flow. *Circ Res.* 1956;4(1):85–90.
46. Nakaoka H, Imataka K, Amano M, et al. Plasma levels of atrial natriuretic factor in patients with congestive heart failure. *N Engl J Med.* 1985;313(14):892–893.
47. Raine AE, Erne P, Burgisser E, et al. Atrial natriuretic peptide and atrial pressure in patients with congestive heart failure. *N Engl J Med.* 1986;315(9):533–537.
48. Sato F, Kamoi K, Wakiya Y, et al. Relationship between plasma atrial natriuretic peptide levels and atrial pressure in man. *J Clin Endocrinol Metab.* 1986;63(4):823–827.
49. Linden RJ, Kappagoda CT. Atrial receptors. *Monogr Physiol Soc.* 1982;39:1–363.
50. Zucker IH, Gorman AJ, Cornish KG, et al. Impaired atrial receptor modulation or renal nerve activity in dogs with chronic volume overload. *Cardiovasc Res.* 1985;19(7):411–418.
51. Volpe M, Tritto C, De Luca N, et al. Failure of atrial natriuretic factor to increase with saline load in patients with dilated cardiomyopathy and mild heart failure. *J Clin Invest.* 1991;88(5):1481–1489.
52. Epstein FH, Post RS, McDowell M. The effects of an arteriovenous fistula on renal hemodynamics and electrolyte excretion. *J Clin Invest.* 1953;32(3):233–241.
53. Gilmore JP. Contribution of baroreceptors to the control of renal function. *Circ Res.* 1964;14:301–317.
54. Pearce JW, Sonnenberg H. Effects of spinal section and renal denervation on the renal response to blood volume expansion. *Can J Physiol Pharmacol.* 1965(43):211–224.
55. Gilmore JP, Daggett WM. Response of the chronic cardiac denervated dog to acute volume expansion. *Am J Physiol.* 1966;210(3):509–512.
56. Knox FG, Davis BB, Berliner RW. Effect of chronic cardiac denervation on renal response to saline infusion. *Am J Physiol.* 1967;213(1):174–178.
57. Schedl HP, Bartter FC. An explanation for and experimental correction of the abnormal water diuresis in cirrhosis. *J Clin Invest.* 1967(46):1297–1308.
58. Guyton A, Scanlon CJ, Armstrong GG. Effects of pressoreceptor reflex and Cushing's reflex on urinary output. *Fed Proc.* 1952(11):61–62.
59. Davis JO. The control of renin release. *Am J Med.* 1973;55(3):333–350.
60. Anderson RJ, Cronin RE, McDonald KM, et al. Mechanisms of portal hypertension-induced alterations in renal hemodynamics, renal water excretion, and renin secretion. *J Clin Invest.* 1976;58(4):964–970.
61. Schrier RW, Berl T, Anderson RJ, et al. Nonosmolar control of renal water excretion. In: Andreoli T, Grantham J, Rector F, eds. *Disturbances in Body Fluid Osmolality.* Bethesda, MD: American Physiological Society; 1977:149–178.
62. Baker DG, Coleridge HM, Coleridge JC, et al. Search for a cardiac nociceptor: stimulation by bradykinin of sympathetic afferent nerve endings in the heart of the cat. *J Physiol.* 1980;306:519–536.
63. Zucker IH, Panzenbeck MJ, Barker S, et al. PGI2 attenuates baroreflex control of renal nerve activity by a vagal mechanism. *Am J Physiol.* 1988;254(3 Pt 2):R424–R430.
64. Panzenbeck MJ, Tan W, Hajdu MA, et al. PGE2 and arachidonate inhibit the baroreflex in conscious dogs via cardiac receptors. *Am J Physiol.* 1989;256(4 Pt 2):H999–H1005.
65. Dzau VJ, Packer M, Lilly LS, et al. Prostaglandins in severe congestive heart failure. Relation to activation of the renin-angiotensin system and hyponatremia. *N Engl J Med.* 1984;310(6):347–352.
66. Sklar AH, Schrier RW. Central nervous system mediators of vasopressin release. *Physiol Rev.* 1983;63(4):1243–1280.
67. Berl T, Henrich WL, Erickson AL, et al. Prostaglandins in the beta-adrenergic and baroreceptor-mediated secretion of renin. *Am J Physiol.* May 1979;236(5):F472–F477.
68. Thomas JA, Marks BH. Plasma norepinephrine in congestive heart failure. *Am J Cardiol.* 1978;41(2):233–243.
69. Levine TB, Francis GS, Goldsmith SR, et al. Activity of the sympathetic nervous system and renin-angiotensin system assessed by plasma hormone levels and their relation to hemodynamic abnormalities in congestive heart failure. *Am J Cardiol.* 1982;49(7):1659–1666.
70. Hasking JG, Esler MD, Jennings GL, et al. Norepinephrine spillover to plasma in patients with congestive heart failure: evidence of increased overall and cardiorenal sympathetic nervous activity. *Circulation.* 1986(73):615–621.
71. Davis D, Baily R, Zelis R. Abnormalities in systemic norepinephrine kinetics in human congestive heart failure. *Am J Physiol.* 1988;254(6 Pt 1):E760–E766.
72. Abraham WT, Hensen J, Schrier RW. Elevated plasma noradrenaline concentrations in patients with low-output cardiac failure: dependence on increased noradrenaline secretion rates. *Clin Sci (Lond).* 1990;79(5):429–435.
73. Cohn JN. Sympathetic nervous system in heart failure. *Circulation.* 2002;106(19):2417–2418.
74. Leimbach WN, Jr., Wallin BG, Victor RG, et al. Direct evidence from intraneural recordings for increased central sympathetic outflow in patients with heart failure. *Circulation.* 1986;73(5):913–919.
75. Francis GS, Benedict C, Johnstone DE, et al. Comparison of neuroendocrine activation in patients with left ventricular dysfunction with and without congestive heart failure. A substudy of the Studies of Left Ventricular Dysfunction (SOLVD). *Circulation.* 1990;82(5):1724–1729.
76. Chidsey CA, Braunwald E, Morrow AG. Catecholamine excretion and cardiac stores of norepinephrine in congestive heart failure. *Am J Med.* 1965;39:442–451.
77. Cohn JN, Levine TB, Olivari MT, et al. Plasma norepinephrine as a guide to prognosis in patients with chronic congestive heart failure. *N Engl J Med.* 1984;311(13):819–823.
78. Latini R, Masson S, Staszewsky L, et al. Valsartan for the treatment of heart failure. *Expert Opin Pharmacother.* 2004;5(1):181–193.
79. The Cardiac Insufficiency Bisoprolol Study II (CIBIS-II): a randomised trial. *Lancet.* 1999;353(9146):9–13.
80. Hjalmarson A, Goldstein S, Fagerberg B, et al. Effects of controlled-release metoprolol on total mortality, hospitalizations, and well-being in patients with heart failure: the Metoprolol CR/XL Randomized Intervention Trial in congestive heart failure

(MERIT-HF). MERIT-HF Study Group. *JAMA*. 2000;283(10): 1295–1302.

81. Packer M, Bristow MR, Cohn JN, et al. The effect of carvedilol on morbidity and mortality in patients with chronic heart failure. U.S. Carvedilol Heart Failure Study Group. *N Engl J Med*. 1996;334(21):1349–1355.
82. Brod J, Fejfar Z, Fejfarova MH. The role of neuro-humoral factors in the genesis of renal haemodynamic changes in heart failure. *Acta Med Scand*. 1954;148(4):273–290.
83. Gill JR, Jr., Mason DT, Bartter FC. Adrenergic nervous system in sodium metabolism: effects of guanethidine and sodium-retaining steroids in normal man. *J Clin Invest*. 1964;43:177–184.
84. DiBona GF, Herman PJ, Sawin LL. Neural control of renal function in edema-forming states. *Am J Physiol*. 1988;254(6 Pt 2): R1017–R1024.
85. Bello-Reuss E, Trevino DL, Gottschalk CW. Effect of renal sympathetic nerve stimulation on proximal water and sodium reabsorption. *J Clin Invest*. 1976(57):1104–1107.
86. Meyers BD, Deen WM, Brenner BM. Effects of norepinephrine and angiotensin II on the determinants of glomerular ultrafiltration and proximal tubule fluid reabsorption in the rat. *Circ Res*. 1975(37):101–110.
87. Ichikawa I, Pfeffer JM, Pfeffer MA, et al. Role of angiotensin II in the altered renal function of congestive heart failure. *Circ Res*. 1984;55(5):669–675.
88. DiBona GF. Neurogenic regulation of renal tubular sodium reabsorption. *Am J Physiol*. 1977;233(2):F73–F81.
89. Carpenter CC, Davis JO, Holman JE, et al. Studies on the response of the transplanted kidney and the transplanted adrenal gland to thoracic inferior vena caval constriction. *J Clin Invest*. 1961;40:196–204.
90. Lifschitz MD, Schrier RW. Alterations in cardiac output with chronic constriction of thoracic inferior vena cava. *Am J Physiol*. 1973;225(6):1364–1370.
91. Merrill AJ, Morrison JL, Brannon ES. Concentration of renin in renal venous blood in patients with chronic heart failure. *Am J Med*. 1946(1):468–472.
92. Francis GS, Goldsmith SR, Levine TB, et al. The neurohumoral axis in congestive heart failure. *Ann Intern Med*. 1984;101(3): 370–377.
93. Bristow MR, Abraham WT. Anti-adrenergic effects of angiotensin converting enzyme inhibitors. *Eur Heart J*. 1995;16(Suppl K): 37–41.
94. Lee WH, Packer M. Prognostic importance of serum sodium concentration and its modification by converting-enzyme inhibition in patients with severe chronic heart failure. *Circulation*. 1986;73(2):257–267.
95. Ichikawa I, Brenner BM. Importance of efferent arteriolar vascular tone in regulation of proximal tubule fluid reabsorption and glomerulotubular balance in the rat. *J Clin Invest*. 1980;65(5): 1192–1201.
96. Liu FY, Cogan MG. Angiotensin II: a potent regulator of acidification in the rat early proximal convoluted tubule. *J Clin Invest*. 1987;80(1):272–275.
97. Eiam-Ong S, Hilden SA, Johns CA, et al. Stimulation of basolateral Na(+)-HCO3-cotransporter by angiotensin II in rabbit renal cortex. *Am J Physiol*. 1993;265(2 Pt 2):F195–F203.
98. Pierpont GL, Francis GS, Cohn JN. Effect of captopril on renal function in patients with congestive heart failure. *Br Heart J*. 1981;46(5):522–527.
99. Cody RJ, Atlas SA, Laragh JH, et al. Atrial natriuretic factor in normal subjects and heart failure patients. Plasma levels and renal, hormonal, and hemodynamic responses to peptide infusion. *J Clin Invest*. 1986;78(5):1362–1374.
100. Hensen J, Abraham WT, Durr JA, et al. Aldosterone in congestive heart failure: analysis of determinants and role in sodium retention. *Am J Nephrol*. 1991;11(6):441–446.
101. Hensen J, Abraham WT, Lesnefsky EJ, et al. Atrial natriuretic peptide kinetic studies in patients with cardiac dysfunction. *Kidney Int*. 1992;41(5):1333–1339.
102. Riegger GA, Liebau G, Kochsiek K. Antidiuretic hormone in congestive heart failure. *Am J Med*. 1982;72(1):49–52.
103. Pruszczynski W, Vahanian A, Ardaillou R, et al. Role of antidiuretic hormone in impaired water excretion of patients with congestive heart failure. *J Clin Endocrinol Metab*. 1984;58(4): 599–605.
104. Bichet DG, Kortas C, Mettauer B, et al. Modulation of plasma and platelet vasopressin by cardiac function in patients with heart failure. *Kidney Int*. 1986;29(6):1188–1196.
105. Goldsmith SR, Francis GS, Cowley AW, Jr., et al. Hemodynamic effects of infused arginine vasopressin in congestive heart failure. *J Am Coll Cardiol*. 1986;8(4):779–783.
106. Goldsmith SR, Francis GS, Cowley AW, Jr. Arginine vasopressin and the renal response to water loading in congestive heart failure. *Am J Cardiol*. 1986;58(3):295–299.
107. Creager MA, Faxon DP, Cutler SS, et al. Contribution of vasopressin to vasoconstriction in patients with congestive heart failure: comparison with the renin-angiotensin system and the sympathetic nervous system. *J Am Coll Cardiol*. 1986;7(4): 758–765.
108. Nicod P, Biollaz J, Waeber B, et al. Hormonal, global, and regional haemodynamic responses to a vascular antagonist of vasopressin in patients with congestive heart failure with and without hyponatraemia. *Br Heart J*. 1986;56(5):433–439.
109. Naitoh M, Suzuki H, Murakami M, et al. Effects of oral AVP receptor antagonists OPC-21268 and OPC-31260 on congestive heart failure in conscious dogs. *Am J Physiol*. 1994;267(6 Pt 2): H2245–H2254.
110. Handelman W, Lum G, Schrier RW. Impaired water excretion in high output cardiac failure in the rat. *Clin Res*. 1979(27):173A.
111. Abraham WT, Oren RM, Crisman TS. Effects of an oral, nonpeptide, selective V2 receptor vasopressin antagonist in patients with chronic heart failure. *J Am Coll Cardiol*. 1997;(29(Suppl A):169A.
112. Ishikawa S, Saito T, Okada K, et al. Effect of vasopressin antagonist on water excretion in inferior vena cava constriction. *Kidney Int*. 1986;30(1):49–55.
113. Yared A, Kon V, Brenner BM, et al. Role for vasopressin in rats with congestive heart failure. *Kidney Int*. 1985(27):337.
114. Gheorghiade M, Gattis WA, O'Connor CM, et al. Effects of tolvaptan, a vasopressin antagonist, in patients hospitalized with worsening heart failure: a randomized controlled trial. *JAMA*. 2004;291(16):1963–1971.
115. Xu DL, Martin PY, Ohara M, et al. Upregulation of aquaporin-2 water channel expression in chronic heart failure rat. *J Clin Invest*. 1997;99(7):1500–1505.
116. Dunn FL, Brennan TJ, Nelson AE, et al. The role of blood osmolality and volume in regulating vasopressin secretion in the rat. *J Clin Invest*. 1973;52(12):3212–3219.
117. McMurray JJ, Ray SG, Abdullah I, et al. Plasma endothelin in chronic heart failure. *Circulation*. 1992(85):504–509.
118. Teerlink JR, Loffler BM, Hess P, et al. Role of ednothelin in the maintenance of blood pressure in conscious rats with chronic heart failure. Acute effects of the endothelin receptor antagonist Ro 47–0203 (bosentan). *Circulation*. 1994;90(5): 2510–2518.
119. Pacher R, Stanek B, Hulsmann M, et al. Prognostic impact of big endothelin-1 plasma concentrations compared with invasive hemodynamic evaluation in severe heart failure. *J Am Coll Cardiol*. 1996;27(3):633–641.
120. Nord EP. Renal actions of endothelin. *Kidney Int*. 1993;44(2): 451–463.
121. Bates ER, Shenker Y, Grekin RJ. The relationship between plasma levels of immunoreactive atrial natriuretic hormone and hemodynamic function in man. *Circulation*. 1986;73(6):1155–1161.
122. Burnett JC, Jr., Kao PC, Hu DC, et al. Atrial natriuretic peptide elevation in congestive heart failure in the human. *Science*. 1986;231(4742):1145–1147.
123. Hirata Y, Ishii M, Matsuoka H, et al. Plasma concentrations of alpha-human atrial natriuretic polypeptide and cyclic GMP in patients with heart disease. *Am Heart J*. 1987;113(6): 1463–1469.
124. Michel JB, Arnal JF, Corvol P. Atrial natriuretic factor as a marker in congestive heart failure. *Horm Res*. 1990;34(3–4):166–168.
125. Mukoyama M, Nakao K, Saito Y, et al. Increased human brain natriuretic peptide in congestive heart failure. *N Engl J Med*. 1990;323(11):757–758.
126. Atlas SA, Kleinert HD, Camargo MJ, et al. Purification, sequencing and synthesis of natriuretic and vasoactive rat atrial peptide. *Nature* 1984;309(5970):717–719.
127. Currie MG, Geller DM, Cole BR, et al. Bioactive cardiac substances: potent vasorelaxant activity in mammalian atria. *Science*. 1983;221(4605):71–73.

128. Molina CR, Fowler MB, McCrory S, et al. Hemodynamic, renal and endocrine effects of atrial natriuretic peptide infusion in severe heart failure. *J Am Coll Cardiol.* 1988;12(1):175–186.
129. Atarashi K, Mulrow PJ, Franco-Saenz R, et al. Inhibition of aldosterone production by an atrial extract. *Science* 1984;224(4652): 992–994.
130. Samson WK. Cardiac hormones and neuroendocrine function. *Adv Exp Med Biol.* 1990;274:177–190.
131. Saito Y, Nakao K, Arai H, et al. Atrial natriuretic polypeptide (ANP) in human ventricle. Increased gene expression of ANP in dilated cardiomyopathy. *Biochem Biophys Res Commun.* 1987;148(1):211–217.
132. Hosoda K, Nakao K, Mukoyama M, et al. Expression of brain natriuretic peptide gene in human heart. Production in the ventricle. *Hypertension.* 1991;17(6 Pt 2):1152–1155.
133. Drexler H, Hirth C, Stasch HP, et al. Vasodilatory action of endogenous atrial natriuretic factor in a rat model of chronic heart failure as determined by monoclonal ANF antibody. *Circ Res.* 1990;66(5):1371–1380.
134. Munagala VK, Burnett JC, Jr., Redfield MM. The natriuretic peptides in cardiovascular medicine. *Curr Probl Cardiol.* 2004; 29(12):707–769.
135. Publication Committee for the VMAC Investigators T. Intravenous nesiritide vs nitroglycerin for treatment of decompensated congestive heart failure: a randomized controlled trial. *JAMA.* 2002(287):1531–1540.
136. Biollaz J, Nussberger J, Porchet M, et al. Four-hour infusions of synthetic atrial natriuretic peptide in normal volunteers. *Hypertension.* 1986;8(6 Pt 2):II96–II105.
137. Borenstein HB, Cupples WA, Sonnenberg H, et al. The effect of a natriuretic atrial extract on renal haemodynamics and urinary excretion in anaesthetized rats. *J Physiol.* 1983;334: 133–140.
138. Dunn BR, Ichikawa I, Pfeffer JM, et al. Renal and systemic hemodynamic effects of synthetic atrial natriuretic peptide in the anesthetized rat. *Circ Res.* 1986;59(3):237–246.
139. Kim JK, Summer SN, Durr JA, et al. Enzymatic and binding effects of atrial natriuretic factor in glomeruli and nephrons. *Kidney Int.* 1989(35):799–805.
140. Koseki C, Hayashi Y, Torikai S, et al. Localization of binding sites for alpha-rat atrial natriuretic polypeptide in rat kidney. *Am J Physiol.* 1986;250(2 Pt 2):F210–F216.
141. Healy DP, Fanestil DD. Localization of atrial natriuretic peptide binding sites within the rat kidney. *Am J Physiol.* 1986(250): F573–F578.
142. Lee ME, Miller WL, Edwards BS, et al. Role of endogenous atrial natriuretic factor in acute congestive heart failure. *J Clin Invest.* 1989;84(6):1962–1966.
143. Abraham WT, Hensen J, Kim JK, et al. Atrial natriuretic peptide and urinary cyclic guanosine monophosphate in patients with chronic heart failure. *J Am Soc Nephrol.* 1992; 2(12):1697–1703.
144. Abraham WT, Lauwaars ME, Kim JK, et al. Reversal of atrial natriuretic peptide resistance by increasing distal tubular sodium delivery in patients with decompensated cirrhosis. *Hepatology.* 1995;22(3):737–743.
145. Kistorp C, Raymond I, Pedersen F, et al. N-terminal pro-brain natriuretic peptide, C-reactive protein, and urinary albumin levels as predictors of mortality and cardiovascular events in older adults. *JAMA.* 2005;293(13):1609–1616.
146. Swain JA, Heyndrickx GR, Boettcher DH, et al. Prostaglandin control of renal circulation in the unanesthetized dog and baboon. *Am J Physiol.* 1975;229(3):826–830.
147. Walker RM, Massey TE, McElligott TF, et al. Acetaminophen-induced hypothermia, hepatic congestion, and modification by N-acetylcysteine in mice. *Toxicol Appl Pharmacol.* 1981;59(3): 500–507.
148. Walshe JJ, Venuto RC. Acute oliguric renal failure induced by indomethacin: possible mechanism. *Ann Intern Med.* 1979;91(1): 47–49.
149. Riegger GA, Kahles HW, Elsner D, et al. Effects of acetylsalicylic acid on renal function in patients with chronic heart failure. *Am J Med.* 1991;90(5):571–575.
150. Shlipak MG, Massie BM. The clinical challenge of cardiorenal syndrome. *Circulation.* 2004;110(12):1514–1517.
151. Bongartz LG, Cramer MJ, Doevendans PA, et al. The severe cardiorenal syndrome: 'Guyton revisited.' *Eur Heart J.* 2005;26(1): 11–17.
152. Hillege HL, Girbes AR, de Kam PJ, et al. Renal function, neurohormonal activation, and survival in patients with chronic heart failure. *Circulation.* 2000;102(2):203–210.
153. Forman DE, Butler J, Wang Y, et al. Incidence, predictors at admission, and impact of worsening renal function among patients hospitalized with heart failure. *J Am Coll Cardiol.* 2004;43(1):61–67.
154. Kitzman DW, Little WC, Brubaker PH, et al. Pathophysiological characterization of isolated diastolic heart failure in comparison to systolic heart failure. *JAMA.* 2002;288(17):2144–2150.
155. DiBona GF. The sympathetic nervous system and hypertension: recent developments. *Hypertension.* 2004;43(2):147–150.
156. Esler M, Rumantir M, Kaye D, et al. Sympathetic nerve biology in essential hypertension. *Clin Exp Pharmacol Physiol.* 2001;28(12): 986–989.
157. Esler M, Kaye D. Increased sympathetic nervous system activity and its therapeutic reduction in arterial hypertension, portal hypertension and heart failure. *J Auton Nerv Syst.* 1998;72(2–3):210–219.
158. Zucker IH, Schultz HD, Li YF, et al. The origin of sympathetic outflow in heart failure: the roles of angiotensin II and nitric oxide. *Prog Biophys Mol Biol.* 2004;84(2–3):217–232.
159. Hundley WG, Kitzman DW, Morgan TM, et al. Cardiac cycle-dependent changes in aortic area and distensibility are reduced in older patients with isolated diastolic heart failure and correlate with exercise intolerance. *J Am Coll Cardiol.* 2001;38(3): 796–802.
160. Chen CH, Nakayama M, Nevo E, et al. Coupled systolic-ventricular and vascular stiffening with age: implications for pressure regulation and cardiac reserve in the elderly. *J Am Coll Cardiol.* 1998;32(5):1221–1227.
161. Kawaguchi M, Hay I, Fetics B, et al. Combined ventricular systolic and arterial stiffening in patients with heart failure and preserved ejection fraction: implications for systolic and diastolic reserve limitations. *Circulation.* 2003;107(5):714–720.
162. Konstam MA, Udelson JE, Anand IS, et al. Ventricular remodeling in heart failure: a credible surrogate endpoint. *J Card Fail.* 2003;9(5):350–353.
163. Tsuruda T, Boerrigter G, Huntley BK, et al. Brain natriuretic peptide is produced in cardiac fibroblasts and induces matrix metalloproteinases. *Circ Res.* 2002;91(12):1127–1134.
164. Cataliotti A, Boerrigter G, Costello-Boerrigter LC, et al. Brain natriuretic peptide enhances renal actions of furosemide and suppresses furosemide-induced aldosterone activation in experimental heart failure. *Circulation.* 2004;109(13):1680–1685.
165. Wang DJ, Dowling TC, Meadows D, et al. Nesiritide does not improve renal function in patients with chronic heart failure and worsening serum creatinine. *Circulation.* 2004;110(12):1620–1625.
166. Sackner-Bernstein JD, Skopicki HA, Aaronson KD. Risk of worsening renal function with nesiritide in patients with acutely decompensated heart failure. *Circulation.* 2005;111(12):1487–1491.
167. Chen HH, Grantham JA, Schirger JA, et al. Subcutaneous administration of brain natriuretic peptide in experimental heart failure. *J Am Coll Cardiol.* 2000;36(5):1706–1712.
168. Levy D, Garrison RJ, Savage DD, et al. Prognostic implications of echocardiographically determined left ventricular mass in the Framingham Heart Study. *N Engl J Med.* 1990;322(22):1561–1566.
169. Francis GS, Cohn JN, Johnson G, et al. Plasma norepinephrine, plasma renin activity, and congestive heart failure. Relations to survival and the effects of therapy in V-HeFT II. The V-HeFT VA Cooperative Studies Group. *Circulation.* 1993;87(6 Suppl): VI40–VI48.
170. Barr CS, Lang CC, Hanson J, et al. Effects of adding spironolactone to an angiotensin-converting enzyme inhibitor in chronic congestive heart failure secondary to coronary artery disease. *Am J Cardiol.* 1995;76(17):1259–1265.
171. Brooks VL. Interactions between angiotensin II and the sympathetic nervous system in the long-term control of arterial pressure. *Clin Exp Pharmacol Physiol.* 1997;24(1):83–90.
172. Weber KT. Aldosterone in congestive heart failure. *N Engl J Med.* 2001;345(23):1689–1697.
173. Myers BD, Deen WM, Brenner BM. Effects of norepinephrine and angiotensin II on the determinants of glomerular ultrafiltra-

tion and proximal tubule fluid reabsorption in the rat. *Circ Res.* 1975;37(1):101–110.
174. Schrier RW, De Wardener HE. Tubular reabsorption of sodium ion: influence of factors other than aldosterone and glomerular filtration rate. 2. *N Engl J Med.* 1971;285(23):1292–1303.
175. Castrop H, Schweda F, Mizel D, et al. Permissive role of nitric oxide in macula densa control of renin secretion. *Am J Physiol Renal Physiol.* 2004;286(5):F848–F857.
176. He XR, Greenberg SG, Briggs JP, et al. Effects of furosemide and verapamil on the NaCl dependency of macula densa-mediated renin secretion. *Hypertension.* 1995;26(1):137–142.
177. Lindenfeld J. Prevalence and outcomes of anemia in heart failure. *Am Heart J.* 2005. In press.
178. McMurray JJ. What are the clinical consequences of anemia in patients with chronic heart failure? *J Card Fail.* 2004;10(Suppl 1):S10–S12.
179. Levin A, Thompson CR, Ethier J, et al. Left ventricular mass index increase in early renal disease: impact of decline in hemoglobin. *Am J Kidney Dis.* 1999;34(1):125–134.
180. Silverberg DS, Wexler D, Iaina A. The role of anemia in the progression of congestive heart failure. Is there a place for erythropoietin and intravenous iron? *J Nephrol.* 2004;17(6):749–761.
181. van der Meer P, Voors AA, Lipsic E, et al. Prognostic value of plasma erythropoietin on mortality in patients with chronic heart failure. *J Am Coll Cardiol.* 2004;44(1):63–67.
182. Volpe M, Tritto C, Testa U, et al. Blood levels of erythropoietin in congestive heart failure and correlation with clinical, hemodynamic, and hormonal profiles. *Am J Cardiol.* 1994;74(5):468–473.
183. Okonko DO, Anker SD. Anemia in chronic heart failure: pathogenetic mechanisms. *J Card Fail.* 2004;10(Suppl 1):S5–S9.
184. Maiese K, Li F, Chong ZZ. New avenues of exploration for erythropoietin. *JAMA.* 2005;293(1):90–95.
185. Fisher JW. Erythropoietin: physiology and pharmacology update. *Exp Biol Med (Maywood).* 2003;228(1):1–14.
186. Calvillo L, Latini R, Kajstura T. Recombinant human erythropoietin protects the myocardium from ischemia-reperfusion injury and promotes beneficial remodeling. *Proc Natl Acad Sci USA.* 2003;100:2802–2806.
187. Anker SD, Ponikowski PP, Clark AL, et al. Cytokines and neurohormones relating to body composition alterations in the wasting syndrome of chronic heart failure. *Eur Heart J.* 1999;20(9):683–693.
188. Sekiguchi K, Li X, Coker M, et al. Cross-regulation between the renin-angiotensin system and inflammatory mediators in cardiac hypertrophy and failure. *Cardiovasc Res.* 2004;63(3):433–442.
189. Knotek M, Rogachev B, Wang W, et al. Endotoxemic renal failure in mice: role of tumor necrosis factor independent of inducible nitric oxide synthase. *Kidney Int.* 2001;59(6):2243–2249.
190. Bryant D, Becker L, Richardson J, et al. Cardiac failure in transgenic mice with myocardial expression of tumor necrosis factor-alpha. *Circulation.* 1998;97(14):1375–1381.
191. Hernandez-Presa M, Bustos C, Ortego M, et al. Angiotensin-converting enzyme inhibition prevents arterial nuclear factor-kappa B activation, monocyte chemoattractant protein-1 expression, and macrophage infiltration in a rabbit model of early accelerated atherosclerosis. *Circulation.* 1997;95(6):1532–1541.
192. Butler J, Forman DE, Abraham WT, et al. Relationship between heart failure treatment and development of worsening renal function among hospitalized patients. *Am Heart J.* 2004;147(2):331–338.
193. McCurley JM, Hanlon SU, Wei SK, et al. Furosemide and the progression of left ventricular dysfunction in experimental heart failure. *J Am Coll Cardiol.* 2004;44(6):1301–1307.
194. Abdallah JG, Schrier RW, Edelstein C, et al. Loop diuretic infusion increases thiazide-sensitive Na(+)/Cl(−)-cotransporter abundance: role of aldosterone. *J Am Soc Nephrol.* 2001;12(7):1335–1341.
195. Weber KT. Furosemide in the long-term management of heart failure: the good, the bad, and the uncertain. *J Am Coll Cardiol.* 2004;44(6):1308–1310.
196. Ahokas RA, Sun Y, Bhattacharya SK, et al. Aldosteronism and a proinflammatory vascular phenotype: role of Mg^{2+}, Ca^{2+}, and H_2O_2 in peripheral blood mononuclear cells. *Circulation.* 2005;111(1):51–57.
197. Cohn JN, Archibald DG, Ziesche S, et al. Effect of vasodilator therapy on mortality in chronic congestive heart failure. Results of a Veterans Administration Cooperative Study. *N Engl J Med.* 1986;314(24):1547–1552.
198. Francis GS, Siegel RM, Goldsmith SR, et al. Acute vasoconstrictor response to intravenous furosemide in patients with chronic congestive heart failure. Activation of the neurohumoral axis. *Ann Intern Med.* 1985;103(1):1–6.
199. Bayliss J, Norell M, Canepa-Anson R, et al. Untreated heart failure: clinical and neuroendocrine effects of introducing diuretics. *Br Heart J.* 1987;57(1):17–22.
200. Packer M, Lee WH, Kessler PD, et al. Prevention and reversal of nitrate tolerance in patients with congestive heart failure. *N Engl J Med.* 1987;317(13):799–804.
201. Katz RJ, Levy WS, Buff L, et al. Prevention of nitrate tolerance with angiotension converting enzyme inhibitors. *Circulation.* 1991;83(4):1271–1277.
202. Taylor AL, Ziesche S, Yancy C, et al. Combination of isosorbide dinitrate and hydralazine in blacks with heart failure. *N Engl J Med.* 2004;351(20):2049–2057.
203. Waagstein F, Bristow MR, Swedberg K, et al. Beneficial effects of metoprolol in idiopathic dilated cardiomyopathy. Metoprolol in Dilated Cardiomyopathy (MDC) Trial Study Group. *Lancet.* 1993;342(8885):1441–1446.
204. Bristow MR, Gilbert EM, Abraham WT, et al. Carvedilol produces dose-related improvements in left ventricular function and survival in subjects with chronic heart failure. MOCHA Investigators. *Circulation.* 1996;94(11):2807–2816.
205. Captpril Multicenter Research Group T. A placebo-controlled trial of captopril in refractory chronic congestive heart failure. *J Am Coll Cardiol.* 1983(2):755–763.
206. CONSENSUS Trial Study Group T. Effects of enalapril on mortality in severe congestive heart failure. Results of the Cooperative North Scandinavian Enalapril Survival Study (CONSENSUS). The CONSENSUS Trial Study Group. *N Engl J Med.* 1987;316(23):1429–1435.
207. SOLVD Investigators T. Effect of enalapril on survival in patients with reduced left ventricular ejection fractions and congestive heart failure. The SOLVD Investigators. *N Engl J Med.* 1991;325(5):293–302.
208. Cohn JN. Future directions in vasodilator therapy for heart failure. *Am Heart J.* 1991;121(3 Pt 1):969–974.
209. Suki WN. Renal hemodynamic consequences of angiotensin-converting enzyme inhibition in congestive heart failure. *Arch Intern Med.* 1989;149(3):669–673.
210. Tobian I, Coffee K, Ferriera D, et al. The effect of renal perfusion pressure on net transport out of distal tubular urine as studied with stop-flow technique. *J Clin Invest.* 1964(43):118–128.
211. Anand I, McMurray J, Cohn JN, et al. Long-term effects of darusentan on left-ventricular remodelling and clinical outcomes in the Endothelin-A Receptor Antagonist Trial in Heart Failure (EARTH): randomised, double-blind, placebo-controlled trial. *Lancet.* 2004;364(9431):347–354.
212. Packer M, McMurray J, Massie BM, et al. Clinical effects of endothelin receptor antagonism with bosentan in patients with severe chronic heart failure: results of a pilot study. *J Card Fail.* 2005;11(1):12–20.
213. Agostoni P, Marenzi G, Lauri G, et al. Sustained improvement in functional capacity after removal of body fluid with isolated ultrafiltration in chronic cardiac insufficiency: failure of furosemide to provide the same result. *Am J Med.* 1994;96(3):191–199.
214. Fauchauld P. Effects of ultrafiltration of body fluid and transcapillary collioid osmotic gradient in hemodialysis patients, improvements in dialysis therapy. *Contrib Nephrol.* 1989(74):170–175.

Differential Diagnosis of Congestive Heart Failure

Risk Factors for Heart Failure

16

Javed Butler

"If you wish to speak to me, you should first define your terms."
—Master Pangloss to Candide in Voltaire's *Candide*

RISK FACTOR DETERMINATION: A RISKY BUSINESS

Beyond a few high-impact and obvious conditions such as myocardial infarction or hypertension, which clearly are associated with the development of heart failure, determination of risk factors for any disease entity is a difficult task. The literature is filled with claims of risk association between various exposures and disease states that are difficult to prove conclusively. Moreover, these associations are often used for unintended purposes (e.g., medical/legal reasons, publicity, and media attention). A perfect example would be the proposed link between silicone breast implants and the risk for connective tissue diseases in women, a debate that has now been active for over a decade without resolution (1,2).

What strength of association is needed between an exposure and a disease for that exposure to be labeled as a risk factor? How much data do we need to be certain? How many times does it have to be reproduced? These questions are difficult to answer. If the risk factor claim is made hastily, without completely understanding the subtleties and nuances, scientific progress can be delayed for a long time. After all, for several decades beta-blockers were considered to be contraindicated in patients with heart failure! On the other hand, waiting too long for the ultimate confirmation of risky exposures can lead to continuing potentially hazardous exposure and ongoing public health concerns. The cardiovascular risk associated with the use of cyclo-oxygenase II inhibitors, commonly used for arthritis, is an example of such a case. Though the increased risk of cardiovascular disease with their use was first described several years ago, these drugs were not taken off the market until 2005 (3).

Risk factor determination is always a progressive and evolving field as understanding of the disease process broadens and the treatment options evolve. Today's risk factors may be obsolete tomorrow as either the treatment or patient profiles change over time, or better colinear associations are discovered, rendering any given established risk factor relatively insignificant. In this respect, heart failure presents an even bigger challenge as this condition is a clinical syndrome and not a narrowly defined disease process. Thus, different risk factors may predict the risk for varying aspects of this syndrome, adding to the complexity of risk factor determination.

Difficulties in Assessing Risk Factors for Heart Failure

Figure 16-1 gives a general conceptual overview of the difficulties in determining risk factors for heart failure.

Risk Factor or Risk Marker

A correlation between a variable and a disease process may represent a so-called true–true but unrelated epiphenomenon, a marker of disease progression, or a directly contributing pathological relationship to the progression of disease. For example, activation of the renin-angiotensin-aldosterone system (RAAS) is seen with advancing heart failure, and elevated angiotensin II

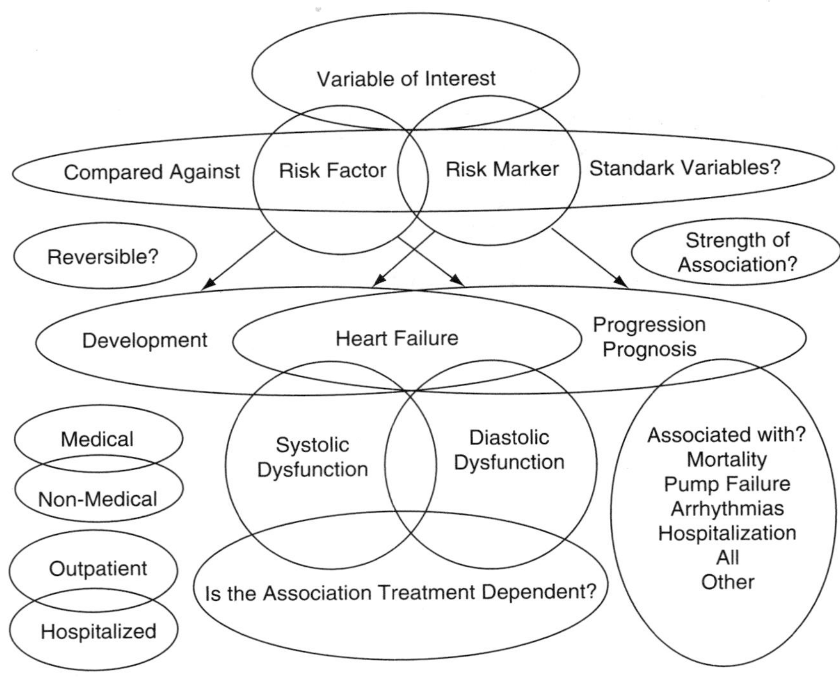

Figure 16-1 Conceptual model for risk factor assessment.

or aldosterone levels are associated with worse outcomes. Mechanistically, this pathogenic link is plausible considering the role that these neurohormones play in apoptosis, fibrosis, remodeling, and the risk for arrhythmias and pump failure (4–6). On the other hand, with advancing heart failure, activation of the natriuretic peptide system is also seen and the levels of B-type natriuretic peptide (BNP), similar to angiotensin II and aldosterone levels, correlate with severity of disease. However, natriuretic peptides are not considered risk factors for heart failure but are markers of severity (7,8). In fact, recombinant natriuretic peptides are used to treat acutely decompensated heart failure. Although this example may be rather clear, the ability to differentiate is not always the case. For example, whether or not C-reactive protein (CRP) is a risk marker or risk factor for progression of coronary artery disease has been debated for many years. We are still awaiting the results of a clinical trial targeting CRP as a therapeutic target to conclude this debate (9,10).

Risk for What?

Like most chronic disease, heart failure can present at various stages with a wide spectrum of manifestations. With respect to risk factors and heart failure, the most important aspects of this spectrum are whether a risk factor is related to the development or progression (and, in turn, prognosis) of heart failure. Some risk factors are associated with both (e.g., diabetes), whereas others may be more specific for either development (e.g., certain chemotherapy agents) or progression (e.g., conduction abnormalities) of heart failure. Similarly, risk factors may vary in their importance with respect to different outcomes (e.g., pump failure versus sudden cardiac death).

Type of Heart Failure

Since heart failure is a syndrome and not a specific, single disease entity, another level of complexity is what type of heart failure the risk is associated with. Is the risk factor pertinent to systolic or diastolic dysfunction? Although diastolic dysfunction is less well-studied, there appears to be considerable overlap between risk factors. For example, hypertension is recognized as being a cause of both systolic and diastolic dysfunction. In contrast, excessive alcohol consumption is associated with a higher risk for systolic dysfunction but no such link is currently known for diastolic dysfunction. Similarly, many other forms of heart failure may have unique risk factors (e.g., thiamine deficiencies and risk for high-output heart failure or idiopathic pulmonary fibrosis and risk for isolated right heart failure).

Is the Risk Factor Modifiable?

Another important consideration is whether or not the risk factor is reversible. Many risk factors are of interest from the epidemiological perspective but have no therapeutic value (e.g., age and gender), whereas others are treatable (e.g., dyslipidemia). Similarly, risk factors can be medical (e.g., hypertension,) or nonmedical (related to patients' demographics or lifestyle choices, such as obesity). Usually, the former are more easily treatable.

Is the Risk Factor Treatment-Dependent?

Medical therapy is fast-changing, as is the relationship between risk factors and outcomes. Certain risk factors, such as advancing age, are immune to therapy while others, such as exercise capacity, are not. Several recent reports have suggested that as prognoses for patients with heart failure have improved with newer therapies and devices, the outcomes for patients with similar peak exercise oxygen consumption level have also improved over time (11–13). This is primarily because several of these therapies that improve outcomes do not impact peak exercise oxygen consumption (e.g., beta-blockers and defibrillators) (14). Thus, the importance of risk factors needs continuous re-evaluation as medical therapy advances.

Statistical Considerations

Before one can be certain of the association between an exposure and the risk of a disease, there are many statistical considerations that have to be satisfied. For example, the independent prognostic power of any risk factor depends largely on what it is compared against. A very simplistic example would be a statistically higher risk of lung cancer among people who carry matches or lighters with them and, hence, we can conclude that these are risk factors for lung cancer. Obviously this will only be the case if one ignores cigarette smoking in the equation. This is the Achilles' heel of the literature on risk factor determination. Because different investigators control for a varying array of variables, ranging from none to extensive, in different patient populations the generalizability of such reports is difficult to ascertain. If such results were to be replicated in other studies with different patient populations (e.g., elderly versus middle-aged) or in association with other copredictors, even if such risk factors remain positive, it is almost certain their strength of association would be different. Since the risk factor analysis is important not only from a qualitative perspective but also to quantify outcomes, these statistical considerations cannot be ignored. Similarly, whether the data are validated, what proportion of outcomes are explained by the risk factors, how well the risk factor predicts outcomes across the spectrum of risks, and so forth are all important considerations when determining risk factors.

Practicality and Feasibility

The most important characteristic of a risk factor is whether or not it is clinically useful. For example, cardiac norepinephrine spillover is a strong but clinically irrelevant risk factor. Measurement of plasma norepinephrine, a potent risk factor which can be measured only by an expensive and difficult-to-obtain test, is another example. Simple measurement of heart rate, however, can give significant clues as to the degree of sympathetic activity. Similarly, a detailed history can generally give a reasonable sense whether the peak exercise oxygen consumption is severely or modestly depressed. For decisions such as transplant listing, this may not be enough, but for routine clinical management in the community this may be an adequate way of risk-stratifying patients, especially when used in conjunction with New York Heart Association class symptoms.

In short, there is no single risk factor that is totally accurate or perfect. In order to assess a patient's risk for development of heart failure or to determine prognosis in patients who already manifest the condition, a careful history and physical examination and measurement of left ventricular function remains the cornerstone. Information obtained from the history and physical should then be used in conjunction with other tests tailored to the patient and the purpose of investigation. This chapter will focus on risk factors for development and progression of heart failure associated with primarily systolic dysfunction as they are seen in the outpatient setting.

RISK FACTORS FOR DEVELOPMENT OF HEART FAILURE

Table 16-1 gives an overview of risk factors for heart failure development.

Demographics

A higher risk of development of heart failure with increasing age and among males has been consistently shown in the literature (15–22). The higher risk in men may be at least partially related to the greater prevalence of coronary heart disease. Low socioeconomic status has also been associated with an increased heart failure risk (23). Though not clear, the association between low socioeconomic status and the risk for heart failure may be related to poor access to health care, compliance issues, or a higher prevalence of other heart failure risk factors (24,25).

Lifestyle-Related

Alcohol Consumption

Relationship between alcohol abuse and development of heart failure is well-known (26,27). This may be related to both the direct myocardial toxicity of alcohol and the higher risk of hypertension development with excessive alcohol use (28–30). However, some data suggest that moderate alcohol consumption may lower the risk of heart failure development (31). This may be related to the lower risk of diabetes, myocardial infarction, and favorable changes in the lipid profile, platelet function, and blood clotting associated with moderate alcohol intake (32–36).

Tobacco and Coffee Consumption

Data regarding the risk for heart failure development with smoking (after controlling for other risk factors) are conflicting (23,37,38). Theoretically, such a relationship is conceivable as smoking is associated with abnormalities that, in turn, increase heart failure risk (e.g., insulin resistance, endothelial dysfunction, oxidative stress, and possible direct myocardial toxicity) (39–42). Similarly, excessive coffee intake has been associated with an increased risk of heart failure (38).

Dietary Sodium Intake

An association between excessive dietary salt intake and risk for heart failure has been reported (43). This may be related to ventricular function abnormalities, hypertension,

TABLE 16-1
RISK FACTORS FOR DEVELOPMENT OF HEART FAILURE

Demographic
Age
Gender
Low socioeconomic status
Lifestyle-related
Tobacco and coffee consumption
Alcohol consumption
Dietary sodium intake
Recreational drug use
Comorbidities
Hypertension
Left ventricular hypertrophy
Myocardial infarction
Obesity
Diabetes mellitus
Valvular heart disease
Renal insufficiency
Dyslipidemia
Sleep apnea
Tachycardia
Impaired lung function
Depression
Echocardiographic
Ventricular dimension
Ventricular mass
Diastolic filling impairment
Pharmacological
Chemotherapeutic agents
Nonsteroidal anti-inflammatory drugs
Thiazolidinediones?
Doxazosin
Biochemical
Albuminuria
Homocysteine
Tumor necrosis factor alpha
Interleukin-6
C-reactive protein
Insulin-like growth factor-I
Natriuretic peptides
Genetic risk factors
Genetic polymorphism

development of left ventricular hypertrophy, or water retention associated with excessive salt intake (43–47).

Recreational Drug Use

Cocaine abuse has been associated with development of heart failure. This has been shown in both acute and chronic settings. It may be related to either development of premature coronary disease, vasospasm, or cocaine's effect on cardiac contractility (48–50). Other agents, particularly methamphetamines, have also been associated with increased heart failure risk.

Biochemical Markers

Albuminuria

In the Heart Outcomes Prevention Evaluation study, presence of microalbuminuria was associated with a threefold increase in the risk of heart failure hospitalization (51). Microalbuminuria is associated with other cardiovascular risks such as hypertension, ventricular hypertrophy, and serum acute phase reactants, which may be important in heart failure development (52–54).

Homocysteine

The Framingham Heart Study has shown that elevated plasma homocysteine levels are associated with almost a 75% increase in risk for heart failure development (55). This may be related to the link between high homocysteine serum levels and oxidative stress and cardiac fibrosis, endothelial dysfunction, and coronary atherosclerosis—all factors important in development of heart failure (56–59).

Tumor Necrosis Factor-α

In recent analyses, after adjustment for other risk factors, every tertile increment in tumor necrosis factor-α (TNF-α) levels was associated with a 60% increase in risk of heart failure (60). TNF-α is a proinflammatory cytokine produced by myocardial macrophages and is associated with myocardial dysfunction and cell death (61). TNF-α has several negative pleiotropic effects and also negative inotropic properties that may be responsible for excessive heart failure risk (62,63); it is also associated with progression of heart failure (64).

Interleukin-6

Similar to TNF-α, interleukin-6 (IL-6) is also a proinflammatory cytokine associated with an excessive risk of development of heart failure (60). Both of these cytokines are associated with ventricular remodeling, fetal gene expression, and myocyte hypertrophy and apoptosis (65). In transgenic mice models, overexpression of IL-6 and its receptor has been associated with left ventricular dilatation (66).

C-Reactive Protein

Data from the Framingham Heart Study also suggest that an increase in CRP level by 5 mg/dL is associated with a greater than twofold increased risk of heart failure, and subjects who simultaneously also had elevated serum IL-6 and TNF-α values had a fourfold increase in risk (60). Whether this increased risk is due to high CRP levels and atherosclerosis risk or through activation of other proinflammatory cytokines is not known.

Insulin-Like Growth Factor-I

Insulin-like growth factor-I (IGF-I) is expressed in various tissues and has been shown to have a positive inotropic effect; it also decreases the rate of apoptosis (67,68). IGF-I may also cause vasodilation, decreasing impedance to cardiac emptying (69). Data from the Framingham Heart Study have linked a serum IGF-I level below 140 mg/L with a doubling of the risk of heart failure development (70).

Natriuretic Peptides

In the Framingham Heart Study, increased levels of plasma BNP and N-terminal atrial natriuretic peptide (N-ANP) were associated with an increased risk of heart failure. As shown in Figure 16-2, BNP levels above the 80th percentile (20 pg/mL for men and 23.3 pg/mL for women) were associated with a threefold increase in heart failure risk (71). BNP and N-ANP are secreted by the cardiac myocytes in response to stretch and have several beneficial physiological effects (72,73). The increased risk for heart failure related to elevated natriuretic peptides is not readily explained. However, this association may be due to the presence of subclinical heart failure, which results in elevation of these hormones.

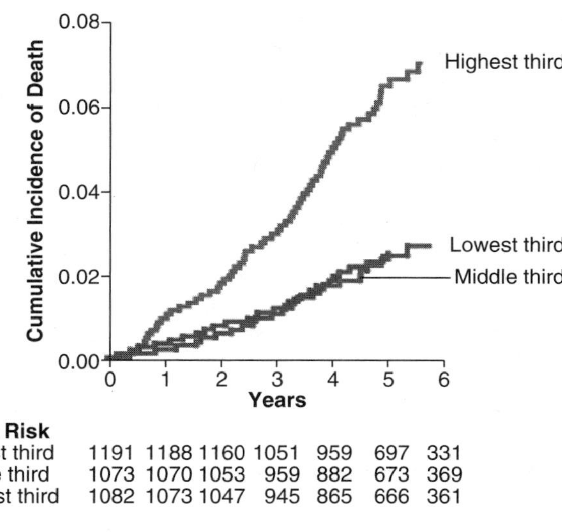

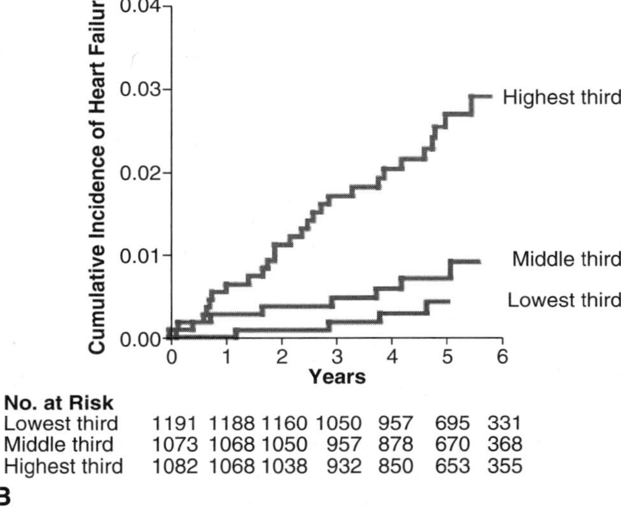

Figure 16-2 Cumulative incidence of death **(A)** and heart failure **(B)** according to the plasma B-type natriuretic peptide level at baseline. The lowest third, middle third, and highest third of plasma B-type natriuretic peptide levels were 4.0 pg/mL or less, 4.1 to 12.7 pg/mL, and 12.8 pg/mL, respectively, for men and 5.9 pg/mL or less, 6.0 to 15.7 pg/mL, and 15.8 pg/mL or more, respectively, for women. Follow-up results are truncated after 6 years (Reprinted from Wang TJ, Larson MG, Levy D, et al. Plasma natriuretic peptide levels and the risk of cardiovascular events and death. *N Engl J Med.* 2004;350:655–663, with permission from the Massachusetts Medical Society.)

Echocardiographic Parameters

Asymptomatic dilatation of the left ventricle, along with increases in left end-diastolic or end-systolic diameter, has been linked to a higher risk of developing heart failure (74). Similar to elevated natriuretic peptides, whether or not this represents the initial stages of left ventricular dysfunction is unknown. One may also include in this category asymptomatic left ventricular dysfunction as a risk factor for developing the syndrome of heart failure (75). Increased left ventricular mass, which is a correlate of left ventricular hypertrophy as assessed by electrocardiogram, is also related to a higher risk for heart failure development (76). Finally, multiple left ventricular diastolic filling abnormalities, such as alterations in the E/A wave ratio, have been associated with a higher heart failure risk (76). These different echocardiographic parameters may act in concert to predict the risk and may be related to the activation of the neurohormonal axis in patients with cardiac structural changes, even in the absence of symptoms (77).

Comorbidities

Hypertension

There is perhaps no better-documented risk factor for predicting the future risk for heart failure development than hypertension, which confers a two- to threefold higher risk (16–21,78). All three components of hypertension (systolic, diastolic, and pulse pressure) have been associated with this higher risk (79,80). Interestingly, the risk of developing heart failure related to a wide pulse pressure is not completely explained by either systolic hypertension or diastolic pressure lowering by medications, suggesting that a combination of elevated systolic and reduced diastolic pressures may confer additional risk related to increased pulse pressure (79).

The mechanism by which hypertension confers the risk for development of heart failure is well-described in the literature and is related to myocyte hypertrophy, increased fibrosis, reduced contractile proteins, eventual neurohormonal activation, and, ultimately, remodeling of the ventricle (81–83). It is therefore not surprising that treatment of hypertension substantially reduces the risk of heart failure development, although different drugs may have varying effect, including higher risk with the use of doxazosin (84,85).

Myocardial Infarction

Similar to hypertension, myocardial infarction is a well-known risk factor for heart failure in terms of its overall association, but it confers a much higher magnitude of risk (on the order of 15-fold or more) (16–21). Therefore, myocardial infarction can be considered the most potent risk factor for heart failure. Also, similar to hypertension, the mechanisms of development of heart failure after an infarction are complex and include cellular slippage, dilatation of the infracted area, subsequent hypertrophy of the unaffected myocytes, excess collagen deposition and fibrosis, apoptosis, and, ultimately, systemic neurohormonal activation and its subsequent consequences (86).

Left Ventricular Hypertrophy

Left ventricular hypertrophy on electrocardiogram, independent of hypertension, is associated with a higher risk of heart failure (87). On a relative scale, this risk appears to be higher in younger subjects than older. The increased risk is likely mediated through multifactorial mechanisms, including a direct effect on myocardium in terms of increased oxygen demand and reduced coronary reserve, higher risk of apoptosis, and also (indirectly) by increasing the risk of coronary artery disease and myocardial infarction (88–90). Regression of left ventricular hypertrophy with medication is associated with an overall reduction of risk for cardiovascular outcomes, and it probably also leads to a reduction in the risk for heart failure (91).

Valvular Heart Disease

Various cardiac valvular abnormalities are associated with an increased risk of heart failure development (92). Whether this presents in the form of pressure overload (e.g., aortic stenosis) or volume overload (e.g., mitral regurgitation), the initial compensatory mechanisms, such as hypertrophy or ventricular dilatation, eventually affect contractility and development of heart failure (93). Timely surgical intervention can substantially improve cardiac function and reduce the risk for heart failure (94).

Diabetes Mellitus

Diabetes mellitus, especially in women and in patients with asymptomatic left ventricular dysfunction, has been associated with a three- to fivefold increased risk of developing heart failure (17–20,95,96). This excess risk may be related to accelerated atherosclerosis, endothelial dysfunction, microvascular diseases, and autonomic dysfunction associated with diabetes (97). Even a modest increase of 1% in glycosylated hemoglobin (HgbAlc) leads to a >10% risk of heart failure hospitalization or death (98).

Overweight

Although debated for some time, being overweight or obese is now a well-established risk factor for heart failure (99). As shown in Figure 16-3, for both men and women there is a worsening gradient for adverse outcomes with increasing body mass index (BMI). This relationship was seen even after adjusting the data for differences in groups with respect to age, lipid levels, smoking and alcohol consumption, and history of hypertension, diabetes, and myocardial infarction. Similar to diabetes, elevated BMI tends to be associated with other high-risk vascular disease traits, but obesity is also associated with potential changes in cardiac structure and function, neurohormonal changes, preload and afterload, and other comorbidities such as renal diseases. Whether this risk is reversible or not has not been elucidated.

Lipid Abnormalities

Hypertriglyceridemia and an increased total cholesterol to high-density lipoprotein (HDL) level are associated with a higher risk of heart failure (100). This may be related to increased atherosclerotic cardiovascular diseases, left ventricular hypertrophy, or cardiac function abnormalities seen in patients with dyslipidemias (101,102). Interestingly, in at least one controlled clinical trial in patients with coronary artery disease, lipid lowering was associated with a 21% reduction in the risk of developing heart failure (103).

Renal Insufficiency

Elevated serum creatinine (1.5 mg/dL in men and 1.3 mg/dL in women) or reduced creatinine clearance (less than 60 mL/minute) is related to a higher risk for new-onset heart failure, even after adjusting for traditional risk factors for heart failure; this risks tends to increase with worsening renal function (104). However, even milder degrees of renal insufficiency are also associated with a progression of asymptomatic systolic dysfunction to symptomatic heart failure (105). Many pathophysiological changes that occur in patients with renal insufficiency can contribute to this excess risk, including hypervolemia, oxidative stress, neurohormonal and cytokine activation, anemia, hypertension, and abnormalities in coagulation cascade (106–109).

Sleep-Disordered Breathing

In both humans and animals, sleep-disordered breathing is associated with a risk for heart failure (110–112). In an epidemiological study consisting of a survey of over 6,400 individuals, the presence of an apnea-hypopnea index (AHI) was associated with a greater than twofold increased risk of heart failure (113). The physiological basis for this increased risk is complicated. Apnea can lead to negative swings in intrathoracic pressure, in turn leading to increase in afterload. A reduced oxygen level and an elevated carbon dioxide level can increase sympathetic activation (114). Hypoxia-induced pulmonary vasoconstriction and increased right ventricular pressure may compromise left ventricular filling. Obstructive sleep apnea also elevates sympathetic activity and hypertension, leading to a higher heart failure risk (115,116). Treatment of sleep apnea in smaller studies has

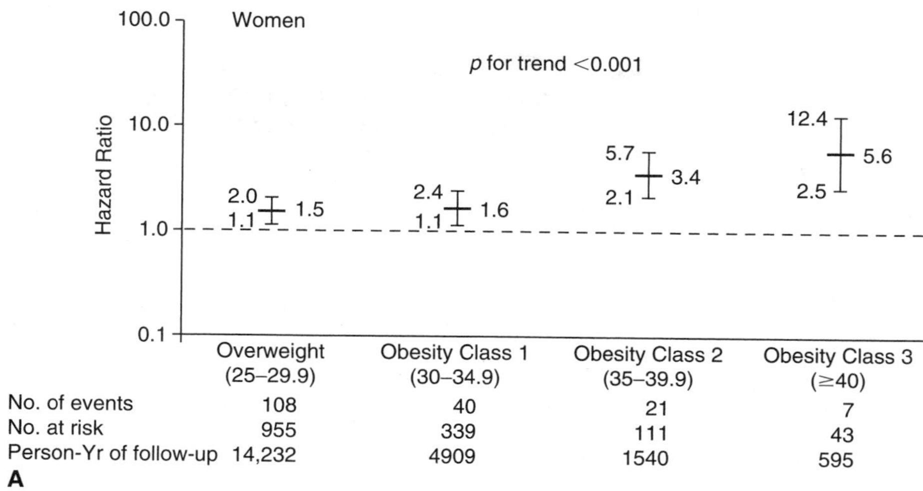

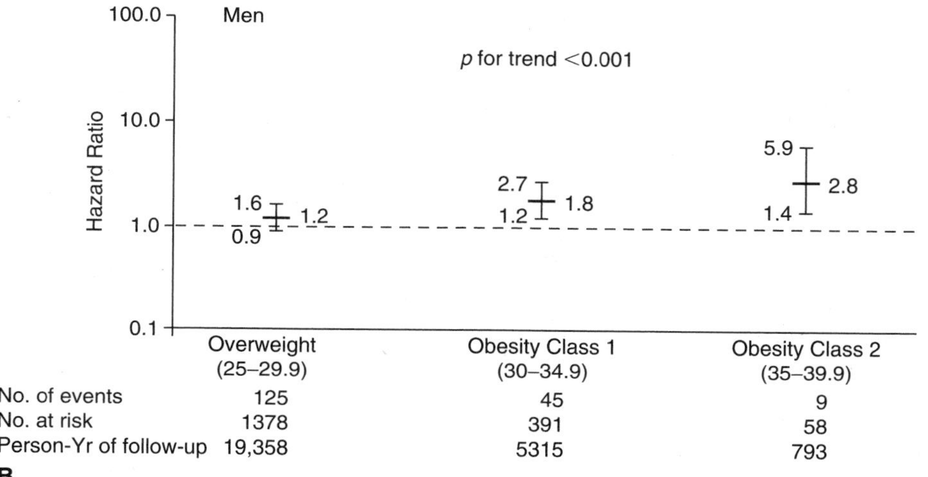

Figure 16-3 Risk of heart failure in obese subjects, according to category of body mass index (BMI) at the baseline examination. I bars represent the 95% confidence intervals for the hazard ratios. Hazard ratios were adjusted for age, total serum cholesterol level, cigarette smoking, alcohol consumption, and presence or absence of valve disease, hypertension, diabetes mellitus, electrocardiographic evidence of left ventricular hypertrophy, and myocardial infarction at baseline. Normal weight (BMI, 18.5 to 24.9) was the reference category. Hazard ratios on the y-axis are shown on a logarithmic scale. Data for men in obesity class 3 are not provided because of the small sample (eight subjects) (Reprinted from Kenchaiah S, Evans JC, Levy D, et al. Obesity and the risk of heart failure. *N Eng J Med.* 2002; 347:305–313.)

been associated with improved outcomes in terms of reduction in blood pressure and sympathetic activity and improved left ventricular function (117,118).

Tachycardia

Tachycardia-induced cardiomyopathy is a well-known entity. In the Framingham Heart Study, a 10-beats-per-minute increase in heart rate was associated with a >10% higher risk for heart failure development (92). Whether this represents existing left ventricular dysfunction and tachycardia in compensation to reduced stroke volume or inappropriate activation of the neurohormonal system is not known.

Pulmonary Function Abnormalities

Data regarding pulmonary function abnormalities and development of heart failure are conflicting. Forced vital capacity and forced expiratory volume in the first second have been associated with an increased risk in some but not other studies (16,119). The most difficult aspect of ascertaining the relationship between heart failure risk and abnormal pulmonary function is the potential for misclassification based on symptoms. However, pulmonary abnormalities are associated with other high-risk cardiovascular diseases and structural cardiac abnormalities, and a direct link is possible (120,121).

Depression and Stress

Social and emotional factors are known to precipitate hospitalization among heart failure patients (122). Depressed elderly patients have been shown to have a twofold higher risk of developing heart failure (123). Gender differences, with a higher risk in women as compared to men, have been described in the literature (124). Although a greater part of this excess risk may be attributable to compliance, an association between stress and depression with sympathetic activation, arrhythmias, and immune system modulation has been described (125–128). Whether treatment of depression prevents the development of heart failure is not known.

Pharmacological Risk Factors

Chemotherapeutic agents such as doxorubicin and cyclophosphamide can cause myocardial damage, which results in left ventricular dysfunction and heart failure (129,130). This risk exists not only in the acute treatment phase but also may occur several months after the exposure to these agents; there generally tends to be a higher risk with increasing cumulative dose (131,132). The heart failure risk associated with the antihypertensive agent doxazosin has been described earlier. Although the link between new-onset heart failure with nonsteroidal anti-inflammatory drugs (NSAIDs) is now clear, in patients on diuretic therapy the use of these agents has clearly been shown to worsen the risk of heart failure hospitalization. This may be related to alterations in renal function or inhibition of prostaglandin synthesis and resulting sodium and water retention (133,134). Finally, the association between use of thiazolidinediones and decompensation of heart failure requiring hospitalization has been challenged based on the potential benefit of insulin sensitization in the heart failure patient. There is currently an ongoing trial assessing the careful use of these agents in patients with heart failure, and additional data are needed to clarify the role of these drugs (135).

Genetics and Heart Failure Risk

Genetic factors and their relationship with heart failure are described in various chapters in this book and a detailed discussion of genetic basis of heart failure is beyond the scope of this chapter. However, several polymorphisms have been associated with a higher risk of development of heart failure. Two such genetic polymorphisms have been evaluated as potential candidates for development of heart failure. This first is related to deletion of four amino acids in positions 322 to 325 of the gene coding for a2C-adrenergic receptors (a2CDel322–325) in the cardiac sympathetic nerve endings, and the other occurs due to the presence of arginine in position 389 of the gene coding for b1-adrenergic receptors (b1Arg389) on the myocytes (136). African-Americans who were homozygous for a2Cdel322–325 alone had a fivefold increased risk of heart failure. Homozygosity for b1Arg389 alone was not associated with an excess heart failure risk, while those who were homozygous for a2Cdel322–325 and b1Arg389 had a 10-fold increased risk for heart failure. Several other genetic markers have been described as being associated with either risk of heart failure [e.g., overexpression of protein kinase C-alpha (PKC-α)] or genetic polymorphisms that have been linked with heart failure risk factors such as hypertension and obesity (137). Similarly, angiotensin-converting enzyme (ACE) and angiotensin II type 1 receptor gene polymorphisms have been evaluated as being associated with risk for left ventricular remodeling (138).

Risk Factors for Heart Failure Progression and Outcomes

As shown in Table 16-2, many risk factors have been associated with outcomes in heart failure patients. It is difficult

TABLE 16-2
RISK FACTORS ASSOCIATED WITH HEART FAILURE PROGRESSION AND OUTCOMES

Clinical
Etiology
Age
Gender
Symptom duration
NYHA class
Weight
Heart rate
Mean arterial pressure
S_3 gallop
Jugular venous pressure
Cardiothoracic ratio
Renal function
Serum sodium
Troponin T
History of diabetes
Anemia
Echocardiographic
Ejection fraction
Exercise ejection fraction
Ventricular dimensions
Sphericity index
Prolonged isovolumic relaxation
Restrictive mitral filling
Changes in E/A ratio
Mitral regurgitation
Contractile reserve
Left ventricular mass
Exercise Tolerance
Exercise duration
Peak O_2 consumption
VE/VCO_2
Anaerobic threshold 6-minute walk test
Hemodynamics
Cardiac index
Pulmonary artery pressure
Pulmonary wedge pressure
Pulmonary vascular resistance
Stroke work index
Right atrial pressure
A–V oxygen difference
Coronary sinus O_2 content
Electrophysiological
Conduction delay
Atrial arrhythmia
Family history of sudden death
Presence of late potentials
QT dispersion
T wave alternans
Neurohormonal
Renin-angiotensin system
Angiotensin II
Aldosterone
Plasma renin activity
Sympathetic nervous system
Norepinephrine
Epinephrine
Heart rate variability
Norepinephrine spillover
Natriuretic factors
Atrial natriuretic peptide

(Continued)

TABLE 16-2
RISK FACTORS ASSOCIATED WITH HEART FAILURE PROGRESSION AND OUTCOMES

B-type natriuretic peptide
N-terminal-pro-ANP
Cytokines and others
TNF-α
Interleukin-6
Endothelin
ICAM-1 and Neuropeptide Y
Arginine vasopressin

to truly ascertain their relative value, as different studies have focused on either individual risk factors or a random combination of these, but there is no study that has compared all of them simultaneously.

Clinical

Etiology

Pathophysiologically, because ischemic and nonischemic cardiomyopathies are distinctly different entities it is therefore reasonable to expect varying outcomes for patients with these two broad disease process categories. Several studies have suggested a worse prognosis with ischemic cardiomyopathy, especially with respect to ventricular arrhythmias and sudden cardiac death (139–142). However, data are conflicting in this respect and other studies have either not found any significant differences in outcomes between patients with ischemic or non-ischemic cardiomyopathy, or have found a better survival among those with ischemic cardiomyopathy (143,144). Whether these differences are related to varying patient characteristics, other comorbidities, medical therapy, or other as-yet undefined characteristics is not known. However, this debate remains important because differences in outcomes to medical therapy have been seen in analyses of several clinical trials (e.g., with amlodipine in the Prospective Randomized Amlodipine Survival Evaluation [PRAISE] trial and with bisoprolol in the Cardiac Insufficiency Bisoprolol Study [CIBIS] trial, where substantial outcomes benefits were seen with nonischemic but not ischemic cardiomyopathy) (145–146). Similarly, some, but not all, studies have shown a greater improvement in ejection fraction with beta-blocker therapy among patients with nonischemic cardiomyopathy (147–149). Overall, this area remains controversial.

Age

Similar to the risk of developing heart failure, advancing age also is a strong risk factor for adverse outcomes and mortality among heart failure patients. In the Framingham Heart Study, there was a 27% increase in risk for mortality for men and a 61% increase for women with heart failure per decade increment in age (150). Data from the Centers for Disease Control and Prevention and from the National Health and Nutrition Examination Survey (NHANES) survey show similar results (151,152).

Gender

Both the Framingham and the NHANES studies have shown that women with heart failure survive longer than men (150,151).

Diabetes

Gender difference is noted in the Framingham Heart Study with respect to diabetes and heart failure mortality, with diabetes increasing the risk in women but not in men (hazard ratio 1.70; CI 1.21–2.38) (150). In the Studies of Left Ventricular Dysfunction (SOLVD) trial, diabetes was a risk factor for adverse outcomes among heart failure patients in both the placebo and the ACE inhibitor-treated groups (153).

Race

Significant differences in outcomes among various clinical trials between white and African-American patients have been demonstrated. This is primarily in relation to the medical therapy response. In the Beta-Blocker Evaluation of Survival Trial (BEST), where prospective stratification based on race was performed to balance the two groups, there was a higher mortality among African-American but not white patients stratified to bucindolol (154). Similar racial differences in outcomes have been observed in the Vasodilator-Heart Failure (V-HeFT) and SOLVD trials, suggesting a potential difference in response to neurohormonal antagonistism between the races (155,156). However, chance finding of a subgroup analysis cannot be ruled out. In addition, part of these differences may be explained on the basis of differences in heart failure etiology, socioeconomic status and access to health care, or polymorphisms in the adrenergic or the RAAS seen between the two races (157,158).

Physical Examination

As shown in Figure 16-4, Drazner et al., using the SOLVD data, showed that after adjusting for the several other risk factors and treatment assignment in the trial, presence of an S_3 gallop or elevated jugular venous pressure was independently predictive of a higher risk for heart failure hospitalization, death, or pump failure-related death among patients with heart failure (159).

Systolic Blood Pressure

Systolic blood pressure has been suggested to have prognostic information with respect to heart failure outcomes (160,161). One study demonstrated that for patients on beta-blockers for heart failure due to dilated cardiomyopathy, systolic pressure tended to be the best baseline predictor of improvement in left ventricular function with therapy (162). Whether systolic blood pressure is a colinear surrogate of better ejection fraction or whether it has independent prognostic value is debatable.

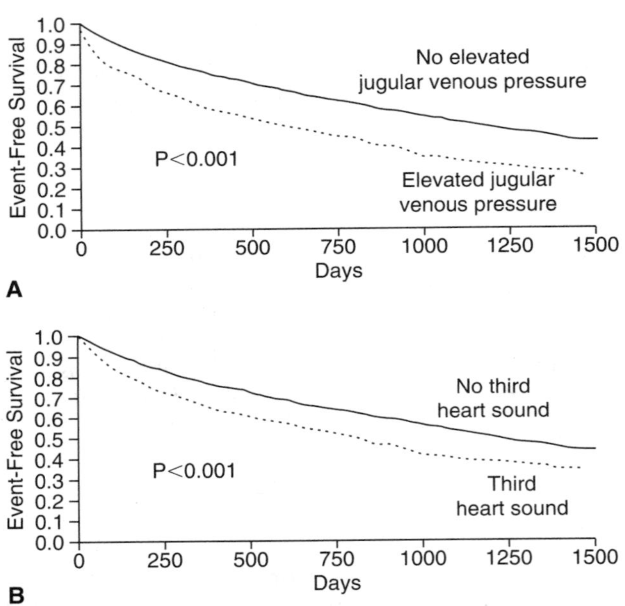

Figure 16-4 Kaplan-Meier analysis of event-free survival according to the presence or absence of elevated jugular venous pressure **(A)** and a third heart sound **(B)**. The endpoint was a composite of death or hospitalization for heart failure. In **A**, the 280 patients with elevated jugular venous pressure were significantly more likely than the 2,199 patients without elevated jugular venous pressure to reach the composite endpoint (p >0.001 by the log-rank test). In **B**, the 597 patients with a third heart sound were significantly more likely than the 1,882 patients without a third heart sound to reach the composite endpoint (p >0.001 by the log-rank test). (Reprinted from Drazner MH, Rame JE, Stevenson LW, et al. Prognostic importance of elevated jugular venous pressure and a third heart sound in patients with heart failure. *N Engl J Med.* 2001;345:574–581, with permission from the Massachusetts Medical Society.)

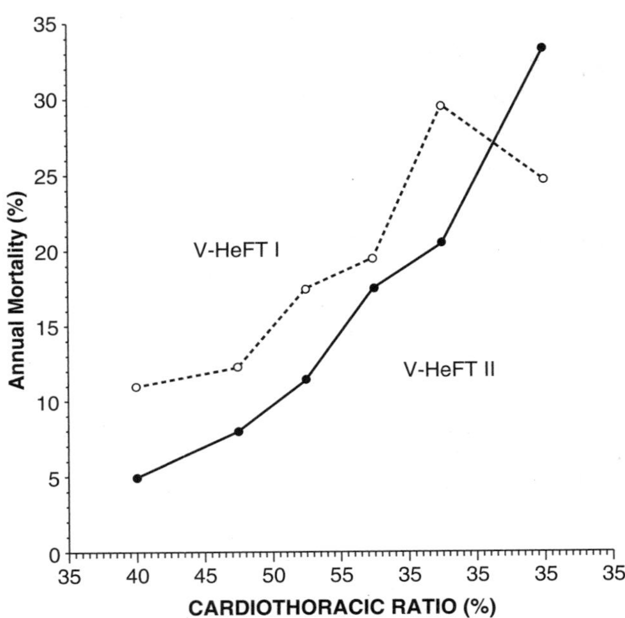

Figure 16-5 Graph showing annual mortality rates for cardiothoracic ratio for 5% cutoff points. (Reprinted from Cohn JN, Johnson GR, Shabetai R, et al., for the V-HeFT VA Cooperative Studies Group. Ejection fraction, peak exercise oxygen consumption, cardiothoracic ratio, ventricular arrhythmias, and plasma norepinephrine as determinants of prognosis in heart failure. *Circulation.* 1993;87:VI5–VI16, with permission.)

Cardiothoracic Ratio

Enlarged cardiothoracic ratio on chest X-ray has been shown to predict worse prognosis in patients with heart failure independent of left ventricular ejection fraction or volumes (143). Figure 16-5 shows the annual mortality rate in relation to cardiothoracic ratio and shows almost a linear association between the two in both the V-HeFT I and II studies. It is intriguing why an enlarged cardiothoracic ratio has independent predictive value beyond ejection fraction; it may be related to either biventricular or atrial enlargement, leading to a widening ratio on x-ray and, hence, a worse prognosis.

Anemia and Renal Function

Recently, there has been significant interest in the role of anemia and renal function in progression of heart failure and their impact on prognosis. Both renal insufficiency and anemia are common among patients with heart failure, although the true prevalence is difficult to estimate due to the varying definitions used to define them, especially anemia. Different studies have suggested a prevalence of anemia ranging from 10% to 60% in the outpatient population (163–167). Multiple post hoc analyses of large clinical trial data and other studies have now confirmed worse prognosis for heart failure patients with anemia and/or renal insufficiency, in conjunction and also independent of each other (168–172). Worsening prognosis with anemia appears to be multifactorial in pathogenesis and is independent of renal function (173). Several small studies have now shown that treatment of anemia in heart failure patients leads to improved symptoms and exercise tolerance, and reduced hospitalization rate and diuretic requirement (174–177). Larger studies assessing treatment of anemia and its impact on heart failure outcomes are currently under way. Although no specific renal insufficiency in heart failure treatments are on the horizon, newer diuretic agents are being developed that are not associated with worsening glomerular filtration rate (e.g., adenosine antagonist). Such drugs are currently under investigation.

Echocardiographic Parameter

One of the strongest and most reproducible risk factors for adverse outcomes among patients with heart failure is left ventricular ejection fraction (143,161). As shown in Figure 16-6, studying the impact of ejection fraction on mortality in the Digitalis Investigator Group trial, Curtis et al. found that among heart failure patients in sinus rhythm, higher left ventricular ejection fractions were associated with a linear decrease in mortality up to an ejection fraction of 45%. However, increases above 45% were not associated with further reductions in mortality (178). This relationship persisted after controlling for other risk factors including age, heart failure etiology, symptom severity, cardiothoracic ratio, gender, diabetes, blood pressure, renal function blood pressure, and medication use. Deaths from worsen-

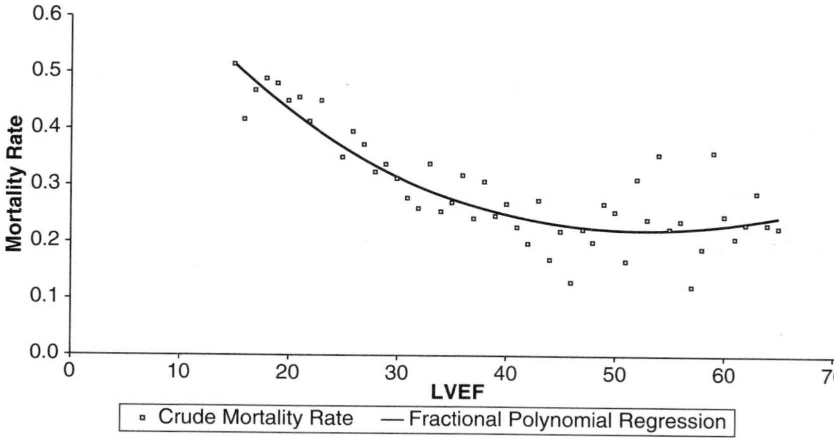

Figure 16-6 Linear trend for left ventricular ejection fraction (LVEF) as a continuous variable and unadjusted all-cause mortality. Each point represents the mortality rate associated with each LVEF point. (Reprinted from Curtis JP, Sokol SI, Wang Y, et al. The association of left ventricular ejection fraction, mortality, and cause of death in stable outpatients with heart failure. *J Am Coll Cardiol.* 2003;42:736–742, with permission from the American College of Cardiology Foundation.)

ing heart failure and due to arrhythmias were more common in patients with lower ejection fraction.

Although ejection fraction is, overall, a strong predictor of outcomes, as patients' symptoms advance it becomes a less-accurate predictor of outcomes, especially among patients with advanced New York Heart Association Class III–IV symptoms (179,180). For example, in the Cooperative North Scandinavian Enalapril Survival Study (CONSENSUS) trial, patients on ACE inhibitor therapy exhibited no correlation between mortality and ejection fraction, within the relatively narrow range of ejection fraction that was present in patients who were included in the study (181). Similarly, the degree to which ejection fraction changes over time, with or without treatment, may also predict the risk for future outcomes. However, this must be taken with caution. For example, both the V-HeFT I and V-HeFT II trials showed that patients who improved their ejection fractions had better outcomes than those who did not. However, in the V-HeFT II trial, patients on vasodilator combination improved their ejection more than those on ACE inhibitor therapy, but outcomes were better for patients on ACE inhibitors (182,183). Thus, although the general principle applies, there seems to be a significant treatment interaction in terms of ejection fraction and mortality risk.

The physiological idea behind improved ejection fraction and better outcomes is related to the presumptions that patients who improve their ejection fraction have potentially viable but dysfunctional myocardium as compared to those patients who do not, and that the latter have irreversible myocyte damage and replacement with scar tissue. This concept is also suggested by certain data that correlate outcomes to dobutamine-induced improvement of ejection fraction as assessed by echocardiogram (184,185).

Left ventricular volumes are also considered risk factors because they represent the markers for the pathological remodeling of the left ventricle and, in turn, worsening failure (186). Irrespective of the preload and afterload, greater left ventricular volumes correlate with more extensive remodeling and greater impairment in ejection fraction. Both the left ventricular end-diastolic volume and end-systolic volume have been shown to be risk factors for adverse outcomes in univariate analysis; data from multivariate analysis have been inconsistent (161,187). This may be because ejection fraction gives similar information and is a more potent predictor of outcomes.

Right ventricular function is very sensitive to changes in pulmonary pressures, which, in turn, correlate with worsening left ventricular function (188). Thus, right ventricular failure (unless primary) represents chronic, more severe disease; not surprisingly, several investigators have noted that right ventricular ejection fraction, both at rest and with exercise, has significant prognostic value and appears to be a strong risk factor for adverse outcomes (189,190).

Parameter of diastolic function in heart failure patients as assessed by Doppler echocardiography also carries prognostic value. These include restrictive mitral filling pattern, and a high E wave to A wave (E/A) ratio has been shown to have some predictive value (191,192). Similarly, left ventricular mass correlates well with ventricular remodeling and was a strong predictor of death or hospitalization in the SOLVD study (187).

Exercise Capacity

Worsening exercise tolerance in terms of either fatigue or shortness of breath is the most common manifestation of heart failure. Initially felt to be due to primarily cardiac dysfunction, at this point it is well-documented that the etiology for exercise tolerance among heart failure patients is multifactorial, including cardiac, pulmonary, and skeletal muscle dysfunction. Metabolic exercise testing and assessment of peak exercise oxygen consumption have been shown to be among the most reliable predictors of outcomes among patients with heart failure (193,194). Also, peak exercise oxygen consumption, unlike ejection fraction, continues to be a good predictor of outcomes among patients with advanced symptoms and, hence, it remains one of the key criteria for listing of patients for cardiac transplantation (195,196).

Several recent reports have suggested that as prognosis for patients with heart failure has improved with newer therapies and devices, the outcomes for patients with similar peak VO_2 levels have also improved over time (11–13). This is primarily because several of these therapies that improve outcomes do not impact peak VO_2 (e.g., beta-blockers and defibrillators). For example, reviewing data on over 2,000 heart failure patients who underwent peak exercise oxygen consumption assessment at the Cleveland Clinic Foundation, O'Neill et al. showed that although peak exercise oxygen consumption continues to be a predictor of outcomes among heart failure patients, the relative prognosis of patients taking beta-blockers is significantly better as compared to those who are not taking them, despite similar exercise capacity (Fig. 16-7). A decrease of 1 mL/minute/kg in peak exercise oxygen consumption resulted in an increased risk of death (hazard ratio 1.13; 95% CI 1.09–1.17) among patients not receiving beta-blockers; in patients receiving beta-blockers, the hazard ratio was 1.27 with a 95% CI of 1.18–1.36. The results were similar when combined endpoint of death or transplantation was considered. This relationship was stable until peak exercise oxygen consumptions values went to less than 10 mL/minute/kg, where the survival rates were equally poor irrespective of beta-blocker use. Nevertheless, peak exercise oxygen consumption remains one of the most important predictors for stratifying risk among heart failure patients.

Other exercise parameters that have been correlated with adverse outcomes risk include exercise duration, anaerobic threshold, and the ratio of ventilation to CO_2 production (VE/VCO_2) (197,198). Similarly, other submaximal exercise protocols such as the 6-minute walk test

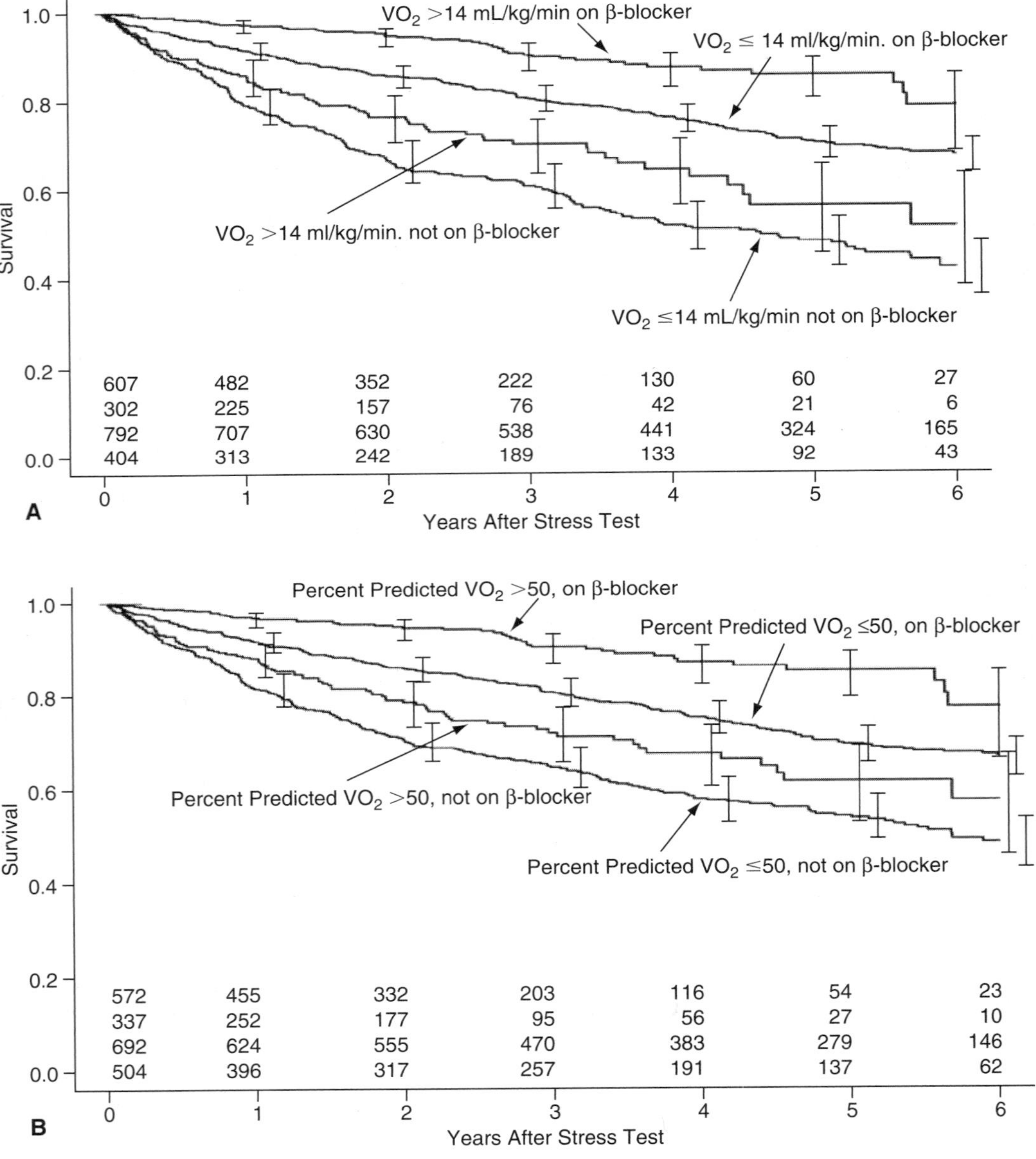

Figure 16-7 Survival according to peak oxygen uptake **(A)** or percent-predicted peak oxygen uptake **(B)** and beta-blocker use. Kaplan-Meier plot with Greenwood confidence intervals. Cardiac transplantation was considered as a time-dependent covariate. (Reprinted from O'Neill JO, Young JB, Pothier CE, et al. Peak oxygen consumption as a predictor of death in patients with heart failure receiving β-blockers. *Circulation.* 2005;111:2313–2318, with permission.)

have also been used to assess prognosis, but none of these tests provides the same degree of information and reliability as peak exercise oxygen consumption (198).

The most subjective assessment of functional capacity in patients with heart failure is New York Heart Association functional class. Despite its subjectivity, it has been remarkably reproducible over the years with respect to assessing the risk for patients with heart failure (144,161,199). However, within a functional class there can be large variations in outcomes; part of that may be because subjective functional class can be changed in the short term with diuretics without changing the underlying disease process.

Hemodynamic Characteristics

Multiple hemodynamic characteristics, in either univariate or multivariate analysis in different studies, have been found to be predictive of adverse outcomes among patients with heart failure, including pulmonary artery pressures, right atrial pressure, pulmonary capillary wedge pressure, and cardiac index (161,200,201). However, the most reliable and consistent risk factor for adverse outcomes in multiple multivariate-adjusted analyses has been elevated pulmonary capillary wedge pressure. Although coronary sinus oxygen content has been linked to outcomes, this may be a surrogate for cardiac index (202). It may also be related to altered myocardial demand or efficiency. The most accurate assessment of cardiac reserve may be the actual measurement of cardiac output response to dynamic exercise. For example, in one study, exercise cardiac output response was found to be the strongest predictor of outcomes after adjusting for left ventricular ejection fraction, peak exercise oxygen consumption, and pulmonary capillary wedge pressure (203). However, this test is expensive and cumbersome, with significant risks to the patient, and therefore does not have wide applicability.

Electrophysiological Characteristics

Because defining sudden cardiac death in patients has been difficult, different studies have quoted varying figures for the proportion of patients with heart failure who die of sudden cardiac death (204). Both the U.S. Carvedilol Heart Failure Trials and the Metoprolol CR/XL Randomized Intervention Trial in Heart Failure (MERIT-HF) reparted approximately half the patients' deaths as sudden cardiac death, the vast majority of which were ventricular arrhythmic in nature (149,205). Interestingly, the proportional risk of sudden cardiac death is higher in patients with less-advanced symptoms (205). Thus, there has been a significant interest in assessing electrophysiological risk factors to predict the risk for sudden cardiac death.

Symptomatic ventricular arrhythmias as assessed by the presence of presyncope, syncope, or resuscitated sudden death (not related to acute ischemia) are related to the risk of sudden death (143,206). Although data are less convincing for asymptomatic, nonsustained ventricular tachycardia, in the VHeFT II and the PROMISE trials the presence of ventricular couplets or tachycardia on Holter monitoring was a predictor of sudden death risk (207–208).

Other electrophysiological markers that predict a higher risk of mortality among patients with heart failure include interventricular conduction defect and the presence of atrial fibrillation/flutter (161,201). Prolonged corrected QT interval (QTc) dispersion represents heterogenous myocardial repolarization and predicts a higher risk among both ischemic and nonischemic cardiomyopathy patients (more so in the ischemic patients) (209,210). Finally, presence of T wave alternans predicts arrhythmia-free survival and identifies high risk for malignant ventricular arrhythmias (211).

Neurohormonal Characteristics

As shown in Figure 16-8, assessment of sympathetic nervous system activity as assessed by noreinephrine level correlated strongly with mortality in both univariate and multivariate analysis in several clinical trials (181,183,212,213). A more direct measure of cardiac adrenergic activity as assessed by cardiac norepinephrine spillover is more predictive of cardiac risk as compared to serum norepinephrine levels; however, this is not a universally available tool (214). Another indirect measure of sympathetic activity in heart failure is heart rate variability, which is also correlated with adverse mortality risk among heart failure patients (215–217).

Similar to the sympathetic nervous system are activation of the RAAS as assessed by plasma renin activity, angiotensin II and aldosterone levels, and, indirectly, serum sodium concentration (62–64,143,181,218–221). Serum norepinephrine levels seem to be more predictive of outcomes, however, as compared to RAAS markers (143).

There is considerable interest in the natriuretic peptides (ANP and BNP) with respect to heart failure prognosis and risk. The role of these peptides is discussed in detail in another chapter. Similar to the development risk, cytokines TNF-α (or the soluble receptor) and IL-6 are elevated in heart failure and play a significant role in its progression (222–225). Another neurohormone that correlates well with functional class in heart failure patients is left ventricular remodeling, and its outcome is endothelin

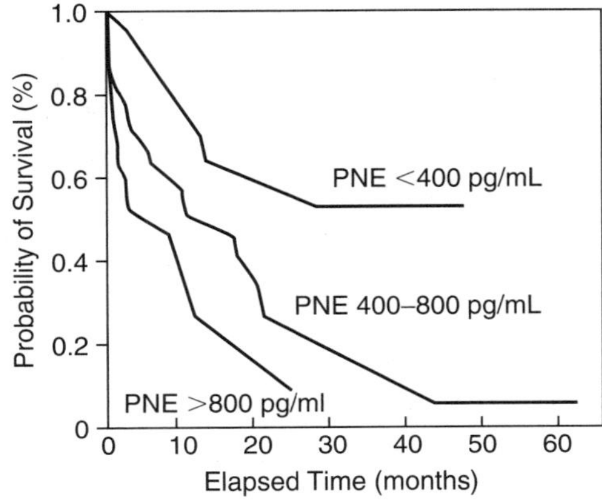

Figure 16-8 Predictive effect of plasma norepinephrine (PNE) levels on the survival of patients with chronic heart failure. (Reprinted from Cohn JN, Levine TB, Olivari MT, et al. Plasma norepinephrine as a guide to prognosis in patients with chronic congestive heart failure. *N Engl J Med.* 1984;311:819–823, with permission from the Massachusetts Medical Society.)

(226–228). Finally, there are data pertaining to other factors suggested to have prognostic value in heart failure patients (e.g., intercellular adhesion molecule-1, plasma neuropeptide Y, arginine vasopressin, and plasma levels of troponin T) (229). More data are needed to identify their role more clearly.

Prognosis Determination in Heart Failure

The preceding discussion briefly lists a variety of risk factors that have been correlated with either development or progression of heart failure, or both. Although a general knowledge of these is helpful in qualitatively assessing heart failure risk on a population basis, quantitative assessment of individual patient risk is not possible with this approach. Quantitative assessment of an individual patient's risks for mortality is, however, very important for many reasons, the first and foremost being the patient's ability to make end-of-life personal decisions. Beyond that, accurate prediction of prognosis is also important to assess the need for advanced therapies that are costly and potentially risky (e.g., cardiac transplantation and left ventricular-assist device placement).

Cardiac transplantation poses special problems due to the significant mismatch between availability of donor organs and the need for them (230,231). Unlike off-the-shelf technology where costs are the major concern, with cardiac transplantation a poor decision can affect not one but two lives—the patient who undergoes transplantation who does not do well (or did not need the transplant in the first place) and the one who, in turn, could have received the organ and enjoyed additional survival. For example, robust research efforts have been dedicated to assess the risk for sudden cardiac death in patients with heart failure in order to define the ideal population for defibrillator implantation. Electrophysiological testing, Holter monitor findings, use of signal-averaged electrocardiograms, assessment of T wave alternans, and so forth have all been reported to modestly help in defining such a population, but all these are far from perfect (232–234). Therefore, the current standard of care is to not try to further narrowly define the risk but, rather, to implant these devices in a broader group of high-risk patients (i.e., those with an ejection fraction of <36%). This is only possible when considering such off-the-shelf therapies, but this nonspecific approach is impractical when deciding upon organ donation for cardiac transplantation.

The primary objective of heart transplantation is to improve survival and functional capacity. Consequently, patients are listed for transplantation only when it is presumed that they will live longer and function better after transplantation than they would with medical therapy. A variety of criteria have been developed in an attempt to identify such patients. The most widely utilized criteria are based on peak exercise oxygen consumption. Specifically, peak exercise oxygen consumption of less than 14 mL/minute/kg is thought to identify patients who will have a survival benefit with heart transplantation (235–238). This was primarily based on the study by Mancini et al. at the University of Pennsylvania, who noted that patients with a peak exercise oxygen consumption less than 14 mL/minute/kg had a 1-year survival rate that was less than that expected post-transplant (239).

Although subjective symptoms of exercise tolerance, such as assessment of New York Heart Association class symptoms, or less-objective measures, such as the 6-minute walk test, correlate well with prognosis, peak exercise oxygen consumption offers several advantages over these measures. Primarily, exercise tolerance can be reduced due to multiple reasons beyond cardiac limitations (e.g., deconditioning or pulmonary problems). Peak exercise oxygen consumption provides objective evidence as to the cardiac reserve at the time of maximum exercise and thus correlates more reproducibly with prognosis. The impact of medical therapy on outcomes in association with peak exercise oxygen consumption has been discussed earlier. Although no official guidelines have since been published, it is likely that in the near future, the threshold for transplant listing may change from a peak exercise oxygen consumption of <14 mL/minute/kg to more stringent criteria, perhaps 10 mL/minute/kg.

To further improve upon the prognosis determination for the purpose of transplant listing, Chomsky et al. at Vanderbilt University assessed the importance of actually measuring exercise hemodynamics directly in these patients (203). They reported that cardiac output response to exercise further refines the risk assessment among heart failure patients. The normal cardiac output response was derived from data previously reported by Higginbotham et al. (240). In their analysis, within the group of patients with a reduced cardiac output response to exercise, two subgroups with significantly different prognoses could be defined on the basis of peak exercise oxygen consumption (Fig. 16-9). In patients with a peak exercise oxygen consumption of >10 mL/minute/kg, 1-year survival rate was 81%, compared to patients with a peak exercise oxygen consumption of ≤10 mL/min/kg who had a 1-year survival rate of only 38% (p <0.0009). In patients with a normal cardiac output response to exercise, there was no significant difference in the survival of patients based on peak exercise oxygen consumption, although the relatively few patients with a peak exercise oxygen consumption of ≤10 mL/minute/kg (n = 15) tended to have a lower survival. These data would suggest that in the presence of a preserved cardiac output response to exercise, even patients who have a reduced peak exercise oxygen consumption can be safely managed medically with periodic reassessment. Although this is a very attractive risk stratification scheme that seems to give information beyond that of peak exercise oxygen consumption, this approach is unfortunately more expensive, cumbersome, and risky for the patient, and is not feasible to do at most centers except in specialized laboratories.

The most practical approach to risk stratification beyond the information gained by peak exercise oxygen consumption alone was adapted by Aaronson et al., who combined the information obtained by several predictors of risk in heart failure (241). Creating a regression analysis using parameter estimates from seven different variables, they developed and validated a model named the Heart Failure Survival Score. The seven risk factors selected were related to several different aspects of heart failure progression and included heart rate (sympathetic activation), serum sodium concentration (RAAS activation), etiology (ischemia), QRS duration (risk of sudden cardiac death), ejection fraction (degree of remodeling), peak exercise oxygen consumption (exercise capacity), and blood pressure (hemodynamics). The range of scores

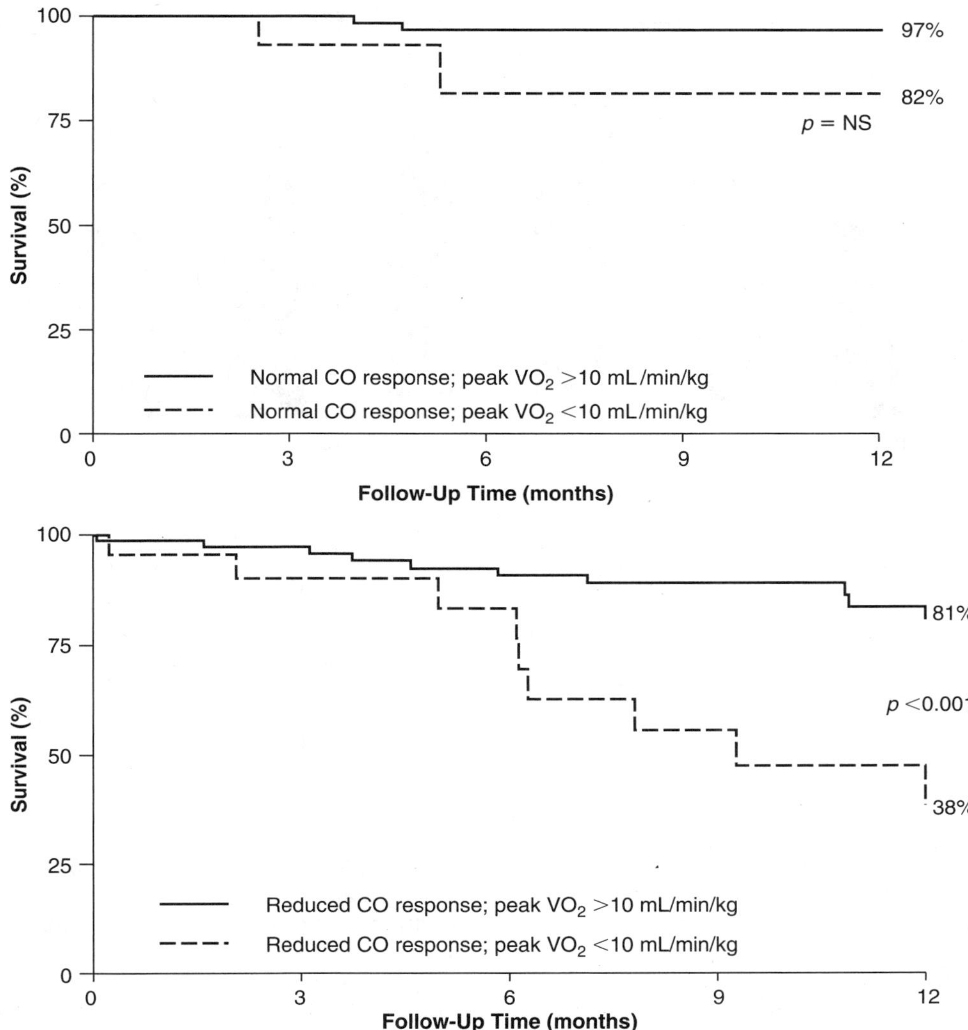

Figure 16-9 Survival curves for patients grouped both by peak VO_2 and cardiac output (CO) response. **Top**, normal CO response to exercise. **Bottom**, reduced CO response to exercise. (Reprinted from Chomsky DB, Lang CC, Rayos GH, et al. Hemodynamic exercise testing. A valuable tool in the selection of cardiac transplantation candidates. *Circulation.* 1996,94:3176–3183, with permission.)

was then divided into three groups, which predicted intermediate-term low, medium, and high risk of mortality.

The utility of the Heart Failure Survival Score has been recently challenged. Assessing the patients in the pre-beta-blocker and beta-blocker era of heart failure therapy, Butler et al. showed a significant improvement in outcomes among patients with a high-risk Heart Failure Survival Score in the current era, as shown in Figure 16-10 (11). Although the debate continues as to whether the quantitative information from the Heart Failure Survival Score is valid in the current era of therapy as compared to when these models were derived, it appears to continue to give valuable information regarding risk assessment for patients with advanced heart failure (242). However, since the development of the Heart Failure Survival Score, several other important risk factors for heart failure progression have been highlighted, most notably renal function and anemia (168–172,243–245). Similarly, other serologic tests such as BNP levels are now routinely used, which give prognostic information (71). Thus, with advances in medical therapy for heart failure, and with these newly described risk factors, the time seems ripe for updating the Heart Failure Survival Score.

One of the major problems with assessing prognosis and transplant eligibility in these studies is the fact that effect of treatment on modifying the outcomes was not taken into consideration. As discussed earlier in this chapter, treatment may significantly modify the quantitative relationship between a risk predictor and an outcome. To assess the impact of contemporary medical therapy including devices and their interaction with traditional risk factors in assessing heart failure prognosis, Levy et al have

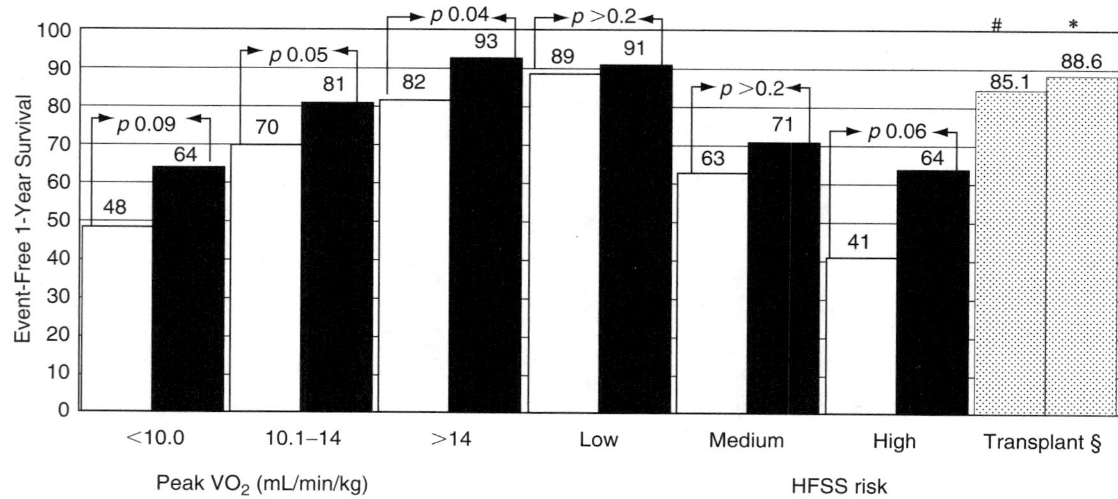

Figure 16-10 Improvement in 1-year event-free survival was noted for patients in the current era of heart failure management for all peak exercise oxygen consumption (VO_2) groups. Patients with a high-risk Heart Failure Survival Score (HFSS) showed the most improvement in survival. Survival for the intermediate-risk peak VO_2 group was comparable to that after transplantation. Open bars, ~past era; solid bars, ~current era; *, Vanderbilt Heart Failure Program; §, 1-year posttransplant survival; #, United Network for Organ Sharing 1990 to 2000. (Reprinted from Butler J, Khadim G, Paul KM, et al. Selection of patients for cardiac transplantation in the current era of heart failure therapy. *J Am Coll Cardiol.* 2004 43;787–793, with permission from the American College of Cardiology Foundation.)

developed a risk prediction model which incorporates both the established and some newer clinical risk predictors, and drug and devices therapy in 1125 patients (246). These variables include clinical predictors (age, gender, functional class, weight, ejection fraction, blood pressure, and heart failure etiology), laboratory data (hemoglobin, lymphocyte count, uric acid, total cholesterol, and serum sodium concentration), and medical therapy (ACE inhibitors, angiotensin receptor blockers, beta-blockers, statins, allopurinol, aldosterone antagonists, and diuretics, and defibrillator and bi-ventricular pacemaker). Moreover, if the patient is not on optimal medical therapy, the baseline risk estimates can be modified as medical and device therapy is altered. The resulting model (Seattle Heart Failure Model) was then validated on five different large heart failure clinical trials databases on a total of over 9,000 patients. The authors show an excellent correlation between the predicted and actual survival with their model in all of the five validation datasets for 1-, 2-, and 3-year survival. The accuracy of the model was excellent with the receiver operating characteristic curve (ROC curve) comparable to the Framingham coronary heart disease risk model. The Seattle Heart Failure Score is likely to significantly impact on how heart failure patients' prognosis is determined.

There is also a growing interest in short-term heart failure prognosis determination as compared to the previously mentioned strategies that predict risks for mostly intermediate- and long-term outcomes. In this respect, some promising work is being done with the use of impedance cardiography (247). Similarly, there are now attempts to develop a risk model for hospital outcome among patients admitted with decompensated heart failure. Although this has been attempted in the past, now with the help of large, multicenter registry databases it is more feasible to develop such models (248). Fonarrow et al. recently published a simple model based on four admission measures that defines hospitalized patients as low-versus high-risk (249).

REFERENCES

1. Wong O. A critical assessment of the relationship between silicone breast implants and connective tissue diseases. *Reg Toxicol Pharmacol.* 1996; 23:74–85.
2. Brinton LA, Buckley LM, Dvorkina O, et al. Risk of connective tissue disorders among breast implant patients. *Am J Epidemiol.* 2004;160:619–627.
3. Mukherjee D, Nissen SE, Topol EJ. Risk of cardiovascular events associated with selective COX-2 inhibitors. *JAMA.* 2001; 286(8):954–959.
4. Francis GS, Cohn JN, Johnson G, et al. Plasma norepinephrine, plasma renin activity, and congestive heart failure: relations to survival and the effects of therapy in V-HeFt II. *Circulation* 1993;87(suppl VI):VI40–VI48.
5. Cohn JN, Rector TS. Prognosis of congestive heart failure and predictors of mortality. *Am J Cardiol.* 1988;62(2):25A–30A.
6. Swedberg K, Eneroth P, Kjekshus J, et al. Hormones regulating cardiovascular function in patients with severe congestive heart failure and their relation to mortality. *Circulation* 1990;82:1730–1736.
7. Tsutamoto T, Wada A, Maeda K, et al. Attenuation of compensation of endogenous cardiac natriuretic peptide system in chronic heart failure: prognostic role of plasma brain natriuretic peptide concentration in patients with chronic symptomatic left ventricular dysfunction. *Circulation.* 1997;96:509–516.
8. Wang TJ, Larson MG, Levy D, et al. Plasma natriuretic peptide levels and the risk of cardiovascular events and death. *N Engl J Med.* 2004;350:655–663.

9. Tracy RP, Lemaitre RN, Psaty BM, et al. Relationship of C-reactive protein to risk of cardiovascular disease in the elderly. *Arterioscler Thromb Vasc Biol.* 1997;17:1121–1127.
10. Ridker PM, Cushman M, Stampfer MJ, et al. Inflammation, aspirin, and the risk of cardiovascular disease in apparently healthy men. *N Engl J Med.* 1997;336:973–979.
11. Butler J, Khadim G, Paul KM, et al. Selection of patients for cardiac transplantation in the current era of heart failure therapy. *J Am Coll Cardiol.* 2004;43:787–793.
12. Zugck C, Haunstetter A, Kruger C, et al. Impact of beta-blocker treatment on the prognostic value of currently used risk predictors in congestive heart failure. *J Am Coll Cardiol.* 2002;39:1615–1622
13. O'Neill JO, Young JB, Pothier CE, et al. Peak oxygen consumption as a predictor of death in patients with heart failure receiving β-blockers. *Circulation.* 2005;111:2313–2318.
14. Bristow MR, Gilbert EM, Abraham WT, et al. Carvedilol produces dose-related improvements in left ventricular function and survival in subjects with chronic heart failure. MOCHA Investigators. *Circulation.* 1996;94:2807–2816.
15. McKee PA, Castelli WP, McNamara PM, et al. The natural history of congestive heart failure: the Framingham study. *N Engl J Med.* 1971;285:1441–1446.
16. Remes J, Reunanen A, Aromaa A, et al. Incidence of heart failure in eastern Finland: a population-based surveillance study. *Eur Heart J.* 1992;13:588–593.
17. Ho KK, Pinsky JL, Kannel WB, et al. The epidemiology of heart failure: the Framingham Study. *J Am Coll Cardiol.* 1993;22:6A–13A.
18. Kimmelstiel CD, Konstam MA. Heart failure in women. *Cardiology.* 1995;86:304–309.
19. Senni M, Tribouilloy CM, Rodeheffer RJ, et al. Congestive heart failure in the community: a study of all incident cases in Olmsted County, Minnesota, in 1991. *Circulation.* 1998;98:2282–2289
20. Chae CU, Pfeffer MA, Glynn RJ, et al. Increased pulse pressure and risk of heart failure in the elderly. *JAMA.* 1999;281:634–639.
21. Chen YT, Vaccarino V, Williams CS, et al. Risk factors for heart failure in the elderly: a prospective community-based study. *Am J Med.* 1999;106:605–612.
22. Gottdiener JS, Arnold AM, Aurigemma GP, et al. Predictors of heart failure in the elderly: the Cardiovascular Health Study. *J Am Coll Cardiol.* 2000;35:1628–1637.
23. He J, Ogden LG, Bazzano LA, et al. Risk factors for congestive heart failure in US men and women: NHANES I epidemiologic follow-up study. *Arch Intern Med.* 2001;161:996–1002.
24. Hypertension Detection and Follow-up Program Cooperative Group. Educational level and 5-year all-cause mortality in the Hypertension Detection and Follow-up Program. *Hypertension.* 1987;9:641–646.
25. Chaturvedi N, Stephenson JM, Fuller JH. The relationship between socioeconomic status and diabetes control and complications in the EURO DIAB IDDM Complications Study. *Diabetes Care.* 1996;19:423–430.
26. Urbano-Marquez A, Estruch R, Navarro-Lopez F, et al. The effects of alcoholism on skeletal and cardiac muscle. *N Engl J Med.* 1989;320:409–415.
27. Rubin E, Urbano-Marquez A. Alcoholic cardiomyopathy. *Alcohol Clin Exp Res.* 1994;18:111–114.
28. Marmot MG, Elliott P, Shipley MJ, et al. Alcohol and blood pressure: the INTERSALT study. *BMJ.* 1994;308:1263–1267.
29. Gillman MW, Cook NR, Evans DA, et al. Relationship of alcohol intake with blood pressure in young adults. *Hypertension* 1995;25:1106–1110.
30. Lee WK, Regan TJ. Alcoholic cardiomyopathy: is it dose-dependent? *Congest Heart Fail.* 2002;8:303–306.
31. Walsh CR, Larson MG, Evans JC, et al. Alcohol consumption and risk for congestive heart failure in the Framingham Heart Study. *Ann Intern Med.* 2002;136:181–191.
32. Ajani UA, Hennekens CH, Spelsberg A, et al. Alcohol consumption and risk of type 2 diabetes mellitus among US male physicians. *Arch Intern Med.* 2000;160:1025–1030.
33. Gaziano JM, Buring JE, Breslow JL, et al. Moderate alcohol intake, increased levels of high-density lipoprotein and its subfractions, and decreased risk of myocardial infarction. *N Engl J Med.* 1993;329:1829–1834.
34. Camargo CA, Jr., Stampfer MJ, Glynn RJ, et al. Moderate alcohol consumption and risk for angina pectoris or myocardial infarction in US male physicians. *Ann Intern Med.* 1997;126:372–375.
35. Rubin R. Effect of ethanol on platelet function. *Alcohol Clin Exp Res.* 1999;23:1114–1118.
36. Ridker PM, Vaughan DE, Stampfer MJ, et al. Association of moderate alcohol consumption and plasma concentration of endogenous tissue-type plasminogen activator. *JAMA.* 1994;272:929–933.
37. Abramson JL, Williams SA, Krumholz HM, et al. Moderate alcohol consumption and risk of heart failure among older persons. *JAMA.* 2001;285:1971–1977.
38. Wilhelmsen L, Rosengren A, Eriksson H, et al. Heart failure in the general population of men—morbidity, risk factors and prognosis. *J Intern Med.* 2001;249:253–261.
39. Facchini FS, Hollenbeck CB, Jeppesen J, et al. Insulin resistance and cigarette smoking. *Lancet.* 1992;339:1128–1130.
40. Michael PR. Cigarette smoking, endothelial injury and cardiovascular disease. *Int J Exp Pathol.* 2000;81:219–230.
41. Burke A, Fitzgerald GA. Oxidative stress and smoking-induced vascular injury. *Prog Cardiovasc Dis.* 2003;46:79–90.
42. Gvozdjakova A, Kucharska J, Gvozdjak J. Effect of smoking on the oxidative processes of cardiomyocytes. *Cardiology.* 1992;81:81–84.
43. He J, Ogden LG, Bazzano LA, et al. Dietary sodium intake and incidence of congestive heart failure in overweight US men and women: first National Health and Nutrition Examination Survey epidemiologic follow-up study. *Arch Intern Med.* 2002;162: 1619–1624.
44. Sugimoto K, Fujimura A, Takasaki I, et al. Effects of renin-angiotensin system blockade and dietary salt intake on left ventricular hypertrophy in Dahl salt-sensitive rats. *Hypertens Res.* 1998;21:163–168.
45. Kupari M, Koskinen P, Virolainen J. Correlates of left ventricular mass in a population. Focus on lifestyle and salt intake. *Circulation.* 1994;89:1041–1050.
46. Schmieder RE, Messerli FH, Garavaglia GE, et al. Dietary salt intake. A determinant of cardiac involvement in essential hypertension. *Circulation.* 1988;78:951–956.
47. Langenfeld MR, Schobel H, Veelken R, et al. Impact of dietary sodium intake on left ventricular diastolic filling in early essential hypertension. *Eur Heart J.* 1998;19:951–958.
48. Karch SB, Billingham ME. The pathology and etiology of cocaine-induced heart disease. *Arch Pathology Lab Med.* 1988;112:225–230.
49. Goldenberg SP, Zeldis SM. Fatal acute congestive heart failure in a patient with idiopathic hemochromatosis and cocaine use. *Chest.* 1987;92:374–375.
50. O'Keefe DD, Grantham RN, Beierholm EA, et al. Cocaine and the contractile response to catecholamines in right ventricular failure. *Am J Physiol.* 1977;233:H399–H403.
51. Gerstein HC, Mann JF, Yi Q, et al. Albuminuria and risk of cardiovascular events, death and heart failure in diabetic and non-diabetic individuals. *JAMA.* 2001;286:421–426.
52. Agrawal B, Berger A, Wolf K, et al. Microalbuminuria screening by reagent strip predicts cardiovascular risk in hypertension. *J Hypertens.* 1996;14:223–228.
53. Dell'Omo G, Giorgi D, Di Bello V, et al. Blood pressure independent association of microalbuminuria and left ventricular hypertrophy in hypertensive men. *J Intern Med.* 2003;254:76–84.
54. Pickup JC, Mattock MB, Chusney GD, et al. NIDDM as a disease of the innate immune system: association of acute-phase reactants and interleukin-6 with metabolic syndrome X. *Diabetologia.* 1997;40:1286–1292.
55. Vasan RS, Beiser A, D'Agostino RB, et al. Plasma homocysteine and risk for heart failure in adults without prior myocardial infarction. *JAMA.* 2003;289:1251–1257.
56. Loscalzo J. The oxidant stress of hyperhomocystinemia. *J Clin Invest.* 1996;98:5–7.
57. Blacher J, Demuth K, Guerin AP, et al. Association between plasma homocysteine concentrations and cardiac hypertrophy in end-stage renal disease. *J Nephrol.* 1999;12:248–255.
58. Symons JD, Mullick AE, Ensunsa JL, et al. Hyperhomocysteinemia evoked by folate depletion: effects on coronary and carotid arterial function. *Arterioscler Thromb Vasc Biol.* 2002;22:772–80.
59. Welch GN, Loscalzo J. Homocysteine and atherothrombosis. *N Engl J Med.* 1998;338:1042–1050.
60. Vasan RS, Sullivan LM, Roubenoff R, et al. Inflammatory markers and risk of heart failure in elderly subjects without prior myocardial infarction: the Framingham Heart Study. *Circulation.* 2003;107:1486–91.

61. Meldrum DR. Tumor necrosis factor in the heart. *Am J Physiol.* 1998;274:R577–R595.
62. Gulick T, Chung MK, Pieper SJ, et al. Interleukin 1 and tumor necrosis factor inhibit cardiac myocyte beta-adrenergic responsiveness. *Proc Natl Acad Sci USA.* 1989;86:6753–6757.
63. Yokoyama T, Vaca L, Rossen RD, et al. Cellular basis for the negative inotropic effects of tumor necrosis factor-alpha in the adult mammalian heart. *J Clin Invest.* 1993;92:2303–2312.
64. Levine B, Kalman J, Mayer L, et al. Elevated circulating levels of tumor necrosis factor in severe chronic heart failure. *N Engl J Med.* 1990;323:236–241.
65. Baumgarten G, Knuefermann P, Mann DL. Cytokines as emerging targets in the treatment of heart failure. *Trends Cardiovasc Med.* 2000;10:216–223.
66. Hirota H, Yoshida K, Kishimoto T, et al. Continuous activation of gp130, a signaltransducing receptor component for interleukin 6-related cytokines, causes myocardial hypertrophy in mice. *Proc Natl Acad Sci USA.* 1995;92:4862–4866.
67. Welch S, Plank D, Witt S, et al. Cardiac-specific IGF-1 expression attenuates dilated cardiomyopathy in tropomodulin-overexpressing mice. *Circulation Res.* 2002;90:641–648.
68. Wang L, Ma W, Markovich R, et al. Regulation of cardiomyocyte apoptotic signaling by insulin-like growth factor I. *Circulation.* 1998;83:516–522.
69. Vecchione C, Colella S, Fratta L, et al. Impaired insulin-like growth factor I vasorelaxant effects in hypertension. *Hypertension.* 2001;37:1480–1485.
70. Vasan RS, Sullivan LM, D'Agostino RB, et al. Serum insulin-like growth factor I and risk for heart failure in elderly individuals without a previous myocardial infarction: the Framingham Heart Study. *Ann Intern Med.* 2003;139:642–648.
71. Wang TJ, Larson MG, Levy D, et al. Plasma natriuretic peptide levels and the risk of cardiovascular events and death. *N Engl J Med.* 2004;350:655–663.
72. Levin ER, Gardner DG, Samson WK. Natriuretic peptides. *N Engl J Med.* 1998;339:321–328.
73. Brunner F, Wolkart G. Relaxant effect of C-type natriuretic peptide involves endothelium and nitric oxide-cGMP system in rat coronary microvasculature. *Cardiovasc Res.* 2001;51:577–584.
74. Vasan RS, Larson MG, Benjamin EJ, et al. Left ventricular dilatation and the risk of congestive heart failure in people without myocardial infarction. *N Engl J Med.* 1997;336: 1350–1355.
75. Wang TJ, Evans JC, Benjamin EJ, et al. Natural history of asymptomatic left ventricular systolic dysfunction in the community. *Circulation.* 2003; 108:977–982.
76. Aurigemma GP, Gottdiener JS, Shemanski L, et al. Predictive value of systolic and diastolic function for incident congestive heart failure in the elderly: the cardiovascular health study. *J Am Coll Cardiol.* 2001;37:1042–1048.
77. Cohn JN, Ferrari R, Sharpe N. Cardiac remodeling—concepts and clinical implications: a consensus paper from an international forum on cardiac remodeling. On behalf of an International Forum on Cardiac Remodeling. *J Am Coll Cardiol.* 2000;35:569–582.
78. Levy D, Larson MG, Vasan RS, et al. The progression from hypertension to congestive heart failure. *JAMA.* 1996;275:1557–1562.
79. Vaccarino V, Holford TR, Krumholz HM. Pulse pressure and risk for myocardial infarction and heart failure in the elderly. *J Am Coll Cardiol.* 2000;36:130–138.
80. Haider AW, Larson MG, Franklin SS, et al. Systolic blood pressure, diastolic blood pressure, and pulse pressure as predictors of risk for congestive heart failure in the Framingham Heart Study. *Ann Intern Med.* 2003;138:10–16.
81. Frohlich ED, Apstein C, Chobanian AV, et al. The heart in hypertension. *N Engl J Med.* 1992;327:998–1008.
82. Vasan RS, Levy D. The role of hypertension in the pathogenesis of heart failure. A clinical mechanistic overview. *Arch Intern Med.* 1996;156:1789–1796.
83. Frohlich ED. State of the art lecture. Risk mechanisms in hypertensive heart disease. *Hypertension.* 1999;34:782–789.
84. Psaty BM, Smith NL, Siscovick DS, et al. Health outcomes associated with antihypertensive therapies used as first-line agents. A systematic review and meta-analysis. *JAMA.* 1997;277:739–745.
85. Davis BR, Cutler JA, Furberg CD, et al. Relationship of antihypertensive treatment regimens and change in blood pressure to risk for heart failure in hypertensive patients randomly assigned to doxazosin or chlorthalidone: further analyses from the ALLHAT Trial. *Ann Intern Med.* 2002;137:313–320.
86. Pfeffer MA, Braunwald E. Ventricular remodeling after myocardial infarction. Experimental observations and clinical implications. *Circulation.* 1990;81:1161–1172.
87. Kannel WB, Levy D, Cupples LA. Left ventricular hypertrophy and risk of cardiac failure: insights from the Framingham Study. *J Cardiovasc Pharmacol.* 1987;10(Suppl 6):S135–S140.
88. Marcus ML, Harrison DG, Chilian WM, et al. Alterations in the coronary circulation in hypertrophied ventricles. *Circulation* 1987;75:I19–I25.
89. Kannel WB, Gordon T, Castelli WP, et al. Electrocardiographic left ventricular hypertrophy and risk of coronary heart disease. The Framingham study. *Ann Intern Med.* 1970;72:813–822.
90. Beache GM, Herzka DA, Boxerman JL, et al. Attenuated myocardial vasodilator response in patients with hypertensive hypertrophy revealed by oxygenation-dependent magnetic resonance imaging. *Circulation.* 2001;104:1214–1217.
91. Kenchaiah S, Pfeffer MA. Cardiac remodeling in systemic hypertension. *Med Clin N Am.* 2004;88:115–130.
92. Kannel WB, D'Agostino RB, Silbershatz H, et al. Profile for estimating risk of heart failure. *Arch Intern Med.* 1999;159:1197–1204.
93. Carabello B, Crawford FA, Jr. Valvular heart disease. *N Engl J Med.* 1997;337:32–41.
94. Bonow RO, Carabello B, de Leon AC, et al. Guidelines for the management of patients with valvular heart disease: executive summary. *Circulation.* 1998;98:1949–1984.
95. Kannel WB, Hjortland M, Castelli WP. Role of diabetes in congestive heart failure: the Framingham study. *Am J Cardiol.* 1974;34:29–34.
96. Shindler DM, Kostis JB, Yusuf S, et al. Diabetes mellitus, a predictor of morbidity and mortality in the Studies of Left Ventricular Dysfunction (SOLVD) Trials and Registry. *Am J Cardiol.* 1996;77:1017–1020.
97. Bonow RO, Mitch WE, Nesto RW, et al. Prevention conference VI: diabetes and cardiovascular disease: writing group V: management of cardiovascular-renal complications. *Circulation.* 2002;105:e159–164.
98. Iribarren C, Karter AJ, Go AS, et al. Glycemic control and heart failure among adult patients with diabetes. *Circulation.* 2001; 103:2668–2673.
99. Kenchaiah S, Evans JC, Levy D, et al. Obesity and the risk of heart failure. *N Engl J Med.* 2002;347:305–313.
100. Kannel WB, Ho K, Thom T. Changing epidemiological features of cardiac failure. *Br Heart J.* 1994;72:S3–S9.
101. Schillaci G, Vaudo G, Reboldi G, et al. High-density lipoprotein cholesterol and left ventricular hypertrophy in essential hypertension. *J Hypertens.* 2001;19:2265–2270.
102. Horio T, Miyazato J, Kamide K, et al. Influence of low high-density lipoprotein cholesterol on left ventricular hypertrophy and diastolic function in essential hypertension. *Am J Hypertens.* 2003;16:938–944.
103. Kjekshus J, Pedersen TR, Olsson AG, et al. The effects of simvastatin on the incidence of heart failure in patients with coronary heart disease. *J Card Fail.* 1997;3:249–254.
104. Fried LF, Shlipak MG, Crump C, et al. Renal insufficiency as a predictor of cardiovascular outcomes and mortality in elderly individuals. *J Am Coll Cardiol.* 2003;41:1364–1372.
105. Dries DL, Exner DV, Domanski MJ, et al. The prognostic implications of renal insufficiency in asymptomatic and symptomatic patients with left ventricular systolic dysfunction. *J Am Coll Cardiol.* 2000;35:681–689.
106. Mourad JJ, Girerd X, Boutouyrie P, et al. Increased stiffness of radial artery wall material in end-stage renal disease. *Hypertension.* 1997;30:1425–1430.
107. Hillege HL, Girbes AR, de Kam PJ, et al. Renal function, neurohormonal activation, and survival in patients with chronic heart failure. *Circulation.* 2000;102:203–210.
108. Shlipak MG, Fried LF, Crump C, et al. Elevations of inflammatory and procoagulant biomarkers in elderly persons with renal insufficiency. *Circulation.* 2003;107:87–92.
109. Herbelin A, Urena P, Nguyen AT, et al. Elevated circulating levels of interleukin-6 in patients with chronic renal failure. *Kidney Int.* 1991;39:954–960.

110. Chaudhary BA, Ferguson DS, Speir WA, Jr. Pulmonary edema as a presenting feature of sleep apnea syndrome. *Chest.* 1982;82: 122–124.
111. Fletcher EC, Proctor M, Yu J, et al. Pulmonary edema develops after recurrent obstructive apneas. *Am J Respir Crit Care Med.* 1999;160:1688–1696.
112. Shahar E, Whitney CW, Redline S, et al. Sleep-disordered breathing and cardiovascular disease: cross-sectional results of the Sleep Heart Health Study. *Am J Respir Crit Care Med.* 2001;163:19–25.
113. McEvoy RD. Obstructive sleep apnea and heart failure: two unhappy bedfellows. *Am J Respir Crit Care Med.* 2004; 169: 329–331.
114. Hedner JA, Wilcox I, Laks L, et al. A specific and potent pressor effect of hypoxia in patients with sleep apnea. *Am Rev Respir Dis.* 1992;146:1240–1245.
115. Sajkov D, Wang T, Saunders NA, et al. Continuous positive airway pressure treatment improves pulmonary hemodynamics in patients with obstructive sleep apnea. *Am J Respir Crit Care Med.* 2002;165:152–158.
116. Peppard PE, Young T, Palta M, Skatrud J. Prospective study of the association between sleep-disordered breathing and hypertension. *N Engl J Med.* 2000;342:1378–1384.
117. Kaneko Y, Floras JS, Usui K, et al. Cardiovascular effects of continuous positive airway pressure in patients with heart failure and obstructive sleep apnea. *N Engl J Med.* 2003;348:1233–1241.
118. Mansfield DR, Gollogly NC, Kaye DM, et al. Controlled trial of continuous positive airway pressure in obstructive sleep apnea and heart failure. *Am J Respir Crit Care Med.* 2004;169: 361–366.
119. Kannel WB, Seidman JM, Fercho W, et al. Vital capacity and congestive heart failure. *Circulation.* 1974;49:1160–1166.
120. Marcus EB, Curb JD, MacLean CJ, et al. Pulmonary function as a predictor of coronary heart disease. *Am J Epidemiol.* 1989;129: 97–104.
121. Enright PL, Kronmal RA, Smith VE, et al. Reduced vital capacity in elderly persons with hypertension, coronary heart disease, or left ventricular hypertrophy. *Chest.* 1995;107:28–35.
122. Perlman LV, Ferguson S, Bergum K, et al. Precipitation of congestive heart failure: social and emotional factors. *Ann Intern Med.* 1971;75:1–7.
123. Abramson J, Berger A, Krumholz HM, et al. Depression and risk of heart failure among older persons with isolated systolic hypertension. *Arch Intern Med.* 2001;161:1725–1730.
124. Williams SA, Kasl SV, Heiat A, et al. Depression and risk of heart failure among the elderly: a prospective community-based study. *Psychosom Med.* 2002;64:6–12.
125. Veith RC, Lewis N, Linares OA, et al. Sympathetic nervous system activity in major depression. Basal and desipramine-induced alterations in plasma norepinephrine kinetics. *Arch Gen Psychiatry.* 1994;51:411–422.
126. Rozanski A, Bairey CN, Krantz DS, et al. Mental stress and the induction of silent myocardial ischemia in patients with coronary artery disease. *N Engl J Med.* 1988;318:1005–1012.
127. Pasic J, Levy WC, Sullivan MD. Cytokines in depression and heart failure. *Psychosom Med.* 2003;65:181–193.
128. DiMatteo MR, Lepper HS, Croghan TW. Depression is a risk factor for noncompliance with medical treatment: meta-analysis of the effects of anxiety and depression on patient adherence. *Arch Intern Med.* 2000;160:2101–2107.
129. Lee BH, Goodenday LS, Muswick GJ, et al. Alterations in left ventricular diastolic function with doxorubicin therapy. *J Am Coll Cardiol.* 1987;9:184–188.
130. Nousiainen T, Vanninen E, Jantunen E, et al. Concomitant impairment of left ventricular systolic and diastolic function during doxorubicin therapy: a prospective radionuclide ventriculographic and echocardiographic study. *Leuk Lymphoma.* 2002;43:1807–1811.
131. Swain SM, Whaley FS, Ewer MS. Congestive heart failure in patients treated with doxorubicin: a retrospective analysis of three trials. *Cancer.* 2003;97:2869–2879.
132. Gottlieb SL, Edmiston WA, Jr., Haywood LJ. Late doxorubicin cardiotoxicity. *Chest.* 1980;78:880–882.
133. Heerdink ER, Leufkens HG, Herings RM, et al. NSAIDs associated with increased risk of heart failure in elderly patients on diuretics. *Arch Intern Med.* 1998;158:108–112.
134. Page J, Henry D. Consumption of NSAIDs and the development of congestive heart failure in elderly patients: an under recognized public health problem. *Arch Intern Med.* 2000;160: 777–784.
135. Masoudi FA, Inzucchi SE, Wang Y, et al. Thiazolidinediones, metformin, and outcomes in older patients with diabetes and heart failure. *Circulation.* 2005;111:583–590.
136. Small KM, Wagoner LE, Levin AM, et al. Synergistic polymorphisms of beta 1- and alpha2C-adrenergic receptors and the risk of congestive heart failure. *N Engl J Med.* 2002;347:1135–1142.
137. Braz JC, Gregory K, Pathak A, et al. PKC-alpha regulates cardiac contractility and propensity toward heart failure. *Nat Med.* 2004;10:248–254.
138. Benetos A, Gautier S, Ricard S, et al. Influence of angiotensin-converting enzyme and angiotensin II type 1 receptor gene polymorphisms on aortic stiffness in normotensive and hypertensive patients. *Circulation.* 1996;94:698–703.
139. Likoff MJ, Chandler SL, Kay HR. Clinical determinants of mortality in chronic congestive heart failure secondary to idiopathic dilated or to ischemic cardiomyopathy. *Am J Cardiol.* 1987;59: 634–638.
140. Myerburg RJ, Kessler KM, Bassett AL, Castellanos A. A biological approach to sudden cardiac death: structure, function, and cause. *Am J Cardiol.* 1989;63:1512–1516.
141. Kao W, Costanzo MR. Prognosis determination in patients with advanced heart failure. *J Heart Lung Transp.* 1997;16:S2–S6.
142. Franciosa JA, Wilen M, Ziesche S, et al. Survival in men with severe chronic left ventricular failure due to either coronary heart disease or idiopathic dilated cardiomyopathy. *Am J Cardiol.* 1983;51:831–836.
143. Cohn JN, Johnson GR, Shabetai R, et al., for the V-HeFT VA Cooperative Studies Group. Ejection fraction, peak exercise oxygen consumption, cardiothoracic ratio, ventricular arrhythmias, and plasma norepinephrine as determinants of prognosis in heart failure. *Circulation.* 1993;87:VI5–VI16.
144. Gradman A, Deedwania F, Cody R, et al., for the Captopril-Digoxin Study Group. Predictors of total mortality and sudden death in mild to moderate heart failure. *J Am Coll Cardiol.* 1989;14:564–570.
145. Packer M, O'Connor CM, Ghali JK, et al., for the Prospective Randomized Amlodipine Survival Evaluation Study Group. Effect of amlodipine on morbidity and mortality in severe chronic heart failure. *N Engl J Med.* 1996;335:1107–1114.
146. CIBIS Investigators and Committees. A randomized trial of beta-blockade in heart failure: the Cardiac Insufficiency Bisoprolol Study. *Circulation.* 1994;90:1765–1773.
147. Bristow MR, Gilbert EM, Abraham WT, et al., for the MOCHA Investigators. Carvedilol produces dose-related improvements in left ventricular function and survival in subjects with chronic heart failure. *Circulation.* 1996;94:2807–2816.
148. Woodley SL, Gilbert EM, Anderson JL, et al. b-Blockade with bucindolol in heart failure due to ischemic vs idiopathic dilated cardiomyopathy. *Circulation.* 1991;84:2426–2441.
149. Packer M, Bristow MR, Cohn JN, et al., for the U.S. Carvedilol Heart Failure Study Group. Effect of carvedilol on morbidity and mortality in chronic heart failure. *N Engl J Med.* 1996;334: 1349–1355.
150. Ho KKL, Anderson KM, Kannel WB, et al. Survival after the onset of congestive heart failure in Framingham Heart Study Subjects. *Circulation.* 1993;88:107–115.
151. Schocken DD, Arrieta MI, Leaverton PE, et al. Prevalence and mortality rate of congestive heart failure in the United States. *J Am Coll Cardiol.* 1992;20:301–306.
152. Mortality from congestive heart failure in United States: 1980–1990. *MMWR.* 1994;43:77–81.
153. Shindler DM, Kostis JB, Yusuf S, et al., for the SOLVD Investigators. Diabetes mellitus, a predictor of morbidity and mortality in the Studies of Left Ventricular Dysfunction (SOLVD) trials and registry. *Am J Cardiol.* 1996;77:1017–1020.
154. Domanski MJ. Beta-Blocker Evaluation of Survival Trial (BEST). *J Am Coll Cardiol.* 2000;35(suppl A):202A.
155. Carson P, Ziesche S, Johnson G, et al, for the Vasodilator-Heart Failure Trial Study Group. Racial differences in response to therapy for heart failure: analysis of the Vasodilator-Heart Failure trials. *J Card Fail.* 1999;5:178–187.

156. Dries DL, Exner DV, Gersh BJ, et al. Racial differences in the outcome of left ventricular dysfunction. *N Engl J Med.* 1999;340: 609–616.
157. Wagoner LE, Hoit BD, Hornung RW, et al. Genetic polymorphisms of the human b2 adrenergic receptor (b2AR) predict survival in patients with heart failure. *Circulation.* 1997;96(I):I92.
158. Bloem LJ, Manatunga AK, Pratt JH. Racial difference in the relationship of an angiotensin I-converting enzyme gene polymorphism to serum angiotensin I-converting enzyme activity. *Hypertension.* 1996;27:62–66.
159. Drazner MH, Rame JE, Stevenson LW, et al. Prognostic importance of elevated jugular venous pressure and a third heart sound in patients with heart failure. *N Engl J Med.* 2001;345: 574–581.
160. Baim DS, Colucci WS, Monrad ES, et al. Survival of patients with severe congestive heart failure treated with oral milrinone. *J Am Coll Cardiol.* 1986;7:661–670.
161. Grzybowski J, Bilinska ZT, Ruzyllo W, et al. Determinants of prognosis in nonischemic dilated cardiomyopathy. *J Card Fail.* 1996;2:77–85.
162. Eichhorn EJ, Heesch CM, Risser RC, et al. Predictors of systolic and diastolic improvement in patients with dilated cardiomyopathy treated with metoprolol. *J Am Coll Cardiol.* 1995;25: 154–162.
163. Androne AS, Katz SD, Lund L, et al. Hemodilution is common in patients with advanced heart failure. *Circulation.* 2003;107: 226–229.
164. Mozaffarian D, Nye R, Levy WC. Anemia predicts mortality in severe heart failure: the Prospective Randomized Amlodipine Survival Evaluation (PRAISE). *J Am Coll Cardiol.* 2003;41: 1933–1939.
165. Sharma R, Francis DP, Pitt B, et al. Haemoglobin predicts survival in patients with chronic heart failure: a substudy of the ELITE II trial. *Eur Heart J.* 2004;25:1021–1028.
166. Anand I, McMurray JJ, Whitmore J, et al. Anemia and its relationship to clinical outcome in heart failure. *Circulation.* 2004;110:149–154.
167. Cohn JN, Tognoni G. Valsartan Heart Failure Trial Investigators. A randomized trial of the angiotensin-receptor blocker valsartan in chronic heart failure. *N Engl J Med.* 2001;345:1667–1675.
168. Al-Ahmad A, Rand WM, Manjunath G, et al. Reduced kidney function and anemia as risk factors for mortality in patients with left ventricular dysfunction. *J Am Coll Cardiol.* 2001;38: 955–962.
169. Horwich TB, Fonarow GC, Hamilton MA, et al. Anemia is associated with worse symptoms, greater impairment in functional capacity and a significant increase in mortality in patients with advanced heart failure. *J Am Coll Cardiol.* 2002;39:1780–1786.
170. Anker SD, Coats AJS, Roecker EB, et al. Hemoglobin level is associated with mortality and hospitalization in patients with severe chronic heart failure: results from the COPERNICUS study. *J Am Coll Cardiol.* 2004;43:A216.
171. Komajda M, Cleland JG, DiLenarda A, et al. Clinical profile and outcome of anaemic patients with chronic heart failure in the COMET trial. *J Cardiac Fail.* 2004;10:S84.
172. McClellan WM, Flanders WD, Langston RD, et al. Anemia and renal insufficiency are independent risk factors for death among patients with congestive heart failure admitted to community hospitals: a population-based study. *J Am Soc Nephrol.* 2002:13: 1928–1936.
173. Felker GM, Adams KF, Jr., Gattis WA, et al. Anemia as a risk factor and therapeutic target in heart failure. *J Am Coll Cardiol.* 2004;44: 959–966.
174. Silverberg DS, Wexler D, Sheps D, et al. The effect of correction of mild anemia in severe, resistant congestive heart failure using subcutaneous erythropoietin and intravenous iron: a randomized controlled study. *J Am Coll Cardiol.* 2001;37:1775–1780.
175. Silverberg DS, Wexler D, Blum M, et al. The effect of correction of anaemia in diabetics and non-diabetics with severe resistant congestive heart failure and chronic renal failure by subcutaneous erythropoietin and intravenous iron. *Neph Dialysis Transp.* 2003:18:141–146.
176. Silverberg DS, Wexler D, Blum M, et al. The use of subcutaneous erythropoietin and intravenous iron for the treatment of the anemia of severe, resistant congestive heart failure improves cardiac and renal function and functional cardiac class, and markedly reduces hospitalizations. *J Am Coll Cardol.* 2000;35: 1737–1744.
177. Mancini DM, Katz SD, Lang CC, et al. Effect of erythropoietin on exercise capacity in patients with moderate to severe chronic heart failure. *Circulation.* 2003;107:294–299.
178. Curtis JP, Sokol SI, Wang Y, et al. The association of left ventricular ejection fraction, mortality, and cause of death in stable outpatients with heart failure. *J Am Coll Cardiol.* 2003;42:736–742.
179. Wilson JR, Schwartz JS, Sutton MS, et al. Prognosis in severe heart failure: relation to hemodynamic measurements and ventricular ectopic activity. *J Am Coll Cardiol.* 1983;2:403–410.
180. Eriksson SV, Kjekshus J, Offstad J, et al. Patients' characteristics in cases of chronic severe heart failure with different degrees of left ventricular systolic dysfunction. *Cardiology.* 1994;85:137–144.
181. Swedberg K, Eneroth P, Kjekshus J, et al. for the CONSENSUS Trial Study Group. Hormones regulating cardiovascular function in patients with severe congestive heart failure and their relation to mortality. *Circulation.* 1990;82:1730–1736.
182. Cintron C, Johnson G, Francis G, et al. Prognostic significance of serial changes in left ventricular ejection fraction in patients with heart failure. *Circulation.* 1993;87:VI17–VI23
183. Cohn JN, Johnson G, Ziesche S, et al. A comparison of enalapril with hydralazine-isosorbide dinitrate in the treatment of chronic congestive heart failure. *N Engl J Med.* 1991;325:303–310.
184. Ramahi TM, Samady H, Zahler R, et al. Prognostic value of dobutamine-induced augmentation of left ventricular ejection fraction in patients with dilated cardiomyopathy. *Circulation* 1997;96:I390.
185. Williams MJ, Odabashian J, Lauer MS, et al. Prognostic value of dobutamine echocardiography in patients with left ventricular dysfunction. *J Am Coll Cardiol.* 1996;27:132–139.
186. Cohn JN. Structural basis for heart failure: ventricular remodeling and its pharmacological inhibition. *Circulation.* 1995;91: 2504–2507.
187. Quinones MA, Greenberg BH, Kopelen HA, et al., for the SOLVD Investigators. Echocardiographic predictors of clinical outcome in patients with left ventricular dysfunction enrolled in the SOLVD registry and trials: significance of left ventricular hypertrophy. *J Am Coll Cardiol.* 2000;35:1237–1244.
188. Konstam MA, Cohen SR, Salem DN, et al. Comparison of left and right ventricular end-systolic pressure-volume relations in congestive heart failure. *J Am Coll Cardiol.* 1985;5:1326–1334.
189. Polak J, Holman L, Wynne J, et al. Right ventricular ejection fraction: an indicator of increased mortality in patients with congestive heart failure associated with coronary artery disease. *J Am Coll Cardiol.* 1983;2:217–224.
190. Di Salvo TG, Mathier M, Semigran MJ, et al. Preserved right ventricular ejection fraction predicts exercise capacity and survival in advanced heart failure. *J Am Coll Cardiol.* 1995;25:1143–1153.
191. Xie GY, Berk MR, Smith MD, et al. Prognostic value of Doppler transmitral flow patterns in patients with congestive heart failure. *J Am Coll Cardiol.* 1993;22:808–815.
192. Pinamonti B, Lenarda AD, Sinagra G, et al, and the Heart Muscle Disease Study Group. Restrictive left ventricular filling pattern in dilated cardiomyopathy assessed by Doppler echocardiography: clinical, echocardiographic and hemodynamic correlations and prognostic implications. *J Am Coll Cardiol.* 1993;22:808–815.
193. Mancini DM, Eisen H, Kussmaul W, et al. Value of peak exercise oxygen consumption for optimal timing of cardiac transplantation in ambulatory patients with heart failure. *Circulation.* 1991;83:778–786.
194. Kao W, Winkel EM, Johnson MR, et al. Role of maximal oxygen consumption in establishment of heart transplant candidacy for heart failure patients with intermediate exercise tolerance. *Am J Cardiol.* 1997;79:1124–1127.
195. Mudge GH, Goldstein S, Addonizio, et al. 24th Bethesda conference: Cardiac transplantation. Task Force 3: Recipient guidelines/prioritization. *J Am Coll Cardiol.* 1993;22:21–31.
196. Costanzo MR, Augustine S, Bourge R, et al. Selection and treatment of candidates for heart transplantation. *Circulation.* 1995;92:3593–3612.
197. MacGowan GA, Janosko K, Cecchetti A, et al. Exercise-related ventilatory abnormalities and survival in congestive heart failure. *Am J Cardiol.* 1997;79:1264–1266.

198. Bittner V, Weiner DH, Yusuf S, et al., for the SOLVD Investigators. Prediction of mortality and morbidity with a 6-minute walk test in patients with left ventricular dysfunction. *JAMA*. 1993;270: 1702–1707.
199. Baim DS, Colucci WS, Monrad ES, et al. Survival of patients with severe congestive heart failure treated with oral milrinone. *J Am Coll Cardiol*. 1986;7:661–670.
200. Glover DR, Littler WA. Factors influencing survival and mode of death in severe chronic ischaemic cardiac failure. *Br Heart J*. 1987;57:125–132.
201. Unverferth DV, Magorien RD, Moeschberger ML, et al. Factors influencing the one-year mortality of dilated cardiomyopathy. *Am J Cardiol*. 1984;54:147–152.
202. White M, Rouleau JL, Ruddy TD, et al. Decreased coronary sinus oxygen content: a predictor of adverse prognosis in patients with severe congestive heart failure. *J Am Coll Cardiol*. 1991;18: 1631–1637.
203. Chomsky DB, Lang CC, Rayos GH, et al. Hemodynamic exercise testing. A valuable tool in the selection of cardiac transplantation candidates. *Circulation*. 1996;94:3176–3183.
204. Narang R, Cleland JGF, Erhardt L, et al. Mode of death in chronic heart failure: a request and proposition for more accurate classification. *Eur Heart J*. 1996;7:1390–1403.
205. MERIT-HF Study Group. Effect of metoprolol CR/XL in chronic heart failure: Metoprolol CR/XL Randomised Intervention Trial in Congestive Heart Failure (MERIT-HF). *Lancet*. 1999;353: 2001–2007.
206. Echt DS, Liebson PR, Mitchell LB, et al., and the CAST Investigators. Mortality and morbidity in patients receiving encainide, flecainide or placebo: the Cardiac Arrhythmia Suppression Trial. *N Engl J Med*. 1991;324:781–788.
207. Fletcher RD, Cintron GB, Johnson G, et al., for the V-HeFT II VA Cooperative Studies Group. Enalapril decreases prevalence of ventricular tachycardia in patients with chronic congestive heart failure. *Circulation*. 1993;87:VI49–VI55.
208. Teerlink JR, Jalaluddin M, Anderson S, et al., on behalf of the PROMISE Investigators. Ambulatory ventricular arrhythmias in patients with heart failure do not specifically predict an increased risk of sudden death. *Circulation*. 2000;101: 40–46.
209. de Bruyne MC, Hoes AW, Kors JA, et al. QTc dispersion predicts cardiac mortality in the elderly: the Rotterdam Study. *Circulation*. 1998;97:467–472.
210. Galinier M, Vialette J-C, Cabrol FP, et al. QT interval dispersion as a predictor of arrhythmic events in congestive heart failure: importance of etiology. *Eur Heart J*. 1998;19: 1054–1062.
211. Armoundas AA, Rosenbaum DS, Ruskin JN, et al. Prognostic significance of electrical alternans versus signal averaged electrocardiography in predicting the outcome of electrophysiological testing and arrhythmia-free survival. *Heart*. 1998;80: 251–256.
212. Cohn JN, Levine TB, Olivari MT, et al. Plasma norepinephrine as a guide to prognosis in patients with chronic congestive heart failure. *N Engl J Med*. 1984;311:819–823.
213. Francis GS, Cohn JN, Johnson G, et al., for the V-HeFT VA Cooperative Studies Group. Plasma norepinephrine, plasma renin activity, and congestive heart failure: relations to survival and the effects of therapy in V-HeFt II. *Circulation*. 1993;87(suppl VI):VI40–VI48.
214. Kaye DM, Lefkovits J, Jennings GL, et al. Adverse consequences of high sympathetic nervous activity in the failing human heart. *J Am Coll Cardiol*. 1995;26:1257–1263.
215. Fauchier L, Babuty D, Cosnay P, et al. Heart rate variability in idiopathic dilated cardiomyopathy: characteristics and prognosis value. *J Am Coll Cardiol*. 1997;30:1009–1014.
216. Jiang W, Hathaway WR, McNulty S, et al. Ability of heart rate variability to predict prognosis in patients with advanced heart failure. *Am J Cardiol*. 1997;80:808–811.
217. Szabo BM, van Veldhuisen DJ, van der Veer N, et al. Prognostic value of heart rate variability in chronic congestive heart failure secondary to idiopathic or ischemic dilated cardiomyopathy. *Am J Cardiol*. 1997;79:978–980.
218. Francis GS, Cohn JN, Johnson G, et al., for the V-HeFT VA Cooperative Studies Group. Plasma norepinephrine, plasma renin activity, and congestive heart failure: relations to survival and the effects of therapy in V-HeFt II. *Circulation*. 1993;87: VI40–VI48.
219. Cohn JN, Rector TS. Prognosis of congestive heart failure and predictors of mortality. *Am J Cardiol*. 1988;62(2):25A–30A.
220. Lee WH, Packer M. Prognostic importance of serum sodium concentration and its modification by converting-enzyme inhibition in patients with severe chronic heart failure. *Circulation* 1986;73:257–267.
221. Klein L, O'Connor C, Leimberger J, et al. Lower serum sodium is associated with increased short-term mortality in hospitalized patients with worsening heart failure: results from the Outcomes of a Prospective Trial of Intravenous Milrinone for Exacerbations of Chronic Heart Failure (OPTIME-CHF) study. *Circulation* 2005;111:2454–2460.
222. Torre-Amione G, Kapadia S, Benedict C, et al. Proinflammatory cytokine levels in patients with depressed left ventricular ejection fraction: a report from the Studies of Left Ventricular Dysfunction (SOLVD). *J Am Coll Cardiol*. 1996;27:1201–1206.
223. Ferrari R, Bachetti T, Confortini R, et al. Tumor necrosis factor soluble receptors in patients with various degrees of congestive heart failure. *Circulation*. 1995;92:1479–1486.
224. Tsutamoto T, Hisanaga T, Wada A, et al. Interleukin-6 spillover in the peripheral circulation increases with the severity of heart failure, and the high plasma level of interleukin-6 is an important prognostic predictor in patients with congestive heart failure. *J Am Coll Cardiol*. 1998;31:391–398.
225. Mann DL. The effect of tumor necrosis factor-alpha on cardiac structure and function: a tale of two cytokines. *J Card Fail*. 1996;2:S165–S172.
226. Rodeheffer RJ, Lerman A, Heublein DM, et al. Increased plasma concentrations of endothelin in congestive heart failure in humans. *Mayo Clin Proc*. 1992;67:719–724.
227. Mulder P, Richard V, Derumeaux G, et al. Role of endogenous endothelin in chronic heart failure: effect of long-term treatment with an endothelin antagonist on survival, hemodynamics, and cardiac remodeling. *Circulation*. 1997;96:1976–1982.
228. Galatius-Jensen S, Wroblewski H, Emmeluth C, et al. Plasma endothelin in congestive heart failure: a predictor of cardiac death? *J Card Fail*. 1996;2:71–76.
229. Tsutamoto T, Hisanaga T, Fukai D, et al. Prognostic value of plasma soluble intercellular adhesion molecule-1 and endothelin-1 concentration in patients with chronic congestive heart failure. *Am J Cardiol*. 1995;76:803–808.
230. Costanzo MR, Augustine S, Bourge R, et al. Selection and treatment of candidates for heart transplantation. A statement for health professionals from the Committee on Heart Failure and Cardiac Transplantation of the Council on Clinical Cardiology, American Heart Association. *Circulation*. 1995;92: 3593–3612.
231. Gridelli B, Remmuzzi G. Strategies for making more organs available for transplantation. *N Eng J Med* 2000;343:404–410.
232. Gold MR. Spencer W. T wave alternans for ventricular arrhythmia risk stratification. *Curr Opin Cardiol*. 2003;18:1–5.
233. Cleland JG, Chattopadhyay S, Khand A, et al. Prevalence and incidence of arrhythmias and sudden death in heart failure. *Heart Fail Rev*. 2002:7:229–242.
234. Elming H, Brendorp B, Kober L, et al. QTc interval in the assessment of cardiac risk. *Cardiac Electrophysiol Rev*. 2002;6:289–294.
235. Deng MC, Smits JM, Packer M. Selecting patients for heart transplantation: which patients are too well for transplant? *Curr Opin Cardiol*. 2002;17:137–144.
236. Mudge GH, Goldstein S, Addonizio, et al. 24th Bethesda conference: Cardiac transplantation. Task Force 3: Recipient guidelines/prioritization. *J Am Coll Cardiol*. 1993;22:21–31.
237. Stevenson LW. Selection and management of candidates for heart transplantation. *Curr Opin Cardiol*. 1996;11:166–173.
238. Hunt SA, Baker DW, Chin MH, et al. ACC/AHA guidelines for the evaluation and management of chronic heart failure in the adult. *Circulation*. 2001;104:2996–3007.
239. Mancini DM, Eisen H, Kussmaul W, et al. Value of peak exercise oxygen consumption for optimal timing of cardiac transplantation in ambulatory patients with heart failure. *Circulation*. 1991;83:778–786
240. Higginbotham MB, Morris KG, Williams RS, et al. Regulation of stroke volume during submaximal and maximal upright exercise in normal man. *Circulation Res*. 1986;58:281–291.

241. Aaronson KD, Schwartz JS, Chen TM, et al. Development and prospective validation of a clinical index to predict survival in ambulatory patients referred for cardiac transplant evaluation. *Circulation.* 1997;95:2660–2667.
242. Koelling TM, Joseph S, Aaronson KD. Heart failure survival score continues to predict clinical outcomes in patients with heart failure receiving beta-blockers. *J Heart Lung Transp.* 2004;23; 1414–1422.
243. Forman DE, Butler J, Wang Y, et al. Incidence, predictors and impact of worsening renal function among patients hospitalized with heart failure. *J Am Coll Cardiol.* 2004;43;61–67.
244. Hillege HL, Girbes AR, de Kam PJ, et al. Renal function, neurohormonal activation, and survival in patients with chronic heart failure. *Circulation.* 2000;102:203–210.
245. Dries DL, Exner DV, Domanski MJ, et al. The prognostic implications of renal insufficiency in asymptomatic and symptomatic patients with left ventricular systolic dysfunction. *J Am Coll Cardiol.* 2000;35:681–689.
246. Levy WC, Mozaffarian D, Linker DT, et al. The Seattle heart failure model: prediction of survival in heart failure. *Circulation.* In press.
247. Moshkovitz Y, Kaluski E, Milo O, et al. Recent developments in cardiac output determination by bioimpedance: comparison with invasive cardiac output and potential cardiovascular applications. *Curr Opin Cardiol.* 2004:19:229–237.
248. Butler J, Hanumanthu SK, Chomsky DB, et al. Frequency of low risk hospital admission for heart failure. *Am J Cardiol.* 1998;81:41–44.
249. Fonarow GC, Adams KF, Jr., Abraham WT, et al. ADHERE Scientific Advisory Committee, Study Group, and Investigators. Risk stratification for in-hospital mortality in acutely decompensated heart failure: classification and regression tree analysis. *JAMA.* 2005;293:572–580.

Heart Failure Secondary to Coronary Artery Disease

17

Roger M. Mills, Jr. **Mouaz Al-Mallah**

This chapter reviews current important basic and clinical aspects of heart failure that occur as a consequence of coronary artery disease (CAD). Table 17-1 outlines some common clinical presentations of this problem. Medical management of end-stage ischemic cardiomyopathy and interventions for the complications of acute myocardial infarction (MI) are covered in another chapter; this chapter will concentrate on the pathophysiology and diagnosis of heart failure associated with potentially reversible myocardial ischemia.

In the United States, CAD remains the most common identifiable process underlying heart failure (1). In the ADHERE database, with over 100,000 heart failure admissions, 55% of patients have evidence of CAD (2). Once overt heart failure occurs, the prognosis for patients with established CAD is poor, with an average annual mortality rate of 30% to 40% (3–5). In older studies, patients who developed heart failure due to CAD had a significantly worse prognosis than those whose heart failure results from nonischemic pathology. Franciosa et al. followed 182 patients with chronic left heart failure and reported 1- and 2-year mortality rates of 46% and 69%, respectively, in patients with CAD as compared with 23% and 48%, respectively, in those with idiopathic dilated cardiomyopathy (6). Similarly, in a study of 201 patients with advanced heart failure, Likoff et al. found a 6-month mortality rate of 65% in patients with ischemic disease versus 40% in the noncoronary group (7). In a series of 860 patients with known or suspected CAD evaluated at the Mayo Clinic, Chuah et al. reported that a history of heart failure was the most important clinical predictor of cardiac events (hazard ratio 4.26) (8). In a study of 3,787 patients who underwent catheterization at Duke University Medical Center, Bart et al. found significantly higher 5-year mortality rates in ischemic versus nonischemic cardiomyopathy. The 5-year adjusted Kaplan-Meier survival statistic was 0.59 for ischemic and 0.69 for nonischemic patients ($p < 0.0001$) (9) (Fig. 17-1).

This difference persisted despite vasodilator therapy, as demonstrated by the Veterans Administration Cooperative study data shown in Figure 17-2, which compared heart failure patients with coronary and noncoronary causes treated with vasodilators versus the then-conventional therapy or placebo. The impact of today's state-of-the-art therapy with neurohormonal blockade, antiplatelet agents, revascularization, and arrhythmia control devices on the prognosis of patients with coronary disease and heart failure has not been documented. However, the Duke Cardiovascular Disease Database observational data strongly support the concept that surgical revascularization benefits patients with impaired left ventricular function and CAD (10).

The approach to diagnosis and management of heart failure associated with coronary disease should focus on assessing the possibility that mechanical revascularization with percutaneous transluminal coronary angioplasty (PTCA) or coronary artery bypass grafting (CABG) might relieve ischemia, alleviate symptoms, and improve both cardiac function and clinical outcome. In this setting, a comprehensive approach might include ventricular remodeling, mitral valve repair, epicardial lead placement for resynchronization, and cardiac restraint device placement as well as revascularization, followed by long-term neurohormonal blockade, antiplatelet and lipid-lowering therapy, and consideration for implantable cardioverter defibrillator (ICD) placement.

Keeping this clinical strategy in mind, this chapter will first review the pathophysiology of ischemia to clarify how

TABLE 17-1
SYNDROMES OF HEART FAILURE WITH CORONARY ARTERY DISEASE

Ischemia
- Diastolic dysfunction, normal heart size
  - "Flash" pulmonary edema with multivessel CAD
  - Exertional dyspnea due to ischemia
- Both systolic and diastolic dysfunction
  - Stunned and hibernating myocardium
  - Transient coronary occlusion during unstable angina or PTCA
- Anatomic disruption
  - Ischemic mitral regurgitation
  - Ventricular septal defect
  - Left ventricular aneurysm
- Chronic scarring
  - Systolic dysfunction with cardiac enlargement
  - Ischemic cardiomyopathy

PTCA, percutaneous transluminal coronary angioplasty.

reduction in coronary blood flow produces hemodynamic dysfunction. A discussion of the role of echocardiography, radionuclide imaging, stress testing, and catheterization laboratory studies in the evaluation of the heart failure patients with known or suspected CAD follows. The brief final section of the chapter offers suggestions for evidence-based decision making and the choice of therapy.

PHYSIOLOGY OF ISCHEMIC LEFT VENTRICULAR DYSFUNCTION

Coronary Blood Flow and Myocardial Oxygen Demand

Atherosclerosis in the coronary arterial tree manifests as clinical CAD when it produces either reversible or irreversible myocardial oxygen supply–demand imbalance. Understanding heart failure due to CAD requires an appreciation of the precise coupling of coronary blood flow with myocardial oxygen demand and myocardial function. This coupling, normally mediated through the integrated responses of coronary endothelium and vascular smooth muscle (11,12), allows coronary blood flow to increase markedly in response to augmented myocardial metabolic demands. This phenomenon is described as coronary flow reserve.

Coronary flow reserve can be measured directly in open-chest laboratory animal experiments using a mechanical snare to constrict the proximal (conduit) vessel and an electromagnetic flow meter to measure distal flow. In this setting, coronary flow at rest and after maximal

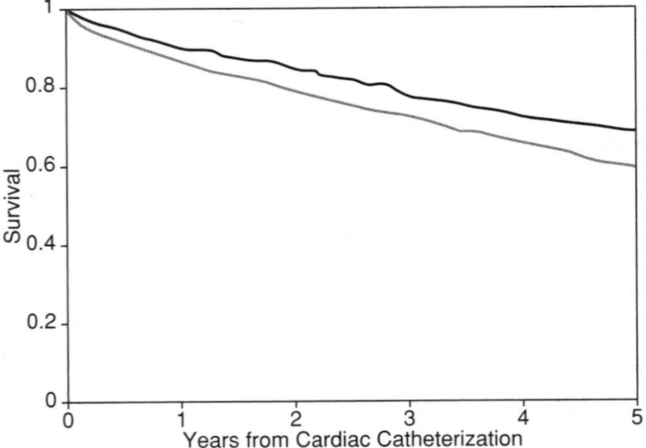

Figure 17-1 Adjusted Kaplan-Meier survival estimates for patients with nonischemic (**solid line**) and ischemic (**dashed line**) cardiomyopathy (p <0.0001). (Adapted from Bart BA, Shaw LK, McCants CB, et al. Clinical determinants of mortality in patients with angiographically diagnosed ischemic or non-ischemic cardiomyopathy. *J Am Coll Cardiol.* 1997;30:1002–1008.)

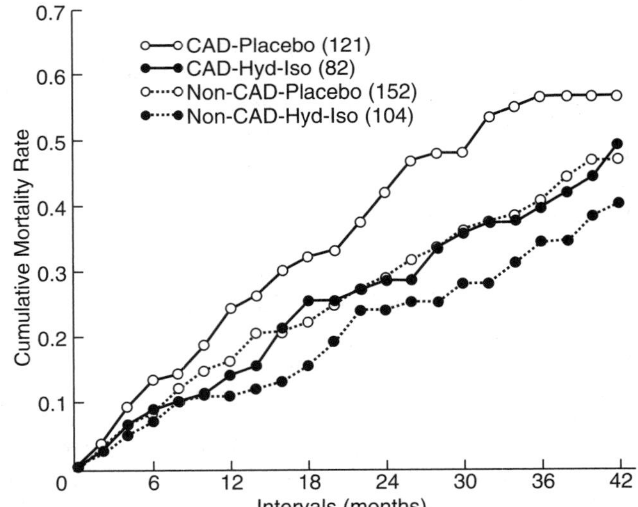

Figure 17-2 Cumulative mortality among patients with (n = 203) and without (n = 256) coronary artery disease (CAD) treated with placebo or hydralazine-isosorbide dinitrate (*Hyd-Iso*). (Reproduced from Tillisch J, Brunken R, Marshall R, et al. Reversibility of cardiac wall motion abnormalities predicted by positron tomography. *N Engl J Med.* 1986;314:884–888.)

coronary resistance vessel vasodilation can be compared while imposing various degrees of proximal epicardial conduit vessel stenosis. Using this technique and intracoronary injections of radiographic contrast as a vasodilator stimulus, Gould et al. (13) demonstrated that coronary flow with unobstructed vessels increased four- to fivefold with maximal vasodilation. Although resting blood flow did not fall until an 85% proximal stenosis was imposed, the normal four- to fivefold coronary flow reserve was impaired by imposing as little as 35% to 40% proximal stenosis. In further studies, these measurements appeared valid with either single or multiple stenoses, and the investigators proposed coronary flow reserve as a physiological measure that described the overall function of the artery as a unit (13,14).

In human studies, coronary flow reserve may be measured using subselective intracoronary Doppler flow velocity catheters. Although the Doppler flow catheter directly measures blood flow velocity, if the studies are performed with maximal vasodilation of the epicardial arteries, then changes in flow velocity are proportional to changes in flow volume. Sample Doppler tracings are shown in Figure 17-3. In addition, the combination of Doppler flow measurement guidewires and intravascular ultrasound (IVUS) catheters allows simultaneous direct measurement of coronary lumen diameter and flow velocity for calculation of coronary flow volumes. Using the Doppler technique alone, Wilson et al. demonstrated 3.5-fold increases over resting flow velocity with intracoronary radiographic contrast injections, fivefold increases with dipyridamole (15), and fivefold increases with papaverine (16) in patients with angiographically normal coronary arteries. These studies convincingly demonstrated coronary flow reserve in humans of a magnitude similar to that seen in the laboratory animal preparations described above.

Figure 17-4 illustrates the concept that as obstructive CAD progresses, coronary flow reserve declines to levels where ischemia and functional impairment occur with only modest increases in myocardial oxygen demand. In a variety of circumstances, the combined effect of atherosclerotic plaque and associated intravascular thrombus may reduce myocardial perfusion below levels required to prevent ischemia during daily activities or even at rest, and no coronary flow reserve exists.

Myocardial Dysfunction with Ischemia

When coronary flow reserve is inadequate, myocardial hypoperfusion results in cellular hypoxia. Because cardiac muscle is an obligate aerobic system with minimal anaerobic energy sources, this leads to biochemical, electrical, and mechanical dysfunction. This is summarized in Table 17-2.

Biochemical Dysfunction

Earlier studies of myocardial ischemia emphasized the rapid changes in intermediary metabolism that occur in association with ischemia. Jennings et al. studied high-energy phosphate metabolism after coronary occlusion in quick-frozen sections of canine hearts (17). They showed a shift from aerobic to anaerobic metabolism beginning within 8 to 10 seconds after coronary ligation. After 40 to 60 minutes of coronary ligation, their studies demonstrated marked loss of high-energy phosphate and low tissue pH, with characteristic ultrastructural changes, including cell swelling with mitochondrial and sarcolemma

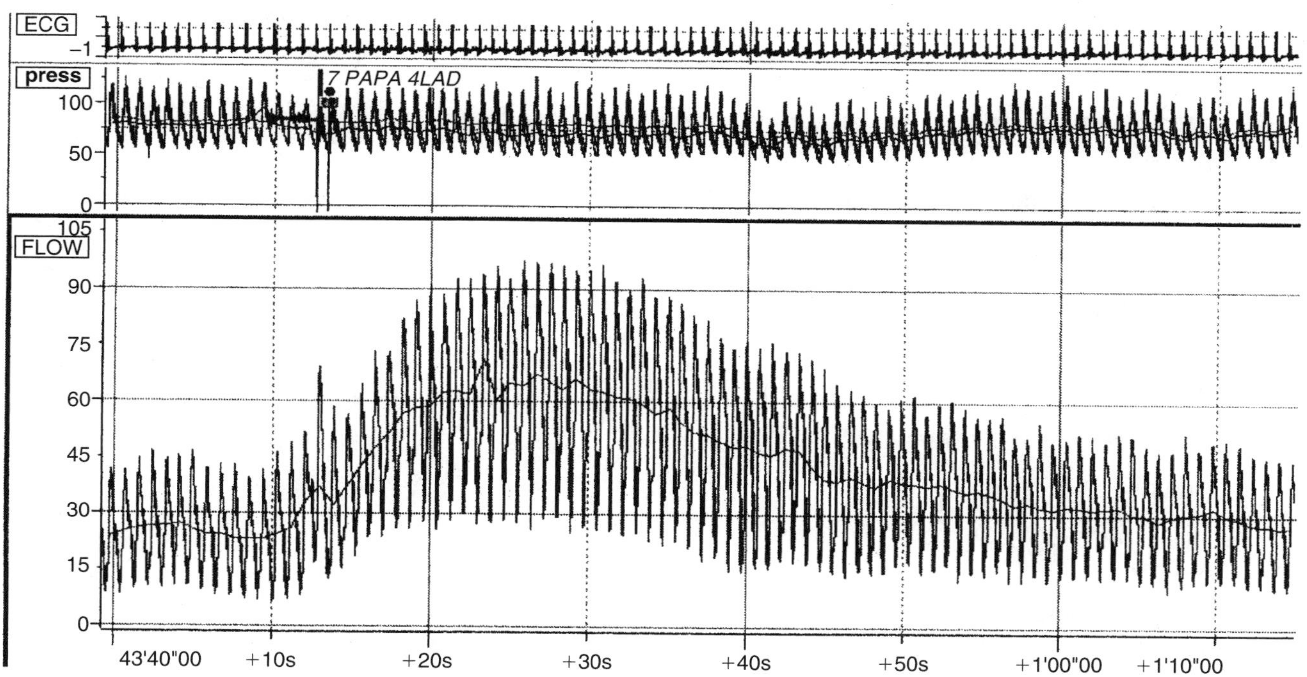

Figure 17-3 Coronary flow reserve (CFR) tracings in a patient with a nonobstructive left anterior descending (LAD) lesion. CFR = 66/21; LAD = 3.1.

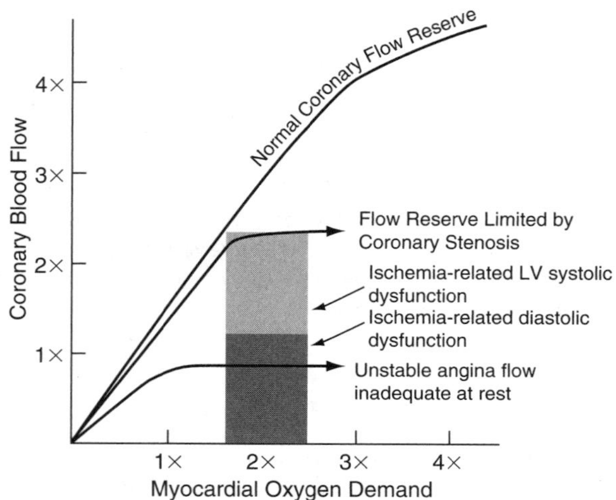

Figure 17-4 Decreasing coronary flow reserve with progressive coronary obstruction.

damage. Clinical studies confirm that myocardial ischemia results in lactate production and a shift to free fatty acids (FFAs) as a preferred metabolic substrate.

Investigators using gene chip technology have characterized extensive changes in structural and regulatory proteins associated with myocardial ischemia and heart failure. The relatively large tissue samples removed at the time of left ventricular assist device (LVAD) implantation and acquisition of the explanted heart after transplant have facilitated these studies. Razeghi et al. from Houston have shown that mechanical unloading causes downregulation of numerous gene regulators of energy metabolism genes (18). Tan et al. at the Cleveland Clinic used gene chips to demonstrate unique patterns of gene expression in failing hearts (19). Margulies has recently reviewed a number of studies to support the concept that relief of mechanical loading on the heart triggers multiple signaling pathways that allow myocardial recovery (20).

Finally, large clinical trials have documented significant elevation of B-type natriuretic peptide (BNP) levels in acute coronary syndromes (21–23). The observed BNP levels can best be explained by increased synthesis and suggest that ischemia as well as mechanical loading stimulates BNP production (24).

In summary, profound metabolic changes occur with myocardial ischemia, including not only shifts in the substrates and products of energy metabolism, but also changes in structural and regulatory proteins and increases in BNP production.

Electrical Dysfunction

With the development of thrombolytic therapy and subsequently of primary angioplasty for management of acute coronary syndromes (ACS), reperfusion has displaced arrhythmia control as the focus of management. In the chronic setting, patients with left ventricular systolic dysfunction and ejection fraction (LVEF) less than 35% benefit from ICD devices, whereas patients with LVEF over 35% do not. These findings, and the association of larger fixed perfusion defects with inducible arrhythmia (25), suggest that scar, not ischemia, is the primary substrate for life-threatening arrhythmia in chronic CAD. Nonetheless, ischemia clearly increases susceptibility to arrhythmia. Stambler et al. (26) studied 20 patients with coronary disease who had no sustained ventricular tachycardia (VT) on baseline electrophysiological testing. With dobutamine infusion, induction of VT was associated with ischemia in nine subjects. The authors concluded that ischemia may contribute to ventricular arrythmia induction in some individuals. Ischemia increases QT dispersion, a marker for malignant ventricular arrhythmia (27), and preconditioning decreases QT dispersion (28). In an animal model, swine with total left anterior descending

TABLE 17-2
MYOCARDIAL DYSFUNCTION WITH ISCHEMIA

A. Biochemical Dysfunction
   a. Lactate production
   b. Shift to FFA as a proffered metabolic substrate
   c. Changes in structural and regulatory proteins
   d. Increases in β-adrenergic receptor density
   e. Elevated BNP concentration
B. Electrical Dysfunction
   a. Increased susceptibility to arrhythmia
   b. QT dispersion
   c. QT prolongation
C. Mechanical Dysfunction
   a. Diastolic dysfunction
   b. Systolic dysfunction
D. Ischemic Preconditioning
   a. Increases in endogenous adenosine
   b. Activation of potassium-adenosine triphosphate (K^+-ATP) channels
   c. Reductions in ischemia-related apoptosis

BNp, B-type natriuretic peptide.

coronary occlusions and hibernating myocardium had a high rate of sudden death due to ventricular fibrillation, suggesting that chronically ischemic myocardium results in "enhanced vulnerability to lethal arrhythmias and sudden cardiac death." (29) In addition, Halkin et al. reported few cases of post-MI torsades de points that is related to an acquired long QT syndrome post-MI (30). Kenigsberg et al. reported that QT prolongation is the most consistent electrocardiographic change seen in patients with balloon occlusion of the coronary artery (31). These data all suggest that, given a susceptible anatomic substrate, ischemia may indeed contribute to significant electrical instability.

Mechanical Dysfunction

The active energy requiring steps in myocyte contraction occur with transport of calcium back into the sarcoplasmic reticulum after actin–myosin interaction. Predictably, limited energy supplies first impair relaxation; only later does failure of contraction occur. In human studies, diastolic function appears to be more sensitive to ischemia than systolic function. Bonow et al. studied filling dynamics using radionuclide angiography in 26 patients with single-vessel CAD and normal left ventricular (LV) systolic function (32). After PTCA, the filling rate improved from 2.5 ± 0.6 to 3.0 ± 0.6 end-diastolic volume/sec and time to peak filling rate decreased from 178 ± 30 to 162 ± 20 milliseconds. These findings suggest that diastolic function may be measurably impaired while overall systolic function remains normal. Piscione et al. studied LV function during balloon occlusion of a coronary artery in 10 patients with normal LV function undergoing PTCA (33). With high-fidelity pressure records and LV angiography during the PTCA, they demonstrated impairment of relaxation within 20 seconds after onset of ischemia associated with impaired peak segmental shortening, as well.

In a dog model where ischemia was induced by 3 minutes of rapid pacing in the presence of moderate coronary stenosis, Takano and Glantz found that decreases in LV contractility were the best determinant of alterations in the LV end-diastolic pressure–volume relationship. They emphasized that coronary flow, myocardial supply and demand balance, and LV contractility (systolic function) were critical factors in altered diastolic function, while noting that in both canine and human hearts systolic function was only mildly depressed when the upward shift of the diastolic pressure–volume relationship was observed (34).

Ultimately, ischemia does depress systolic function. Development of a reversible LV wall motion disorder during exercise or pharmacologic stress as shown by echocardiography, radionuclide ventriculography, or magnetic resonance imaging (MRI) (35) represents the impairment of myocardial contraction associated with tissue hypoxia. Measures that include both the extent and severity of the wall motion abnormalities may improve the prognostic significance of stress echo studies (36).

Ischemic Preconditioning

Paradoxically, although ischemia produces significant impairment of cardiac function, repeated brief episodes of ischemia appear to protect against some of the detrimental consequences of ischemia-reperfusion injury (37–39). Among the mechanisms proposed to account for this phenomenon (ischemic preconditioning) are increases in endogenous adenosine, activation of potassium-adenosine triphosphate (K^+-ATP) channels, and reductions in ischemia-related apoptosis. Preconditioning produced by episodes of tachycardia reduced infarct size in a canine model, and adenosine receptor blockade with 8-phenyltheophylline abolished the observed protective effects (40). Cleveland et al. confirmed the phenomenon of ischemic preconditioning in human right atrial tissue obtained at the time of surgery and demonstrated that long-term exposure to oral hypoglycemic agents prevented preconditioning (41). Their data suggest that preconditioning activates K^+-ATP channels. Piot et al. have recently shown that ischemic preconditioning decreases apoptosis in rat hearts in vivo, lending additional support to the hypothesis that triggering of programmed cell death may be another important consequence of ischemia (42).

Nicoradil, a drug with both nitrate-like actions and K^+-ATP channel-opener activity, appears to simulate the effects of preconditioning. Nicorandil is available in Europe and Japan, and many Japanese investigators have used the controlled circumstances of balloon angioplasty to evaluate the effects of nicorandil (43). Two recent trials, including 32 patients undergoing PTCA in one and 44 undergoing PTCA in the other, demonstrated enhanced myocardial tolerance to ischemia (typical of preconditioning) with nicorandil as compared to saline controls (44,45). The bulk of the nicorandil data support the concept that preconditioning involves activation of K^+-ATP channels

Disturbingly, Dekker et al. (46) have reported a study of the effects of ischemic preconditioning on cellular electrical coupling in rabbit papillary muscle preparations from normal and failing hearts. In this model, ischemic preconditioning produced detrimental effects in failing papillary muscle, advancing the onset of irreversible damage. Aging (47) and diabetes (48) also appear to reduce the impact of preconditioning, although nicorandil may restore preconditioning responsiveness in the elderly (49). These observations suggest that the effects of repeated episodes of ischemic preconditioning may differ according to clinical circumstances.

In summary, under normal physiological circumstances myocardial blood flow exquisitely matches myocardial oxygen demand and can increase four- to fivefold in response to demand. As CAD diminishes physiological flow reserve, ischemia may result from either increases in oxygen demand or decreases in oxygen supply. Ischemia rapidly produces profound changes in intermediary energy metabolism, resulting in impaired diastolic and systolic function. In addition, chronic ischemia leads to altered gene expression, changes in structural and regulatory proteins, and initiation of cellular mechanisms leading to apoptosis and fibrosis. Furthermore, chronic ischemia causes increases in β-adrenergic receptor density, and both acute and chronic ischemia lead to increased myocardial production of BNP. In a self-protective adaptation, repeated brief episodes of ischemia may induce preconditioning, probably related to K^+-ATP channel opening, reducing the extent of myocardial injury.

Myocardial Stunning and Hibernation

Myocardial stunning and hibernation, clinically important concepts in understanding heart failure due to CAD, represent a recent and dramatic paradigm shift in our approach to coronary disease. Before the introduction of these concepts, ischemic injury was thought of as an acute, self-limited process with only two possible outcomes: complete recovery of normal function or cellular necrosis with infarction and subsequent scar formation. In fact, ischemic LV dysfunction is far more complex. Impaired contraction may occur as a result of isolated or repetitive episodes of ischemia followed by reperfusion, as in unstable angina. This mechanical dysfunction is referred to as *myocardial stunning*. Contractile failure may also develop as a pathophysiological adaptation to chronic ischemia; the descriptive term *hibernating myocardium* has been used in this chronic setting (50–55).

As originally proposed, *stunning* implied a prolonged, albeit transient, state of impaired function following a momentary event. Imagine a boxer stunned after a violent blow to the head; within a few hours, he regains his full capacities. In contrast, *hibernating* indicated a prolonged state of metabolic downregulation with markedly reduced activity; for example, imagine a bear who will survive the long cold winter by sleeping curled in her den (56).

The concept of myocardial stunning is outlined in Figure 17-5. Myocardial stunning may occur after a single, prolonged episode or repetitive, brief episodes of coronary hypoperfusion, as demonstrated by increased diastolic stiffness after repeated balloon occlusions during PTCA. Wijns et al. (57) studied the effects of three to ten balloon inflations lasting 15 to 75 seconds on diastolic performance and demonstrated decreased diastolic function lasting up to 12 minutes after the final inflation, whereas systolic function returned quickly to normal. Impaired systolic function also occurs with repeated episodes of ischemia, as demonstrated by Nixon et al. (58). Stunned myocardium retains the ability to contract under inotropic stimulation or postextrasystolic potentiation (59). After successful thrombolysis, ejection fraction (EF) may remain depressed shortly after treatment but improves substantially 10 to 14 days later. Stack et al. (60) showed improvement in LVEF from 40% ± 8% to 48% ± 6% 16 days after successful lytic therapy; Reduto et al. (61) also demonstrated a similar improvement, 46% ± 14% to 55% ± 10% in 10 days.

Kim et al. have reviewed recent laboratory studies of the pathogenesis of stunning (62). In large-animal models, stunning produces significant changes in gene and protein regulation, with upregulation of an array of survival genes. Biopsy specimens from patients undergoing cardiac surgery also suggest important differences in stunned and hibernating tissue as compared to normal control samples, with increased cyclic adenosine monophosphate (cAMP) in hibernating myocardium and increased levels of heat shock protein 72 in stunned tissue (63). These data demonstrate that, at a very basic level, stunning produces more profound changes than just a brief alteration in intermediary metabolism; in fact, gene expression is altered to favor protection of the threatened myocardium.

Hibernating myocardium describes chronic contractile dysfunction at rest occurring in response to marked

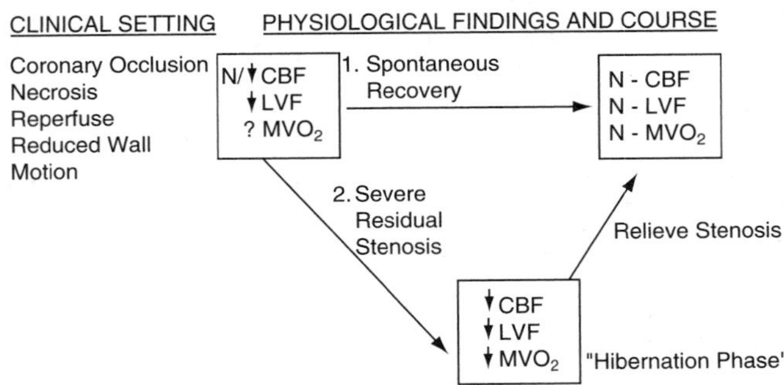

Figure 17-5 When a severe coronary stenosis reduces coronary flow without necrosis, there may be a downregulation of myocardial function. The decrease in myocardial contractility reduces myocardial energy demands; hence, no necrosis occurs. Thus, the physiologic findings in the course of this clinical phenomenon would be reduced coronary blood flow, reduced LV function, and reduced myocardial oxygen demands. There are three possible consequences given these findings. The first, spontaneous recovery with which coronary blood flow may normalize due to collateral flow relief of coronary spasm, will result in return of LV myocardial oxygen requirements and function. The second possibility is to relieve the stenosis. Under these circumstances coronary blood flow normalizes immediately, but LV function may recover immediately or its recovery may be delayed. If its recovery is delayed, the findings (basically, a normal coronary blood flow with reduced LV function and, presumably, myocardial oxygen demand) resemble those seen in myocardial stunning, which occurs after MI is reperfused. Thus, the hibernating myocardium may go through a delayed recovery phase, which we have termed a *stunned phase*. With time, spontaneous recovery should occur. A third possibility would be if the relationship between the reduced coronary blood flow and reduced myocardial oxygen demand is disturbed by further reduction in coronary blood flow for an increase in myocardial oxygen consumption; myocardial necrosis may ensue. Under these circumstances the necrosed myocardium may be reperfused, in which case coronary blood flow is normalized; this myocardial region also may go through a stunned phase before spontaneous recovery. N, normal.

impairment of flow reserve. Resting myocardial blood flow in hibernating segments is close to normal, but extremely limited flow reserve leads to myocardial ischemia with minimal activity and to chronic ventricular dysfunction (64). The dysfunction is reversible by revascularization (65). This concept is diagrammed in Figure 17-6. Keller et al. have studied the effects of reduced coronary flow on myocardial metabolism in the isolated perfused rat heart using nuclear magnetic resonance spectroscopy (66). Their data indicate that modest decreases in coronary flow reduce contractile performance and myocardial oxygen consumption before any observable decrease in adenosine triphosphate (ATP) or myocardial pH occurs, and before significant lactate production begins. These balanced reductions in ventricular performance and oxygen consumption without the traditional metabolic markers of ischemia were felt to provide a model for hibernating myocardium, in that reduction of contractility appeared to be directly related to reduced tissue oxygen delivery.

Evidence confirming that restoration of flow to hibernating myocardium results in restoration of function continues to accumulate (67). Topol et al. demonstrated improved wall thickening by transesophageal echo immediately after surgical revascularization in 20 patients undergoing CABG

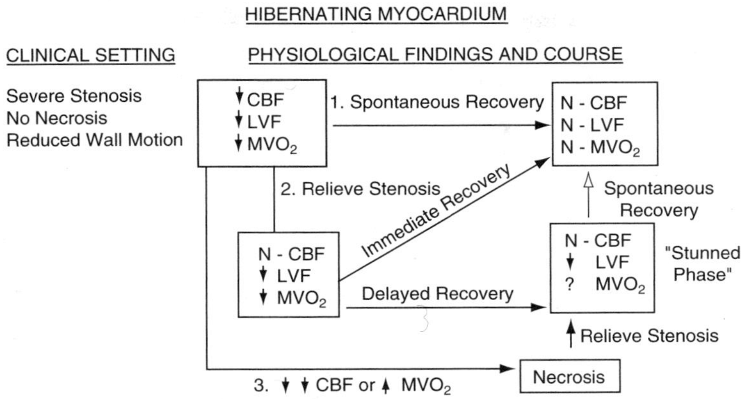

HIBERNATING MYOCARDIUM

CLINICAL SETTING

Severe Stenosis
No Necrosis
Reduced Wall Motion

PHYSIOLOGICAL FINDINGS AND COURSE

↓CBF
↓LVF
↓MVO_2

1. Spontaneous Recovery

N - CBF
N - LVF
N - MVO_2

2. Relieve Stenosis

Immediate Recovery

Spontaneous Recovery

N - CBF
↓ LVF
↓ MVO_2

Delayed Recovery

N - CBF
↓ LVF
? MVO_2

"Stunned Phase"

↑Relieve Stenosis

3. ↓ ↓ CBF or ↑ MVO_2

Necrosis

Figure 17-6 Stunned myocardium occurs in the clinical setting of severe, acute-onset coronary occlusion, which results in necrosis of myocardium in the region at risk. The occlusion is relieved when the myocardium is reperfused; however, reduced myocardial wall motion exists in the region at risk in the viable myocardium. Physiologically, coronary blood flow may be normal or slightly reduced in this stunned region, LV function is reduced, and myocardial consumption may be reduced. There are two possible consequences or courses to these findings. The first is spontaneous recovery, in which case coronary blood flow normalizes as LV function normalizes and myocardial oxygen consumption normalizes. However, in the course of a persistent, severe residual coronary stenosis that persists after reperfusion, there may be delayed recovery. Hence, the stunned myocardium may progress to a phase that is indistinguishable from the hibernating myocardium (i.e., reduced coronary blood flow, reduced LV function, and reduced oxygen consumption). Thus, stunned myocardium may go through a hibernation phase. With time, the hibernation phase may undergo delayed recovery as coronary blood flow is normalized and the stenosis is relieved. N, normal.

(68). Tillisch et al. showed improved wall motion after revascularization in 35 of 41 ischemic myocardial segments with preserved glucose uptake on positron emission tomography, whereas 24 of 26 segments without glucose uptake failed to improve (69). In a 3-year follow-up study of 70 patients with CAD and depressed LV function who underwent CABG, Pagley et al. found that the extent of viable myocardium, as determined by preoperative thallium 201 scintigraphy, was the only independent predictor of cardiac event-free survival (70). Meluzin et al. showed that in revascularized patients with CAD and moderate or severe LV dysfunction, the presence of a large amount of dysfunctional but viable myocardium identified patients with the best prognosis (71) (Fig. 17-7). In a meta-analysis of 24 studies involving 3,088 patients with depressed LV function, patients with documented viability by thallium perfusion imaging, positron emission tomography (PET) scanning, or dobutamine echocardiography had a significant 80% reduction in annual mortality with revascularization (3.2% versus 16% for medical therapy). The degree of LV dysfunction was directly related to the magnitude of benefit (72).

Table 17-3 shows the difference between stunned and hibernating myocardium (73). However, extensive data now suggest that, in contrast to the conceptual models, stunned and hibernating myocardium frequently coexist, and differentiating chronic hibernation from repetitive stunning may be extremely difficult. The degree of impairment of coronary flow reserve may well be the conceptual link between stunning and hibernating myocardium (64). In an animal model with a single epicardial stenosis, 52 miniswine had blood flow and fluorodeoxyglucose PET studies as well as dobutamine stress echocardiography. Of 303 myocardial segments studied, 182 were classified as hibernating and 92 as stunned. Hibernating segments showed greater resting ischemia and poorer resting wall motion. Hibernation and stunning frequently occurred in different segments of the same vessel distribution (74).

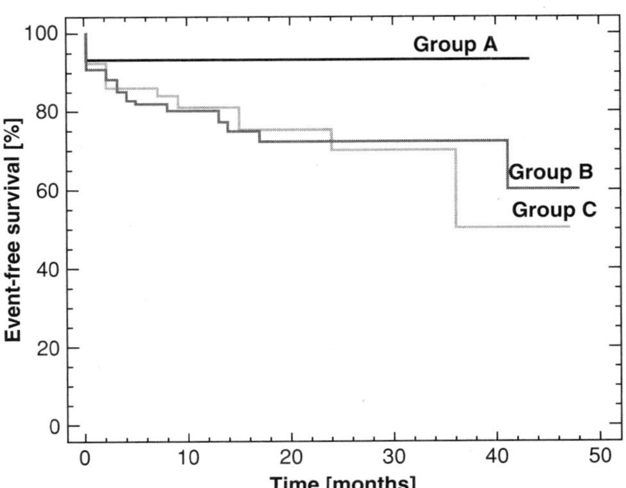

Figure 17-7 Kaplan-Meier curves showing survival free of cardiac events (including death, nonfatal MI, unstable AP requiring hospitalization, and hospitalization for heart failure) in patients with left ventricular dysfunction. Group A comprised patients with a large amount of dysfunctional but viable myocardium (six or more dysfunctional but viable myocardial segments); group B included patients with a small amount of dysfunctional by viable myocardium (two to five dysfunctional but viable segments); and group C comprised patients in whom dysfunctional myocardium was irreversibly damaged.

TABLE 17-3
DIFFERENTIATION BETWEEN HIBERNATION AND STUNNING

	Stunned	Hibernating
Response to inotropes	↑ then ↓↓	↑
Glycolysis	↓↓	↓
Rest blood flow	↓	Normal
Coronary flow reserve	↓↓	↓
Post revascularization Recovery	↑↑	↑↑

Adapted from Redwood SR, Ferrari R, Marber MS. Myocardial libernation and stunning: from physiological principles to clinical practice. *Heart.* 1998;80:218–222.

As in many other areas of heart failure, recent basic investigations have focused on changes in gene expression and proteins in hibernating tissue. In biopsy specimens from surgical patients, myocardial segments that showed recovery of function with revascularization had higher expression of the embryonal form of smooth myosin heavy chain and a higher ratio of α-smooth muscle actin to collagen compared to segments that did not recover. Tenascin, a marker of remodeling activity, was also higher in the segments that recovered (75). In both patients and animal models, Depre et al. have shown upregulation of genes and the product proteins involved in antiapoptosis (76).

Extensive clinical and laboratory evidence supports the concepts of myocardial stunning and hibernation (77). In many patients with heart failure due to CAD, the interaction of these mechanisms in the context of chronic CAD leads to potentially reversible sustained depression of myocardial function and initiates the neurohormonal spiral of clinical heart failure. Most important, successful revascularization may lead to prompt functional improvement and better long-term outcomes.

Remodeling: Recovery and Healing of Ischemia-Related Injury

The process of alteration in ventricular geometry following ischemic myocardial injury is complex, but for simplicity of discussion can be divided into two different phases: infarct expansion and ventricular remodeling. Although neither of these occurs during active ischemia, both contribute to the progression of clinical heart failure following myocardial infarction.

Infarct Expansion

Infarct expansion describes the increase in ventricular size that occurs as a result of acute stretching, thinning, and dilation of the injured myocardial segment. Erlebacher et al. studied 27 patients with acute anterior MI with two-dimensional echocardiography and localized early LV dilation to the infarct zone (78). In follow-up, six of eight patients with infarct expansion were New York Heart Association (NYHA) Class II or worse, but only one of seven without infarct expansion had limiting symptoms. Expansion early after infarction is more common in Q-wave infarction than non-Q-wave infarction, and in first infarctions as compared with reinfarctions (79).

Ventricular Remodeling

In contrast to the acute and localized process of infarct expansion, remodeling refers to chronic global shape changes in the LV following a regional injury (Figs. 17-8 and 17-9) (80). Remodeling begins early after MI and continues well beyond the usually recognized convalescent phase. McKay et al. studied 30 patients with a first MI acutely and at 2 weeks after MI with LV angiography (81). In patients showing a more than 20% increase in LV end-diastolic volume at 2 weeks, the endocardial perimeter of the infarct segment increased 13% and the noninfarcted segments 19%, suggesting that early dilation is associated with later remodeling of the entire LV. Jeremy et al. first studied 50 MI patients with serial radionuclide angiograms over 6 months (82). Eleven patients had dilated LVs within 10 days and 10 more had dilated by 6 months. Eight of these 21 patients, all of whom had anterior MI, showed progressive dilation with a decrease in LVEF from 35% ± 6% to 24% ± 10%. Risk factors for progressive dilation included larger infarct size, early infarct expansion, persistently occluded infarct-related artery, and myocardial dysfunction due to ischemia.

Open-Artery Hypothesis

Clinical studies after thrombolytic therapy of MI have suggested a significant improvement in long-term survival with restoration of antegrade flow in the infarct-related artery, even when reperfusion occurs after the time when cell death would have occurred. In patients who were reperfused late after MI, LV function did not improve but mortality was reduced from 36% in patients with partial or no reperfusion to 5% in patients with complete restoration of flow. Similar clinical findings were evident with even later therapy (83).

In a rat model (84), after ligation of the left coronary artery, no difference in infarct size was demonstrated between animals with ligature release at 2 hours and those with permanent ligation. However, infarct expansion was significantly inhibited in the reperfused group, with fewer than 20% showing marked expansion as against 60% in the permanent ligation group.

These clinical and laboratory findings underlie the "open artery hypothesis" (i.e., patients benefit from a

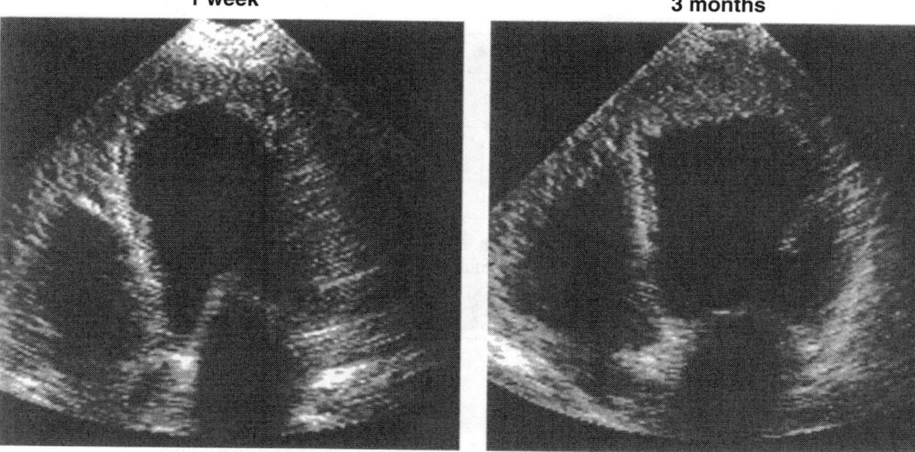

Figure 17-8 Left ventricular (LV) remodeling after transmural anteroseptal myocardial infarction (MI): two-dimensional echocardiographic evaluation at 1 week and 3 months. (Adapted from Sutton MG, Sharpe N. Left ventricular remodeling after myocardial infarction: pathophysiology and therapy. *Circulation.* 2000;101:2989–2990.)

patent infarct-related artery, even if restoration of antegrade flow occurs after the time when revascularization could salvage myocardium). It seems likely that the significant benefits from continued patency are mediated by reduction in infarct expansion and remodeling associated with the restoration of blood flow.

Pharmacologic Modification of Remodeling

Early pharmacologic intervention to block neurohormonal activation after myocardial infaction reduces ventricular remodeling and now represents the standard of care. LeJemtel et al. have reviewed the role of angiotensin-converting enzyme (ACE) inhibition and β-adrenergic blockade in attenuating and reversing remodeling (85), and Jugdutt has extensively reviewed the evidence that nitrates also may favorably influence this process (86). More recently, both laboratory studies and clinical trials have shown benefit from direct aldosterone inhibition with spironolactone or eplerenone. In a rat model, eplerenone, either alone or in addition to ACE inhibition, reduced the rise in left ventricular end-diastolic pressure (LVEDP) and left ventricular end-diastolic volume (LVEDV) seen in control animals and prevented increases in collagen type I along with a variety of other metabolic changes associated with myocardial hypertrophy and fibrosis (87). In a series of 57 patients studied acutely after a first MI, cardiac extraction of aldosterone was correlated with biochemical markers of fibrosis and with LVEDV index after 1 month (88). In a subsequent clinical trial, the investigators studied 134 patients with a first anterior acute MI. In these patients, the combination of spironolactone and ACE inhibitor prevented remodeling more effectively than an ACE inhibitor alone (89). The evidence to date indicates that ventricular remodeling represents the anatomic consequences of neurohormonal activation, largely mediated by direct effects of aldosterone on the heart. This process links the initial acute ischemic insult to long-term structural changes in heart failure, and the prospect of meaningful pharmacologic intervention is truly exciting.

Negative Feedback Cycles Associated with Ischemia and Heart Failure

Patients with cardiac failure due to CAD often deteriorate clinically in gradually worsening cycles. Impairment of systolic and, particularly, diastolic function further compromises subendocardial perfusion because elevation of LV diastolic pressure diminishes the diastolic transcoronary perfusion gradient (90). When abnormal resistance to diastolic flow is imposed by epicardial conduit vessel disease, this impairment of diastolic perfusion becomes even more severe (Fig. 17-10). Loss of diastolic perfusion time associated with compensatory tachycardia further compromises myocardial perfusion as stroke volume decreases (91–94). Atrial pacing in patients with CAD and normal resting LV function can induce wall motion abnormalities and lactate production (94). Ferro et al. have shown the importance of diastolic perfusion time as an index of myocardial oxygen supply in exercise stress and atrial pacing studies of ischemic threshold (95). Testing upright and supine, with and without therapy and pacing stress, diastolic perfusion time and ischemic threshold remained relatively constant. These observations, along with extensive laboratory studies reviewed by Crawford (96), suggest that heart rate-related limitation of subendocardial blood flow may be an important mechanism in the pathogenesis of exercise-induced ischemia. Under stress, the poorly perfused and poorly functioning ventricle enters into a negative feedback cycle of worsening ischemia-related dysfunction (Fig. 17-11).

In this setting, primary pump dysfunction leads to activation of multiple neurohormonal mechanisms that further

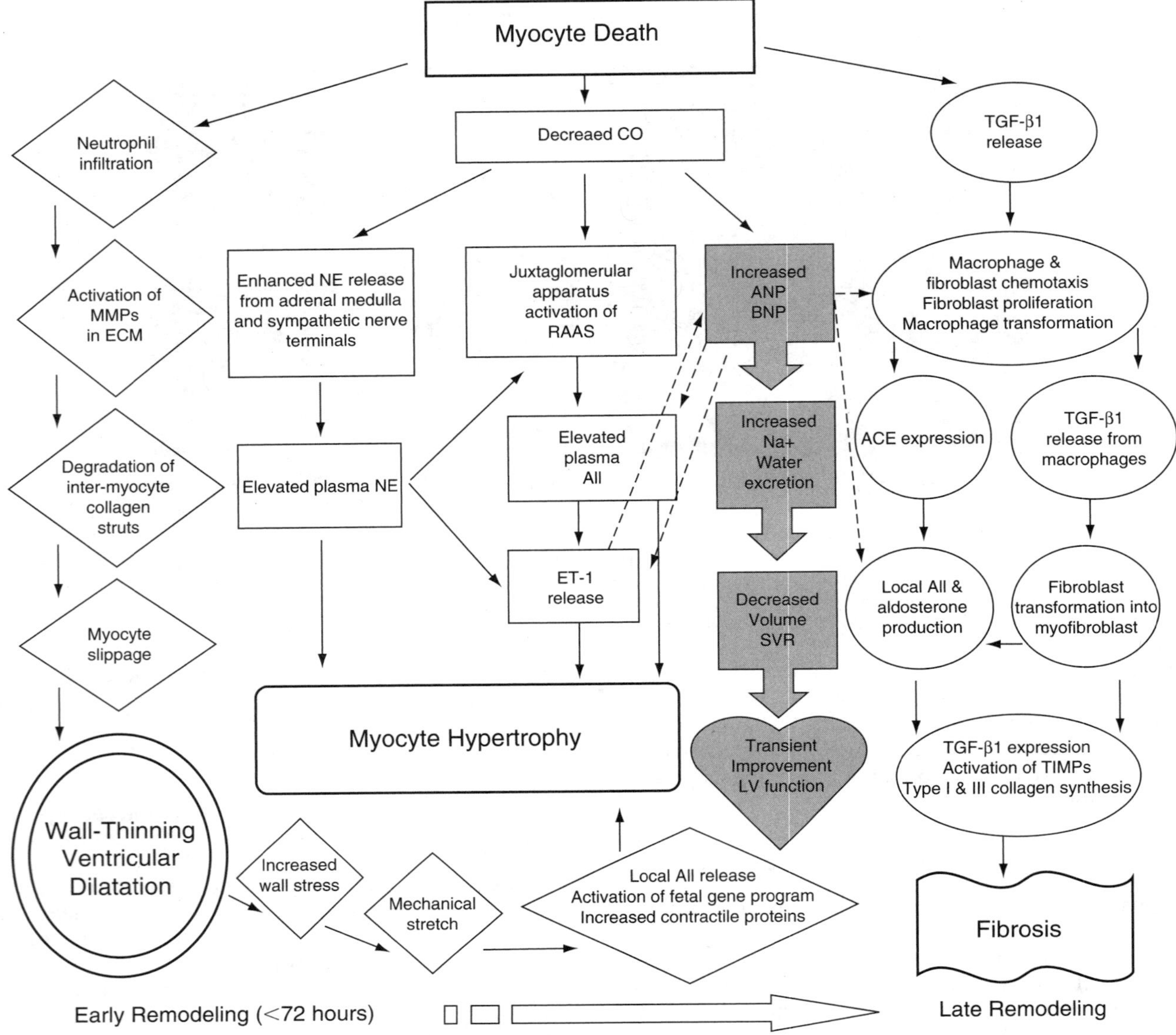

Figure 17-9 Diagrammatic representation of the many factors involved in the pathophysiology of ventricular remodeling. (Adapted from Sutton MG, Sharpe N. Left ventricular remodeling after myocardial infarction: pathophysiology and therapy. *Circulation*. 2000; 101:2989–2990.)

adversely load the failing heart. With better understanding of the pathophysiology of heart failure, it has become clear that the heart has a major role in regulation of salt and water balance. When salt and water retention impose the additional loads of increased systemic vascular resistance and high filling pressures on a heart limited by systolic and diastolic dysfunction, overt heart failure ensues.

ACQUISITION OF CLINICAL DATA

Cinical decisions in the management of heart failure due to CAD are primarily influenced by three parameters:

1. An estimate of the relative proportions of:
   a. Viable but ischemic myocardium
   b. Nonviable myocardium
   c. Viable nonischemic myocardium
2. The technical feasibility of successful mechanical revascularization
3. The extent and severity of comorbidities in the individual patient

Each patient's assessment requires acquisition and integration of relevant clinical, noninvasive, and catheterization data. Two principles should guide this activity. First, Bayesian analysis requires understanding that the data derived from any test reflect the pretest likelihood of disease as well as the sensitivity and specificity of the test. Second, the cost and risk of acquiring information that will not be acted upon are unacceptable. Table 17-4 outlines the assessment of these patients.

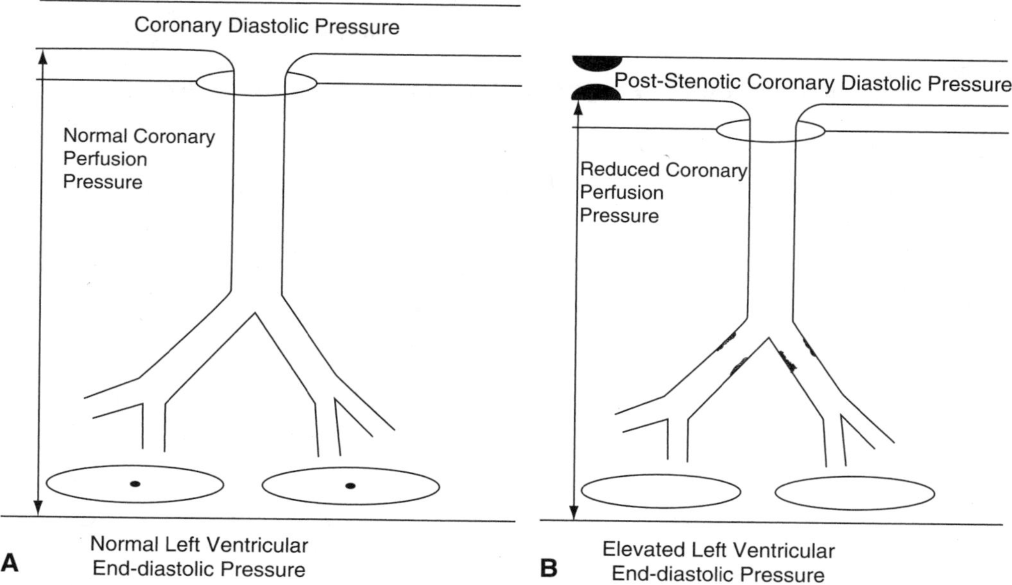

Figure 17-10 Reduction in myocardial perfusion due to coronary artery stenosis and elevated LV diastolic pressure.

Clinical Assessment

History and Physical Examination

The dire natural history of heart failure due to CAD justifies a thorough search for opportunities to intervene in most patients. A meticulous history and physical examination remain the foundation of the clinical assessment. Typical exertional angina pectoris remains an important clue to the possibility of reversible ischemia. On the other hand, the absence of angina does not exclude silent ischemia as a cause of impaired LV function. Diabetic patients, hypertensives, and the elderly often have asymptomatic ischemia and unrecognized infarction. In diabetic patients with coronary disease undergoing treadmill exercise testing, Ranjadayalan et al. demonstrated increased time from onset of 0.1 mm ST-segment depression to angina (97). They suggested that repetitive asymptomatic ischemic episodes in these patients might predispose them to heart failure.

In order to put risk–benefit issues into context, a complete history should always include an assessment of the patient's NYHA functional classification. Mortality increases dramatically with the transition from stable NYHA Class I–II status to Class II–IV symptoms.

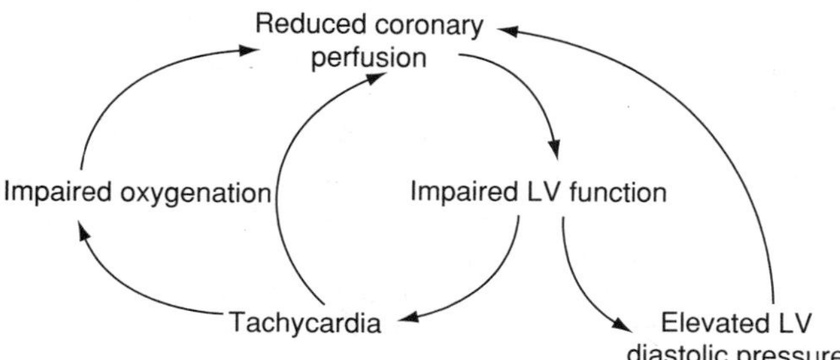

Figure 17-11 Negative feedback cycles in coronary disease with LV dysfunction.

The physical examination must include accurate vital signs: height, weight, blood pressure in both arms, an ankle-brachial index, and body mass index. The examiner should focus on assessment of filling pressures and LV function, as well as a search for associated comorbidities such as peripheral vascular disease, chronic pulmonary disease, thyroid disease, and anemia. Critical observations include assessment of jugular venous pressure and pulses, including hepatojugular reflux. Jugular V-waves are often the best clue to tricuspid regurgitation. Careful precordial palpation may require patience and placing the patient in the left lateral decubitus position in order to appreciate the sustained impulse characteristic of resting LV dysfunction (98). Documentation of the presence or absence of diastolic filling sounds, evaluation of the intensity of the pulmonic second sound, and appreciation of mitral and tricuspid regurgitant murmurs will also provide clues as to resting hemodynamics and ventricular function. Associated cardiac disease, particularly aortic valve stenosis, may be very difficult to appreciate in low-flow states.

Electrocardiogram

The standard resting 12-lead electrocardiogram (ECG) provides useful information in many patients with heart failure due to CAD. Prolonged QRS duration (>140 milliseconds) suggests that resynchronization should be considered. Uncontrolled tachycardia or a rapid ventricular response to atrial fibrillation may contribute to reversible ischemic cardiac dysfunction by increasing myocardial oxygen requirements and decreasing diastolic perfusion time. Definite Q-wave infarction confirms the clinical diagnosis of CAD. However, in a small series of 17 patients, 57% of pathological Q-wave infarction regions showed PET evidence of glucose uptake consistent with reversibility (99). Q-waves associated with persistent ST-segment elevations are highly specific for focal wall motion disorders (ventricular aneurysm) (100), but even this ECG pattern does not exclude

TABLE 17-4
EVALUATION OF CONGESTIVE HEART FAILURE SECONDARY TO CORONARY ARTERY DISEASE

A. History and physical examination
  a. Check for angina, coronary disease risk factors, functional capacity estimation
  b. Accurate vital signs: height, weight, blood pressure in both arms, an ankle-brachial index, and body mass index
  c. Jugular venous pressure and pulses, including hepatojugular reflux
  d. Precordial palpation
  e. Check for diastolic filling sounds, evaluation of the intensity of the pulmonic second sound, and appreciation of mitral and tricuspid regurgitant murmurs
B. ECG
  a. Rhythm
  b. QRS duration
  c. Q-waves
C. Chest X-ray
  a. Cardiac enlargement
  b. Pulmonary congestion
D. Assessment of viability
  a. Dobutamine echo
  b. Nuclear (SPECT or PET)
  c. MRI
E. Echocardiography
  a. LV function
  b. Wall motion abnormalities
  c. Mitral regurgitation
  d. Aortic stenosis
  e. Pulmonary artery pressure
  f. Aneurysms
F. Exercise testing
  a. Functional capacity assessmment
G. Electrophysiological evaluation
  a. Cardiac resynchronization therapy
  b. Implantable defibrillators
  c. Rhythm abnormalities management
H. Cardiac catheterization
  a. Coronary artery evaluation
  b. Right heart catheterization (volume status)
  c. Pulmonary artery resistance assessment

myocardial viability in the infarct distribution; in a series of 132 patients with chronic anterior Q-wave infarction, 63% of those with chronic ST-elevation and 56% of those without had viable myocardium in the infarct zone (101).

Chest X-Ray

The posteroanterior (PA) and lateral chest x-ray may give confirmatory evidence of cardiac enlargement and pulmonary congestion when abnormalities are present, but chronic heart failure patients may have severe LV systolic dysfunction and passive pulmonary hypertension with remarkably benign chest films. A normal cardiac silhouette with pulmonary congestion suggests radiographic evidence of diastolic dysfunction, possibly due to CAD and reversible ischemia.

Noninvasive Assessment of Myocardial Viability

All major guidelines for heart failure management support an initial quantitative evaluation of LV function (102). Beyond that first step, the noninvasive laboratory assessment of patients with heart failure due to CAD should be planned to objectively demonstrate viability and ischemia with clinically useful reproducibility, specificity, and sensitivity in a cost-effective manner. This requires choosing from a variety of imaging options including echocardiography, radionuclide techniques, and MRI.

Contractile reserve is the echocardiographic surrogate for metabolic activity. Contractile reserve indicates an improvement in systolic function in a hypocontractile segment in response to low-dose (5–15 μg/kg per minute) dobutamine infusion. Hypocontractile function at rest with initial low-dose improvement and then deterioration of function with higher dobutamine doses constitutes a biphasic response, consistent with hibernating myocardium. In the echocardiographic laboratory, sets of similar images obtained at rest, with low-dose and high-dose dobutamine, and after infusion are compared, usually by visually inspecting a split-screen display of the same echo projection with all four states at once. Image quality depends on technical expertise, and accurate interpretation is dependent on physician experience. Technical improvements, including myocardial contrast and tissue Doppler techniques, may soon offer further improvement in echocardiographic viability assessment.

Using radionuclide techniques, decreased resting regional myocardial blood flow may be demonstrated on perfusion images, usually obtained by single-photon emission computed tomographic (SPECT) imaging of thallium 201 or technetium 99m MIBI. A second set of metabolic images is then required to assess viability of the hypoperfused areas. Metabolic images may be generated with one of two approaches. By allowing the original tracer to redistribute into myocardium with or without a second reinjection, where it binds to mitochondrial membranes in viable tissue, a late viability image can be obtained for a rest/redistribution study. Alternatively, a positron imaging agent, usually fluorine 18 fluorodeoxyglucose (FDG), actively accumulated by viable myocardium, can be used to produce PET viability images for a perfusion/metabolic study. In either situation, the end-product of the study will be two sets of images that are compared for concordant or discordant segmental defects. Again, image comparability depends on careful technique and interpretation depends on physician experience.

Despite an extensive clinical literature on viability assessment, in a systematic review Bax et al. found only 37 studies published between 1980 and early 1997 with sufficient detail for calculating sensitivity and specificity to compare imaging techniques (103). Their sensitivity/specificity analysis showed that sensitivity for prediction of functional recovery after revascularization is high for all techniques reviewed. Specificity was highest, however, for low-dose dobutamine echo (LDDE) and was lowest for the thallium studies. They concluded that the available evidence favors the use of LDDE as the technique of first choice for prediction of regional functional recovery. It is important to emphasize that no studies with FDG-SPECT and perfusion imaging were included in this review. Figure 17-12 shows the sensitivity and specificity of dobutamine stress echocardiography (DSE) and nuclear imaging (Nuclear) techniques based on pooled data from 11 studies ($n = 325$ patients) that performed a direct comparison between DSE and nuclear imaging to predict improvement in regional LV function after revascularization. The sensitivity of the nuclear techniques was significantly higher as compared to DSE, whereas the specificity of DSE was significantly higher (104).

Bax et al. also evaluated the combination of ^{201}Th SPECT perfusion images and FDG-SPECT metabolic images (with hyperinsulinemic euglycemic clamping) in 55 patients with LV dysfunction. They found that 19 patients with three or more viable dysfunctional myocardial segments had significant increases in LVEF, from 28% ± 8% to 35% ± 9%, after revascularization (CABG or PTCA). In 36 patients with fewer than three viable dysfunctional segments, LVEF remained unchanged after revascularization. They concluded that FDG-SPECT imaging effectively identified patients in whom LV function improved after revascularization (105).

Srinvasan et al. have compared FDG uptake measured by PET with FDG-SPECT and thallium-SPECT in 28 patients with CAD and impaired LVEF (33% ± 15%). They found good overall concordance and concluded that FDG-SPECT significantly increased sensitivity for viability detection as compared with thallium (106). In a companion editorial review, Udelson concluded that ^{201}Th/18-FDG perfusion/metabolic SPECT data had more powerful predictive value for functional recovery in dysfunctional myocardium than did thallium reinjection or LDDE studies (107).

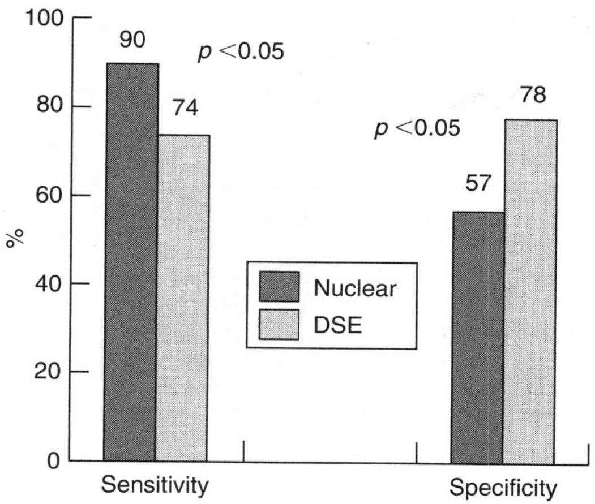

Figure 17-12 Sensitivity and specificity of dobutamine stress echocardiography (DSE) and nuclear imaging (Nuclear) techniques (based on pooled data from 11 studies ($n = 325$ patients) that performed a direct comparison between DSE and nuclear imaging to predict improvement in regional LV function after revascularization. The sensitivity of the nuclear techniques was significantly higher as compared to DSE, whereas the specificity of DSE was significantly higher. (From Bax JJ, Poldermans D, Elhendy A, et al. Sensitivity, specificity, and predictive accuracies of various noninvasive techniques for detecting hibernating myocardium. *Curr Probl Cardiol.* 2001;26:141–186.)

MRI techniques can also be used in viability assessment, using dobutamine stress (33), strain maps (108), or radiofrequency tissue tagging (109). Hyperenhancement on delayed enhancement MRI indicates irreversible ischemic injury (110). In short, cardiac MRI appears to have great potential for noninvasive assessment of ischemic heart disease. The primary limitations today are related to the cost of the equipment and limited availability of the technique.

In practice, institutional factors, including availability of imaging equipment and the technical expertise of echocardiographic interpretation, often influence the selection of methods for viability assessment. Nonetheless, viability assessment is critically important. It is estimated that 50% of patients with ischemic heart disease and severely impaired left ventricles have hibernating myocardium (111). Calhoun et al. found that over half of a series of patients with CAD referred for heart transplantation, and over 60% of CAD patients referred for heart failure evaluation, had evidence of substantial myocardial viability using nuclear techniques (112). In an evaluation of 103 patients where PET and SPECT imaging were compared to determine management strategies, no difference in event-free survival was demonstrated between management based on FDG-PET data and that based on stress/rest sestamibi SPECT findings (113).

TABLE 17-5
EXERCISE TOLERANCE TESTING IN HEART FAILURE DUE TO CORONARY ARTERY DISEASE

Diagnostic testing
- Poor exercise tolerance limits usefulness
- Digitalis, diuretics both decrease sensitivity/specificity of ECG changes

Management tool
- Provides quantification of physical capacity (oxygen uptake)
- May help clarify role of inadequate flow reserve in pathogenesis of symptoms
- Quantitates pharmacologic control of heart rate and blood pressure during exercise
- May reassure patient about safety of moderate exercise
- Provides guidelines for exercise prescription

The ability to assess overall ventricular function, evaluate valve function, and estimate hemodynamic status at reasonable cost gives echocardiography great appeal as a primary imaging modality. In a recent study of 100 patients with ischemic cardiomyopathy who had undergone dobutamine stress echocardiography and revascularization, patients with more viable segments had less LV remodeling, improvement of heart failure symptoms, and fewer cardiac events (114). These data support both the concept of revascularization for ischemic LV dysfunction and the utility of echocardiographic assessment. Dobutamine echocardiography offers a reasonable alternative approach to nuclear studies for viability assessment with excellent sensitivity and specificity.

Exercise Testing for Functional Evaluation

As a management tool, when the diagnosis of CAD has been angiographically confirmed, the exercise test is invaluable in the functional assessment of the patient. The information generated includes overall exercise capacity and an evaluation of heart rate/blood pressure product required to evoke ischemia (115–117). Furthermore, with the addition of relatively straightforward online measurements of oxygen consumption, the functional assessment during exercise can be expanded to include determination of maximum oxygen consumption. A substantial body of data, comprehensively reviewed by Jennings and Esler, indicates that functional capacity in patients with heart failure does not correlate with resting hemodynamics or LVEF (116). For example, several studies have shown no correlation between overall functional capacity and pulmonary capillary wedge pressures at rest or during exercise (117,118). As many as one-fifth of patients with impaired systolic function do not show clinical heart failure (119), and in many series as many as half the patients with clinical heart failure do not show impaired systolic function. Thus, the choice and assessment of interventions in heart failure due to CAD require an initial assessment of functional capacity. Table 17-5 compares and contrasts standard exercise tolerance testing as a diagnostic procedure and as a management tool. Figure 17-13 compares the clinical versus functional approaches to the assessment of heart failure, using maximal oxygen uptake. We agree with Stevenson and Miller that functional assessment with determination of maximal oxygen uptake is mandatory for all but the most critically ill cardiac transplant candidates (120).

Electrophysiogical Evaluation

The electrophysiological evaluation of heart failure patients with CAD is beyond the scope of this chapter and is addressed more fully elsewhere in this text. However, as previously noted, control of ventricular rate, particularly in patients with CAD, is critical to effective management of heart failure, and prevention of sudden arrhythmic death in patients at risk is critical to optimal long-term outcomes.

Implantable defibrillator devices are clearly superior to antiarrhythmical drugs for prevention of sudden death in clinical trials. Electrophysiological consultation should be part of the management of almost all our patients. When revascularization is planned, our practice has been to involve the consulting electrophysiologist before surgery to discuss placing epicardial leads for later resynchronization therapy if indicated, and to plan for reassessment after the initial postsurgical recovery.

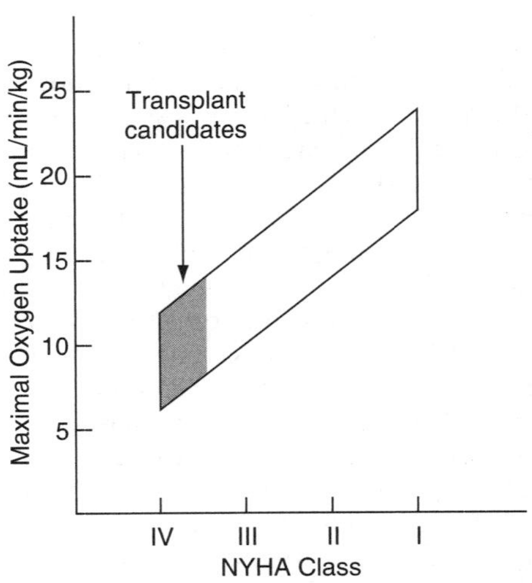

Figure 17-13 Comparison of assessment of heart failure using the NYHA classification versus functional assessment with maximal oxygen uptake.

In heart failure patients with established atrial fibrillation, poor ventricular rate control often contributes to refractory symptoms. Ambulatory monitoring will frequently document wide swings in heart rate ("brady-tachy" response to atrial fibrillation). In this setting, the clinical, pharmacologic, and economic benefits of atrioventricular-nodal ablation and VVI-R pacing are well-established. A recent study suggests that restoration and maintenance of sinus rhythm by catheter ablation without the use of drugs in patients with congestive heart failure and atrial fibrillation significantly improved cardiac function, symptoms, exercise capacity, and quality of life (121).

Catheterization Laboratory Assessment

The continued technical improvement of two-dimensional and Doppler echocardiography, and the use of both intravenous and oral drugs with striking hemodynamic effects, have significantly altered the role of the catheterization laboratory in assessment of patients with heart failure. For many patients, echocardiography adequately defines both LV systolic function and the severity of mitral regurgitation.

In patients with severe congestive symptoms, the risks and benefits of using radiographic contrast with its risk of renal dysfunction and volume shifts must be considered (122). Important procedural preventive measures include the use of low-osmotic contrast and reduction of total contrast volume. For example, contrast ventriculography can often be omitted from the catheterization when echo or nuclear data are adequate to quantify ejection fraction. Recent studies have also shown benefit from pretreatment with N-acetylcysteine (123) and from careful hydration with intravenous solutions of sodium bicarbonate (124). In view of the profound impact of renal dysfunction on prognosis in heart failure (125), every effort to protect renal function in the catheterization laboratory is warranted.

A complete coronary examination should be performed, and in patients undergoing catheterization for evaluation of heart failure a right heart catheterization is indicated. Assessments of any transvalvular pressure gradients should be made with the realization that in low-output states small gradients may reflect important valvular obstruction. Inotropes may be required to increase cardiac output acutely and allow more accurate assessment. Low cardiac outputs determined by the indicator dilution technique should be confirmed at least by measurement of pulmonary artery oxygen saturations, if not by a formal Fick method cardiac output measurement. If pulmonary hypertension with elevated pulmonary vascular resistance is present, acute administration of oxygen, vasodilators, and/or inotropes should be considered following pre-existing local protocols to assess reversibility.

If the laboratory has appropriate radiographic equipment, a digital subtraction screening examination of the abdominal aorta and renal and iliac arteries adds substantially to the assessment of many patients with heart failure due to CAD. Useful anatomic data include the state of the renal arteries, the presence or absence of aneurysmal disease in the aorta, and determination of suitability for intra-aortic balloon pump support.

Common pitfalls in the catheterization laboratory assessment include failure to adequately evaluate the proximal subclavian artery in patients with left internal thoracic artery grafts, failure to appreciate the importance of modest systolic pressure gradients across the aortic valve in low-output states, and failure to obtain right heart pressures, particularly when LV diastolic pressures are significantly elevated. The cardiac catheterization study of a heart failure patient must be carefully planned and the catheterization team should clinically evaluate each patient before his or her study (126).

CLINICAL AND SURGICAL DECISIONS

An algorithm for clinical assessment of patients with heart failure due to CAD is outlined in Figure 17-14. Responsible clinicians know that information not acted upon is so-called noise, and avoid generating inappropriate data. If a patient's noncardiac comorbidities preclude intervention, then extensive and expensive evaluation is inappropriate. On the other hand, the benefits of percutaneous revascularization with stent technology and the improvements in functional status with cardiac resynchronization may be dramatic, even in relatively frail elderly patients. The benefits of restoring sufficient cardiac compensation for a member of an older functional couple to remain comfortable and reasonably active in a home environment cannot be overstated.

The growing understanding of the impact of easily measured comorbidities, particularly impaired renal function and peripheral vascular disease, on heart failure outcomes has put even more emphasis on thorough clinical assessment. In an era when targeting costly, high-risk interventions to those individuals most likely to benefit has become critical, multiple lines of evidence suggest that patients with advanced noncardiac disease should not undergo complex procedures. Thoughtful evaluation of the clinical problem, candid discussion with the patient and family, and active involvement of the primary care physi-

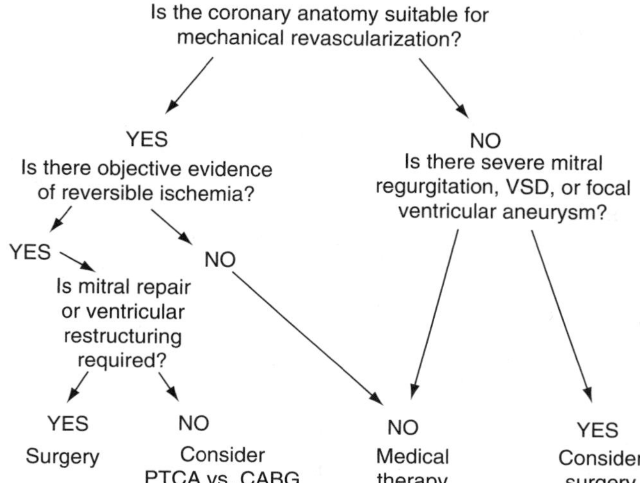

Figure 17-14 A practical approach to the management of heart failure due to CAD.

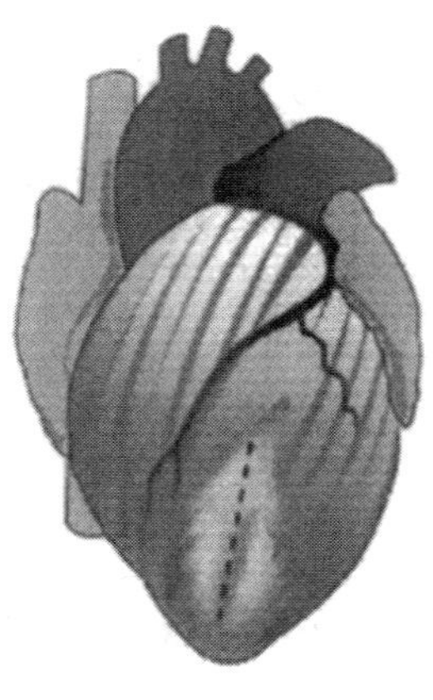

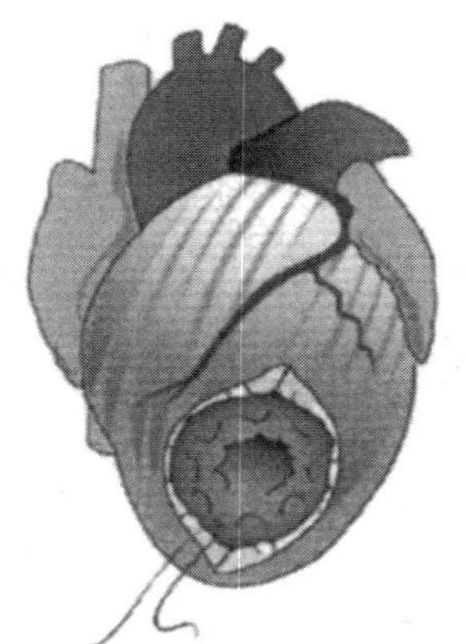

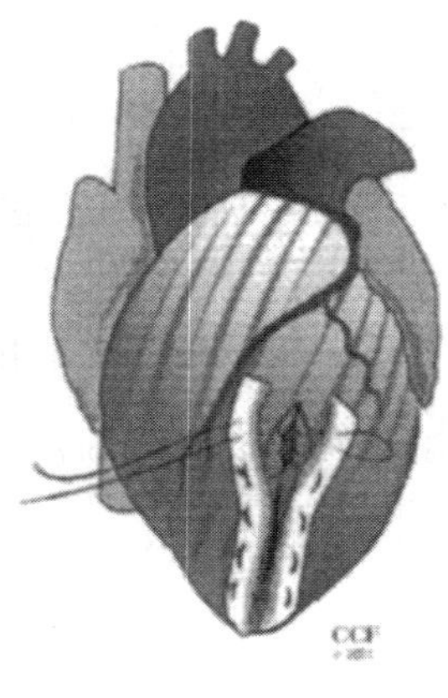

Figure 17-15 Dor procedure. The surgeon makes a small incision into the left ventricle and finds the exact location of the dead or scarred tissue, then places two or more rows of circular stitches around the border of the dead tissue to separate it from healthy muscle tissue. Stitches are then pulled together (like a purse string) to permanently separate the dead tissue from the rest of the heart. (From www.clevelandclinic.org/heartcenter/pub/heartfailure/acorn.htm.)

cian in decision making usually lead to reasonable management decisions.

Surgical Considerations

A number of excellent clinical studies support the contention that revascularization, not resection of nonviable myocardium, provides surgical benefit. Faxon et al. (127) reported the Coronary Artery Surgery Study data on 664 medical and 467 surgical patients with angiographically documented LV aneurysm. In the surgical group, 238 underwent LV resection, most with revascularization, and 229 had revascularization without resection. Medical and surgical survival rates were similar for patients with single- and double-vessel disease. Despite an overall operative mortality of 7.9%, surgical patients with triple-vessel disease had 62% survival at 6 years versus 47% survival in the medical group. LV resection, however, did not influence survival or heart failure symptoms. Akins (128) reported a series of 100 consecutive patients undergoing surgical aneurysmectomy. In 93 patients with anterior aneurysms, survival at just over 3 years was 91.2% in those with associated revascularization and 72% in those without. Louagie et al. (129) reported on 109 patients with heart failure and post-infarct LV aneurysms. Forty-nine had LV resection and 60 were treated medically with no difference in 5-year survival; however, the researchers concluded that left anterior descending revascularization and relief of ischemia were critical to improvement.

A newer approach, surgical infarct exclusion or the Dor procedure, differs from earlier surgical aneurysmectomy techniques in that left ventricular reconstruction with a patch technique attempts to return the ventricle to a more normal size and shape (Fig. 17-15). The difficulties of obtaining long-term data and prospective randomized outcomes data for surgical approaches are formidable. In an observational series of 1,174 referrals for transplant evaluation, 3-year survival in the 217 patients transplanted and the 200 who underwent a variety of nontransplant surgeries, including various combinations and permutations of revascularization, valve repair, and infarct exclusion, was similar at 82% (130).

Another new surgical technique, placement of a passive containment device to prevent progressive cardiac dilation, is currently under investigation. Preliminary data (131) suggest that the device is both safe and effective (Fig. 17-16).

Hemodynamically significant mitral regurgitation occurs frequently in advanced systolic heart failure (132). Dramatic advances in mitral valve repair have led to development of operations combining revascularization with valve repair for ischemic mitral regurgitation. In an analysis of 482 patients with ischemic mitral regurgitation who underwent surgery at the Cleveland Clinic, a relatively better-risk group did significantly better with valve repair. In contrast, outcomes were poor with either technique in the poor-risk group. Overall, the authors felt that about 70% of patients were benefited by valve repair. Failure to use an internal thoracic artery graft, lateral wall motion abnormality, and complex mitral regurgitant jet substantially decreased the benefit of the surgery (133).

After a complete diagnostic assessment, the critical clinical task is integration of data from all sources to determine

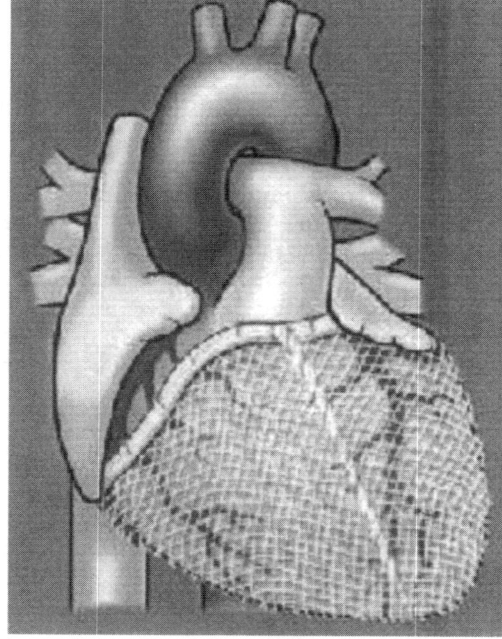

Figure 17-16 A passive containment device, called an Acorn device, to prevent progressive cardiac dilation. (From www.cleveladclinic.org/heartcenter/pub/heartfailure/acorn.htm.)

if there is a role for mechanical revascularization in management. Are there suitable target lesions for PTCA or target vessels for CABG, and is the myocardium in those target distributions likely to be viable? Data from echocardiography, the nuclear laboratory, and the cardiac catheterization laboratory must ultimately fit into an overall functional, metabolic, and anatomic picture. Nothing can substitute for personally reviewing the images and discussing them with the subspecialists involved, including the interventionist or surgeon who may be asked to actually take on the responsibility for revascularization. The objective should be to offer the benefits of PTCA, CABG, or more advanced complex procedures to those patients with impaired LV function who have a reasonable chance of benefit, and to avoid the risks of intervention in those who are unlikely to enjoy improvement.

In a recent editorial, Bach has concisely and elegantly reviewed the concept of myocardial viability and posed a sound argument for revascularization in most patients with good surgical target vessels (134). The management of heart failure due to coronary disease, however, should rest on a solid understanding of the pathophysiology and evidence-based interventions. The authors hope that this chapter will provide that background for their readers.

REFERENCES

1. Gheorgiade M, Bonow RO. Coronary artery disease and chronic heart failure. *Circulation.* 1998;97:282–289.
2. Fonarow GC, ADHERE Scientific Advisory Committee. The Acute Decompensated Heart Failure National Registry (ADHERE): opportunities to improve care of patients hospitalized with acute decompensated heart failure. *Rev Cardiovasc Med.* 2003;(4 Suppl 7):S21–S30.
3. Smith WM. Epidemiology of congestive heart failure. *Am J Cardiol.* 1985;55:3A–8A.
4. Bigger JT. Why patients with congestive heart failure die: arrhythmias and sudden cardiac death. *Circulation.* 1987;75:IV28–IV35.
5. Parmley WW. Pathophysiology and current therapy of congestive heart failure. *J Am Coll Cardiol.* 1989;13:771–785.
6. Franciosa JA, Wilen M, Ziesch S, et al. Survival in men with severe chronic left ventricular failure due to either coronary heart disease or idiopathic dilated cardiomyopathy. *Am J Cardiol.* 1983;51:831–836.
7. Likoff MJ, Chandler SL, Kay HR. Clinical determinants of mortality in chronic congestive heart failure secondary to idiopathic dilated or ischemic cardiomyopathy. *Am J Cardiol.* 1987;59:634–638.
8. Chuah SC, Pellikka PA, Roger VL, et al. Role of dobutamine stress echocardiography in predicting outcome in 860 patients with known or suspected coronary artery disease. *Circulation.* 1998;97:1474–1480.
9. Bart BA, Shaw LK, McCants CB, et al. Clinical determinants of mortality in patients with angiographically diagnosed ischemic or non-ischemic cardiomyopathy. *J Am Coll Cardiol.* 1997;30:1002–1008.
10. O'Connor CM, Velazquez EJ, Gardner LH, et al. Comparison of coronary artery bypass grafting versus medical therapy on long-term outcome in patients with ischemic cardiomyopathy (a 25-year experience from the Duke Cardiovascular Disease Databank). *Am J Cardiol.* 2002;90:101–107.
11. Chilian WC, NHLBI Workshop participants. Coronary microcirculation in health and disease. *Circulation.* 1997;95:522–528.
12. Cannon RO. Does coronary endothelial dysfunction cause myocardial ischemia in the absence of obstructive coronary artery disease? *Circulation.* 1997;96:3251–3254.
13. Gould KL, Lipscomb K, Hamilton GW. Physiologic bases for assessing critical coronary stenosis. *Am J Cardiol.* 1974;33:87–94.
14. Gould KL, Lipscomb K. Effects of coronary stenoses on coronary flow reserve and resistance. *Am J Cardiol.* 1974;34:48–55.
15. Wilson RF, Laughlin DE, Ackell PH, et al. Transluminal, subselective measurement of coronary artery blood flow velocity and vasodilator reserve in man. *Circulation.* 1985;72:82–92.
16. Wilson RF, White CW. Intracoronary papaverine: an ideal coronary vasodilator for studies of the coronary circulation in conscious humans. *Circulation.* 1986;73:444–451.
17. Jennings RB, Murry CE, Steenbergen C, et al. Development of cell injury in sustained acute ischemia. *Circulation.* 1990; 82(Suppl II):2–12.
18. Razeghi P, Young ME, Ying J, et al. Downregulation of metabolic gene expression in failing human heart before and after mechanical unloading. *Cardiology.* 2002;97:203–209.
19. Tan FL, Moravec CS, Li J, et al. The gene expression fingerprint of human heart failure. *Proc Nat Acad Sci USA.* 2002; 99:11387–11392.
20. Margulies KB. Reversal mechanisms of left ventricular remodeling: lessons from left ventricular assist device experiments. *J Card Fail.* 2002;8:S500–S505.
21. DeLemos JA, Morrow DA, Bentley JH, et al. The prognostic value of B-type natriuretic peptide in patients with acute coronary syndromes. *N Engl J Med.* 2001;345:1014–1021.
22. Jernberg T, Stridsberg M, Venge P, et al. N-terminal pro-brain natriuretic peptide on admission for early risk stratification of patients with chest pain and no ST-segment elevation. *J Am Coll Cardiol.* 2002;40:437–445.
23. Mega JL, Morrow DA, DeLemos JA, et al. B-type natriuretic peptide at presentation and prognosis in patients with ST-segment elevation myocardial infarction: an ENTIRE-TIMI-23 substudy. *J Am Coll Cardiol.* 2004;44:335–339.
24. Goetz JP. Pro-BNP-derived peptides in cardiac disease. *Scand J Clin Lab Invest.* 2004;64:497–510.
25. Gradel C, Jain D, Batsford WP, et al. Relationship of scar and ischemia to the results of programmed electrophysiological stimulation in patients with coronary artery disease. *J Nucl Cardiol.* 1997;4:379–386.
26. Stambler BS, Akosah KO, Mohanty PK, et al. Myocardial ischemia and induction of sustained ventricular tachyarrhythmias: evaluation using dobutamine stress echocardiography-electrophysiologic testing. *J Cardiovasc Electrophysiol.* 2004;15:901–907.
27. Yunus A, Gillis AM, Traboulsi M, et al. Effect of coronary angioplasty on precordial QT dispersion. *Am J Cardiol.* 1997;79: 1339–1342.
28. Okishige K, Yamashita K, Yoshinaga H, et al. Electrophysiologic effects of ischemic preconditioning on QT dispersion during coronary angioplasty. *J Am Coll Cardiol.* 1996;28:70–73.
29. Canty JM, Jr., Suzuki G, Banas MD, et al. Hibernating myocardium: chronically adapted to ischemia but vulnerable to sudden death. *Circ Res.* 2004;94:1142–1149.
30. Halkin A, Roth A, Lurie I, et al. Pause-dependent torsade de pointes following acute myocardial infarction: a variant of the acquired long QT syndrome. *J Am Coll Cardiol.* 2001;38: 1168–1174.
31. Kenigsberg DN, Khanal S, Krishnan S. QT prolongation is the most consistent electrocardiographic change seen in patients during balloon occlusion of the coronary artery with percutaneous coronary intervention. *J Am Coll Cardiol.* 2004;43(5): A415.
32. Bonow RO, Vitale DF, Bacharach SL, et al. Asynchronous left ventricular regional function and impaired global diastolic filling in patients with coronary artery disease: reversal after coronary angioplasty. *Circulation.* 1985;71:297–307.
33. Piscione F, Hugenholtz PG, Serruys PW. Impaired left ventricular filling dynamics during percutaneous transluminal coronary angioplasty for coronary artery disease. *Am J Cardiol.* 1987;59: 29–37.
34. Takano H, Glantz SA. Left ventricular contractility predicts how the end-diastolic pressure-volume relation shifts during pacing-induced ischemia in dogs. *Circulation.* 1995;91: 2423–2434.
35. Schalla S, Klein C, Paetsch I, et al. Real time MR image acquisition during high dose dobutamine hydrochloride stress for detecting left ventricular wall-motion abnormalities in

patients with coronary arterial disease. *Radiology.* 2002; 224:845–851.
36. Yao SS, Qureshi E, Syed A, et al. Novel stress echocardiographic model incorporating the extent and severity of wall motion abnormality for risk stratification and prognosis. *Am J Cardiol.* 2004;94:715–719.
37. Murray CE, Jennings RB, Reimer KA. Development of cell injury in sustained ischemia. *Circulation.* 1990;S2(Suppl II):2–12.
38. Yellon DM, Alkhulaifi AM, Pugsley WB. Preconditioning the human myocardium. *Lancet.* 1993;342:276–277.
39. Ottani F, Galvani M, Ferrini D, et al. Prodromal angina limits infarct size. A role for ischemic preconditioning. *Circulation* 1995;91:291–297.
40. Domenech RJ, Macho P, Velez D, et al. Tachycardia preconditions infarct size in dogs. *Circulation.* 1998;97:786–794.
41. Cleveland JC, Meldrum DR, Cain BS, et al. Oral sulfonylurea hypoglycemic agents prevent ischemic preconditioning in human myocardium. *Circulation.* 1997;96:29–32.
42. Piot C, Padmanaban D, Ursell PC, et al. Ischemic preconditioning Decreases apoptosis in rate hearts in vivo. *Circulation.* 1997;96:1598–1604.
43. Eeckhout E. Nicorandil: a drug for many purposes: too good to be true? *Eur Heart J.* 2003;24:1282–1284.
44. Sakai K, Yamagata T, Teragawa H, et al. Nicorandil enhances myocardial tolerance to ischemia without progressive collateral recruitment during coronary angioplasty. *Circ J.* 2002;66:317–322.
45. Matsuo H, Watanabe S, Segawa T, et al. Evidence of pharmacologic preconditioning during PTCA by intravenous pretreatment with ATP-sensitive K+ channel opener nicorandil. *Eur Heart J.* 2003;24:1296–1303.
46. Dekker LRC, Rademaker H, Vermeulen JT, et al. Cellular uncoupling during ischemia in hypertrophied and failing rabbit ventricular myocardium. *Circulation.* 1998;97:1724–1730.
47. Bartling B, Friedrich I, Silber RE, et al. Ischemic preconditioning is not cardioprotective in senescent human myocardium. *Ann Thorac Surg.* 2003;76:105–111.
48. Ghosh S, Standen NB, Galinianes M. Failure to precondition pathological human myocardium. *J Am Coll Cardiol.* 2001;37: 711–718.
49. Lee TM, Su SF, Chou TF, et al. Loss of preconditioning by attenuated activation of myocardial ATP sensitive potassium channels in elderly patients undergoing coronary angioplasty. *Circulation.* 2002;105:334–40.
50. Braunwald E, Kloner RA. The stunned myocardium: prolonged, postischemic ventricular dysfunction. *Circulation.* 1982;66: 1146–1149.
51. Zhao M, Zang H, Robinson TF, et al. Profound structural alterations of the extracellular collagen matrix in postischemic dysfunctional ("stunned") but viable myocardium. *J Am Coll Cardiol.* 1987;10:1322–1334.
52. Patel B, Kloner RA, Przyklenk K, et al. Post-ischemic myocardial "stunning." A clinically relevant phenomenon. *Ann Intern Med.* 1988;108:626–628.
53. Rahimtoola SH. The hibernating myocardium. *Am Heart J.* 1989;117:211–221.
54. Kloner RA, Przyklenk K, Patel B. Altered myocardial states: the stunned and hibernating myocardium. *Am J Med.* 1989;86 (Suppl IA):14–22.
55. Bolli R. Mechanism of myocardial stunning. *Circulation.* 1990;82:723–738.
56. Nelson OL, McEwan MM, Robbins CT, et al. Evaluation of cardiac function in active and hibernating grizzly bears. *J Am Vet Med Assoc.* 2003;223:1170–1175.
57. Wijns W, Serruys PW, Slager CJ, et al. Effect of coronary occlusion during percutaneous transluminal angioplasty in humans on left ventricular chamber stiffness and regional diastolic pressure-radius relations. *J Am Coll Cardiol.* 1986; 7:455–463.
58. Nixon JV, Brown CN, Smitherman TC. Identification of transient and persistent segmental wall motion abnormalities in patients with unstable angina by two-dimensional echocardiography. *Circulation.* 1982;65:1497–1503.
59. Patel B, Kloner RA, Przyklenk K, et al. Post-ischemic myocardial "stunning." A clinically relevant phenomenon. *Ann Intern Med.* 1988;108:626–628.
60. Stack RS, Phillips HR III, Grierson DS, et al. Functional improvement of jeopardized myocardium following intracoronary streptokinase infusion in acute myocardial infarction. *J Clin Invest.* 1983:72:84–95.
61. Reduto LA, Freund GC, Gaetal JM, et al. Coronary artery reperfusion in acute myocardial infarction: beneficial effects of intracoronary streptokinase on left ventricular salvage and performance. *Am Heart J.* 1981;102:1168–1177.
62. Kim SJ, Depre C, Vatner SF. Novel mechanisms mediating stunned myocardium. *Heart Fail Rev.* 2003;8:143–153 .
63. Luss H, Schafers M, Neumann J, et al. Biochemical mechanisms of hibernation and stunning in the human heart. *Cardiovasc Res.* 2002;56:411–421.
64. Camici PG, Dutka DP. Repetitive stunning, hibernation, and heart failure: contribution of PET to establishing a link. *Am J Physiol.* (*Heart Circ Physiol.*) 2001;280:H929–H936.
65. Rahimtoola SH. Importance of diagnosing hibernating myocardium: how and in whom? *J Am Coll Cardiol.* 1997; 30:1701–1706.
66. Keller AN, Cannon PJ, Wolny AC. Effective graded reductions of coronary pressure and flow on myocardial metabolism performance: a model of hibernating myocardium. *J Am Coll Cardiol.* 1991;17:1661–1670.
67. Rahimtoola SH. Importance of diagnosing hibernating myocardium: how and in whom [Comment]. *J Am Coll Cardiol.* 1997;7:1693–1700.
68. Topol EJ, Weiss JL, Guzman PA, et al. Immediate improvement of dysfunctional myocardial segments after coronary revascularization: detection by intraoperative transesophageal echocardiography. *J Am Coll Cardiol.* 1984;4:1123–1134.
69. Tillisch J, Brunken R, Marshall R, et al. Reversibility of cardiac wall motion abnormalities predicted by positron tomography. *N Engl J Med.* 1986;314:884–888.
70. Pagley PR, Beller GA, Watson DD, et al. Improved outcome after coronary bypass surgery in patients with ischemic cardiomyopathy and residual myocardial viability. *Circulation.* 1997;96: 793–800.
71. Meluzín J, Černy J, Frélich M, et al. Prognostic value of the amount of dysfunctional but viable myocardium in revascularized patients with coronary artery disease and left ventricular dysfunction. *J Am Coll Cardiol.* 1998;32:912.
72. Allman KC, Shaw LJ, Hachamovitch R, et al. Myocardial viability testing and impact of revascularization on prognosis in patients with coronary artery disease and left ventricular dysfunction: a meta-analysis. *J Am Coll Cardiol.* 2002;39(7):1151–1158.
73. Redwood SR, Ferrari R, Marber MS. Myocardial hibernation and stunning: from physiological principles to clinical practice. *Heart.* 1998;80: 218–222.
74. Hughes GC, Landolfo CK, Yin B, et al. Is chronically dysfunctional yet viable myocardium distal to a coronary stenosis hypoperfused? *Ann Thorac Surg.* 2001;72:163–168.
75. Frangogiannis NG, Shimoni S, Chang SM, et al. Active interstitial remodeling: an important process in the hibernating human myocardium. *J Am Coll Cardiol.* 2002;39:1468–1474.
76. Depre C, Kim SJ, John AS, et al. Program of cell survival underlying human and experimental hibernating myocardium. *Circ Res.* 2004;95:433–440.
77. Kloner RA, Bolli R, Marban E, et al. Medical and cellular implications of stunning, hibernation, and preconditioning, an NHLBI workshop. *Circulation.* 1998;97:1848–1867.
78. Erlebacher JA, Weiss JL, Weisfeldt ML, et al. Early dilation of the infarcted segment in acute transmural myocardial infarction: role of infarct expansion in acute left ventricular enlargement. *J Am Coll Cardiol.* 1984;4:201–208.
79. Pepine CJ. New concepts in the pathophysiology of acute myocardial ischemia and infarction and their relevance to contemporary management. *Cardiovasc Clin.* 1989;20: 3–18.
80. Sutton MG, Sharpe N. Left ventricular remodeling after myocardial infarction: pathophysiology and therapy. *Circulation.* 2000;101:2989–2990.
81. McKay RG, Pfeffer MA, Pasternak RC, et al. Left ventricular remodeling after myocardial infarction: a corollary to infarct expansion. *Circulation.* 1986;74;693–702.

82. Jeremy RW, Allman KC, Bautovitch G, et al. Patterns of left ventricular dilation during the six months after myocardial infarction. *J Am Coll Cardiol.* 1989;13:304–310.
83. Braunwald E. Myocardial reperfusion, limitation of infarct size, reduction of left ventricular dysfunction, and improved survival. *Circulation.* 1989;79:441–444.
84. Hochman JS, Choo H. Limitation of infarct expansion by reperfusion independent of myocardial salvage. *Circulation.* 1987;75:299–306.
85. LeJemtel TH, Galveo M, Sonnenblick E. Beta-adrenergic blockade reverses while ACE inhibition attenuates left ventricular remodeling in patients with chronic heart failure. *Heart Fail.* 1998;14:57–63.
86. Jugdutt BI. Nitrates and left ventricular remodeling. *Am J Cardiol.* 1998;8:57A–67A.
87. Fraccarollo D, Galuppo P, Hildemann S, et al. Additive improvement of left ventricular remodeling and neurohormonal activation by aldosterone receptor blockade with eplerenone and ACE inhibition in rats with myocardial infarction. *J Am Coll Cardiol.* 2003;42:1666–1673.
88. Hayashi M, Tsutamoto T, Wada A, et al. Relationship between transcardiac extraction of aldosterone and ventricular remodeling in patients with first acute myocardial infarction: extracting aldosterone through the heart promotes ventricular remodeling after acute myocardial infarction. *J Am Coll Cardiol.* 2001;38:1375–1382.
89. Hayashi M, Tsutamoto T, Wada A, et al. Immediate administration of mineralocorticoid receptor anagonist spironolactone prevents post-infarct left ventricular remodeling associated with suppression of a marker of myocardial collagen synthesis in patients with first anterior acute myocardial infarction. *Circulation.* 2003;107:2559–2565.
90. Strauer BE. Functional dynamics of the left ventricle in hypertensive hypertrophy and failure. *Hypertension.* 1984;6:1141–1172.
91. Parker JO, Ledwich JR, West RO, et al. Reversible cardiac failure during angina pectoris. *Circulation.* 1969;39:745–757.
92. Dwyer EM, Jr. Left ventricular pressure-volume alterations and regional disorders of contraction during myocardial ischemia induced by atrial pacing. *Circulation.* 1970;42:1111–1122.
93. Pasterac A, Gorlin R, Sonnenblick EH, et al. Abnormalities of ventricular motion induced by atrial pacing in coronary artery disease. *Circulation.* 1972;45:1195–1205.
94. Kessler KM. Heart failure with normal systolic function. *Arch Intern Med.* 1988;148:2109–2111.
95. Ferro G, Spinelli L, Duillio L, et al. Diastolic perfusion time at ischemic threshold in patients with stress-induced ischemia. *Circulation.* 1991;84:49–56.
96. Crawford MH. Exercise-induced myocardial ischemia importance of coronary blood flow. *Circulation.* 1991;84:424–425.
97. Ranjadayalan K, Umachandran V, Ambepityia G, et al. Prolonged anginal perceptual threshold in diabetes: effect on exercise capacity and myocardial ischemia. *J Am Coll Cardiol.* 1990;16:1120–1124.
98. Mills RM, Kastor JA. Quantitative grading of cardiac palpation. *Arch Intern Med.* 1973;132:831–834.
99. Tillisch J, Brunken R, Marshall R, et al. Reversibility of cardiac wall-motion abnormalities predicted by positron tomography. *N Engl J Med.* 1986;314:884–888.
100. Mills RM, Young E, Gorlin R, et al. Natural history of ST segment elevation after acute myocardial infarction. *Am J Cardiol.* 1975; 35:609–614.
101. Saber W, Obenza-Nishime E, Brunken RC, et al. Does chronic ST segment elevation following Q wave myocardial infarction exclude tissue viability? *Cardiology.* 2003;100:11–16.
102. Young JB, Mills RM. Chapter 12. In: *Clinical Management of Heart Failure.* 2nd ed. West Islip, NY: Professional Communications, Inc.; 2004.
103. Bax JJ, Wijns W, Cornel JH, et al. Accuracy of currently available techniques for prediction of functional recovery after revascularization in patients with left ventricular dysfunction due to chronic coronary artery disease: comparison of pooled data. *J Am Coll Cardiol.* 1997;30:1451–1460.
104. Bax JJ, Poldermans D, Elhendy A, et al. Sensitivity, specificity, and predictive accuracies of various non-invasive techniques for detecting hibernating myocardium. *Curr Probl Cardiol.* 2001;26:141–186.
105. Bax JJ, Cornel JH, Visser FC, et al. Prediction of improvement of contractile function in patients with ischemic ventricular dysfunction after revascularization by fluorine-18 flurodeoxyglucose single-photon emission computed tomography. *J Am Coll Cardiol.* 1997;30:377–383.
106. Srinvasan G, Kitsiou AN, Bacharach SL, et al. Fluorodeoxyglucose single photon emission computed tomography. Can it replace PET and thallium SPECT for the assessment of myocardial viability? *Circulation.* 1998;97:843–838.
107. Udelson JE. Steps forward in the assessment of myocardial viability in left ventricular dysfunction. *Circulation* 1998;97: 833–838.
108. Castillo E, Lima JA, Bluemke DA. Regional myocardial function: advances in MR imaging and analysis. *Radiographics.* 2003;23: S127–S140.
109. Maniar HS, Cupps BP, Potter DD, et al. Ventricular function after coronary artery bypass grafting: evaluation by magnetic resonance imaging and myocardial strain analysis. *J Thorac Cardiovasc Surg.* 2004;128:76–82.
110. Srichai MD, Schvartzman PR, Sturm B, et al. Extent of myocardial scarring on nonstress delayed-contrast-enhancement cardiac magnetic resonance imaging correlates directly with degrees of rest regional dysfunction in chronic ischemic heart disease. *Am Heart J.* 2004;148:342–348 .
111. Al-Mohammad A, Mahy IR, Norton MY, et al. Prevalence of hibernating myocardium in patients with severely impaired ischaemic left ventricles. *Heart.* 1998;80:559–564.
112. Calhoun WB, Mills RM, Drane WE. Clinical importance of viability assessment in chronic ischemic heart failure. *Clin Cardiol.* 1996;5:367–369.
113. Siebelink HM, Blanksma PK, Crijns HJ, et al. No difference in cardiac event-free survival between positron emission tomography-guided and single-photon emission computed tomography-guided patient management: a prospective, randomized comparison of patients with suspicion of jeopardized myocardium. *J Am Coll Cardiol.* 2001;37:81–88.
114. Rizzello V, Poldermans D, Boersma E, et al. Opposite patterns of left ventricular remodeling after coronary revascularization in patients with ischemic cardiomyopathy: role of myocardial viability. *Circulation.* 2004;110:2383–2388 .
115. Szlachcic J, Massie BM, Kramer BL, et al. Correlates and prognostic implication of exercise capacity in chronic congestive heart failure. *Am J Cardiol.* 1985;55:1037–1042.
116. Jennings GL, Esler MD. Circulatory regulation at rest and exercise and the functional assessment of patients with congestive heart failure. *Circulation.* 1990;81:II5–II13.
117. Franciosa JA. Why patients with heart failure die: hemodynamic and functional determinants of survival. *Circulation.* 1987;75: IV20–IV27.
118. Mancini DM, LeJemtel TH, Factor S, et al. Central and peripheral components of cardiac failure. *Am J Med.* 1986;80(Suppl 2B):2–12.
119. Marantz PR, Topin JN, Wasserthiel-Smoller S, et al. The relationship between left ventricular systolic function and congestive heart failure diagnosed by clinical criteria. *Circulation.* 1988;77:607–612.
120. Stevenson LW, Miller LW. Cardiac transplantation as therapy for heart failure. *Curr Prob Cardiol.* 1991;16:219–305.
121. Hsu LF, Jaïs P, Sanders P, et al. Catheter ablation for atrial fibrillation in congestive heart failure. *N Engl J Med.* 2004;351: 2373–2383.
122. Gami AS, Garovic VD. Contrast nephropathy after coronary angiography. *Mayo Clin Proc.* 2004;79:211–219.
123. Birck R, Krzossok S, Markowetz F, et al. Acetylcysteine for prevention of contrast nephropathy: meta-analysis. *Lancet.* 2003; 362: 598–603.
124. Merten GJ, Burgess WP, Gray LV, et al. Prevention of contrast-induced nephropathy with sodium bicarbonate; a randomized controlled trial. *JAMA.* 2004;291:2328–2334.
125. Dries DL, Exner DV, Domanski MJ, et al. The prognostic implications of renal insufficiency in asymptomatic and symptomatic patients with left ventricular dysfunction. *J Am Coll Cardiol.* 2000;35:681–689.
126. Mills RM, Jr., Young JB. Cardiac catheterization in the evaluation of the pre- and post-transplant patient. In: Pepine CJ,

Hill JA, Lambert CR, eds. *Diagnostic and Therapeutic Cardiac Catheterization*. 2nd ed. Baltimore: Williams & Wilkins; 1994.
127. Faxon DP, Myers WO, McCabe CH, et al. The influence of surgery on the natural history of angiographically documented left ventricular aneurysm: the Coronary Surgery Study. *Circulation*. 1986;74: 110–118.
128. Akins CW. Resection of left ventricular aneurysm during hypothermic fibrillatory arrest without aortic occlusion. *J Thorac Cardiovasc Surg*. 1986;91:610–618.
129. Louagie Y, Alouini T, Lesperance J, et al. Left ventricular aneurysm with predominating congestive heart failure. A comparative study of medical and surgical treatment. *J Thorac Cardiovasc Surg*. 1987;94:571–581.
130. Mahon NG, O'Neill JO, Young JB, et al. Contemporary outcomes of outpatients referred for cardiac transplantation evaluation to a tertiary heart failure center: impact of surgical alternatives. *J Card Fail*. 2004;10:273–278.
131. Lembke A, Wiese TH, Dushe S, et al. Effects of passive cardiac containment on left ventricular structure and function: verification by volume and flow measurements. *J Heart Lung Transplant*. 2004;23:11–19.
132. Patel JB, Borgeson DD, Barnes ME, et al. Mitral regurgitation in patients with advanced systolic heart failure. *J Card Fail*. 2004;10:285–291.
133. Gillinov AM, Wierup PN, Blackstone EH, et al. Is repair preferable to replacement for ischemic mitral regurgitation? *J Thorac Cardiovasc Surg*. 2001;122:1125–1141.
134. Bach DS. Viability, prognosis, revascularization, and Pascal. *J Am Coll Cardiol*. 2003;42:2106–2108.

The Cardiomyopathic and Inflammatory Diseases

18

Jeffrey David Hosenpud *Bart L. Cox*

The concept of primary myocardial disease was first suggested in the late nineteenth century by Krehl, who described several cases of "chronic myocarditis" in which autopsied hearts demonstrated myocardial degeneration, hypertrophy, and inflammation (1). The term primary myocardial disease was coined by Josserand and Gallavardin at the beginning of this century (2). However, it was not until 1957 that the term cardiomyopathy was introduced by Brigden to describe myocardial disease of unknown etiology occurring in the absence of coronary disease (3). Subsequently, in 1968, the terminology was specifically defined by the World Health Organization as myocardial disease excluding vascular, hypertensive, and valvular disease. Cardiomyopathy was further subclassified as primary or secondary, depending on whether its causes were unknown or known (4). The definition was further refined in 1980 by a combined task force of the World Health Organization and the International Society and Federation of Cardiology, which exchanged the term secondary cardiomyopathy for specific heart-muscle disease (5). Despite these very specific definitions, the term cardiomyopathy is used by most to denote primary myocardial disease, either of specific or unknown etiology. Unfortunately, it is used by many as a synonym for ventricular dysfunction of any cause (e.g., ischemic cardiomyopathy, valvular cardiomyopathy). For the purposes of this chapter, the term cardiomyopathy will be used to denote diseases of the myocardium of either known or unknown etiology.

Traditionally, the cardiomyopathies have been grouped according to anatomical-physiological rather than etiological features These categories include dilated, hypertrophic, and restrictive cardiomyopathy. The dilated form is most common, and the restrictive form least common. Although this classification does not take into account underlying etiologies, more often than not specific etiologies tend to fall into specific anatomical groupings. Furthermore, this anatomical classification is quite helpful in the medical management of patients with cardiomyopathy, as is described later. Finally, prognosis is more closely linked to anatomical-physiological class rather than specific etiology in most cases.

DILATED CARDIOMYOPATHY

Pathophysiology and Mechanisms of Disease

The primary myocardial defect in patients with dilated cardiomyopathy is an abnormality in contraction. As a result of reduction in myocardial contractility, the heart dilates out of proportion to the degree of hypertrophy, resulting in four-chamber enlargement with relatively thin cardiac walls (6). This increase in radius relative to wall thickness increases myocardial wall stress (7) and decreases subendocardial coronary flow (8), leading to further cardiac dysfunction. Figure 18-1 demonstrates a typical echocardiogram from a patient with dilated cardiomyopathy. The M-mode echocardiogram shows the left ventricle (LV) to be markedly enlarged and systolic function reduced. The two-dimensional echocardiogram from the same patient demonstrates that all four chambers are enlarged.

In most cases of dilated cardiomyopathy, the mechanism(s) for the initial myocardial insult are unknown. Furthermore, it is unclear whether the defect is one of primary individual myocardial cell loss or cell dysfunction followed ultimately by myocardial cell loss and

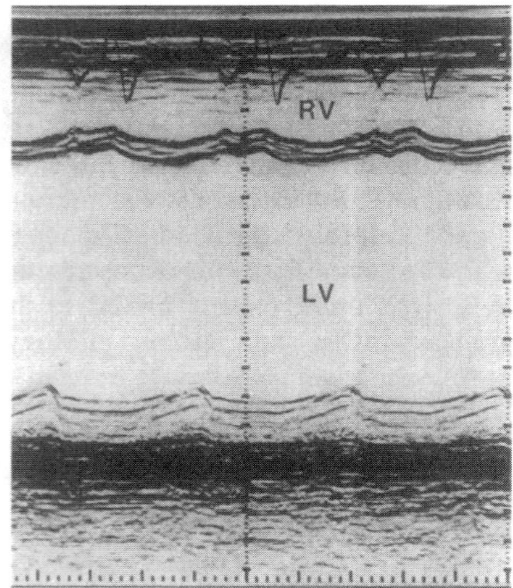

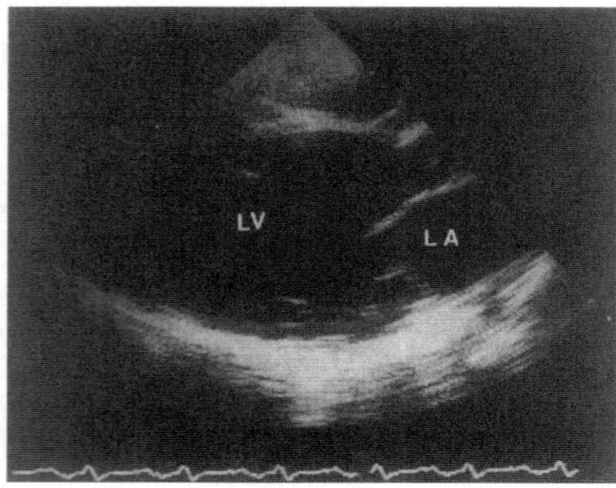

Figure 18-1 An M-mode **(top)** and two-dimensional **(bottom)** echocardiogram from a patient with dilated cardiomyopathy. Note the large chamber sizes and poor systolic contraction. LV, left ventricle; RV, right ventricle; LA, left atrium.

replacement with fibrous connective tissue. A host of molecular, biochemical, and cellular abnormalities have been described in patients with dilated cardiomyopathy. These include alterations in calcium handling by the sarcoplasmic reticulum (9), a reduction β_1-receptor density (10,11), alterations in Gs and Gi proteins (12,13), alterations in cholinergic receptor density and function (14), and expression of altered or fetal myosin subtypes (15). It is not clear, however, whether any of these noted abnormalities is specific to dilated cardiomyopathy or is a more general manifestation of cardiac dilatation and failure.

As previously noted, as early as the late nineteenth century it was hypothesized that cardiomyopathy is the result of chronic inflammatory disease (1). About 80 years later, the concept that dilated cardiomyopathy might be the result of an acute, subacute, or chronic myocarditis again received attention (16). The hypothesis put forth was that a myocardial insult, be it an acute viral infection or toxin, somehow altered the antigenicity of the myocardium so that it was mistaken for foreign tissue and an autoimmune attack was elicited (17). The problem with this hypothesis is that the pieces of the puzzle have been difficult to prove in a convincing way despite major research efforts to support them.

In terms of the initial insult, it has long been appreciated that the coxsackie group B virus is an important pathogen in acute viral myocarditis, and this has provided an excellent model for the study of acute myocarditis in animals. Furthermore, in some murine strains, acute coxsackievirus myocarditis leads to a more chronic myocarditis and cardiac dilation suggestive of dilated cardiomyopathy (18). The difficulty in linking coxsackievirus to human dilated cardiomyopathy has been the inability to identify the virus in cardiac tissue. Serology is nonspecific (19), viral cultures are rarely positive (20), and electron microscopy for viral particles is difficult to interpret. With the recent growth of molecular biological techniques, new methods for viral diagnosis have become available. Bowles et al. (21) utilized in vitro nucleic acid hybridization to study whether enterovirus RNA is present in the myocardium of patients with dilated cardiomyopathy (21). Of the 40 patients studied, 21 had dilated cardiomyopathy and 19 were controls who had heart failure secondary to either coronary disease or congenital heart disease. Enterovirus RNA was detected in the myocardium of 6 of the 21 patients with dilated cardiomyopathy and only one of the controls.

A number of studies have investigated the immunological milieu in dilated cardiomyopathy. Limas and Limas (22) found that HLA-DR4 was represented in 40% of patients with dilated cardiomyopathy, but in only 24% of controls. Koike (23) investigated cell-mediated immune function in 18 patients with dilated cardiomyopathy. In these patients, phytohemagglutinin (PHA)-mediated lymphocyte blastogenesis was reduced; the ratio of $CD4^+$ (helper) to $CD8^+$ (suppressor) lymphocytes was higher; the PHA-mediated release of interleukin-2 (IL-2), a T-cell growth factor, was enhanced; and the number of activated lymphocytes (positive for IL-2 receptor) was reduced in comparison with controls. These data would suggest an inherited predisposition to immunological disease.

Antimyocardial antibodies have been extensively studied during the past several years. However, a link between the presence of antibody and an alteration in cardiac function or metabolism has not been established. In previous studies by Schultheiss et al. (24), an antibody directed against the adenosine diphosphate-adenosine triphosphate (ADP-ATP) carrier protein of the mitochondrial membrane was described in patients with dilated cardiomyopathy. The regulation of β_1-receptors on myocardium in patients with heart failure has been well-described (10). The mechanism for this downregulation is felt to be a negative feedback related to chronically elevated levels of circulating catecholamines, presumably a nonspecific mechanism related to the degree of heart failure. Limas et al. (25) demonstrated that a high percentage of patients with dilated cardiomyopathy, especially those in whom HLA-DR4 was represented, had circulating anti-β_1-receptor autoantibodies. An additional mechanism for modulating cell surface β-receptors specific to dilated cardiomyopathy could therefore be hypothesized.

Mechanisms for the development of dilated cardiomyopathy other than those involving immunological abnormalities have been investigated. Based on their experimental data derived from the Syrian hamster, Factor et al. (27) postulated that some forms of dilated cardiomyopathy are secondary to small-vessel disease and specifically to microvascular spasm. This mechanism is presumed to play an important role in the dilated cardiomyopathy associated with pheochromocytoma (28). A study by Treasure et al. (29) demonstrated that the endothelium-dependent dilation of the coronary microvasculature is impaired in patients who have dilated cardiomyopathy in comparison with controls. Van Hoeven and Factor (30) reviewed endomyocardial biopsy specimens from 145 patients with dilated cardiomyopathy and demonstrated small-vessel thickening in 56% of these patients. This was not a specific finding, however, as a significant proportion of patients with hypertension, diabetes, unexplained arrhythmias, and chest pain syndromes had similar changes.

Direct myocardial toxicity is suggested for alcohol-induced cardiomyopathy (31) and is clearly present in anthracycline-induced dilated cardiomyopathy (31–33). Although alcohol is a potent depressant of myocardial function in the muscle bath, the variable effects of alcohol on the myocardium in vivo are poorly understood. Although several mechanisms (to be discussed later) have been suggested for anthracycline cardiotoxicity, there is at least a dose-related effect of anthracyclines on cardiac function.

What is becoming increasingly clear is that many of the idiopathic dilated cardiomyopathies have a genetic basis and, with more extensive screening, appear to be familial. This is a fairly new concept as, historically, most considered dilated cardiomyopathy to be sporadic in nature, unlike well-defined genetic diseases such as hypertrophic cardiomyopathy, which will be discussed later in this chapter. In fact, familial disease was found in as high as 48% of patients with apparent idiopathic cardiomyopathy when cardiac enlargement by echocardiography was used as a marker for early cardiomyopathy (34). Other studies using echo and other screening have suggested prevalences in the 25% to 35% range depending on the criteria used (35,36).

A recent review of the subject of familial dilated cardiomyopathy discusses these prior investigations as well as the specific genetic abnormalities identified to date. Ninety percent of familial dilated cardiomyopathy appear to be inherited with autosomal dominance, with 16 gene mutations identified. Defects in the lamin A/C or β-myosin heavy chain account for between 5% to 10%, with abnormalities in actin and desmin being less common (37). X-linked familial cardiomyopathy usually secondary to defects in the dystrophin gene may account for between 5% and 10% of familial dilated cardiomyopathy and is usually also associated with skeletal muscle involvement (muscular dystrophies). Rarely, autosomal recessive inheritance patterns have been described, as in one family with a mutation in the cardiac troponin I gene (37).

In most cases, proof of a genetic cause of a cardiomyopathy has a limited impact on the treatment of the index patient. Gene therapy, referring to the introduction of altered or foreign genes into human tissues for the purpose of correcting a genetic defect, is not now feasible for most genetic cardiomyopathies, and there are serious logistic reasons to question whether such treatment will ever be possible or desirable. However, the demonstration that a cardiomyopathy is genetic in origin has important implications beyond those of clinical management, such as the need for family screening to identify other affected persons, or for genetic counseling of affected patients who wish to have children.

Specific Causes or Associations and Dilated Cardiomyopathy

Table 18-1 provides a partial listing of the causes of and conditions associated with dilated cardiomyopathy. Although the list is extensive, in the vast majority of patients there will be no obvious cause of disease.

Duchenne and Becker Muscular Dystrophy, and X-Linked Cardiomyopathy

Duchenne muscular dystrophy, described in 1868 as a "hypertrophic paraplegia of infancy" (38), is an X-linked recessive neuromuscular disorder that affects primarily boys. Clinical manifestations are usually evident by age 5. Progressive muscle weakness is usually first evident in the lower extremities, with involvement of proximal muscles being more marked than that of distal muscles. Calf muscles, and sometimes other muscles as well, become enlarged, partly owing to true muscle hypertrophy and partly because of infiltration of the muscle with fat. Joint contractures develop and walking becomes more and more difficult. Respiratory muscle weakness leads to pulmonary infection and respiratory failure. Intellectual impairment may also occur. Laboratory findings include elevation of creatine kinase and electromyographic abnormalities (39).

Genetic mapping techniques led in 1986 to the cloning and identification of the gene for Duchenne muscular dystrophy (40,41). As previously noted, the product of this gene, called dystrophin (42), is a rod-shaped cytoskeletal protein that is normally found on the cytoplasmic surface of the sarcolemma (43,44). It is known to bind on its amino-terminal end to actin (45) and on its carboxy-terminal end to a membrane-spanning group of proteins called the dystrophin-associated glycoprotein complex (46,47). One

TABLE 18-1
REPORTED CAUSES OF AND ASSOCIATIONS WITH DILATED CARDIOMYOPATHY

Idiopathic
Idiopathic dilated cardiomyopathy
Idiopathic arrhythmogenic right ventricular dysplasia
Valvular disease (mitral regurgitation, aortic regurgitation, aortic stenosis); (valvular cardiomyopathy)
Peripartum or postpartum dysfunction
Familial (hereditary)
Autosomal dominant
Autosomal recessive
X-chromosomal
Polymorphism
Chronic hypertension (hypertensive cardiomyopathy)
Hypersensitivity myocarditis
Toxic
Antiretroviral agents (zidovudine, didanosine, zalcitabine)

of the extracellular components of this complex, named α-dystroglycan, binds to the extracellular matrix protein laminin (48). The result is that dystrophin acts as a link between the cytoskeleton and the extracellular matrix (49). It is therefore theorized that the function of dystrophin is to stabilize the sarcolemma and to protect it from the mechanical stresses of muscle contraction (50).

In patients with Duchenne muscular dystrophy, dystrophin is almost entirely absent from the muscle cell membrane (51,52). The absence of dystrophin from the sarcolemma is thought to expose the membrane to mechanical stress, which leads to abnormal ion fluxes, loss of force transduction across the membrane, and perhaps disruption of the membrane itself (53–55). Genetic studies have demonstrated that a variety of mutations, including deletions, duplications, and point mutations (56–58), can all lead to dystrophin deficiency.

Cardiac involvement has long been recognized to be a feature of Duchenne muscular dystrophy (59,60). Electrocardiograms are often abnormal in childhood (61) and echocardiography demonstrates that LV dysfunction is the rule by age 18 (62,63). Symptomatic congestive heart failure is less common, partly because the patient's progressive motor debility places decreasing demands on cardiac function (64).

The extent of cardiac involvement does not correlate well with the severity of the skeletal muscle disorder (65). The myocardial dysfunction is most marked in the posterobasal LV free wall (66,67); not only is this region of the heart hypokinetic but also its echodensity often appears to be increased, suggestive of fibrosis (68). These observations have led to the hypothesis that myofiber orientation and force distribution in the posterior LV differ from those of the anterior wall, leading to greater and earlier damage to the sarcolemma in the posterior wall in the absence of dystrophin (69). The focal nature of the ventricular dysfunction seen on noninvasive imaging corresponds to the histopathological findings, which include myofibrillar loss and fibrosis most pronounced in the posterobasal LV (70,71). These observations may also explain the typical electrocardiographic features, which include tall R waves in leads V_1 and V_2 and deep, narrow Q waves in the lateral and sometimes inferior leads (72). Although dilated cardiomyopathy is the most common form of disease seen in Duchenne muscular dystrophy, hypertrophic cardiomyopathy is seen in some patients (73). Arrhythmias and conduction disturbances have also been described (74). Because cardiac involvement may contribute to morbidity and may at times be the cause of death, regular screening for cardiac manifestations is recommended (75).

Becker muscular dystrophy is a less-severe form of X-linked muscular dystrophy. The clinical manifestations are similar to those of Duchenne muscular dystrophy but they occur later in life and progress more slowly (76,77). With the identification of the Duchenne muscular dystrophy gene and its protein product, it has been demonstrated that Becker muscular dystrophy is also a consequence of mutations in dystrophin (78,79). Typically, mutations causing Becker muscular dystrophy result in the production of a structurally abnormal dystrophin protein; in contrast, mutations causing Duchenne muscular dystrophy result in a severe quantitative deficiency of the protein (80,81). The clinical course and degree of cardiac involvement in Becker muscular dystrophy are much more variable than in Duchenne muscular dystrophy (82,83). Data suggest that even among sibling pairs with identical dystrophin mutations, the onset of cardiomyopathy is variable and unpredictable (84), and the cardiac dysfunction may precede the evidence of skeletal muscle weakness (85). Cardiac failure is actually a more common cause of death in Becker muscular dystrophy than in Duchenne muscular dystrophy. This may be because the skeletal muscle function of patients with Becker muscular dystrophy is relatively well-preserved, so that they remain more active and place a heavier work load on the myocardium, which leads to a more rapid progression of cardiomyopathy (86,87).

In 1993, Towbin et al. (88) reported that the family originally described by Berko and Swift, as well as another family with X-linked dilated cardiomyopathy, showed evidence of genetic linkage to the 5′ portion of the dystrophin gene locus. This report provided the first evidence that a dilated cardiomyopathy without any skeletal muscle manifestations could be caused by an abnormality of dystrophin. Since then, numerous other families with dystrophin mutations and isolated dilated cardiomyopathy have been described (89–92). Some of these reports have also investigated the abundance and structure of dystrophin in the heart and skeletal muscle of the subject families; both qualitative (93) and quantitative (94) dystrophin abnormalities have been detected. Absence of cardiac membrane-associated dystrophin can be seen with normal skeletal muscle findings (95,96).

A family history in which only the male relatives have dilated cardiomyopathy may be the first clue that a patient has a dystrophinopathy; however, some women may be affected as manifesting carriers, as previously noted (97). Furthermore, as many as a third of cases of Duchenne muscular dystrophy represent de novo mutations with no family history (98). Therefore, a diagnosis may be difficult to make based on kindred analysis alone. Creatine kinase levels are almost always elevated in patients with a dystrophin disorder; such elevations should prompt further investigation of skeletal muscle function, possibly a cardiac and skeletal muscle biopsy, and consideration of dystrophin gene or protein analysis (99).

Other Muscular Dystrophies

Several other muscular dystrophies are known to have a significantly frequent association with cardiac involvement. Emery-Dreifuss muscular dystrophy is an X-linked disorder that, in contrast to Duchenne muscular dystrophy, is characterized by an absence of calf hypertrophy and a distinct pattern of muscle wasting referred to as humeroperoneal (proximal muscles of the upper extremities and distal muscles of the lower extremities are the most affected) (100,101). Joint contractures are a prominent feature of this condition, especially at the elbows, Achilles tendons, and posterior cervical muscles (102). The most common forms of cardiac involvement are rhythm disturbances, including atrial fibrillation or flutter and conduction block (103). However, dilated cardiomyopathy has also been described (104,105) and cardiac transplantation for cardiac failure has been reported (106). Genetic mapping of the relevant region of the X chromosome has led to the identification of the responsible gene (107). The protein product of this gene has been named emerin. It has been demonstrated to localize to the inner membrane of the nucleus (108) but its function has not yet been determined. A disorder that is clinically indistinguishable from Emery-Dreifuss muscular dystrophy, but with an autosomal dominant mode of inheritance, has also been described (109).

Limb-girdle muscular dystrophy refers to a group of disorders, some with autosomal dominant and some with autosomal recessive transmission, that typically are characterized by proximal muscle weakness and wasting that progresses to involve all extremities; the face is spared (110). Conduction system disease has been described in limb-girdle muscular dystrophy type I, and dilated cardiomyopathy has been reported (111–113).

Mitochondrial Myopathies

The mitochondria are the site of oxidative phosphorylation, the metabolic process that generates most of the ATP produced by eukaryotic cells. Pyruvic acid, the product of glycolysis, is taken up into the mitochondrial matrix and reacts with coenzyme A (CoA) to form acetyl CoA. The enzymes of the citric acid cycle, mostly in solution in the mitochondrial matrix, oxidize the acetyl group of acetyl CoA to carbon dioxide and, in the process, reduce nicotinamide adenine dinucleotide (NAD) to NADH and flavin adenine dinucleotide (FAD) to $FADH_2$. Protein complexes on the inner mitochondrial membrane then transport electrons from NADH and $FADH_2$ through the cytochrome system to oxygen. The energy accumulated during this process is used to create high-energy phosphate bonds, which can then be used for all the metabolic requirements of the cell (114). Muscle and nerve cells, which rely heavily on oxidative metabolism to supply their high energy demands, typically contain large numbers of mitochondria (115). Genetic abnormalities of mitochondrial function, especially of oxidative phosphorylation, therefore tend to affect the nervous system, skeletal muscle, and the heart, although they may affect a wide variety of other organ systems as well (116). Mitochondria have their own genome, a circular molecule of DNA that is distinct from the nuclear chromosome. Mitochondrial DNA encodes several of the component polypeptides of the enzymatic pathway for oxidative phosphorylation; in addition, it encodes a set of distinct mitochondrial ribosomal RNAs and transfer RNAs, which are necessary for translation of the mitochondrial genes (117). The replication, transcription, and translation of mitochondrial DNA occur independently of the analogous nuclear processes. Each mitochondrion typically contains several copies of the mitochondrial genome, and each cell usually contains numerous mitochondria. Thus, the stoichiometry of mitochondrial genetic information is quite different from the strict diploidy of nuclear genes. Mutations may occur in one or several copies of the mitochondrial DNA but not in others. When cells divide, the daughter cells may inherit unequal numbers of mitochondria, some bearing mutations and others identical to the germline (118).

Mitochondrial DNA is maternally inherited—children inherit virtually all their mitochondrial genes from their mother, not their father (119). This is a consequence of the fact that the great majority of the mitochondria in a developing embryo are acquired from the ovum; the sperm contains very few mitochondria. As a result, mutations of mitochondrial DNA are transmitted from mother to child, whereas paternal mitochondrial mutations are not transmitted (120). This maternal pattern of inheritance is distinct from the usual mendelian categories and may be the first evidence leading to clinical recognition of a mitochondrial disorder (121,122). However, because some of the enzymatic components involved in oxidative phosphorylation are encoded in the nucleus, genetic defects of mitochondrial function may also exhibit mendelian inheritance (123). Furthermore, abnormalities of mitochondrial DNA have been identified that exhibit autosomal dominant inheritance, which suggests that nuclear genes responsible for the regulation of mitochondrial DNA synthesis are affected (124,125). Finally, because mitochondrial DNA has an exceptionally high mutation rate, many cases of mitochondrial disease occur in the absence of any family history (126).

The diseases of oxidative phosphorylation are clinically diverse, with heterogenous manifestations. There is a wide variety of possible mutations, including point mutations, deletions, insertions, and multiple sequence anomalies. These genetic alterations may be transmitted in varying copy numbers to different tissues and organs, and the requirements of the tissues and organs themselves for the energy produced by oxidative metabolism may vary. Over time, additional mutations may accumulate in the mitochondria of some tissues but not others (127,128). As a result, it is difficult to establish a useful classification system for mitochondrial diseases (129,130). Nonetheless, several distinct phenotypes have been identified and are used in describing individual patients with disorders of oxidative phosphorylation (131–133).

An example of this is the Kearns-Sayre syndrome, which was first described in 1958 (134). The diagnosis is defined by onset before the age of 20, external ophthalmoplegia, ptosis, and pigmentary retinopathy. In addition, a number of other clinical features may be present, including heart block, skeletal muscle weakness, cerebellar dysfunction, deafness, and elevated cerebrospinal fluid protein (135–137). Conduction disturbances in Kearns-Sayre syndrome include left anterior hemiblock, right bundle-branch block, Mobitz type II second-degree atrioventricular block, and complete heart block (138,139). Permanent pacemakers have prolonged survival significantly in Kearns-Sayre syndrome type II. Dilated cardiomyopathy has been reported in Kearns-Sayre syndrome (140,141) and patients have undergone successful cardiac transplantation (142,143).

On skeletal muscle biopsy in Kearns-Sayre syndrome, myocytes stained with the Gomori trichrome stain show a characteristic pattern, with the eosinophilic mitochondria clumped in shaggy clusters around the periphery of the cell. This appearance has given rise to the term ragged red fibers to describe the histology of Kearns-Sayre syndrome and other mitochondrial disorders. Under the electron microscope, the mitochondria themselves are seen to be abnormal; they are often enlarged, elongated, or fused, with loss of the usual folding pattern of the internal cristae, and they may contain crystalline inclusion bodies sometimes described as having a so-called railway track or parking lot appearance, in reference to their highly regular, blocklike array. Mitochondria in the myocardium have also been shown to be abnormal in patients with cardiac involvement, although the inclusion bodies have typically been more amorphous and unlike the rectilinear crystals noted in skeletal muscle.

Arrhythmogenic Right Ventricular Dysplasia

Arrythmogeneic right ventricular dysplasia (ARVD) is a primary myocardial disorder characterized by fatty infiltration of the right ventricle, progressive loss of myocytes, inflammatory infiltrate, thinning and dilatation of the ventricular wall, and replacement fibrosis. The right ventricle is affected predominantly; however, both interventricular septal and left ventricular involvement have been reported. Usually manifested by ventricular arrhthymias with left bundle configuration, electrocardiographic abnormalities (including an epsilon wave and sudden-death heart failure) are a less-common feature. The fibrofatty infiltration progresses to yield systolic dysfunction of the right ventricle and, in advanced cases, the left ventricle as well. A negative endomyocardial biopsy does not exclude the diagnosis, and consensus diagnostic criteria include endomyocardial biopsy, echocardiography, electrocardiography, and magnetic resonance imaging (MRI). ARVD is a genetic disorder. Eight loci have been mapped and three genes identified. Autosomal dominant transmission is the most common transmission, but an autosomal recessive has been reported (144–148).

Alcohol-Induced Cardiomyopathy

The major difficulty with this diagnosis is that cardiomyopathy is a relatively uncommon event and alcohol abuse is a common condition. Clinically and histologically, the overt response to general medical therapy is not significantly different in these patients than in those with idiopathic cardiomyopathy. Alcohol abuse has been identified as a significant risk factor in cardiomyopathy with a frequency of between 20% and 30% (149,150).

It is clear that high blood levels of alcohol produce mildly negative inotropism (151,152). Furthermore, several animal studies have investigated the effects of prolonged alcohol administration. In primates, long-term alcohol administration results in myocytolysis and fibrosis (153). In dogs, cardiac fibrosis is produced, leading mainly to measurable myocardial dysfunction (154,155). In a hamster model, long-term alcohol administration resulted in a reduction in myocardial high-energy phosphates (156).

The specific mechanisms by which alcohol might produce myocardial dysfunction have also been investigated. Cellular events that have been described with long-term alcohol exposure include impaired sarcoplasmic reticular uptake of calcium (157), inhibition of myosin ATPase (158), elevation of intracellular Na^+ and water (159), inhibition of the Na^+,K^+-ATPase (160), and alterations in the incorporation of membrane fatty acid and phospholipids (155,161).

The expression of alcohol-induced cardiomyopathy is obviously quite variable. There is evidence to suggest that excessive alcohol consumption is likely to be present for a minimum of 10 years before the onset of heart failure (162–164), that men are more susceptible than women (165), and that concurrent smoking, hypertension, and malnutrition may be contributing factors. Furthermore, there appear to be differences between persons in organ susceptibility to alcohol, as chronic cirrhosis is unlikely to develop in those with cardiomyopathy (166).

An interesting, likely unrelated phenomenon occurred in the 1960s when cobalt was added to beer as a foam-stabilizing agent in a few areas of Europe and Canada. An acute and aggressive form of cardiomyopathy developed in heavy beer drinkers that was attributable to the cobalt (167,168). When this element was no longer used, no further cases of this form of cardiomyopathy were reported.

There is some evidence to suggest that abstaining from alcohol has a beneficial effect on prognosis in alcohol-induced cardiomyopathy. In one study of 64 patients, approximately one-third discontinued excessive alcohol use. This subgroup had a 9% mortality rate during the subsequent 4 years, contrasted with a 57% mortality rate in the remainder who continued drinking (31). A second but smaller study (31 patients) supported these findings (169).

Cocaine and Cardiomyopathy

Long-term cocaine abuse may result in the development of a dilated cardiomyopathy. Termed cocaine-induced cardiomyopathy, cocaine's direct toxicity to the myocardium may be responsible. These direct effects include provocation of coronary spasm, increased catecholamine release, enhanced platelet aggregation, decreased fibrinolysis, and upregulation of tissue plasminogen activator inhibitors (predisposing the abuser to coronary thrombosis) (170–172). Hypersensitivity myocarditis due to cocaine or associated contaminants may be another mechanism (173). Finally, cocaine may induce lethal arrhythmias. Similar to alcoholic cardiomyopathy, abstinence is crucial in therapy and cessation-related reversal of dysfunction has been reported (174).

Treatment with β-blockade was popular in the 1980s; however, reports of cocaine-induced hypertension or myocardial ischemia were thought to be due to use of β-blockers and the resulting unopposed α-receptors. Thus, treatment with β-blockers decreased. While no significant data exist, utilization of labetalol or carvedilol (both of which have α- and β-receptor antagonist activities) may warrant further investigation (175).

Diabetic Cardiomyopathy

Diabetic cardiomyopathy as a unique entity has only recently been recognized. In 1972, Rubler et al. (176) presented data from four patients with Kimmelstiel-Wilson disease and dilated cardiomyopathy in the absence of coronary, valvular, or other cardiomyopathic risk factors. Supportive data have included a retrospective analysis from the Framingham Heart Study demonstrating a 2.4-

fold higher incidence of heart failure in diabetics on insulin (177) and a higher-than-expected incidence of diabetes in a population of patients with idiopathic dilated cardiomyopathy (178). Potential pathogenetic mechanisms for diabetic cardiomyopathy have included increased vascular permeability resulting in increased glycosylation of collagen (179), alterations in intracellular Ca^{2+} kinetics (180), and microvascular damage (181) akin to that of diabetic retinopathy and nephropathy.

The clinical presentation of diabetic cardiomyopathy is not unlike that of idiopathic dilated cardiomyopathy. In a series of 16 diabetics with cardiomyopathy, cardiac volumes, LV filling pressures, and ventricular mass were increased in all patients and cardiac index was reduced in approximately half (178). These findings were confirmed in a small series that also demonstrated a decrease in myocardial compliance (182). Several investigators have demonstrated that diabetics have abnormal cardiac function based on systolic time intervals (183–185). Seneviratne noted these abnormalities to be present only in diabetic patients with evidence of other microangiopathy (retinopathy or nephropathy) (184).

Histopathologically, hearts from diabetic patients with dilated cardiomyopathy are similar to those from nondiabetic patients. Some investigators have reported, in addition to the hypertrophy and interstitial fibrosis, an increase in interstitial material positive for periodic acid-Schiff (PAS), consistent with glycoprotein (186). Other investigators have reported hyalin thickening of small vessels in the myocardium (187).

Peripartum Cardiomyopathy

The syndrome of unexplained heart failure in women postpartum was detailed in the mid-1930s by a number of investigators (188,189) but had been suggested even earlier. The disease was initially described as occurring primarily in the postpartum period, but it is now clear that it can present as early as the end of the middle of the third trimester or as late as several months after delivery. Most commonly, however, signs and symptoms of heart failure occur postpartum (190).

The etiology of peripartum cardiomyopathy is unknown, although several factors have been associated with development of the disease. As the disease appears to be more common in less-affluent populations, nutritional deficiencies during pregnancy have been postulated (191,192). Other suggested associations have included toxemia of pregnancy (192), immunologic factors such as the development of antiheart antibodies (193), genetic susceptibility (194,195), and drug-induced hypersensitivity (196).

Although the general clinical signs, symptoms, and histology (except for patients with myocarditis) are no different from those of patients with idiopathic dilated cardiomyopathy, prior series suggested certain associated factors, including race (with a much higher incidence in African-Americans), advanced maternal age, multiparity, and twin pregnancies (190,197). A more recent series of 123 patients suggested otherwise. While patients were somewhat older (mean age of 31), most (67%) were white, gestational hypertension was present in almost half of the patients, and tocolytic therapy was used in 19%; only 13% were twin pregnancies (198).

This entity is undoubtedly distinct from other forms of dilated cardiomyopathy, as evidenced by three well-documented phenomena. First, as previously stated, the onset of disease in most cases is close to the postpartum period (197). Second, relatively speaking, the prognosis of peripartum cardiomyopathy is excellent compared with the prognosis in other forms of dilated cardiomyopathy. With current medical therapy based on the most recent series of patients, 54% of patients had normalization of their ejection fraction (198). Third, the disease appears to recur during subsequent pregnancies in a portion of patients, even those who have completely recovered from their first episode (194,199).

Anthracycline-Induced Cardiomyopathy

This form of toxin-induced cardiomyopathy may affect anywhere from 5% to 20% of patients receiving the agent, depending on a variety of risk factors and total dose. This is a unique form of cardiomyopathy that has provided several insights into toxin-induced cardiac disease and global cardiac function for the following reasons: First, as a toxin, anthracycline appears to affect certain cardiac cells but not others, according to electron microscopic studies (200,201). The number of affected cells appears to be related to total dose. This is presumably a different phenomenon from that noted in other forms of dilated cardiomyopathy, in which the insult or defect appears to affect cardiac tissue more diffusely. Second, there appears to be a threshold effect, in which gross cardiac function remains normal until a certain percentage of cells has been affected; cardiac function can then deteriorate precipitously (202). This would suggest a partial redundancy in the number of contractile units (myocytes) in the heart, similar to that in the functioning units of other organs (e.g., glomeruli).

Several hypotheses have been proposed to explain the cardiotoxic effect of anthracyclines. Oxygen free radicals, lipid peroxidation, altered arachidonic acid metabolism, a direct interaction with the calcium release from sarcoplasmic reticulum, and metabolite action on the calcium pump from sarcoplasmic reticulum have all been implicated in the cardiotoxic effects (203).

The clinical presentation of cardimyopathy secondary to anthracycline toxicity is not dissimilar to that of dilated cardiomyopathy of other etiologies. It has been reported as early as a week following the last dose of doxorubicin but can present even years after chemotherapy (204). It has been suggested that the shorter the latency period, the greater the severity and the poorer the ultimate prognosis (204). Most studies have suggested that cardiac toxicity is uncommon in cumulative doses of less than 450 mg/m^2 in the absence of other risk factors (204). When risk factors are present (which include advancing age, mediastinal radiation, concomitant cardiotoxic chemotherapy, underlying cardiac disease, and large bolus therapy) cardiac toxicity has been noted at substantially lower total doses (204–208).

Although a variety of cardiovascular studies have been advocated to follow patients for cardiac toxicity, the most sensitive appears to be endomyocardial biopsy (202). This can in part be attributed to the threshold phenomenon previously described. Histopathologic findings include disruption of myofibrils and dissolution of myofilaments, extensive vacuolization secondary to swelling of the sarcoplasmic reticulum, mitochondrial pleomorphism, and dissociation of the tight junctions (200,201). These findings are graded according to the number of cells affected and severity of the changes. Most noninvasive studies, such as echocardiography, radionuclide angiography, and systolic time intervals, rely on systolic cardiac function, which may not fall despite significant histological evidence of toxicity (209). It is conceivable that diastolic function might provide more sensitive data for following these patients.

While anthracycline cardiac toxicity has been reduced, first, by more careful monitoring of toxicity and a better understanding of risk factors, patients with impaired LV dysfunction should probably receive anthracyclines only as a last resort. Even with normal LV function, once the total dose of doxorubicin exceeds 450 mg/m^2 (or less if risk factors are present), histological monitoring by endomyocardial biopsy is warranted before additional drug is administered. A high-grade biopsy specimen should preclude additional anthracycline exposure irrespective of LV systolic function. Second, it appears that toxicity can be reduced by reducing peak levels of the drug, so that protocols have been changed from monthly large infusions to weekly smaller infusions and even daily continuous intravenous administration. It has been observed that larger total doses can be achieved, efficacy is not impaired, and toxicity is lessened (209).

Trastuzumab (Herceptin)-Induced Cardiomyopathy

Trastuzumab is a relatively new monoclonal antibody directed against the HER2/erbB2 recepter that is overexpressed on many breast carcinomas (CA). It is being used more commonly in both the adjuvant as well as treatment settings for breast CA and, not infrequently, in combination with doxorubicin and other anthracyclines. In a subset of individuals, trastuzumab induces a resersible cardiomyopathy. The mechanism of cardiac toxicity is unknown, but the cardiomyocyte does express low levels of HER2/erbB2. In vitro data suggest that despite these low levels, the cardiac receptor appears to be uniquely susceptible to trastuzumab in the subset of individuals where there is an interaction between trastuzumab and the cardiac HER2/erbB2 receptor (210). In most patients the cardiac dysfunction is reversible with discontinuation of therapy (210).

Left Ventricular Dysfunction Associated with Inflammation

A number of infectious agents and two major inflammatory conditions have been associated with left ventricular dysfunction. These are outlined in Table 18-2.

Viral Myocarditis

Viral myocarditis follows a pattern. The virus is usually introduced through the respiratory or gastrointestinal tract. In the first stage (the first 3 days), viremia results in acute myocarditis by way of myocardial invasion, viral replication, nuclear transmission, release to the cell surface, and subsequent infection of other cells. The first response to myocarditis is a nonspecific immune response. Nuclear factor kappa B (NF-κB), an intracellular transcription factor

TABLE 18-2
PRINCIPAL ETIOLOGICAL AGENTS ASSOCIATED WITH MYOCARDITIS

Viral Infections

Adenovirus, arbovirus, coxsackievirus, cytomegalovirus, echovirus, encephalomyocarditis virus, hepatitis virus, human immunodeficiency virus, infectious mononucleosis, influenza, mumps, *Mycoplasma pneumoniae,* poliomyelitis, psittacosis, respiratory syncytial virus, rabies, rubella, rubeola, vaccinia, varicella, variola, yellow fever

Rickettsial Infections

Rocky Mountain spotted fever, Q fever, scrub typhus, typhus

Bacterial Infections

Streptococcal, staphylococcal, pneumococcal, meningococcal, *Haemophilus,* gonococcal, brucellosis, diphtheria, salmonellosis, tuberculosis, tularemia

Spirochetal Infections

Leptospirosis, Lyme disease, relapsing fever, syphilis

Parasitic Infections

Cysticercosis, schistosomiasis, toxoplasmosis, trichinosis, trypanosomiasis, visceral larva migrans

Fungal Infections

Aspergillosis, actinomycosis, blastomycosis, candidiasis, coccidioidomycosis, cryptococcosis, histoplasmosis which produces cytokines, nitric oxide, and intracellular adhesion molecules, is virus-activated. The inflammatory response to cardiac viral infection involves all three substances resulting from NF-κB. Lung or gut infection results in cytokine expression, which may lead to a cardiac immune response. The invasion of myocytes results in cell necrosis and macrophage activation. Macrophage activation results in cytokine expression, including tumor necrosis factor-alpha (TNF-α), interleukins, and interferon (211–216).

The second stage (subacute myocarditis, days 3 to 14) is an immunologic response and consists of the infiltration of mononuclear cells, B lymphocytes, and cytotoxic T cells. Natural killer cells limit viral replication and release perforin, forming lesions on the infected cells' membrane surfaces, thus sparing noninfected cells from injury. Macrophages and dendritic cells ingest viral agents and are responsible for the initial cell-mediated response to viral myocarditis by releasing proteases, cytokines, perforin, and interleukins. Nitric oxide (NO) is increased in macrophages in the setting of myocarditis. NO plays a role in this phase, which may be beneficial or detrimental by enhancing or suppressing myocardial function. In animal models, NO may contribute to the progression of myocyte damage (217–221).

The third stage (chronic myocarditis, days 14 to 90) is marked by fibrosis, cardiac dilatation, and heart failure. Possible mechanisms of progression to dilated cardiomyopathy include viral persistence, apoptosis, coronary microvascular spasm, and autoimmunity. Persistence of virus (although the virus cannot multiply, it may be housed in the skeletal muscle) coupled with an activated immune system is the first possible mechanism. Apoptosis (programmed cell death) is a second possible mechanism of progression to dilated cardiomyopathy and may be triggered by certain viruses. Coronary microvascular spasm results in myocyte necrosis. Finally, a third possible mechanism is the role of autoimmunity in this progression by way of antibody to viral proteins crossreacting with normal heart architecture (222–225).

Clinical manifestations are variable, ranging from the asymptomatic patient to cardiogenic shock. Cardiac involvement occurs days to weeks subsequent to a viral illness. The clinical presentation of cardiac inflammation consists of symptoms due to heart failure, arrhythmia, and embolic events. Myocarditis-associated syncope may be due to ventricular arrhythmias or atrioventricular (AV) block. The AV block is usually transient. Sudden cardiac death due to myocarditis has been reported. Patients note symptoms of a preceding viral illness followed by myalgias, fever, palpitations, dyspnea, and chest pain. Chest pain may be pleuritic due to simultaneous pericardial inflammation, typical of myocardial ischemia, or atypical. The cardiac exam demonstrates tachycardia, gallops, murmurs of AV valve regurgitation, or possibly a pericardial friction rub. A presentation identical to acute myocardial infarction may occur including chest pain, ST elevation, elevation of the MB fraction of focal or diffuse wall motion abnormalities, a normal coronary angiogram, and biopsy-proven myocarditis. Both viral arteritis of the coronary arteries and vasospasm have been reported. Ventricular microaneurysms due to myocarditis are diagnosed by LV biopsy in the setting of preserved systolic function and nonsustained ventricular tachycardia (226–235).

Laboratory findings are nondiagnostic. The white blood cell count is usually elevated, and eosinophilia and elevation of the erythrocyte sedimentation rate are sometimes noted. Cardiac-specific troponin I is elevated in up to one-third of patients, while CK-MB is increased in 10% of patients. The electrocardiogram demonstrates ST-T wave changes, supraventricular or ventricular ectopy, atrial fibrillation, conduction abnormalities, low voltage, and prolongation of the QTc interval. Rarely, an acute infarct pattern is seen. The most frequent electrocardiogram finding is sinus tachycardia. Cytokine elevation, including IL-6, TNG, and IgG3 may be seen in patients with progressive ventricular dysfunction (236–238).

Echocardiographic findings include ventricular thrombi, increased wall thickness, and systolic dysfunction with possible segmental wall motion abnormalities. MRI may identify myocarditis-induced tissue alterations (239–243).

Endomyocardial biopsy can confirm the diagnosis if the clinical diagnosis is confusing. The diagnosis of active myocarditis requires an inflammatory infiltrate of the myocardium with necrosis and/or degeneration of adjacent myocytes not typical of the ischemic damage associated with coronary artery disease (244).

Supportive therapy for heart failure in general is utilized in the setting of myocarditis. Patients should limit their physical activity. Diuretics are used for relief of congestive signs and symptoms. Steroids prolong viremia in rats. Supportive care with angiotensin-converting enzyme (ACE) inhibitors should be employed. Digoxin, which increases the expression of cytokines in animal studies, is used both cautiously and at a low dose due to concern for precipitating vascular spasm. Data regarding the use of calcium channel antagonists are lacking (245–247).

Immunosuppressive therapy has been evaluated in studies with discouraging results. Intravenous immunoglobulin was not shown to be beneficial in a trial of 62 patients with heart failure, only 16 of whom had myocarditis per the Dallas criteria (248).

The Myocarditis Treatment Trial evaluated the response to conventional therapy versus prednisone in combination with either cyclosporine or azathioprine in patients with biopsies compatable with myocarditis (nonviral) per the Dallas criteria. No difference was found in any group in terms of ejection fraction increase, mortality, or disease attenuation. Parillo reported the effect of prednisone in 102 patients with established dilated cardiomyopathy (not viral myocariditis), finding no lasting improvement in ejection fraction after 9 months. Routine use of immunosuppressive therapy cannot be recommended. Antiviral therapy is currently being investigated (249,250).

Rickettsial Myocarditis

Myocarditis due to rickettsial disease is common, although usually subclinical. ST-T wave changes are frequently noted. Vasculitis and perivascular inflammation are pathologic features, and peripheral vascular abnormalities (with or without accompanying myocarditis) are responsible for circulatory collapse. Rickettsial infections responsible for myocarditis include Q fever (*Rickettsia burnettii*), Rocky Mountain spotted fever (*R. rickettsii*), and scrub typhus (*R. tsutsugamushi*) (251–255).

Bacterial Myocarditis

Bacterial myocarditis is rare and has been associated with a number of gram-positive and gram-negative organisms. These include but are not limited to organisms responsible for brucellosis, clostridial disease, diptheria, Legionnaire disease, mycoplasma, psittacosis, *Salmonella*, *Streptococcus*, and tuberculosis (256–263).

Spirochetal Infections

Spirochetal infections causing myocarditis include syphilis, relapsing fever, and leptospirosis. Leptospirosis, a cause of fatal myocarditis, occurs with ST-T wave changes noted on the surface ECG in half of all cases.

Lyme disease is caused by *Borrelia burgdorferi*, a spirochete introduced by a tick bite. Erythema chronicum migrans, the characteristic rash of Lyme disease, first appears, with subsequent neurological or cardiac manifestations appearing weeks to months later. Cardiac involvement is seen in approximately in 10% of cases and presents as variable degrees of AV block, ventricular tachycardia, myopericarditis, bundle-branch block, LV dysfunction, transient ST-T wave changes, and syncope due to complete heart block. Endomyocardial biopsy may demonstrate active myocarditis and (rarely) spirochetes. Immune-mediated mechanisms may be involved. The prognosis is good and most patients recover completely. Treatment includes hospitalizing those patients with second- or third-degree AV block and placement of a temporary pacemaker, which may be necessary for a week or longer. While the efficacy of antibiotics has not been established, both intravenous (ceftriaxone or penicillin G) and oral agents have been used. Corticosteroid therapy after treatment with tetracycline may be helpful in treating carditis, but treatment with steroids to ameliorate heart block is controversial (264–270).

Protozoal Myocarditis: Trypanosomiasis (Chagas Disease)

Chagas disease, the most common cause of heart failure in the world, is caused by the bite of the reduviid bug, which harbors the protozoan *Trypanosoma cruzi*. Especially prevalent in Central and South America, the disease is characterized by three phases: acute, latent, and chronic. After inoculation, the protozoa multiply and affect multiple tissues via hematogenous spread. Both the endocardium and epicardium are involved in this acute phase and cardiac injury appears to be mediated by both humoral- and cell-mediated immunity. Clinical manifestations of this acute phase include myocarditis and heart failure, diaphoresis, myalgias, hepatosplenomegaly, and occasionally death. Most patients recover from this phase and an asymptomatic, latent phase is then entered. Approximately 20 years later, 30% of patients manifest the chronic disease findings, including thromboembolic phenomenon, heart failure, cardiomegaly (sometimes right-sided more than left-sided), and sudden death.

Radiographic findings include cardiomegaly. On laboratory exam, the serum aldolase is elevated. Echocardiographic findings include impaired systolic function, diastolic filling abnormalities, posterior wall hypokinesis, apical aneurysm, and dilated chambers. The electrocardiogram may demonstrate right bundle-branch block, left anterior fasicular block, ventricular ectopy, and atrial fibrillation. Ventricular arrhythmias are frequently seen in chronic disease and sudden death may appear before heart failure (271–276).

Serodiagnostic techniques found useful include complement fixation test, indirect immunofluorescent antibody test, and hemagluttination test. Xenodiagnosis utilizing the reduviid bug is widely used (277).

Treatment includes the following: amiodarone for ventricular ectopy and implantable cardioverter defibrillator (ICD) implantation for life-threatening arrhythmias; anticoagulation for thromboembolism in certain cases permanent pacemaker implantation for complete heart block; standard therapy for heart failure; antiparasitic agents (such as nifurtimox) during the acute phase; possible immunosuppressive therapy; and heart transplantation (278–282).

Fungal Infections of the Heart

Fungal myocarditis may be due to infections with the actinomycosis, aspergillosis, blastomycosis, candidiasis, coccidioidmycosis, cryptococcosis, histoplasmosis, and mucormycosis. Patients at risk for myocardial fungal involvement include those receiving chemotherapy, steroids, radiation, or immunosuppressive therapy. Other predisposing factors include cardiac surgery, intravenous drug abuse, and human immunodeficiency virus (HIV) infection. Direct extension from the lungs or mediastinum or hematogenous dissemination may result in fungal myocarditis. Fungal mycelia may obstruct coronary arteries (283–290).

Giant Cell Myocarditis

Giant cell myocarditis is rare, aggressive, progressive, resistant to treatment, and usually fatal. An immune or autoimmune origin is possible. Patients present with a rapid onset of fever, chest pain, rapidly progressive heart failure, and occasionally arrhythmia (ventricular arrhythmias poorly responsive to medical therapy) or complete heart block. The average age affected is 43, with reported cases ranging in age from 6 weeks to 88 years. The gender incidence is equal and 90% of patients affected are white. Associated autoimmune disorders are noted in 20% of patients (291–294).

The diagnosis is established by endomyocardial biopsy, which has 80% sensitivity. Histiological findings include diffuse myocyte necrosis and a mixed inflammatory infiltrate including eosinophils, multinucleated giant cells without granuloma formation, histiocytes, and T lymphocytes (both helper and suppressor) (295).

Giant cell myocarditis is usually fatal; Cooper et al. (290) reported that the average length of survival without immunosuppressive therapy was 3 months. Steroid therapy alone yielded minimal improvement. Combining azathiaprine, OKT3, and cyclosporine improved the survival to longer than 1 year. No formal recommendations have been made regarding immunosuppression regimens, as data from large scale trials are lacking. Both ventricular assist device implantation and placement of an intraortic ballon pump may be necessary while awaiting transplantation. When transplanted, recurrence of the giant cells has been reported in less than 25% of recipients and is usually treated with intensification of immunosuppressive therapy (296–300).

Sarcoidosis

Sarcoidosis, a systemic granulomatous disease of unknown cause, is characterized by lung, skin, and reticuloendothelial infiltration. The pathological feature is the noncaseating granuloma, which may occur in many organs. An initial inflammatory infiltrate includes T lymphocytes and cytokine-secreting macrophages. The macrophages differentiate into giant cells, which aggregate and form clusters. Pulmonary involvement, affected in over 90% of patients, may lead to right-heart failure. Primary cardiac involvement has been found at autopsy in 20% to 30% of patients. Sarcoid granulomas replace portions of myocardial walls and, frequently, sudden death occurs. Clinical manifestations of cardiac sarcoid include heart failure, conduction disturbances, syncope, and atrial and ventricular arrhythmias. Cardiac sarcoid show features of restrictive and/or dilated cardiomyopathy. Diagnosis with endomyocardial biopsy is possible but a negative biopsy does not rule out the disease. An echocardiogram may demonstrate wall motion abnormalities, and MRI is sometimes helpful. Treatment with corticosteroids reverses the electrocardiographic abnormalities and cardiac symptoms in many patients. Ventricular tachycardia may optimally be treated with an ICD. Heart transplantation has been utilized with a low recurrence rate in the allograft. Prognosis of cardiac sarcoidosis is variable to poor (300–306).

Clinical Features of Dilated Cardiomyopathy

Irrespective of underlying etiology, most patients with dilated cardiomyopathy present in similar fashion, albeit in a continuum of heart failure. In general, patients present with progressive symptoms of exercise limitation; the duration of symptoms can range from days to months or years. Dyspnea with exertion, orthopnea, paroxysmal nocturnal dyspnea, and (less commonly) chest discomfort similar to typical angina can be presenting symptoms. Early in the course of the disease, left-sided symptoms seem to predominate and it is only later that evidence of right ventricular (RV) failure appears. This is a curious feature, as the myopathic process presumably involves both ventricles. Coexistent symptoms or even modes of presentation include the onset of ventricular or atrial arrhythmias and systemic embolization. Physical findings, especially in the acute setting, are typically those generally associated with heart failure, such as sinus tachycardia, elevated jugular venous pressure, pulmonary rales, a third and likely a fourth heart sound, mitral insufficiency, and (in the most severe cases) hepatic congestion and peripheral edema. In a study by Fuster et al. (149) of 104 patients with dilated cardiomyopathy, the mean time between initial symptoms and presentation to a physician was 1.3 years. At the time of diagnosis, 87% of patients had cardiomegaly, 80% had electrocardiographic abnormalities, a full 73% presented in overt heart failure, and 4% presented with evidence of systemic embolization. In a similar study of 68 patients with dilated cardiomyopathy by Schwarz et al. (150), all had symptoms of congestive heart failure [65% New York Heart Association (NYHA) functional Class II, 35% NYHA Class III], 82% had cardiomegaly, 97% had electrocardiographic abnormalities, and 47% experienced episodes of chest pain.

Table 18-3 provides a summary of several clinical series of patients with dilated cardiomyopathy. Typically, the ejection fraction is reduced to approximately half of normal values, the LV and (in severe cases) RV filling pressures are twice normal, and cardiac index is reduced. This, coupled with an increased heart rate, implies an even greater reduction of stroke volume. Differences between the series likely reflect referral patterns in a given community and earlier or later stages of the disease process.

Therapy

Therapy for patients with dilated cardiomyopathy is primarily directed toward the treatment of congestive heart failure. This is extensively addressed elsewhere in this text. In brief, digitalis glycosides, diuretics, ACE inhibitors, β-blockers, and possibly angiotensin II receptor antagonists are the mainstays of therapy, in regard to both relief of symptoms and improvement of prognosis. For asymptomatic patients who present with dilated cardiomyopathy, data from the Studies of Left Ventricular Dysfunction (SOLVD) trial and early data from the β-blocker experience suggest that treatment with ACE inhibitors and β-blockers should be instituted early.

The prevention and management of other complications of LV dysfunction, including arrhythmias and thromboembolism, likewise need to be addressed. The issue of management of ventricular arrhythmias has been simplified substantially with the publication of several trials

TABLE 18-3
HEMODYNAMICS IN DILATED CARDIOMYOPATHY

Parameter	Series 1	Series 2	Series 3
Ejection fraction	0.27	0.30	0.26
LV filling pressure (mm Hg)	20	20	22
Cardiac index (L/min/m^2)	1.9	2.5	2.5

Series 1, adult, from Bione S, Maestrini E, Rivella S, et al. Identification of a novel X-linked gene responsible for Emery-Dreifuss muscular dystrophy. *Nat Genet.* 1994;8:323–327; Series 2, adult, from Merchat MP, Zdonczyk D, Gujrati M. Cardiac transplantation in female Emery-Dreifuss muscular dystrophy. *J Neurol.* 1990;237:316–319; Series 3, pediatric, from Yoshioka M, Saida K, Itagaki Y, Kamiya T. Follow-up study of cardiac involvement in Emery-Dreifuss muscular dystrophy. *Arch Dis Child.* 1989;64:713–715.
LV, left ventricular.

demonstrating a survival benefit with the use of defibrillators in patients with ejection fractions at or below 35%. The prevention of thromboembolism is also critical in patients with dilated cardiomyopathy. Again, based on the authors' experience, patients should be given the anticoagulant warfarin in any one of the following situations: (a) the ejection fraction is less than 25%; (b) there is a history of thromboembolism; (c) the patient is in atrial fibrillation (an indication by itself); or (d) the underlying disease is peripartum cardiomyopathy, especially in the first few months following delivery.

Prognosis

There has been a substantial change in the prognosis of patients with dilated cardiomyopathy and heart failure in general. This is in large part due to the standard practice of administering neurohumoral blocking agents to stabilize or improve cardiac function and the use of prophylactic ICDs to treat malignant arrhythmias. While historically the 1-year survival in dilated cardiomyoapthy could be as low as 60% to 70% (149,307–309), a recent study of 458 patients comparing the benefits of prophylactic ICDs to medication alone (85% of all patients on β-blockers) demonstrated a 1-year survival rate of 93.8% in those on medication alone and 97.4% in those receiving medication plus an ICD (310). Table 18-4 lists factors that can influence prognosis in dilated cardiomyopathy, but many of these risk factors are based on historical data.

TABLE 18-4
PREDICTORS OF OUTCOME IN DILATED CARDIOMYOPATHY

Left ventricular enlargement
Right ventricular enlargement
Left and right ventricular ejection fraction
Elevated left ventricular filling pressures
Persistent S3 gallop
Right-sided heart failure
Pulmonary hypertension
Moderate to severe mitral regurgitation
Electrocardiographic findings: first- or second-degree atrioventricular block or left bundle-branch block
Recurrent ventricular tachycardia
Reduced heart rate variability
Late potentials of QRS in signal-averaged CKG
Myocytolysis on endomyocardial biopsy
Elevated levels of neurohormones (brain natiuretic peptide, norepinephrine, plasma renin activity, endothelin-1)
Elevated levels of cytokines (tumor necrosis factor-alpha and interleukin-6)
Elevation of serum creatine kinase MB, troponin T, troponin I levels
Peak oxygen consumption <10 to 12 mL/kg/min
Reduced contractile response with dobutamine
Serum sodium <137 mmol/L
Advanced New York Heart Association class
Advanced age (>64 years)

RESTRICTIVE CARDIOMYOPATHY

Pathophysiology

The primary myocardial defect in patients with restrictive cardiomyopathy (RCM) is an abnormality of diastolic relaxation, which results in restricted ventricular filling, high filling pressures, and (despite normal or nearly normal systolic function) a reduced stroke volume secondary to a reduction in total ventricular volume (311). As a result, diastolic pressure at any given diastolic volume is increased in comparison with the normal heart (Fig. 18-2). In addition to the shift in the pressure–volume relationship to the left, the rate of rise in pressure for any given change in volume is greater in the restrictive myopathic heart (312).

The characteristic LV and RV filling pressures are depicted in Figure 18-3. Initially, after the ventricle empties, filling occurs rapidly but then plateaus early in diastole as the limits of ventricular compliance are reached. This dip-and-plateau configuration is also seen in constrictive pericarditis, making separation of these entities sometimes difficult. More careful analysis of these filling characteristics has demonstrated that in constrictive pericarditis, most ventricular filling occurs within the first half of diastole. In contrast, in restrictive myopathy only about half of ventricular filling occurs during this time (313,314). An explanation for these differences is that in constriction, filling is relatively normal until the constraints of the pericardium are met, whereas in restrictive disease, filling is abnormal throughout the diastolic period. In contrast to constrictive pericarditis, myocardial restriction usually results in differences in RV and LV filling pressures (315). In addition, in severe restrictive disease, filling pressures even at the onset of diastole are elevated, suggesting that both ventricles empty incompletely (316). In contrast, in pericardial constriction, the initial diastolic pressure can be low (317). In mild cases of RCM or in patients who have been excessively volume-depleted with diuretic therapy, the restrictive physiology may be occult and volume manipulation or exercise may be required for it to become manifest (316).

The mechanisms responsible for the reduction in ventricular compliance vary depending on the specific disease process. Potential mechanisms include an intrinsically abnormal myocardium; infiltration of the myocardium with nonmyocardial materials, such as collagen or abnormal protein; endomyocardial disease; and space-occupying lesions

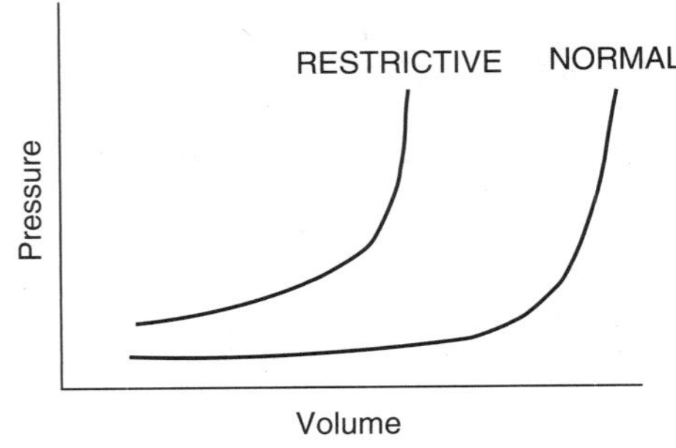

Figure 18-2 Theoretical ventricular pressure–volume relationships in ventricles with normal and restricted physiology. Not only is ventricular pressure greater for a given volume in the restricted heart, but the rate of rise in pressure for a given increase in volume is also increased (reduced compliance).

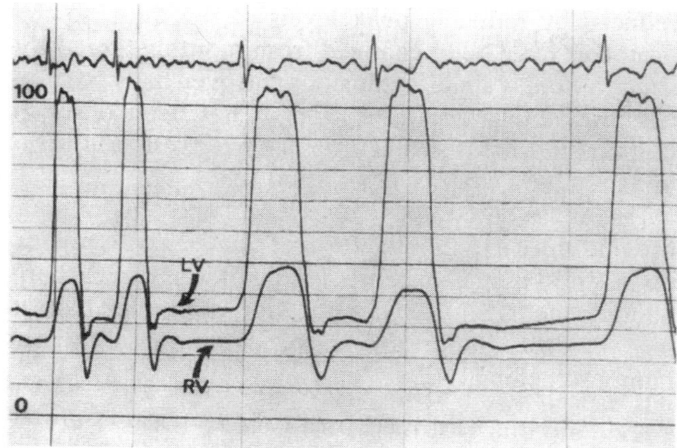

Figure 18-3 LV and RV pressure tracings in a patient with restrictive cardiomyopathy. Filling pressures are elevated in both chambers but not equalized. Note the early diastolic "dip" followed rapidly by a "plateau" in the pressure pulse. This "square root" sign is also seen in constrictive pericarditis. (Reproduced with permission from Hosenpud JD. *Restrictive Cardiomyopathy [Progress in Cardiology 1989]*. Philadelphia: Lea & Febiger; 1989:92.)

(thrombus or tumor) that reduce the total ventricular volumes. These potential etiologies are further delineated next.

Differential Diagnosis and Specific Etiologies

Table 18-5 lists most of the reported causes of restrictive cardiomyopathy. Features of idiopathic RCM and RCM associated with amyloidosis and endocardial fibrosis will be discussed further; other causes will be only briefly mentioned.

Idiopathic

It appears that in restrictive cardiomyopathy, as in dilated cardiomyopathy, no specific etiology can be found in many patients (311,315,316,318). The histopathological findings in cases of primary or idiopathic RCM are nonspecific and generally include myocardial cell hypertrophy and an increase in interstitial fibrosis. A primary defect in myocardial cell relaxation is presumably present. The clinical and hemodynamic findings of patients with idiopathic RCM are presented in Table 18-6; these are based on compiled data from seven separate series (311,315,316,318–321). The mean age at presentation is similar to that in other forms of idiopathic cardiomyopathy, with a very large age range. There is an almost equal distribution between male and female patients. Despite the fact that dyspnea is one of the most frequent complaints, only a minority of patients have objective evidence of pulmonary interstitial or alveolar edema. Chest pain that is atypical of angina is the second-most frequent complaint in these patients, followed by fatigue. Filling pressures, as expected, are elevated but resting cardiac output tends to be normal. Ejection fractions are normal and, as expected, LV end-diastolic volumes tend to be small as a consequence of the restrictive process.

TABLE 18-6
CLINICAL AND HEMODYNAMIC CHARACTERISTICS OF 34 PATIENTS WITH PRIMARY RESTRICTIVE CARDIOMYOPATHY*

Age	
Mean, 39 y	Range, 1 to 77 yrs
Sex	
19 (56%) male	15 (44%) female
Symptomatology	
Chest pain	56%
Fatigue	50%
Dyspnea	61%
Clinical Findings	
Jugular venous distention	62%
Rales	19%
S_3	48%
S_4	32%
Ascites	25%
Edema	32%
Hemodynamics⁺	
Right atrial (mm Hg)	12 ± 6
Pulmonary wedge (mm Hg)	21 ± 7
Cardiac index (L/min/m^2)	2.9 ± 1.0
LV EDVI (mL/m^2)	67 ± 18
LV ejection fraction	0.68 ± 0.10

*Compiled data from seven studies (Manilal S, Nguyen TM, Sewry CA, et al. The Emery-Dreifuss muscular dystrophy protein, emerin, is a nuclear membrane protein. *Hum Mol Genet.* 1996;5:801–808; Bialer MG, McDaniel NL, Kelly TE. Progression of cardiac disease in Emery-Dreifuss muscular dystrophy. *Clin Cardiol.* 1991;14:411; Moxley RT. The myotonias: their diagnosis and treatment. *Compr Ther.* 1996;22:8–21; Phillips MF, Harper PS. Cardiac disease in myotonic dy trophy. *Cardiovasc Res.* 1997; 33:13–22; Perloff JK, Stevenson WG, Roberts NK, et al. Cardiac involvement in myotonic muscular dystrophy (Steinert's disease): a prospective study of 25 patients. *Am J Cardiol.* 1984;54:1074–1087; Moorman JR, Coleman RE, Packer DL, et al. Cardiac involvement in myotonic muscular dystrophy. *Medicine.* 1985;64:371–387; Child JS, Perloff JK. Myocardial myotonia in myotonic muscular dystrophy. *Am Heart J.* 1995;129:982–990.)
⁺Results expressed as mean + 1 SD.
LV EDVI, left ventricular end-diastolic volume index.

TABLE 18-5
REPORTED CAUSES OF RESTRICTIVE CARDIOMYOPATHY

Primary (idiopathic)	Tumor infiltration
Amyloidosis	Storage diseases
Endocardial fibrosis	Anthracyclines
Eosinophilic heart disease	Radiation
Hemochromatosis	Cardiac transplant
Sarcoidosis	

Reprinted with permission from Hosenpud JD. Restrictive Cardiomyopathy *(Progress in Cardiology 1989)*. Philadelphia: Lea & Febiger; 1989.

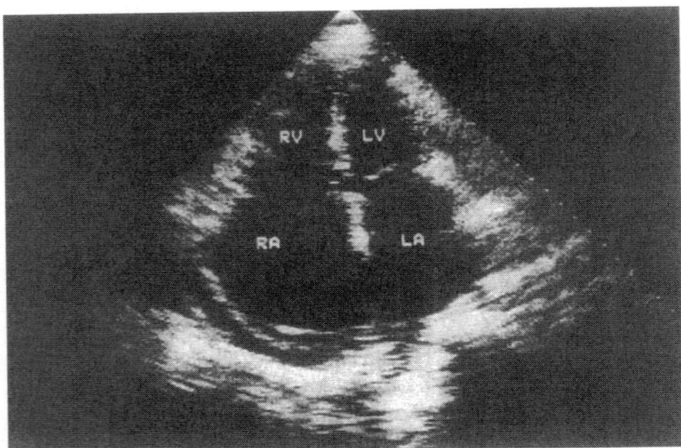

Figure 18-4 Echocardiogram from a patient with restrictive cardiomyopathy (apical four-chamber view). Note the small left (*LV*) and right (*RV*) chamber sizes and the relatively normal wall thicknesses. The left (*LA*) and right (*RA*) atria are markedly enlarged. (Reproduced with permission from Hosenpud JD. *Restrictive Cardiomyopathy [Progress in Cardiology 1989]*. Philadelphia: Lea & Febiger; 1989:95.)

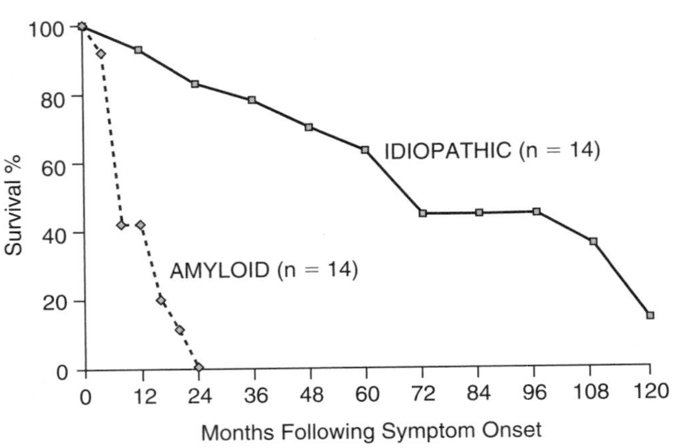

Figure 18-6 Actuarial survival data in primary restrictive cardiomyopathy compiled from several studies (312,313,316,317,319,320). Short and intermediate survival is reasonable; however, ultimate survival following onset of symptoms is approximately 10% at 10 years. In contrast, actuarial survival of patients with amyloid heart disease from compiled data (325–329,334) is extremely poor. There is essentially no survival beyond 24 months from the onset of cardiac symptoms.

The charactristic gross anatomical findings in these patients are small left and right ventricles, with ventricular wall thickness normal or mildly increased and atria moderately to severely enlarged. Figure 18-4 presents an echocardiographic apical four-chamber view from a patient with primary restrictive cardiomyopathy. Histopathologically, prominent interstitial fibrosis as seen in Figure 18-5 is a prominent finding (311,316,322).

In contrast to patients with dilated cardiomyopathy, who have an extremely high 1- and 2-year mortality, as shown in Figure 18-6, patients with primary RCM appear to have a better early prognosis (approximate 10% mortality at 1 year). Ultimately, however, the prognosis is poor, with only 10% of patients surviving at 10 years.

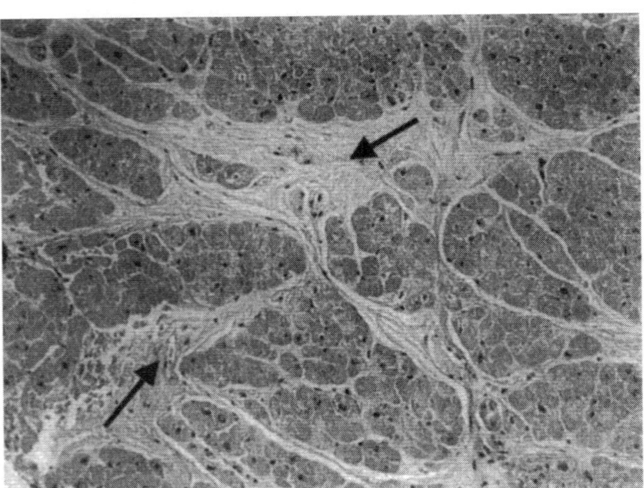

Figure 18-5 Endomyocardial biopsy specimen (hematoxylin and eosin, 255×) from a patient with primary restrictive cardiomyopathy, showing extensive interstitial fibrosis (**arrows**) and relatively normal myocytes. (Reproduced with permission from Hosenpud JD. *Restrictive Cardiomyopathy [Progress in Cardiology 1989]*. Philadelphia: Lea & Febiger; 1989:95.)

Amyloidosis

A second frequently reported cause of RCM is amyloid protein deposition into the myocardial interstitium. Amyloid is a generic term for the deposition of a variety of fibrous proteins arranged spatially in a β-pleated sheet configuration. It is this spatial configuration that gives amyloid its characteristic staining properties in tissue. There are four types of amyloidosis, and cardiac involvement is most common in primary amyloidosis (AL type). Primary amyloidosis is caused by plasma cell production of immunoglobulin light chains, often related to multiple myeloma. Serum protein electrophoresis demonstrates monoclonal gammopathy. Secondary amyloidosis is attributable to the deposition of a nonimmunoglobulin protein termed AA (323). Secondary amyloidosis is due to chronic infection or autoimmune disease. The third type of amyloidosis is familial (324). Senile amyloidosis, the fourth form, is due to the production of either an atrial natiuretic-like protein or transthyretin.

Restrictive ventricular filling in cardiac amyloidosis is thought to result from amyloid fiber deposition in the cardiac interstitium, replacing normal contractile elements. The deposition may be widespread or localized to conduction tissue, valves, pericardium, or coronary arteries. Coronary artery infiltration may result in ischemia, leading to systolic dysfunction. The deposition of insoluble fibers in cardiac chambers results in increased wall thickness. The amyloid-affected myocardium is firm and noncompliant.

Table 18-7 presents data compiled from case reports and small series of patients with amyloidosis for whom individual clinical and follow-up data were available (314,325–329). Myeloma, plasmacytoma, or other plasma cell dyscrasias are present overall in 45% of cases of cardiac amyloidosis. Based on the age distribution for plasma cell diseases, one would expect and the data confirm an overall older group of patients with this form of RCM than with primary disease. The remaining cases of

TABLE 18-7

CLINICAL CHARACTERISTICS OF 14 PATIENTS WITH AMYLOID CARDIOMYOPATHY*

Age	
Mean, 56 y	Range, 44 to 86 y
Sex	
50% male	50% female
Symptomatology	
Chest pain	0%
Fatigue	73%
Dyspnea	100%
Clinical Findings	
Jugular venous distention	83%
Rales	58%
S_3	91%
S_4	50%
Ascites	55%
Edema	92%
Hemodynamics+	
Right atrial (mm Hg)	14 ± 4
Pulmonary wedge (mm Hg)	20 ± 3
Cardiac index (L/min/m^2)	2.1 ± 0.4
LV EDVI (mL/m^2)	60 ± 14
LV ejection fraction	0.57 ± 0.10

*Compiled data from seven studies (Emery AEH. X-linked muscular dystrophy with early contractures and cardiomyopathy (Emery Dreifuss type). *Clin Genet.* 1987;32:360–367; Harley HG, Rundle SA, MacMillian JC, et al. Size of the unstable CTG repeat sequence in relation to phenotype and parental transmission in myotonic dystrophy. *Am J Hum Genet.* 1993;52:1164–1174; Timchenko L, Monckton DG, Caskey CT. Myotonic dystrophy: an unstable CTG repeat in a protein kinase gene. *Semin Cell Biol.* 1995;6:13–19; Melacini P, Villanova C, Menagazzo E, et al. Correlation between cardia involvement and CTG trinucleotide repeat length in myotonic dystrophy. *J Am Coll Cardiol.* 1995;25:239–245; Wang J, Pegoraro E, Menagazzo E, et al. Myotonic dystrophy: evidence for a possible dominant-negative RNA mutation. *Hum Mol Genet.* 1995;4:599–606; and Cox GF, Kunkel LM. Dystrophies and heart disease. Curr *Opin Cardiol.* 1997;12:329–343.)
+Results expressed as mean + 1 SD.
LV EDVI, left ventricular end-diastolic volume index.

cardiac amyloidosis, with few exceptions, are manifestations of systemic disease, and amyloid deposition is found in various other organs. Patients with amyloid heart disease tend to be more symptomatic, are more often clinically in congestive heart failure, and have reduced cardiac indices; in contrast, normal cardiac outputs are seen in primary RCM.

The gross anatomical findings in amyloid heart disease are similar to those in primary restrictive cardiomyopathy, with some notable differences. Both LV and RV wall thicknesses on echocardiography tend to be symmetrically increased and there is hypokinesis of the intraventricular septum. The atrioventricular valves are also involved and can appear thickened on echocardiography. Finally, a particular granular and speckled pattern of the myocardium has been described (330–332). Unfortunately, this particular finding can be quite variable depending on gain settings and the particular machine used. Therefore, the diagnosis of amyloid should not be confirmed or ruled out based on the echocardiographic tissue characteristics. Figure 18-7 demonstrates the histopathology of an endomyocardial biopsy specimen from a patient with severe RCM secondary to amyloid infiltration. The amyloid protein is deposited throughout the interstitium, surrounding individual myocytes, with larger deposition in the perivascular areas. If one views amyloid in tissue under polarized light, a characteristic green birefringence is present.

Reviewing Figure 18-6, it is clear that the prognosis of patients having RCM secondary to amyloidosis is extremely poor in comparison with the prognosis of those having idiopathic restrictive disease, with no survival beyond 2 years of symptoms. These prognostic data are further supported by a larger, single study of patients with amyloid heart disease and congestive heart failure, whose median survival was 6 months (333).

Endomyocardial Fibrosis

Endomyocardial fibrosis with or without eosinophilia, first described by Loeffler in 1930 (334), is another frequently cited cause of RCM. Since Loeffler's original two patients, more than 100 cases have been reported. It has been suggested that eosinophilic damage to the endocardium is the primary etiology in all cases of endomyocardial fibrosis, and that those patients without documented eosinophilia are presenting at a later stage of the disease (335). The mechanism of injury appears to be a direct toxic effect of eosinophilic secretory products (granule basic proteins) on the myocardium (336). The pattern of injury appears to progress through three stages: the necrotic stage, characterized by an eosinophilic endomyocarditis and arteritis; a

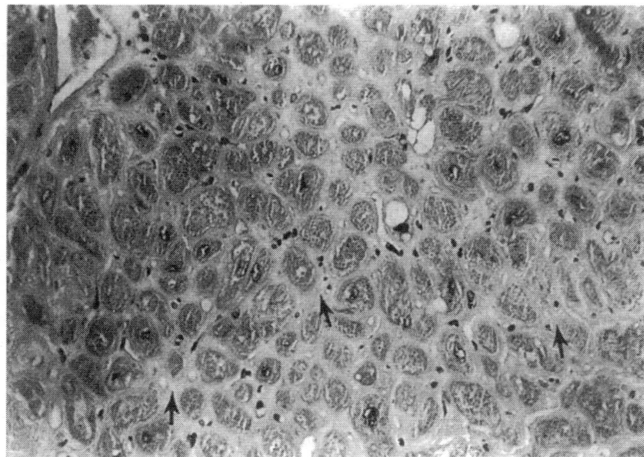

Figure 18-7 Endomyocardial biopsy specimen (hematoxylin and eosin, 250×) from a patient with amyloid heart disease, showing extensive deposits of amorphous material surrounding individual myocytes (**arrows**) within the interstitium. (Reproduced with permission from Hosenpud JD. *Restrictive Cardiomyopathy [Progress in Cardiology 1989]*. Philadelphia: Lea & Febiger; 1989:98.)

mural thrombosis stage, during which platelets and thrombin are deposited along the damaged endothelium; and finally a fibrotic stage, in which the endocardial thrombus and damaged endothelium are replaced by fibrous tissue (337,338).

The mechanisms of the resulting restrictive hemodynamic findings in patients with endomyocardial fibrosis may differ depending on the stage of the disease process. During the thrombotic stage, in addition to the endomyocardial damage, ventricular thrombi may be so large that the remaining ventricular chamber volume is inadequate to sustain cardiac output. In the fibrotic stage, the thick endocardial peel presumably prevents normal diastolic relaxation.

The cardiovascular clinical findings in endomyocardial fibrosis are basically identical to those found in other forms of RCM and include symptoms and signs of biventricular congestive heart failure (339–342). The prognosis appears to be quite variable and probably depends on the underlying disease process. Although eosinophilia can be present for a prolonged period of time before the appearance of cardiac symptoms (343), the prognosis appears to be poor once cardiac symptoms develop (343–345). In studies in which aggressive therapy is directed simultaneously to reducing the total eosinophil count, treating the congestive heart failure, and in some cases surgically stripping the endomyocardium and replacing valves, the outcome may be modified (337,339,341).

Other Causes

RCM due to Fabry disease is the result of an accumulation of glycosphingolipids in the lysosomes of the cardiac tissues. RCM is also caused by Gaucher disease (cardiac tissues accumulate cerbrosides), hemochromatosis (excessive iron deposition in cardiac tissue), glycogen storage disease, sarcoidosis (noncaseating granulomatous involvement of the heart), collagen vascular disease, coronary arteritis, and genetic connective tissue disease. Endocardial plaques (usually involving right-heart structures) and RCM are due to excessive serotonin and 5-HIAA in the carcinoid syndrome. Malignant infiltration of the heart with metastatic tumors may produce RCM, especially when the pericardium is involved. Iatrogenic etiologies of constriction include chest radiation, anthracycline and methysergide toxicity, and L-tryptophan-containing oils. Cardiac allografts commonly demonstrate a restrictive pattern of filling and, in a minority of patients, this may persist for at least 1 year (346–350).

Therapy

Specific Therapy

Because no specific etiology for primary RCM is known, there is obviously no specific treatment. Modest evidence is now available to suggest that the treatment of myeloma and plasma cell dyscrasias may alter the course of cardiac amyloidosis. The effect of melphalan and prednisone has been studied in two major trials. Kyle et al. (354) studied 220 patients with the AL (primary) form of amyloidosis who were randomized to three treatment protocols: colchicine, melphalan and prednisone, or colchicine plus melphalan and prednisone. The median survival of patients in the colchicine group was 8.5 months, in those receiving melphalan plus prednisone it was 18 months, and in those receiving melphalan plus prednisone plus colchicine it was 17 months. Skinner et al. (355) reported that the median survival was significantly longer for patients with cardiac amyloidosis and congestive heart failure who received melphalan and prednisone (12 months) than it was for controls (5 months). Since the liver produces transthyretin in the familial form of amyloidosis, liver transplant may improve survival. As discussed earlier, aggressive therapy of eosinophilic systemic disease may influence the endomyocardial damage (341) and, once damage is present, aggressive surgical therapy may improve cardiac performance (339). There have been isolated reports of aggressive total-body iron removal influencing cardiac function in patients with hemochromatosis (352), and of corticosteroid therapy improving cardiac performance in patients with sarcoidosis and other granulomatous diseases of the myocardium (351).

Generic Therapy

Generic therapy for restriction is extremely difficult once severe cardiovascular compromise is present. Diuretics are a mainstay of therapy, but cautious use is required. As the diastolic ventricular pressure–volume relationship in RCM is quite steep, small changes in volume can produce large changes in filling pressures. The decrease in myocardial compliance requires higher filling pressures for adequate ventricular filling, so a reduction in filling pressures to alleviate symptoms of congestion may produce dramatic falls in cardiac output. Systolic performance in patients with RCM is usually normal and may in some patients be at the upper range of normal. This finding limits the use of inotropic agents, and digitalis specifically may have a role only in rhythm control, as many patients with restriction and atrial dilation have atrial arrhythmias. In addition, patients with amyloid heart disease may be hypersensitive to the toxic effects of digitalis (333).

Vasodilator therapy, although a mainstay of treatment for most forms of heart failure, may be of very limited use in restrictive disease. In restriction, stroke volume is dependent on high filling pressures and is usually fixed at peak pressures. As cardiac dilation is seldom present, this component of wall stress would not play a major role. The expected response in patients with RCM to vasodilator therapy would be a reduction in preload, reducing filling and stroke volume, and a potentially profound reduction in arterial pressure secondary to both arteriolar dilation and the fall in cardiac output. Furthermore, the beneficial effects of calcium-channel blockers in hypertrophic cardiomyopathy have not been demonstrated in RCM. Because most calcium antagonists are vasodilators, the effects anticipated with vasodilator therapy would also be anticipated with calcium channel antagonists. In addition, both verapamil and diltiazem produce direct suppressant effects on sinus node function that results in a slowing of heart rate, and they have negative inotropic properties (356). In patients whose stroke volume is fixed and whose cardiac output is dependent on heart rate, it is evident that the effects of calcium-channel blockers are potentially more deleterious than beneficial. Furthermore, in both the infiltrative diseases and those in which the endomyocardium is primarily affected, one would expect the myocardial diastolic properties to be relatively normal. Therapy for RCM is therefore limited, for all practical purposes, to diuretic therapy for mild to moderate symptoms and cardiac transplantation for severe disease.

HYPERTROPHIC CARDIOMYOPATHY

Pathophysiology and Mechanisms of Disease

Hypertrophic cardiomyopathy (HCM), initially described by Teare in 1958 (357), has since that time been surrounded by controversy and is still poorly understood. This lack of understanding is reflected in the several primarily descriptive names of the disease, including hypertrophic obstructive cardiomyopathy, idiopathic hypertrophic subaortic stenosis, asymmetric septal hypertrophy, and muscular subaortic stenosis—all related to the concept that obstruction of the outflow tract is a principal pathophysiological mechanism. However, this aspect of the disease is controversial. In fact, most students of primary myocardial disease feel that although outflow tract obstruction may be present, the principal abnormality is that of impaired ventricular compliance, which is likely a consequence of the inappropriate myocardial hypertrophy. Hence, HCM, now the most commonly used terminology, is likely the most appropriate.

What is clear is that a distinctive pattern of hypertrophy involving the ventricular septum out of proportion to the other ventricular walls (asymmetric septal hypertrophy) is present in the majority of patients. Microscopically, the myocardial fibers in the areas of hypertrophy are disorganized without evidence of the usual orientation parallel to the lines of stress. This has been referred to as myofibril disarray. In addition to asymmetric septal hypertrophy, most patients have evidence of a pressure gradient across the aortic outflow tract, caused primarily by the mitral valve moving anteriorly during systole and abutting the septum. This condition is termed systolic anterior motion (358). The specific controversies surrounding the measured pressure gradient will be discussed later.

HCM appears to be inherited in an autosomal dominant pattern in between 50% and 75% of cases, with the remainder being sporadic (359,360). As with other autosomal dominant diseases, penetrance and phenotype (even within a given family) can be quite variable. As previously stated, most patients manifest asymmetric septal hypertrophy and a measured gradient. However, others (even within the same family) manifest a more concentric hypertrophy or asymmetric septal hypertrophy without obstruction (Fig. 18-8). It is now clear that HCM is the result of a number of specific mutations in one of four genes that encode cardiac sarcomere proteins. These include the β-myosin heavy chain gene on chromosome 14, the α-tropomyosin gene on chromosome 15, the myosin binding protein on chromosome 11, and the cardiac troponin T gene on chromosome 1 (361–364). More

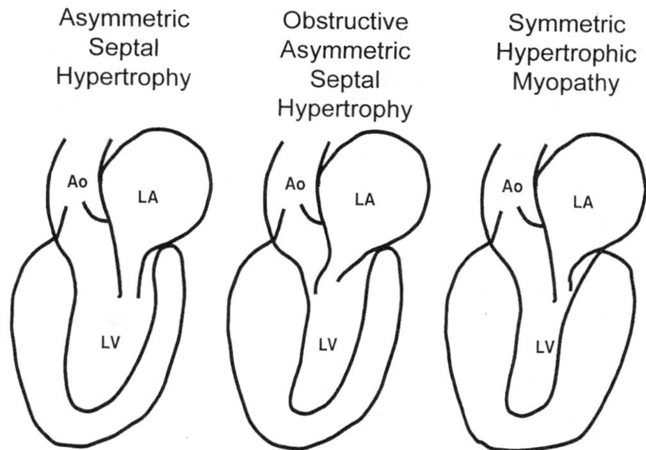

Figure 18-8 The presentation of hypertrophic cardiomyopathy is highly variable, even within the same family. A patient can present with hypertrophy localized primarily to the septum with or without obstruction. When present, obstruction occurs at the level of the anterior mitral leaflet, or a more diffuse pattern of hypertrophic disease involves the entire LV.

than 70 specific mutations have been identified and are predominantly those of a missense type. The variability in disease onset, severity, and prognosis before the identification of specific mutations had appeared to be quite mysterious. Although one anticipates with further information an improved ability to prognosticate based on the specific abnormal protein involved and the functional severity of the mutation, variabilities in presentation (even within families) suggest that nongenetic factors may influence the course of disease.

Figure 18-9 demonstrates the typical M-mode and two-dimensional echocardiographic findings from a patient with HCM and an outflow tract gradient. As previously stated, the gradient is produced when the anterior leaflet of the mitral valve abuts the septum in late systole. This outflow tract obstruction, similar to that of fixed aortic valvular disease, was assumed to be the basis of the primary morbidity in this disease. It was Criley et al. (365) who first suggested that the outflow tract gradients seen in patients with HCM are caused by the extremely powerful and rapid contraction of the ventricle and the resulting cavity obliteration. This school proposed that the primary morbidity in HCM is secondary to abnormal diastolic function and ventricular stiffness rather than obstruction (366–368). Arguments for and against the importance of obstruction peppered the medical literature for the next 15 years, with proponents of the "obstruction school" citing the beneficial effects of septal myectomy and the reduction in gradients after administration of β-blockers and calcium-channel blockers as supportive evidence (369,370).

The opposing school countered with evidence suggesting that most of the ejection from the LV occurred before the development of the gradient and cavity obliteration seen in most patients (365,371). The counter-explanation for surgical improvement was the creation of a larger ventricular chamber that improved LV filling; β-blockers slowed heart rate and reduced contractility (improving diastolic function) and calcium antagonists both reduced

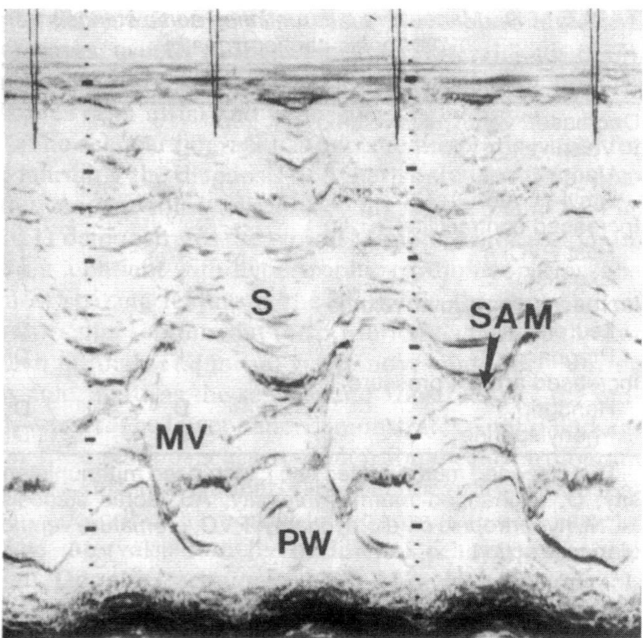

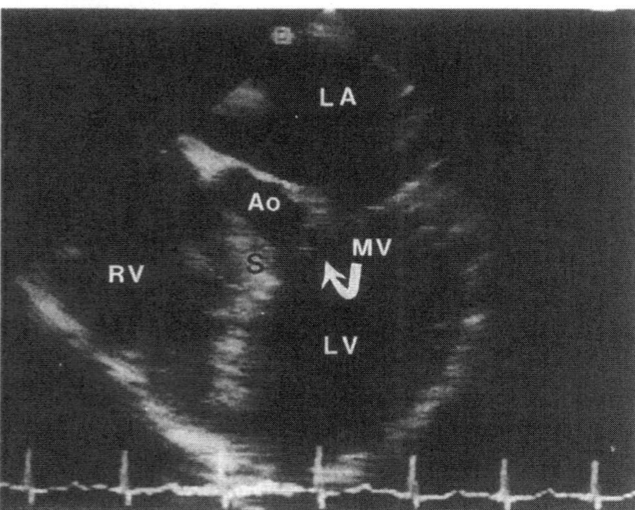

Figure 18-9 Typical M-mode **(top)** and transesophageal **(bottom)** echocardiograms seen in patients with hypertrophic cardiomyoapthy. With the onset of systole, the mitral valve (*MV*) exhibits systolic anterior motion (*SAM*) and abuts the ventricular septum (*S*), causing an outflow tract gradient. LV, left ventricle; RV, right ventricle; PW, posterior wall; LA, left atrium; Ao, aorta.

contractility and possibly directly altered the diastolic properties of the myocardium. Finally, there did not appear to be any difference in symptoms or ultimate prognosis between patients who had or did not have an outflow tract gradient (371,372).

Clinical Features of Hypertrophic Cardiomyopathy

Symptoms

The principal symptoms of patients with HCM are dyspnea, chest pain, and syncope (373–376). Exertional dyspnea is certainly the most common symptom and has been reported in more than 90% of patients with the disease (377). The dyspnea is likely a consequence of high filling pressures (especially during exercise), secondary to the reduced myocardial compliance (363–368). It is clear that this symptom (along with chest pain and syncope) does not correlate with the presence or amount of the outflow tract gradient (378,379).

Angina is the next most frequent symptom and can occur in up to 75% of patients (380). Moreover, myocardial infarction has been documented in 15% of patients at autopsy (381). The infarction can, on rare occasions, involve the entire subendocardium, resulting in complete shelling of the entire LV subendocardium. The mechanism of the angina and myocardial necrosis is felt to be a combination of inadequate subendocardial coronary blood flow to meet the needs of the marked hypertrophy, direct subendocardial vascular compression caused by high systolic and diastolic LV cavity pressures, and abnormal regulation of the coronary microcirculation (381–386).

Syncope or near-syncope has been reported in up to 50% of patients with HCM (374–376). Although initially thought to be secondary to the outflow tract gradient through mechanisms similar to that seen in valvular aortic stenosis, it is clear now that there is no relationship between syncopal symptoms and the severity of outflow tract gradients (374–376,379,387). According to findings from Holter monitor and treadmill exercise studies demonstrating frequent ventricular and atrial arrhythmias and overt ventricular tachycardia in up to 40% of patients, the syncope is most certainly arrhythmic in etiology in most cases (388–391). According to electrophysiological studies, the propensity for ventricular tachyarrhythmias may be a consequence of disordered electrophysiological properties of the abnormally hypertrophied ventricle (392). The sole mechanism for atrial arrhythmias may be the elevated ventricular filling pressures, which result in atrial stretch (390,391). Other abnormalities, including associated atrioventricular bypass tracts, have been reported (393).

Finally, in a minority of patients and usually late in the disease, systolic ventricular function deteriorates and more characteristic symptoms of heart failure supervene. Signs and symptoms of both LV and RV dysfunction can occur, especially if patients lose sinus rhythm and atrioventricular synchrony (374,378).

Overall, patients with HCM are less symptomatic than patients with other forms of cardiomyopathy. A full 30% of patients will be asymptomatic, as evidenced by recent, well-publicized stories of athletes who died suddenly during sporting events, being subsequently found to have HCM. Another 50% of patients are NYHA functional Class II, and it is a rare patient who presents with functional Class IV symptoms (375,394).

Clinical Findings

Clinical findings in patients without resting or exercise outflow tract gradients can be entirely normal or may be confined to signs of elevated LV filling pressures (fourth heart sound). In the more advanced stages (especially with loss of sinus rhythm and progressive ventricular dysfunc-

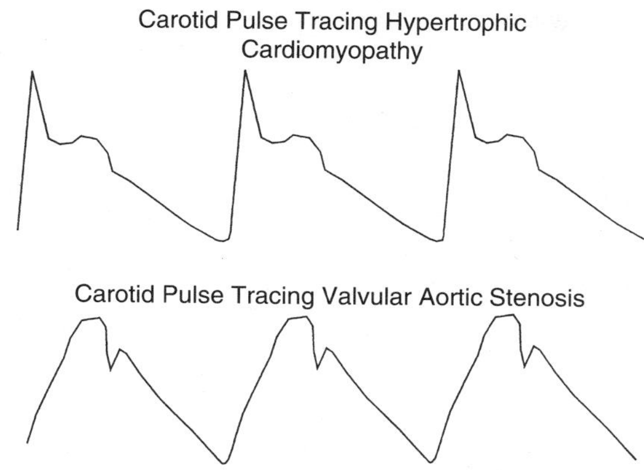

Figure 18-10 The carotid impulse in patients with hypertrophic cardiomyopathy demonstrates a characteristic rapid initial upstroke followed by a "dip-and-plateau" configuration resulting from the abrupt cessation of blood flow secondary to the anterior motion of the mitral valve. This contrasts with the delayed upstroke and prominent dicrotic notch (especially with low cardiac output) seen in patients with native aortic stenosis.

tion), signs of both systemic and pulmonary venous congestion can be present. In patients with a resting or provoked outflow tract gradient, the clinical examination findings can be diagnostic. In Figure 18-10, the carotid impulse from a patient with HCM is contrasted with the carotid impulse from a patient with valvular aortic stenosis. Unlike the carotid impulse of the patient with aortic stenosis, which is reduced in amplitude and delayed in timing, the carotid impulse of the patient with HCM is rapid in upstroke, bifid, and followed by a prominent dicrotic notch. This "spike-and-dome" pulse tracing is secondary to rapid ventricular emptying caused by enhanced contractility, followed by abrupt reduction of flow secondary to mitral valve anterior motion (systolic anterior motion), which occludes the outflow tract.

The jugular venous pressure is typical of patients with reduced ventricular compliance. As long as the patient remains in sinus rhythm, the A wave is large, and usually the V wave is normal unless significant tricuspid regurgitation is present.

As the outflow tract gradient is dynamic, the murmur in patients with HCM is quite characteristic and can be altered by a series of bedside maneuvers or pharmacologic interventions. Table 18-8 contrasts the murmur of HCM with that of fixed aortic stenosis. In general, the murmur is heard best along the left sternal border and usually does not radiate well into the carotid arteries. In contrast to what is observed in valvular aortic stenosis, any maneuver that reduces preload and, hence, ventricular size accentuates the murmur because of an earlier abutment of the mitral valve against the septum and an increase in the outflow tract gradient. Conversely, any maneuver that increases ventricular size, such as raising the legs or squatting, will reduce the intensity of the murmur. As in aortic stenosis, an increase in contractility or reduction in afterload (after ventricular premature beat, amyl nitrate) will increase the intensity of the murmur. In contrast to what occurs in aortic stenosis, however, these latter maneuvers will actually decrease the pulse pressure as assessed by carotid or brachial palpation because of the earlier occurrence of systolic anterior motion. Finally, in addition to the outflow tract murmur, many patients (especially those with moderate to severe systolic anterior motion of the mitral valve) will have coexistent mitral insufficiency of varying degrees.

TABLE 18-8
MANEUVERS DIFFERENTIATING AORTIC STENOSIS FROM HYPERTROPHIC CARDIOMYOPATHY

Maneuver	AS	HCM
Decreased ventricular volume	—	—
Valsalva	D	I
Upright posture	U	I
Amyl nitrate	—	—
Increased contractility	—	—
Post-PVC	I	I
Exercise	I	I
Increased ventricular volume	—	—
Leg elevation	I	D
Pregnancy	I	D
Increased arterial pressure	—	—
Handgrip	D	D
Phenylephrine	D	D

D, decreased murmur intensity; I, increased murmur intensity; U, unchanged murmur intensity; AS, aortic stenosis; HCM, hypertrophic cardiomyopathy; PVC, premature ventricular contraction.

Invasive and Noninvasive Studies

The electrocardiogram in patients with HCM most often demonstrates LV hypertrophy (374), left atrial (LA) enlargement, and abnormal Q waves, usually in the inferior and lateral leads (395). As previously mentioned, Holter monitoring demonstrates both atrial and ventricular arrhythmias.

The echocardiogram has become the primary tool for confirming the diagnosis of HCM. As previously discussed, the upper panel of Figure 18-9 demonstrates the typical M-mode echocardiogram from a patient with HCM. The most striking feature is the markedly thickened intraventricular septum, but the posterior wall is also thicker than normal. The mitral valve moves anteriorly during systole, abutting the septum and obstructing the outflow tract. The lower panel demonstrates similar findings on a transesophageal two-dimensional echocardiogram from a different patient. Other echocardiographic features described have included abnormalities in diastolic time intervals, both by traditional echocardiographic and Doppler techniques (396–401). Shaver et al. (402), studying 84 patients with HCM, demonstrated abnormally prolonged isovolumic relaxation periods in 31 of the 84.

The hemodynamic findings of patients with HCM and outflow tract gradients are well-described (403–405). Figure 18-11 is a representation of LV and aortic pressure tracings corresponding to the above clinical findings of the phenomenon first described by Brokenbrough. The systolic contraction immediately following a premature ventricular complex is augmented, which results in higher

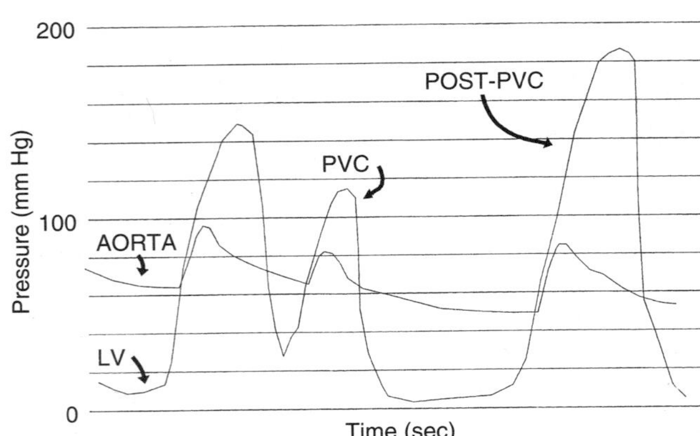

Figure 18-11 A representation of the aortic and LV pressure tracing in a patient with hypertrophic cardiomyopathy. The so-called Brokenbrough effect is produced when a premature ventricular contraction (PVC) causes postsystolic potentiation of the subsequent beat. The increase in contractility increases the intraventricular pressure, the outflow tract gradient increases, and pulse pressure actually falls.

intraventricular pressure. This augmentation of ventricular pressure results in an earlier anterior motion of the mitral valve, a larger outflow tract gradient, and a fall in aortic pressure in comparison with a normal beat. As previously described the same maneuvers used at the bedside to change loading conditions and volume of the ventricle alter a resting gradient or can provoke a gradient that is not present at rest (404). With careful hemodynamic monitoring during LV pullback, the gradient can usually be found within the LV outflow tract before the aortic valve is crossed. Other associated hemodynamic findings include elevations in both LV and RV filling pressures, a corresponding accentuation of the wave in both ventricles and, in a minority of patients in the later stages of disease, a reduction in cardiac output (406).

Angiographic findings include asymmetric septal hypertrophy; a small, hypercontractile ventricle, often associated with a completely obliterated cavity (evidence against hemodynamically important obstruction); and hypertrophied papillary muscles. Mitral regurgitation can range from mild to severe. The shape of the ventricle in systole has been referred to as an inverted cone because of the massive hypertrophy and cavity obliteration that encroach on the outflow tract (403–406).

Therapy

Because HCM is an autosomal dominant disorder, a screening echocardiogram in first-degree relatives is recommended, with re-evaluation of family members every 5 years or earlier should signs and symptoms so warrant. Risk stratification for sudden cardiac death and therapy aimed at relief of symptoms are essential. Nonobstructive HCM is treated medically for symptom relief due to diastolic dysfunction. Dual-chamber pacing and septal debulking (either surgical or catheter-based with alcohol) may not be indicated in patients without obstruction. General measures of therapy for obstructive HCM include infective endocarditis prophylaxis, anticoagulation in the setting of atrial fibrillation, and avoiding dehydration, alcohol, and isometric or anaerobic exercise. Exertional symptoms are treated medically with maximally tolerated doses of β-blockers, rate-slowing calcium-channel blockers, or disopyramide, used alone or in combination. Septal debulking, either surgically or with catheter-based alcohol infusion, is appropriate in patients with outflow tract obstruction and symptoms refractory to medical therapy. Dual-chamber pacing may be considered in those patients with refractory symptoms due to obstruction and contraindications to septal debulking.

Medical Management

As early as 1964, Harrison et al. (407) reported the potential benefits of *β*-blocking agents on the hemodynamics of patients with HCM. Since that time, several studies have demonstrated the efficacy of these agents, both in reducing symptoms and improving hemodynamics. Most hemodynamic studies demonstrated a reduction in the outflow tract gradient with *β*-blockade and suggested that the improvement in symptoms was secondary to such reduction (408,409). Other, more likely mechanisms include the reduction in contractility, which in turn reduces myocardial oxygen demand both at rest and during exercise; the reduction of heart rate, which allows for an increase in diastolic time and filling; and possibly a reduction in the amount of mitral regurgitation. Initial studies suggested that *β*-blockade might improve diastolic function (410,411) but subsequent careful studies of diastolic indices have not supported this (412,413). Finally, β-blockers may effect the generation of ventricular arrhythmias, especially during exercise and stress when catecholamine levels are elevated. Although the initial response to β-blockers in many patients is quite good, the long-term response has been less satisfactory, with many patients experiencing fatigue and depression, especially if high doses of β-blockers are required.

In contrast to what has been observed with β-blockers, a large body of work has demonstrated the efficacy and sustained response of patients with HCM to treatment with calcium-channel blockers (414–418). Although several of the calcium-channel blockers have been demonstrated to be efficacious, most of the experience has been with verapamil. Rosing et al. (415) demonstrated that verapamil improved exercise performance by an average of 45% in 19 patients with HCM. In this study, there was no correlation between improvement in exercise performance and change in outflow tract gradient, which was reduced by an average of 35 mm Hg. The efficacy of calcium-channel blockers, similar to that of the *β*-blockers, can be attributed to a combination of factors, including a reduction in contractility and a reduction in heart rate. However, there is reproducible evidence that calcium-channel blockers, unlike the β-blockers, improve diastolic function in this disease. Shaffer et al. (419) demonstrated that verapamil improved two indices of diastolic function (peak filling rate and time to peak filling rate) and improved exercise performance in 10 children (aged 7 to 18 years) for an average treatment period of 1.8 years. The mechanisms responsible for improved relaxation potentially include an improvement in coronary flow to reduce subendocardial ischemia, a possible improvement in ventricular synchrony, and an improvement in both preload and afterload (420–422). There is also experimental evidence that abnormal cardiac hypertrophy results in altered calcium flux and an intracellular calcium overload state (364). In experimentally induced calcium overload, verapamil improves relaxation in cultured myocardial cells (423).

More recent studies have demonstrated a hemodynamically beneficial effect of the antiarrhythmic agent amiodarone (424). The mechanisms responsible for this efficacy are unclear but they may be the negative inotropic effects of this agent along with vascular dilation. There also may be the added benefit of suppression of ventricular arrhythmias. This agent has been demonstrated to improve symptoms of patients refractory to both β-blockers and calcium-channel blockers (425).

In patients with elevated filling pressures, careful use of diuretic therapy is indicated. As in the treatment of restrictive cardiomyopathy, one is hampered by the need to reduce resting filling pressures enough to eliminate symptoms of congestion but not enough to reduce ventricular filling. This is particularly difficult in patients who are in chronic atrial fibrillation, as atrial contraction in this disease can be responsible for as much as 50% of ventricular filling.

Arrhythmia management is a major concern in patients with HCM. Patients may become severely symptomatic with loss of atrial synchrony, as alluded to earlier. It is reasonable to attempt to convert atrial arrhythmias either electrically or pharmacologically and try to maintain sinus rhythm in patients who become symptomatic with loss of atrioventricular synchrony. Amiodarone has been demonstrated to be beneficial in controlling both atrial and ventricular arrhythmias in patients with HCM.

Finally, attempts to prevent comorbidity should be undertaken. In patients with intermittent or persistent atrial fibrillation, systemic anticoagulation is indicated; in patients with a systolic murmur consistent with systolic anterior motion, endocarditis prophylaxis is required.

Pacing

Implantation of a dual-chamber pacemaker has been performed in symptomatic patients with hypertrophic obstructive cardiomyopathy to relieve symptoms and reduce the outflow gradient. The proposed mechanism involved pacemaker initiation of the electrical impulse in the RV apex, thereby altering the contraction sequence of the basal interventricular septum, resulting in a reduction in outflow gradient. Additional rationale included chronic remodeling and optimizing AV delay to allow full benefit of so-called atrial kick.

Earlier cohort studies suggested a substantial improvement in symptoms and outflow tract gradient, but recent and more rigorous trials utilizing a blinded placebo group demonstrated patients reporting symptomatic improvement during the period without pacemaker activity. While some patients report benefit from pacemaker implantation, most demonstrate no longstanding clinical improvement. The average residual gradient after pacing is still 30 to 50 mm Hg, and randomized crossover trials demonstrate both a strong placebo effect and, in the majority of patients, no improvement in objective measures of exercise capacity. While some patients demonstrate active, pacing-induced reduction in gradient and improvement of exercise capacity, there are no known parameters to suggest which patients will derive benefit from pacemaker implantation. Older patients may be more likely to have a prolonged benefit.

Even more equivocal is the indication for pacemaker implantation in patients without a resting outflow gradient. A retrospective comparison of surgical myectomy with dual-chamber pacing suggested superior symptom relief and exercise tolerance with surgical myectomy. Thus, dual-chamber pacing is limited to patients with contraindications to other therapies, those with low resting heart rates precluding use of β-blockers or rate-slowing calcium-channel blockers, or those with indications for bradycardia pacing independent of HCM (426–430).

Alcohol-Induced Septal Ablation

A newer approach to debulking the septum involves infusion of 100% alcohol down the septal perforator artery supplying the septum at the point of mitral leaflet–septal contact, inducing a controlled infarction of the affected portion of the seputm. Alcohol infusion induces local akinesis of the septum initially, widening the outflow tract and decreasing the gradient. Weeks to months later, postinfarct remodeling induces thinning of the involved portion of the septum, again widening the outflow tract. Three to 12 months later, both improved hemodynamics and symptom relief have been reported, including significant reduction or elimination of the gradient, improved exercise capacity, and improved NYHA functional class.

No randomized trials comparing septal myectomy with septal ablation have been conducted. No data have been generated thus far regarding survival, prevention of sudden cardiac death, or onset of heart failure. Initially, the complication rate, including infarction and need for permanent pacemaker implantation, was approximately 25%. Other complications include ventricular perforation, large myocardial infarction, ventricular septal defect, and intractable ventricular fibrillation. More recent experience has reduced the need for permanent pacemaker implantation to approximately 10%. Advantages of septal ablation over myectomy include shorter hospital stay and avoidance of general anesthetic and sternotomy. Disadvantages include inability to address coexistent abnormalities (such as coronary artery disease, abnormal papillary muscle anatomy, fixed subaortic obstruction, midventricular obstruction, and intrinsic mitral valve disease); uncertainty regarding long-term effects of iatrogenic infarction; need for permanent pacing in 10% of patients; and failure of the procedure in 15% to 20% of the patients due to lack of suitable septal arteries in the area needing to be addressed. Septal ablation may be a potential alternative to surgical myectomy in those patients with a significant outflow tract gradient and symptoms refractory to medical therapy (431–437).

Surgical Management

In the first report of surgical therapy for HCM, presented by Morrow and Brockenbrough in 1961 (447), a subaortic ventriculomyotomy was performed on two patients, following which a reduction in outflow tract gradient and clinical improvement were noted. Since that time, the procedure has been modified and a large number of patients refractory to medical management have undergone the procedure (448). The overall operative mortality ranges from 0% to 26%, depending on the series, with additional late mortality (449). Maron et al. (369) reported on 124 patients who underwent septal myotomy-myectomy at the National Institutes of Health, with an operative mortality of 8%. In 88% of the patients, clinical improvement was noted in the first 6 months after surgery and this improvement persisted in 70% of the initial group.

Figure 18-12 demonstrates the completed septal myotomy-myectomy procedure. The mechanisms by which improvement occurs following this operation are not clear. There is no doubt that the procedure reduces the resting outflow tract gradient (369). It is also well-documented that the clinical results of the operation do not correlate with the preoperative gradient or hemodynamics (369). If reduction in the gradient is the principal mechanism for improvement, then the reduction in LV pressures could be seen to reduce myocardial oxygen demand, improve coronary flow, and possibly improve diastolic function by reducing ischemia. Alternatively, septal myotomy-myectomy does increase the size of the ventricular chamber. This size increase in and of itself may improve filling characteristics and increase stroke volume and cardiac output.

The current recommendations for septal myotomy-myectomy are that it be undertaken only for patients who are refractory to medical management and who have an outflow tract gradient of at least 50 mm Hg. Because there is no evidence that surgical therapy prolongs survival or has an impact on arrhythmias in these patients, symptoms alone must justify the surgical risks.

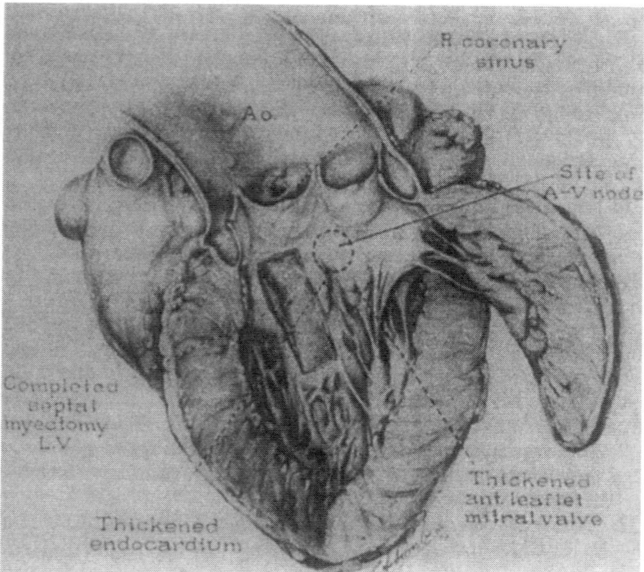

Figure 18-12 A completed septal myectomy is demonstrated. (Reproduced with permission from *J Thoracic Cardiovasc Surg.* 1978;76:429.)

Implantable Cardioverter Defibrillator Therapy and the Risk of Sudden Death

The substrate for sudden cardiac death (SCD) in HCM may lie in the histology. The myofibril disarray, with the chaotic arrangement of myocytes (especially in the septum) probably provides an unstable electrical environment, increasing the chance of re-entrant ventricular tachyarrhythmias. Coupled with intermittent episodes of ischemia due to small-vessel disease and narrowed intramural coronary arteries and subsequent replacement fibrosis, this environment provides a nidus for malignant arrhythmias. SCD is most common in patients younger than age 25 to 30 years who have had no or mild symptoms. The risk decreases in midlife but never disappears; thus, reaching a certain age does not render one immune from the risk of SCD. The identification of those at risk for SCD is controversial. Major risk factors for SCD in HCM include previous cardiac arrest with ventricular fibrillation; spontaneous sustained ventricular tachycardia (VT), family history of premature sudden death (particularly in a first-degree relative and/or multiple relatives); unexplained syncope (defined as one or more episode and particularly if recurrent, exertional, or in the young); LV wall thickness $\geq$30 mm; abnormal blood pressure response to exercise (defined as a fall or failure to rise $\geq$25 mm Hg during maximum upright exercise testing in patients $<$50 years of age); or nonsustained VT on Holter monitoring (defined as greater than or equal to three consecutive complexes at a rate $\geq$120 bpm) (438–445).

A retrospective analysis of ICD use in secondary prevention strategies has shown that an appropriate ICD discharge occurred within 10 years after implantation in 70% to 80% of patients. The use of a defibrillator as a primary prevention strategy demonstrated an appropriate device discharge in 20% of patients (446).

It is unsettled how many major risk factors a given patient must possess before a prophylactic ICD can be justified. The American College of Cardiology/American Heart Association (ACC/AHA) guidelines designate previous cardiac arrest with ventricular fibrillation (VF) as a Class I indication for device implantation.

Prognosis

Figure 18-13 demonstrates the survival of four patient groups presented in three studies (369,372,450). In a large cohort of patients from the United Kingdom in which 184 patients were adults at the time of diagnosis and 27 were children, the overall 10-year actuarial survival was above 80% in the adults and less than 60% in the pediatric group (260). In a large surgical series from the National Institutes of Health, the 10-year actuarial survival was somewhat lower than the adult series, but above 70% (369). However, in a meta-analysis of both surgical and medical approaches to this disease, Canedo and Frank (449) compared 255 surgically treated and 184 medically treated patients with HCM and could demonstrate no differences in outcome between groups. In a selected series of 33 patients who had experienced cardiac arrest and were successfully resuscitated, the outcome was substantially poorer than in the general adult experience, with a 10-year actuarial survival of less than 65% (450). Finally, an interesting study from Spirito et al. (451) pointed

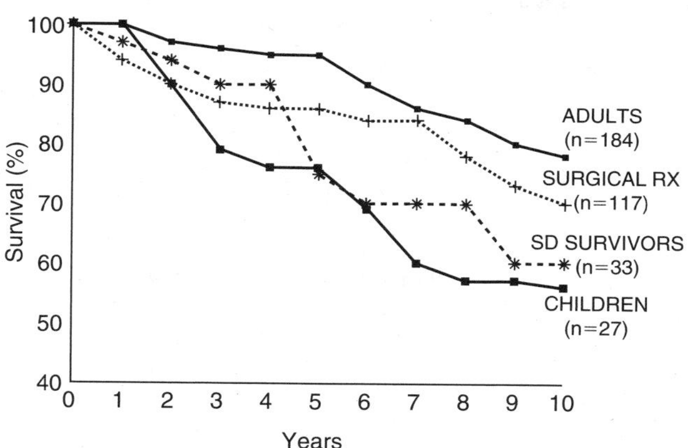

Figure 18-13 Survival in four groups of patients with hypertrophic cardiomyopathy (370,373,375). There appears to be no difference in survival between adult patients treated medically and those treated surgically. High-risk groups appear to be children and those with a prior history of cardiac arrest.

out the difficulty of determining the natural history of a disease by using data from recognized referral centers for that disease. In a group of 25 out-patients with the diagnosis of HCM and a mean follow-up period of 4.4 years, there were no deaths or evidence of clinical deterioration documented. Therefore, the prognosis appears particularly good in the relatively asymptomatic patient with this disease.

Aside from mortality, there is a real incidence of morbid events in patients with HCM. In approximately 5% of patients, endocarditis will develop; another 5% to 10% of patients will experience systemic emboli, approximately 10% to 15% will eventually have atrial fibrillation, and approximately 5% to 10% will have myocardial decompensation and symptoms of heart failure. Recognizing such comorbid events in this patient population and directing preventive therapy (antibiotic prophylaxis, anticoagulation) when available will, it is hoped, reduce the incidence of these complications.

CONCLUSIONS

The cardiomyopathies are a heterogenous group of diseases with multiple associations but disease mechanisms that are largely unknown. The anatomical classification of cardiomyopathies, albeit primitive, allows for some insight into etiology and association and definite insights into medical management and prognosis. Clearly, the hypertrophic cardiomyopathies are primarily genetic in etiology and it is becoming more obvious that a large proportion of the dilated myopathies may have a genetic cause. While direct therapy is currently unavailable for most of the diseases, generic management of heart failure has certainly improved substantially. A better understanding of the genetic mutations involved in many of our patients may ultimately lead to more directed care.

REFERENCES

1. Krehl L. Beitrag zur Kentniss der idiopathischen Herzmuskelerkrankungen. *Dtsch Arch F Klin Med.* 1891;48: 414–431.
2. Josserand E, Gallavardin L. De l'asystole progressive des jeunes sujets par myocardite subaigue primitive. *Arch Gen Med.* 1901;6:684–704.
3. Brigden W. Uncommon myocardial diseases. The noncoronary cardiomyopathies. *Lancet.* 1957;2:1243–1249.
4. Fejfar Z. Accounts of international meetings: idiopathic cardiomegaly. *Bull World Health Organ.* 1968;28:979–992.
5. WHO/ISFC Task Force. Report of the WHO/ISFC Task Force on the Definition and Classification of Cardiomyopathies. *Br Heart J.* 1980;44:672–673.
6. Douglas PS, Morrow R, Ioli A, et al. Left ventricular shape, afterload and survival in idiopathic dilated cardiomyopathy. *J Am Coll Cardiol.* 1989;13:311–315.
7. Grossman W, Jones D, McLaurin LP. Wall stress and patterns of hypertrophy in the human left ventricle. *J Clin Invest.* 1975;56:56–64.
8. O'Keefe DD, Hoffman JIE, Cheitlin R, et al. Coronary blood flow in experimental canine left ventricular hypertrophy. *Circ Res.* 1978;43:43–51.
9. Limas CJ, Olivari MT, Goldenberg IF, et al. Calcium uptake by cardiac sarcoplasmic reticulum in human dilated cardiomyopathy. *Cardiovasc Res.* 1987;21:601–605.
10. Bristow MR, Ginsburg R, Minobe W, et al. Decreased catecholamine sensitivity and beta-adrenergic-receptor density in failing human hearts. *N Engl J Med.* 1982;307: 205–211.
11. Heilbrunn SM, Shah P, Bristow MR, et al. Increased beta-receptor density and improved hemodynamic response to catecholamine stimulation during long-term metoprolol therapy in heart failure from dilated cardiomyopathy. *Circulation.* 1989;79:483–490.
12. Feldman AM, Cates AE, Veazey WB, et al. Increase of the 40,000-mol. wt. pertussis toxin substrate (G protein) in the failing human heart. *J Clin Invest.* 1988;82:189–197.
13. Bohm M, Gierschik P, Jakobs KH, et al. Increase of Gi alpha in human hearts with dilated but not ischemic cardiomyopathy. *Circulation.* 1990;82:1249–1265.
14. Bohm M, Ungerer M, Erdmann E. Beta adrenoceptors and M-cholinoceptors in myocardium of hearts with coronary artery disease or idiopathic dilated cardiomyopathy removed at cardiac transplantation. *Am J Cardiol.* 1990;66:880–882.
15. Walsh RA, Henkel R, Robbins J. Cardiac myocin heavy- and light-chain gene expression in hypertrophy and heart disease. *Heart Failure* 1990–91;6:238–243.
16. Robinson JA, O'Connell JB. *Myocarditis: Precursor of Cardiomyopathy.* Lexington, MA: Collamore Press; 1983.
17. Hosenpud JD. Chronic idiopathic myocarditis: controversies in causes and therapy. *Cardiovasc Rev Rep.* 1988;9:31–37.
18. Reyes MP, Lerner AM. Coxsackievirus myocarditis: with special reference to acute and chronic effects. *Prog Cardiovasc Dis.* 1985;27:373–394.
19. Woodruff JF. Viral myocarditis. *Am J Pathol.* 1980;101:427–479.
20. Daly K, Richardson PJ, Olsen EGJ, et al. Acute myocarditis: role of histological and virological examination in the diagnosis and assessment of immunosuppressive treatment. *Br Heart J.* 1984;51:30–35.
21. Bowles NE, Rose ML, Taylor P, et al. End-stage dilated cardiomyopathy: persistence of enterovirus RNA in myocardium at cardiac transplantation and lack of immune response. *Circulation.* 1989;80:1128–1136.
22. Limas CJ, Limas C. HLA antigens in idiopathic dilated cardiomyopathy. *Br Heart J.* 1989;62:379–383.
23. Koike S. Immunological disorders in patients with dilated cardiomyopathy. *Jpn Heart J.* 1989;30:799–807.
24. Schultheiss HP, Schulze K, Kuhl U, et al. The ADP/ATP carrier as a mitochondrial auto-antigen: facts and perspectives. *Ann NY Acad Sci.* 1986;488:44–64.
25. Limas CJ, Limas C, Kubo SH, et al. Anti-beta receptor antibodies in human dilated cardiomyopathy and correlation with HLA-DR antigens. *Am J Cardiol.* 1990;65:483–487.
26. Hosenpud JD, Campbell SM, Mendelson DJ. Interleukin-1 induced myocardial depression in an isolated perfused beating heart preparation. *J Heart Transplant.* 1989;8:460–464.
27. Factor SM, Minase T, Cho S, et al. Microvascular spasm in the cardiomyopathic Syrian hamster: a preventable cause of focal myocardial necrosis. *Circulation.* 1982;66:342–354.
28. Leonard DA, Sonnenblick EH, LeJemtel TH. Endocrine cardiomyopathies. *Heart Failure.* 1985;July/August:179–186.

29. Treasure CB, Vita JA, Cox DA, et al. Endothelium-dependent dilation of the coronary microvasculature is impaired in dilated cardiomyopathy. *Circulation.* 1990;81:772–779.
30. van Hoeven KH, Factor SM. Endomyocardial biopsy diagnosis of small vessel disease: a clinicopathologic study. *Int J Cardiol.* 1990;26:103–110.
31. Demakis JG, Proskey A, Rahimtoola SH, et al. The natural course of alcoholic cardiomyopathy. *Ann Intern Med.* 1974;80:293–297.
32. Kantrowitz NE, Bristow MR. Cardiotoxicity of antitumor agents. *Prog Cardiovasc Dis.* 1984;27:195–200.
33. Bristow MR, Mason JW, Billingham ME, et al. Dose-effect and structure-function relationships in doxorubicin cardiomyopathy. *Am Heart J.* 1981;102:709–718.
34. Gruenig E, Tasman JA, Kuecherer H, et al. Frequency and phenotypes of familial dilated cardiomyopathy. *J Am Coll Cardiol.* 1998;31:186–194.
35. Mestroni L, Mianid, DiLenarda A, et al. Clinical and pathologic study of familial dilated cardiomyopathy. *Am J Cardiol.* 1990;65: 1449–1453.
36. Michels VV, Moll PP, Miller FA, et al. The frequency of familial dilated cardiomyopathy in a series of patients with idiopathic dilated cardiomyopathy. *N Engl J Med.* 1992;326:77–82.
37. Burkett EL, Hershberger RE. Clinical and genetic issues in familial cardiomyopathy. *J Am Coll Cardiol.* 2005;45:969–981.
38. Emery AEH, Emery MLH. *The History of a Genetic Disease: Duchenne Muscular Dystrophy or Meryon's Disease.* London: The Royal Society of Medicine Press; 1995.
39. Emery AEH. *Duchenne Muscular Dystrophy.* 2nd ed. Oxford: Oxford University Press; 1993.
40. Monaco AP, Neve RL, Colletti-Feener C, et al. Isolation of candidate cDNAs for portions of the Duchenne muscular dystrophy gene. *Nature.* 1986;323:646–650.
41. Koenig M, Hoffman EP, Bertelson CJ, et al. Complete cloning of the Duchenne muscular dystrophy (DMD) cDNA and preliminary genomic organization of the DMD gene in normal and affected individuals. *Cell.* 1987;50:509–517.
42. Hoffman EP, Brown RJ, Kunkel LM. Dystrophin: the protein product of the Duchenne muscular dystrophy locus. *Cell.* 1987;51:919–928.
43. Koenig M, Monaco AP, Kunkel LM. The complete sequence of dystrophin predicts a rod-shaped cytoskeletal protein. *Cell.* 1988;53:219–226.
44. Bonilla E, Samitt CE, Miranda AF, et al. Duchenne muscular dystrophy: deficiency of dystrophin at the muscle cell surface. *Cell.* 1988;54:447–452.
45. Levine BA, Moir AJG, Patchell VB, et al. The interaction of actin with dystrophin. *FEBS Lett.* 1990;263:159–162.
46. Campbell KP, Kahl SD. Association of dystrophin and an integral membrane glycoprotein. *Nature.* 1989;338:259–262.
47. Ervasi JM, Campbell KP. Membrane organization of the dystrophin-glycoprotein complex. *Cell.* 1991;66:1121–1131.
48. Ibraghimov-Beskrovnaya O, Ervasti JM, Leveille KJ, et al. Primary structure of dystrophin-associated glycoproteins linking dystrophin to the extracellular matrix. *Nature.* 1992;355:696–702.
49. Ervasti JM, Campbell KP. A role for the dystrophin-glycoprotein complex as a transmembrane linker between laminin and actin. *J Cell Biol.* 1993;122:809–823.
50. Petrof BJ, Shrager JB, Stedman HH, et al. Dystrophin protects the sarcolemma from stresses developed during muscle contraction. *Proc Natl Acad Sci USA.* 1993;90:3710–3714.
51. Nye RE, Lovejoy FW, Yu PN. Clinical and hemodynamic studies of myocardial fibrosis. *Circulation.* 1957;16:332–338.
52. Hoffman EP, Fischbeck KH, Brown RH, et al. Characterization of dystrophin in muscle-biopsy specimens from patients with Duchenne's and Becker's muscular dystrophy. *N Engl J Med.* 1988;318:1363–1368.
53. Franco-Obregon A, Jr., Lansman JB. Mechanosensitive ion channels in skeletal muscle from normal and dystrophic mice. *J Physiol.* 1994;481:299–309.
54. Worton R. Muscular dystrophies: diseases of the dystrophin-glycoprotein complex. *Science.* 1995;270:755–756.
55. Michalak M, Opas M. Functions of dystrophin and dystrophin-associated proteins. *Curr Opin Neurol.* 1997;10:436–442.
56. den Dunnen JT, Grootscholten PM, Bakker E, et al. Topography of the Duchenne muscular dystrophy (DMD) gene: FIGE and cDNA analysis of 194 cases reveals 115 deletions and 13 duplications. *Am J Hum Genet.* 1989;45:835–847.
57. Roberts RG, Gardner RJ, Bobrow M. Searching for the 1 in 2,400,000: a review of dystrophin gene point mutations. *Hum Mutat.* 1994;4:1–11.
58. Doriguzzi C, Palucci L, Mongini T, et al. Systematic use of dystrophin testing in muscle biopsies: results in 201 cases. *Eur J Clin Invest.* 1997;27:352–358.
59. Globus JH. The pathologic findings in heart muscle in progressive muscular dystrophy. *Arch Neurol Psychiatry.* 1923;9:59–72.
60. Perloff JK, de Leon AC, O'Doherty D. The cardiomyopathy of progressive muscular dystrophy. *Circulation.* 1966;33:625–648.
61. Skyring A, McKusick VA. Clinical, genetic and electrocardiographic studies in childhood muscular dystrophy. *Am J Med Sci.* 1961;242–254.
62. Hunsaker RH, Fulkerson PK, Barry FJ, et al. Cardiac function in Duchenne's muscular dystrophy. Results of 10-year follow-up study and noninvasive tests. *Am J Med.* 1982;73:235–238.
63. Nigro G, Comi LI, Plitano L, et al. The incidence and evolution of cardiomyopathy in Duchenne muscular dystrophy. *Int J Cardiol.* 1990;26:271–277.
64. Melacini P, Vianello A, Villanova C, et al. Cardiac and respiratory involvement in advanced-stage Duchenne muscular dystrophy. *Neuromuscul Disord.* 1996;6:367–376.
65. Brockmeier K, Schmitz L, von Moers A, et al. X-chromosomal (p21) muscular dystrophy and left ventricular diastolic and systolic function. *Pediatr Cardiol.* 1998;19:139–144.
66. Kovick RB, Fogelman AM, Abbasi AD, et al. Echocardiographic evaluation of posterior left ventricular wall motion in muscular dystrophy. *Circulation.* 1975;52:447–454.
67. De Kermadec JM, Becane HM, Chenard A, et al. Prevalence of left ventricular systolic dysfunction in Duchenne muscular dystrophy: an echocardiographic study. *Am Heart J.* 1994;127:618–623.
68. Miyoshi K. Echocardiographic evaluation of fibrous replacement in the myocardium of patients with Duchenne muscular dystrophy. *Br Heart J.* 1991;66:452–455.
69. Cziner DG, Levin RI. The cardiomyopathy of Duchenne's muscular dystrophy and the function of dystrophin. *Med Hypotheses.* 1993;40:169–173.
70. Frankel KA, Rosser RJ. The pathology of the heart in progressive muscular dystrophy. *Hum Pathol.* 1976;7:375–386.
71. Sanyal SK, Johnson WW, Thapar MK, et al. An ultrastructural basis for the electrocardiographic alterations associated with Duchenne's muscular dystrophy. *Circulation.* 1978;57:1122–1129.
72. Perloff JK, Roberts WC, de Leon AC, et al. The distinctive electrocardiogram of Duchenne's progressive muscular dystrophy. *Am J Med.* 1967;42:179–188.
73. Nigro G, Comi LI, Politano L, et al. The incidence and evolution of cardiomyopathy in Duchenne muscular dystrophy. *Int J Cardiol.* 1990;26:271–277.
74. Perloff JK. Cardiac rhythm and conduction in Duchenne's muscular dystrophy. *J Am Coll Cardiol.* 1984;3:1263–1268.
75. Quinlivan RM, Lewis P, Marsden P, et al. Cardiac function, metabolism and perfusion in Duchenne and Becker muscular dystrophy. *Neuromuscul Disord.* 1996;6:237–246.
76. Emery AE, Skinner R. Clinical studies in benign (Becker type) X-linked muscular dystrophy. *Clin Genet.* 1976;10:189–201.
77. Ringel SP, Carroll JE, Schold SC. The spectrum of mild X-linked recessive muscular dystrophy. *Arch Neurol.* 1977;34:408–416.
78. Kunkel LM, Hejtmancik JF, Caskey CT. Analysis of deletions in DNA from patients with Becker and Duchenne muscular dystrophy. *Nature.* 1986;322:73–77.
79. Hoffman EP, Kunkel LM. Dystrophin abnormalities in Duchenne/Becker muscular dystrophy. *Neuron.* 1989;2:1019–1029.
80. Monaco AP, Bertelson CJ, Leichti-Gallati S, et al. An explanation for the phenotypic differences between patients bearing partial deletions for the DMD locus. *Genomics.* 1988;2:90–95.
81. Beggs AH, Hoffman EP, Snyder JR, et al. Exploring the molecular basis for variability among patients with Becker muscular dystrophy: dystrophin gene and protein studies. *Am J Hum Genet.* 1991;49:54–67.
82. Comi GP, Prelle A, Bresolin N, et al. Clinical variability in Becker muscular dystrophy. Genetic, biochemical and immunohistochemical correlates. *Brain.* 1994;117:1–14.
83. Melacini T, Fanin M, Danieli GA, et al. Cardiac involvement in Becker muscular dystrophy. *J Am Coll Cardiol.* 1993;22:1927–1934.
84. Hoogerwaard EM, de Voogt WG, Wilde AAM, et al. Evolution of cardiac abnormalities in Becker muscular dystrophy over a 13-year period. *J Neurol.* 1997;244:657–663.

85. Yu Y, Yamabe H, Fujita H, et al. Cardiac involvement in a family with Becker muscular dystrophy. *Intern Med.* 1995;34:919–923.
86. Sait M, Kawai H, Akaike M, et al. Cardiac dysfunction with Becker muscular dystrophy. *Am Heart J.* 1996;132:642–647.
87. Melacini P, Fanin M, Danieli GA, et al. Myocardial involvement is very frequent among patients affected with subclinical Becker's muscular dystrophy. *Circulation.* 1996;94:3168–3175.
88. Towbin JA, Hejtmancik F, Brink P, et al. X-linked dilated cardiomyopathy. Molecular genetic evidence of linkage to the Duchenne muscular dystrophy (dystrophin) gene at the Xp21 locus. *Circulation.* 1993;87:1854–1865.
89. Muntoni F, Cau M, Ganau A, et al. Deletion of the dystrophin muscle-promoter region associated with X-linked dilated cardiomyopathy. *N Engl J Med.* 1993;329:921–925.
90. Milasin J, Muntoni F, Severini GM, et al. A point mutation in the 5′ splice site of the dystrophin gene first exon responsible for X-linked dilated cardiomyopathy. *Hum Mol Genet.* 1996;5:73–79.
91. Franz WM, Cremer M, Herrmann R, et al. X-linked dilated cardiomyopathy. Novel mutation of the dystrophin gene. *Ann NY Acad Sci.* 1996;752:470–491.
92. Bies RD, Maeda M, Roberds SL, et al. A 5′ dystrophin duplication mutation causes membrane deficiency of α-dystroglycan in a family with X-linked cardiomyopathy. *J Mol Cell Cardiol.* 1997;29:3175–3188.
93. Towbin JA, Hejtmancik F, Brink P, et al. X-linked dilated cardiomypathy. Molecular genetic evidence of linkage to the Duchenne muscular dystrophy (dystrophin) gene at the Xp21 locus. *Circulation.* 1993;87:1854–1865.
94. Franz WM, Cremer M, Herrmann R, et al. X-linked dilated cardiomyopathy. Novel mutation of the dystrophin gene. *Ann NY Acad Sci.* 1996;752:470–491.
95. Milasin J, Muntoni F, Severini GM, et al. A point mutation in the 5′ splice site of the dystrophin gene first exon responsible for X-linked dilated cardiomyopathy. *Hum Mol Genet.* 1996;5:73–79.
96. Bies RD, Maeda M, Roberds SL, et al. A 5′ dystrophin duplication mutation causes membrane deficiency of α-dystroglycan in a family with X-linked cardiomyopathy. *J Mol Cell Cardiol.* 1997;29:3175–3188.
97. Moser H, Emery AEH. The manifesting carrier in Duchenne muscular dystrophy. *Clin Genet.* 1974;5:271–284.
98. Abbs S, Roberts RG, Mathew CG, et al. Accurate assessment of intragenic frequency within the Duchenne muscular dystrophy gene. *Genomics.* 1990;7:602–606.
99. Beggs AH. Dystrophinopaty, the expanding phenotype. Dystrophin abnormalities in X-linked dilated cardiomyopathy. *Circulation.* 1997;95:2344–2347.
100. Emery AEH, Dreifuss FE. Unusual type of benign X-linked muscular dystrophy. *J Neurol Neurosurg Psychiatry.* 1966; 29:338–342.
101. Hopkins LC, Jackson JA, Elsas LJ. Emery-Dreifuss humeroperoneal muscular dystrophy: an X-linked myopathy with unusual contractures and bradycardia. *Ann Neurol.* 1981;10:230–237.
102. Emery AEH. X-linked muscular dystrophy with early contractures and cardiomyopathy (Emery-Dreifuss type). *Clin Genet.* 1987;32:360–367.
103. Bialer MG, McDaniel NL, Kelly TE. Progression of cardiac disease in Emery-Dreifuss muscular dystrophy. *Clin Cardiol.* 1991; 14:411.
104. Yoshioka M, Saida K, Itagaki Y, Kamiya T. Follow-up study of cardiac involvement in Emery-Dreifuss muscular dystrophy. *Arch Dis Child.* 1989;64:713–715.
105. Bialer MG, McDaniel NL, Kelly TE. Progression of cardiac disease in Emery-Dreifuss muscular dystrophy. *Clin Cardiol.* 1991;14: 411–416.
106. Merchat MP, Zdonczyk D, Gujrati M. Cardiac transplantation in female Emery-Dreifuss muscular dystrophy. *J Neurol.* 1990;237:316–319.
107. Bione S, Maestrini E, Rivella S, et al. Identification of a novel X-linked gene responsible for Emery-Dreifuss muscular dystrophy. *Nat Genet.* 1994;8:323–327.
108. Manilal S, Nguyen TM, Sewry CA, et al. The Emery-Dreifuss muscular dystrophy protein, emerin, is a nuclear membrane protein. *Hum Mol Genet.* 1996;5:801–808.
109. Witt TN, Garner CG, Pongratz D, et al. Autosomal dominant Emery-Dreifuss syndrome: evidence of a neurogenic variant of the disease. *Eur Arch Psychiatry Neurol Sci.* 1988;237:230–236.
110. Panegyres PK, Mastaglia Fl, Kakulas BA. Limb-girdle syndromes: clinical, morphological and electrophysiological studies. *J Neurol Sci.* 1990;95:201–218.
111. Hosio A, Kotake H, Saito M, et al. Cardiac involvement in a patient with limb-girdle muscular dystrophy. *Heart Lung.* 1987;16:439–441.
112. Kawashima S, Ulno M, Kondo T, et al. Marked cardiac involvment in limb girdle muscular dystrophy. *Am J Med Sci.* 1990;299:411–414.
113. van der Kooi AT, Ledderhof TM, de Voogt WG, et al. A newly recognized autosomal dominant limb girdle muscular dystrophy with cardiac involvement. *Ann Neurol.* 1996;39:636–642.
114. Darnell J, Lodish H, Baltimore D. *Molecular Cell Biology.* 2nd ed. New York: WH Freeman; 1990.
115. DiMauro S, Bonilla E, Davidson M, et al. Mitochondria in neuromuscular disorders. *Biochim Biophys Acta.* 1998;1366:199–210.
116. John DR. Mitochondrial DNA and disease. *N Engl J Med.* 1995;33:638–644.
117. Anderson S, Bankier AT, Barrell BG, et al. Sequence and organization of the human mitochondrial genome. *Nature.* 1981;290:457–465.
118. Wallace DC. Diseases of the mitochondrial DNA. *Annu Rev Biochem.* 1992;61:1175–1212.
119. Giles RE, Blanc H, Cann HM, et al. Maternal inheritance of mitochondrial DNA. *Proc Natl Acad Sci USA.* 1980;77: 6715–6719.
120. Shoffner JM, Wallace DC. Mitochondrial genetics: principles and practice. *Am J Hum Genet.* 1992;51:1179–1186.
121. Kelly DP, Strauss AW. Inherited cardiomyopathies. *N Engl J Med.* 1994;330:913–919.
122. Warner TT, Schapira AHV. Genetic counseling in mitochondrial diseases. *Curr Opin Neurol.* 1997;10:408–412.
123. Shoffner JM, Wallace DC. Oxidative phosphorylation diseases: disorders of two genomes. *Adv Hum Genet.* 1990;19:267–330.
124. Zeviani M, Servidei S, Gellera C, et al. An autosomal dominant disorder with multiple deletions of mitochondrial DNA starting at the D-loop region. *Nature.* 1989;339:309–311.
125. Suomalainen A, Kaukonen J, Amati P, et al. An autosomal locus predisposing to deletions of mitochondrial DNA. *Nat Genet.* 1995;9:146–151.
126. Wallace DC. Mitochondrial DNA sequence variation in human evolution and disease. *Proc Natl Acad Sci USA.* 1994;91: 8739–8746.
127. Wallace DC. Diseases of the mitochondrial DNA. *Annu Rev Biochem.* 1992;61:1175–1212.
128. Wallace DC. Mitochondrial diseases: genotype versus phenotype. *Trends Genet.* 1993;9:128–133.
129. Rowland LP, Hays AP, DiMauro S, et al. Diverse clinical disorders associated with morphological abnormalities of mitochondria. In: G Scarlato, C Cerri, eds. *Mitochondrial Pathology in Muscle Diseases.* Padova: Piccin; 1983: 142–158.
130. Petty RKH, Harding AE, Morgan-Hughes JA. The clinical features of mitochondrial myopathy. *Brain.* 1986;109:915–938.
131. John DR. Mitochondrial DNA and disease. *N Engl J Med.* 1995;333:638–644.
132. Trijbels JMF, Sengers RCA, Ruitenbeek W, et al. Disorders of the mitochondrial respiratory chain: clinical manifestation and clinical approach. *Eur J Pediatr.* 1988;148:92–97.
133. Schon EA, Hirano M, DiMauro S. Mitochondrial encephalomyopathies: clinical and molecular analysis. *J Bioenerg Biomembr.* 1994;26:291–299.
134. Kearns TP, Sayre GP. Retinitis pigmentosa, external ophthalmoplegia, and complete heart block. *Arch Ophthalmol.* 1958;60:280–289.
135. Petty RKH, Harding AE, Morgan-Hughes JA. The clinical features of mitochondrial myopathy. *Brain.* 1986;109:915–938.
136. DiMauro S, Bonilla E, Lombes A, et al. Mitochondrial encephalomyopathies. *Neurol Clin.* 1990;8:483–506.
137. Pavlakis SG, Rowland LP, DeVivo DC, et al. Mitochondrial myopathies. In: Plum F, ed. *Advances in Contemporary Neurology.* Philadelphia: FA Davis Co. 1988:95–133.
138. Roberts NK, Perloff JK, Kark RAP. Cardiac conduction in the Kearns-Sayre syndrome (a neuromuscular disorder associated with progressive external ophthalmoplegia and pigmentary retinopathy). *Am J Cardiol.* 1979;44:1396–1400.
139. Charles R, Holt S, Kay JM, et al. Myocardial ultrastructure and the development of atrioventricular block in Kearns-Sayre syndrome. *Circulation.* 1981;63:214–219.

140. Channer KS, Channer JL, Campbell MJ, et al. Cardiomyopathy in the Kearns-Sayre syndrome. *Br Heart J.* 1988; 59:486–490.
141. Tveskov C, Angelo-Nielsen K. Kearns-Sayre syndrome and dilated cardiomyopathy. *Neurology.* 1990;40:553–554.
142. Channer KS, Channer JL, Campbell MJ, et al. Cardiomyopathy in the Kearns-Sayre syndrome. *Br Heart J.* 1988; 59:486–490.
143. Tranchant C, Mousson B, Bohr M, et al. Cardiac transplantation in an incomplete Kearns-Sayre syndrome with mitochondrial DNA deletion. *Neuromuscul Disord.* 1993;3:561–566.
144. Severini GA, Krajinovic M, Pinamonti B, et al. A new locus for arrhythmogenic right ventricular dysplasia on the long arm of chromosome 14. *Genomics.* 1996;31:193–200.
145. Coonar AS, Protonotarios N, Tsatsopoulou A, et al. Gene for arrhythmogenic right ventricular cardiomyopathy with diffuse nonepidermolytic palmoplantar keratoderma and woolly hair (Naxos disease) maps to 17q21. *Circulation.* 1998;97:2049–2058.
146. Li D, Ahmad F, Gardner MJ, et al. The locus of a novel gene responsible for arrhythmogenic right ventricular dysplasia characterized by early onset and high penetrance maps to chromosome 10p12-p14. *Am J Hum Genet.* 2000;66:148–156.
147. Ahmad F, Li D, Karibe A, et al. Localization of a gene responsible for arrhythmogenic right ventricular dysplasia to chromosome 3p23. *Circulation.* 1998;98:2791–2795.
148. Tiso N, Stephan DA, Nava A, et al. Identification of mutations in the cardiac ryanodine receptor gene in families affected with arrhythmogenic right ventricular cardiomyopathy type 2 (ARVD2). *Hum Mol Genet.* 2001;10:189–194.
149. Fuster V, Gersh BJ, Giuliani ER, et al. The natural history of idiopathic dilated cardiomyopathy. *Am J Cardiol.* 1981;47: 525–531.
150. Schwarz F, Mall G, Zebe H, et al. Determinants of survival in patients with congestive cardiomyopathy: quantitative morphologic findings and left ventricular hemodynamics. *Circulation.* 1984;70:923–928.
151. Regan TJ, Levinson GE, Oldewurtel HA, et al. Ventricular function in noncardiacs with alcoholic fatty liver: role of ethanol in the production of cardiomyopathy. *J Clin Invest.* 1969;48:397–407.
152. Lang RM, Borow KM, Neumann A, et al. Adverse cardiac effects of acute alcohol ingestion in young adults. *Ann Intern Med.* 1985;102:742–747.
153. Vasdev SC, Chakravarti RN, Subrahmanyam D, et al. Myocardial lesions induced by prolonged alcohol feeding in rhesus monkeys. *Cardiovasc Res.* 1975;9:134–140.
154. Regan TJ, Khan MI, Ettinger PO, et al. Myocardial function and lipid metabolism in the chronic alcoholic animal. *J Clin Invest.* 1974;54:740–752.
155. Thomas G, Haider B, Oldewurtel HA, et al. Progression of myocardial abnormalities in experimental alcoholism. *Am J Cardiol.* 1980;46:233–241.
156. Wu S, White R, Wikman-Coffelt J, et al. The preventive effect of verapamil on ethanol-induced cardiac depression: phosphorus-31 nuclear magnetic resonance and high-pressure liquid chromatographic studies of hamsters. *Circulation.* 1987;75: 1058–1064.
157. Segal LD, Rendig SV, Mason DT. Alcohol-induced cardiac hemodynamic and Ca^{2+} flux and dysfunctions are reversible. *J Mol Cell Cardiol.* 1981;13:443–455.
158. Sarma JSM, Ikeda S, Fischer R, et al. Biochemical and contractile properties of heart muscle after prolonged alcohol administration. *J Mol Cell Cardiol.* 1976;8:951–972.
159. Polimeni PI, Hoeschen O, Hoeschen LE. In vivo effects of ethanol on the rat myocardium: evidence for a reversible, nonspecific increase of sarcolemmal permeability. *J Mol Cell Cardiol.* 1983;15:113–122.
160. Noren GR, Staley NA, Einzig S, et al. Alcohol-induced congestive cardiomyopathy: an animal model. *Cardiovasc Res.* 1983;17:81–87.
161. Reitz RC, Helsabeck E, Mason DP. Effects of chronic alcohol ingestion on the fatty acid composition of the heart. *Lipids.* 1973;8:80–84.
162. Burch GE, Giles, TD. Alcoholic cardiomyopathy: concept of the disease and its treatment. *Am J Med.* 1971;50:141–145.
163. Koide T, Machida K, Nakanishi A, et al. Cardiac abnormalities in chronic alcoholism. An evidence suggesting association of myocardial abnormality with chronic alcoholism in 107 Japanese patients admitted to a psychiatric ward. *Jpn Heart J.* 1972;13:418–427.
164. McDonald CD, Burch GE, Walsh JJ. Alcoholic cardiomyopathy managed with prolonged bed rest. *Ann Intern Med.* 1971; 74:681–691.
165. Wu CF, Sudhakar M, Jaferi G, et al. Preclinical cardiomyopathy in chronic alcoholics: a sex difference. *Am Heart J.* 1976;91:281–286.
166. Lefkowitch JH, Fenoglio JJ, Jr. Liver disease in alcoholic cardiomyopathy: evidence against cirrhosis. *Hum Pathol.* 1983; 14:457–463.
167. Morin Y, Daniel P. Quebec beer-drinkers' cardiomyopathy: etiological considerations. *Can Med Assoc J.* 1967;97:926–928.
168. Sullivan J, Parker M, Carson SB. Tissue cobalt content in "beer drinkers' myocardiopathy." *J Lab Clin Med.* 1968;71:893–896.
169. Shugoll GI, Bowen PJ, Moore JP, et al. Follow-up observations and prognosis in primary myocardial disease. *Arch Intern Med.* 1972;129:67–72.
170. Mann DL, Kent RL, Parsons B, et al. Adrenergic effects on the biology of the adult mammalian cardiocyte. *Circulation.* 1992;85:790–804.
171. Shin G, Rice P. Cocaine use and acute coronary syndromes. *Lancet.* 2001;358:1367–1368.
172. Chakko S, Myerburg R. Cardiac complications of cocaine abuse. *Clin Cardiol.* 1995;18:67–72.
173. Virmani R, Robinowitz M, Smialek JE, et al. Cardiovascular effects of cocaine: an autopsy study of 40 patients. *Am Heart J.* 1988;115:1068–1076.
174. Henzlova MJ, Smith SH, Prchal VM, et al. Apparent reversibility of cocaine-induced congestive cardiomyopathy. *Am Heart J.* 1991;122:577–579.
175. Leikin J. Cocaine and beta-adrenergic blockers: a remarriage after a decade-long divorce? *Crit Care Med.* 1999;27:688–689.
176. Rubler S, Dglugash J, Yuceoglu YZ, et al. New type of cardiomyopathy associated with diabetic glomerulosclerosis. *Am J Cardiol.* 1972;30:595–602.
177. Kannel WB, Hjortland M, Castelli WP. Role of diabetes in congestive heart failure: the Framingham study. *Am J Cardiol.* 1974;34:29–34.
178. Hamby RI, Zoneraich S, Sherman S. Diabetic cardiomyopathy. *JAMA.* 1974;229:1749–1754.
179. Brownlee M, Cerami A, Viassara H. Advanced glycosylation end products in tissue and the biochemical basis of diabetic complications. *N Engl J Med.* 1988;318:1315–1321.
180. Ganguly PK, Pierce GN, Dhalla KS, et al. Defective cardiac sarcoplasmic reticular calcium transport in diabetic cardiomyopathy. *Am J Physiol.* 1983;244:E528–E535.
181. Factor SM, Minase T, Cho S, et al. Coronary microvascular abnormalities in the hypertensive-diabetic rat. A primary cause of cardiomyopathy? *Am J Pathol.* 1984;116:9–20.
182. Regan TJ, Lyons MM, Ahmed SS, et al. Evidence for cardiomyopathy in familial diabetes mellitus. *J Clin Invest.* 1977;60:885–899.
183. Ahmed SS, Jaferi GA, Narang RM, et al. Preclinical abnormaility of left ventricular function in diabetes mellitus. *Am Heart J.* 1975;89:153–158.
184. Seneviratne BIB. Diabetic cardiomyopathy: the preclinical phase. *BMJ.* 1977;1:1444–1446.
185. Sykes CA, Wright AD, Malins JM, et al. Changes in systolic time intervals during treatment of diabetes mellitus. *Br Heart J.* 1977;39:255–259.
186. Blumenthal HT, Alex M, Goldenberg S. A study of lesions of the intramural coronary branches in diabetes mellitus. *Arch Pathol.* 1960;70:27–42.
187. Silver MD, Huckell VS, Lorber M. Basement membranes of small cardiac vessels in patients with diabetes and myxedema: preliminary observations. *Pathology.* 1977;9:213–220.
188. Hull E, Hafkesbring E. Toxic post-partal failure. *New Orleans Med Surg J.* 1937;89:556–557.
189. Gouley BA, McMillan TM, Bellet S. Idiopathic myocardial degeneration associated with pregnancy and especially the puerperium. *Am J Med Sci.* 1937;194:185–199.
190. Homans DC. Peripartum cardiomyopathy. *N Engl J Med.* 1985;312:1432–1437.
191. Metcalfe J. The maternal heart in the postpartum period. *Am J Cardiol.* 1963;12:439–440.
192. Demakis JG, Rahimtoola SH. Peripartum cardiomyopathy. *Circulation.* 1971;44:964–968.
193. Rand RJ, Jenkins DM, Scott DG. Maternal cardiomyopathy of pregnancy causing stillbirth. *Br J Obstet Gynaecol.* 1975;82:172–175.

194. Walsh JJ, Burch GE, Black WC, et al. Idiopathic myocardiopathy of the puerperium (postpartal heart disease). *Circulation.* 1965;32:19–31.
195. Pierce JA, Price BO, Joyce JW. Familial occurrence of postpartal heart failure. *Arch Intern Med.* 1963;111:651–655.
196. Brown AK, Doukas N, Riding WD, et al. Cardiomyopathy and pregnancy. *Br Heart J.* 1967;29:387–393.
197. Julian DG, Szekely P. Peripartum cardiomyopathy. *Prog Cardiovasc Dis.* 1985;27:223–240.
198. Elkayam U, Akhter MW, Singh H, et al. Pregnancy-associated cardiomyopathy. *Circulation.* 2005;111:2050–2055.
199. Meadows WR. Idiopathic myocardial failure in the last trimester of pregnancy and the puerperium. *Circulation.* 1957;15:903–914.
200. Billingham ME, Mason JW, Bristow MR, et al. Anthracycline cardiomyopathy monitored by morphologic changes. *Cancer Treat Rep.* 1978;62:865–872.
201. Ferrans VJ. Overview of cardiac pathology in relation to anthracycline cardiotoxicity. *Cancer Treat Rep.* 1978;62:955–961.
202. Mason JW, Bristow MR, Billingham ME, et al. Invasive and noninvasive methods of assessing adriamycin cardiotoxic effects in man: superiority of histopathologic assessment using endomyocardial biopsy. *Cancer Treat Rep.* 1978;62:857–864.
203. Olson RD, Mushlin PS. Doxorubicin cardiotoxicity: analysis of prevailing hypotheses. *FASEB J.* 1990;4:3076–3086.
204. Saltiel E, McGuire W. Doxorubicin (adriamycin) cardiomyopathy. *West J Med.* 1983;139:332–341.
205. Minow RA, Benjamin RS, Lee ET, et al. Adriamycin cardiomyopathy: risk factors. *Cancer.* 1977;39:1397–1402.
206. Billngham ME, Bristow MR, Glatstein E, et al. Adriamycin cardiotoxicity: endomyocardial biopsy evidence of enhancement by irradiation. *Am J Surg Pathol.* 1977;1:17–23.
207. Billingham ME. Endomyocardial changes in anthracycline-treated patients with and without irradiation. *Front Radiat Ther Oncol.* 1979;13:67–81.
208. Torti FM, Bristow MR, Howes AE, et al. Reduced cardiotoxicity of doxorubicin delivered on a weekly schedule. *Ann Intern Med.* 1983;99:745–756.
209. Bristow MR, Lopez MB, Mason JW, et al. Efficacy and cost of cardiac monitoring in patients receiving doxorubicin. *Cancer.* 1982;50:32–41.
210. Schneider JW, Chang AY, Garratt A. Trastuzumab cardiotoxicity: speculations regarding pathophysiology and targets for further study. *Sem Oncol.* 2002;29:22–28.
211. Liu PP, Opavsky MA. Viral myocarditis: receptors that bridge the cardiovascular with the immune system? *Circ Res.* 2000;86:253.
212. Knowlton KU, Badorff C. The immune system in viral myocarditis: maintaining the balance. *Circ Res.* 1999;85:559.
213. Liu PP, Le J, Nian M. Nuclear factor-kappa B decoy: infiltrating the heart of the matter in inflammatory heart disease. *Circ Res.* 2001;89:850.
214. Aretz HT, Billingham ME, Edwards WD, et al. Myocarditis: a histopathologic definition and classification. *Am J Cardiovasc Pathol.* 1987;1:3.
215. Eriksson U, Kurrer MO, Schmitz N, et al. Interleukin-6-deficient mice resist development of autoimmune myocarditis associated with impaired upregulation of complement C3. *Circulation.* 2003;107:320.
216. Watanabe K, Nakazawa M, Fuse K, et al. Protection against autoimmune myocarditis by gene transfer of interleukin-10 by electroporation. *Circulation.* 2001;104:1098.
217. Kawai C. From myocarditis to cardiomyopathy: mechanisms of inflammation and cell death. Learning from the past for the future. *Circulation.* 1999;99:1091.
218. Gebhard JR, Perry CM, Harkins S, et al. Coxsackie B3-induced myocarditis: perforin exacerbates disease, but plays no detectable role in virus clearance. *Am J Pathol.* 1998;153:417.
219. Godeny EK, Gauntt CJ. Interferon and natural killer cell activity in coxsackie virus B3-induced murine myocarditis. *Eur Heart J.* 1987;8(Suppl):433.
220. Diefenbach A, Schindler H, Donhauser N, et al. Type 1 interferon (IFN alpha/beta) and type 2 nitric oxide synthase regulate the innate immune response to a protozoan parasite. *Immunity.* 1998;8:77–87.
221. Zaragoza C, Ocampo C, Saura M, et al. The role of inducible nitric oxide synthase in the host response to coxsackievirus myocarditis. *Proc Natl Acad Sci USA.* 1998;95:2469–2474.
222. Kawai C. From myocarditis to cardiomyopathy: mechanisms of inflammation and cell death: learning from the past for the future. *Circulation.* 1999;99:1091.
223. Wessely R, Henke A, Zell R, et al. Low-level expression of a mutant coxsackieviral cDNA induces a myocytopathic effect in culture: an approach to the study of enteroviral persistence in cardiac myocytes. *Circulation.* 1998;98:450.
224. Rao I, Debbas M, Sabbatini P, et al. The adenovirus EIA proteins induce apoptosis, which is inhibited by the EIB 19-kDa and Bcl-2 proteins. *Proc Natl Acad Sci USA.* 1992;89:7742
225. Sole MJ, Liu P. Viral myocarditis: a paradigm for understanding the pathogenesis and treatment of dilated cardiomyopathy. *J Am Coll Cardiol.* 1993;22:99A.
226. Kimby A, Sodermark T, Volpe U, et al. Stokes-Adams attacks requiring pacemaker treatment in three patients with acute nonspecific myocarditis. *Acta Med Scand.* 1980;207:177.
227. Badorff C, Zeiher AM, Hohnloser SH. Torsade de pointes tachycardia as a rare manifestation of acute enteroviral myocarditis. *Heart.* 2001;86:489.
228. Theleman KP, Kuiper JJ, Roberts WC. Acute myocarditis (predominately lymphocytic) causing sudden death without heart failure. *Am J Cardiol.* 2001;88:1078.
229. Maron BJ, Shirani J, Poliac LC, et al. Sudden death in young competitive athletes: clinical, demographic, and pathological profiles. *JAMA.* 1996;276:199.
230. Dec GW. Introduction to clinical myocarditis. In: Cooper LT, ed. *Myocarditis: From Bench to Bedside*. Totowa, NJ: Humana Press; 2003:257–281.
231. Angelini A, Calzolari V, Calabrese F, et al. Myocarditis mimicking acute myocardial infarction: role of endomyocardial biopsy in the differential diagnosis. *Heart.* 2000;84:245.
232. Sarda L, Colin P, Boccara F, et al. Myocarditis in patients with clinical presentation of myocardial infarction and normal coronary angiograms. *J Am Coll Cardiol.* 2001;37:786.
233. Burch G, Shewey L. Viral coronary arteritis and myocardial infarction. *Am Heart J.* 1976;92:11.
234. Ferguson D, Farwell A, Bradley W, et al. Coronary artery vasospasm complicating acute myocarditis. *West J Med.* 1988; 148:664.
235. Chimenti C, Calabrese F, Thiene G, et al. Inflammatory left ventricular microaneurysms as a cause of apparently idiopathic ventricular tachyarrhythmias. *Circulation.* 2001;104:168.
236. Smith SC, Ladenson JH, Mason JW, et al. Elevations of cardiac troponin I associated with myocarditis: experimental and clinical correlates. *Circulation.* 1997;95:163.
237. Torre-Amione G, Kapadia S, Benedict C, et al. Proinflammatory cytokine levels in patients with depressed left ventricular ejection fraction: a report from the Studies of Left Ventricular Dysfunction (SOLVD). *J Am Coll Cardiol.* 1996;27:1201.
238. Toyozaki T, Hiroe M, Saito T, et al. Levels of soluble Fas in patients with myocarditis, heart failure of unknown origin, and in healthy volunteers. *Am J Cardiol.* 1998;81:798.
239. Pinamonti B, Alberti E, Cigalotto A, et al. Echocardiographic findings in myocarditis. *Am J Cardiol.* 1988; 62:285.
240. Felker GM, Boehmer JP, Hruban RH, et al. Echocardiographic findings in fulminant and acute myocarditis. *J Am Coll Cardiol.* 2000;36:227.
241. Chandraratna P, Nimalasuriya A, Reid C, et al. Left ventricular asynergy in acute myocarditis. *JAMA.* 1983;250:1428.
242. Gagliardi M, Bevilacqua M, Di Renzi P, et al. Usefulness of magnetic resonance imaging for diagnosis of acute myocarditis in infants and children, and comparison with endomyocardial biopsy. *Am J Cardiol.* 1991;68:1089.
243. Aretz HT, Billingham ME, Edwards WD, et al. Myocarditis: a histopathologic definition and classification. *Am J Cardiovasc Pathol.* 1987;1:3.
244. Rezkalla SH, Raikar S, Kloner RA. Treatment of viral myocarditis with focus on captopril. *Am J Cardiol.* 1996;77:634.
245. Matsumori A, Igata H, Ono K, et al. High doses of digitalis increase the myocardial production of proinflammatory cytokines and worsen myocardial injury in viral myocarditis: a possible mechanism of digitalis toxicity. *Jpn Circ J.* 1999;63:934.
246. Wang WZ, Matsumori A, Yamada T, et al. Beneficial effects of amlodipine in a murine model of congestive heart failure induced by viral myocarditis: a possible mechanism through inhibition of nitric oxide production. *Circulation.* 95:245.

247. McNamara DM, Holubkov R, Starling RC, et al. Controlled trial of intravenous immune globulin in recent-onset dilated cardiomyopathy. *Circulation.* 2001;103:2254.
248. Mason JW, O'Connell JB, Herskowitz A, et al. A clinical trial of immunosuppressive therapy for myocarditis. *N Engl J Med.* 1995;333:269.
249. Parillo JE, Cunnion RE, Epstein SE, et al. A prospective, randomized, controlled trial of prednisone for dilated cardiomyopathy. *N Engl J Med.* 1989;321:1061
250. Fournier PE, Etienne J, Harle JR, et al. Myocarditis, a rare but severe manifestation of Q fever: report of 8 cases and review of the literature. *Clin Infect Dis.* 2001;32:1440.
251. Raoult D, Tissot-Dupont H, Foucault C, et al. Q fever 1985–1998: clinical and epidemiologic features of 1,383 infections. *Medicine* (Baltimore) 2000;79:109.
252. Marin-Garcia J, Barrett FF. Myocardial function in Rocky Mountain spotted fever: echocardiographic assessment. *Am J Cardiol.* 1983;51:341.
253. Yotsukura M, Aoki N, Fukuzumi N, et al. Review of a case of Tsutsugamushi disease showing myocarditis and confirmation of rickettsia by endomyocardial biopsy. *Jpn Circ J.* 1991;55:149.
254. Tsay RW, Chang FY. Serious complications in scrub typhus. *J Microbiol Immunol Infect.* 1998;31:240.
255. Jubber AS, Gunawardana DR, Lulu AR. Acute pulmonary edema in *Brucella* myocarditis and interstitial pneumonitis. *Chest* 1990;97:1008.
256. Stevens DL, Troyer BE, Merrick DT, et al. Lethal effects and cardiovascular effects of purified alpha- and theta-toxins from *Clostridium perfringens. J Infect Dis.* 1988;157:272.
257. Loukoushkina EF, Bobko PV, Kolbasova EV, et al. The clinical picture and diagnosis of diphtheritic carditis in children. *Eur J Pediatr.* 1998;157:528.
258. Armengol S, Domingo C, Mesalles E. Myocarditis: a rare complication during Legionella infection. *J Int Cardiol.* 1992;37:418.
259. Agarwala BN, Ruschhaupt DG. Complete heart block from *Mycoplasma pneumoniae* infection. *Pediatr Cardiol.* 1991;12:233.
260. Odeh M, Oliven A. Chlamydial infections of the heart. *Eur J Clin Microbiol Infect Dis.* 1992;11:885.
261. Neuwirth C, François C, Laurent N, et al. Myocarditis due to *Salmonella virchow* and sudden infant death. *Lancet.* 1999;354:1004.
262. Afzal A, Keohane M, Keeley E, et al. Myocarditis and pericarditis with tamponade associated with disseminated tuberculosis. *Can J Cardiol.* 2000;16:4.
263. Haywood GA, O'Connell S, Gray HH. Lyme carditis: a United Kingdom perspective. *Br Heart J.* 1993;70:15.
264. Asch ES, Bujak DI, Weiss M, et al. Lyme disease: an infectious and postinfectious syndrome. *J Rheumatol.* 1994;21:454.
265. Ledford DK. Immunologic aspects of vasculitis and cardiovascular disease. *JAMA.* 1997;278:1962.
266. Nagi KS, Joshi R, Thakur RK. Cardiac manifestations of Lyme disease: a review. *Can J Cardiol.* 1996;12:503.
267. Stanek G, Klein J, Bittner R, et al. Isolation of *Borrelia burgdorferi* from the myocardium of a patient with long-standing cardiomyopathy. *N Engl J Med.* 1990;322:249.
268. Nowakowski JN, Nadelman RB, Sell R, et al. Long-term follow-up of patients with culture-confirmed Lyme disease. *Am J Med.* 2003;115:91.
269. Rahn DW, Malawista SE. Lyme disease: recommendations for diagnosis and treatment. *Ann Intern Med.* 1991;14:472.
270. Hagar JM, Rahimtoola SH. Chagas' heart disease. *Curr Probl Cardiol.* 1995;20:825.
271. Parada H, Carrasco HA, Anez N, et al. Cardiac involvement is a constant finding in acute Chagas' disease: a clinical, parasitological and histopathological study. *Int J Cardiol.* 1997;60:49.
272. Rossi MA, Bestetti RB. The challenge of chagasic cardiomyopathy: the pathologic roles of autonomic abnormalities, autoimmune mechanisms and microvascular changes, and therapeutic implications. *Cardiology* 1995;86:1.
273. Carrasco HA, Alarçon M, Olmos L, et al. Biochemical characterization of myocardial damage in chronic Chagas' disease. *Clin Cardiol.* 1997;20:865.
274. Faul JL, Hoang K, Schmoker J, et al. Constrictive pericarditis due to coccidioidomycosis. *Ann Thorac Surg.* 1999;68:1407.
275. Bestetti RB, Dalbo CM, Freitas QC, et al. Noninvasive predictors of mortality for patients with Chagas' heart disease: a multivariate stepwise logistic regression study. *Cardiology.* 1994;84:261.
276. Ferreira AW, de Avila SD. Laboratory diagnosis of Chagas' heart disease. *Rev Paul Med.* 1995;113:767.
277. de Paola AA, Gondin AA, Hara V, et al. Medical treatment of cardiac arrhythmias in Chagas' heart disease. *Rev Paul Med.* 1995;113:858.
278. Muratore C, Rabinovich R, Iglesias R, et al. Implantable cardioverter defibrillators in patients with Chagas' disease: are they different from patients with coronary disease? *Pacing Clin Electrophysiol.* 1997;20:194.
279. Braga JC, Labrunie A, Villaca F, et al. Thromboembolism in chronic Chagas' heart disease. *Rev Paul Med.* 1995;113:862.
280. Apt W, Aguilera X, Arribada A, et al. Treatment of chronic Chagas' disease with itraconazole and allopurinol. *Am J Trop Med Hyg.* 1998;59:133.
281. Bocchi EA, Bellotti G, Mocelin AO, et al. Heart transplantation for chronic Chagas' heart disease. *Ann Thorac Surg.* 1996;61:1727.
282. Bashour TT, Gord C, Baladi N, et al. Intracardiac actinomycosis. *Am Heart J.* 1997;133:467.
283. Berarducci L, Ford K, Olenick S, et al. Invasive intracardiac aspergillosis with widespread embolization. *J Am Soc Echocardiogr.* 1993;6:539.
284. Serody JS, Mill MR, Detterbeck FC, et al. Blastomycosis in transplant recipients: report of a case and review. *Clin Infect Dis.* 1993;16:54.
285. Franklin WG, Simon AB, Sodeman TM. Candida myocarditis without valvulitis. *Am J Cardiol.* 1976;38:924.
286. Faul JL, Hoang K, Schmoker J, et al. Constrictive pericarditis due to coccidioidomycosis. *Ann Thorac Surg.* 1999;68:1407.
287. Lafont A, Wolff M, Marche C, et al. Overwhelming myocarditis due to *Cryptococcus neoformans* in an AIDS patient. *Lancet.* 1987;2:1145.
288. Kirchner SG, Hernanz-Schulman M, Stein SM, et al. Imaging of pediatric mediastinal histoplasmosis. *Radiographics.* 1991;11:365.
289. Virmani R, Connor DH, McAllister HA. Cardiac mucormycosis: a report of five patients and review of 14 previously reported cases. *Am J Clin Pathol.* 1982;78:42.
290. Cooper, LT Jr., Berry GJ, Shabetai R. Idiopathic giant-cell myocarditis: natural history and treatment. Multicenter Giant Cell Myocarditis Study Group Investigators. *N Engl J Med.* 1997;336:1860.
291. Nash CL, Panaccione R, Sutherland LR, et al. Giant cell myocarditis, in a patient with Crohn's disease, treated with etanercept: a tumour necrosis factor-alpha antagonist. *Can J Gastroenterol.* 2001;15:607.
292. Hyogo M, Kamitani T, Oguni A, et al. Acute necrotizing eosinophilic myocarditis with giant cell infiltration after remission of idiopathic thrombocytopenic purpura. *Intern Med.* 1997;36:894.
293. Frustaci A, Cuoco L, Chimenti C, et al. Celiac disease associated with autoimmune myocarditis. *Circulation.* 2002; 105:2611.
294. Shields RC, Tazelaar HD, Berry GJ, et al. The role of right ventricular endomyocardial biopsy for idiopathic giant cell myocarditis. *J Card Fail.* 2002 Apr;8(2):74–78.
295. Frustaci A, Chimenti C, Pieroni M, et al. Giant cell myocarditis responding to immunosuppressive therapy. *Chest.* 2000;117:905.
296. Pinderski LJ, Fonarow GC, Hamilton M, et al. Giant cell myocarditis in a young man responsive to T-lymphocyte cytolytic therapy. *J Heart Lung Transplant.* 2002;221:818.
297. Menghini VV, Savcenko V, Olson LJ, et al. Combined immunosuppression for the treatment of idiopathic giant cell myocarditis. *Mayo Clin Proc.* 1999;74:1221.
298. Davies RA, Veinot JP, Smith S, et al. Giant cell myocarditis: Clinical presentation, bridge to transplantation with mechanical circulatory support, and long-term outcome. *J Heart Lung Transplant.* 2002;21:674.
299. Scott RL, Ratliff NB, Starling RC, et al. Recurrence of giant cell myocarditis in cardiac allograft. *J Heart Lung Transplant.* 2001;20:375.
300. Shimada T, Shimada K, Sakane T, et al. Diagnosis of cardiac sarcoidosis and evaluation of the effects of steroid therapy by gadolinium-DTPA-enhanced magnetic resonance imaging. *Am J Med.* 2001;110:520.
301. Okura Y, Dec GW, Hare JM, et al. A clinical and histopathologic comparison of cardiac sarcoidosis and idiopathic giant cell myocarditis. *J Am Coll Cardiol.* 2003;41:322.

302. Shabetai R. Sarcoidosis and the heart. *Curr Treat Options Cardiovasc Med.* 2000;2:385.
303. Uemura A, Morimoto S, Hiramitsu S, et al. Histologic diagnostic rate of cardiac sarcoidosis: evaluation of endomyocardial biopsies. *Am Heart J.* 1999;328:299.
304. Chandra M, Silverman ME, Oshinski J, et al. Diagnosis of cardiac sarcoidosis aided by MRI. *Chest.* 1996;110:562.
305. Schaedel H, Kirsten D, Schmidt A, et al. Sarcoid heart disease: results of follow-up investigations. *Eur Heart J.* 1991;12:26.
306. Valentine HA, Tazelaar HD, Macoviak J, et al. Cardiac sarcoidosis: response to steroids and transplantation. *J Heart Transplant.* 1987;5:244.
307. Figulla HR, Rahlf G, et al. Spontaneous hemodynamic improvement or stabilization and associated biopsy findings in patients with congestive cardiomyopathy. *Circulation.* 1985;71:1095–1104.
308. Taliercio CP, Seward JB, Driscoll DJ, et al. Idiopathic dilated cardiomyopathy in the young: clinical profile and natural history. *J Am Coll Cardiol.* 1985;6:1126–1131.
309. Griffin ML, Hernandez A, Martin TC, et al. Dilated cardiomyopathy in infants and children. *J Am Coll Cardiol.* 1988; 11:139–144.
310. Kadish A, Dyer A, Daubert JP, et al. Defibrillators in Non-Ischemic Cardiomyopathy Treatment Evaluation (DEFINITE) Investigators, Prophylactic defribrillator implantation in patients with nonischemic dilated cardiomyopathy. *N Engl J Med.* 2004;350(21):2151–2158.
311. Chew CYC, Ziady GM, Raphael MJ, et al. Primary restrictive cardiomyopathy, non-tropical endomyocardial fibrosis and hypereosinophilic heart disease. *Br Heart J.* 1977;39:399–413.
312. Benotti JR, Grossman W. Restrictive cardiomyopathy. *Annu Rev Med.* 1984;35:113–125.
313. Janos GG, Arjunan K, Meyer RA, et al. Differentiation of constrictive pericarditis and restrictive cardiomyopathy using digitized echocardiography. *J Am Coll Cardiol.* 1983;1: 541–549.
314. Tyberg TI, Goodyer AVN, Hurst VW III, et al. Left ventricular filling in differentiating restrictive amyloid cardiomyopathy and constrictive pericarditis. *Am J Cardiol.* 1981;47:791–796.
315. Benotti JR, Grossman W, Cohn PF. Clinical profile of restrictive cardiomyopathy. *Circulation.* 1980;61:1206–1212.
316. Hosenpud JD, Niles NR. Clinical hemodynamic and endomyocardial biopsy findings in idiopathic restrictive cardiomyopathy. *West J Med.* 1986;144:303–306.
317. Montgomery JF. Pericarditis. *West J Med.* 1975;127:295–308.
318. Siegel RJ, Shah PK, Fishbein MC. Idiopathic restrictive cardiomyopathy. *Circulation.* 1984;70:165–169.
319. Mehta AV, Ferrer PL, Pickoff AS, et al. M-mode echocardiographic findings in children with idiopathic restrictive cardiomyopathy. *Pediatr Cardiol.* 1984;5:273–280.
320. Sapire DW, Casta A, Swischuk LE, et al. Massive dilatation of the atria and coronary sinus in a child with restrictive cardiomyopathy and persistence of the left superior vena cava. *Cathet Cardiovasc Diagn.* 1983;9:47–53.
321. Erath HG, Graham TP, Jr., Smith CW, et al. Restrictive cardiomyopathy in an infant with massive biatrial enlargement and normal ventricular size and pump function. *Cathet Cardiovasc Diagn.* 1978;4:289–296.
322. Arbustini E, Buonanno C, Trevi G, et al. Cardiac ultrastructure in primary restrictive cardiomyopathy. *Chest.* 1983; 84: 236–238.
323. Glenner GG. Amyloid deposits and amyloidosis. *N Engl J Med.* 1980;302:1283–1292.
324. Olofsson BO, Bjerle P, Osterman G. Hemodynamic and angiocardiographic observations in familial amyloidosis with polyneuropathy. *Acta Med Scand.* 1982;212:77–81.
325. Maule WF, Martin RH. Primary cardiac amyloidosis: an angiocardiographic clue to early diagnosis. *Ann Intern Med.* 1983; 98:177–180.
326. Kern MJ, Lorell BH, Grossman W. Cardiac amyloidosis masquerading as constrictive pericarditis. *Cathet Cardiovasc Diagn.* 1982;8:629–635.
327. Edhag O, Helmers C, Samnegard H, et al. Two cases of myocardial disease simulating constrictive pericarditis. *Scand J Thorac Cardiovasc Surg.* 1977;11:225–227.
328. Meaney E, Shabetai R, Bhargava V, et al. Cardiac amyloidosis, constrictive pericarditis in restrictive cardiomyopathy. *Am J Cardiol.* 1976;38:547–556.
329. Naggar CZ. Rapid amyloid infiltration of the heart. *Am J Cardiol.* 1986;80:276–278.
330. Child JS, Krivokapich J, Abbasi AS. Increased right ventricular wall thickness on echocardiography in amyloid infiltrative cardiomyopathy. *Am J Cardiol.* 1979;44:1391–1395.
331. Child JS, Levisman JA, Abbasi AS, et al. Echocardiographic manifestations of infiltrative cardiomyopathy. *Chest.* 1976;70:726–731.
332. Pierard L, Verheugt FWA, Meltzer RS, et al. Echocardiographic aspects of cardiac amyloidosis. *Acta Cardiol.* 1981;36:455–461.
333. Kyle RA, Greipp PR. Amyloidosis (AL): clinical and laboratory features in 229 cases. *Mayo Clin Proc.* 1983;58:665–683.
334. Loeffler W. Endocarditis parietalis fibroplastica Mit Bluteosinophiline. *Schweiz Med Wochnschr.* 1930;66:817–820.
335. Roberts WC, Ferrans VJ. Pathologic anatomy of the cardiomyopathies. Idiopathic dilated and hypertrophic types, infiltrative types, and endomyocardial disease with and without eosinophilia. *Hum Pathol.* 1975;6:287–342.
336. Spry CJF, Tai P-C, Davies J. The cardiotoxicity of eosinophils. *Postgrad Med J.* 1983;59:147–151.
337. Fauci AS, Harley JB, Roberts WC, et al. The idiopathic hypereosinophilic syndrome. *Ann Intern Med.* 1982;97:78–92.
338. Olsen EGJ. Pathological aspects of endomyocardial fibrosis. *Postgrad Med J.* 1983;59:135–139.
339. Cherian G, Vijayaraghavan G, Krishnaswami S, et al. Endomyocardial fibrosis: report on the hemodynamic data in 29 patients and review of the results of surgery. *Am Heart J.* 1983; 105:659–666.
340. Olsen EGJ, Spry CJF. Relation between eosinophilia and endomyocardial disease. *Prog Cardiovasc Dis.* 1985;27: 241–254.
341. Parrillo JE, Borer JS, Henry WL, et al. The cardiovascular manifestations of the hypereosinophilic syndrome. *Am J Med.* 1979;67:572–582.
342. Kudenchuk PJ, Hosenpud JD, Fletcher S. Eosinophilic endomyocardiopathy. *Clin Cardiol.* 1986;9:344–348.
343. Solley GO, Maldonado JE, Gleich GJ, et al. Endomyocardiopathy with eosinophilia. *Mayo Clin Proc.* 1976;51:697–708.
344. Benvenisti DS, Ultmann JE. Eosinophilic leukemia. Report of 5 cases and review of the literature. *Ann Intern Med.* 1969;71: 732–736.
345. Chusid MJ, Dale DC, West BC, et al. The hypereosinophilic syndrome: analysis of 14 cases and review of the literature. *Medicine.* 1975;54:1–27.
346. Frustaci A, Chimenti C, Ricci R, et al. Improvement in cardiac function in the cardiac variant of Fabry's disease with galactose-infusion therapy. *N Engl J Med.* 2001;345:25.
347. Linhart A, Magage S, Palecek T, et al. Cardiac involvement in Fabry disease. [Review] *Acta Paediatr.* 2002;91(439):15–20.
348. Perrot A, Osterziel KJ, Beck M, et al. Fabry disease: focus on cardiac manifestations and molecular mechanisms. *Herz.* 2002;27:699.
349. Goffbrand AV. Diagnosing myocardial iron overload. *Eur Heart J.* 2001;22:2140.
350. Okura Y, Dec GW, Hare JM, et al. A clinical and histopathologic comparison of cardiac sarcoidosis and idiopathic giant cell myocarditis. *J Am Coll Cardiol.* 2003;41:322.
351. Ratner SJ, Fenoglio JJ, Jr., Ursell PC. Utility of endomyocardial biopsy in the diagnosis of cardiac sarcoidosis. *Chest.* 1986;90:528–533.
352. Cutler DJ, Isner JM, Bracey AW, et al. Hemochromatosis heart disease: an unemphasized cause of potentially reversible restrictive cardiomyopathy. *Am J Med.* 1980;69:923–928.
353. Schoenfeld MH, Supple EW, Dec GW Jr., et al. Restrictive cardiomyopathy versus constrictive pericarditis: role of endomyocardial biopsy in avoiding unnecessary thoracotomy. *Circulation.* 1987;75:1012–1017.
354. Kyle RA, Gertz MA, Greipp PR, et al. A trial of three regimens for primary amyloidosis: colchicine alone, melphalan and prednisone, and melphalan, prednisone and colchicine. *N Engl J Med.* 1997;336:1202–1207.
355. Skinner M, Anderson J, Simms R, et al. Treatment of 100 patients with primary amyloidosis: a randomized trial of melphalan, prednisone, and colchicine versus colchicine only. *Am J Med.* 1996;100:290–298.
356. Braunwald E. Mechanism of action of calcium-channel-blocking agents. *N Engl J Med.* 1982;307:1618–1627.

357. Teare D. Asymmetrical hypertrophy of the heart in young patients. *Br Heart J.* 1958;20:1–8.
358. Maron BJ, Epstein SE. Hypertrophic cardiomyopathy. *Am J Cardiol.* 1980;45:141–154.
359. Clark CE, Henry WL, Epstein SE. Familial prevalence and genetic transmission of idiopathic hypertrophic subaortic stenosis. *N Engl J Med.* 1973;289:709–714.
360. Maron BJ, Nichols PF, Pickle LW, et al. Patterns of inheritance in hypertrophic cardiomyopathy: assessment by M-mode and two-dimensional echocardiography. *Am J Cardiol.* 1984;53:1087–1094.
361. Watkins H, Rosenzweig A, Hwang D-S, et al. Characteristics and prognostic implications of myosin missense mutations in familial hypertrophic cardiomyopathy. *N Engl J Med.* 1992; 326:1108–1114.
362. Schwartz K, Carrier L, Guicheney P, et al. Molecular basis of familial cardiomyopathies. *Circulation.* 1995;91:532–540.
363. Marian AJ, Roberts R. Recent advances in the molecular genetics of hypertrophic cardiomyopathy. *Circulation.* 1995;92:1336–1347.
364. Rosenzweig A, Watkins H, Hwang D-S, et al. Preclinical diagnosis of familial hypertrophic cardiomyopathy by genetic analysis of blood lymphocytes. *N Engl J Med.* 1991;325:1753–1760.
365. Criley JM, Lewis KB, White RI, Jr., et al. Pressure gradients without obstruction: a non concept of "hypertrophic subaortic stenosis." *Circulation.* 1965;32:881–887.
366. Stewart S, Mason DT, Braunwald E. Impaired rate of left ventricular filling in idiopathic subaortic stenosis and valvular aortic stenosis. *Circulation.* 1968;37:8–14.
367. Sanderson JE, Gibson DG, Brown DJ, et al. Left ventricular filling in hypertrophic cardiomyopathy: an angiographic study. *Br Heart J.* 1977;39:661–670.
368. Hanrath P, Mathey DG, Siegert R, et al. Left ventricular relaxation and filling pattern in different forms of left ventricular hypertrophy: an echocardiographic study. *Am J Cardiol.* 1980;45:15–23.
369. Maron BJ, Merrill WH, Freier PA, et al. Long-term clinical course and symptomatic status of patients after operation for hypertrophic subaortic stenosis. *Circulation.* 1978;57:1205–1213.
370. Epstein SE, Henry WL, Clark CE, et al. Asymmetric septal hypertrophy. *Ann Intern Med.* 1974;81:650–680.
371. Goodwin JF. An appreciation of hypertrophic cardiomyopathy. *Am J Med.* 1980;68:797–800.
372. McKenna W, Deanfield J, Faruqui A, et al. Prognosis in hypertrophic cardiomyopathy: role of age and clinical, electrocardiographic and hemodynamic features. *Am J Cardiol.* 1981;47:532–538.
373. Brock R. Functional obstruction of the left ventricle (acquired aortic subvalvular stenosis). *Guy's Hosp Rep.* 1957;106:221–238.
374. Braunwald E, Lambrew CT, Rockoff SD, et al. Idiopathic hypertrophic subaortic stenosis. I. A description of the disease based upon an analysis of 64 patients. *Circulation.* 1964;29/30(Suppl IV):3–119.
375. Swan DA, Bell B, Oakley CM, et al. Analysis of symptomatic course and prognosis and treatment of hypertrophic obstructive cardiomyopathy. *Br Heart J.* 1971;33:671–685.
376. Fiddler GI, Tajik AJ, Weidman WH, et al. Idiopathic hypertrophic subaortic stenosis in the young. *Am J Cardiol.* 1978;42:793–799.
377. Nishimura RA, Giuliani ER, Brandenburg RO. Hypertrophic cardiomyopathy. *CVR&R.* 1983;4:931–962.
378. Shah PM, Adelman AG, Wigle ED, et al. The natural (and unnatural) history of hypertrophic obstructive cardiomyopathy. *Circ Res.* 1974;34/35(Suppl II):II179–II195.
379. Adelman AG, Wigle ED, Ranganathan N, et al. The clinical course in muscular subaortic stenosis. A retrospective and prospective study of 60 hemodynamically proved cases. *Ann Intern Med.* 1972;77:515–525.
380. Stewart S, Schreiner B. Coexisting idiopathic hypertrophic subaortic stenosis and coronary artery disease. Clinical implication and operative management. *J Thorac Cardiovasc Surg.* 1981; 82:278–280.
381. Maron BJ, Epstein SE, Roberts WC. Hypertrophic cardiomyopathy and transmural myocardial infarction without significant atherosclerosis of the extramural coronary arteries. *Am J Cardiol.* 1979;43:1086–1112.
382. Pichard AD, Meller J, Teichholz LE, et al. Septal perforator compression (narrowing) in idiopathic hypertrophic subaortic stenosis. *Am J Cardiol.* 1977;40:310–314.
383. Kostis JB, Moreyra AE, Natarajan N, et al. The pathophysiology and diverse etiology of septal perforator compression. *Circulation.* 1979;59:913–919.
384. St. John Sutton MG, Tajik AJ, Smith HC, et al. Angina in idiopathic hypertrophic subaortic stenosis: a clinical correlate of regional left ventricular dysfunction: a videometric and echocardiographic study. *Circulation.* 1980;61:561–568.
385. Pitcher D, Wainwright R, Maisey M, et al. Assessment of chest pain in hypertrophic cardiomyopathy using exercise thallium-201 myocardial scintigraphy. *Br Heart J.* 1980;44:650–656.
386. Weiss MB, Ellis K, Sciacca RR, et al. Myocardial blood flow in congestive and hypertrophic cardiomyopathy: relationship to peak wall stress and mean velocity of circumferential fiber shortening. *Circulation.* 1976;54: 484–494.
387. Hardarson T, de la Calzada CS, Curiel R, et al. Prognosis and mortality of hypertrophic obstructive cardiomyopathy. *Lancet.* 1973;2:1462–1467.
388. Canedo MI, Frank MJ, Abdulla AM. Rhythm disturbances in hypertrophic cardiomyopathy: prevalence, relation to symptoms and management. *Am J Cardiol.* 1980;45:848–855.
389. Ingham RE, Rossen RM, Goodman DJ, et al. Treadmill arrhythmias in patients with idiopathic hypertrophic subaortic stenosis. *Chest.* 1975;68:759–764.
390. McKenna WJ, England D, Doi YL, et al. Arrhythmia in hypertrophic cardiomyopathy. I. Influence on prognosis. *Br Heart J.* 1981;46:168–172.
391. Maron BJ, Savage DD, Wolfson JK, et al. Prognostic significance of 24-hour ambulatory electrocardiographic monitoring in patients with hypertrophic cardiomyopathy: a prospective study. *Am J Cardiol.* 1981;48:252–257.
392. Cosio FG, Moro C, Alonso M, et al. The Q-waves of hypertrophic cardiomyopathy. An electrophysiologic study. *N Engl J Med.* 1980;302:96–99.
393. Goodwin JF, Kirkler DM. Arrhythmia as a cause of sudden death in hypertrophic cardiomyopathy. *Lancet.* 1976;2: 937–940.
394. Frank S, Braunwald E. Idiopathic hypertrophic subaortic stenosis: clinical analysis of 126 patients with emphasis on the natural history. *Circulation.* 1968;37:759–788.
395. Prescott R, Quinn JS, Littman D. Electrocardiographic changes in hypertrophic subaortic stenosis which stimulates myocardial infarction. *Am Heart J.* 1963;66:42–48.
396. St. John Sutton MG, Tajik AJ, Gibson DG, et al. Echocardiographic assessment of left ventricular filling and septal and posterior wall dynamics in idiopathic hypertrophic subaortic stenosis. *Circulation.* 1978;57:512–520.
397. Hanrath P, Mathey D, Siegert R, et al. Left ventricular relaxation and filling pattern in different forms of left ventricular hypertrophy. An echocardiographic study. *Am J Cardiol.* 1980; 45:15–23.
398. Sanderson JE, Traill TA, St. John Sutton MG, et al. Left ventricular relaxation and filling in hypertrophic cardiomyopathy. An echocardiographic study. *Br Heart J.* 1978;40:596–601.
399. Murgo JP, Alter BR, Dorethy JF, et al. Dynamics of left ventricular ejection in obstructive and nonobstructive hypertrophic cardiomyopathy. *J Clin Invest.* 1980;66:1369–1382.
400. Stewart S, Mason DT, Braunwald E. Impaired rate of left ventricular filling in idiopathic hypertrophic subaortic stenosis and valvular aortic stenosis. *Circulation.* 1968;37:8–14.
401. Wigle ED, Marquis Y, Auger P. Muscular subaortic stenosis: initial left ventricular inflow tract pressure in the assessment of intraventricular pressure differences in man. *Circulation.* 1967;35:1110–1117.
402. Shaver JA, Salerni R, Curtiss EI, et al. Clinical presentation and noninvasive evaluation of the patient with hypertrophic cardiomyopathy. *Cardiovasc Clin.* 1989;19:149–192.
403. Adelman AG, McLoughlin MJ, Marquis Y, et al. Left ventricular cineangiographic observations in muscular subaortic stenosis. *Am J Cardiol.* 1969;24:689–697.
404. Whalen RE, Cohen AL, Sumner RG, et al. Demonstration of the dynamic nature of idiopathic hypertrophic subaortic stenosis. *Am J Cardiol.* 1963;11:8–17.
405. Simon AR, Ross J, Jr., Gault JH. Angiographic anatomy of the left ventricle and mitral valve in idiopathic hypertrophic subaortic stenosis. *Circulation.* 1967;36:852–867.
406. Murgo JP. The hemodynamic evaluation in hypertrophic cardiomyopathy: systolic and diastolic dysfunction. *Cardiovasc Clin.* 1989;19:193–220.
407. Harrison DC, Braunwald E, Glick G, et al. Effects of beta adrenergic blockade on the circulation., with particular reference to observations in patients with hypertrophic subaortic stenosis. *Circulation.* 1964;29:84–98.

408. Flamm MD, Harrison DC, Hancock EW. Muscular subaortic stenosis. Prevention of outflow obstruction with propranolol. *Circulation.* 1968;38:846–858.
409. Stenson RE, Flamm MD, Jr., Harrison DC, et al. Hypertrophic subaortic stenosis. Clinical and hemodynamic effects of long-term propranolol therapy. *Am J Cardiol.* 1973;31:763–773.
410. de la Calzada CS, Ziady GM, Hardarson T, et al. Effect of acute administration of propranolol on ventricular function in hypertrophic obstructive cardiomyopathy measured by non-invasive techniques. *Br Heart J.* 1976;38:798–803.
411. Swanton RH, Brooksby IAB, Jenkins BS, et al. Hemodynamic studies of beta blockade in hypertrophic obstructive cardiomyopathy. *Eur J Cardiol.* 1977;5:327–341.
412. Speiser KW, Krayenbuehl HP. Reappraisal of the effect of acute beta-blockade on left ventricular filling dynamics in hypertrophic obstructive cardiomyopathy. *Eur Heart J.* 1981;2:21–29.
413. Hess OM, Grimm J, Krayenbuehl HP. Diastolic function in hypertrophic cardiomyopathy: effects of propranolol and verapamil on diastolic stiffness. *Eur Heart J.* 1983;4(Suppl F):47–56.
414. Kaltenbach M, Hopf R, Kober G, et al. Treatment of hypertrophic obstructive cardiomyopathy with verapamil. *Br Heart J.* 1979;42:35–42.
415. Rosing DR, Condit JR, Maron BJ, et al. Verapamil therapy: a new approach to the pharmacologic treatment of hypertrophic cardiomyopathy. III. Effects of long-term administration. *Am J Cardiol.* 1981;48:545–553.
416. Rosing DR, Idanpaan-Heikkla U, Maron BJ, et al. Use of calcium channel blocking drugs in hypertrophic cardiomyopathy. *Am J Cardiol.* 1985;55:185B–195B.
417. Bonow RO, Dilsizian V, Rosing DR, et al. Verapamil-induced improvement in left ventricular diastolic filling and increased exercise tolerance in patients with hypertrophic cardiomyopathy: short and long term effects. *Circulation.* 1985;72:853-864.
418. Rosing DR, Kent KM, Maron BJ, et al. Verapamil therapy: a new approach to the pharmacologic treatment of hypertrophic cardiomyopathy. II. Effects on exercise capacity and symptomatic status. *Circulation.* 1979;60:1208–1213.
419. Shaffer EM, Rocchini AP, Spicer RL, et al. Effects of verapamil on left ventricular diastolic filling in children with hypertrophic cardiomyopathy. *Am J Cardiol.* 1988;61:413–417.
420. Bonow RO, Vitale DF, Maron BJ, et al. Regional left ventricular asynchrony and impaired global filling in hypertrophic cardiomyopathy: effect of verapamil. *J Am Coll Cardiol.* 1987;9:1108–1116.
421. Bonow RO, Ostrow HG, Rosing DR, et al. Verapamil effects on left ventricular systolic and diastolic function in patients with hypertrophic cardiomyopathy: pressure-volume analysis with a non-imaging scintillation probe. *Circulation.* 1983;68:1062–1073.
422. Ito Y, Suko J, Chidsey CA. Intracellular calcium and myocardial contractility. V. Calcium uptake of sarcoplasmic reticulum fractions in hypertrophied and failing rabbit hearts. *J Mol Cell Cardiol.* 1974;6:237–247.
423. Lorell BH, Barry WH. Effects of verapamil on contraction and relaxation of cultured chick embryo ventricular cells during calcium overload. *J Am Coll Cardiol.* 1984;3:341–348.
424. Paulus WJ, Nellens P, Heyndrickx GR, et al. Effects of long-term treatment with amiodarone on exercise hemodynamics and left ventricular relaxation in patients with hypertrophic cardiomyopathy. *Circulation.* 1986;74:544–554.
425. Leon MB, Rosing DR, Maron BJ, et al. Amiodarone in patients with hypertrophic cardiomyopathy and refractory cardiac symptoms: an alternative to current medical therapy [Abstract]. *Circulation.* 1984;70(Suppl II):II18.
426. Morrow AG, Brockenbrough EC. Surgical treatment of idiopathic hypertrophic subaortic stenosis: technic and hemodynamic results of subaortic ventriculomyotomy. *Ann Surg.* 1961;154:181–189.
427. Morrow AG. Hypertrophic subaortic stenosis. *J Thorac Cardiovasc Surg.* 1978;76:423–430.
428. Maron BJ, Nishimura RA, McKenna WJ, et al. Assessment of permanent dual chamber pacing as a treatment for drug-refractory symptomatic patients with obstructive hypertrophic cardiomyopathy. A randomized, double-blind, crossover study (M-PATHY). *Circulation.* 1999;99:2927.
429. Nagueh SF, Lakkis NM, Middleton KJ, et al. Changes in left ventricular diastolic function 6 months after nonsurgical septal reduction therapy for hypertrophic obstructive cardiomyopathy. *Circulation.* 1999;99:344.
430. Kappenberger L, Linde C, Daubert C, et al. Pacing in hypertrophic obstructive cardiomyopathy. A randomized crossover study. PIC study group. *Eur Heart J.* 1997;18:1249.
431. Gadler F, Linde C, Daubert C, et al. Significant improvement of quality of life following atrioventricular synchronous pacing in patients with hypertrophic obstructive cardiomyopathy. Data from 1 year of follow-up. PIC study group. Pacing in Cardiomyopathy. *Eur Heart J.* 1999;20:1044
432. Linde C, Gadler F, Kappenberger L, et al. Placebo effect of pacemaker implantation in obstructive hypertrophic cardiomyopathy. PIC study group. Pacing in Cardiomyopathy. *Am J Cardiol.* 1999;83:903
433. Knight C, Kurbaan AS, Seggewiss H, et al. Nonsurgical septal reduction for hypertrophic obstructive cardiomyopathy: outcome in the first series of patients. *Circulation.* 1997;95:2075–2081.
434. Faber L, Meissner A, Ziemssen P, et al. Percutaneous transluminal septal myocardial ablation for hypertrophic obstructive cardiomyopathy: long-term follow-up of the first series of 25 patients. *Heart.* 2000;83:326–331.
435. Gietzen FH, Leuner CJ, Obergassel L, et al. Role of transcoronary ablation of septal hypertrophy in patients with hypertrophic cardiomyopathy, New York Heart Association functional class III or IV, and outflow obstruction only under provocable conditions. *Circulation.* 2002;106:454–459.
436. Gietzen FH, Leuner CJ, Raute-Kreinsen U, et al. Acute and long-term results after transcoronary ablation of septal hypertrophy (TASH). Catheter interventional treatment for hypertrophic obstructive cardiomyopathy. *Eur Heart J.* 1999;20: 1342–1354.
437. Knight CJ. Five years of percutaneous transluminal septal myocardial ablation. *Heart.* 2000;83:255–256.
438. Lakkis N, Plana JC, Nagueh S, et al. Efficacy of nonsurgical septal reduction therapy in symptomatic patients with obstructive hypertrophic cardiomyopathy and provocable gradients. *Am J Cardiol.* 2001;88:583–586.
439. Shamim W, Yousufuddin M, Wang D, et al. Nonsurgical reduction of the interventricular septum in patients with hypertrophic cardiomyopathy. *N Engl J Med.* 2002;347:1326–1333.
440. Elliot PM, Gimeno B, Jr., Mahon NG, et al. Relation between severity of left ventricular hypertrophy and prognosis in patients with hypertrophic cardiomyopathy. *Lancet* 2001;357: 420–424.
441. Spirito P, Bellone P, Harris KM, et al. Magnitude of left ventricular hypertrophy and risk of sudden death in hypertrophic cardiomyopathy. *N Engl J Med.* 2000; 342:1778–1785.
442. McKenna WJ, Chetty S, Oakley CM, et al. Arrhythmia in hypertrophic cardiomyopathy: exercise and 48 hour ambulatory electrocardiographic assessment with and without beta adrenergic blocking therapy. *Am J Cardiol.* 1980;45:1–5.
443. McKenna WF, England D, Doi YL, et al. Arrhythmia in hypertrophic cardiomyopathy. I. Influence on prognosis. *Br Heart J.* 1981;46:168–172.
444. Shah PM, Adelman AG, Wigle ED, et al. The natural (and unnatural) history of hypertrophic obstructive cardiomyopathy. *Circ Res.* 1974;35(2)(Suppl II):179–195.
445. Fay WP, Talierco CP, Ilstrup DM, et al. Natural history of hypertrophic cardiomyopathy in the elderly. *J Am Coll Cardiol.* 1990; 16:821–826.
446. Maron BJ, Roberts WC, Edwards JE, et al. Sudden death in patients with hypertrophic cardiomyopathy: characterization of 26 patients with functional limitation. *Am J Cardiol.* 1978;41: 803–810.
447. McKenna WJ, Deanfield JE. Hypertrophic cardiomyopathy: an important cause of sudden death. *Arch Dis Child.* 1984; 59:971–975.
448. Maron BJ, Shen WK, Link MS, et al. Efficacy of implantable cardioverter-defibrillators for the prevention of sudden death in patients with hypertrophic cardiomyopathy. *N Engl J Med.* 2000;342:365–373.
449. Canedo MI, Frank MJ. Therapy of hypertrophic cardiomyopathy: medical or surgical? Clinical and pathophysiologic considerations. *Am J Cardiol.* 1981;48:383–388.
450. Cecchi F, Maron BJ, Epstein SE. Long-term outcome of patients with hypertrophic cardiomyopathy successfully resuscitated after cardiac arrest. *J Am Coll Cardiol.* 1989;13:1283–1288.
451. Spirito P, Chiarella F, Carratino L, et al. Clinical course and prognosis of hypertrophic cardiomyopathy in an outpatient population. *N Engl J Med.* 1989; 320:749–755.

Congestive Heart Failure as a Consequence of Valvular Heart Disease

19

William J. McKenna   Denis Pellerin   Niall G. Mahon
Barry H. Greenberg

The management of patients with congestive heart failure (CHF) has become an international health care problem in the ever-aging population. In the United States, nearly 5 million people suffer from heart failure (HF) and fewer than 3,000 are offered transplantation due to limitations of age and the persistent and worsening shortage of donors.

Although the current epidemic of HF in developed countries is chiefly attributable to coronary disease and hypertension, valvular heart disease remains responsible for a significant proportion of cases (1). Valvular heart disease is a mechanical problem and, ideally, it warrants a mechanical solution. The art and science of managing valvular disease consist of determining the optimal time for surgery. In patients with valvular disease, the consequences of volume or pressure overload on left ventricular (LV) cavity size and function are the main prognosis indicators. The development of HF is usually the result of a severe impairment of valvular function that overwhelms the physiologic compensatory mechanisms that are activated for response to the increased load on the heart. Once HF has occurred, valvular heart disease is associated with a dramatic worsening of prognosis. Thus, prevention, prompt recognition, and appropriate treatment of HF in patients with valvular heart disease are of the utmost importance.

In this chapter, we will review specific issues related to chronic and acute HF as a consequence of valvular lesions of the left side of the heart. General principles and major issues of management are discussed. For further details, the reader is referred to the guidelines for the management of patients with valvular heart disease of the American College of Cardiology/American Heart Association (ACC/AHA) Task Force (2). Congestive HF secondary to valvular disease of the right side of the heart is discussed in another chapter in this text.

CELLULAR AND MOLECULAR CONSEQUENCES OF CHRONIC VALVULAR DISEASE

Volume overload stretches the myocardium and induces LV dilatation. Pressure overload increases wall stress and wall thickness. Cellular and molecular consequences of chronic valvular disease, including physiological response to pressure or/and volume overload, and progression from hypertrophy with small cavity to dilatation and dysfunction are not fully understood.

Because the cells of adult heart muscle are terminally differentiated and have lost their capacity to divide, wall thickness is increased through individual myocyte hypertrophy. This is a dynamic process resulting from an imbalance between protein synthesis and degradation, in which an increased number of sarcomeres provides a short-term adaptive response to overload. In this process, fetal muscle-specific gene products may reappear but, as the cell cycle remains blocked, cell division is not achieved (3). In chronic valve disease, pressure overload leads to concentric hypertrophy and volume overload leads to dilatation and eccentric hypertrophy. A notable difference between these two patterns is the spatial arrangement of the sarcomeres; in concentric hypertrophy they are arranged in parallel (increasing the cellular thickness), while in eccentric hypertrophy they are disposed in series (increasing the cellular length). Although the molecular basis of these responses is not well-known, two basic triggering mechanisms appear to be involved: neurohormonal and mechanical stretch activation (Fig. 19-1).

In neurohormonal activation associated with overload in vivo, the plasma concentrations of adrenergic agonists,

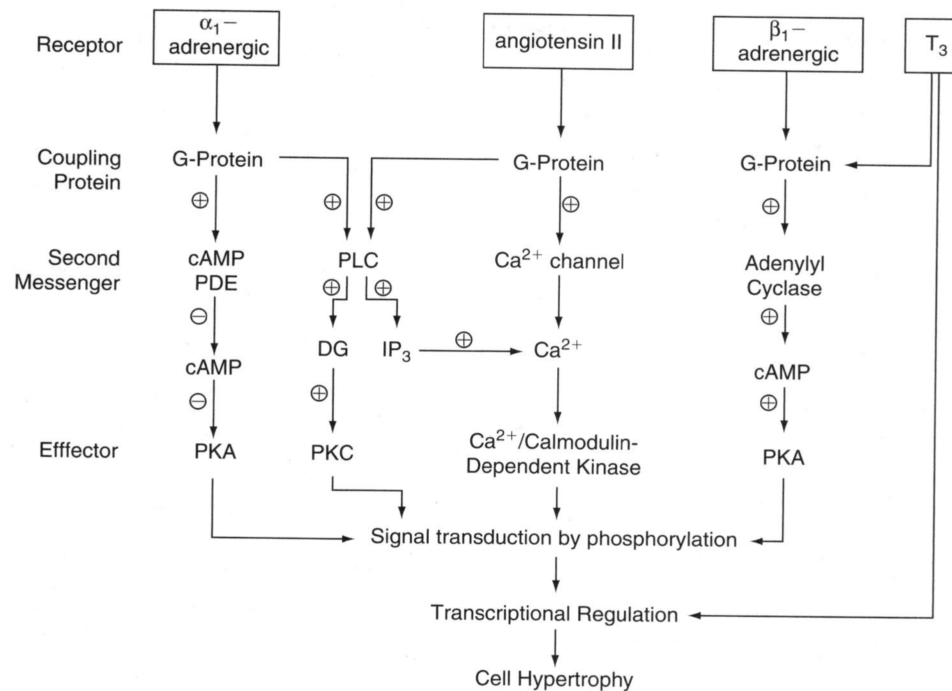

Figure 19-1 Molecular mechanisms of hypertrophy. (Reproduced from Morgan HE, Baker KM. Cardiac hypertrophy: mechanical, neural, and endocrine dependence. Circulation. 1991;83:13–25, with permission.)

thyroxin, and angiotensin (Ang) increase. The activation of angiotensin II (Ang II) type 1 (AT_1) and of α- and β-receptors by their endogenous agonists Ang II, adrenaline, and noradrenaline triggers the activation of the G-protein system, through metabolic pathways in which cyclic adenosine monophosphate (cAMP), Ca^{2+}, phospholipase C, and other mediators, lead to the activation of protein kinases. These act by phosphorylating DNA binding proteins, reversing the inhibition that they exert over DNA transcription. This leads to expression of sequences coding for contractile proteins, ribosomal RNA, and oncogenes. Thus, protein synthesis and cell hypertrophy are initiated (4). Thyroid hormone levels are also increased as a consequence of neurohormonal activation. Thyroid hormone may act either through activation of the G-protein system, which triggers a similar response to that observed with Ang or α- or β-receptor agonists, or through activation of its receptor located in specific DNA sequences on target genes, which leads to the activation of contractile protein synthesis (3). In addition, both pressure and volume overload enhance mechanical stretch and cell deformation, thereby inducing activation of stretch-activated ion channels and G-proteins. This in turn activates protein kinase, which causes hypertrophy by the mechanisms previously outlined.

The consequence of these responses is enhanced metabolic activity and increase in the number of sarcomeres, which provide a short-term adaptation to overload. However, several of the growth factors that accelerate protein synthesis, including the proto-oncogenes c-myc and c-fos and the peptide transforming growth factor-β (TGF-β), have recently been shown to be capable of stimulating programmed cell death. This may be one of the mechanisms by which the unnatural growth triggered by overload also leads to accelerated myocyte death and impairment of contractility. Prevention of apoptosis may be one of the benefits of neurohormonal inhibition (5).

QUANTIFICATION OF LEFT VENTRICULAR PERFORMANCE IN PATIENTS WITH CHRONIC VALVULAR DISEASE

Evaluation of ventricular performance has important prognosis and therapeutic implications. Assessment of ventricular performance includes LV systolic function, volume, mass, LV geometry, LV diastolic function and pressure, and regional performance. Ventricular ejection fraction varies with heart rate, preload, afterload, and ventricular geometry even in the absence of changes in myocardial contractility.

Echocardiography is central to the diagnosis and follow-up of patients with valvular disease. Preoperative echocardiographic LV ejection fraction (LVEF) was the most powerful predictor of late survival in patients with chronic mitral regurgitation (MR) (6). According to American Society of Echocardiography (ASE) guidelines, echo evaluation of LVEF is best measured by biplane apical Simpson's rule. However, this method has suboptimal reproducibility related to endocardial definition. Contrast cavity opacification markedly improves endocardial border delineation in patients with suboptimal image quality. A recent multicenter study showed that contrast echocardiography significantly improved interobserver agreement on LVEF compared with conventional echocardiography (7). Contrast echocardiography reaches a level comparable to magnetic resonance imaging (MRI) and is better than those obtained by cineventriculography (7). Other limitations of two-dimensional echo such as correct image plane orientation and true long axis of the ventricle are overcome by three-dimensional echo. Contrast cavity opacification can be combined with three-dimensional echo for further improvement of LVEF accuracy and reproducibility. In addition, recently described indices of global LV systolic performance are not dependent on endocardial definition and are less dependent on loading conditions: *dP/dt* calculated from MR flow recordings, early diastolic mitral annular velocity, and peak systolic strain rate.

Ventricular volumes are also calculated with biplane apical Simpson's rule. LV end-systolic volume seems to be less dependent on loading conditions and has been shown to be a strong prognostic factor and criterion for surgical indication in chronic aortic regurgitation (AR) and MR. Noninvasive hemodynamic assessment, including estimation of LV filling pressure, pulmonary artery systolic pressure (PASP), right atrial pressure, and cardiac output, can also be performed. Echocardiography is the investigation of choice to assess valve morphology, etiology, coexistence of other valvular disease, in addition to the changes in LV dimensions, wall thickness, and function (8,9). Quantification of valvular disease severity is obtained with the use of Doppler techniques. Multiplane transesophageal study is helpful when there is poor image quality with transthoracic echocardiography and to assess the mechanism and suitability for valve repair in mitral regurgitation. In addition, echo is practical for serial evaluations and guides the decision-making process for surgical referral. Transesophageal echocardiography is helpful to define valve anatomy, and mechanism of dysfunction, and is being used intraoperatively to assess results of mitral valve (MV) repair and for hemodynamic monitoring. History, physical examination, ECG, and exercise performance must also be taken into account.

During cardiac catheterization, direct measurement of transvalvular gradient, cardiac output, pressures in the cardiac chambers, ejection fraction, and LV dimensions can be performed. In patients with significant valve disease, cardiac catheterization, contrast ventriculography, and coronary angiography should be performed preoperatively when valve dysfunction is more than moderate, there is multiple valve disease, there are discrepancies between clinical and echo findings, and in patients who have angina or risk factors for coronary disease or who are older than 40 years of age (10,11).

Radionuclide angiography with gated pool imaging or first-pass angiography may be used to assess severity of regurgitation, LV volumes, and ejection fraction. MRI, when available, may be useful to assess the severity of valve regurgitation and ventricular volumes, particularly in patients with a poor ultrasonic acoustic window (12) when ultrasound contrast agents cannot be used and when the patient is not a transesophageal echocardiography candidate.

AORTIC STENOSIS WITH LEFT VENTRICULAR SYSTOLIC DYSFUNCTION

Etiology

In adults, degenerative or senile aortic stenosis (AS) has become the leading indication for valve replacement (13). In a large population above 65 years of age, advanced age, male sex, smoking, hypertension, height, and elevated low-density-lipoprotein (LDL) cholesterol were associated with AS or aortic sclerosis, suggesting that risk factors for AS or aortic sclerosis may be similar to risk factors for atherosclerosis (14). Degenerative disease associated with a bicuspid aortic valve accounts for 50% of cases of AS. Degenerative disease in a tricuspid aortic valve accounts for 12% of cases (15). In developed countries, rheumatic fever now accounts for fewer than 20% of cases of AS and is almost always associated with coexistent MV disease (16). Uncommon causes of AS in adults include atherosclerosis (in association with severe hypercholesterolemia and advanced atherosclerotic lesions in the aorta and great vessels), ochronosis, Paget bone disease, and advanced chronic renal failure.

Onset of Symptoms and Outcome

Symptoms appear late in the natural history of AS and are an ominous development (Fig. 19-2). The median untreated survival rates once angina pectoris or syncope has occurred are 5 and 3 years, respectively. HF occurs late in the natural history of the condition and is associated with the worst prognosis, the mean life expectancy then being less than 2 years (17). For patients with severe AS, the onset of the symptoms of angina, syncope, or CHF indicates the need for aortic valve replacement (17,18). The outcome is excellent after surgery in patients who have recently become symptomatic. Because sudden death can occur soon after the onset of symptoms, patients should be instructed to report changes in their clinical status. In cases in which the symptomatic status is unclear, supervised exercise testing may be helpful. The risk of exercise testing in these patients is lower than in those with classic symptoms of AS (19). If exercise performance is poor, surgical treatment should be considered (20). It should be noted that ST segment shifts during the exercise test may be related to LV hypertrophy.

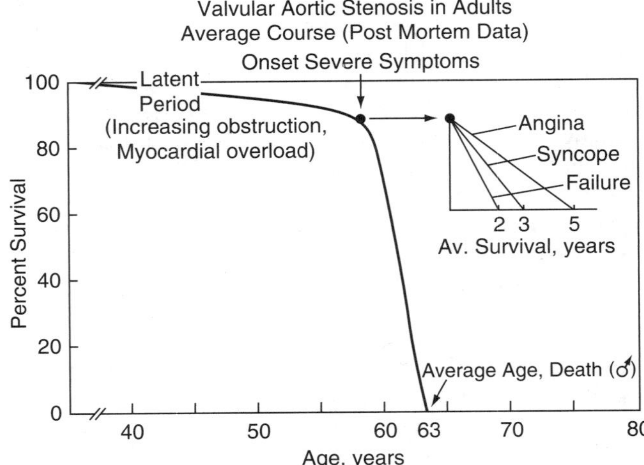

Figure 19-2 Natural history of AS. (Reproduced from Ross J, Jr., Braunwald E. Aortic stenosis. Circulation. 1968;38:61–67, with permission.)

The rate of progression of AS from mild to severe forms has been shown to be quite variable between patients (21). In general, aortic area as calculated by the Gorlin formula decreases by about 0.1 cm^2 per year (22,23) and Doppler-derived transvalvular gradient increases by 7 mm Hg per year (24). Therefore, mild AS may become severe within a few years. Several clinical features, including a degenerative etiology and the presence of risk factors for coronary disease, appear to be associated with more rapid progression, but no variable is predictive of the rate and pattern of progression in an individual patient (25).

Pathophysiology

AS causes pressure overload (Fig. 19-3). Diastolic dysfunction precedes systolic dysfunction; thus, when congestive symptoms do arise, systolic function is usually normal. The hallmark adaptation to pressure overload is hypertrophy. This may be regarded as an attempt to normalize wall stress by increasing wall thickness. These adaptive phenomena parallel the progression of AS and help maintain systolic function within the normal range. In severe AS, however, the capacity to increase cardiac output during exercise may be impaired and end-systolic stress is not completely normalized (26). Furthermore, hypertrophy, which is associated with increased collagen deposition, causes increased LV stiffness resulting in reduced LV compliance and diastolic dysfunction (27). There is an upward shift of the pressure–volume relationship so that LV pressure is increased at any given diastolic volume. Elevated end-diastolic pressure may be transmitted to the pulmonary vascular bed, causing exertional congestive symptoms.

Patients with Aortic Stenosis, Low Cardiac Output, and Low Gradient

Some patients present with advanced CHF and reduced EF. Although reduced systolic function is usually an indicator of worse prognosis in most types of heart disease, it is less ominous for patients with AS. For those patients whose ejection performance is reduced because of the high afterload presented by the obstructing valve (afterload mismatch) and for whom the LV can still generate a mean Ao-LV gradient >30 mm Hg, prognosis is excellent following aortic valve replacement (26,28,29). In contrast, patients with AS, low gradient, and severe LV contractile dysfunction have a poor prognosis (28–31), with 21% operative risk and only 50% survival at 4 years (31). Nonetheless, many patients in this category do benefit from surgery (32).

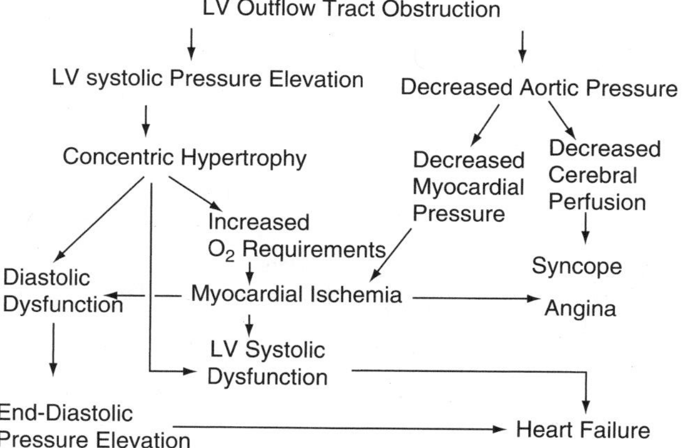

Figure 19-3 Pathophysiology of AS.

Severe and calcified AS with low cardiac output is defined as aortic valve area <1 cm^2 or <0.6 cm^2/m^2 with LV systolic dysfunction (LVEF <40%) and mean transvalvular gradient <40 mm Hg (33,34). Calculation of aortic valve area at rest cannot distinguish between patients with severe AS and patients with mild AS. In both cases, the calculated aortic valve area may be low (35–37). Surgical candidates can be selected using hemodynamic manipulation performed either in the echocardiographic or catheterization laboratories to distinguish between patients with severe valvular obstruction from those with only mild obstruction and aortic pseudostenosis (38,39).

Using echocardiography, patients with low EF and low gradient should be studied at rest and then following infusion of dobutamine. Dobutamine infusion starts at 5 μg/kg per minute and is progressively increased by 2.5-μg/kg/per/minute increments every 5 minutes and stopped when heart rate increase is ≥10 beats per minute. Therefore, inotropic effect is obtained with low risk of inducing ischemia (33). Noninvasive hemodynamic study with infusion of dobutamine detects aortic valve area changes during increase in stroke volume on the one hand, and also detects contractile reserve on the other hand. Contractile reserve with dobutamine stress is defined as 20% increase in stroke volume. Because the LV outflow tract diameter is unchanged, this is equivalent to a 20% increase in aortic velocity time integral (VTI). There are three possible responses to dobutamine stress (39):

1. Contractile reserve with increase in transvalvular gradient. Aortic valve area does not change or increases by less than 0.3 cm^2 or to a valve area <1.0 cm^2, indicating the presence of truly severe aortic stenosis with preserved contractile reserve.
2. Contractile reserve without significant increase in transvalvular gradient. Aortic valve area increases by more than 0.3 cm^2 or to a valve area >1.0 cm^2, indicating nonischemic or ischemic cardiomyopathy with aortic pseudostenosis.
3. There is no contractile reserve with dobutamine and quantification of aortic stenosis severity cannot be performed. Such patients have a poor prognosis regardless of the type of treatment and of stenosis severity (33,40).

Using an invasive approach, nitroprusside can be infused during cardiac catheterization (38,41,42). If the stenotic valve is the primary and main obstruction to outflow, infusion of a vasodilator will decrease total peripheral resistance but flow cannot increase through the stenotic valve. There will be a fall in downstream pressure and an increase in gradient with little change in output. In this case, aortic valve area does not increase or may even decrease. A major risk in the use of sodium nitroprusside to make this determination is the potential for fall in downstream pressure in patients with true severe stenosis.

Thus, the drug must be used with caution, increasing the dose in tiny increments while monitoring hemodynamics carefully. On the other hand, if the valve is not severely stenotic (aortic pseudostenosis), then vasodilatation decreases total peripheral resistance, resulting in increased flow through the mildly stenotic valve; the gradient changes little and the valve area increases substantially. Coronary angiography can be performed during the same session.

Management

There is no major role for medical therapy in the management of AS. If the patient is asymptomatic, no treatment is required, and if the patient is symptomatic, surgery is indicated. Reduction of both preload and afterload can be detrimental and associated with hypotension and prerenal failure. For this reason, angiotensin-converting enzyme (ACE) inhibitors are generally contraindicated in AS and diuretics must be used with caution. In patients who are not surgical candidates, digoxin and diuretics may transiently relieve symptoms but no long-term benefit has been shown. Medications may also be of value in maintaining sinus rhythm in cases associated with atrial fibrillation.

Balloon aortic valvotomy is not indicated in adults because the rate of serious complications of the procedure exceeds 10% and the mortality 18 months after the procedure is similar to that observed in an untreated population. However, it may improve the clinical and hemodynamic status of very sick patients for a short time and serve as a bridge to aortic valve replacement in critically ill patients (43).

Aortic valve replacement remains the treatment of choice. Even octogenarian patients who are otherwise fit have been shown to do well following surgical treatment (44–47). When aortic valve replacement is indicated, there is increased risk of surgery if another valve has to be replaced or repaired, if coronary artery bypass grafts or aortic root replacement are required, and if the patient has renal failure or poor general condition. In patients with AS and low gradient, the presence of a contractile reserve under dobutamine is a strong indicator of favorable outcome after aortic valve replacement. Although the absence of contractile reserve is not a contraindication for surgery, it should be combined with other operative risk factors to assess the risk–benefit ratio. In patients with aortic stenosis and low gradient, presence of contractile reserve under dobutamine and mean transvalvular gradient <20 mm Hg before aortic valve replacement were two independent prognostic factors of 30-day surgical mortality after aortic valve replacement (40). In addition, preserved contractile reserve was associated with symptomatic improvement and better long-term survival after aortic valve replacement.

Patient–prosthesis mismatch is responsible for higher mortality and poorer regression of LV hypertrophy when smaller valve sizes with larger gradients are inserted in patients with low LVEF (31,48–50). If the patient begins with only a 25-mm Hg transvalvular gradient, a residual gradient of 10 mm Hg represents 40% of the original gradient. Patient–prosthesis mismatch is defined by an effective orifice area ≤ 0.8 cm^2/m^2 (50,51). The risk of mismatch is real in patients with severe AS because they have a smaller aortic annular size due to the underlying pathological process. Tables indicating the size of each prosthetic valve according to body surface area (BSA) are useful. If the surgeon cannot insert an appropriate-sized prosthetic valve according to the reference tables, options include stentless bioprosthetic valves, new mechanical valves with best hemodynamic profile, homografts, the Ross procedure, and aortic root enlargement (52).

CHRONIC AORTIC REGURGITATION

Etiology

The causes of AR may be divided into those that affect the aortic valve and those that affect the aortic root. Of patients undergoing surgery, rheumatic disease has been shown to account for approximately 25%, endocarditis for 20%, and aortic root disease for 42% (53).

The prevalence of rheumatic AR is declining; it generally coexists with AS and rheumatic mitral disease (54). Infective endocarditis, which typically affects bicuspid, rheumatic, or otherwise structurally abnormal valves, often presents as an acute or subacute hemodynamic deterioration that requires rapid identification and management (Fig. 19-4). The regurgitant jet may impact and infect the anterior leaflet of the MV, worsening the natural history of the disease (55). Other valvular causes of aortic insufficiency include deterioration of a bioprosthetic valve, thoracic trauma causing cusp rupture (56), myxomatous degeneration, and collagen vascular diseases. Bicuspid aortic valves are predominantly associated with AS but in some cases AR may coexist or predominate. Other congenital diseases, such as ventricular septal defects, subaortic stenosis, and rupture of fenestrated aortic cusps, are rare causes of AR.

Conditions causing AR through dilatation of the aortic root are age-related or degenerative aortic dilatation, cystic medial necrosis of the aorta, Marfan syndrome, hypertension, syphilis, aortic dissection, ankylosing spondylitis, Behçet syndrome, Reiter disease, and Takayasu disease.

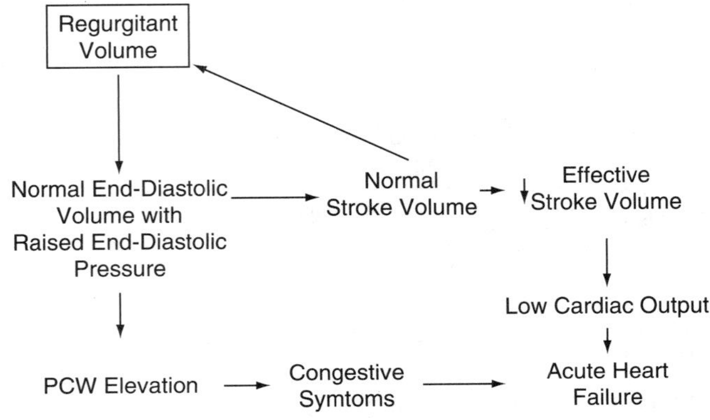

Figure 19-4 Pathophysiology of acute AR.

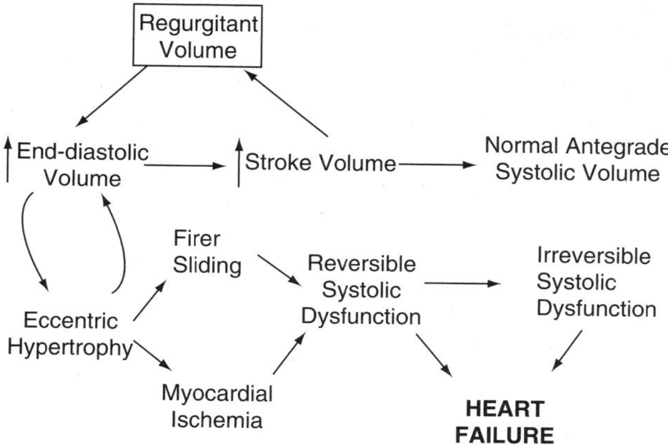

Figure 19-5 Pathophysiology of chronic AR.

Pathophysiology

Chronic AR is responsible for combined volume and pressure overload of the LV (Fig. 19-5). However, if the AR progresses slowly, several adaptive phenomena occur, allowing cardiac output and LV end-diastolic pressure to remain within the normal range even during strenuous exercise (Fig. 19-6). Cardiac chamber dilatation is the most important of these adaptive changes. Dilatation of the LV and pericardium allow a rightward shift of the pressure–volume relationship, so that any given volume of blood can be accommodated at a lower pressure than in a normal-size chamber (57). As a consequence of the increased end-diastolic volume, an increase in stroke volume is achieved, mediated by a normal performance of each myocardial segment on an enlarged circumference (58). For this reason, although the regurgitant fraction can reach 50% to 80% of the total stroke volume, the effective antegrade stroke volume remains within normal range. Because the increase in ventricular diastolic volume is proportional to the increase in stroke volume, there is no change in EF. The increase in wall stress caused by increased ventricular volumes is accompanied by compensatory eccentric LV hypertrophy. In AR, the molecular mechanisms of hypertrophy are thought to be similar to those described for AS. The replication of sarcomeres is mainly in series, leading to dilatation as well as hypertrophy.

There is a transitional stage in which the LV progressively dilates and acquires a more spherical geometry, accompanied by increasing LV diastolic pressures and systolic wall stress. Subsequently, LVEF decreases, which eventually leads to symptoms of HF. These changes may be produced either by an increase in regurgitant fraction or by a decline in LV contractility related to fibrosis, sliding of muscle fibers, ischemia, or apoptosis (3,5). The progression of LV dysfunction is slow. In follow-up studies (59–61) of asymptomatic patients with severe AR, LV dilatation, and preserved EF, only 4% to 5% of patients per year needed surgical treatment.

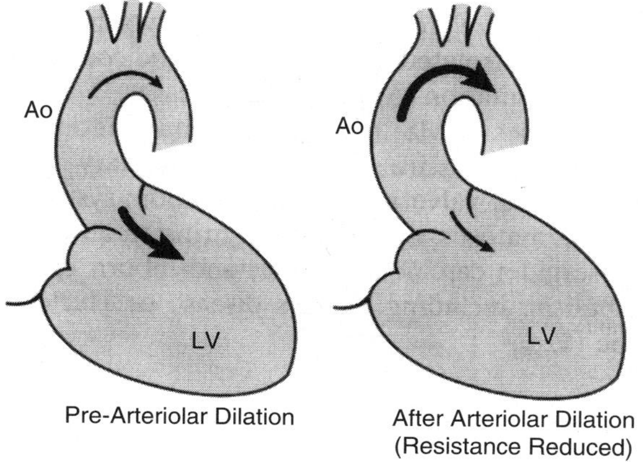

Figure 19-6 Distribution of stroke volume in aortic insufficiency. By decreasing impedance to forward flow, arteriolar dilation can increase cardiac output and reduce regurgitant flow. (Reproduced from Greenberg BH. Medical therapy for patients with aortic insufficiency [Review]. *Cardiol Clin.* 1991;9(2):255–270, with permission.)

Clinical Features

During the compensated phase, patients with chronic AR may remain asymptomatic for years. Symptoms of HF usually develop insidiously. The clinical features of chronic AR are described in classic texts. Infective endocarditis is the main cause of rapid worsening of AR.

Assessment

Echocardiography is the investigation of choice to assess the severity of AR, its etiology, and its effects on LV dimensions and function (8,9). In addition, it is of considerable importance in the follow-up of patients with chronic AR. Echocardiographic criteria for surgical referrals are discussed later. Three-dimensional echo provides refined structural evaluation of the valve.

During cardiac catheterization, the severity of AR may be assessed by characterizing the degree of LV opacification. LV diastolic pressure, resting cardiac output, and LVEF, end-systolic and end-diastolic diameters and volumes can be measured (11). The indications for cardiac catheterization are similar to those for AS.

Management

The distribution of blood flow in AR is sensitive to manipulations that alter the impedance to flow in the systemic circulation. Vasodilator therapy, by reducing afterload, may reduce the regurgitant fraction and LV end-diastolic volume and pressure (Figs. 19-7 and 19-8) (62–67).

Patients who are symptomatic or who have LV dysfunction should be referred for aortic valve replacement (68). Symptomatic patients should undergo surgery even in the presence of normal LV dimensions and function. Symptoms caused by AR are strong predictors of clinical prognosis. Patients with an EF of less than 50% at rest should undergo surgery (2). In a study of 246 patients with moderate to severe AR, the adverse event rate was 2.5% in 113 asymptomatic patients and 25% per year in symptomatic New York Heart Association (NYHA) Class III and IV patients (69). Independent predictors of survival were age, symptom severity, comorbidity, LV end-systolic diameter index, and atrial fibrillation. An initial conservative strat-

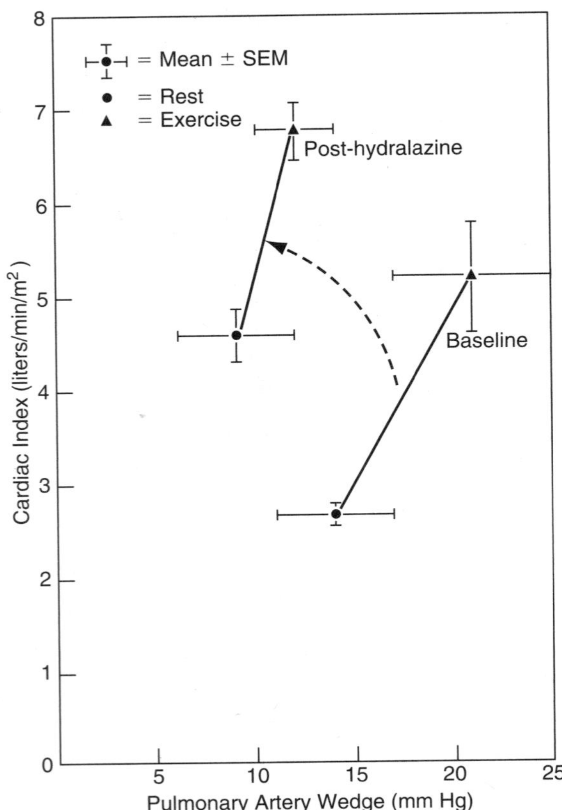

Figure 19-7 Effects of oral hydralazine on rest and exercise hemodynamic variables in ten patients with chronic, severe aortic insufficiency. (Reproduced from Greenberg BH. Medical therapy for patients with aortic insufficiency. [Review] *Cardiol Clin.* 1991;9(2):255–270, with permission.)

egy may be appropriate for patients with LV enlargement and preserved systolic function. Parameters associated with a poor postoperative prognosis are an end-systolic dimension greater than 55 mm (68) (Fig. 19-9); an end-systolic volume greater than 60 mL/m^2, a shortening fraction below 28% (70), and ratio of LV end-systolic dimension to

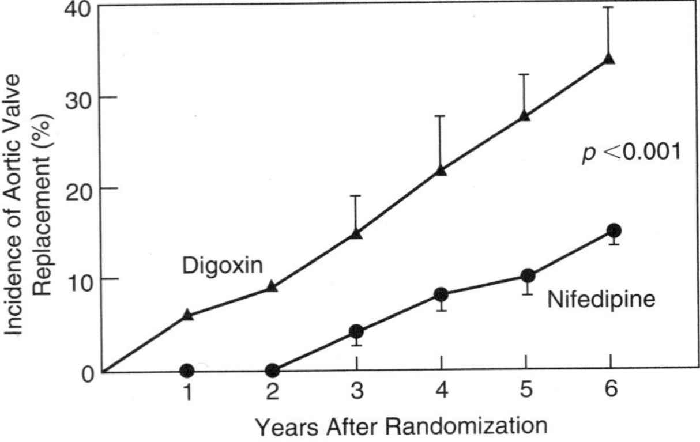

Figure 19-8 Cumulative annual incidence of progression to aortic valve replacement in nifedipine- and digoxin-treated patients with severe AR. (Reproduced from Scognamiglio R, Rahimtoola SH, Fasoli G, et al. Nifedipine in asymptomatic patients with severe aortic regurgitation and normal left ventricular function. *N Engl J Med.* 1994;331(11):689–694, with permission.)

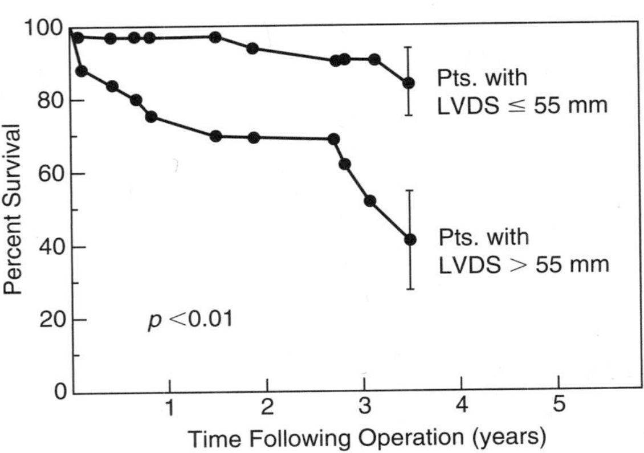

Figure 19-9 End-systolic LV dimension as a marker of postoperative prognosis. (Reproduced from Bonow RO, Rosing DR, Kent KM, et al. Timing of operation for chronic aortic regurgitation. [Review] *Am J Cardiol.* 1982;50(2):325–336, with permission.)

BSA greater than 26 mm/cm^2 (71). Current ACC/AHA guidelines recommend valve replacement for patients with severe LV dilatation (end-diastolic dimension greater than 75 mm or end-systolic dimension greater than 55 mm) (2). These guidelines were published in 1998 and cut-off values of parameters are likely to decrease in the next version. Women undergoing surgery have a worse long-term postoperative outcome than do men and may warrant earlier intervention than is currently recommended (72). In cases of severe dysfunction (EF less than 30%), the operative mortality is high (reaching 10% or more), but overall prognosis is better than with conservative management (73). Duration of LV dysfunction has an impact on outcome. Frank LV dysfunction present for less than 1 year does not carry the same ominous prognosis as does a prolonged period of LV dysfunction (74,75).

The standard surgical treatment is aortic valve replacement with either a biological or mechanical prosthesis (76), with replacement of the aortic root in cases of severe aortic dilatation or dissection. Pulmonary autografting (Ross procedure) or aortic valve reconstruction may be performed in selected cases (77,78). In asymptomatic patients, the EF and LV dimensions usually improve following surgery and may even return to normal ranges. Post operative improvement is usually apparent within 8 months. In patients with severe LV dysfunction and LVEF <25% due to AR, aortic valve surgery is unlikely to be beneficial (2) and cardiac transplantation should be considered.

MITRAL STENOSIS

Etiology

Mitral stenosis (MS) is almost invariably rheumatic in etiology. However, because of extensive use of antibiotics in the treatment of streptococcal infection, its prevalence is diminishing (79). MS is more frequent in women (two-thirds of all cases) (80) and coexists with MR in 40% of cases.

Rare causes of MS include congenital abnormalities of leaflets, commissures, chords, and papillary muscles;

mitral valve annular calcification; systemic lupus erythematosus and associated syndromes; rheumatoid arthritis; treatment with methysergide; carcinoid tumors; and inborn errors of metabolism, including Fabry disease or Hurler syndrome (81).

Pathophysiology

The anatomical changes of commissural fusion, fibrosis and calcification of cusps, annulus, and subvalvular apparatus progress slowly during years following the onset of acute rheumatic fever. Although severe stenosis may develop in tropical countries within 2 years (82), in temperate countries symptoms develop in the third or fourth decade (83).

Although a gradient may be measured with MV areas of 2 cm^2 or less, left atrial (LA) pressure is not raised until the area is smaller than 1.5 cm^2. With areas of 1 to 1.5 cm^2, LA pressure may be normal at rest but rises during exercise, which leads to exertional symptoms (Fig. 19-10). With areas of 1 cm^2 or less, cardiac output is reduced and pulmonary pressures are raised (56). Thus, patients exhibit symptoms of low cardiac output, such as fatigue or weakness, and have a reduction in exercise capacity that is proportional to the degree of elevation of pulmonary artery pressure (84) as a consequence of raised pulmonary venous pressures. This may cause pulmonary arteriolar constriction, which leads to further elevations in pulmonary artery pressure. Moreover, in advanced cases, organic obliterative changes in the pulmonary vascular beds can develop and exacerbate pulmonary hypertension (85). The development of moderate pulmonary hypertension is usually well-tolerated. However, if pulmonary pressure becomes severe and exceeds 60 mm Hg, right ventricular (RV) pressure overload occurs, leading to failure of the right side of the heart (86). When the RV begins to fail, the time course of clinical deterioration accelerates considerably. As RV stroke volume diminishes, the amount of blood traversing the pulmonary circulation to the LA is reduced, and LA pressure may be reduced in this setting with significant drop in cardiac output because high levels of LA pressure are required to force blood across the stenotic MV. The onset of RV failure also leads to the development of systemic congestion.

The increase in hydrostatic pressure results in transudation of fluid from the intravascular to the extravascular lung spaces. This is accompanied by a compensatory hypertrophy of pulmonary lymphatics and obliterative changes in the vascular wall, which reduce the amount of pulmonary edema that develops and explain why signs and symptoms of pulmonary congestion may be absent in some patients with long-standing MS despite LA pressure exceeding 30 to 35 mm Hg (87) (Fig. 19-10).

Two conditions, in particular, have been associated with the onset of clinically evident congestive HF in previously asymptomatic patients with MS: the onset of atrial fibrillation and pregnancy. The presence of atrial fibrillation is more likely in advanced disease (88) and often marks a turning point in the clinical course of the disease. Atrial systolic contraction is an important mechanism for forcing blood across a stenotic MV (89). When atrial fibrillation occurs, LA pressure increases rapidly and cardiac output falls. The problem is accentuated by the increase in heart rate, which decreases the diastolic filling period. This augments the transmitral gradient and elevates LA pressures further. During pregnancy, plasma volume and cardiac output increase 30% to 50% by week 20 to 24. With a relatively fixed obstruction at the level of the MV, this flow increase brings about an increase in the transvalvular gradient and LA pressure. As a result, pulmonary congestive symptoms or even pulmonary edema may develop for the first time during this period. Emotional stress, exercise, or infection may also precipitate congestive HF in patients with MS.

In some patients with MS, LV systolic function may be globally impaired through poorly understood mechanisms. Possible causes include chronically increased afterload (a consequence of depressed cardiac output), extension of the scarring rheumatic process from the MV into the posterobasal segments of the LV, limited LV distensibility, variable diastolic suction, diastolic ventricular interaction, and myocardial atrophy resulting from reduced ventricular work (90,91). MS is often associated with AR or MR leading to volume overload.

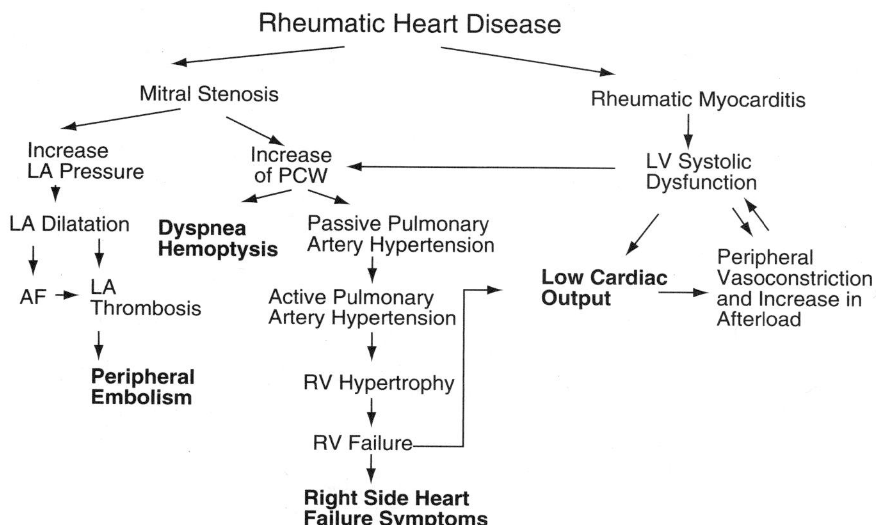

Figure 19-10 Pathophysiology of MS.

Once symptoms have occurred, the clinical course is slowly but relentlessly downhill. In the presurgical era, functional Class III patients had a 5-year survival of only 62% and functional Class IV patients a 5-year survival of 15% (92).

Clinical Features

In addition to symptoms of left-sided HF, patients may complain of cough and wheezing related to bronchial hyperreactivity secondary to mucosal edema and dilatation of bronchial vessels (93,94). Events such as fever, respiratory infections, strenuous exercise, pregnancy, atrial fibrillation with rapid ventricular rate, or other tachycardia can precipitate pulmonary edema. Symptoms of right-sided HF follow the development of pulmonary hypertension. Hemoptysis is a typical symptom that may be induced by physical exercise; it is caused by rupture of pulmonary or bronchopulmonary venules as a consequence of pulmonary venous hypertension. Thromboembolic complications are associated with atrial fibrillation, large LA, and low cardiac output. Chest pain may be secondary to pulmonary hypertension or coronary embolism (Fig. 19-11).

Assessment

Radiological findings of LA and pulmonary artery enlargement without cardiac dilatation may raise the suspicion for MS. Echocardiographic evaluation includes quantification of MV area, assessment of leaflet mobility, extent of commissural fusion, leaflet and annular calcification (95,96), and subvalvular apparatus abnormalities. These parameters are combined into the Wilkins score. Echocardiographic evaluation also includes quantification of MR severity, LA size, PASP, and detection of other valvular disease. Enlarged LA >6 cm is associated with suboptimal MV area increase after mitral commissurotomy (97). Detection of LA and left atrial appendage thrombus by transesophageal echocardiography is mandatory even in patients in sinus rhythm (98) for the selection of candidates for percutaneous balloon mitral commissurotomy.

The indications for catheterization in patients with MS are multiple valvular diseases, discrepancy between clinical and echocardiographic findings, and suspected coronary artery disease. Exercise echocardiography is useful to assess symptoms and PASP in patients with MV area between 1.0 and 1.5 cm^2.

Medical Management

Although symptomatic obstruction is best treated by mechanical relief of stenosis, medical therapy plays an important role in the management of MS. This includes the use of antiarrhythmic agents for the restoration and maintenance of sinus rhythm or for rate control in established atrial fibrillation, and the use of anticoagulants to prevent systemic embolism. Diuretics are helpful for the control of symptoms of cardiac failure but must be administered cautiously, as patients with MS may experience a reduction in cardiac output when diuresis reduces LA pressure below a critical level. Aggravating factors such as anemia should be identified and treated.

Indications for Intervention

Survival of patients with MS according to functional class and treatment is shown in Figure 19-11 (99). If the MV area is larger than 1.5 cm^2, the risk-to-benefit ratio of intervention is unfavorable (100). Intervention in the form of percutaneous balloon mitral commissurotomy or surgical commissurotomy is indicated in patients with MV areas less than 1 cm^2, in patients who are symptomatic on medical therapy with MV areas between 1 and 1.5 cm^2, and when PASP is >50 mm Hg at rest or >60 mm Hg during exercise. Although intervention is indicated for patients with established pulmonary hypertension, operative risks are higher (101). Following intervention, pulmonary arterial pressure falls in almost all patients, regardless of previous levels (102). There are several other circumstances in which intervention may be considered:

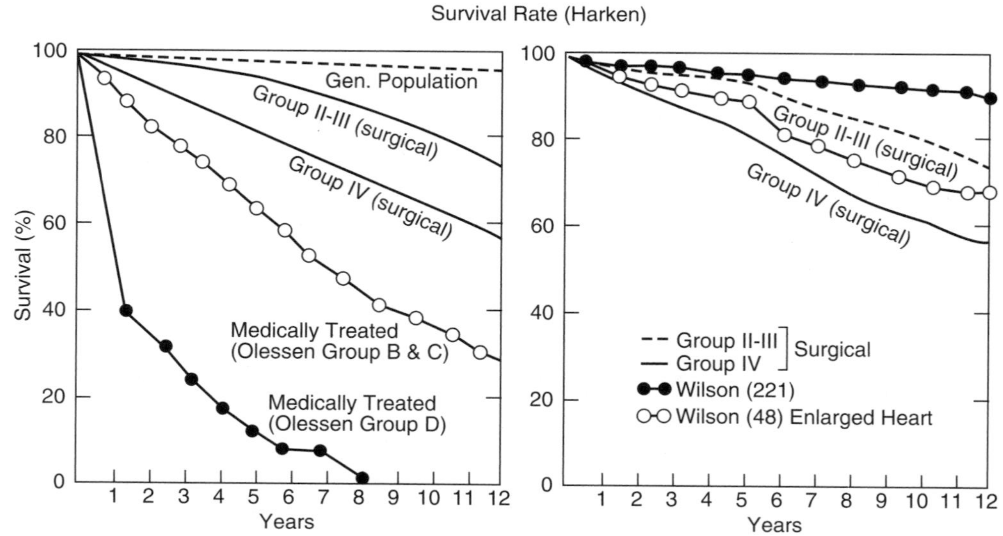

Figure 19-11 Natural history of MS. (Reproduced from Ross J Jr., Braunwald E. Aortic stenosis. *Circulation*. 1968;38:61–67, with permission.)

1. To prevent recurrent embolism in patients with previous thromboembolic episodes. Percutaneous or surgical mitral commissurotomy is indicated because of the risks for thromboembolism associated with prosthetic valves (103–105).
2. To facilitate successful cardioversion and maintenance of sinus rhythm in patients with moderate to severe MS and recent onset of atrial fibrillation (106).
3. Before pregnancy in women at high risk for deterioration, or during pregnancy in patients in whom cardiac failure has developed.

Surgical options include mitral commissurotomy with or without open heart surgery and MV replacement. Perioperative and long-term survival are related to preoperative LV function (107). Overall 5-year survival are 80% to 85%. Patients in functional Class III or lower have an operative mortality of 2%, whereas patients in Class IV have a mortality of 25% (108). Although only 60% to 80% of patients are suitable for closed mitral commissurotomy, results in this group are excellent, survival and freedom from operation at 10 years being 95% and 90%, respectively. Uncontrolled data suggested that early commissurotomy in patients with moderate stenosis and few symptoms may improve long-term survival and decrease the rate of complications and repeated intervention (109).

Percutaneous balloon mitral commissurotomy is a noninvasive alternative that can effectively increase MV area, decrease LA pressure and pulmonary vascular resistance and pressures, increase cardiac output, and improve functional class (110–112). Selection of symptomatic patients with severe MS before percutaneous balloon mitral commissurotomy is based on mobile mitral leaflets, no major calcification of the leaflets or subvalvular apparatus, MR no greater than mild+, no LA and left atrial appendage thrombus, no significant aortic valve disease, and no severe tricuspid regurgitation. Transthoracic echocardiography also plays a crucial role during balloon mitral commissurotomy, including guidance of transseptal puncture, position of balloon across the mitral orifice, quantification of changes in MV area and MR, and detection of pericardial effusion. The medium-term results are good and, in most series, more than 70% of patients do not require repeat intervention during follow-up periods of 4 to 5 years. Factors predictive of events during follow-up are age, higher NYHA functional class before the procedure, valve morphology, high pulmonary vascular resistance, and valve area after valvulotomy (113,114). Complications of balloon mitral commissurotomy include tears of mitral valve leaflets due to large balloon size resulting in moderate to severe MR, systemic embolization (0% to 4%), bleeding, cardiac perforation, and tamponade. In the National Heart, Lung, and Blood Institute (NHLBI) balloon valvuloplasty registry, the incidence of serious complications was 12% with 1% in-hospital deaths (115). In centers with skilled, experienced operators, valvuloplasty has become the procedure of choice in patients with favorable valve morphology in the absence of significant MR or LA thrombus, and in those in whom anticoagulation may be problematic (for example, lupus anticoagulant) or when surgery is contraindicated.

CHRONIC MITRAL REGURGITATION

Etiology

The mitral functional unit is a complex structure that comprises the mitral leaflets, annulus, chordae tendineae, papillary muscles, and ventricular myocardium. Disruption of any of these components may lead to MR.

With the decreased incidence of rheumatic fever, degenerative MV disease (including MV prolapse) has become the principal cause of MR in developed countries (116–118). Ischemic heart disease is an increasingly important cause of MR, with some degree of regurgitation present in up to 30% of patients undergoing coronary bypass grafting (119). Other causes include LV dysfunction of any etiology, mitral annular calcification, infective endocarditis, and hypertrophic cardiomyopathy. Less-common causes include thoracic trauma, Marfan syndrome, Ehlers-Danlos syndrome, pseudoxanthoma elasticum, infiltrative diseases, carcinoid syndrome, radiation therapy, rheumatoid arthritis, scleroderma, and systemic lupus erythematosus (81). Congenital malformations include MV clefts or fenestrations, parachute MV, abnormalities in association with endocardial cushion defects, endocardial fibroelastosis, transposition of the great arteries, and anomalous origin of the left coronary artery.

Pathophysiology

The origin and mechanisms of MR in patients with CHF can be divided into valvular origin and ventricular origin. The mechanism of MR has a crucial role in patient management. MR of valvular origin relates to primary abnormalities of the structure of the MV, including MV prolapse or flail of degenerative origin, leaflet perforation due to infectious endocarditis, and leaflet mobility restriction and retraction secondary to rheumatic disease (120). MR of ventricular origin relates to geometric remodeling of the LV without structural abnormalities of the MV leaflets. Progressive LV dilatation and dysfunction seem to play a larger role in MR severity than does an ischemic or nonischemic origin. LV dilatation results in further increases in mitral annular diameter, papillary muscle displacement, and MV tethering with restricted leaflet closure (121–123). This may create a vicious circle in which MR begets more MR (124). MR of ventricular origin, also called functional MR, is a complication of end-stage cardiomyopathy and is associated with poor prognosis. We will now focus on MR of ventricular origin in patients with CHF.

The LV responds to volume overload by dilatation (Fig. 19-12). Thus, wall stress tends to increase and reach normal or supernormal levels. This is counterbalanced by the addition of new sarcomeres, leading to eccentric hypertrophy (125). The result is the transformation of the LV into a compliant chamber that is adapted to deliver a large stroke volume (126). In chronic compensated MR, only LV end-diastolic volume, mass, and stroke volume are increased. There is little or no increase in ventricular diastolic or pulmonary venous pressure, in part because of concomitant dilatation and augmentation of LA compliance. This compensated state may be maintained for years with few or no symptoms of HF. The progression to the

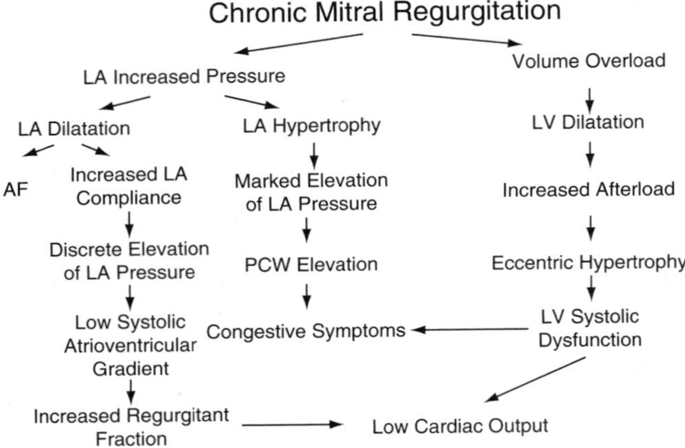

Figure 19-12 Pathophysiology of MR.

decompensated stage begins with either an increase in severity of MR, further chamber dilatation, or both. This decompensated stage is characterized by progressive ventricular enlargement with a rise in diastolic pressure, increased systolic wall stress, and reduced fiber shortening and EF. Progressive atrial enlargement, atrial fibrillation, and pulmonary hypertension occur. When LV function is severely depressed, response to surgery is poor.

After myocardial infarction, despite successful early reperfusion, late LV dilatation develops in 20% of patients and leads to CHF (127,128). Ventricular geometry is a surrogate for myocardial fibers orientation and there is a close interaction between LV geometry and function. In normal subjects, the LV has an ellipsoid shape and myofibers have an oblique orientation at midcavity and apex with a 60-degree angle to the longitudinal axis. CHF progression is associated to a spherical LV shape with horizontally oriented fibers and modified apical shape. Ischemic LV dysfunction fails to produce severe MR without LV dilatation or distortion. MR jet is usually central if there is homogenous LV dilatation. However, it may be eccentric after large myocardial infarction with displacement and dysfunction of one papillary muscle, thin and akinetic walls facing remote, noninfarcted myocardium with remaining motion. Detection of leaflets abnormalities is crucial and is performed through assessment of mitral leaflet morphology and structure with scallop-by-scallop evaluation.

The degree of LA enlargement in MR is variable. At one extreme of the spectrum, the LA may suffer marked dilatation, usually coupled with an increased compliance. Atrial fibrillation is usually present and, consequently, the contribution of atrial contraction in ventricular filling is lost. Accordingly, large regurgitant volumes will cause little elevation of LA pressure and patients may not have marked symptoms of pulmonary congestion. However, an inadequate cardiac output is observed because the LA becomes a preferred low-pressure outlet for LV ejection (129). Other patients with severe MR have only moderate LA dilatation, remain in sinus rhythm, and have marked elevations in atrial pressure and signs of pulmonary congestion. Changes associated with reactive pulmonary hypertension may occur (130). The mechanisms of these differential responses are poorly understood.

Clinical Features

Although patients with chronic MR may be asymptomatic for years, once symptoms have appeared, the presence of LV dysfunction is often irreversible. The clinical features of HF in chronic MR are usually mild in the earliest stages and progressively worsen during the natural history of the disease. LV dysfunction may be present in asymptomatic patients.

Assessment

As with other lesions, the chest roentgenogram may demonstrate atrial enlargement and mitral calcification, indicating the possible role of MV disease in patients with HF; conversely, an enlarging cardiac silhouette may indicate the development of LV dysfunction in a patient with MR.

Echocardiography has a central role in MR assessment. The goals are to quantify MR severity, valve analysis which requires a systematic approach including functional analysis according to leaflet motion, segmental scallop-by-scallop analysis and evaluation of the amount and quantity of leaflet tissue available, measurement of annular diameter size, detection of commissural jet, leaflets and annular calcification, subvalvular apparatus abnormalities, and detection of associated lesions such as AR (which has a role in the determination of the mode of cardioplegia), aortic root dilatation, marked calcifications of ascending aorta, severe tricuspid regurgitation, and atrial septal defect. The mechanism and etiology of the regurgitation must be determined. Consequences of MR on cavity size and function, and PASP are also evaluated. These objectives can be achieved by transthoracic echocardiography in many cases. Extension of color regurgitant jet into the left atrium cannot be used as a criterion of severe MR, due to severe underestimation of regurgitant volume with adherent or eccentric jets and overestimation with free jets. Criteria for severe MR have been described (131). Vena contracta width measurement and proximal isovelocity surface area (PISA) measurement are the most reliable methods.

Functional MR can be quantified during bicycle exercise in patients with HF (132). When dyspnea is responsible for stopping exercise in these patients, increase in PASP is correlated to increase in mitral regurgitant volume. In addition, exercise-induced changes in MR in patients with chronic, ischemic LV dysfunction are a prognostic factor (133).

A multiplane, transesophageal echocardiography study is necessary when transthoracic echocardiography image quality is poor or when severe MR requires surgery. Information given by transthoracic echocardiography determines the timing of the transesophageal echocardiography assessment. Transesophageal echocardiography assesses feasibility of repair, predicts the techniques to be used, and provides a road map to guide the repair. It is crucial that the members of a team (cardiologists, echocardiographers, surgeons, and anesthetists) use the same nomenclature and classification of disease. Transesophageal echocardiography assessment in the operating theater is performed before surgery to detect additional abnormalities since last evaluation and after repair when off pump and appropriate loading conditions to assess morphological analysis of the leaflets, adequate leaflet coaptation, residual MR and MS, regional wall motion abnormalities, and changes in EF.

Coronary angiography is indicated when there is more than moderate MR of ischemic origin in patients with CHF. If ischemia is suspected, coronary angiography should be performed prior to mitral surgery to identify the extent of native coronary disease or to assess the patency of grafts in those patients who have had prior revascularization. Myocardial viability and contractile reserve assessment is mandatory when marked hypokinetic or akinetic areas are detected by transthoracic echocardiography in patients with low LVEF to determine if a preoperative percutaneous or a concomitant surgical revascularization procedure is warranted (134). Nuclear perfusion scintigraphy, dobutamine stress echocardiography, dynamic contrast MRI, and positron emission tomographic scanning have emerged as reliable methods to identify preoperative myocardial viability and predict postoperative function recovery with improved survival.

MRI may be used to evaluate the severity of MR and ventricular volumes. Good correlation with results of invasive tests has been observed (135). Radionuclide angiography with gated pool imaging or first-pass angiography may be used to assess severity of regurgitation, LV dimensions, and EF, and to determine the timing of surgery (136).

Medical Management

In chronic MR the administration of vasodilators has a beneficial effect by reducing afterload and preload and leading to a reduction of LV dimension (Fig. 19-13). This causes a reduction of the regurgitant fraction, particularly in patients with dynamic papillary muscle dysfunction secondary to either ischemia or dilated cardiomyopathy (137). In patients with symptomatic MR of mixed etiologies treated for 1 year with quinapril, Schon et al. (138) found a reduction in end-diastolic LV volume and regurgitant volume and an improvement in hemodynamic variables during exercise. Although according to physiological considerations vasodilators might be expected to benefit asymptomatic patients, there are no long-term studies demonstrating such a benefit. One study, in which captopril was used in asymptomatic patients, did not detect any reduction in LV volumes following 6 months of therapy (62). In symptomatic patients, diuretics may be helpful and digoxin may be used for the control of atrial fibrillation.

Surgical Management

Although increased survival has been shown with medical therapy in patients with CHF, mortality at 3 years after presentation is more than 50% (139,140). Further reduction in survival has been shown in patients with CHF and MR (141). Prior to surgical intervention, an aggressive regimen of diuretic and vasodilator therapy to minimize ventricular afterload and normalize circulating volume is required. For patients with severe HF, a brief period of inotropic therapy for ventricular resuscitation may be necessary preoperatively. Inability to be weaned from this support may be indicative of severe myocardial dysfunction and poor overall prognosis with any surgical therapy other than mechanical ventricular assistance or transplantation. Moreover, markedly elevated pulmonary artery pressures, RV failure, or debilitating ascites should be considered relative contraindications for mitral surgery.

In chronic MR of valvular origin, the best markers of postsurgical outcome are LVEF and end-systolic LV diameter, which is less dependent on preload than are EF and end-diastolic diameter (142). An end-systolic diameter larger than 45 mm is associated with an adverse prognosis. Patients with severe, long-standing LV dysfunction are best treated medically and may be candidates for biventricular pacing (Fig. 19-14).

In patients with functional MR secondary to ischemic or other cardiomyopathies, MR exacerbates the volume overload of the already dilated ventricle and leads to a vicious

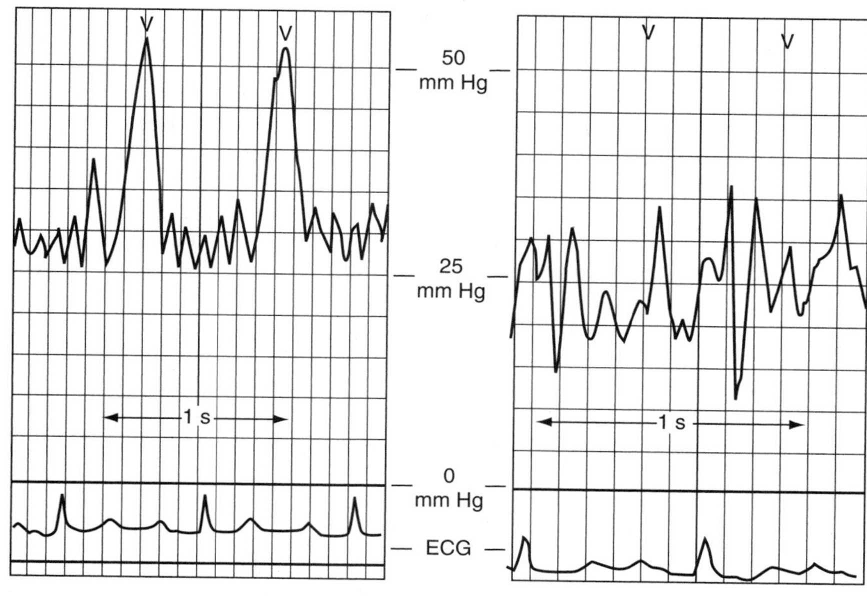

Figure 19-13 Effects of hydralazine on v waves caused by MR. (Reproduced from Greenberg BH, Rahimtoola SH. Vasodilator therapy for valvular heart disease. *JAMA*. 1981;246:249–272.)

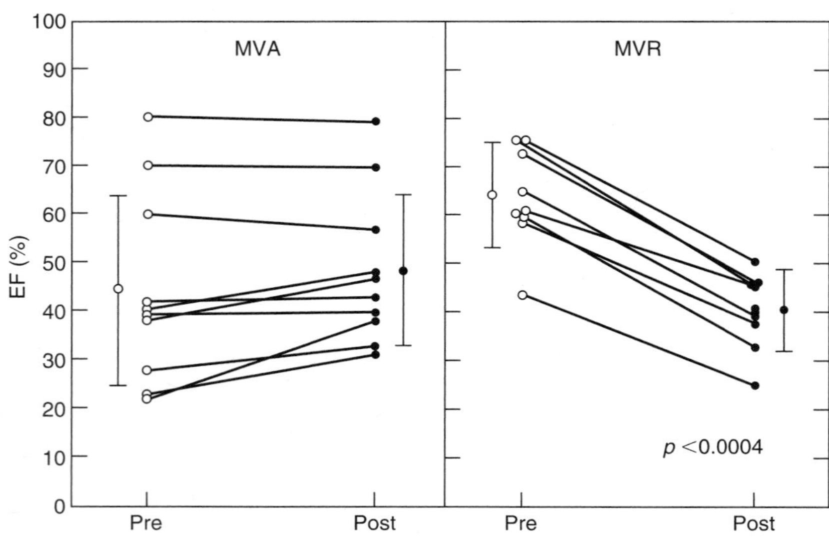

Figure 19-14 Levels of ventricular dysfunction in patients with mitral valve repair compared with levels in patients with mitral valve replacement. (Reproduced from Goldman ME, Mora F, Guarino T, et al. Mitral valvuloplasty is superior to valve replacement for preservation of left ventricular function: an intraoperative two-dimensional echocardiographic study. *J Am Coll Cardiol.* 1987;10(3):568–575, with permission.)

cycle of further dilatation and worsening MR. Five-year survival of patients with EF ≤35% is 50% to 65% in patients with severe CHF after coronary artery bypass grafts alone (143–145). Ventricular volume (not EF) is the major determinant of survival in severe ischemic cardiomyopathy. After myocardial infarction, patients with LV end-systolic volume index >60 mL/m^2 have a fivefold increase in mortality compared with those with normal volume (146,147). Nonmedical options in patients with severe CHF include biventricular pacing, MV annuloplasty using undersized flexible ring (Bolling procedure), endoventricular circular reconstruction with patch plasty (Dor operation) or without patch plasty (McCarthy operation), and an external remodeling jacket. Other techniques such as partial left ventriculectomy (Batista operation) and cardiomyoplasty are now rarely performed based on the absence of compelling evidence to recommend these approaches. Maze procedure/cryoablation at the limit of endocardial resection may be usefully combined with other surgical procedures in selected cases.

Bolling et al. (148) reported a series of 145 patients with end-stage cardiomyopathy and refractory, severe MR treated by geometric mitral reconstruction with an undersized flexible annuloplasty ring to recreate the coaptation zone. All patients were in NYHA functional Class III or IV HF despite receiving maximal medical therapy. Patients had severe LV systolic dysfunction as defined by an EF of less than 25%, with a mean of 14%. On immediate postoperative echocardiograms, the mean transmitral gradient was only 3 ± 1 mm Hg. The overall operative mortality has been 3.5%. There were five 30-day mortalities. Only five patients required intra-aortic balloon counterpulsation (3.5%) and no patient required mechanical LV assistance. Mean follow-up was 38 months. There have been 27 late deaths: 12 from sudden ventricular arrhythmias, nine from progression of CHF without MR, three related to complications from other operative procedures, two that progressed to transplantation, and one suicide. The 1-, 2-, and 5-year actuarial survival rates were 82%, 71%, and 57%, respectively. At 24-month assessment, all patients were in NYHA Class I or II. Their mean EF had increased from 14% to 26%. NYHA symptoms were reduced. Echocardiographically, there were improvements in regurgitant fraction, end-diastolic volume, cardiac output, and sphericity index. Although significant undersizing of the mitral annulus was employed to overcorrect for the zone of coaptation, no systolic anterior motion of the anterior leaflet or MS was noted in these patients. No patients required coronary revascularization (148). Similar results have been reported by other groups (149–152). Further evaluation of this promising approach is ongoing. Although percutaneous implantation of mitral ring has been described, studies are needed to determine the feasibility of this approach (153).

In patients with previous anterior myocardial infarction and large anterior-antero septal akinetic/dyskinetic area, without akinesia of remote, noninfarcted walls, large LV dilatation (LV end-systolic volume index ≥60 mL/m^2), and low EF (<35%), endoventricular circular reconstruction with patch plasty and end-diastolic volume balloon sizing (Dor operation, surgical anterior ventricular endocardial restoration) or without patch (McCarthy operation) have been shown to be beneficial. LV reconstruction should always be associated with complete coronary revascularization and mitral annuloplasty ring if moderate or worse MR. Results of endoventricular circular patch plasty surgery have been reported in 439 patients from 11 centers with a mean follow-up of 18 months. There were associated coronary artery bypass grafts in 89%, MV repair in 22%, and MV replacement in 4% of patients. LVEF index improved from 29% to 39% and LV end-systolic volume index improved from 109 to 69 mL/m^2. Hospital mortality was 6.6% and 18-month survival was 88% in cases of combined procedures. MV replacement showed poor survival rate, even with chordae preservation. Eighteen-month freedom from hospital readmission for CHF was 85% (154). The registry of endoventricular circular patch plasty surgery, including 1,198 postmyocardial infarction CHF patients between 1998 and 2003, reported 5.3% hospital mortality. This technique was combined with coronary artery bypass grafts in 95% of patients, MV repair in 22%, and MV replacement in 1%. Five-year survival was 68.6%

and 5-year freedom from hospital readmission for CHF was 78%. Patients with dyskinesia before surgery showed better survival at 5 years than did patients with akinesia (80% versus 65%) (155). However, optimal indications and timing for LV reconstruction are not well-defined.

Additional approaches include external remodeling jackets, which have been shown to improve LVEF, LV end-diastolic diameter, and 36-month survival (156). Further evaluation of this device is ongoing.

Finally, surgical options in patients with severe, nonischemic cardiomyopathy include MV annuloplasty ring if there is more than moderate MR, and external remodeling jackets. Indications might be contraindication to heart transplantation and nonresponder to biventricular pacing.

ADDITIONAL PARAMETERS TO BE TAKEN INTO ACCOUNT FOR PATIENT MANAGEMENT AND SURGICAL DECISION-MAKING

Valvular origin may be difficult to establish as the main cause of severe LV dysfunction when previous medical history is unknown. Discordance between valvular disease severity and LV dysfunction raises the question of associated cardiomyopathy of nonvalvular origin. An ischemic origin can be suspected when regional wall motion abnormalities are detected during transthoracic echocardiography. Idiopathic dilated cardiomyopathy can be suspected when there is a family history of cardiomyopathy and mild to moderate valvular disease.

The aim of surgery is recovery of function and improved long-term prognosis with acceptable hospital mortality. Detection and evaluation of comorbidity factors, multiple valvular disease, and aortic root size are mandatory. Surgical risk significantly increases in cases of double valve replacement, combined coronary artery bypass grafts or aortic root replacement, poor general condition, and renal failure. In symptomatic patients who are not candidates for valve surgery and for heart transplantation, assessment of ventricular dysynchrony may be performed to select potential responders for biventricular pacing.

Patients with chronic, multiorgan diseases such as systemic lupus erythematosus must be carefully evaluated to detect future difficulties with oral anticoagulation therapy. Oral anticoagulation should be avoided in patients with lupus anticoagulant and these patients should have biological prosthetic valves when valve replacement is indicated.

ACUTE HEART FAILURE

Detection of severe valvular dysfunction is difficult during acute HF, especially when previous medical history is unknown, because there is rapid heart rate and low cardiac output. The murmur is often absent or soft and classical clinical findings (e.g., peripheral signs of AR) are absent. Clinical diagnostic criteria include new onset of third heart sound, and increased pulse pressure. In the context of cardiac failure, chest roentgenogram at bedside may detect LA and pulmonary artery enlargement without LV dilatation, which may raise the suspicion of MS. In acute MR there are signs of pulmonary congestion but cardiac size is usually normal. Dilatation of the ascending aorta and aortic valve calcification may suggest the diagnosis of AS. Transthoracic echocardiography is also limited by tachycardia and low cardiac output. Color flow mapping often markedly underestimates regurgitation severity, which should be based on valvular morphology assessed from gray-scale images; for example, heavy aortic valve calcification may indicate severe AS and MV flail may suggest severe MR. When valvular dysfunction is suspected or when the mechanism of acute HF is not clear, transesophageal echocardiography examination is mandatory. Mechanical ventilation may be required before performing the transesophageal echocardiography study during acute HF. Recent onset of atrial fibrillation with rapid heart rate, pregnancy, pulmonary infection, severe hypertension, and severe anemia may induce HF in chronic, significant valvular disease.

Acute Aortic Regurgitation

The etiology of acute AR includes aortic dissection, acute endocarditis with valve perforation, and thoracic trauma. In significant, acute AR, the normal LV is relatively noncompliant and has a limited capacity to accommodate an increased diastolic volume. As the volume load in the chamber increases, the ventricle begins to ascend onto the steep, upward portion of the pressure–volume relationship. This causes premature closure of the MV during diastole and pulmonary congestion with acute pulmonary edema. Furthermore, because compensatory mechanisms have not developed, there is no significant increase in forward stroke volume and effective stroke volume (forward volume minus regurgitant volume) and cardiac output may fall dramatically. In this setting, it is important to note that once the steep, ascending portion of the pressure–volume curve has been reached, diastolic pressures may increase rapidly with only small increases in volume. Thus, the volume overload in the LV that gives rise to mild congestive HF may not be much smaller than the volume that gives rise to fulminant pulmonary edema. For this reason, the appearance of mild CHF, rather than being reassuring, should be viewed with the utmost concern. Catecholamine-induced vasoconstriction increases impedance to forward flow and increases the severity of regurgitant flow, worsening the hemodynamic situation and hastening the development of cardiac failure (Fig. 19-4).

In acute, symptomatic AR, treatment with vasodilators should be initiated. Nitroprusside produces significant reductions in arterial pressure and LV end-diastolic pressure and volume, and an increase in the systolic EF and cardiac index. Diuretics are useful for the relief of pulmonary congestion and inotropic drugs also may be useful in some situations. Surgical treatment should not be delayed.

Acute Mitral Regurgitation

The etiology of acute MR includes chordal rupture, infectious endocarditis with valve perforation, thoracic trauma, or rupture of papillary muscle head during acute myocardial infarction. Chordal rupture with flail leaflet was found to be the most frequent cause of acute and severe MR and related HF in patients with unknown MV disease, and the most frequent cause of unexpected rapid aggravation in patients with known MR. Initially, impedance to LV emptying is reduced as blood is ejected into the low-pressure LA (157). Because the compliance of this chamber is normal, a sudden increase in LA pressure occurs with a large, sharp v wave on pulmonary wedge pressure tracings. This raised pressure is transmitted to the pulmonary circulation and results in severe pulmonary congestion. In acute MR, the height of the v wave is a good indicator of valve lesion severity. The magnitude of the v wave is less closely related to the severity of the disease in chronic MR, as LA dilatation dampens the increase in pressure because of regurgitant flow. In patients with systolic LV dysfunction, pulmonary edema may be related to increase in MR volume and PASP during exercise in the absence of acute ischemia, arrhythmia, and severe aortic valve disease (158).

In acute MR, medical treatment must be initiated immediately to stabilize the patient for definitive treatment. The use of vasodilators such as nitroprusside or nitroglycerin in critically ill patients may be life-saving. Diuretics are also of benefit in the acute situation. Early surgical treatment is generally mandatory but carries a higher mortality than does elective surgery. Patients with a ruptured head of papillary muscle who can be stabilized medically and with intra-aortic counterpulsation may benefit from a delay to avoid surgery during the acute phase of myocardial infarction.

CONCLUSION

In this chapter, we have emphasized the pathophysiological mechanisms leading to congestive HF in valvular disease. An understanding of these mechanisms facilitates optimal patient management.

As a general rule, when LV function is severely depressed, response to surgery is poor. Exceptions are severe AS with contractile reserve during dobutamine infusion, more-than-moderate MR of ventricular origin, and more than 10% of viable myocardium detected by stress echocardiography or nuclear perfusion scintigraphy.

In the future, diagnostic procedures such as three-dimensional echocardiography and MRI will be available in most centers. These may identify more specific and early signs of LV dysfunction and promote the development of new management algorithms in valvular heart disease. Mitral and aortic valve repairs are being increasingly used with the advantages of avoiding prosthesis-related risks and decreasing operative morbidity and mortality. Finally, as more becomes known about the cellular and molecular bases of myocardial dysfunction, it is likely that novel strategies for preventive therapy to preserve LV function will become available.

REFERENCES

1. Ho KK, Anderson KM, Kannel WB, Grossman W, et al. Survival after the onset of congestive heart failure in Framingham Heart Study subjects. *Circulation.* 1993;88:107–115.
2. Bonow RO, Carabello B, de Leon AC, Jr., et al. Guidelines for the management of patients with valvular heart disease. Executive summary. A report of the American College of Cardiology/American Heart Association Task Force on Practice Guidelines (Committee on Management of Patients with Valvular Heart Disease). *Circulation.* 1998;98:1949–1984.
3. Katz AM. The cardiomyopathy of overload: an unnatural growth response in the hypertrophied heart. *Ann Intern Med.* 1994;121:363–371. 1994
4. Morgan HE, Baker KM. Cardiac hypertrophy. Mechanical, neural, and endocrine dependence. *Circulation.* 1991;83:13–25.
5. Taketani S, Sawa Y, Taniguchi K, et al. C-myc expression and its role in patients with chronic aortic regurgitation. *Circulation.* 1997;96:II83–II87; discussion II87–II89.
6. Enriquez-Sarano M, Tajik AJ, et al. Echocardiographic prediction of survival after surgical correction of organic mitral regurgitation. *Circulation.* 1994;90:830–837.
7. Hoffmann R, von Bardeleben S, ten Cate F, et al. Assessment of systolic left ventricular function. A multi-centre comparison of cineventriculography, cardiac magnetic resonance imaging, unenhanced and contrast-enhanced echocardiography. *Eur Heart J.* 2005;26:607–616.
8. Simpson IA, de Belder MA, Kenny A, et al. How to quantitate valve regurgitation by echo Doppler techniques. British Society of Echocardiography. *Br Heart J.* 1995;73:1–9.
9. Dolan MS, Castello R, St. Vrain JA, et al. Quantitation of aortic regurgitation by Doppler echocardiography: a practical approach. *Am Heart J.* 1995;129:1014–1020.
10. Ugartemendia C, Esplugas E. [Which patients with heart valve diseases require invasive evaluation?]. *Rev Esp Cardiol.* 1995;48: 215–222.
11. Grossman W. Profiles in valvular heart disease. In: Baim DS, Grossman W, eds. *Cardiac Catheterization, Angiography and Intervention.* Baltimore: Williams & Wilkins; 1995: 735–756.
12. Sondergaard L, Lindvig K, Hildebrandt P, et al. Quantification of aortic regurgitation by magnetic resonance velocity mapping. *Am Heart J.* 1993;125:1081–1090.
13. Roberts WC. Valvular, subvalvular and supravalvular aortic stenosis: morphologic features. *Cardiovasc Clin.* 1973;5:97–126.
14. Stewart BF, Siscovick D, Lind BK, et al. Clinical factors associated with calcific aortic valve disease. Cardiovascular Health Study. *J Am Coll Cardiol.* 1997;29:630–634. 1997
15. Davies MJ. *Pathology of Cardiac Valves.* London: Butterworth-Heinemann; 1980.
16. Boudoulas H, Vavuranakis M, Wooley CF. Valvular heart disease: the influence of changing etiology on nosology. *J Heart Valve Dis.* 1994;3:516–526.
17. Ross J, Jr., Braunwald E. Aortic stenosis. *Circulation.* 1968;38:61–67.
18. Kelly TA, Rothbart RM, Cooper CM, et al. Comparison of outcome of asymptomatic to symptomatic patients older than 20 years of age with valvular aortic stenosis. *Am J Cardiol.* 1988;61:123–130.
19. Areskog NH. Exercise testing in the evaluation of patients with valvular aortic stenosis. *Clin Physiol.* 1984;4:201–208.
20. Carabello BA. Indications for valve surgery in asymptomatic patients with aortic and mitral stenosis. *Chest.* 1995;108: 1678–1682.
21. Faggiano P, Aurigemma GP, Rusconi C, et al. Progression of valvular aortic stenosis in adults: literature review and clinical implications. *Am Heart J.* 1996;132:408–417.
22. Otto CM, Pearlman AS, Gardner CL. Hemodynamic progression of aortic stenosis in adults assessed by Doppler echocardiography. *J Am Coll Cardiol.* 1989;13:545–550.
23. Faggiano P, Ghizzoni G, Sorgato A, et al. Rate of progression of valvular aortic stenosis in adults. *Am J Cardiol.* 1992;70:229–233.
24. Peter M, Hoffmann A, Parker C, et al. Progression of aortic stenosis. Role of age and concomitant coronary artery disease. *Chest.* 1993;103:1715–1719.
25. Roger VL, Tajik AJ, Bailey KR, et al. Progression of aortic stenosis in adults: new appraisal using Doppler echocardiography. *Am Heart J.* 1990;119:331–338.

26. Huber D, Grimm J, Koch R, et al. Determinants of ejection performance in aortic stenosis. *Circulation.* 1981;64:126–134.
27. Hess OM, Ritter M, Schneider J, et al. Diastolic stiffness and myocardial structure in aortic valve disease before and after valve replacement. *Circulation.* 1984;69:855–865.
28. Carabello BA, Green LH, Grossman W, et al. Hemodynamic determinants of prognosis of aortic valve replacement in critical aortic stenosis and advanced congestive heart failure. *Circulation.* 1980;62:42–48.
29. Lund O. Preoperative risk evaluation and stratification of long-term survival after valve replacement for aortic stenosis. Reasons for earlier operative intervention. *Circulation.* 1990;82:124–139.
30. Brogan WC, 3rd, Grayburn PA, Lange RA, et al. Prognosis after valve replacement in patients with severe aortic stenosis and a low transvalvular pressure gradient. *J Am Coll Cardiol.* 1993;21:1657–1660.
31. Connolly HM, Oh JK, Schaff HV, et al. Severe aortic stenosis with low transvalvular gradient and severe left ventricular dysfunction: result of aortic valve replacement in 52 patients. *Circulation.* 2000;101:1940–1946.
32. Pereira JJ, Lauer MS, Bashir M, et al. Survival after aortic valve replacement for severe aortic stenosis with low transvalvular gradients and severe left ventricular dysfunction. *J Am Coll Cardiol.* 2002;39:1356–1363.
33. Monin JL, Monchi M, Gest V, et al. Aortic stenosis with severe left ventricular dysfunction and low transvalvular pressure gradients. Risk stratification by low-dose dobutamine echocardiography. *J Am Coll Cardiol.* 2001;37:2101–2107.
34. Nishimura RA, Grantham JA, Connolly HM, et al. Low-output, low-gradient aortic stenosis in patients with depressed left ventricular systolic function: the clinical utility of the dobutamine challenge in the catheterization laboratory. *Circulation.* 2002;106:809–813.
35. Wranne B, Baumgartner H, Flachskampf F, et al. Stenotic lesions. *Heart.* 1996;75:36–42.
36. Blitz LR, Herrmann HC. Hemodynamic assessment of patients with low-flow, low-gradient valvular aortic stenosis. *Am J Cardiol.* 1996;78:657–661.
37. Burwash IG, Thomas DD, Sadahiro M, et al. Dependence of Gorlin formula and continuity equation valve areas on transvalvular volume flow rate in valvular aortic stenosis. *Circulation.* 1994;89:827–835.
38. Cannon JD, Jr., Zile MR, Crawford FA, Jr., et al. Aortic valve resistance as an adjunct to the Gorlin formula in assessing the severity of aortic stenosis in symptomatic patients. *J Am Coll Cardiol.* 1992;20:1517–1523.
39. deFilippi CR, Willett DL, Brickner ME, et al. Usefulness of dobutamine echocardiography in distinguishing severe from nonsevere valvular aortic stenosis in patients with depressed left ventricular function and low transvalvular gradients. *Am J Cardiol.* 1995;75:191–194.
40. Monin JL, Quere JP, Monchi M, et al. Low-gradient aortic stenosis: operative risk stratification and predictors for long-term outcome. A multicenter study using dobutamine stress hemodynamics. *Circulation.* 2003;108:319–324.
41. Carabello BA. Selection of patients with aortic stenosis for operation: the asymptomatic patient and the patient with poor LV function. *Adv Cardiol.* 2002;39:49–60.
42. Ford LE, Feldman T, Chiu YC, et al. Hemodynamic resistance as a measure of functional impairment in aortic valvular stenosis. *Circ Res.* 1990;66:1–7.
43. Carabello BA, Crawford FA, Jr. Valvular heart disease. *N Engl J Med.* 1997;337:32–41.
44. Logeais Y, Langanay T, Roussin R, et al. Surgery for aortic stenosis in elderly patients. A study of surgical risk and predictive factors. *Circulation.* 1994;90:2891–2898.
45. Ruygrok PN, Barratt-Boyes BG, Agnew TM, et al. Aortic valve replacement in the elderly. *J Heart Valve Dis.* 1993;2:550–557.
46. Elayda MA, Hall RJ, Reul RM, et al. Aortic valve replacement in patients 80 years and older. Operative risks and long-term results. *Circulation.* 1993;88:II11–II16.
47. Sprigings DC, Forfar JC. How should we manage symptomatic aortic stenosis in the patient who is 80 or older? *Br Heart J.* 1995;74:481–484.
48. Milano AD, De Carlo M, Mecozzi G, et al. Clinical outcome in patients with 19-mm and 21-mm St. Jude aortic prostheses: comparison at long-term follow-up. *Ann Thorac Surg.* 2002;73:37–43.
49. Arom KV, Goldenberg IF, Emery RW. Long-term clinical outcome with small size Standard St. Jude Medical valves implanted in the aortic position. *J Heart Valve Dis.* 1994;3:531–536.
50. Blais C, Dumesnil JG, Baillot R, et al. Impact of valve prosthesis–patient mismatch on short-term mortality after aortic valve replacement. *Circulation.* 2003;108:983–988.
51. Pibarot P, Dumesnil JG. Hemodynamic and clinical impact of prosthesis-patient mismatch in the aortic valve position and its prevention. *J Am Coll Cardiol.* 2000;36:1131–1141.
52. Castro LJ, Arcidi JM, Jr., Fisher AL, et al. Routine enlargement of the small aortic root: a preventive strategy to minimize mismatch. *Ann Thorac Surg.* 2002;74:31–36; discussion 36.
53. Guiney TE, Davies MJ, Parker DJ, et al. The aetiology and course of isolated severe aortic regurgitation: a clinical, pathological, and echocardiographic study. *Br Heart J.* 1987;58:358–368.
54. Becker AE, Anderson RH. *Cardiac Pathology. An Integrated Text and Colour Atlas.* Edinburgh: Churchill Livingstone; 1983: 4.2–4.29.
55. Treasure T. When to operate in chronic aortic valvar regurgitation. *Br J Hosp Med.* 1993;49:613,616–622,626–619.
56. Parmley LF, Manion WC, Mattingly TW. Nonpenetrating traumatic injury of the heart. *Circulation.* 1958;18:371–396.
57. Stouffer GA, Uretsky BF. Hemodynamic changes of aortic regurgitation. *Am J Med Sci.* 1997;314:411–414.
58. Ross J, Jr. Adaptations of the left ventricle to chronic volume overload. *Circ Res.* 1974;35(Suppl II):64–70.
59. Bonow RO, Rosing DR, McIntosh CL, et al. The natural history of asymptomatic patients with aortic regurgitation and normal left ventricular function. *Circulation.* 1983;68:509–517.
60. Siemienczuk D, Greenberg B, Morris C, et al. Chronic aortic insufficiency: factors associated with progression to aortic valve replacement. *Ann Intern Med.* 1989;110:587–592.
61. Bonow RO, Lakatos E, Maron BJ, et al. Serial long-term assessment of the natural history of asymptomatic patients with chronic aortic regurgitation and normal left ventricular systolic function. *Circulation.* 1991;84:1625–1635.
62. Wisenbaugh T, Sinovich V, Dullabh A, et al. Six month pilot study of captopril for mildly symptomatic, severe isolated mitral and isolated aortic regurgitation. *J Heart Valve Dis.* 1994;3:197–204.
63. Greenberg B, Massie B, Bristow JD, et al. Long-term vasodilator therapy of chronic aortic insufficiency. A randomized double-blinded, placebo-controlled clinical trial. *Circulation.* 1988;78:92–103.
64. Lin M, Chiang HT, Lin SL, et al. Vasodilator therapy in chronic asymptomatic aortic regurgitation: enalapril versus hydralazine therapy. *J Am Coll Cardiol.* 1994;24:1046–1053.
65. Schon HR, Dorn R, Barthel P, et al. Effects of 12 months quinapril therapy in asymptomatic patients with chronic aortic regurgitation. *J Heart Valve Dis.* 1994;3:500–509.
66. Gaasch WH, Sundaram M, Meyer TE. Managing asymptomatic patients with chronic aortic regurgitation. *Chest.* 1997;111: 1702–1709.
67. Scognamiglio R, Fasoli G, Ponchia A, et al. Long-term nifedipine unloading therapy in asymptomatic patients with chronic severe aortic regurgitation. *J Am Coll Cardiol.* 1990;16:424–429.
68. Bonow RO, Rosing DR, Kent KM, et al. Timing of operation for chronic aortic regurgitation. *Am J Cardiol.* 1982;50:325–336.
69. Dujardin KS, Enriquez-Sarano M, Schaff HV, et al. Mortality and morbidity of aortic regurgitation in clinical practice. A long-term follow-up study. *Circulation.* 1999;99:1851–1857.
70. Henry WL, Bonow RO, Rosing DR, et al. Observations on the optimum time for operative intervention for aortic regurgitation. II. Serial echocardiographic evaluation of asymptomatic patients. *Circulation.* 1980;61:484–492.
71. Gaasch WH, Carroll JD, Levine HJ, et al. Chronic aortic regurgitation. Prognostic value of left ventricular end-systolic dimension and end-diastolic radius/thickness ratio. *J Am Coll Cardiol.* 1983;1:775–782.
72. Klodas E, Enriquez-Sarano M, et al. Surgery for aortic regurgitation in women. Contrasting indications and outcomes compared with men. *Circulation.* 1996;94:2472–2478.
73. Bonow RO, Nikas D, Elefteriades JA. Valve replacement for regurgitant lesions of the aortic or mitral valve in advanced left ventricular dysfunction. *Cardiol Clin.* 1995;13:73–83, 85.

74. Bonow RO, Rosing DR, Maron BJ, et al. Reversal of left ventricular dysfunction after aortic valve replacement for chronic aortic regurgitation: influence of duration of preoperative left ventricular dysfunction. *Circulation.* 1984;70:570–579.
75. Bonow RO, Dodd JT, Maron BJ, et al. Long-term serial changes in left ventricular function and reversal of ventricular dilatation after valve replacement for chronic aortic regurgitation. *Circulation.* 1998;78:1108–1120.
76. Treasure T. Which prosthetic valve should we choose? *Curr Opin Cardiol.* 1995;10:144–149.
77. Yacoub M, Rasmi NR, Sundt TM, et al. Fourteen-year experience with homovital homografts for aortic valve replacement. *J Thorac Cardiovasc Surg.* 1995;110:186–193; discussion 193–184.
78. Duran CM. Present status of reconstructive surgery for aortic valve disease. *J Card Surg.* 1993;8:443–452.
79. Massell BF, Chute CG, Walker AM, et al. Penicillin and the marked decrease in morbidity and mortality from rheumatic fever in the United States. *N Engl J Med.* 1988;318:280–286.
80. Chiang CW, Kuo CT, Chen WJ, et al. Comparisons between female and male patients with mitral stenosis. *Br Heart J.* 1994;72:567–570.
81. Waller BF, Howard J, Fess S. Pathology of mitral valve stenosis and pure mitral regurgitation—Part I. *Clin Cardiol.* 1994;17:330–336.
82. Chopra P, Tandon HD, Raizada V, et al. Comparative studies of mitral valves in rheumatic heart disease. *Arch Intern Med.* 1983;143:661–666.
83. Bowe JC, Bland F, Sprague HB, et al. Course of mitral stenosis without surgery: 10- and 20-year perspectives. *Ann Intern Med.* 1960;741–748.
84. Song JK, Kang DH, Lee CW, et al. Factors determining the exercise capacity in mitral stenosis. *Am J Cardiol.* 1996;78:1060–1062.
85. Haworth SG, Hall SM, Panja M. Peripheral pulmonary vascular and airway abnormalities in adolescents with rheumatic mitral stenosis. *Int J Cardiol.* 1988;18:405–416.
86. Wroblewski E, James F, Spann JF, et al. Right ventricular performance in mitral stenosis. *Am J Cardiol.* 1981;47:51–55.
87. Davies SW, Bailey J, Keegan J, et al. Reduced pulmonary microvascular permeability in severe chronic left heart failure. *Am Heart J.* 1992;124:137–142.
88. Moreyra AE, Wilson AC, Deac R, et al. Factors associated with atrial fibrillation in patients with mitral stenosis: a cardiac catheterization study. *Am Heart J.* 1998;135:138–145.
89. Stott DK, Marpole DG, Bristow JD, et al. The role of left atrial transport in aortic and mitral stenosis. *Circulation.* 1970;41:1031–1041.
90. Snyder RW, Jr., Lange RA, Willard JE, et al. Frequency, cause and effect on operative outcome of depressed left ventricular ejection fraction in mitral stenosis. *Am J Cardiol.* 1994;73:65–69.
91. Gaasch WH, Folland ED. Left ventricular function in rheumatic mitral stenosis. *Eur Heart J.* 1991;12(Suppl B):66–69.
92. Olesen KH. The natural history of 271 patients with mitral stenosis under medical treatment. *Br Heart J.* 1962;24:349–357.
93. Nishimura Y, Maeda H, Yokoyama M, et al. Bronchial hyperreactivity in patients with mitral valve disease. *Chest.* 1990;98:1085–1090.
94. Rolla G, Bucca C, Caria E, et al. Bronchial responsiveness in patients with mitral valve disease. *Eur Respir J.* 1990;3:127–131.
95. Reid CL, Otto CM, Davis KB, et al. Influence of mitral valve morphology on mitral balloon commissurotomy: immediate and six-month results from the NHLBI Balloon Valvuloplasty Registry. *Am Heart J.* 1992;124:657–665.
96. Reid CL, Chandraratna PA, Kawanishi DT, et al. Influence of mitral valve morphology on double-balloon catheter balloon valvuloplasty in patients with mitral stenosis. Analysis of factors predicting immediate and 3-month results. *Circulation.* 1989;80:515–524.
97. Alfonso F, Macaya C, Iniguez A, et al. Comparison of results of percutaneous mitral valvuloplasty in patients with large (greater than 6 cm) versus those with smaller left atria. *Am J Cardiol.* 1992;69:355–360.
98. Bansal RC, Heywood JT, Applegate PM, et al. Detection of left atrial thrombi by two-dimensional echocardiography and surgical correlation in 148 patients with mitral valve disease. *Am J Cardiol.* 1989;64:243–246.
99. Roy SB, Gopinath N. Mitral stenosis. *Circulation.* 1968;38:68–76.
100. Fowler NO, van der Bel-Kahn JM. Indications for surgical replacement of the mitral valve, with particular reference to common and uncommon causes of mitral regurgitation. *Am J Cardiol.* 1979;44:148–157.
101. Vincens JJ, Temizer D, Post JR, et al. Long-term outcome of cardiac surgery in patients with mitral stenosis and severe pulmonary hypertension. *Circulation.* 1995;92:II137–II142.
102. Braunwald E, Braunwald NS, Ross J Jr., et al. Effects of mitral-valve replacement on the pulmonary vascular dynamics of patients with pulmonary hypertension. *N Engl J Med.* 1965;273: 509–514.
103. Cormier B, Vahanian A, Iung B, et al. Influence of percutaneous mitral commissurotomy on left atrial spontaneous contrast of mitral stenosis. *Am J Cardiol.* 1993;71:842–847.
104. Vahanian A. Percutaneous mitral commissurotomy. *Eur Heart J.* 1996;17:1465–1469.
105. Essop MR. Relief of rheumatic mitral stenosis: when and how? *Am J Cardiol.* 1994;73:85–87.
106. Dittrich HC, Erickson JS, Schneiderman T, et al. Echocardiographic and clinical predictors for outcome of elective cardioversion of atrial fibrillation. *Am J Cardiol.* 1989;63:193–197.
107. Arom KV, Nicoloff DM, Kersten TE, et al. Ten years' experience with the St. Jude Medical valve prosthesis. *Ann Thorac Surg.* 1989;47:831–837.
108. Appelbaum A, Kouchoukos NT, Blackstone EH, et al. Early risks of open heart surgery for mitral valve disease. *Am J Cardiol.* 1976;37:201–209.
109. Eguaras MG, Garcia Jimenez MA, et al. Early open mitral commissurotomy: long-term results. *J Thorac Cardiovasc Surg.* 1993;106:421–426.
110. Carroll JD, Feldman T. Percutaneous mitral balloon valvotomy and the new demographics of mitral stenosis. *JAMA.* 1993;270: 1731–1736.
111. Hung JS, Chern MS, Wu JJ, et al. Short- and long-term results of catheter balloon percutaneous transvenous mitral commissurotomy. *Am J Cardiol.* 1991;67:854–862.
112. Ruiz CE, Allen JW, Lau FY. Percutaneous double balloon valvotomy for severe rheumatic mitral stenosis. *Am J Cardiol.* 1990;65:473–477.
113. Palacios IF, Tuzcu ME, Weyman AE, et al. Clinical follow-up of patients undergoing percutaneous mitral balloon valvotomy. *Circulation.* 1995;91:671–676.
114. Herrmann HC, Ramaswamy K, Isner JM, et al. Factors influencing immediate results, complications, and short-term follow-up status after Inoue balloon mitral valvotomy: a North American multicenter study. *Am Heart J.* 1992;124:160–166.
115. A report from the NHLBI Balloon Valvuloplasty Registry. Complications and mortality of percutaneous balloon mitral commissurotomy. *Circulation.* 1992;85:2014–2024.
116. Agozzino L, Falco A, de Vivo F, et al. Surgical pathology of the mitral valve: gross and histological study of 1,288 surgically excised valves. *Int J Cardiol.* 1992;37:79–89.
117. Joy J, Kartha CC, Balakrishnan KG. Non-myxomatous mitral valve prolapse: a clinical and pathological study. *Cardiology* 1989;76:249–254.
118. Luxereau P, Dorent R, De Gevigney G, et al. Aetiology of surgically treated mitral regurgitation. *Eur Heart J.* 1991;12(Suppl B):2–4.
119. Izumi S, Miyatake K, Beppu S, et al. Mechanism of mitral regurgitation in patients with myocardial infarction: a study using real-time two-dimensional Doppler flow imaging and echocardiography. *Circulation.* 1987;76:777–785.
120. Pellerin D, Brecker S, Veyrat C. Degenerative mitral valve disease with emphasis on mitral valve prolapse. *Heart.* 2002;88(Suppl 4):iv20–iv28.
121. Liel-Cohen N, Guerrero JL, Otsuji Y, et al. Design of a new surgical approach for ventricular remodeling to relieve ischemic mitral regurgitation: insights from 3-dimensional echocardiography. *Circulation.* 2000;101:2756–2763.
122. Nesta F, Otsuji Y, Handschumacher MD, et al. Leaflet concavity: a rapid visual clue to the presence and mechanism of functional mitral regurgitation. *J Am Soc Echocardiogr.* 2003;16:1301–1308.
123. Levine RA, Schwammenthal E. Ischemic mitral regurgitation on the threshold of a solution: from paradoxes to unifying concepts. *Circulation.* 2005;112:745–758.

124. Braunwald E, Turi ZG. Pathophysiology of mitral valve disease. In: Wells FC, Shapiro LM, eds. *Mitral Valve Disease*. London: Butterworth-Heinemann;1996: 20–37.
125. Eckberg DL, Gault JH, Bouchard RL, et al. Mechanics of left ventricular contraction in chronic severe mitral regurgitation. *Circulation*. 1973;47:1252–1259.
126. Corin WJ, Murakami T, Monrad ES, et al. Left ventricular passive diastolic properties in chronic mitral regurgitation. *Circulation*. 1991;83:797–807.
127. Gaudron P, Eilles C, Kugler I, et al. Progressive left ventricular dysfunction and remodeling after myocardial infarction. Potential mechanisms and early predictors. *Circulation*. 1993;87:755–763.
128. Migrino RQ, Young JB, Ellis SG, et al. End-systolic volume index at 90 to 180 minutes into reperfusion therapy for acute myocardial infarction is a strong predictor of early and late mortality. The Global Utilization of Streptokinase and t-PA for Occluded Coronary Arteries (GUSTO)-I Angiographic Investigators. *Circulation*. 1997;96:116–121.
129. Braunwald E, Awe WC. The syndrome of severe mitral regurgitation with normal left atrial pressure. *Circulation*. 1963;27:29–35.
130. Braunwald E. Mitral regurgitation: physiologic, clinical and surgical considerations. *N Engl J Med*. 1969;281:425–433.
131. Zoghbi WA, Enriquez-Sarano M, Foster E, et al. Recommendations for evaluation of the severity of native valvular regurgitation with two-dimensional and Doppler echocardiography. *J Am Soc Echocardiogr*. 2003;16:777–802.
132. Lebrun F, Lancellotti P, Pierard LA. Quantitation of functional mitral regurgitation during bicycle exercise in patients with heart failure. *J Am Coll Cardiol*. 2001;38:1685–1692.
133. Lancellotti P, Troisfontaines P, Toussaint AC, et al. Prognostic importance of exercise-induced changes in mitral regurgitation in patients with chronic ischemic left ventricular dysfunction. *Circulation*. 2003;108:1713–1717.
134. Marwick TH, Zuchowski C, Lauer MS, et al. Functional status and quality of life in patients with heart failure undergoing coronary bypass surgery after assessment of myocardial viability. *J Am Coll Cardiol*. 1999;33:750–758.
135. Hundley WG, Li HF, Willard JE, et al. Magnetic resonance imaging assessment of the severity of mitral regurgitation. Comparison with invasive techniques. *Circulation*. 1995;92:1151–1158.
136. Rigo P. Quantification of mitral insufficiency by radionuclide techniques. *Eur Heart J*. 1991;12(Suppl B):15–18.
137. Yoran C, Yellin EL, Becker RM, et al. Dynamic aspects of acute mitral regurgitation. Effects of ventricular volume, pressure and contractility on the effective regurgitant orifice area. *Circulation*. 1979;60:170–176.
138. Schon HR, Schroter G, Barthel P, et al. Quinapril therapy in patients with chronic mitral regurgitation. *J Heart Valve Dis*. 1994;3:303–312.
139. Tavazzi L. Epidemiology of dilated cardiomyopathy: a still undetermined entity. *Eur Heart J*. 1997;18:4–6.
140. Hunt SA. Current status of cardiac transplantation. *JAMA*. 1998;280:1692–1698.
141. Blondheim DS, Jacobs LE, Kotler MN, et al. Dilated cardiomyopathy with mitral regurgitation: decreased survival despite a low frequency of left ventricular thrombus. *Am Heart J*. 1991;122:763–771.
142. Carabello BA. Clinical assessment of systolic dysfunction. *ACC Curr J Rev*. 1994:25–29.
143. Alderman EL, Fisher LD, Litwin P, et al. Results of coronary artery surgery in patients with poor left ventricular function (CASS). *Circulation*. 1983;68:785–795.
144. Trachiotis GD, Weintraub WS, Johnston TS, et al. Coronary artery bypass grafting in patients with advanced left ventricular dysfunction. *Ann Thorac Surg*. 1998;66:1632–1639.
145. Shah PJ, Hare DL, Raman JS, et al. Survival after myocardial revascularization for ischemic cardiomyopathy: prospective ten-year follow-up study. *J Thorac Cardiovasc Surg*. 2003;126: 1320–1327.
146. White HD, Norris RM, Brown MA, et al. Left ventricular end-systolic volume as the major determinant of survival after recovery from myocardial infarction. *Circulation*. 1987;76:44–51.
147. Yamaguchi A, Ino T, Adachi H, et al. Left ventricular volume predicts postoperative course in patients with ischemic cardiomyopathy. *Ann Thorac Surg*. 1998;65:434–438.
148. Bolling SF, Pagani FD, Deeb GM, et al. Intermediate-term outcome of mitral reconstruction in cardiomyopathy. *J Thorac Cardiovasc Surg*. 1998;115:381–386; discussion 387–388.
149. Calafiore AM, Gallina S, Di Mauro M, et al. Mitral valve procedure in dilated cardiomyopathy: repair or replacement? *Ann Thorac Surg*. 2001;71:1146–1152; discussion 1152–1143.
150. Chen FY, Adams DH, Aranki SF, et al. Mitral valve repair in cardiomyopathy. *Circulation*. 1998;98:II124–II127.
151. Bishay ES, McCarthy PM, Cosgrove DM, et al. Mitral valve surgery in patients with severe left ventricular dysfunction. *Eur J Cardiothorac Surg*. 2000;17:213–221.
152. Bitran D, Merin O, Klutstein MW, et al. Mitral valve repair in severe ischemic cardiomyopathy. *J Card Surg*. 2001;16:79–82.
153. Kaye DM, Byrne M, Alferness C, et al. Feasibility and short-term efficacy of percutaneous mitral annular reduction for the therapy of heart failure-induced mitral regurgitation. *Circulation*. 2003;108:1795–1797.
154. Athanasuleas CL, Stanley AW, Jr., Buckberg GD, et al. Surgical Anterior Ventricular Endocardial Restoration (SAVER) in the dilated remodeled ventricle after anterior myocardial infarction. RESTORE Group. Reconstructive endoventricular surgery, returning torsion original radius elliptical shape to the LV. *J Am Coll Cardiol*. 2001;37:1199–1209.
155. Athanasuleas CL, Buckberg GD, Stanley AW, et al. Surgical ventricular restoration in the treatment of congestive heart failure due to post-infarction ventricular dilation. *J Am Coll Cardiol*. 2004;44:1439–1445.
156. Pilla JJ, Blom AS, Brockman DJ, et al. Ventricular constraint using the acorn cardiac support device reduces myocardial akinetic area in an ovine model of acute infarction. *Circulation*. 2002;106:I207–I211.
157. Urschel CW, Covell JW, Sonnenblick EH, Ross J, Jr., et al. Myocardial mechanics in aortic and mitral valvular regurgitation: the concept of instantaneous impedance as a determinant of the performance of the intact heart. *J Clin Invest*. 1968;47:867–883.
158. Pierard LA, Lancellotti P. The role of ischemic mitral regurgitation in the pathogenesis of acute pulmonary edema. *N Engl J Med*. 2004;351:1627–1634.

20 Congestive Heart Failure Secondary to Congenital Heart Disease

Yuk M. Law *David J. Sahn*

The management of patients with congestive heart failure (CHF) secondary to congenital heart disease must be examined at three interrelated levels: age, pathophysiological basis, and impact of surgery. For ease of reference and simplicity, this chapter will be organized by age. Although one pathophysiological state or surgery may predominate at one age, this interrelationship and its effects on medical management is a continuum through the different age groups.

As opposed to adults with heart failure from cardiomyopathy with systolic dysfunction, sufficient clinical trials in children with heart failure from cardiomyopathy or patients with congenital heart disease have not been done. However, because the success of modern treatment is pathophysiology-based, these different groups may still share certain common mechanistic pathways. Hence, it is important to understand the pathophysiological basis of their circulatory compromise so the proper extrapolation of data can be made in the management of the congenital patient.

Table 20-1 lists the pathophysiological categories of heart failure seen in congenital heart disease. Unlike many of the disorders in adults with acquired heart disease (for which the development of major symptoms of CHF is necessary to warrant the risk of surgery), most congenital heart defects are corrected or palliated before the development of significant symptoms. Furthermore, since many patients can only be palliated, the strategic planning of interventions is critical, making the accurate diagnosis, monitoring, and coordination of medical, percutaneous, and surgical treatment paramount. When CHF supervenes late in the course of the disease, the opportunity for intervention (short of transplantation) may be primarily medical and supportive. Indeed, the indication for heart transplantation in children under one year of age is congenital heart disease, most of these patients deemed irreparable. The opposite is true for adolescents, and young adults, where cardiomyopathy is the main indication (Fig. 20-1).

FETUS

Fetal CHF is recognized as hydrops by the obstetrician or ultrasonographer. The fetus develops massive fluid accumulation in serous cavities and soft tissue and rapidly increases in size by examination and is large for dates. Ultrasound identifies the fetus as the source of the abnormal growth. Currently, at least 20% of the etiologies are cardiovascular (1) (Table 20-2). Because the mortality ranges from 50% to 98% in hydrops fetalis, early identification can allow pregnancy termination. Conversely, otherwise-healthy fetuses with readily correctable problems might be treated, for example, by surgical correction of urinary tract obstruction or chemical cardioversion of tachyarrhythmias. The possibility of fetal cardiac corrective surgery continues to be explored; however, these procedures are not yet ready for human trials (2,3). Percutaneous catheter balloon dilatation to promote growth of a strangulated ventricle and alleviate heart failure in critical pulmonic and aortic stenosis has not been successful (2). More recent interest is being placed on averting the lethal outcome before surgery in neonates with hypoplastic left heart syndrome and a highly restrictive patent foramen ovale by percutaneous balloon dilatation of the fetal foramen. In one study, the outcome was not improved in seven fetuses (4).

Fetal tachyarrhythmias, which can be easily diagnosed by fetal echocardiography (Fig. 20-2), have been the most

TABLE 20-1
HEART FAILURE IN CONGENITAL HEART DISEASE BASED ON PATHOPHYSIOLOGICAL STATES

Volume overload
Semilunar and atrioventricular valvar regurgitation
Left-to-right shunt
Pressure overload
Systemic or pulmonary arterial stenosis
Semilunar valve stenosis
Pulmonary vascular disease
Systolic dysfunction
Diastolic dysfunction
Noncompliant ventricle
Pulmonary venous obstruction
Restrictive ASD in complete mixing lesions of single ventricles

ASD, atrioventricular septum. From Holzgreve W, Holzgreve B, Curry CR. Nonimmune hydrops fetalis: diagnosis and management. Semin Perinatol. 1985;9:52–67.

amenable to treatment in utero. The variety of arrhythmias encountered is shown in Table 20-3 (5). The vulnerability of the fetus to tachyarrhythmias has a physiological basis (6): as the fetal myocardium matures, calcium release and uptake shifts from sarcolemma to sarcoplasmic reticulum with the development of that organelle. Thus, the immature myocardium may be less able to relax at elevated heart rates due to the lack of development of the sarcoplasmic reticulum. Fetal muscle is also stiffer than neonatal or adult heart muscle and exhibits a reversed E wave to A wave (E/A) ratio on inflow Doppler imaging. This may result from the relative lack of fibril in the immature myocyte.

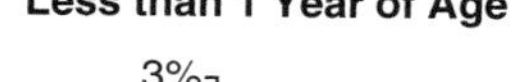

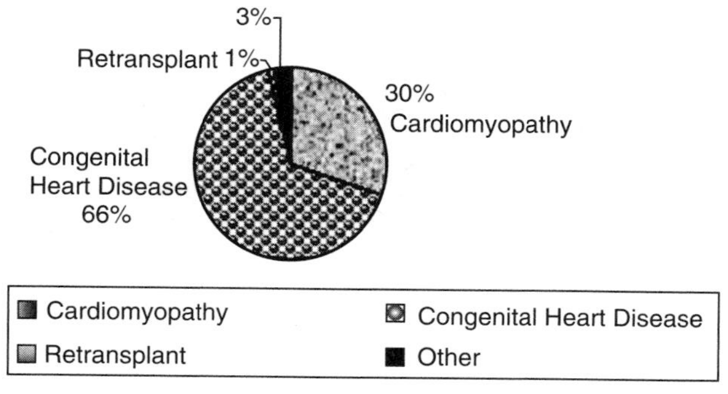

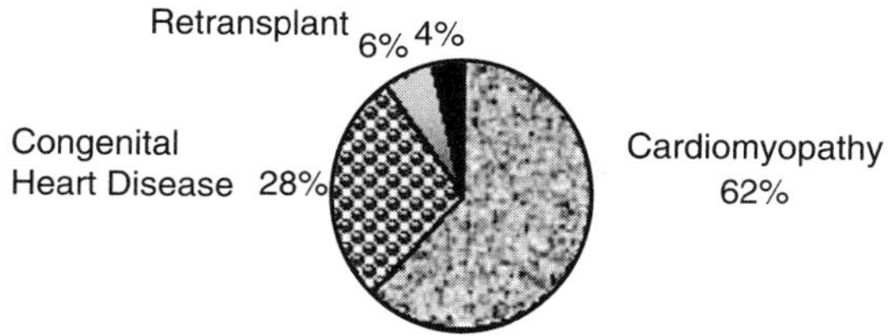

Figure 20-1 Heart transplants by cardiac diagnosis in infants and adolescents.

TABLE 20-2
CAUSES OF NONIMMUNE HYDROPS

Causes	Cases of Hydrops in Study
Cardiovascular	21
Arrhythmia	6
Chromosomal	16
Malformation syndromes	11
Twin–twin transfusions	10
Pulmonary	8
Hematological	6
Infection	4
Urinary	3
Gastrointestinal	3
Miscellaneous	6
Unknown	16
Total	**103**

From Kleinman CS, Copel JA, Weinstein EM, et al. In utero diagnosis and treatment of fetal supraventricular tachycardia. Semin Perinatol. 1985;5:113–129.

Thus, fetal tachycardia can diminish ventricular filling, even at elevated pressures.

Transplacental antiarrhythmic therapy is frequently employed to convert supraventricular tachycardia or to control the rate in atrial flutter or fibrillation. In Kleinman et al.'s series of 16 patients with atrial tachyarrhythmias, 15 were controlled with digoxin, verapamil, propranolol, procainamide, or their combination (5). The decision to treat is based on evidence of fetal distress (hydrops) and knowledge that premature delivery may have considerable complications. Thus, delivery is recommended only for failure of in utero rhythm management.

NEONATE AND INFANT

The transition from intrauterine life to a terrestrial existence is accompanied by a cardiovascular revolution (6). Oxygen consumption is doubled because of the need for movement, respiration, digestion, and thermal regulation. Increase in the left ventricular (by 200%) and right ventricular (50%) output, as well as oxygenation of arterial blood, enables this demand to be met. With the onset of neonatal respiration, pulmonary vascular resistance falls and pulmonary venous return raises left atrial pressure, closing the foramen. Ligation of the cord eliminates the placental and venosus shunts. The patent ductus arteriosus (PDA) closes in response to elevated oxygen levels by 48 hours, and the fetal circulation has acquired the characteristics it will retain for the rest of life. However, if anatomic abnormalities exist, the circulation may not be able to adapt and heart failure may ensue. The early infancy period has by far the greatest incidence of CHF in the pediatric population (7). The common causes of heart failure during this period are listed in Table 20-4.

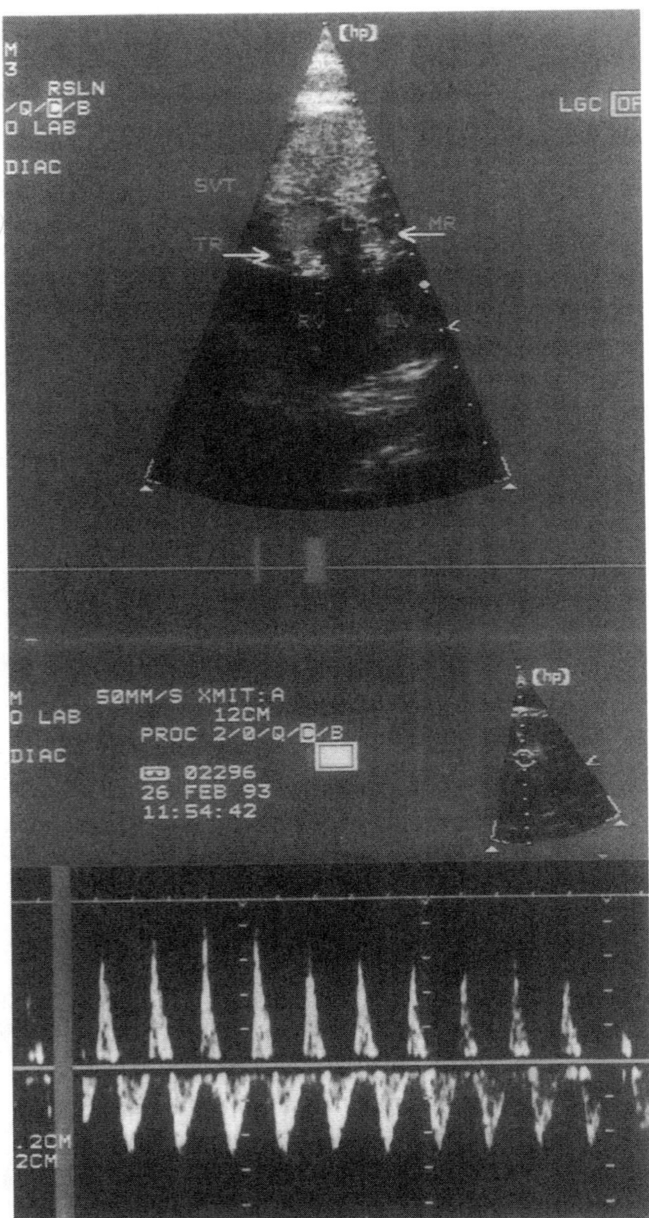

Figure 20-2 Fetal supraventricular tachycardia (SVT) with mitral regurgitation (MR) and tricuspid regurgitation (TR), precursors of hydrops.

TABLE 20-3
FETAL ARRHYTHMIAS

Causes	Cases of Arrythmia in Study
First-degree AV block	15
Supraventricular tachycardia	15
Ventricular tachycardia	2
Complete heart block	8
Atrial flutter	3
Atrial fibrillation	2
Sinus bradycardia	2
Total	**47**

AV, atrioventricular.

The persistence of the fetal circulation pathway in the premature or term infant (right-to-left shunting at the foramen ovale or PDA) is usually associated with important pulmonary disease such as congenital diaphragmatic hernia, sepsis, pneumonia, or meconium aspiration, resulting in persistent pulmonary hypertension of the newborn (8). These infants are hemodynamically compromised with combined cardiopulmonary failure and require pressor, inotropic, or ventilatory support, sometimes culminating in extracorporeal membranous oxygenation circulatory assist. In fact, this is the only indication for which inhaled nitric oxide is approved (9). Pulmonary disease can prevent the normal fall in pulmonary vascular resistance with birth, but other pulmonary diseases, such as premature lungs, are exquisitely sensitive to overperfusion through the PDA and heart failure is commonly seen, even with small shunts. Ductal closure using prostaglandin inhibition or surgery is then required.

Severe obstruction to flow through the left heart and aorta becomes manifest as heart failure shortly after birth because of the separation of the parallel circulation of the fetus into series circulation with the closure of the fetal shunts. In hypoplastic left heart syndrome, severe mitral stenosis, critical aortic stenosis, or coarctation of the aorta (Fig. 20-3), the right ventricle (RV) must supply blood to the body using the PDA in utero and postnatally (Fig. 20-4). These infants are critically ill and need prompt diagnosis and, if feasible, surgical palliation. Some of these infants are not recognized to have heart disease and are discharged from the nursery only to present in cardiogenic shock as outpatients when the ductus closes. This is one lesion whereby prenatal diagnosis by fetal echocardiography has utmost utility.

TABLE 20-4
COMMON CAUSES OF CONGESTIVE HEART FAILURE IN INFANTS WITH CONGENITAL HEART DISEASE

Preterm	Term neonates	Infants
Patent ductus arteriosus	Hypoplastic left heart	Large VSD
	Coarctation of aorta	Atrioventricular septal defect (AV canal)
	Severe aortic stenosis	D-TGA with VSD
	Atrial arrhythmias	Truncus arteriosus
		Anomalous pulmonary venous return with obstruction

VSD, ventricular septal defect; AV, atrioventricular; D-TGA, dextro-transposition of the great vessels.

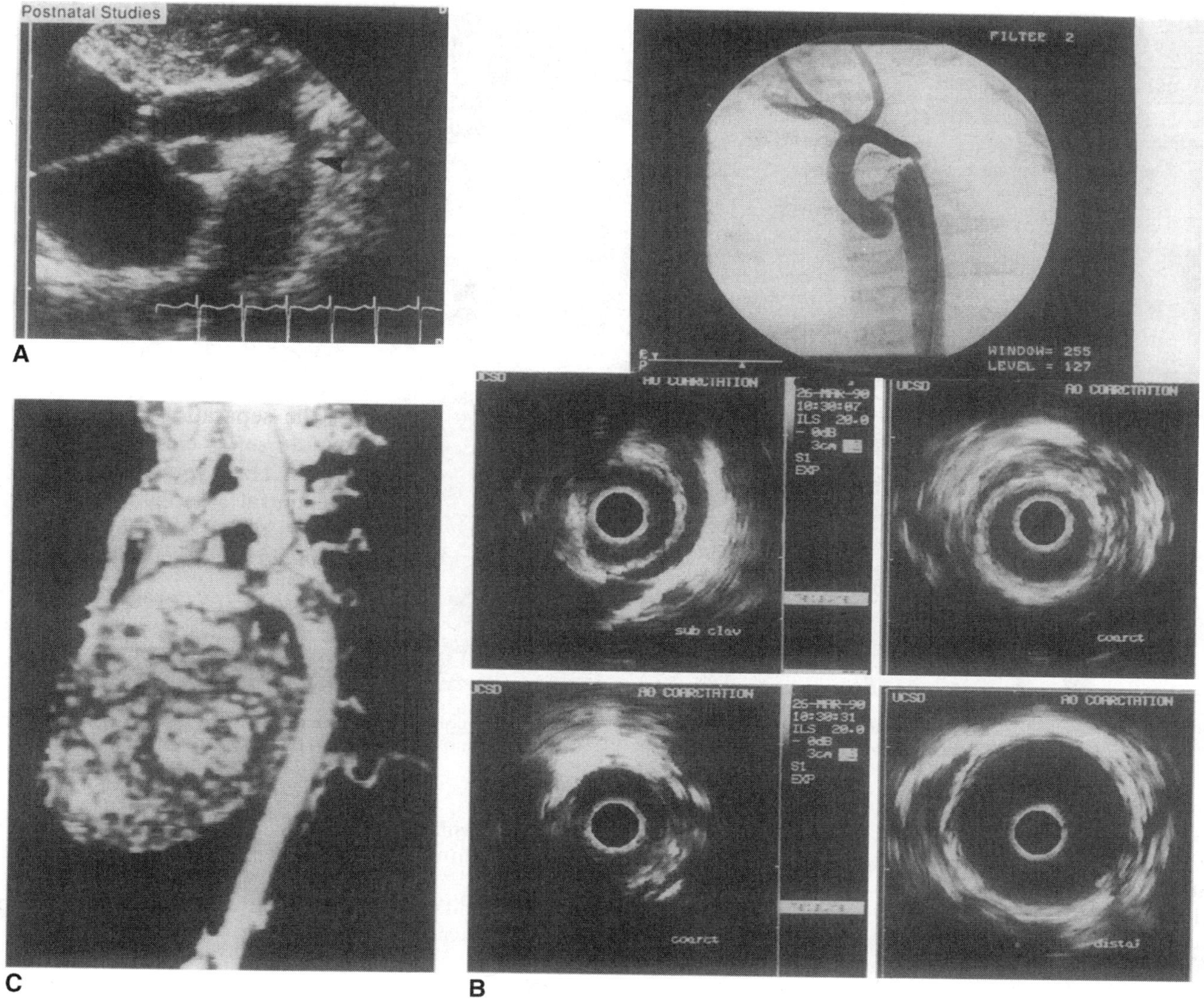

Figure 20-3 Severe coarctation imaged by ultrasound **(A)**, intravascular echography and angiography **(B)**, and three-dimensional reconstruction of magnetic resonance flow data **(C)**.

The progressive decline in pulmonary vascular resistance following birth invites increasing pulmonary blood flow when unrestricted communication exists between the high-pressure left ventricle (LV) or aorta and the RV or pulmonary artery. Although the systemic ventricle normally doubles its output at birth, pulmonary blood flow may exceed systemic blood flow by fourfold with large defects. In this setting, the systemic ventricle will be overloaded with pulmonary venous return and CHF ensues. These infants may appear well at birth when the pulmonary vascular resistance is still relatively high, and the defect may go unnoticed. In addition, the programmed fall in pulmonary vascular resistance can be retarded by increased flow and pressures, delaying the threshold of clinical presentation until weeks later. The lesions most commonly responsible for this form of high-output heart failure are large defects of the ventricular septum (VSD) or atrioventricular septum (ASD) (Fig. 20-5). Dextra-transposition of the great arteries (D-TGA) with a large VSD and truncus arteriosus may also produce heart failure with progressive fall in pulmonary vascular resistance, but cyanosis is usually the presenting sign. Total anomalous pulmonary venous return with obstruction can also present with cyanosis but florid pulmonary edema will predominate. It should be noted that ASDs, regardless of size, rarely result in heart failure at this age. Shunting at the atrial level is dependent on diastolic rather than systolic or arterial pressure differences. Left-to-right shunting occurs only to the extent that the RV is larger and more compliant than the LV. Therefore, overt heart failure in an infant with an ASD requires careful inspection for additional left-sided lesions (10). In addition, RV diastolic pressure cannot exceed LV diastolic pressure; thus, RV failure is rare unless severe pulmonary hypertension is present or until late in the natural history of this lesion.

Paroxysmal supraventricular tachycardia (SVT) may also cause CHF in infants. Whether the mechanism is dual atrioventricular (AV) nodal pathways or Wolf-Parkinson-White syndrome, the rapid ventricular response may be

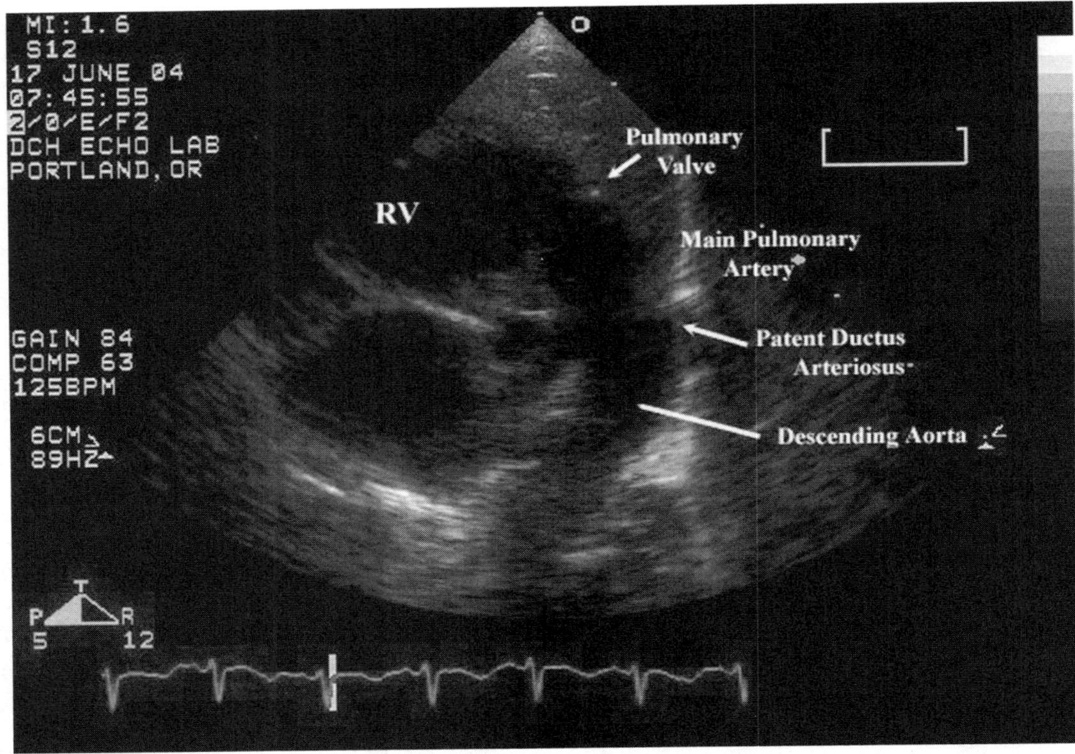

Figure 20-4 Right ventricle acts as "left ventricular assist" through the patent ductus arteriosus in hypoplastic left heart syndrome, a ductal-dependent lesion causing heart failure in neonates.

poorly tolerated. Attention should be directed toward conversion to and maintenance of sinus rhythm, and delineation of any underlying cardiac abnormalities by echocardiography. Ebstein anomaly and cardiac tumors are known to be associated with SVT.

Other less-common causes of heart failure include congenital anomalies of the coronary arteries, mitral stenosis (Fig. 20-6), and supramitral stenosis from cor triatriatum. Anomalous origin of the left main or left anterior descending coronary arteries from the pulmonary artery (Fig. 20-7), or as a single right coronary artery (Fig. 20-8), usually

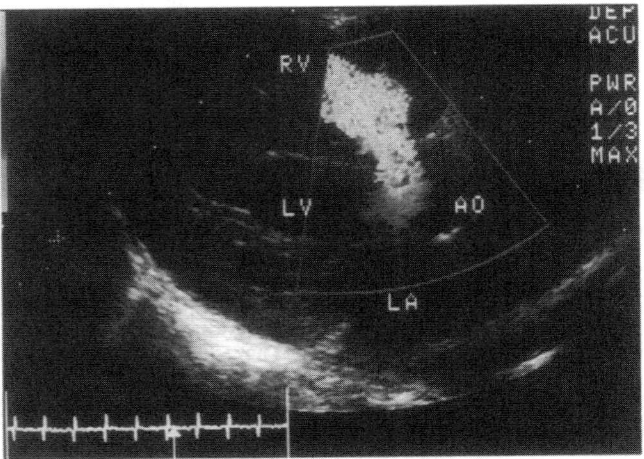

Figure 20-5 Moderate sized perimembranous ventricular septal defect (VSD) with color Doppler indicating a left-to-right shunt.

presents with ischemia or infarction. Primary heart muscle and inflammatory diseases finish the list of differential diagnoses.

Congenital cardiomyopathies can present with insidious or acute heart failure. Although these are too lengthy to describe here in detail, it is especially important in this age group that the diagnostic workup must consider cytogenetic aberrations, syndromes, neuromuscular diseases, and abnormal metabolic/endocrine pathways. Neonatal enterovirus infection can be devastating and can cause myocarditis. Maternal lupus antibody–mediated congenital complete heart block (11) is a unique pediatric entity that can also cause heart failure, even with prompt pacemaker implantation. Evidence points to prenatal maternal anti-SSA/Ro and anti-SSB/La antibodies attacking only fetal cardiomyocytes, leading to myocarditis or cardiomyopathy, as the disease does not exist in adults with lupus (12).

Diagnosis of heart failure in infants relies on echocardiography but it is nevertheless important to recognize the clinical manifestations (Table 20-5). Because young infants do not "walk up stairs," a simple-to-use heart failure severity scale is difficult to develop; attempts have been made but none has been widely adopted (13–15). This further impedes the ability to systematically study the progression and success of various medical interventions. Of promise are heart failure biomarkers, such as B-type natriuretic peptide (BNP), used as a surrogate classification scale (16–19), but the proper accuracy studies must still be performed. Since the major functional activities in infants are feeding and growing, growth may be another accepted endpoint in future heart failure studies in this population.

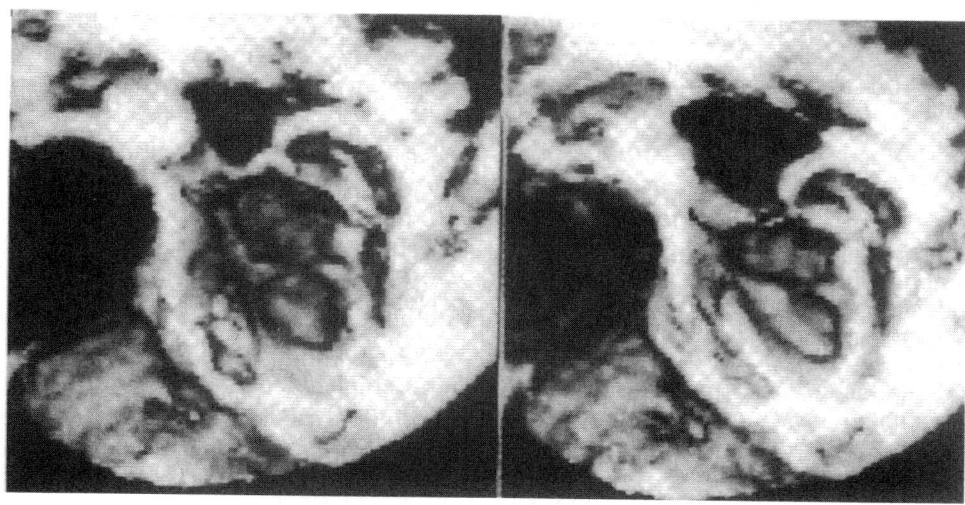

Figure 20-6 Three-dimensional echocardiographic reconstruction of severe congenital mitral stenosis in an infant.

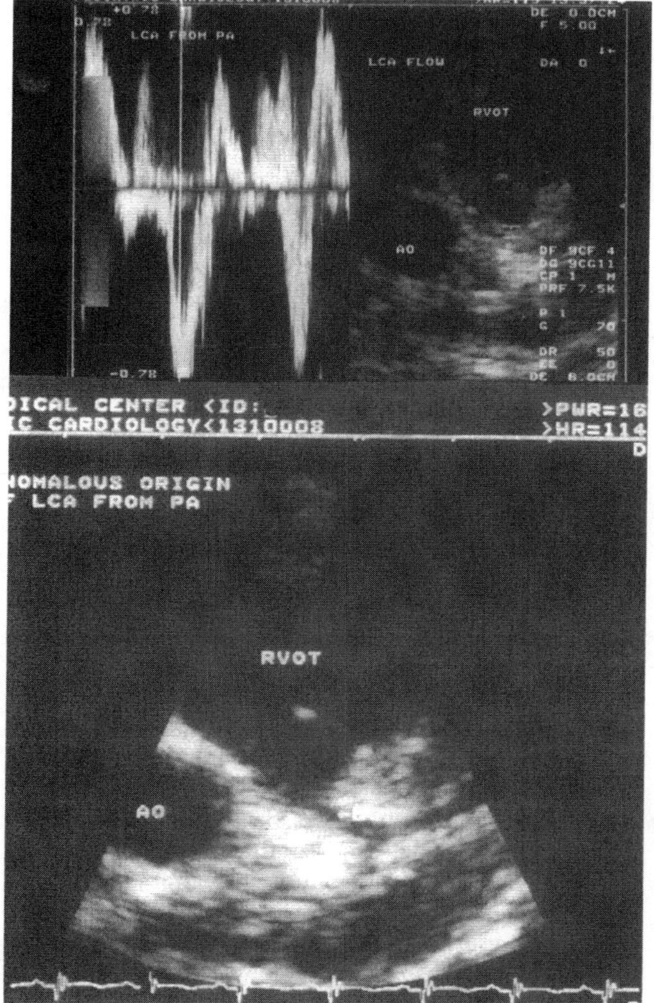

Figure 20-7 Anomalous left coronary artery from the pulmonary artery, transthoracic echocardiography. Cardinal findings are a dilated right coronary artery, identification of an aberrant vascular structure from the pulmonary artery, and reversal of flow direction in the left coronary artery when collaterals have developed.

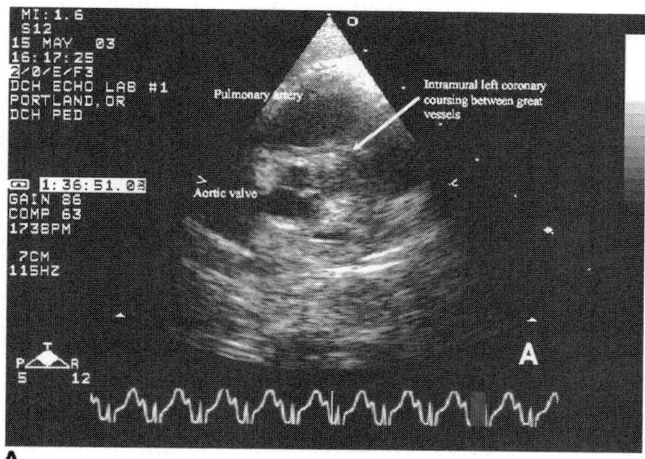

A

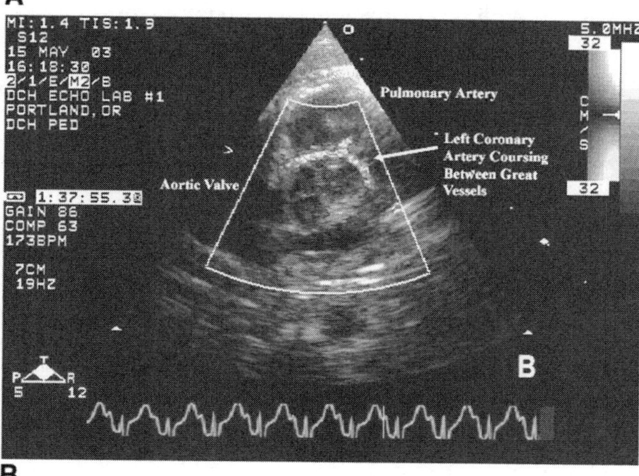

B

Figure 20-8 Anomalous origin of left coronary artery: single coronary arising from right-facing aortic sinus, resulting in an intramural left coronary artery traversing between both great vessels **(A)**. Color Doppler echocardiography shows direction of flow is from right to left **(B)**. (Images courtesy of Dr. Mary Rice, Oregon Health & Science University, Portland.)

TABLE 20-5
RECOGNITION OF CONGESTIVE HEART FAILURE IN INFANTS

Poor weight gain, failure to thrive
Feeding intolerance, gastroesophageal reflux
Tachypnea, grunting, flaring, retractions, rales, and wheezing (asthma)
Tachycardia, decreased pulses
Hyperdynamic precordium, ventricular lift
Loud single S_2, S_3, or S_4 heart sounds, diastolic rumble
Diaphoresis, cool extremities, mottling, pallor
Decreased urination
Irritability or lethargy
Hepatomegaly
Facial and eyelid edema
Bulging fontanels
Cardiomegaly, increased vascularity, pulmonary edema, bronchial thickening on X-ray

The management of infants with CHF should not be delayed; CHF is an emergency if there is hemodynamic compromise. Attention must be quickly directed to stabilization of respiratory, acid–base, and hemodynamic variables, followed immediately by anatomic definition of the underlying cardiovascular abnormalities by echocardiography. Surgical therapy is urgent, when appropriate. With improvement in echocardiography, catheterization and angiography are seldom needed. The general approach in this age group is not significantly different from that in other age groups. The major exceptions are (a) manipulation of the PDA; (b) cautious use of vasodilators; (c) insufficient evidence-based trial data; and (d) planning of intervention with surgery in mind. Relaxation of ductal constriction by prostaglandin E_1 in hypoplastic left heart syndrome allows the right ventricle to continue its fetal role of supplying systemic blood flow, thus improving systemic perfusion. With severe juxtaductal coarctation, ductal relaxation (even if the ductus cannot be made patent) can sometimes allow enough antegrade flow across the coarctation. Conversely, premature infants with respiratory failure from left heart failure may benefit from ductal constriction with prostaglandin inhibition with indomethacin.

Vasodilator therapy for afterload or preload reduction is effective therapy for cardiac dysfunction caused by cardiomyopathy, ischemia, postcardiotomy, or severe aortic or mitral valve regurgitation (20). However, the high prevalence of heart failure caused by shunts and multilevel lesions in infants requires a secure anatomic diagnosis before empiric therapy is begun. Theoretically, systemic afterload reduction should help left-to-right shunt heart failure. However, properly controlled studies to assess its benefits beyond the acute setting are lacking.

Similarly, the proven benefits of beta-blocker therapy in adults with heart failure may also benefit selected infants with chronic heart failure. Studies have shown elevated catecholamine, inflammatory cytokine, and renin-angiotensin-aldosterone system (RAAS) levels in some congenital lesions (21–24). One controlled study was able to demonstrate the salutary effect of neurohormone inhibition in infants with shunt-related heart failure (25,26). Akin to the adult patient with systolic dysfunction, digoxin has been incorporated into the pediatric practice and theory of heart failure management, but its effectiveness has never been convincingly demonstrated. Under careful monitoring, patients who remain symptomatic after optimization may receive additional benefits from it. Nevertheless, diuretics to decongest pulmonary symptoms remain the cornerstone of pharmacologic therapy. Refer to *The Harriet Lane Handbook* (27) for pediatric dosing of standard cardiovascular drugs. Inotropes are rarely needed for high-output heart failure except in postoperative management or as rescue from cardiogenic shock. Milrinone has finally been shown to be advantageous in postcardiac surgery support of infants (28).

CHILD AND ADOLESCENT

The initial occurrence of CHF in a child with congenital heart disease without prior corrective or palliative surgery is uncommon. Therefore, in the diagnostic workup of CHF in this age group, acquired heart disease must be strongly considered. A description of acquired causes is beyond the scope of this book; nevertheless, several congenital defects may present with CHF in childhood or adolescence. As congenital heart repairs are now done earlier in life, infants who were repaired or palliated will also present in this age group with CHF secondary to the progression of residual abnormalities or to late postoperative complications.

Unoperated Patients

It must be remembered that this is a widely diverse group in terms of congenital heart disease (Table 20-6). Some individuals did not undergo an operation because their lesion was subclinical at an earlier age. Others simply are not amenable or would not be better off with any palliation. Also, some patients never had access to care, although this is less-often encountered in Western countries. The last two groups largely contribute to those who go on to develop Eisenmenger syndrome.

Pulmonary Hypertension and Eisenmenger Syndrome

Progressive pulmonary vascular obstructive disease occurs with high pressure and flow in the pulmonary circuit. This results from left-to-right shunting because of ventricular or great vessel communication. Although associated, atrial shunting alone is not usually the sole cause of severe pulmonary hypertension. With severely elevated and fixed pulmonary vascular resistance, pulmonary artery pressures equal systemic pressures and right-to-left shunting occurs, culminating with significant cyanosis and Eisenmenger syndrome. Pulmonic and tricuspid insufficiency is usually seen. In general, patients with Eisenmenger syndrome remain free of CHF much longer than those with idiopathic pulmonary hypertension, probably because the disease process is different and the former have biventricular assist

TABLE 20-6

CAUSES OF CONGESTIVE HEART FAILURE IN CHILDREN AND ADOLESCENTS (UNOPERATED)

Myocardial dysfunction
Myocardial dysfunction caused by severe cyanosis
Morphological right ventricle as systemic ventricle
Valvar abnormalities
Aortic insufficiency
Mitral regurgitation
Atrioventricular valve regurgitation with single ventricle
Mitral stenosis
Tricuspid insufficiency with Ebstein anomaly or CTGA
Subaortic stenosis
Volume overload from shunting
Atrial septal defects
Miscellaneous
Eisenmenger syndrome
Endocarditis

CTGA, Congenitally corrected transposition of the great arteries.

and pop-off across their defects. Therefore, intervention (short of heart–lung transplantation) is uncommon. However, children who have high resistance but reversible right-to-left shunting may still be able to have their defect closed if they demonstrate reasonable pulmonary vasoreactivity. The initial episode of heart failure may be heralded by atrial flutter, fibrillation, or ectopic tachycardia.

Severe Cyanosis

With complex congenital heart disease, it is often difficult to determine exactly which mechanisms led to ventricular dysfunction. Excessive pressure and volume loads are frequently present for a long duration. It is likely that reduced oxygenation to the developing myocardium also contributes to the subendocardial ischemia, necrosis, and fibrosis that ultimately result in ventricular dysfunction and heart failure in complex congenital lesions.

Ebstein's Anomaly

Apical displacement of the tricuspid valve in Ebstein's anomaly is associated with tricuspid insufficiency and varying amounts of dysfunction of the remainder of the atrialized right ventricle (Fig. 20-9). As right atrial pressure rises, cyanosis may occur because of a patent foramen ovale or, less commonly, ASD. Fortunately, in the absence of pulmonary hypertension the regurgitation is well-tolerated in healthy youngsters. As with Eisenmenger syndrome, CHF may be precipitated by an atrial arrhythmia, usually fibrillation or flutter. Kent bundles are quite frequent in Ebstein's anomaly, and re-entry paroxysmal SVT is often seen.

Congenitally Corrected Transposition of the Great Arteries (CTGA)

Although this abnormality may be unrecognized and children with it may live a near-normal life span, some will develop left-sided CHF in childhood or adolescence. The main clinical problems are the development of AV block and systemic ventricle dysfunction with associated AV valve regurgitation. Neither the morphological right ventricle nor the tricuspid valve is ideally suited for long-term function at systemic pressures. Thus, as with other dysfunctional RVs such as in Ebstein's anomaly, D-TGA after atrial switch, and single right ventricle hearts, pump and heart failure develop with time. In CTGA, there is an increased risk of sudden cardiac death in the setting of ventricular dysfunction (29).

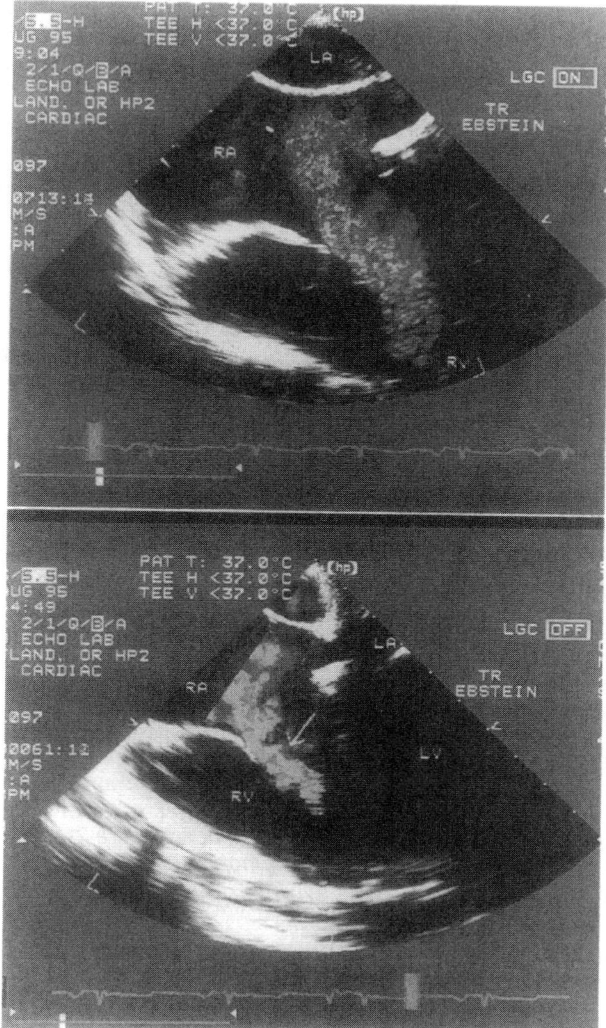

Figure 20-9 Ebstein's anamoly, intraoperative transesophageal echocardiogram (TEE) view.

Mitral Regurgitation

The mitral valve is more resistant to pressure and volume overload than the tricuspid valve but is not immune to these stressors. Unfortunate individuals with tricuspid atresia or other single ventricle malformations who were not palliated can develop mitral valve insufficiency because of the increased volume load from the obligatory mixing of deoxygenated with oxygenated blood. Congenitally abnormal mitral valves, such as an isolated cleft (the most subtle of the wide spectrum of endocardial cushion defects), can cause progressive regurgitation leading to annular dilation and ventricular enlargement, further preventing proper coaptation. Timing for repair depends on the state of the myocardial function, presence of pulmonary hypertension, and heart failure symptoms. Controversy does exist on whether the younger LV can recover and withstand regurgitation better than what is known from the adult experience (30,31).

Endocarditis

Infection of the heart and great vessels in patients with congenital heart disease is most common in locations with high-velocity jets and turbulence. Thus, restrictive VSDs, PDAs, surgically created systemic-to-pulmonary shunts, aortic and truncal valve disease, aortic coarctation, systemic AV valve regurgitation, and moderate to severe pulmonary stenosis are all indicatiors of a high risk for infection. CHF usually occurs because of destruction of the systemic side valve leaflet. However, pulmonary embolization and tricuspid valve destruction with endocarditis involving a small VSD can also present with severe right heart failure. Conduction delay and frank, complete heart block have also been observed.

Subaortic Stenosis

The recognition of subaortic stenosis is not difficult by echocardiography. Its substrate can be an isolated fibrous ridge, a membrane that attaches to the mitral valve, or a muscular protrusion into the left ventricular outflow tract. After resection, recurrence is common, making the decision to intervene difficult. Similar to aortic stenosis or native coarctation of the aorta, heart failure in an otherwise healthy individual is uncommon from childhood to adolescence.

Mitral Stenosis

Congenital mitral stenosis typically occurs with other left-side restrictive lesions such as endocardial fibroelastosis, hypoplastic aortic arch, coarctation, stenotic aortic valve, or hypoplastic left heart syndrome. While many patients may have had these other lesions repaired early in life, some will have mitral stenosis in isolation and only later will require mitral valve repair for symptomatic heart failure or pulmonary hypertension. An arcade-like supporting apparatus, a single papillary muscle, and a double orifice from a connecting bridge of tissue are some of the pathologies seen in congenital mitral stenosis. The development of pulmonary edema with exercise is similar to adults with the same pathophysiology. Pulmonary hypertension can be quite advanced if the defect was hemodynamically significant early in life and is associated with other lesions. Prosthetic mitral valve replacement and lifelong anticoagulation are inevitably needed since repair or dilatation cannot be applied to such lesions. Diuretics and beta-blockade can temporize symptoms in the short term.

Atrial Septal Defect

An ASD, particularly of the sinus venosus or primum type, can cause overt heart failure in this age group. The symptoms can be subtle and some parents recognize the true activity level of their child only after the defect is closed. Percutaneous device closure of secundem defects is highly successful. Occasionally, sinus venosus defects are missed by transthoracic echocardiography, necessitating MRI, angiography, or transesophageal echography to explain the dilated right side. In superior sinus venosus ASD, the right upper pulmonary vein inevitably drains to the superior vena cava (SVC) and it must be incorporated in the repair to baffle its flow back to the left atrium.

Operated Patients

Causes of CHF in surgically treated children and adolescents are shown in Table 20-7. The list of operations for congenital heart disease is daunting, and most can have CHF as an unnatural or natural occurrence following the procedure. Because definitive corrective repair is not always possible or cannot be sustained indefinitely, some of the causes overlap with those of the unoperated patient. Nevertheless, operated patients with heart failure can be divided into major groups of dysfunction for recognition and management.

Myocardial Dysfunction

Myocardial necrosis, scarring, and dysfunction occur after surgery because of intraoperative injury (ischemia or incision) or excessive postoperative loading conditions. Advances in myocardial preservation have greatly reduced intraoperative myocardial damage. It is now possible to arrest the myocardium physiologically for extended periods of time. The greatest limitation in vivo is obtaining adequate cooling of both ventricles in the face of complicated anatomy. Right ventriculotomy is still performed for resection of infundibular stenosis in tetralogy of Fallot (TOF), but most simple VSDs and some TOF conditions are now repaired through the tricuspid valve. Coronary artery laceration is uncommon but remains a concern.

TABLE 20-7

CAUSES OF CONGESTIVE HEART FAILURE IN CHILDREN AND ADOLESCENTS (OPERATED)

- Myocardial dysfunction
  - Perioperative ischemic injury
  - Ventriculotomy
  - Preoperative myocardial disease
  - Coronary artery injury
- Volume overload
  - Valvular regurgitation
  - Persistent VSD
  - Large bronchial collaterals
  - Large systemic arterial-to-pulmonary artery shunt
- Prosthetic dysfunction
- Single ventricle circulation status post-Fontan procedure
- Morphological right ventricle as systemic ventricle
- Pulmonary hypertension
- Endocarditis
- Arrhythmias

VSD, ventricular septal defect.

Unfortunately, myocardial dysfunction may be present before surgery because of the combined assaults of pressure and volume overload in the face of cyanosis over time. Unsatisfactory results have pressed cardiologists and surgeons to intervene as soon as is technically feasible to effect definitive repair of congenital defects. Because of this practice, the number of patients with postoperative myocardial dysfunction has dropped dramatically, and short- and long-term prognoses have improved accordingly.

Volume Overload

Volume overload occurs after surgery for many reasons. Surgeons create systemic arterial-to-pulmonary shunts to hypoperfused lungs that cannot be treated definitively. Even the perfect-sized anastomosis necessarily increases the work of the systemic ventricle, and eventually it may fail. Shunts that are too large may cause heart failure early in the perioperative period or result in subclinical injury that surfaces later. Uncorrected, an excessively large shunt may also damage the pulmonary vasculature. The purpose of surgical shunts today is to temporize defects that are destined for single ventricle repair or where the pulmonary arteries are very hypoplastic. In the former scenario, an intermediary stage known as a Glenn or bidirectional cavopulmonary connection is performed, whereby the SVC is connected to the pulmonary artery so that the ventricle can be unloaded and allowed to de-remodel before the inferior vena cava (IVC) is also incorporated in the pulmonary circuit (Fontan completion). If not thus staged, the previously overloaded and hypertrophied ventricle may exhibit diastolic dysfunction and impede blood return from the pulmonary circuit after the Fontan connection, resulting in a low–cardiac-output heart failure state (32–34).

Previously installed systemic–pulmonary shunts may also be difficult to remove during definitive surgery (e.g., a Pott shunt from the left pulmonary artery [LPA] to the aorta). Naturally occurring bronchial artery collaterals may provide substantial and necessary pulmonary blood flow in cyanotic individuals before correction, but they can also be too diffuse and difficult to locate at the time of definitive surgery. With the rerouting of systemic venous return to the lungs, persistent collaterals can result in overcirculation and heart failure. Careful delineation of collaterals is part of any preoperative assessment and postoperative workup of the patient with persistent heart failure. The interventionalist may subsequently embolize collaterals not addressed at surgery. Patients remaining in recalcitrant heart failure after transplant, from significant residual collaterals from their pretransplant cyanotic congenital heart condition, have been reported (35).

All four valves may leak after surgery and result in or contribute to CHF. Generally, tricuspid and pulmonary regurgitation are better-tolerated than are mitral and aortic regurgitation. However, in the face of RV volume overload, RV pressure overload from pulmonary valve, pulmonary artery, or pulmonary vascular constriction, volume overload will be less well-tolerated in this setting. Unsuccessful repair of the valve in Ebstein anomaly may result in recurrent right heart failure, even with normal pulmonary artery pressures.

Late right heart failure following TOF repair is usually multifactorial, including myocardial dysfunction from presurgical pressure overload, ventriculotomy, patch aneurysm, and wide-open pulmonary insufficiency (Fig. 20-10). It is difficult to serially assess RV volume and function to decide when valve replacement should be performed, especially in borderline or asymptomatic patients. With the advent of cardiac magnetic resonance imaging and emerging outcome data on valve replacement (36,37), the trend is toward earlier pulmonic valve replacement. Because hypoplastic or distorted pulmonary arteries downstream will accentuate the RV dysfunction, coordination of the relief of the stenoses with the interventionalist must be considered if such lesions are lurking. Mitral or systemic AV valve regurgitation may be associated with failed repair of a cleft mitral valve (Fig. 20-11), D-TGA after atrial baffling, CTGA, single ventricle anatomy (Fig. 20-12), or tricuspid atresia following Fontan repair.

Aortic insufficiency may follow surgical or balloon valvotomy, Ross procedure, arterial switch for D-TGA, VSD closure, an incompetent truncal valve, or TOF repair. Persistence of a VSD may cause CHF after an operation to relieve pulmonary valve, subvalvar, or artery stenosis or atresia.

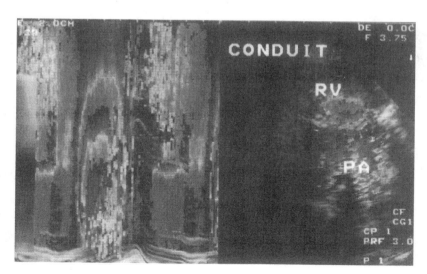

Figure 20-10 Conduit after tetralogy of Fallot (TOF) repair with wide-open pulmonary regurgitation on color M-mode.

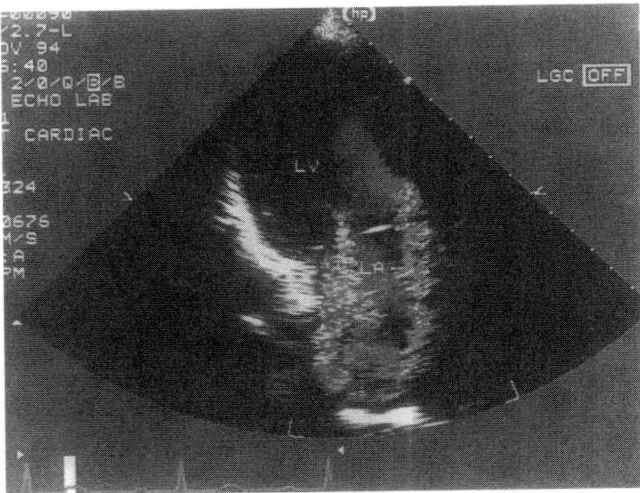

Figure 20-11 Moderate mitral regurgitation after repair of atrioventricular canal.

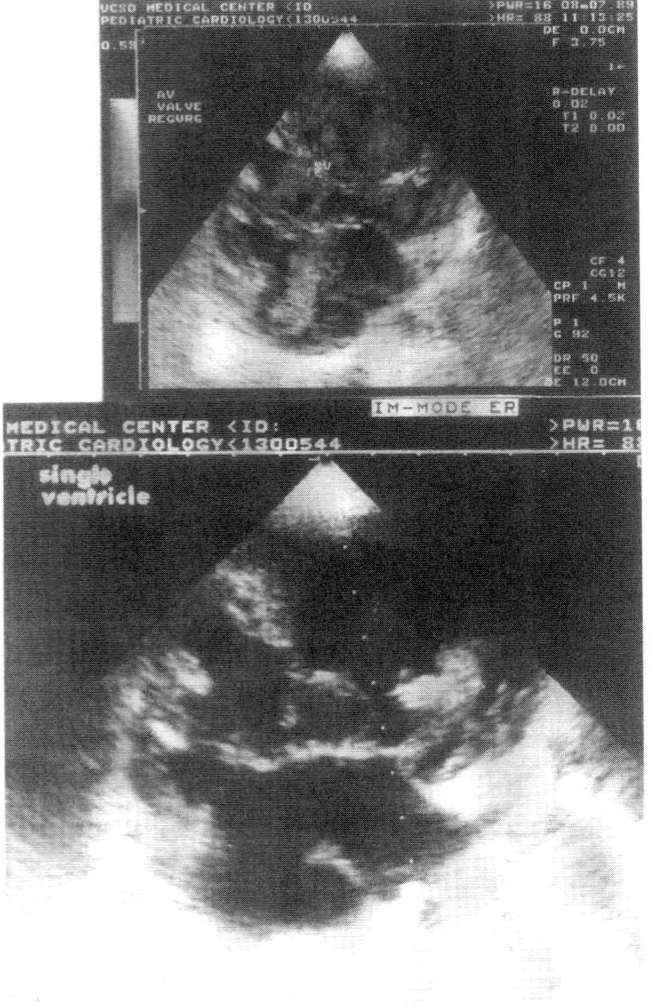

Figure 20-12 Atrioventricular valve regurgitation in a single ventricle.

Prosthetic Dysfunction

Prosthetic dysfunction results when biological or artificial valves or conduits fail or are outgrown. Heart failure tends to be more insidious and less severe. However, acute prosthesis failure can be critical. Insertion of prosthetic material into a patient represents a new disease whose natural history may or may not be known (38). There was tremendous enthusiasm for porcine prosthetic valves in the 1970s; the major attraction for children was the lack of need for anticoagulation compared to a mechanical valve. However, children and young adults proved to have accelerated calcification and degeneration of these prostheses, whether they were placed in anatomic valve positions or conduits. These prostheses are now avoided in this age group. Enthusiasm has shifted to the use of cryopreserved homografts, which are implanted in the aortic or pulmonic position or in conduits between the right ventricle and pulmonary artery. The durability of these valves is certainly greater than glutaraldehyde-preserved tissue but the ultimate fate of these devices in patients remains to be determined.

Mechanical prostheses require coumarin anticoagulation to reduce the incidence of thromboembolic complications. Despite anticoagulation (and related to poor anticoagulation), these prostheses may develop thrombotic obstruction. Prostheses in the tricuspid position are most vulnerable, with the mitral intermediate and aortic position being the least susceptible. Material failure of currently implanted prostheses is rare.

Conduit obstruction may also occur because of the development of pseudointimal proliferation, thrombosis of the conduit or associated valve, or fibrocalcific degeneration of an associated bioprosthesis.

Bioprosthesis dysfunction is usually associated with fibrocalcific degeneration of the leaflets. This process results in mixed stenosis and regurgitation of the valve.

Occasionally, a leaflet will tear and the manifestation of dysfunction may be acute, severe regurgitation.

Patient prosthesis mismatch occurs as a natural consequence of growth when a child must have a heart valve or conduit placed that may be too small for that individual after puberty. Unfortunately, a hypoplastic annulus or great vessel may also require that a small prosthesis be placed in even fully grown young adults.

The Fontan Procedure

The Fontan procedure connects the right atrium directly to the pulmonary arteries or, through an overflow chamber, to the pulmonary valve for patients with single ventricle or tricuspid atresia. Recognizing that a dilated atrium is associated with recalcitrant atrial arrhythmias, evolution of surgical techniques has led to the direct cavopulmonary anastomosis with a lateral tunnel within the right atrium, excluding most of this chamber. The newest Fontan strategies exclude the atrium completely by fashioning an extracardiac tubular graft from the IVC to the pulmonary artery. Without an effective pulmonary ventricle, mean right atrial (or central venous) and pulmonary artery pressures are the same and must be higher than the left atrial pressure. To be successful, left ventricular systolic and diastolic function and mitral valve function must be normal and pulmonary vascular resistance must be low. Hence, it is important to not keep a systemic arterial–pulmonary shunt beyond early infancy, as is staging to a Glenn before completing the division of the circulation. Even then, it can be difficult to predict who will have a perfect Fontan circulation. The main reason is the dynamic changes that occur in each component of the circulation when the IVC flow (greater than 50% of cardiac return) is abruptly added to the pulmonary circuit without a pump.

Heart failure is manifested early on as low cardiac output dependent on inotropic and mechanical ventilatory support. A fenestration created at surgery between the Fontan tunnel and left atrium can alleviate congestion and enable venous return to the systemic ventricle so cardiac output can be maintained, but at the cost of hypoxemia. Some patients can achieve a steady state to come off support but may remain in right heart failure with ascites or transudative or chylous pleural effusions for an extended period of time. More long-term manifestations of this unique form of heart failure include transaminitis, portal hypertension and liver dysfunction, protein-losing enteropathy, plastic bronchitis, atrial arrhythmias, thromboembolism (Fig 20-13), and poor somatic growth (39,40). In fact, even patients with an uneventful Fontan have a noticeably higher mortality and morbidity rate over time (39).

Although well-controlled prospective studies examining the development and treatment of heart failure in this patient population are not available, numerous studies have shown Fontan or single ventricle patients to have functional limitations related to the cardiovascular system. When challenged, decreased cardiac performance is seen and, in essence, such patients start off after the Fontan in NYHA functional class I (41–45). Furthermore, residual pressure and volume loading (outflow obstruction, systemic arterial-pulmonary collaterals, or AV volume regurgitation) must be avoided and may require surgical intervention, often years after a Fontan procedure.

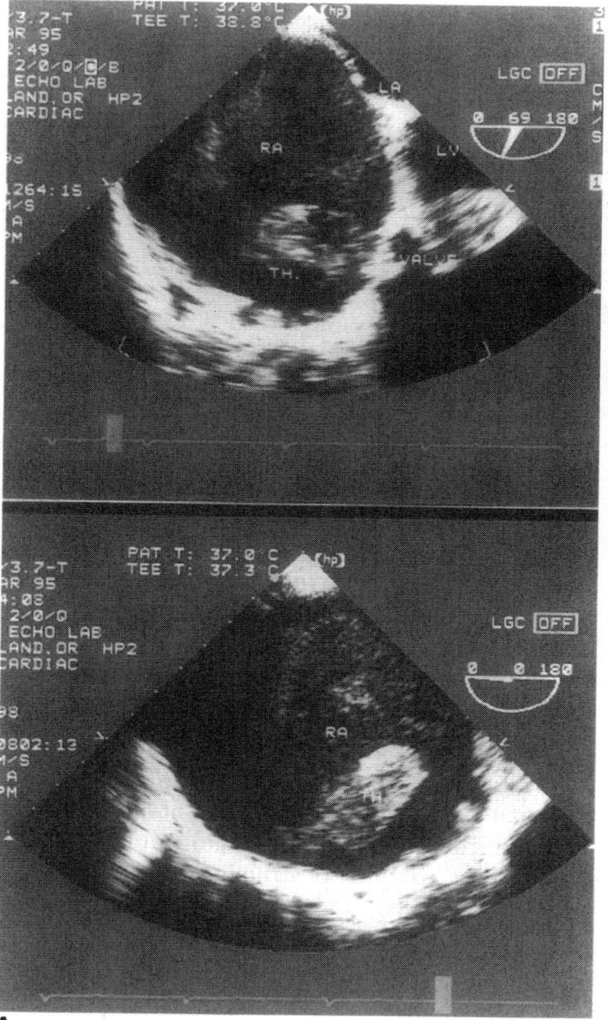

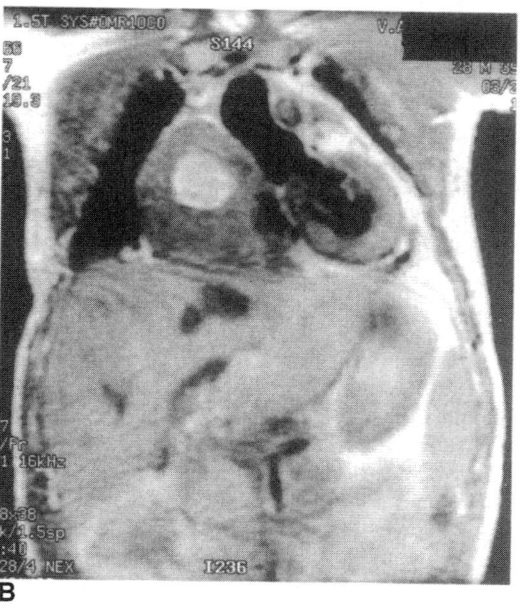

Figure 20-13 Obstruction by thrombus of an atriopulmonary Fontan in a patient who was not on anticoagulation and who presented with atrial flutter/fibrillation: transesophageal echocardiography **(A)** and MRI **(B)**.

Endocarditis

Endocarditis remains a threat for any prosthetic valve, with an incidence of approximately 1% per year. Small residual VSDs and mild aortic and mitral insufficiency are also fertile grounds for endocarditis in the postsurgical patient and may result in leaflet destruction and acute or chronic CHF.

Arrhythmias

Arrhythmias are precipitating causes of CHF in patients with borderline ventricular systolic function, patients with stiff ventricles dependent on atrial booster pump function, and patients with the Fontan procedure. Patients with atrial baffling procedures (Mustard, Senning), a Fontan procedure, or CTGA (operated or unoperated) are also at increased risk for atrial arrhythmias. Thus, atrial flutter in a patient with D-TGA who has had previous Mustard repair may be poorly tolerated because of systemic ventricular dysfunction. Likewise, atrial tachycardia in a patient with TOF repair with moderate residual outflow tract obstruction and insufficiency may develop right heart failure. Atrial arrhythmias remain a major cause of CHF in these patients. Moreover, sudden cardiac death, presumably secondary to primary ventricular arrhythmias or secondary to rapid ventricular response to atrial tachycardia, is concerning (29), particularly in TOF (46), congenitally corrected transposition (29), and D-TGA patients corrected by the atrial switch operation (47). Similar to adults with cardiomyopathy, poor ventricular systolic function appears to be an associated risk factor.

Congenital or acquired complete heart block may also become a manifest problem in this age group. Although the bradycardia and lack of atrial–ventricular synchrony may well be tolerated for years, the concurrent insults of ventricular dysfunction and prosthetic heart valve or other postsurgical changes may promote CHF. Restoration of atrial–ventricular synchrony with heart rate responsive to a normally innervated atrium or to patient activity may be indicated. For example, the Fontan patient should benefit from atrial–ventricular synchrony to enhance diastolic function. Interventricular or intraventricular resynchronization may also be an attractive therapeutic tool. Morphological RV dysfunction on the pulmonary or systemic side is difficult to treat. Commonly accompanied by previous ventriculotomy, septal dyskinesis from a VSD patch, volume overload, and AV or ventricular conduction delay, electromechanical dyssynchrony can be a therapeutic target. Small studies have shown acute hemodynamic benefits (48,49) and medium-term improvement in strictly systemic RV heart failure patients (50). Similar to the unfolding cardiomyopathy resynchronization case, proper patient selection and clinical heart failure benefits must be demonstrated. Unlike in adults with cardiomyopathy, RV pacing in congenital patients can be more feasible with a single ventricular lead or can be done at time of surgery.

Pulmonary Hypertension

Pulmonary hypertension secondary to either pulmonary arteriolar changes associated with volume and pressure overload or multiple pulmonary arterial stenoses may remain after otherwise successful corrective surgery. In this setting, the competence of the pulmonary and tricuspid valves, as well as pulmonary ventricular function, are critical, or right heart failure may ensue. Significant pulmonary arterial hypertension can also develop from congenital or postsurgical pulmonary vein stenosis. The latter variety may be more favorable if a technical problem can be fixed by revising the pulmonary venous–atrium anastomosis. Intrinsic pulmonary vein stenosis in isolation or with other defects (typically, complex single ventricle or heterotaxy syndrome) portends a worst prognosis as this is typically a progressive process and surgical or percutaneous angioplasty is not effective. Sometimes, even unilateral pulmonary venous obstruction (e.g. Scimitar syndrome) can lead to severe pulmonary hypertension and RV failure, probably via interlung communication by secreted vasoactive substances (51).

Diagnosis and Management

The recognition of CHF in children and adolescents with or without prior surgical intervention makes full use of patient history, physical examination, laboratory database, and echocardiography. Usually, the diagnosis can be made securely at the bedside, with confirmation of left heart failure by chest X-ray, linkage to a mechanism established from the past history, and echocardiographic findings (Table 20-8). Occasionally, cardiac catheterization may be necessary if pulmonary hypertension is suspected, for further delineation of the anatomic abnormalities, or if a hemodynamic correlation is needed as the final arbiter. This may be more necessary in children because of the difficulty in eliciting a precise history. Finally, the application of plasma natriuretic peptides has great appeal, too, because of the confounding factors involved in evaluating a child. There is no doubt that BNP levels are also elevated in children with heart failure with or without congenital heart disease (19,52,53); the importance will be in demonstrating its utility in the appropriate patient populations for diagnosis and monitoring.

The management of CHF in children and adolescents with congenital heart disease is outlined in Table 20-9. Management begins with a thorough understanding of the previous and current underlying anatomy (natural and surgical), physiology, and function of the cardiovascular system. Most of these patients will have had multiple interactions with the medical system, including prior surgery. It is imperative that old records documenting prior findings at catheterization, surgery, and echocardiography be available and understood. Where surgical therapy has the possibility of improved survival or reduced morbidity, it should be judiciously applied. For failed conduits or prostheses, reoperation is usually the only option. When increased pulmonary vascular resistance, ventricular dysfunction, valvar incompetence, arrhythmia, or endocarditis is present, initial medical management is usually indicated.

Drug therapy is similar to adults with cardiomyopathy. The main difference is that prospective, placebo-controlled, randomized trials with meaningful clinical endpoints are largely lacking in the pediatric and congenital populations. For example, digitalis remains the mainstay of therapy for heart failure, despite lack of evidence for its clinical efficacy,

TABLE 20-8

RECOGNITION OF CONGESTIVE HEART FAILURE IN CHILDREN AND ADOLESCENTS

Weight loss or arrested weight gain, anorexia, nausea
Weight gain
Dyspnea
Excessive absences from school
Lack of interest in playing with peers
Reduced exercise tolerance
Tachycardia
Tachypnea
Elevated central venous pressure
Precordial bulge, ventricular lift
S_3 or S_4 heart sounds
Rales
Hepatomegaly, facial or extremity edema, ascites
Cardiomegaly, pulmonary congestion on chest x-ray
Arrhythmias on ECG
Abnormal anatomy and function on echocardiography

ECG, electrocardiography

particularly in shunt-related heart failure where systolic function is normal. The effects of diuretic therapy are self-evident when congestion is present but long-term benefits have never been established. Afterload reduction with angiotensin-converting enzyme (ACE) inhibitors must be considered integral therapy in patients with systemic ventricular dysfunction or systemic valvar regurgitant lesions. The only exception is in severe pulmonary hypertension. Although without solid data to justify this approach, extrapolation from trials in adults with CHF seems warranted. Because of the ease with which therapy with ACE inhibitors can be carried out, the burden of proof might be on those practitioners who recommend against such empiric treatment. Because of its ability to prevent remodeling and slow progression, many have also adopted a pre-emptive strategy in single ventricle and systemic morphological right ventricle patients as the risk of eventual heart and pump failure is high in these patients.

TABLE 20-9

MANAGEMENT OF CONGESTIVE HEART FAILURE IN CHILDREN AND ADOLESCENTS WITH CONGENITAL HEART DISEASE

Obtain complete records of previous anatomic studies or operations
Obtain complete current anatomic-functional data with echocardiography, MRI, and, if necessary, catheterization
Repair surgically correctable lesions
Reoperate on incomplete or failed repairs, failed or outgrown prostheses
Correct arrhythmias
Provide atrioventricular resynchronization
Optimize preload and afterload
Exclude or treat endocarditis
Optimize medical regimen

Early postoperative elevation of neurohormones has been demonstrated (54,55), but ambulatory values and correlation with outcomes have not been established to define this pre-emptive approach as being evidence-based. As for any vasoactive agent, careful incremental increases and monitoring are needed in pediatric patients. A goal of diuretic therapy would be to obtain the lowest possible filling pressures for decongestion without decreasing cardiac output. This is particularly true in Fontan patients, as they exhibit relative diastolic or AV valve stenosis physiology at baseline. Spironolactone appears to work well in eliminating the need for potassium supplements in children who require loop diuretics. Adverse effects directly related to the above drugs, such as cough or gynecomastia, are extremely uncommon in children. The use of beta-blockade, described elsewhere in this text, has also been adopted in pediatric patients with primary dilated cardiomyopathy (56,57), even as results of a highly anticipated trial are forthcoming (58). However, its use has not been studied except in shunt-related, high-output heart failure in infants (25). Critically ill patients may require inotropic and parenteral vasodilator support.

The group of patients with pulmonary ventricle failure without left side dysfunction may also benefit from pulmonary-specific vasoactive agents. Epoprostenol infusion places patients with a shunt at higher risk for stroke and systemic hypotension. Bosentan, an oral agent approved for idiopathic pulmonary arterial hypertension, is undergoing evaluation for use in pulmonary arterial hypertension with congenital heart disease (59,60). Perhaps more vasoactive is sildenafil, which inhibits phosphodiesterase-5 (rich in the pulmonary vasculature), and is now approved for use in the treatment of pulmonary arterial hypertension (Venice classification Group I) in adults (61,62). What is intriguing is finally the availability of a convenient pulmonary-specific vasodilator, since many congenital patients can benefit from afterload reduction on this side of the circulation as well, with or without pulmonary hypertension (e.g., patients with Fontan construction, Fallot tetralogy, Eisenmenger syndrome, postoperative VSDs, or Ebstein's anomaly).

ADULT

Causes of heart failure from congenital heart disease in unoperated and previously operated patients are shown in Tables 20-10 and 20-11, respectively. Adults with congenital heart disease are a rapidly increasing patient population (63). This has occurred because of the increasing survival of patients with congenital heart disease palliated or corrected earlier in life. Although extracardiac defects such as patent ductus and coarctation were approached in the 1930s and 1940s, intracardiac repair awaited the advent of the heart/lung machine in the 1950s. Ventricular septal defects and TOF were first repaired in 1955, and D-TGA in 1959. The first Fontan procedure was performed in 1971. Thus, a large number of young adults are emerging with operated congenital heart disease (Fig. 20-14). Adults with inoperable or deferred surgery also exist and, at the UCLA Adult Congenital Heart Disease Clinic, occur in numbers equal to those who have had previous surgery (64). Thus, the spectrum of adults with congenital heart disease is broad.

TABLE 20-10
CAUSES OF HEART FAILURE IN ADULTS WITH CONGENITAL HEART DISEASE (UNOPERATED)

Eisenmenger syndrome
Fibrocalcific degeneration of abnormal aortic valve
Systemic ventricular dysfunction and/or tricuspid regurgitation in CTGA
Atrial septal defect with mitral regurgitation secondary to myxomatous mitral valve
Congenital MR
Arrhythmia
Endocarditis
Other degenerative diseases (CAD, hypertension, etc.)
Drug, alcohol abuse
Pregnancy

CTGA, congenitally corrected transposition of the great arteries; MR CAD, coronany artery disease.

The mechanisms for development of CHF in adults with congenital heart disease are similar to those for children and adolescents. In addition, adults have had more time to develop other degenerative diseases that contribute to the development of CHF. These include diabetes, hypertension, coronary artery disease, and renal insufficiency. Pulmonary vascular obstructive disease frequently runs its final course in the fourth and fifth decades of life. Dystrophic fibrosis and calcification of congenitally abnormal aortic valves progress rapidly in some young adults, bringing either important aortic stenosis or insufficiency or their combination to the clinical threshold. Previously asymptomatic patients with ASD may be pushed into CHF by the development of mitral regurgitation or hypertension. Finally, adults have access to cardiotoxic drugs including alcohol, cocaine, and tobacco, which may aggravate myocardial, coronary, or vascular disease.

TABLE 20-11
CAUSES OF CONGESTIVE HEART FAILURE IN ADULTS WITH CONGENITAL HEART DISEASE (OPERATED)

Myocardial dysfunction
Valvular regurgitation
Persistent left-to-right shunt
Pulmonary vascular disease
Prosthetic dysfunction
Status post-Fontan
Arrhythmia
Endocarditis
Other degenerative diseases (coronary artery disease, hypertension, etc.)
Drug, alcohol abuse

Case Studies

Man (Aged 22) with Previous Mustard Operation for D-TGA

This young man recently moved to our area. He had a balloon septostomy and then atrial septectomy shortly after birth. The Mustard procedure was performed at age 3. Over the last several years, he has had multiple hospital admissions for CHF, atrial tachyarrhythmias, and hemoptysis. He was unemployed and essentially homeless. He binged alcohol and smoked. Recent evaluation at our institution by echocardiography and catheterization showed severe systemic ventricular dysfunction and moderate-to-severe systemic AV valve regurgitation. The arrhythmias were identified as atrial flutter and paroxysmal SVT. Inpatient treatment with intravenous nitroprusside, furosemide, and digitalis was begun. He responded and was discharged on digitalis, furosemide, and enalapril but was later readmitted with hemoptysis. An aortogram showed a large bronchial collateral to the right lung (a previously documented site of bleeding), and this was embolized with cessation of bleeding.

He was counseled regarding the importance of compliance and refraining from use of alcohol or tobacco. He responded dramatically, with normalization of jugular venous pressure, resolution of S_3 gallop, and improvement from functional class IV to II status. While visiting relatives, he again binged alcohol and had a recurrence of SVT and decompensated heart failure.

This young man illustrates the sequelae of congenital heart disease and its surgical treatment. He has systemic ventricular dysfunction and atrioventricular valve regurgitation related to the anatomic unsuitability of the morphological right ventricle and tricuspid valve under systemic load and work conditions. He has atrial arrhythmias associated with the extensive atrial suture line from the Mustard procedure. However, if comorbid conditions and behavior are modified, these problems can be controlled. Initially, we thought his prognosis was bleak, with transplantation imminent. Currently, he may have many more years of service from his heart.

Woman (Aged 20) with Previous Repair of Tetralogy of Fallot

A classic Blalock-Taussig shunt was placed shortly after birth to improve pulmonary blood flow. Definitive repair by ventricular septal defect closure, infundibular resection, and transpulmonary annular tract patch were performed at age 5 years. She did well as a child. As a teenager, she exhibited a cardiothoracic ratio of 60%, prolonged QRS of 140 milliseconds, dilated RV and RA, moderate tricuspid valve regurgitation (TR), and free pulmonary insufficiency (PI) with RV pressure less than half systemic. She was able to perform regular daily activities, including attending school and physical education. She was not counseled on family planning in regard to her cardiac condition and she became pregnant after graduation. She was much fatigued, had peripheral edema and intermittent atrial tachycardias, and was finally referred to our adult congenital and perinatal service. Diuretics, digitalis, and meticulous salt, fluid, and nutritional management improved her symptoms.

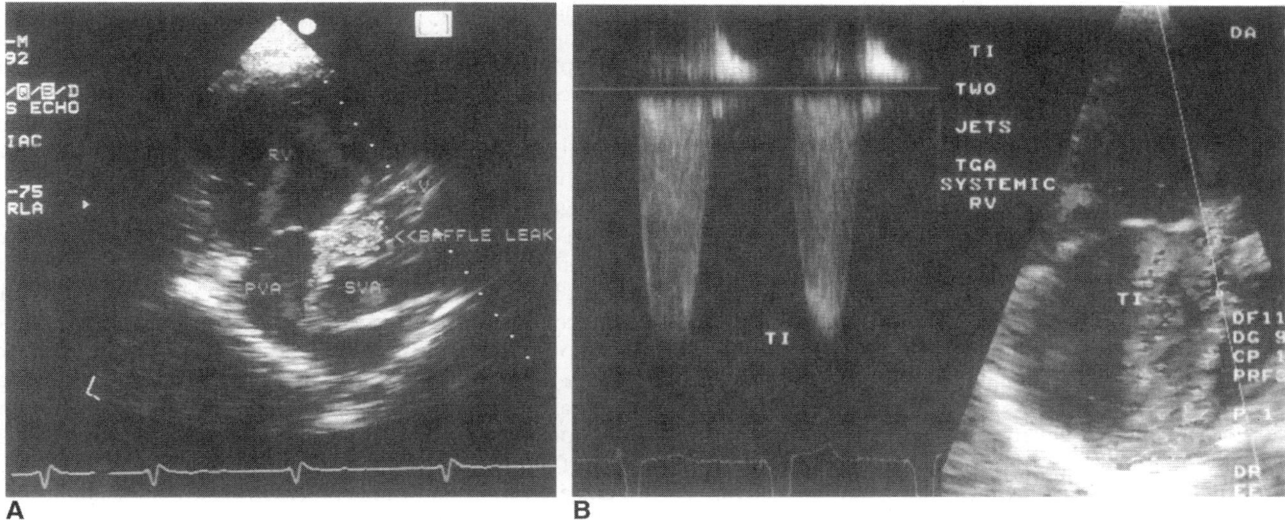

Figure 20-14 Two adults after Mustard atrial repair of D-TGA. One has a left-to-right baffle leak from the pulmonary vein atrium (PVA) the into systemic vein atrium (SVA) **(A)**; the other has moderate tricuspid valve regurgitation (TR) and early decompensation of morphological RV function **(B)**.

After normal fetal echocardiograms during the second trimester, she delivered a healthy infant without complications. However, she has never regained her baseline condition, NYHA class I. She was anticoagulated for chronic atrial flutter and her cardiothoracic ratio increased to 75%. She was also showing early signs of cachexia.

Social workers intervened and were able to arrange for temporary placement of her infant with a family member. After 1 week of fine-tuning with parenteral agents, she underwent pulmonary and tricuspid valve replacement with bioprosthetic valves, atrial reduction, and a maze procedure. Preoperatively and postoperatively, her RV and RA were akinetic, and "smoke" was seen on echocardiography. She had a tumultuous postoperative period with renal and hepatic dysfunction. She also had ventricular tachycardia and slow junctional rhythm and, after going on amiodarone, went on to receive a dual chamber epicardial system with the intention of ventricular pacing to reduce her QRS to 120 from 160 milliseconds.

Although most patients with TOF repair are functional class I or II, some will have significant RV dysfunction and arrhythmias. Eventually, right heart failure occurs and, in this case, was precipitated by pregnancy. It is unclear if preemptive valve replacement before pregnancy would have changed her course and increased the chance of RV recovery.

Man (Aged 37) with Congenitally Corrected Transposition

As an infant, he had a loud murmur thought to be consistent with pulmonary stenosis. Pulmonary valve commissurotomy was performed, and corrected transposition (CTGA) was found unexpectedly. Follow-up catheterization as a child showed pulmonary ventricular pressure of 90 mm Hg from subpulmonic stenosis, but the pulmonary arteries could not be entered. Systemic ventricular function was reduced. After being lost to follow-up, he resurfaced with exertional dyspnea and fatigue, and could not keep up with his work. Chest x-ray showed cardiomegaly and pulmonary edema, and echocardiography confirmed the previous anatomy and showed severe systemic ventricular dysfunction associated with moderate systemic AV valve regurgitation and aortic insufficiency. The pulmonary ventricular function was normal and outflow tract gradient remained at 50 mm Hg. He was referred to our Adult Congenital Heart Clinic. Therapy was begun with hydrochlorothiazide, digoxin, and enalapril. He responded and improved from NYHA class III to II, but because he has no insurance, he now must be unemployed to qualify for Medicaid.

One year ago, he had multiple respiratory infections associated with his children's illnesses. Pulmonary infiltrates were intermittently identified. Several courses of antibiotics were given after blood cultures were negative. His clinical condition deteriorated with increasing dyspnea, fatigue, edema, hepatomegaly, abnormal liver function tests, and renal dysfunction. He was admitted to the hospital. Because of mitral–pulmonary valve continuity, a right heart catheterization was done instead of placement of a thermodilution catheter at bedside. Severely high RV and LV filling pressures with a cardiac index of 1 to 5 L/minute/m^2 was confirmed. Parenteral therapy with dobutamine, furosemide, and milrinone improved his output and promoted a diuresis. Repeat echocardiography confirmed severe, systemic ventricular dysfunction. Follow-up right heart catheterization 1 week later showed improvement in hemodynamics with the pulmonary vascular resistance less than 2 Wood units. He remained inotropic-dependent and was referred for heart transplantation evaluation and received an organ as status 1A.

This man had exhausted the reserve of his systemic morphological RV by the fourth decade of his life. Because he had CTGA, he was never exposed to cyanosis and his only previous surgery was a brief pump run for pulmonary valve commissurotomy. Thus, the morphological RV may not be well-suited for long-term service as the systemic ventricle.

This may particularly be the case with a coexisting abnormality such as subpulmonic stenosis (65). In this patient the pulmonary circuit was never overperfused and his pulmonary vascular resistance was low enough to allow heart transplantation alone. For many patients with end-stage congenital heart disease who could not be more definitively palliated (e.g., closure of high-pressure shunts, diffuse pulmonary arterial stenoses), pulmonary vascular disease will also be present and heart–lung transplantation will be the only recourse.

CONCLUSION

The management of patients with congenital heart disease and CHF has primarily been the responsibility of the pediatrician, the neonatologist, and the pediatric cardiologist. As previously noted, prompt therapy and diagnosis accompanied by sophisticated surgical or interventional correction or palliation have improved the outcome for many of these children who have grown to the adult age. The seamless transition of these patients to an affiliated adult facility under a multidisciplinary approach (pediatric and adult cardiologists and surgeons, social workers, psychiatrists, nutritionists) will be important for these complicated patients, many of whom are defining the natural history of a new disease. Opportunities for offering life-prolonging surgical therapy are more difficult to find in adults with congenital heart disease, and these opportunities cannot be missed. Strategies for early and effective medical management of ventricular dysfunction and valvar regurgitation need to be devised and implemented. Likewise, one can argue that pre-emptive ventricular and pulmonary vascular protection from remodeling for high-risk patients should start even before heart failure develops, as the natural history of this young population can continue to unfold for many decades. A proposed strategy for the prevention of heart failure in patients with congenital heart disease is shown in Table 20-12.

The pediatric cardiologist, surgeon, and pediatric interventionalist have already put early recognition and management into successful practice. Optimizing myocardial preservation and minimizing myocardial incisions are continually reducing surgical injury. Pending further information, it seems reasonable for the pediatric heart failure specialist to extrapolate from studies of other patient groups regarding the potential life-prolonging benefits and morbidity reduction of early and aggressive neurohormonal inhibition. The rapid progression of electrophysiological techniques (physiological pacing, ablation, resynchronization), which can maintain sinus rhythm and electromechanical association, also needs to be integrated into the management. More novel approaches such as oral pulmonary-specific vasodilators, natriuretic peptides as biomarkers and therapy (nesiritide, [66–68]), and beta-blockers in complex anatomical conditions may also make their way into the congenital heart disease practice. Despite these efforts, this aging population will produce a large number of patients with end-stage heart or pulmonary disease (69) and may require organ replacement. Unfortunately, because of organ shortage, poor outcomes in heart–lung transplantation, and constraints of insurance coverage, we may not be able to rely solely on transplantation for all who qualify for this technology.

TABLE 20-12

STRATEGIES TO PREVENT HEART FAILURE IN CONGENITAL HEART DISEASE

Early recognition and elimination of cyanosis, pressure, and volume overload
Elimination of surgical injury
Early afterload reduction and neurohormonal blockade for ventricles at risk,[a] such as:
Fontan procedure
Congenitally corrected transposition (CTGA)
S/P Mustard or Senning procedure for transposition
Regurgitant lesions not appropriate for surgery
Aggressive maintenance of sinus rhythm, AV synchrony[a] and possibly interventricular synchrony[a]

[a]Unproven for this population. AV, atrioventricular.

REFERENCES

1. Holzgreve W, Holzgreve B, Curry CR. Nonimmune hydrops fetalis: diagnosis and management. *Semin Perinatol.* 1985;9: 52–67.
2. Kohl T. Fetal echocardiography: new grounds to explore during fetal cardiac intervention. *Pediatr Cardiol.* 2002;23: 334–346.
3. Tworetzky W, Marshall AC. Fetal interventions for cardiac defects. *Pediatr Clin N Am.* 2004;51:1503–1513.
4. Marshall AC, Van Der Velde ME, Tworetzky W, et al. Creation of an atrial septal defect in utero for fetuses with hypoplastic left heart syndrome and intact or highly restrictive atrial septum. *Circulation.* 2004;110:253–258.
5. Kleinman CS, Copel JA, Weinstein EM, et al. In utero diagnosis and treatment of fetal supraventricular tachycardia. *Semin Perinatol.* 1985;5:113–129.
6. Thornburg KL, Morton MJ. Development of the cardiovascular system. In: Thornburg GD, Harding R, eds. *Textbook of Fetal Physiology.* Oxford: Oxford University Press; 1994: 95–130.
7. Friedman WF. Congenital heart disease in infancy and childhood. In: Braunwald E, ed. *Heart Disease.* Philadelphia: WB Saunders; 1997: 877–955.
8. Kinsella JP, Abman SH. Recent developments in the pathophysiology and treatment of persistent pulmonary hypertension of the newborn. *J Pediatr.* 1995;126:853–864.
9. The Neonatal Inhaled Nitric Oxide Study Group. Inhaled nitric oxide in full-term and nearly full-term infants with hypoxic respiratory failure. *N Engl J Med.* 1997;336:597–604.
10. Manning PB, Mayer JE, Jr., Sanders SP, et al. Unique features and prognosis of primum ASD presenting in the first year of life. *Circulation.* 1994;90:II30–II35.
11. Buyon JP, Rupel A, Clancy RM. Neonatal lupus syndromes. *Lupus.* 1994;13:705–712.
12. Nield LE, Silverman ED, Taylor GP, et al. Maternal anti-Ro and anti-La antibody-associated endocardial fibroelastosis. *Circulation.* 2002;105:843–848.
13. Ross RD, Bollinger RO, Pinsky WW. Grading the severity of congestive heart failure in infants. *Pediatr Cardiol.* 1992;13: 72–75.
14. Connolly D, Rutkowski M, Auslender M, et al. The New York University Pediatric Heart Failure Index: a new method of quantifying chronic heart failure severity in children. *J Pediatr.* 2001;138:644–648.
15. Ross RD. Grading the graders of congestive heart failure in children. *J Pediatr.* 2001;38:618–620.
16. Westerlind A, Wahlander H, Lindstedt G, et al. Clinical signs of heart failure are associated with increased levels of natriuretic peptide types B and A in children with congenital heart defects or cardiomyopathy. *Acta Paediatrica* 2004;93:340–345.

17. Suda K, Matsumura M, Matsumoto M. Clinical implication of plasma natriuretic peptides in children with ventricular septal defect. *Pediatr Int*. 2003;45:249–254.
18. Ohuchi H, Takasugi H, Ohashi H, et al. Stratification of pediatric heart failure on the basis of neurohormonal and cardiac autonomic nervous activities in patients with congenital heart disease. *Circulation*. 2003;108:2368–23676.
19. Law YM, Keller BB, Feingold BM, et al. Usefulness of plasma B-type natriuretic peptide to identify ventricular dysfunction in pediatric and adult patients with congenital heart disease. *Am J Cardiol*. 2005;95:474–478.
20. Friedman WF, George BL. Treatment of congestive heart failure by altering loading conditions of the heart. *J Pediatr*. 1985;106: 697–706.
21. Ross RD, Daniels SR, Schwartz DC, et al. Plasma norepinephrine levels in infants and children with congestive heart failure. *Am J Cardiol*. 1987;59:911–914.
22. Ross RD, Daniels SR, Schwartz DC, et al. Return of plasma norepinephrine to normal after resolution of congestive heart failure in congenital heart disease. *Am J Cardiol*. 1987;60:1411–1413.
23. Buchhorn R, Ross RD, Bartmus D, et al. Activity of the renin-angiotensin-aldosterone and sympathetic nervous system and their relation to hemodynamic and clinical abnormalities in infants with left-to-right shunts. *Int J Cardiol*. 2001;78:225–230.
24. Wu JR, Chang HR, Huang TY, et al. Reduction in lymphocyte beta-adrenergic receptor density in infants and children with heart failure secondary to congenital heart disease. *Am J Cardiol*. 1996;77:170–174.
25. Buchhorn R, Hulpke-Wette M, Hilgers R, et al. Propranolol treatment of congestive heart failure in infants with congenital heart disease: The CHF-PRO-INFANT Trial. Congestive heart failure in infants treated with propanolol. *Int J Cardiol*. 2001;79:167–173.
26. Buchhorn R, Bartmus D, Siekmeyer, et al. Beta-blocker therapy of severe congestive heart failure in infants with left to right shunts. *Am J Cardiol*. 1998;81:1366–1368.
27. Siberry GK, Iannone R, eds. *The Harriet Lane Handbook*, 15th ed. St. Louis: Mosby; 2000: 654,669-692,697,698,704,725,776,791, 829,851.
28. Hoffman TM, Wernovsky G, Atz AM, et al. Efficacy and safety of milrinone in preventing low cardiac output syndrome in infants and children after corrective surgery for congenital heart disease. *Circulation*. 2003;107:996–1002.
29. Oechslin EN, Harrison DA, Connelly MS. Mode of death in adults with congenital heart disease. *Am J Cardiol*. 2000;86: 1111–1116.
30. Krishnan US, Gersony WM, Berman-Rosenzweig E, Apfel HD. Late left ventricular function after surgery for children with chronic symptomatic mitral regurgitation. *Circulation*. 1997;96:4280–4285.
31. Lee JY, Noh CI, Bae EJ, et al. Preoperative left ventricular end systolic dimension as a predictor of postoperative ventricular dysfunction in children with mitral regurgitation. *Heart*. 2003;89: 1243–1244.
32. Freedom RM, Nykanen D, Benson LN. The physiology of the bidirectional cavopulmonary connection. *Ann Thorac Surg*. 1998;66: 664–667.
33. Walker SG, Stuth EA. Single-ventricle physiology: perioperative implications. *Semin Ped Surg*. 2004;3:188–202.
34. de Leval MR. The Fontan circulation: What have we learned? What to expect. *Pediatr Cardiol*. 1998;19:316–320.
35. Krishnan US, Lamour JM, Hsu DT, et al. Management of aortopulmonary collaterals in children following cardiac transplantation for complex congenital heart disease. *J Heart Lung Transp*. 2004;23:564–569.
36. Therrien J, Siu SC, McLaughlin PR, et al. Pulmonary valve replacement in adults late after repair of tetralogy of Fallot: are we operating too late? *J Am Coll Cardiol*. 2000;36:1670–1675.
37. Vliegen HW, van Straten A, de Roos A, et al. Magnetic resonance imaging to assess the hemodynamic effects of pulmonary valve replacement in adults late after repair of tetralogy of Fallot. *Circulation*. 2002;6:1703–1707.
38. Haas G, Laks H, Perloff JK. The selection, use, and long-term effects of prosthetic materials. In: Perloff JK, Child JS, eds. *Congenital Heart Disease in Adults*. Philadelphia: WB Saunders; 1991: 213–223.
39. Fontan F, Kirklin JW, Fernandez G. Outcome after a "perfect" Fontan operation. *Circulation*. 1990;81:1520–1536.
40. Marino BS. Outcomes after the Fontan procedure. *Curr Opin Pediatr*. 2002;14:620–626.
41. Driscoll DJ, Offord KP, Feldt RH. Five- to fifteen-year follow-up after Fontan operation. *Circulation*. 1992;85(2):469–496.
42. Harrison DA, Liu P, Walters JE et al. Cardiopulmonary function in adult patients late after Fontan repair. *J Am Coll Cardiol*. 1995;26:1016–1021.
43. Driscoll DJ, Danielsson GK, Puga FJ, et al. Exercise tolerance and cardiorespiratory response to exercise after the Fontan operation for tricuspid atresia or functional single ventricle. *J Am Coll Cardiol*. 1986;7:1087–1094.
44. Durongpisitkul K, Driscoll DJ, Mahoney DW, et al. Cardiorespiratory response to exercise after modified Fontan operation: determinants of performance. *J Am Coll Cardiol*. 1997;29:785–790.
45. Troutman WB, Barstow TJ, Galindo AJ, et al. Abnormal dynamic cardiorespiratory responses to exercise in pediatric patients after the Fontan procedure. *J Am Coll Cardiol*. 1998;31:668–673.
46. Gatzoulis MA, Balaji S, Webber SA, et al. Risk factors for arrhythmia and sudden cardiac death late after repair of tetralogy of Fallot: a multicentre study. *Lancet*. 2000;356:975–981.
47. Williams WG, Trusler GA, Kirklin JW, et al. Early and late results of a protocol for simple transposition leading to an atrial switch (Mustard) repair. *J Thorac Cardiovasc Surg*. 1988;95:717–726.
48. Janousek J, Vojtovic P, Hucin B, et al. Resynchronization pacing is a useful adjunct to the management of acute heart failure after surgery for congenital heart defects. *Am J Cardiol*. 2001;88:145–152.
49. Dubin AM, Feinstein JA, Reddy M, et al. Electrical resynchronization: a novel therapy for the failing right ventricle. *Circulation*. 2003;107:2287–2289.
50. Janousek J, Tomek V, Chaloupecky V, et al. Cardiac resynchronization therapy: a novel adjunct to the treatment and prevention of systemic right ventricular failure. *J Am Coll Cardiol*. 2004;44:1927–1931.
51. Huddleston CB, Exil V, Canter CE, et al. Scimitar syndrome presenting in infancy. *Ann Thor Surg*. 1999;67:154–159.
52. Nir A, Bar-Oz B, Perles Z, et al. N-terminal pro-B-type natriuretic peptide: reference plasma levels from birth to adolescence. Elevated levels at birth and in infants and children with heart diseases. *Acta Paediatrica*. 2004;93:603–607.
53. Mir TS, Marohn S, Laer S, et al. Plasma concentrations of N-terminal pro-brain natriuretic peptide in control children from the neonatal to adolescent period and in children with congestive heart failure. *Pediatrics*. 2002;110:e76.
54. Mainwaring RD, Lamberti JJ, Carter TL Jr, et al. Renin, angiotensin II, and the development of effusions following bidirectional Glenn and Fontan procedures. *J Cardiac Surg*. 1995;10:111–118.
55. Mainwaring RD, Lamberti JJ, Moore JW, et al. Comparison of the hormonal response after bidirectional Glenn and Fontan procedures. *Ann Thorac Surg*. 1994;57:59–63.
56. Shaddy RE, Tani LY, Gidding SS, et al. Beta-blocker treatment of dilated cardiomyopathy with congestive heart failure in children: a multi-institutional experience. *J Heart Lung Transp*. 1999; 18:269–274.
57. Bruns LA, Chrisant MK, Lamour JM, et al. Carvedilol as therapy in pediatric heart failure: an initial multicenter experience. *Pediatrics*. 2001;138:505–511.
58. Shaddy RE, Curtin EL, Sower B, et al. The Pediatric Randomized Carvedilol Trial in Children with Heart Failure: rationale and design. *Am Heart J*. 2002;144:383–389.
59. Apostolopoulou SC, Manginas A, Cokkinos DV, et al. Effect of the oral endothelin antagonist bosentan on the clinical, exercise, and haemodynamic status of patients with pulmonary arterial hypertension related to congenital heart disease. *Heart*. 2005;10:1136.
60. Barst RJ, Ivy D, Dingemanse J, et al. Pharmacokinetics, safety, and efficacy of bosentan in pediatric patients with pulmonary arterial hypertension. *Clin Pharmacol Ther*. 2003;73:372–382.
61. Madden BP, Sheth A, Ho TB, et al. Potential role for sildenafil in the management of perioperative pulmonary hypertension and right ventricular dysfunction after cardiac surgery. *Br J Anaesthes*. 2004;93:155–156.
62. Sastry BK, Narasimhan C, Reddy NK, et al. Clinical efficacy of sildenafil in primary pulmonary hypertension: a randomized,

placebo-controlled, double-blind, crossover study. *J Am Coll Cardiol.* 2004;43:1149–1153.
63. Perloff JK. A brief historical perspective. In: Perloff JK, Child JS, eds. *Congenital Heart Disease in Adults.* Philadelphia: WB Saunders; 1991: 3–17.
64. Perloff JK. The UCLA congenital heart disease program. *Am J Cardiol.* 1986;57:1190–1192.
65. Connelly MS, Liu PP, Williams WG, et al. Congenitally corrected transposition of the great arteries in the adult: functional status and complications. *J Am Coll Cardiol.* 1996;27: 1238–1243.
66. Marshall J, Berkenbosch JW, Russo P, et al. Preliminary experience with nesiritide in the pediatric population. *J Intens Care Med.* 2004;19:164–170.
67. Feingold B, Law YM. Nesiritide use in pediatric patients with congestive heart failure. *J Heart Lung Transp.* 2004;23: 1455–1459.
68. Munagala VK, Burnett JC, Redfield MN. The natriuretic peptides in cardiovascular medicine. *Curr Probl Cardiol.* 2004;29:707–769.
69. Piran S, Veldtman G, Siu S, et al. Heart failure and ventricular dysfunction in patients with single or systemic right ventricles. *Circulation.* 2002;105:1189–1194.

Right Heart Failure

21

Marvin A. Konstam   Sunny Srivastava   James E. Udelson

Right heart failure may result from dysfunctional right ventricular (RV) myocardium, excessive load imposed on the right ventricle during systole and/or diastole, or obstruction to RV inflow. The clinical expression of right heart failure is similar regardless of cause and is mediated via a combination of elevated systemic venous pressure and depressed cardiac output, with resulting sodium and water retention. The primary manifestations are edema, fatigue, and breathlessness. In addition, the failed right ventricle may adversely influence left ventricular (LV) performance through ventricular interaction and thus may promote signs and symptoms of left heart failure.

In this chapter, we review (a) the pathophysiology and clinical manifestations of right heart failure; (b) assessment of RV function; (c) the various specific causes of right heart failure; (d) the physiology and clinical implications of ventricular interdependence; (e) the manner in which RV performance may relate to the clinical expression of left heart failure; and (f) therapy for right heart failure.

PATHOGENESIS AND CLINICAL MANIFESTATIONS OF RIGHT HEART FAILURE

Right heart failure may be separated into diastolic failure, defined as abnormal elevation in right heart filling pressure, and systolic failure, defined as abnormally low RV forward output. In the absence of a perturbation in the serial nature of left and right heart output (as with intracardiac shunt), depression of right heart forward flow is a necessary accompaniment of a primary reduction in left heart output. This interaction is mediated through an increase in RV afterload and/or relative reduction in right heart inflow.

Load Dependence of Right Ventricular Function

Right ventricle volume and systolic function are exquisitely sensitive to changes in load. The thin RV free wall, normally no more than 4 mm in thickness (1), renders the right ventricle more compliant during both diastole and systole than is the left ventricle (Fig. 21-1) (2–6). That is, increases in diastolic pressure or in systolic pressure are accompanied by relatively large increments in diastolic volume and in end-systolic volume, respectively. The relation between RV afterload and systolic function may be expressed quantitatively through the RV end-systolic pressure–volume relation (Fig. 21-2) (5–8). The slope of this relation represents RV chamber elastance or the ability to sustain contractile performance in response to changes in systolic load. It has been found to increase in response to inotropic stimulation (5). The ventricular systolic pressure–volume slope is shallower for the right ventricle than for the left ventricle because, for the thin-walled right ventricle, a given change in pressure translates into a greater change in wall stress than for the thick-walled left ventricle (6).

A clinically relevant corollary of these observations is that, relative to the left ventricle, the right ventricle is less suited to accommodate to pressure overload but is more suited to accommodate to volume overload. The sensitivity of RV volume to changes in pressure during diastole is responsible for the ability of the RV to accommodate to substantial increases in preload with relatively small increases in systemic venous pressure. However, the

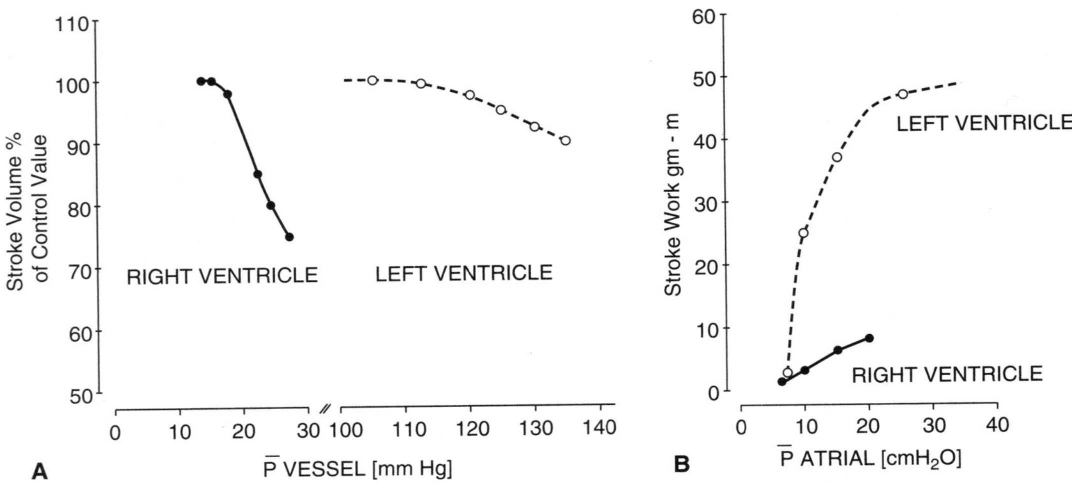

Figure 21-1 **(A)** Effects of increasing afterload and preload on right and left ventricular function. Data were obtained by constricting the main pulmonary artery or aorta in dogs. **B** demonstrates the effect of increasing preload. (Reprinted from McFadden ER Jr., Braunwald E. Cor pulmonale. In: Braunwald E, ed. *Heart Disease. A Textbook of Cardiovascular Medicine.* Philadelphia: WB Saunders; 1988.)

sensitivity of RV end-systolic volume to changes in end-systolic pressure is responsible for the fact that reduction in RV ejection fraction (RVEF) and clinical findings of right heart failure are more commonly manifestations of abnormal afterload, caused by left heart failure or pulmonary vascular pathology, than of intrinsic pathology of the RV myocardium (9–14) (Fig. 21-3). Conversely, RVEF may be maintained in the normal range despite moderate myocardial derangement as long as it is ejecting into a low-resistance circulation. Canine studies indicate that in the setting of acute pulmonary hypertension, inadequacy of RV coronary flow to meet the increased metabolic demand contributes to reduction in RV systolic performance (15).

The development of RV hypertrophy in response to chronic pressure overload results in reduction in wall stress for any given intracavitary pressure. As hypertrophy progresses, the mechanical characteristics of the right ventricle become more similar to those of the left ventricle, retaining systolic function in the face of heightened pulmonary artery (PA) pressure but requiring higher filling pressure to maintain preload and forward flow. In patients with pul-

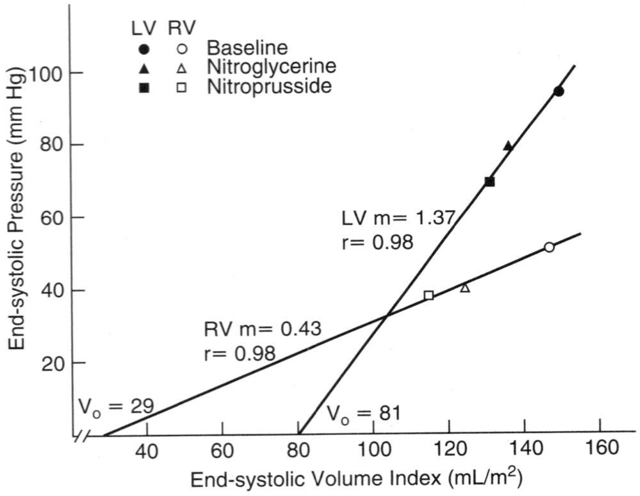

Figure 21-2 Comparison of left and right ventricular end-systolic pressure–volume relations (group mean data with linear regression lines) derived from 10 patients with biventricular failure secondary to healed myocardial infarction or dilated cardiomyopathy. Pulmonary or systemic arterial end-systolic (dicrotic notch) pressures are plotted against radionuclide-derived right or left ventricular end-systolic volumes, respectively, at baseline and during infusion of nitroglycerin and nitroprusside. The shallower slope of the right ventricular relationship indicates less right ventricular systolic stiffness compared with the left ventricle. That is, identical changes in systolic pressure effect greater changes in systolic performance for the right ventricle than for the left ventricle. (Reprinted from Konstam MA, Levine HJ. Effects of afterload and preload on right ventricular systolic performance. In: Konstam MA, Isner JM, eds. *The Right Ventricle.* Boston: Kluwer; 1988.)

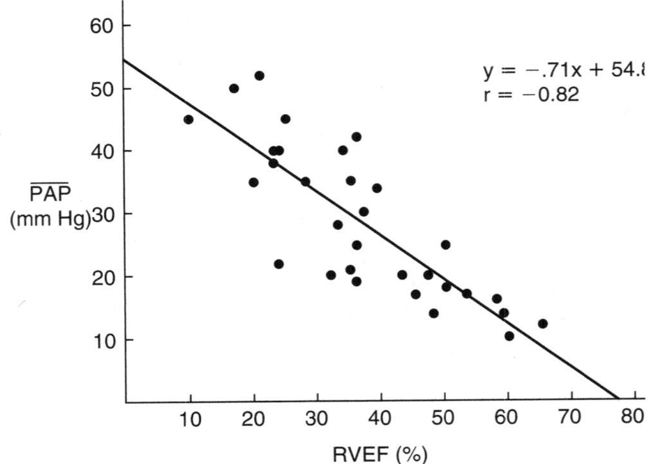

Figure 21-3 Relation between RVEF and mean pulmonary artery pressure (PAP) in patients with diagnoses of coronary artery disease or valvular heart disease. (Reprinted from Korr KS, Gandsman EJ, Winkler ML, et al. Hemodynamic correlates of right ventricular ejection fraction measured with gated radionuclide angiography. *Am J Cardiol.* 1982;49:71–77.)

monary hypertension, the degree to which RV hypertrophy develops and serves to maintain systolic function depends, in part, on the rapidity and age of onset of the hemodynamic stimulus. With progressive hypertrophy, RV systolic function may deteriorate, possibly because of intrinsic myocardial contractile dysfunction associated with cardiac hypertrophy. This occurrence is controversial, with some but not all studies of experimentally induced RV hypertrophy showing reduction of intrinsic contractility (16–20). These studies have documented intrinsic contractile derangement during the early stages of pressure-overload hypertrophy, as indicated by reduction in the maximum unloaded velocity and in the maximum rate of tension development of isolated myocardium. However, in time, these abnormalities have generally been observed to revert toward normal. Alternatively, a limitation in coronary flow reserve has been documented in animal models and in patients with RV myocardial hypertrophy, and may result in ischemic contractile dysfunction (21,22).

Depending on the rate and extent of progression of RV pressure overload (of any etiology), RV hypertrophy may be inadequate to maintain a normal level of systolic stress. As RV systolic stress becomes excessive (perhaps compounded by intrinsic RV myocardial contractile dysfunction), ejection performance declines. Under these conditions, the right ventricle generally distends during diastole, in part representing a compensatory mechanism by which preload is recruited to maintain stroke volume. The RV distension is accelerated by the advent of tricuspid regurgitation (TR), which tends to thwart the compensatory Starling mechanism. Thus, in a variety of circumstances, RV pressure overload and volume overload coexist.

Clinical Findings in Right Heart Failure

In clinical practice, systolic and diastolic right heart failure, regardless of cause, often coincide. The clinical expression of right heart failure depends on a combination of elevated systemic venous pressure and depressed cardiac output. Clinical findings depend on the chronicity of hemodynamic derangement. Acute right heart failure, as caused by RV infarction, is characterized by signs and symptoms of depressed cardiac output and elevated jugular venous pressure, often with prominent v-wave and *y*-descent. Other findings that may be present include RV S_3 gallop, a murmur of TR, and the Kussmaul sign (23–26). Edema has not had time to develop. Acute severe pulmonary embolism presents a similar picture (27–29). Additional signs of chronic pulmonary hypertension with RV hypertrophy—RV heave, RV S_4 gallop, prominent jugular venous A-wave—may or may not be present because hypertrophy has not had time to develop, and the normal thin-walled right ventricle is limited in the level of PA pressure that it can generate (30,31).

With chronic right heart failure of any cause, edema becomes a prominent feature (32). In addition to peripheral edema and ascites, edema of the visceral organs contributes to alteration in hepatic, renal, and intestinal function. Pleural effusions develop as a result of impediment to parietal pleural drainage. Other clinical signs depend on the etiology of right heart failure. For example, pulmonary vascular disease or recurrent pulmonary emboli are associated with signs of pulmonary hypertension and RV hypertrophy: RV heave, loud pulmonic component of the second heart sound, and RV S_4 gallop (27–29).

Systemic Neurohormonal Responses

Systemic neurohormonal activation plays an important role in mediating the clinical manifestations of right heart failure. The development of edema (discussed later) is supported by renal sodium retention provoked by reduced forward cardiac output and perturbation of neuroendocrine activity (33). These mechanisms are described in detail elsewhere in this volume. In brief, reduction in cardiac output directly reduces glomerular filtration rate, diminishing tubular sodium delivery. Activation of the renin-angiotensin-aldosterone axis stimulates sodium-potassium exchange (34,35). In the setting of right heart failure, increased renin secretion, leading to enhanced vasoconstriction and sodium retention, is accentuated by augmented adrenergic activity (35). The latter is supported by impairment of baroreceptor function (36).

An increase in right atrial (RA) pressure stimulates release of atrial natriuretic peptide (ANP), and patients with heart failure have been found to have a two- to tenfold increase in circulating levels of ANP compared with normals (37–40). However, in patients with heart failure, end-organ responsiveness to ANP is severely reduced (41). This feature accounts for further reduction in glomerular filtration rate through glomerular afferent arteriolar constriction and may accelerate tubular sodium resorption.

Differential Neurohormonal Responses in the Left and Right Ventricles

Cardiac neurohormonal stimulation and response are differentially regulated across the two ventricles in a manner that appears to be linked to the nature of the hemodynamic derangement. In a rat model of LV infarction and failure, regional sympathetic activity, as assessed by ventricular norepinephrine turnover, is increased within the left ventricle but not the right ventricle (42). Increased regional sympathetic activity may be responsible for the finding of differentially reduced β-receptor density and diminished adenylyl cyclase activity within the left but not the right ventricle within the same animal model (43). On the other hand, in this model of left heart failure, RV myocardial concentrations of both norepinephrine and epinephrine are increased, whereas similar increases have not been observed in other organs (42). These observations may imply a specific increase in RV uptake of circulating catecholamines in the setting of left heart failure. In contrast to the rat myocardial infarction (MI) model, heart failure in the spontaneously hypertensive rat has been found to be associated with preferential downregulation in RV β-receptor density (44).

Experimentally induced right heart failure has been found to diminish RV norepinephrine uptake-1 carrier density and norepinephrine uptake activity (Fig. 21-4) (45). This abnormality appears to be directly related to a

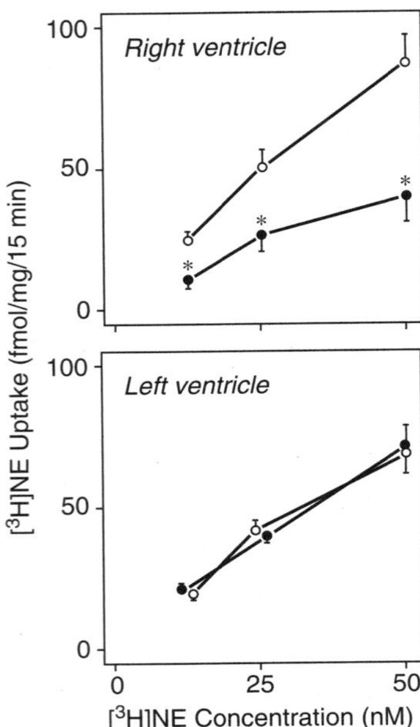

Figure 21-4 Specific ^{3}H uptake activity (representing tissue ^{3}H-norepinephrine [NE] uptake), at three concentrations of ^{3}H-NE, using fresh tissue slices taken from the right and left ventricular free walls of sham-operated dogs **(open circles)** and dogs with experimentally induced right heart failure **(closed circles)**. In dogs with right heart failure, there is reduction in NE uptake within right ventricular, but not left ventricular, myocardium. (Reprinted from Liang CS, Fan TH, Sullebarger JT, et al. Decreased adrenergic neuronal uptake activity in experimental right heart failure. A chamber specific contributor to beta-adrenoceptor downregulation. *J Clin Invest.* 1989;84:1267–1275.)
*Significant difference from sham-operated group.

regional perturbation of cardiac function, perhaps because of altered myocardial stress, as it was not evident within the LV myocardium in a model with isolated right heart failure (45). Reduced norepinephrine uptake may, in part, be responsible for excess exposure of myocardial β receptors to circulating and neuronally released norepinephrine, thereby yielding reduced norepinephrine sensitivity.

Thus, regulation of RV sympathetic activity and of signal transduction pathways is complex, is influenced by differences in the hemodynamic state, and is distinct from regulatory mechanisms occurring in the left ventricle.

Pathogensis of Edema

Edema of peripheral tissues and systemic organs, a prominent feature of chronic right heart failure (32), generally requires both elevation of central venous pressure and a stimulus for renal sodium and water retention. Because detectable edema requires an increase of approximately 5 L of extracellular fluid in an adult human (46), hemodynamic derangement must be prolonged before edema becomes apparent. Additional factors may accelerate the development of edema. Normally, competent venous valves and muscular activity in anatomically dependent zones tend to mitigate against transudation of intravascular fluid to the extravascular compartment. Potential factors that may provoke or accentuate tissue edema include incompetence of peripheral venous valves, muscular inactivity, and reduced plasma oncotic pressure.

Manifestations of right heart failure are not merely the direct effect of altered RV hemodynamics. Rather, the right heart interfaces with, and contributes to, a perturbed neurohormonal milieu. A vicious cycle is established, with altered RV systolic and diastolic performance leading to vascular, renal, and neuroendocrine abnormalities, leading to further right heart dysfunction as a result of progressively abnormal RV loading conditions.

In patients with heart failure, excess pleural fluid is most common when elevations of pulmonary venous pressure and central venous pressure coincide. Pleural fluid is drained (a) by parietal pleural lymphatic vessels that empty into the systemic veins, as well as (b) via visceral pleural communication to the pulmonary venous system (47–49). Therefore, in the presence of left heart failure or right heart failure in isolation, one drainage route is likely to compensate for failure of the alternate route. In studies of patients with chronic cor pulmonale and elevated RA pressure, in the absence of left heart failure, pleural effusions have not been frequently observed (50). However, pleural effusion has been ascribed to systemic venous hypertension without pulmonary venous hypertension in the setting of acute RV MI (25,51). It is likely that in patients with chronic right heart failure, without left heart failure, alternative pleural drainage routes, which are not operative acutely, are ultimately recruited.

Clinical findings published in the 1940s tended to support the view that pleural effusions secondary to heart failure occurred predominantly on the right (52–54). However, more recent postmortem and clinical studies have indicated that between 70% and 90% of patients with heart failure and pleural effusions manifest bilateral pleural fluid (55,56). In the small number of patients with unilateral effusions, the ratio of right-sided to left-sided effusions is approximately 2 to 1. Differences between the findings of older versus newer literature have been attributed to implementation of potent diuretics (56). In patients in whom pleural effusions occur in association with primary pericardial disease, the pleural fluid has been observed to be predominantly left-sided (57). It has been speculated that this finding may be directly related to the presence of pericardial inflammation (57). Pleural effusions caused by heart failure are predominantly transudative, being primarily the product of abnormal hydrostatic forces. In some studies, diuresis has been observed to transform the chemical composition of pleural fluid to that of a "pseudoexudate" (58), although others have found this occurrence to be unusual (59).

In patients with heart failure, failure of systemic organs predominantly results from a combination of increased venous pressure and reduced arterial perfusion. Tissue ischemia tends to accelerate formation of interstitial edema through capillary membrane injury. In turn, edema contributes to tissue ischemia through an increase in interstitial pressure, thus impeding blood flow. A vicious cycle is established that may be acutely exacerbated by an abrupt increase in venous pressure and/or an abrupt reduction in perfusion pressure. These events may lead to chronic renal dysfunction, sometimes with superimposed acute tubular necrosis. Similarly, severe right heart failure is frequently associated with chronic hepatic dysfunction as a result of the combination of edema, ischemia, and impediment to venous drainage, with chronic elevation in serum transaminase as well as alkaline phosphatase and bilirubin. The latter is often predominantly indirect, indicating a deficiency in conjugation. Acute severe liver injury is common and may or may not be preceded by abrupt overt elevation in systemic venous pressure. Severe elevation in serum transaminase may occur and may be associated with a cholestatic picture. It is not uncommon that these findings are confused with acute viral hepatitis or chronic primary liver disease until it is appreciated that central venous pressure is elevated. Furthermore, because venous pressure may fluctuate and because abrupt reduction of hepatic arterial perfusion, rather than abrupt increase in hepatic venous pressure, may be the direct stimulus to liver necrosis, systemic venous pressure may not be severely elevated at the time when hepatic injury is clinically recognized.

Anorexia, malabsorption, and reduced responsiveness to oral medications have been attributed to intestinal edema in patients with right heart failure. However, cachexia in heart failure is likely to be multifactorial, resulting from a combination of anorexia, malabsorption, relatively increased metabolic demand, and possibly humoral factors (60–64). Recently, patients with heart failure and cachexia have been found to have increased circulating levels of tumor necrosis factor, which may play a causative role in this syndrome (65).

ASSESSMENT OF RIGHT VENTRICULAR FUNCTION

In the past, the importance of the right ventricle in cardiac disease had been largely underestimated. It is now well known that right ventricular volume, mass, and function influence outcomes of many cardiac disease syndromes, such as MI, chronic heart failure, and a variety of congenital malformations.

Quantification of ventricular function is technically more difficult and less exact for the right ventricle than for the left ventricle. While the elliptical left ventricle resembles a more convenient volumetric model, the RV has a complex, crescentic shape that defies a conventional geometric description. This is compounded by coarse trabeculations, a separate infundibulum, a thinner myocardium, geometric complexity with discrete inflow and outflow portions, as well as variations in right ventricular shape which occur with altered loading conditions (66).

The RV chamber is bounded by a free wall and a thick-walled septum that occupies most of the posterior and medial surfaces of the chamber. The RV body, or inflow region, is normally concave around the intrerventricular septum. Contraction resembles the movement of a rounded bellow, the walls of which approach each other in a parallel manner during systole. Across the base of these bellow is the crista supraventricularis, which is a thick muscle bundle that closes the bellows during normal systolic contraction. The other walls are thin and their trabeculae act as chords to assist in bellows closure during systole. Therefore, unlike what is seen in the left ventricle, wall motion observed in one region of the RV may in fact be due to muscle contraction occurring at a distance from that wall (67).

As mentioned previously, the RV often changes its shape and its motion patterns substantially in the setting of pressure and/or volume overload. Paradoxical septal motion seen with prolonged pressure overload consists of septal endocardial and epicardial movement toward the RV during systole, rather than its normal pattern toward the center of the LV cavity (though wall thickening is preserved). In patients with volume overload, the curvature of the interventricular septum is displaced toward the left ventricle at end-diastole, concave toward the right ventricle because of the increased diastolic load. At end-systole, the ventricles return toward a more normal configuration, resulting in motion of the septum toward the RV (68–76).

For all of these reasons, the RV is poorly amenable to geometric modeling for the purpose of volume measurement. Despite these difficulties, numerous studies have examined imaging modalities to estimate relative change in RV volume through the cardiac cycle and thus to measure RVEF.

Most studies investigating RV function have found the range of normal ejection fractions to be lower than that of the left ventricle. The lower limit of RVEF has generally been found to be in the range of 40% to 45%. This finding indicates that normal end-diastolic and end-systolic volumes are larger for the right ventricle than for the left ventricle, with the upper limit of normal for RV end-diastolic volume estimated as 120 mL/m^2 (77).

Right ventricular function may be assessed by the use of any modality with the capability of estimating relative changes in RV volume; this is a field that has changed rapidly over the past 5 to 10 years. Several modalities have been investigated, including contrast ventriculography, radionuclide ventriculography, echocardiography, magnetic resonance imaging, and cine computerized tomography.

Contrast Ventriculography

Contrast ventriculography, performed by the catheter administration of radiocontrast media, was the first method employed for visualization of the right ventricle. This technique had long been the gold standard for assessment of RV volumes and functional measurements. In order to estimate ventricular volumes, this method typically requires an assumption of a geometric model for approximating the overall ventricular shape. Additionally, Simpson's rule can be used, where the ventricle is divided into a series of segments and the volume of each segment is derived after approximating its shape. There are several factors that diminish the accuracy of these methods, however. First, it is more difficult to accurately delineate the borders of the ventricular cavity at end-systole as a result of the heavy trabeculations. Secondly, the previously mentioned tendency for the RV shape to be significantly changed as a result of various pathological states and their resulting altered loading conditions render any geometric models to essentially be rough estimates of cavity shape. Finally, as opposed to the LV which retains its elliptical shape during systole, the RV cavity contour may be significantly different at end-systole when compared to end-diastole (78–80).

There are other pitfalls of contrast ventriculography to consider, as well. Even though right heart catheterization carries less of a risk than left heart catheterization, the test is still an invasive procedure. Furthermore, injection of contrast media into the right ventricle is not without risk, especially in those with RV disease or elevated pulmonary pressures. The procedure is time-consuming and often requires the employment of rigorous methodology. As a result of all of these factors, it cannot be routinely utilized for repeated measurements in a serial manner when following patients who would otherwise not need a right heart catheterization (79).

Radionuclide Ventriculography

Radionuclide ventriculography (RVG) is a method that was first introduced in the early 1970s. It uses intravascular agents that emit gamma radiation subsequently detected by an external device to visualize the cardiac chambers. Two applications of RVG have generally been used to assess RV volume and function. These include first-pass radionuclide ventriculography and equilibrium radionuclide angiography (ERNA).

The first-pass method is well-suited for visualization of the right heart because it precedes pulmonary and systemic tracer circulation and, as a result, there is an absence of background or chamber overlap. Even though there is a lack of dependence on geometric assumptions, there are still significant problems with the first-pass method. Only several cardiac cycles can be incorporated into the study and, as a result, accuracy may be diminished in the setting of motion or arrhythmia. In addition, the advantage of minimal background activity is lost when repeated studies are needed in the setting of acute interventions (78). Although widely used in the past for calculations of intracardiac shunting, most laboratories have little experience with this technique in the contemporary era.

ERNA is a method with several advantages to first-pass imaging. It is a technique that allows image acquisition to occur over several minutes. Numerous cardiac cycles are incorporated into the study by electrocardiographic gating, thus increasing the temporal resolution as well as reducing the likelihood that the presence of a transient arrhythmia will diminish the accuracy of the study. It should also be noted that there is a high degree of correlation with first-pass scintigraphy for RVEF as well as minimal intraobserver variation (81), but there still exists the problem of overlap between the RV and its surrounding chambers. The overlap between the right and left ventricle is minimized in the left anterior oblique (LAO) view and a modified LAO view helps to minimize the overlap between the RA and RV. Furthermore, overlap may be exacerbated in conditions where the RA or RV is enlarged (78,82). RVG is noninvasive, easy to perform, not time-consuming, and has a fairly high level of accuracy and reproducibility that is not subject to a patient's body habitus, as is often the case with echocardiography, for example.

There are some disadvantages to RVG that must be considered when contemplating the ideal imaging modality for the RV. While it is suitable to evaluate the size and performance of the RV, it lacks the ability to evaluate wall thickness and RV mass. In addition, there is exposure to ionizing radiation, especially when applied in a serial manner for follow-up studies. This technique also suffers from attenuation artifacts as well as difficulty in minimizing the overlap of the RA and RV. As a result, there is an underestimation of EF when compared with values obtained via contrast ventriculography (67,83). Nonetheless, although absolute volumes and EF may be systematically overestimated and underestimated, respectively, *changes* in those parameters in serial studies over time, as in a clinical trial examining the effect of a therapy on the RV in heart failure, for example, may be robust.

Echocardiography

In the past, M-mode, two dimensional, and Doppler echocardiography were the only ultrasound-guided approaches available to clinicians for visualization of cardiac structures. These techniques have been useful in the evaluation of the size and function of the left ventricle but their use has been somewhat limited in assessing the right ventricle. More recently, however, three-dimensional echocardiography has become an increasingly available and promising tool, more applicable to the unusual structure of the right ventricle.

Because of the complex geometry and the peculiar changes seen with volume or pressure overload for the right ventricle that have been outlined earlier, it is difficult to derive any quantitative indices of RV function by two-dimensional echocardiography (78). This technique has been able to provide information regarding RV volume and can reliably differentiate RV volume overload from a normal right ventricle. Assessment of RV function has been limited by difficulties in defining the endocardium properly, as well as the complex RV geometry that has been previously outlined. As a result, routine two-dimensional echocardiographic assessment of the right ventricle has been somewhat limited and has largely been qualitative (84,85).

Doppler echocardiography has provided the ability to accurately assess RV systolic pressures, as RV pressure overload is generally associated with functional tricuspid regurgitation. The systolic pressure gradient between the RV and the RA may be estimated by the modified Bernoulli formula, $4V^2$, where V is the peak velocity of the regurgitant tricuspid jet. Addition of an estimated RA pressure yields an accurate assessment of RV systolic pressure (86).

Three-dimensional echocardiography is a relatively new and promising technique that permits noninvasive imaging of the RV in real time. It overcomes some of the limitations of two-dimensional echo by reconstructing the ventricle without the need for geometric assumptions or standardized imaging planes. It combines multiple intersecting planes, thereby improving the consistency of border detection (87,88). Studies have shown that three-dimensional echo is a reliable method to assess end-diastolic volumes of normal and diseased right ventricles and it has the ability to take into account variations of RV anatomy (89). End-systolic volumes are less accurate, and this is probably due to the fact that RV trabeculations are more pronounced in systole than in diastole and, as a result, may influence identification of the endocardial borders. RV mass measurements are thought to be less accurate as well, likely due to the difficulties encountered in obtaining two-dimensional transthoracic datasets which include the entire epicardium, especially at the apex and the apical free wall of the RV (90).

In addition to the difficulties in assessing end-systolic volumes and RV mass, there remain technical challenges to wider use of three-dimensional echocardiography. Data acquisition and image reconstruction are still time-consuming and burdensome. One improvement may take the form of improved automatic border detection software; however, cost is still somewhat prohibitive. An advantage of three-dimensional echocardiography, however, is that volumetric data may be assessed without cardiac or respiratory gating in real time and the technique is completely noninvasive, theoretically allowing image acquisition with a handheld transducer and a portable machine.

Computed Tomography

The improvement seen in spatial and temporal resolution with multidetector row CT (MDCT) compared to spiral and electron beam CT has opened up many new possibilities in cardiac imaging. With multidetector scanning, it is possible to acquire high-resolution, three-dimensional images of the heart and great vessels. Cardiac CT is especially useful in evaluating the myocardium, coronary arteries, pulmonary veins, thoracic aorta, pericardium, and cardiac masses. In addition, studies have shown that assessment of global right ventricular function with cardiac 16-detector-row CT is possible and reproducible (91); however, much of the research has been focused on MDCT and its ability to detect coronary artery disease. Nonetheless, studies have now shown that CT assessment of RV volume is reasonably precise and reproducible, as is assessment of RV mass (Fig. 21-5) (92,93).

With regard to RV function, there is good correlation with magnetic resonance imaging (MRI) for RV stroke volume and RVEF. End-systolic and end-diastolic RV volumes have also shown fairly good correlation with MRI studies, but there appears to be a slight overestimation of these volumes with MDCT. This is likely due to the limited temporal resolution of MDCT compared with MR imaging (91). This latter limitation may be attenuated as more advanced CT technology with 32- and 64-detector-row CT scanners becomes more widely available; however, there is a paucity of data at this time focusing on the assessment of RV function with this more advanced technology.

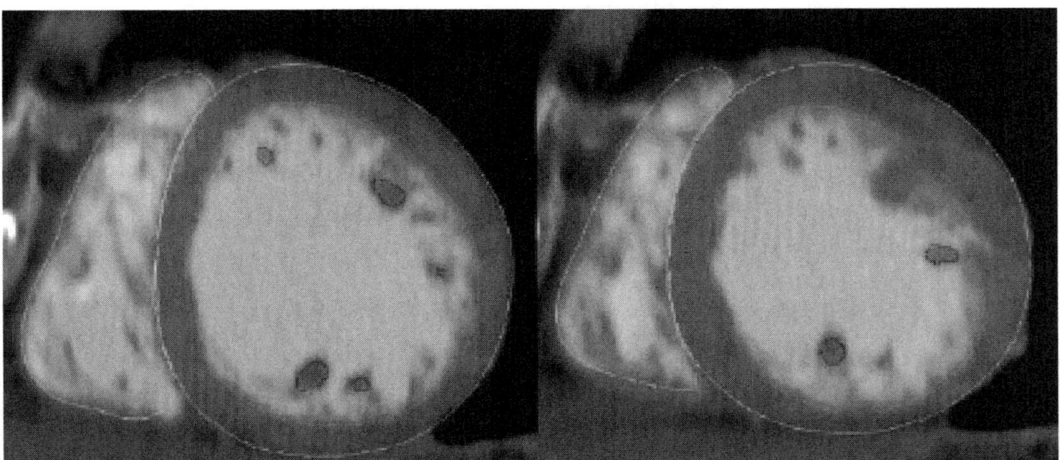

A

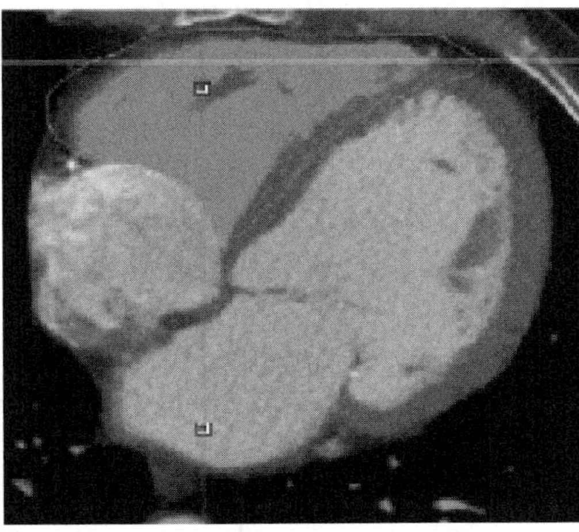

B

Figure 21-5 (A) Representative short axis view of the right and left ventricles by multidetector computed tomography (MDCT) at end diastole and end systole with the endocardial borders outlined. **(B)** Axial MDCT image with the right ventricle as the region of interest, shaded gray. (Reprinted from Koch K, Oellig F, Oberholzer K, et al. Assessment of right ventricular function by 16-detector-row CT: comparison with magnetic resonance imaging. *Eur Radiol.* 2005;15:312–318.)

MDCT is clearly an evolving technology, but it does not represent the test of choice when assessing RV volume and mass at this time. The presence of a regular cardiac rhythm is essential for optimum acquisition and, with 16-slice equipment, the necessary breath-hold of 20 to 25 seconds and the contrast load can be too burdensome for some patients. As 64-slice technology becomes more widespread, requiring only 5 seconds of breath-hold, research into this area will likely advance, as it will facilitate the study of patients with heart failure. Moreover, as more implantable cardiac defibrillators are placed and such patients become ineligible for MRI examination, the role of cardiac CT will likely grow substantially in the near future for evaluation of ventricular volumes and function.

Magnetic Resonance Imaging

Cardiac magnetic resonance (CMR) imaging has become a sophisticated diagnostic technique for cardiovascular imaging that utilizes high intensity magnetic fields and radiofrequency to generate three-dimensional/tomographic images, resulting in studies with high resolution and excellent contrast. There are several available techniques within the MRI system, but two are the mainstay of clinical CMR: spin echo imaging and cine MRI. Spin echo imaging depicts tissue structures of the heart as bright and the blood pool as dark; it is largely employed for the evaluation of anatomy and structure, assessing myocardial mass or regions of infarction, as well as identifying the fatty infiltration seen in arrhythmogenic RV dysplasia, for instance (94). The other technique, cine MRI, generates images in which the blood pool is bright and the cardiac structures are dark; it is used primarily to evaluate ventricular function and volumes, valvular lesions, and to detect intracardiac masses. This stark contrast between blood and tissue allows accurate assessment of the ventricular wall, function, and size of the chamber.

CMR has demonstrated substantial accuracy and reproducibility in assessing LV volumes, function, and mass. Because of the aforementioned geometric difficulties in assessing the RV, CMR is an ideal modality to examine the RV because of the three-dimensional volume acquisition of the chamber (83), and the complete tomographic interrogation of the three-dimensional structure in the absence of overlap (Fig. 21-6). CMR of RV volumes has shown excellent correlation with other techniques such as contrast ventriculography and RVG (95). It has also shown good interstudy reproducibility for RV function, which is key when monitoring a patient's response to a therapeutic intervention over a long period of time or for use in clinical trials (83).

One distinct advantage of CMR is that RV volume measurements can be performed irrespective of the ventricular shape and, as a result, CMR is now considered to be the gold standard of RV volume assessment (89). In addition, CMR can provide any desired imaging plane without the need for contrast or ionizing radiation. It is a noninvasive, safe, and repeatable technique. Furthermore, there is no problem with the poor acoustic windows that can be encountered in echocardiography. Despite the need for expensive nonportable equipment, as well as a long and complicated examination, CMR can now be considered the preferred noninvasive modality for determining RV volume, mass, and function.

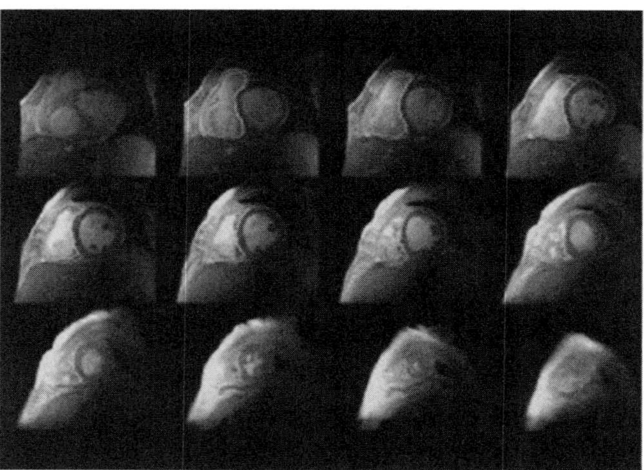

Figure 21-6 Representative cardiac magnetic resonance (CMR) images: contiguous end-diastolic short axis images covering both ventricles from base to apex in a patient with a dilated cardiomyopathy. The epicardial and endocardial boundaries are easily traced for mass and end-diastolic volume calculations. End-systolic volumes, end-diastolic volumes, and ejection fraction can be calculated once the full coverage images are obtained. (Reprinted from Grothues F, Moon J, Bellenger N, et al. Interstudy reproducibility of right ventricular volumes, function, and mass with cardiovascular magnetic resonance. *Am Heart J.* 2004;147(2):218–223, with permission.)

ETIOLOGIES OF RIGHT VENTRICULAR FAILURE

Table 21-1 presents a differential diagnosis of right heart failure, broadly subdivided into primary myocardial dysfunction, pressure overload, and volume overload. As previously mentioned, these pathophysiological states often coexist. The most common cause of RV pressure overload, left heart failure, is further discussed in a later section. In addition, RV failure may be simulated by disorders that impede inflow into the right ventricle. These disorders include tricuspid stenosis, cardiac tamponade, pericardial constriction, and restrictive myopathy. Although this category is not discussed here in detail, restrictive myopathies are covered in the Cardiomyopathy section.

Right Ventricular Myocardial Dysfunction

Right Ventricular Myocardial Infarction

The clinical syndrome of RV MI was first described in the 1970s as a syndrome involving diminished cardiac output with clear lungs and jugular venous distension (23,25,96). Since those initial descriptions, the described clinical spectrum of RV involvement in myocardial infarction has broadened considerably (97–99). Pathologically, infarction involving the right ventricle most often is an accompaniment of infarction involving the posterior free wall of the left ventricle and the posterior portion of the ventricular septum (96). The extent of involvement of the RV

TABLE 21-1
DIFFERENTIAL DIAGNOSIS OF RIGHT HEART FAILURE

I. RV myocardial dysfunction
  A. RV myocardial infarction
  B. Dilated cardiomyopathy
  C. RV dysplasia

II. Primary RV pressure overload
  A. Left ventricular failure
  B. Mitral valve disease
  C. Atrial myxoma
  D. Pulmonary veno-occlusive disease
  E. Cor pulmonale
    1. Obstructive lung disease
    2. Primary pulmonary hypertension
    3. Pulmonary emboli
  F. Pulmonic stenosis
    1. Supravalvular
    2. Valvular
    3. Subvalvular
  G. Ventricular septal defect
  H. Aortopulmonary communication

III. Primary RV volume overload
  A. Pulmonic regurgitation
  B. Tricuspid regurgitation
  C. Atrial septal defect
  D. Partial anomalous pulmonary venous return

IV. Impediment to RV inflow
  A. Tricuspid stenosis
  B. Cardiac tamponade
  C. Pericardial constriction
  D. Restrictive cardiomyopathy

RV, right ventricular.

free wall is variable and does not necessarily correlate with the degree of hemodynamic perturbation. Profoundly abnormal hemodynamics may be observed in the presence of an anatomically small extent of RV involvement with infarction. Less common pathologically is involvement of the anterolateral RV free wall with anterior infarctions (99). These infarctions tend to be anteroseptal, extensive, and associated with moderate to severe reduction in LV ejection fraction (99). Hemodynamically relevant RV infarction almost always signifies evidence of right coronary occlusion proximal to the RV free wall branches (100).

Elevation of jugular venous pressure in a patient with an electrocardiographic inferior infarction usually indicates RV infarction. Right precordial leads often document RV infarction, with ST elevation in leads V_3R and V_4R (98). RVG or echocardiography may demonstrate RV dilation with regional and global RV functional abnormalities (101). Hemodynamic measurements in the setting of acute RV infarction most commonly reveal elevation of RA and RV diastolic pressure, which are often equilibrated with PA diastolic and PA wedge pressures, a pattern similar to pericardial constriction (23,34,96). The RA pressure wave form often resembles an M or a W, with y descent deeper than x descent. In some patients, however, these findings are not seen, and low pressures may be observed in both the right atrium and the pulmonary wedge position. In such patients, the hemodynamic abnormalities may be brought out by volume loading (102). The constellation of hemodynamic findings seen in RV infarction appears to require the presence of an intact pericardium. In animal models of RV infarction, the hemodynamic abnormalities improve markedly following pericardiotomy (103).

The outcome of patients sustaining an MI with RV involvement appears to be dependent on the extent of LV infarction, as the presence or absence of hemodynamic or noninvasive evidence of RV dysfunction in acute myocardial infarction does not influence the long-term prognosis (104). Serial noninvasive studies of patients with RV myocardial infarction document the common occurrence of improvement in RV performance over the weeks to months following an RV infarct (101,105). The occurrence of recovery of RV function in the contemporary treatment era appears to be importantly influenced by reperfusion. In a study by Bowers et al. of patients with acute RV infarction undergoing primary percutaneous angioplasty, successful reperfusion was associated with rapid and profound recovery of RV function (106). In contrast, those patients without successful reperfusion did not recover RV function, had more evidence of clinical RV infarction syndrome, and a higher mortality. Occasionally, patients with large RV MI will manifest a syndrome of chronic severe right heart failure with TR.

Cardiomyopathy, Myocardial Infiltration, and Metabolic Disease

In most cases of dilated cardiomyopathy, right heart failure results, at least in part, from left heart involvement with resulting excessive RV afterload. However, the RV myocardium may be involved in the cardiomyopathic process to an extent that may be less than, similar to, or greater than involvement of the left ventricle. In some such cases, the clinical manifestations of myocardial involvement will be predominantly those of right heart failure.

There have been reports of cardiomyopathy predominantly involving the right ventricle (107). A quantitative histological analysis performed in patients dying of dilated cardiomyopathy demonstrated that the cell diameter of myocytes in the RV free wall was often as enlarged as those in the LV free wall, and the myocyte cell diameter in both locations was significantly greater than that in control myocytes (108). Furthermore, the percent volume fibrosis in the RV free wall was greater than that of controls. Although these data do not prove primary involvement of the RV myocardium (i.e., these changes may have occurred from long-standing excess in afterload), they suggest that in some patients with cardiomyopathy, the RV may be importantly involved histologically.

Cardiac amyloidosis most often presents with clinical manifestations of biventricular failure. Left-sided involvement is commonly heralded by a restrictive cardiomyopathy with abnormal diastolic compliance characteristics. Prominent manifestations relating to right-sided failure are often seen. Edema and ascites may be exacerbated by concomitant nephrotic syndrome. In a histologic study of 54 necropsy patients with cardiac amyloidosis, the majority of patients had amyloid deposits involving the myocardium of both ventricles as well as gross involvement of the tricuspid leaflets (in over 80% of patients) and gross involvement of pulmonic leaflets (in over 50% of patients) (109). Thus, amyloid deposition is an infiltrative cardiomyopathy that may importantly involve the right ventricle directly. Evidence of RV failure or disproportionate RV dilation (e.g., ratio of LV to RV end-diastolic chamber areas ≤2) (110) in patients with cardiac amyloidosis carries a grim prognosis, with one series showing greater than 70% mortality within 6 months (111) and another showing a median survival of 4 months (110). It is uncertain to what extent this association with worse outcome is related to direct RV involvement with amyloid deposition as opposed to altered RV function from severe derangement in LV hemodynamics. There is, to date, no proven treatment regimen to reverse the infiltrative abnormalities of cardiac amyloidosis.

Primary or secondary hemachromatosis may involve the heart, and particularly the right ventricle, with iron deposition and toxic damage to myocytes (112). Clinically, hemochromatosis may appear as either a restricted or a dilated cardiomyopathy (112). Once heart disease secondary to iron deposition is clinically manifest, the course of the disease is often progressive and refractory to therapy. In some cases, however, a degree of reversal of the hemodynamic derangement and improvement in ventricular function may be seen with repeated phlebotomy or following treatment with the iron-chelating agent deferoxamine (113,114).

Although sarcoidosis of the heart is most often associated with abnormalities of the cardiac conduction system, myocardial involvement and clinical evidence of heart failure are also seen (115). RV myocardial involvement by the granulomatous process was observed in almost half of the specimens in a necropsy study of patients with clinically manifest cardiac sarcoidosis (115). Sudden death, syncope, paroxysmal arrhythmias, and heart failure are the common clinical syndromes of cardiac sarcoidosis. Survival is variable; in some cases the initial clinical presentation of cardiac involvement is sudden death (115). In contrast, survival over 10 years has been reported (116,117). Treatment can be problematic, as arrhythmias may be refractory to conventional pharmacologic management. Symptoms associated with conduction system abnormalities are treated with permanent pacing. The use of steroids is controversial. There may be improvement in conduction abnormalities, arrhythmias, and ventricular function by steroid-induced reduction in the inflammatory granulomatous burden (118), but some evidence exists that this approach may facilitate ventricular aneurysm formation (115).

Within the spectrum of hypereosinophilic syndromes, there exist several types that involve the heart. Loffler's original description of endomyocardial fibrosis involved two patients who, at autopsy, were found to have extensive fibrous thickening of the mural endocardium of both the right and left ventricles (119). Loffler referred to this as endocarditis parietalis fibroplastica. Among patients with the variant known as endomyocardial fibrosis, the mural endocardial fibrosis and overlying thrombosis are usually limited to the inflow tracts of both ventricles with frequent involvement of the ventricular aspect of the posterior mitral and tricuspid leaflets. Among patients described as having cardiac involvement with the hypereosinophilic syndrome at the National Institutes of Health, RV mural endocardial thickening was noted in 13 of 16 autopsied patients (119). Most schemes now classify the spectrum of endomyocardial disease and eosinophilia into two varieties (120). The so-called temperate region syndrome is characterized by endomyocardial disease, which is also accompanied by a systemic illness and eosinophilia. In this type, almost 100% of the patients have biventricular endomyocardial involvement. Cardiomegaly and mitral regurgitation are often present, although heart failure may or may not be manifest. A beneficial effect on clinical symptoms and survival has been seen with medical therapy consisting of steroids and cytotoxic drugs (particularly hydroxyurea) early in the course of the disease, as well as surgical therapy for the fibrotic endomyocardial disease with restrictive physiology (119,120).

The second type of endomyocardial disease with eosinophilia, referred to as the tropical variety, may be a late manifestation of what was initially a temperate region variant. The tropical syndrome tends to have no systemic illness, may or may not have eosinophilia, and demonstrates biventricular endomyocardial involvement in approximately 75% of patients. Isolated involvement of the right ventricle is found in this syndrome in 20% of cases (120). Generally, patients with this type of endomyocardial disease demonstrate a progressive downhill course, although prolonged survival has been reported (121). Predominant right heart involvement seems to be associated with more prolonged survival. Surgical endocardiectomy with associated valve replacement or repair offers symptomatic relief, although operative mortality is high with this complex operation (122,123).

Carcinoid syndrome is an endocrinopathy that, in its more severe forms, will often have important right heart involvement. Among 21 patients with clinically important carcinoid heart disease studied at necropsy, 12 had gross RV mural endocardial involvement with carcinoid plaques (124). In all 21 patients, both the tricuspid and the pulmonic valves were involved. In over 70% of patients, all of the involvement with carcinoid plaques was limited to the right side of the heart. Such carcinoid plaques are composed of an unusual type of fibrous tissue devoid of elastic fibrils within which are contained smooth muscle cells and mucopolysaccharide. Most often, these plaques are located on the downstream aspect of the valve, which results in a distinct physiological abnormality for each valve involved (124). Tricuspid regurgitation is far more common than tricuspid stenosis. In contrast, pulmonic stenosis is the predominant lesion resulting from involvement of the pulmonic valve. In selected cases, percutaneous tricuspid and/or pulmonic balloon valvuloplasty may be a useful palliative treatment. The prognosis in patients with carcinoid heart disease is generally related to the extent of the primary carcinoid tumor rather than the extent of cardiac involvement.

Signs and symptoms of RV failure may be noted in patients with massive obesity. Although abnormal RV performance may be caused by pulmonary hypertension resulting from hypoventilation or chronic pulmonary emboli, gross and histologic myocardial abnormalities have been described (125). All 12 patients in one autopsy study of patients with massive obesity had dilated right ventricles, many of which demonstrated evidence of cellular hypertrophy. Three of the 12 patients demonstrated clear-cut fatty infiltration within the RV myocardium, both by gross observation and by microscopy.

Right Ventricular Dysplasia

Right ventricular dysplasia comprises a spectrum of RV morphologic abnormalities, with clinical manifestations ranging from little or no derangement of RV performance to severe right heart failure (126). The functional abnormalities range from subtle areas of hypokinesis (127) to severe generalized hypokinesis of a parchment-thin right ventricle, referred to as the Uhl anomaly (128). Right ventricular dysplasia may be associated with ventricular or supraventricular arrhythmias. Characteristically, ventricular tachycardia in arrhythmogenic RV dysplasia has a left bundle branch morphology with right axis deviation, indicating its origin from the right ventricle. In patients with RV dysplasia, symptoms depend on the extent and functional importance of RV myocardial involvement as well as on the presence and rate of the tachyarrhythmia. The natural history of this condition is not known. RV dysplasia must be distinguished from the Ebstein anomaly, atrial septal defect (ASD), partial anomalous pulmonary venous return, congenital absence of the left pericardium, RV infarction, or primary or secondary TR.

Right ventricular dysplasia is often diagnosed only at autopsy or heart transplant. In a series of 42 patients, pathological examination revealed LV involvement, with fibrofatty infiltration, either histologically or macroscopically, in 76% (129). Those with LV involvement had a higher incidence of heart failure and of clinically overt ventricular arrhythmias and had hearts that weighed more, with a greater degree of RV thinning and inflammatory infiltrates. Thus, there is evidence that this condition should no longer be considered a disorder exclusively affecting the right ventricle.

In patients with ventricular arrhythmias, antiarrhythmic therapy has met with varying success, although fatal dysrhythmias are relatively uncommon. When antiarrhythmic therapy is not efficacious, surgical therapy has been advocated. The right ventricle is dissected from its LV attachments and reattached such that a scar forms around the suture line and does not allow the arrhythmic focus to spread to the left ventricle (130).

Right Ventricular Pressure Overload States

Cor Pulmonale

Cor pulmonale refers to the combination of pressure overload, hypertrophy, and dilation of the right ventricle in the face of pulmonary hypertension. The latter may result from lung disease, such as chronic obstructive pulmonary disease, or from a primary abnormality in the pulmonary vasculature such as primary pulmonary hypertension.

In contrast to conventional thought, normal pulmonary vessels have been found experimentally to be intrinsically stiffer than systemic vessels. The ability of the pulmonary vascular bed to accept increases in cardiac output (and thus flow) without important increments in pressure and RV afterload predominantly relates to the ability of the pulmonary vasculature to recruit portions of the vasculature that are underperfused at rest. This large amount of vascular reserve explains why substantial reductions in the size of the pulmonary vascular bed must occur before clinically relevant pulmonary hypertension develops. Even so, other factors must be involved in the pathophysiolgy of pulmonary hypertension caused by chronic lung disease, beyond reduction in the size of the vascular bed. For example, in emphysema, despite reduction in the number of alveolar vessels by pulmonary parenchymal destruction, it is unusual for cor pulmonale to be present until late in the course of the disease. Additional factors contributing to pulmonary hypertension in patients with obstructive lung disease include hypoxia, hypoxemia, and acidosis, resulting in pulmonary vasoconstriction, and polycythemia, resulting in hyperviscosity.

In the presence of these abnormalities of the pulmonary vascular bed, the pulmonary vasculature cannot accept increases in cardiac output during stress without substantial increases in PA pressure (Fig. 21-7) (131). The resulting reduction in RV systolic function is associated with limitation in cardiac output response to exercise.

Cor pulmonale is relatively common in patients with chronic bronchitis, in whom the disease is characterized by chronic productive cough, frequent respiratory infections, hypoxemia and hypercapnea at rest, and elevated hematocrit. Diffusion capacity is relatively maintained because anatomic destruction of alveolae is not a prominent feature. Hypoxic vasoconstriction results from extensive ventilation-perfusion mismatching. Pulmonary hypertension at rest may be marked and worsened further with modest degrees of exertion, resulting in overt right heart failure. The degree of reduction in RVEF correlates with the magnitude of pulmonary hypertension, which is, in turn, related to the degree of hypoxemia and hypercapnea.

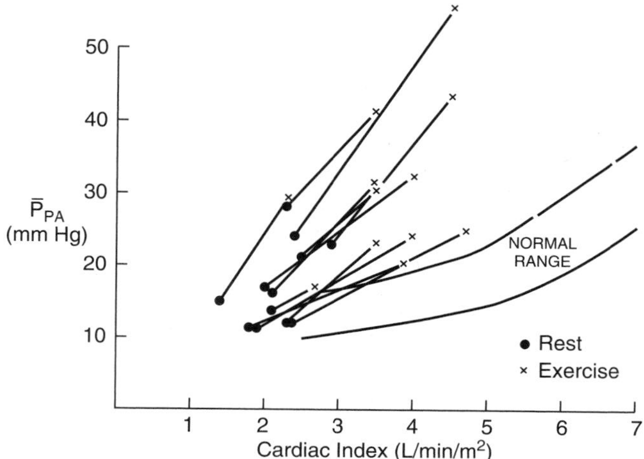

Figure 21-7 Relationship of resting and exercise cardiac index versus mean pulmonary artery pressure (PPA) in 12 patients with chronic obstructive pulmonary disease. Normal range represents values taken from 75 normal subjects. (Reprinted from Mahler DA, Brent BN, Like J, et al. Right ventricular performance and central circulatory hemodynamics during upright exercise in patients with chronic obstructive pulmonary disease. *Am Rev Respir Dis.* 1984; 130:722–729, with permission.)

In contrast, in patients with emphysema, cough and sputum production are not prominent, and hyperventilation can generally maintain arterial oxygen tension in a relatively normal range despite a widened alveolar-arterial oxygen gradient. Thus, pulmonary hypertension in general is less prominent despite variable degrees of pulmonary vascular destruction. Signs and symptoms of right heart failure and noninvasive evidence of abnormalities in RV ejection performance are relatively late events.

Mitral Stenosis

Pulmonary hypertension in patients with mitral stenosis is multifactorial, resulting from a combination of elevated left atrial pressure, reactive pulmonary vasoconstriction, potentially reversible pulmonary arteriolar medial hypertrophy, and fixed obliterative pulmonary vascular changes.

In patients with mild mitral stenosis, PA pressure is usually normal or only slightly elevated at rest, resting RV systolic performance is normal, and symptoms of right heart failure are absent. However, PA pressure may rise markedly during exercise, causing excessive RV afterload and reduced RV systolic function (11,12,132,133). As the severity of the valvular abnormality worsens, PA pressure may become elevated at rest and occasionally may exceed systemic pressure. Under such conditions, signs and symptoms of right heart failure frequently accompany reduction in resting RVEF. The magnitude of the change in EF with exercise is related to the degree of elevation in PA pressure (134).

In patients with mitral stenosis, once a substantial degree of precapillary obstructive change occurs within the pulmonary circulation, clinical findings of reduced cardiac output and right heart failure predominate. On one hand, these vascular changes tend to mitigate against transudation of fluid into the pulmonary extravascular space. On the other hand, RV afterload becomes excessive, resulting in RV systolic failure, RV dilation, TR, and manifestations of systemic venous hypertension.

Improvement in RV function following correction of mitral stenosis results directly from alleviation of mitral valve obstruction and from regression of pulmonary vascular medial hypertrophy. Remodeling of RV architecture with diminished RV dilation, in combination with diminished PA pressure, results in improvement in forward cardiac output as a result of both augmented RV ejection performance with the relief of afterload and a reduction in TR.

Pulmonic Stenosis

The majority of cases of pulmonic stenosis result from congenital abnormalities of the pulmonic valve, either with fusion and variable thickening of the normal tricuspid leaflet or, much less commonly, a bicuspid valve. In addition, patients with Noonan syndrome may demonstrate dysplastic changes of the pulmonic valve. Secondary hypertrophy of the RV infundibulum may occur with advancing age in adults with valvular pulmonic stenosis and contribute to RV systolic pressure overload.

Mild to moderate pulmonic stenosis may remain asymptomatic throughout life. However, in patients with more severe stenosis, symptoms such as dyspnea and fatigue, particularly with exercise, may occur as a result of the inability of the right ventricle to augment cardiac output with increased demand (135). With severe outflow obstruction, RV hypertrophy may not suffice to maintain normal wall stress. Reduction in forward output will be exacerbated by TR, and signs and symptoms of right heart failure will appear. Exertional syncope or lightheadedness may occur, although sudden death is rare (136). Angina pectoris may occur because of the increased demand on the right ventricle in concert with an inability of RV vasodilator reserve to maximally increase coronary perfusion.

Noninvasive studies are able to document the severity of the valvular obstruction and consequent preservation or impairment of RV function. When a QR complex is present in lead V_1 of the electrocardiogram, the pressure gradient across the pulmonic valve generally exceeds 80 mm Hg. Doppler interrogation of the RV outflow tract and proximal PA can quantify the gradient based on the flow velocity across the valve (137). This technique is useful for serial assessment of asymptomatic patients as well as for determining the degree of postoperative improvement and potential onset of pulmonic regurgitation.

Pulmonic valvuloplasty now appears to be the initial treatment of choice for patients with right heart failure from valvular pulmonic stenosis (138). The degree to which RV hemodynamics and function return to normal is related to the relative contribution of afterload mismatch and of intrinsic myocardial dysfunction to the original hemodynamic syndrome. In some patients, RV end-diastolic pressure may remain elevated following relief of outflow tract obstruction, presumably because of a degree of interstitial fibrosis that had resulted from the long-standing pressure overload. In patients with a significant contribution of subvalvular stenosis, relief of the valvular obstruction may not improve symptoms and, in fact, may worsen obstruction at the infundibular level. The treatment of choice for such patients is surgical relief of both the valvular abnormality and the infundibular obstruction.

Right Ventricular Volume Overload States

Tricuspid Regurgitation

By far the most common etiology of TR is derangement of valve function caused by (a) excessive RV systolic pressure, or (b) dilation of the right ventricle with secondary enlargement of the tricuspid annulus. Rheumatic heart disease may directly affect the tricuspid valve, almost always in combination with anatomical or clinical involvement of at least two other valves. Other nonrheumatic etiologies that may be associated with TR include infective endocarditis (particularly in intravenous drug abusers), Ebstein anomaly, Marfan syndrome, and carcinoid syndrome. Cardiac tumors, in particular right atrial myxoma, may be associated with functional TR.

Tricuspid regurgitation is common in patients with major RV infarction (139) and may substantially exacerbate the clinical syndrome, contributing to reduction in forward flow and to RV dilation with severe elevation in central venous pressure. In RV infarction, valve dysfunction may be caused by RV distension alone. Alternatively, the papillary apparatus may be dysfunctional because of ischemic injury.

In the absence of pulmonary hypertension, TR usually causes no clinical symptoms. In the setting of pulmonary hypertension, TR exacerbates the clinical expression of right heart failure. In patients with heart failure of any etiology, functional TR may result in an effective descending limb of the Starling curve. As the right ventricle distends, TR worsens and forward output decreases. In severe TR, the physical exam reflects ventricularization of the RA pressure wave form, with a prominent V wave in the jugular venous profile. The murmur of TR usually increases during inspiration, a finding known as the Rivero-Carvello sign. Echocardiography can aid in the grading of TR, and Doppler interrogation of the TR jet allows estimation of the PA peak systolic pressure (86). Specific surgical correction of a regurgitant tricuspid valve is usually not needed; rather, both medical and surgical therapy are directed at the underlying cause of RV pressure overload. However, when significant primary abnormality of the tricuspid valve exists, or when pulmonary hypertension cannot be fully reversed, surgical palliation of TR may be performed by insertion of a Carpentier ring (140), which diminishes annular dilation and improves valvular coaptation.

Atrial Septal Defect

An atrial-level left-to-right shunt is characterized by chronic RV volume overload. The magnitude of shunt flow is related primarily to the relative compliance of the right and left ventricles. The RV chamber, already capable of accommodating volume flow because of its chamber compliance characteristics, can increase its capacity further through dilation as well as some degree of hypertrophy to maintain normal levels of wall stress despite its greater chamber radius. In the absence of pulmonary vascular obstructive changes, the majority of patients with ASDs remain asymptomatic throughout life. Symptoms may intervene in later life as a result of a gradual elevation in PA pressure in association with increasing left-to-right shunting, as LV compliance diminishes. Pulmonary hypertension transforms an ASD from a condition of pure RV volume overload to one of combined pressure and volume overload.

In patients with ASDs, signs and symptoms of right heart failure may result directly from left-sided abnormalities in the absence of RV failure because left atrial pressure is transmitted directly into the systemic venous circulation via the interatrial shunt. In this setting, mitral regurgitation may manifest elevated jugular venous pressure, with a prominent regurgitant pressure wave, in the absence of TR.

A minority of patients develop pulmonary vascular obstructive disease, resulting in pulmonary hypertension, reduced RV compliance, reversal of shunt flow, reduction in pulmonary flow, and cyanosis (Eisenmenger syndrome). The right-to-left flow reduces the degree of right heart failure by reducing the degree of RV volume load, which would otherwise coincide with the worsening pressure load. In this circumstance, surgical closure is no longer feasible because it would result in abrupt worsening of right heart failure. In contrast, there have been several reports regarding patients with pulmonary hypertension who have had modest clinical improvement following the induction of right-to-left shunting by balloon septostomy. Although this procedure produces or worsens cyanosis, it relieves RV volume overload and augments forward flow.

In one study, RV systolic function was found to be reduced in a group of patients with ASDs and normalized following surgical repair (141). However, in another study (142), RVEF was found to be higher in patients with ASDs than in patients with comparable elevations in PA pressure but without left-to-right shunt. In the latter study, following surgical repair, RV volume normalized, but EF decreased. Thus, RV volume overload tends to increase EF, although under these circumstances, EF overestimates the intrinsic level of RV contractility and may mask myocardial dysfunction.

VENTRICULAR INTERDEPENDENCE: EFFECT OF RIGHT HEART FAILURE ON THE LEFT HEART

The potential exists for direct interaction between the two ventricles through direct transseptal pressure transmission and/or alteration in intrapericardial pressure (77, 143–148). A distended right heart may aggravate or possibly induce left heart failure via direct ventricular interaction. Abnormally elevated RV systolic or diastolic load has been shown to induce perturbations in septal geometry and in the mechanics of septal contribution to LV filling and ejection (68–76). Under most circumstances, changes in intrapericardial pressure match changes in RA pressure (149). Elevations in RA pressure therefore reduce LV transmural (or distending) pressure at any given level of LV intracavitary pressure. Alternatively, for transmural pressure to be maintained, intracavitary pressure must rise. During diastole, transmural pressure determines the degree of LV filling, whereas an increase in intracavitary pressure is the stimulus for pulmonary venous hypertension and transudation of fluid into the pulmonary interstitium. Thus, RV and RA distension may adversely alter observed LV compliance characteristics (i.e., the relation between intracavitary pressure and volume). In contrast to changes in intrinsic distensibility of LV myocardium, which are associated with changes in the slope of the LV diastolic pressure–volume relation, increased LV chamber stiffness resulting from ventricular interaction is characterized by a parallel shift in the LV compliance curve (143–145,150). In addition, increased RA pressure may reduce LV compliance through myocardial vascular engorgement (erectile effect), resulting from an increase in coronary venous pressure (151). These effects may cause reduction in LV filling with an attendant decrease in stroke volume via the Starling mechanism or an increase in the stimulus to develop pulmonary edema.

Volume loading in pigs producing increases in RV end-diastolic pressure from 3 to 9 mm Hg resulted in ventricular interdependence during both systole and diastole, as examined through the ratio of change in either systolic or diastolic pressures between the two ventricles (152) during sudden LV unloading. Compared with normal pigs, pigs with pacing-induced heart failure showed exaggeration of this ventricular interdependence during systole but not during diastole. The ventricular interdependence effect of volume loading was present during both systole and diastole, whether or not the pericardium was intact. Thus, any syndrome associated with acute RV volume overload may be expected to impact on LV performance during both systole and diastole.

Acute severe right heart dilation, such as occurs with RV MI, may present a hemodynamic picture that is similar to pericardial constriction with near-equalization of RA and PA wedge pressures, prominent atrial *y*-descent, and "dip and plateau" of ventricular pressure contours during diastole (25). These findings suggest intrapericardial constraint on left heart filling imposed by the distended right heart. If these direct interventricular forces were not in effect, cardiac output would be sustained as long as LV intracavitary pressures were maintained in a physiological range. However, because increased intrapericardial pressure renders LV intracavitary pressure an underestimate of transmural distending pressure, there is an apparent downward displacement of the LV Starling curve, and supranormal PA wedge pressure is needed to sustain a normal LV stroke volume.

In patients with right heart failure, withdrawal of the RV constraint on LV filling appears to contribute to vasodilator-induced augmentation of stroke volume and reduction in pulmonary venous pressure (148,150). In the presence of right heart failure, nitroprusside induces a parallel downward shift in the LV pressure–volume or pressure–dimension curve (Fig. 21-8) (150). Presumably, this shift results from a change in the relation between LV intracavitary pressure and transmural distending pressure as nitroprusside reduces RA (and therefore intrapericardial) pressure through venodilation. Similarly, the effect of acute angiotensin-converting enzyme (ACE) inhibition on the rate of LV diastolic filling is related to the state of the right ventricle. We observed that enalaprilat has no effect on LV peak filling rate in patients with isolated LV failure. However, enalaprilat augments LV peak filling rate in patients with LV systolic dysfunction and RV dilation, presumably by withdrawing the RV constraint to LV filling (Fig. 21-9) (77).

Thus, it appears reasonable to presume that right heart failure may induce or exacerbate left heart failure through direct ventricular interaction and that the manner and magnitude of response to therapeutic intervention may be influenced by this interaction.

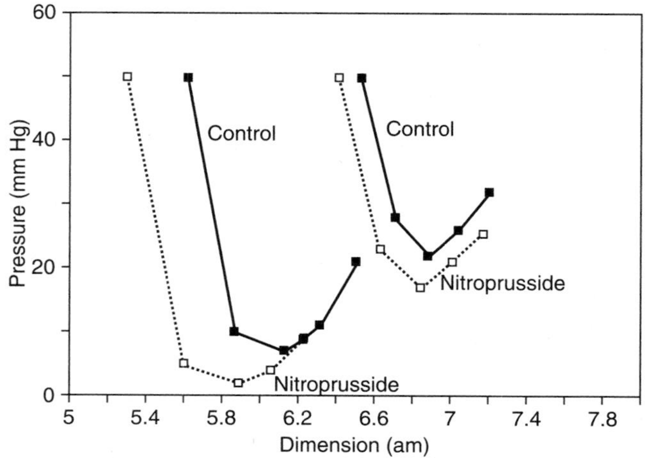

Figure 21-8 The average left ventricular diastolic pressure–dimension relations before and after nitroprusside. **Panel on left** represents data from patients with normal right atrial pressure (n = 5), in whom nitroprusside caused left ventricular dimension and pressure to decrease along a constant pressure–volume relation. **Panel on right** represents data from patients with elevated right atrial pressure (n = 5), in whom nitroprusside caused a reduction in intracavitary pressure out of proportion to the change in chamber size (i.e., a downward shift in the diastolic pressure–volume relation), suggesting an effect related to pericardial constraint and/or ventricular interaction. (Reprinted from Carroll JD, Land RM, Neumann AL, et al. The differential effects of positive inotropic and vasodilator therapy on diastolic properties in patients with congestive cardiomyopathy. *Circulation.* 1986;74:815–825, with permission.)

ROLE OF THE RIGHT HEART IN LEFT HEART FAILURE

The maintenance or loss of normal right heart performance has been linked to the clinical expression of left heart failure in a number of respects. In a population of patients with depressed LV systolic performance, RVEF has been observed to be positively correlated with functional capacity (153) (Fig. 21-10) and with survival (154,155). Among a subset of patients in the Survival and Ventricular Enlargement (SAVE) trial with post-MI LV dysfunction who underwent quantitative echocardiography, the RV fractional area change was a strong predictor of mortality, cardiovascular mortality, and subsequent development of

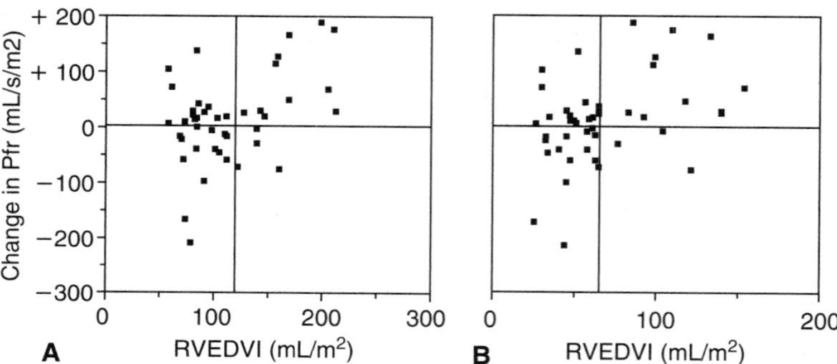

Figure 21-9 Relationship of enalaprilat-induced change in left ventricular peak filling rate (PFR) versus **(A)** baseline right ventricular (RV) end-diastolic volume index (EDVI) and versus **(B)** baseline RV end-systolic volume index (ESVI). **Vertical lines** mark the upper limits of normal for RV volumes. Enalaprilat had no consistent effect on PFR in patients with normal RV volumes but increased PFR in the majority of patients with enlarged RV volumes. (Reprinted from Konstam MA, Kronenberg MW, Udelson JE, et al. Effect of acute angiotensin converting enzyme inhibition on left ventricular filling in patients with congestive heart failure. Relation to right ventricular volumes. *Circulation* 1990;81(Suppl III):III-115–III-122, with permission.)

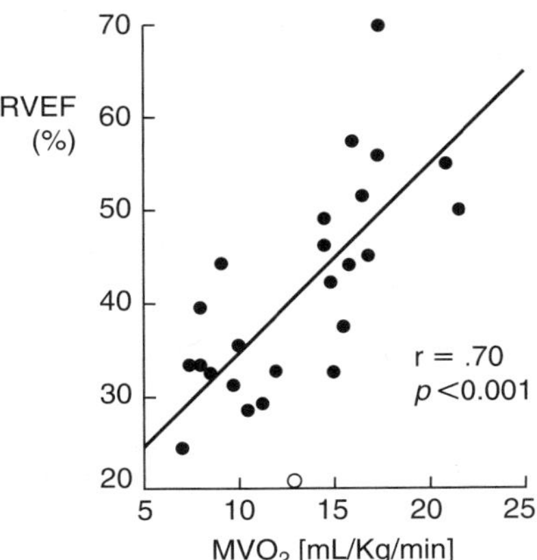

Figure 21-10 The correlation between resting right ventricular ejection fraction (RVEF) and maximum oxygen consumption (MVO2) in 25 patients with congestive heart failure caused by left ventricular systolic dysfunction. (Reprinted from Baker BJ, Wilen MM, Boyd CM, et al. Relation of right ventricular ejection fraction to exercise capacity in chronic left ventricular failure. *Am J Cardiol.* 1984;54:596–599, with permission.)

overt heart failure (156). In addition, the state of RV systolic function is linked to the nature of symptomatology in patients with left heart failure. The relationship of RV performance to clinical manifestations and outcomes in the setting of left heart failure is multifactorial.

As previously discussed, RV systolic performance is strongly influenced by systolic load. During vasodilator administration in patients with left heart failure, a linear relation exists between the fractional or absolute reductions in PA dicrotic notch pressure and RV end-systolic volume (6,7,10). This close association between RV systolic performance and afterload is likely to be a major mediator of the relation between RVEF and functional capacity. As left heart failure progresses, RV afterload is augmented and RV stroke volume and EF decrease. As RV systolic failure ensues, RV dilation must occur in order to maintain forward stroke volume. This defense mechanism is thwarted by the development of TR, which may establish a vicious cycle of progressive right heart failure, cardiac output reduction, salt and water retention, left heart failure, and further increments in RV afterload.

We have compared the ventricular mechanisms for augmentation of cardiac output during cycle exercise in patients with symptomatic versus asymptomatic LV systolic dysfunction (157). In asymptomatic patients, despite exhaustion of contractile reserve, stroke volume increases during exercise through augmentation of LV end-diastolic volume (i.e., recruitment of preload reserve). In contrast, in patients with symptomatic heart failure, preload reserve appears to be exhausted, with no detectable change in LV end-diastolic volume during exercise, and increases in cardiac output are totally dependent on tachycardia. Right heart failure may relate to these phenomena in at least two ways. First, the failing right ventricle may not be capable of augmenting PA perfusion pressure during exercise sufficiently to increase LV preload. Second, as previously discussed, the failed right ventricle may directly impede left heart filling through ventricular interdependence. Thus, in a number of respects, RV performance is likely to impact directly on functional capacity.

In a large cohort of patients with LV systolic dysfunction and heart failure, a multivariate analysis indicated that the strongest identifiable correlate of rapid-onset pulmonary edema without associated overt myocardial ischemia was RVEF (158). Compared to the remainder of the population, patients with rapid-onset pulmonary edema manifested substantially higher RVEFs, with many patients having hypercontractile right ventricles. These observations may be explained on the basis of variation in the manner in which the right ventricle responds to left heart failure. As previously discussed, in the majority of patients with left heart failure, the thin-walled, compliant right ventricle succumbs to increased afterload, fails to maintain normal pump function, and dilates during diastole. It is limited in the degree to which it may augment PA pressure and therefore sustain an increase in pulmonary capillary pressure in the face of an expanded intravascular volume. Instead, under such conditions, the failed right ventricle distends further during systole and diastole and may fail to maintain its forward stroke volume. However, it contributes to a buffering of intravascular volume, thus mitigating against abrupt changes in pulmonary capillary pressure. It appears likely that in some patients with left heart failure, the right ventricle hypertrophies before dilating and is capable of maintaining systolic performance in the face of augmented afterload. In response to increased intravascular volume, the right ventricle might move up a relatively steep Starling curve and augment PA pressure sufficiently to sustain a substantial augmentation of pulmonary capillary pressure. A hypertrophied, hypercontractile right ventricle tends to maintain forward output but is associated with a reduced capacity to buffer acute changes in intravascular volume and may predispose the patient to rapid-onset pulmonary edema. The precise determinants of RV hypertrophy remain to be elucidated.

Thus, in a variety of ways, the maintenance or failure of RV performance is closely linked to various aspects of the clinical expression of left heart failure, beyond manifestations of right heart failure per se. It is likely that, in some respects, RV performance and clinical symptomatology are coincident by-products of altered RV load produced by left heart failure. In other respects, primary variability in RV performance may directly influence the clinical presentation.

THERAPY

In this section, we review physiological and practical aspects of the treatment of right heart failure. Treatment for right heart failure is directed largely at (a) optimizing RV loading conditions, and (b) minimizing the peripheral effects of right heart failure. Most therapeutic modalities strive toward both of these goals in concert. Efforts to optimize load differ somewhat, depending on the primary pathological stimulus to abnormal load. In addition, we discuss the role of inotropic agents.

Optimizing Right Ventricular Preload

Optimization of RV preload generally represents the most appropriate primary intervention in patients with right heart failure. The direction of change to be instituted depends on the clinical circumstance and the predominant clinical manifestation of right heart failure, namely, low output or systemic venous hypertension. In patients with severe acute right heart failure, as caused by acute RV infarction, or postoperative RV dysfunction, volume loading should be instituted to increase RV filling pressure (25,159) and thus force the right ventricle to ascend its relatively shallow Starling curve. However, two cautions to this approach should be stated. First, excessive RV dilation may worsen functional TR, thus establishing an effective descending Starling curve limb and reducing forward output. Second, in the setting of acute RV dilation, PA wedge pressure may not adequately reflect true LV filling pressure. This caveat is a result of ventricular interdependence and pericardial restraint on left heart filling. Stated differently, as the right heart distends and RA pressure increases, intrapericardial pressure increases as well, and LV transmural, or distending, pressure diverges from intracavitary pressure (149). Thus, even in the absence of primary LV systolic dysfunction, forward output will be less than anticipated for a given level of PA wedge pressure. For these reasons, as volume loading is instituted, its effect on forward output must be tracked. Because in the setting of right heart distension with tricuspid regurgitation, thermodilution cardiac output measurements may be spurious, it may be helpful to monitor an alternative indicator of forward output such as mixed venous oxygen saturation.

Maintenance of atrial contribution to RV filling represents an important means for optimizing RV preload in the setting of acute right heart failure. Significant clinical deterioration may occur with the onset of atrial fibrillation or initiation of ventricular pacing for bradyarrhythmias. Thus, in these circumstances, consideration should be given to emergent cardioversion or institution of dual-chamber pacing (160).

In patients with chronic right heart failure, diuretics act to reverse sodium and water retention, reduce central venous pressure, and relieve edema (161,162). Diuretics may also improve forward output by relieving RV distension and thus reducing the degree of functional TR. In addition to loop diuretics, spironolactone is often effective in reducing the edema associated with right heart failure because a hyperrenin, hyperaldosterone state is almost universal in patients with right heart failure and contributes substantially to sodium retention.

Nitrates have been found to exert salutary hemodynamic effects and to improve exercise performance in patients with various forms of heart failure, including patients with cor pulmonale and primary right heart failure (163–169). Nitrates exert a venodilator effect, acting to recruit venous capacitance and thus reduce systemic venous hypertension. In addition, nitrates have been found to augment exercise capacity in patients with heart failure, an effect that may be mediated via arterial dilation with reduction in LV afterload (164). Alternatively, to the extent that RV distension impedes left heart filling through ventricular interdependence, a reduction in RV diastolic pressure may contribute to the effect of nitrates on functional capacity (150).

Reduction of Right Ventricular Systolic Load

As previously discussed, the most effective way to augment RV systolic performance is reduction of afterload (7,168,170,171). Thus, any intervention that reduces RV systolic load will tend to augment forward output and presumably improve functional capacity. In patients with left heart failure, this effect is best achieved by reducing left heart filling pressure and pulmonary venous pressure. Thus, systemic arteriolar dilators, which augment LV stroke volume and reduce the stimulus for augmenting LV preload, serve to secondarily reduce RV afterload and augment RV systolic performance. In addition, most systemic arteriolar dilators also act as pulmonary vasodilators, thus reducing the additional afterload imposed on the right ventricle by pulmonary vasoconstriction. This group of agents includes α-adrenergic antagonists, calcium channel antagonists, ACE inhibitors, and direct-acting vasodilators, including nitrates. Thus, in addition to directly impacting on RV diastolic failure through venodilation, nitrates influence RV systolic failure by reducing pulmonary venous pressure and pulmonary vascular resistance.

Despite the fact that angiotensin II has little, if any, direct effect on systemic venous tone, ACE inhibitors may benefit patients with systolic or diastolic right heart failure via a variety of mechanisms (171). For reasons previously cited, RV afterload may be reduced. In addition, reduction in plasma aldosterone reduces the stimulus to renal sodium retention.

Reduction of Right Ventricular Afterload in Cor Pulmonale

Efforts to minimize RV afterload require special additional considerations in the setting of right heart failure caused by pulmonary vascular pathology. These considerations differ depending on whether obstruction to pulmonary blood flow results from hypoxic vasoconstriction, thromboembolism, or primary vascular pathology, as in the case of primary pulmonary hypertension.

In most cases of cor pulmonale related to chronic obstructive pulmonary disease (COPD), reversible vasoconstriction evoked by hypoxia plays a role. Under such circumstances, efforts should be directed primarily toward maximizing oxygenation. In patients with COPD, use of supplemental oxygen has been found to improve hemodynamics, functional status, and survival (167,172–175). The latter effect appears to be related to reversibility of pulmonary hypertension (174).

In patients with COPD, bronchodilators may improve RV function and reduce signs and symptoms of right heart failure through a number of mechanisms. Both β-adrenergic agonists and phosphodiesterase inhibitors potentially exert their clinical effects through a combination of bronchodilation, direct pulmonary vasodilation, and inotropic action. In patients with COPD, terbutaline has been found to reduce pulmonary vascular resistance, increase cardiac output, and improve RVEF without significant change in P_aO_2 (174–177). Pulmonary artery pressure tends to remain unchanged. Theophylline has been found to reduce PA pressure and vascular resistance and to increase RVEF (177–181).

Several classes of direct and indirect vasodilators have been employed, with variable success, in patients with COPD and pulmonary vascular disease. The likelihood of clinical efficacy is probably related to the degree to which active vasoconstriction contributes to pulmonary hypertension. In patients with COPD, several studies have documented augmentation of cardiac output by hydralazine (182–185). However, benefit in terms of other hemodynamic functional parameters has been variable, with some investigators finding an increase in PA pressure and worsening of hypoxia and dyspnea (183), possibly related to an adverse change in ventilation-perfusion relationships. Calcium-channel antagonists have been found to blunt hypoxic pulmonary vasoconstriction (186), increase cardiac output, and reduce pulmonary vascular resistance and PA pressure (187). However, some investigators have identified a worsening of hypoxemia with administration of calcium-channel blockers, which has been attributed to augmented blood flow to poorly ventilated areas of lung (188). In a rat model, the ACE inhibitor captopril has been found to reduce the degree to which hypoxia induces pulmonary vascular pathology and RV hypertrophy (189). In patients with COPD, the hemodynamic benefits of ACE inhibitors have been found to be minor (190,191), although long-term clinical data are lacking.

In the setting of right heart failure caused more directly by pulmonary vascular disease, as caused by primary pulmonary hypertension, Eisenmenger syndrome, or long-standing mitral valve disease, a variety of vasodilators have been advocated. Although individual patients have been reported to manifest hemodynamic efficacy, in general vasodilator therapy is considerably less rewarding than in the setting of left heart failure and must be undertaken with caution (192,193). In such patients, the reflex systemic vasoconstriction associated with reduced cardiac output is more responsive to vasodilators than is the morphologically altered pulmonary circulation. Therefore, all available vasodilators have the potential for inducing abrupt severe hypotension in patients with fixed pulmonary vascular disease. Systemic vasodilation may initiate a vicious cycle, with reduced coronary perfusion pressure, diminished RV contractile function, and further hypotension. If vasodilator therapy is to be attempted, it should be initiated under careful hemodynamic monitoring to confirm hemodynamic benefit and facilitate rapid drug withdrawal with necessary countermeasures, including volume expansion and/or administration of α-adrenergic agonists, in the event of hypotension.

Recent attention has focused on the use of endothelin receptor antagonists for the treatment of patients with pulmonary hypertension. Animal model and clinical data suggest benefit, and studies demonstrate improvement in RV function accompanying the reduction in PA pressure and RV afterload. Miyauchi et al. reported preservation of normal central venous pressure and ANP levels (as markers of right ventricular function and hemodynamics) after pretreatment with an endothelin A receptor antagonist in monocrotaline-induced pulmonary hypertension in rats (194). In human studies, the endothelin receptor antagonist bosentan, now approved for clinical use in pulmonary hypertension, has been shown to improve RV structure (reduced dilatation) and function, in association with improvements in clinical parameters such as 6-minute walk testing (195). These data represent a promising treatment avenue for preventing RV dysfunction secondary to pulmonary vascular disease.

Inotropic Agents

The role of inotropic agents in right heart failure has received considerable debate and has not been definitively clarified. In patients with left heart failure, the effect of amrinone on RV systolic performance has been found to be entirely explainable on the basis of reduced RV afterload caused by a combination of improved LV performance and pulmonary vasodilation (196). In contrast, dobutamine has been found to significantly augment RV contractility in patients with COPD, as shown by end-systolic pressure–volume analysis (10). In patients with LV failure, the effect of dobutamine on RV systolic performance has been found to be greater than that of milrinone for a given reduction in RV afterload, suggesting that some of dobutamine's hemodynamic effects may be mediated by augmented RV contractility (197).

In the clinical setting, it is difficult to sort out the degree to which improvement in RV systolic performance results from augmentation of RV contractility, as opposed to direct and/or indirect effects on RV load. For example, both β-adrenergic agents and amrinone have a vasodilator effect on the pulmonary circulation (198). Digoxin and the selective β_1 agonist dobutamine have little or no direct pulmonary vasodilator effect. However, in patients with left heart failure, the LV inotropic effect results in reflex withdrawal of vasoconstrictor stimuli, resulting in reduction of pulmonary as well as systemic vascular resistance. Therefore, even in the absence of a direct pulmonary vasodilator effect, inotropic agents may reduce RV systolic load. When these effects are present, it is likely that they predominate in determining the RV systolic functional response.

The clinical role of digitalis glycosides in patients with cor pulmonale has received considerable debate (199–204). Several studies have documented some hemodynamic improvement in such patients, consisting of augmented cardiac output, stroke volume, and stroke work, with reduction in RV filling pressure (200,201). However, digitalis glycosides may increase pulmonary vascular resistance by direct vasoconstrictor effects (202,203). The net hemodynamic benefit of these agents appears to be less than that of other classes of agents. For example, the benefit of digitalis has been found to be less than that of oxygen (204). For this reason, and because of the relatively high incidence of adverse effects, digitalis is not generally recommended for the management of cor pulmonale in the absence of concomitant supraventricular arrhythmia or LV failure.

Treatment of Postoperative Right Ventricular Failure

Following cardiopulmonary bypass, right heart failure is common and results from ischemic injury to the right ventricle or from pulmonary vascular injury. RV dysfunction may result from antecedent RV infarction or from acute RV ischemic insult secondary to inadequate RV myocardial protection, particularly in the setting of right coronary arterial occlusive disease. The RV failure may be provoked or exacerbated by pre-existing pulmonary vascular disease, as induced by chronic valvular or congenital heart disease. In addition, acute RV failure may complicate cardiac transplantation (205), particularly in the setting of pulmonary vascular obstructive disease combined with an inadequately sized donor heart.

In patients with postoperative RV failure, attention should first be directed toward optimizing oxygenation and acid-base status to minimize pulmonary vasoconstriction, maintaining adequate volume status to optimize RV preload, and maintaining the atrial contribution to RV filling (see earlier) (206,207). The potent pulmonary vasodilators prostacyclin and prostaglandin E_1 may be valuable (208–210), although their effects may be limited by concomitant systemic vasodilation. Both β-adrenergic agents and amrinone may exert substantial clinical benefit through combined inotropic and pulmonary vasodilator effects (198,211,212). If these various measures prove inadequate to sustain forward output, urgent consideration should be given to mechanical support of the right ventricle. Such support may take the form of PA balloon counterpulsation (213–215) or, preferably, a mechanical assist pump (205,216,217). Such devices may be life-sustaining until RV mechanical function recovers.

REFERENCES

1. Suzuki J, Sakamoto T, Takenaka K, et al. Assessment of the thickness of the right ventricular free wall by magnetic resonance imaging in patients with hypertrophic cardiomyopathy. *Br Heart J.* 1988;60:440–445.
2. Laks MM, Garner D, Swan HJC. Volumes and compliances measured simultaneously in the right and left ventricles of the dog. *Circ Res.* 1967;20:565.
3. Abel FL, Waldhausen JA. Effects of alterations in pulmonary vascular resistance on right ventricular function. *J Thorac Cardiovasc Surg.* 1967;54:886.
4. Sarnoff SJ, Berglund D. Ventricular function. I. Starling's law of the heart studied by means of simultaneous right and left ventricular function curves in the dog. *Circulation.* 1954;9:706.
5. Maughan WL, Shoukas AA, Sagawa K, et al. Instantaneous pressure-volume relationship of the canine right ventricle. *Circ Res.* 1979;44:309–315.
6. Konstam MA, Cohen SR, Salem DN, et al. Comparison of left and right ventricular end-systolic pressure-volume relations in congestive heart failure. *J Am Coll Cardiol.* 1985;5:1326–1334.
7. Konstam MA, Salem DN, Isner JM, et al. Vasodilator effect on right ventricular function in congestive heart failure and pulmonary hypertension: end-systolic pressure-volume relationship. *Am J Cardiol.* 1984;54:132–136.
8. Friedman BJ, Lozner EC, Curfman GD, et al. Characterization of the human right ventricular pressure-volume relation: effect of dobutamine and right coronary artery stenosis. *J Am Coll Cardiol.* 1984;4:999–1005.
9. Iskandrian AS, Hakki AH, Ren BF, et al. Correlation among right ventricular preload, afterload and ejection fraction in mitral valve disease: radionuclide, echocardiographic and hemodynamic evaluation. *J Am Coll Cardiol.* 1984;6:1403–1411.
10. Brent BN, Berger HJ, Matthay RA, et al. Physiologic correlates of right ventricular ejection fraction in chronic obstructive pulmonary disease: a combined radionuclide and hemodynamic study. *Am J Cardiol.* 1982;50:255–262.
11. Wroblewski E, James F, Spann JF, et al. Right ventricular performance in mitral stenosis. *Am J Cardiol.* 1981;47:51–55.
12. Winzelberg GC, Boucher CA, Pohost GM, et al. Right ventricular function in aortic and mitral valve disease. *Chest.* 1981;79:520–528.
13. Korr KS, Gandsman EJ, Winkler ML, et al. Hemodynamic correlates of right ventricular ejection fraction measured with gated radionuclide angiography. *Am J Cardiol.* 1982;49:71–77.
14. Konstam MA, Weiland DS, Conlon TP, et al. Hemodynamic correlates of left ventricular versus right ventricular radionuclide volumetric responses to vasodilator therapy in congestive heart failure secondary to ischemic or dilated cardiomyopathy. *Am J Cardiol.* 1987;59:1131–1137.
15. Vlahakes GJ, Turley K, Hoffman JIE. The pathophysiology of failure in acute right ventricular hypertension: hemodynamic and biochemical correlations. *Circulation.* 1981;63:87–95.
16. Spann JF, Buccino RA, Sonnenblick EH, et al. Contractile state of cardiac muscle obtained from cats with experimentally produced ventricular hypertrophy and heart failure. *Circ Res.* 1967;21:341–354.
17. Kaufmann RL, Homburger H, Wirth H. Disorder in excitation-contraction coupling of cardiac muscle from cats with experimentally produced right ventricular hypertrophy. *Circ Res.* 1971; 28:346–357.
18. Bing OHL, Matsushita S, Fanburg BL, et al. Mechanical properties of rat cardiac muscle during experimental hypertrophy. *Circ Res.* 1973;28:234–245.
19. Williams JF, Potter RD. Normal contractile state of hypertrophied myocardium after pulmonary artery constriction in the cat. *J Clin Invest.* 1974;54:1266–1272.
20. Cooper G, Tomanek RJ, Ehrhardt JC, et al. Chronic progressive pressure overload of the cat right ventricle. *Circ Res.* 1981;48: 488–497.
21. Murray PA, Vatner SF. Reduction of maximum coronary vascular response to exercise in dogs with severe right ventricular hypertrophy. *J Clin Invest.* 1981;67:1314–1323.
22. Doty D, Wright C, Eastham C, et al. Coronary reserve in atrial septal defect. *Circulation.* 1980;62(Suppl III):III–115.
23. Cohn JN, Gwha NH, Broder MI, et al. Right ventricular infarction. Clinical and hemodynamic features. *Am J Cardiol.* 1974;33:209–214.
24. Sharpe DN, Botvinick EH, Shames DM, et al. The noninvasive diagnosis of right ventricular infarction. *Circulation.* 1978; 57:483–490.
25. Lorell B, Leinbach RC, Pohost GM, et al. Right ventricular infarction. *Am J Cardiol.* 1979;43:465–471.
26. Dell'Italia LJ, Starling MR, O'Rourke RA. Physical examination for exclusion of hemodynamically important right ventricular infarction. *Ann Intern Med.* 1983;99:608–611.
27. Dalen JE, Haffajee CI, Alpert JS 3rd, et al. Pulmonary embolism, pulmonary hemorrhage and pulmonary infarction. *N Engl J Med.* 1977;296:1431–1435.
28. Sharma GV, Schoolman M, Cella G, et al. Pulmonary embolism. Part I. *Circulation.* 1983;67:245–247.
29. Sharma GV, Schoolman M, Cella G, et al. Pulmonary embolism. Part II. *Circulation.* 1983;67:474–477.
30. Dalen JE, Haynes FW, Hoppin FG, et al. Cardiovascular responses to experimental pulmonary embolism. *Am J Cardiol.* 1967;20:3–9.
31. Dobell AR. Capability of the right ventricle. *Can J Cardiol.* 1988;4:12–16.
32. Jaenike JR, Waterhouse C. The nature and distribution of cardiac edema. *Lab Clin Med.* 1958;52:384–393.
33. Davis JO. The mechanism of salt and water retention in cardiac failure. *Hosp Pract.* 1970;5:63–76.
34. Davis JO, Freeman RH. Mechanisms regulating renin release. *Physiol Rev.* 1976;56:1–56.
35. Zanchetti A, Stella A. Neural control of renin release. *Clin Sci Mol Med.* 1975;48:215s–223s.
36. Ferguson DW, Abboud FM, Mark AL. Selective impairment of baroreflex-mediated vasoconstrictor responses in patients with ventricular dysfunction. *Circulation.* 1984;69:451–460.
37. Cody RJ, Atlas SA, Laragh JH, et al. Atrial natriuretic factor in normal subjects and heart failure patients. *J Clin Invest.* 1986;78:1362–1374.
38. Raine AEG, Erne P, Burgisser E, et al. Atrial natriuretic peptide and atrial pressure in patients with congestive heart failure. *N Engl J Med.* 1986;315:533–537.
39. Creager MA, Hirsch AT, Nabel EG, et al. Responsiveness of atrial natriuretic factor to reduction in right atrial pressure in patients with chronic congestive heart failure. *J Am Coll Cardiol.* 1988;11:1191–1198.
40. Keller N, Sykulski R, Thamsborg G, et al. Changes in atrial natriuretic factor during preload reduction with nitroglycerin in patients with congestive heart failure. *Clin Physiol.* 1988; 8:57–64.
41. Koepke JP, DiBona GF. Blunted natriuresis to atrial natriuretic peptide in chronic sodium-retaining disorders. *Am J Physiol.* 1987;252:F865–F871.

42. Ganguly PK, Dhalla KS, Shao Q, et al. Differential changes in sympathetic activity in left and right ventricles in congestive heart failure after myocardial infarction. *Am Heart J.* 1997; 133:340–345.
43. Sethi R, Dhalla KS, Beamish RE, et al. Differential changes in left and right ventricular adenylyl cyclase activities in congestive heart failure. *Am J Physiol.* (Heart Circ Physiol.) 1997; 272(41): H884–H893.
44. Atkins FL, Bing OHL, DiMauro PG, Conrad CH, Robinson KG, Brooks WW. Modulation of left and right ventricular beta-adrenergic receptors from spontaneously hypertensive rats with left ventricular hypertrophy and failure. *Hypertension* 1995;26: 78–82.
45. Liang CS, Fan TH, Sullebarger JT, et al. Decreased adrenergic neuronal uptake activity in experimental right heart failure. A chamber specific contributor to beta-adrenoceptor downregulation. *J Clin Invest.* 1989;84:1267–1275.
46. Braunwald E. Clinical manifestations of heart failure. In: Braunwald E, ed. *Heart Disease.* Philadelphia: WB Saunders; 1988.
47. Remetz MS, Cleman MW, Cabin HS. Pulmonary and pleural complications of cardiac disease. *Clin Chest Med.* 1989;10: 545–592.
48. Wiener-Kronish JP, Berthiaume Y, Albertine KH. Pleural effusions and pulmonary edema. *Clin Chest Med.* 1985;6:509–519.
49. Wiener-Kronish JP, Matthay MA, Callen PW, et al. Relationship of pleural effusions to pulmonary hemodynamics in patients with congestive heart failure. *Am Rev Respir Dis.* 1985;132: 1253–1256.
50. Wiener-Kronish JP, Goldstein R, et al. Lack of association of pleural effusion with chronic pulmonary arterial and right atrial hypertension. *Chest.* 1987;92:967–970.
51. Isner JM. Right ventricular myocardial infarction. In: Konstam MA, Isner JM, eds. *The right ventricle.* Boston: Kluwer; 1988.
52. White PD, August S, Michael CR. Hydrothorax in congestive heart failure. *Am J Med Sci.* 1947;214:243–247.
53. McPeak EM, Levine SA. The preponderance of right hydrothorax in congestive heart failure. *Ann Intern Med.* 1946;25:916–927.
54. Bedford DE, Lovibond JL. Hydrothorax in heart failure. *Br Heart J.* 1941;3:93–111.
55. Race GA, Scheifley CH, Edwards JE. Hydrothorax in congestive heart failure. *Am J Med.* 1957;22:83–90.
56. Weiss JM, Spodick DH. Laterality of pleural effusions in chronic congestive heart failure. *Am J Cardiol.* 1984;53:951.
57. Weiss JM, Spodick DH. Association of left pleural effusion with pericardial disease. *N Engl J Med.* 1983;308:696–697.
58. Chakko SC, Caldwell SH, Sforza PP. Treatment of congestive heart failure. Its effect on pleural fluid chemistry. *Chest.* 1989; 95:798–802.
59. Shinto RA, Light RW. Effects of diuresis on the characteristics of pleural fluid in patients with congestive heart failure. *Am J Med.* 1990;88:230–234.
60. Pittman JG, Cohen P. The pathogenisis of cardiac cachexia. *N Engl J Med.* 1964;271:403–409,453–460.
61. Resnick H Jr, Friedman B. Studies on the mechanism of the increased oxygen consumptin in patients with cardiac disease. *J Clin Invest.* 1935;14:551–562.
62. Berkowitz D, Croll MN, Likoff W. Malabsorption as a compilcation of congestive heart fiure. *Am J Cardiol.* 1963;11:43–47.
63. Estes NAM, Levine HJ. Cardiac cachexia. *Med Grand Rounds.* 1982;1:188–200.
64. Carr JG, Stevenson LW, Walden JA, et al. Prevalence and hemodynamic correlates of malnutrition in severe congestive heart failure secondary to ischemic or idiopathic dilated cardiomyopathy. *Am J Cardiol.* 1989;63:709–713.
65. Levine B, Kalman J, Mayer L, et al. Elevated circulating levels of tumor necrosis factor in severe chronic heart failure. *N Engl J Med.* 1990;323:236–241.
66. Levine RA, Gibson TC, Aretz T, et al. Echocardiographic measurement of right ventricular volume. *Circulation.* 1984; 69:497.
67. Ratner S, Huang P, Friedman M, et al. Assessment of right ventricular anatomy and function by quantitative radionuclide ventriculography. *JACC.* 1989;13(2):354–359.
68. Diamond MA, Dillon JC, Haine CL, et al. Echocardiographic features of atrial septal defect. *Circulation.* 1971;43:129–135.
69. Tajik AJ, Gau GT, Ritter DG, et al. Echocardiographic pattern of right ventricular diastolic volume overload in children. *Circulation.* 1972;46:36–43.
70. Meyer RA, Schwartz DC, Benzing G, et al. Ventricular septum in right ventricular volume overload. *Am J Cardiol.* 1972;30: 349–353.
71. Kerber RE, Dippel WF, Abbound FM. Abnormal motion of the interventricular septum in right ventricular volume overload. *Circulation.* 1973;48:86–96.
72. Hagen AD, Francis GS, Sahn DJ, et al. Ultrasound evaluation of systolic anterior septal motion in patients with and without right ventricular volume overload. *Circulation.* 1974;50:248–254.
73. Pearlman AS, Clark CE, Henry WL, et al. Determinants of ventricular septal motion. Influence of relative right and left ventricular size. *Circulation.* 1976;54:83–91.
74. Visner MS, Arentzen CE, O'Connor MJ, et al. Alterations in left ventricular three-dimensional dynamic geometry and systolic function during acute right ventricular hypertension in the conscious dog. *Circulation.* 1983;67:353–365.
75. Badke FR. Left ventricular dimensions and function during exercise in dogs with chronic right ventricular pressure overload. *Am J Cardiol.* 1984;53:1187–1193.
76. Feneley M, Gavaghan T. Paradoxical and pseudoparadoxical interventricular septal motion in patients with right ventricular volume overload. *Circulation.* 1986;74:230–238.
77. Konstam MA, Kronenberg MW, Udelson JE, et al. Effect of acute angiotensin converting enzyme inhibition on left ventricular filling in patients with congestive heart failure. Relation to right ventricular volumes. *Circulation* 1990;81(Suppl III):III-115–III-122.
78. Konstam MA, Pandian N. Assessment of right ventricular function. In: Konstam MA, Isner J, eds. *The Right Ventricle.* Boston: Kluwer; 1988.
79. Boxt LM. Radiology of the right ventricle. *Radiol Clin North Am.* 1999;37(2):379–400.
80. Gentzler RD, Briselli MF, Gault JH. Angiographic estimation of right ventricular volume in man. *Circulation.* 1964;50:324–330
81. Maddahi J, Berman DS, Matsuoka DT, et al. A new technique for assessing right ventricular ejection fraction using rapid multiple-gated equilibrium cardiac blood pool scintigraphy. *Circulation.* 1979;60:581–589.
82. Konstam MA, Kahn PC, Curran BH, et al. Equilibrium (gated) radionuclide ejection fraction measurement in the pressure or volume overloaded right ventricle. *Chest.* 1984;86:681–687.
83. Grothues F, Moon J, Bellenger N, et al. Interstudy reproducibility of right ventricular volumes, function, and mass with cardiovascular magnetic resonance. *Am Heart J.* 2004;147(2): 218–223.
84. Kaul S, Tei C, Hopkins JM, et al. Assessment of right ventricular function using two dimensional echocardiography. *Am Heart J.* 1984;107:526–531.
85. Bommer W, Weinert L, Neumann A, et al. Determination of right atrial and right ventricular size by two dimensional echocardiography. *Circulation.* 1979;60:91.
86. Yock P, Popp R. Noninvasive estimation of right ventricular systolic pressure by Doppler ultrasound in tricuspid regurgitation. *Circulation* 1984;70:657.
87. Schindera S, Mehwald P, Sahn, D, et al. Accuracy of real time three-dimensional echocardiography for quantifying right ventricular volume. *J Ultrasound Med.* 2002;21:1069–1075.
88. Jiang L, Siu S, Handschumaher M, et al. Myocardial imaging: three dimensional echocardiography: In vivo validation for right ventricular volume and function. *Circulation.* 1994;89: 2342–2350.
89. Vogel M, White P, Redington A. In vitro validation of right ventricular volume measurement by three dimensional echocardiography. *Br Heart J.* 1995;74(10):460–463.
90. Vogel M, Gutberlet M, Dittrich S, et al. Comparison of transthoracic three dimensional echocardiography with magnetic resonance imaging in the assessment of right ventricular volume and mass. *Heart.* 1997;78(2):127–130.
91. Koch K, Oellig F, Oberholzer K, et al. Assessment of right ventricular function by 16-detector-row CT: comparison with magnetic resonance imaging. *Eur Radiol.* 2005;15:312–318.
92. Reiter S, Ruberger J, Feiring A, et al. Precision of measurements of right and left ventricular volume by cine computed tomography. *Circulation.* 1986;74:890–900.
93. Hajduczok Z, Weiss R, Stanford R, Marcus M. Determination of right ventricular mass in humans and dogs with ultrafast cardiac computed tomography. *Circulation.* 1990;82(1):202–212.

94. Menghetti L, Basso C, Nava A, et al. Spin-echo nuclear magnetic resonance for tissue characterization in arrhythmogenic right ventricular cardiomyopathy. *Heart.* 1996;76:67.
95. Langmore D, Underwood S, Hounsfiled G, et al. Dimensional accuracy of magnetic resonance in studies of the heart. *Lancet.* 1985; i:1360–1362.
96. Isner JM, Roberts WC. Right ventricular infarction complicating left ventricular infarction secondary to coronary heart disease. Frequency, location, associated findings and significance from analysis of 236 necropsy patients with acute or healed myocardial infarction. *Am J Cardiol.* 1978;42:885–894.
97. Ratliff NB, Hackel DB. Combined right and left ventricular infarction: pathogenesis and clinicopathologic correlations. *Am J Cardiol.* 1980;45:217–221.
98. Chou TC, Fowler NO, Gabel M, et al. Electrocardiographic and hemodynamic changes in experimental right ventricular infarction. *Circulation.* 1983;67:1258–1267.
99. Cabin HS, Clubb S, Wackers FJ, et al. Right ventricular myocardial infarction with anterior wall left ventricular infarction: an autopsy study. *Am Heart J.* 1987;113:16–23.
100. Weinshel AJ, Isner JM, Salem DN, et al. The coronary anatomy of right ventricular myocardial infarction: relationship between the site of right coronary occlusion and origin of the right ventricular free wall branches. *Circulation.* 1983;68:III-351.
101. Shah PK, Maddahi J, Berman DS, et al. Scintigraphically detected predominant right ventricular dysfunction in acute myocardial infarction: clinical and hemodynamic correlates and implications for therapy and prognosis. *J Am Coll Cardiol.* 1985;6: 1264–1272.
102. Lopez-Sendon J, Coma-Canella I, Gamello C. Sensitivity and specificity of hemodynamic criteria in the diagnosis of right ventricular infarction. *Circulation.* 1981;64:515–525.
103. Goldstein JA, Vlahakes GJ, Verrier ED, et al. The role of right ventricular systolic dysfunction and elevated intrapericardial pressure in the genesis of low output in experimental right ventricular infarction. *Circulation.* 1982;65:513–522.
104. Haines DE, Beller GA, Watson DD, et al. A prospective clinical, scintigraphic, angiographic and functional evaluation of patients after inferior myocardial infarction with and without right ventricular dysfunction. *J Am Coll Cardiol.* 1985;6:995.
105. Dellitalia LJ, Starling MR, Crawford MH, et al. Right ventricular infarction identification by hemodynamic measurements before and after volume loading and correlation with non-invasive techniques. *J Am Coll Cardiol.* 1984;4:931.
106. Bowers TR, O'Neill WW, Grines C, et al. Effect of reperfusion on biventricular function and survival after right ventricular infarction. *N Engl J Med.* 1998;338:933–940
107. Ibsen HHW, Baandrup U, Simonsen EE. Familial right ventricular dilated cardiomyopathy. *Br Heart J.* 1985;54:156–159.
108. Unverferth DV, Baker PB, Swift SE, et al. Extent of myocardial fibrosis and cellular hypertrophy in dilated cardiomyopathy. *Am J Cardiol.* 1986;57:816–821.
109. Roberts WC, Waller BF. Cardiac amyloidosis causing cardiac dysfunction: analysis of 54 necropsy patients. *Am J Cardiol.* 1983;52:137–146.
110. Patel AR, Dubrey SW, Mendes LA, et al. Right ventricular dilation in primary amyloidosis: an independent predictor of survival. *Am J Cardiol.* 1997;80:486–492.
111. Johnson RA, Palacios I, Harrington WJ, et al. Nondilated cardiomyopathies. In Stollerman G, et al., eds. *Advances in Internal Medicine.* Chicago: Year Book Medical Publishers; 1984.
112. Buja LM, Roberts WC. Iron in the heart. Etiology and significance. *Am J Med.* 1971;51:209–221.
113. Cutler DJ, Isner JM, Bracey AW, et al. Hemachromatosis heart disease. An unemphasized cause of potentially reversible restrictive cardiomyopathy. *Am J Med.* 1980;69:923.
114. Short EM, Winkle RE, Billingham ME. Myocardial involvement in idiopathic hemachromatosis. Morphologic and clinical improvement following venesection. *Am J Med.* 1981;70: 1275.
115. Roberts WC, McAllister HA, Ferrans VJ. Sarcoidosis of the heart. *Am J Med.* 1977;63:86–108.
116. Fleming HH. Sarcoid heart disease. *BMJ.* 1986;292:1095.
117. Koide T, Itoyzma S, Kato K, et al. Cardiac sarcoidosis with 12-year survival. *Jpn Heart J.* 1982;23:263.
118. Ishikawa T, Kondoh H, Nagakaw S, et al. Steroid therapy in cardiac sarcoidosis: increased left ventricular contractility concomitant with electrocardiographic improvement after prednisolone. *Chest.* 1984;85:445.
119. Fauci AS, Harley JB, Roberts WC, et al. The idiopathic hypereosinophilic syndrome. *Ann Intern Med.* 1982;97:78–92.
120. Olsen EGJ, Spry CJF. Relation between eosinophilia and endomyocardial disease. *Prog Cardiovasc Dis.* 1985;27:241.
121. Davies JNP, Coles RM. Some considerations regarding obscure disease affecting the mural endocardium. *Am Heart J.* 1960; 59:606.
122. Cherian G, Vijayaraghavan G, Krishnaswami S, et al. Endomyocardial fibrosis: report on the hemodynamic data in 29 patients and review of the results of surgery. *Am Heart J.* 1983; 105:659.
123. Metras D, Coulibaly AO, Ouattara K. The surgical treatment of endomyocardial fibrosis: results in 55 patients. *Circulation.* 1985;72:II-274.
124. Ross EM, Roberts WC. The carcinoid syndrome: comparison of 21 necropsy subjects with carcinoid heart disease to 15 necropsy subjects without carcinoid heart disease. *Am J Med.* 1985;79:339–354.
125. Warnes CA, Roberts WC. The heart in massive (more than 300 pounds or 136 kilograms) obesity: analysis of 12 patients studied at necropsy. *Am J Cardiol.* 1984;54:1087–1091.
126. Marcus FI, Fontaine GH, Guiraudon G, et al. Right ventricular dysplasia: a report of 24 adult cases. *Circulation.* 1982; 65:384.
127. Robertson JH, Brady GH, German LD, et al. Comparison of two-dimensional echocardiographic and angiographic findings in arrhythmogenic right ventricular dysplasia. *Am J Cardiol.* 1985;55:1506.
128. Diggelmann U, Baur HR. Familial Uhl's anomaly in the adult. *Am J Cardiol.* 1984;53:1402.
129. Corrado D, Basso C, Thiene G, et al. Spectrum of clinicopathologic manifestations of arrhythmogenic right ventricular cardiomyopathy/dysplasia: a multicenter study. *J Am Coll Cardiol.* 1997;30:1512–1520.
130. Guiraudon GM, Klein GJ, Gulamhusein SS, et al. Total disconnection of the right ventricular free wall: surgical treatment of right ventricular tachycardia associated with right ventricular dysplasia. *Circulation.* 1983;67:464.
131. Mahler DA, Brent BN, Like J, et al. Right ventricular performance and central circulatory hemodynamics during upright exercise in patients with chronic obstructive pulmonary disease. *Am Rev Respir Dis.* 1984;130:722–729.
132. Cohen M, Horowitz SF, Machac J, et al. Response of the right ventricle to exercise in isolated mitral stenosis. *Am J Cardiol.* 1985;55:1054–1058.
133. Grose R, Strain J, Yipinatosoi T. Right ventricular function in valvular heart disease: relation to pulmonary artery pressure. *J Am Coll Cardiol.* 1983;2:225–232.
134. Johnston DL, Kostuk WJ. Left and right ventricular function during symptom-limited exercise in patients with isolated mitral stenosis. *Chest* 1986;89:186.
135. Krabill KA, Wang Y, Einzig S, et al. Rest and exercise hemodynamics in pulmonary stenosis: comparison of children and adults. *Am J Cardiol.* 1985;56:360.
136. Johnson LW, Grossman W, Dalen JE, et al. Pulmonic stenosis in the adult: long-term follow-up results. *N Engl J Med.* 1972;287:1159.
137. Johnson GL, Kwan IL, Handshoe S, et al. Accuracy of combined two-dimensional echocardiography and continuous wave recordings in the estimation of pressure gradient in right ventricular outlet obstruction. *J Am Coll Cardiol.* 1984;3:1013.
138. Locke J, Keane J, Ferllows K. The use of catheter intervention procedures for congenital heart disease. *J Am Coll Cardiol.* 1986;7:1421.
139. McAllister RG, Friesinger GC, Sinclair-Smith BC. Tricuspid regurgitation following inferior myocardial infarction. *Arch Intern Med.* 1976;136:905.
140. Carpentier A, Deloche A, Dauptain A. A new reconstructive operation for correction of tricuspid and mitral insufficiency. *J Thorac Cardiovasc Surg.* 1971;61:1.
141. Liberthson RR, Boucher CA, Strauss HW, et al. Right ventricular function in adult atrial septal defect: preoperative and postoper-

ative assessment and clinical implications. *Am J Cardiol.* 1981; 47:56–60.
142. Konstam MA, Idoine J, Wynne J, et al. Right ventricular function in pulmonary hypertensive adults with and without atrial septal defects. *Am J Cardiol.* 1983;51:1144–1148.
143. Ludbrook PA, Byrne JD, McKnight RC. Influence of right ventricular hemodynamics on left ventricular diastolic pressure-volume relations in man. *Circulation.* 1979;59:21–31.
144. Ross J. Acute displacement of the diastolic pressure-volume curve of the left ventricle: role of the pericardium and the right ventricle. *Circulation.* 1979;59:32–37.
145. Lorell BH, Palacios I, Daggett WM, et al. Right ventricular distension and left ventricular compliance. *Am J Physiol.* 1981;240: H87–H89.
146. Lavine SJ, Tami L, Jawad I. Pattern of left ventricular diastolic filling associated with right ventricular enlargement. *Am J Cardiol.* 1988;62:444–448.
147. Smith ER, Tyberg JV. Ventricular interdependence. In: Konstam MA, Isner JM, eds. *The right ventricle.* Boston: Kluwer; 1988.
148. Dittrich HC, Chow LC, Nicod PH. Early improvement in left ventricular diastolic function after relief of chronic right ventricular pressure overload. *Circulation.* 1989;80:823–830.
149. Tyberg JV, Taichman GC, Smith ER, et al. The relation between pericardial pressure and right atrial pressure: an intraoperative study. *Circulation.* 1986;73:428–432.
150. Carroll JD, Land RM, Neumann AL, et al. The differential effects of positive inotropic and vasodilator therapy on diastolic properties in patients with congestive cardiomyopathy. *Circulation.* 1986;74:815–825.
151. Watanabe J, Levine MJ, Bellotto F, et al. Effects of coronary venous pressure on left ventricular diastolic distensibility. *Circ Res.* 1990;67:923–932.
152. Farrar DJ, Chow E, Brown CD. Isolated systolic and diastolic ventricular interactions in pacing-induced dilated cardiomyopathy and effects of volume loading and pericardium. *Circulation.* 1995;92:1284–1290.
153. Baker BJ, Wilen MM, Boyd CM, et al. Relation of right ventricular ejection fraction to exercise capacity in chronic left ventricular failure. *Am J Cardiol.* 1984;54:596–599.
154. Polak JF, Holman BL, Wynne J, et al. Right ventricular ejection fraction: an indicator of increased mortality in patients with congestive heart failure associated with coronary artery disease. *J Am Coll Cardiol.* 1983;2:217–224.
155. Brill DM, Konstam MA, Vivino PG, et al. Importance of right ventricular systolic function as an independent predictor of mortality in patients with congestive heart failure. *Circulation.* 1989;80:II-649.
156. Zornoff LA, Skali H, Pfeffer MA, SAVE Investigators. Right ventricular dysfunction and risk of heart failure and mortality after myocardial infarction. *J Am Coll Cardiol.* 2002;39: 450–455.
157. Konstam MA, Kronenberg MW, Udelson JE, et al, for the SOLVD Investigators. Preload reserve: a determinant of clinical status in patients with left ventricular systolic dysfunction. *J Am Coll Cardiol.* 1991;17:89A.
158. Brill DM, Konstam MA, Vivino PG, et al. Rapid-onset pulmonary edema in patients with left ventricular systolic dysfunction: a syndrome related to right ventricular ejection fraction. *J Am Coll Cardiol.* 1989;13:179A.
159. Goldstein JA, Vlahakes GJ, Verrier ED, et al. Volume loading improves low cardiac output in experimental right ventricular infarction. *J Am Coll Cardiol.* 1978;2:270–278.
160. Isner JM, Fisher GP, Del Negro AA, et al. Right ventricular infarction with hemodynamic decompensation due to transient loss of active atrial augmentation: successful treatment with atrial pacing. *Am Heart J.* 1981;102:792–794.
161. Taylor SH. Diuretics in cardiovascular therapy. Perusing the past, practicing in the present, preparing for the future. *Z Kardiol.* 1985;74(Suppl 2):2–12.
162. Heinemann HO. Right-sided heart failure and the use of diuretics. *Am J Med.* 1978;64:367–370.
163. Franciosa JA, Nordstrom LA, Cohn JN. Nitrate therapy for congestive heart failure. *JAMA.* 1978;240:443–446.
164. Leier CV, Huss P, Magorien RD, et al. Improved exercise capacity and differing arterial and venous tolerance during chronic isosorbide dinitrate therapy for congestive heart failure. *Circulation.* 1983;67:817–822.
165. Armstrong PW. Pharmacokinetic-hemodynamic studies of transdermal nitroglycerin in congestive heart failure. *J Am Coll Cardiol.* 1987;9:420–425.
166. Packer M, Halperin JL, Brooks KM, et al. Nitroglycerin therapy in the management of pulmonary hypertensive disorders. *Am J Med.* 1984;76:67–75.
167. Morrison D, Caldwell J, Lakshminaryan S, et al. The acute effects of low flow oxygen and isosorbide dinitrate on left and right ventricular ejection fractions in chronic obstructive pulmonary disease. *J Am Coll Cardiol.* 1983;2:652–660.
168. Brent BN, Berger HJ, Matthay RA, et al. Contrasting acute effects of vasodilators (nitroglycerin, nitroprusside, and hydralazine) on right ventricular performance in patients with chronic obstructive pulmonary disease and pulmonary hypertension: a combined radionuclide-hemodynamic study. *Am J Cardiol.* 1983;51:1682–1689.
169. Banahy DT, Tobis JM, Aronow WS, et al. Effects of isosorbide dinitrate on pulmonary hypertension in chronic obstructive pulmonary disease. *Clin Pharmacol Ther.* 1979;25:541–548.
170. Geggel RL, Dozor AJ, Fyler DC, et al. Effect of vasodilators at rest and during exercise in young adults with cystic fibrosis and chronic cor pulmonale. *Am Rev Respir Dis.* 1985;131:531–536.
171. Zielinski J, Hawrylkiewicz I, Gorecka D, et al. Captopril effects on pulmonary and systemic hemodynamics in chronic cor pulmonale. *Chest.* 1986;90:562–565.
172. Wilson RH, Hoseth W, Dempsey ME. The effects of breathing of 99.6% oxygen on pulmonary vascular resistance and cardiac output in patients with pulmonary emphysema and chronic hypoxia. *Ann Intern Med.* 1955;42:629–637.
173. Abraham AS, Cole RB, Bishop JM. Reversal of pulmonary hypertension by prolonged oxygen administration in patients with chronic bronchitis. *Circ Res.* 1968;23:147–157.
174. Ashutosh K, Mead G, Dunsky M. Early effects of oxygen administration on prognosis in chronic obstructive pulmonary disease and cor pulmonale. *Am Rev Respir Dis.* 1983;127:399–404.
175. Stark RD, Finnegan P, Bishop JM. Daily requirement of oxygen to reverse pulmonary hypertension in patients with chronic bronchitis. *Br Med J.* 1972;3:724–728.
176. Brent BN, Mahler DA, Berger HJ, et al. Augmentation of right ventricular performance in chronic obstructive pulmonary disease by terbutaline: a combined radionuclide and hemodynamic study. *Am J Cardiol.* 1982;50:313–319.
177. Teule GJ, Majid PA. Hemodynamic effects of terbutaline in chronic obstructive airways disease. *Thorax.* 1980;35:536–542.
178. Rutherford JD, Vatner SF, Braunwald E. Effects of mechanisms of action of aminophylline on cardiac function and regional blood flow distribution in conscious dogs. *Circulation.* 1981;63: 378–387.
179. Parker JO, Ashekian PB, DiGiorgi S, et al. Hemodynamic effects of aminophylline in chronic obstructive pulmonary disease. *Circulation.* 1967;35:365–372.
180. Matthay RA, Berger HJ, Toke J, et al. Effects of aminophylline upon right and left ventricular performance in chronic obstructive pulmonary disease. Noninvasive assessment by radionuclide angiocardiography. *Am J Med.* 1978;65:903–910.
181. Matthay RA, Berger HJ, Davies R, et al. Improvement in cardiac performance by oral long-acting theophylline in chronic obstructive pulmonary disease. *Am Heart J.* 1982;104: 1022–1026.
182. Keller CA, Shepard JW, Chun DS, et al. Effects of hydralazine on hemodynamics, ventilation, and gas exchange in patients with chronic obstructive pulmonary disease and pulmonary hypertension. *Am Rev Respir Dis.* 1984;130:606–611.
183. Tuxen DV, Powles ACP, Mathur PN, et al. Detrimental effects of hydralazine in patients with chronic air-flow obstruction and pumlonary hypertension. *Am Rev Respir Dis.* 1984;129:388–395.
184. Dal Nogare AR, Rubin L. The effects of hydralazine on exercise capacity in pulmonary hypertension secondary to chronic obstructive pulmonary disease. *Am Rev Respir Dis.* 1986; 133:385–389.
185. Rubin LJ, Peter RH. Hemodynamics at rest and during exercise after oral hydralazine in patients with cor pulmonale. *Am J Cardiol.* 1981;47:116–122.

186. Simmoneau G, Escourrou P, Puroux P, et al. Inhibition of hypoxic pulmonary vasoconstriction by nifedipine. *N Engl J Med.* 1981;304:1582–1585.
187. Sturani C, Bassein L, Schiavani M, et al. Oral nifedipine in chronic cor pulmonale secondary to severe chronic obstructive pulmonary disease (COPD). *Chest.* 1983;84:135–142.
188. Melot C, Hallemans R, Naeije R, et al. Deleterious effect of nifedipine on pulmonary gas exchange in chronic obstructive pulmonary disease. *Am Rev Respir Dis.* 1984;130:612–616.
189. Zakheim RM, Mattioli L, Molteni A, et al. Prevention of pulmonary vascular changes of chronic alveolar hypoxia by inhibition of angiotensin I converting enzyme in the rat. *Lab Invest.* 1975;33:57–61.
190. Bertoli L, LoCicero S, Busnardo I, et al. Effects of captopril on hemodynamics and blood gases in chronic obstructive lung disease with pulmonary hypertension. *Respiration.* 1986;49:251–256.
191. Boschetti E, Tantucci C, Cocchieri M, et al. Acute effects of captopril in hypoxic pulmonary hypertension. Comparison with transient oxygen administration. *Respiration.* 1985;48:296–302.
192. Packer M, Greenberg B, Massie B, et al. Deleterious effects of hydralazine in patients with pulmonary hypertension. *N Engl J Med.* 1982;306:1326–1332.
193. Packer M. Vasodilator therpy for primary pulmonary hypertension. Limitations and hazards. *Ann Intern Med.* 1985;103:258–270.
194. Miyauchi T, Sato R, Sakai S, et al. Endothelin-1 and right-sided heart failure in rats: effects of an endothelin receptor antagonist on the failing right ventricle. *J Cardiovasc Pharmacol.* 2000;36(5 Suppl 1):S327–S330.
195. Galie N, Hinderliter AL, Torbicki A, et al. Effects of the oral endothelin-receptor antagonist bosentan on echocardiographic and Doppler measures in patients with pulmonary arterial hypertension. *J Am Coll Cardiol.* 2003;41:1380–1386.
196. Konstam MA, Cohen SR, Salem DN, et al. Amrinone effect on right ventricular function: predominance of afterload reduction. *Circulation.* 1986;74:359–366.
197. Eichhorn EJ, Konstam MA, Weiland DS, et al. Differential effects of milrinone and dobutamine on right ventricular preload, afterload, and systolic performance in congestive heart failure secondary to ischemic or idiopathic dilated cardiomyopathy. *Am J Cardiol.* 1987;60:1329–1333.
198. Hill NS, Rounds S. Amrinone dilates pulmonary vessels and blunts hypoxic vasoconstriction in isolated rat lungs. *Proc Soc Exp Biol Med.* 1983;173:205–212.
199. Green LH, Smith TW. The use of digitalis in patients with pulmonary disease. *Ann Intern Med.* 1977;87:419–465.
200. Ferrer MI, Harvey RM, Cathcart RT, et al. Some effects of digoxin upon the heart and circulation in man. Digoxin in cor pulmonale. *Circulation.* 1950;1:161–186.
201. Jezek V, Schrijen F. Haemodynamic effect of deslanoside at rest and during exercise in patients with chronic bronchitis. *Br Heart J.* 1973;35:2–8.
202. Kim YS, Aviado DM. Digitalis and the pulmonary circulation. *Am Heart J.* 1961;62:680–686.
203. Linde LM, Goldberg SJ, Gaal P, et al. Pulmonary and systemic hemodynamic effects of cardiac glycosides. *Am Heart J.* 1968;76:356–364.
204. Berglund E, Widimsky J, Malmberg R. Lack of effect of digitalis in patients with pulmonary disease with and without heart failure. *Am J Cardiol.* 1963;11:477–482.
205. Fonger JD, Borkon AM, Baumgartner WA, et al. Acute right ventricular failure following heart transplantation: improvement with prostaglandin E_1 and right ventricular assist. *Heart Transplant.* 1986;5:317–321.
206. Spence PA, Weisel RD, Salerno TA. Right ventricular failure. Pathophysiology and treatment. *Surg Clin North Am.* 1985;65:689–697.
207. Payne DD, Cleveland RJ. Perioperative right heart dysfunction. In: Konstam MA, Isner JM, eds. *The Right Ventricle.* Boston: Kluwer; 1988.
208. Esmore DS, Spratt PM, Branch JM, et al. Right ventricular assist and prostacyclin infusion for allograft failure in the presence of high pulmonary vascular resistance. *J Heart Transplant.* 1990;9: 136–141.
209. D'Ambra MN, LaRaia PJ, Philbin DM, et al. Prostaglandin E_1. A new therapy for refractory right heart failure and pulmonary hypertension after mitral valve replacement. *J Thorac Cardiovasc Surg.* 1985;89:567–572.
210. Armitage JM, Hardesty RL, Griffith BP. Prostaglandin E_1: an effective treatment of right heart failure after orthotopic heart transplantation. *J Heart Transplant.* 1987;6:348–351.
211. Deeb GM, Bolling SF, Guynn TP, et al. Amrinone versus conventional therapy in pulmonary hypertensive patients awaiting cardiac transplantation. *Ann Thorac Surg.* 1989;48: 665–669.
212. Hess W, Arnold B, Veit S. The haemodynamic effects of amrinone in patients with mitral stenosis and pulmonary hypertension. *Eur Heart J.* 1986;7:800–807.
213. Jett GK, Siwek LG, Picone AL, et al. Pulmonary artery balloon counterpulsation for right ventriuclar failure. *J Thorac Cardiovasc Surg.* 1983;86:364–372.
214. Flege JB, Jr., Wright CB, et al. Successful balloon counterpulsation for right ventricular failure. *Ann Thorac Surg.* 1984;37:167–168.
215. Symbas PN, McKeown PP, Santora AH, et al. Pulmonary artery counterpulsation for treatment of intra-operative right ventricular failure. *Ann Thorac Surg* 1985;39:437–440.
216. Dembitsky WP, Daily PO, Raney AA, et al. Temporary extracorporeal support of the right ventricle. *J Thorac Cardiovasc Surg.* 1986;91:518–525.
217. O'Neill MJ, Jr., Pierce WS, Wisman CB, et al. Successful management of right ventricular failure with the ventricular assist pump following aortic valve replacement and coronary artery bypass grafting. *J Thorac Cardiovasc Surg.* 1984;87:106–111.

Heart Failure in Cardiac Tamponade, Constrictive Pericarditis, and Restrictive Cardiomyopathy

22

Ralph Shabetai

Constrictive pericarditis and cardiac tamponade both manifest as specific forms of heart failure with preserved systolic function. While cardiac tamponade is usually managed by intensivists or interventional cardiologists, the syndrome of constrictive pericarditis shares many features of right heart failure of other etiologies, especially restrictive cardiomyopathy, and therefore is particularly relevant to heart failure, particularly diastolic heart failure. I have therefore emphasized constrictive pericarditis and its differential diagnosis from restrictive cardiomyopathy in this chapter.

CARDIAC TAMPONADE

Definition

The definition of cardiac tamponade is pericardial fluid under increased pressure that compresses the heart, thereby impeding diastolic filling, and does not permit change in total cardiac volume. Systolic function of the left ventricle as judged by its ejection fraction (LVEF) is not impaired, and often is increased because of the increase in adrenergic and sympathetic tone that accompanies cardiac tamponade. Cardiac tamponade is thus an important but uncommon cause of diastolic heart failure.

Almost every pericardial disease may be effusive and any effusion may accumulate faster than it can be absorbed and therefore may stretch the pericardium. When the pericardium is stretched it becomes increasingly stiff and eventually inextensible because the pressure volume and stress–strain curves of normal pericardium are J-shaped (Fig. 22-1). Once the pericardium has been tightly stretched, the volume of the pericardial cavity becomes fixed; this invariant pericardial volume underlies much of the pathophysiology of cardiac tamponade. Nevertheless, studies of diastolic heart failure or heart failure with preserved systolic function have shown that in these patients analysis of myocardial function discloses impairment of clinically insignificant myocardial function. This may be true for some cases of tamponade as well, but the issue has not been investigated and, in any case, is not sufficient to contribute to heart failure.

Etiology

Chief offenders include pericardial injury, occurring either at the same time as tamponade, or earlier, as in a postpericardial injury syndrome. Other causes include inflammation of any cause, neoplastic pericardial disease, acute viral or idiopathic pericarditis, tuberculous pericarditis, and mediastinal radiation. Acquired immunodeficiency syndrome (AIDS) frequently causes pericardial effusion but tamponade is uncommon unless there is a superimposed infection to which these patients are liable. The effusion is often small but is associated with poor prognosis unrelated to hemodynamics (1).

By the time patients with cardiac tamponade seek medical care their tamponade is acute, but this event may occur either immediately after a penetrating pericardial injury or be delayed for weeks or more in the case of trauma that may be blunt, as in steering wheel accidents or a blow from a fast, hard ball. Cardiac tamponade should be considered in any patient with unexplained hemodynamic deterioration after cardiac surgery. This event may occur hours after the operation has been concluded but may be delayed, sometimes until after the patient has been discharged home.

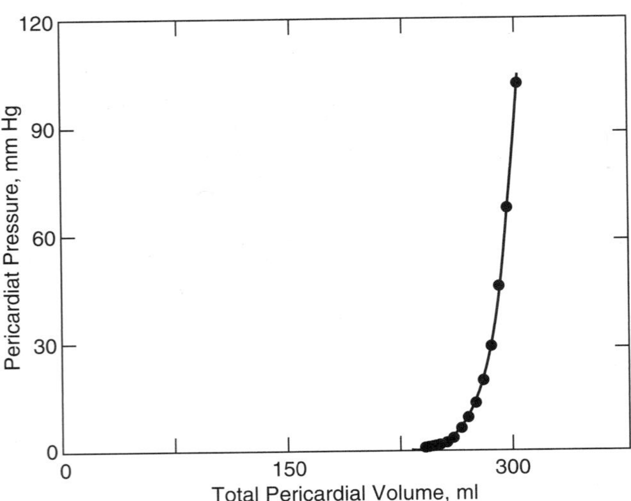

Figure 22-1 Fresh postmortem canine pericardial pressure–volume curve.

Pathophysiology

The clinical and laboratory findings are explained by the pathophysiology. Once the pericardium has been tightly stretched, it becomes inextensible; therefore, total pericardial volume cannot vary. The consequence is that if one cardiac chamber or side of the heart increases in volume, the opposite one must decrease. Attention in this regard has been focused on the ventricles and is termed ventricular interaction or interdependence. The clinical manifestation of increased ventricular interaction is pulsus paradoxus (2), a greater than normal decline in systemic arterial systolic and pulse pressures, the latter reflecting decreased stroke volume. Diastolic pressure variation remains normal. While ventricular interaction is the predominant cause of pulsus paradoxus in tamponade, other mechanisms, described elsewhere (2), contribute.

Because of the multiplicity of mechanisms, pulsus paradoxus in the two circuits is almost, but not always, precisely 180 degrees out of phase, such that peak systolic pressure of one ventricle is highest when that of the opposite ventricle is lowest. This phase relationship is known as ventricular discordance. It is another manifestation of ventricular interdependence and, as we shall see later, also occurs in constrictive pericarditis where it is of critical importance in the differential diagnosis from restrictive cardiomyopathy, in which it is absent. The major hemodynamic signs of cardiac tamponade are a pulsus paradoxus in both the systemic and pulmonary circulation, and a large increase in the amount that inspiration decreases filling of the left ventricle and increases that of the right. These abnormalities are readily detected by cardiac catheterization or echo-Doppler cardiography (3).

Another fundamental pathophysiological feature is that, in spite of even severe tamponade, the inspiratory decline in intrathoracic pressure is transmitted (although not completely) to the pericardium and heart; therefore, systemic venous return increases, much as it does in normal subjects (2,4,5). Because the pericardial volume cannot increase, the consequent increase in right ventricular volume is accomplished entirely by bulging the septum from right to left, encroaching on left ventricular volume. Cardiac volume is redistributed, not changed. The drop in central venous pressure with inspiration has the same mechanism as in normal subjects but is greater because of ventricular interaction. It can be detected at the bedside by inspecting the jugular pulse; also, the reciprocal changes in left and right ventricular dimensions and areas are readily seen on M-mode and two-dimensional echocardiograms. Because inspiration lowers pressure in the pulmonary veins that lie in the thorax but outside the pericardium, whereas the left ventricle lies entirely within the pericardium, inspiration lowers pulmonary wedge pressure more than left ventricular diastolic pressure (Fig. 22-2). This reduction in the pressure gradient for left ventricular filling makes a further contribution to diminished left ventricular volume during inspiration.

Raised pericardial pressure compresses the thin-walled atria (6) and right ventricle (7) but usually the left ventricle is hardly, if at all, directly compressed. Thus, the chief mechanism that reduces left ventricular volume is ventricular interaction, but diminished pulmonary venous return by the compressed right ventricle makes a contribution. Echocardiography clearly demonstrates compression of the right atrium (8) and collapse of the right ventricular cavity in early diastole (9,10), a time when its pressure is minimal. The pathophysiology and, hence, the clinical features of tamponade in most medical patients in whom effusion develops slowly differ importantly from those of surgical patients in whom effusion is often virtually instantaneous (11).

Total cardiac volume is minimal during ventricular ejection and is maximal in late diastole; therefore, tamponade is slightly less severe during the ejection period and is most severe in late diastole. Venous return, instead of taking place both in the ejection period (noted clinically as the x descent of venous pressure) and immediately after the atrio-ventricular valves open (noted by the y descent) (Fig. 22-3), is confined to the period of ejection (12). The jugular pulse, therefore, shows a prominent x descent but no y descent (Fig. 22-4).

Cardiac tamponade may be acute or chronic and causes characteristic clinical and hemodynamic signs. Atypical variants also occur, the most important of which are low-pressure tamponade, sometimes referred to as occult tamponade, and regional tamponade in which the fluid is loculated and therefore does not exert pressure circumferentially, but over a localized area of the heart. In some patients, cardiac tamponade and constrictive pericarditis occur together, a syndrome known as effusive-constrictive pericarditis. These variants will be discussed later in the chapter.

The hemodynamics of tamponade, owing to rupture of an aortic aneurysm of the heart or laceration of a coronary vessel or bypass graft, differ from those of postpericardial injury and other causes of tamponade as a result of the extreme rapidity of the effusion, because the pericardium is stretched in inverse proportion to the rate of effusion. When effusion is virtually instantaneous, pericardial stretch is minimal; therefore, the effusion cannot be large but pericardial pressure is extremely high and causes rapidly progressive shock (Figs. 22-5 and 22-6). An effusion that accumulates more slowly progressively stretches

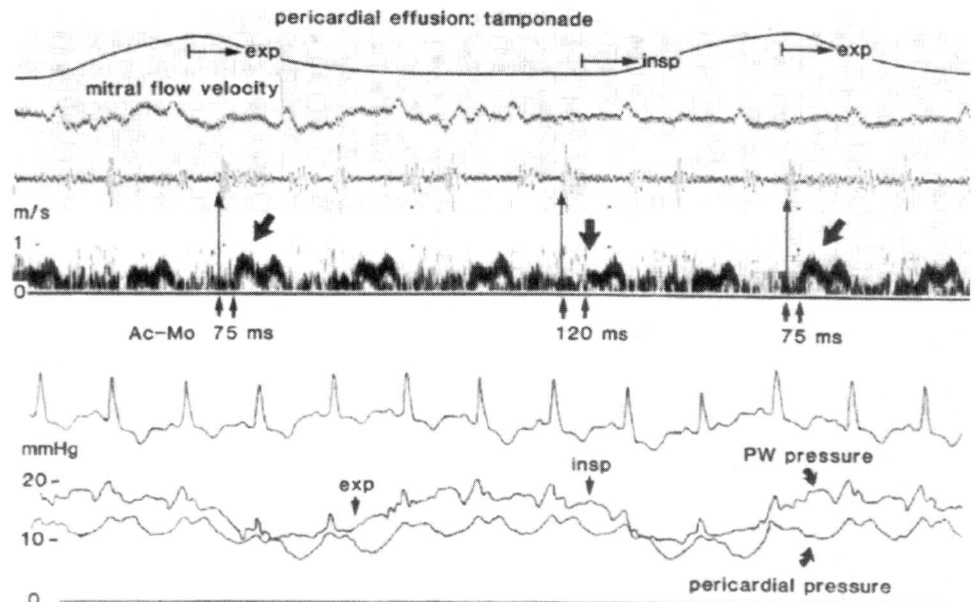

Figure 22-2 Reciprocal respiratory variation of mitral and tricuspid inflow velocities in a patient with severe cardiac tamponade. **(Top panel)** Tracings from above down: respirometer, mitral inflow velocity, ECG. The **three heavy arrows** show, sequentially, apnea, the onset of inspiration, and expiration. The **small arrows** mark isovolumic relaxation times. **(Lower panel)** Pulmonary wedge and pericardial pressures. Note that with inspiration, the pressure gradient from pulmonary wedge to pericardium (and thus presumably ventricular diastolic pressure) falls. (From Appleton CP, Hatle LK, Popp RL. Cardiac tamponade and pericardial effusion: respiratory variation in transvalvular flow velocities studied by Doppler echocardiography. *J Am Coll Cardiol.* 1988;11:1020–1030.)

the pericardium, causing it to remodel with increased compliance.

Cases seen in the practice of medicine are usually less acute [medical tamponade, (11)]; therefore, the effusion is considerably larger, causing radiological cardiomegaly, and pericardial pressure elevation is less severe but high enough to cause clinically significant cardiac tamponade (Fig. 22-7).

Typical Medical Tamponade

Clinical Examination

The history often discloses factors mentioned under Etiology, previously discussed. The predominant symptom is dyspnea, often with orthopnea, and many patients report fullness in the chest. In the more severe cases, the patients note lightheadedness or presyncope that eventually progresses to cardiogenic shock and death, unless treated.

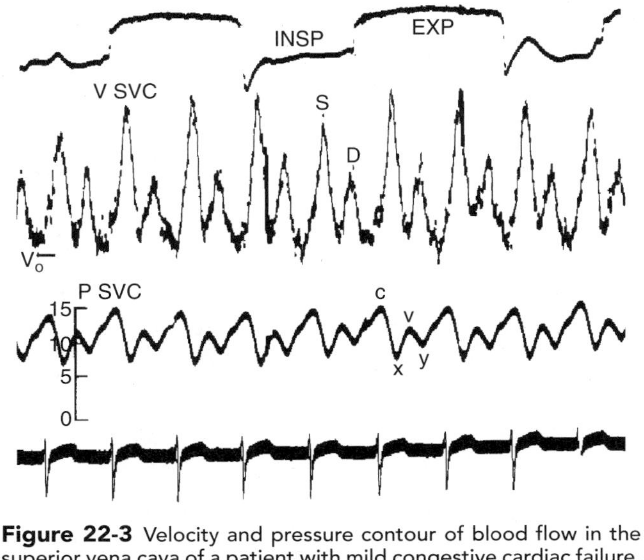

Figure 22-3 Velocity and pressure contour of blood flow in the superior vena cava of a patient with mild congestive cardiac failure. V_o indicates zero flow. V SVC and P SVC are velocity and pressure, respectively, in the superior vena cava. The predominant peak (S) is systolic and corresponds with the *x* descent of pressure. The second and smaller peak (D) corresponds with the *y* trough. (Reproduced from Shabetai R. The role of the pericardium in the pathophysiology of heart failure. In: Hosenpud JD, Greenberg BH, eds. *Congestive Heart Failure.* 2nd ed. Philadelphia: Lippincott Williams & Wilkins; 2000: 157–187.)

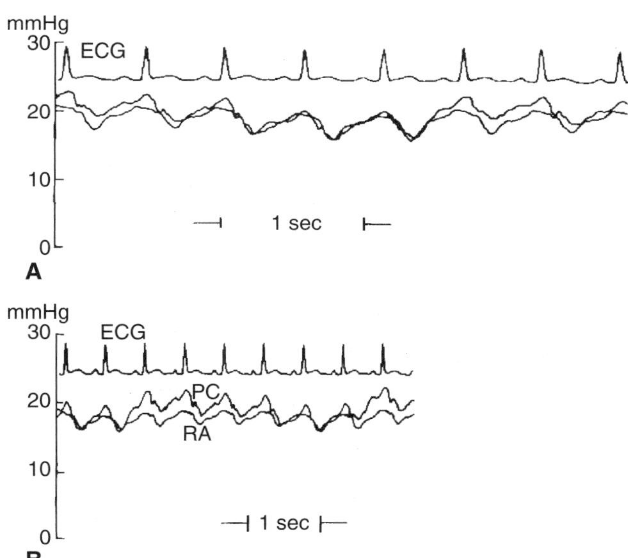

Figure 22-4 Pressure equilibration and right atrial pressure contour in cardiac tamponade. **(A)** Right atrial and pericardial pressures. **(B)** Right atrial and pulmonary capillary wedge pressures. Note absence of the *y* descent of right atrial pressure. (Reproduced from Shabetai R. The role of the pericardium in the pathophysiology of heart failure. In: Hosenpud JD, Greenberg BH, eds. *Congestive Heart Failure.* 2nd ed. Philadelphia: Lippincott Williams & Wilkins; 2000:157–187.)

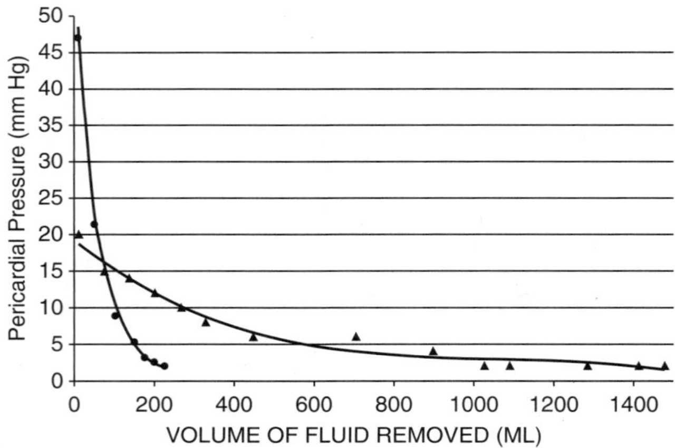

Figure 22-5 Pericardial pressure–volume curve records from a case of hyperacute cardiac tamponade (illustrated in Fig. 22-6) and from a case of cardiac tamponade complicating acute pericarditis. The curve from hyperacute tamponade shows the small volume of the effusion and a rapid decline in pericardial pressure when a small volume of fluid was withdrawn. (Reproduced from Shabetai R. Cardiac tamponade. In: Shabetai R. *The Pericardium*. Norwell, MA: Kluwer Academic Publishers; 2003:121–166.)

On examination, the patient is in distress. In milder cases, the systemic arterial blood pressure is normal but, with increasing severity, falls progressively. In severe cases, signs of low cardiac output and reduced perfusion are present.

Sinus tachycardia is seen in almost all patients, allowing for at least partial maintenance of cardiac output. One exception is subacute tamponade, due to the pericardial effusion associated with hypothyroidism, in which the underlying disease tends to produce bradycardia. Patients with early tamponade have elevated jugular pressure but are fully neurohormonally compensated and therefore do not have tachycardia. A pericardial rub may be heard in patients with inflammatory pericarditis (13).

The jugular venous pressure is almost always elevated. The *x* descent (the first inward deflection of the internal jugular pulse during systole due to atrial relaxation and downward displacement of the tricuspid valve with ventricular ejection) is preserved. However, the *y* descent (the second inward deflection of the internal jugular pulse due to diastolic inflow of blood into the right ventricle) is attenuated or absent (12) because of the limited or absent late diastolic filling of the right ventricle.

Pulsus paradoxus, defined as decrease in systolic blood pressure exceeding 10 mm Hg on inspiration, is a common finding in moderate to severe tamponade. To measure pulsus paradoxus, a sphygmomanometer is employed for blood pressure measurement in the standard fashion except that the cuff is deflated more slowly than usual. During deflation, the first Korotkoff sounds are audible only during expiration but, with further deflation, Korotkoff sounds are heard throughout the respiratory cycle. The difference between the systolic pressure, at which the first Korotkoff

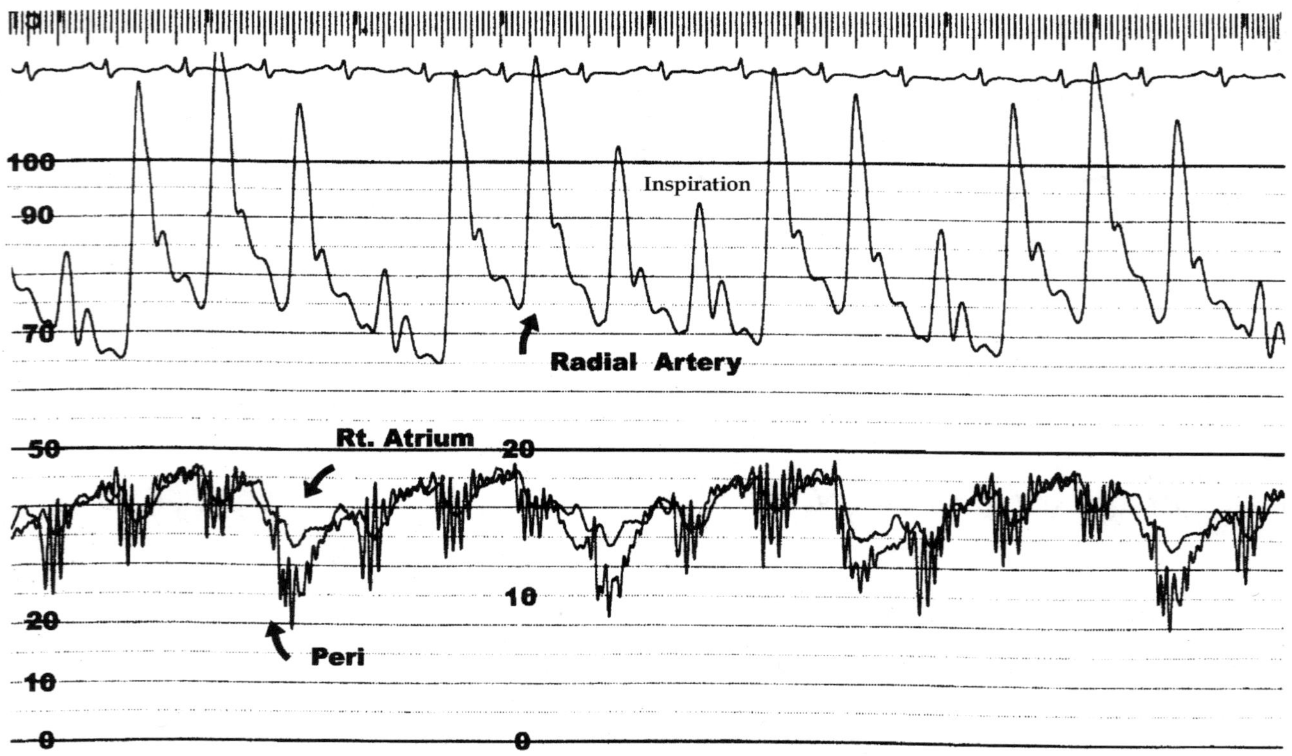

Figure 22-6 Hyperacute cardiac tamponade. Tamponade was caused by puncture of a vein graft. Pulsus paradoxus is extreme. With some inspirations, the pulse pressure falls to 10 mm Hg and mean right atrial pressure is close to 40 mm Hg. Pericardial pressure is equal to right atrial, except that it falls below it at the onset of inspiration. The sanguineous effusion was small. (Reproduced from Shabetai R. Cardiac tamponade. In: Shabetai R. *The Pericardium*. Norwell, MA: Kluwer Academic Publishers; 2003:121–166.)

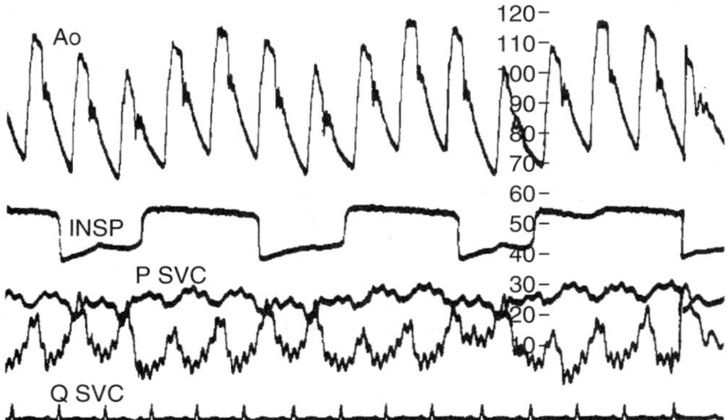

Figure 22-7 Cardiovascular pressures recorded from a patient with moderately severe cardiac tamponade. From above down, aorta showing pulsus paradoxus without hypotension, respirometry, superior caval pressure (P SVC) and velocity (Q SVC), ECG. (From Shabetai R, Fowler NO, Guntheroth WG. The hemodynamics of cardiac tamponade and constrictive pericarditis. *Am J Cardiol.* 1970;26:480–489.)

sounds are heard during expiration, and the pressure at which they are heard throughout the respiratory cycle quantifies pulsus paradoxus.

In a number of conditions pulsus paradoxus is usually absent despite cardiac tamponade. Pulsus paradoxus occurs in the absence of pre-existing heart disease because the diastolic pressure in both ventricles is identical, being equal to pericardial pressure. Compliance of the two ventricles is thus equalized. Pre-existing heart disease prevents this equalization of ventricular diastolic compliance and pulsus paradoxus is therefore absent. Common examples include hypertension and chronic renal disease, in which the left ventricle is hypertrophied and therefore is stiffer than normal (14). Right ventricular hypertrophy prevents the pulsus paradoxus of tamponade in the same manner (15). The volume of a large left-to-right shunt through an atrial septal defect (ASD) does not vary with the respiratory cycle because it has no extrathoracic component and greatly exceeds systemic venous return; therefore, pulsus paradoxus is absent (16). Because the volume of severe aortic regurgitation is constant throughout respiration, pulsus paradoxus is absent in this condition, too. In some of these cases, a left ventricular diastolic pressure higher than pericardial pressure is an additional factor preventing pulsus paradoxus. Rupture of an aortic aneurysm into the pericardium is an important example of acute tamponade in which pulsus paradoxus may be absent. Tamponade may stop hemorrhage from the ruptured myocardium, allowing time for surgical repair. Pericardiocentesis should not be performed but, if it is deemed life-saving, the volume of blood aspirated should be kept to the minimal possible amount.

Electrocardiogram

The electrocardiogram (ECG) changes usually are not specific. Occasionally, ST segment or PR depression indicating acute pericarditis is present. Sinus tachycardia is usual. Cardiac tamponade is a sensitive but not specific cause of low voltage (17). When the effusion is massive, electrical alternans may ensue (18,19) but lacks specificity except when it includes alternation of the P and T waves as well as the QRS complex. The combination of pericardial effusion and low voltage should alert physicians and medical staff to the possibility of cardiac tamponade.

Chest Radiogram

The cardio-pericardial silhouette is increased without selective enlargement of any specific chamber. The lung fields are less congested than in cases of heart failure of other etiology, except when accompanied by severe tricuspid regurgitation. An unexplained increase in the silhouette and hemodynamic deterioration also suggest cardiac tamponade.

Echocardiogram

Pericardial effusion is a sine qua non for cardiac tamponade. In most cases of medical tamponade the effusion is substantial. Echocardiography is the optimal means of establishing the absence or presence of pericardial effusion and is indicated whenever pericardial effusion or cardiac tamponade is suspected; this indication has been endorsed by several published guidelines (20).

Echocardiography not only provides evidence of the size, distribution, and nature of the effusion but also of the likelihood of the patient having tamponade. Right atrial compression (8) and early diastolic ventricular collapse (9) are readily identified by this means. M-mode shows reciprocal respiratory variation of the magnitude of the left and right ventricular diastolic dimensions; the timing of ventricular collapse can be shown to be in diastole by simultaneous imaging of the open mitral or closed aortic valve. Increased diameter of the inferior vena cava and absent or less than 50% collapse with inspiration or a sniff are nicely documented by M-mode (21).

Two-dimensional Doppler echocardiography furnishes valuable additional information. Compression of the right heart chambers and, less commonly, of the left (22), especially the atrium (23), is identified in several image planes. Just as patients with cardiac tamponade who also have heart disease may not show pulsus paradoxus (14,16), likewise coexisting heart disease may prevent the expected compression of the right atrium and ventricle (24). Similarly, severe right heart failure may greatly elevate right ventricular diastolic and right atrial pressures, such that if the patient develops cardiac tamponade, the right heart diastolic pressures exceed pericardial pressure and, thus, collapse of the right heart chambers is prevented.

Like the inferior vena cava, the hepatic veins are engorged. Thus, the study provides ample proof of plethora in the majority of cases of at least moderate severity. Low-pressure tamponade is a significant exception to this rule (25).

Doppler interrogation of the atrio-ventricular orifices provides clear evidence of ventricular interdependence in that respiratory variation is greatly increased. During inspiration, the mitral E wave normally declines by up to 10%, but in tamponade may fall by as much as 45% (3,26). Reciprocal and somewhat larger changes are seen in the tricuspid E wave. Pulsus paradoxus is documented by decreased aortic stroke volume during inspiration.

Cardiac Catheterization

From the foregoing, it is apparent that the diagnosis can be readily made without cardiac catheterization, and usually is; therefore, technical details are not given here but have been published elsewhere (27). It is, however, relevant to re-emphasize here that accurate calibration of pressure transducers is critical for demonstrating diastolic pressure equalization. Relevant pressures should be recorded simultaneously, preferably superimposed and at high gain. Left- and right-sided pressures should also be recorded at low gain so as to visualize the phase relation of peak systolic pressures in the systemic and pulmonary circulation throughout several respiratory cycles. Finally, in this regard a respirometer tracing is very useful but, if one is not available, pulmonary wedge pressure should be recorded with other pressures of interest as a marker of the phase of respiration.

An example of the findings from a typical case of cardiac tamponade in a patient with viral or idiopathic pericarditis is shown in Figure 22-7. Even coexisting heart disease is easily recognized and evaluated noninvasively. However, right heart catheterization should, in my opinion, be included with pericardiocentesis to ascertain that pericardial pressure has been restored to near normal and to exclude effusive-constrictive pericarditis, in which pericardiocentesis normalizes pericardial (but not right atrial and pulmonary) wedge pressures (28,29).

Left ventriculography is no longer performed for the diagnosis or evaluation of cardiac tamponade, but construction of pressure–volume loops (usually using a volume-sensing catheter) is a useful research tool. A beautiful example of a left ventricular pressure–volume loop using opaque contrast medium on a canine model of tamponade, showing elevated diastolic pressure, hypotension, and low stroke volume, was published in 1968 (30) (Fig. 22-8).

Before a significant volume of fluid has been aspirated, the right atrial, pulmonary wedge, pericardial right ventricular, and pulmonary arterial diastolic pressures are all elevated and are just about equal to each other. In typical medical tamponade (11), the pressures are usually in the range of 15 to 25 mm Hg. The right atrial (and central venous) pressure shows a normal fall with inspiration, and the normal bimodal waveform with x and y descents is replaced by a waveform in which the y descent is replaced by a progressive upslope leading to end-diastole (12) (Fig. 22-9).

Treatment

The appropriate treatment depends on the severity of tamponade that varies from subclinical, through mild and moderate, to severe (14,26). Mild tamponade (i.e., with pericardial pressure less then 10 mm Hg) often can be managed without pericardiocentesis. Such patients are managed as hospital in-patients where they are monitored for evidence of progression in the severity of tamponade that first is evident by further rise in the jugular pressure, decreased blood pressure, and some subjective discomfort. If the tamponade was caused by a reversible process such as acute pericarditis, it should vanish after a few days of anti-inflammatory treatment.

Moderate tamponade (i.e., with pericardial pressure about 10 to 15 mm Hg) normally indicates the need for elective drainage of pericardial fluid. Pericardial pressure higher than that means the tamponade is severe and that

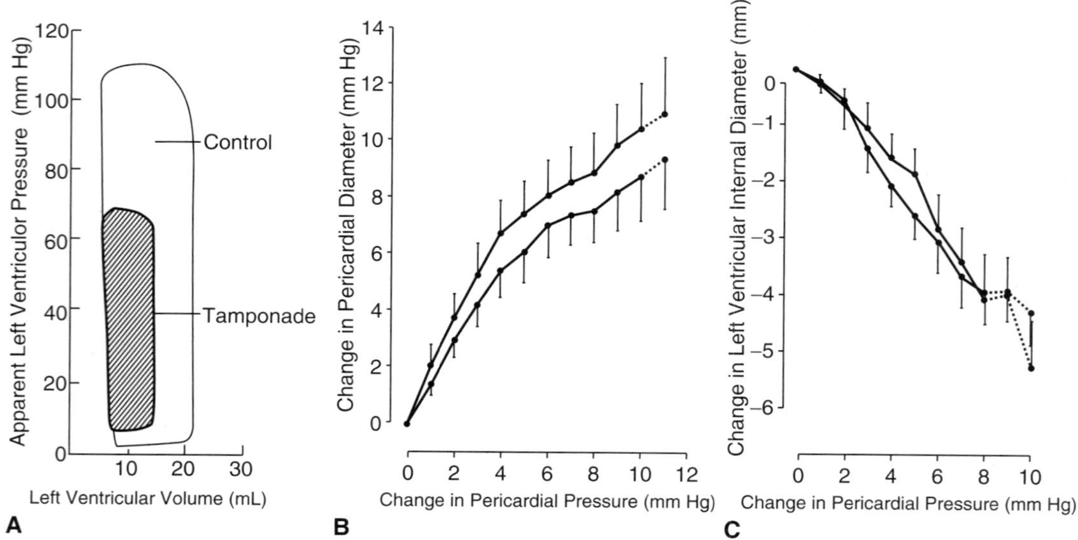

Figure 22-8 **(A)** Left ventricular pressure–volume loops before and after acute tamponade induced in a dog. Cardiac volumes, stroke volume, and systolic pressure are drastically reduced and diastolic pressure has increased. (From Craig RJ, Whalen RE, Behar VS, et al. Pressure and volume changes of the left ventricle in acute pericardial tamponade. *Am J Cardiol.* 1968;22:65–74, with permission.) **(B)** Changes in pericardial diameter. **(C)** Left ventricular internal dimension during induction of experimental cardiac tamponade. **Upper graph**, end-diastole; **Lower graph**, end-systole. (From Pegram BL, Kardon MB, Bishop VS. Changes in left ventricular internal diameter with increasing pericardial pressure. *Cardiovasc Res.* 1975;9:707–714.)

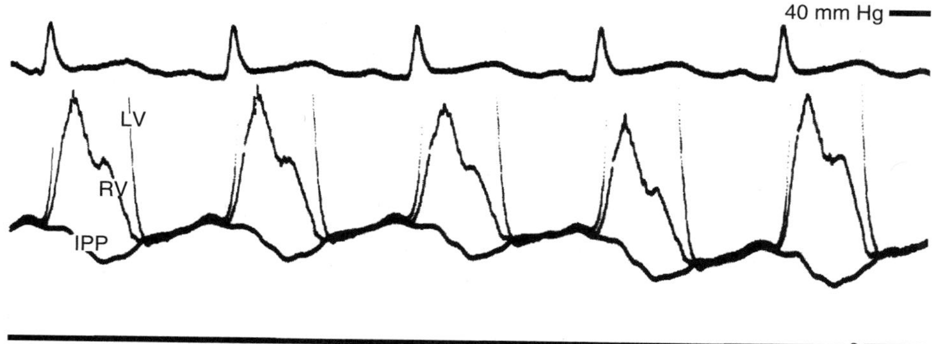

Figure 22-9 Cardiac tamponade. Pressure recordings from the left and right ventricles and the pericardium. Diastolic pressures equilibrate at 17 mm Hg. Note that the diastolic pressures rise throughout diastole and are unlike the dip-and-plateau pattern of constrictive pericarditis. (From Reddy PS. Hemodynamics of cardiac tamponade in man. In: Reddy PS, Leon DF, Shaver JA, eds. *Pericardial Disease*. New York: Raven Press; 1982:161–185.)

drainage is urgent or needs to be performed as an emergency procedure. When the cause of clinically manifest tamponade is not apparent, a search for the etiology is required and includes examination of the pericardial fluid and, less often, pericardial biopsy.

Tamponade that ensues immediately after pericardial injury (e.g., during a cardiac intervention) requires immediate emergency relief because a small volume of blood can quickly raise pericardial pressure to life-threatening values (Figs. 22-5 and 22-6). Skilled interventional cardiologists can tap these small effusions (31,32). When this fails, they can access the pericardium through a subxiphoid incision. Catheter techniques, reversal of anticoagulation and fibrinolysis, and life-support measures can stop the bleeding and stabilize the patient. Removal of only some of the blood dramatically improves the patient because it substantially lowers the pericardial pressure (Fig. 22-6).

Methods of Pericardial Drainage

The most common method is pericardiocentesis using an intrapericardial thin-walled pigtail catheter, guided into place using echocardiography or fluoroscopy. Best results are obtained when the pericardial catheter remains in place until drainage drops to 50 mL per day. The techniques have been described elsewhere (32–35). Some internists and surgeons favor open drainage via a subxiphoid incision. While this is a minority view for tamponade with a large effusion, it is a good option for effusions less than 1 cm from the skin and for effusions showing echocardiographic or CAT scan evidence of organization, and when pericardial biopsy is deemed essential. The operation can be performed under local anesthesia and allows easy access to pericardial tissue for biopsy. Balloon pericardiotomy can be accomplished by inflating a large balloon in the pericardial space and then pulling it out of the pericardium, creating a tear that permits pericardial fluid to drain into the pleural or peritoneal cavity where it is readily absorbed (36,37). This method was used primarily for neoplastic pericardial effusion but is now employed less frequently. When draining a malignant pericardial effusion, the catheter can be left in place for the instillation of any of a variety of sclerosing agents, although some investigators report that prolonged catheter drainage alone encourages adhesive sealing of the pericardial cavity.

Low-Pressure Cardiac Tamponade

Patients who are severely hypovolemic because of traumatic hemorrhage, hemodialysis or ultrafiltration, or overdiuresis at presentation may have low-pressure tamponade in which the intracardiac diastolic pressures are 6 to 8 mm Hg or less (25) (Fig. 22-10). The hemodynamic significance of these effusions can be demonstrated on echocardiography by right heart chamber collapse and exaggerated respiratory variations in transvalvular flows during quiet breathing. Pulsus paradoxus may be present.

Patients receiving hemodialysis may present a unique therapeutic dilemma because, in such cases, hypervolemia may be caused either by associated cardiac disease or by insufficient dialysis, whereas normovolemia or hypovolemia may be an expression of low-pressure tamponade. Echocardiography settles the question. Fortunately, cardiac tamponade complicating hemodialysis (which used to be a frequent event in hemodialysis units) has become uncommon since the introduction of improved dialysis membrane.

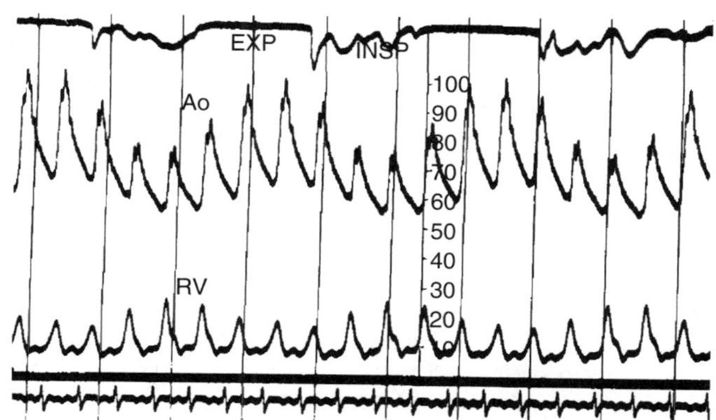

Figure 22-10 Low-pressure cardiac tamponade. This woman was brought to our attention because of hypotension and obvious pulsus paradoxus on clinical examination. The findings at cardiac catheterization were diagnostic of low-pressure cardiac tamponade. Right ventricular diastolic pressure was only 10 mm Hg. Aortic systolic pressure was 100 mm Hg at expiration, but 75 mm Hg in inspiration. The heart rate was rapid. Aortic and right ventricular peak systolic pressures were discordant, being just about 180 degrees out of phase. (From Shabetai R, Fowler NO, Guntheroth WG. The hemodynamics of cardiac tamponade and constrictive pericarditis. *Am J Cardiol*. 1970;26:480–489.)

Regional Cardiac Tamponade

A loculated, eccentric effusion or localized hematoma can produce regional tamponade in which only selected chambers are compressed. As a result, the typical physical, hemodynamic, and echocardiographic signs of tamponade are usually absent. Regional tamponade has been created in animal models (38,39). In patients, regional tamponade is most often seen after pericardial incision for surgical exposure of the heart; clinical suspicion should be heightened in these settings. Establishing the diagnosis is challenging, often requiring transesophageal echocardiography and other advanced imaging techniques.

Effusive Constrictive Pericarditis

This topic, discussed under Constrictive Pericarditis, below, presents features of both cardiac tamponade and constrictive pericarditis (28,40).

CONSTRICTIVE PERICARDITIS

Definition

Constrictive pericarditis is a clinical syndrome resulting from a disease, injury, or other insult that induces morphological changes such that the pericardium loses its normal compliance and becomes a firm, noncompliant structure that impedes ventricular diastolic filling and, when sufficiently severe, reduces ventricular volume. In the majority of cases, the pathology is that of chronic inflammation with extensive replacement fibrosis and sometimes calcification (41). Less commonly, the pericardium is extensively invaded by neoplasm (primary or secondary) and, rarely, is infiltrated by amyloid. In many of the cases, pericardial thickness is substantially increased but it is important to know that this is not a universal finding. The pericardium is adherent to the superficial myocardium. A recent review from the Mayo Clinic reported that surgical pathology obtained between 1993 and 1999 found 143 cases of constrictive pericarditis among 361 cases. Fibrosis was found in 96% of these but calcification in only 35%. Pericardial thickness was normal in 4% (42).

Like cardiac tamponade, constrictive pericarditis is a compressive disorder of the heart that impairs the diastolic function of both ventricles, but usually systolic function is preserved. Whereas the compressive force in cardiac tamponade is exerted by pericardial fluid under increased pressure, compression in constrictive pericarditis is caused by abnormal restraint imposed by the pericardium itself. This difference in the nature of compression underlies differences in the pathophysiology of the two disorders discussed in Pathophysiology, later. Because both are compressive disorders of the heart, however, the two disorders share many important pathophysiological effects.

Constrictive pericarditis is of even greater importance than cardiac tamponade to heart failure specialists because the symptoms and many of the physical signs and laboratory abnormalities are identical to those of right heart failure of other etiology. Too often, the diagnosis is long-delayed while patients are evaluated for left heart failure, cor pulmonale, or valvular heart disease as the cause of their severe right heart failure. Constrictive pericarditis should always be included in the differential diagnosis of the reason for unexplained right heart failure. Constrictive pericarditis prevents dilation of the atria and ventricles; therefore, the plasma levels of atrial and brain natriuretic peptides are not much increased, accounting for fluid retention (43).

Etiology

The reported prevalence of constrictive pericarditis varies considerably with demography, the era in which the data were published, and the special interest of the clinic or institution making the report. Clinical investigation often fails to reveal the cause, in part because the initial insult to the pericardium frequently preceded clinical presentation by many years. In most published series, therefore, the disease is labeled as idiopathic in a substantial proportion of cases. A large number of diseases may result in constrictive pericarditis; some of the more conspicuous of these are listed in the following.

Neoplasm

Malignant disease of the pericardium may take the form of acute pericarditis, pericardial effusion, cardiac tamponade, or constrictive pericarditis. Some cases have constrictive pericarditis but without obliteration, and have effusive-constrictive pericarditis (44). Bronchogenic and mammary carcinoma and, especially, mesothelioma are particularly apt to cause constrictive pericarditis. Malignant melanoma more often involves the myocardium than the pericardium. All malignant tumors have the potential to metastasize to the pericardium.

Ionizing Radiation

Mediastinal radiation, usually given as therapy for malignant disease (but occasionally by accident), is an important cause of constrictive pericarditis and myocardial radiation injury (45,46). In earlier series published when radiotherapy for Hodgkin disease began to be widely applied, radiation accounted for a substantial proportion of cases of constrictive pericarditis. Constrictive pericarditis is often preceded by acute pericarditis and subsequent pericardial effusion.

Infection

A common cause of acute pericarditis is viral infection, especially coxsackie but also adenovirus, hepatitis C, and mumps. Fortunately, viral pericarditis only seldom causes subsequent constrictive pericarditis and the same is true for recurrent pericarditis.

Several infections may cause severe constrictive pericarditis (actually, any living organism may infect the pericardium); some do so commonly, others rarely or mostly limited to immunocompromised patients. Important among infections that may lead to constrictive pericarditis are purulent pericarditis of any cause, tuberculosis in which fully developed constriction may be preceded by effusive-constrictive pericarditis, and a number of fungal infections, including histoplasmosis, blastomycosis, candidiasis, and coccidiodomycosis.

Trauma

Constrictive pericarditis, often severe, may be a sequel to prior blunt trauma, with or without evident myocardial contusion. Steering wheel and other vehicular accidents and a forceful impact from a hard ball are potent examples. Less commonly, blunt trauma creates an intrapericardial hematoma causing local constriction.

Collagen Vascular Diseases

Almost all of the collagen vascular diseases may be complicated by constrictive pericarditis (47), but chief among them are rheumatoid arthritis, lupus erythematosus, progressive systemic sclerosis, and the CREST syndrome (acronym for calcinosis, Raynaud syndrome, esophageal dysmotility, sclerodactyly, and telangiectasia). Rheumatoid arthritis is perhaps the most common of these troublesome conditions to develop constrictive pericarditis. Constrictive pericarditis has also been documented in dermatomyositis and lupus erythematosus.

Prior Cardiac Surgery

Cardiac surgery has emerged as an important cause of constrictive pericarditis. Although this complication is reported in only 0.1 to 0.3 of cardiac operations, the large number of cardiac operations performed annually translates into a large prevalence. It is important, therefore, to suspect postoperative constrictive pericarditis in cases with unexplained hemodynamic deterioration soon or, less commonly, long after a cardiac operation. Extensive adhesions, a well-known bane of surgeons performing a subsequent cardiac operation, are far more common than constriction. Constrictive pericarditis may also complicate invasive diagnostic and therapeutic cardiac interventions.

Prior Pericarditis

All types of pericarditis have the potential to cause constrictive pericarditis, but this potential usually is not realized. In this category, postpericardial injury syndrome, acute pericarditis, and recurrent pericarditis are included.

Uncommon Causes

Sarcoidosis may involve the pericardium but this involvement is much less common than myocardial and only rarely is clinically evident. Likewise, cardiac amyloidosis is essentially a disease of the myocardium causing restrictive cardiomyopathy with severe heart failure, but amyloid may also be found in the pericardium. Constrictive pericarditis may occur in asbestosis and cholesterol pericarditis, and in the hypereosinophilic syndrome. Of particular concern to heart failure and transplant cardiologists, constrictive pericarditis may occur in a cardiac allograft (48) and may be responsible for short deceleration time and increased E wave to A wave (E/A) ratio of mitral inflow. The rare association of constrictive pericarditis is unexplained. Mulibrey nanism is a familial disorder found in Finland that causes both restrictive cardiomyopathy and constrictive pericarditis (49).

Drug-Induced

The use of a number of prescription drugs has been associated with the subsequent appearance of constrictive pericarditis. Relevant to heart failure specialists is the association of hydralazine with constrictive pericarditis.

Pathophysiology

Like cardiac tamponade, constrictive pericarditis creates a globally increased cardiac restraint that causes equal elevation of ventricular diastolic and atrial pressures. Also, because the abnormal constraint of constrictive pericarditis is not pandiastolic (it commences only after the completion of early rapid filling), the contour of ventricular diastolic and atrial pressures is quite distinct from that of cardiac tamponade. Early rapid filling is faster than normal owing to the faster ventricular relaxation. After ventricular filling has been halted by the rigid pericardium, ventricular diastolic pressure does not increase but, instead, plateaus at the level attained by the end of early rapid filling. The abnormally fast early rapid filling is represented by a sharp negative deflection of ventricular pressure in early diastole, followed by a level plateau for the remainder of diastole. This highly distinctive waveform of ventricular diastolic pressure is known as "dip and plateau," or the "square root sign" (50) (Figs. 22-11 and 22-12). The waveform of the atrial pressure consequently also differs markedly from that of cardiac tamponade, in which the *y* descent is absent. In constrictive pericarditis, both the *x* and *y* descents are more prominent than normal and become the major deflections on atrial pressure recordings (Fig. 22-13).

The scarred pericardium does not allow variation in intrapericardial volume; however, the nature of the restraint is different, being the inelastic pericardial scar, not

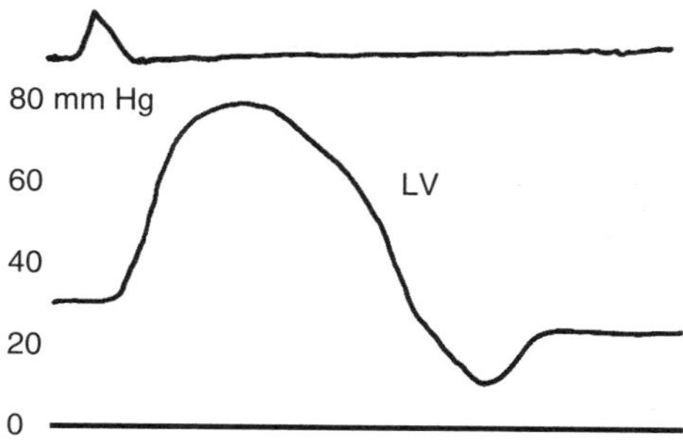

Figure 22-11 Left ventricular pressure recorded in a case of severe chronic constrictive pericarditis using a catheter tip micromanometer. High-fidelity measurements display with great accuracy the shape of the pressure changes with time. The early dip appears less prominent than when recorded using a conventional fluid-filled catheter and an external transducer. LV, left ventricle (Reproduced from Shabetai R. Constrictive pericarditis. In: Shabetai R. *The Pericardium*. Norwell, MA: Kluwer Academic Publishers; 2003: 191–252.)

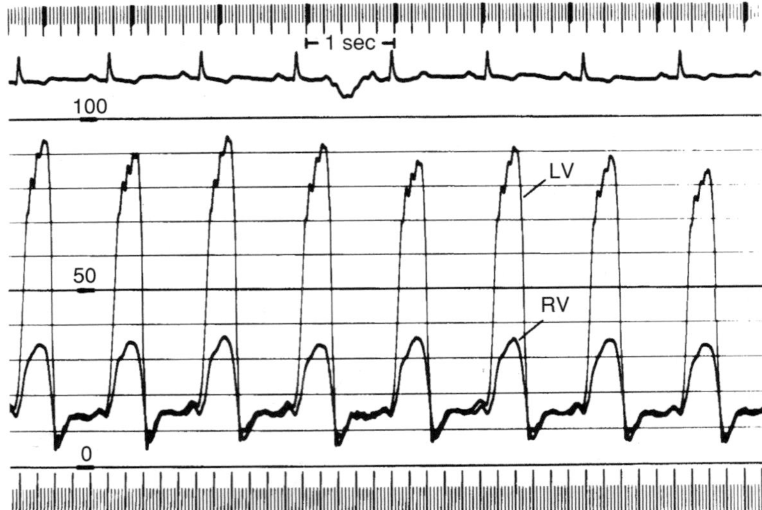

Figure 22-12 Simultaneously recorded pressures from the left and right ventricles using a critically damped fluid-filled system. Note the equalization of diastolic pressures, the dip-and-plateau pattern of diastolic pressure, and discordance of peak systolic pressure of the two ventricles. LV and RV, left and right ventricles. (Reproduced from Shabetai R. Constrictive pericarditis. In: Shabetai R. *The Pericardium*. Norwell, MA: Kluwer Academic Publishers; 2003:191–252.)

fluid under high pressure. The constricting pericardium does not allow transmission of respiratory variation of intrathoracic pressure to the cardiac chambers. There are three consequences of ventricular diastolic and atrial pressures that do not decrease when the patient inspires, First, systemic venous return is not augmented by inspiration (5,13). Second, inspiration, by decreasing pulmonary venous pressure but not changing left ventricular diastolic pressure, lowers the pressure gradient for left heart filling and therefore decreases pulmonary venous return (13). Finally, inspiration can increase flow from, but not beyond, the extra-thoracic great veins; therefore, a deep inspiration increases jugular pressure—the Kussmaul venous sign. With normal inspiration, the jugular mean pressure remains constant during respiration—a *forme fruste* Kussmaul sign.

From the foregoing, it is clear that in both tamponade and constriction, right ventricular volume increases while that of the left ventricle decreases because of heightened ventricular interaction, but the mechanism differs in each. In constriction, the primary event is the inspiratory decline in left ventricular volume, which allows the right ventricle to occupy the vacated intrapericardial space. Conversely, in cardiac tamponade it is increased systemic venous return (2).

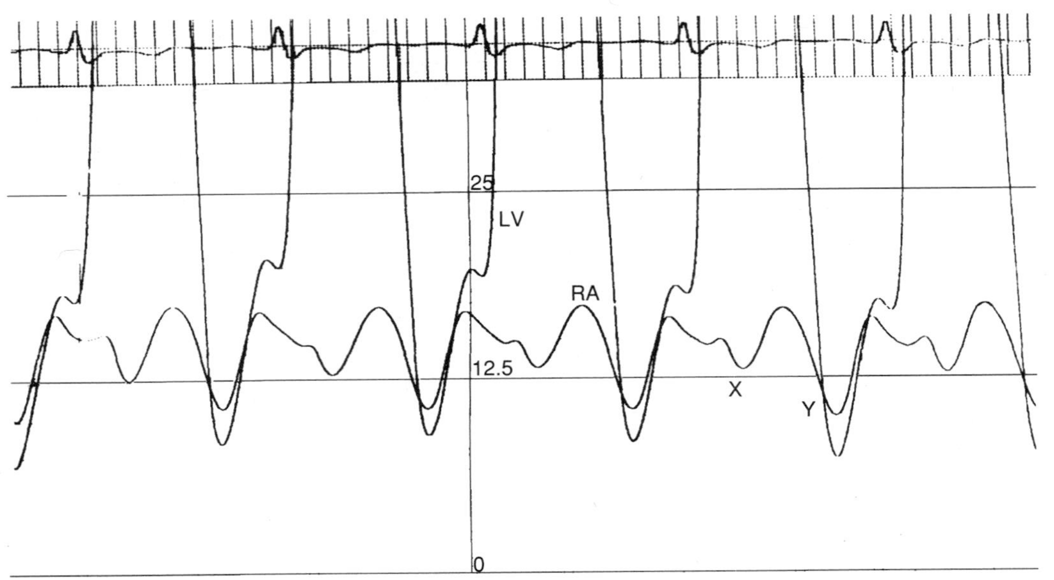

Figure 22-13 Simultaneous records of left ventricular and right atrial pressures using a fluid-filled recording system in a case of constrictive pericarditis. Note the prominent *x* and *y* descents of right atrial (RA) pressure, the early diastolic dip of left ventricular (LV) diastolic pressure, and the absence of a plateau of pressure after the dip owing to tachycardia. (Reproduced from Shabetai R. Constrictive pericarditis. In: Shabetai R. *The Pericardium*. Norwell, MA: Kluwer Academic Publishers; 2003:191–252.)

Heart failure cardiologists know that the Kussmaul sign is not unique to constrictive pericarditis; it is present in any severe right heart failure and in severe tricuspid regurgitation.

The elevated ventricular diastolic pressures generate congestion but the atria and ventricles are not stretched as they are in heart failure; therefore, absence of greatly elevated atrial (51) and brain natriuretic peptide contributes to the severity of congestion (43). Much of the plasma volume is shifted to the systemic circulation, causing predominantly right heart failure with prominent congestion of systemic organs.

Clinical Findings

The mildest cases may well be asymptomatic and their physical examination may reveal nothing abnormal other than an increase in jugular pressure up to approximately 10 cm. As constriction worsens, venous pressure slowly rises and is accompanied by peripheral edema and eventually anasarca. In severe cases, ascites is often present and edema can be massive. Commonly, a patient newly diagnosed at this stage will rapidly lose 20 or more pounds when given a loop diuretic.

History

When constriction is moderate or severe, the chief complaints are distension of the abdomen, swelling of the legs, and weight gain, often correctly attributed by the patient to fluid retention. Patients also complain of breathlessness on exertion and decreased exercise tolerance, but swelling is usually the main complaint. Chest pain is unusual. The patient must be carefully questioned for previous chest trauma, therapeutic radiation procedures or surgical operations requiring pericardial invasion, and tuberculosis or histoplasmosis or other fungal infection. Drugs such as mesalamine or mythergicide have also been reported as causes of constrictive pericarditis. It is important to inquire about rheumatic and collagen vascular diseases.

Physical Examination

In mild cases, the examination is unremarkable save for a slightly elevated level of jugular pulsation with a dominant *y* wave, easily recognized because it is seen in between carotid pulsations. The more severe the constrictive process, the higher the jugular pressure is, frequently 20 cm or more. Signs of fluid overload also increase with severity, unless the patient has been treated with high-dose diuretics for right heart failure. Ascites is a prominent feature and often is tense and out of proportion to peripheral edema; the latter, however, may also be impressive, extending to the thighs and scrotum. In advanced cases, the cardiac rhythm is atrial fibrillation. No cardiac murmur is pathognomonic of constrictive pericarditis, but about one-third of the patients have a loud, crisp third heart sound, known as pericardial knock (52). Early diastolic filling is extremely fast, such that the heart completely fills the pericardial space that exists from systole to the first third of diastole. After it has done so, its expansion is abruptly halted, generating the pericardial knock. If the ascites is not too tense, the congested liver is palpable and pulsates synchronously with the jugular pulse (53). In truly advanced disease, cutaneous markers of liver insufficiency such as palmar erythema, spider angiomata, and jaundice can be observed.

Chest X-Ray

The chest X-ray is helpful when it shows circumferential pericardial calcification but is otherwise not diagnostic. The atria are somewhat enlarged, but not as greatly as they are in restrictive cardiomyopathy because they are restrained by the pericardial scar. Pulmonary congestion, if present, is not severe.

Electrocardiogram

The tracing shows the diffuse inversion of the T wave characteristic of chronic pericarditis. Abnormal depolarization is absent except in a minority of cases in which the epicardial coronary arteries are encroached upon by pericardial scarring, or when left or right bundle branch block, atrioventricular conduction delay, or even pathological Q waves may be present (54). Far more commonly, abnormal depolarization is caused by myocardial disease; this finding is useful when differentiating between restrictive cardiomyopathy and constrictive pericarditis.

Imaging

Increased pericardial thickness, a pathophysiological feature of most but not all cases, can be detected and be readily and accurately measured by transesophageal echocardiography (55), computer assisted tomography (56–58) (Fig. 22-14), and magnetic resonance imaging (59). Cine computerized tomography is also an accurate technique for diagnosing constrictive pericarditis (60). The choice of which of these techniques to use for this purpose is a matter of local preference and expertise. All three techniques also provide diagnostic information regarding cardiac chamber size and function, the size of the liver, and dimensions of the great veins.

Transthoracic echocardiography documents systemic plethora; the inferior vena cava is dilated and often reaches a diameter in excess of 2.5 cm and, during inspiration, either fails to diminish in diameter or the change is less than 50% (Fig. 22-15). Thus, in addition to the best anatomical visualization of the pericardium, functional abnormalities consistent with constrictive pericarditis are displayed. Transthoracic echocardiography is much less applicable for assessing pericardial structure because pericardial thickness or calcification must be substantial before the image is diagnostic for constrictive pericarditis. Furthermore, increased pericardial brightness may simply have been caused by setting the sensitivity too high when the pericardium is normal. With severe constriction and a grossly thickened pericardium, tethering of the pericardium to the myocardium is disclosed by synchronous anterior motion of both pericardium and myocardium.

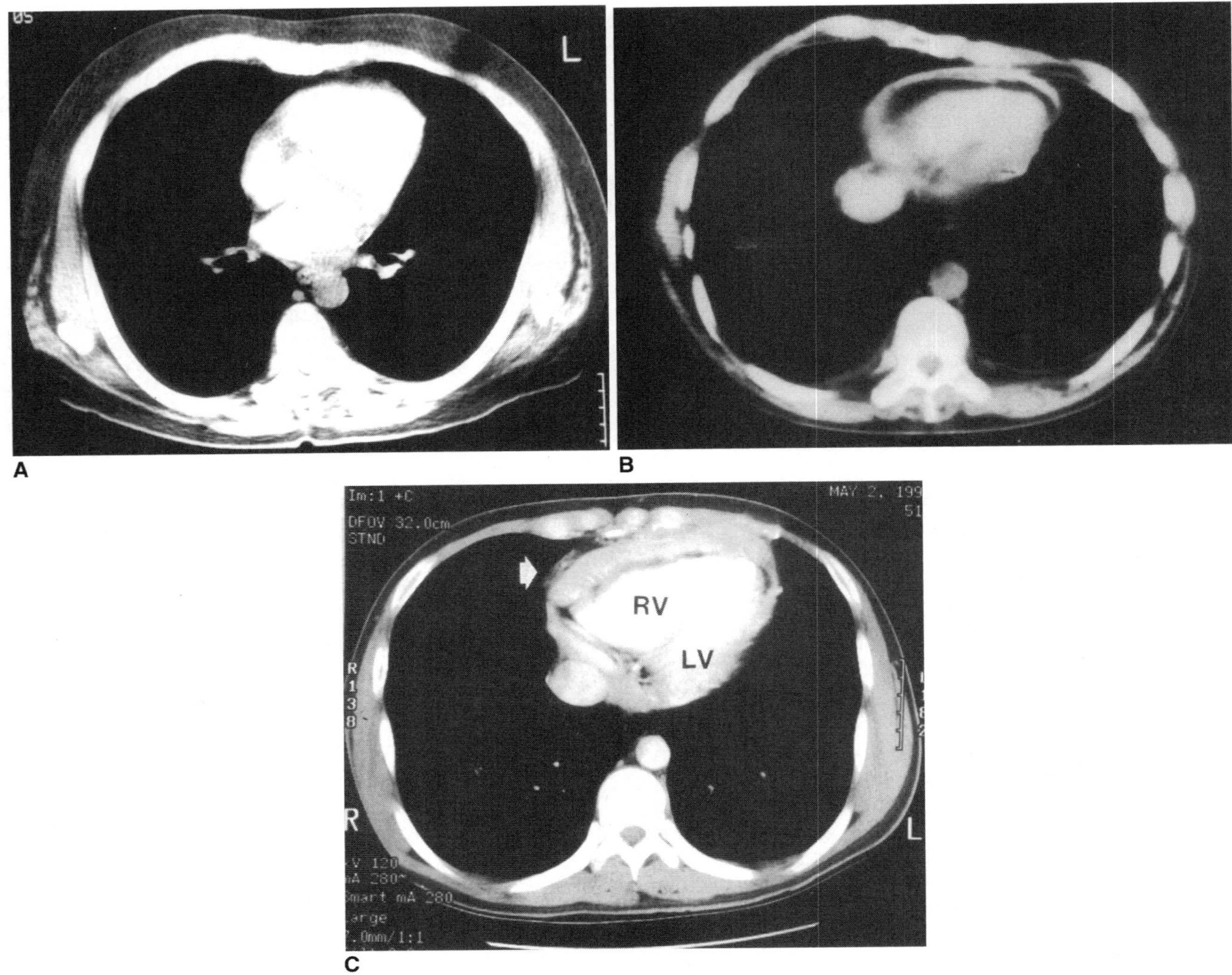

Figure 22-14 Computerized tomograms to demonstrate pericardial morphology. **(A)** Subject with no evidence of pericardial disease. The thin pericardium was not visualized because of absent epicardial fat. **(B)** Pericardium from a case of fungal constrictive pericarditis. The pericardium is thick. **(C)** Massive pericardial thickness from a case of constriction by malignant mesothelioma. (Reproduced from Shabetai R. Constrictive pericarditis. In: Shabetai R. *The Pericardium*. Norwell, MA: Kluwer Academic Publishers; 2003:191–252.)

Doppler Interrogation

Standard techniques for recording ventricular stroke input and output document their increased respiratory variation (61), as previously discussed under Pathophysiology. Transmitral inflow velocity varies about 10% in normal adults breathing quietly, but increases up to 40% in many patients with constrictive pericarditis. This sign of increased ventricular interaction may be absent in patients with high preload but can be restored by interventions that lower preload, such as head-up tilt (62). Respiratory variation in pulmonary venous flow exceeds that of transatrio-ventricular flow (63). Stroke volume may also show excessive decline during inspiration, but less often than in cardiac tamponade.

Cardiac Catheterization

The major findings are those explained under Pathophysiology, previously discussed. In summary, they are as follows:

- LV and RV diastolic pressures elevated and equal to each other.
- Dip-and-plateau configuration of ventricular diastolic pressures.
- RA pressure: prominent *x* and *y* descents, mean does not vary with inspiration, but *y* is deeper on inspiration.
- Respiratory variation of peak ventricular pressures are close to being 180 degrees out of phase.

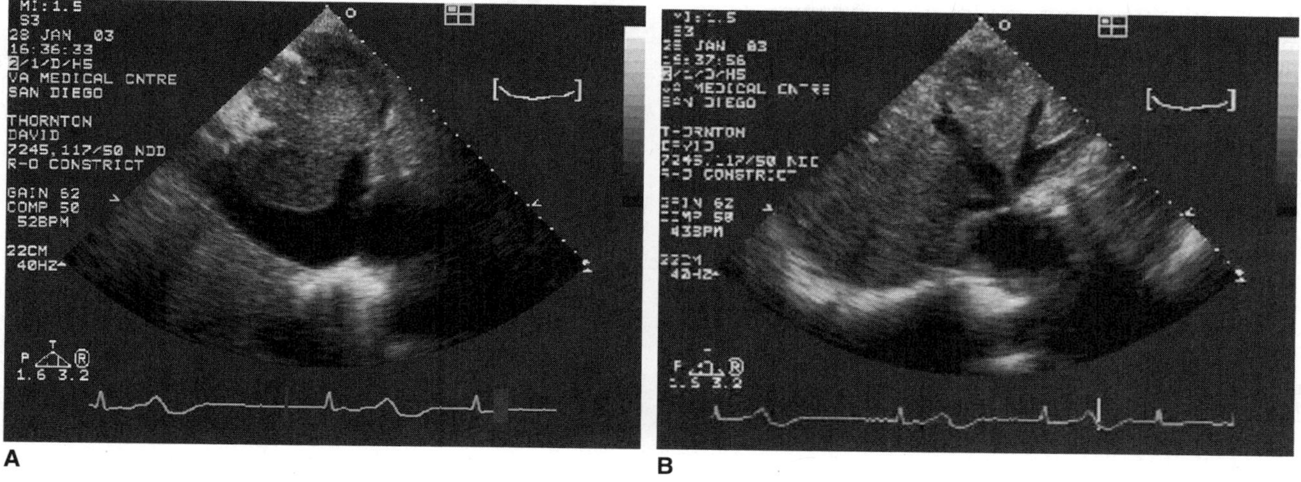

Figure 22-15 Plethora shown on the transthoracic echocardiogram of a patient with severe idiopathic constrictive pericarditis. **(A)** Hugely dilated inferior vena cava. The vein did not collapse on inspiration or sniffing. **(B)** Dilated hepatic veins; they showed systolic retrograde flow by Doppler. (Reproduced from Shabetai R. Constrictive pericarditis. In: Shabetai R. *The Pericardium*. Norwell, MA: Kluwer Academic Publishers; 2003:191–252.)

- Pulmonary hypertension: systolic PA pressure is approximately 40 mm Hg.
- Stroke volume is low.
- In severe cases, cardiac output is also low.

DIFFERENTIAL DIAGNOSIS

For cardiologists, the important task is to exclude restrictive cardiomyopathy. Other physicians, if they do not carefully assess the jugular pressure, may mistake constrictive pericarditis for anasarca that is not owing to cardiac or pericardial disease. Notable examples are hepatic (64) and renal diseases.

Restrictive Cardiomyopathy

This serious malady of the myocardium causes severe ventricular diastolic dysfunction and mimics constrictive pericarditis in many ways. A systematic analysis of the clinical and laboratory abnormalities may establish the correct diagnosis. Often, however, noninvasive or even invasive hemodynamic investigation is required because the history and past history were not informative. In the vast majority of cases, it is then clear whether the patient has cardiomyopathy or pericardial disease, but the possibility of the patient having both requires expert clinical judgement. This important differential diagnosis is usually left to a heart failure specialist or to individuals with a special interest in pericardial disease.

History

The history may be highly informative. Prior pericarditis or pericardial effusion, pericardial injury, and/or past or present illness associated with pericardial disease obviously strongly points to constrictive pericarditis. Conversely, amyloidosis and multiple myeloma favor restrictive cardiomyopathy, and therapeutic radiation and chemotherapy suggest mixed pericardial constriction and myocardial restriction. Patients who have had prior cardiac surgery constitute another group who may have mixed myocardial and pericardial disease. These patients may have features atypical of constrictive pericarditis (e.g., too much left atrial enlargement if the earlier operation was performed for mitral stenosis).

Physical Examination

The physical examination does not help to distinguish between the two entities. This is the reason why, when the history and past medical history offer no clues pointing either to constrictive pericarditis or restrictive cardiomyopathy, the correct diagnosis rests entirely with the laboratory findings.

Electrocardiogram

In contrast to the physical examination, the ECG can be very helpful. Low voltage is a fairly common finding in restrictive cardiomyopathy. The combination of low voltage and apparent hypertrophy by echocardiography is particularly likely in restrictive cardiomyopathy. Here the apparent hypertrophy is due to amyloid infiltration of the myocardium. Ventricular depolarization and conduction abnormalities strongly support the diagnosis of restrictive cardiomyopathy. As mentioned under the Electrocardiographic section of Constrictive Pericarditis, myocardial penetration by fibrosis or calcium in that disease occasionally causes changes in the ECG, usually seen in restrictive cardiomyopathy (54). However, abnormalities confined to repolarization are consistent with either restrictive cardiomyopathy or constrictive pericarditis. In summary, the ECG is not diagnostic for either condition but depolarization abnormalities and conduction disturbances make restrictive cardiomyopathy considerably more probable. Atrial fibrillation develops late in the course of constrictive pericarditis but also is a common feature of restrictive cardiomyopathy. P mitrale precedes the onset of established atrial tachycardia in constrictive pericarditis, whereas the P wave of restrictive cardiomyopathy reflects biatrial enlargement. Ventricular tachycardia strongly favors restrictive cardiomyopathy.

Chest X-ray

Obvious atrial enlargement on the chest film is common in restrictive cardiomyopathy but, although the atrial pressures are comparable in the two diseases, constrictive pericarditis limits the increase in atrial volume. Patchy pericardial calcification is not helpful but a ring of calcium around the heart is diagnostic of constrictive pericarditis.

Echocardiogram

Transthoracic images may be helpful. In favor of restrictive cardiomyopathy is the glittering appearance of cardiac amyloidosis and greatly enlarged atria. In many cases of restrictive cardiomyopathy, ventricular systolic function is preserved but, when the disease is far advanced, the patient may have severe systolic as well as diastolic functional impairment. Significant global hypokinesis is rare in constrictive pericarditis. A greatly thickened or calcified pericardium, sometimes tethered to the myocardium, excludes restrictive cardiomyopathy. Transesophageal images showing increased pericardial thickness indicate constrictive pericarditis but, in some cases, remain normal in spite of severe constriction.

Doppler Interrogation

Several Doppler techniques are critically important (65–68). In restrictive cardiomyopathy, ventricular interaction is not increased; therefore, respiratory variation in transatrio-ventricular and pulmonary blood flow velocities remains normal. Tissue Doppler is very helpful in determining when the transmitral E/A ratio and a short deceleration time are caused by increased myocardial versus pericardial stiffness. In constrictive pericarditis both the velocity of mitral inflow in early diastole (denoted by the E wave) and the corresponding motion of the mitral annulus are increased, reflected by the tissue Doppler E′. In restrictive cardiomyopathy, transmitral early diastolic velocity is also high but, because myocardial shortening and lengthening are severely restricted, E′ is diminutive (65–67) (Fig. 22-16). Likewise, color M-mode Doppler, which measures myocardial velocity gradient, shows that the transit of

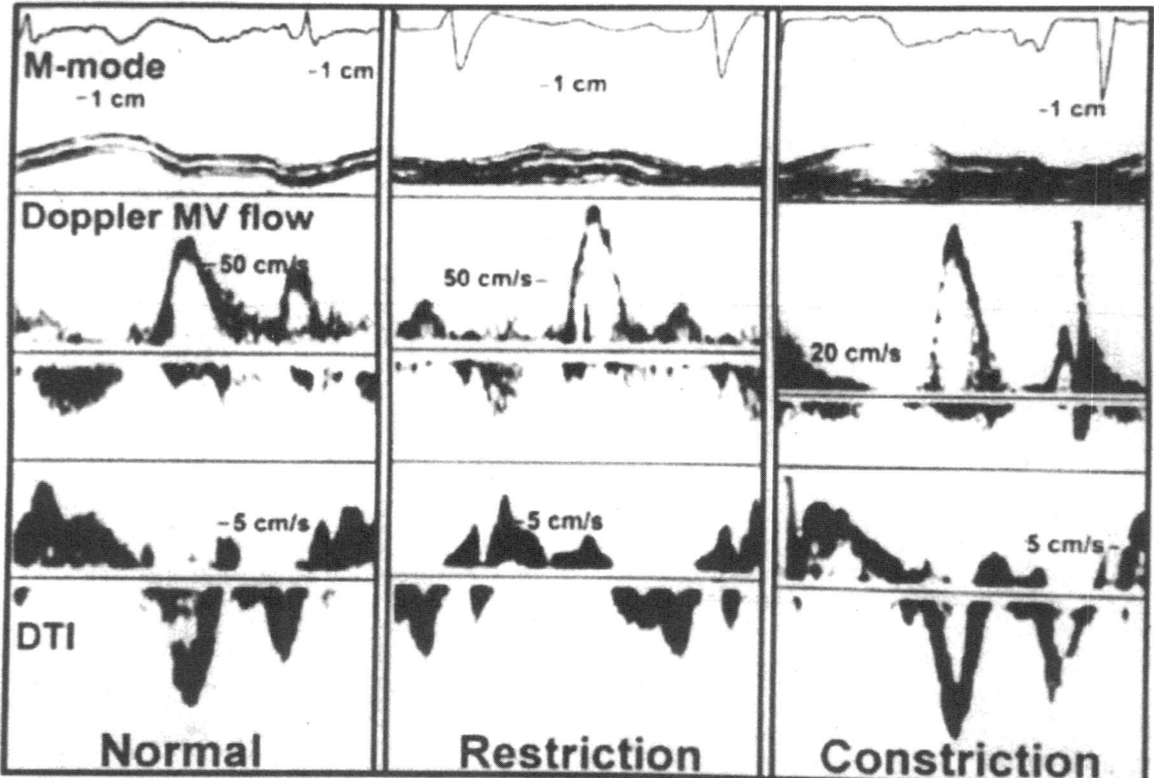

Figure 22-16 Doppler, transmitral and tissue. M-mode echocardiogram **(top)**, transmitral velocity **(middle)**, and tissue Doppler **(bottom)**. Compared with normal, in constrictive pericarditis, transmitral and tissue velocities show more rapid filling and short deceleration time. In restriction, transmitral velocity is rapid but tissue velocity is slow. **Arrows** depict E and E′. (From Garcia MJ, Thomas JD, Klein AL. New Doppler echocardiographic applications for the study of diastolic function. *J Am Coll Cardiol.* 1998;32:865–875.)

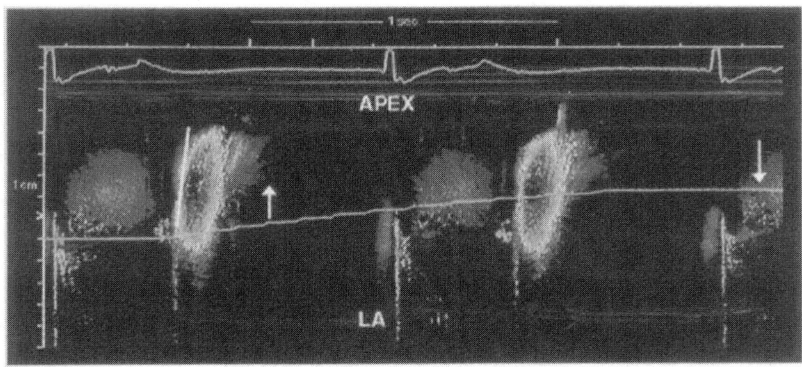

A

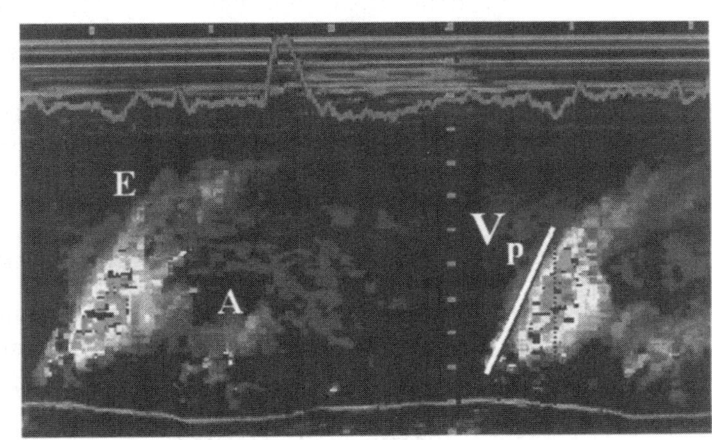

B

Figure 22-17 Color M-mode Doppler from left atrium toward the ventricular apex, comparing constrictive pericarditis **(A)**, in which flow is rapid, and restrictive cardiomyopathy **(B)**, in which it is slow. Isovolumic flow in restriction is rapid **(yellow line)**. (From Rajagopalan N, Garcia MJ, Rodriguez L, et al. Comparison of new Doppler echocardiographic methods to differentiate constrictive pericardial heart disease and restrictive cardiomyopathy. *Am J Cardiol.* 2001;87:86–94.)

blood from the mitral orifice to the apex is rapid in constrictive pericarditis but is slower than normal in restrictive cardiomyopathy (67) (Fig. 22-17).

Cardiac Catheterization

The highest peak of left systolic pressure is almost exactly in phase with that of the right ventricle in patients with restrictive cardiomyopathy, not out-of-phase as in constrictive pericarditis. In constrictive pericarditis, the highest peak ventricular systolic pressure is synchronous with the lowest peak systolic pressure of the opposite ventricle (68). This phenomenon is termed ventricular discordance (Fig. 22-12). Left ventricular diastolic and pulmonary wedge pressures decline by an equal amount in restrictive cardiomyopathy but, in constrictive pericarditis, the decline in left ventricular pressure is less than that of the pulmonary wedge pressure (69). The dip-and-plateau pattern of ventricular diastolic pressure with the plateaus equally elevated is found in restrictive cardiomyopathy and constrictive pericarditis (Fig. 22-18), but a plateau higher on the left signifies restrictive cardiomyopathy (Fig. 22-19).

Most of the findings obtained by cardiac catheterization are identical in constrictive pericarditis and restrictive cardiomyopathy.

An important exception regarding the different effect of respiration on pulmonary wedge and left ventricular pressures has already been pointed out. Heart failure specialists

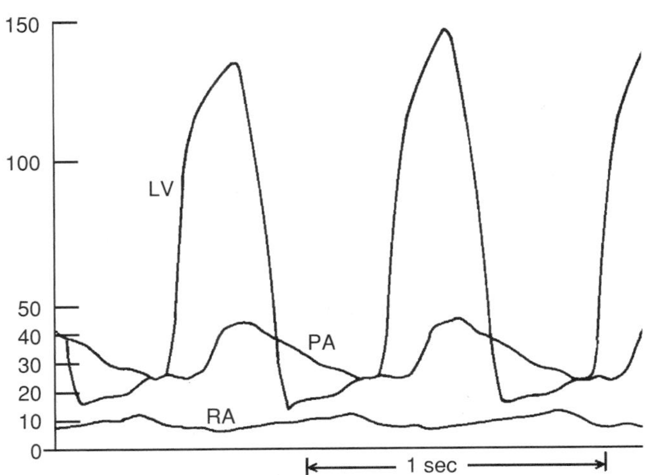

Figure 22-18 Restrictive cardiomyopathy. Pressure recorded from the left ventricle (LV), pulmonary artery (PA), and right atrium (RA). The pressures at end-diastole are 25 mm Hg in the LV and PA but 8 mm Hg in the RA. This pressure difference is incompatible with typical constrictive pericarditis. Equally elevated pressures in diastole, however, may be present in both constrictive pericarditis and restrictive cardiomyopathy. (Reproduced from Meaney E, Shabetai R, Bhargava V, et al. Cardiac amyloidosis, constrictive pericarditis and restrictive cardiomyopathy. *Am J Cardiol.* 1976;38:547–556.)

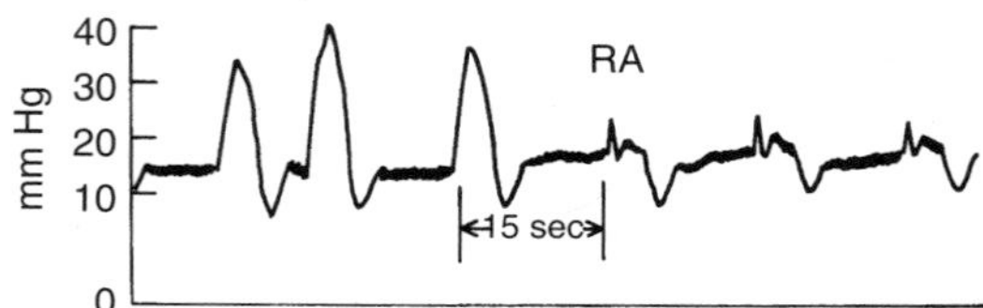

Figure 22-19 Pressures recorded from the right ventricle (RV) and as the catheter was withdrawn into the right atrium (RA) in a woman with cardiac amyloidosis. The figure is an example of diastolic pressure values and waveforms indistinguishable from those in constrictive pericarditis. (Reproduced from Meaney E, Shabetai R, Bhargava V, et al. Cardiac amyloidosis, constrictive pericarditis and restrictive cardiomyopathy. *Am J Cardiol.* 1976;38:547–556.)

may be called upon to decide if a patient has restrictive cardiomyopathy or constrictive pericarditis and perform cardiac catheterization to help make this determination. Whenever possible, the study should include high-quality recordings over several respiratory cycles of simultaneously measured left ventricular and pulmonary wedge pressures at high gain to determine the effect of inspiration.

Endomyocardial Biopsy

Newer, noninvasive imagery has decreased the need for biopsy but, where doubt persists, and in some cases with both cardiomyopathy and pericardiopathy, endomyocardial biopsy may provide data helpful in deciding whether or not to recommend pericardiectomy. In the unlikely event that, after comprehensive investigation, the cause of diastolic dysfunction remains in doubt, endomyocardial biopsy may disclose unsuspected myocardial disease (70). If the biopsy is normal, it is safe to diagnose constrictive pericarditis but, if extensive myocardial necrosis and fibrosis are present, the outcome from this operation is very likely to be less than satisfactory.

Mixed Constrictive Pericarditis and Restrictive Cardiomyopathy

Some patients have both constrictive pericarditis and restrictive cardiomyopathy; in such cases the echo-Doppler findings can be atypical (71). The best-known example is combined radiation injury of the heart and pericardium, but other patients may have pre-existing cardiomyopathy. In patients whose constrictive pericarditis is a complication of cardiac surgery, cardiomyopathy related to ischemic or valvular heart disease may be present. Constrictive pericarditis is an uncommon complication in patients with a cardiac allograft (72), some of whom also have independent diastolic dysfunction due to graft vasculopathy. Although respiratory variation of ventricular inflow from the left atrium and pulmonary veins may be attenuated, in these patients (for the purpose of recognizing the combination) their clinical findings are more important than the laboratory findings. Not surprisingly, pericardiectomy benefits these patients less than those with isolated constrictive pericarditis. It is important to assess the severity of the myocardial component, for which purpose endomyocardial biopsy may be needed, as mentioned previously.

Treatment

The standard treatment, with the exceptions previously noted, is pericardiectomy (73). In the preoperative period, diuretic dosing often needs to be reduced to ensure that the patient is not hypovolemic at the time of operation. With improved technique, the mortality rate for this operation has fallen to 5%; therefore, the risk–benefit ratio is favorable. Because not every otherwise excellent cardiac surgeon has extensive experience with pericardiectomy for constrictive pericarditis, patients are often rightly referred to centers with a special interest in these cases. Cardiopulmonary bypass apparatus is set up routinely but does not always have to be used. The pericardiectomy should be as complete as technically possible, with excision of both diseased visceral and parietal pericardium. The systemic venous pressure drops substantially as soon as it is evident that the heart has been freed, but several additional months pass before it returns to normal (74). Persisting ventricular diastolic dysfunction suggests a significant element of increased myocardial stiffness.

Poor outcome after pericardiectomy has been well-documented when the operation was performed for radiation-induced constrictive pericarditis (74,75). Patients should be informed of this fact before being asked to consent to the operation. Some patients develop heart failure postoperatively; it is self-limiting but treatment may be required for several months.

Atypical Constrictive Pericarditis

Transient Constriction

In patients with acute pericarditis or effusive-constrictive pericarditis, constrictive pericarditis may be only a transient phenomenon caused by pericardial edema and exudate (76,77). It may resolve spontaneously but is best treated with anti-inflammatory agents. It may be seen with acute pericarditis of any etiology and usually resolves within 3 months. When evidence of constriction is found in this setting, pericardiectomy should be withheld and performed only if significant constriction lasts longer than 3 months.

Effusive-Constrictive Pericarditis

In the case of transient constrictive pericarditis, the morphological changes that decrease pericardial compliance are transient, whereas in effusive-constrictive pericarditis the pericardial pathology may be either irreversible fibrosis or transient inflammation. The effusion is seldom large; the importance of this syndrome is that relief of tamponade leaves the patient with significant constrictive pericarditis (40,77). Clues to the diagnosis, when present, include tuberculous or neoplastic etiology and impaired respiratory variation of right atrial pressure with the presence of an unexpected *y* descent. Frequently, the diagnosis is unsuspected until it is discovered during hemodynamic monitoring of pericardiocentesis (Fig. 22-20). In uncomplicated tamponade, pericardiocentesis lowers pericardial pressure to a normal subatmospheric level during inspiration and restores right atrial pressure to normal. If the pericardial pressure normalizes but the right atrial wedge pressures remain elevated, the patient has effusive-constrictive pericarditis.

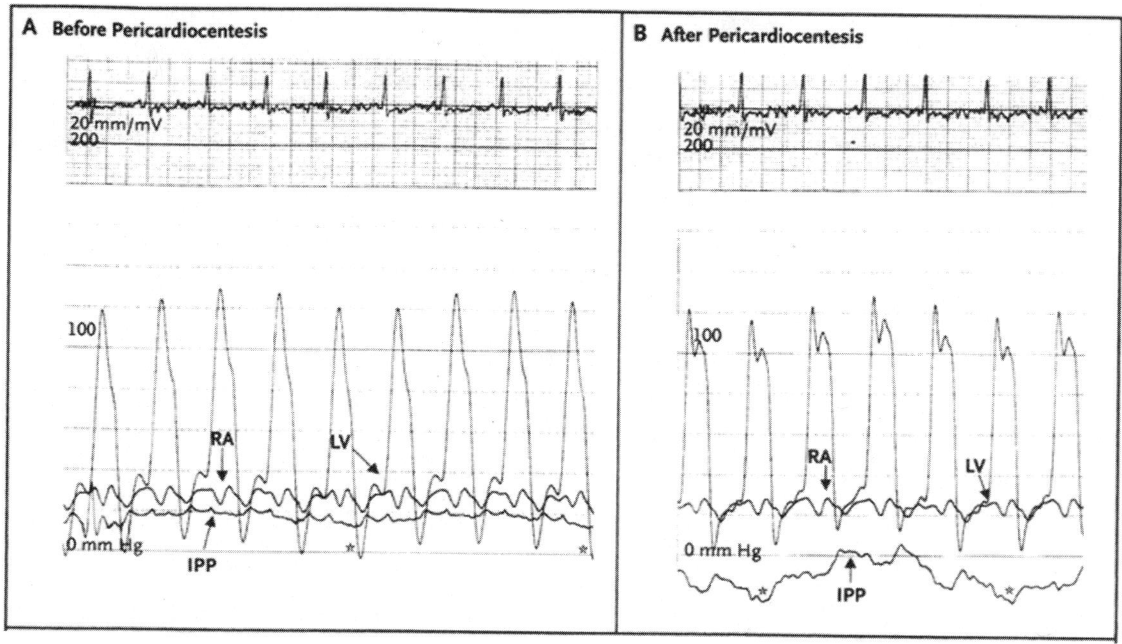

Figure 22-20 Effusive-constrictive pericarditis. Hemodynamic findings obtained during pericardiocentesis in a patient with effusive constrictive pericarditis. **(A)** The intrapericardial pressure IPP) is 21 mm Hg, and the right atrial (RA) and left ventricular (LV) pressures are 35 mm Hg. **(B)** After pericardiocentesis, pericardial pressure is subatmospheric, whereas left ventricular diastolic and right atrial pressures are little changed and a dip-and-plateau morphology of ventricular diastolic pressure is present. *, end-inspiration. (Reproduced from Sagrista-Sauleda J, Angel J, Sanchez A, et al. Effusive-constrictive pericarditis. *N Engl J Med.* 2004;350:469–475.)

REFERENCES

1. Heidenreich PA, Eisenberg MJ, Kee LL, et al. Pericardial effusion in AIDS: incidence and survival. *Circulation.* 1995;92:3229–3234.
2. Shabetai R, Fowler NO, Fenton JC, et al. Pulsus paradoxus. *J Clin Invest.* 1965;44:1882–1898.
3. Appleton CP, Hatle LK, Popp RL. Cardiac tamponade and pericardial effusion: respiratory variation in transvalvular flow velocities studied by Doppler echocardiography. *J Am Coll Cardiol.* 1988;11:1020–1030.
4. Gabe IT, Mason DT, Gault JH, et al. Effect of respiration on venous return and stroke volume in cardiac tamponade. *Br Heart J.* 1970;32:592.
5. Shabetai R, Fowler NO, Guntheroth WG. The hemodynamics of cardiac tamponade and constrictive pericarditis. *Am J Cardiol.* 1970;26:480–489.
6. Fowler NO, Gabel M. The hemodynamic effects of tamponade: mainly the result of atrial, not ventricular, compression. *Circulation.* 1985;71:154–157.
7. Ditchey R, Engler RL, LeWinter MM, et al. The role of the right heart in acute cardiac tamponade in dogs. *Circ Res.* 1981;48: 701–710.
8. Gillam LD, Guyer DE, Gibson TC, et al. Hydrodynamic compression of the right atrium: a new echocardiographic sign of cardiac tamponade. *Circulation.* 1983;68:294–301.
9. Schiller NB, Botvinick EH. Right ventricular compression as a sign of cardiac tamponade. An analysis of echocardiographic ventricular dimensions and their clinical implications. *Circulation.* 1977;56:774–779.
10. Klopfenstein HS, Schuchard GH Wann LS, et al. The relative merits of pulsus paradoxus and right ventricular diastolic collapse in the early detection of cardiac tamponade: an experimental echocardiographic study. *Circulation.* 1985;71:829–833.
11. Guberman BA, Fowler NO, Engel PJ, et al. Cardiac tamponade in medical patients. *Circulation.* 1981;64:633–640.
12. DeCristofaro D, Liu CK. The haemodynamics of cardiac tamponade and blood volume overload in dogs. *Cardiovasc Res.* 1969;3:292–298.
13. Troughton RW, Asher, CR, Klein, AL. Pericarditis. *Lancet* 2004;363:717.
14. Reddy PS, Curtiss EI, O'Toole JD, et al. Cardiac tamponade: hemodynamic observations in man. *Circulation.* 1978;58:265–272.
15. Plotnick GD, Rubin DC, Feliciano Z, et al. Pulmonary hypertension decreases the predictive accuracy of echocardiographic clues for cardiac tamponade. *Chest.* 1995;107:919–924.
16. Winer HE, Kronzon I. Absence of paradoxical pulse in patients with cardiac tamponade and atrial septal defects. *Am J Cardiol.* 1979;44:378–380.
17. Bruch C, Schmermund A, Dagres N, et al. Changes in QRS voltage in cardiac tamponade and pericardial effusion: reversibility after pericardiocentesis and after anti-inflammatory drug treatment. *J Am Coll Cardiol.* 2001;38:219–226.
18. Chou, TC. *Electrocardiography in Clinical Practice: Adults and Pediatrics.* 4th ed. Philadelphia: WB Saunders; 1996.
19. Spodick. DH. Acute cardiac tamponade. *N Engl J Med.* 2003; 349:684.
20. Cheitlin MD, Alpert JS, Armstrong WF, et al. ACC/AHA guidelines for the clinical application of echocardiography: a report of the American College of Cardiology/American Heart Association Task Force on Practice Guidelines (Committee on Clinical Application of Echocardiography). Developed in collaboration with the American Society of Echocardiography. *Circulation.* 1997;95:1686.
21. Himelman RB, Kircher B, Rockey DC, et al. Inferior vena cava plethora with blunted respiratory response: a sensitive echocardiographic sign of tamponade. *J Am Coll Cardiol.* 1988;12:1470.
22. Fusman, B, Schwinger ME, Charney R, et al. Isolated collapse of left-sided heart chambers in cardiac tamponade: demonstration by two-dimensional echocardiography. *Am Heart J.* 1991;121:613.
23. Reydel B, Spodick DH. Frequency and significance of chamber collapses during cardiac tamponade. *Am Heart J.* 1990;119:1160.

24. Pai RK, Kedia A, Hsu PY, et al. AIDS associated with severe cor pulmonale and large pericardial effusion with cardiac tamponade. *Cardiol Rev*. 2004;12:49–55.
25. Antman EM, Cargill V, Grossman W. Low-pressure cardiac tamponade. *Ann Intern Med*. 1979;91:403–406.
26. Shaver JA, Reddy PS, Curtiss EI, et al. Noninvasive/invasive correlates of exaggerated ventricular interdependence in cardiac tamponade. *J Cardiol*. 2001;37(Suppl 1):71–76.
27. Shabetai R. Cardiac tamponade. In: Shabetai R. *The Pericardium*. 2nd ed. Norwell, MA: Kluwer Academc Publishers; 2003.
28. Hancock EW. Subacute effusive-constrictive pericarditis. *Circulation*. 1971;43:183–192.
29. Hancock EW. Effusive constrictive pericarditis. In: Reddy PS, Leon DF, Shaver JA, eds. *Pericardial Diseases*. New York: Raven Press; 1980: 357–369.
30. Craig RJ, Whalen RE, Behar VS, et al. Pressure and volume changes of the left ventricle in acute pericardial tamponade. *Am J Cardiol*. 1968;22:65–74.
31. Tsang TS, Freeman WK, Barnes ME, et al. Rescue echocardiographically guided pericardiocentesis for cardiac perforation complicating catheter-based procedures. The Mayo Clinic experience. *J Am Coll Cardiol*. 1998;32:1345–1350.
32. Shabetai R. Pericardiocentesis. In: Shabetai R. *The Pericardium*. 2nd ed. Norwell, MA: Kluwer Academic Publishers; 2003.
33. Tsang TS, Freeman WK, Sinak LJ, et al. Echocardiographically guided pericardiocentesis: evolution and state-of-the-art technique. *Mayo Clin Proc*. 1998;73:647–652.
34. Tsang TS, Oh JK, Seward JB. Diagnosis and management of cardiac tamponade in the era of echocardiography. *Clin Cardiol*. 1999;22:446–452.
35. Tsang TS, Seward JB. Pericardiocentesis under echocardiographic guidance. *Eur J Echocardiogr*. 2001;2:68.
36. Palacios IF, Tuzcu EM, Ziskind AA, et al. Percutaneous balloon pericardial window for patients with malignant pericardial effusion and tamponade. *Cathet Cardiovasc Diagn*. 1991;22:244–249.
37. Ziskind AA, Pearce AC, Lemmon CC, et al. Percutaneous balloon pericardiotomy for the treatment of cardiac tamponade and large pericardial effusions: description of technique and report of the first 50 cases. *J Am Coll Cardiol*. 1993;21:1–5.
38. Fowler NO, Gabel M. The hemodynamic effects of tamponade: mainly the result of atrial, not ventricular, compression. *Circulation*. 1985;71:154–157.
39. Fowler NO, Gabel M. Regional cardiac tamponade: a hemodynamic study. *J Am Coll Cardiol*. 1987;10:164–169.
40. Hancock EW. On the elastic and rigid forms of constrictive pericarditis. *Am Heart J*. 1980;100:917–923.
41. Ling LH, Oh JK, Breen JF, et al. Calcific constrictive pericarditis: is it still with us? *Ann Intern Med*. 2000;132:444–450.
42. Oh KY, Shimizu M, Edwards WD, et al. Surgical pathology of the parietal pericardium: a study of 344 cases (1993–1999). *Cardiovasc Pathol*. 2001;10:157–168.
43. Anand IS, Ferrari R, Kalra GS, et al. Pathogenesis of edema in constrictive pericarditis. Studies of body water and sodium, renal function, hemodynamics, and plasma hormones before and after pericardiectomy. *Circulation*. 1991;83:1880–1887.
44. Mann T, Brodie BR, Grossman W, et al. Effusive-constrictive hemodynamic pattern due to neoplastic involvement of the pericardium. *Am J Cardiol*. 1978;41:781–788.
45. Lee PJ, Mallik R. Cardiovascular effects of radiation therapy: practical approach to radiation therapy-induced heart disease. *Cardiol Rev*. 2005;13:80–86.
46. Stewart JR, Fajardo LP, Gillette SM, et al. Radiation injury to the heart. *Int J Radiation Oncology Biol Phys*. 1995;31:1205–1211.
47. Cooper DK, Cleland WP, Bentall HH. Collagen diseases as a cause of constrictive pericarditis. *Thorax*. 1978;33:368–371.
48. Hinkamp TJ, Sullivan HJ, Montoya A, et al. Chronic cardiac rejection masking as constrictive pericarditis. *Ann Thorac Surg*. 1994;57:1579–1583.
49. Cumming GR, Kerr D, Ferguson CC. Constrictive pericarditis with dwarfism in two siblings (Mulibrey nanism). *J Pediatr*. 1976;88:569–572.
50. Hansen AT, Eskildsen P, Gotzsche H. Pressure curves from the right auricle and the right ventricle in chronic constrictive pericarditis. *Circulation*. 1951;3:881–888.
51. Leya FS, Arab D, Joyal D, et al. The efficacy of brain natriuretic peptide levels in differentiating constrictive pericarditis from restrictive cardiomyopathy. *J Am Coll Cardiol*. 2005;45:1900–1902.
52. Mounsey P. The early diastolic sound of constrictive pericarditis. *Br Heart J*. 1955;17:143–152.
53. Magna P, Vythilingum S, Mitha AS. Pulsatile hepatomegaly in constrictive pericarditis. *Br Heart J*. 1984;52:465–467.
54. Levine HD. Myocardial fibrosis in constrictive pericarditis: electrocardiographic and pathologic observations. *Circulation*. 1973;48:1268–1281.
55 Ling LH, Oh JK, Tei C, et al. Pericardial thickness measured with transesophageal echocardiography: feasibility and potential clinical usefulness. *J Am Coll Cardiol*. 1997;29:1317–1323.
56. Silverman PM, Harell GS. Computed tomography of the normal pericardium. *Invest Radiol*. 1983;18:141–144.
57. Silverman PM, Harell GS, Korobkin M: Computed tomography of the abnormal pericardium. *AJR*. 1983;140:1125–1129.
58. Romberger JA. Electron beam (ultrafast) computed tomography for the evaluation of cardiac disease and function. 2005.
59. Soulen RL, Stark DD, Higgins CB. Magnetic resonance imaging of constrictive pericardial disease. *Am J Cardiol*. 1985;55: 480–484.
60. Oren RM, Grover-McKay M, Stanford W, et al. Accurate preoperative diagnosis of pericardial constriction using cine computed tomography. *J Am Coll Cardiol*. 1993;22:832–838.
61. Oh JK, Hatle LK, Seward JB, et al. Diagnostic role of Doppler echocardiography in constrictive pericarditis. *J Am Coll Cardiol*. 1994;23:154–162.
62. Oh JK, Tajik AJ, Appleton CP, et al. Preload reduction to unmask the characteristic Doppler features of constrictive pericarditis. A new observation. *Circulation*. 1997;95:796–799.
63. Tabata T, Kabbani SS, Murray RD, et al. Difference in the respiratory variation between pulmonary venous and mitral inflow Doppler velocities in patients with constrictive pericarditis with and without atrial fibrillation. *J Am Coll Cardiol*. 2001;37: 1936–1943.
64. Van der Merwe S, Dens J, Daenen W, et al. Pericardial disease is often not recognised as a cause of chronic severe ascites. *J Hepatol*. 2000;32:164–169.
65. Rajagopalan N, Garcia MJ, Rodriguez L, et al. Comparison of new Doppler echocardiographic methods to differentiate constrictive pericardial heart disease and restrictive cardiomyopathy. *Am J Cardiol*. 2001;87:86–94.
66. Ha JW, Oh JK, Ling LH, et al. Annulus paradoxus: transmitral flow velocity to mitral annular velocity ratio is inversely proportional to pulmonary capillary wedge pressure in patients with constrictive pericarditis. *Circulation*. 2001;104:976–978.
67. Palka P, Lange A, Donnelly JE, et al. Differentiation between restrictive cardiomyopathy and constrictive pericarditis by early diastolic Doppler myocardial velocity gradient at the posterior wall. *Circulation*. 2000;102:655.
68. Garcia MJ, Thomas JD, Klein AL. New Doppler echocardiographic applications for the study of diastolic function. *J Am Coll Cardiol*. 1998;32:865–875.
69. Hurrell DG, Nishimura RA, Higano ST, et al. Value of dynamic respiratory changes in left and right ventricular pressures for the diagnosis of constrictive pericarditis. *Circulation*. 1996;93: 2007–2013.
70. Schoenfeld MH, Supple EW, Dec GW, Jr., et al. Restrictive cardiomyopathy versus constrictive pericarditis: role of endomyocardial biopsy in avoiding unnecessary thoracotomy. *Circulation*. 1987;75:1012–1017.
71. Erciyes D, Mousseaux E, Cabanes L, et al. Pericardial and myocardial adiastole in rheumatoid polyarthritis. *Arch Mal Coeur Vaiss*. 1999;92:1381–1384.
72. Roca J, Manito N, Castells E, et al. Constrictive pericarditis after heart transplantation: report of two cases. *Heart Lung Transp*. 1995;14:106–110.
73. Bertog SC, Thambidorai SK, Parakh K, et al. Constrictive pericarditis: etiology and cause-specific survival after pericardiectomy. *J Am Coll Cardiol*. 2004;43:1445–1452.
74. Senni M, Redfield MM, Ling LH, et al. Left ventricular systolic and diastolic function after pericardiectomy in patients with constrictive pericarditis: Doppler echocardiographic findings

and correlation with clinical status. *J Am Coll Cardiol*. 1999;33: 1182–1188.
75. Sagrista-Sauleda J, Permanyer-Miralda G, Candell-Riera J, et al. Transient cardiac constriction: an unrecognized pattern of evolution in effusive acute idiopathic pericarditis. *Am J Cardiol*. 1987;59:961–966.
76. Haley JH, Tajik AJ, Danielson GK, et al. Transient constrictive pericarditis: causes and natural history. *J Am Coll Cardiol*. 2004;43:271–275.
77. Sagrista-Sauleda J, Angel J, Sanchez A, et al. Effusive-constrictive pericarditis. *N Engl J Med*. 2004;350:469–475.

Pharmacologic Therapy of Heart Failure

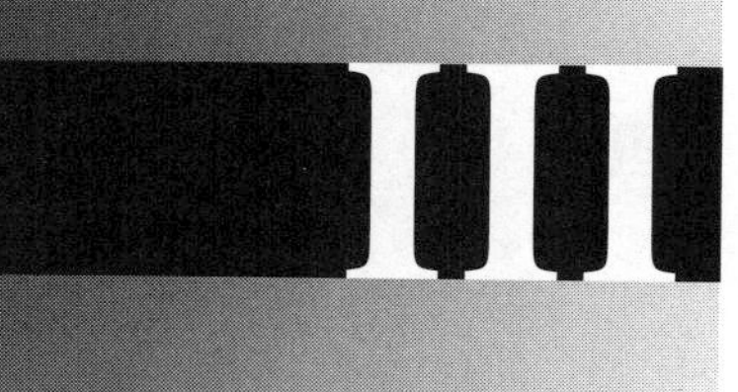

23

Clinical Pharmacokinetics in Congestive Heart Failure

Paul Nolan **Alan S. Nies** **Paul E. Fenster**

Pharmacokinetics is the study of drug movement in the body from the time of dosing to the time at which all of the drug has been eliminated. Knowledge of pharmacokinetics is key to the design of dosing regimens for optimizing a drug's therapeutic effect. Drug movement across short distances, such as from the lumen of the gastrointestinal tract into the intestinal mucosa or across a cell membrane in the body, is not dependent on blood flow. Intuitively, the circulation must be an important determinant of a drug's movement over longer distances. However, only in the past two decades has there been an attempt to model and quantify the effect of changes in circulatory function on various pharmacokinetic parameters (1–4). It is now known that all aspects of pharmacokinetics (i.e., absorption, distribution, and elimination) are critically dependent on the circulation. Changes produced by heart failure that would be expected to influence these pharmacokinetic parameters include (a) reduced blood flow to sites of drug absorption such as skin, subcutaneous tissue, or intestine; (b) interstitial edema at sites of absorption in the intestine or skin; (c) delayed gastric emptying due to increased sympathetic and reduced parasympathetic tone; (d) reduced blood flow to tissues that normally store drug in the body, such as fat and muscle; (e) reduced blood flow to the liver; (f) hepatocellular damage due to hypoxia or congestion; and (g) reduced blood flow to the kidney with resulting changes in renal function (5–7). Data exist for some model compounds regarding the influence of an altered circulation on pharmacokinetic variables, and from these data certain generalizations can be made to guide therapy with drugs for which data do not yet exist. This chapter starts with the basics. A description of the important aspects of pharmacokinetics as they relate to the circulation is followed by information on specific drugs that are important for the treatment of patients with congestive heart failure (CHF).

PHARMACOKINETIC PRINCIPLES

Absorption

To produce systemic effects, drugs must be delivered into the central circulation (Table 23-1). When a drug is delivered directly into the vascular space, all of the drug administered is available to produce its effect. For other routes of administration, the drug must pass a variety of barriers before it is able to gain access to the circulation. This absorption process will delay delivery of drug to its site of action and in some circumstances will reduce the total quantity of drug reaching the circulation. At a minimum, a single cell layer, the capillary endothelium, must be traversed even when a drug is administered intramuscularly. Much more complex is absorption after oral administration where several cell layers must be crossed before the drug reaches the portal circulation, after which the drug must make it through the liver before it reaches the systemic circulation. Many β-adrenergic receptor antagonists, calcium-channel blockers, antiarrhythmic agents, and nitrates are substantially metabolized by the liver before they reach the systemic circulation. This presystemic or first-pass elimination accounts for the much larger oral dose required to produce the same effect as an intravenous dose. Bioavailability is the term that quantifies the amount of a dose that actually reaches the systemic circulation and varies on a scale from 0 (none of the drug reaches the circulation) to 1 (100% of the dose reaches the systemic

TABLE 23-1
INFLUENCE OF HEART FAILURE ON PHARMACOKINETIC FACTORS INFLUENCING THE PLASMA CONCENTRATION OF DRUGS

	Effects of Heart Failure	Consequences	Examples
Absorption oral	Delayed but extent not usually affected	Steady-state concentration unaffected but peak concentration reduced and delayed	Furosemide and bumetamide delivered later and in lower concentration to tubular fluid
Percutaneous	May be reduced	Reduced blood concentration	Nitroglycerin levels reduced
V_D	May be reduced if large	Increased plasma concentration after a loading dose, but concentration at steady state is unaffected; shortens $t_{1/2}$	Lidocaine and procainamide loading doses must be reduced
Hepatic blood flow	Reduced	Reduced clearance and increased concentration at steady state of high-clearance drugs that are administered parenterally. Steady-state concentration of orally administered drugs is unaffected.	Lidocaine maintenance infusion rate must be reduced
Hepatic metabolic capacity	May be reduced by ischemia and/or congestion	Reduced clearance and increased concentration at steady state of drugs that undergo phase I metabolism (oxidation, reduction, dealkylation). This affects low-clearance drugs given by any route and high-clearance drugs given orally. Phase II metabolism (conjugation) usually unaffected. Increased $t_{1/2}$ (*see also* V_D).	Theophylline and quinidine maintenance doses may need to be reduced. Plasma concentration of these drugs should be used to guide dosing.
Renal function	May be reduced	Reduced clearance and increased concentration at steady state of drugs cleared mainly by the kidney. Increased $t_{1/2}$ (*see also* V_D).	Procainamide, digoxin, enalapril, and lisinopril maintenance doses may need to be reduced in proportion to the reduction in creatinine clearance. For procainamide, the concentration of both the parent drug and its active metabolite (acecainide) must be monitored.

V_D, apparent volume of distribution.

circulation). A reduction of bioavailability after oral administration of a drug indicates either poor absorption or presystemic elimination (8).

Most drugs are absorbed from their site of administration by passive diffusion, with the driving force for absorption being the concentration of drug in contact with the absorbing surface. Thus, the rate of absorption can be manipulated by controlling the dissolution of drug from the dosage form. This principle has been useful for designing drug preparations that delay and prolong absorption after oral, intramuscular, subcutaneous, or percutaneous sites of administration. In this way drugs that have short durations of action can be used for chronic therapy with relatively infrequent dosing. Depot preparations for intramuscular use (e.g., penicillin and progesterone) slowly release drug, which then is dissolved in tissue fluids and absorbed into the circulation, sustaining an effect over days or weeks. Long-acting oral preparations (e.g., calcium-channel blockers, procainamide, and theophylline) release drug slowly from the dosage form. For these oral preparations, the duration of sustained absorption is limited to 12 to 24 hours by the transit time of the gastrointestinal tract. Percutaneous absorption is achieving increasing use for a few, highly potent, lipid-soluble drugs. The duration of absorption is limited by the ability to incorporate sufficient drug into the patch that is applied to the skin. The absorption of percutaneous clonidine is sustained over a week; nitroglycerin is administered daily. The advantages of these sustained-release preparations are that they are more convenient and thus have the ability to enhance compliance, and they produce a relatively constant blood level so that toxicity associated with the peaks and inefficacy associated with troughs of blood concentration are avoided.

With preparations other than oral, drug can reach the systemic circulation without having to pass through the liver and be subjected to hepatic presystemic metabolism. This can improve the bioavailability for a drug, such as nitroglycerin, which is essentially metabolized completely by the liver after oral administration. However, presystemic metabolism may not be avoided entirely because skin also may metabolize nitroglycerin before it reaches the circulation during percutaneous absorption. A disadvantage is that interindividual variation in absorption is increased with the sustained-release preparations; with oral dosage forms, sustained-release preparations are more likely to be affected by changes in gastrointestinal motility such that increases in motility can reduce the total quantity of drug absorbed. Another disadvantage that is unrelated to pharmacokinetics is the increased potential for the development of tolerance to the drug's effect when blood levels are sustained relatively constant over long periods of time. This has been of particular interest with the use of percutaneous nitroglycerin, which is discussed elsewhere in this book.

Factors other than drug concentration are important for absorption, particularly in disease states such as CHF (5). Resistance of the absorbing surface to diffusion is a function of the area available for absorption as well its permeability to the drug. Blood flow to the absorption site also is important to remove drug and thereby maximize the concentration gradient across the absorbing surface (9). For drugs that dissolve readily from the dosage form and diffuse rapidly across cells, blood flow to the site of absorption may be rate-limiting. For most drugs, however, the rate of drug delivery from the dosage preparation or the resistance of the absorbing surface to diffusion is the rate-limiting step in absorption such that alterations in blood flow become less important. In CHF, edema and a reduction of blood flow at the absorbing site have the potential to reduce bioavailability and/or alter the time course of drug absorption (10). After oral dosing, most drugs are absorbed across the mucosa of the small intestine so that a delay in gastric emptying can retard absorption. This most commonly delays and decreases the height of the peak concentration in the blood. In heart failure, the sympathetic nervous system is activated and the parasympathetic nervous system is depressed. In the gastrointestinal tract these consequences of heart failure reduce peristaltic activity and delay gastric emptying. Thus, several features of heart failure, including edema formation, a reduction of blood flow, and a delay in gastric emptying, would be predicted to reduce the rate or extent (i.e., the bioavailability) of absorption of some drugs (11). It is important to recognize the consequences of a reduction in the rate or extent of drug absorption. For drugs such as digoxin and theophylline that are administered chronically and for which the target blood levels must remain within a certain range for therapeutic effect, a delay in the rate without a decrease in the extent of absorption is of little or no importance. In fact, a delay in absorption will result in a more constant blood concentration than would be achieved if the dose were absorbed rapidly. However, the rate of absorption can be important if the circulating drug concentration must reach a threshold level or if the rate of drug delivery to the site of action is a critical determinant of the drug's effect. This is the case for furosemide, which has a renal response that is determined by the rate as well as the extent of drug reaching the tubular fluid (12). A reduction in the rate of oral absorption is one mechanism accounting for the resistance to the diuretic effect of oral furosemide in patients with heart failure.

In contrast to the relative unimportance of a reduction in rate of absorption for most drugs, a reduction in extent of absorption (bioavailability) will be of importance for all drugs affected because the steady-state concentration of the drug in the plasma will be reduced. The limited amount of data available in CHF indicates that the extent of drug absorption by the gastrointestinal tract usually is affected only minimally and unpredictably. However, the rate of drug absorption from the gut often is delayed, probably as a consequence of a delay in gastric emptying, although edema of the gut wall and a diminished blood flow also could play a role. With transdermal nitroglycerin, there is some evidence that bioavailability is variably reduced in patients with severe CHF, probably as a consequence of subcutaneous edema and reduced dermal blood flow.

Distribution

Once absorbed into the blood, drugs are distributed throughout the body, initially to the well-perfused tissues, including the vasculature, heart, and brain, and then to the less well-perfused tissues, including fat and skeletal muscle. The extent of uptake into tissues depends on the ability of the tissues to bind or partition the drug relative to the binding or partitioning in the plasma. The pharmacokinetic term that describes the distribution of drugs is called the apparent volume of distribution (V_D). V_D is defined as the volume that would be required to contain an amount of drug at the concentration achieved in plasma, and therefore is a constant that describes the ratio of the amount of drug in the body (Amt) to the resulting plasma concentration (C_p):

$$V_D = \frac{Amt}{C_P} \tag{23-1}$$

Depending on the rate of drug entry into the circulation, the body often behaves as if it were composed of two or more compartments that each have their own V_D. Drug is introduced initially to a smaller V_D (often designated as the central compartment) and only more gradually is distributed to a larger V_D (often called the peripheral compartment). Thus, immediately after an intravenous bolus of a drug such as lidocaine, the drug concentration in the blood is high, but the drug rapidly disappears from the central compartment as it is distributed to the peripheral compartment. The drug concentration then decreases more gradually as drug is eliminated from the body.

The two phases have been called the initial distribution phase followed by the elimination phase. The most important phase for chronic drug therapy is the elimination phase, during which drug is in equilibrium between the blood and the tissues of the body, and the concentration of drug in the blood therefore bears a consistent relationship to drug at the site of action. Therefore, the V_D describing this apparent volume of the peripheral compartment is the most clinically relevant value for most drugs and is the V_D listed in tables describing drug pharmacokinetics. Whether the drug concentration in plasma during the distribution phase is predictive of drug effects is dependent on the individual drug. For many drugs such as lidocaine that quickly reach their site of action, plasma concentrations achieved during the distribution phase are associated with therapeutic or toxic effects on the well-perfused tissues such as the heart and brain. On the other hand, for a few drugs like digoxin, the plasma concentrations during the distribution phase are not predictive of drug effects. Only after 4 to 8 hours is there sufficient time for equilibrium to occur such that digoxin in the blood reflects drug at the site of action. A common error in the interpretation of digoxin concentrations in plasma is to ascribe meaning to the high values obtained when blood is sampled within 4 to 6 hours after a dose of digoxin (13). Although concentrations of 4 to 10 ng/mL may be present at this time, they have no predictive value because they are not in equilibrium with digoxin at its site of action.

The V_D is an apparent volume that is rarely related to an actual volume, and it is a common mistake to attempt to label the V_D as plasma volume, extracellular water, or some other actual fluid space. For drugs that are bound to tissues, the V_D can be much larger than any real volume contained in any fluid space in the body. For instance, digoxin has a V_D of the peripheral compartment of 7 L/kg in normal individuals. Thus, an intravenous dose of 0.5 mg digoxin will be distributed in a peripheral compartment that has an apparent volume of about 500 L in a 70-kg patient, resulting in a plasma concentration of 1 µg/L or 1 ng/mL. A large V_D is the quantitative expression of the fact that drug in the body is present in the tissues at a higher concentration than in the blood. Even drugs that have a V_D similar to a body fluid compartment are rarely distributed everywhere at the same concentration.

The physiological determinants of the V_D are the relative affinities of the tissues and the plasma for the drug and the state of the circulation (2,5,14). Binding of drug to plasma proteins acts to retain drug in the plasma because it limits the amount of unbound drug that can distribute to the tissues. Displacement of drug from plasma proteins will increase its V_D because there is an increase in the fraction of drug that is unbound, which will leave the central compartment. Drug binding to plasma proteins can be affected by diseases and other drugs. Uremia can reduce the binding of some drugs to plasma albumin because retained acidic metabolites can compete for binding sites. Nephrotic syndrome and hepatic disease can reduce the albumin concentration and thereby reduce the binding of drugs to plasma proteins. CHF usually is not associated with changes in binding to plasma proteins unless it is also accompanied by renal or hepatic failure. However, the state of the circulation itself is apparently an important determinant of the V_D. This is probably related to the fact that drug is not as readily delivered to the tissues when the circulation is impaired (15). During heart failure, intense peripheral vasoconstriction restricts access of drug to poorly perfused tissues that make up the peripheral compartment of the V_D. Thus, drugs that are extensively distributed out of the plasma, and therefore have a large V_D, may have a contraction of the V_D in patients with heart failure. This is perhaps counterintuitive on first glance because the edema present in patients with heart failure might suggest that the V_D should be increased. However, this is a fallacy based on thinking of the V_D as a real volume. One model compound for which the V_D has been shown to be increased is aminopyrine, a substance that actually does seem to distribute only in body water (16). For most drugs the following rule generally holds: if the V_D is large (1 L/kg or more) then the V_D may be reduced in patients with heart failure; for drugs with small V_D (<1 L/kg), there is little or no change in V_D with heart failure. Lidocaine is the best-studied example of a drug that has a reduced V_D of the central and peripheral compartments by about 50% in patients with heart failure (17).

The size of a loading dose (LD) is determined by the volume of distribution of the drug. The concept is that sufficient drug must be given such that after the distribution phase, the plasma concentration is in the desired range ($C_{desired}$). Generally, the V_D of the peripheral compartment is the constant used to calculate an LD delivered into the circulation by rearranging Equation 23-1:

$$LD = V_D \times C_{desired} \tag{23-2}$$

For many drugs the calculated LD must be administered slowly to allow time for distribution so that the very high concentrations resulting from the initial distribution into the small V_D of the central compartment are avoided. In the presence of heart failure, LDs of some drugs must be reduced to account for the reduced V_D in this condition. For lidocaine, therefore, the loading boluses in a patient with heart failure should be about half the standard doses because the V_D for lidocaine is reduced by half in such patients.

Elimination

Most drugs are eliminated from the body by the liver, the kidney, or both organs. For a few drugs, elimination occurs in the lung, the blood, or in other tissues. For most drugs, the elimination rates are directly proportional to the concentration of drug in the plasma, a process mathematically described as first-order elimination. The most useful concept for describing the variables that are physiologically important for drug elimination is drug clearance. Drug clearance usually is defined as the volume of fluid (blood or plasma) completely cleared of drug in a unit of time, so clearance has units of flow. Clearance was a concept originally used by renal physiologists to describe renal function. Creatinine clearance is the volume of plasma that is completely cleared of creatinine per minute and is calculated as the urinary elimination rate of creatinine divided by the plasma creatinine concentration. By analogy, drug clearance (Cl) can be considered as the rate of drug elimination (R_e) normalized to the plasma concentration (C_p) (4):

$$Cl = \frac{R_e}{C_p} \tag{23-3}$$

The total body drug clearance is the sum of all the individual organ clearances (renal clearance plus hepatic clearance plus lung clearance plus clearance by all other means).

Physiologically, clearance is equal to the product of blood flow (Q) to the eliminating organ and the extraction ratio (E), which is the fraction of the drug in the blood removed during a single passage through the organ:

$$Cl = Q \times E \qquad (23\text{-}4)$$

Clearance is thus an index of the efficiency of drug removal from the blood and is not influenced by the distribution of drug in the body. Equation 23-4 implies that hepatic drug clearance (Cl_H) would be related directly to hepatic blood flow. However, this is not the case because the extraction ratio is not a constant. Hepatic extraction of drug from the blood is a function of (a) hepatic blood flow, (b) the inherent ability of the liver to irreversibly remove drug from the blood, and (c) the binding of drug to the plasma proteins and the cellular components of blood (2,3). A number of models of hepatic elimination have been proposed (4). The most useful is the well-stirred model, which assumes that drug available to the eliminating processes of the liver is in equilibrium with hepatic venous blood (1). Based on this model, the following relationship can be derived:

$$Cl_H = QE = Q\left[\frac{f_B Cl^u_{int}}{Q + f_B Cl^u_{int}}\right] = Q\left(\frac{Cl_{int}}{Q + Cl_{int}}\right) \qquad (23\text{-}5)$$

where f_B is the free (unbound) fraction of drug in the blood and Cl^u_{int} is the intrinsic hepatic clearance, an index of the ability of the liver to remove unbound drug from liver water by metabolizing enzymes and transport processes. Because binding of drug to plasma proteins is not changed by heart failure, $f_B Cl^u_{int}$ can be combined into a single term, Cl_{int}, which represents the ability of the liver to remove drug from blood rather than from liver water. Although Equation 23-5 appears formidable, it is useful for predicting the changes in hepatic drug clearance that occur when hepatic blood flow is impaired in CHF. It is instructive to consider two drug types that represent the limits of this equation. First consider a drug with a very high intrinsic hepatic clearance. In this case, Cl_{int} is much larger than hepatic blood flow, and so the extraction ratio $[Cl_{int}/(Q + Cl_{int})]$ is very high and approaches 1. Thus, hepatic drug clearance (Eq. 23-5) approaches hepatic blood flow. Drugs that have this type of Cl_{int} are called high-clearance drugs and include lidocaine, propranolol, nifedipine, diltiazem, and verapamil. When given intravenously, their clearance is dependent on hepatic blood flow. Because of the very high hepatic extraction, such drugs are subject to a high first-pass hepatic extraction and consequently have poor oral bioavailability. Contrast this with the situation when Cl_{int} is much less than hepatic blood flow. In this case the extraction ratio approaches $[Cl_{int}/Q]$, and hepatic drug clearance therefore approaches Cl_{int} and is independent of hepatic blood flow. Such drugs are called low-clearance drugs and include warfarin, theophylline, quinidine, and mexiletine. Thus, the model predicts that the hepatic clearance of drugs with a high hepatic extraction ratio and, hence, a high hepatic clearance are very sensitive to changes in hepatic blood flow, whereas the clearance of drugs with a low extraction ratio and consequently a low hepatic clearance are insensitive to changes in blood flow. This is because the extraction of these low-clearance drugs is inversely proportional to hepatic blood flow so that as blood flow is reduced, the extraction ratio increases nearly proportionally, and clearance, which is the product of blood flow and extraction, is therefore little changed. This is illustrated graphically in Figure 23-1. Figure 23-1A illustrates the hepatic clearance (solid line) and hepatic extraction ratio (dashed line) versus hepatic blood flow for a high-clearance drug that has a hepatic extraction of 0.9 at a normal liver blood flow of 1,500 mL per minute. Cl_{int} is assumed to remain constant as hepatic blood flow changes. As hepatic blood flow varies from 400 mL per minute to 2,000 mL per minute, the actual hepatic clearance for the high-clearance drug varies almost proportionally and the extraction ratio remains relatively constant. In Figure 23-1B, the effect of changes in hepatic blood flow on the actual hepatic clearance (solid line) and extraction ratio (dashed line) is depicted for a low-clearance drug that has a hepatic extraction ratio of 0.1 at a normal liver blood flow of 1,500 mL per minute. Here the hepatic clearance remains relatively constant as liver

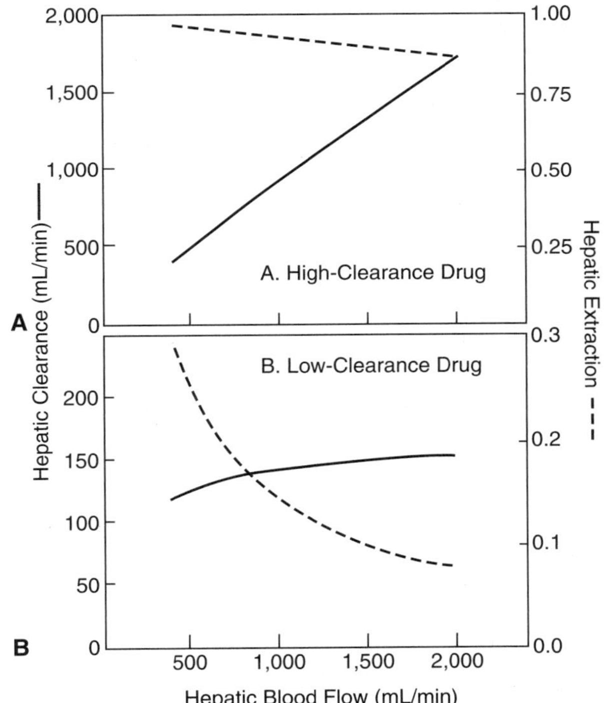

Figure 23-1 The effect of changes in hepatic blood flow on the actual hepatic clearance (**solid line**) and extraction ratio (**dashed line**) of two drugs that are metabolized entirely by the liver. A high-clearance drug (E = 0.9 at a liver blood flow of 1,500 mL per minute) is shown **(A)** and a low-clearance drug (E = 0.1 at a liver blood flow of 0.1 mL per minute) is shown **(B).** Liver blood flow is varied over the range of 400 to 2,000 mL per minute. (Modified from Wilkinson GR, Shand DG. A physiological approach to hepatic drug clearance. *Clin Pharmacol Ther.* 1975;18:377–390.)

blood flow changes because the extraction of the low-clearance drug is increased as hepatic blood flow is reduced (2,3).

A similar series of arguments can be applied to changes in hepatic function related to high- and low-clearance drugs. In the model, changes in hepatic function are reflected by changes in Cl_{int}. Thus, the hepatic clearance of low-clearance drugs is influenced primarily by changes in hepatic function and is relatively independent of changes in blood flow, and vice versa for high-clearance drugs. Severe CHF can produce hepatocellular damage from hypoperfusion or congestion, which will result in a reduction of Cl_{int}. Therefore, because heart failure can reduce hepatic function as well as hepatic blood flow, the hepatic clearance of both high-clearance and low-clearance drugs can be affected, but for different reasons.

A powerful prediction from the model that is not intuitively obvious is that the average plasma concentration of an orally administered drug that is eliminated solely by hepatic metabolism is not affected by changes in hepatic blood flow, even if the drug is a high-clearance drug. This is because a change in hepatic blood flow will alter the extraction of drug not only on the first pass through the liver but also on each subsequent pass, and these influences cancel each other. As shown in Figure 23-2, a reduction in hepatic blood flow will increase the first-pass hepatic extraction (E) of a high-clearance drug (Eq. 23-5), reducing the amount of an oral dose reaching the systemic circulation and thereby reducing the peak plasma concentration achieved after the dose. However, this reduced amount of drug is then cleared less well because of the decrease in hepatic blood flow (Eq. 23-5), which, if V_D is unchanged, will prolong the drug's half-life. This reduction in hepatic clearance exactly counters the reduced amount escaping hepatic extraction on the first pass, resulting in no change in average plasma concentration. Mathematically, the apparent clearance of a hepatically metabolized drug administered orally (Cl_O) is the hepatic clearance (Cl_H) divided by the fraction of the dose escaping first-pass hepatic extraction (1 – E). By substituting in Equation 23-5 and solving for Cl_O, one derives the surprising fact that:

$$Cl_O = Cl_{int,} \qquad (23\text{-}6)$$

indicating that the apparent clearance for a drug given orally is independent of hepatic blood flow and only dependent on the Cl_{int}, which is the functional capacity of the liver to remove drug from blood. Clinically, Equation 23-6 suggests that if heart failure produces changes in steady-state blood levels for any given oral dosing regimen of a drug that is solely eliminated by hepatic metabolism, then there must be a reduction in hepatocellular function. It is only for intravenous infusions of high-clearance drugs, such as lidocaine, that hepatic blood flow has a significant effect on steady-state blood levels.

Renal clearance of drugs is much simpler and more predictable than hepatic drug clearance. Fortunately, drug clearance by the kidney is proportional to glomerular filtration rate even if the drug is cleared by tubular secretion and/or reabsorption rather than by filtration. Thus, by estimating or measuring creatinine clearance, one can determine the effect of renal dysfunction on renal drug clearance, and dosage adjustments can be made accordingly (8).

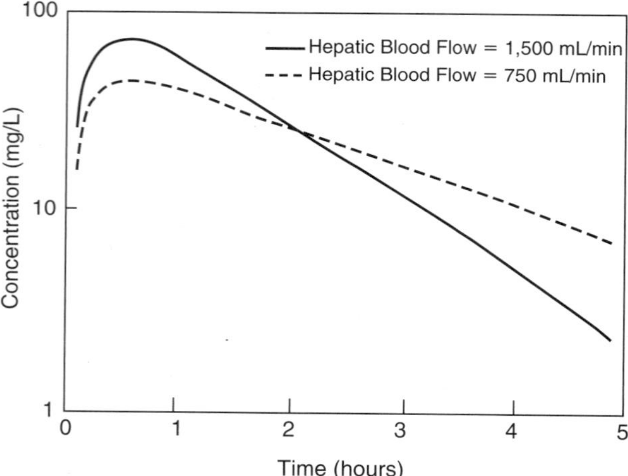

Figure 23-2 The effect of a change in hepatic blood flow on the plasma concentration-time profile of a high-clearance drug (E = 0.9 at a liver blood flow of 1,500 mL per minute) that is metabolized entirely by the liver and is administered orally at time 0. The curve with a normal liver blood flow is depicted by the **solid line**, and the curve with a liver blood flow of half normal (750 mL per minute) is depicted by the **dashed line**. When liver blood flow is reduced, the peak plasma concentration is reduced, indicating an increased hepatic presystemic elimination. However, once in the circulation, the drug is eliminated less rapidly because the hepatic blood flow is reduced. As a result of these two effects of a reduction in hepatic blood flow, the average plasma concentration (i.e., the area under the curve) is unchanged. (Modified from Wilkinson GR, Shand DG. A physiological approach to hepatic drug clearance. *Clin Pharmacol Ther.* 1975;18:377–390.)

Half-Life

The most commonly used pharmacokinetic term is drug half-life ($t_{1/2}$), which is the time required to reduce the plasma concentration of drug by half. Half-life often is used to characterize drug elimination. However, it frequently is not appreciated that half-life is actually a hybrid term that is dependent on two independent variables, drug clearance (Cl) and V_D:

$$t_{\frac{1}{2}} = \frac{0.693V_D}{Cl} \qquad (23\text{-}7)$$

Thus, at any given clearance, more time will be required (i.e., a longer half-life) to clear the body of drug if there is a large V_D than if the V_D is smaller. If clearance is reduced, half-life will be prolonged as long as V_D is not changed. Thus, a change in half-life cannot be used as an index of efficiency of drug elimination unless the apparent volume of distribution is unchanged. Cardiac failure can reduce the clearance as well as the volume of distribution of some drugs; therefore, half-life is a particularly poor index of changes in drug elimination in this disease state. The best example is that of lidocaine, which has a reduction of both clearance and V_D of about 50% in some patients with heart failure. However, because of the relationship in Equation 23-7, half-life may not be changed. Nonetheless, the loading doses and maintenance doses of lidocaine must be reduced to avoid toxicity. If only half-life is measured, there will be no clue to the major changes in kinetics that have occurred in this illness.

Half-life is important for the time course of drug elimination and accumulation. If drug administration ceases, only half the drug leaves the body in one half-life, half the remaining drug is eliminated in the second half life, and so forth. Thus, if 100% is present at time 0, 50% will be present after one half-life, 25% after two half-lives, 12.5% after three half-lives, 6.25% after four half-lives, and 3.125% after five half-lives. In theory, an infinite time is needed to rid the body of all drug; in practice, three to five half-lives are needed to effectively eliminate drug.

When drugs are given as a continuous infusion or as repeated intermittent doses, drug accumulates in the body until a steady state is achieved. The rate of drug accumulation depends on drug half-life and is the mirror image of the rate of drug elimination previously discussed. Thus, accumulation to half of the ultimate steady-state level occurs in one half-life, but it takes three half-lives to achieve 87.5% of steady state and five half-lives to reach 96.875% of steady state. For practical purposes, steady state is achieved when 90% of the ultimate accumulation occurs. For drugs with a long half-life accumulation occurs slowly, and an LD may be necessary to achieve therapeutic effects quickly. However, regardless of whether a loading dose is given, the final steady state achieved is independent of the loading dose or the half-life and is determined solely by the maintenance dose and the drug clearance (discussed later). The concept of accumulation applies equally well to a continuous infusion or to intermittent doses. Because smaller doses are given more frequently, the variation in peaks and troughs diminishes, but the average blood level reached at steady state is independent of dose frequency and is determined only by the dose per unit time and the clearance.

Half-life also describes the time course of changes in drug concentration when the dose or infusion rate is changed. Using the same reasoning as previously discussed, three to five half-lives will be required to achieve a new steady state. Thus, the consequences of changing doses or infusion rates are delayed, and this delay is dependent on the half-life.

Maintenance Doses

When the amount of drug administered and absorbed over a period of time (dose/time, D/t) is the same as the amount of drug eliminated during the same time (elimination rate, R_e), steady state has been achieved. From the definition of clearance in Equation 23-3, it can be readily appreciated that both the dose/time and the elimination rate are equal to drug clearance multiplied by the steady-state plasma concentration (C_{ss}):

$$R_e = \frac{D}{t} = Cl \times C_{ss} \qquad (23\text{-}8)$$

Thus, drug clearance and the dose/time are the sole determinants of the concentration of drug in the blood and the amount of drug in the body at steady state. Importantly, the steady-state concentration is independent of the V_D or the half-life. For drugs given intravenously, hepatic clearance is dependent on both hepatic blood flow and hepatic function, which therefore influence the steady-state concentration. For drugs given orally, the hepatic portion of drug clearance is independent of hepatic blood flow and only dependent on the liver's metabolic capacity (Eq. 23-5). Equation 23-8 can be used to calculate the dose required to achieve a given plasma concentration of the drug if clearance is known. As an example, the clearance of lidocaine in an average adult without heart failure or hepatic disease is about 800 mL per minute. Thus, achieving a therapeutic plasma concentration of 3 mg/L will require an infusion of 2.4 mg per minute. In a patient with heart failure and reduced hepatic blood flow, lidocaine clearance may be reduced to 400 mL per minute, and thus an infusion rate of 1.2 mg per minute will be all that is necessary to achieve the same therapeutic level of 3 mg/L.

EFFECT OF HEART FAILURE ON PHARMACOKINETICS OF SPECIFIC DRUGS

Antiarrhythmic Drugs

Quinidine

Much of the early data on quinidine kinetics in heart failure are confusing because of nonspecific assay methodology (9,18). Oral absorption can be delayed in some patients with heart failure, and the V_D (normally 2.7 L/kg) may be reduced such that quinidine concentrations peak later and are higher after an oral dose in patients with heart failure (19,20). Quinidine is largely metabolized by the liver as a low-clearance drug (normally 4.7 mL/min/kg). However, if heart failure is severe enough to cause hepatocellular dysfunction, the clearance of quinidine will be reduced so that higher blood levels will result from usual oral doses (21,22). Quinidine's half-life (normally 6 to 7 hours), however, is not changed in most patients with heart failure because of an equivalent reduction in V_D and clearance. However, an occasional patient with severe heart failure and hepatic dysfunction with markedly depressed hepatic quinidine clearance will have a prolonged half-life (23).

Quinidine has pharmacokinetic drug interactions with a number of drugs. Its metabolism can be induced by several common enzyme inducers, including phenobarbital (24), phenytoin (24), and rifampin (25), resulting in an increase in hepatic clearance as a consequence of an increase in Cl_{int}. Quinidine plasma concentration therefore will decrease as a result of this interaction and may fall below the therapeutic range. Cimetidine (26), verapamil (27), and amiodarone (28) can reduce the metabolism of quinidine and thereby reduce its clearance, resulting in an increase in steady-state quinidine levels. Quinidine and verapamil also produce additive effects on the vasculature, and the combination can result in severe hypotension (29). Importantly, quinidine can reduce the clearance of digoxin (30) and, to a lesser extent, digitoxin (31), increasing the blood levels of these glycosides. Finally, quinidine can block the enzyme that accounts for the rapid metabolism of encainide and propafenone in 93% of the population who are extensive metabolizers of these drugs (32,33).

The consequences of this interaction are complex because both encainide and propafenone have active metabolites, and whether dosage adjustments are required is not clear.

Procainamide

Procainamide is normally well-absorbed from the gastrointestinal tract, but in the presence of severe heart failure absorption may be delayed and/or incomplete. The V_D of procainamide (normally 1.9 L/kg) has been found to be reduced in some patients with heart failure (34), but this has not been a universal finding (35). Procainamide is metabolized to an active metabolite, N-acetylprocainamide (NAPA, acecainide), which has class III antiarrhythmic activity. The metabolism rate is genetically determined, with about half of the American population being fast and half slow acetylators. In all patients with normal renal function, 60% to 80% of procainamide and essentially all of the acetylated metabolite is excreted in the urine. Hepatic clearance of procainamide is low and not affected much by liver blood flow. The major determinant of the drug's clearance, therefore, is the renal function (36). When renal function is diminished, the acetylated metabolite accumulates more than the parent drug, and this can be the case in heart failure-induced renal dysfunctions (37). Thus, for optimum patient management, the blood concentrations of both procainamide and acecainide should be monitored. In the absence of renal dysfunction, patients with heart failure do not have any consistent changes in procainamide clearance and therefore require drug doses similar to patients without heart failure to maintain therapeutic concentrations of the drug in the blood (35).

Cimetidine (26), ranitidine (26), trimethoprim (38), and amiodarone (28) can reduce the renal clearance of procainamide and its active metabolite NAPA, resulting in increased plasma concentration of both at any given dose of procainamide.

Disopyramide

Disopyramide is contraindicated in patients with heart failure because of its potent negative inotropic effects (39–41). Therefore, there are not many studies of its kinetics in this situation. Oral absorption of disopyramide is not changed by heart failure. The clearance of disopyramide (normally 1.2 mL/min/kg) is about 55% renal, with the remainder being hepatic metabolism. Clearance can be reduced in heart failure, and half-life (normally 6 hours) can be prolonged, especially if there is renal dysfunction (42). The V_D of disopyramide is relatively small (normally 0.6 L/kg) and is unchanged in heart failure.

The most important interactions with disopyramide are with other negatively inotropic drugs such as β-adrenergic receptor antagonists that can add to the cardiac depression produced by disopyramide. A few pharmacokinetic interactions with potential clinical importance have been reported, including a reduction of disopyramide clearance with hepatic P450-inducing drugs (43), such as phenobarbital, phenytoin, or rifampin, and inhibition of disopyramide metabolism with erythromycin (44).

Moricizine

Moricizine is well-absorbed after oral administration but undergoes first-pass metabolism that reduces the bioavailability to 35% to 40%. It has a high hepatic clearance (20 mL/min/kg), no renal clearance, a large V_D (3 L/kg), and a short half-life of 2 to 6 hours (45,46). There may be active metabolites because there is no apparent correlation between blood levels and effects, and the onset of antiarrhythmic effect is substantially delayed from the time of the peak plasma concentration. Whether heart failure influences the pharmacokinetics of moricizine is unknown.

Few drug interactions have been reported with moricizine. Cimetidine inhibits the metabolism of moricizine (47). Because active metabolites as well as the parent drug may be important to the effects of moricizine, it is impossible to predict the outcome of such an interaction but it does not appear to have much clinical importance. Moricizine may enhance the metabolism and reduce the plasma concentration of theophylline (47).

Lidocaine

Lidocaine was used frequently as an example in the discussion earlier because it has been well-studied in patients with heart failure. Its V_D (normally 1.5 L/kg) is reduced by as much as 50% and its clearance (normally 11 mL/min/kg), which is entirely hepatic, is reduced by 50% or more, largely because of the decreased hepatic blood flow as a consequence of a low cardiac output (17,48–50). The half-life may be prolonged or it may be unchanged. As a consequence of these changes, lidocaine loading doses and maintenance infusion rates should be reduced by half in patients with heart failure and signs of toxicity must not be overlooked. Blood concentrations of lidocaine may be helpful in determining the proper maintenance dose in individual patients.

Drug interactions with lidocaine are relatively rare. β-adrenergic receptor antagonists can reduce hepatic blood flow and some also may reduce the Cl_{int} of lidocaine, resulting in a reduction of lidocaine clearance of 15% to 45% (51). Cimetidine also has been reported to reduce lidocaine clearance (26). This is probably because of cimetidine's effect on hepatic drug metabolism (i.e., the Cl_{int} of lidocaine). Cimetidine also may reduce hepatic blood flow in some circumstances.

Mexiletine

Oral absorption of mexiletine is not affected by heart failure. Its V_D is large (normally 4.9 L/kg). The drug is metabolized almost entirely by the liver as a low- to moderate-clearance drug (normally 6.3 mL/min/kg). Heart failure does not affect mexiletine clearance unless it is severe, in which case half-life (normally 9 to 12 hours) can be prolonged (52).

Mexiletine's hepatic clearance can by enhanced by the enzyme inducers rifampin (53) or phenytoin (54). Smokers have a higher clearance than nonsmokers (55). Mexiletine can reduce the clearance of theophylline, occasionally resulting in theophylline toxicity (56).

Tocainide

Tocainide pharmacokinetics is little changed by mild to moderate heart failure (57). The drug is well-absorbed and is eliminated by the liver (60%) and the kidneys (40%). Some studies suggest a reduction in clearance (normally 2.6 mL/min/kg) in severe heart failure associated with renal dysfunction, and there also may be a reduction in the V_D (normally 3.0 L/kg) with no change in half-life (normally 14 hours). However, the interpatient variability of half-life in a group of patients with heart failure is large and some patients can have a markedly prolonged half-life (58,59).

Tocainide does not interact with many other drugs. The results of one study in healthy volunteers suggested that cimetidine can inhibit the absorption of tocainide (60) and the results of another suggested that rifampin may increase the hepatic metabolism of tocainide (61), but the clinical significance of these studies is uncertain.

Sotalol

Sotalol is a β-adrenoreceptor blocker with antiarrhythmic properties. The β-blocking effect is noncardioselective and occurs at low doses. In patients with impaired left ventricular function, sotalol reduces the cardiac index and increases the pulmonary capillary wedge pressure. Therefore, sotalol is either avoided in patients with heart failure or is used only with slow upward titration of the dose and careful monitoring of clinical status.

Sotalol is 90% to 100% bioavailable after oral administration. Peak plasma levels are reached in 2.5 to 4 hours. The mean elimination half-life is 12 hours. Sotalol is not metabolized and is eliminated by the kidneys (62). Therefore, the dose should be decreased, by prolonging the interval between doses, when creatinine clearance is less than 60 mL per minute (63).

Flecainide

Because of its negative inotropic activity, flecainide usually is not given to patients with severe heart failure (64). Flecainide is well-absorbed and has a high bioavailability after oral administration. Its clearance is relatively low (5.6 mL/min/kg), its V_D is large (4.9 L/kg), it is metabolized to inactive metabolites, and renal elimination accounts for about 40% of the dose. The average half-life in patients with heart failure (19 hours) is somewhat longer than in normal individuals (14 hours), which may be due to a reduction in the renal elimination of the drug (65,66). An occasional patient with heart failure can have a markedly reduced clearance and prolonged half-life (67,68). Blood levels of flecainide correlate with effects and toxicity and can be used to guide dosage in patients with arrhythmias.

Cimetidine, quinidine, and amiodarone reduce the hepatic metabolism of flecainide, thus decreasing clearance and increasing plasma concentrations at steady state. Flecainide may slightly increase the serum levels of digoxin. The clinical significance of these interactions is not known (66).

Propafenone

Although well-absorbed, propafenone undergoes extensive first-pass metabolism in 93% of the population to active metabolites, which reduces the bioavailability of propafenone to 10% to 15% (69). The drug is a weak β-adrenergic receptor antagonist (69,70). This property, along with its negative inotropic effect, suggests that propafenone must be given with caution to patients with decompensated heart failure (71,72). Propafenone has a high, but variable, hepatic clearance and a half-life of 2 to 10 hours in the extensive metabolizers (69). In the poor metabolizers, who make up 7% of the population, the hepatic clearance is low and the half-life is much longer (12 to 32 hours). There are no data on the changes in pharmacokinetics produced by heart failure.

Rifampin has been reported to increase the clearance of propafenone and to reduce its antiarrhythmic effect (73). Propafenone can increase digoxin concentration in normal volunteers and patients, perhaps increasing the effects of digoxin (74,75). The metabolism of warfarin may be inhibited by propafenone, thereby increasing the anticoagulant effect (76). The metabolism of propranolol and metoprolol can be inhibited by propafenone, resulting in increased concentrations of these β-adrenergic antagonists (77). Quinidine can reduce the metabolism of propafenone to one of its active metabolites but the clinical significance of this observation is unknown (69).

Amiodarone

Amiodarone has a low and variable oral bioavailability, which may be due in part to first-pass metabolism by the gut mucosa. The V_D of amiodarone is extremely large (66 L/kg), which, combined with a low clearance (1.9 mL/min/kg, entirely hepatic), results in a very long half-life of 1 to 2 months (78). It is unlikely that heart failure will alter the pharmacokinetics of amiodarone but this has not been specifically studied.

Amiodarone interacts with many other drugs to inhibit their metabolism or excretion (78,79). This results in a reduced clearance and increased plasma concentration of the other drug. Drugs documented to be affected include digoxin, flecainide, phenytoin, warfarin, quinidine, encainide, procainamide, diltiazem, and benzodiazepines. Undoubtedly, this list is not complete. A good rule is to assume that amiodarone will reduce the clearance of all other drugs coadministered and to monitor carefully blood levels and/or effects when amiodarone is added to any other drug regimen.

Inotropic Drugs

Digoxin

Digoxin in tablet form is absorbed slowly from the gut to the extent of about 65% to 70%. CHF does not consistently alter the rate or extent of absorption (80,81) but absorption can be delayed in some patients with heart failure, particularly after a myocardial infarction (82). This is probably related to a change in bowel motility. The V_D of

7 L/kg is similar in patients with or without heart failure. Because the drug is predominantly eliminated by the kidney, the clearance of the drug and the half-life are not altered unless renal function is affected by heart failure. Thus, renal function can be used as a guide to selecting the maintenance dose of digoxin in heart failure.

A number of drugs reduce digoxin clearance and increase plasma digoxin concentration; these drugs include quinidine, amiodarone, verapamil, flecainide, and propafenone (30,75,83,84). The best-studied and probably most important and consistent of these interactions is that of quinidine and digoxin (30). When a patient who is receiving digoxin is begun on quinidine, the maintenance dose of digoxin should be reduced by half. The plasma digoxin concentration should be monitored but it is not worthwhile to obtain a level sooner than 5 days (about three half-lives of digoxin) after beginning the quinidine, unless clinical signs and symptoms warrant it. The next most significant of these interactions is that with amiodarone (85,86). Amiodarone may increase digoxin absorption by an unknown mechanism as well as reduce digoxin clearance. This interaction may be gradual as the body load of amiodarone gradually increases. The dose of digoxin need not be reduced initially but the plasma digoxin concentration should be monitored weekly for 2 weeks to determine if there is an interaction occurring that requires a dosage adjustment. For the interaction of digoxin with the other drugs listed, a single blood level drawn 1 week after beginning the interacting drug should be adequate to determine whether the digoxin dosage needs to be adjusted.

Dobutamine

Used as an acute inotropic agent, dobutamine is given intravenously and titrated to produce a specific effect. In patients with CHF, dobutamine has a small V_D (0.2 L/kg) that may be somewhat larger in patients with edema, a large clearance (2,350 mL/min/m^2) that is independent of cardiac output or liver blood flow, and a short half-life (2.37 minutes) (87). With drugs such as dobutamine, knowledge of pharmacokinetic changes in disease is not particularly helpful because the drug is given until it produces the hemodynamic endpoint desired (88). Pharmacokinetic drug interactions are not important for the use of dobutamine.

Amrinone

The first of the phosphodiesterase inhibitors, amrinone is used intravenously for its acute inotropic and vasodilator effects. Although well-absorbed orally, amrinone is not used for chronic therapy because of its toxicities. The drug has a V_D of 1.3 L/kg (89) that is not altered in heart failure (88). It is cleared by renal and hepatic mechanisms. Part of hepatic metabolism is by N-acetylation at a genetically determined rate. About half the U.S. population are fast acetylators and have a substantially increased total clearance (9 mL/kg per minute) and shorter half-life (2 hours) compared with the slow acetylators (4 mL/kg per minute and 4.4 hours) (90). Clearance is reduced by about half and half-life is doubled in patients with heart failure (88,91,92). Whether this is due to reduced hepatic or renal function is not known. Pharmacokinetic drug interactions are not important in the use of amrinone.

Milrinone

Milrinone is another phosphodiesterase inhibitor. It can be administered orally or intravenously. The oral bioavailability of amrinone in normal volunteers is over 0.9. Patients with severe heart failure have delayed absorption and slightly reduced bioavailability (0.75). The V_D of milrinone is 0.25 to 0.45 L/kg and is little affected by heart failure (88,92). The drug is eliminated mainly by the kidneys, with a total clearance of 6 mL/min/kg that is reduced by half in patients with heart failure who have renal dysfunction. The half-life of milrinone is 0.9 hour in normal individuals and twice as long in patients with severe heart failure (93). Drug interaction with milrinone is not known to be of importance.

Diuretics

Furosemide

Furosemide pharmacokinetics and pharmacodynamics have been particularly well-studied in CHF. The oral absorption of furosemide is considerably delayed in patients with severe heart failure so that the peak concentration achieved is lower and occurs later. However, contrary to general belief, the extent of absorption (normal bioavailability of 0.5) is not consistently changed in patients with heart failure (94,95). The V_D is small (0.15 to 0.2 L/kg) and is not changed in heart failure (94). Sixty percent of the absorbed dose is eliminated by the kidneys. The renal clearance (normally 1 mL/min/kg) is reduced in patients with heart failure who have a reduced creatinine clearance, but the nonrenal clearance is unchanged (94). The half-life (normally 90 minutes) is increased up to twice of normal in patients with heart failure because of the reduction in renal clearance (94,96). Because the response to furosemide requires the drug to gain access to the tubular fluid, patients who have diminished renal function due to heart failure will have a reduced response to the diuretic. However, other factors also are important, such as the time course of delivery of furosemide into the tubular fluid; therefore, the delay in oral absorption of furosemide also is a factor in the diminished response to the drug that is sometimes seen in patients with severe heart failure (12,97,98). For a prompt diuretic response, intravenous drug is preferred.

Part of furosemide's diuretic effect and its ability to increase venous capacitance after intravenous administration are inhibited by nonsteroidal anti-inflammatory drugs (NSAIDs) that inhibit prostaglandin synthesis (99). Another important interaction is enhanced otic or renal toxicity with aminoglycosides.

Bumetanide

Although bumetanide is about 40 times more potent and is better-absorbed (normal bioavailability is 0.8) than furosemide, there is no important reason to choose one of these diuretics over the other for use in patients with CHF

(98,100,101). Heart failure affects the absorption, clearance, and half-life of bumetanide to the same extent as furosemide (102). Thus, absorption is delayed but the extent of absorption is not affected (103). Bumetanide's V_D of 0.15 L/kg is unchanged in heart failure, but its renal clearance (normally 2.6 mL/min/kg) may be reduced and its half-life (normally 0.8 hour) prolonged two- to threefold in patients with heart failure who have renal dysfunction, similar to the effect of heart failure on the kinetics of furosemide. Drug interactions with bumetanide are the same as with furosemide.

Torsemide

Torsemide acts within the ascending limb of the loop of Henle. The diuretic effect correlates better with the rate of excretion of the drug in the urine than with the plasma concentration of drug.

Torsemide is nearly completely absorbed after oral administration and the bioavailability is 80% to 90%. The elimination half-life is 3 to 4 hours in normal subjects and is prolonged to approximately 6 hours in patients with heart failure. Torsemide is 50% to 80% metabolized in the liver. The half-life is not prolonged in patients with renal insufficiency, although renal insufficiency may impair delivery of the drug to the tubular fluid.

In heart failure patients, the rate of absorption of drug is slowed, so the maximal diuretic effect may occur more than 4 hours after drug ingestion. In addition, the responsiveness of the nephron to loop diuretics may be diminished. The diuretic response may be optimized by giving the usual doses, but dosing more frequently.

Torsemide and salicylates compete for secretion by renal tubules, so the risk of salicylate toxicity is increased when high doses of salicylates are coadministered with torsemide.

Indomethacin partially inhibits the natriuretic effect of torsemide. Probenecid reduces the diuretic effect of torsemide by reducing secretion of torsemide into the proximal tubule.

Hydrochlorothiazide

Hydrochlorothiazide absorption may be diminished in some patients with CHF but this drug has not been studied extensively. Hydrochlorothiazide is cleared almost entirely by the kidney so that its clearance (normally 5 mL/min/kg) is reduced and its half-life (normally 2.5 hours) is prolonged in patients who have CHF with renal dysfunction (7,104).

In general, drug interactions are not important with thiazide diuretics. Lithium clearance may be reduced in patients with heart failure, particularly if they are on thiazide diuretics, which can result in lithium toxicity in patients receiving lithium carbonate therapy (105).

Metolazone

Metolazone inhibits sodium reabsorption, primarily at the cortical diluting site but also in the proximal convoluted tubule. The increased delivery of sodium to the distal tubule causes increased potassium excretion. These mechanisms of action are similar to those of thiazide diuretics. A diuretic effect begins approximately 1 hour after oral ingestion of metolazone and may persist for 24 hours. The duration of effect is longer at higher doses.

Concurrent administration of metolazone and furosemide may produce a marked diuresis, even in patients refractory to the effect of each diuretic given alone. This combination also may cause marked losses of sodium, potassium, and chloride, so careful monitoring is necessary.

Angiotensin-Converting Enzyme Inhibitors

Angiotensin-converting enzyme (ACE) inhibitors are well-established as the cornerstone of pharmacologic therapy of heart failure. These drugs slow the progression of left ventricular dysfunction and decrease mortality and the need for hospitalization in heart failure patients. An ACE inhibitor is therefore indicated in most patients with left ventricular dysfunction, even in the absence of clinical heart failure. In heart failure patients, the dose of ACE inhibitor should be slowly titrated up to the maximal recommended dose. Some reduction in blood pressure is common, especially with the first few doses. Patients at risk for excessive hypotension include those with more severe heart failure or hyponatremia, those on high-dose diuretic therapy, those who have recently undergone intensive diuresis, and those with volume depletion of any etiology. These patients should be followed closely during initiation of ACE inhibitor treatment.

There are a few important drug interactions with ACE inhibitors. The decrease in aldosterone caused by ACE inhibitors diminishes the excretion of potassium by the kidneys. Therefore, potassium supplements, potassium-containing salt substitutes, and potassium-retaining diuretics (e.g., amiloride, spironolactone, triamterene) may be used only with great caution because hyperkalemia may develop rapidly. NSAIDs reduce the antihypertensive effects of ACE inhibitors, especially captopril (106).

Most ACE inhibitors have a biexponential course of elimination, with most of the drug eliminated during the earlier phase. The second phase of elimination usually has a much longer half-life. This phase is due to slow release of the ACE inhibitor from the binding to the ACE. This later phase usually does not contribute to the accumulation of the drug.

Captopril

The oral bioavailability of captopril is about 65% and this does not appear to be altered by heart failure. The V_D of 0.8 L/kg may be increased in heart failure (107). The normal half-life is 2 hours and the total clearance is 12 mL/min/kg, which is 40% renal. The renal clearance can be reduced and half-life prolonged if renal insufficiency is present. The metabolites of captopril, which is a sulfhydryl-containing compound, include mixed disulfides that may act as a reservoir for the active drug (108). Captopril metabolism is not influenced by heart failure. Heart failure may increase the response to captopril and other converting enzyme inhibitors, but this is not due to a pharmacokinetic change. Rather, it is related to the fact that plasma renin activity often is elevated in patients with heart failure (109).

Enalapril

Unlike captopril, enalapril is a prodrug that must be activated by hydrolysis to enalaprilic acid, a diacid that is the active compound (110). The absorption of enalapril is about 70%, and about 55% of that is hydrolyzed to the diacid so that 35% to 40% of an oral dose is converted into active compound (111,112). Most of the diacid is eliminated in the urine with a half-life of 11 hours. CHF does not alter these pharmacokinetic parameters, although if renal dysfunction is present, the clearance will be reduced and the active metabolite will accumulate (111).

Lisinopril

Lisinopril is a lysine analog of enalaprilic acid, which, unlike most ACE inhibitors, does not require activation before it can inhibit ACE. After oral administration lisinopril is absorbed slowly (peak level at 6 hours) and incompletely (about 30%). The drug is cleared solely by the kidneys with a half-life of about 12 hours. The clearance of lisinopril is correlated with creatinine clearance, both of which are reduced in the elderly (113,114). Patients with CHF may have a reduced total absorption of lisinopril as well as a reduced renal clearance; because of these two opposing effects, the plasma concentration achieved after oral dosing may not be altered much by heart failure (115). However, some patients with heart failure and marked renal dysfunction may achieve higher than expected plasma concentrations with the usual doses (113,114). The half-life is similar in normal individuals and patients with heart failure despite the reduced drug clearance, suggesting that the V_D may be reduced in these patients (115).

Benazepril

Benazepril is a prodrug that is converted to the active metabolite benazeprilat in the liver. Benazeprilat appears in the blood within 30 minutes of oral ingestion and reaches a peak concentration in about 1 to 2 hours. Both benazepril and benazeprilat are eliminated by the kidneys.

Levels of benazeprilat are not altered in hepatic dysfunction, so no dose adjustment is needed. A low starting dose and slow upward titration are recommended in renal insufficiency with a serum creatinine greater than 3 mg/dL.

Fosinopril

Fosinopril is a prodrug that is converted to the diacid fosinoprilat. Fosinoprilat is eliminated approximately equally by the liver and kidney. No dosage adjustment is needed in renal insufficiency but lower starting doses are recommended in patients with severe hepatic impairment.

Moexipril

Moexipril is a prodrug that is converted to moexiprilat. Food intake reduces the absorption by 40% to 50%, so the drug should be taken in a fasting state. In patients with moderate or severe renal or hepatic impairment, moexipril treatment may be initiated at very low dosage, with slow upward titration.

Perindopril

Perindopril is a prodrug that is converted in the liver to perindoprilat. Peak plasma concentrations of perindoprilat occur 3 to 7 hours after perindopril administration. The clearance of perindoprilat is substantially reduced in either heart failure or renal failure, so treatment should be initiated at low doses and slowly titrated upward.

Quinapril

Quinapril is a prodrug that is converted in the liver to the active diacid metabolite quinaprilat. The peak plasma concentration of quinaprilat occurs approximately 2 hours after oral ingestion. Quinaprilat is almost completely eliminated by renal excretion. Therefore, treatment should be initiated at very low doses in patients with either renal insufficiency or severe heart failure.

Ramipril

Ramipril is a prodrug that is converted in the liver to the active diacid ramiprilat. Peak plasma levels of ramiprilat occur 2 to 4 hours after oral ingestion. Ramiprilat is eliminated by both renal and biliary excretion. In either heart failure or renal insufficiency patients, treatment should be initiated at low dosage.

Trandolapril

Trandolapril is a prodrug that is converted to the active diacid metabolite trandolaprilat. Peak trandolaprilat plasma levels occur 4 to 10 hours after oral ingestion. About one-third of trandolaprilat is eliminated in the urine, and two-thirds in feces. The initial dosage should be low in patients with heart failure or renal insufficiency or hepatic impairment.

Angiotensin II Receptor Antagonists

Angiotensin II receptor antagonists competitively block the angiotensin II type 1 receptor. Losartan, valsartan, irbesartan, and candesartan are marketed angiotensin II receptor antagonists, approved by the U.S. Food and Drug Administration for the treatment of hypertension. Losartan was compared with captopril in the treatment of heart failure in the elderly (ELITE study) (116). The all-cause mortality rate during 48 weeks of active treatment was 4.8% in the losartan group versus 8.7% in the captopril group, a 46% reduction ($p = 0.035$). Losartan was better-tolerated than captopril: 12.2% of losartan-treated patients discontinued treatment due to adverse effects, compared with 20.8% of captopril-treated patients. This favorable effect on survival was not confirmed in a clinical trial comparing enalapril with candesartan and with the combination of the two drugs in heart failure patients (RESOLVD pilot study). This study showed no significant differences in survival among the treatment groups, nor in symptoms of heart failure, nor in measures of quality of life. However, the combination drug treatment was associated with the smallest increase in left ventricular volumes and the greatest increase in ejection fraction after 43 weeks of treatment. These studies suggest angiotensin receptor blockers may have a role in the treatment of heart failure, either as an alternative to ACE inhibitors or in combination with them.

With all angiotensin receptor blockers, as with ACE inhibitors, caution is necessary when administering these drugs to patients with heart failure. In these patients, renal function may be dependent on the activity of the renin-angiotensin-aldosterone system. Inhibiting this system may be associated with oliguria or progressive renal dysfunction. Consequently, careful monitoring of clinical and renal status is necessary.

Losartan

Losartan undergoes substantial first-pass metabolism by cytochrome P450 enzymes, and about 14% of an oral dose is converted to an active metabolite, E-3174. The metabolite is responsible for most of the angiotensin II receptor antagonism associated with losartan treatment. The elimination half-life of losartan is about 2 hours and that of E-3174 is about 6 to 9 hours.

Heart failure patients are often elderly and may have associated renal or hepatic insufficiency. Studies comparing elderly hypertensive individuals with young healthy subjects show no significant changes in the pharmacokinetics of losartan, but there is a 30% increase in plasma concentrations of E-3174. However, this is not associated with any change in antihypertensive efficacy or in safety. Therefore, no dosage adjustment is necessary in elderly patients.

In renal failure, the renal clearances of losartan and E-3174 are reduced, but the plasma concentrations of E-3174 are not changed (117). Therefore, no dosage adjustment is needed in the setting of renal impairment. In patients with cirrhosis, the clearance of losartan is reduced about 50%, resulting in fourfold to fivefold higher plasma concentrations, and 1.5- to twofold higher plasma levels of E-3174, compared with healthy subjects (118). Therefore, losartan should be used with caution in patients with severe hepatic insufficiency, and a lower than usual initial dose would be appropriate.

Cimetidine slightly increases, and phenobarbital slightly reduces, the area under the concentration versus time curve for losartan, but these interactions are not likely to be of clinical significance.

Valsartan

Valsartan has a bioavailability of about 25% and an elimination half-life of about 6 hours. Approximately 83% of orally administered valsartan is eliminated in the feces, mostly as unchanged drug. Only about 20% is recovered as metabolites. In the elderly, the half-life of valsartan is 35% longer and the area under the concentration versus time curve is 70% higher, but the clinical effects are comparable with those in younger patients. Therefore, no dosage adjustment is necessary.

Because only a small fraction of a dose of valsartan is eliminated by the kidneys, no dosage adjustment is needed in mild or moderate renal insufficiency, whether due to intrinsic renal disease or secondary to decreased cardiac output. There is little information on the kinetics of valsartan in severe renal impairment, so caution is advised in dosing in this setting.

Similarly, because valsartan is eliminated mostly as unchanged drug, changes in hepatic function should have little effect on kinetics. However, caution is advised, by starting with lower than usual doses in patients with severe hepatic impairment. No clinically important drug interactions with valsartan have been identified.

Candesartan

Candesartan is administered orally as candesartan cilexetil, a prodrug that is hydrolyzed to candesartan during absorption. The bioavailability of candesartan, after administration of candesartan cilexetil, is 15%. The peak serum concentration is reached 3 to 4 hours after tablet ingestion. Most of the candesartan is excreted unchanged in the urine and feces. The elimination half-life is approximately 9 hours.

The plasma concentrations of candesartan are approximately 50% higher in patients over the age of 65, compared with younger subjects given the same dose. Plasma concentrations are approximately doubled in patients with severe renal impairment. Despite the pharmacokinetic alterations, no adjustment of initial dose is recommended in these patients.

Other Vasodilators

Hydralazine

Hydralazine is acetylated to an inactive metabolite during its absorption after oral dosing. The acetylation rate is genetically determined, with about 50% of the U.S. population being slow or fast acetylators. The bioavailability of hydralazine is 16% in the fast acetylators and 35% in the slow acetylators. The systemic clearance of hydralazine is very high (normally 56 mL/min/kg) and approaches cardiac output. The V_D is 1.5 L/kg and the half-life is 1 hour. CHF does not consistently alter the kinetics of hydralazine (119) but some patients with heart failure have been described who have a reduced clearance and an increased half-life (120). Hydralazine is not subject to known pharmacokinetic drug interactions.

Nitrates

There is a poor correlation between the plasma levels of the nitrates and the clinical effects because of the complex pharmacokinetics, the formation of active metabolites, and the rapid development of tolerance to these drugs when they are administered continuously (121,122). After oral administration, less than 1% of nitroglycerin reaches the circulation, and activity seen after oral dosing is likely due to dinitrate metabolites (123–125). Sublingual bioavailability averages 31% (126) and transdermal bioavailability from ointment is variable but substantial (70%), despite some presystemic metabolism by the skin (127). Transdermal bioavailability, particularly from patches, seems to be reduced in some patients with heart failure, possibly related to tissue edema or poor subcutaneous blood flow (128,129). Nitroglycerin has a very large metabolic clearance (200 mL/min/kg), which may be depressed in some patients with severe heart failure (130). However, because there is a poor correlation between the therapeutic effects or toxicity and the plasma levels, these changes are of limited clinical relevance.

Isosorbide dinitrate is well-absorbed orally but is only 25% bioavailable because of substantial first-pass elimination. Its clearance is high (normally 45 mL/min/kg), the V_D is 1.5 L/kg, and the half-life is 0.8 hour. Isosorbide dinitrate is metabolized to active metabolites (isosorbide 2-mononitrate and isosorbide 5-mononitrate), which have longer half-lives than the parent compound. Neither the pharmacokinetics of isosorbide dinitrate nor its metabolites are altered by heart failure (7,121).

Drug interactions with nitrates are not of clinical importance. There is some interest in the possibility that N-acetylcysteine can reduce the development of tolerance to nitrates but this is not a clinically significant drug interaction.

β-Adrenergic Blockers

Chronic heart failure is associated with activation of the sympathetic nervous system. Norepinephrine can have direct and indirect adverse effects on the failing heart and circulation, and higher circulating levels of norepinephrine are a marker of a worse prognosis in heart failure. These findings stimulated research on the role of β-adrenergic blockers in the treatment of heart failure; this topic is discussed elsewhere in this text. The largest clinical experience with β-blockers in heart failure is with carvedilol, metoprolol, bisoprolol, and bucindolol.

Several clinical, pharmacologic, and pharmacokinetic factors affect the dosing of, and response to, β-blockers in heart failure. These include the severity of left ventricular dysfunction, heart rate, blood pressure, renal function, hepatic function, volume status, degree of sympathetic nervous system activation, and concomitant medications. A consequence of this complex interplay of multiple factors is that dosing of β-blockers in heart failure must be slowly and carefully titrated and individualized, regardless of the pharmacokinetic properties of the individual drug.

Carvedilol

Carvedilol is a racemic mixture in which the S(−) enantiomer has nonselective β-blocking activity and both R(+) and S(−) enantiomers have α-blocking activity. Carvedilol has a bioavailability of approximately 30%, due to significant hepatic first-pass metabolism by cytochrome P450 enzymes. The elimination half-life is 7 to 10 hours. In heart failure, the area under the plasma concentration versus time curve is increased, by as much as 100% in severe heart failure. However, the elimination half-life is not significantly altered. Taking carvedilol with food slows the rate of absorption; this is helpful in heart failure to reduce the risk of orthostatic hypotension.

Drugs that induce or inhibit cytochrome P450 enzymes may affect carvedilol pharmacokinetics. Rifampin decreases the area under the plasma concentration versus time curve by about 70%, whereas cimetidine increases it by about 30%. Other drugs that inhibit cytochrome P450 CYP2D6, and therefore would be expected in increased plasma carvedilol levels, include quinidine, propafenone, and fluoxetine.

In heart failure, the recommended starting dose of carvedilol is 3.125 mg twice daily. The patient should be followed closely, with no dosage change for 2 weeks. The β-blocking effects may initially worsen the clinical status and additional diuretic may be needed. Alternatively, the α-blocking effects may cause vasodilation and hypotension, necessitating a reduction in dose of concomitant ACE inhibitor or other vasodilators. If tolerated, the carvedilol dose may be doubled every 2 weeks, up to a maximum of 50 mg twice daily. If excessive bradycardia (heart rate below 55 beats per minute) develops, the dose of carvedilol should be decreased.

Metoprolol

Metoprolol is a β_1-selective adrenoreceptor blocker with no intrinsic sympathomimetic activity. Following oral administration, plasma levels of metoprolol are highly variable, due in part to significant hepatic first-pass metabolism. The elimination of half-life is 3 to 7 hours; however, the duration of β-blocking and clinical effects is much longer. Due to the variability in pharmacokinetics and in clinical response, careful dose titration is especially important in heart failure patients.

In the larger heart failure clinical trials with metoprolol, the initial oral dose was 5 mg twice daily (131) or 6.25 mg twice daily (132), with slow upward titration over approximately 6 weeks to 100 or 150 mg daily. In the Metoprolol CR/XL Randomised Intervention Trial in Heart Failure (MERIT-HF), mortality and serious adverse events were significantly reduced by the addition of metoprolol in patients with moderate to severe chronic heart failure, most of whom were already receiving standard treatment with digoxin, diuretic, and ACE inhibitors.

Bisoprolol

Bisoprolol is a β_1-selective adrenoreceptor blocker without intrinsic sympathomimetic activity. The bioavailability of an oral dose is about 80%. The elimination half-life is 9 to 12 hours. Bisoprolol is eliminated equally by renal excretion of unchanged drug and by metabolism to inactive products. Because of this balanced clearance, the half-life is prolonged only twofold in patients with severe renal or hepatic insufficiency (133,134).

In the Cardiac Insufficiency Bisoprolol Study (CIBIS) (135), 641 patients with New York Heart Association (NYHA) functional Class III or IV heart failure received, in addition to standard therapy, either bisoprolol or placebo. The dosing regimen was 1.25 mg daily, which was increased after 48 hours to 2.5 mg daily, and after 1 month to 5 mg daily. On this regimen, bisoprolol was well-tolerated. In CIBIS-II, bisoprolol was slowly titrated up to 10 mg daily in patients with NYHA Class III or IV heart failure. The all-cause mortality rate was 11.8% over approximately 2 years compared with 17.3% in the placebo control. This beneficial effect was highly statistically significant.

Bucindolol

Bucindolol is a nonselective β-blocker with mild vasodilator effects. Bucindolol is well-absorbed after oral administration but undergoes extensive first-pass hepatic metabolism. The bioavailability is 30% and the elimination half-life is approximately 2.5 to 5.5 hours.

In heart failure clinical trials, bucindolol has been administered initially in a dose of 3.0 to 12.5 mg twice daily, with slow upward titration to 100 mg twice daily.

Other Drugs

Theophylline

Theophylline is a drug with a narrow therapeutic window for which there is a good correlation between the plasma concentration and therapeutic and toxic effects. The drug is well-absorbed orally with or without heart failure. Theophylline is a low-clearance drug (normally 0.65 mL/min/kg) that is eliminated entirely by hepatic metabolism. The V_D is 0.5 L/kg, and the half-life is 9 hours. Heart failure with hepatic congestion and pulmonary edema can reduce the clearance by half and prolong the half-life by twofold or more (136). Because of substantial interpatient variability, plasma levels must be used for safe and effective intravenous use of theophylline, not only in patients with heart failure but with all patients receiving the drug.

Theophylline is subject to many important drug interactions affecting its metabolic clearance (137,138). Theophylline clearance is inhibited by cimetidine, erythromycin, verapamil, ciprofloxacin and other fluoroquinolones, mexiletine, thiabendazole, and troleandomycin. Any of these drugs can increase theophylline plasma concentration and produce theophylline toxicity. Inducers of theophylline clearance, thereby reducing plasma concentrations, are barbiturates, carbamazepine, phenytoin, and rifampin. Smokers also have an increased theophylline clearance rate and require larger doses to achieve therapeutic concentrations and effects.

Warfarin

The effect of heart failure on the pharmacokinetics of warfarin has not been carefully examined. Warfarin is a mixture of two stereoisomers; S-warfarin is more potent than R-warfarin. There are no data regarding the influence of heart failure on the kinetics of the isomers of warfarin. Increased sensitivity to the anticoagulant effect of warfarin has been reported in CHF (139) but this may not be due to an alteration in the pharmacokinetics of warfarin because no effect of heart failure on warfarin half-life has been found (140,141). Although the limitations of half-life as an index of drug elimination must be kept in mind, warfarin has a small V_D (0.14 L/kg) that is unlikely to be affected by heart failure, so that an unchanged half-life (normally 37 hours) probably indicates that clearance (normally 0.045 mL/min/kg) is not changed by heart failure. Nonetheless, because of the increased sensitivity in some patients, the initial doses should be small and the dose titrated to the desired effect on prothrombin time.

Many drugs interact with warfarin to increase or decrease its metabolism or effect (142,143). Some of these drugs have differential effects on the two isomers of warfarin. Drugs that affect the S isomer produce the greatest change in the effects of warfarin. The most important drugs that reduce the clearance of warfarin and thereby enhance its hypoprothrombinemic effect are amiodarone, cimetidine, some sulfonamides (e.g., sulfamethoxazole), ciprofloxacin and other fluoroquinolones, disulfiram, erythromycin, metronidazole, phenylbutazone, and sulfinpyrazone. Clofibrate and some anabolic steroids also increase warfarin's anticoagulant effect but by poorly understood mechanisms that do not involve warfarin's metabolism. Drugs that increase the clearance of warfarin and reduce its hypoprothrombinemic effect include barbiturates, phenytoin, rifampin, and carbamazepine. Many other drugs have been the subject of case reports that suggest an interaction with warfarin but the clinical significance of these is uncertain.

GENERAL PHARMACOKINETIC PRINCIPLES TO GUIDE THERAPY IN HEART FAILURE

Based on the concepts outlined, a few generalizations can be made regarding the influence of CHF on pharmacokinetics.

1. Oral absorption of drugs that are normally rapidly absorbed in the upper small intestine may be delayed, but the extent of absorption is less likely to be affected. Drugs that are normally slowly absorbed will be influenced less by heart failure.
2. Transdermal drug absorption can be delayed and the extent of absorption may be reduced as a consequence of a reduction in blood flow and subcutaneous edema.
3. The V_D of drugs that are extensively distributed is likely to be reduced such that smaller loading doses will be required to produce therapeutic effects. For drugs with relatively small V_D, heart failure will not produce much change in the V_D, which may even increase slightly.
4. Hepatic clearance of high-clearance drugs will be reduced as a consequence of the reduced hepatic blood flow. This is of particular importance for those drugs given intravenously, such as lidocaine. With severe heart failure accompanied by hepatocellular damage, the intrinsic hepatic clearance of drugs will be reduced. This will result in higher blood levels at a given intravenous dose of low-clearance drugs and higher blood levels after oral dosing for both low- and high-clearance drugs, so that smaller maintenance doses will be required for therapy.

5. Renal clearance of drugs and their metabolites will be influenced only if renal function is depressed by heart failure.
6. Drug half-life may or may not be prolonged in patients with heart failure, depending on the effects of the disease on the V_D and clearance. Half-life is a poor indicator of the effects of heart failure on drug elimination.
7. For many drugs used in heart failure, the doses are titrated to effect. This is true for the inotropic agents, diuretics, vasodilators, and oral anticoagulants. For such drugs, pharmacokinetic changes produced by heart failure are of less clinical relevance because the individual patient's response, rather than the blood levels, is the primary guide to therapy.
8. For some drugs, the real endpoint of therapy may be difficult to determine and plasma levels become a useful surrogate endpoint to guide dosage adjustment. Theophylline is the prime example, where successful intravenous therapy requires the frequent monitoring of plasma levels to aid in adjustment of the infusion rate as heart failure or infection progresses or improves. Determination of plasma levels also is useful for many antiarrhythmic drugs (quinidine, procainamide, disopyramide, mexiletine, tocainide, lidocaine, and flecainide). However, some antiarrhythmic drugs are metabolized to several active metabolites so that plasma concentration measurements, at least as performed currently, are not helpful (e.g., encainide and propafenone). The utility of plasma level monitoring for digoxin therapy is less clear. In most patients, routine monitoring of digoxin plasma concentrations is not worthwhile. However, in patients where noncompliance, renal dysfunction, drug interaction, or drug overdose is suspected, the measurement of plasma digoxin concentration may be helpful for patient management. The timing of blood sampling is important in interpretation of the results of a blood level measurement. In general, the most useful concentration is that determined at steady state (at least three half-lives after the last dosage adjustment) and obtained just prior to a dose (trough level) or during a continuous infusion (as with theophylline and lidocaine). In the interpretation of blood level data, it is important to remember that the plasma concentration is only one piece of information about the drug in an individual patient and, by itself, cannot be diagnostic of adequate therapy or toxicity of a drug.
9. Although some of the changes produced by heart failure may be anticipated, the interpatient variability may exceed the alteration produced by heart failure. The principles outlined are derived from populations with heart failure and can only give an approximation of initial dosing recommendations for a single patient. Thereafter, the drug's therapeutic effect or the blood concentrations produced by the dosing regimen must be evaluated and the dose adjusted based on the individual patient's response.

REFERENCES

1. Rowland M, Benet LZ, Graham GG. Clearance concepts in pharmacokinetics. *J Pharmacokinet Biopharm*. 1973;1:123–136.
2. Wilkinson GR, Shand DG. A physiological approach to hepatic drug clearance. *Clin Pharmacol Ther*. 1975;18:377–390.
3. Nies AS, Shand DG, Wilkinson GR. Altered hepatic blood flow and drug disposition. *Clin Pharmacokinet*. 1976;1:135–155.
4. Wilkinson GR. Clearance approaches in pharmacology. *Pharmacol Rev*. 1987;39:1–47.
5. Benowitz NL, Meister W. Pharmacokinetics in patients with cardiac failure. *Clin Pharmacokinet*. 1976;1:389–405.
6. Williams RL, Benet LZ. Drug pharmacokinetics in cardiac and hepatic disease. *Annu Rev Pharmacol Toxicol*. 1980;20:389–413.
7. Shammas FV, Dickstein K. Clinical pharmacokinetics in heart failure. An updated review. *Clin Pharmacokinet*. 1988;15:94–113.
8. Nies AS. Principles of drug therapy. In: Wyngaarden JB, Smith LH, Jr., eds. *Cecil's Textbook of Medicine*. 19th ed. Philadelphia: WB Saunders; 1991.
9. Winne D. The influence of villous counter current exchange on intestinal absorption. *J Theoret Biol*. 1975;53:145–176.
10. Berkowitz D, Droll MN, Likoff W. Malabsorption as a complication of congestive heart failure. *Am J Cardiol*. 1963;11:43–47.
11. Benet LZ, Greither A, Meister W. Gastrointestinal absorption of drugs in patients with congestive heart failure. In: Benet LZ, ed. *The Effect of Disease States on Pharmacokinetics*. Washington, D.C.: American Pharmaceutical Association Academy of Pharmaceutical Sciences; 1976: 33–50.
12. Kaojarern S, Day B, Brater DC. The time course of delivery of furosemide into urine: an independent determinant of overall response. *Kidney Int*. 1982;22:69–74.
13. Gibb I, Cowan JC, Parnham AJ, Thomas TH. Use and misuse of a digoxin assay service. *BMJ*. 1986;293:678–680.
14. Benowitz N, Forsyth RP, Melmon KL, et al. Lidocaine disposition kinetics in monkey and man. I. Prediction by a perfusion model. *Clin Pharmacol Ther*. 1974;16:87–98.
15. Benowitz N, Forsyth RP, Melmon KL, et al. Lidocaine disposition kinetics in monkey and man. II. Effects of hemorrhage and sympathomimetic drug administration. *Clin Pharmacol Ther*. 1974;16:99–109.
16. Hepner GW, Vesell ES, Tantum KR. Reduced drug elimination in congestive heart failure. Studies using aminopyrine as a model drug. *Am J Med*. 1978;65:271–276.
17. Thomson PD, Rowland M, Melmon KL. The influence of heart failure, liver disease, and renal failure on the disposition of lidocaine in man. *Am Heart J*. 1971;82:417–421.
18. Woosley RL. Pharmacokinetics and pharmacodynamics of antiarrhythmic agents in patients with congestive heart failure. *Am Heart J*. 1987;114:1280–1290.
19. Bellet S, Roman LR, Boza A. Relation between serum quinidine levels and renal function. Studies in normal subjects and patients with congestive failure and renal insufficiency. *Am J Cardiol*. 1971;27:368–371.
20. Crouthamel WG. The effect of congestive heart failure on quinidine pharmacokinetics. *Am Heart J*. 1975;90:335–339.
21. Conrad KA, Molk BL, Chidsey CA. Pharmacokinetic studies of quinidine in patients with arrhythmias. *Circulation*. 1977;55:1–7.
22. Ochs HR, Greenblatt DJ, Woo E. Clinical pharmacokinetics of quinidine. *Clin Pharmacokinet*. 1980;5:150–168.
23. Kessler KM, Lowenthal DT, Warner H, et al. Quinidine elimination in patients with congestive heart failure or poor renal function. *N Engl J Med*. 1974;290:706–709.
24. Data JL, Wilkinson GR, Nies AS. Interaction of quinidine with anticonvulsant drugs. *N Engl J Med*. 1976;294:699–702.
25. Twum-Barima Y, Carruthers SG. Quinidine-rifampin interaction. *N Engl J Med*. 1981;304:1466–1469.
26. Baciewicz AM, Baciewicz FA, Jr. Effect of cimetidine and ranitidine on cardiovascular drugs. *Am Heart J*. 1989;118:144–154.
27. Edwards DJ, Lavoie R, Beckman H, et al. The effect of coadministration of verapamil on the pharmacokinetics and metabolism of quinidine. *Clin Pharmacol Ther*. 1987;41:68–73.
28. Saal AK, Werner JA, Greene HL, et al. Effect of amiodarone on serum quinidine and procainamide levels. *Am J Cardiol*. 1984;53:1264–1267.
29. Maisel AS, Motulsky HJ, Insel PA. Hypotension after quinidine plus verapamil. Possible additive competition at alpha-adrenergic receptors. *N Engl J Med*. 1985;312:167–170.
30. Bigger JT, Jr., Leahey EB, Jr. Quinidine and digoxin. An important interaction. *Drugs*. 1982;24:229–239.

31. Kuhlmann J, Dohrmann M, Marcin S. Effects of quinidine on pharmacokinetics and pharmacodynamics of digitoxin achieving steady-state conditions. *Clin Pharmacol Ther*. 1986;39: 288–294.
32. Funck-Brentano C, Kroemer HK, Pavlou H, et al. Genetically determined interaction between propafenone and low dose quinidine: role of active metabolites in modulating net drug effect. *Br J Clin Pharmacol*. 1989;27:435–444.
33. Turgeon J, Pavlou HN, Wong W, et al. Genetically determined steady-state interaction between encainide and quinidine in patients with arrhythmias. *J Pharmacol Exp Ther*. 1990;255: 642–649.
34. Koch-Weser J, Klein SW. Procainamide dosage schedules, plasma concentrations, and clinical effects. *JAMA*. 1971;215:1454–1460.
35. Kessler KM, Kayden DS, Estes DM, et al. Procainamide pharmacokinetics in patients with acute myocardial infarction or congestive heart failure. *J Am Coll Cardiol*. 1986;7:1131–1139.
36. Benet LZ, Williams RL. Appendix II. Design and optimization of dosage regimens: pharmacokinetic data. In: Gilman AG, Rall TW, Nies AS, Taylor P, eds. *Goodman and Gilman's The Pharmacological Basis of Therapeutics*. 8th ed. New York: Pergamon; 1990: 1650–1735.
37. Drayer DE, Lowenthal DT, Woosley RL, et al. Cumulation of N-acetylprocainamide, an active metabolite of procainamide, in patients with impaired renal function. *Clin Pharmacol Ther*. 1977;22:63–69.
38. Vlasses PH, Kosoglou T, Chase SL, et al. Trimethoprim inhibition of the renal clearance of procainamide and N-acetylprocainamide. *Arch Intern Med*. 1989;149:1350–1353.
39. Kowey PR, Friedman PL, Podrid PJ, et al. Use of radionuclide ventriculography for assessment of changes in myocardial performance induced by disopyramide phosphate. *Am Heart J*. 1982;104:769–774.
40. Di Bianco R, Gottdiener JS, Singh SN, et al. A review of the effects of disopyramide phosphate on left ventricular function and the peripheral circulation. *Angiology*. 1987;38:174–183.
41. Podrid PJ, Schoeneberger A, Lown B. Congestive heart failure caused by oral disopyramide. *N Engl J Med*. 1980;302:614–617.
42. Landmark K, Bredesen JE, Thaulow E, et al. Pharmacokinetics of disopyramide in patients with imminent to moderate cardiac failure. *Eur J Clin Pharmacol*. 1981;19:187–192.
43. Aitio ML, Mansury L, Tala E, et al. The effect of enzyme induction on the metabolism of disopyramide in man. *Br J Clin Pharmacol*. 1981;11:279–285.
44. Ragosta M, Weihl AC, Rosenfeld LE. Potentially fatal interaction between erythromycin and disopyramide. *Am J Med*. 1989;86:465–466.
45. Woosley RL, Morganroth J, Fogoros RN, et al. Pharmacokinetics of moricizine HCl. *Am J Cardiol*. 1987;60:35F–39F.
46. Fitton A, Buckley MM-T. Moricizine: a review of its pharmacological properties, and therapeutic efficacy in cardiac arrhythmias. *Drugs*. 1990;40:138–167.
47. Siddoway LA, Schwartz SL, Barbey JT, et al. Clinical pharmacokinetics of moricizine. *Am J Cardiol*. 1990;65:21D–25D.
48. Stenson RE, Constantino RT, Harrison DC. Interrelationships of hepatic blood flow, cardiac output, and blood levels of lidocaine in man. *Circulation*. 1971;43:205–211.
49. Thomson PD, Melmon KL, Richardson JA, et al. Lidocaine pharmacokinetics in advanced heart failure, liver disease and renal failure in humans. *Ann Intern Med*. 1973;78:499–508.
50. Zito RA, Reid PR. Lidocaine kinetics predicted by indocyanine green clearance. *N Engl J Med*. 1978;298:1160–1163.
51. Schneck DW, Luderer JR, Davis D, et al. Effects of nadolol and propranolol on plasma lidocaine clearance. *Clin Pharmacol Ther*. 1984;36:584–587.
52. Campbell RWF. Mexiletine. *N Engl J Med*. 1987;316:29–34.
53. Pentikainen PJ, Koivula IH, Hiltunen HA. Effect of rifampicin treatment on the kinetics of mexiletine. *Eur J Clin Pharmacol*. 1982;23:261–266.
54. Begg EJ, Chinwah PM, Webb C, et al. Enhanced metabolism of mexiletine after phenytoin administration. *Br J Clin Pharmacol*. 1982;14:219–223.
55. Grech-Belanger O, Gilbert M, Turgeon J, et al. Effect of cigarette smoking on mexiletine kinetics. *Clin Pharmacol Ther*. 1985;37:638–643.
56. Stanley R, Comer T, Taylor JL, et al. Mexiletine–theophylline interaction. *Am J Med*. 1989;86:733–734.
57. MacMahon B, Bakshi M, Branagan P, et al. Pharmacokinetics and hemodynamic, effects of tocainide in patients with acute myocardial infarction complicated by left ventricular failure. *Br J Clin Pharmacol*. 1985;19:429–434.
58. Mohiuddin SM, Esterbrooks D, Hilleman DE, et al. Tocainide kinetics in congestive heart failure. *Clin Pharmacol Ther*. 1983; 34:596–603.
59. Graffner C, Conradson TB, Hofvendahl S, et al. Tocainide kinetics after intravenous and oral administration in healthy subjects and in patients with acute myocardial infarction. *Clin Pharmacol Ther*. 1980;27:64–71.
60. North DS, Mattern AL, Kapil RP, et al. The effect of histamine$_2$ receptor antagonists on tocainide pharmacokinetics. *J Clin Pharmacol*. 1988;28:640–643.
61. Rice TL, Patterson JH, Celestin C, et al. Influence of rifampin on tocainide pharmacokinetics in humans. *Clin Pharm*. 1989;8:200–205.
62. Schnelle K, Klein G, Schinz A. Studies on the pharmacokinetics and pharmacodynamics of the beta-adrenergic blocking agent sotalol in normal man. *J Clin Pharmacol*.1979;19:516–522.
63. Blair AD, Burgess ED, Maxwell BM, et al. Sotalol kinetics in renal insufficiency. *Clin Pharmacol Ther*. 1981;29:457–463.
64. de Paola AA, Horowitz LN, Morganroth J, et al. Influence of left ventricular dysfunction on flecainide therapy. *J Am Coll Cardiol*. 1987;9:163–168.
65. Conard GJ, Ober RE. Metabolism of flecainide. *Am J Cardiol*. 1984;53:41B–51B.
66. Roden DM, Woosley RL. Flecainide. *N Engl J Med*. 1986; 315:36–41.
67. Nitsch J, Neyses L, Kohler U, et al. [Elevated plasma flecainide concentrations in heart failure]. *Dtsch Med Wochenschr*. 1987;112:1698–1700.
68. Cavilli A, Maggioni AP, Marchi S, et al. Flecainide half-life prolongation in 2 patients with congestive heart failure and complex ventricular arrhythmias. *Clin Pharmacokinet*. 1988; 14:187–188.
69. Funck-Brentano C, Kroemer HK, Lee JT, et al. Propafenone. *N Engl J Med*. 1990;322:518–525.
70. Burnett DM, Gal J, Zahniser NR, et al. Propafenone interacts stereoselectively with β_1 and β_2-adrenergic receptors. *J Cardiovasc Pharmacol*. 1988;12:615–619.
71. Harron DWG, Brogden RN. Propafenone. A review of its pharmacodynamic and pharmacokinetic properties and therapeutic use in the treatment of arrhythmias. *Drugs*. 1987;34:617–647.
72. Ravid S, Podrid PJ, Lampert S, et al. Congestive heart failure induced by six of the newer antiarrhythmic drugs. *J Am Coll Cardiol*. 1989;14:1326–1330.
73. Castel JM, Cappiello E, Leopaldi D, et al. Rifampicin lowers plasma concentrations of propafenone and its antiarrhythmic effect. *Br J Clin Pharmacol*. 1990;30:155–156.
74. Nolan PE, Jr., Marcus FI, Erstad BL, et al. Effects of coadministration of propafenone on the pharmacokinetics of digoxin in healthy volunteer subjects. *J Clin Pharmacol*. 1989;29:46–52.
75. Calvo MV, Martin-Suarez A, Martin Luengo C, et al. Interaction between digoxin and propafenone. *Ther Drug Monit*. 1989; 11:10–15.
76. Kates RE, Yee YG, Kirsten EB. Interaction between warfarin and propafenone in healthy volunteer subjects. *Clin Pharmacol Ther*. 1987;42:305–311.
77. Wagner F, Kalusche D, Trenk D, et al. Drug interaction between propafenone and metoprolol. *Br J Clin Pharmacol*. 1987; 24:213–220.
78. Mason JW. Amiodarone. *N Engl J Med*. 1987;316:455–466.
79. Wilson JS, Podrid PJ. Side effects from amiodarone. *Am Heart J*. 1991;121:158–171.
80. Applefeld MM, Adir J, Crouthamel WG, et al. Digoxin pharmacokinetics in congestive heart failure. *J Clin Pharmacol*. 1981;21:114–120.
81. Ohnhaus EE, Vozeh S, Nuesch E. Absorption of digoxin in severe right heart failure. *Eur J Clin Pharmacol*. 1979;15:115–120.
82. Korhonen UR, Jounela AJ, Pakarinen AJ, et al. Pharmacokinetics of digoxin in patients with acute myocardial infarction. *Am J Cardiol*. 1979;44:1190–1194.

83. Marcus FL. Pharmacokinetic interactions between digoxin and other drugs. *J Am Coll Cardiol.* 1985;5:82A–90A.
84. Brodie MJ, Feely J. Adverse drug interactions. *Br Med J.* 1988;296:845–849.
85. Nademanee K, Kannan R, Hendrickson J, et al. Amiodarone-digoxin interaction: clinical significance, time course of development, potential pharmacokinetic mechanisms and therapeutic implications. *J Am Coll Cardiol.* 1984;4:111–116.
86. Robinson K, Johnston A, Walker S, et al. The digoxin-amiodarone interaction. *Cardiovasc Drugs Ther.* 1989;3:25–28.
87. Kates RE, Leier CV. Dobutamine pharmacokinetics in severe heart failure. *Clin Pharmacol Ther.* 1978;24:537–541.
88. Rocci ML, Jr., Wilson H. The pharmacokinetics and pharmacodynamics of newer inotropic agents. *Clin Pharmacokinet.* 1987;13:91–109.
89. Park GB, Kershner RP, Angellotti J, et al. Oral bioavailability and intravenous pharmacokinetics of amrinone in humans. *J Pharm Sci.* 1983;72:817–819.
90. Hamilton RA, Kowalsky SF, Wright EM, et al. Effect of the acetylator phenotype on amrinone pharmacokinetics. *Clin Pharmacol Ther.* 1986;40:615–619.
91. Wilson H, Rocci ML Jr., Weber KT, et al. Pharmacokinetics and hemodynamics of amrinone in patients with chronic cardiac failure of diverse etiology. *Res Commun Chem Pathol Pharmacol.* 1987;56:3–19.
92. Edelson J, Stroshane R, Benziger DP, et al. Pharmacokinetics of the bipyridines amrinone and milrinone. *Circulation.* 1986; 73(Suppl III):145–152.
93. Benotti JR, Lesko LJ, McCue JE, et al. Pharmacokinetics and pharmacodynamics of milrinone in chronic congestive heart failure. *Am J Cardiol.* 1985;56:685–689.
94. Brater DC, Seiwell R, Anderson S, et al. Absorption and disposition of furosemide in congestive heart failure. *Kidney Int.* 1982;22:171–176.
95. Vasco MR, Brown-Cartwright D, Knochel JP, et al. Furosemide absorption altered in decompensated congestive heart failure. *Ann Intern Med.* 1985;102:314–318.
96. Chaturvedi PR, O'Donnell JP, Nicholas JM, et al. Steady state absorption kinetics and pharmacodynamics of furosemide in congestive heart failure. *Int J Clin Pharmacol Ther Toxicol.* 1987;25:123–128.
97. Brater DC, Chennavasin P, Seiwell R. Furosemide in patients with heart failure: shift in dose-response curves. *Clin Pharmacol Ther.* 1980;28:182–186.
98. Brater DC. Resistance to loop diuretics. Why it happens and what to do about it. *Drugs.* 1985;30:427–443.
99. Favre L, Glasson P, Riondel A, et al. Interaction of diuretics and non-steroidal anti-inflammatory drugs in man. *Clin Sci.* 1983;64:407–415.
100. Brater DC. Disposition and response to bumetanide and furosemide. *Am J Cardiol.* 1986;57:20A–25A.
101. Ward A, Heel RC. Bumetanide. A review of its pharmacodynamic and pharmacokinetic properties and therapeutic use. *Drugs.* 1984;28:426–464.
102. Cook JA, Smith DE, Cornish LA, et al. Kinetics, dynamics, and bioavailability of bumetanide in healthy subjects and patients with congestive heart failure. *Clin Pharmacol Ther.* 1988;44: 487–500.
103. Brater DC, Day B, Burdette A, et al. Bumetanide and furosemide in heart failure. *Kidney Int.* 1984;26:183–189.
104. Beermann B, Groschinsky-Grind M. Pharmacokinetics of hydrochlorothiazide in patients with congestive heart failure. *Br J Clin Pharmacol.* 1979;7:579–583.
105. Kerry RJ, Ludlow JM, Owen G. Diuretics are dangerous with lithium. *BMJ.* 1980;281:371.
106. Breckenridge AM. Drug interactions with ACE inhibitors. *J Hum Hypertens.* 1989;3:133–138.
107. Duchin KL, McKinstry DN, Cohen AL, et al. Pharmacokinetics of captopril in healthy subjects and in patients with cardiovascular diseases. *Clin Pharmacokinet.* 1988;14:241–259.
108. Brogden RN, Todd PA, Sorkin EM. Captopril. An update of its pharmacodynamic and pharmacokinetic properties, and therapeutic use in hypertension and congestive heart failure. *Drugs.* 1988;36:540–600.
109. Belz GG, Kirch W, Kleinbloesem CH. Angiotensin-converting enzyme inhibitors. Relationship between pharmacodynamics and pharmacokinetics. *Clin Pharmacokinet.* 1988;15:295–318.
110. Todd PA, Heel RC. Enalapril. A review of its pharmacodynamic and pharmacokinetic properties, and therapeutic use in hypertension and congestive heart failure. *Drugs.* 1986;31:198–248.
111. Dickstein K, Till AE, Aarsland T, et al. The pharmacokinetics of enalapril in hospitalized patients with congestive heart failure. *Br J Clin Pharmacol.* 1987;23:403–410.
112. Dickstein K. Pharmacokinetics of enalapril in congestive heart failure. *Drugs.* 1986;32:40–44.
113. Gautam PC, Vargas E, Lye M. Pharmacokinetics of lisinopril (MK521) in healthy young and elderly subjects and in elderly patients with cardiac failure. *J Pharm Pharmacol.* 1987;39: 929–931.
114. Thomson AH, Kelly JG, Whiting B. Lisinopril population pharmacokinetics in elderly and renal disease patients with hypertension. *Br J Clin Pharmacol.* 1989;27:57–65.
115. Till AE, Dickstein K, Aarsland T, et al. The pharmacokinetics of lisinopril in hospitalized patients with congestive heart failure. *Br J Clin Pharmacol.* 1989; 27:199–204.
116. Pitt B, Segal R, Martinez FA, et al. Randomised trial of losartan versus captopril in patients over 65 with heart failure (Evaluation of Losartan In The Elderly study, ELITE). *Lancet.* 1977;349: 747–752.
117. Sica DA, Lo MV, Shaw W, et al. The pharmacokinetics of losartan in renal insufficiency. *J Hypertens.* 1995;13(Suppl 1):49–52.
118. Christ DD. Human plasma protein binding of the angiotensin II receptor antagonist losartan potassium (DUP-753/MK954) and its pharmacologically active metabolite E-3174. *J Clin Pharmacol.* 1995;35:515–520.
119. Mulrow JP, Crawford MH. Clinical pharmacokinetics and therapeutic use of hydralazine in congestive heart failure. *Clin Pharmacokinet.* 1989;16:86–89.
120. Hanson A, Johansson BW, Wernersson B, et al. Pharmacokinetics of oral hydralazine in chronic heart failure. *Eur J Clin Pharmacol.* 1983;25:467–473.
121. Thadani U, Whitsett T. Relationship of pharmacokinetic and pharmacodynamic properties of the organic nitrates. *Clin Pharmacokinet.* 1988;15:32–43.
122. Bogaert MG. Clinical pharmacokinetics of organic nitrates. *Clin Pharmacokinet.* 1983;8:410–421.
123. Lee FW, Salmonson T, Metzler CH, et al. Pharmacokinetics and pharmacodynamics of glyceryl trinitrate and its two dinitrate metabolites in conscious dogs. *J Pharmacol Exp Ther.* 1990; 255:1222–1229.
124. Nakashima E, Rigod JF, Lin ET, et al. Pharmacokinetics of nitroglycerin and its dinitrate metabolites over a thirtyfold range of oral doses. *Clin Pharmacol Ther.* 1990;47:592–598.
125. Noonan PK LZ. The bioavailability of oral nitroglycerin. *J Pharm Sci.* 1986;75:241–243.
126. Noonan PK, Benet LZ. Incomplete and delayed bioavailability of sublingual nitroglycerin. *Am J Cardiol.* 1985;55:184–187.
127. Nakashima E, Noonan PK, Benet LZ. Transdermal bioavailability and first-pass skin metabolism: a preliminary evaluation with nitroglycerin. *J Pharmacokinet Biopharm.* 1987;15:423–437.
128. Armstrong PW. Pharmacokinetic-hemodynamic studies of transdermal nitroglycerin in congestive heart failure. *J Am Coll Cardiol.* 1987;9:420–425.
129. Armstrong PW, Armstrong JA, Marks GS. Pharmacokinetic-hemodynamic studies of nitroglycerin ointment in congestive heart failure. *Am J Cardiol.* 1980;46:670–676.
130. Armstrong PW, Armstrong JA, Marks GS. Pharmacokinetic-hemodynamic studies of intravenous nitroglycerin in congestive cardiac failure. *Circulation.* 1980;62:160–166.
131. Waagstein F, Bristow MR, Swedberg K, et al. Beneficial effects of metoprolol in idiopathic dilated cardiomyopathy. *Lancet.* 1993;342:1441–1446.
132. Fisher ML, Gottlieb SS, Plotnick GD, et al. Beneficial effects of metoprolol in heart failure associated with coronary artery disease: a randomized trial. *J Am Coll Cardiol.* 1994;23: 943–950.
133. Kirch W, Rose I, Demers HG, Leopold G, Pabst J, Ohnhaus EE. Pharmacokinetics of bisoprolol during repeated oral administra-

tion to healthy volunteers and patients with kidney or liver disease. *Clin Pharmacokinet.* 1987;13:110–117.
134. Payton CD, Fox JG, Pauleau NF, et al. The single dose pharmacokinetics of bisoprolol (10 mg) in renal insufficiency: the clinical significance of balanced clearance. *Eur Heart J.* 1987;8(Suppl M):15–22.
135. CIBIS Investigators. A randomized trial of β-blockade in heart failure. The Cardiac Insufficiency Bisoprolol Study (CIBIS). *Circulation.* 1994;90:1765–1773.
136. Piafsky KM, Sitar DS, Rangno RE, et al. Theophylline kinetics in acute pulmonary edema. *Clin Pharmacol Ther.* 1977;21: 310–316.
137. Upton RA. Pharmacokinetic interactions between theophylline and other medication. 1. *Clin Pharmacokinet.* 1991;20:66–80.
138. Upton RA. Pharmacokinetic interactions between theophylline and other medication. 2. *Clin Pharmacokinet.* 1991;20: 135–150.
139. O'Reilly RA, Aggeler PM. Determinants of the response to oral anticoagulant drugs in man. *Pharmacol Rev.* 1970;22:35–96.
140. Ristola P, Pyorala K. Determinants of the response to coumarin anticoagulants in patients with acute myocardial infarction. *Acta Med Scand.* 1972;192:183–188.
141. Kelly JG, O'Malley K. Clinical pharmacokinetics of oral anticoagulants. *Clin Pharmacokinet.* 1979;4:1–15.
142. O'Reilly RA. Warfarin metabolism and drug-drug interactions. *Adv Exp Med Biol.* 1987;214:205–212.
143. Serlin MJ, Breckenridge AM. Drug interactions with warfarin. *Drugs.* 1983;25:610–620.

Traditional Diuretics and Other Diuresing Agents

24

Stephen S. Gottlieb

Diuretic medications are deemed essential for the treatment of most patients with heart failure, particularly when congestion is present. The underlying abnormality present in patients with heart failure leads to neurohormonal activation as well as salt and water retention. Thus, medicines that increase sodium and water excretion can be extremely effective. Indeed, symptoms of congestive heart failure may be completely relieved by this simple and inexpensive intervention. However, the adverse consequences associated with the use of diuretic medications are rarely considered. Knowledge of potential problems as well as benefits can lead to safer and more effective use of these agents.

EFFECTS OF DIURETICS ON CARDIAC PERFORMANCE

Diuretics have the ability to decrease many of the symptoms associated with heart failure. The presence of systemic congestion leads to abdominal fullness, bloating, and peripheral edema. Whereas the former leads to gastrointestinal (GI) symptoms (and may impair the absorption of nutrients and medications), the latter is often painful and can greatly limit mobility. Pulmonary congestions leads to the subjective complaint of dyspnea (starting with exertion and progressing to rest) and, when advanced, can impair oxygenation. Diuretics can dramatically improve these symptoms by enhancing the urinary excretion of salt and water. Although this may occur without increasing cardiac index (1), diuretic medications also have been reported to improve cardiac performance at rest and during exercise (2). No direct inotropic effect has been ascribed to any diuretic but there are multiple explanations as to why diuresis may acutely increase cardiac performance.

It is possible that some of the benefits seen with diuretics are secondary to a reduction in systemic vascular resistance. Diuretic-induced reductions in extravascular pressure may directly lead to vasodilation. Improved heart failure status could also lead to a reduction in neurohormonal activation and a withdrawal of the vasoconstriction that is mediated by most of the neurohormonal agents that are increased in heart failure. In addition, venous capacitance increases within 5 minutes of furosemide administration, suggesting an acute mechanism of vasodilation as well (3). In contrast to the decreased peripheral resistance frequently observed following diuresis, however, some of the neurohormonal changes associated with diuretics may cause vasoconstriction. Thus, blood pressure may acutely increase with diuretics, with the beneficial hemodynamic effects of diuresis only developing later (4). Nevertheless, in most patients chronic diuretic use causes decreased symptoms of heart failure, improved cardiac performance, and vasodilation (5). The decreased afterload probably explains many of the reported improvements in cardiac index and other load-dependent indexes of cardiac performance following diuresis (6). The importance of afterload reduction as the cause of the improved cardiac performance is supported by the finding that the increased stroke volume often seen with diuretics is closely related to decreases in systemic vascular resistance, but not to decreases in preload (7).

Despite the importance of afterload reduction, there are some actions on preload that also could improve cardiac performance. The abnormal valvular and papillary muscle geometry caused by ventricular enlargement can lead to abnormal mitral valve function and significant regurgitation (8). Even abnormal atrial geometry may lead to mitral regurgitation (9). Decreases in ventricular (and perhaps atrial) size could therefore increase forward flow by reducing backward flow. The importance of reversing mitral regurgitation has been clearly demonstrated using vasodilators (10). Presumably, diuretic-induced volume reduction also decreases mitral regurgitation and thereby increases cardiac output. This concept could explain why diuretics may improve cardiac output in patients with congestive heart failure but not in individuals with normal cardiac size and function (11).

Although frequently hypothesized, it is unlikely that a decreased preload shifts the ventricle to a more optimal position on Starling's curve. A descending limb of the curve has only been noted at extremely high pressures (above 60 mm Hg) (12), and sarcomere length in a dilated canine heart is close to optimal (13). However, it is likely that decreased systolic wall stress with reduced left ventricular size (the Laplace effect) is beneficial. Not only would a decreased afterload improve cardiac performance but the lower filling pressures associated with diuretics might limit ischemia (14). Neurohormonal activation and a consequent positive inotropic effect could be another possible explanation of the improved cardiac performance frequently noted with the administration of diuretics to patients with heart failure.

Diuretics, of course, can lead to decreased cardiac output if the left ventricular filling pressure is decreased excessively. In contrast to the upper end of Starling's curve, the lower end of the curve is clinically important and it has been demonstrated to be operative in humans (15). Although neurohormonal activation may minimize the effects of the Starling phenomenon in normal individuals, in the severely compromised heart failure patient overdiuresis may cause devastating effects and should be avoided.

The chronic effects of diuretics on cardiac function may be different than the acute effect. Indeed, there is evidence that chronic furosemide may lead to decreased cardiac function. In a study of rats with pacing-induced cardiomyopathy, those animals randomized to receive furosemide experienced more cardiac dilatation and decreased contractility than those who received placebo (16). These animals also demonstrated activation of the renin-angiotensin-aldosterone axis (Fig 24-1).

NEUROHORMONAL EFFECTS

Neurohormonal activation is important to the pathophysiology of congestive heart failure. It may reflect the severity of disease as well as alter its natural history. These issues are discussed in other chapters but are important to any discussion of diuretics because neurohormones may be affected by their administration. Whether these neurohormonal changes directly cause benefit or harm, or whether they merely reflect changes in physiology, is often debated.

Renin-Angiotensin-Aldosterone System

Stimulation of the renin-angiotensin-aldosterone system (RAAS) is commonly found in patients with congestive heart failure, is associated with increased mortality, and may have both beneficial and detrimental effects. Although stimulation of this system is usually assumed to be secondary to the severity of illness, increased angiotensin II concentrations and plasma renin activity actually often reflect the intensity of diuretic treatment. Renin release may be caused by volume contraction and stimulation of baroreceptors and the macula densa (17). Thus, it is not surprising that many studies document increased plasma renin activity and plasma concentrations of angiotensin II in heart failure patients and animals following diuretic therapy (18,19) (Fig. 24-1). Indeed, concentrations may be normal in heart failure patients not treated with diuretics (18,20).

Aldosterone concentrations are similarly affected by diuretics. Normal concentrations prior to treatment may be

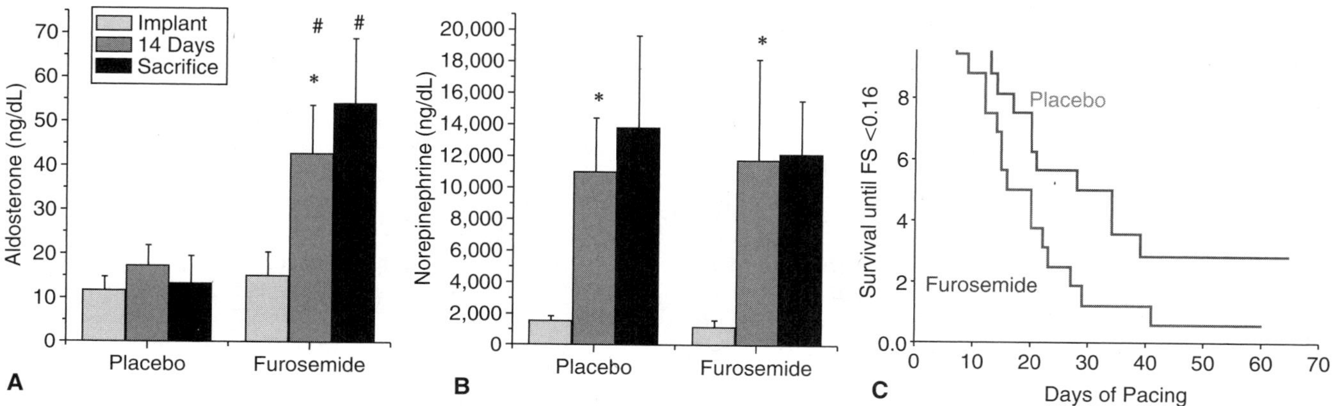

Figure 24-1 Neurohormonal concentrations before and after pacing induced cardiomyopathy in animals receiving placebo or furosemide (**Panels A** and **B**). Note that norepinephrine concentrations increased in both groups but aldosterone only increased in those animals receiving furosemide. The animals receiving furosemide also experienced more rapid deterioration in cardiac function (**Panel C**). (Adapted from McCurley JM, Hanlon SU, Wei SK, et al. Furosemide and the progression of left ventricular dysfunction in experimental heart failure. *J Am Coll Cardiol.* 2004;44:1301–1307.)

followed by increases with diuresis (20,21). Interestingly, patients with elevated aldosterone concentrations prior to treatment with diuretics may exhibit decreases following their administration (18). The varying response of aldosterone may reflect the conflicting consequences of the effects of diuretics on the severity of illness and their effects on delivery of sodium to the distal tubule. The importance of both of these factors is suggested by a report that patients with elevated baseline aldosterone concentrations demonstrate decreased concentrations with initial diuretic treatment (and improvement in symptoms), but increased concentrations as dry weight approaches and less sodium is delivered to the renal tubule (22).

The increased angiotensin II and aldosterone caused by diuretic administration may have adverse effects. For example, aldosterone stimulates collagen production (23) and aldosterone antagonists probably have an impact unrelated to actions on electrolytes or diuresis. Indeed, it is likely that the impact of furosemide on the RAAS may explain the decreased contractility caused by furosemide in the rat pacing cardiomyopathy study previously mentioned (16). The implications of the effects of diuretics on the renin-angiotensin-aldosterone axis are presumably mitigated by our interventions with angiotensin-converting enzyme (ACE) inhibitors and spironolactone. Nevertheless, it is possible that RAAS stimulation, even in the presence of antagonists, can cause adverse effects.

Arginine Vasopressin

Following diuretic administration, both stimulation and inhibition of the release of arginine vasopressin (ADH) have been reported. The complex regulation of ADH is probably responsible for these conflicting studies. Arginine vasopressin concentrations are affected by both osmotic and baroreceptor stimuli, and diuretics could increase the concentrations because of actions on these parameters. However, the physiological effects of diuretics are not extensive enough to cause a consistent increase in ADH. Although the decreased blood volume and increased plasma osmolality noted with furosemide (24) might be expected to result in increased arginine vasopressin concentrations, a decrease in volume of 10% is needed to stimulate the baroreceptors and the relative iso-osmotic diuresis observed following the use of most diuretics should not alter ADH concentrations. It is therefore unclear whether diuretics directly cause the increased ADH concentrations often found in individuals with left ventricular dysfunction.

Indirect effects of diuretics, however, could impact on arginine vasopressin regulation; changes in the activity of other neurohormonal systems may alter ADH concentrations. For example, angiotensin II may directly affect its release; this mechanism may explain the increased ADH concentration noted with acute diuresis, even if the diuresis is iso-osmotic and there is no change in oncotic pressure (4). In contrast, normalization of the hemodynamic status with diuresis may return arginine vasopressin concentrations to the normal range (18). Most likely, alterations in arginine vasopressin secretion are not important consequences of diuretic administration.

Atrial Natriuretic Peptide and Brain Natriuretic Peptide

An individual's volume status is related to secretion of atrial natriuretic peptide (ANP) and brain natriuretic peptide (BNP). Atrial stretch and ventricular distension cause release of these peptides which, in turn, may cause natriuresis and vasodilation (25,26). Diuretics would therefore be expected to lead to lower concentrations and to mitigation of the peptide's diuretic and vasodilatory effects. However, decreased natriuretic peptide concentrations have not been noted following diuretic administration (19) and the high concentrations seen in patients with severe heart failure appear to have little clinical effect, suggesting that downregulation of receptor sites may prevent most of the response to natriuretic peptides in these patients (27). While highly prognostic (28), hemodynamic tolerance to chronic marked elevations in concentration has suggested that any impact of diuresis on natriuretic peptide secretion may be clinically unimportant in these individuals (29). Indeed, the recent ESCAPE (Evaluation Study of Congestive Heart Failure and Pulmonary Artery Catheterization Effectiveness) trial showed a poor relationship between the change in BNP and the change in pulmonary capillary wedge pressure.

Prostaglandins

Prostaglandins affect the vasculature, and diuretic medications may alter prostaglandin concentrations by both direct and indirect means. Therefore, diuretics may exert beneficial or detrimental actions via this little-appreciated mechanism. For example, furosemide, which increases venous capacitance, does not have the same effect in the presence of indomethacin concentrations known to inhibit prostaglandin production (30). This suggests that its direct actions on prostaglandin production, such as stimulation of the renal production of prostaglandin E_2 (PGE_2), may have important therapeutic effects. Indeed, the clinical importance of the effects of furosemide on prostaglandin synthesis has been noted in disorders other than congestive heart failure. In premature infants, for example, furosemide increases the incidence of patent ductus arteriosus, presumably via prostaglandin stimulation (31). Other diuretics also may cause alterations in prostaglandin production; various diuretics increase the production of prostacyclin (PGI_2) from arachidonic acid in aortic smooth muscle cells (32). Although the actions of diuretics on prostaglandins is rarely recognized, it is conceivable that some of the beneficial effects observed with diuretics may result from increased concentrations of prostaglandins.

The use of nonsteroidal anti-inflammatory drugs (NSAIDs) may therefore affect the actions of diuretics, especially regarding renal function. Renal prostaglandins help to maintain renal blood flow in the presence of countervailing influences. Thus, if diuresis leads to neurohormonal activation, limiting renal plasma flow, prostaglandins may be essential for the maintenance of renal function. The combination of diuretics and NSAIDs would then decrease renal plasma flow and glomerular filtration. Indeed, in normal individuals in whom diuretics and aspirin individually had no effect on renal function, the combination caused marked decreases in the glomerular filtration rate (33). In patients with congestive heart failure and compromised renal plasma flow, the effects might be even greater.

Catecholamines

In contrast to investigations of the renin-angiotensin system, studies of the sympathetic nervous system have consistently reported increased norepinephrine concentrations in patients with heart failure prior to treatment with diuretics (19,20). Also in contrast to the renin-angiotensin system, catecholamine concentrations frequently decrease coincident with the symptomatic improvement caused by diuresis (Fig. 24-1) (20); norepinephrine concentrations are a sensitive reflector of poor cardiac performance (34). This decrease in catecholamines could be an extremely important benefit of diuretic therapy. If catecholamines are responsible for arrhythmogenesis or cardiac deterioration, as is commonly believed (35), diuretics (or any intervention that improves left ventricular performance) may lead to improved myocardial function and survival.

DIURETIC-INDUCED ELECTROLYTE ABNORMALITIES

In addition to the neurohormonal effects, diuretics also have important metabolic actions. Volume contraction leads to avid sodium reabsorption and (when secondary to diuretics other than carbonic anhydrase inhibitors and potassium-sparing agents) bicarbonate reabsorption and metabolic alkalosis. Uric acid excretion is inhibited by the commonly used diuretic medications, and this explains the high prevalence of gout in patients with congestive heart failure. The most problematic consequences of diuretic usage, however, are marked and potentially serious direct and indirect effects on electrolytes. Diuretic medications disturb electrolyte homeostasis, most notably altering potassium, magnesium, sodium, and calcium concentrations. The implications of most of these alterations remain controversial.

Potassium

Most diuretics (other than potassium-sparing agents) increase sodium delivery to the distal renal tubule, where potassium is excreted as sodium is reabsorbed; potassium depletion may therefore result. Although even acute diuresis may cause hypokalemia, total body potassium depletion is associated with the duration of diuretic use (36). Yet, the hypokalemia commonly observed in patients with heart failure cannot be attributed to diuretics alone because hypokalemia is more frequently noted in patients receiving these medications for heart failure than in those receiving them for hypertension. Metabolic alkalosis resulting from intensive diuresis, decreased sodium intake, and neurohormonal activation may contribute to the hypokalemic effects of diuretics in patients with heart failure. Activation of the sympathetic nervous system and elevated aldosterone concentrations are also common in patients with severe heart failure and can lead to hypokalemia. Importantly, these factors may stimulate the kaliuretic actions of diuretics even when they do not directly increase potassium excretion. For example, diuretics may potentiate the hypokalemia caused by epinephrine or albuterol (37,38). Thus, although diuretics themselves do not necessarily cause marked hypokalemia, in combination with the abnormal physiology of patients with congestive heart failure most diuretics may induce potassium depletion.

Hypokalemia can cause symptoms such as muscle aches, but of most concern are the potential arrhythmogenic effects of this state. In the hypertension literature the effect of hypokalemia on mortality has been controversial (39,40) but it is generally accepted that hypokalemia increases the risk of arrhythmias in patients with heart failure. Most investigators assume that studies of hypertensive patients are not relevant to patients with congestive heart failure because of marked differences in anatomy and physiology. Although the concern about the dangers of hypokalemia in patients with heart failure is based on indirect evidence, it is convincing. For example, hypokalemia increases the frequency of early after-depolarizations caused by quinidine (41) and the risk of arrhythmias associated with digoxin (42). Low serum potassium concentrations are also associated with increased risk of arrhythmias following a myocardial infarction (43). More important than the degree of hypokalemia, however, is probably the rate of change of the serum potassium (44); hypokalemia associated with rapid diuresis may be more detrimental than that associated with chronic use of diuretics.

When discussing diuretics, the risks of hyperkalemia are frequently neglected. Not only may the use of potassium-sparing agents lead to hyperkalemia, but the routine prescription of potassium supplements with initiation of diuretics also can cause this fatal complication. Poor renal function, concomitant use of angiotensin-converting enzyme (ACE) inhibitors and/or aldosterone antagonists, and excessive potassium intake can produce hyperkalemia and consequent ventricular arrhythmias and sudden death (45). Therefore, the serum potassium concentration should be monitored carefully in all patients receiving diuretics.

Considering the problems associated with abnormal potassium concentrations, it is wise to keep the serum concentration above 4.0 mEq/L, but within the normal range. Although potassium-sparing diuretics or ACE inhibitors may be used to help achieve this goal, it should be realized that the combination of these two interventions increases the risk of hyperkalemia. Salt substitutes contain potassium and also should be considered as a cause of hyperkalemia in patients receiving potassium-sparing agents. The use of any diuretic mandates close follow-up of the patient in order to maintain the potassium concentration within the normal range.

Magnesium

Although reports of the prevalence of magnesium deficiency in patients with congestive heart failure range from 7% to more than 37%, the true prevalence is disputed for many reasons (46). First, there is no gold standard measurement of magnesium deficiency. Determination of the serum magnesium concentration is easy but it may not reflect total body stores of the electrolyte. Serum, myocardial, lymphocyte, and muscle magnesium concentrations do not correlate (47) and the concentration (if any) that is most clinically relevant is unknown. There are other factors that also prevent determination of the true prevalence of magnesium deficiency. Diverse definitions of normal magnesium concentrations, differing nutritional intake, and analyses of patients with varying severity of disease have led to wide-ranging estimates of the prevalence of magnesium depletion. Nevertheless, investigations consistently demonstrate that a large percentage of patients with heart failure are magnesium-deficient.

It is often assumed that diuretics are the cause of magnesium depletion in patients with heart failure, and chronic diuretic use probably does lead to magnesium depletion (48), with the duration of therapy an important determinant of the extent of depletion (36). However, other factors also affect magnesium excretion. Some studies suggest that low magnesium concentrations are common in heart failure patients even prior to treatment with diuretics (49), possibly caused by aldosterone-induced magnesium excretion (50). In contrast, other neurohormonal mechanisms may limit the excretion of magnesium caused by diuretics; renal denervation leads to increased magnesium excretion following the administration of diuretics (51). Despite these confounding factors, it is likely that diuretics are the predominant cause of hypomagnesemia in congestive heart failure patients.

The clinical implications of magnesium depletion in patients with congestive heart failure are controversial. There are reports of various symptoms related to hypomagnesemia, ranging from muscle weakness to depression (52). It is also possible that magnesium depletion impairs cardiac performance, either by directly reducing cardiac contractility (53) or by causing peripheral vasoconstriction (54). However, the consequence of most concern is the possibility that magnesium depletion causes ventricular arrhythmias and sudden death.

There are reasons to suspect that magnesium depletion increases the frequency of ventricular arrhythmias. A low magnesium concentration decreases the threshold needed to induce ventricular tachycardia and ventricular fibrillation in normal and digitalis-treated dogs (55), and hypomagnesemia potentiates the development of digitalis-induced arrhythmias (56). Furthermore, administration of intravenous magnesium suppresses early after-depolarizations and ventricular tachycardia induced by cesium in dogs (57) and may prevent the clinical occurrence of ventricular tachycardia in patients (58,59). These actions of magnesium may be related to its function as a critical cofactor in the cellular functions that regulate intracellular electrolyte concentrations (60). Hypomagnesemia also may exacerbate the development of hypokalemia and cause arrhythmias indirectly (61).

Despite the multiple reasons to suspect that hypomagnesemia may be clinically important, this hypothesis has not been proven. Some studies suggest an association of hypomagnesemia and arrhythmias (62), whereas others do not (63). There are no large, prospective, well-controlled studies evaluating the significance of magnesium and there is no proof that magnesium supplementation is beneficial. It is thus presently unknown whether the actions of diuretics on magnesium excretion need to be countered. However, magnesium administration should be considered in the settings of intractable ventricular arrhythmias or refractory hypokalemia coincident with hypomagnesemia.

Sodium

Hyponatremia may be observed in patients with heart failure and it is often ascribed to diuretic therapy. Although heart failure patients not on diuretics can experience hyponatremia secondary to total body fluid overload (not sodium depletion) (64), diuretics clearly can exacerbate hyponatremia. Direct renal actions lead to sodium excretion, which, in the presence of inappropriately elevated arginine vasopressin concentrations (perhaps partially caused by the diuretic itself), may lead to hyponatremia (65–67). Usually, however, the diuresis associated with potent diuretics is relatively iso-osmotic and does not cause hyponatremia. Indeed, only patients receiving diuretics will experience reversal of hyponatremia with ACE inhibition (68). Similarly, loop diuretics inhibit the ability of the medullary interstitium to concentrate and therefore may correct the hyponatremia associated with syndrome of inappropriate antidiuretic hormone. Therefore, diuretics, which may cause hyponatremia, also may correct hyponatremia induced by severe heart failure.

Hyponatremia itself generally does not cause symptoms in patients with congestive heart failure. It is gradual in onset, so nervous system complications do not occur. There is no evidence that chronic hyponatremia is dangerous and needs to be treated. Even though hyponatremia is rarely directly deleterious, it does reflect stimulation of the renin-angiotensin system and has prognostic implications (69). It also may reflect overdiuresis, a situation in which it should be accompanied by evidence of renal dysfunction, hypotension, or other clinical problems and which can be treated, if necessary, by adjustment of diuretics. In contrast to the chronic development of hyponatremia, acute hyponatremia (although rare) could be dangerous. When secondary to overdiuresis, it is easily corrected with modification of the treatment regimen and without administration of sodium. When severe hyponatremia progresses despite diuretic modification, a syndrome of inappropriate ADH secretion should be considered.

Calcium

Diuretic medications alter urinary calcium excretion in various ways. Some diuretics, such as furosemide, increase calcium excretion (70), whereas others, such as thiazides, depress it (71). The combination of these medications may minimize changes (e.g., metolazone decreases furosemide-induced calciuria) (72). Whether these urinary changes reflect important physiological perturbations is unknown because compensatory actions, such as alteration of parathyroid hormone secretion, may occur and prevent clinical harm. Because the measurement of low serum concentrations of calcium may not adequately reflect ionized calcium or intracellular concentrations, it is difficult to determine the significance of altered calcium excretion.

Nevertheless, there are reasons to be concerned that diuretic-induced alterations of calcium concentrations could have important physiological effects. Myocardial function is dependent on calcium and, although total serum calcium concentration does not correlate with cardiac performance, the influence of ionized calcium concentrations on myocardial function has been suggested (73). There is even a case report of myocardial function varying with the serum ionized calcium concentration. It was hypothesized that myocardial function in severely ill patients is particularly dependent on calcium concentration because of β-receptor downregulation (74). However, at present it is unclear if the actions of diuretics on calcium excretion alter myocardial function.

RENAL EFFECTS

Alterations in glomerular filtration are commonly noted following the administration of diuretic medications, and frequently they mandate modification of the treatment regimen. Most often, the indirect actions consequent to intravascular sodium and volume depletion explain these renal effects of diuretics, but direct renal actions also may have important ramifications. If the volume contraction is severe or chronic enough, the physiological alterations that maintain blood pressure can cause decreased glomerular filtration and, ultimately, renal failure. Neurohormonal activation is the most likely cause of the resultant renal dysfunction. The importance of neurohormonal factors is suggested by the commonly noted diuresis that occurs with reclining. The increased glomerular filtration rate and sodium, potassium, and volume excretion in patients who are reclining (as compared to standing) is associated with less stimulation of the sympathetic and renin-angiotensin-aldosterone systems when reclining (76).

Diuresis need not lead to intravascular depletion (77). Plasma volume may actually increase, perhaps secondary to increased venous capacitance, decreased capillary hydrostatic pressure, and increased colloid pressure. In such patients, effects of diuretics on glomerular filtration may be secondary to direct actions on renal vascular resistance and renal plasma flow. For example, renal vascular resistance has been reported to increase following the administration of hydrochlorothiazide (78). However, renal vascular resistance also may decrease following the administration of diuretics. Renal artery vasodilation with furosemide and ethacrynic acid probably explains the acute increases in both renal plasma flow and glomerular filtration caused by these agents (79). Increased prostaglandin production, reflected by increased urinary excretion of PGE_2 and PGF_{2a}, may be the cause of these acute renal effects (78). The possible influence of diuretic administration on intrarenal adenosine, known to be increased in patients with heart failure, is also being investigated (80).

There are some data to suggest that persistent use of diuretics leads to decreased efficacy (75). While decreased gastrointestinal absorption or delivery to the nephron is often explained as the cause of tolerance, the physiological actions of diuretics may be even more important. For example, the renal actions of diuretics may be limited by direct neurohormonal activation in the kidneys. Such concepts provide rationale for alternative means of fluid removal.

PRACTICAL IMPLICATIONS OF THE MULTIPLE EFFECTS OF DIURETICS

There is no doubt that diuretic medications are and will continue to be a primary tool in the treatment of congestive heart failure. The rapid and dramatic clinical effects caused by these agents will continue to mandate their prescription. However, the obvious symptomatic benefits derived from the correct use of diuretics have blinded us to a careful evaluation of their risks and benefits. An analysis of the multiple neurohormonal, electrolyte, renal, and cardiac performance effects of diuretics should alter the way we prescribe these and concomitant medications. Although not all of the answers are in, the data increasingly suggest that we can achieve an optimal level of diuresis while minimizing adverse effects.

The neurohormonal effects of diuretics are probably very important. For example, the activation of the renin-angiotensin system by diuretics may be detrimental; blockade of the renin-angiotensin system improves symptoms and survival. This suggests that ACE inhibitors should be started in the early stages of heart failure, when initiation of diuretics increases plasma renin activity. Studies of the effect of ACE inhibitors on survival in the early stages of heart failure should be analyzed to test the effect of these drugs in patients receiving diuretics as compared with those not receiving diuretics. In contrast to the actions on the renin-angiotensin system, however, diuretics act to inhibit the sympathetic nervous system in patients with mild heart failure. This might raise questions as to the presumed benefits of β-blockade in the early stages of congestive heart failure.

Extent of Diuresis

Measurement of activation of neurohormonal systems may be the indicator of the optimal level of diuresis for which we have searched. Although presently the absence of peripheral edema is the most widely used gauge of adequate diuresis, it may make more sense to analyze the physiological parameters reflected by neurohormones. With initiation of diuresis, catecholamine and aldosterone concentrations decrease coincident with the observed improvement of symptoms. However, the concentrations of these neurohormones increase as dry weight is approached. Perhaps the lowest level of neurohormonal activation is the best indicator of optimal volume status.

Even if the optimal extent of diuresis is not certain, clinical experience provides us with tools to assess fluid status. Lung sounds are poor indicators of optimal fluid status; clear lungs do not necessarily indicate adequate diuresis, and diuresis may not resolve the occurrence of rales. Rather, assessment of total body fluid (using peripheral edema, ascites, and sacral edema as guides) is easy and should indicate the necessity for diuresis. Nevertheless, inadequate diuresis is probably the most common mistake made in the treatment of congestive heart failure. Many physicians are reluctant to aggressively treat patients with diuretics. Hospitalized patients are often diuresed enough to eliminate pulmonary edema but they are then sent home despite obvious total body fluid overload. With inadequate diuretic doses at home, increased edema and severe symptoms soon return.

A patient should be diuresed until no edema is present or other complications occur. Decreased renal function or increased blood urea nitrogen (BUN)/serum creatinine ratio following diuresis is usually a reflection of the rate of diuresis, and not the extent. Hospitalized, massively overloaded patients can usually be diuresed safely, losing approximately 1 kg per day, with slight deterioration in renal function. An increasing serum creatinine predicts a poor outcome in patients hospitalized for heart failure (81). It predicts both prolonged hospitalization and increased mortality. At present, however, it is not known if worsening renal function causes a worse outcome or reflects worse underlying heart failure. Similarly, although BUN predicts a worse outcome, whether this reflects the severity of illness or abnormalities caused by diuresis is not proven (82). At present, an elevated BUN concentration can usually be ignored in such circumstances; the patient is being intentionally intravascularly depleted while being diuresed and there are no proven therapies to prevent adverse outcomes of diuretic therapy. Even a slightly elevated serum creatinine concentration can usually be tolerated. When the patient's weight stabilizes with the resolution of intravascular depletion, the indexes of renal function will generally improve. However, BUN and creatinine concentrations that are elevated from baseline, but stable, are usually tolerated if the resultant fluid status results in improved symptomatology.

Prevention of Complications

Although renal dysfunction usually does not occur with diuretic use, significant increases in serum creatinine concentrations and decreases in glomerular filtration rate can be worrisome. When this occurs, simple measures usually resolve the problem. A slower rate of diuresis is often sufficient. It also may be advisable to limit the use of ACE inhibitors while aggressively diuresing a patient. Patients who develop renal failure with ACE inhibition are usually sodium and volume intravascularly depleted (83), and initiation of ACE inhibitors after the patient is euvolemic may prevent the renal failure that occasionally occurs with the combination of these drugs and diuretics.

The various electrolyte abnormalities that can occur with diuretic use have been discussed, but it is only the potassium concentration, according to general wisdom, that must be kept within the normal range (usually >4.0 mEq/L). Even with aggressive diuresis, this can be accomplished with frequent measurement of serum concentrations and appropriate potassium replacement. Intravenous magnesium is also often given to normalize serum concentrations. Unfortunately, oral magnesium supplements tend to be poorly absorbed and of minimal utility. Methods that counteract the underlying causes of potassium loss may more efficiently and safely prevent hypokalemia as well as other potentially important electrolyte abnormalities.

The potassium-sparing diuretics are not potent but may be very helpful for electrolyte conservation. ACE inhibition may similarly prevent the electrolyte depletion associated with most diuretics. However, the effects of the combined use of these two modalities may be unpredictable and patients need to be followed carefully in such a situation. Although such a combination may be helpful for maintaining a normal potassium concentration in some patients with refractory hypokalemia, it may lead to hyperkalemia in other patients. Spironolactone (and eplerenone) are now commonly used at low doses for their cardiac effects. Higher doses can be used for synergistic diuretic effects, with careful attention paid to serum potassium.

The best means of keeping patients euvolemic would be the avoidance of the causes of fluid and sodium retention. Decreased sodium intake can decrease the need for high doses of diuretics and should be encouraged in all patients, but fluid restriction is rarely beneficial. Although the hyponatremia and fluid overload associated with congestive heart failure make fluid restriction appealing, such an approach is rarely successful. First, the drive to drink water is strong and it is virtually impossible to successfully fluid-restrict a patient. Second, diuresis can be successful without fluid restriction. Third, hyponatremia rarely causes problems and excessive hyponatremia can be successfully treated by modifying the diuretic regimen.

COMPARISONS OF DIURETICS

There are many excellent reviews of the pharmacokinetics and pharmacodynamics of the various diuretic medications (84–86). These are summarized in Table 24-1. Figure 24-2 demonstrates the four areas where these agents work; the efficacy and side effects of most agents can in large part be ascribed to the sites of action of the drugs. However, the efficacy of any particular agent also depends on the particular pharmacokinetics of that agent, and congestive heart failure significantly alters the pharmacokinetics of most medications. Gastrointestinal absorption, volume of distribution, and delivery of the drug to its active site may be altered with congestive heart failure (87). In addition, the efficacy of any agent is limited by the severity of heart failure. Diuresis cannot exceed the filtered sodium level and the renal function is often limited by the multiple physiological alterations that occur in heart failure. Effective use

TABLE 24-1
COMPARISON OF DIURETIC MEDICATIONS LISTED ACCORDING TO SITE OF ACTION

Diuretic	FENa$^+$ (max, %)	Dosage (mg/day)	Onset of Action		Action Duration		Peak Oral Effect (h)	Comments
			Oral (h)	IV (min)	Oral (h)	IV (h)		
Ascending loop of Henle								
Furosemide	20–25	40–400	1	5	6–8	2–3	1–3	
Bumetanide	20–25	1–5	0.5	5	4–6	4–6	1–3	
Torsemide	20–25	10–200	1	10	6–8	6–8	1–3	
Ethacrynic acid	20–25	50–100	0.5	5	6–8	3	2	High ototoxicity risk, but (unlike other loop diuretics) can be used in sulfa-allergic patients
Early Distal Tubule								
Metolazone	5–8	2.5–20	1	—	12–24	—	2–4	Greatest potential for potassium loss; also slight actions in proximal tubule
Chlorthalidone	5–10	25–200	2	—	24–48	—	6	Ineffective when GFR <30
Hydrochlorothiazide	5–8	25–100	2	—	12	—	4	Ineffective when GFR <30
Chlorothiazide	5–8	500–1,000	1	15–30	8	—	4	Ineffective when GFR <30
Late Distal Tubule								
Spironolactone	2	50–400	48–72	—	48–72	—	1–2 days	Efficacy dependent on aldosterone presence
Triamterene	2	75–300	2	—	12–16	—	6–8	
Amiloride	2	5–10	2	—	24	—	6–16	
Proximal Tubule								
Acetazolamide	4	250–375	1	30–60	8	3–4	2–4	Efficacy limited by the metabolic acidosis it causes

FENa$^+$ (max, %), maximal natriuretic effect (maximum fractional excretion of filtered sodium); GFR, glomerular filtration rate.

of diuretics in patients with congestive heart failure mandates knowledge of the actions of the drugs in these particular patients.

The loop diuretics are the agents most frequently used in patients with heart failure because of efficacy and potency, and there appear to be minimal clinically significant differences between furosemide, bumetanide, and torsemide (88,89). However, inadequate doses of these agents are often prescribed in heart failure patients. Because loop diuretics are secreted in the proximal tubule and act from the luminal side of the loop of Henle, increasing doses of these drugs are needed as glomerular filtration rate decreases. The effective doses of these agents in normal individuals, therefore, are often inadequate in patients with heart failure who frequently exhibit decreased renal function. Physicians should not hesitate to use doses at the upper end of the therapeutic range in patients refractory to lower doses. Comparisons of loop diuretics are problematic, as it is difficult to know what are comparable doses. Thus, the implications of a study that showed increased efficacy with torsemide (as compared to furosemide) are uncertain (90). Similarly, it is difficult to know if a small study that showed less fibrosis with torsemide reflects true differences between diuretics on neurohormonal activation and fibrosis (91).

There are other reasons why high doses of loop diuretics may be needed in patients with heart failure. Contrary to popular belief, it appears as if the total bioavailability of the drugs is the same in these individuals as in normal controls, but the time course of oral absorption may vary (88). Therefore, poor absorption is not the mechanism of decreased activity of diuretic medications in heart failure. Rather, the increased time of absorption can result in lower peak plasma concentrations of loop diuretics in some patients and high oral doses of the agents may be needed to achieve a therapeutic effect. The lower peak serum concentration, however, indicates that the risk of ototoxicity from a large oral dose of loop diuretics given to a patient with heart failure is no higher than a lower dose given to a normal individual. In contrast, a big dose when given intravenously will result in higher peak concentrations as well as both increased efficacy and increased risk of toxicity.

Alterations in pharmacokinetics of loop diuretics in fluid-overloaded patients is probably less frequent than is generally assumed. We have documented that marked diuresis alters the pharmacokinetics of both furosemide and torsemide in only a small percentage of patients. Although the time to maximum concentration decreased following diuresis, the maximum concentration did not

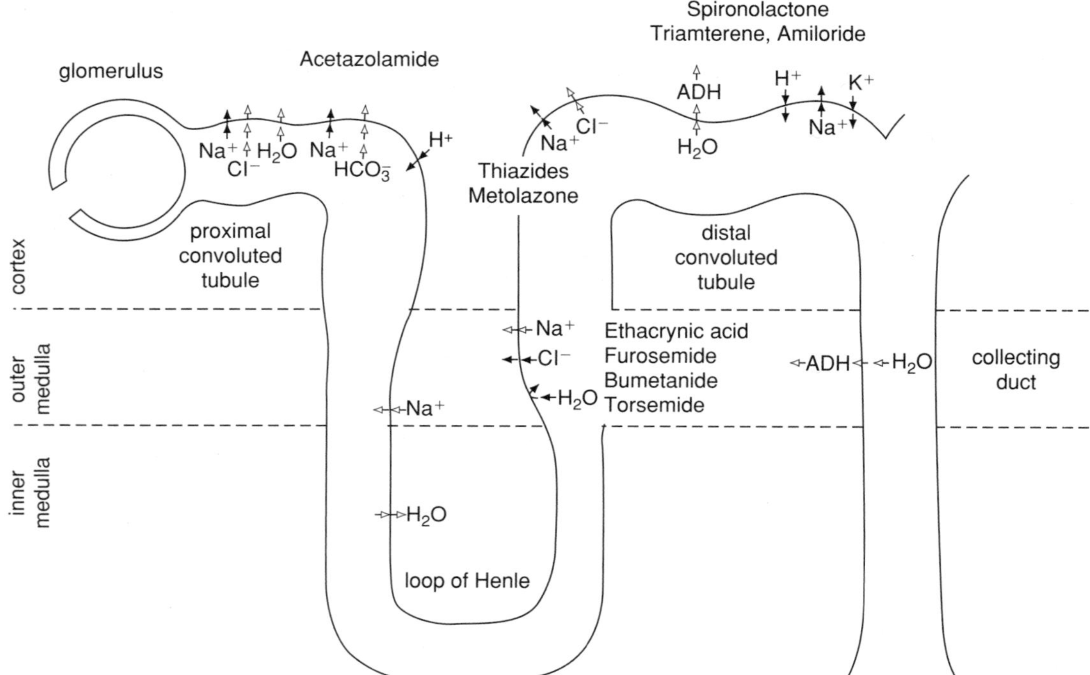

Figure 24-2 Fluid and electrolyte transport within the nephron, with sites of action of most commonly used diuretics. The **solid arrow** indicates active transport, and the **open arrow** indicates passive reabsorption. (Adapted from Puschett JB. Physiologic basis for the use of new and older diuretics in congestive heart failure. *Cardiovasc Med.* 1977;2:119–134.)

change in most patients (89). This suggests that the use of adequate doses of oral diuretics in edematous patients may be successful, thereby permitting home treatment with oral diuretics and avoiding the cost of hospitalizations or home intravenous administration services.

The mechanism of action of loop diuretics means that treatment of heart failure, which often increases renal flow and the clearance of the drug, may increase the efficacy of diuretic medications; the ability of the direct-acting vasodilator hydralazine to increase furosemide clearance and diuresis has indeed been demonstrated (92). Diuretic doses should be evaluated and adjusted frequently when the patient's overall status and fluid state are changing.

The thiazides are rarely used in patients with heart failure, for a number of reasons. First and foremost, they are not as potent as the loop diuretics and therefore are not desirable when extensive diuresis is necessary. Second, renal clearance decreases in patients with congestive heart failure (93), and thiazides are ineffective when the glomerular filtration rate is below approximately 30 mL per minute. Third, thiazide diuretics cause a greater decrease in potassium than loop diuretics for the same quantity of diuresis (39).

Spironolactone is not a potent diuretic, partially because its actions are countered by a compensatory increase in aldosterone concentration (94). Other potassium-sparing agents are therefore often used when a potent agent is desired. However, the consequences of the antagonism of aldosterone by spironolactone may be important in many ways. Spironolactone conserves potassium; it can help maintain serum potassium concentration in a patient who excretes a large quantity of the electrolyte. Like other potassium-sparing agents, it is also often used for its synergistic effects when combined with other diuretic medications. Not only does spironolactone limit potassium excretion, it also reportedly prevents the exacerbation of hypokalemia, which is normally associated with epinephrine infusion (37). Spironolactone also may be able to prevent digoxin toxicity, not only by conserving potassium but also perhaps by directly countering the actions of digoxin (95). A metabolite of spironolactone, canrenone, may even have direct effects on the sodium-potassium pump (96). Spironolactone also has been reported to decrease digoxin clearance but many of these reports may be secondary to interference in the assay, and increased digoxin levels have not always been found following spironolactone administration (97). More important are the direct cardiac effects that probably led to the mortality benefit seen in RALES (Randomized Aldactone Evaluation Study) (98).

The toxicities of the commonly used diuretic agents are listed in Table 24-2. Some, such as the effects on acid–base status and potassium, are avoidable if the patient is observed carefully and diuretic dosage adjusted as necessary. Others are more rare, but the potential of diuretics to cause these problems needs to be remembered.

COMBINATION OF DIURETICS

It is often difficult to attain effective diuresis in patients with heart failure. The physiological stimulus to retain fluid may be strong enough to overwhelm the diuretic

TABLE 24-2
COMMON TOXICITIES ASSOCIATED WITH DIURETIC USE

Hypersensitivity Reactions
Various skin rashes (most agents)
Interstitial nephritis (furosemide, thiazides)
Pancreatitis (thiazides)
Deafness
Loop diuretics
Renal Calculi
Acetazolamide
Triamterene
Hyperuricemia, Gout
Thiazides
Loop diuretics
Gynecomastia
Spironolactone
Carbohydrate Intolerance
Thiazides
Furosemide, bumetanide
Potassium Abnormalities
Hypokalemia (loop diuretics, thiazides)
Hyperkalemia (spironolactone, triamterene, amiloride)
Acid–base Abnormalities
Acidosis (acetazolamide, spironolactone, triamterene, amiloride)
Alkalosis (loop diuretics, thiazides)

Adapted from Dirks JH, Sutton RAL, eds. *Diuretics: Physiology, Pharmacology, and Clinical Use*. Philadelphia: WB Saunders; 1986.

actions of any single agent. Thus, potent diuretics (such as the loop diuretics) may be rendered ineffective by distal reabsorption. In contrast, agents that act distally, such as potassium-sparing agents, may not be potent enough to yield the desired results. In such patients, the synergistic effects of combining diuretics can have many beneficial consequences.

The combination of loop diuretics and metolazone has proven to be particularly potent (99–101). With the combined use of these agents, effective diuresis may be produced in patients who have been resistant to other interventions. However, it may take days to see the results of the addition of metolazone because of the pharmacokinetics of the drug. It is also important to realize that the hypokalemia resulting from the combined use of loop diuretics and metolazone may be severe; serum potassium concentrations need to be watched especially carefully in these patients. The other useful method of combining diuretics is to add a potassium-sparing agent to the diuretic regimen. Not only does this potentiate the diuretic actions of the original regimen, it also prevents extreme potassium loss and simplifies electrolyte management.

OTHER METHODS

Because fluid retention develops from the abnormal hemodynamic status of patients with heart failure, enhancement of that status is an obvious means of improving diuresis. Inotropes are often used in patients with poor renal function and fluid overload, even though their routine use in hospitalized patients with heart failure has been shown to not be beneficial (102). The data concerning low-dose dopamine are contradictory. While some studies suggest renal benefit, increased renal function could be secondary to increased cardiac function. Indeed, a recent meta-analysis demonstrated no improvement in mortality, prevention of acute renal failure, or need for dialysis when dopamine was given in various patient groups (103).

Continuous infusions of loop diuretics have been advocated (104,105) but other studies have shown no differences in efficacy of intermittent and continuous furosemide administration (106,107). Although continuous infusion can certainly be tried in patients with inadequate diuresis to bolus administration, the prolonged half-life of these agents in heart failure minimizes the potential advantages. In fact, the elimination half-life of loop diuretics is increased two to three times in patients with heart failure as compared with normal individuals. However, a continuous infusion is often used for convenience (as opposed to repeated bolus dosing) and can eliminate the time after the diuretic is excreted and metabolized when compensatory sodium and fluid retention occur.

When all else fails, ultrafiltration may improve the fluid status of a patient. Perhaps the many actions of diuresis on cardiac performance and neurohormones explain the reports of the chronic benefit of this intervention. Ultrafiltration is discussed further in another chapter.

Nesiritide is a vasodilator approved for the use in patients with congestive heart failure for symptomatic relief and hemodynamic improvement. Its renal effects, however, are questionable. The pivotal VMAC (Vasodilation in the Management of Acute CHF) trial, for example, showed no increase in urine output in patients receiving nesiritide (although lower doses of furosemide were given) (108). In a randomized, placebo-controlled crossover trial, there was no improvement in glomerular filtration rate, renal plasma flow, urine output, or sodium excretion in hospitalized patients with increasing creatinine either when nesiritide was first given or after a 24-hour infusion (109).

There are other studies that suggest that nesiritide may actually decrease renal function. A retrospective analysis from the Cleveland Clinic showed a 15% incidence of a decreased glomerular filtration rate of at least 50% in patients who received nesiritide (110). A meta-analysis of randomized studies showed a higher incidence of renal dysfunction in patients receiving the drug (111). While the renal actions of nesiritide are still unclear, it is likely that the lower blood pressure caused by nesiritide may lead to worsening renal function in at least some patients.

INVESTIGATIONAL AGENTS

Investigation of the cause of water retention in patients with heart failure has long focused on neurohormonal activation. It is thus not surprising that various neurohormonal antagonists are being studied as possible effective and safe diuretics. For example, a nonpeptide arginine vasopressin selective

V_2 receptor antagonist increased urine flow while increasing serum sodium concentration in patients with congestive heart failure (112). Similarly, dual V_{1A} and V_2 vasopressin receptor antagonists appear to acutely increase urine output in patients with heart failure (113). The chronic effects are less clear. In an animal model, there was marked aquaretic effects of a selective V_2 vasopressin antagonist and continued aquaresis with chronic administration. However, the chronic effects were clearly and markedly decreased from the acute effects. Perhaps more importantly, however, the animals increased their fluid intake to match the aquaresis, leading to no decrease in weight (114). In a study of heart failure patients, the diuretic effect of another V_2 antagonist, tolvaptan, was decreased after the first dose. While a weight lower than baseline continued through hospitalization, by 60 days there was no difference between patients receiving active drug and those receiving placebo (115). Vasopressin antagonists acutely appear to limit the need for conventional diuretics. Whether this will be of long-term benefit needs to be evaluated.

The possible importance of adenosine as an important regulator of renal function has been recognized. Plasma adenosine concentrations are increased in patients with congestive heart failure (116), and adenosine has been shown to decrease renal blood flow (by increasing vasoconstriction in resistance arteries) in these patients (80). Adenosine A_1 antagonists may increase both glomerular filtration rate and urine flow in healthy individuals (117) and they have started to be evaluated in patients with heart failure. There is preliminary information that an A_1 antagonist can lead to mild diuresis without decreasing renal function. Perhaps more importantly, when combined with furosemide, the antagonist appeared to have an additive diuretic effect without causing any decrease in renal dysfunction (118). If this proves to be true, the control of volume without an adverse effect on renal dysfunction would be an important addition to the treatments available to physicians taking care of heart failure patients.

CONCLUSIONS

Diuretic medications are valuable tools in our armamentarium for the treatment of congestive heart failure. They acutely improve symptoms and cardiac performance by multiple mechanisms. However, their chronic ramifications have not been adequately evaluated. Neurohormonal, electrolytic, and renal effects may have unintended consequences. Increased study and application of the results of these studies to the clinical arena should provide a more rational approach to the magnitude of diuresis and choice of diuretics prescribed for patients with congestive heart failure.

REFERENCES

1. Achhammer I, Podszuz T. Effect of furosemide on pulmonary and cardiac haemodynamics after treatment of chronic heart failure. In: Puschett JB, Greenberg A, eds. *Diuretics III: Chemistry, Pharmacology, and Clinical Applications*. New York: Elsevier Science; 1990: 331–333.
2. Stampfer M, Epstein SE, Beiser GD, et al. Hemodynamic effects of diuresis at rest and during intense upright exercise in patients with impaired cardiac function. *Circulation*. 1968;37:900–911.
3. Dikshit K, Vyden JK, Forrester JS, et al. Renal and extrarenal hemodynamic effects of furosemide in congestive heart failure after acute myocardial infarction. *N Engl J Med*. 1973;288: 1087–1090.
4. Francis GS, Siegel RM, Goldsmith SR, et al. Acute vasoconstrictor response to intravenous furosemide in patients with chronic congestive heart failure. *Ann Intern Med*. 1985;103:1–6.
5. Biddle TL, Yu PN. Effect of furosemide on hemodynamics and lung water in acute pulmonary edema secondary to myocardial infarction. *Am J Cardiol*. 1979;43:86–90.
6. Hutcheon D, Nemeth E, Quinlan D. The role of furosemide alone or in combination with digoxin in the relief of symptoms of congestive heart failure. *J Clin Pharmacol*. 1980;20:59–68.
7. Wilson JR, Reichek N, Dunkman WB, et al. Effect of diuresis on the performance of the failing left ventricle in man. *Am J Med*. 1981;70:234–239.
8. Perloff JK, Roberts WC. The mitral apparatus: functional anatomy and mitral regurgitation. *Circulation*. 1972;46: 227–239.
9. Stevenson LW, Dadourian BJ, Child JS, et al. Mitral regurgitation after cardiac transplantation. *Am J Cardiol*. 1987;60:119–122.
10. Stevenson LW, Brunken RC, Belil D, et al. Afterload reduction with vasodilators and diuretics decreases mitral regurgitation during upright exercise in advanced heart failure. *J Am Coll Cardiol*. 1990;15:174–180.
11. Ramirez A, Abelmann WH. Hemodynamic effects of diuresis by ethacrynic acid. *Arch Intern Med*. 1968;121:320–326.
12. MacGregor CD, Covell JW, Mahler F, et al. Relations between afterload, stroke volume, and the descending limb of Starling's curve. *Am J Physiol*. 1975;227:884–890.
13. Ross J, Jr., Sonnenblick EH, Taylor RR, et al. Diastolic geometry and sarcomere length in the chronically dilated canine left ventricle. *Circ Res*. 1971;28:49–61.
14. Nechwatal W, Stange A, Sigel H, et al. Der Einfluss von Piretanid auf die zentrale Hamodynamik und Belastungstoleranz von Patienten mit angina pectoris. *Herz Kreislauf*. 1982;14:91–96.
15. Ross J Jr. The assessment of myocardial performance in man by hemodynamic and cineangiographic technics. *Am J Cardiol*. 1969;23:511–515.
16. McCurley JM, Hanlon SU, Wei SK, et al. Furosemide and the progression of left ventricular dysfunction in experimental heart failure. *J Am Coll Cardiol*. 2004;44:1301–1307.
17. Keeton TK, Campbell WB. The pharmacologic alteration of renin release. *Pharmacol Rev*. 1980;32:81–227.
18. Broqvist M, Dahlstrom U, Karlberg BE, et al. Neuroendocrine response in acute heart failure and the influence of treatment. *Eur Heart J*. 1989;10:1075–1083.
19. Francis GS, Benedict C, Johnstone DE, et al. for the SOLVD Investigators. Comparison of neuroendocrine activation in patients with left ventricular dysfunction with and without congestive heart failure: a substudy of the Studies of Left Ventricular Dysfunction (SOLVD). *Circulation*. 1990;82:1724–1729.
20. Bayliss J, Norell M, Canepa-Anson R, et al. Untreated heart failure: clinical and neuroendocrine effects of increasing diuretics. *Br Heart J*. 1987;57:17–22.
21. Verho M, Heintz B, Nelson K, et al. The effects of piretanide on catecholamine metabolism, plasma renin activity and plasma aldosterone: a double-blind study versus furosemide in healthy volunteers. *Curr Med Res Opin*. 1985;7:461–467.
22. Knight RK, Miall PA, Hawkins LA, Dacombe J, Edwards CRW, Hamer J. Relation of plasma aldosterone concentration to diuretic treatment in patients with severe heart disease. *Br Heart J*. 1979;42:316–325.
23. Weber KT, Brilla CG. Pathological hypertrophy and cardiac interstitium: fibrosis and renin-angiotensin-aldosterone system. *Circulation*. 1991;83:1849–1865.
24. Bayliss PH, DeBeer FC. Human plasma vasopressin response to potent loop-diuretic drugs. *Eur J Clin Pharmacol*. 1981; 20:343–346.
25. Genest J. The atrial natriuretic factor. *Br Heart J*. 1986;56: 302–316.
26. Edwards BS, Zimmerman RS, Burnett JC. Jr. Atrial natriuretic factor: physiologic actions and implications in congestive heart failure. *Cardiovasc Drugs Ther*. 1987;1:89–100.

27. Schiffrin EL. Decreased density for binding sites of atrial natriuretic peptide on platelets of patients with severe congestive heart failure. *Clin Sci*. 1988;74:213–218.
28. Gottlieb SS, Kukin ML, Ahern D, et al. Prognostic importance of atrial natriuretic peptide in patients with chronic heart failure. *J Am Coll Cardiol*. 1989;13:1534–1539.
29. Riegger GAJ, Elsner D, Kromer EP, et al. Atrial natriuretic peptide in congestive heart failure in the dog: plasma levels, cyclic guanosine monophosphate, ultrastructure of atrial myoendocrine cells, and hemodynamic, hormonal, and renal effects. *Circulation*. 1988;77:398–406.
30. Johnston GD, Hiatt WR, Nies AS, et al. Factors modifying the early non-diuretic vascular effects of furosemide in man. *Circ Res*. 1983;53:630–635.
31. Green TP, Thompson TR, Johnson DE, et al. Furosemide promotes patent ductus arteriosus in premature infants with the respiratory distress syndrome. *N Engl J Med*. 1983;308: 743–748.
32. Dorian B, Larrue J, Defeudis FV, et al. Activation of prostacyclin synthesis in cultured aortic smooth muscle cells by diuretic-antihypertensive drugs. *Biochem Biophys Res Commun*. 1984;33: 2265–2269.
33. Multher RS, Potter DM, Bennett WM. Aspirin-induced depression of glomerular filtration rate in normal humans: role of sodium balance. *Ann Intern Med*. 1981;94:317–321.
34. Kao W, Gheorghiade M, Hall V, et al. Relation between plasma norepinephrine and response to medical therapy in congestive heart failure secondary to coronary artery disease or idiopathic dilated cardiomyopathy. *Am J Cardiol*. 1989;64: 609–613.
35. Packer M, Lee WH, Kessler PD, et al. Role of neurohormonal mechanisms in determining survival in patients with severe chronic heart failure. *Circulation*. 1987;75:IV80–IV92.
36. Abraham AS, Meshulam Z, Rosenmann D, et al. Influence of chronic diuretic therapy on serum, lymphocyte and erythrocyte potassium, magnesium and calcium concentrations. *Cardiology*. 1988;75:17–23.
37. Whyte KF, Whitesmith R, Reid JL. The effect of diuretic therapy on adrenaline-induced hypokalemia and hypomagnesemia. *Eur J Clin Pharmacol*. 1988;34:333–337.
38. Lipworth BJ, McDevitt DG, Struthers AD. Prior treatment with diuretic augments the hypokalemic and electrocardiographic effects of inhaled albuterol. *Am J Med*. 1989;86:653–657.
39. Morgan DB, Davidson C. Hypokalemia and diuretics: an analysis of publications. *Br Med J*. 1980;280:905–908.
40. Papademetriou V, Burris JF, Notargiacomo A, et al. Thiazide therapy is not a cause of arrhythmia in patients with systemic hypertension. *Arch Intern Med*. 1988;148:1272–1276.
41. Roden DM, Hoffman BF. Action potential prolongation and induction of abnormal automaticity by low quinidine concentrations in canine Purkinje fibers: relationship of potassium and cycle length. *Circ Res*. 1985;56:857–867.
42. Steiness E, Olesen KH. Cardiac arrhythmias induced by hypokalemia and potassium loss during maintenance digoxin therapy. *Br Heart J*. 1976;38:167–172.
43. Dyckner T, Helmers C, Lundman T, et al. Initial serum potassium level in relation to early complications and prognosis in patients with acute myocardial infarction. *Acta Med Scand*. 1975;197:207–210.
44. Pelleg A, Mitamura H, Price R, et al. Extracellular potassium ion dynamics and ventricular arrhythmias in the canine heart. *J Am Coll Cardiol*. 1989;13:941–950.
45. Packer M, Lee WH. Provocation of hyper- and hypokalemic sudden death during treatment with and withdrawal of converting enzyme inhibition in severe chronic congestive heart failure. *Am J Cardiol*. 1986;57:347–348.
46. Gottlieb SS. Importance of magnesium in congestive heart failure. *Am J Cardiol*. 1989;63:39G–42G.
47. Ralston MA, Murnane MR, Kelley RE, et al. Magnesium content of serum, circulating mononuclear cells, skeletal muscle, and myocardium in congestive heart failure. *Circulation*. 1989;80: 573–580.
48. Dorup I, Skajaa K, Clausen T, et al. Reduced concentrations of potassium, magnesium, and sodium-potassium pumps in human skeletal muscle during treatment with diuretics. *BMJ*. 1988;296:455–458.
49. Lim P, Jacob E. Magnesium deficiency in patients on long-term diuretic therapy for heart failure. *BMJ*. 1972;3:60–62.
50. Mulder H, Schopman W, van der Lely AJ, et al. Acute change in plasma renin activity, plasma aldosterone concentration and plasma electrolyte concentrations following furosemide administration in patients with congestive heart failure—interrelationships and diuretic response. *Horm Metab Res*. 1987;19:80–83.
51. Girchev RA, Natcheff ND. Excretory function after renal denervation and administration of diuretic to unanesthetized dogs. *Biomed Biochim Acta*. 1988;6:507–514.
52. Sheehan J, White A. Diuretic-associated hypomagnesemia. *BMJ*. 1982;285:1157–1159.
53. Polimeni PI, Page E. Magnesium in heart muscle. *Circ Res*. 1973;33:367–374.
54. Dagirmanjian R, Goldman H. Magnesium deficiency and distribution of blood in the rat. *Am J Physiol*. 1970;218:1464–1467.
55. Ghani MF, Rabah M. Effect of magnesium chloride on electrical stability of the heart. *Am Heart J*. 1977;94:600–602.
56. Flink EB. Hypomagnesemia in patients receiving digitalis. *Arch Intern Med*. 1985;145:625–626.
57. Bailie DS, Inoue H, Kaseda S, et al. Magnesium suppression of early afterdepolarizations and ventricular tachyarrhythmias induced by cesium in dogs. *Circulation*. 1988;6:1395–1402.
58. Iseri LT, Freed J, Bures AR. Magnesium deficiency and cardiac disorders. *Am J Med*. 1975;58:837–846.
59. Ramee SR, White CJ, Svinarich JT, et al. Torsades des pointe and magnesium deficiency. *Am Heart J*. 1985;109:823–828.
60. White RE, Hartzell HC. Magnesium ions in cardiac function: regulator of ion channels and second messengers. *Biochem Pharmacol*. 1989;38:859–867.
61. Shils ME. Experimental human magnesium deficiency. *Medicine*. 1969;48:61–85.
62. Gottlieb SS, Baruch L, Kukin ML, et al. Prognostic importance of the serum magnesium concentration in patients with congestive heart failure. *J Am Coll Cardiol*. 1990;16:827–831.
63. Ralston MA, Murnane MR, Unverferth DV, et al. Serum and tissue magnesium concentrations in patients with heart failure and serious ventricular arrhythmias. *Ann Intern Med*. 1990;113:841–846.
64. Anand IS, Ferrari R, Kalra GS, et al. Edema of cardiac origin. Studies of body water and sodium, renal function, hemodynamic indexes, and plasma hormones in untreated congestive cardiac failure. *Circulation*. 1989;80:299–305.
65. Gross P, Ketteler M, Hausmann C, et al. Role of diuretics, hormonal derangements, and clinical setting of hyponatremia in medical patients. *Klin Wochenschr*. 1988;66:662–669.
66. Kennedy RM, Earley LE. Profound hyponatremia resulting from a thiazide-induced decrease in urinary diluting capacity in a patient with primary polydypsia. *N Engl J Med*. 1970;282: 1185–1186.
67. Schrier RW, Berl T, Anderson RJ. Osmotic and nonosmotic control of vasopressin release. *Am J Physiol*. 1979;236:F321–F332.
68. Dzau VJ, Hollenberg NK. Renal response to captopril in severe heart failure: role of furosemide in natriuresis and reversal of hyponatremia. *Ann Intern Med*. 1984;100:777–782.
69. Lee WH, Packer M. Prognostic importance of serum sodium concentration and its modification by converting-enzyme inhibition in patients with severe chronic heart failure. *Circulation* 1986;73:257–267.
70. White MG, van Gelder J, Estes G. The effect of loop diuretics on the excretion of Na^+, Ca^{2+}, Mg^{2+}, and Cl^-. *J Clin Pharmacol*. 1981;21:610–614.
71. Breslau N, Moses AM, Weiner IM. The role of volume contraction in the hypocalciuric action of chlorothiazide. *Kidney Int*. 1976;10:164–170.
72. Marone C, Muggli F, Lahn W, et al. Pharmacokinetic and pharmacodynamic interaction between furosemide and metolazone in man. *Eur J Clin Invest*. 1985;15:253–257.
73. Bristow MR, Schwartz HD, Binetti G, et al. Ionized calcium and the heart: elucidation of *in vivo* concentration-response relationships in the open-chest dog. *Circ Res*. 1977;41:565–574.
74. Ginsburg R, Esserman LJ, Bristow MR. Myocardial performance and extracellular ionized calcium in a severely failing human heart. *Ann Intern Med*. 1983;98:603–606.
75. Agostoni P, Marenzi G, Lauri G, et al. Sustained improvement in functional capacity after removal of body fluid with isolated ultrafiltration in chronic cardiac insufficiency: failure

of furosemide to provide the same result. *Am J Med.* 1994; 96:191–199.
76. Ring-Larsen H, Henriksen JH, Wilken C, et al. Diuretic treatment in decompensated cirrhosis and congestive heart failure: effect of posture. *BMJ.* 1986; 292:1351–1353.
77. Schuster CJ, Weil MH, Besso J, et al. Blood volume following diuresis induced by furosemide. *Am J Med.* 1984;76:585–592.
78. Hook JB, Blatt AH, Brody MJ, et al. Effects of several saluretic-diuretic agents on renal hemodynamics. *J Pharmacol Exp Ther.* 1966;154:667–673.
79. Kim KE, Onesti G, Moyer J, et al. Ethacrynic acid and furosemide: diuretic and hemodynamic effects and clinical uses. *Am J Cardiol.* 1971;27:407–415.
80. Elkayam U, Mehra A, Cohen G, et al. Renal circulatory effects of adenosine in patients with chronic heart failure. *J Am Coll Cardiol.* 1998;32:211–215.
81. Gottlieb SS, Abraham W, Butler J, et al. The prognostic importance of different definitions of worsening renal function in congestive heart failure. *J Card Fail.* 2002; 8:136–141.
82. Fonarow GC, Adams KF, Jr., Abraham WT, et al., ADHERE Scientific Advisory Committee, Study Group, and Investigators. Risk stratification for in-hospital mortality in acutely decompensated heart failure: classification and regression tree analysis. *JAMA.* 2005;293:572–580.
83. Hricik DE. Captopril-induced renal insufficiency and the role of sodium balance. *Ann Intern Med.* 1985;103:222–223.
84. Sica DA, Gehr T. Diuretics in congestive heart failure. *Cardiol Clin.* 1989;7:87–96.
85. Brater DC. Pharmacology of diuretics. *Am J Med Sci.* 2000;319:38–50.
86. Dirks JH, Sutton RAL, eds. *Diuretics: Physiology, Pharmacology, and Clinical Use.* Philadelphia: WB Saunders; 1986.
87. Tilstone WJ, Dargie H, Dargie EN, et al. Pharmacokinetics of metolazone in normal subjects and in patients with cardiac or renal failure. *Clin Pharmacol Ther.* 1976;16:322–329.
88. Brater DC, Day B, Burdette A, et al. Bumetanide and furosemide in heart failure. *Kidney Int.* 1984;26:183–189.
89. Gottlieb SS, Khatta M, Wentworth D, et al. The effects of diuresis on the pharmacokinetics of the loop diuretics furosemide and torsemide in patients with heart failure. *Am J Med.* 1998;104: 533–538.
90. Cosín J, Díez J. Torasemide in chronic heart failure: results of the TORIC study. *Eur J Heart Fail.* 2002;4:507–513.
91. Lopez B, Querejeta R, Gonzalez A, et al. Effects of loop diuretics on myocardial fibrosis and collagen type I turnover in chronic heart failure. *J Am Coll Cardiol.* 2004;43:2028–2035.
92. Nomura A, Yasuda H, Minami M, et al. Effect of furosemide in congestive heart failure. *Clin Pharmacol Ther.* 1981;30:177–182.
93. Beermann B, Groschinsky-Grind M. Pharmacokinetics of hydrochlorothiazide in patients with congestive heart failure. *Br J Clin Pharmacol.* 1979;7:579–583.
94. Nicholls MG, Espiner EA, Hughes H, et al. Effect of potassium-sparing diuretics on the renin-angiotensin-aldosterone system and potassium retention in heart failure. *Br Heart J.* 1976;38: 1025–1039.
95. Waldorff S, Hansen PB, Egeblad H, et al. Interactions between digoxin and potassium-sparing diuretics. *Clin Pharmacol Ther.* 1983;33:418–423.
96. Garay RP, Diez J, Nazaret C, et al. The interaction of canrenone with the Na^+, K^+ pump in human red blood cells. *Arch Pharmacol.* 1985;329:311–315.
97. Finnegan TP, Spence JD, Cape RD. Potassium sparing diuretics: interaction with digoxin in elderly men. *J Am Geriatr Soc.* 1984;32:129–131.
98. Pitt B, Zannad F, Remme WJ, et al. The effect of spironolactone on morbidity and mortality in patients with severe heart failure. *N Engl J Med.* 1999;341:709–717.
99. Kiyingi A, Field MJ, Pawsel CC, et al. Metolazone in treatment of severe refractory congestive heart failure. *Lancet* 1990;335:29–31.
100. Ghose RR, Gupta SK. Synergistic actions of metolazone with "loop" diuretics. *BMJ.* 1981;812:1432–1433.
101. Channer KS, McLean KA, Lawson-Matthew P, et al. Combination diuretic treatment in severe heart failure: a randomized controlled trial. *Br Heart J.* 1994;71:146–150.
102. Cuffe MS, Califf RM, Adams KF, Jr., et al. Short-term intravenous milrinone for acute exacerbation of chronic heart failure: a randomized controlled trial. *JAMA.* 2002;287,:1541–1547.
103. Kellum JA, M Decker J. Use of dopamine in acute renal failure: a meta-analysis. *Crit Care Med.* 2001;29:1526–1531.
104. Lawson DH, Gray JMB, Henry DA, et al. Continuous infusion of furosemide in refractory oedema. *BMJ.*1978;2:476.
105. Dormans TP, van Meyel JJ, Gerlag PG, et al. Diuretic efficacy of high dose furosemide in severe heart failure: bolus injection versus continuous infusion. *J Am Coll Cardiol.* 1996;28: 376–382.
106. Schuller D, Lynch JP, Fine D. Protocol-guided diuretic management: comparison of furosemide by continuous infusion and intermittent bolus. *Crit Care Med.* 1997;25:1969–1975.
107. Aaser E, Gullestad L, Tollofsrud S, et al. Effect of bolus injection versus continuous infusion of furosemide on diuresis and neurohormonal activation in patients with severe congestive heart failure. *Scand J Clin Lab Invest.* 1997;57:361–367.
108. Publication Committee for the VMAC Investigators. Intravenous nesiritide vs nitroglycerin for treatment of decompensated congestive heart failure: a randomized controlled trial. *JAMA.* 2002;287:1531–1540.
109. Wang DJ, Dowling TC, Meadows D, et al. Nesiritide does not improve renal function in patients with chronic heart failure and worsening serum creatinine. *Circulation.* 2004;110:1620–1625.
110. Tang WHW, Barcelona R, Young JB, et al. Hypotension associated with nesiritide infusion in patients with decompensated heart failure is related to large volume diuresis: implications for monitoring and dose adjustments. *J Am Coll Cardiol.* 2004;43(5 Suppl A):192A.
111. Sackner-Bernstein JD, Skopicki HA, Aaronson KD. Risk of worsening renal function with nesiritide in patients with acutely decompensated heart failure. *Circulation.* 2005;111:1487–1491.
112. Abraham WT, Oren TS, Crisman TS, et al. Effects of an oral, non-peptide, selective V_2 receptor vasopressin antagonist in patients with chronic heart failure. *J Am Coll Cardiol.* 1997;29:169A.
113. Udelson JE, Smith WB, Hendrix GH, et al. Acute hemodynamic effects of conivaptan, a dual V(1A) and V(2) vasopressin receptor antagonist, in patients with advanced heart failure. *Circulation.* 2001;104:2417–2423.
114. Lacour C, Galindo G, Canals F, et al, Aquaretic and hormonal effects of a vasopressin V(2) receptor antagonist after acute and long-term treatment in rats. *Eur J Pharmacol.* 2000;394:131–138.
115. Gheorghiade M, Gattis WA, O'Connor CM, et al. Effects of tolvaptan, a vasopressin antagonist, in patients hospitalized with worsening heart failure: a randomized controlled trial. *JAMA.* 2004;291:1963–1971.
116. Funaya H, Kitakaze M, Node K, et al. Plasma adenosine levels increase in patients with chronic heart failure. *Circulation.* 1997;95:1363–1365.
117. Balakrishnan VS, Coles GA, Williams JD. A potential role for endogenous adenosine in control of human glomerular and tubular function. *Am J Physiol.* 1993;265:F504–F510.
118. Gottlieb SS, Brater DC, Thomas I, et al. BG9719 (CVT-124), an A_1 adenosine receptor antagonist, protects against the decline in renal function observed with diuretic therapy. *Circulation.* 2002;105:1348–1353.
119. Puschett JB. Physiologic basis for the use of new and older diuretics in congestive heart failure. *Cardiovasc Med.* 1977; 2:119–134.

Digitalis Glycosides

25

Paul J. Hauptman *Ralph A. Kelly*

HISTORICAL PERSPECTIVES

Cardiac glycosides have played a prominent role in the therapy of congestive heart failure since William Withering codified their use in his classic monograph on the efficacy of the leaves of the common foxglove plant (*Digitalis purpurea*) in 1785. Nevertheless, a controversy has existed about whether the risks of digitalis preparations outweigh their benefits, particularly in patients with heart failure in sinus rhythm (1). The standard for clinical use of the cardiac glycosides in modern medicine was reflected in a debate between two eminent clinicians, who were also the co-editors of *The Oxford Medicine*, Henry Christian and James Mackenzie. Mackenzie advocated the use of digitalis preparations only in those patients with heart failure who also had atrial arrhythmias, prompting the following response from Christian (2):

> My views evidently differ from those of my fellow editor of the *Oxford Medicine*. The views of Sir James MacKenzie have been concurred in by numerous observers, with the result that there is a growing feeling that, unless the pulse is absolutely irregular and rapid, little is to be gained from digitalis therapy. My own experience is so directly contrary to this that is seems worthwhile to restate the views already expressed by me. . . . My own view with regard to digitalis, as a rule, is that it has a striking effect on those changes in the patient which are brought on by cardiac insufficiency, and this effect appears irrespective of whether or not the pulse is irregular.

Within the United States, at least, Christian's views prevailed until several retrospective and uncontrolled trials in the 1970s pointed to a lack of efficacy of digitalis preparations in many patients for whom they were prescribed. This debate became more relevant with the availability of other less-toxic remedies for heart failure, most notably the introduction of loop diuretics in the 1960s, the development of new classes of vasodilators in the 1980s, and the advent of the β-adrenergic antagonists (β-blockers) in the 1990s. Although a number of prospective controlled trials (discussed in detail later) that document the safety and efficacy of digitalis in patients with moderate and severe congestive heart failure have been published, controversy over the role of digoxin gained intensity with the recognition that serum digoxin levels may be important and the persistence of uncertainty about the potential lack of clinical efficacy in certain patient subgroups.

In this chapter, we begin with a brief overview of the basic pharmacology of the actions of cardiac glycosides. This is followed by a review of the pharmacokinetics of digoxin with important drug interactions. The data justifying the use of digoxin in patients with moderate to severe congestive heart failure are reviewed in some detail, followed by a description of the mechanisms underlying the toxic manifestations of this class of drugs and their treatment. We also offer a section on contemporary practice that includes a discussion of the place digoxin has in the published guidelines of various professional societies. Readers interested in citations prior to 1990, particularly those citations that address the basic pharmacology of the cardiac glycosides, are referred to the first edition of this text.

CARDIAC GLYCOSIDES: NATURAL SOURCES AND CHEMICAL STRUCTURE

The terms *digitalis* and *cardiac glycosides* are used in this chapter to refer to any of the steroid or steroid glycoside compounds that exert characteristic positive inotropic and electrophysiological effects on the heart. Although there are important differences in pharmacokinetics among the more than 300 known compounds with these properties, their pharmacologic actions are fundamentally similar. They are found in plants and in the venom and skin of certain toads. Clinically useful preparations are derived from the leaves and seeds of plants in the genera *Digitalis* and *Strophanthus*. Digitoxin is derived from the leaves of *D. purpurea*, and digoxin is derived (after a mild alkaline hydrolysis step) from those of *D. lanata*, as are lanatoside C and deslanoside. From the seeds of *S. gratus* comes ouabain, a hydrophilic, relatively rapidly acting cardiac glycoside. Currently, digoxin is by far the most commonly prescribed of these drugs due to the ready availability of techniques for measuring serum levels, flexibility in its routes of administration, and its intermediate duration of action.

A detailed description of sources of cardiac glycosides, their chemistry, and structure–activity relationships are extensively considered in standard texts (3,4). The steroid nucleus common to all cardiac glycosides contains an α, β-unsaturated lactone ring attached at the C-17 position. Without the sugar moieties, the steroid and unsaturated lactone part of the molecule is called a *genin* or an *aglycon*. The genins are usually less potent and have more transient actions due to altered pharmacokinetics than do the parent glycosides. It is apparent from structure–activity comparisons that the cardioactive glycosides demonstrate considerable variation in the structure of the steroid nucleus, as well as the sugar substituents attached at the C-3 position. Digitoxin differs from digoxin only by the absence of a hydroxyl group at C-12. This absent hydroxyl group reduces the hydrophilicity of the compound and results in markedly different metabolism and protein binding compared with digoxin.

MECHANISM OF ACTION

Positive Inotropic Effect

By the late 1920s, it became clear that digitalis preparations caused a positive inotropic effect on the intact ventricle, resulting in an increase in the rate of increase of intracavitary pressure during isovolumic systole at constant heart rate and aortic pressure. This effect could be demonstrated in normal, as well as failing, cardiac muscle. Cardiac glycoside administration caused the ventricular function (Frank-Starling) curve of the intact heart to shift upward and to the left, so that more stroke work is generated at a given filling pressure. This was found to be true of both right and left ventricles, and of atrial as well as ventricular myocardium. Force–velocity curves for isolated cardiac muscle are shifted in parallel upward and to the right by cardioactive steroids. These effects appear to be sustained during in vivo administration of digitalis, for periods of weeks to months, without any evidence of desensitization or tachyphylaxis. The time to peak force generation and the relaxation rates are altered little by subtoxic doses or concentrations of cardioactive steroids, but the positive inotropic effect observed is highly dependent on contraction frequency, declining on either side of an intermediate frequency that yields the maximal inotropic response.

It is now generally believed that digitalis compounds bring about an increase in the availability of activator Ca^{2+} in heart cells and that this increase in intracellular Ca^{2+} activity is sufficient to explain both the inotropic and arrhythmogenic effects of these drugs (3,5,6). Importantly, it is also now accepted that the increase in intracellular Ca^{2+} is a consequence of the direct effect of cardiac glycosides on transmembrane Na^+ transport (3–7).

Inhibition of Na,K-ATPase

All cardioactive steroids share the properties of being potent and highly specific inhibitors of the intrinsic membrane protein Na,K-adenosine triphosphatase (Na,K-ATPase). The plasma membrane Na,K-ATPase, the molecular machinery that comprises the cellular sodium pump, is representative of a family of evolutionarily ancient enzymes in which membrane ion translocation is coupled to the hydrolysis of a high-energy ATP phosphate. Indeed, Jens Skou of Denmark was awarded the 1997 Nobel Prize in Chemistry for his discovery in the 1950s and 1960s of the enzyme activity he termed the Na^+,K^+-ATPase, which he characterized in giant neurons of shellfish (8,9). The α or catalytic subunit component of the sodium pump, the roughly 100-kDa integral membrane protein that almost certainly contains the Na^+, K^+, and ATP binding sites of the intact enzyme, has been highly conserved in eukaryotes for the establishment and maintenance of transmembrane Na^+ and K^+ gradients. Unique to the Na,K-ATPase is the presence of an approximately 40-kDa glycosylated subunit termed the γ subunit, the function of which is as yet unknown. This subunit, too, has been highly conserved as indicated by nucleotide sequence analysis from phylogenetically diverse species ranging from the electric fish *Torpedo californica* to humans (10,11). A third, small hydrophobic subunit termed τ is not necessary for association, membrane targeting, or function of α/β subunits but appears to regulate activation of Na,K pumps by K^+ (12–14).

Aside from its α,β-heterodimer structure, another characteristic of the Na,K-ATPase that is unique among the P-type ATPases is the presence of a binding site on the extracytoplasmic face of the α subunit for the cardiac glycosides (15,16). Although the binding affinity varies among isoforms of the enzyme and from species to species, the ability of the enzyme to bind and to be inhibited by cardiac glycosides has been very highly conserved; it is so highly conserved, in fact, that cardiac glycoside binding is a sine qua non for identifying functional Na,K-ATPase and is used to define the contribution of the sodium pump to plasmalemmal monovalent cation fluxes. One cardiac glycoside binding site facing the extracellular surface is present per α chain. Optimal binding requires Na^+, Mg^{2+}, and ATP and is inhibited by extracellular K^+. Cardiac glycoside binding results in complete inhibition of enzymatic and transport functions of each Na,K-ATPase site occupied.

In addition to a wealth of evidence from animal, whole heart, isolated muscle, single cell, and molecular studies, inhibition of the sodium pump in atrial tissue of patients treated with conventional doses of digoxin also has been demonstrated. Indeed, the highly selective action of the cardiac glycosides to bind to the digitalis binding site on the extracellular face of the α subunit of Na,K-ATPase has engendered much speculation about the possible existence of endogenous ligands, simply because the amino acid sequence and conformation that form their binding site has been so highly conserved over many phyla and millennia. Although many intriguing data exist, there is, as yet, no proof that any endogenous digitalis exists that has a well-defined biological role in regulating Na,K-ATPase function.

Three isoforms of the α subunit of Na,K-ATPase have been identified. Several investigators (17,18) have suggested, based on high-resolution immunocytochemical staining techniques using antibodies specific for each isoform, that each α subunit isoform subserves a distinct subcellular role. The α_1 subunit appears to regulate bulk cytosolic Na^+, whereas α_2- and α_3-containing Na,K-ATPases appear to be localized to areas of the sarcolemma in close apposition to the endoplasmic reticulum (i.e., sarcoplasmic reticulum in muscle) (18). Because the isoforms differ in their affinities for cardiac glycosides (indeed, it was this property that led to their original discovery), the subcellular targeting of each α subunit isoform may impact importantly on the pharmacology of these drugs.

Na^+–Ca^{2+} Exchange and Increased Intracellular Calcium

Compelling direct evidence supporting cardiac glycoside-induced increases in intracellular Na^+ concentration or activity ($[Na^+]_i$) is available from studies of cardiac cells impaled with Na^+-sensitive microelectrodes. The relationship of $[Na^+]_i$ to tension development is direct and remarkably steep. Data from these and other experiments support the view that inhibition of active cellular Na^+ transport results in augmentation of myocyte Ca^{2+} content, which, in turn, produces a positive inotropic response. This is analogous to the increase in contractility that follows an increase in $[Na^+]_i$ due to increased contraction frequency, a phenomenon termed *treppe* or *Bowditch staircase*. The mechanism of both digitalis-induced positive inotropy and the staircase phenomenon appears to involve an altered balance between intracellular Na^+ and Ca^{2+}. The transmembrane Na^+ influx occurring with each action potential, in the presence of diminished outward Na^+ pumping due to digitalis, leads to the increased intracellular Na^+ concentration proposed to promote increased intracellular Ca^{2+} stores, either through enhanced Ca^{2+} entry, reduced Ca^{2+} efflux, or both. These effects are thought to be mediated via Na^+–Ca^{2+} exchange. At rapid heart rates, Na^+ influx in the presence or absence of digitalis may be sufficiently great to approach the maximum inotropically effective intracellular Na^+. This is consistent with the diminished effects of cardiac glycosides at high contraction frequencies.

Studies with spontaneously contracting, isolated, and cultured ventricular cells have demonstrated direct correlations between ouabain-induced enhancement of the contractile state, inhibition of Na^+ and K^+ transport, and increased cellular content of both Na^+ and Ca^{2+} (7). These data support the hypothesis that inhibition of the Na^+ pump by digitalis leads to a positive inotropic response and are consistent with modulation of Ca^{2+} content by Na^+ via the Na^+–Ca^{2+} exchange carrier mechanism (Fig. 25-1). A similar effect can be achieved by decreasing

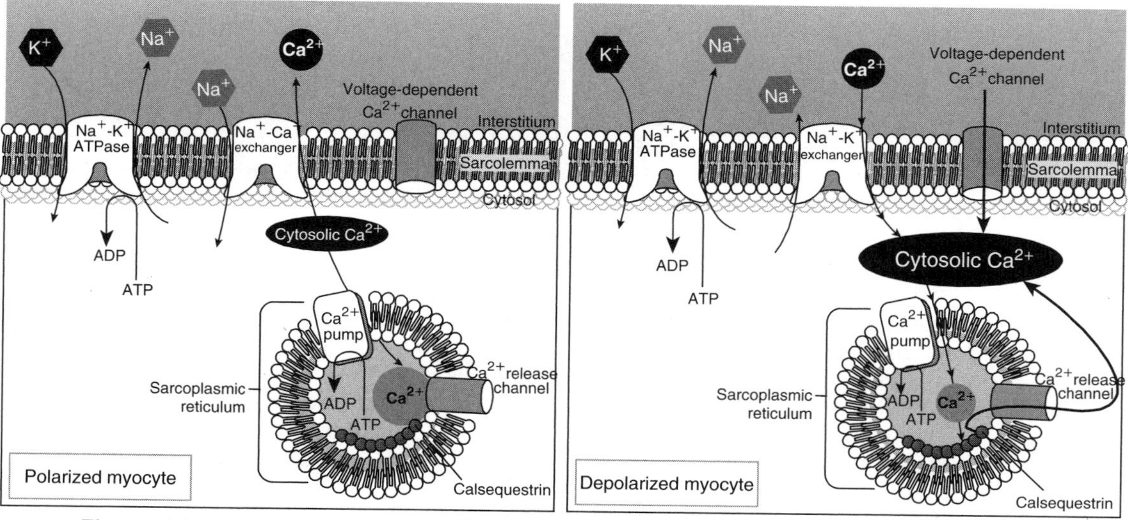

Figure 25-1 The figure illustrates the flux of sodium (Na^+), potassium (K^+), and calcium (Ca^{2+}) across the plasmalemmal membrane and sarcoplasmic reticular membrane, during diastole (left panel) and systole (right panel). Digitalis glycosides such as digoxin bind to the Na^+-K^+-ATPase, and decrease the flux of potassium into, and sodium out of, the cell, resulting in increased levels of intracellular Na^+. This increase in intracellular Na+ results, among other effects, in increased Na^+/Ca^{2+} exchange, a subsequent rise in intracellular Ca^{2+}, including SR calcium content, which results in a modest increase in contractile force during each cardiac cycle. Other mechanisms of action of the cardiac glycosides at drug levels achieved using clinically relevant dosing algorithms have been postulated, including direct effects on ryanodine receptors.

extracellular [K^+], which can produce equivalent positive inotropic effects accompanied by inhibition of Na^+ and K^+ transport and an increase in intracellular [Na^+] and intracellular calcium activity, $[Ca^{2+}]_i$, via Na^+–Ca^{2+} exchange (19). Direct evidence for an increase in $[Ca^{2+}]_i$ following digitalis comes from studies using the Ca^{2+}-activated photoprotein aequorin, as well as Ca^{2+}-specific fluorescent probes such as fura-2 and indo-1. During the inotropic effect of digitalis, there is a close association between the increase in peak systolic aequorin luminescence, which is directly related to intracellular [Ca^{2+}] over the relevant range, and the increase in twitch force.

The immediate positively inotropic effect of cardiac glycosides, measured either in the intact heart in a conscious dog model or in isometrically contracting papillary muscle strips, is achieved with remarkable energy transfer efficiency and little oxygen wasting (20). When compared with β-adrenergic agonists or a cyclic adenosine monophosphate phosphodiesterase inhibitor, ouabain caused no significant change, for the same degree of tension development, in the tension-time integral per unit initial heat, an index of the economy of isometric contraction in an isolated muscle preparation. Interestingly, Peng et al. (21) have shown that ouabain-induced net influx of Ca^{2+} induces *c-fos* and other early response gene transcription. Huang et al. (22,23) also have demonstrated that sodium pump inhibition can lead to cardiac myocyte hypertrophy in vitro, accompanied by a characteristic phenotypic shift to a fetal gene program in these cells. Whether these observations in cell culture preparations are relevant to the clinical pharmacology of these drugs in humans is not known.

Electrophysiological Effects

As with the positive inotropic effect of these drugs, the major effect on cardiac rhythm of digitalis preparations is believed to be due to inhibition of the sodium pump. The 80- to 90-mV transmembrane resting potential of cardiac cells is maintained by Na^+ and K^+ gradients (particularly the latter), which in turn are dependent on the integrity of the active Na,K pump mechanism. There is general agreement that inhibition of Na,K-ATPase underlies the direct toxic effects of digitalis preparations on cardiac rhythm, and thus represents an extension of the drugs' therapeutic effects. Cells in various parts of the heart show differing sensitivities to digitalis, and both direct and neurally mediated effects must be dissected before conclusions can be drawn about the mechanisms involved. For example, digoxin does not produce significant changes in atrial effective or functional refractory periods in denervated hearts, nor does it change sinus node cycle length. These findings point to the importance of the autonomic nervous system in the regulation of automaticity and conduction by digitalis. Indeed, at the lower concentrations associated with therapeutic levels of digoxin, the drugs decrease automaticity and increase maximum diastolic potential (effects that can be blocked by atropine), whereas higher concentrations decrease diastolic potentials and increase automaticity.

Similarly, the toxic arrhythmogenic effect of the cardiac glycosides is due to a combination of direct effects on the myocardium and neurally mediated increases in autonomic activity. During exposure to high concentrations of digitalis, isolated myocardial preparations demonstrate small, unstimulated depolarizations and contractions following action potentials. These oscillatory events coincide with the development of digitalis-toxic arrhythmias in intact animals exposed to similar levels of digitalis. Both systolic and diastolic $[Ca^{2+}]_i$ increase during digitalis-induced arrhythmias, increases that were first inferred from changes in tension, leading to the idea that intracellular calcium overload contributes to the observed arrhythmogenic effects. These occur presumably because $[Ca^{2+}]_i$ increases progressively until the sarcoplasmic reticulum (the major intracellular organelle responsible for Ca^{2+} sequestration) is no longer capable of retaining all the Ca^{2+} taken up with each depolarization. Spontaneous cycles of Ca release and reuptake then ensue, resulting in after depolarizations and after contractions. The after-depolarization is the result of a Ca^{2+}-activated transient outward current and is thought to be the macroscopic manifestation of Ca-activated nonspecific cation channels, plus Na–Ca exchange current (I_{TO}). This formulation has been confirmed by Hancox and Levi in rabbit atrioventricular nodal tissue (24). Interestingly, mice that lack a functioning endothelial nitric oxide synthase (eNOS) isoform gene are more susceptible to digitalis-induced increases in I_{TO} and after-depolarizations (Han, Kubota, and Kelly, unpublished observations [25]). This implicates local, cardiac myocyte-derived nitric oxide (NO) in the regulation of transmembrane Ca^{2+} currents in digitalis-treated animals (25–27).

Neurally Mediated Actions of Cardiac Glycosides

It is important to understand the pathophysiology of heart failure and the role of digitalis glycosides in modifying the abnormal autonomic nervous system activity characteristic of advanced heart failure, including altered baroreflex activity. The responsiveness of the baroreflex system is diminished in congestive heart failure. Because stimulation of this reflex normally inhibits sympathetic outflow, the result of diminished baroreflex activity in these patients is increased sympathetic nerve activity, as well as increased vasopressin.

Mason et al. (28) observed that intravenous ouabain increased mean arterial pressure, forearm vascular resistance, and venous tone in normal human subjects, probably due to direct but transient effects on vascular smooth muscle. In contrast, patients with heart failure responded with a decline in heart rate and other effects that were consistent with enhanced baroreflex responsiveness. Direct effects of cardiac glycosides on carotid baroreflex responsiveness to changes in carotid sinus pressure have been reported in isolated baroreceptor preparations from animals with experimentally induced heart failure. Ferguson et al. (29) demonstrated in patients with moderate to severe heart failure that infusion of deslanoside increased forearm blood flow and cardiac index and decreased heart rate, concomitant with a marked decrease in skeletal muscle sympathetic nerve activity measured as an indicator of centrally mediated sympathetic nervous system activity. Indeed, the neurohormonal effects are quite broad; in addition to attenuation of carotid sinus baroreceptor discharge sensitivity, digoxin has vasomimetic and sympathoinhibitory effects and effects that decrease serum norepinephrine, plasma renin activity, and possibly aldosterone (30). Based on these and other observations, reduced neurohumoral activation may be the most significant mechanism contributing to the efficacy of cardiac glycosides in the treatment of patients with heart failure, and may occur at blood levels of these drugs that are below those necessary to achieve a direct inotropic effect (31).

CLINICAL PHARMACOLOGY

Pharmacokinetics

Although a number of cardiac glycoside preparations remain available, digoxin is the most commonly prescribed; only its pharmacology will be described here in detail. The reader should refer to the first edition of this text for a description of the pharmacology of other cardiac glycosides that remain in clinical use.

Digoxin is excreted exponentially, with an elimination half-life of 36 to 48 hours in patients with normal renal function, resulting in the loss of about one-third of body stores daily. The drug is excreted for the most part unchanged, although some patients excrete detectable quantities of the inactive metabolite dihydrodigoxin, which arises through bacterial biotransformation in the gut lumen. Renal excretion of digoxin is proportional to the glomerular filtration rate (and, hence, to creatinine clearance). In patients with prerenal azotemia, digoxin clearance may correlate more closely with urea clearance, suggesting that the drug may undergo some degree of tubular reabsorption.

With daily maintenance therapy, a steady state is reached when daily losses are matched by daily intake. For patients not previously given digoxin, institution of daily maintenance therapy without a loading dose results in development of steady-state plateau concentrations after four to five half-lives, or about 7 days, in subjects with normal renal function. If the half-life of the drug is prolonged, the length of time before a steady state is reached on a daily maintenance dose would also be prolonged proportionately. Because of the high degree of tissue binding of digoxin (i.e., a large volume of distribution, averaging 4 to 7 L/kg), the drug is not effectively removed from the body by dialysis. Serum digoxin levels and pharmacokinetics are essentially the same before and after the loss of large amounts of adipose tissue in massively obese subjects, suggesting that a patient's estimated lean body mass should be used in the calculation for maintenance dosing. Finally, the steady-state volume of distribution of digoxin (Vd_{ss}) is decreased in chronic renal failure, and therefore loading doses of digoxin as well as maintenance doses should be decreased in these patients (32).

In patients with advanced heart failure, initiation of therapy with vasodilators tends to increase renal digoxin clearance (probably by increasing cardiac output) and may necessitate adjustment of the maintenance digoxin dosage. Infants and children absorb and excrete digoxin in much the same way as adults do, although recent evidence suggests that secretion at the renal tubular level may be quantitatively more important in children before puberty. Digoxin doses in neonates and infants are substantially larger than those in adults when adjusted for weight or per square meter of body surface area. These higher doses result in relatively higher serum digoxin concentrations, which are generally well-tolerated. Digoxin does cross the placenta and fetal umbilical cord venous blood levels of the drug are similar to maternal blood levels. There is no contraindication for use of digoxin during pregnancy or during lactation.

Numerous studies over several decades have documented incomplete absorption of digoxin following oral administration, with the bioavailability of currently marketed tablet preparations averaging about 65% to 75%. Individual patient variation, interactions with other concurrently administered drugs, and the characteristics of the digoxin preparation ingested are all known to affect the drug's bioavailability. Patients with malabsorption syndromes often absorb digoxin poorly and erratically. However, patients with pancreatic insufficiency, despite steatorrhea, appear to absorb the drug normally. Administration of digoxin after meals is likely to delay absorption, thus diminishing peak serum levels, but absolute bioavailability is not affected to any noteworthy degree. Absorption of digoxin tends to be reduced by drugs that increase motility, particularly if a particular formulation releases the active drug slowly. In addition, nonabsorbable substances such as cholestyramine and nonabsorbable antacids, when taken concurrently with digoxin, can interfere with gastrointestinal absorption of digoxin.

Digoxin Dosing Schedules

There is usually no need to treat patients with a loading dose of digoxin except in the setting of certain supraventricular arrhythmias when other drugs useful in treating these arrhythmias are contraindicated or have not been effective. This is due to the narrow therapeutic window of cardiac glycosides, which often makes it difficult to judge accurately an effective loading dose of digoxin that also will minimize the risk of toxicity. Often the patients who would benefit most from the addition of a cardiac glycoside are also those at greatest risk of exhibiting toxic effects of these drugs. Nevertheless, if a loading dose is to be given (assuming a bioavailability of 75% to 80% for most digoxin tablet formulations), between 0.9 and 1.8 mg given in divided doses over 24 hours will result in plasma levels that approximate those achieved by either 0.25 or 0.50 mg of digoxin, respectively, given daily for about a week in patients with normal renal function. Lean body mass should be used in the calculation of both loading and maintenance digoxin doses. In adults, intravenous loading doses of 0.50 to 0.75 mg per 45 kg (i.e., 100 pounds) of body weight, in divided doses over 24 hours, are unlikely to cause toxicity and can be supplemented as required by the patient's clinical condition. The loading dose of digoxin should be reduced in patients with renal insufficiency due to a reduction in the drug's volume of distribution in this condition, as previously noted.

The calculation of the regular maintenance dose is determined by the drug's clearance rate from the body, which, in the case of digoxin, is closely related to the rate of clearance of creatinine. A reasonable approximation of the daily percentage loss of digoxin is given by:

$$\text{\% daily loss} = 14 + \frac{\text{creatinine clearance in mL/min}}{5}$$

The daily maintenance dose (33,34) is calculated by multiplying the percentage daily loss times the loading dose given that resulted in effective therapeutic drug levels (adjusting for reduced bioavailability if the maintenance dose is to be given orally, but the loading dose was given intravenously).

Drug Interactions

Concomitant drug administration may directly alter the pharmacokinetics of digitalis preparations, or indirectly alter their action on the heart by pharmacodynamic interactions (Table 25-1). Quinidine reduces both the renal and nonrenal elimination of digoxin and decreases its volume of distribution. The net result is an increase in serum digoxin concentration that averages twofold in patients given conventional doses of quinidine. Unfortunately, individual responses to quinidine may vary and close surveillance of clinical status and the serum digoxin concentration is warranted. Procainamide and disopyramide do not appear to alter serum digoxin levels, but verapamil does increase the serum digoxin concentration by an average of 35%, again by decreasing digoxin's volume of distribution and clearance rate. Nifedipine and diltiazem have no reproducible effect on digoxin clearance. Both short-term and long-term amiodarone administration has been found to increase the steady-state digoxin concentration, and maintenance doses of digoxin should be decreased by half (or more). Newly introduced drugs will require close surveillance for interactions with cardiac glycosides (35,36). Furthermore, over-the-counter drugs and nutraceuticals (37,38) also may interact with digoxin clearance.

Other examples of pharmacodynamic interactions include concomitantly administered diuretic agents that may increase the incidence of digitalis toxicity both by decreasing the glomerular filtration rate due to volume depletion and by inducing a variety of electrolyte disturbances, including hypokalemia, hypomagnesemia, and (for thiazide diuretics) hypercalcemia. Also, concurrent administration of some antiarrhythmic agents may increase the possibility of proarrhythmic events, an outcome that is often unpredictable in an individual patient.

Several anesthetic agents, such as cyclopropane and succinylcholine, may demonstrate additive or synergistic proarrhythmic effects when coadministered with digitalis. Experimental studies demonstrate that catecholamine-induced increases in ventricular automaticity add to the arrhythmogenic effects of digitalis. Therefore, it is reason-

TABLE 25-1
PHARMACOKINETIC AND PHARMACODYNAMIC INTERACTIONS WITH DIGOXIN

Drug	Mechanism	Clinical Management
Cholestyramine, kaolin-pectin, neomycin, sulfasalazine	Decrease absorption	Give digoxin 8 h before agent, or use solution or gel form
Antacids	Unclear	Temporal dispersion of doses
Bran	Decreases absorption	Temporal dispersion of doses
Propafenone, quinidine, verapamil, amiodarone	Decrease renal digoxin clearance, volume of distribution, or both	Decrease digoxin by 50% and monitor serum digoxin levels as necessary
Thyroxine	Increases volume of distribution and renal clearance	Monitor serum digoxin levels
Erythromycin, omeprazole, tetracycline	Increase digoxin absorption	Monitor serum digoxin levels
Albuterol	Increases volume of distribution	Monitor serum digoxin levels
Captopril, diltiazem, nifedipine, nitrendipine	Variable moderate decrease in digoxin clearance, volume of distribution, or both	
Cyclosporine	May decrease renal function	Monitor serum digoxin levels frequently
β-blockers, verapamil, diltiazem, flecainide, disopyramide, bepridil	Diminish SA or AV junctional conduction of automaticity	Monitor ECG for evidence of SA or AV block
Kaliuretic diuretics	Decrease serum and tissue K^+, increase automaticity, and promotes inhibition of Na^+,K^+-ATPase by digoxin	Monitor ECG for arrhythmias consistent with digoxin toxicity
Sympathomimetic drugs	Increase automaticity	Monitor ECG for arrhythmia
Verapamil, diltiazem, β-adrenergic blocking agents	Diminish cardiac contractile state	Discontinue or lower dose of Ca^{2+} channel or β-adrenergic blocker

AV, atrioventricular; ECG, electrocardiogram.

able to assume that sympathomimetic agents increase the likelihood of enhanced automaticity of atrial and ventricular tissue in patients receiving digitalis.

CARDIAC GLYCOSIDES AND HEART FAILURE

Despite the fact that digitalis has been used for the treatment of symptoms of congestive heart failure for over 200 years, it was not until early in the twentieth century that a series of clinical observations led to the recognition that these drugs could be useful in patients with normal sinus rhythm.

Digitalis in Patients with Congestive Heart Failure in Sinus Rhythm: Early Clinical Trials

Clinical studies appeared in the 1960s and 1970s that questioned Christian's assertion that patients in sinus rhythm with heart failure clearly benefited from digitalis. These studies suggested that many patients receiving chronic maintenance doses of digoxin did not benefit from the drug (42,43). A number of small, double-blinded, placebo-controlled trials involving 22 to 30 patients appeared in the period from 1980 to 1992, yielding conflicting results (44–46).

Changes in quantitative measures of contractile function in these and other studies were variably correlated with symptoms or exercise performance, where such correlations were sought. In general, patients with more severe contractile dysfunction demonstrated the most pronounced beneficial response to digoxin. This was particularly evident in a study by Gheorghiade et al. (47), in which marked improvements in mean cardiac output (+48%), left ventricular filling pressure (−36%), and ejection fraction (+8%) were observed in the subset of patients who remained in overt failure after diuretic and vasodilator treatment, whereas no significant further improvement was observed in the subset of patients who were relatively well-compensated at the completion of the diuretic-vasodilator treatment period.

Several larger, multicenter trials also appeared at the beginning of the 1990s. The digoxin and xamoterol study examined 433 patients (the majority had New York Heart Association [NYHA] Class I or II failure). Xamoterol is a partial β_1-selective adrenergic agonist with some antagonist activity (48). Patients were randomized to placebo, xamoterol, or digoxin in a 1:2:1 ratio; diuretics were continued but were limited to no more than 80 mg per day of furosemide or equivalent. Three hundred patients completed the double-blind phase with valid exercise tests at entry and at 3 months. Digoxin did not improve exercise duration or work done on a bicycle ergometer. However, although both digoxin and xamoterol demonstrated a significant improvement in symptoms compared with placebo, xamoterol was subsequently shown to cause excess mortality in patients with heart failure.

The captopril-digoxin trial compared captopril, digoxin, and placebo during maintenance diuretic therapy in 196 patients, 85% of whom were judged to be in NYHA Class I or II (49). Patients who did not tolerate withdrawal from digoxin were not randomized, thus excluding the subset of patients who were presumably the most likely to demonstrate benefit from digoxin. Two major conclusions emerged from this trial: digoxin (but not captopril) significantly improved the left ventricular ejection fraction, and digoxin and captopril were both similarly effective in reducing morbidity (by about half) compared with placebo in terms of increased diuretic requirements and hospitalization and emergency room visits.

The milrinone-digoxin trial randomly assigned 230 patients in sinus rhythm with moderately severe heart failure to treatment with digoxin, oral milrinone, both drugs, or placebo added to baseline diuretic therapy (50). After 3 months, digoxin improved exercise tolerance by 14% ($p < 0.05$) compared with placebo. There was a marked benefit of digoxin over placebo or milrinone as judged by the frequency of decompensation within the initial 2 weeks and at 3 months. There also was a significantly lower incidence of ventricular ectopy in the digoxin-treated group, compared with those patients randomized to receive milrinone. Oral milrinone was subsequently documented to increase mortality in patients with heart failure.

Digoxin Withdrawal Trials

The PROVED (Prospective Randomized Study of Ventricular Failure and Efficacy of Digoxin) (51) and RADIANCE (Randomized Assessment of Digoxin on Inhibition of Angiotensin-Converting Enzyme) (52) trials were two prospective, multicenter, placebo-controlled trials that examined the effects of withdrawal of digoxin in patients with stable, mild to moderate heart failure (i.e., NYHA Class II and III) and systolic ventricular dysfunction (i.e., a left ventricular ejection fraction of ≤0.35%). All patients studied were in sinus rhythm. The target serum digoxin concentration in both studies during the baseline run-in phase was 0.9 to 2.0 ng/mL, achieved with an average digoxin dose of 0.38 mg per day. Patients in the RADIANCE trial also received concurrent therapy with an angiotensin-converting enzyme (ACE) inhibitor. When patients were randomly assigned to either continue active digoxin therapy or to withdraw from active therapy and receive a matching placebo, 40% of patients in PROVED and 28% of patients in RADIANCE who received placebo noted a significant worsening of heart failure symptoms compared with 20% and 6%, respectively, in patients who continued to receive active drug. This absolute risk reduction of 20% in digoxin-treated patients constituted a substantial treatment effect. Maximal treadmill exercise tolerance also declined significantly in patients withdrawn from digoxin in both trials, despite continuation of other medical therapies for heart failure, notably ACE inhibitors in RADIANCE (52). In addition, the benefits of digoxin (compared to withdrawal) were seen over the range of serum levels of drug, somewhat in contrast to the conclusions derived from the post hoc analysis of the Digoxin Investigation Group (DIG) trial (53) (see The Digoxin Investigation Group Trial, later). Overall, however, none of the withdrawal trials had the statistical power to detect an effect of digoxin therapy on the survival of patients with heart failure.

There are limited data on digoxin withdrawal in the β-blocker era (54). Although theoretically more likely to work, given redundancy in sympatholytic effects, digoxin withdrawal in patients on β-blockers has not been subjected to rigorous study and there are no multicenter efforts that provide any useful information.

Other Clinical Trial Data

Many short- and long-term, controlled and uncontrolled clinical trials, reviewed in detail by Rahimtoola and Tak (55) and Jaeschke et al. (56), have suggested that digoxin results in an impressive array of benefits, including increases in left ventricular function, prolongation of exercise time, and improvement in clinical status. Nevertheless, there are, once again, conflicting results for some therapeutic endpoints, and the conclusions that can be drawn from these and other relatively recent trials are quite limited. For example, in a trial of ibopamine, an orally bioavailable dopamine analog, control patients treated with digoxin and diuretics alone (most with moderate, NYHA Class II failure) exhibited an increase in exercise time and a decrease in blood norepinephrine levels at 6 months, but there was no change in the heart failure score (57). In the SPRINT trial, a secondary prevention study of the efficacy of nifedipine in patients following a myocardial infarction, digoxin use was associated with a significant increase in mortality. This finding held even after accounting for an increased prevalence of comorbidities in digoxin-treated patients, although patients with advanced heart failure symptoms, who might have been expected to receive the most benefit from digoxin, were excluded by design (58).

Trials designed for other purposes can also provide some indirect insight into digoxin use and effects, albeit with the understanding that the data are retrospectively reviewed and subject to bias. For example, in an analysis of the U.S. Carvedilol studies and the Australia/New Zealand Heart Failure Study (ANZ) (59), the effect of digoxin on outcomes in patients on carvedilol or placebo was examined. Patients on digoxin were younger and more likely to have symptoms consistent with an advanced NYHA class, a lower ejection fraction, and higher basal heart rate compared to patients not on digoxin. With the endpoints of hospitalization or the combination of all-cause hospitalization and all-cause mortality, digoxin had no additive (or negative) effects, though the fact that the patients on digoxin were sicker at baseline might have masked a positive effect.

In other clinical trials, digoxin use has been variable, limiting the ability of investigators to infer any definitive conclusions about the effects of digoxin. Several recent trials outline the issues: in the Randomized Aldactone Evaluation Study (RALES) (60), use of digoxin occurred in 73% of the cohort at baseline; in the Valsartan Heart Failure Trial (VAL-HeFT) (61), 67%; and in the Candesartan in Heart Failure Assessment of Reduction in Mortality and morbidity (CHARM) study (62), 43%. In the Atrial Fibrillation Follow-Up Investigation of Rhythm Management (AFFIRM) trial (63), first-line medical therapy for rate control included digoxin alone in 16%, digoxin in combination with β-adrenergic blockers in 14% and digoxin in combination with calcium-channel blockers in 14%; however, this was not a heart failure cohort.

The Digoxin Investigation Group Trial

A number of lingering controversies over the role of digoxin were to be resolved by the well-publicized, large, multicenter DIG trial, composed of two studies in a total of 302 centers in the United States and Canada (64,65). The main trial required that patients be in sinus rhythm, with documented left ventricular ejection fraction of ≤0.45%, and heart failure as determined by preset signs, symptoms, and/or radiographic criteria. Prior or ongoing therapy with digoxin was admissible because of concern by the investigators that limiting the trial to patients not currently receiving digoxin therapy would select for a group of patients who would likely be less ill, and thus have a lower event rate. Thus, the DIG trial also comprised a group of patients who would be randomized to receive placebo, thus incorporating a digoxin withdrawal trial into the DIG study.

The use of ACE inhibitors was not mandated but strongly encouraged; additional drugs could be added at the discretion of the investigator; and follow-up was established at 4 weeks, 4 months, and then every subsequent 4 months. The primary endpoint was all-cause mortality and secondary endpoints were mortality from cardiovascular causes, mortality from worsening heart failure, and hospitalization from worsening heart failure or other causes. Among the 6,800 patients enrolled in this main trial, there were no differences in baseline characteristics between active drug and placebo group.

After a mean follow-up of 37 months (range 28 to 58 months), there were no differences in all-cause or cardiovascular mortality. There was a trend toward a reduction in death from heart failure with a relative risk of 0.88 (95% CI crossing unity). Importantly, there was a decreased risk of hospitalization for heart failure in the digoxin-treated group, with a relative risk for patients on digoxin of 0.72 (95% CI 0.66–0.79). This effect was sufficiently large so that, when combined with the mortality endpoints, it remained statistically significant (Fig. 25-2). A higher percentage of deaths or hospitalizations due to heart failure (45.3%) occurred in patients previously on digoxin and randomized to placebo (a digoxin withdrawal group) compared with patients who were not previously on (and did not receive) the drug (32%). The effect of digoxin was similar (risk ratio of 0.74 and 0.77, respectively) when corrected for prior digoxin use. However, the reduction in relative risk was also greater for patients with ejection fractions less than 25% and for more advanced symptoms as measured by the NYHA classification. The heart failure survival and hospitalization curves appear to separate early after randomization, especially in the patient subgroup in which digoxin was withdrawn, supporting the conclusions reached in the PROVED (51) and RADIANCE (52) trials.

There were more hospitalizations for suspected digoxin toxicity but the effect was not sufficiently great to overcome the overall effect of digoxin to decrease hospitalizations. Hospitalizations for other reasons (including myocardial infarction, unstable angina, need for revascu-

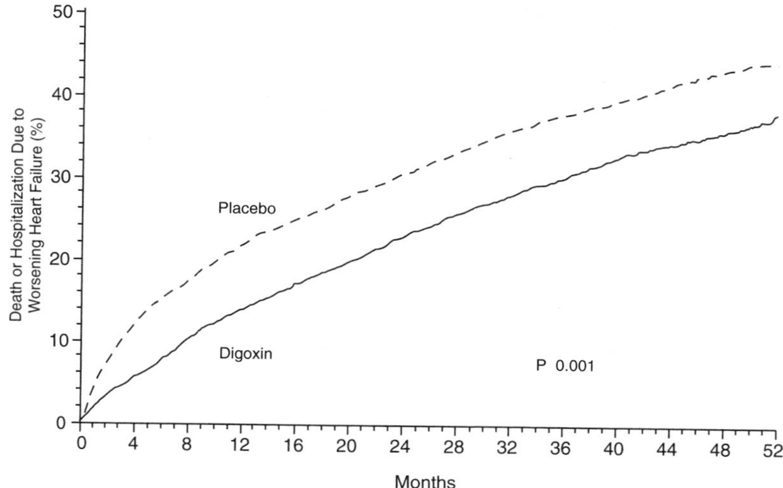

Figure 25-2 Incidence of death or hospitalization due to worsening heart failure in the digoxin and placebo groups for patients in the DIG study. (Reproduced from The Digitalis Investigation Group. The effect of digoxin on mortality and morbidity in patients with heart failure. *N Engl J Med.* 1997; 336:525–533.

larization, or cerebrovascular accident) were not different between active drug and placebo groups. Overall, there were nearly 10% fewer total cardiovascular hospitalizations (1,694 or 49.9% versus 1,850 or 54.4%) as well as fewer hospitalizations for each digoxin-treated patient. Nevertheless, fewer deaths from other cardiac causes were noted in the placebo group. This category included deaths presumed to result from arrhythmias without worsening heart failure, and deaths due to atherosclerotic coronary disease, low-output states, and cardiac surgery. Out-of-hospital deaths presumed to be due to an arrhythmia was not a prespecified endpoint and no data have been published from the trial for this separate group.

Open-label digoxin was given to more patients on placebo than on digoxin (22.0% versus 14.2%). In the subgroup of patients with recorded digoxin levels, over 88% were within the prescribed therapeutic range of 0.5 to 2.0 ng/mL at 1 month. However, a serum level measured at 1 month from randomization correlated with outcomes (Fig. 25-3) (53). Serum levels were divided into three ranges: 0.5 to 0.8, 0.9 to 1.1, and ≥1.2 ng/mL. Crude all-cause mortality rates were lower in the lowest dose range in treated patients and, when compared to placebo, the lowest serum levels appeared to have a favorable mortality profile that persisted after multivariable adjustment for covariates. Patients with the lowest serum level were, as expected, hospitalized less frequently for suspected digoxin toxicity. These findings provide indirect evidence in support of the concept that the primary mode of action that contributes to efficacy is its neurohormonal modulating effects and that this effect is achieved at lower serum digoxin levels.

Despite the improvement in hospitalization, the DIG trial failed to show an impact on quality of life (66), using a subset of patients in the trial that had reasonably similar baseline characteristics. Measurements with a variety of instruments including the Minnesota Living with Heart Failure Questionnaire and several domains from the SF-36 were obtained at baseline, 4 months, and 12 months. Imputation for missing scores using both the worst score and best score methods did not change the results. The explanations for the lack of improvement are many: the study involved less than 10% of all patients enrolled; the effects of digoxin, if mild, may have been diluted by the general improvement in quality of life measures typically seen in both placebo and actively treated patients in

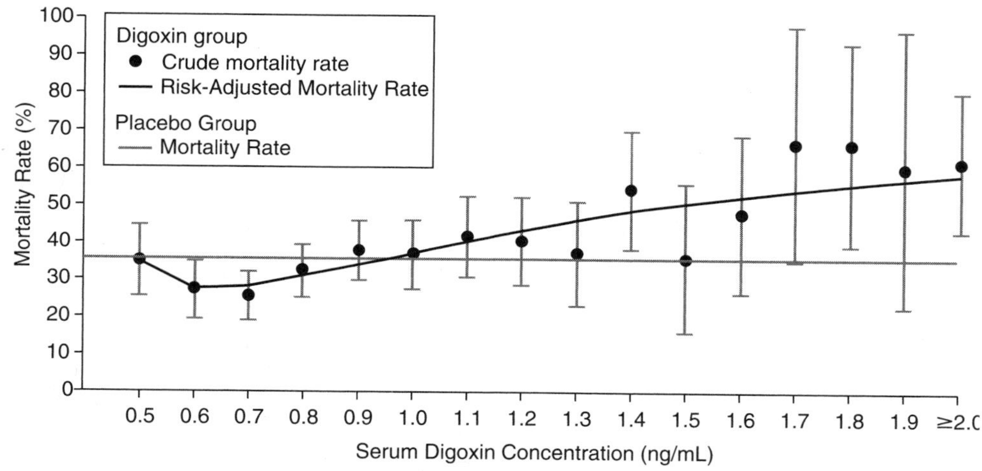

Figure 25-3 Association of serum digoxin concentrations and outcomes in the DIG trial. (Reproduced from Rathore SS, Curtis JP, Wang Y, et al. Association of serum digoxin concentration and outcomes in patients with heart failure. *JAMA.* 2003;289:871–878.)

double-blinded, placebo-controlled trials; the adjustment of patients to the symptoms of heart failure (an important point since the subset in whom Quality of Life was measured had a shorter duration of heart failure compared with the DIG population at large) may have blunted differences between digoxin and placebo; the instruments used may not be sensitive to change in this population; the effect on quality of life could be limited to those patients with serum digoxin levels in the lower range; and the substudy was underpowered to detect meaningful differences among the most symptomatic patients (e.g., NYHA Classes III and IV), who reported worse general health, poorer physical functioning, and more depression.

Despite the comprehensive data set that emerges from the DIG trial, potential confounders and changing trends in the management of heart failure patients between the time the trial was conceived and final patient enrollment limit our ability to resolve all outstanding controversies with digoxin. For example, although the prevention of hospitalizations with digoxin was a critical endpoint, the shift toward disease management, which began to occur as the trial progressed, may have brought about a decrease in hospitalization rates for all patients with heart failure, independent of digoxin use. In the final years of the trial, confounding also may have occurred due to increasing use of other agents known to suppress neurohormonal activation in heart failure, most notably β-adrenergic blockers. It is this aspect that most likely evokes the strongest resistance to incorporation of the findings of the DIG trial into wide acceptance, though published guidelines (see Guidelines on the Use of Digoxin, later) continue to favor digoxin use in defined groups largely based on the DIG trial data set.

After the DIG Trial

Following the publication of the DIG trial data and the results of subgroup analyses, there have been few additional studies of digoxin and no original prospective trials. In a meta-analytic review of digoxin trials (67) that were double-blinded and placebo-controlled with at least 20 patients followed for a minimum of 7 weeks, the odds ratio for mortality was 0.98 (95% CI 0.89–1.09); for hospitalization it was 0.68 (95% CI 0.61–0.75). However, the majority of the patients in the analysis were derived from the DIG trial; hence the numbers parallel what was seen in that trial. Outside the framework of clinical trials, data may be less rigorously derived but nonetheless important if the trends are consistent with the trial data. One study, designed to evaluate the utility of prognostic markers in heart failure (68), demonstrated a higher mortality in patients on digoxin compared to patients not managed with digoxin when digoxin use was adjusted for important variables such as patient age, NYHA class, and diuretic dose. However, the retrospective nature of these analyses is problematic since there is no way to control for bias.

THERAPEUTIC DRUG MONITORING: RELEVANCE OF DIGOXIN LEVELS

As previously suggested, cardiac glycosides may function by diminishing the overactivity of the sympathetic nervous system, as demonstrated in studies of direct nerve recordings, cardiac norepinephrine spillover, heart rate variability studies, and changes in plasma norepinephrine, aldosterone, and renin levels (69–76).

Data supporting the concept that the favorable impact of digoxin on neurohormonal axes is achieved at low serum levels (whereas the classic positively inotropic effects are observed at higher levels without any further neurohormonal benefits) come from several small clinical studies, in addition to the post hoc DIG trial analysis (53). Gheorghiade et al. (77) showed that increasing the dose from a mean of 0.2 to 0.39 mg per day (corresponding to an increase in serum levels from 0.67 to 1.22 ng/mL) resulted in an increase in ejection fraction but no change in exercise tolerance or decline in venous norepinephrine levels. Slatton et al. (78) enrolled 19 men in sinus rhythm with NYHA Class II or III failure and studied them at baseline, then at 2 weeks after digoxin therapy at 0.125 mg per day, and again 2 weeks after another dose escalation to 0.25 mg daily. Although average heart rate and heart rate variability did change at the low dose compared with the baseline, no further changes were observed at the higher dose. Krum et al. (70) showed that after 4 to 8 weeks of digoxin therapy in patients with Class I to III failure, plasma norepinephrine levels declined and abnormalities in heart rate variability improved, but only the latter correlated with serum digoxin levels.

The possibility that a gradient of effect may exist could explain why patients with high digoxin levels (>1.1 ng/mL) had a higher mortality rate in the Prospective Randomised Milrinone Survival Evaluation (PROMISE) trial (which examined the efficacy and safety of oral milrinone) independent of ejection fraction (79). Indeed, the issue of appropriate dosing appears to be as relevant for digoxin as it is with ACE inhibitors (80) and possibly β-adrenergic antagonists (81) in heart failure. In the case of digoxin, the relatively narrow therapeutic window and the difficulty of predicting individual patient responsiveness complicate the debate over dose or serum levels. Regardless, judicious use of digitalis in appropriate patient subgroups and recognition of concomitant medications or disease states that could affect digoxin pharmacokinetics, as well as early recognition of potential toxicity, remain essential for safe and effective dosing of this class of drugs (55,82).

DIGITALIS TOXICITY

Although the appropriateness of digoxin administration as a first-line agent to patients with mild congestive heart failure remains controversial, the data previously reviewed suggest that cardiac glycosides are efficacious in some patients with moderate to severe left ventricular dysfunction. However, it is this particular group of subjects (many of whom are elderly with underlying ischemic heart disease and often diseases of other organ systems, as well) who are at greatest risk for digoxin toxicity. The most prevalent and dangerous manifestations of digoxin overdosing are the toxic electrophysiological effects of the drug.

Electrophysiological Abnormalities

The effect of therapeutic serum levels of the cardiac glycosides in patients in sinus rhythm is often a minor slowing of the atrial rate, due to a diminution of adrenergic tone as a result of enhanced cardiac performance and to a direct effect of the drug on baroreceptor activity. The effects of the cardiac glycosides on the atrioventricular node (slowing conduction and prolonging atrioventricular nodal refractoriness) constitute a major antiarrhythmic action of these drugs and are largely mediated by enhanced parasympathetic and decreased adrenergic tone. At toxic levels, however, the direct actions of these drugs on atrioventricular nodal tissue prolong the atrioventricular nodal refractory period, and this effect (along with the heightened parasympathetic tone) may lead to advanced atrioventricular junctional conduction block.

The electrocardiographic manifestations of digoxin toxicity, while numerous, are too nonspecific in most instances to be diagnostic. At higher doses, junctional pacemakers may begin to discharge at increasing frequency, resulting in a nonparoxysmal atrioventricular junctional tachycardia. This is recognized clinically as a paradoxic regularization of the ventricular rate in patients with persistent atrial fibrillation. Common supraventricular arrhythmias associated with digitalis toxicity include atrioventricular nodal re-entrant tachycardias and tachycardias that originate due to enhanced atrial automaticity. Although paroxysmal atrial tachycardia with block is often recognized as being a classic digitalis-toxic arrhythmia, there are no electrocardiographic features that clearly distinguish whether this supraventricular arrhythmia is or is not due to digitalis.

Almost every variety of ventricular arrhythmia has been associated with digitalis toxicity. The most common manifestation is an increase in the frequency of ventricular premature beats of any morphology, with either fixed or varying coupling intervals to preceding supraventricular beats. One uncommon ventricular arrhythmia that is associated with digoxin toxicity is ventricular bigeminy with alternating left- and right-axis deviation. Rarely, bidirectional or fascicular ventricular tachycardia may occur, an arrhythmia that is suggestive of digitalis toxicity. Another characteristic but less-specific pattern is multiform and repetitive ventricular premature beats occurring during atrial fibrillation.

Although there is no one electrocardiographic abnormality that is pathognomonic of digitalis excess, the combination of enhanced automaticity and impaired conduction (e.g., atrioventricular block accompanied by an accelerated junctional pacemaker) is highly suggestive of toxicity, even in patients whose serum levels are within the accepted therapeutic range.

Increased Sensitivity to Toxic Manifestations of Digitalis: Risk Factors

Disturbances of potassium homeostasis clearly influence the action of digitalis. The ability of potassium depletion to increase the risk of digoxin toxicity is due to several factors. The enhanced automaticity of cardiac tissue in response to toxic levels of cardiac glycosides is increased by hypokalemia in experimental animals, whereas the appearance of delayed after-depolarizations that could reach threshold is antagonized by hyperkalemia. Although most of these electrophysiological effects of hypokalemia have been observed in vitro or in experimental animal preparations, clinical experience suggests that such electrophysiological effects likely also occur in humans.

In contrast to hypokalemia, when the serum potassium concentration is normal or elevated (>5.5 mEq/L), any further increase in extracellular potassium will necessarily result in a further depolarization of myocardial conduction tissue. This effect may be most pronounced in atrioventricular nodal tissue, where conduction is relatively slow, leading to an exacerbation of digitalis-induced conduction delays. Thus, extracellular potassium exhibits a bimodal effect on atrioventricular conduction depending on the extracellular concentration; hypokalemia may exacerbate digitalis-induced atrioventricular block, whereas hyperkalemia may worsen nodal conduction delays of any etiology. For this reason, potassium should be administered cautiously to any patient with first- or second-degree atrioventricular block, as well as third-degree block, and facilities for external or transvenous cardiac pacing should be readily available. Potassium is particularly efficacious for treatment of cardiac glycoside-induced ventricular arrhythmias such as supraventricular tachycardia (SVT) with atrioventricular (AV) block and may be effective even when the serum potassium concentration is in the normal range (Table 25-2).

Disturbances in serum levels of other electrolytes also can influence myocardial sensitivity to digitalis, although less profoundly than K^+ concentration. Administration of Mg^{2+} salts suppresses digitalis-induced arrhythmias, and hypomagnesemia appears to predispose to digitalis toxicity. Magnesium depletion may become clinically important in patients chronically treated with diuretic agents, as well as in those with gastrointestinal disease, diabetes mellitus, or poor nutritional status.

TABLE 25-2
GUIDELINES FOR POTASSIUM ADMINISTRATION CONCURRENT WITH CHRONIC CARDIAC GLYCOSIDE THERAPY

Indications

Serum potassium <3.5 mEq/L
Combined diuretic/cardiac glycoside therapy

Use particular caution with the following:

Concurrent administration of
- Potassium-sparing diuretics
- β-adrenergic antagonists
- Angiotensin-converting enzyme inhibitors
- Angiotensin II receptor (AT_1) antagonists
- Nonsteroidal anti-inflammatory drugs

Chronic renal insufficiency (GFR <20 mL/min)
Hyporeninism (type IV RTA; diabetes mellitus)

GFR, glomerular filtration rate; RTA, renal tubular acidosis.

Elevated serum Ca^{2+} levels increase ventricular automaticity and this effect is at least additive to, and perhaps synergistic with, the effects of digitalis. Administering intravenous calcium parenterally to digitalized patients may provoke lethal ventricular arrhythmias.

The interactions of cardiac glycosides with acid–base disturbances are complex. Perturbations in potassium homeostasis that follow a shift in blood pH will affect myocardial binding of cardiac glycosides. Similarly, acid–base status will influence the serum levels of ionized Ca^{2+}, with subsequent effects on automaticity. Whether acid–base balance, independent of these changes, alters myocardial sensitivity to digitalis is unclear.

Treatment of Digitalis Toxicity

The key to successful treatment is early recognition that an arrhythmia may be related to digitalis intoxication. The more common manifestations, including occasional ectopic beats, marked first-degree atrioventricular block, or atrial fibrillation with a slow ventricular response, require only temporary withdrawal of the drug, electrocardiographic monitoring (if indicated), and subsequent adjustment of the dosage schedule to prevent recurrence. Rhythm disturbances that impair cardiac output require more active intervention. Ventricular tachycardia due to digitalis intoxication demands immediate, vigorous treatment. Sinus bradycardia, sinoatrial arrest, and AV block of the second or third degree are sometimes treated effectively with atropine. On occasion, electrical pacing is required. Nonparoxysmal accelerated AV junctional rhythms with rates greater than 90 bpm, or those associated with exit block, ought to be followed closely and treated actively if hemodynamic impairment is evident. AV junctional escape rhythms may simply be monitored if the rate is satisfactory.

Potassium

Hyperkalemia can occur as a consequence of massive digitalis overdose, usually following attempted suicide, but rarely complicates the more common forms of digitalis toxicity in patients with underlying heart disease. Administration of potassium salts is recommended for ectopic ventricular arrhythmias, even when the serum potassium is within the normal range. Potassium also may improve digitalis-induced AV block in the presence of hypokalemia, although it should be given cautiously, with continuous electrocardiographic monitoring, and with either an external pacemaker or facilities for transvenous pacing close at hand.

Antiarrhythmics

Drugs useful for treatment of digitalis-induced ventricular arrhythmias include phenytoin and lidocaine, each of which has relatively little effect on the sinus node or on sinoatrial, AV, or His-Purkinje conduction. Phenytoin may improve sinoatrial or AV conduction under some circumstances. Both quinidine and procainamide can depress AV and sinoatrial conduction, as well as occasionally exhibiting proarrhythmic effects in the presence of digitalis-toxic arrhythmias. β-adrenergic antagonists also may exacerbate atrioventricular conduction disturbances due to digitalis, although they are likely to be effective in decreasing catecholamine-induced automaticity. β-adrenergic antagonists also shorten the refractory period of atrial and ventricular muscle and slow conduction velocity, effects that would tend to improve some digitalis-induced arrhythmias. Use of a short-acting β-blocker, such as esmolol, may be appropriate initially if indicated in severely ill patients monitored in an intensive care unit.

Electrical Cardioversion

In the absence of digitalis-induced arrhythmias, synchronous direct-current (DC) cardioversion is safe, particularly if lower energy levels are used. Electrical cardioversion is potentially hazardous when severe arrhythmias are due to digitalis toxicity and should be avoided if other measures are available and effective.

Binding Resins and Hemodialysis

Selected cardiac glycosides such as digitoxin, which undergo some enterohepatic circulation, may be trapped by binding resins during transit through the gut lumen. Both cholestyramine and colestipol can reduce serum digitoxin levels by this means, but the decrease is not of sufficient magnitude or rapidity to affect life-threatening toxicity. Hemodialysis is ineffective both in the case of digitoxin toxicity, due to its extensive binding by serum proteins, and in the treatment of digoxin toxicity, due to the drug's large volume of distribution.

Digoxin-Specific Fab Fragments

The widespread availability of Fab fragments of high-affinity polyclonal digoxin-specific antibodies provides the clinician with a means of rapidly and selectively reversing digoxin toxicity with little risk of adverse effects (83). Fab fragments of antidigoxin antibodies also have been used to reverse life-threatening digitoxin toxicity. The use of Fab fragments, as opposed to intact immunoglobulin G molecules, results in rapid clearance of the antibody fragment-digitalis complex, a property that reduces the immunogenicity of this foreign (i.e., sheep) protein. Digoxin-specific Fab fragments also have a large volume of distribution and result in rapid binding of digoxin from myocardial and other tissue binding sites (Table 25-3).

Over 20 years of experience with the polyclonal ovine antidigoxin Fab preparations has confirmed the safety and efficacy of this preparation (83–85). Final results from a multicenter prospective trial of Fab fragments for acute, life-threatening digitalis toxicity (86) and data from an observational postmarketing surveillance study have been published (87). The ages of patients treated in the prospective trial ranged from neonates within a few hours of birth

TABLE 25-3

CALCULATION OF DOSE OF ANTIDIGOXIN FAB FRAGMENTS

Step 1. Estimate total body digitalis content (in mg)

A. Acute digitalis poisoning:
Estimating amount ingested acutely (mg) × 0.80

B. Known or suspected toxicity during chronic digoxin therapy:

$$\frac{\text{Serum digoxin concentration} \times (5.6) \times (\text{weight in kg})}{1{,}000}$$

Step 2. Calculate dose of Fab fragments, by either:

A. $\frac{\text{Mol. mass Fab frag.} = 50{,}000 \times 64 \times \text{total body dig content}}{\text{Mol. mass digoxin} = 781}$

= dose of Fab fragments (mg)

or, if using a standard formulation (e.g., "Digibind," 65K),

B. $\frac{\text{Estimated total body load of digoxin (mg)}}{0.6\ (\text{mg/vial})}$

= "Digibind" dose (number of vials)

to adults aged 94 years. The average serum digoxin level at the time that antidigoxin Fab was administered was 8.0 ng/mL. The mean time to an initial response was 19 minutes and a complete response was usually observed within 90 minutes. Approximately 90% of patients (133 of 150 subjects) exhibited a complete or partial response to Fab, whereas failure to respond was usually attributable to either inadequate dosing or to a moribund clinical status at the time of Fab administration. The most prominent adverse effect, observed in 4% of patients, was the rapid development of hypokalemia, presumably resulting from the rapid reactivation of sodium pump activity in skeletal muscle and other tissues after digoxin binding to Fab, as well as to the administration of potassium-chelating resins and other treatments for hyperkalemia that preceded infusion of Fab fragments. No allergic complications were observed. A number of patients have now been treated with antidigoxin Fab fragments on two or more occasions without incident.

Neither the prospective trial of the use of Fab fragments of digoxin-specific antibodies nor the surveillance study of the postmarketing use of the antibody preparation addressed the issue of whether this drug ought to be given to patients with moderate digoxin toxicity. The efficacy of antidigoxin Fab fragments as a diagnostic agent in patients with suspected digitalis toxicity has not been studied, nor is it likely that a prospective clinical trial of sufficient magnitude to examine this issue will be initiated. Nevertheless, the good safety record of the antidigoxin Fab preparation, and its specificity and clear efficacy, argue for the use of this agent in the treatment of known cases of advanced and potentially life-threatening digitalis toxicity [the history of the development of the digoxin radioimmunoassay and digoxin-specific Fab antibodies by Tom Smith, Vincent Butler, and Ed Haber in the 1960s and 1970s has been reviewed by Kelly et al. (88)].

DIGOXIN IN CONTEMPORARY CLINICAL PRACTICE

Physician surveys have suggested that cardiologists rely on digoxin as part of the management of congestive heart failure to a greater degree than do internists or family practitioners, independent of the severity of the illness (89). However, skepticism about the ability of digoxin to save lives is long-standing. Hlatky et al. (90) reported that only about one-third of physicians surveyed in 1986 believed that there was a survival benefit with digoxin. This may partially explain current practice patterns, which suggest that despite an overall trend toward increasing pharmacotherapy for heart failure the use of digoxin is either decreasing or is largely unchanged. According to data from the Studies of Left Ventricular Dysfunction (SOLVD) Registry (91), only 45% of patients in that study were on digoxin at enrollment. Use of digoxin correlated with the severity of left ventricular dysfunction (65% of patients with an ejection fraction of <0.20% compared with 30% of patients with an ejection fraction between 0.36% and 0.45%). A study of practice at an academic medical center demonstrated that the use of digoxin in patients with left ventricular systolic dysfunction did not change significantly between 1990 and 1995 despite the publication of the PROVED and RADIANCE trials during this period of time, whereas important increases were seen in the overall use of ACE inhibitors, other vasodilator therapy, and β-adrenergic blockers (92). Reis et al. (93) also have shown that the use of digoxin differs among internal medicine specialties. Data from the ADHERE Registry demonstrate a decline in digoxin use from late 2001 to late 2004 (94). In addition, data from a prescription database (95) suggest a decline in digoxin and an increase in beta adrenergic antagonist use among patients at the time of discharge from a hospitalization for heart failure during the period 1989 to 2000. While the decrease in digoxin use was modest (2.4 percentage points per year) compared with the increase in β-blocker use, the change in digoxin prescriptions was especially significant in the latter 5 years and among patients with coronary disease or hypertension.

There may be important geographical differences in digoxin dosing, as well. Saunders et al. (96) reported on their screening of prescription databases from the United States, France, and the United Kingdom and found that digoxin dosing in the United Kingdom was significantly lower than in either the United States or France.

Any evaluation of digoxin in contemporary practice must recognize that the drug may not be appropriate in certain subgroups. Accordingly, the two categories of greatest focus have been the elderly and women.

Gender

The role for digoxin according to gender is controversial. A retrospective post hoc analysis from the DIG trial (97) suggests that women in the trial were generally older, had higher ejection fractions, higher basal heart rates, higher systolic blood pressures, and more advanced symptoms than did the men, but they had a lower overall mortality rate. Women on digoxin had a higher overall mortality rate (4.2% in absolute terms) compared to women on placebo, with a hazard ratio after multivariable adjustment of 1.23 (95% CI 1.02–1.47; $p = 0.014$) (Table 25-4). Similarly, the effect on hospitalization was blunted in women (95% CI crossed unity). In the subset of patients in whom a digoxin level was measured, the median level was slightly higher in women at 1 month compared with men but was similar at 12 months; similarly, the likelihood of a level of greater than 2.0 ng/mL was no different. In contrast, data from a Swedish hospital demonstrated both higher rates of adverse reactions to digoxin and higher serum levels in women (98).

Age

The use of digoxin in the elderly can present special challenges, due mostly to the increased risk of toxicity. This can occur because of polypharmacy as well as physiological factors, including lower lean body mass and decreased glomerular filtration rate (GFR) (30). In the DIG trial, increasing age was an independent predictor of both poor outcome and suspected digoxin toxicity (99). However, no clear relationship between age and digoxin use was seen with respect to the clinical endpoints. In a study of elderly patients transferred to a nursing facility following a heart failure hospitalization, the subsequent mortality of patients treated with digoxin but no ACE inhibitor was compared with those on ACE inhibitor but no digoxin (100). The former were older and had greater functional impairment, more ischemic heart disease, and a higher likelihood of being underweight. These factors may very well explain a significant proportion of the higher mortality rate in the digoxin group. Given the uncertainty over the relative balance between risk and benefit in this cohort and the finding of frequent inappropriate administration (101,102), digoxin use in the elderly is a less-reasonable alternative than was previously thought. Indeed, a study of physician self-reported prescribing practices suggests that there is heightened concern about the risk of digoxin toxicity in the elderly cohort (90).

TABLE 25-4
DIGOXIN-ASSOCIATED RISK OF DEATH AND HOSPITALIZATION AMONG MEN AND WOMEN

Variable	Death from Any Cause	Death from Cardiovascular Cause	Death from Worsening Heart Failure	Hospitalization for Worsening Heart Failure	Hospitalization for Other Causes	Death from Worsening Heart Failure or Hospitalization for Worsening Heart Failure in Ancillary Trial
Men						
Unadjusted hazard ratio* (95% CI)	0.95 (0.87–1.04)	0.98 (0.88–1.08)	0.83 (0.71–0.97)	0.68 (0.62–0.75)	1.16 (1.06–1.27)	0.67 (0.45–0.99)
Adjusted hazard ratio (95% CI)†	0.93 (0.85–1.02)	0.96 (0.87–1.06)	0.79 (0.68–0.92)	0.66 (0.60–0.73)	1.17 (1.07–1.28)	0.72 (0.48–1.07)
Women						
Unadjusted hazard ratio (95% CI)	1.17 (0.97–1.40)	1.18 (0.97–1.44)	1.07 (0.80–1.42)	0.85 (0.71–1.01)	1.14 (0.96–1.36)	0.95 (0.67–1.36)
Adjusted hazard ratio (95% CI)†	1.23 (1.02–1.47)	1.24 (1.02–1.52)	1.17 (0.87–1.56)	0.87 (0.72–1.04)	1.15 (0.97–1.37)	0.92 (0.64–1.31)
Interaction between Sex and Digoxin‡						
Unadjusted *p* value	0.047	0.097	0.14	0.039	0.87	0.19
Adjusted *p* value†	0.014	0.035	0.026	0.011	0.91	0.32

*Hazard ratios represent the risk of the outcome among patients randomly assigned to digoxin as compared with patients randomly assigned to placebo and were obtained with the use of a Cox proportional-hazards model.
† Values were adjusted for age, race, body-mass index, left ventricular ejection fraction, cardiothoracic ratio, New York Heart Association functional class, number of signs and symptoms of heart failure, serum creatinine level, systolic blood pressure, and presence or absence of diabetes, prior digoxin use, and concomitant use of diuretics, nitrates, and vasodilators.
‡ p values are for the sex-and-digoxin-therapy interaction term entered in the Cox proportional-hazards model.
From Saunders KB, Amerasinghe AKCP, Saunders KL. Dose of digoxin prescribed in the UK compared with France and the USA. *Lancet.* 1997;349:833–836.

Pharmacoeconomic Analyses

The economic impact of treating heart failure with digoxin has not been as rigorously analyzed as it has been with ACE inhibitors (103,104). Ward et al. (105), using data from the digoxin withdrawal studies, demonstrated that significant cost savings would be realized if digoxin therapy were continued in otherwise stable heart failure patients. Other investigators have examined the potential costs of care associated with digoxin toxicity (106–108), although it has been pointed out that judicious monitoring and targeted use of widely available antidigoxin immunotherapy should lower the costs of this complication. Weintraub et al. (108) have estimated that continuation of digoxin in a stable HF patient (based on the withdrawal trials) is cost-effective as long as the hospitalization rate for suspected digoxin toxicity does not exceed 33%. Although no data are yet forthcoming directly from the DIG trial on the potential savings from decreased hospitalizations due to heart failure, estimates have been generated by Mark (103). Before any formal pharmacoeconomic analysis is performed, however, the debate about the magnitude of this beneficial effect (109,110) needs to be resolved.

Guidelines on the Use of Digoxin

The guidelines of the Heart Failure Society of America (111) provide several recommendations for digoxin use: the drug should be considered for patients who have symptoms of heart failure (with an emphasis on NYHA Class II and III) and, in the majority of cases, the dose should be between 0.125 mg and 0.25 mg daily. In the American College of Cardiology/American Heart Association (ACC/AHA) practice guidelines for heart failure (112), digoxin is given a Class IIa indication (weight of evidence or opinion in favor of usefulness/efficacy) for patients with Stage C heart failure but a Class II indication (evidence and/or general agreement that a procedure is not useful/effective and in some cases may cause harm) for the Stage B (asymptomatic LV dysfunction) patient. The recent guidelines of the Task Force on Acute Heart Failure of the European Society of Cardiology (113) provide no formal recommendations in the acute setting. Indeed, as suggested by Gheorghiade (30), use of intravenous digoxin may paradoxically worsen heart failure.

Digoxin in the New Millennium

Despite uncertainties about efficacy in contemporary usage, it is unlikely that another study will be performed to resolve the outstanding clinical issues in the post-DIG trial era. The effort and costs required to enroll patients in a non-industry-sponsored trial with sufficient power of a generically available drug are prohibitive. Furthermore, as standard drug therapy for heart failure improves, a larger number of patients will be required to show an effect on survival. Other endpoints would need to be developed (115,116) and validated that would more accurately reflect the underlying pathophysiology of ventricular remodeling.

Therefore, the future of digoxin remains uncertain. Arguments have been made that there are multiple reasons to consider removing the drug from the contemporary care of patients with heart failure. The higher likelihood of toxicity in patients with renal insufficiency (117), and in older patients whose decline in GFR is often underappreciated, is an ongoing concern. Even with a focus on in-hospital quality initiatives (118), digoxin toxicity may be missed. The lack of impact on quality of life remains a distinct limitation, especially in a disease that is marked by significant symptomatic burden and functional limitations. Lack of definitive efficacy with β-blockers, uncertainty about use in the elderly and women, the high likelihood for inappropriate use or (at the very least) inappropriate dosing, and a very narrow therapeutic window are also considerations.

Nevertheless, as noted, the guidelines continue to demonstrate a consensus about digoxin use from a distance; that is, digoxin is indicated for patients with impaired LV systolic function who are in sinus rhythm and who remain symptomatic (NYHA Classes II and III) despite the use of ACE inhibitor and β-adrenergic antagonist. For the patient presenting with new onset of symptoms, the argument can be made that digoxin serves a role by virtue of its modest sympatholytic effects, especially at a time when the initiation of β-blocker may be delayed (e.g., until euvolemia and hemodynamic stability are achieved). Targeting digoxin use to those patients with severe symptoms, a marked reduction in LV ejection fraction, or rapid, poorly controlled atrial fibrillation in the setting of LV dysfunction, is likewise prudent. For patients with heart failure and preserved or nearly preserved LV function, the role for digoxin is less clear and probably should be avoided. Elderly patients, especially women and those with impairment of renal function or cachexia, should be monitored closely; indeed, the risk-to-benefit ratio likely favors nonuse in this population. For the average patient, a dose of 0.125 mg daily is suggested without loading; for the patient with risk factors for digoxin toxicity, a dose of 0.125 mg every other day or three times weekly can be a viable alternative.

In the setting of the maturation of newer therapies for heart failure and the focus on survival as the important outcome, the likelihood is that the digitalis debate, as well as the use of this venerable class of drugs, will fade in intensity, albeit without a clear declaration of victory by either proponents or detractors. For the former, it will be difficult to give up on a drug with such a long history in the annals of therapeutics. With that said, it may indeed be true that, as stated by Packer, "As the list of therapeutic agents that prolong life grows, the use of digitalis will inevitably wane. . . . This is not a prediction of doom and gloom; it is merely a reflection of the natural evolution of medical practice" (119).

REFERENCES

1. Withering W. An account of the foxglove and some of its medical uses, with practical remarks on dropsy, and other disease. In: Willius FA, Keys TE, eds. *Classics of Cardiology*. Vol. I. New York: Henry Schuman, Dover Publications; 1941: 231–252.

2. Christian HA. Digitalis effects in chronic cardiac cases with regular rhythm in contrast to auricular fibrillation. *Med Clin North Am*. 1922;5:117–119.
3. Eisner DA, Smith TW. The Na-K pump and its effectors in cardiac muscle. In: Fozzard HA, Haber E, Katz AM, Morgan HE, eds. *The Heart and Cardiovascular System*. New York: Raven; 1991: 863–902.
4. Thomas R, Gray P, Andrews J. Digitalis: its mode of action, receptor, and structure-activity relationships. In: Testa B, ed. *Advances in Drug Research*. Vol. 19. New York: Academic; 1989.
5. Marban E, Tsien RW. Enhancement of cardiac calcium current during digitalis inotropy: positive feedback regulation by intracellular calcium. *J Physiol (Lond)*. 1982;329:589–614.
6. Wier WG, Hess P. Excitation-contraction coupling in cardiac Purkinje fibers. Effects of cardiotonic steroids on the intracellular $[Ca^{2+}]$ transient, membrane potential, and contraction. *J Gen Physiol*. 1984;83:395–415.
7. Barry WH, Hasin Y, Smith TW. Sodium pump inhibition, enhanced Ca-influx via Na-Ca exchange, and positive inotropic response in cultured heart cells. *Circ Res*. 1985;56:231–241.
8. Skou JC. The Na,K-pump. *Methods Enzymol*. 1988;156:1–28.
9. Surridge C. Nobel prizes honor biologists' work on protein energy converters. *Nature*. 1997;389:771.
10. Shull GE, Schwartz A, Lingrel JB. Amino-acid sequence of the catalytic subunit of the $(Na^+$-$K^+)$ATPase deduced from a complementary DNA. *Nature*. 1985;316:691–695.
11. Shull GE, Lane LK, Lingrel JB. Amino-acid sequence of the beta-subunit of the $(Na^+$-$K^+)$ATPase deduced from a cDNA. *Nature*. 1986;321:429–431.
12. Geering K, Beggah A, Good P, et al. Oligomerization and maturation of Na,K-ATPase-functional interaction of the cytoplasmic NH_2 terminus of the subunit with the α subunit. *J Cell Biol*. 1996;133:1193–1204.
13. Beguin P, Wang XY, Firsov D, et al. The subunit is a specific component of the Na,K-ATPase and modulates its transport function. *EMBO J*. 1997;16:4250–4260.
14. Geering K. Na,K-ATPase. *Curr Opin Nephrol Hypertens*. 1997;6: 434–439.
15. Palasis M, Kuntzweiler TA, Arguello JM, et al. Ouabain interactions with the H5-H6 hairpin of the Na,K-ATPase reveal a possible inhibition mechanism via the cation binding domain. *J Biol Chem*. 1996;271:14176–14182.
16. Croyle ML, Woo AL, Lingrel JB. Extensive random mutagenesis analysis of the Na^+/K^+-ATPase α subunit identifies known and previously unidentified amino acid residues that alter ouabain sensitivity–implications for ouabain binding. *Eur J Biochem*. 1997;248:488–495.
17. Juhaszova M, Blaustein MP. Na^+ pump low and high ouabain affinity α subunit isoforms are differently distributed in cells. *Proc Natl Acad Sci USA*. 1997;94:1800–1805.
18. McDonough AA, Zhang YB, Shin V, et al. Subcellular distribution of sodium pump isoform subunits in mammalian cardiac myocytes. *Am J Physiol*. 1996;39:C1221–C1227.
19. Mullerehmsen J, Frank K, Brixius K, et al. Increase in force of contraction by activation of the Na^+/Ca^{2+} exchanger in human myocardium. *Br J Clin Pharmacol*. 1997;43:399–405.
20. Hasenfuss G, Mulieri LA, Allen PD, et al. Influence of isoproterenol and ouabain on excitation-contraction coupling, cross-bridge function and energetics in failing human myocardium. *Circulation*. 1996;94:3155–3160.
21. Peng M, Huang L, Xie Z, et al. Partial inhibition of Na^+/K^+-ATPase by ouabain induces the Ca^{2+}-dependent expressions of early-response genes in cardiac myocytes. *J Biol Chem*. 1996;271:10372–10378.
22. Huang LY, Li H, Xie ZJ. Ouabain-induced hypertrophy in cultured cardiac myocytes is accompanied by changes in expression of several late response genes. *J Mol Cell Cardiol*. 1997;29: 429–437.
23. Huang LY, Kometiani P, Xie ZJ. Differential regulation of Na/K-ATPase α subunit isoform gene expressions in cardiac myocytes by ouabain and other hypertrophic stimuli. *J Mol Cell Cardiol*. 1997;29:3157–3167.
24. Hancox JC, Levi AJ. Actions of the digitalis analogue strophanthidin on action potentials and L-type calcium current in single cells isolated from the rabbit atrioventricular node. *Br J Pharmacol*. 1996;118:1447–1454.
25. Han X, Kubota I, Feron O, et al. Muscarinic cholinergic regulation of cardiac myocyte $I_{Ca\text{-}L}$ is absent in mice with targeted disruption of endothelial nitric oxide synthase (eNOS). *Proc Natl Acad Sci USA*. 1998;95:6510–6515.
26. Kelly RA, Balligand J-L, Smith TW. Nitric oxide and cardiac function: a review. *Circ Res*. 1996;79:363–380.
27. Kelly RA, Han X. Nitrovasodilators have (small) direct effects on cardiac contractility. Is this important? *Circulation*. 1997; 96:2493–2495.
28. Mason DT, Braunwald E, Karsh RB, et al. Studies on digitalis. X. Effects of ouabain on forearm vascular resistance and venous tone in normal subjects and in patients in heart failure. *J Clin Invest*. 1964;43:532–543.
29. Ferguson DW, Berg WJ, Sanders JS, et al. Sympathoinhibitory responses to digitalis glycosides in heart failure patients. Direct evidence from sympathetic neural recordings. *Circulation*. 1989;80:65–77.
30. Gheorghiade M, Kirkwood F, Adams KF, et al. Digoxin in the management of cardiovascular disorders. *Circulation*. 2004;109: 2959–2964.
31. Gheorghiade M, Ferguson D. Digoxin. A neurohormonal modulator in heart failure? *Circulation* 1991;84:2181.
32. Cheng JW, Charland SL, Shaw LM, et al. Is the volume of distribution of digoxin reduced in patients with renal dysfunction? Determining digoxin pharmacokinetics by fluorescence polarization immunoassay. *Pharmacotherapy*. 1997;17:584–590.
33. Jelliffe RW, Brooker G. A nomogram for digoxin therapy. *Am J Med*. 1974;57:63–68.
34. Hougen TJ. Use of digoxin in the young. In: Smith TW, ed. *Digitalis Glycosides*. Orlando: Grune & Stratton; 1985: 169–208.
35. Juurlink DN, Mamdani MM, Kopp A, et al. A population-based assessment of the potential interaction between serotonin-specific reuptake inhibitors and digoxin. *British J Clin Pharm*. 2005;59(1):102–107.
36. Zhou H, Parks V, Pata A, et al. Absence of a clinically relevant interaction between etanercept and digoxin. *J Clin Pharm*. 2004;44(11):1244–1251.
37. Dasgupta A, Szelei-Stevens KA. Neutralization of free digoxin-like immunoreactive components of oriental medicines Dan Shen and Lu-Shen-Wan by the Fab fragment of antidigoxin antibody (Digibind). *Am J Clin Pathology*. 2004;121(2):276–281.
38. Mueller SC, Uehleke B, Woehling H, et al. Effect of St. John's wort dose and preparations on the pharmacokinetics of digoxin. *Clin Pharm and Therapeutics*. 2004;75(6):546–557.
39. Matsumori A, Ono K, Nishio R, et al. Modulation of cytokine production and protection against lethal endotoxemia by the cardiac glycoside ouabain. *Circulation*. 1997;96: 1501–1506.
40. Foey AD, Crawford A, Hall ND. Modulation of cytokine production by human mononuclear cells following impairment of Na,K-ATPase activity. *Biochim Biophys Acta*. 1997;1355:43–49.
41. Arstall MA, Kelly RA. The role of nitric oxide in ventricular dysfunction. *J Cardiac Fail*. 1998;4:249–260.
42. Starr I, Luchi RJ. Blind study on the action of digitoxin on elderly women. *Am Heart J*. 1969;78:740–751.
43. Dobbs SN, Kenyon WI, Dobbs RJ. Maintenance digoxin after an episode of heart failure. Placebo controlled trial in outpatients. *BMJ*. 1977;1:749–752.
44. Fleg L, Gottlieb SH, Lakatta EG. Is digoxin really important in compensated heart failure? *Am J Med*. 1982;73:244–250.
45. Taggart AJ, Johnston GD, McDevitt DG. Digoxin withdrawal after cardiac failure in patients with sinus rhythm. *J Cardiovasc Pharmacol*. 1983;5:229–234.
46. Lee DC-S, Johnson RA, Bingham JB, et al. Heart failure in outpatients. A randomized trial of digoxin versus placebo. *N Engl J Med*. 1982;306:699–705.
47. Gheorghiade M, St. Clair J, St. Clair C, et al. Hemodynamic effects of intravenous digoxin in patients with severe heart failure initially treated with diuretics and vasodilators. *J Am Coll Cardiol*. 1987;9:849–857.
48. German and Austrian Xamoterol Study Group. Double-blind placebo-controlled comparison of digoxin and xamoterol in chronic heart failure. *Lancet*. 1988;1:489–493.
49. Captopril-Digoxin Multicenter Research Group. Comparative effects of therapy with captopril and digoxin in patients with mild to moderate heart failure. *JAMA*. 1988;259:539–544.

50. DiBianco R, Shabetai R, Kostuk W, et al. A comparison of oral milrinone, digoxin, and their combination in the treatment of patients with chronic heart failure. *N Engl J Med.* 1989; 320:677–683.
51. Uretsky BF, Young JB, Shahidi E, et al. Randomized study assessing the effect of digoxin withdrawal in patients with mild to moderate chronic congestive heart failure: results of the PROVED trial. *J Am Coll Cardiol.* 1993;22:955–962.
52. Packer M, Gheorghiade M, Young JB, et al. Withdrawal of digoxin from patients with chronic heart failure treated with angiotensin-converting enzyme inhibitors. *N Engl J Med.* 1993; 329:1–7.
53. Rathore SS, Curtis JP, Wang Y, et al. Association of serum digoxin concentration and outcomes in patients with heart failure. *JAMA.* 2003;289:871–878.
54. Shammas NW, Harris ML, McKinney D, et al. Digoxin withdrawal in patients with dilated cardiomyopathy following normalization of ejection fraction with beta blockers. *Clin Cardiol.* 2001;24(12):786–787.
55. Rahimtoola SH, Tak T. The use of digitalis in heart failure. *Curr Prob Cardiol.* 1996;21:787–853.
56. Jaeschke R, Oxman A, Guyatt G. To what extent do congestive heart failure patients in sinus rhythm benefit from digoxin therapy? A systematic overview and meta-analysis. *Am J Med.* 1990;88:279–286.
57. Brouwer J, Van Veldhuisen DJ, Manintveld AJ, et al. Heart rate variability in patients with mild to moderate heart failure: effects on neurohormonal modulation by digoxin and ibopamine. *J Am Coll Cardiol.* 1995;26:983–990.
58. Leor J, Goldbourt U, Behar S, et al. Digoxin and mortality in survivors of acute myocardial infarction: observations in patients at low and intermediate risk. The SPRINT Study Group. Secondary Prevention Reinfarction Israel Nifedipine Trial. *Cardiovasc Drug Ther.* 1995;9:609–617.
59. Eichhorn EJ, Lukas MA, Wu B, et al. Effect of concomitant digoxin and carvedilol therapy on mortality and morbidity in patients with chronic heart failure. *Am J Cardiol.* 2000;86(9): 1032–1035.
60. Pitt B, Zannad F, Remme WJ, Cody R, et al. The effect of spironolactone on morbidity and mortality in patients with severe heart failure. Randomized Aldactone Evaluation Study Investigators. *N Engl J Med.* 1999;341:709–717.
61. Cohn JN, Tognoni G. Valsartan Heart Failure Trial Investigators. A randomized trial of the angiotensin-receptor blocker valsartan in chronic heart failure. *N Engl J Med.* 2001;345:1667–1675.
62. Pfeffer MA, Swedberg K, Granger CG, et al. CHARM Investigators and Committees. Effects of candesartan on mortality and morbidity in patients with chronic heart failure: the CHARM overall programme. *Lancet.* 2003;362:759–766.
63. Olshansky B, Rosenfeld LE, Warner AL, et al., AFFIRM Investigators. The Atrial Fibrillation Follow-Up Investigation of Rhythm Management (AFFIRM) study: approaches to control rate in atrial fibrillation. *J Am Coll Cardiol.* 2004;43(7):1201–1208.
64. The Digitalis Investigation Group. The effect of digoxin on mortality and morbidity in patients with heart failure. *N Engl J Med.* 1997;336:525–533.
65. The Digitalis Investigation Group. Rationale, design, implementation, and baseline characteristics of patients in the DIG trial: a large, simple, long-term trial to evaluate the effect of digitalis on mortality in heart failure. *Controlled Clin Trials.* 1996;17: 77–97.
66. Lader E, Egan D, Hunsberger S, et al. The effect of digoxin on the quality of life in patients with heart failure. *J Card Fail.* 2003;9(1):4–12.
67. Hood WB, Dans AL, Guyatt GH, et al. Digitalis for treatment of congestive heart failure in patients in sinus rhythm: a systematic review and meta-analysis. *J Card Fail.* 2004;10(2):155–164.
68. Lindsay SJ, Kearney MT, Prescott RJ, et al. Digoxin and mortality in chronic heart failure. UK Heart Investigation. *Lancet* 1999;354(9183):1003.
69. Newton GE, Tong JH, Schofield AM, et al. Digoxin reduces cardiac sympathetic activity in severe congestive heart failure. *J Am Coll Cardiol.* 1996;28:155–161.
70. Krum H, Bigger JT, Jr., Goldsmith RL, et al. Effect of long-term digoxin therapy on autonomic function in patients with chronic heart failure. *J Am Coll Cardiol.* 1995;2:289–294.
71. van Veldhuisen DJ, Man in 'T Veld AJ, Dunselman PHJM, et al. Double-blind placebo-controlled study of ibopamine and digoxin in patients with mild to moderate heart failure: results of the Dutch Ibopamine Multicenter Trial (DIMT). *J Am Coll Cardiol.* 1993;22:1564–1573.
72. Leier CV. Positive inotropic therapy: an update and new agents. *Curr Prob Cardiol.* 1996;21:527–581.
73. Sackner-Bernstein JD, Mancini DM. Rationale for treatment of patients with chronic heart failure and adrenergic blockade. *JAMA.* 1995;274:1462–1467.
74. Tsutamoto T, Wada A, Maeda K, et al. Digitalis increases brain natriuretic peptide in patients with severe congestive heart failure. *Am Heart J.* 1997;134:910–916.
75. Khoury AM, Davila DF, Bellabarba G, et al. Acute effects of digitalis and enalapril on the neurohormonal profile of chagasic patients with severe congestive heart failure. *Int J Cardiol.* 1996; 57:21–29.
76. Flapan AD, Goodfield NE, Wright RA, et al. Effects of digoxin on time domain measures of heart rate variability in patients with stable chronic cardiac failure—withdrawal and comparison group studies. *Int J Cardiol.* 1997;59:29–36.
77. Gheorghiade M, Hall VB, Jacobsen G, et al. Effects of increasing maintenance dose of digoxin on left ventricular function and neurohormones in patients with chronic heart failure treated with diuretics and angiotensin-converting enzyme inhibitors. *Circulation.* 1995;92:1801–1807.
78. Slatton ML, Irani WN, Hall SA, et al. Does digoxin provide additional hemodynamic and autonomic benefit at higher doses in patients with mild to moderate heart failure and normal sinus rhythm? *J Am Coll Cardiol.* 1997;29:1206–1213.
79. Yusuf S, Garg R, Held P, et al. Need for a large randomized trial to evaluate the effect of digitalis on morbidity and mortality in congestive heart failure. *Am J Cardiol.* 1992;69:64G–70G.
80. Packer M. Do ACE inhibitors prolong life in patients with heart failure treated in clinical practice? *J Am Coll Cardiol.* 1996;28:1323–1327.
81. Bristow MR, O'Connell JB, Gilbert EM, et al. Dose-response of chronic β-blocker treatment in heart failure from either idiopathic dilated or ischemic cardiomyopathy. *Circulation* 1994; 89:1632–1642.
82. Borron SW, Bismuth C, Muszynski J. Advances in the management of digoxin toxicity in the older patient. *Drugs Aging.* 1997;10:18–33.
83. Kelly RA, Smith TW. Antibody therapies for drug overdose. In: Austen KF, Burakoff SJ, Rosen FS, Strom TR, eds. *Therapeutic Immunology.* Vol. 27. Boston: Blackwell Scientific; 1996: 353–362.
84. Ujhelyi MR, Robert S. Pharmacokinetic aspects of digoxin-specific Fab therapy in the management of digitalis toxicity. *Clin Pharmacokinet.* 1995;28:483–493.
85. Renard C, Grenelerouge N, Beau N, et al. Pharmacokinetics of digoxin-specific Fab: effects of decreased renal function and age. *Br J Clin Pharmacol.* 1997;44:135–138.
86. Antman EM, Wenger TL, Butler VP, Jr., et al. Treatment of 150 cases of life-threatening digitalis intoxication with digoxin-specific Fab antibody fragments: final report of a multicenter study. *Circulation.* 1990;81:1744–1752.
87. Hickey AR, Wenger TL, Carpenter VP, et al. Digoxin immune Fab therapy in the management of digitalis intoxication: safety and efficacy results of an observational surveillance study. *J Am Coll Cardiol.* 1991;17:590–598.
88. Kelly RA, Smith TW. 1936 to 1997. *Can J Cardiol.* 1997;13: 1052–1056.
89. Chin MH, Friedmann PD, Cassel CK, et al. Differences in generalist and specialist physicians' knowledge and use of angiotensin-converting enzyme inhibitors for congestive heart failure. *J Gen Intern Med.* 1997;12:523–530.
90. Hlatky MA, Fleg JL, Hinton PC, et al. Physician practice in the management of congestive heart failure. *J Am Coll Cardiol.* 1986;4:966–970.
91. Bourassa MG, Gurné O, Bangdiwala SI, et al. Natural history and patterns of current practice in heart failure. *J Am Coll Cardiol.* 1993;32:14A–19A.
92. Rich MW, Brooks K, Luther P. Temporal trends in the pharmacotherapy of congestive heart failure at an academic medical center: 1990–1995. *J Am Coll Cardiol.* 1997;29:323A.

93. Reis SE, Holubkov R, Edmundowicz D, et al. Treatment of patients admitted to the hospital with congestive heart failure: specialty-related disparities in practice patterns and outcomes. *J Am Coll Cardiol.* 1997;30:733–738.
94. Hauptman PJ, Hussain ZM. Patterns of digoxin use and digoxin toxicity in the post-DIG trial era. *J Cardiac Fail.* 2005;11:S165.
95. Smith NL, Chan JD, Rea TD, et al. Time trends in the use of beta-blockers and other pharmacotherapies in older adults with congestive heart failure. *Am Heart J.* 2004;148:710–717.
96. Saunders KB, Amerasinghe AKCP, Saunders KL. Dose of digoxin prescribed in the UK compared with France and the USA. *Lancet.* 1997;349:833–836.
97. Rathore SS, Wang Y, Krumholz HM. Sex-based differences in the effect of digoxin for the treatment of heart failure. *N Engl J Med.* 2002;347(18):1403–1411.
98. Hallbert P, Michaelsson K, Melhus H. Digoxin for the treatment of heart failure. *N Engl J Med.* 2003;348:661–663.
99. Rich MW, McSherry F, Williford WO, et al. Digitalis Investigation Group. Effect of age on mortality, hospitalizations and response to digoxin in patients with heart failure: the DIG study. *J Am Coll Cardiol.* 2001;38(3):806–813.
100. Gambassi G, Lapane KL, Sgadari A, et al. Effects of angiotensin-converting enzyme inhibitors and digoxin on health outcomes of very old patients with heart failure. *Arch Intern Med.* 2000;160(1):53–60.
101. Ahmed A, Allman RM, DeLong JF. Inappropriate use of digoxin in older hospitalized heart failure patients. *J Gerontol A Biol Sci Med Sci.* 2002;57(2):M138–M143.
102. Haas GJ, Young JB. Inappropriate use of digoxin in the elderly: how widespread is the problem and how can it be solved? *Drug Safety* 1999;20(3):223–230.
103. Mark DB. Economics of treating heart failure. *Am J Cardiol.* 1997;80:33H–38H.
104. McMurray J, Davie A. The pharmacoeconomics of ACE inhibitors in chronic heart failure. *Pharmacoeconomics.* 1996;9: 188–197.
105. Ward RE, Gheorghiade M, Young JB, et al. Economic outcomes of withdrawal of digoxin therapy in adult patients with stable congestive heart failure. *J Am Coll Cardiol.* 1995;26: 93–101.
106. Gandhi AJ, Vlasses PH, Morton DJ, et al. Economic impact of digoxin toxicity. *Pharmacoeconomics.* 1997;12:175–181.
107. Mauskopf JA, Wenger TL. Cost-effectiveness analysis of the use of digoxin immune Fab (ovine) for treatment of digoxin toxicity. *Am J Cardiol.* 1991;68:1709–1714.
108. Weintraub WS, Cole J, Tooley JF. Cost and cost-effectiveness studies in heart failure research. *Am Heart J.* 2002;143:565–576.
109. Packer M. End of the oldest controversy in medicine. Are we ready to conclude the debate on digitalis? *N Engl J Med.* 1997; 336:575–576.
110. Waagstein F, Bristow MR, Swedberg K, et al. Beneficial effects of metoprolol in idiopathic dilated cardiomyopathy. *Lancet.* 1993;342:1441–1446.
111. Heart Failure Society of American. HFSA guidelines for management of patients with heart failure caused by left ventricular systolic dysfunction—pharmacological approaches. *J Cardiac Fail.* 1999;5:357–382.
112. Hunt A, Baker DW, Chin MH, et al. ACC/AHA 2005 Guideline update for the evaluation and management of chronic heart failure in the adult. A report of the American College of Cardiology/American Heart Association Task Force on Practice Guideline. Committee to Revise the 1995 Guidelines for the Evaluation and American College of Cardiology web site. Available at: *http://www.acc.org/clinical/guidelines/failure/hf_index.htm.* Accessed January 31, 2006.
113. Task Force on Acute Heart Failure of the European Society of Cardiology. Executive summary of the guidelines on the diagnosis and treatment of acute heart failure. *Eur Heart J.* 2005;26: 384–416.
114. Massie BM, Abdalla I. Heart failure in patients with preserved left ventricular systolic function: do digitalis glycosides have a role? *Prog Cardiovasc Dis.* 1998;40:357–369.
115. Hauptman PJ. Measurement of end points in heart failure trials: jousting at windmills? *Mount Sinai J Med.* 2004;71:298–304.
116. Packer M. Proposal for a new clinical end point to evaluate the efficacy of drugs and devices in the treatment of chronic heart failure. *J Cardiac Fail.* 2001;7:176–182.
117. Shlipak MG, Smith GL, Rathore SS, et al. Renal function, digoxin therapy, and heart failure outcomes: evidence from the digoxin intervention group trial. *J Am Soc Nephrol.* 2004;15:2195–2203.
118. Galanter WL, Polikaitis A, DiDomenico RJ. A trial of automated safety alerts for inpatient digoxin use with computerized physician order entry. *J Am Med Inform Assoc.* 2004;11:270–277.
119. Packer M. Digoxin in patients with heart failure. *N Engl J Med.* 1997;337:131.

26 Inhibition of the Renin-Angiotensin-Aldosterone System in Chronic Heart Failure: Rationale, Results, and Current Recommendations

John R. Teerlink Kiran K. Khush Barry M. Massie

Our understanding of the pathophysiology of chronic heart failure has progressed significantly, from simple pump failure, to an expanded cardio-renal model, to our currently accepted neurohormonal model (1). We now recognize the vital role that neurohormonal activation plays in the initiation and progression of heart failure (HF), even in the absence of further direct insults. The renin-angiotensin-aldosterone system (RAAS) lies at the heart of this neurohormonal cascade, and our understanding of the complex, important roles played by angiotensin II and aldosterone continues to evolve. While the hemodynamic and renal effects of these hormones are now well-characterized, their cellular and molecular effects continue to be a source of intense investigation.

Clinical observations, leading to clinical trials using a variety of neurohormonal antagonists which have improved symptoms and outcomes of HF patients, have given direction to basic investigations clarifying the physiological and cellular mechanisms by which these endogenous neurohormones and their antagonists produce their deleterious and beneficial effects. This chapter will review the role of the RAAS in the pathophysiology of HF, with an emphasis on the rationale for the use of RAAS inhibitors, clinical trial results, and current treatment recommendations.

RATIONALE FOR BLOCKADE OF THE RENIN-ANGIOTENSIN-ALDOSTERONE SYSTEM IN HEART FAILURE

Hemodynamic Alterations in Heart Failure

The characteristic hemodynamic abnormalities in patients with HF are a reduction in stroke volume and cardiac output, and concomitant elevation of left and right ventricular filling pressures, either at rest or with activity (2). These changes are accompanied by an increase in systemic vascular resistance and redistribution of regional blood flow, thereby contributing to the typical signs and symptoms of HF, such as fluid retention and inadequate blood flow to vital organs including the kidneys and exercising muscle. Such physiological alterations result in dyspnea, exercise intolerance, fatigue, and edema. Neurohormonal activation plays a central role in causing these abnormalities, which in turn can be alleviated by blocking these responses.

Neurohormonal Activation in Heart Failure

HF represents a highly complex syndrome in which myocardial injury leads to neurohormonal activation and subsequent ventricular remodeling (3) (Fig. 26-1). In the neurohormonal model, HF develops as a result of the overexpression of peptide molecules which exert toxic long-term effects on the cardiovascular system (1,4,5). In the acute phase of HF, neurohormonal activation may help maintain adequate cardiac output and peripheral perfusion. Sustained neurohormonal activation, however, eventually results in increased cardiac wall stress, ventricular dilatation, and adverse remodeling (6,7). A variety of endogenously produced substances, including norepinephrine, angiotensin II, aldosterone, endothelin, and tumor necrosis factor-alpha (TNF-α), have been implicated as biologically active molecules which contribute to disease progression in the failing heart.

Therefore, although the early approaches to treating HF, such as positive inotropic agents and diuretics, provide symptomatic relief and hemodynamic improvement, they have relatively limited impact on its natural history. In contrast, inhibition of the activated RAAS and sympathetic nervous system prevents or slows ventricular remodeling—a process closely linked to the progression of HF, discussed elsewhere in this text—and consequently has beneficial effects on its natural history

The Endocrine Renin-Angiotensin-Aldosterone System

As described in another chapter of this text, the activation of the RAAS in acute and chronic HF is triggered by reduced stroke volume or cardiac output, with resultant impairment of renal blood flow and perfusion pressure. The cascade is initiated by the release of renin from the juxtaglomerular cells of the kidney in response to renal hypoperfusion and sympathetic activation (8). Angiotensinogen produced by the liver is then cleaved by renin to yield the inactive decapeptide angiotensin I (Ang I). Circulating Ang I is then converted to angiotensin II (Ang II) in the lungs and other tissues by angiotensin-converting enzyme (ACE). Ang II exerts its biological effects by binding to Ang II receptors in target organs and tissues (Fig. 26-2).

In the kidneys, Ang II causes sodium and water retention and vasoconstriction of efferent arterioles of the glomerulus, thereby increasing blood pressure and sodium reabsorption. Ang II concomitantly stimulates the secretion of aldosterone by the adrenal cortex and arginine vasopressin by the posterior pituitary gland, both of which contribute to extracellular volume expansion and sympathetic activation. At a molecular level, Ang II stimulates myocyte hypertrophy, apoptosis, fibroblast proliferation, collagen deposition, and interstitial fibrosis (7). Furthermore, evidence now implicates the RAAS in the development of atherosclerosis (9), which indirectly may negatively impact on the natural history of HF patients. These disparate effects, in sum, promote the development of left ventricular dysfunction, vascular abnormalities, and the clinical syndrome of HF (Fig. 26-3).

The Cardiac Renin-Angiotensin-Aldosterone System

Until relatively recently, the classical endocrine RAAS was considered to be the mediator of the cardiovascular effects of angiotensin and aldosterone. However, experimental evidence now provides strong support for the existence of a local cardiac RAAS (10,11). The individual components of the RAAS are present within cardiac and vascular myocytes and fibroblasts, leading to production of neurohormones such as Ang II and aldosterone within the myocardium itself. These mediators act in an autocrine and paracrine manner, independent of the effects of circulating renin, thereby contributing to local cardiac injury.

The discovery of local expression and activation of the RAAS in both the myocardium and vasculature has prompted investigation into the tissue-specific affinity of different ACE inhibitors (ACEIs), and whether tissue-specificity confers any clinical benefit. Although some ACEIs have a higher tissue affinity than others (12,13), there is no evidence that the commonly used agents differ in their clinical effects and the relative clinical importance of the cardiac tissue RAAS remains unclear.

Angiotensin-Converting Enzyme

ACE is a zinc metallopeptidase that catalyzes the conversion of Ang I to Ang II. This enzyme, which is primarily tissue-based, is induced in virtually all states of cardiac injury, including volume overload (14,15), myocardial

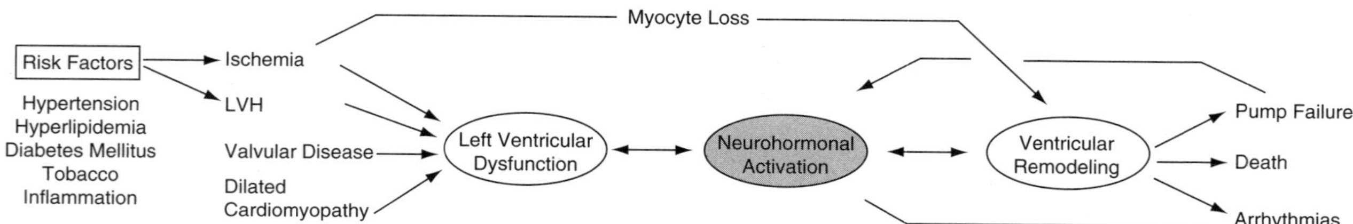

Figure 26-1 Pathophysiology of heart failure. Neurohormonal activation, through the renin-angiotensin-aldosterone system and other sympathetic axes, is central to the development and progression of heart failure. LVH, left ventricular hypertrophy.

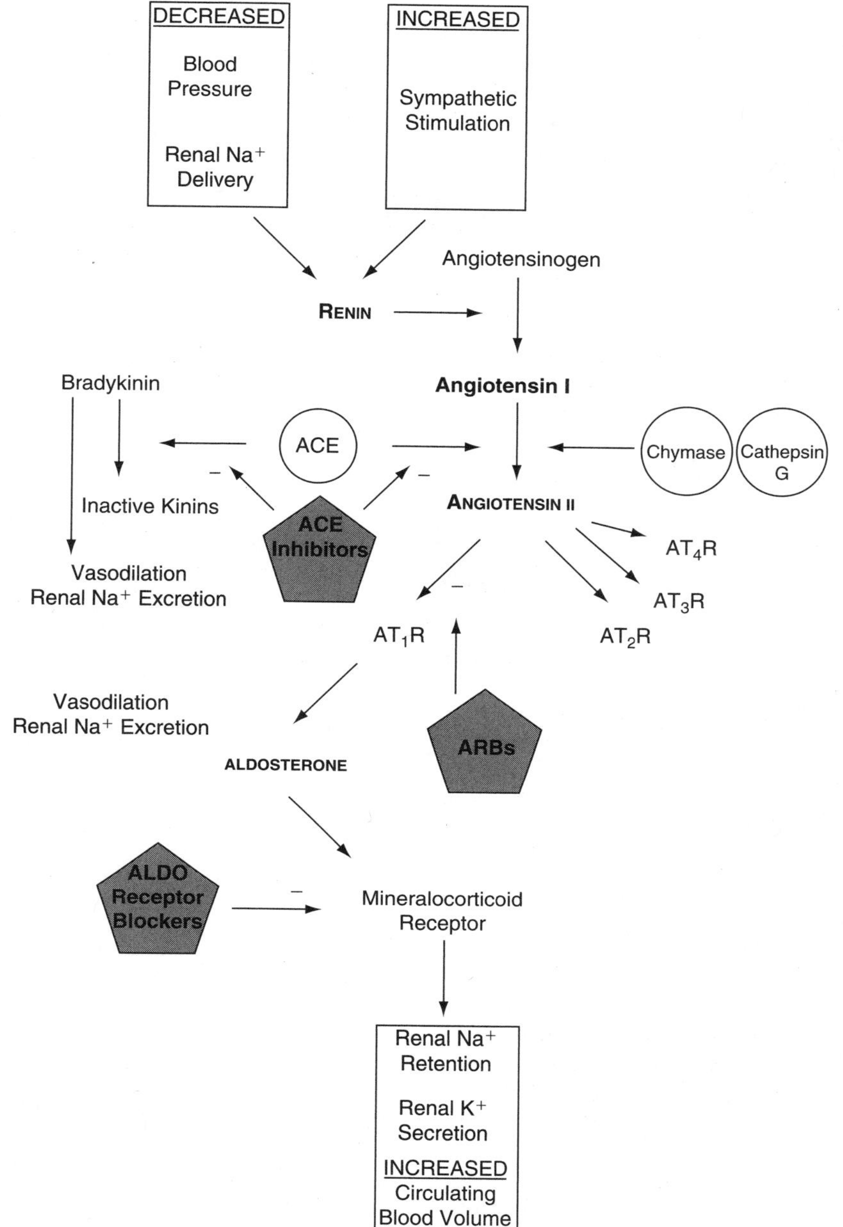

Figure 26-2 The renin-angiotensin-aldosterone system, including sites of pharmacologic inhibition of this neurohormonal axis. Na+, sodium; K+, potassium; ACE, angiotensin-converting enzyme; ATR, angiotensin receptor; ARB, angiotensin receptor blocker; ALDO, aldosterone; BK, bradykinin.

infarction (MI) (16,17), and HF. Its actions, which are triggered by elevated left ventricular wall stress, regulate the balance between competing vasoconstrictive and vasodilatory systems. While the RAAS causes vasoconstriction and salt retention via the actions of Ang II and aldosterone, the kallikrein-kinin system leads to vasodilation and natriuresis through the effects of bradykinin (18). Bradykinin, which is degraded by ACE (also known as kininase II), is a potent vasodilator that stimulates endothelial cells to release prostaglandins, which in turn enhance nitric oxide production (19). Reduced prostaglandin release may thereby adversely affect the clinical outcomes of HF patients. Inhibition of ACE ultimately slows the progression of cardiovascular diseases by improving endothelial function, exerting antiproliferatory and antimigratory effects on smooth muscle cells, neutrophils, and monocytes (20,21), and by exerting antithrombotic effects (13).

Pharmacology of Renin-Angiotensin-Aldosterone System Manipulation

The introduction of the first oral ACEIs in the 1980s represented a major breakthrough in the management of HF

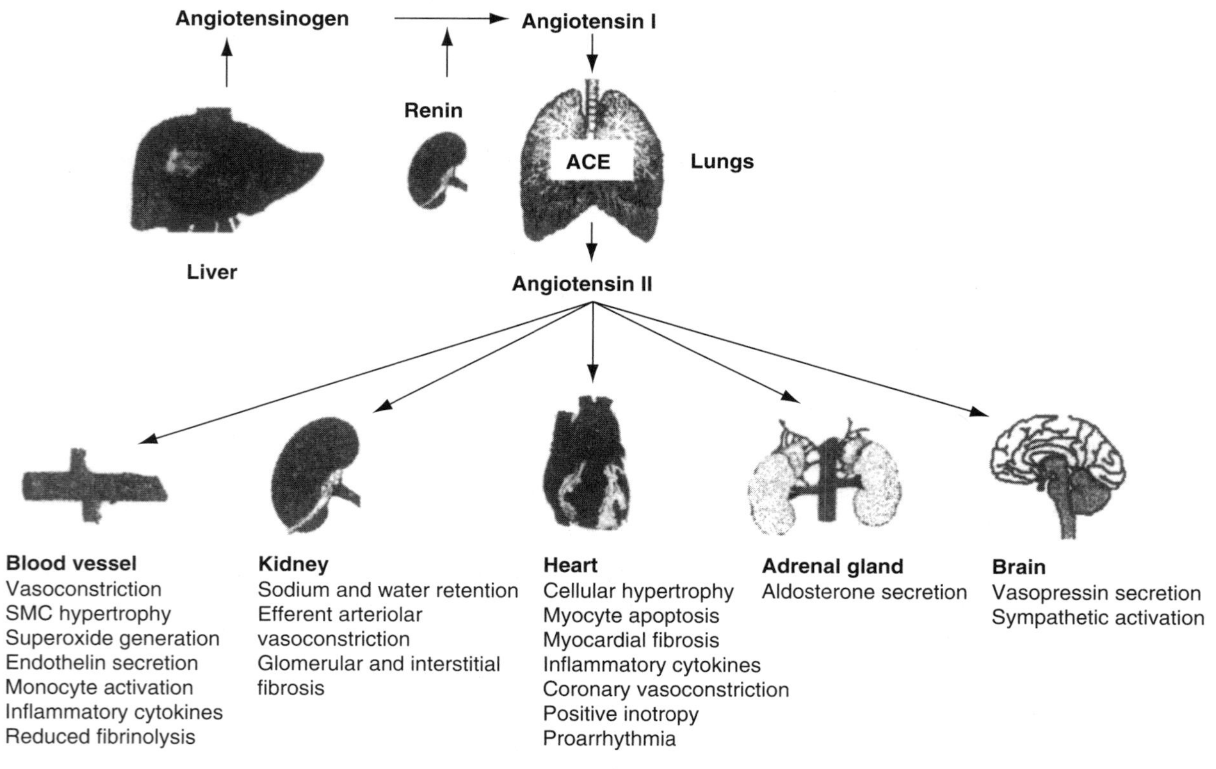

Figure 26-3 Pathophysiology of the renin-angiotensin-aldosterone system, demonstrating the end-organ effects of Ang II. (Reproduced from Givertz MM. Manipulation of the renin-angiotensin system. *Circulation*. 2001;104:e14–e18, with permission.) SMC, smooth muscle cell.

patients. Several large, randomized, placebo-controlled studies in patients with left ventricular systolic dysfunction, treated with diuretics, proved that this class of drugs can improve symptoms and decrease morbidity and mortality in patients with mild, moderate, or even severe HF, regardless of its etiology. These drugs, which block the conversion of Ang I to Ang II, decrease the formation of Ang II and the Ang II-mediated release of aldosterone. ACE inhibitors also inhibit the breakdown of bradykinin, resulting in increased plasma concentrations of nitric oxide and vasodilating prostaglandins (22). Inhibition of Ang II and aldosterone production eventually leads to a decrease in sodium and water retention and adverse cardiac remodeling. Cardiac preload and afterload are concomitantly reduced, leading to an improvement in hemodynamic status (23).

ANGIOTENSIN-CONVERTING ENZYME INHIBITORS

Angiotensin-Converting Enzyme Inhibitors: Hemodynamic Effects

The initial studies with ACEIs focused on their hemodynamic effects (24–27). These studies demonstrated significant decreases in mean arterial pressure and systemic vascular resistance, increases in cardiac output and stroke volume, and reductions in left and right ventricular filling pressures, as well as end-diastolic volumes. Similar changes were noted during exercise. Interestingly, rather than promoting a reflex tachycardia, ACEIs were shown to cause a modest decrease in heart rate (24). This effect may be due to a withdrawal of sympathetic tone in the setting of ACEI therapy. Importantly, the hemodynamic effects of ACEIs were maintained during chronic therapy. Sustained hemodynamic effects, as well as increased exercise capacity, maximal work load, and oxygen consumption were observed following 3 months of treatment with captopril, compared to those who were given placebo (Table 26-1) (27).

Angiotensin-Converting Enzyme Inhibitors and Vascular Protection

The importance of ACE inhibition on prevention of vascular events was initially demonstrated in several large, placebo-controlled trials which enrolled patients with HF and myocardial infarction (MI) (28,29). Patients receiving ACEIs had an unexpected 11% to 25% lower rate of recurrent MI compared to placebo. This led to the vascular hypothesis, which suggests a preventive effect of ACEIs in a wide variety of patients with a history of stroke or transient ischemic attacks, coronary artery disease, peripheral arterial disease, diabetes mellitus, renal disease, and hypertension with additional risk factors, even in the absence of left ventricular dysfunction (Fig. 26-4).

TABLE 26-1
EFFECTS OF ACE INHIBITORS ON HEMODYNAMICS AND LEFT VENTRICULAR REMODELING

Hemodynamic Effects	Effects on Remodeling	Other Significant Effects
Rest		
↓ left and right venticular filling pressures	↓ LV hypertrophy	↑ LV ejection fraction
↓ mean arterial pressure	↓ fibrosis	Improved exercise tolerance
↓ right and left ventricular end-diastolic volume	↓ LV dilation	↑ maximal work load
↓ cardiac index		↑ oxygen consumption with exercise
↓ stroke work index		Improved NYHA functional class
↓ systemic vascular resistance		
Mild decrease in heart rate		↑ symptoms of heart failure
Exercise		
↑ cardiac output and stroke output		
Less increase in arterial pressure, pulmonary artery pressure, and ventricular filling pressure		

NYHA, New York Heart Association.

Angiotensin-Converting Enzyme Inhibitors in Chronic Heart Failure

In the first multicenter, randomized, placebo-controlled clinical trial of an ACEI, the Captopril Multicenter study (26), 92 patients with HF refractory to digitalis and diuretics were randomized to captopril or placebo. After 12 weeks, 80% of the patients treated with captopril experienced a clinical improvement, compared to 27% of those given placebo. The captopril group demonstrated a significant improvement in New York Heart Association (NYHA) functional class, a 24% increase in exercise tolerance, and a significant increase in left ventricular ejection fraction (LVEF) when compared to placebo. The improvement seen in exercise tolerance was gradual and sustained throughout the follow-up period (26). Albeit small, this study initiated the era of ACEI therapy for chronic HF.

The next major breakthrough in HF therapy was the demonstration that ACEIs not only improve hemodynamics and symptoms but also long-term prognosis. In a series of trials, ACEIs were shown to decrease morbidity and mortality in patients with mild, moderate, and severe symptoms, regardless of HF etiology (26,30–32). The first mortality trial was CONSENSUS I (Cooperative North Scandinavian Enalapril Survival Study), in which patients with severe NYHA Class IV HF were randomized to enalapril or placebo. After 20 months, the patients treated with enalapril experienced a 27% reduction in overall mortality and a 50% decrease in mortality due to progressive HF (33) (Fig. 26-5). The SOLVD (Studies of Left Ventricular Dysfunction) Treatment trial extended the indications for ACEI therapy by demonstrating a significant mortality benefit in patients with less-severe HF (NYHA Class II–III) than those enrolled in CONSENSUS I (Fig. 26-6) (34).

A systematic review of the trials of ACEI therapy in patients with chronic HF pooled the data from 7,105 patients enrolled in 32 randomized, controlled studies which remain the primary source of data on these agents (35). This comprehensive analysis demonstrated a 23% reduction in mortality and a 35% reduction in the combined endpoint of mortality or hospitalization for HF in patients treated with ACEIs (Table 26-2). The reduction in mortality was primarily due to fewer deaths from progressive HF, and patients with poor LV function appeared to

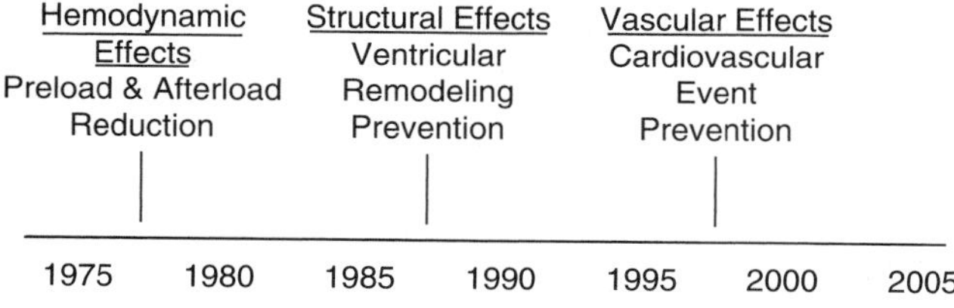

Figure 26-4 Evolving paradigms for the use of angiotensin-converting enzyme inhibitors for the treatment of heart failure.

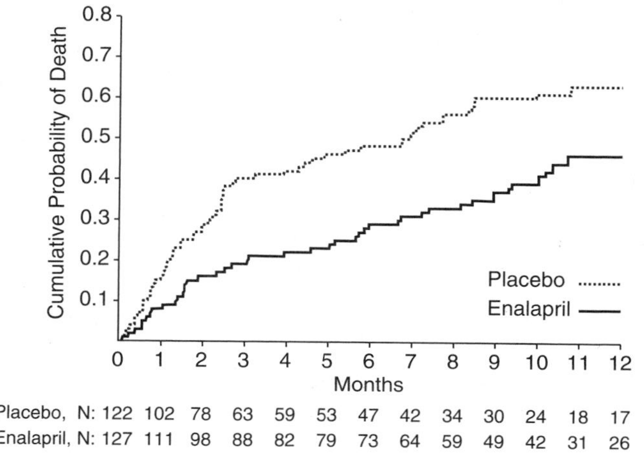

Figure 26-5 Kaplan-Meier survival curve from the CONSENSUS study. (Reproduced from The CONSENSUS Trial Study Group. Effects of enalapril on mortality in severe congestive heart failure. Results of the Cooperative North Scandinavian Enalapril Survival Study [CONSENSUS]. *N Engl J Med.* 1987;316:1429–1435, with permission.)

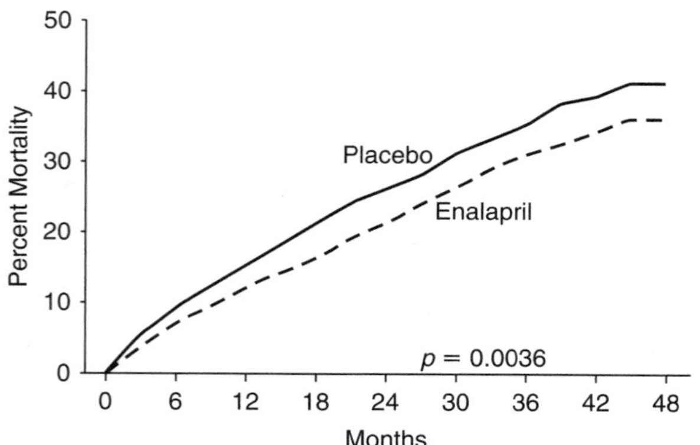

Figure 26-6 Kaplan-Meier survival curve from SOLVD-Treatment study. (Reproduced from the SOLVD Investigators. Effect of enalapril on survival in patients with reduced left ventricular ejection fractions and congestive heart failure. *N Engl J Med.* 1991;325:293–302, with permission.)

gain the most benefit. This review also suggested that, while the greatest effects were seen during the initial 3 months of ACEI therapy, additional benefits accrued during prolonged treatment.

Importantly, ACEI therapy proved superior to treatment with other vasodilators, although their hemodynamic effects may be similar. In the V-HeFT II trial, treatment with enalapril reduced mortality by 28% compared to combination therapy with isosorbide dinitrate and hydralazine (36). These findings suggest that neurohormonal antagonism with RAAS blockers favorably influences the natural history of HF and has significant beneficial effects beyond hemodynamic improvement alone.

Angiotensin-Converting Enzyme Inhibitors: Effects on Left Ventricular Remodeling

As described elsewhere in this text, HF is characterized by progressive and deleterious LV remodeling. A large body of evidence implicates Ang II and aldosterone in the remodeling process, and ACEIs have been shown to prevent pathological hypertrophy, myocardial fibrosis, and progressive left ventricular dilation. These favorable effects of ACEIs were elegantly demonstrated in the rat coronary ligation model developed by Pfeffer et al. (37). In this model, MI was induced by occlusion of the left anterior descending (LAD) artery, which subsequently resulted in left ventricular systolic dysfunction (LVSD) and HF. Pfeffer et al. demonstrated that long-term ACE inhibition with captopril prevented or attenuated progressive LV dilation and deterioration of systolic function, and improved survival (38).

These initial animal studies paved the way for human studies investigating the effects of ACEI therapy on LV remodeling (Fig. 26-7). Pfeffer et al. performed a double-blind, placebo-controlled, randomized trial in patients with their first MI and LVEF $<45\%$ (39). After administration of captopril for 12 months, LV end-diastolic volume had increased by 21 ± 8 mL in patients randomized to placebo, compared to 10 ± 6 mL in patients randomized to the ACEI ($p < 0.02$). The antiremodeling effects of captopril were most apparent in a subset of patients at exceptionally high risk due to persistent occlusion of the LAD artery. Thus, ACE inhibition with captopril appeared to prevent or attenuate the process of left ventricular remodeling which commonly occurs after MI. This beneficial effect provided the rationale for future trials of ACEI therapy on clinical endpoints in patients with HF.

Angiotensin-Converting Enzyme Inhibitors After Myocardial Infarction

Several well-designed randomized, controlled trials demonstrated the favorable effects of ACEIs when given prophylactically after MI. ACE inhibition appears to attenuate ventricular dilation, reduce hospitalizations for HF, prevent recurrent ischemic events, and increase survival.

The post-MI ACEI trials may be considered to fall into two categories: those studying the effects of ACE inhibition in patients with clinical HF and/or LVD, and those studying the short-term effects of ACEIs in unselected post-MI patients. The former category includes the Survival and Ventricular Enlargement trial (SAVE) (28), the Acute Infarction Ramipiril Efficacy Study (AIRE) (29), the Survival of Myocardial Infarction Long-term Evaluation study (SMILE) (40), and the Trandolapril Cardiac Evaluation study (TRACE) (41). These trials demonstrated impressive benefits of ACEI therapy, with risk reductions for all-cause mortality of 19%, 27%, 24%, and 22%, respectively.

The second category of post-MI trials involved the use of ACEIs for several weeks to 6 months in unselected patients. These studies, which include GISSI-3 (42), ISIS-4 (43), and the Chinese Cardiac Study (44), demonstrated mortality risk reductions of 12%, 7%, and 5%, respectively (Table 26-3). These landmark trials, which demonstrated the consistent, significant benefits of ACEIs, provided evidence for the routine use of ACEIs in all post-MI patients, regardless of HF symptoms or degree of left ventricular dysfunction. The one exception, CONSENSUS II (45), studied intravenous enalaprilat administered immediately after admission for acute MI, followed by oral enalapril, and demonstrated an adverse trend in mortality. This finding has been attributed to potentially deleterious effects of the early decline in blood pressure, especially in patients without evidence of HF. Thus, it appears that patients with poor left ventricular function or large areas of infarction appear to gain the most benefit, as this is the group at highest risk for adverse left ventricular remodeling and future cardiovascular events, and that in these patients early and sustained ACE inhibition is warranted.

Angiotensin-Converting Enzyme Inhibitors in Asymptomatic Left Ventricular Dysfunction

The SOLVD-Prevention (46) study, which was performed in parallel with the SOLVD-Treatment study, enrolled patients with asymptomatic LVD. In many ways, SOLVD-Prevention can be viewed in the context of the post-MI studies in that most patients had prior MIs and were still susceptible to further remodeling and the development of clinical HF. In this study, administration of enalapril delayed the development of clinical HF (22.3 months versus 8.3 months in placebo-treated patients) and significantly reduced the risk for HF hospitalizations. This was associated with less LV dilatation (47) in a population with serial measurements of LV

TABLE 26-2
EFFECTS OF ACE INHIBITORS ON MORTALITY IN PATIENTS WITH CHRONIC HEART FAILURE

Trial	ACE Inhibitor	NYHA Class	Subjects (N)	LV Ejection Fraction	Starting Dose	Target Dose	Mean Follow-Up	Mortality			Other Effects
								ACE-I (%)	Controls (%)	RR (95% CI)	
Captopril Multicenter Research Group[20]	Captopril	II-III	92	≤ 40%	25 mg tid	100 mg tid	12 weeks	n/a	n/a	n/a	↑ Exercise capacity, imp NYHA class, improved LV EF
CONSENSUS I[33]	Enalapril	IV	253	n/a	5 mg bid	20 mg bid	188 days	39	54	0.56 (9.34–0.91)	Imp NYHA class, reduced heart size, reduced need for other meds
SOLVD-Treatment[34]	Enalapril	II-III	2,569	≤ 35%	2.2–5 mg bid	10 mg bid	41 months	35	40	0.82 (0.70–0.97)	↓ HF hospitalizations
Meta-analysis[35] (Garg and Yusuf)	n/a	II-IV	7,105	≤40%	n/a	n/a	n/a	16	22	0.77 (0.67–0.88)	Less progression of HF and deceased HF hospitalizations

ACE, Angiotensin Converting Enzyme; NYHA, New York Heart Association; LV, Left Ventricular; HF, Heart failure; CONSENSUS, Cooperative North Scandinavian Enalapril Survival Study; SOLVD, Studies of Left Ventricular Dysfunction; n/a, not applicable or data not available.

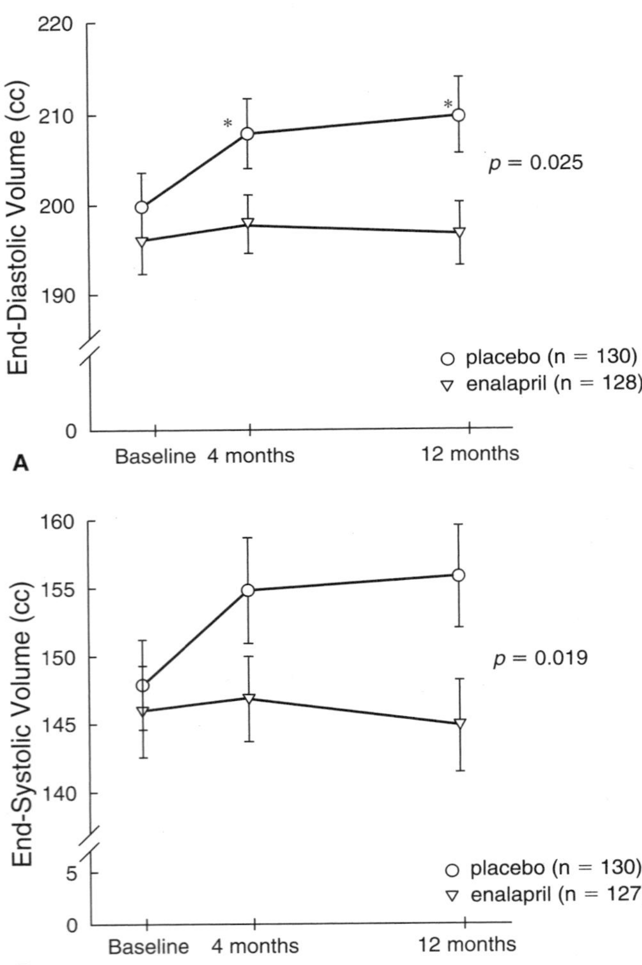

Figure 26-7 The echocardiographic substudy of SOLVD was designed to assess the effects of enalapril on changes in LV volumes and mass over a 1-year period. Changes in LV end-diastolic **(A)** and end-systolic **(B)** volumes are demonstrated. Enalapril significantly attenuated remodeling in this subset of the SOLVD patient population. (Reproduced from Greenberg B, Quinones MA, Koipillai C, et al. Effects of long-term enalapril therapy on cardiac structure and function in patients with left ventricular dysfunction. Results from the SOLVD echocardiography substudy. *Circulation.* 1995;91:2573–2581, with permission.)

volumes. There was also a nonsignificant trend toward improved survival. Of note, after 10 years of follow-up those patients randomized to enalapril demonstrated a significant improvement in long-term survival (48). The SOLVD-Prevention study lent further support to the growing body of evidence that ACEIs are beneficial in all patients with reduced LV systolic function.

Angiotensin-Converting Enzyme Inhibitors in Patients at High Risk for the Development of Left Ventricular Dysfunction

Given the consistent benefit derived from ACE inhibition in patients with HF, further research efforts addressed the utility of ACE blockade as primary prevention in patients deemed at to be high-risk for the development of LVSD. The first major trial to address this issue was the HOPE (Heart Outcomes Prevention Evaluation) (49) study, which enrolled patients with documented coronary, cerebrovascular, or peripheral vascular disease. HOPE randomized 9,541 patients to ramipril (10 mg per day) or placebo, and followed them for the development of HF, cardiovascular events, or stroke. This positive trial was terminated early due to the impressive 23% relative risk reduction for the development of HF in the ramipril-treated group (9.2% versus 11.7%, $p = 0.002$). The ramipril arm also had a 22% reduction in the primary endpoint of cardiac death, nonfatal MI, or stroke.

The HOPE study was followed by the EUROPA (EUropean trial on Reduction Of cardiac events with Perindopril in stable coronary Artery disease) (50) trial, which also assessed the effects of ACE inhibition in patients with stable coronary heart disease and no known history of HF. In EUROPA, 13,665 patients with prior MI, history of coronary revascularization, a positive stress test, or angiographic coronary artery disease were randomized to perindopril or placebo for a mean of 4.2 years. Only 8% of patients assigned to perindopril, compared to 10% of placebo-treated patients, experienced the primary endpoint of cardiovascular death, MI, or cardiac arrest (RRR 20%, 95% CI 9%–29%; $p = 0.0003$). The results of EUROPA, combined with HOPE, led to the widespread use of ACEIs in patients known with coronary artery disease or other high-risk features, even in the absence of LVSD.

The recently completed PEACE (Prevention of Events with Angiotensin Converting Enzyme inhibition) (51) study, in which low-risk patients with known coronary artery disease and LVEF >40% were randomized to trandolapril or placebo, failed to reproduce the findings of HOPE and EUROPA. At 5 years follow-up, there was no significant difference in the combined primary endpoint of cardiovascular death, MI, or coronary revascularization between the two groups, although the point estimate for all-cause mortality was similar to that seen in HOPE and EUROPA (Fig. 26-8). The lack of significant benefit in the ACEI-treated patients is perhaps explained by the low-risk nature of the patients studied [average LVEF = 58% and blood pressure (BP) = 133/78 mm Hg] and the much more aggressive medical management that they received, compared to the earlier studies, with 90% treated with antiplatelet agents, 60% receiving beta-blockers, and 70% on lipid-lowering therapy. Thus, the additional benefit of ACE inhibition may be diminished in low-risk patients who are maximally treated with other anti-ischemic, anti-remodeling therapies. Nonetheless, ACEIs remain a mainstay of therapy for prevention of HF in high-risk patients and are usually given concurrently with other proven medications (Table 26-4).

Indications, Adverse Effects, and Contraindications for Angiotensin-Converting Enzyme Inhibitor Use

As previously reviewed, there is a large body of evidence supporting the routine use of ACEIs in patients with mild, moderate, and severe HF. ACEIs confer hemodynamic and

TABLE 26-3
EFFECTS OF ACE INHIBITORS ON MORTALITY IN PATIENTS WITH POST-MILV DYSFUNCTION

Trial	ACE Inhibitor	Subjects (N)	Study Population	Starting Dose	Target Dose	Follow-Up	Mortality			Other Effects
							ACE-I (%)	Controls (%)	RR (95% CI)	
SAVE[28]	Captopril	2,231	3–16 days post-MI, EF ≤ 40%	6.25 mg tid	25–50 mg tid	42 months	20	25	0.81 (0.68–0.97)	↓ HF in post-MILV dysfunction, ↓ recurrent MI
AIRE[29]	Ramipril	2,006	3–10 days post-MI, clinical HF	2.5 mg bid	5 mg bid	15 months	17	23	0.73 (0.60–0.89)	↓ Worsening HF in post-MIHF
TRACE[41]	Trandalopril	1,749	3–7 days post-MI, EF ≤ 35%	1 mg qd	4 mg qd	24–50 months	35	42	0.78 (0.67–0.91)	↓ Sudden death, ↓ worsening HF
SMILE[40]	Zofenopril	1,556	Within 24 hours of acute MInot receiving thrombolytics	7.5 mg bid	30 mg bid	12 months	10	14	0.71 (0.49–0.94)	↓ Development of severe HF
GISSI-3[42]	Lisinopril	18,895	Within 24 hours of acute MI	5 mg qd	10 mg qd	6 weeks	6.3	7.1	0.88 (0.79–0.99)	↓ Major cardiovascular events
ISIS-4[43]	Captopril	58,050	Within 24 hours of acute MI	6.25 mg	50 mg bid	5 weeks	7.2	7.7	$p = 0.02$	
Chinese Cardiac Study[44]	Captopril	13,634	With 36 hours of acute MI	6.25 mg	12.5 mg tid	4 weeks	9.1	9.6	$p = 0.30$	
CONSENSUS II[45]	Enalapril	6,090	Within 24 hours of acute MI	2.5 mg bid	20 mg qd	6 months	10.2	9.4	1.1 (0.93–1.29)	

ACE, Angiotensin Converting Enzyme; MI, Myocardial Infarction; LV, Left Ventricular; HF, Heart Failure; SAVE, Survival and Ventricular Enlargement; AIRE, Acute Infarction Ramipril Efficacy; TRACE, Trandolapril Cardiac Evaluation; SMILE, Survival of Myocardial Infarction Long-term Evaluation; GISSI, Gruppo Italiano per lo Studio della Sopravivenza nell'Infarto Miocardico; ISIS, International Study of Infarct Survival; CONSENSUS, Cooperative North Scandinavian Enalapril Survival Study.

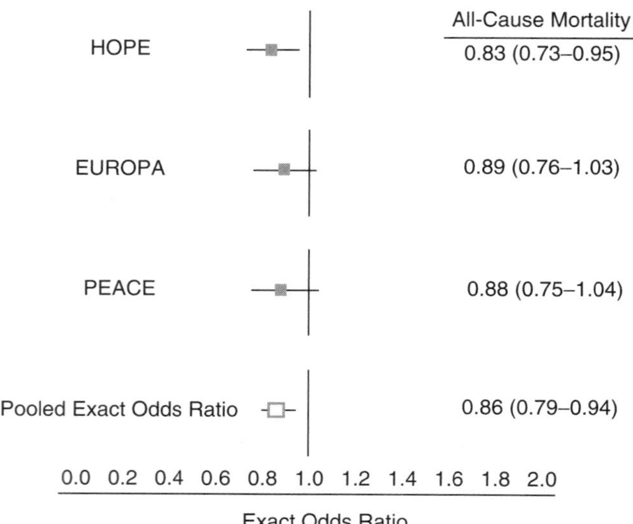

Figure 26-8 Meta-analysis of all-cause mortality from the HOPE, EUROPA, and PEACE studies. (Reproduced from Shelton RJ, Velavan P, Nikitin NP, et al. Clinical trials update from the American Heart Association meeting: ACORN-CSD, primary care trial of chronic disease management, PEACE, CREATE, SHIELD, A-HeFT, GEMINI, vitamin E meta-analysis, ESCAPE, CARP, and SCD-HeFT cost-effectiveness study. *Eur J Heart Fail.* 2005;7:127–135, with permission.)

symptomatic improvement, prevent progression of LV dysfunction, and provide a strong mortality benefit for patients with HF due to LVSD, especially in patients with LVEF ≤35%. Patients with asymptomatic systolic dysfunction experience a reduction in the progression to clinical HF and, most likely, a modest improvement in long-term survival. There is strong evidence supporting the use of ACEIs in the setting of acute MI, particularly when clinical HF, systolic dysfunction, or large infarction is present, in order to improve survival, prevent the occurrence or worsening of HF, and to prevent recurrent cardiovascular events. Finally, ACEIs are also effective in preventing vascular events in other high-risk groups of patients.

ACEIs are absolutely contraindicated during pregnancy due to their known teratogenic effects. They are also contraindicated in patients with hypotension due to cardiogenic shock or early following acute MI, and in patients with any history of ACEI-induced angioedema. ACEIs should generally be avoided in patients with systolic BP <80 to 90 mm Hg, serum creatinine >3 mg/dL, bilateral renal artery stenosis, or serum potassium >5.2 mmol/L except in selected patients with very close monitoring and very strong indications. Patients with borderline BP, renal function, or potassium levels and those with associated diabetes should be monitored closely, with repeat measurements no later than 1 week after initiation of therapy. Patients with mild to moderate renal insufficiency, on the other hand, generally tolerate ACEI therapy and often experience slower rates of progressive renal dysfunction when treated with these agents (52,53).

Cough is a common reason cited for discontinuation of ACEI therapy, and the incidence of ACEI-induced cough is often overestimated. Rigorous clinical trials in which patients have been re-challenged have estimated a <5% true incidence of cough in patients treated with ACEIs. It is important to recognize that cough may develop due to pulmonary vascular congestion. A recent study demonstrated a decrease in dry cough upon increasing enalapril dose—a benefit that was accompanied by an improvement in clinical symptoms and decreased neurohormonal stimulation (54). In the case of persistent or troublesome cough, ACEIs should be discontinued and replaced with an angiotensin receptor blocker (ARB).

Angioedema is a potentially life-threatening complication of ACEI therapy, with an incidence of 0.1% to 0.2% (55). Typically, angioedema involves the face or upper airway. The pathophysiology of ACEI-induced angioedema is poorly understood, although one study demonstrated significant elevations in plasma bradykinin levels during acute attacks of captopril-induced angioedema (56). ARBs, which do not significantly increase bradykinin levels, have generally been found to be safe to use in patients with ACEI-induced angioedema unless it has been life-threatening; indeed, angioedema has been reported only rarely with ARB therapy and a direct causal link has not been proven.

Several factors that often lead to inappropriate withdrawal of ACEI therapy deserve mention. Levels of serum creatinine often rise after initiation of ACEI therapy in patients with severe HF (57), independent of baseline renal function. Only a small fraction of these patients requires discontinuation of therapy, however, and creatinine levels often slowly return to baseline, even in the absence of dose adjustment (58). Measures to reduce renal complications while initiating ACEI therapy include starting with low doses, avoiding concomitant use of NSAIDs, and avoiding volume depletion. If, on the other hand, serum creatinine continues to rise, the presence of renal artery stenosis should be excluded. In addition to mild increases in serum creatinine, the lack of apparent therapeutic benefit after several weeks of therapy should not lead to drug discontinuation. The short-term effects of ACEIs, such as hemodynamic improvement, are distinct from their long-term benefits (59). Indeed, the benefits of ACEI therapy may not be apparent for several months (26). Persistence is thus advised when initiating ACEI therapy, always bearing in mind that hyperkalemia (K >5.5), renal failure, angioedema, severe hypotension, and pregnancy are absolute contraindications to the use of these drugs.

Angiotensin-Converting Enzyme Inhibitor Dose in Patients with Heart Failure

The dose of ACEIs used in clinical trials is generally higher than those used in standard practice, perhaps due to concerns of precipitating renal insufficiency or hypotension at high doses. The issue of ACEI dosing was formally evaluated in the ATLAS (Assessment of Treatment with Lisinopril and Survival) (60) trial, which randomized patients with predominantly NYHA Class III HF and LVEF <35% to low-dose lisinopril (2.5 to 5.0 mg per day) or high-dose lisinopril (32.5 to 35 mg per day). After 46 months of mean follow-up,

TABLE 26-4

EFFECTS OF ACE INHIBITORS ON MORTALITY IN PATIENTS AT RISK FOR THE DEVELOPMENT OF HEART FAILURE

Trial	ACE Inhibitor	Subjects (N)	Starting Dose	Target Dose	Follow-Up	Background Therapy			Average Initial Blood Pressure (mm Hg)	Overall Mortality			Other Effects
						Antiplatelet	Beta-Blocker	Lipid Lowering		ACE-1 (%)	Controls (%)	RR (95% CI)	
HOPE[49]	Ramipril	9,297	2.5 mg qd	10 mg qd	5 years	76%	40%	29%	139/79	10.4	12.1	0.84 (0.75–0.95)	↓ New-onset HF, MI, revascularization procedures, and cardiac arrest
EUROPA[50]	Perindopril	12,218	2–4 mg qd	8 mg qd	4.2 years	92%	62%	58%	137/82	6.1	6.9	0.89 (0.77–0.98)	↓ Composite endpoint of cardiovascular mortality, MI, or cardiac arrest, ↓ HF hospitalizations
PEACE[51]	Trandolapril	8,290	2 mg qd	4 mg qd	4.8 years	90%	60%	70%	134/78	7.2	8.1	0.89 (0.76–1.04)	No significant difference in outcomes between treatment and placebo groups, but point estimate identical to EUROPA and p-value = 0.13
SOLVD-Prevention[48*]	Enalapril	4,228	2.5 mg bid	10 mg bid	3.1 years	54%	24%		125/78	14.8	15.8	0.92 (0.79–1.08)	↓ Development of clinical HF and rate of HF hospitalizations

ACE, Angiotensin Converting Enzyme; MI, Myocardial Infarction; HF, Heart Failure; HOPE, Heart Outcomes Prevention Evaluation; EUROPA, European trial on Reduction Of cardiac events with Perindopril in stable coronary Artery disease; PEACE, Prevention of Events with Angiotensin Converting Enzyme inhibition.

high-dose lisinopril produced a significant 12% reduction in the combined endpoint of death or all-cause hospitalization, compared to low-dose lisinopril (p = 0.002). Specifically, treatment with high-dose lisinopril reduced HF hospitalizations by 25% and resulted in a trend toward reduced cardiovascular and all-cause mortality in patients with severe HF (LVEF ≤30%). In addition to demonstrating efficacy, the ATLAS trial also demonstrated the excellent safety and tolerability profile of high-dose ACEI therapy (61). Over 90% of patients in both arms of the trial were successfully titrated to their target dose of medication. Despite a higher incidence of hypotension and renal insufficiency in the high-dose group, the incidence of serious adverse effects requiring withdrawal of the study medication was similar in both groups. Thus, a strategy of titrating ACEIs to high doses, preferably the target doses demonstrated to be effective in clinical trials, is safe and beneficial.

Interaction with Aspirin

Aspirin is commonly prescribed to patients with HF, due to the high prevalence of ischemic heart disease in this population (62). However, several post hoc analyses of major ACEI trials have noted lesser benefit of these agents in patients treated with aspirin. The proposed mechanism of such an interaction is the interference by aspirin with the ACEI-mediated increase in prostaglandin synthesis (49,63–65). In a small, prospective, randomized but unblinded study, aspirin was associated with more HF hospitalizations than was either warfarin or no antithrombotic therapy (66). Although no definitive recommendations can be made about the use of aspirin in patients with chronic HF, it is prudent to limit aspirin use to those who have specific indications for this agent—primarily those with prior MI or known coronary disease—and to carefully weigh the benefit versus risk of aspirin (versus the use of another antithrombotic agent) in patients with severe or refractory HF. This issue is discussed in detail elsewhere in this text.

How to Use Angiotensin-Converting Enzyme Inhibitors

As previously noted, ACEIs should be considered first-line therapy for the treatment of patients with clinical HF due to reduced LVSD, patients with asymptomatic LV dysfunction, and for patients who are at high risk for the development of HF due to the presence of coronary, cerebrovascular, or peripheral vascular disease. Treatment should not be deferred in patients with few or no symptoms because of the significant mortality benefit derived from ACEI therapy. In patients with dyspnea or other symptoms or signs of volume retention, ACEIs should be administered along with a diuretic. ACEIs do not prevent fluid retention and should not be substituted for diuretics in this setting (67).

There is now sufficient evidence, from the clinical trials reviewed previously, that the benefits observed with ACEI therapy are a class effect. In general, ACEIs should be initiated at a low dose, such as captopril 12.5 mg three times daily, enalapril or lisinopril 5 mg once daily, or ramipril 2.5 mg daily. Patients with a pretreatment blood pressure of less than 90 to 100 mm Hg, serum creatinine level >1.6 to 2.0 mg/dL, or those who have recently undergone aggressive diuresis may be started at even lower doses. If patients tolerate ACEI therapy, the drug dose should be gradually increased at 1- to 4-week intervals until the target dose used in clinical trials is reached, unless these doses are not tolerated. Due to the documented benefits of high-dose ACEI therapy, the dose should be increased even if the patient experiences symptomatic improvement at lower doses. Approximately 5% to 10% of patients will develop symptoms of hypotension, such as dizziness, or documented systolic BP <80 to 90 mm Hg. In these patients, the doses of other drugs which may cause hypotension, such as nitrates, alpha-blockers, or other vasodilators, should be reduced or rescheduled so that their peak effects do not coincide with that of the ACEI. It may also be possible to reduce diuretic dosage, watching closely for symptoms or signs of fluid retention.

ANGIOTENSIN RECEPTOR BLOCKERS

Rationale for the Use of Angiotensin Receptor Blockers

It is now clear that there is both a rationale and potential benefit from inhibiting the RAAS at a number of steps along the pathway discussed previously. Circulating Ang II levels initially decrease with short-term ACEI therapy but often return to pretreatment levels with long-term ACE inhibition. This escape phenomenon may be due, in part, to non-ACE pathways of Ang II production. Cathepsin D has been shown to cleave angiotensinogen (68), and chymase has been identified as an important enzyme in Ang I to Ang II conversion, particularly in the human heart (11,69). These alternative mechanisms may explain the slow rise in Ang II levels that occurs after months to years of ACEI therapy (70,71).

Ang II binds to angiotensin receptors in a variety of tissues, including the vascular endothelium and the renal arterioles and glomerulus (72). There are now believed to be four angiotensin receptors, AT_1 through AT_4, which mediate pleiotropical physiologic effects. The AT_1 receptor mediates the classic actions of Ang II, such as vasoconstriction and sodium and water retention, and also plays an important role in cardiovascular remodeling (73). The AT_2 receptor appears to oppose the actions of AT_1 stimulation, with antiproliferative, antigrowth, and vasodilatory effects (74). The roles of the AT_3 and AT_4 receptors remain to be characterized.

An additional approach to blocking the RAAS is through the use of orally active, nonpeptide, Ang II type 1 receptor blockers (ARBs), which bind competitively to AT_1 receptors (75). Although this approach to blocking the RAAS seems more direct, the primary rationale for using ARBs in lieu of ACEIs relates to their lower side-effect profile. Some of the adverse effects, as well as the benefits, of ACEIs are related to increased levels of bradykinin and prostaglandins, which do not occur with ARBs. As a result, these agents can be used in patients with ACEI-induced cough and, with extreme care, in some patients who have experienced angioedema with ACEIs, as long as it has not occurred in a life-threatening manner. In a double-blind, randomized, parallel-group comparison of the ARB losartan, the ACEI lisinopril, and hydrochlorothiazide for 8 weeks in 135 patients, the frequency of cough with losartan therapy was lower than in the lisinopril group and was similar to the group of patients taking hydrochlorothiazide (76). Similarly, in the CHARM-Alternative Study, which randomized 2,028 ACEI-intolerant patients to the ARB candesartan or placebo, only one patient had to discontinue candesartan therapy due to angioedema (77).

Angiotensin Receptor Blockers as Alternatives to Angiotensin-Converting Enzyme Inhibitors

ELITE-I (Evaluation of Losartan in the Elderly) was the first study to compare an ARB and an ACEI with an endpoint of clinical outcomes. In this study, 722 patients, age ≥60 years with LVEF ≤40% were randomized to captopril, titrated to 50 mg thrice daily, or losartan titrated to 50 mg once daily and followed for 1 year. Although this study did not show any difference in its prespecified endpoint of renal function or in HF endpoints, there were somewhat fewer deaths, particularly those classified as sudden, in the losartan arm (78). Therefore, a larger randomized trial, ELITE-II, was designed to test the hypothesis that losartan was superior to captopril with a primary endpoint of survival. The entry criteria and drug doses were identical to ELITE-I (79). This trial not only did not support the favorable post hoc findings of ELITE-I, but the trends in all-cause mortality ($p = 0.16$) and the secondary endpoint of sudden death or resuscitated arrests ($p = 0.08$) favored captopril. Although fewer patients in the losartan group discontinued study therapy due to adverse events (9.7% versus 14.7%, $p < 0.001$), primarily severe cough but also angioedema, the advantage of fewer side effects did not outweigh the trend toward improved survival in the captopril group.

A second trial employing the same agents and doses, OPTIMAAL (Optimal Trial in Myocardial Infarction with Angiotensin II Antagonist Losartan) (80), was conducted in patients with LVD after MI. This study also demonstrated a trend toward lower all-cause mortality in the captopril group, compared to the losartan group (RR 0.87, 95% CI 0.72–1.01; $p = 0.07$), and fewer captopril-treated patients experienced sudden death or a resuscitated cardiac arrest. Unfortunately, it is impossible to determine whether these results reflect the relatively low 50-mg dose of losartan or superiority of ACE inhibition over Ang II blockade.

The only trial that provides a meaningful comparison of these two drug classes is the VALIANT (Valsartan in Acute Myocardial Infarction) trial (81), which compared the effects of an ARB (valsartan) with an ACEI (captopril) after MI. In this trial, post-MI patients with HF, LVSD, or both were randomized to valsartan 320 mg daily (a substantially higher dose in terms of Ang II receptor blockade) or captopril 150 mg daily for 2 years. This study rigorously proved the comparability of these two classes, showing essentially identical rates of mortality and combined car-

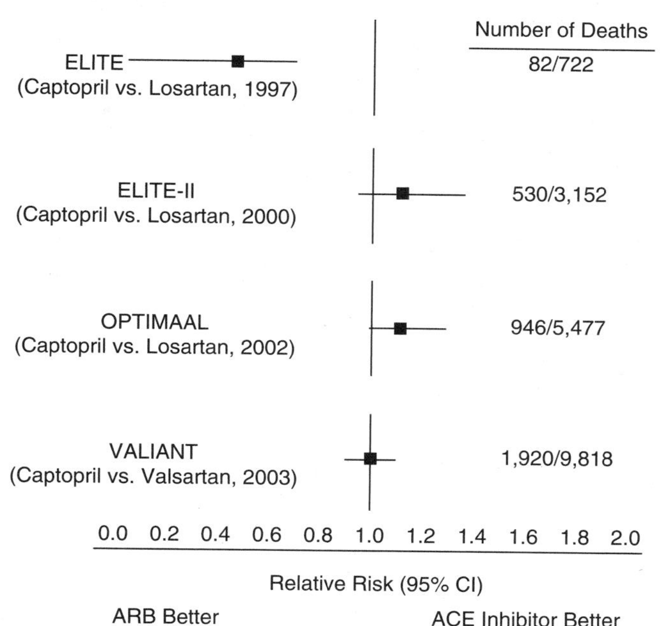

Figure 26-9 Comparison of the efficacy of ACEIs versus ARBs in reducing all-cause mortality in major clinical trials.

diovascular endpoints in patients treated with either of these two agents (Fig. 26-9). The third arm of the VALIANT trial, in which patients were treated with both the ARB and ACEI, will be discussed later.

Angiotensin Receptor Blockers in Combination with Angiotensin-Converting Enzyme Inhibitors

Because ARBs and ACEIs interfere with the RAAS system at different points in the pathway, and Ang II levels remain elevated during chronic ACEI therapy in HF patients, another logical approach is to use these agents in combination. Although a number of small studies showed that combination therapy produced additive hemodynamic effects, this approach was first investigated rigorously in the RESOLVD (Randomized Evaluation of Strategies for Left Ventricular Dysfunction) (82) trial. This study compared the effects of enalapril, several doses of the ARB candesartan, and a combination of the two agents in 768 patients with symptomatic HF due to LVSD. There were no appreciable differences between the therapies with regard to exercise performance, NYHA class, or quality of life. The combination therapy lowered aldosterone levels transiently but this difference disappeared during longer-term follow-up. The most intriguing finding of the RESOLVD study was a reduction in remodeling, as evidenced by prevention of LV dilation, with the two agents in combination versus either agent alone. Although this was an isolated finding in the absence of any improvement in clinical outcomes, it was considered sufficient proof-of-concept to commence large-scale clinical trials with this combination approach (Fig. 26-10).

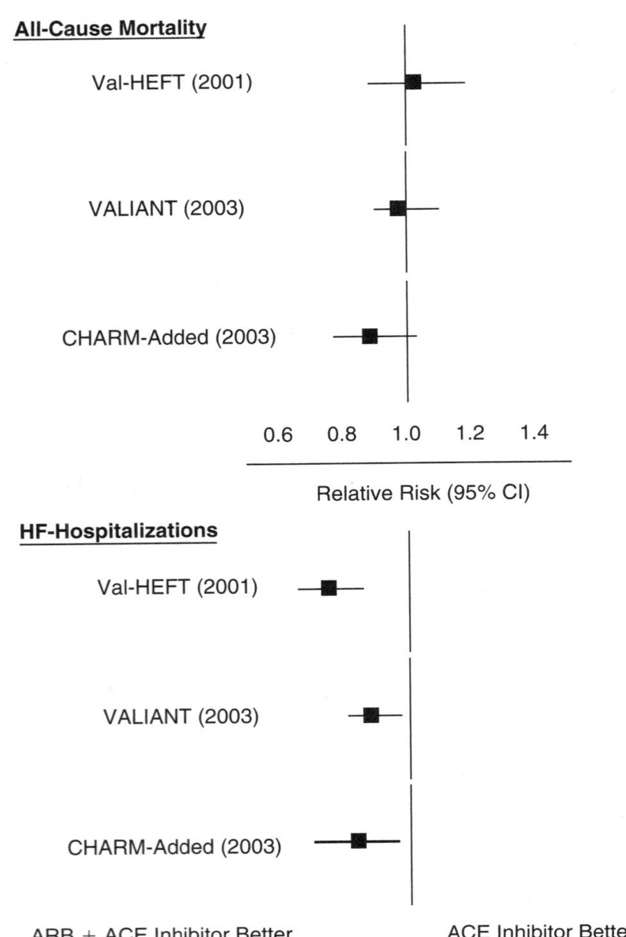

Figure 26-10 Comparison of the effects of ACEIs alone versus a combination of an ACEI and ARB in reducing all-cause mortality and heart failure hospitalizations in major clinical trials.

The first of these studies, Val-HeFT (Valsartan Heart Failure Trial) (83), evaluated whether treatment with valsartan would result in a significant clinical benefit in patients already receiving an ACEI, diuretics, and in some cases digoxin and/or a beta-blocker. The addition of valsartan did not improve mortality but it did reduce the combined endpoint of mortality plus nonfatal cardiovascular events (mainly hospitalizations for HF) by 13.2% (RR 0.87, 97.5% CI 0.77–0.97; $p = 0.009$). Subgroup analyses demonstrated that the small group of patients who were not receiving an ACEI experienced a 33% reduction in mortality and a 54% reduction in morbidity plus mortality when treated with valsartan. However, the larger group of patients already treated with an ACEI and a beta-blocker had a significant 42% *increase* in mortality with the addition of valsartan ($p = 0.009$) and a trend toward an increase in morbidity plus mortality ($p = 0.10$). Thus, although the Val-HeFT study suggested that ARBs are useful alternatives to ACEIs in intolerant patients, it also raised possible concerns about the safety of treatment with multiple neurohormonal agents.

The CHARM-Added trial (84) more recently investigated the effects of combination therapy with an ACEI and ARB in 2,548 patients with NYHA Class II to IV HF and LVEF ≤40% who were randomized to the ARB candesartan, titrated to a high dose of 32 mg daily if tolerated, or placebo. All patients were treated with an ACEI, 55% with a beta-blocker, and 17% with an aldosterone antagonist. Significant reductions in cardiovascular death (HR 0.84, 95% CI 0.72–0.98; $p = 0.029$) and HF hospitalizations (HR 0.83, 95% CI 0.71–0.96; $p = 0.014$) were evident in the combination therapy group; however, there was no significant reduction in all-cause mortality (HR 0.89, 95% CI 0.77–1.02; $p = 0.086$). Importantly, this study clearly alleviates the concerns about using ARBs in combination with both an ACEI and beta-blocker raised by Val-HEFT, since this subgroup (which was much larger in CHARM than Val-HEFT) showed similar or even greater benefit in the much larger group that was receiving both agents as background therapy.

The previously mentioned VALIANT study (81), which compared the clinical effects of valsartan and captopril in post-MI patients, also studied the benefit of combining these two agents. The combination of valsartan plus captopril did not reduce all-cause mortality when compared to captopril alone but did demonstrate small but significantly reduced incidence of hospital admissions for worsening HF (HR 0.89, $p = 0.005$), which was not a major endpoint of this study. The combination arm experienced a significantly higher rate of drug intolerance, renal dysfunction, and hyperkalemia, which led the investigators to conclude that any benefit was outweighed by the higher adverse event rate and that there was no justification for using ARBs together with ACEIs in the early post-MI population.

Angiotensin Receptor Blockers in Patients Intolerant of Angiotensin-Converting Enzyme Inhibitors

The efficacy of ARBs as alternatives in patients who were intolerant of ACEIs was suggested by a subgroup analysis in Val-HeFT. The CHARM-Alternative (77) trial was designed to specifically test this hypothesis in 2,028 patients with symptomatic HF and LVEF ≤40% who were intolerant of ACEIs, by randomizing them to candesartan or placebo. The patients treated with candesartan experienced significant reductions in cardiovascular mortality and hospitalizations for HF when compared to placebo (adjusted HR 0.70, 95% CI 0.60–0.81; $p < 0.0001$). The rate of study-drug discontinuation due to adverse events, such as severe cough and angioedema, was similar in the candesartan (30%) and placebo (29%) groups, suggesting that the ARB was very well-tolerated.

Angiotensin Receptor Blockers in Patients with Heart Failure and Preserved Left Ventricular Function

Approximately half of all patients diagnosed with chronic HF have preserved LV systolic function (35). Although these patients have high rates of mortality and hospital admissions, little is known about effective therapy for this condition. Studies have recently addressed the question of whether RAAS blockade would also benefit this subset of

HF patients. The CHARM-Preserved (85) study investigated the effects of candesartan therapy in patients with clinical HF and LVEF >40%. This trial failed to show a significant benefit of ARB therapy with respect to cardiovascular mortality, but fewer patients treated with candesartan were hospitalized for HF. This trial provided a compelling basis for further studies of neurohormonal antagonism in patients with HF and preserved LV function. The Irbesartan in Heart Failure with Preserved Systolic Function (I-PRESERVE) trial (86) is currently investigating the effects of the ARB irbesartan in 4,100 patients with preserved systolic function and more rigorously defined HF, and should provide a definitive answer to this question upon study completion in 2007.

Using Angiotensin Receptor Blockers

The often conflicting results of the previously mentioned trials raise the possibility that not all ARBs are equally beneficial. The difference in dosing regimens and other pharmacologic properties between the specific agents may account for their disparate clinical effects. For instance, candesartan and valsartan have a much higher affinity for the AT_1 receptor than does losartan (75). However, valsartan's bioavailability is reduced by approximately 40% when taken with food. Losartan, although itself a relatively weak receptor blocker, produces an active metabolite which causes powerful AT_1 receptor blockade (75). These pharmacologic differences may have important clinical consequences: blood pressure studies have shown that a total daily dose of valsartan 160 mg or candesartan 8 mg is more effective than losartan 100 mg daily (75). Similarly, the varying efficacy of different ARB preparations may help explain why CHARM and Val-HEFT, which used relatively potent ARBs, led to reductions in hospital admissions for HF, while ELITE-II and OPTIMAAL, which used low-dose losartan, failed to demonstrate a significant benefit over ACEIs.

Another theory worth mentioning suggests that the blood pressure-lowering effect of ARBs may, in part, explain their clinical benefits (87). ELITE-II, OPTIMAAL, and VALIANT did not demonstrate superiority of ARBs over ACEIs, and all of these studies had similar blood pressure reductions in the two treatment arms. Conversely, CHARM-Added and Val-HEFT demonstrated significant blood pressure-lowering with the addition of an ARB and achieved significant reductions in cardiovascular morbidity or mortality. Thus, the degree to which an ARB lowers blood pressure in patients with HF may account for some of their clinical benefits. This theory is currently being evaluated by the Heart failure End point evaluation with the Angiotensin II Antagonist Losartan (HEAAL) study, which is comparing 50 mg versus 150 mg of losartan daily in ACEI-intolerant patients with HF.

The Role of Angiotensin Receptor Blockers

The role of ARBs as effective alternatives to ACEIs in patients with chronic HF or LVSD following acute MI has been established by the Val-HeFT, CHARM-Alternative, and VALIANT trials. However, the two studies of chronic HF enrolled only patients with prior ACEI intolerance, and the only rigorous trial comparing an ARB and an ACEI, ELITE-II, demonstrated an advantage for the ACEI with regard to survival. Therefore, ACEIs should be considered the agents of choice for this indication, with ARBs clearly indicated in those who do not tolerate ACEIs due to cough, rash, or angioedema. Candesartan, titrated to a target dose of 32 mg daily, is the best-studied agent; however, valsartan, titrated to a target dose of 160 mg twice daily, also may be effective in this setting. In patients with post-MI LVSD, valsartan 160 mg twice daily appears comparable to an ACEI with regard to survival and other clinical outcomes. However, the relative lack of experience with ARBs compared to ACEIs in this population, and the higher cost of ARBs, suggest that an ACEI should be preferred as the first-line RAAS blocker for this indication.

ARBs do appear to provide some additive benefit to ACEIs in the treatment of patients with chronic HF. However, the greater benefit of adding beta-blockers to ACEIs in this setting is clear. ARBs should be considered only as an adjunct to these two agents and there does not appear to be a significant role for ARBs (in combination with ACEIs) in the post-MI patient. Furthermore, the data presented in the next section support the earlier use of aldosterone antagonists in certain settings. There is only limited data to support the combined use of an ARB with an ACEI and an aldosterone antagonist, so this approach should be used with caution and with very careful monitoring of serum potassium levels and renal function.

ALDOSTERONE ANTAGONISTS

Role of Aldosterone in Heart Failure

The pivotal role played by aldosterone in the pathogenesis of HF is now well-recognized (Fig. 26-11). Activation of the RAAS leads to marked elevations in plasma aldosterone levels, which have been shown to correlate with increased mortality (88). Elevated aldosterone levels lead to excessive sodium retention, with expansion of the extracellular volume, worsening hemodynamic conditions, and a fall in cardiac output. Decreased renal blood flow further stimulates the RAAS, causing secondary hyperaldosteronism and further sodium retention. In addition, by contributing to hypokalemia and hypomagnesemia, aldosterone increases the sensitivity of cardiac tissue to arrhythmias, with a resultant increase in sudden death (89,90).

Investigations regarding the role of aldosterone in HF have revealed a number of important mechanisms which may contribute to the progression of this condition and to sudden death. For instance, a growing body of evidence suggests that aldosterone may contribute to endothelial dysfunction, possibly through reduced nitric oxide bioavailability (91). Since the endothelium plays a critical role in the regulation of vascular tone, platelet aggregation, and thrombosis, endothelial dysfunction predicts subsequent cardiovascular events (92). Furthermore, aldosterone contributes to the development of HF by promoting myocardial fibrosis. In vitro studies have demonstrated that administration of aldosterone to cardiac fibroblasts

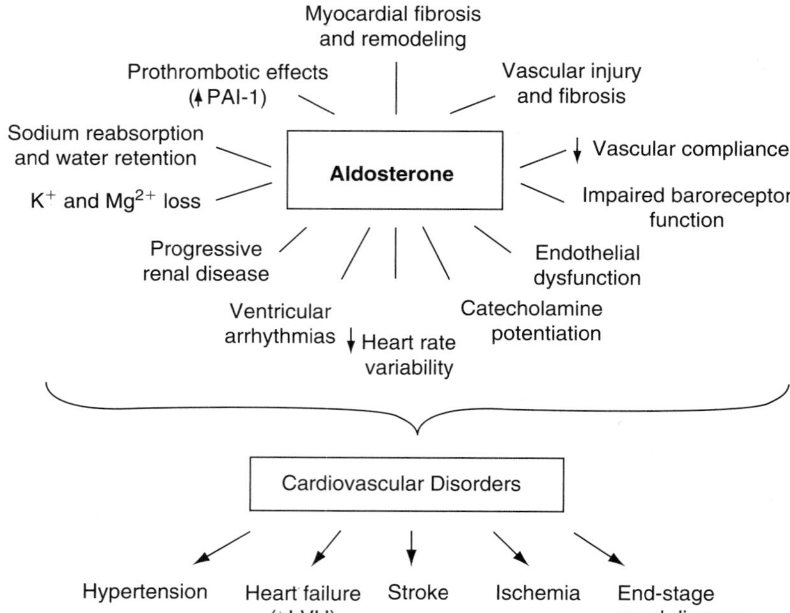

Figure 26-11 Multiple mechanisms by which aldosterone dysregulation may contribute to cardiovascular disease. LVH, left ventricular hypertrophy; PAI-1, plasminogen activator inhibitor-1. (Reproduced from Struthers AD, MacDonald TM. Review of aldosterone and angiotensin-II-induced target organ damage and prevention. *Cardiovasc Res.* 2004;61:663–670, with permission.)

significantly enhances collagen synthesis (93)—a finding that has been confirmed in rat models (94). Clinical studies in patients with essential hypertension who were treated with ACEIs subsequently demonstrated a reduction in LV mass index in patients with suppressed aldosterone production, and no significant difference in those with aldosterone escape (95). Another potentially harmful effect of aldosterone is its ability to blunt the baroreflex response. Administration of aldosterone to dogs (96) and to healthy human volunteers (97) resulted in an elevation in the threshold for baroreflex activation and a reduction in peak discharge rate. Finally, aldosterone has been shown to promote the activation and aggregation of platelets and to enhance arteriolar constriction (98).

The importance of excessive aldosterone production in HF was initially overlooked with the advent of ACEI therapy, which was widely believed to suppress aldosterone production via upstream blockade of the RAAS. However, the early fall in aldosterone levels after initiation of ACEI therapy has proven to be a transient phenomenon, and aldosterone production subsequently rises, leading to aldosterone escape. In a study of 14 patients with chronic HF, aldosterone levels decreased by only 20% after 6 weeks of captopril therapy (99). Similarly, aldosterone levels have been shown to slowly increase in patients treated with ACEIs for essential hypertension (95) or after acute MI (100). Even combination therapy with an ACEI and ARB fails to adequately suppress aldosterone production. The RESOLVD study demonstrated that aldosterone levels decreased significantly after 17 weeks in patients treated with both enalapril and candesartan, compared to those treated with either agent alone, but subsequently returned to baseline levels after 43 weeks, even with maximum doses of both agents (82).

Proposed mechanisms for aldosterone escape include alternative stimuli for aldosterone synthesis (such as adrenocorticotrophic hormone and endothelin), potassium-dependent aldosterone secretion, and reduced aldosterone clearance. Moreover, aldosterone may also be produced by non-ACE pathways, such as those that employ the enzyme chymase in the brain, heart, and blood vessels (101). Regardless of the mechanism, aldosterone exacerbates the tissue-damaging effects of Ang II and exerts a number of detrimental effects in HF (102–105).

The relationship between aldosterone levels and clinical outcomes was assessed in a neurohormonal substudy of the SAVE trial (106). Among 534 subjects randomized to captopril or placebo after MI, mean aldosterone levels were lower in the group of patients who remained free of cardiovascular events over the ensuing 2 years compared to those who died, developed severe HF, or had recurrent ischemia. Multivariate analyses confirmed the authors' hypothesis that aldosterone levels correlate significantly with the risk of a cardiovascular event.

We now know that aldosterone blockade prevents ventricular remodeling and collagen formation in patients with post-MI LVD, and affects a number of other pathophysiological mechanisms which determine long-term prognosis (107). In patients with HF, high levels of collagen precursors are associated with poor outcomes. Levels of these markers, such as pro-collagen III (108), have been shown to decrease during therapy with spironolactone (103). These findings suggest that limitation of excessive extracellular matrix turnover may be one of the extrarenal mechanisms by which spironolactone confers benefits in patients with HF. Another contributing mechanism may involve inhibition of free radical production. Aldosterone has been shown to increase free radical formation, and aldosterone blockade with spironolactone decreases reactive oxygen species, thereby improving endothelial function (91,109). Thus, the benefits conferred by treatment with aldosterone blockers may be partly due to a decrease in collagen synthesis, reduced free radical formation, and increased nitric oxide bioavailability.

Substantial evidence also suggests that aldosterone blockade restores autonomic balance. Aldosterone blockade improves norepinephrine uptake into the myocardium, decreases circulating norepinephrine levels, decreases QT dispersion, reduces ventricular arrhythmias, and improves both baroreceptor function and heart rate variability (108,110). These effects suggest a decrease in sympathetic stimulation and an increase in vagal tone.

The first aldosterone antagonist to be extensively evaluated in clinical studies was spironolactone, which competitively inhibits aldosterone-sensitive sodium channels in the cortical collecting duct of the nephron, thereby causing sodium and free water excretion and potassium retention, as well as receptors in other tissues. A daily dose of 25 mg of spironolactone has proven effective in blocking aldosterone receptors (111), and at higher concentrations spironolactone can inhibit the biosynthesis of aldosterone (112).

Hemodynamic studies have shown that low-dose spironolactone (25 mg daily) produces a significant reduction in diastolic arterial pressure, mean arterial pressure, and systemic vascular resistance. It also significantly diminishes right and left ventricular filling pressures, suggesting that spironolactone improves venous and arterial compliance (113). A randomized, placebo-controlled study of 10 patients with NYHA Class II–III HF who were receiving standard diuretic and ACEI therapy demonstrated that the addition of spironolactone 50 mg daily for 1 month significantly increased forearm blood flow response to acetylcholine, increased nitric oxide bioactivity, and inhibited vascular Ang I conversion in patients with HF (91).

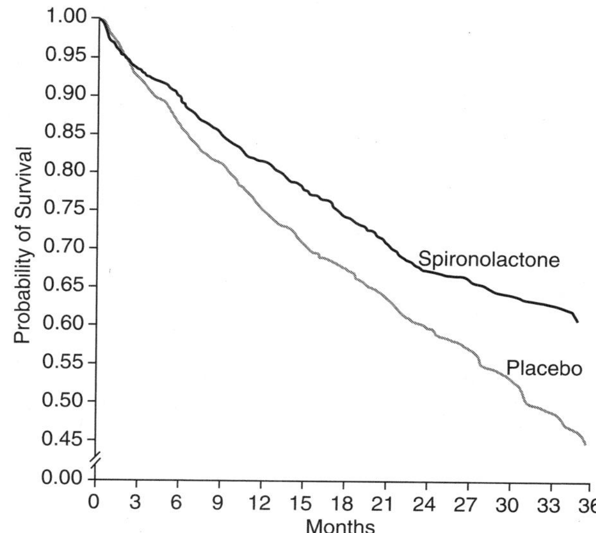

Figure 26-12 Probability of survival among patients in the placebo group and patients in the spironolactone group in the RALES trial. The risk of death was 30% lower among patients in the spironolactone group compared to patients in the placebo group. (Reproduced from Pitt B, Zannad F, Remme WJ, et al. The effect of spironolactone on morbidity and mortality in patients with severe heart failure. *N Engl J Med.* 1999;341:709–717, with permission.)

Aldosterone Antagonists in Chronic Heart Failure

The first clinical trial demonstrating the benefits of aldosterone receptor blockade in HF was the Randomized Aldosterone Evaluation Study (RALES), in which 1,633 patients with NYHA Class III–IV chronic HF, already receiving ACEIs, were randomized to spironolactone versus placebo (111). Patients were initiated on 12.5 or 25 mg of spironolactone daily and were titrated to 25 mg daily, with the possibility of increasing to 50 mg. Patients with a serum creatinine greater than 2.5 mg/dL or serum potassium greater than 5.0 mmol/L were excluded, and these blood tests were monitored closely. The relative risk of death was reduced by 30% over two years (RR 0.7, 95% CI 0.60–0.82; $p < 0.001$) (Fig. 26-12), with a 35% reduction in HF hospitalizations and an improvement in functional class. Of note, although only 11% of the trial participants were receiving beta-blockers, the aldosterone antagonist appeared to confer significant additive benefits in patients already treated with both ACEIs and beta-blockers.

Aldosterone Antagonists in Post-Myocardial Infarction Left Ventricular Dysfunction

Since spironolactone is a nonspecific aldosterone receptor antagonist with estrogenic effects, it can induce breast tenderness and gynecomastia in approximately 10% of male patients and can increase the incidence of sexual dysfunction. As a result, eplerenone, a selective aldosterone antagonist that blocks the mineralocorticoid receptor without inhibiting the glucocorticoid, progesterone, or androgen receptors was developed (107,111). The safety and efficacy of eplerenone as monotherapy or in combination regimens for the treatment of hypertension have been evaluated in a number of clinical trials (114,115). Furthermore, several studies have demonstrated that eplerenone provides end-organ protection. In patients with hypertension and LV hypertrophy, eplerenone 100 mg daily produced reductions in LV mass equivalent to that produced by enalapril 40 mg daily (114). The concomitant use of both agents resulted in additional LV mass reduction.

Eplerenone was recently evaluated in the early post-MI setting, when the antiremodeling actions of aldosterone blockade would be expected to be particularly beneficial. In the EPHESUS (Eplerenone Post-Acute Myocardial Infarction HF Efficacy and Survival Study) trial (107), eplerenone was evaluated in 6,632 high-risk, post-MI patients with LVEF $\leq$40% and either clinical evidence of HF or diabetes, who were randomized to eplerenone or placebo in addition to optimal post-MI therapy. Patients with serum creatinine levels >2.5 mg/dL or serum K^+ >5.0 mmol/L were excluded. Eplerenone was initiated at 25 mg daily within 14 days after MI, and after 4 weeks was increased to a maximum of 50 mg per day. The addition of eplerenone to standard medical therapy after MI resulted in a 15% reduction in mortality (RR 0.85, 95% CI 0.75–0.96; $p = 0.008$) (Fig. 26-13) and a 13% reduction in death from cardiovascular causes, which was readily apparent and greatest during the initial 30 to 60 days post-MI.

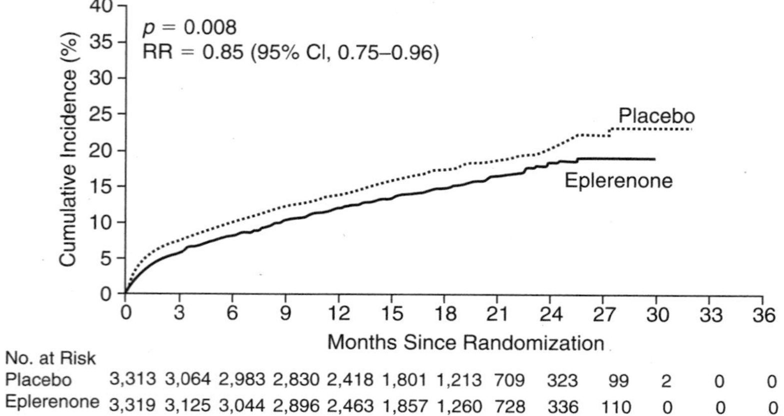

Figure 26-13 Kaplan-Meier estimates of the rate of death from any cause in the EPHESUS trial. RR, relative risk; CI, confidence interval. (Reproduced from Pitt B, Remme W, Zannad F, et al. Eplerenone, a selective aldosterone blocker, in patients with left ventricular dysfunction after myocardial infarction. *N Engl J Med.* 2003;348:1309–1321, with permission.)

The reduction in cardiovascular mortality was in large part due to a 21% reduction in the rate of sudden death from cardiac causes. As in RALES, eplerenone was at least as effective in patients taking both beta-blockers and ACEIs as in those taking only one of these agents. In the 3,300 patients randomized to eplerenone and followed for a mean of 16 months, there was no increased incidence of gynecomastia, breast pain, impotence in males, or menstrual irregularities in females, confirming the relative selectivity of eplerenone for the mineralocorticoid receptor. In summary, the EPHESUS study demonstrated that the addition of an aldosterone blocker, as distinct from an ARB, produces further reductions in morbidity and mortality in well-treated patients in the post-MI setting.

Using Aldosterone Antagonists

We now have convincing evidence that aldosterone antagonists confer a significant benefit in terms of overall mortality, cardiovascular mortality (particularly sudden death), and hospitalizations in patients with moderate to severe HF. The benefits conferred by aldosterone antagonists in the treatment of HF, however, must be carefully weighed against the risks associated with their use, and close monitoring for side effects is mandatory. Serious hyperkalemia was uncommon in RALES (2%) but is seen much more often in clinical practice (116). In EPHESUS, hyperkalemia occurred in 3.4% of patients treated with eplerenone—a significant but relatively low incidence considering that 32% of participants had diabetes, which predisposes to hyperkalemia. Partly balancing this effect was the significantly lower incidence of hypokalemia (0.5% versus 1.5%, $p < 0.001$) with eplerenone.

Several reports have noted higher rates of serious adverse events with the use of aldosterone blockers in nontrial settings, primarily consisting of hyperkalemia or worsening renal function. This is likely due to broader use and less-intensive follow-up (116,117), so it is critical that these agents be used judiciously. With regard to patient selection, patients with serum $K^+ > 5.0$ mEq/L or creatinine levels >2.5 mg/dL should generally not be treated with aldosterone blockers. Diabetics are at higher risk of developing hyperkalemia and worsening renal function than are nondiabetics because of unrecognized renal dysfunction and a propensity to develop type IV renal tubular acidosis. It is also important to note that in RALES, virtually all patients were receiving loop diuretics, which were continued when spironolactone was added. The background of diuretics protects against hyperkalemia, and concomitant reduction or withdrawal of diuretics is likely to be associated with fluid retention and worsening HF since spironolactone in the recommended low doses has only a modest diuretic effect.

Even in appropriate patients, it is critical to use these agents carefully. Renal function and potassium levels should be measured within 1 week after initiation, and even earlier in higher-risk patients with baseline renal dysfunction, potassium levels at the upper limit of normal, and diabetes. Subsequent monitoring should be determined by the stability of renal function and fluid status but should occur at least monthly for the first 3 months and every 3 months thereafter. Downward adjustment or discontinuation of aldosterone antagonists should occur if serum potassium exceeds 5.5 mEq/L (118). The maximum doses in the RALES and EPHESUS trials were 50 mg of spironolactone and 50 mg of eplerenone, respectively, with the latter agent producing less-potent aldosterone blockade on a milligram-to-milligram basis. Higher doses have not been shown to have any greater efficacy and should be avoided.

Choice of Aldosterone-Blocking Agent

The two available aldosterone receptor blockers, spironolactone and eplerenone, have not been compared in patients with HF or recent MI. Both are effective in the doses and patient populations studied. It is likely that spironolactone would also be effective in post-MI patients and, conversely, that eplerenone would be effective in chronic HF. Because of the substantial difference in cost, spironolactone is a logical first choice for these indications, with eplerenone being substituted in patients who develop side effects related to the nonselective properties of spironolactone, such as gynecomastia, breast tenderness, or sexual dysfunction.

CONCLUSIONS AND FUTURE DIRECTIONS

This chapter has reviewed the physiology of the RAAS and its role in the clinical syndrome of HF. The results of numerous clinical trials performed over the past three decades have demonstrated the importance of RAAS activation in the initiation and progression of LV dysfunction and remodeling. ACEIs clearly improve the symptoms and prognosis of patients with symptomatic and asymptomatic LVD, and prevent the development of HF in high-risk patients. Thus, ACEIs should be first-line therapy for patients with mild, moderate, and severe HF due to the weight of clinical evidence supporting their use and their demonstrated cost-effectiveness (119).

ARBs have now emerged as an effective alternative therapy for patients who are intolerant of ACEIs. In ACEI-intolerant patients they produce significant reductions in mortality and other cardiovascular events. The higher cost of ARBs, combined with the lack of evidence demonstrating their superiority, suggest that they be reserved for use in patients with documented side effects from ACEIs, including cough or skin rashes. In addition, combination therapy with an ACEI and ARB appears to provide additional clinical benefits and further protection against LV remodeling in patients with chronic HF, compared to treatment with either agent alone.

Aldosterone antagonists have produced impressive reductions in sudden death and other cardiovascular endpoints in patients with chronic HF and post-MI LV dysfunction. In carefully selected patients, combination therapy with an ACEI, beta blocker, and aldosterone antagonist appears to confer greater mortality benefit than does combined treatment with an ACEI and ARB.

A logical direction for future HF therapies will be the identification of agents that more effectively antagonize neurohormonal activation. For instance, renin inhibitors have recently been developed and have been shown to provide dose-dependent benefits in the treatment of hypertension (120). Similarly, peptide fragments such as angiotensin-(1–7) may antagonize the biological effects of Ang II (121). In vitro studies and clinical testing of these agents will provide new insights into the pathophysiology of HF and will enable us to further prevent and treat this increasingly prevalent condition.

REFERENCES

1. Mann DL. Mechanisms and models in heart failure: a combinatorial approach. *Circulation.* 1999;100:999–1008.
2. Massie BM, Kramer B, Haughom F. Acute and long-term effects of vasodilator therapy on resting and exercise hemodynamics and exercise tolerance. *Circulation.* 1981;64:1218–1226.
3. Klein L, O'Connor CM, Gattis WA, et al. Pharmacologic therapy for patients with chronic heart failure and reduced systolic function: review of trials and practical considerations. *Am J Cardiol.* 2003;91:18F–40F.
4. Tan LB, Jalil JE, Pick R, et al. Cardiac myocyte necrosis induced by angiotensin II. *Circ Res.* 1991;69:1185–1195.
5. Bristow MR. The adrenergic nervous system in heart failure. *N Engl J Med.* 1984;311:850–851.
6. Sutton MG, Sharpe N. Left ventricular remodeling after myocardial infarction: pathophysiology and therapy. *Circulation.* 2000;101:2981–2988.
7. Weber KT. Extracellular matrix remodeling in heart failure: a role for de novo angiotensin II generation. *Circulation.* 1997;96:4065–4082.
8. Givertz MM. Manipulation of the renin-angiotensin system. *Circulation.* 2001;104:E14–E18.
9. Weir MR, Dzau VJ. The renin-angiotensin-aldosterone system: a specific target for hypertension management. *Am J Hypertens.* 1999;12:205S–213S.
10. Re RN. The clinical implication of tissue renin angiotensin systems. *Curr Opin Cardiol.* 2001;16:317–327.
11. Urata H, Nishimura H, Ganten D. Chymase-dependent angiotensin II forming systems in humans. *Am J Hypertens.* 1996;9:277–284.
12. Hernandez-Presa M, Bustos C, Ortego M, et al. Angiotensin-converting enzyme inhibition prevents arterial nuclear factor-kappa B activation, monocyte chemoattractant protein-1 expression, and macrophage infiltration in a rabbit model of early accelerated atherosclerosis. *Circulation.* 1997;95:1532–1541.
13. Napoleone E, Di Santo A, Camera M, et al. Angiotensin-converting enzyme inhibitors downregulate tissue factor synthesis in monocytes. *Circ Res.* 2000;86:139–143.
14. Ruzicka M, Skarda V, Leenen FH. Effects of ACE inhibitors on circulating versus cardiac angiotensin II in volume overload-induced cardiac hypertrophy in rats. *Circulation.* 1995;92:3568–3573.
15. Pieruzzi F, Abassi ZA, Keiser HR. Expression of renin-angiotensin system components in the heart, kidneys, and lungs of rats with experimental heart failure. *Circulation.* 1995;92:3105–3112.
16. Hirsch AT, Talsness CE, Schunkert H, et al. Tissue-specific activation of cardiac angiotensin converting enzyme in experimental heart failure. *Circ Res.* 1991;69:475–482.
17. Fabris B, Jackson B, Kohzuki M, et al. Increased cardiac angiotensin-converting enzyme in rats with chronic heart failure. *Clin Exp Pharmacol Physiol.* 1990;17:309–314.
18. Rajagopalan S, Kurz S, Munzel T, et al. Angiotensin II-mediated hypertension in the rat increases vascular superoxide production via membrane NADH/NADPH oxidase activation. Contribution to alterations of vasomotor tone. *J Clin Invest.* 1996;97:1916–1923.
19. Linz W, Wiemer G, Gohlke P, et al. Contribution of kinins to the cardiovascular actions of angiotensin-converting enzyme inhibitors. *Pharmacol Rev.* 1995;47:25–49.
20. Vaughan DE. Fibrinolytic balance, the renin-angiotensin system and atherosclerotic disease. *Eur Heart J.* 1998;19(Suppl G):G9–G12.
21. Valentin S, Reutlingsperger CP, Nordfang O, et al. Inhibition of factor X activation at extracellular matrix of fibroblasts during flow conditions: a comparison between tissue factor pathway inhibitor and inactive factor VIIa. *Thromb Haemost.* 1995;74:1478–1485.
22. Brown NJ, Ryder D, Gainer JV, et al. Differential effects of angiotensin converting enzyme inhibitors on the vasodepressor and prostacyclin responses to bradykinin. *J Pharmacol Exp Ther.* 1996;279:703–712.
23. Braunwald E, Bristow MR. Congestive heart failure: fifty years of progress. *Circulation.* 2000;102:IV14–IV23.
24. Massie B, Kramer BL, Topic N, et al. Hemodynamic and radionuclide effects of acute captopril therapy for heart failure: changes in left and right ventricular volumes and function at rest and during exercise. *Circulation.* 1982;65:1374–1381.
25. Massie BM, Packer M, Hanlon JT, et al. Hemodynamic responses to combined therapy with captopril and hydralazine in patients with severe heart failure. *J Am Coll Cardiol.* 1983;2:338–344.
26. Captopril Multicenter Research Group. A placebo-controlled trial of captopril in refractory chronic congestive heart failure. *J Am Coll Cardiol.* 1983;2:755–763.
27. Kramer BL, Massie BM, Topic N. Controlled trial of captopril in chronic heart failure: a rest and exercise hemodynamic study. *Circulation.* 1983;67:807–816.
28. Pfeffer MA, Braunwald E, Moye LA, et al. Effect of captopril on mortality and morbidity in patients with left ventricular dysfunction after myocardial infarction. Results of the survival and ventricular enlargement trial. The SAVE Investigators. *N Engl J Med.* 1992;327:669–677.
29. The Acute Infarction Ramipril Efficacy (AIRE) Study Investigators. Effect of ramipril on mortality and morbidity of survivors of acute myocardial infarction with clinical evidence of heart failure. *Lancet.* 1993;342:821–828.

30. Sharpe DN, Murphy J, Coxon R, et al. Enalapril in patients with chronic heart failure: a placebo-controlled, randomized, double-blind study. *Circulation.* 1984;70:271–278.
31. Flather MD, Yusuf S, Kober L, et al. Long-term ACE-inhibitor therapy in patients with heart failure or left-ventricular dysfunction: a systematic overview of data from individual patients. ACE-Inhibitor Myocardial Infarction Collaborative Group. *Lancet* 2000;355:1575–1581.
32. The Captopril-Digoxin Multicenter Research Group. Comparative effects of therapy with captopril and digoxin in patients with mild to moderate heart failure. *JAMA.* 1988;259:539–544.
33. The CONSENSUS Trial Study Group. Effects of enalapril on mortality in severe congestive heart failure. Results of the Cooperative North Scandinavian Enalapril Survival Study (CONSENSUS). *N Engl J Med.* 1987;316:1429–1435.
34. The SOLVD Investigators. Effect of enalapril on survival in patients with reduced left ventricular ejection fractions and congestive heart failure. *N Engl J Med.* 1991;325:293–302.
35. Garg R, Yusuf S. Overview of randomized trials of angiotensin-converting enzyme inhibitors on mortality and morbidity in patients with heart failure. Collaborative Group on ACE Inhibitor Trials. *JAMA.* 1995;273:1450–1456.
36. Cohn JN, Johnson G, Ziesche S, et al. A comparison of enalapril with hydralazine-isosorbide dinitrate in the treatment of chronic congestive heart failure. *N Engl J Med.* 1991;325:303–310.
37. Pfeffer JM, Pfeffer MA, Braunwald E. Influence of chronic captopril therapy on the infarcted left ventricle of the rat. *Circ Res.* 1985;57:84–95.
38. Pfeffer MA, Pfeffer JM, Steinberg C, et al. Survival after an experimental myocardial infarction: beneficial effects of long-term therapy with captopril. *Circulation.* 1985;72:406–412.
39. Pfeffer MA, Lamas GA, Vaughan DE, et al. Effect of captopril on progressive ventricular dilatation after anterior myocardial infarction. *N Engl J Med.* 1988;319:80–86.
40. Ambrosioni E, Borghi C, Magnani B. The effect of the angiotensin-converting-enzyme inhibitor zofenopril on mortality and morbidity after anterior myocardial infarction. The Survival of Myocardial Infarction Long-Term Evaluation (SMILE) Study Investigators. *N Engl J Med.* 1995;332:80–85.
41. Kober L, Torp-Pedersen C, Carlsen JE, et al. A clinical trial of the angiotensin-converting-enzyme inhibitor trandolapril in patients with left ventricular dysfunction after myocardial infarction. Trandolapril Cardiac Evaluation (TRACE) Study Group. *N Engl J Med.* 1995;333:1670–1676.
42. Gruppo Italiano per lo Studio della Sopravvivenza nell'infarto Miocardico. GISSI-3: effects of lisinopril and transdermal glyceryl trinitrate singly and together on 6-week mortality and ventricular function after acute myocardial infarction. *Lancet.* 1994;343:1115–1122.
43. ISIS-4 (Fourth International Study of Infarct Survival) Collaborative Group. ISIS-4: a randomised factorial trial assessing early oral captopril, oral mononitrate, and intravenous magnesium sulphate in 58,050 patients with suspected acute myocardial infarction. *Lancet.* 1995;345:669–685.
44. No authors listed. Oral captopril versus placebo among 13,634 patients with suspected acute myocardial infarction: interim report from the Chinese Cardiac Study (CCS-1). *Lancet.* 1995;345:686–687.
45. Swedberg K, Held P, Kjekshus J, et al. Effects of the early administration of enalapril on mortality in patients with acute myocardial infarction. Results of the Cooperative New Scandinavian Enalapril Survival Study II (CONSENSUS II). *N Engl J Med.* 1992;327:678–684.
46. Effect of enalapril on mortality and the development of heart failure in asymptomatic patients with reduced left ventricular ejection fractions. The SOLVD Investigattors. *N Engl J Med.* 1992;327:685–691.
47. Konstam MA, Kronenberg MW, Rousseau MF, et al. Effects of the angiotensin converting enzyme inhibitor enalapril on the long-term progression of left ventricular dilatation in patients with asymptomatic systolic dysfunction. SOLVD (Studies of Left Ventricular Dysfunction) Investigators. *Circulation.* 1993;88: 2277–2283.
48. Jong P, Yusuf S, Rousseau MF, et al. Effect of enalapril on 12-year survival and life expectancy in patients with left ventricular systolic dysfunction: a follow-up study. *Lancet.* 2003;361:1843–1848.
49. Yusuf S, Sleight P, Pogue J, et al. Effects of an angiotensin-converting-enzyme inhibitor, ramipril, on cardiovascular events in high-risk patients. The Heart Outcomes Prevention Evaluation Study Investigators. *N Engl J Med.* 2000;342:145–153.
50. Fox KM. Efficacy of perindopril in reduction of cardiovascular events among patients with stable coronary artery disease: randomised, double-blind, placebo-controlled, multicentre trial (the EUROPA study). *Lancet.* 2003;362:782–788.
51. Braunwald E, Domanski MJ, Fowler SE, et al. Angiotensin-converting-enzyme inhibition in stable coronary artery disease. *N Engl J Med.* 2004;351:2058–2068.
52. Ruggenenti P, Perna A, Remuzzi G. ACE inhibitors to prevent end-stage renal disease: when to start and why possibly never to stop: a post hoc analysis of the REIN trial results. Ramipril Efficacy in Nephropathy. *J Am Soc Nephrol.* 2001;12:2832–2837.
53. Pisoni R, Faraone R, Ruggenent P, et al. Inhibitors of the renin-angiotensin system reduce the rate of GFR decline and end-stage renal disease in patients with severe renal insufficiency. *J Nephrol.* 2002;15:428–430.
54. Brunner-La Rocca HP, Weilenmann D, Kiowski W, et al. Plasma levels of enalaprilat in chronic therapy of heart failure: relationship to adverse events. *J Pharmacol Exp Ther.* 1999;289:565–571.
55. Vleeming W, van Amsterdam JG, Stricker BH, et al. ACEI-induced angioedema. Incidence, prevention and management. *Drug Saf.* 1998;18:171–188.
56. Nussberger J, Cugno M, Amstutz C, et al. Plasma bradykinin in angio-oedema. *Lancet.* 1998;351:1693–1697.
57. Shlipak MG. Pharmacotherapy for heart failure in patients with renal insufficiency. *Ann Intern Med.* 2003;138:917–924.
58. Ljungman S, Kjekshus J, Swedberg K. Renal function in severe congestive heart failure during treatment with enalapril (the Cooperative North Scandinavian Enalapril Survival Study [CONSENSUS] Trial). *Am J Cardiol.* 1992;70:479–487.
59. Massie BM, Kramer BL, Topic N. Lack of relationship between the short-term hemodynamic effects of captopril and subsequent clinical responses. *Circulation.* 1984;69:1135–1141.
60. Packer M, Poole-Wilson PA, Armstrong PW, et al. Comparative effects of low and high doses of the angiotensin-converting enzyme inhibitor, lisinopril, on morbidity and mortality in chronic heart failure. ATLAS Study Group. *Circulation.* 1999;100:2312–2318.
61. Massie BM, Armstrong PW, Cleland JG, et al. Toleration of high doses of angiotensin-converting enzyme inhibitors in patients with chronic heart failure: results from the ATLAS trial. The Assessment of Treatment with Lisinopril and Survival. *Arch Intern Med.* 2001;161:165–171.
62. Massie BM, Shah NB. Evolving trends in the epidemiologic factors of heart failure: rationale for preventive strategies and comprehensive disease management. *Am Heart J.* 1997;133:703–712.
63. Al-Khadra AS, Salem DN, Rand WM, et al. Antiplatelet agents and survival: a cohort analysis from the Studies of Left Ventricular Dysfunction (SOLVD) trial. *J Am Coll Cardiol.* 1998;31: 419–425.
64. Massie BM, Teerlink JR. Interaction between aspirin and angiotensin-converting enzyme inhibitors: real or imagined. *Am J Med.* 2000;109:431–433.
65. Nguyen KN, Aursnes I, Kjekshus J. Interaction between enalapril and aspirin on mortality after acute myocardial infarction: subgroup analysis of the Cooperative New Scandinavian Enalapril Survival Study II (CONSENSUS II). *Am J Cardiol.* 1997;79:115–119.
66. Cleland JG, Findlay I, Jafri S, et al. The Warfarin/Aspirin Study in Heart failure (WASH): a randomized trial comparing antithrombotic strategies for patients with heart failure. *Am Heart J.* 2004;148:157–164.
67. Grinstead WC, Francis MJ, Marks GF, et al. Discontinuation of chronic diuretic therapy in stable congestive heart failure secondary to coronary artery disease or to idiopathic dilated cardiomyopathy. *Am J Cardiol.* 1994;73:881–886.
68. Katwa LC, Campbell SE, Tyagi SC, et al. Cultured myofibroblasts generate angiotensin peptides de novo. *J. Mol Cell Cardiol.* 1997;29:1375–1386.
69. Balcells E, Meng QC, Johnson WH, Jr., et al. Angiotensin II formation from ACE and chymase in human and animal hearts: methods and species considerations. *Am J Physiol.* 1997;273: H1769–H1774.

70. MacFadyen RJ, Lee AF, Morton JJ, et al. How often are angiotensin II and aldosterone concentrations raised during chronic ACE inhibitor treatment in cardiac failure? *Heart.* 1999;82:57–61.
71. Roig E, Perez-Villa F, Morales M, et al. Clinical implications of increased plasma angiotensin II despite ACE inhibitor therapy in patients with congestive heart failure. *Eur Heart J.* 2000;21:53–57.
72. Meister B, Lippoldt A, Bunnemann B, et al. Cellular expression of angiotensin type-1 receptor mRNA in the kidney. *Kidney Int.* 1993;44:331–336.
73. Weber KT, Brilla CG. Pathological hypertrophy and cardiac interstitium. Fibrosis and renin-angiotensin-aldosterone system. *Circulation.* 1991;83:1849–1865.
74. Nakajima M, Hutchinson HG, Fujinaga M, et al. The angiotensin II type 2 (AT2) receptor antagonizes the growth effects of the AT1 receptor: gain-of-function study using gene transfer. *Proc Natl Acad Sci USA.* 1995;92:10663–10667.
75. Burnier M, Brunner HR. Angiotensin II receptor antagonists. *Lancet.* 2000;355:637–645.
76. Lacourciere Y, Brunner H, Irwin R, et al. Effects of modulators of the renin-angiotensin-aldosterone system on cough. Losartan Cough Study Group. *J Hypertens.* 1994;12:1387–1393.
77. Granger CB, McMurray JJ, Yusuf S, et al. Effects of candesartan in patients with chronic heart failure and reduced left-ventricular systolic function intolerant to angiotensin-converting-enzyme inhibitors: the CHARM-Alternative trial. *Lancet.* 2003;362:772–776.
78. Pitt B, Segal R, Martinez FA, et al. Randomised trial of losartan versus captopril in patients over 65 with heart failure (Evaluation of Losartan in the Elderly Study, ELITE). *Lancet.* 1997;349:747–752.
79. Pitt B, Poole-Wilson PA, Segal R, et al. Effect of losartan compared with captopril on mortality in patients with symptomatic heart failure: randomised trial—the Losartan Heart Failure Survival Study ELITE II. *Lancet.* 2000;355:1582–1587.
80. Dickstein K, Kjekshus J. Effects of losartan and captopril on mortality and morbidity in high-risk patients after acute myocardial infarction: the OPTIMAAL randomised trial. Optimal Trial in Myocardial Infarction with Angiotensin II Antagonist Losartan. *Lancet.* 2002;360:752–760.
81. Pfeffer MA, McMurray JJ, Velazquez EJ, et al. Valsartan, captopril, or both in myocardial infarction complicated by heart failure, left ventricular dysfunction, or both. *N Engl J Med.* 2003;349:1893–1906.
82. McKelvie RS, Yusuf S, Pericak D, et al. Comparison of candesartan, enalapril, and their combination in congestive heart failure: randomized evaluation of strategies for left ventricular dysfunction (RESOLVD) pilot study. The RESOLVD Pilot Study Investigators. *Circulation.* 1999;100:1056–1064.
83. Cohn JN, Tognoni G. A randomized trial of the angiotensin-receptor blocker valsartan in chronic heart failure. *N Engl J Med.* 2001;345:1667–1675.
84. McMurray JJ, Ostergren J, Swedberg K, et al. Effects of candesartan in patients with chronic heart failure and reduced left-ventricular systolic function taking angiotensin-converting-enzyme inhibitors: the CHARM-Added trial. *Lancet.* 2003;362:767–771.
85. Yusuf S, Pfeffer MA, Swedberg K, et al. Effects of candesartan in patients with chronic heart failure and preserved left-ventricular ejection fraction: the CHARM-Preserved Trial. *Lancet.* 2003;362:777–781.
86. Carson P, Massie BM, McKelvie RS, et al. The Irbesartan in Heart Failure with Preserved Systolic Function (I-PRESERVE) Trial: Rationale and Design. *J Card Fail.* 2005;11:576–585.
87. Gring CN, Francis GS. A hard look at angiotensin receptor blockers in heart failure. *J Am Coll Cardiol.* 2004;44:1841–1846.
88. Swedberg K, Eneroth P, Kjekshus J, et al. Hormones regulating cardiovascular function in patients with severe congestive heart failure and their relation to mortality. CONSENSUS Trial Study Group. *Circulation.* 1990;82:1730–1736.
89. Tsuji H, Venditti FJ, Jr., Evans JC, et al. The associations of levels of serum potassium and magnesium with ventricular premature complexes (the Framingham Heart Study). *Am J Cardiol.* 1994;74:232–235.
90. Gottlieb SS, Baruch L, Kukin ML, et al. Prognostic importance of the serum magnesium concentration in patients with congestive heart failure. *J Am Coll Cardiol.* 1990;16:827–831.
91. Farquharson CA, Struthers AD. Spironolactone increases nitric oxide bioactivity, improves endothelial vasodilator dysfunction, and suppresses vascular angiotensin I/angiotensin II conversion in patients with chronic heart failure. *Circulation.* 2000;101:594–597.
92. Heitzer T, Schlinzig T, Krohn K, et al. Endothelial dysfunction, oxidative stress, and risk of cardiovascular events in patients with coronary artery disease. *Circulation.* 2001;104:2673–2678.
93. Brilla CG, Zhou G, Matsubara L, et al. Collagen metabolism in cultured adult rat cardiac fibroblasts: response to angiotensin II and aldosterone. *J. Mol Cell Cardiol.* 1994;26:809–820.
94. Brilla CG, Pick R, Tan LB, et al. Remodeling of the rat right and left ventricles in experimental hypertension. *Circ Res.* 1990;67:1355–1364.
95. Sato A, Saruta T. Aldosterone escape during angiotensin-converting enzyme inhibitor therapy in essential hypertensive patients with left ventricular hypertrophy. *J Int Med Res.* 2001;29:13–21.
96. Wang W. Chronic administration of aldosterone depresses baroreceptor reflex function in the dog. *Hypertension.* 1994;24:571–575.
97. Yee KM, Struthers AD. Aldosterone blunts the baroreflex response in man. *Clin Sci.* (Lond) 1998;95:687–692.
98. Vaughan DE, Lazos SA, Tong K. Angiotensin II regulates the expression of plasminogen activator inhibitor-1 in cultured endothelial cells. A potential link between the renin-angiotensin system and thrombosis. *J Clin Invest.* 1995;95:995–1001.
99. Cleland JG, Dargie HJ, Hodsman GP, et al. Captopril in heart failure. A double blind controlled trial. *Br Heart J.* 1984;52:530–535.
100. Borghi C, Boschi S, Ambrosioni E, et al. Evidence of a partial escape of renin-angiotensin-aldosterone blockade in patients with acute myocardial infarction treated with ACE inhibitors. *J Clin Pharmacol.* 1993;33:40–45.
101. Urata H, Nishimura H, Ganten D. Mechanisms of angiotensin II formation in humans. *Eur Heart J.* 1995;16(Suppl N):79–85.
102. Struthers AD. Aldosterone escape during angiotensin-converting enzyme inhibitor therapy in chronic heart failure. *J Card Fail.* 1996;2:47–54.
103. Zannad F, Alla F, Dousset B, et al. Limitation of excessive extracellular matrix turnover may contribute to survival benefit of spironolactone therapy in patients with congestive heart failure: insights from the randomized aldactone evaluation study (RALES). Rales Investigators. *Circulation.* 2000;102:2700–2706.
104. Weber KT, Villarreal D. Aldosterone and antialdosterone therapy in congestive heart failure. *Am J Cardiol.* 1993;71:3A–11A.
105. Barr CS, Lang CC, Hanson J, et al. Effects of adding spironolactone to an angiotensin-converting enzyme inhibitor in chronic congestive heart failure secondary to coronary artery disease. *Am J Cardiol.* 1995;76:1259–1265.
106. Vantrimpont P, Rouleau JL, Ciampi A, et al. Two-year time course and significance of neurohumoral activation in the Survival and Ventricular Enlargement (SAVE) Study. *Eur Heart J.* 1998;19:1552–1563.
107. Pitt B, Remme W, Zannad F, et al. Eplerenone, a selective aldosterone blocker, in patients with left ventricular dysfunction after myocardial infarction. *N Engl J Med.* 2003;348:1309–1321.
108. MacFadyen RJ, Barr CS, Struthers AD. Aldosterone blockade reduces vascular collagen turnover, improves heart rate variability and reduces early morning rise in heart rate in heart failure patients. *Cardiovasc Res.* 1997;35:30–34.
109. Bauersachs J, Heck M, Fraccarollo D, et al. Addition of spironolactone to angiotensin-converting enzyme inhibition in heart failure improves endothelial vasomotor dysfunction: role of vascular superoxide anion formation and endothelial nitric oxide synthase expression. *J Am Coll Cardiol.* 2002;39:351–358.
110. Yee KM, Pringle SD, Struthers AD. Circadian variation in the effects of aldosterone blockade on heart rate variability and QT dispersion in congestive heart failure. *J Am Coll Cardiol.* 2001;37:1800–1807.
111. Pitt B, Zannad F, Remme WJ, et al. The effect of spironolactone on morbidity and mortality in patients with severe heart failure. Randomized Aldactone Evaluation Study Investigators. *N Engl J Med.* 1999;341:709–717.
112. Jackson EK. Diuretics. In: Hardman JG, Limbird LE, Molinoff PB, et al., eds. *Goodman & Gilman's The Pharmacological Basis of Therapeutics.* 9th ed. New York: McGraw-Hill; 1996: 706–711.

113. Khan NU, Movahed A. The role of aldosterone and aldosterone-receptor antagonists in heart failure. *Rev Cardiovasc Med.* 2004;5:71–81.
114. Pitt B, Reichek N, Willenbrock R, et al. Effects of eplerenone, enalapril, and eplerenone/enalapril in patients with essential hypertension and left ventricular hypertrophy: the 4E-left ventricular hypertrophy study. *Circulation.* 2003;108:1831–1838.
115. White WB, Duprez D, St Hillaire R, et al. Effects of the selective aldosterone blocker eplerenone versus the calcium antagonist amlodipine in systolic hypertension. *Hypertension.* 2003;41:1021–1026.
116. Juurlink DN, Mamdani MM, Lee DS, et al. Rates of hyperkalemia after publication of the Randomized Aldactone Evaluation Study. *N Engl J Med.* 2004;351:543–551.
117. Bozkurt B, Agoston I, Knowlton AA. Complications of inappropriate use of spironolactone in heart failure: when an old medicine spirals out of new guidelines. *J Am Coll Cardiol.* 2003;41:211–214.
118. Hunt SA, Baker DW, Chin MH, et al. ACC/AHA guidelines for the evaluation and management of chronic heart failure in the adult: executive summary. A report of the American College of Cardiology/American Heart Association Task Force on Practice Guidelines (Committee to Revise the 1995 Guidelines for the Evaluation and Management of Heart Failure): Developed in Collaboration With the International Society for Heart and Lung Transplantation; Endorsed by the Heart Failure Society of America. *Circulation.* 2001;104:2996–3007.
119. Paul SD, Kuntz KM, Eagle KA, et al. Costs and effectiveness of angiotensin converting enzyme inhibition in patients with congestive heart failure. *Arch Intern Med.* 1994;154:1143–1149.
120. Gradman AH, Schmieder RE, Lins RL, et al. Aliskiren, a novel orally effective renin inhibitor, provides dose-dependent antihypertensive efficacy and placebo-like tolerability in hypertensive patients. *Circulation.* 2005;111:1012–1018.
121. Ferrario CM, Chappell MC. Novel angiotensin peptides. *Cell Mol Life Sci.* 2004;61:2720–2727.

Vasodilators

27

Uri Elkayam Fahed Bitar Sarkis Kiramijyian
Parta Hatamizadeh Philip F. Binkley Carl V. Leier

The introduction of vasodilator therapy as a major intervention for heart failure occurred when Gould et al. (1) reported in 1969 that the α-adrenergic blocker phentolamine improved hemodynamics and the clinical status of patients with heart failure. Nitroprusside was later noted to augment hemodynamics and improve the clinical condition of patients with heart failure after myocardial infarction (2). The wide recognition of vasodilator therapy as a major intervention for congestive heart failure (CHF) was greatly affected by the introduction of the flow-directed pulmonary artery catheter (3). The report of the Veterans Heart Failure Trial (V-HeFT) in 1986 (4) showed the potential of chronic vasodilation therapy in improving long-term outcome, and recently the African-American Heart Failure Trial (A-HeFT) study (5) demonstrated a powerful effect of vasodilators given in addition to other heart failure therapies in African-Americans with chronic symptomatic CHF. This chapter reviews the principles of administration and the role of vasodilators in the treatment of heart failure.

RATIONALE FOR THE USE OF VASODILATORS IN CONGESTIVE HEART FAILURE

Reduction of Afterload

Ventricular afterload (ventricular wall stress during systole) is raised in most patients with heart failure because of an increase in one or more of its determinants, including ventricular systolic volume, aortic impedance, and systemic vascular resistance. Excessive afterload has an unfavorable effect on ventricular function in heart failure (Fig. 27-1A); the magnitude of this effect is proportional to the degree of ventricular failure (6). Vasodilator therapy is therefore directed at reducing the excessive ventricular afterload or wall stress of the failing heart, which results in augmentation of ventricular systolic function, stroke volume, cardiac output, and overall cardiovascular performance (Fig. 27-1B).

Reduction of Preload

Ventricular preload (cardiomyocyte stretch at end-diastole) increases in most forms of CHF secondary to an expansion of intravascular (and therefore intracardiac) volume via fluid retention by the kidney, neurogenic and hormonal venoconstriction, and elevated afterload. An increase in preload or end-diastolic actin-myosin stretch is generally accompanied by an augmentation of ventricular systolic function (Fig. 27-2A), a phenomenon commonly referred to as the Frank-Starling relationship (7). In patients with severe decompensated ventricular dysfunction, the rise in preload does not elicit a sufficient augmentation of ventricular systolic function because of a flat systolic function-preload curve. For this reason, any increase in ventricular end-diastolic pressure or volume (i.e., preload) is accompanied by only modest augmentation of systolic function and stroke volume (Fig. 27-2B). The persistent depression of stroke work and volume and cardiac output perpetuates the mechanisms responsible for fluid retention, venoconstriction, and excessive afterload, such that preload increases further to high levels (Fig. 27-2C) with accompanying signs and symptoms of congestion.

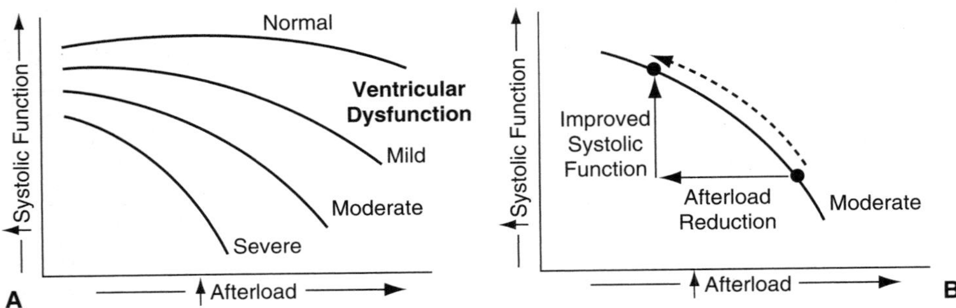

Figure 27-1 **(A)** The relationship between ventricular afterload and systolic function for normal and failing ventricles. (Adapted from Cohn JN, Franciosa JA. Vasodilator therapy of cardiac failure. *N Engl J Med.* 1977;297:27–31,254–258, with permission.) **(B)** Schematic representation of how vasodilator therapy augments ventricular systolic function by reducing ventricular afterload.

Combined Reduction of Afterload and Preload

It shall be noted that although vasodilator drugs are traditionally separated into those that achieve mostly afterload reduction and those that are directed mostly at preload reduction, all agents with predominant afterload-reducing properties also reduce preload via a number of mechanisms, including enhancement of ventricular systolic emptying and, in many patients, reduction of valvular regurgitation. Conversely, the predominantly preload-reducing drugs can favorably affect afterload by reducing ventricular volume.

NITROPRUSSIDE

Nitroprusside is the sodium (or potassium) salt of a complex molecule made up of ferric cyanide (Fe^{2+} and five cyanide groups) and nitric acid. Its effect appears to be mediated largely by production of nitrosothiol in vasculature, which in turn generates cyclic guanosine monophosphate (cGMP) in vascular smooth muscle and evokes relaxation (8).

Nitroprusside has a rapid onset of action, with vasodilating effects detectable within 60 to 90 seconds of initiation of the infusion. Some of the administered nitroprusside decomposes after entering the bloodstream, with the release of cyanide into the circulation (10). Additional cyanide is produced when nitroprusside is metabolized by vascular tissue, which then is further metabolized by the liver to thiocyanate and is slowly cleared by the kidneys (about a 3- to 4-day half-life). Because of its long half-life, thiocyanate can accumulate during prolonged or high-dose nitroprusside infusions or in the setting of renal dysfunction, and can evoke signs and symptoms of thiocyanate toxicity.

Hemodynamic Effects

Nitroprusside reduces the excessively elevated ventricular filling pressures in patients with CHF by multiple mechanisms. The drug diminishes heightened venous tone and thereby increases venous capacitance, with a resultant peripheral shift of central blood volume. By reducing the afterload of both left and right ventricles, nitroprusside decreases ventricular systolic and diastolic volume via greater ventricular systolic emptying and less valvular regurgitation (3,9–12). Nitroprusside may also lower ventricular filling pressure by improving ventricular diastolic properties or negating the restraining effect of the pericardium (by lowering intracardiac pressures and volume) (13,14). Improved renal blood flow may lead to increased diuresis and this may further contribute to preload reduction mediated by nitroprusside (15).

The use of nitroprusside in patients with decompensated heart failure results in a significant fall in systemic blood pressure, right atrial pressure, pulmonary arterial pressure, pulmonary capillary wedge pressure (PCWP), and systemic and pulmonary vascular resistance (Fig. 27-3). These changes are associated with a significant increase in cardiac output and no change in heart rate (9,11).

In the setting of CHF, nitroprusside generally lowers myocardial oxygen consumption as it reduces systolic and diastolic wall stress (16,17). The effect of nitroprusside on coronary hemodynamics has not been extensively studied in human heart failure. The net effect of nitroprusside on coronary blood flow in patients with significant coronary obstructive disease, however, may be determined by multiple factors, including effect on myocardial oxygen demand, coronary vasodilatory effect, and effect on perfusion pressure as well as diastolic filling time (17–19). In addition, nitroprusside may induce a coronary steal phenomenon by producing vasodilation of nonobstructed coronary beds, thus directing blood flow away from the already maximally vasodilated beds downstream from the coronary artery lesions (20,21).

In the setting of human CHF, nitroprusside preferentially reduces limb vascular resistance, with an augmentation of limb blood flow comparable in degree to the rise in cardiac output (22). Renal vascular resistance is also reduced in the therapeutic range of nitroprusside; however, the resultant renal blood flow and renal function are heavily dependent on changes in systemic blood pressure and renal perfusion pressure (15,22). Hepatic-splanchnic vascular resistance and blood flow are not significantly altered during infusion of nitroprusside at therapeutic rates (22).

Neurohormonal Responses

The neurohormonal response to nitroprusside infusion in heart failure varies considerably. Olivari et al. (23) found

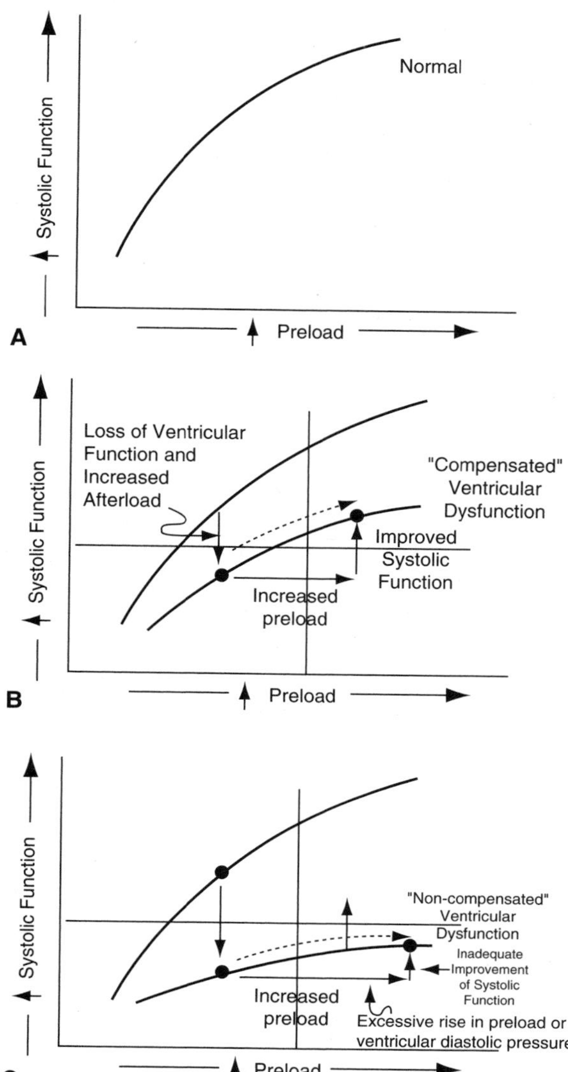

Figure 27-2 **(A)** The Frank-Starling mechanism relating ventricular preload (as determined by ventricular diastolic volume and pressure) to ventricular systolic function. **(B)** Schematic representation how a rise in preload can improve systolic function and bring a patient into the range of compensated ventricular dysfunction following a myocardial insult and resultant rise in afterload. **(C)** With severe loss of ventricular function, the marked rise in preload (to the point of large elevation in ventricular end-diastolic pressure and volume) is not capable of evoking an adequate increase in ventricular systolic function. The patient remains in a decompensated state of cardiac dysfunction, characterized by the clinical and hemodynamic manifestations of low cardiac output and markedly elevated ventricular filling pressures.

disparate responses of norepinephrine (NE) in a population of patients with CHF despite similar resting hemodynamics and comparable hemodynamic responses. One group (Group I) experienced an increase in plasma NE and the other group (Group II) experienced a decrease during the infusion. Group II patients appeared to be in a more advanced and severe stage of heart failure, with a higher mortality. Differences in baroreceptor and mechanoreceptor sensitivity and responsiveness have been suggested as a cause for disparate responses to NE in the two groups. A

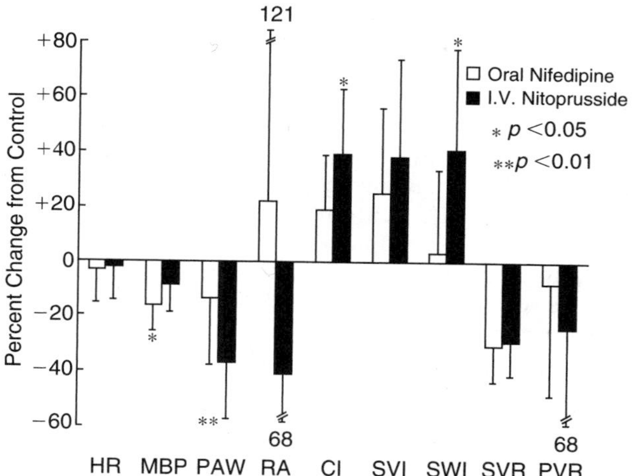

Figure 27-3 Comparison of percent changes from control after nifedipine and nitroprusside therapy. HR, heart rate; MBP, mean blood pressure; PAW, pulmonary artery wedge pressure; RA, mean right atrial pressure; CI, cardiac index; SVI, stroke volume index; SWI, left ventricular stroke work index; SVR, systemic vascular resistance; PVR, pulmonary vascular resistance. (From Elkayam U, Weber L, Torkan B, et al. Comparison of hemodynamic responses to nifedipine and nitroprusside in severe chronic congestive heart failure. *Am J Cardiol.* 1984;53:1321–1325, with permission.)

later study by Johnson et al. (24) examined the effect of diuretics and nitroprusside in 34 patients with decompensated heart failure. This therapy resulted in a significant increase in aldosterone levels and plasma renin activity. There was no significant change in NE levels, while endothelin and plasma atrial natriuretic levels showed a significant fall.

Clinical Application and Administration

Indications

Nitroprusside is most commonly employed in the treatment of acute decompensated heart failure (9,11,24,25), complicated acute myocardial infarction (MI) (26), and acute valvular insufficiency (27). It is also frequently encountered in patients who have undergone cardiopulmonary bypass or other cardiac surgery and it has been shown to be effective for chronic infusion in patients with end-stage CHF awaiting heart transplantation (28). Nitroprusside is also employed in the evaluation of potential recipients of heart transplantation to determine the reversibility of elevated pulmonary vascular resistance (29). A recent report demonstrated a significant improvement of functional class of patients with end-stage heart failure awaiting heart transplantation with chronic infusion of nitroprusside, which was safer and more effective than dobutmaine in relieving symptoms, facilitating unloading therapy, and improving survival (28). Khot et al. (30) examined the effect of nitroprusside in 25 patients with severe aortic stenosis and left ventricular (LV) dysfunction. This therapy, which had been previously considered contraindicated for this patient population, resulted in a significant increase in cardiac output. Based on these results, it was suggested by the authors that nitroprusside may provide a safe and effective bridge to aortic valve replacement in patients with aortic stenosis presenting with severe CHF.

Nitroprusside can effectively augment the hemodynamic effects of other drugs such as dopamine, dobutamine, and similar agents (31,32). Combination pharmacologic support is occasionally employed in the intensive care setting to optimize hemodynamic and clinical responses in patients with severely depressed cardiac output and elevated ventricular filling pressures.

Administration

Nitroprusside is administered intravenously with an infusion pump or microdrip regulator system to ensure controlled, precise dosing. Because of its light-sensitivity, the infusion set should be shielded. In CHF, the initial dose is 0.10 to 0.20 μg/kg per minute; this is gradually advanced as needed to attain the clinical and hemodynamic objectives. The incidence of side effects and toxicity is directly related to the dose and duration of administration. Because of its potent dose-related hemodynamic effect and the difficulties in determining maximal effective dose, nitroprusside is optimally administered with hemodynamic monitoring consisting of pulmonary artery catheterization and a close monitoring of systemic blood pressure.

Potential Adverse Effects and Toxicity

The most commonly encountered adverse effect of nitroprusside administration is systemic hypotension (23,33). When accompanied by a fall in coronary perfusion pressure and a rise in heart rate, nitroprusside-induced hypotension can be detrimental in patients with myocardial ischemia and infarction (20). A worsening renal function has been noted in association with nitroprusside infusions, typically during periods of systemic hypotension or hypoperfusion. Some patients may experience hemodynamic rebound with symptomatic deterioration after the abrupt discontinuation of nitroprusside (34). Gradual discontinuation is therefore recommended in order to achieve a smoother withdrawal.

Nausea, disorientation, confusion, psychosis, weakness, muscle spasm, hyperreflexia, and convulsions are side effects of thiocyanate toxicity, which may occur as plasma thiocyanate concentrations rise above 6 mg (33,35). The early sign of cyanide toxicity is metabolic (lactic) acidosis. Thiocyanate can be removed with hemodialysis and cyanide toxicity has been successfully managed with infusions of thiosulfate, sodium nitrate, and hydroxycobalamin. Conversion of cyanide to prussic acid raises methemoglobin levels and thus lowers the oxygen-carrying capacity of the blood. Thiocyanate and cyanide toxicity are rare during the usual administration of nitroprusside in heart failure (≤3 μg/kg per minute for ≤72 hours).

Nitroprusside can lower systemic arterial oxygen content by causing or exacerbating a pulmonary ventilation-perfusion mismatch, probably via dilatation of pulmonary arterioles in nonventilated areas (36). However, for most patients receiving nitroprusside, oxygen delivery is still augmented during the infusion because of the rise in cardiac output.

Laboratory data suggest that nitroprusside is capable of diverting blood flow from ischemic or threatened myocardium to normal myocardium by dilating the arterioles in the normal region (20,21). This potential for so-called coronary steal suggests a preference of nitroglycerin (NTG) over nitroprusside in patients with occlusive coronary artery disease. Other, far less commonly encountered side effects of nitroprusside include reduced platelet number and function, hypothyroidism (thiocyanate impairs iodine transport), and vitamin B_{12} deficiency (37,38).

ORGANIC NITRATES

Nitrates have been used for more than 100 years in clinical medicine, predominantly in the treatment of angina pectoris. Although not officially approved by the U.S. Food and Drug Administration (FDA) for use in CHF, nitrates have earned a role in the therapeutics of this condition during the past two decades (39,40).

Mechanism of Effect

Organic nitrates are prodrugs that undergo a complex metabolic biotransformation predominantly in the smooth muscle intracellular space (41). This biotransformation leads to the formation of nitric oxide (NO) or a related S-nitrosothiol, which stimulates the enzyme guanylate cyclase and leads to the formation of cyclic guanosine monophosphate (cGMP) in the vascular wall. GMP reduces intracellular calcium levels by decreasing its release from the cytoplasmic reticulum and by reducing its influx from the extracellular space. The decrease in intracellular calcium leads to a venous and arterial vasodilatation, which is the main cardiovascular effect of these drugs. Endothelial production and release of prostacylin may also contribute (42). Nitrates are cleared by extraction in the vasculature, hydrolysis in blood, and the action of glutathione-nitrate reductase in the liver (43).

Intravenous Nitroglycerin

Dose and Administration

Intravenous NTG is available as 5- and 10-mg/mL solutions that are diluted with normal saline or 5% dextrose solutions to provide infusions of 100 mg NTG/250 mL (44). Onset of action is immediate, as is offset when the infusion is stopped. Glass bottles and nonpolyvinyl chloride plastic tubing must be used to avoid a loss of the active drug via absorption onto plastics (45).

Infusion rates are usually initiated at 10 to 20 μg per minute and titrated upward in a stepwise fashion using 10 to 60 μg per minute increments to predetermined endpoints, such as improvement of symptoms, development of the drug-related side effects, change in a systolic blood pressure or pulmonary artery wedge pressure, or a maximum dose of 200 to 500 μg per minute (46,47).

Therapeutic Effects of Nitroglycerin in Patients with Heart Failure

Hemodynamic Effects

The potential hemodynamic effects of a therapeutic dose of NTG in patients with CHF include a substantial reduction in right and left ventricular filling pressure, systemic and pulmonary vascular resistance, and systemic blood pressure (Fig. 27-4). There is little or no change in heart rate, while cardiac output usually increases (46,47). The mechanisms for increased cardiac output include left ventricular and right ventricular afterload reduction, improvement in myocardial ischemia, and reduction in the degree of mitral regurgitation (44,48).

Effect on Mitral Regurgitation

Regurgitation of the mitral valve is common in patients with CHF, usually due to severe dilatation of the left ventricle and the mitral valve annulus. Use of intravenous (IV) NTG in a group of patients with chronic, nonischemic mitral regurgitation resulted in a reduction in LV and diastolic volume and mitral valve regurgitant area as well as a marked improvement in the severity of mitral regurgitation and the hemodynamic profile (48,49).

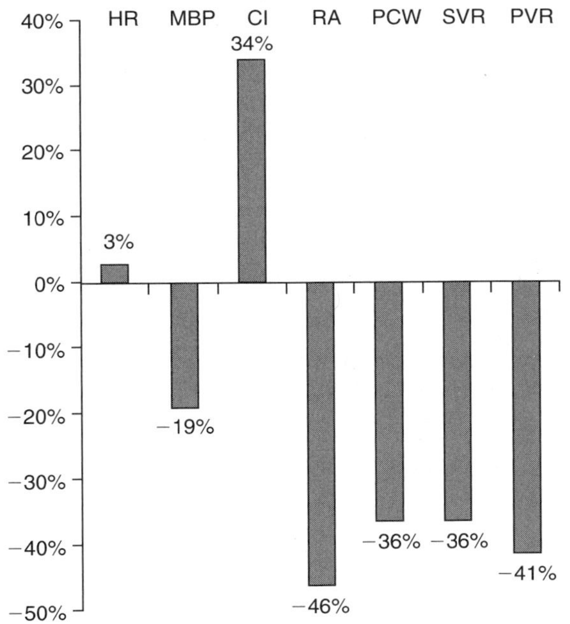

Figure 27-4 Intravenous nitroglycerin in the treatment of decompensated heart failure. CI, cardiac index; HR, heart rate; MBP, mean blood pressure; PCW, pulmonary capillary wedge pressure; PVR, pulmonary vascular resistance; RA, mean right atrial pressure; SVR, systemic vascular resistance. (From Elkayam U. Nitrates in the treatment of congestive heart failure. *Am J Cardiol.* 1996;77; 41C–51C, with permission.)

Neurohormonal Effects

The effect of acute and sustained IV NTG on hormone secretion was studied in nine patients with CHF by Webster et al. (Fig. 27-5) (50). NTG was administered at a dose uptitrated to achieve a 30% to 50% reduction in PCWP (50 to 245 μg per minute) and was associated with a substantial reduction in mean right atrial pressure and PCWP, a mild but significant reduction in systemic blood pressure (85 mm Hg to 78 mm Hg, $p = 0.04$), and no change in heart rate. These hemodynamic changes were associated with a reduction in plasma atrial natriuretic peptide, but also a significant increase in plasma aldosterone, cortisol, and epinephrine levels with a small and statistically significant increase in plasma NE or plasma renin activity.

The effect of IV NTG on arginine-vasopressin, plasma renin activity, aldosterone, and atrial natriuretic peptide was also evaluated by Dupuis et al. (47) in 13 men hospitalized with severe CHF (NYHA Class IV). The hemodynamic changes induced by NTG were accompanied by an increase in arterial epinephrine and plasma renin activity and a decrease in atrial natriuretic peptide. In contrast, there was no change in arterial NE, aldosterone, or arginine-vasopressin. By 6 hours of continuous infusion, arterial epinephrine levels returned to baseline values, possibly due to less-pronounced hypotension; however, plasma renin activity remained elevated and atrial natriuretic peptide remained decreased. Dakak et al. (51) also evaluated the hemodynamic and neurohormonal effects of 12 patients with severe heart failure. NTG dose was 276 ± 100 μg per minute, which resulted in considerable hemodynamic effects that were significantly attenuated due to nitrate tolerance after several hours of continuous infusion. NTG infusion was associated with a substantial increase in plasma renin activity and serum aldosterone, while atrial natriuretic peptide showed a marked but transient decrease in keeping with the development of hemodynamic tolerance.

Effect on Coronary Circulation

No information is available on the effect of IV NTG on coronary blood flow in patients with heart failure. In an unpublished study performed by our group, intracoronary administration of 200 μg NTG in a group of 25 patients with heart failure secondary to idiopathic dilated cardiomyopathy resulted in a significant dilatation of the epicardial coronary artery diameter by 8% ± 4%, as well as an increase in coronary blood flow by 42% ± 12% (44). These data suggest a combined effect of NTG on both the epicardial conductance as well as the resistance of coronary arteries in patients with heart failure due to idiopathic cardiomyopathy.

Effect on Renal Circulation

The effect of IV NTG on the renal circulation in patients with acute decompensated heart failure (ADHF) has not been studied. Infusion of NTG at a rate calculated to achieve blood concentration of 10^{-7}, 10^{-6}, 10^{-5} mol/L into

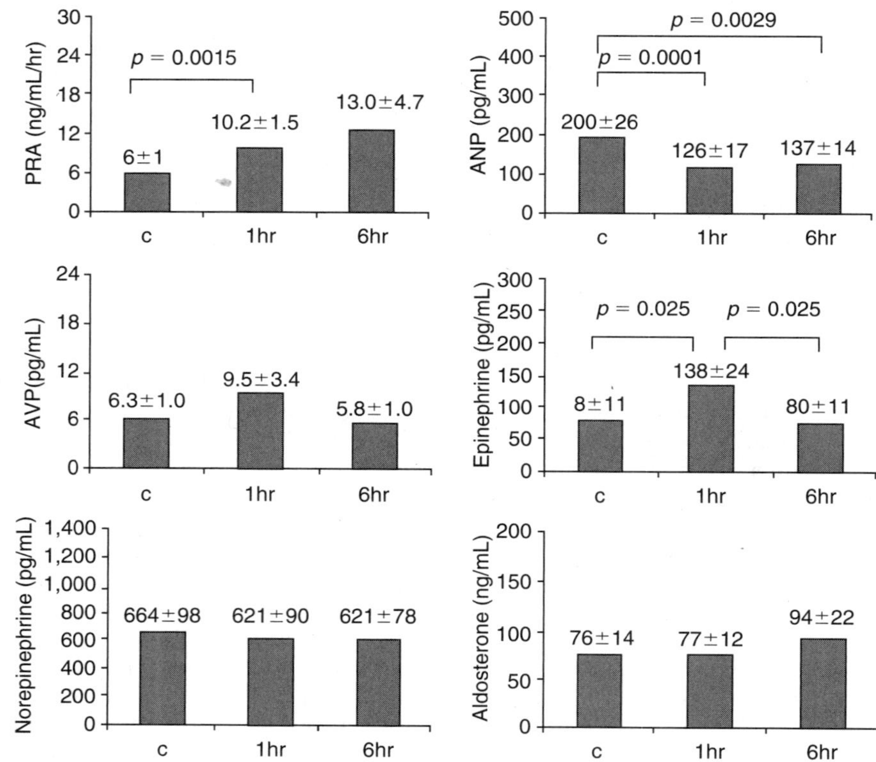

Figure 27-5 Neurohumoral changes during the first 6 hours of nitroglycerin infusion. Arterial epinephrine increased after 1 hour of infusion then returned to the baseline value at 6 hours. Plasma renin activity (PRA) increased and atrial natriuretic peptide (ANP) decreased throughout the first 6 hours of the infusion. There was no significant change in arginine vasopressin (AVP), norepinephrine, and aldosterone during nitroglycerin infusion. (From Dupuis J, Lalonde G, Lemieux R, et al. Tolerance to intravenous NTG in patients with congestive heart failure: role of increased intravascular volume, neurohumoral activation and lack of prevention with N-acetylcysteine. *J Am Coll Cardiol.* 1990;16:923–931, with permission.)

the renal artery in patients with heart failure resulted in a significant dilatation of the main renal artery with no significant effect on renal blood flow (52). These findings suggest a significant vasodilatory effect of NTG on large-conductance renal arteries but not on small-resistance vessels.

Potential Limitations of Intravenous Nitroglycerin in the Treatment of Acute Decompensated Heart Failure

Side Effects

Table 27-1 shows the reported side effects of IV NTG in 216 patients with ADHF, enrolled in the Vasodilatation in the Management of Acute CHF (VMAC) study (53). The most common adverse effect was headache, which was seen in 20% of the patients, followed by asymptomatic hypotension (8%), and nausea (6%).

Nitrate Resistance

A decreased vasodilatatory response and attenuated hemodynamic effect of nitrates have been reported in patients with heart failure. A recent study by Katz et al. (54) showed a twofold increase in femoral artery blood flow velocity with

TABLE 27-1

ADVERSE EFFECTS OF NITROGLYCERIN DURING FIRST 24 HOURS AFTER THE START OF THERAPY IN 216 PATIENTS IN VMAC STUDY

Adverse Effect	Number of Patients	Percent
Cardiovascular		
Hypotension		
Asymptomatic	17	8
Symptomatic	10	5
Nonsustained tidal volume	11	5
Angina pectoris	5	2
Other Adverse Effects		
General headache	44	20
Pain		
General	11	5
Abdominal	11	5
Catheter	11	5
Nausea	13	6
Any Adverse Event	146	68

From the publication Committee for the VMAC Investigators (Vasodilatation in the Management of Acute CHF). Intravenous nesiritide vs NTG for treatment of decompensated congestive heart failure: a randomized controlled trial. *JAMA.* 2002;287: 1531–1540, with permission.

intra-arterial infusion of NTG at a concentration of 10^{-7} mol/L in normal subjects. This response, however, was markedly attenuated in patients with heart failure and could be overcome only by increasing the dose to 10^{-5} mol/L. Potential mechanisms for vascular resistance to NTG include an increase in sodium and water within the vascular wall or an increased mechanical compression caused by accumulation of subcutaneous fluid (55), sulfhydryl group deficiency (56), and neurohormonal stimulation leading to activation of vasoconstrictive mechanisms including catecholamines, angiotensin II, endothelin, and vasopressin, which may attenuate the vasodilatory effect of the drug (57).

Nitrate Tolerance

Early development of tolerance and marked attenuation of initial hemodynamic effects of IV NTG in hospitalized patients with heart failure have been demonstrated by a number of investigators. Elkayam et al. (46), in a randomized, double-blind, placebo-controlled study, documented the early development of tolerance in 31 hospitalized patients with heart failure, which resulted in a significant attenuation of hemodynamic effects (Fig. 27-6). Analysis of individual data showed the development of early tolerance in approximately half of the patients, which could not be predicted by baseline hemodynamic and neurohormonal values. Similar attenuation of hemodynamic effects of IV NTG within several hours of initiation of therapy in hospitalized patients with heart failure has been shown by other investigators (47). Potential mechanisms for the development of early tolerance to NTG effect include the activation of neurohormonal mechanisms (47).

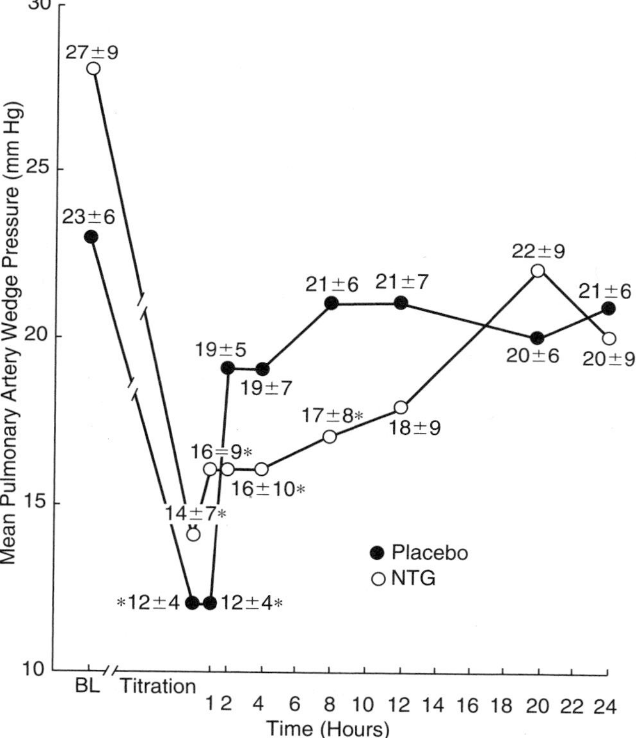

Figure 27-6 Values of mean pulmonary artery wedge pressure (PAWP) as measured at baseline (BL), during nitroglycerin (NTG) titration and during the 24 hours of the study infusion. After titration of NTG, 16 patients were randomly assigned to receive placebo and 15 patients were assigned to receive NTG. (From Elkayam U, Kulick D, McIntosh N, et al. Incidence of early tolerance to hemodynamic effects of continuous infusion of NTG in patients with coronary artery disease and heart failure. *Circulation.* 1987;76:577–584, with permission.)
*$p < 0.05$ versus baseline (BL).

Oral Nitrates

Hemodynamic Effects

Oral nitrates result in a substantial reduction in resting RV and LV filling pressures, systemic vascular resistance, and systemic blood pressure (56,58). There is little or no change in heart rate, and cardiac output is usually increased because of the reduction in LV afterload, decrease in pulmonary vascular resistance, improvement in myocardial ischemia, and reduction in the degree of mitral regurgitation (59).

The hemodynamic benefit of organic nitrates in patients with chronic CHF is also seen during both dynamic and isometric exercise. Hecht et al. (60) showed a significant decrease in PCWP, mean pulmonary arterial pressure, mean systemic arterial pressure, heart rate, systemic vascular resistance, and pulmonary vascular resistance, along with an increase in cardiac index, stroke volume index, and stroke work index during dynamic exercise in patients with chronic CHF. Elkayam et al. (61) studied the hemodynamic effect of nitrate therapy during isometric exercise in a similar patient population and showed nitrate-mediated prevention of unfavorable hemodynamic changes, including an increase in RV and LV filling pressure, pulmonary pressures, and systemic vascular resistance with a reduction in stroke volume and stroke work index.

Effect on Mitral Regurgitation

Regurgitation of the mitral valve is found in a large number of patients with CHF because of severe dilation of the left ventricle and the mitral valve annulus. Studies have shown a favorable effect of nitrates in patients with mitral regurgitation, with reduction in LV end-diastolic volume and mitral valve regurgitation area as well as marked improvement in the severity of mitral regurgitation and the hemodynamic profile (62). Similar nitrate-mediated hemodynamic improvement in patients with mitral regurgitation was shown during isometric exercise (61).

Hamilton et al. (62) showed a significant reduction in mitral and tricuspid valvular regurgitation after approximately 3 days of intensive vasodilator therapy, mainly with angiotensin-converting enzyme (ACE) inhibitors and oral isosorbide dinitrate (ISDN). Mitral and tricuspid regurgitation were significantly reduced as determined by two-dimensional and Doppler echocardiography with color-flow imaging in 14 patients with advanced heart failure secondary to dilated cardiomyopathy. This reduction was sustained after an average follow-up of 6 ± 2 months. In addition, mean left and right atrial volumes were reduced with initial therapy and showed a further decrease at 6 months.

Effect on Exercise Tolerance

Two early studies evaluated, in a randomized, double-blind fashion, the effect of a 3-month therapy that used oral ISDN on both maximal exercise time (63,64) and oxygen consumption in patients with chronic CHF, and showed a significant favorable effect of therapy. More recently, Elkayam et al. (65) published the results of a study regarding the effect of high-dose (50 to 100 mg), intermittent (12 hours per day) transdermal NTG in patients with chronic CHF, already treated by standard therapy that included ACE inhibitors, and showed a significant and sustained effect of therapy on maximal treadmill exercise time.

Potential Limitations of Oral Nitrate Therapy in Heart Failure

Side Effects

In a recent study (65), 46% of patients with moderate CHF developed headache during treatment with large-dose (2 to 4 mg per hour) transdermal NTG. Only 13% of the patients, however, discontinued therapy because of this side effect.

Nitrate Resistance

In a previous hemodynamic evaluation of the commonly used single ISDN dose (40 mg) in 99 consecutive patients with moderate and severe CHF (66), lack of hemodynamic response was found in almost half of the patients. A significantly higher mean right atrial pressure was found in nonresponders compared with responders. A dose increase to 80 or 120 mg in the nonresponders overcame resistance in 42% of the patients. Overall, almost half of the patients did not respond to the commonly recommended dose of 40 mg of ISDN and almost 25% did not respond at all, even to doses as high as 120 mg.

Nitrate Tolerance

The temporary nature of nitrate-mediated hemodynamic effects with a marked attenuation occurring within the first 24 hours of therapy has been shown by numerous investigators (67). One study showed early development of tolerance with the use of frequent dosing (every 4 to 6 hours) of oral ISDN given to patients with chronic heart failure (68).

HYDRALAZINE

Hydralazine (HYD), a hydrazinophthalazine and a potent dilator of arterioles, was introduced as an antihypertensive agent more than 40 years ago. Its vascular effects have earned it a role in the management of CHF.

Basic Pharmacology, Metabolism, and Pharmacokinetics

HYD likely produces vasodilation through a modulating effect on intracellular calcium kinetics, and a HYD-induced elevation of cyclic adenosine monophosphate (cAMP) or cGMP has been proposed (69). In addition, indirect mechanisms, including HYD-induced alterations in sympathetic nervous system tone, release of prostanoids, and inhibition of thromboxane A_2 biosynthesis have also been suggested (70–72). HYD is rapidly and almost totally absorbed from the gastrointestinal tract, with peak plasma concentration occurring 30 to 60 minutes after ingestion (69,72,73). HYD undergoes significant first-pass metabolism by the liver, which accounts for a bioavailability of 10% to 35% (69,74). More than 90% of administered HYD is cleared by the liver and the remainder by renal excretion. The HYD molecule is metabolized by acetylation, oxidative reactions, ring hydroxylation, and glucuronide conjugation (69,74). In genetically slow acetylators, higher plasma concentrations are achieved and much of the metabolism of HYD is shifted from acetylation to primary oxidative reactions and hydroxylation (69,73,74). Eighty to ninety percent of circulating HYD is protein-bound. Elimination half-life is 0.5 to 2.0 hours and the clearance rate can range from 30 to 150 mL/kg per minute. Whether CHF influences the pharmacokinetics of HYD has not been convincingly resolved (73–75).

Cardiovascular Pharmacology in Congestive Heart Failure

Central Hemodynamic Effects

HYD, a potent arteriolar vasodilator, decreases systemic and pulmonic vascular resistance. The resultant fall in RV and LV afterload evokes an overall improvement in ventricular performance, with augmentation of stroke volume, stroke work, and cardiac output (76). After the administration of HYD or most other vasodilators in heart failure, the augmented stroke volume averts the development of significant systemic hypotension and reflex tachycardia. Hemodynamic effects in human heart failure generally become apparent by 20 minutes, peak at 60 to 120 minutes, and wane from 6 to 8 hours after oral dosing.

It has also been demonstrated in human heart failure that HYD also elicits a positive inotropic response (77). Enhancement of sympathetic nervous system tone appears to be the mechanism explaining much of the positive inotropic properties of HYD, although direct myocardial stimulation has not been convincingly excluded (78).

The powerful arteriolar vasodilating effects of HYD make it one of the drugs of choice for decreasing of the amount of valvular regurgitation across any incompetent heart valve (61,79) and the degree of left-to-right shunting in atrial and ventricular septal defects (80,81). In these conditions, HYD can lower ventricular filling pressures considerably despite its modest vasodilating, preload-reducing capabilities. The inotropic effect of HYD may be clinically relevant and may explain the successful withdrawal of dobutamine from end-stage heart failure patients with the help of HYD (82).

Myocardial Energetics and Coronary Blood Flow

In contrast to most vasodilating agents and ACE inhibitors, HYD (because of its potential to increase myocardial contractibility as well as heart rate) can increase myocardial oxygen consumption to a mild degree (83). For patients with occlusive coronary artery disease, the rise in myocardial oxygen demand with HYD may not be matched in all regions of the ventricular wall with an adequate increase in coronary blood flow and myocardial perfusion and may result in myocardial ischemia.

Regional Blood Flow

HYD significantly increases blood flow to limb musculocutaneous structures in patients with CHF; the increase is dose-related, generally proportional to the rise in cardiac output, and maintained during long-term administration (84). The augmentation of limb flow at rest may not be accompanied by an increase in nutritional flow to working muscle during exercise (85). Hepatic-splanchnic blood flow tends to increase during HYD therapy in heart failure, although the change is less than the concomitant elevation in cardiac output (84).

HYD is one of the few drugs used in heart failure management that is capable of substantially reducing renal vascular resistance and increasing renal blood flow (86). The rise in renal blood flow is dose-related and proportional to the elevation in cardiac output, and it persists during long-term therapy. The effects of HYD on other parameters of renal function are far less dramatic with glomerular filtration rate, cation (Na+ and K+) excretion, and water clearance either not changing or increasing only modestly (86,87). It has been suggested that HYD may enhance the renal clearance of digoxin and furosemide (88,89).

Exercise Hemodynamics

Most of the resting favorable central hemodynamic responses noted following administration of HYD in a patient with CHF also persist during exercise (90). With initial dosing, this transfer of favorable hemodynamic effects generally does not achieve an increase in exercise capacity. This may be partly explained by the inability of HYD to enhance nutritional blood flow of working skeletal muscle during exercise.

Potential Undesirable Properties and Effects

HYD also manifests the pharmacologic phenomena of drug resistance and tolerance. Patients with a high mean RA pressure (>10 mm Hg) and LV minor axis smaller than 60 mm during diastole appear to be hemodynamically more resistant to oral HYD (91,92). Pharmacodynamic tolerance to HYD may occur during long-term administration, although the prevalence and predisposing factors for the development of this problem have not been established (93). Interestingly, the sudden withdrawal of HYD has been reported to precipitate severe congestive failure in isolated instances (89).

Side effects of HYD include hypotension, headache, and dizziness, as well as gastrointestinal symptoms, arthralgias, or a systemic lupus erythematosus-like illness. It should be noted, however, that problems of drug-induced arthralgias, rheumatoid manifestations, and lupus erythematosus are relatively uncommon in CHF compared to hypertension.

HYD can evoke symptoms and signs of myocardial ischemia and cause infarction in heart failure patients with occlusive coronary artery disease (94). These events are due to positive inotropic effects of HYD and its tendency to enhance sympathetic nervous system tone, as well as to hypotension and tachycardia, which are occasionally evoked by HYD.

Hydralazine–Nitrate Combination

The use of nitrates in combination with HYD was initially based on a hemodynamic of achieving a combined effect on LV preload and afterload (95). The HYD–nitrate combination causes a greater reduction in systemic vascular resistance and a greater increase in stroke volume and cardiac output than nitrates alone and a greater reduction in ventricular filling pressures than HYD alone. The V-HeFT studies (4,96) evaluated the effect of ISDN in combination with HYD on survival in mildly to moderately symptomatic patients with CHF. In the V-HeFT I study (4), the use of oral ISDN at a maximum dose of 160 mg per day with HYD (300 mg per day) resulted in a reduction in mortality compared to control patients treated with placebo or with prazosin, a vasodilator with an alpha-adrenergic blocking activity (Fig. 27-7). At 1 year, the cumulative mortality rate in the patients receiving the HYD–ISDN combination was reduced by 38% compared to placebo (12.1% versus 19.5%). The difference in mortality between the two groups persisted for 3 years.

The V-HeFT II study (96) was designed to compare the effects of direct vasodilation with HYD–ISDN to that of the ACE inhibitor enalapril (maximum dose, 20 mg per day). The results of this study demonstrated that enalapril had a

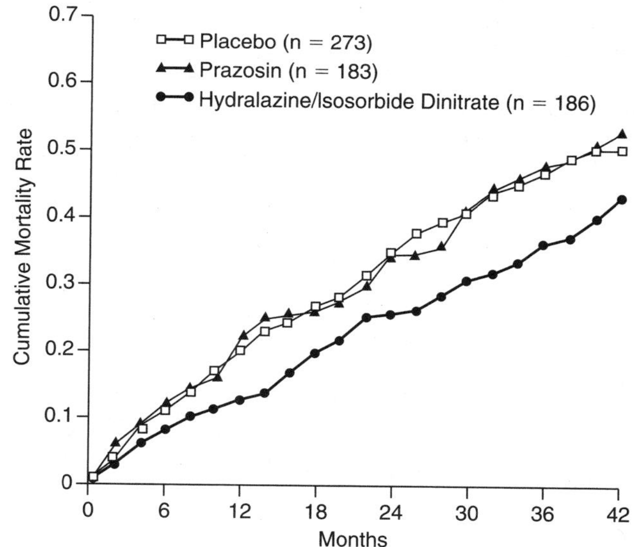

Figure 27-7 A cumulative mortality from time of randomization to placebo, prazosin or isosorbide dinitrate/hydralazine in the Vasodilator Heart Failure Trial (V-HeFT) I; $p = 0.093$ on the log-rank test and $p = 0.046$ on the generalized Wilcoxon test, which gives more weight to treatment differences occurring in the earlier part of the mortality curves and less weight to the latter part of the curves, where the numbers are smaller. (From Cohn JN, Archibald DG, Ziesche S, et al. Effect of vasodilator therapy on mortality in chronic congestive heart failure. Results of a Veterans Administration Cooperative Study. *N Engl J Med.* 1986;314:1547–1552, with permission.)

larger effect on survival than did oral HYD–ISDN in combination, given to mildly to moderately symptomatic patients with CHF. Lower mortality in the enalapril group was due to a lower incidence of sudden death, while mortality due to worsening heart failure was similar. The results of these studies clearly demonstrated that ACE inhibition in symptomatic patients with heart failure provided a stronger protective effect than did direct vasodilation. The improvement in survival with HYD–ISDN in comparison with placebo, however, indicated that this drug combination is a useful alternative in patients with chronic CHF who do not tolerate ACE inhibitors.

Effect on Exercise Tolerance

The results of the V-HeFT trials demonstrated a small but significant ($p < 0.05$) improvement in peak oxygen consumption in patients treated with HYD–ISDN (97). Improvement in peak oxygen consumption with this drug combination was seen for the first 6 months of the follow-up period and was greater than the effects of enalapril.

Effect on Left Ventricular Ejection Fraction

Data from V-HeFT II (98) demonstrated a significant improvement in left ventricular ejection fraction (LVEF) with the combination of HYD–ISDN. Similar to the effect on peak oxygen consumption, the effect of this drug combination was superior to that of enalapril. A relationship was demonstrated between improvement in LVEF and survival in patients treated with HYD–ISDN. In patients whose LVEF rose by 10% or more, there was a very favorable effect on long-term survival (80% at 5 years), whereas survival was only 30% at 5 years in patients whose LVEF remained unchanged or decreased during the first 6 months of the study. Thus, although patients with CHF achieved a greater survival benefit from enalapril, the combination of HYD–ISDN improved exercise tolerance and LVEF significantly more than did enalapril in these patients.

Effect of Hydralazine on Nitrate Tolerance

Multiple studies have clearly demonstrated that frequent administration of oral nitrate or continuous administration of IV or topical nitrates resulted in early development of nitrate tolerance with marked attenuation of the initial hemodynamic effect. It is therefore not surprising that various strategies have been proposed and attempted for the prevention of nitrate tolerance. These strategies included concomitant administration of sulfhydryl groups, ACE inhibitors, or diuretics (99). However, these methods have not been proven beneficial in patients with CHF. Intermittent nitrate therapy allowing a daily nitrate washout interval of at least 12 hours has been effective in the prevention of nitrate tolerance (71,100); however, this regimen is limited by its inability to provide continuous and interrupted therapeutic effect. Interaction between HYD and nitrates was first reported by Unger et al. (101), who demonstrated potentiation of NTG response with HYD incubation in isolated aortic rings rendered tolerant in vivo to NTG. Münzel et al. (102) later showed the ability of HYD to inhibit vascular superoxide production and prevent nitrate tolerance in vitro. The results of these investigations suggested that the antioxidant properties of HYD may be responsible for the prevention of nitrate tolerance.

Two studies performed approximately 10 and 15 years ago, one in an in vivo animal model of CHF (103) and the other in patients with CHF (104), also demonstrated that concomitant administration of HYD was useful in the prevention of nitrate tolerance. In the first study, infusion of NTG to CHF rats produced a reduction in LV end-diastolic pressure (64% ± 3%). However, with continuation of NTG infusion the initial hemodynamic effect was not maintained and LV end-diastolic pressure returned to near baseline values within 6 hours as a result of the development of tolerance. Co-administration of HYD given intravenously prevented the development of nitrate tolerance and the initial reduction in LV end-diastolic pressure with NTG was maintained throughout the 10-hour infusion period.

Because of the potential therapeutic value of these study results, a similar experiment to evaluate the effect of oral HYD on the development of nitrate tolerance was conducted in 28 patients with chronic CHF (NYHA functional Class III or IV) (104). Patients were randomized to receive a continuous infusion of NTG for 24 hours either alone (14 patients; Group 1) or concomitantly with oral HYD (14 patients; Group 2) given at a dose of 75 mg 4 times daily and started at least 24 hours before the study. NTG was started in both groups at a rate of 20 μg per minute, which was increased in increments of 20 to 60 μg per minute every 5 minutes to achieve at least a 30% reduction in mean pulmonary artery wedge pressure. Continuous infusion of NTG alone resulted in a gradual and significant attenuation of the initial effect of therapy (Group 1) on mean pulmonary artery pressure and mean pulmonary artery wedge pressure. In contrast, in Group 2 concomitant administration of oral HYD prevented NTG-induced hemodynamic tolerance and resulted in persistent effects on mean pulmonary artery and pulmonary wedge pressures throughout the study period. In addition, the initial effect on blood pressure reduction was attenuated at 24 hours in Group 1 (Fig. 27-8). The results of this study supported the observation made by Bauer and Fung (103) in animals, indicating the ability of HYD to prevent early development of nitrate tolerance and maintain nitrate-mediated favorable hemodynamic effects.

Effect of Hydralazine–Isosorbide Dinitrate in African-Americans with Congestive Heart Failure in V-HeFT Trials

African-Americans comprised 180 out of 642 patients in V-HeFT I and 215 out of 804 patients in V-HeFT II (105). A retrospective analysis of the outcome of African-Americans compared with whites in V-HeFT I (Fig. 27-9) showed a significantly lower annual mortality rate in African-American patients (56%) who were treated with HYD–ISDN compared with placebo (9.7% versus 17.3%, $p = 0.04$). The use of HYD–ISDN was also associated with a greater effect on oxygen consumption, which increased by 1.25 mL/kg per minute in African-Americans, compared

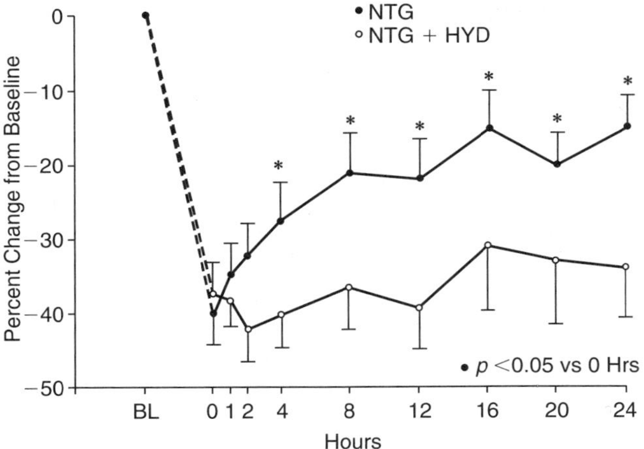

Figure 27-8 Values of mean pulmonary artery wedge pressure as measured over time during continuous administration of nitroglycerin (NTG) alone or nitroglycerin concomitantly with oral hydralazine (HYD) 75 mg, 4 times daily. (From Elkayam U. Nitrates in the treatment of congestive heart failure. *Am J Cardiol.* 1996;77;41C–51C, with permission.)

to a decrease of 0.4 mL/kg per minute with placebo. The difference between the two groups was borderline significant. Despite a superior effect of enalapril on survival in the overall V-HeFT II study population, the effect of HYD–ISDN was comparable to that of enalapril in African-American patients (12.9% versus 12.8%, p = NS). In addition, compared with enalapril, HYD–ISDN significantly improved quality of life for African-Americans ($p < 0.043$). When peak oxygen consumption was analyzed using a longitudinal model that took into account all data collected during the entire year, HYD–ISDN performed slightly better than enalapril compared with baseline ($p < 0.067$). Collectively, these results demonstrated that HYD–ISDN combination was more effective than placebo and was as effective as enalapril in reducing mortality in African-Americans compared with whites. It was also significantly more effective at improving quality of life than enalapril in those patients, despite only modest improvement in oxygen consumption.

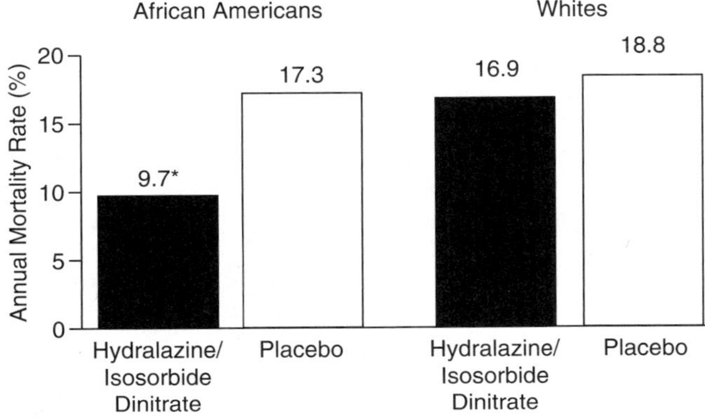

Figure 27-9 Annual mortality rate in the Vasodilator Heart Failure Trial I among African-Americans and whites treated with isosorbide dinitrate/hydralazine or placebo. (From Carson P, Ziesche S, Johnson G, et al. Racial differences in response to therapy for heart failure: analysis of the Vasodilator-Heart Failure trials. Vasodilator-Heart Failure Trial Study Group. *J Card Fail.* 1999;5: 178–187, with permission.)
$^{*}p = 0.04$.

African-American Heart Failure Trial

This study (A-HeFT) was performed on the basis of the above-mentioned retrospective analyses, suggesting that African-American patients respond favorably to a combination of ISDN and HYD (105). The study was designed to evaluate the efficacy of a fixed dose of ISDN plus HYD in African-American patients who had symptomatic CHF (Class III–IV) and with dilated ventricles and who were receiving background therapy that included neurohormonal blockers (5). The study was terminated early on the recommendation of the independent Data and Safety Monitoring Board after 1,050 of the planned 1,100 patients had undergone randomization, owing to a significantly higher mortality rate in the placebo group than in the group given HYD–ISDN (10.2% versus 6.2%, $p = 0.02$) (Fig. 27-10) at the end of a mean follow-up duration of 10 months (range: 0 to 18 months). The data showed the emergence of survival difference at approximately 180 days, which widened progressively thereafter ($p = 0.01$ by the log-rank test).

The primary endpoint for the trial was a composite score made up of weighted values for death from any cause; first hospitalization for CHF during the 18-month follow-up period; and change in the quality of life at 6 months. At the termination of the trial, the primary composite score was significantly better in the HYD–ISDN group ($p = 0.01$). In addition, all three components of the primary composite score were separately affected, with a 42% reduction in all-cause mortality, 33% reduction of the rate of first hospitalization for CHF ($p = 0.001$), and improvement in the quality of life ($p = 0.02$).

Calcium-Channel Blockers

Since calcium-channel blockers (CCBs) are vasodilators and have an anti-ischemic effect, these drugs have been

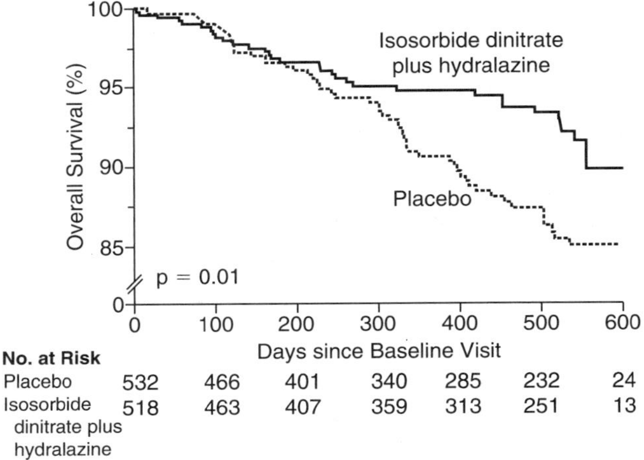

Figure 27-10 Kaplan-Meier estimation of overall survival. (Reprinted from Taylor AL, Zliesche S, Yancy C, et al. Combination of isosorbide dinitrate and hydralazine in blacks with heart failure. *N Engl J Med.* 2004;351:2049–2057, with permission.)

investigated in numerous studies for the treatment of CHF (106). A large number of studies involving the majority of available CCBs have not been able to establish a therapeutic role for this group of agents but have provided information on their safety in patients with heart failure.

CLINICAL EXPERIENCE WITH CALCIUM ANTAGONISTS IN HEART FAILURE

First-Generation Calcium-Channel Blockers

Nifedipine

Initial evaluation by several investigators (107–109) reported hemodynamic improvement after a single-dose administration of nifedipine given either orally or sublingually in patients with acute or chronic CHF. Hemodynamic changes included a reduction in systemic vascular resistance (SVR) and mean blood pressure and augmentation of cardiac output and stroke volume. Lack of change in both RV and LV filling pressures in most studies (110) verified the predominant arteriolar and negligible venous effect of the drug. Further evaluation in larger groups of patients, however, demonstrated that nifedipine was also associated with a cardiodepressant effect (110,111).

Comparison of nifedipine with nitroprusside (112) demonstrated a smaller augmentation in cardiac output and a larger decrease in systemic blood pressure with nifedipine despite a similar reduction in SVR. These hemodynamic changes were associated with a decrease in the first derivative of LV pressure (dP/dT) (113). In addition, a similar reduction in SVR with HYD and nifedipine in patients with CHF (114) resulted in a significantly smaller augmentation of stroke volume, cardiac output, and LV stroke work index with nifedipine, demonstrating the clinical relevance of its negative inotropic effect. Further evaluation of nifedipine in two large series of patients showed acute hemodynamic and clinical deterioration after a single dose of 20 to 50 mg in about 20% of the patients (111,115). In addition, a strong relationship was found between an unfavorable acute hemodynamic response to nifedipine and long-term mortality (115), supporting a hypothesis that hemodynamic deterioration after nifedipine administration was more likely to occur in patients with more severe heart failure. Evaluation of the acute neurohormonal effect of nifedipine in patients with CHF (116,117) demonstrated a significant activation of the renin system without a change in aldosterone level, which was most likely due to inhibition of calcium-mediated secretion of aldosterone in the renal macula densa.

The long-term effect of nifedipine in patients with heart failure due to LV systolic dysfunction was evaluated several years ago in two randomized trials. In the first study (118), a symptomatic and functional improvement and enhancement of exercise tolerance were seen with captopril but not with nifedipine. In the second study, Elkayam et al. (119) demonstrated a significantly higher incidence of CHF worsening, necessitating an increase in diuretic dose, a hospitalization, or both, in patients treated with nifedipine either alone or in combination with ISDN as compared to ISDN alone.

In summary, in spite of a strong vasodilatory effect, numerous studies have demonstrated an unfavorable effect of nifedipine on hemodynamic as well as clinical status in patients with CHF due to LV systolic dysfunction.

Diltiazem

The unfavorable results reported with the use of nifedipine in patients with chronic heart failure led to the attempts to use diltiazem, a first-generation calcium antagonist with a lesser myocardial depressant effect (120). Hemodynamic evaluation of this agent in patients with severe, chronic CHF demonstrated either no change or improvement in hemodynamic profile (121–123) and no change in plasma renin activity and catecholamines (123). In addition, another report also demonstrated a safe and effective use of intravenous diltiazem for heart rate control in patients with atrial fibrillation and LV systolic dysfunction (124). However, occasional hemodynamic deteriorations reported in some patients receiving oral diltiazem (123) presented the first indication of a potential hazard of this drug as well.

The chronic use of diltiazem in patients with CHF resulted in conflicting findings. Figulla et al. (125) reported improvement in cardiac function, exercise capacity, and subjective status without deleterious effects on transplant listing-free survival with diltiazem in patients with dilated cardiomyopathy. Different results, however, were found in a large, multicenter post-infarction trial (126), which showed an association between diltiazem and increased incidence of cardiac events in patients with evidence of pulmonary congestion on chest radiogram or those with radionuclide ejection fraction less than 40% and anterolateral Q wave infarction. In contrast, in 1,909 patients without pulmonary congestion, diltiazem therapy resulted in a lower incidence of cardiac events. A further evaluation of the development of CHF in this study (127) showed that patients with pulmonary congestion, anterolateral Q wave infarction, or reduced ejection fraction (<40%) at baseline were more likely to develop CHF during follow-up. This trial conclusively demonstrated the hazard involved in the chronic use of diltiazem in patients with LV systolic dysfunction due to coronary artery disease and myocardial infarction.

Verapamil

The experience related to the use of verapamil in heart failure has been limited because of the known negative inotropic effect of the drug. In a small study, Ferlinz and Gallo (128) demonstrated symptomatic deterioration in four of ten patients with CHF on long-term verapamil therapy in spite of acute hemodynamic improvement. The Danish study of the effect of verapamil on death or reinfarction (129) in survivors of acute MI demonstrated a significant reduction in mortality and cardiac events in patients without (but not with) chronic heart failure. This study excluded 13% of the patients with CHF not controlled with furosemide. Although the investigators concluded that (in contrast to diltiazem) verapamil had no detrimental effect in patients with CHF, one cannot exclude the possibility that the favorable effect of verapamil reported in patients without CHF was offset by a detrimental effect of the drug in patients with CHF.

Second-Generation Calcium-Channel Blockers

Nisoldipine

Small studies in patients with symptomatic CHF (130) demonstrated a nisoldipine-mediated decreased SVR and mean systemic arterial pressure and increased stroke volume and LVEF at rest and during exercise, and reduced exercise values of LV filling pressure. There was no change in plasma NE and renin levels. In spite of hemodynamic improvement (130), there was no change in exercise duration after both acute and chronic nisoldipine therapy (131). A further evaluation of chronic administration (2 months) of nisoldipine in patients with CHF, however, resulted in hospitalization of 70% of the patients because of worsening of CHF despite initial improvement in hemodynamic profile.

In summary, available information demonstrates a strong vasodilatory effect of nisoldipine in patients with CHF resulting in decreased LV afterload, and augmentation of cardiac output, and LVEF in some patients. These changes, however, resulted in either no or small changes in exercise capacity. In spite of initial hemodynamic improvement, clinical deterioration may occur, indicating a potential risk associated with the chronic use of nisoldipine in patients with chronic CHF.

Nicardipine

Evaluations of the effect of nicardipine in small groups of patients with CHF suggested favorable acute and short-term effects with a decrease in SVR and pulmonary artery wedge pressure, an increase in cardiac index both at rest and during exercise, and an improvement in LVEF (132–134). Gheorghiade et al. (135) evaluated the long-term effect of nicardipine (20 to 30 mg every 8 hours) given over 4 months in patients with chronic CHF, and found clinical worsening in 60% of the patients compared to only 20% of patients receiving placebo ($p = 0.06$).

In summary, in spite of reported favorable effects of nicardipine on hemodynamic profile and both systolic as well as diastolic LV functions, long-term administration of this drug may result in a significant clinical deterioration in patients with chronic CHF.

Felodipine

Felodipine was reported to have negligible negative inotropic effects and high selectivity for smooth muscle (136). The short-term administration of felodipine in patients with CHF during the resting state resulted in a reduction of SVR and blood pressure along with elevated LV filling pressure and an increase in cardiac output (137). Studies examining the long-term effects of felodipine in chronic CHF also reported hemodynamic benefits both at rest and during exercise (138,139).

The largest experience with the use of felodipine in patients with heart failure has been provided by the V-HeFT III study (140). This study enrolled 451 male patients with heart failure and exercise tolerance limited by dyspnea or fatigue who were treated with diuretics and enalapril and were randomized to receive either felodipine (5 mg BID) or placebo. The analysis of the outcome of the study demonstrated no difference between felodipine and placebo in mortality, both in patients with and without coronary artery disease. Similarly, felodipine did not have an effect on peak exercise capacity 12 weeks after randomization. Plasma norepinephrine was elevated at baseline and demonstrated a similar rise in both the felodipine and the placebo groups. Plasma atrial natriuretic peptide (ANP) was reduced by felodipine, while it was increased in the placebo group. Based on these results, the investigators of the V-HeFT III study concluded that felodipine, when used as adjunctive therapy to ACE inhibitors and diuretics in patients with CHF, may exert a sustained favorable effect on ANP which may be due to its hemodynamic effect, but does not influence either mortality or exercise tolerance in this patient population. It should be noted, however, that any conclusion based on the V-HeFT III study regarding the effect of felodipine on mortality in patients with CHF is limited by the small number of patients included in the trial.

In summary, available information suggests a beneficial hemodynamic effect of felodipine in patients with chronic CHF. However, there is no evidence that these hemodynamic changes can lead to clinical improvement or reduced mortality.

Amlodipine

The effect of amlodipine on outcome of patients with chronic heart failure was evaluated in the two PRAISE (Prospective Randomized Amlodipine Survival Evaluation) studies (141,142). The first study (141) evaluated the effect of chronic treatment with amlodipine in addition to background therapy with digitalis, diuretics, and ACE inhibitors on morbidity and mortality of patients with chronic, severe (NYHA Class IIIb and IV) CHF. The study was prospectively designed to evaluate separately the effect of therapy in patients with ischemic and nonischemic cardiomyopathy. The 1,153 patients were randomized and were followed for 6 to 33 months, with a median follow-up time of 14.5 months. Of these, 732 patients were diagnosed of having ischemic and 421 patients of having nonischemic dilated cardiomyopathy (NIDCM). The results of the study demonstrated an identical effect on the combined endpoint of mortality and morbidity in the subgroup of patients with ischemic cardiomyopathy. In contrast, there was a significant reduction in the combined endpoint in the group of patients with NIDCM. Similarly, all-cause mortality was lower in the patients with NIDCM treated with amlodipine but not in patients with ischemic cardiomyopathy. Based on the results of the PRAISE I study, it seemed that amlodipine had neutral effects on mortality and morbidity in patients with CHF due to ischemic heart disease but offered a substantial favorable effect on survival of patients with CHF due to NIDCM. This latter conclusion, however, could not be confirmed by the PRAISE II study (142), which was a randomized, double-blind, placebo-controlled, multicenter study of 1,652 patients with chronic CHF due to nonischemic cardiomyopathy, LVEF <30%, and NYHA Class IIIb or IV, despite therapy with diuretics, ACE inhibitors, and digoxin. Patients receiving CCBs, beta-blockers, or cardiodepressant, antiarrhythmic drugs were excluded. All-cause mortality was 32% in the placebo group and 34% in the amlodipine group ($p = 0.32$) and, similarly, there was no change in cardiac mortality. All-cause mortality in the combined population of PRAISE I and II studies was 34% in the placebo group and 33% in the amlodipine group (HR 0.98, 95% CI 0.87–1.12; $p = 0.81$). In conclusion, therefore, the PRAISE II study did not confirm the results of the smaller PRAISE I study but did demonstrate that long-term treatment with amlodipine (in addition to standard treatment with diuretics, digoxin, and ACE inhibitors) did not have an unfavorable effect on mortality in patients with severe CHF of nonischemic etiology.

New Class of Calcium Antagonists

Mibefradil

Mibefradil is a chemically novel calcium antagonist and is the only calcium antagonist that is able to block both L- and T-type voltage-operated calcium channels (143). Animal experiments comparing equipotent doses of mibefradil, verapamil, and diltiazem failed to show a negative inotropic effect with mibefradil. In addition, clinical studies showed the effectiveness and safety of mibefradil in patients with chronic, stable angina and hypertension. Based on the above preliminary findings demonstrating potent vasodilatory and anti-ischemic effects in addition to a negative chronotropic effect and a lack of effect on contractility and neurohormonal profile, it was hypothesized that mibefradil could be a suitable addition to standard heart failure therapy (144). For these reasons, the largest CCB CHF trial was designed to evaluate the efficacy and safety of this drug in the treatment of chronic CHF (MACH-1 Mortality Assessment of Congestive Heart Failure) (144). This study was a multicenter, double-blind, placebo-controlled trial that randomized 2,591 patients with chronic CHF (NYHA Class II–IV) and LVEF <35% who were symptomatic on optimal-dose loop diuretics and ACE inhibitors. The results of the study showed no significant effect of mibefradil on overall mortality and a trend toward increased mortality with mibefradil in the first 3 months after drug initiation. Patients with more severe heart failure and, in particular, those receiving amiodarone appeared to be at highest risk for increased mortality. While MACH-1 was being carried out, it became apparent that mibefradil interacted significantly with other commonly used drugs, including the statins. As a result, the manufacturer voluntarily withdrew the drug from the market.

Currently, the CCBs are not recommended for the treatment of patients with heart failure and impaired systolic function. Their direct negative inotropic effects, together with their capacity to activate neurohormonal systems, may lead to clinical deterioration. In targeted groups of patients with heart failure, such as patients with hypertension or angina where the use of CCBs may be considered, drugs with neutral effect (felodipine and amlodipine) should be used in addition to standard heart failure therapy.

NESIRITIDE

Pharmacokinetics and Elimination

Nesiritide is a sterile, purified preparation of human B-type natriuretic peptide (BNP). It is manufactured from *Escherichia coli* using recombinant DNA technology and has the same 32-amino-acid sequence as the endogenous BNP produced by the ventricular myocardium. The intravenous administration of nesiritide results in a biphasic disposition from the plasma. The mean terminal elimination half-life of nesiritide in patients with heart failure is approximately 18 minutes (145). At steady state, plasma BNP levels increase from baseline endogenous levels by approximately threefold to sixfold with nesiritide infusion doses ranging from 0.01 to 0.03 μg/kg per minute.

Human BNP elimination from the circulation occurs by three independent mechanisms in the following order of decreasing importance (145): (a) by binding to cell surface natriuretic peptide clearance receptors (receptor C) with subsequent cellular internalization and isosome proteolysis; (b) proteolytic cleavage by neutral endopeptidases present within renal tubular cells and vascular cells; and (c) renal filtration clearance of nesiritide. The latter is proportional to body weight and supports weight-adjusted dosing of the drug. Clearance is not influenced significantly by age, gender, race, baseline endogenous BNP concentration, severity of heart failure, or concomitant administration of ACE inhibitors. Although nesiritide is eliminated in part through renal clearance, clinical data do not suggest a need for dose adjustment in patients with renal insufficiency.

Clinical Experience

Prior to its approval for clinical use, nesiritide was studied in 10 clinical trials (145) that included almost 1,000 patients, the majority of them at NYHA functional Class III or IV heart failure. The mean age of the studied population was 60 years and 56% of all patients were women. Five of the trials were randomized, multicenter, placebo- or active-controlled studies in which 772 patients with decompensated heart failure received continuous infusions of nesiritide at doses ranging from 0.01 to 0.03 μg/kg per minute. Agents used for comparison in the active-controlled studies were primarily dobutamine and NTG (146,147). Most patients (70%) were given nesiritide infusion for at least 24 hours, while 48% received the drug for 24 to 48 hours, and 22% for longer than 48 hours. In controlled trials, nesiritide was used either alone or in combination with diuretics, digoxin, oral ACE inhibitors, anticoagulants, oral nitrates, statins, class III antiarrhythmic agents, beta-blockers, dobutamine, calcium-channel blockers, angiotensin II receptor antagonists, and dopamine (3,4). Nesiritide has been studied in a broad range of patients including the elderly, women, African-Americans, and patients with history of various cardiovas-

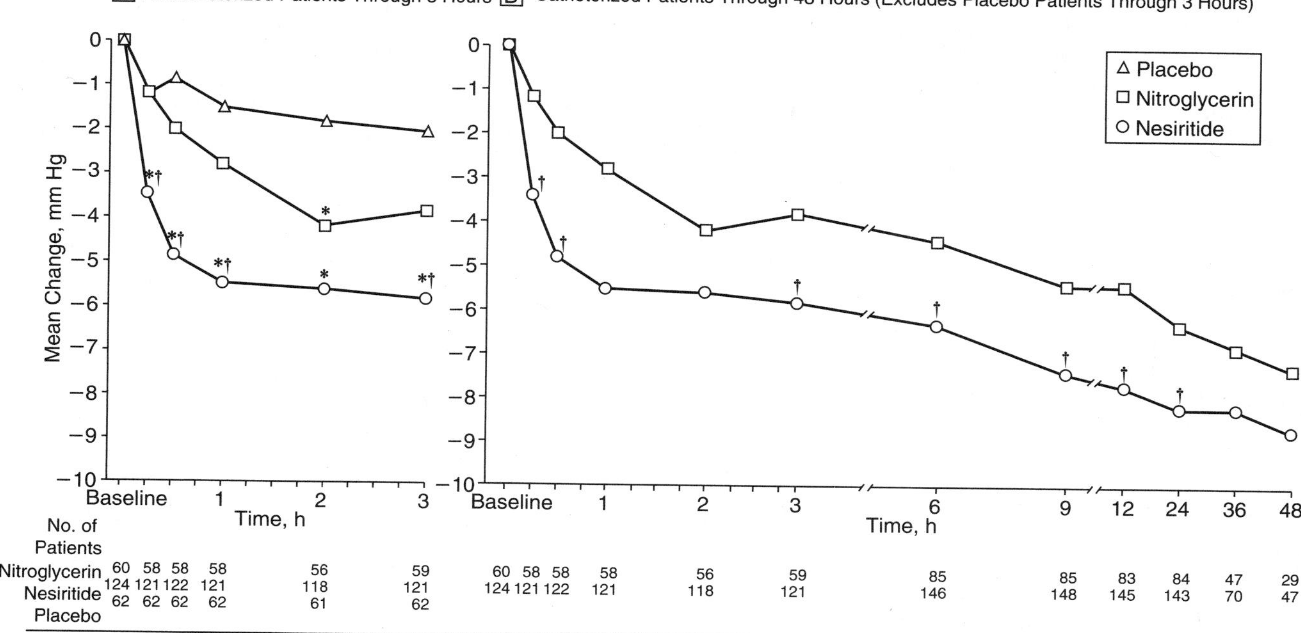

Asterisk indicates $P < 0.05$ for nesiritide or nitroglycerin compared with placebo; dagger, $P < 0.05$ for nesiritide compared with nitroglycerin.

Figure 27-11 Changes from baseline in pulmonary capillary wedge pressure in nitroglycerine, nesiritide and placebo groups. (From Publication Committee for the VMAC Investigators [Vasodilatation in the Management of Acute CHF]. Intravenous nesiritide vs nitroglycerin for treatment of decompensated congestive heart failure: a randomized controlled trial. *JAMA.* 2002;287:1531–1540, with permission.)

cular conditions including hypertension, diabetes, post-MI, atrial fibrillation/flutter, nonsustained ventricular tachycardia, LV diastolic dysfunction, and acute coronary syndrome (147).

Hemodynamic Effects

The VMAC trial (Vasodilation in the Management of Acute CHF) (147) provided information on hemodynamic effect of currently recommended doses of nesiritide (Fig. 27-11). This was a multicenter, randomized, double-blind trial designed to compare the clinical effects of nesiritide to those of IV NTG when both were added to standard care in patients with decompensated heart failure. In this trial, 489 patients with dyspnea at rest due to decompensated heart failure were treated with either nesiritde (starting with a bolus of 2 μg/kg and followed by continuous infusion of 0.01 μg/kg per minute) or IV NTG at a dose determined by the investigators. The mean systolic blood pressure for the entire group was 121 ± 22 mm Hg and the mean PCWP was 28 ± 6 mm Hg in 246 patients who received invasive hemodynamic monitoring.

Nesiritide led to a significant reduction in PCWP, which was observed as early as 15 minutes with further effect at 1 hour. The effect of nesiritide on PCWP was superior to that of NTG. The administration of nesiritide was also associated with a significant reduction in right atrial pressure and peripheral vascular resistance. Systolic blood pressure was reduced by 4 ± 11 mm Hg (3%) 15 minutes after initiation of nesiritide infusion, which was comparable to that of NTG (−3 ± 11 mm Hg) at 15 minutes and was less than NTG at 1 hour (3 ± 13 mm Hg versus 6 ± 14 mm Hg, $p < 0.05$ for NTG versus placebo and not significant for nesiritide versus placebo). Nesiritide also had a significant effect on pulmonary vascular resistance and augmented cardiac output. Through 24 hours, nesiritide lowered PCWP to a significantly greater extent than did NTG, with no evidence of attenuation of effect (147,149). At 36 and 48 hours, PCWP continued to be reduced by a greater magnitude with nesiritide than with NTG (148).

Effect on Coronary Hemodynamics

The use of IV nesiritide in a standard dose in 10 patients undergoing cardiac catheterization showed a 52% reduction in right atrial pressure, 19% reduction in pulmonary artery wedge pressure, and 11% reduction in mean systemic blood pressure. Coronary blood flow increased 35% ($p = 0.007$), whereas coronary resistance decreased 23% ($p = 0.036$), and myocardial oxygen uptake decreased 8% ($p = 0.045$) (150). The study thus showed that nesiritide exerts coronary vasodilator effects on both the coronary conductance and resistance arteries; despite a decrease in coronary perfusion pressure, coronary artery blood flow was increased, coronary resistance was decreased, and myocardial oxygen uptake was decreased.

Tachyphylaxis

Tachyphylaxis, which results in a rapid and significant attenuation of hemodynamic effects, has been described with the use of continuous infusion of NTG and limits the usefulness of this drug in the treatment of patients with decompensated heart failure (149). In a study by Mills et al. (151) the hemodynamic effects of nesiritide seen at 1 hour after initiation of drug infusion were sustained throughout the 24-hour infusion time. Similarly, the hemodynamic effect of nesiritide was maintained throughout the 24 hours of the study period in the VMAC study (147). These findings indicate that, unlike NTG, continuous administration of nesiritide is not associated with the development of tolerance to the drug.

Effects on Symptoms

The effects of nesiritide on symptoms of heart failure were evaluated in comparison to placebo and to standard care, which included use of intravenous vasoactive drugs such as NTG, dobutamine, and milrinone. The double-blind use of nesiritide infused for 6 hours in 127 Class III and IV heart failure patients resulted in a superior hemodynamic improvement compared to placebo, which was also associated with a marked improvement in heart failure symptoms, including dyspnea and fatigue (148). Another study compared the effect of nesiritide to that of standard care in a group of 305 patients admitted to hospitals for decompensated heart failure (148). In this study, 57% of patients randomized to standard care received dobutamine, 19% received milrinone, 18% received NTG, and 6% received dopamine. Nesiritide administration was associated with improvement of heart failure symptoms within the first 6 hours in the majority of the patients and the rate of improvement was similar to that seen with standard care. The VMAC study compared the effect of nesiritide with that of placebo and of IV NTG when added to standard heart failure treatment (147). The patients' self-assessed dyspnea score at 3 hours was significantly improved in the nesiritide group compared to placebo ($p < 0.034$), while the effect of NTG on change in dyspnea score at 3 hours was not statistically significant ($p = 0.191$) compared to placebo.

Neurohumoral Effects

In animals with CHF, release of ANP was found to inhibit production of catecholamines, angiotensin II, aldosterone, and endothelin-1, while infusion of antagonists of natriuretic peptide A and B receptors led to a significant increase in the levels of these hormones (145). In the study recently reported by Colucci et al. (148), the administration of nesiritide at doses of 0.015 and 0.03 μg/kg per minute was associated with a significant decrease in plasma aldosterone levels compared to placebo.

Evaluation of neurohormonal effects of nesiritide versus dobutamine was performed in a subset of 82 patients with decompensated CHF (152). This study showed a significant decrease in endothelin-1 levels during nesiritide infusion compared to a significant increase during dobutamine treatment. There was no significant change in plasma levels of norepinephrine, TNF-α, and interleukin-6.

Effect on Urine Output

Reports on the effect of nesiritide on urine output have resulted in conflicting information. In an efficacy trial (148) patients were blindly randomized to either placebo (42 patients), nesiritide at a dose of 0.015 μg/kg per minute (43 patients), or at a dose of 0.03 μg/kg per minute (42 patients), and intravenous diuretics were withheld for 4 hours before baseline measurements and for the first 6 hours of the infusion. The mean urine output over 6 hours was 560 mL and 659 mL, respectively, in the groups assigned to nesiritide and was 380 mL in the placebo group ($p = 0.004$).

In a comparative trial (148) patients were randomized to standard care (including other vasoactive medications) or to nesiritide given as a bolus of 0.3 or 0.6 μg/kg followed by infusion of 0.015 or 0.03 μg/kg per minute, and intravenous diuretics could be added at any time. Intravenous diuretics were given to fewer patients in the groups assigned to nesiritide (84% and 74%, respectively) than in the standard therapy group (96%, $p < 0.001$ for both comparisons). In 10 patients postsurgery for heart transplant with mean serum creatinine value of 2.82 mg/dL and PCWP >22 mm Hg who were refractory to standard medical therapy, the addition of standard-dose nesiritide resulted in a significant and favorable hemodynamic effect and an increase in average 24-hour urine output from 1,625 ± 318 mL to 4,641 ± 692 mL ($p < 0.001$).

In contrast, a study by Wang et al. (153) failed to document an effect of nesiritide added to diuretics on urine output in a group of 15 patients with heart failure and worsening serum creatinine. These results probably indicate a variable effect of nesiritide on urine output, which may be related to the patient population treated and the degree of volume overload.

Effect on Renal Function

A meta-analysis of five randomized clinical trials comparing nesiritide with either placebo or active control suggested an increased risk of worsening renal function in patients with ADHF treated with nesiritide (154). The validity of these findings has been questionable since the studies were not designed to evaluate effect on renal function, information regarding concomitant therapy was not available, and data regarding renal function were incomplete. Further analysis of the same data suggested a dose-related effect of nesiritide on serum creatinine without a significant effect with the standard dose (155), and a strong relationship between nesiritide-associated increase in serum creatinine and the concomitant use of large doses of diuretics (156). In addition, no relationship could be found between nesiritide-associated increase in serum creatinine (>0.5 mg/dL) and 30-day mortality (157). More information from prospective studies will be needed for further understanding of the effect of nesiritide on renal function in patients with ADHF and its clinical implications.

Safety

The most common side effect associated with the administration of currently recommended doses of nesiritide used in the VMAC study (2-μcg/kg bolus followed by infusion of 0.01 μg/kg per minute in the majority of patients) was headache, which was reported by 8% of the patients (147). However, this adverse effect occurred significantly less often in patients treated with nesiritide than in those treated with NTG (20%, $p < 0.001$). Symptomatic hypotension was reported in 4% of the patients treated with nesiritide compared to 5% of those receiving NTG. In another study, decreases in blood pressure were found to be dose-dependent, and symptomatic hypotension was reported in 11% of patients with decompensated heart failure during infusion of 0.015 μg/kg per minute and in 17% patients receiving 0.03 μg/kg per minute (148).

In the VMAC trial (149), symptomatic hypotension reported during the first 24 hours of treatment in the nesiritide patients was of longer duration than in patients receiving NTG (2.2 hours with nesiritide and 0.7 hours with NTG), most likely due to the longer half-life of nesiritide. None of those episodes resulted in adverse sequelae in either treatment group. Most hypotensive episodes were considered mild to moderate and only one subject in each treatment group experienced an event that was classified by the investigator as severe. Most events resolved either spontaneously after a dose decrease or discontinuation or with an intravenous volume challenge of 250 mL or less. The potential for hypotension may be increased by combining nesiritide with other vasodilators. In the VMAC trial, the frequency of symptomatic hypotension during the first 24 hours of treatment in nesiritide patients who received concomitantly an oral ACE inhibitor was 6%, compared to 1% in patients not receiving ACE inhibitors (149). This was similar for NTG patients who were on concomitant ACE inhibitors.

Heart Rate and Arrhythmias

The effect of nesiritide on heart rate and ventricular arrhythmias was evaluated and compared to that of dobutamine in the PRECEDENT study (Prospective, Randomized Evaluation of Cardiac Ectopy with Dobutamine or Natrecor Therapy) (146). In this study, patients received nesiritide administered at one of two doses (0.015 μg/kg per minute or 0.03 μg/kg per minute) or dobutamine at a minimum dose of 5 μg/kg per minute. The effect of the therapy was assessed by Holter monitoring performed for 24 hours during drug infusion, which was compared to recordings for a similar period of time before treatment. The study included 246 patients with NYHA Class III or IV heart failure; 51% of these patients had ischemic cardiomyopathy. In contrast to the dobutamine group, which showed a significant increase in heart rate and proarrhythmic effect, the lower nesiritide dose showed no significant effect on heart rate and a significant decrease in the number of couplets, triplets, and episodes of nonsustained ventricular tachycardia and the higher nesiritide dose was associated with no significant change in heart rate or ventricular ectopic beats. In addition, when using two independent criteria for proarrhythmic effect, dobutamine but not nesiritide was found to be proarrhythmic.

Effect on Short-Term Outcome

A subgroup analysis of 261 patients who were included in two studies comparing effects of dobutamine to nesiritide in hospitalized patients with decompensated heart failure (158) has demonstrated that although there was no difference in length of stay between the two groups, the use of dobutamine was associated with a longer duration of drug infusion compared to nesiritide (median duration of study drug infusion was significantly shorter by 25 h [in those receiving nesiritide 0.015 μg/Kg per minute] and 39 h [nesiritide 0.030 μg/Kg per minute], $p < 0.001$). Dobutamine was also associated with a higher rate of readmission to the hospital during the first 21 days after discharge (20% [dobutamine] versus 8% [nesiritide 0.015 μg/Kg per minute, $p < 0.05$ compared to dobutamine] versus 11% [nesiritide 0.030 μg/Kg per minute, p not significant]). There was also a trend for a higher readmission rate for heart failure (13% versus 4% for both groups, $p = 0.081$). When compared to NTG in the VMAC study, there was no difference in the rate of 30-day readmissions between the nesiritide and the NTG groups (158).

The effect of nesiritide on 6-month mortality was compared to that of dobutamine (158) and NTG (147). Effect of nesiritide on long-term survival compared to that of dobutamine was evaluated in 261 patients, who were treated with either dobutamine (n = 58) or nesiritide in two different doses (0.06 μg/kg per bolus and 0.030 μg/kg per minute infusion in 100 patients, and 0.03 μg/kg per bolus followed by 0.015 μg/kg per minute in 103 patients). Despite similar baseline characteristics, the use of dobutamine was associated with higher mortality compared to patients receiving nesiritide (158). The difference in the 6-month mortality rate between patients receiving dobutamine and nesiritide at 0.015 μg/kg per minute was statistically significant ($p = 0.04$).

A recently published meta-analysis of three of the available randomized, controlled trials evaluating nesiritide has compared 30-day mortality in 485 patients randomized to nesiritide and 377 patients receiving other therapies (159). This analysis found a trend ($p = 0.057$) for higher mortality at 30 days among patients randomized to nesiritide. A later analysis of all six available trials with 30-day mortality data and four with 6-month mortality data, however, failed to demonstrate a significant difference in either 30-day or 6-month mortality between patients with ADHF treated with nesiritide or not (Figs. 27-12 and 27-13) (160). A recent analysis of 15,230 patients with ADHF (161) who were

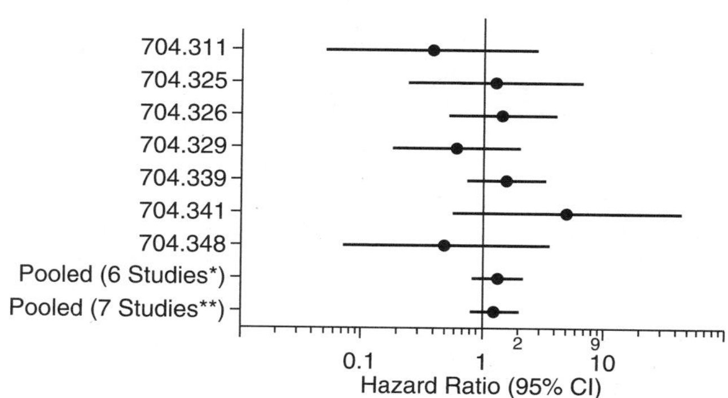

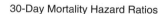

Figure 27-12 Effect on 30-day mortality derived from available randomized studies evaluating the effect of nesiritide. The analysis shows no significant effect of nesiritide on mortality. (From the FDA safety Information and Adverse Event reporting Program [MEDWATCH], Natrecor label, April 2005; www.fda.gov/cder/foi/label/2005/020920s008lbl.pdf.)

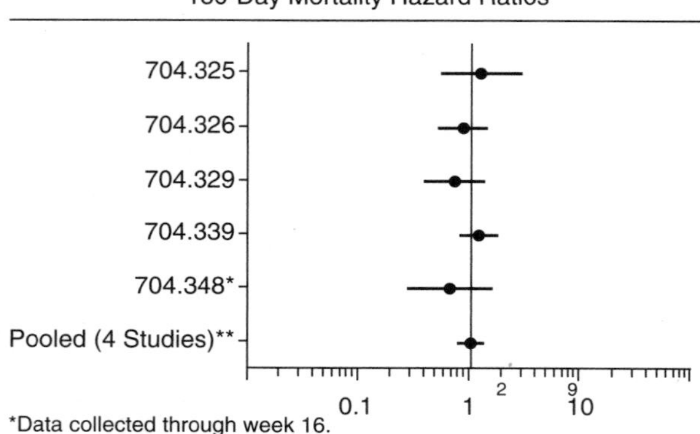

Figure 27-13 Effect on 6-month mortality derived from available randomized studies evaluating the effect of nesiritide. The analysis shows no significant effect of nesiritide on mortality. (From the FDA safety Information and Adverse Event reporting Program [MED-WATCH], Natrecor label, April 2005; www.fda.gov/cder/foi/label/2005/020920s008lbl.pdf.)

included in the ADHERE registry and received vasoactive medications demonstrated a 41% and 53% lower in hospital mortality in patients treated with nesiritide compared to milrinone and dobutamine, respectively ($p < 0.005$) and similar mortality compared to NTG. More information in adequately powered, prospective studies is needed in order to evaluate a possible effect of nesiritide on short- and long-term mortality in patients with ADHF.

REFERENCES

1. Gould L, Zahir M, Ettinger S. Phentolamine and cardiovascular performance. *Br Heart J.* 1969;31:154–162.
2. Franciosa JA, Limas CJ, Guiha NH, et al. Improved left ventricular function during nitroprusside infusion in acute myocardial infarction. *Lancet.* 1972;1:650–654.
3. Cohn JN, Franciosa JA. Vasodilator therapy of cardiac failure. *N Engl J Med.* 1977;297:27–31,254–258.
4. Cohn JN, Archibald DG, Ziesche S, et al. Effect of vasodilator therapy on mortality in chronic congestive heart failure. Results of a Veterans Administration Cooperative Study. *N Engl J Med.* 1986;314:1547–1552.
5. Taylor AL, Zliesche S, Yancy C, et al. Combination of isosorbide dinitrate and hydralazine in blacks with heart failure. *N Engl J Med.* 2004;351:2049–2057.
6. Finkelstein SM, Cohn JN, Collins VR, et al. Vascular hemodynamic impedance in congestive heart failure. *Am J Cardiol.* 1985;55:423–427
7. Starling EH. *Linacre Lecture on the Law of the Heart.* London: Longman; 1918.
8. Tsai SC, Adamik R, Manganiello VC, et al. Effects of nitroprusside and NTG on cGMP content and PGI_2 formation in aorta and vena cava. *Biochem Biophys Res Commun.* 1989;38:61–65.
9. Hamilton MA, Stevenson LW, Child JS, et al. Acute reduction of atrial overload during vasodilator and diuretic therapy in advanced congestive heart failure. *Am J Cardiol.* 1990;65:1209–1212.
10. Goodman DJ, Rossen RM, Holloway EL, et al. Effect of nitroprusside on left ventricular dynamics in mitral regurgitation. *Circulation.* 1974;50:1025–1032.
11. Elkayam U, Weber L, Torkan B, et al. Comparison of hemodynamic responses to nifedipine and nitroprusside in severe chronic congestive heart failure. *Am J Cardiol.* 1984;53:1321–1325.
12. Merillon JP, Fontenier G, Lerallut JF, et al. Aortic input impedance in heart failure: comparison with normal subjects and its changes during vasodilator therapy. *Eur Heart J.* 1984;5:447–455.
13. Herrmann HC, Ruddy TD, Dec GW, et al. Diastolic function in patients with severe heart failure: comparison of the effects of enoximone and nitroprusside. *Circulation.* 1987;75:1214–1221.
14. Lavine SJ, Campbell CA, Held AC, et al. Effect of inotropic and vasodilator therapy on left ventricular diastolic filling in dogs with severe left ventricular dysfunction. *J Am Coll Cardiol.* 1990;15:1165–1172.
15. Cogan JJ, Humphreys MH, Carlson CJ, et al. Renal effects of nitroprusside and HYD in patients with congestive heart failure. *Circulation.* 1980;61:316–323.
16. Hasenfuss G, Holubarsch C, Heiss HW, et al. Myocardial energetics in patients with dilated cardiomyopathy. Influence of nitroprusside and enoximone. *Circulation.* 1989; 80:51–64.
17. Powers ER, Reison DS, Berke A, et al. The effect of nitroprusside on coronary and systemic hemodynamics in patients with severe congestive heart failure. [Abstract] *Circulation.* 1982;66:II211
18. Chatterjee K, Parmley WW, Ganz W, et al. Hemodynamic and metabolic responses to vasodilator therapy in acute myocardial infarction. *Circulation.* 1973;48:1183–1193.
19. Miller RR, Awan NA, Mason DT. Nitroprusside therapy in acute and chronic coronary heart disease. *Am J Med.* 1978;65: 167–172.
20. Awan NA, Miller RR, Vera Z, et al. Reduction of S-T segment elevation with infusion of nitroprusside in patients with acute myocardial infarction. *Am J Cardiol.* 1976;38:435–439.
21. Mann T, Cohn PF, Holman LB, et al. Effect of nitroprusside on regional myocardial blood flow in coronary artery disease. Results in 25 patients and comparison with NTG. *Circulation.* 1978;57:732–738.
22. Leier CV, Bambach D, Thompson MJ, et al. Central and regional hemodynamic effects of intravenous isosorbide dinitrate, NTG, and nitroprusside in patients with congestive heart failure. *Am J Cardiol.* 1981;48:1115–1123.
23. Olivari MT, Levine TB, Cohn JN. Abnormal neurohumoral response to nitroprusside infusion in congestive heart failure. *J Am Coll Cardiol.* 1983;2:411–417.
24. Johnson W, Omland T, Hall C, et al. Neurohormonal activation rapidly decreases after intravenous therapy with diuretics and vasodilators for Class IV heart failure. *J Am Coll Cardiol.* 2002;39:1623–1629.
25. Stevenson LW, Dracup KA, Tillisch JH. Efficacy of medical therapy tailored for severe congestive heart failure in patients transferred for urgent cardiac transplantation. *Am J Cardiol.* 1989;63:461–464.
26. Subramanyam R, Tandon R, Shrivastava S. Hemodynamic effects of sodium nitroprusside in patients with ventricular septal defect. *Eur J Pediatr.* 1982;138:307–310.
27. Miller R, Vismara LA, DeMaria AN, et al. Afterload reduction therapy with nitroprusside in severe aortic regurgitation: improved cardiac performance and reduced regurgitant volume. *Am J Cardiol.* 1976;38:564–567.
28. Capomolla S, Febo O, Opasich C, et al. Chronic infusion of dobutamine and nitroprusside in patients with end-stage heart failure awaiting heart transplantation: safety and clinical outcome. *Eur J Heart Fail.* 2001;3:601–610.
29. Addonizio LJ, Gersony WM, Robbins RC, et al. Elevated pulmonary vascular resistance and cardiac transplantation. *Circulation.* 1987;76:V52–V55.
30. Khot UN, Novaro GM, Popovic ZB, et al. Nitroprusside in critically ill patients with left ventricular dysfunction and aortic stenosis. *N Engl J Med.* 2003;348:1756–1763.
31. Stemple DR, Kleiman JH, Harrison DC. Combined nitroprusside-dopamine therapy in severe chronic congestive heart failure. Dose-related hemodynamic advantages over single drug infusions. *Am J Cardiol.* 1978;42:267–275.
32. Miller RR, Awan NA, Joye JA, et al. Combined dopamine and nitroprusside therapy in congestive heart failure. Greater augmentation of cardiac performance by addition of inotropic stimulation to afterloads reduction. *Circulation.* 1977;55:881–884.
33. Cohn JN, Burke LP. Nitroprusside. *Ann Intern Med* 1979;91: 752–757.
34. Packer M, Meller J, Medina N, et al. Rebound hemodynamic events after the abrupt withdrawal of nitroprusside in patients with severe chronic heart failure. *N Engl J Med.* 1979; 301:1193–1197.

35. Vesey CJ, Cole PV. Blood cyanide and thiocyanate concentrations produced by long-term therapy with sodium nitroprusside. *Br J Anaesth.* 1985;57:148–155.
36. Bencowitz HZ, LeWinter MM, Wagner PD. Effect of sodium nitroprusside on ventilation-perfusion mismatching in heart failure. *J Am Coll Cardiol.* 1984;4:918–922.
37. Mehta J, Mehta P. Platelet function studies in heart disease. Enhanced platelet aggregate formation activity in congestive heart failure: inhibition by sodium nitroprusside. *Circulation.* 1979;60:497–503.
38. Nourok DS, Glassock RJ, Solomon DH, et al. Hypothyroidism following prolonged sodium nitroprusside therapy. *Am J Med Sci.* 1964;248:129–138.
39. Elkayam U, Karralp IS, Wani OR, et al. The role of organic nitrates in the treatment of heart failure. *Prog Cardiovasc Dis.*1999;41:255–264.
40. Bitar F, Akhter MW, Khan S, et al. Survey of the use of organic nitrates for the treatment of chronic congestive heart failure in the United States. *Am J Cardiol.* 2004;94:1465–1468.
41. Ignarro LJ, Lippton H, Edwards JC, et al. Mechanism of vascular smooth muscle relaxation by organic nitrates, nitrites, nitroprusside and nitric oxide: evidence for the involvement of S-nitrosothiols as active intermediates. *J Pharmacol Exp Ther.* 1981;218:739–749.
42. De Caterina R, Dorso CR, Tack-Goldman K, et al. Nitrates and endothelial prostacyclin production: studies in vitro. *Circulation.* 1985;71:176–182.
43. Fung HL. Pharmacokinetic determinants of nitrate action. *Am J Med.* 1984;76(Suppl 6A):22–26.
44. Elkayam U, Bitar F, Akhter MW, et al. Intravenous NTGe in the treatment of decompensated heart failure: potential benefits and limitations. *J Cardiovasc Pharmacol Ther.* 2004;9: 227–241.
45. Mueller RL, Scheidt S. NTG. In: Messerli FG, ed. *Cardiovascular Drug Therapy.* 2nd ed. Philadelphia: WB Saunders; 1996: 865–876.
46. Elkayam U, Kulick D, McIntosh N, et al. Incidence of early tolerance to hemodynamic effects of continuous infusion of NTG in patients with coronary artery disease and heart failure. *Circulation.* 1987;76:577–584.
47. Dupuis J, Lalonde G, Lemieux R, et al. Tolerance to intravenous NTG in patients with congestive heart failure: role of increased intravascular volume, neurohumoral activation and lack of prevention with N-acetylcysteine. *J Am Coll Cardiol.* 1990;16: 923–931.
48. Elkayam U, Roth A, Kumar A, et al. Hemodynamic and volumetric effects of venodilation with NTG in chronic mitral regurgitation. *Am J Cardiol.* 1987;60:1106–1111.
49. Elkayam U. Nitrates in the treatment of congestive heart failure. *Am J Cardiol.* 1996;77;41C–51C.
50. Webster MW, Sharpe DN, Coxon R, et al. Effect of reducing atrial pressure on atrial natriuretic factor and vasoactive hormones in congestive heart failure secondary to ischemic and nonischemic dilated cardiomyopathy. *Am J Cardiol.* 1989;63: 217–221.
51. Dakak N, Makhoul N, Merdler A, et al. Haemodynamic and neurohumoral effects of flosequinan in severe heart failure: similarities and differences compared with intravenous NTG therapy. *Eur Heart J.* 1993;14:836–844.
52. Elkayam U, Cohen G, Gogia H, et al. Renal vasodilatory effect of endothelial stimulation in patients with chronic congestive heart failure. *J Am Coll Cardiol.* 1996;28:176–182.
53. Publication Committee for the VMAC Investigators (Vasodilatation in the Management of Acute CHF). Intravenous nesiritide vs NTG for treatment of decompensated congestive heart failure: a randomized controlled trial. *JAMA.* 2002;287: 1531–1540.
54. Katz SD, Biasucci L, Sabba C, et al. Impaired endothelium-mediated vasodilation in the peripheral vasculature of patients with congestive heart failure. *J Am Coll Cardiol.* 1992;19: 918–925.
55. Magrini F, Niarchos AP. Ineffectiveness of sublingual NTG in acute left ventricular failure in the presence of massive peripheral edema. *Am J Cardiol.* 1980;45:841–847.
56. Mehra A, Shotan A, Ostrzega E, et al. Potentiation of isosorbide dinitrate effects with N-acetylcysteine in patients with chronic heart failure. *Circulation.* 1994;89:2595–2600.
57. Elkayam U, Mehra A, Shotan A, et al. Nitrate resistance and tolerance: potential limitations in the treatment of congestive heart failure. *Am J Cardiol.* 1992;70:98B–104B.
58. Mehra A, Ostrzega E, Shotan A, et al. Persistent hemodynamic improvement with short-term nitrate therapy in patients with chronic congestive heart failure already treated with captopril. *Am J Cardiol.* 1992;70:1310–1314.
59. Elkayam U. Nitrates in heart failure. *Cardiol Clin.* 1994; 12:73–85.
60. Hecht HS, Karahalios SE, Schnugg SJ, et al. Improvement in supine bicycle exercise performance in refractory congestive heart failure after isosorbide dinitrate: radionuclide and hemodynamic evaluation of acute effects. *Am J Cardiol.* 1982; 49:133–140.
61. Roth A, Shotan A, Elkayam U. A randomized comparison between the hemodynamic effects of HYD and NTG alone and in combination at rest and during isometric exercise in patients with chronic mitral regurgitation. *Am Heart J.* 1993;125: 155–163.
62. Hamilton MA, Stevenson LW, Child JS, et al. Sustained reduction in valvular regurgitation and atrial volumes with tailored vasodilator therapy in advanced congestive heart failure secondary to dilated (ischemic or idiopathic) cardiomyopathy. *Am J Cardiol.* 1991;67:259–263.
63. Leier CV, Huss P, Magorien RD, et al. Improved exercise capacity and differing arterial and venous tolerance during chronic isosorbide dinitrate therapy for congestive heart failure. *Circulation.* 1983;67:817–822.
64. Franciosa JA, Goldsmith SR, Cohn JN. Contrasting immediate and long-term effects of isosorbide dinitrate on exercise capacity in congestive heart failure. *Am J Med.* 1980;69:559–566.
65. Elkayam U, Johnson JV, Shotan A, et al. Double-blind, placebo-controlled study to evaluate the effect of organic nitrates in patients with chronic heart failure treated with angiotensin-converting enzyme inhibition. *Circulation.* 1999;99:2652–2657.
66. Kulick D, Roth A, McIntosh N, et al. Resistance to isosorbide dinitrate in patients with chronic heart failure: incidence and attempt at hemodynamic prediction. *J Am Coll Cardiol.* 1988;12:1023–1028.
67. Elkayam U. Tolerance to organic nitrates: evidence, mechanisms, clinical relevance, and strategies for prevention. *Ann Intern Med.* 1991;114:667–677.
68. Elkayam U, Roth A, Mehra A, et al. Randomized study to evaluate the relation between oral isosorbide dinitrate dosing interval and the development of early tolerance to its effect on left ventricular filling pressure in patients with chronic heart failure. *Circulation.* 1991;84:2040–2048.
69. Rudd P, Blaschke TF. Antihypertensive agents and the drug therapy of hypertension. In: Gilman AG, Goodman LS, Rall TW, Murad F, eds. *The Pharmacologic Basis of Therapeutics.* 7th ed. New York: Macmillan; 1985: 784–805.
70. Haeusler G, Gerold M. Increased levels of prostaglandin-like material in the canine blood during arterial hypotension produced by HYD, diHYD and minoxidil. *Naunyn Schmiedebergs Arch Pharmacol.* 1979;310:155–167.
71. Greenwald JE, Wong LK, Rao M, et al. A study of three vasodilating agents as selective inhibitors of thromboxane A_2 biosynthesis. *Biochem Biophys Res Commun.* 1978;84:1112–1118.
72. Worcel M, Saiag B, Chevillard C. An unexpected mode of action for HYD. *Trends Pharmacol Sci.* 1980;1:136–138.
73. Mulrow JP, Crawford MH. Clinical pharmacokinetics and therapeutic use of HYD in congestive heart failure. *Clin Pharmacokinet.* 1989;16:86–89.
74. Crawford MH, Ludden TM, Kennedy GT. Determinants of systemic availability of oral HYD in heart failure. *Clin Pharmacol Ther.* 1985;38:538–543.
75. Hanson A, Johansson BW, Wernersson B, et al. Pharmacokinetics of HYD in chronic heart failure. *Eur J Clin Pharmacol.* 1983;25:467–473.
76. Elkayam U, Weber L, McKay CR, et al. Differences in hemodynamic response to vasodilation due to calcium channel antagonism with nifedipine and direct-acting agonism with HYD in chronic refractory heart failure. *Am J Cardiol.* 1984;54:126–131.
77. Leier CV, Desch CE, Magorien RD, et al. Positive inotropic effects of HYD in human subjects: comparison with prazosin in the setting of congestive heart failure. *Am J Cardiol.* 1980;46:1039–1044.

78. Elkayam U, Roth A, Hsueh W, et al. Neurohumoral consequences of vasodilator therapy with HYD and nifedipine in severe congestive heart failure. *Am Heart J*. 1986;111:1130–1138.
79. McKay CR, Nana M, Kawanishi DT, et al. Importance of internal controls, statistical methods, and side effects in short-term trials of vasodilators: a study of HYD kinetics in patients with aortic regurgitation. *Circulation*. 1985;72:865–872.
80. Kolibash AJ, Magorien RD, Robinson JL, et al. Hemodynamic effects of vasodilator therapy in severe left heart failure combined with large atrial septal defects. *Am J Med*. 1982; 73:439–444.
81. Beekman RH, Rocchini AP, Rosenthal A. Hemodynamic effects of HYD in infants with a large ventricular septal defect. *Circulation*. 1982;65:523–528.
82. Binkley PF, Starling RC, Hammer DF, Leier CV. Usefulness of hydralazine to withdraw from dobutamine in severe congestive heart failure. *Am J Cardiol*. 1991;68:1103–1106.
83. Magorien RD, Brown GP, Unverferth DV, et al. Effects of HYD on coronary blood flow and myocardial energetics in congestive heart failure. *Circulation*. 1982;65:528–533.
84. Magorien RD, Unverferth DV, Leier CV. HYD therapy in chronic congestive heart failure. Sustained central and regional hemodynamic responses. *Am J Med*. 1984;77:267–274.
85. Rubin SA, Chatterjee K, Parmley WW. Metabolic assessment of exercise in chronic heart failure patients treated with short-term vasodilators. *Circulation*. 1980;61:543–548.
86. Elkayam U, Weber L, Campese VM, et al. Renal hemodynamic effects of vasodilation with nifedipine and HYD in patients with heart failure. *J Am Coll Cardiol*. 1984;4:1261–1267.
87. Pierpont GL, Brown DC, Franciosa JA, et al. Effect of HYD on renal failure in patients with congestive heart failure. *Circulation*. 1980;61:323–327.
88. Cogan JJ, Humphreys MH, Carlson CJ, et al. Acute vasodilator therapy increases renal clearance of digoxin in patients with congestive heart failure. *Circulation*. 1981;64:973–976.
89. Nomura A, Yasuda H, Katoh K, et al. HYD and furosemide kinetics. *Clin Pharmacol Ther*. 1982;32:303–306.
90. Chatterjee K, Massie B, Rubin S, et al. Long-term outpatient vasodilator therapy of congestive heart failure. Consideration of agents at rest and during exercise. *Am J Med*. 1978;65:134–145.
91. Packer M, Meller J, Medina N, et al. Dose requirements of HYD in patients with severe chronic congestive heart failure. *Am J Cardiol*. 1980;45:655–660.
92. Packer M, Meller J, Medina N, et al. Importance of left ventricular chamber size in determining the response to HYD in severe chronic heart failure. *N Engl J Med*. 1980;303:250–255.
93. Packer M, Meller J, Medina N, et al. Hemodynamic characterization of tolerance to long-term HYD therapy in severe chronic heart failure. *N Engl J Med*. 1982;306:57–62.
94. Packer M, Meller J, Medina N, et al. Provocation of myocardial ischemic events during initiation of vasodilator therapy for severe chronic heart failure. Clinical and hemodynamic evaluation of 52 consecutive patients with ischemic cardiomyopathy. *Am J Cardiol*. 1981;48:939–946.
95. Pierpont GL, Cohn JN, Franciosa JA. Combined oral HYD-nitrate therapy in left ventricular failure. Hemodynamic equivalency to sodium nitroprusside. *Chest*. 1978;73:8–13.
96. Cohn JN, Johnson G, Ziesche S, et al. A comparison of enalapril with HYD-isosorbide dinitrate in the treatment of chronic congestive heart failure. *N Engl J Med*. 1991;325:303–310.
97. Cohn JN, Archibald D, Johnson G, and the VA Cooperative Study Group. Effects of vasodilator therapy on peak exercise oxygen consumption in heart failure: V-HeFT. [Abstract] *Circulation*. 1987;76:IV443.
98. Cohn JN. Vasodilators in heart failure: conclusions from V-HeFT II and rationale for V-HeFT III. *Drugs*. 1994;47(Suppl 4):47–57.
99. Elkayam U. Nitrates in the treatment of congestive heart failure. *Am J Cardiol*. 1996;77:41C–51C.
100. Packer M, Lee WH, Kessler PD, et al. Prevention and reversal of nitrate tolerance in patients with congestive heart failure. *N Engl J Med*. 1987;317:799–804.
101. Unger P, Berkenboom G, Fontaine J. Interaction between HYD and nitrovasodilators in vascular smooth muscle. *J Cardiovasc Pharmacol*. 1993;21:478–483.
102. Münzel T, Kurz S, Rajagopalan S, et al. HYD prevents NTG tolerance by inhibiting activation of a membrane-bound NADH oxidase. A new action for an old drug. *J Clin Invest*. 1996;98: 1465–1470.
103. Bauer JA, Fung HL. Concurrent HYD administration prevents NTG-induced hemodynamic tolerance in experimental heart failure. *Circulation*. 1991;84:35–39.
104. Gogia H, Mehra A, Parikh S, et al. Prevention of tolerance to hemodynamic effects of nitrates with concomitant use of HYD in patients with chronic heart failure. *J Am Coll Cardiol*. 1995;26:1575–1580.
105. Carson P, Ziesche S, Johnson G, et al. Racial differences in response to therapy for heart failure: analysis of the Vasodilator-Heart Failure trials. Vasodilator-Heart Failure Trial Study Group. *J Card Fail*. 1999;5:178–187.
106. Elkayam U, Shotan A, Mehra A, et al. Calcium channel blockers in heart failure. *J Am Coll Cardiol*. 1993;22:139A–144A.
107. Miller AB, Conetta DA, Bass TA. Sublingual nifedipine: acute effects in severe chronic congestive heart failure secondary to idiopathic dilated cardiomyopathy. *Am J Cardiol*. 1985;55: 1359–1362.
108. Magorien RD, Leier CV, Kolibash AJ, et al. Beneficial effects of nifedipine on rest and exercise myocardial energetics in patients with congestive heart failure. *Circulation*. 1984;70: 884–890.
109. Ludbrook PA, Tiefenbrunn AJ, Sobel BE. Influence of nifedipine on left ventricular systolic and diastolic function. Relationship to manifestations of ischemia and congestive failure. *Am J Med*. 1981;71:683–692.
110. Elkayam U, Weber L, Torkan B, et al. Acute hemodynamic effect of oral nifedipine in severe chronic congestive heart failure. *Am J Cardiol*. 1983;52:1041–1045.
111. Elkayam U, Weber L, McKay C, et al. Spectrum of acute hemodynamic effects of nifedipine in severe congestive heart failure. *Am J Cardiol*. 1985;56:560–566.
112. Elkayam U, Weber L, Torkan B, et al. Comparison of hemodynamic responses to nifedipine and nitroprusside in severe chronic congestive heart failure. *Am J Cardiol*. 1984;53: 1321–1325.
113. Fifer MA, Colucci WS, Lorell BH, et al. Inotropic, vascular and neuroendocrine effects of nifedipine in heart failure: comparison with nitroprusside. *J Am Coll Cardiol*. 1985;5:731–737.
114. Elkayam U, Weber L, McKay CR, et al. Differences in hemodynamic response to vasodilation due to calcium channel antagonism with nifedipine and direct-acting agonism with HYD in chronic refractory congestive heart failure. *Am J Cardiol*. 1984;54:126–131.
115. Packer M, Lee WH, Medina N, et al. Prognostic importance of the immediate hemodynamic response to nifedipine in patients with severe left ventricular dysfunction. *J Am Coll Cardiol*. 1987;10:1303–1311.
116. Prida XE, Kubo SH, Laragh JH, et al. Evaluation of calcium-mediated vasoconstriction in chronic congestive heart failure. *Am J Med*. 1983;75:795–800.
117. Elkayam U, Roth A, Hsueh W, et al Neurohumoral consequences of vasodilator therapy with HYD and nifedipine in severe congestive heart failure. *Am Heart J*. 1986;111:1130–1138.
118. Agostoni PG, De Cesare N, Doria E, et al. Afterload reduction: a comparison of captopril and nifedipine in dilated cardiomyopathy. *Br Heart J*. 1986;55:391–399.
119. Elkayam U, Amin J, Mehra A, et al. A prospective, randomized, double-blind crossover study to compare the efficacy and safety of chronic nifedipine therapy with that of isosorbide dinitrate and their combination in the treatment of chronic congestive heart failure. *Circulation*. 1990;82:1954–1961.
120. Henry PD. Comparative pharmacology of calcium antagonists: nifedipine, verapamil and diltiazem. *Am J Cardiol*. 1980;46: 1047–1058.
121. Walsh RW, Porter CB, Starling MR, et al. Beneficial hemodynamic effects of intravenous and oral diltiazem in severe congestive heart failure. *J Am Coll Cardiol*. 1984;3:1044–1050.
122. Packer M, Lee WH, Medican Y, et al. Comparative negative inotropic effects of nifedipine and diltiazem in patients with severe left ventricular dysfunction. [Abstract] *Circulation*. 1985;72(Suppl III):III275.
123. Kulick DL, McIntosh N, Campese VM, et al. Central and renal hemodynamic effects and hormonal response to diltiazem in severe congestive heart failure. *Am J Cardiol*. 1987;59: 1138–1143.

124. Heywood JT, Graham B, Marais GE, et al. Effects of intravenous diltiazem on rapid atrial fibrillation accompanied by congestive heart failure. *Am J Cardiol.* 1991;67:1150–1152.
125. Figulla HR, Gietzen F, Zeymer U, et al. Diltiazem improves cardiac function and exercise capacity in patients with idiopathic dilated cardiomyopathy. Results of the Diltiazem in Dilated Cardiomyopathy Trial. *Circulation.* 1996;94:346–352.
126. The Multicenter Diltiazem Postinfarction Trial Research Group. The effect of diltiazem on mortality and reinfarction after myocardial infarction. *N Engl J Med.* 1998;319:385–392.
127. Goldstein RE, Boccuzzi SJ, Cruess D, et al. Diltiazem increases late-onset congestive heart failure in postinfarction patients with early reduction in ejection fraction. The Adverse Experience Committee and the Multicenter Diltiazem Postinfarction Research Group. *Circulation.* 1991;83:52–60.
128. Ferlinz J. Gallo CT. Responses of patients in heart failure to long-term oral verapamil administration. [Abstract] *Circulation.* 1984;70(Suppl II):II305.
129. The Danish Study Group on Verapamil in Myocardial Infarction. Secondary prevention with verapamil after myocardial infarction. *Am J Cardiol.* 1990;66:331–401.
130. Minderjahn KP, Hanrath P, Bleifeld W. The influence of nisoldipine on rest and exercise hemodynamics of the left ventricle in chronic left heart insufficiency. *Z Kardiol.* 1983;73(Suppl 1):83.
131. DeiCas L, Metra M, Ferrari R, et al. Acute and chronic hemodynamic effects of the dihydropyridine calcium antagonist nisoldipine on the resting and exercise hemodynamics, neurohumoral parameters and functional capacity of patients with chronic heart failure. *Cardiovasc Drugs Ther.* 1993;7:103–110.
132. Ryman KS, Kubo SH, Lystash J, et al. Effect of nicardipine on rest and exercise hemodynamics in chronic congestive heart failure. *Am J Cardiol.* 1986;58:583–588.
133. Lahiri A, Robinson CW, Kohli RS, et al. Acute and chronic effects of nicardipine on systolic and diastolic left ventricular performance in patients with heart failure: a pilot study. *Clin Cardiol.* 1986;9:257–261.
134. Lahiri A, Rodrigues EA, Carboni GP, et al. Effects of long-term treatment with calcium antagonists on left ventricular diastolic function in stable angina and heart failure. *Circulation.* 1990;81(Suppl III):130–138.
135. Gheorghiade M, Hall V, Goldberg D, et al. Long-term clinical and neurohormonal effects of nicardipine in patients with severe heart failure on maintenance therapy with angiotensin converting enzyme inhibitors [Abstract] *J Am Coll Cardiol.* 1991;17(Suppl A):274A.
136. Ljung B. Vascular selectivity of felodipine. *Drugs.* 1985;29(Suppl 2):46–58.
137. Timmis AD, Campbell S, Monaghan MJ, et al. Acute and metabolic effects of felodipine in congestive heart failure. *Br Heart J.* 1984;51:445–451.
138. Agostoni P, Doria E, Riva S, et al. Acute and chronic efficacy of felodipine in congestive heart failure. *Int J Cardiol.* 1991; 30:89–95.
139. Dunselman PH, Kuntze CE, Van Bruggen A, et al. Efficacy of felodipine in congestive heart failure. *Eur Heart J.* 1989; 10:354–364.
140. Cohn JN, Ziesche S, Smith R, et al. Effect of the calcium antagonist felodipine as supplementary vasodilator therapy in patients with chronic heart failure treated with enalapril: V-HeFT III. Vasodilator-Heart Failure Trial (V-HeFT) Study Group. *Circulation.* 1997;96:856–863.
141. Packer M. Prospective Randomized Amlodipine Survival Evaluation 2. Presented in the 49th American College of Cardiology Meeting, Anaheim, CA. March 2000.
142. Packer M, O'Connor CM, Ghali JK, et al. Effect of amlodipine on morbidity and mortality in severe chronic heart failure. Prospective Randomized Amoldipine Survival Evaluation Study Group. *N Engl J Med.* 1996;335:1107–1114.
143. Schulz R, Post H, Jalowy A, et al. Unique cardioprotective action of the new calcium antagonist mibefradil. *Circulation.* 1999;99:305–311.
144. Levin TB, Peter J, Bermink LM, et al. Effect of mibedfradil, a T-type calcium channel blocker, on morbidity and moratlity in moderate to severe congesgtive heart failure: the MACH-1 Study. *Circulation.* 2000;101:758–764.
145. Elkayam U, Akhter MW, Tummala P, et al. Nesiritide: a new drug for the treatment of decompensated heart failure. *J Cardiovasc Pharmacol Ther.* 2002;7:181–194.
146. Burger AJ, Horton DP, LeJemtel T. Effect of nesiritide (B-type natriuretic peptide) and dobutamine on ventricular arrhythmias in the treatment of patients with acutely decompensated congestive heart failure: the PRECEDENT study. *Am Heart J.* 2002;144:1102–1108.
147. Publication Committee for the VMAC Investigators (Vasodilatation in the Management of Acute CHF). Intravenous nesiritide vs nitroglycerin for treatment of decompensated congestive heart failure: a randomized controlled trial. *JAMA.* 2002;287: 1531–1540.
148. Colucci WS, Elkayam U, Horton DP. Intravenous nesiritide, a natriuretic peptide, in the treatment of decompensated congestive heart failure. Nesiritide Study Group. *N Engl J Med.* 2000;343:246–253.
149. Elkayam U, Akhter MW, Singh H, et al. Comparison of effects on left ventricular filling pressure of intravenous nesiritide and high-dose nitroglycerin in patients with decompensated heart failure. *Am J Cardiol.* 2004;93:237–240.
150. Michaels AD, Klein A, Madden JA, et al. Effects of intravenous nesiritide on human coronary vasomotor regulation and myocardial oxygen uptake. *Circulation.* 2003;107: 2697–2701.
151. Mills RM, LeJemtel TH, Horton DP, et al. Sustained hemodynamic effects of an infusion of nesiritide (human B-type natriuretic peptide) in heart failure: a randomized, double-blind, placebo-controlled clinical trial. Natrecor Study Group. *J Am Coll Cardiol.* 1999;34:155–162.
152. Burger AJ, Horton DP, Elkayam U, et al. Comparison of the effects of dobutamine and nesiritide (B-type natriuretic peptide) on cardiac ectopy in acutely decompensated ischemic versus non-ischemic cardiomyopathy. *J Card Fail.* 2000;6(Suppl 2):49.
153. Wang DJ, Dowling TC, Meadows D. Nesiritide does not improve renal function in patients with chronic heart failure and worsening serum creatinine. *Circulation* 2004;110: 1620–1625.
154. Sackner-Bernstein JD, Skopicki HA, et al. Risk of worsening renal function with nesiritide in patients with acutely decompensated heart failure. *Circulation.* 2005;111:1487–1491.
155. Abraham WT. Serum creatinine elevations in patients receiving nesiritide are related to starting dose. [Abstract] *Circulation.* 2005;112(Suppl):II589.
156. Heywood JT. Combining nesiritide with high-dose diuretics may increase the risk of increased serum creatinine. [Abstract] *Circulation.* 2005;112 (Suppl):II451.
157. Elkayam U. Nesiritide may diminish the increased acute mortality risk associated with worsening renal function. [Abstract] *Circulation.* 2005;112 (Suppl):II675.
158. Silver MA, Horton DP, Ghali JK, et al. Effect of nesiritide versus dobutamine on short-term outcomes in the treatment of patients with acutely decompensated heart failure. *J Am Coll Cardiol.* 2002;39:798–803.
159. Sackner-Bernstein JD, Kowalski M, Fox M, et al. Short-term risk of death after treatment with nesiritide for decompensated heart failure: a pooled analysis of randomized controlled trials. *JAMA.* 2005;293:1900–1905.
160. Abraham WT. Nesiritide does not increase 30-day or 6-month mortality risk. [Abstract] *Circulation.* 2005;112 (Suppl):II676.
161. Abraham WT, Adams KF, Fonarow GC. In-hospital mortality in patients with acute decompensated heart failure requiring intravenous vasoactive medications: an analysis from the Acute Decompensated Heart Failure National Registry (ADHERE). *J Am Coll Cardiol.* 2005;46:57–64.

28 Beta-Blocker Therapy for Heart Failure

Henry Krum

Beta-adrenergic blocking agents (beta-blockers) are now well-established as mandatory therapy in patients with systolic chronic heart failure, unless not tolerated or contraindicated. Use of beta-blockers for the treatment of chronic heart failure has quite literally been a revolution in pharmacological therapy for this condition. These agents have long been contraindicated in the treatment of patients with systolic heart failure, the clinical consequence of impaired myocardial contractile function. However, in the late 1970s and early 1980s Swedish researchers tested the hypothesis that blockade of chronic sympathetic activation might, in fact, be beneficial in this setting. Decades later, we now have an extensive clinical trials database demonstrating the benefits of these agents in improving prognosis, reducing hospitalization, and (particularly in more severe cases) relieving symptoms. This database of placebo-controlled beta-blocker trials in congestive heart failure (CHF) is now more extensive than that for angiotensin-converting enzyme (ACE) inhibitors, which is standard background therapy for this condition. The robustness of this data is reflected by current heart failure guidelines that mandate the use of beta-blockers if tolerated in patients with mild, moderate, and severe symptoms of systolic heart failure, provided the patient has been stabilized and rendered euvolemic.

PATHOPHYSIOLOGICAL CONSIDERATIONS

Role of the Sympathetic Nervous System in Heart Failure

Chronic heart failure is characterized by activation of a number of neurohormonal vasoconstrictor systems including the sympathetic nervous system, the renin-angiotensin system, vasopressin, and, more recently, peptide systems such as endothelin and urotensin-II (1,2). This neurohormonal activation can be viewed as a compensatory response to the reduction in cardiac output and systemic blood pressure that accompanies systolic ventricular dysfunction.

Beta-adrenoceptor agonism activates regulatory G-proteins to increase intracellular cyclic adenosine monophosphate (AMP) via adenylate cyclase stimulation (3). Increased cyclic AMP (cAMP) stimulates downstream protein kinases which, in turn, phosphorylate calcium channels leading to influx of intracellular calcium, and enhancement of coupling of actin and myosin filaments, resulting in inotropy (Fig. 28-1).

While there is generalized sympathetic activation in heart failure, norepinephrine spillover is particularly increased in the heart and kidneys (4). As a consequence of the chronic catecholamine excess that accompanies this activation, there is depletion of catecholamines from storage vesicles in cardiac sympathetic nerve terminals (5), downregulation (decreased density) of beta-adrenoceptors on myocardial cells, and uncoupling of the receptor from adenylate cyclase (3).

In the short term, the sympathetic activation that accompanies heart failure is an important compensatory mechanism providing inotropic support and maintaining cardiac output; indeed, that is the rationale for the use of sympathomimetic amines in patients with acutely decompensated heart failure. However, over longer periods of time this sympathetic activation may be deleterious, thus providing the rationale for use of beta-adrenoceptor-locking agents in this setting. There are several lines of evidence to support the conclusion that long-term sympathetic activation is detrimental in heart failure and

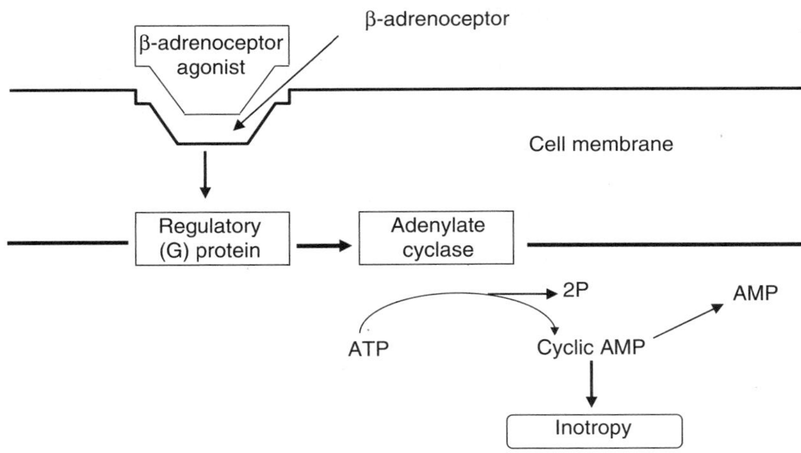

Figure 28-1 The β-adrenegic receptor system. ATP, adenosine triphosphate; AMP, adenosine monophosphate.

contributes to disease progression and adverse clinical outcomes.

Evidence from Mechanistic Studies

Possible detrimental effects of long-term sympathetic activation derived from mechanistic studies in chronic heart failure include direct myocardial toxicity secondary to long-term catecholamine excess (6), requirement for increased myocardial oxygen consumption (7), myocardial beta-adrenoceptor3 downregulation, impaired myocardial function secondary to tachycardia, reduction in threshold for arrhythmogenesis (8), and activation of other vasoconstrictor systems such as the renin-angiotensin improvement in endothelial function and endothelin systems.

Evidence from Clinical Outcome Studies

There are also a number of lines of evidence supporting the deleterious effects of chronic sympathetic activation derived from clinical studies. It has long been observed that patients with diseases associated with chronic catecholamine excess (e.g., pheochromocytoma) present with myocardial disease phenotypically indistinguishable from that of dilated cardiomyopathy (9).

Drugs that augment the effects of catecholamines on the myocardium such as beta-adrenoceptor agonists (10) or type III phosphodiesterase inhibitors (11) are associated with adverse mortality outcomes. This was perhaps best demonstrated in the PROMISE study (11) with long-term oral use of the phosphodiesterase inhibitor, milrinone, associated with significantly impaired survival. Similar outcomes were associated with the partial beta-adrenoceptor agonist, xamoterol (10). In contrast to these dismal results with long-term oral treatment, milrinone remains a useful short-term intravenous therapy, providing inotropic support to the failing myocardium in decompensated heart failure (12). A number of studies have demonstrated a close association between measures of sympathetic activation (peripheral venous plasma norepinephrine levels, whole-body norepinephrine spillover rate, and microneurography) with markers of disease severity and subsequent mortality (13,14).

Finally, the accumulating evidence from studies of beta-adrenoceptor-blockers themselves in heart failure supports the underlying rationale for their use: that blockade of the toxic effects of catecholamines on the myocardium is associated with improved clinical status and survival in these patients.

Rationale for Adrenergic Blockade in Patients with Chronic Heart Failure

The preceding mechanistic and clinical data regarding long-term sympathetic activation in chronic heart failure strongly support a therapeutic role for beta-adrenoceptor-blockers in this condition. Theoretical benefits of beta-adrenoceptor-blockers include direct myocardial protection from the toxic effects of catecholamines, reduction in stimulation of other neurohormonal vasoconstrictor systems, blockade of the proarrhythmic effects of catecholamines and anti-ischemic effects via increased coronary blood flow during diastole, and reduced myocardial oxygen demand.

It has also been proposed that restoration of beta-adrenoceptor density and receptor-adenylate cyclase coupling with the use of these drugs may be a potential mechanism for their beneficial effects. Myocardial beta-adrenoceptor downregulation and receptor-cyclase uncoupling in heart failure may limit contractile function (3,15), and drugs such as metoprolol have been demonstrated to increase beta-adrenoceptor density in this setting (16). However, other beta-adrenoceptor-blocking drugs have been demonstrated to produce significant clinical benefits in this condition (e.g., carvedilol) and are not associated with beta-adrenoceptor upregulation or restoration of receptor-cyclase coupling (17). Thus, although some beta-adrenoceptor-blockers do cause upregulation of beta-adrenoceptors, this is unlikely to be the mechanism of benefit of this group of drugs overall.

PHARMACOLOGY OF BETA-BLOCKERS

Bisoprolol

Bisoprolol is a beta-1 selective agent without additional vasodilatory properties. Its beta-1 to beta-2 ratio makes it a particularly selective agent and thus, in theory, less likely to contribute to bronchoconstriction in individuals with airways disease. The pharmacokinetics of the agent is that of a lipid-insoluble agent with a plasma half-life of 10 to 12 hours, permitting once-daily dosing. The target dose is generally 10 mg per day. Elimination is via both renal and hepatic routes.

Carvedilol

Carvedilol is a moderately lipid-soluble, nonselective (beta-1, beta-2) receptor antagonist without intrinsic sympathomimetic activity (ISA) but with the additional property of alpha-1 blockade, mediating peripheral vasodilation. It also possesses ancillary properties of being antioxidant, antiproliferative, and having antiendothelin actions. Its half-life is 6 to 10 hours and twice-daily dosing is recommended, although a prolonged-release formulation is currently being developed. Elimination is primarily hepatic and dose adjustment is not required in renal impairment. The target dose is 25 mg twice daily (50 mg twice daily in patients >85 kg).

Metoprolol

Metoprolol is a mildly lipid-soluble beta-1 selective agent without ancillary properties or vasodilator activity. It comes in an immediate-release formulation with a half-life of 3 to 5 hours, requiring two- to three-times-daily dosing, as well as an extended-release formulation permitting once-daily dosing. The target dose in heart failure of the extended-release formulation is 200 mg per day.

Nebivolol

Nebivolol is a lipophilic beta-1 selective agent that has additional vasodilator properties mediated via nitric oxide donation. Based on the Study of Effects of Nebivolol Intervention on Outcomes and Rehospitalization in Seniors (SENIORS) study (18), its target dose is 10 mg per day.

Other Beta-Blocking Agents

A number of other beta-blockers have been studied in heart failure, including bucindolol. Bucindolol is a nonselective beta-1 receptor antagonist. There is ongoing debate as to whether bucindolol also possesses ISA (19,20); this has been observed in both animal studies and in failing human myocardium. The significance of the presence of ISA is that of adverse outcomes with agents that possess this property, including the beta-1 partial agonist xamoterol (10), as well as non–beta-blocking agents that act via cAMP, the second messenger of the beta-adrenoceptor vesnarinone (21), flosequinan (22), ibopamine (23).

EFFICACY OF BETA-BLOCKERS IN HEART FAILURE

Studies of Clinical Status/Surrogate Markers

The pioneering clinical observations of Swedish and other investigators (24–26) established the utility of beta-blockers in heart failure. However, many of these early studies were often uncontrolled and involved administration of drugs for only short periods of time. Nevertheless, the clinical experience and data obtained from these trials have subsequently proven invaluable, leading to larger, placebo-controlled studies and the widespread clinical use of these drugs.

Short-term use of beta-adrenoceptor-blockers in these early studies was found to result in neutral or adverse clinical outcomes (27,28) and led many investigators to abandon this therapeutic approach. However, it is now understood that in the context of recovery of the myocardium from chronic catecholamine stimulation, studies of at least 3 months' duration are generally required to demonstrate clinical benefit with these drugs. Early studies were also important in establishing the need for commencement of beta-adrenoceptor-blocker therapy at extremely low doses to avoid sudden interference with the inotropic support provided to the failing myocardium by the increased sympathetic activity that accompanies heart failure.

Since these early trials, a number of longer-term, double-blind, placebo-controlled studies of beta-adrenoceptor-blockers have assessed clinical status in patients with chronic heart failure (28–32). These studies have demonstrated consistent improvements in ejection fraction, usually accompanied by improved patient well-being but with variable effects on exercise tolerance. The lack of consistent benefit of beta-adrenoceptor-blockers on exercise tolerance is a feature of therapy with this drug class and relates to the heart rate-limiting effects of beta-adrenoceptor-blockade during exercise. Heart rate is one of the factors that determines maximal exercise capacity (VO_{2max}) and, as such, it is not surprising that beta-adrenoceptor-blockers do not lead to increases in VO_{2max}, despite the hemodynamic improvements that accompany use of these drugs. These studies also demonstrated that beta-adrenoceptor-blockers inhibit other neurohormonal systems activated in chronic heart failure, such as the renin-angiotensin system (29) and endothelin-1 (33), as well as restoring parasympathetic activity (34), which is impaired in this condition.

The beneficial clinical effects observed with beta-adrenoceptor-blockers in heart failure in single-center studies has led to the more widespread evaluation of these drugs. The Carvedilol U.S. study program (35) addressed multiple questions regarding clinical efficacy of this drug in heart failure: use in delaying progression of heart failure, clinical utility in patients with moderate to severe heart failure, and whether a clinical dose–response relationship existed. The overall findings were concordant with those of the previous single-center studies with the drug. Carvedilol significantly improved left ventricular ejection fraction, New York Heart Association (NYHA) functional class, and physician and patient global assessment of heart failure status. Improvements in left ventricular function were found to be dose-dependent, the greatest benefits being seen in those patients randomized to receive the highest dose of the drug.

Retardation of progression of disease with carvedilol was also noted in the Australian New Zealand Heart Failure Study (36), where a reduction in left ventricular chamber size was observed in mild heart failure patients treated with beta-adrenoceptor-blocker, indicating restoration of ventricular contour toward normal. This finding provided strong a priori evidence that excess catecholamines are important in the ventricular remodeling process in heart failure and that beta-adrenoceptor-blockers can interfere with this remodelling in a clinically significant manner. However, significant improvements in NYHA class were not seen in this very mild group of patients, 30% of whom were already NYHA class I (i.e., asymptomatic) at time of entry into the study.

Studies on Mortality and Hospitalization

Chronic sympathetic activation is associated with adverse mortality outcomes in heart failure. Patients with the highest plasma levels of norepinephrine (a crude marker of sympathetic activation) have the most adverse mortality outcomes. Because sympathetic activation is also a marker of disease severity, the mortality association may simply reflect patients with the most advanced disease having the greatest mortality. As previously described, chronic sympathetic stimulation is associated with proarrhythmia, direct trophic and toxic effects on the myocardium, and activation of other neurohormonal systems, all of which may independently lead to adverse mortality outcomes. Thus, it would be reasonably anticipated that use of these drugs should confer beneficial effects on mortality, providing a powerful rationale for prescribing such drugs in these patients. A number of placebo-controlled studies have now conclusively demonstrated beneficial effects on mortality and hospitalization (Figs. 28-2 and 28-3).

Studies of Carvedilol

U.S. Carvedilol

This was a study of carvedilol versus placebo on a number of surrogate endpoint studies that spanned systolic CHF severity from mild through to severe (35). The pooled mortality result (prespecified) demonstrated a 65% risk reduction, resulting in the Data Safety and Monitoring Board (DSMB) terminating the study early. The magnitude of this benefit appeared to be similar in patients with mild through severe symptoms, regardless of idiopathic, dilated, or ischemic cardiomyopathy etiology. There were only a small number of deaths recorded in the U.S. Carvedilol study, leading some observers to conclude that a definitive mortality effect with beta-adrenoceptor-blockers had not been adequately demonstrated. There were also highly significant effects on hospitalization.

ANZ Carvedilol

Similar observations were made in the ANZ Carvedilol study (36). This was a study of mild heart failure patients, all with ischemic etiology. Although this study was not powered to detect a morbidity/mortality outcome, the findings were a 41% reduction in death or all-cause hospitalization and a 25% reduction in mortality alone.

COPERNICUS Study

This was a placebo-controlled study of carvedilol in patients with advanced heart failure (37). Although NYHA Class was not assessed in COPERNICUS, patients within this subgroup were selected on the basis of advanced heart failure symptoms together with an ejection fraction of >25%. Patients were permitted to have been recently hospitalized and to have received intravenous inotropic therapy within 4 days of randomization. The 2,289 patients were included in the intent-to-treat analysis, with a 35% decrease in mortality at the time the study was stopped early by its DSMB.

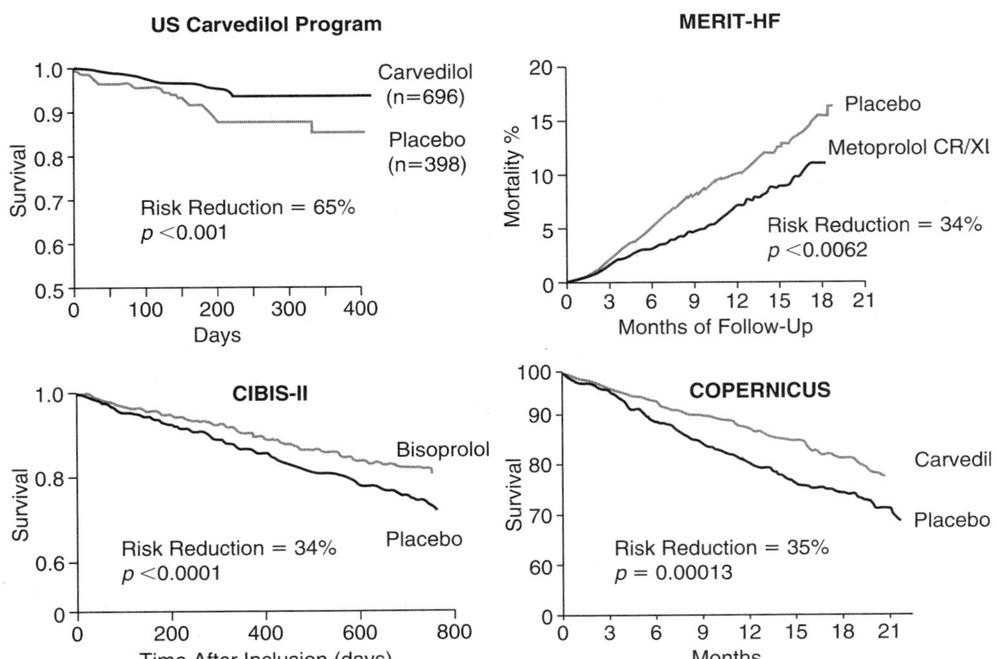

Figure 28-2 Placebo-controlled studies of beta-blocker therapy.

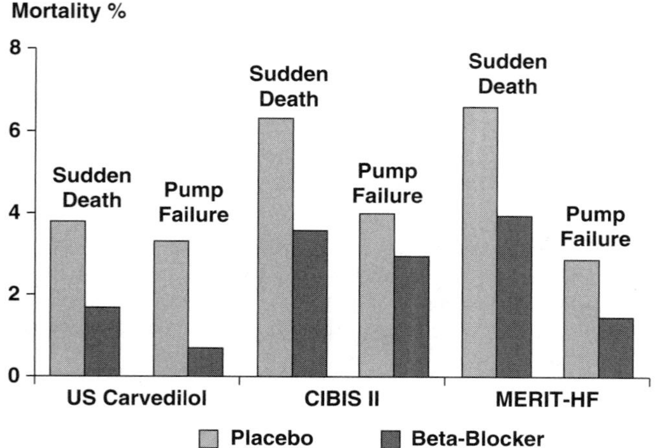

Figure 28-3 Placebo-controlled studies of beta-blocker therapy.

Studies of Bisoprolol

There have been two studies exploring the effects of bisoprolol on mortality in comparison to placebo. These were focused on patients with moderate to severe heart failure.

The first Cardiac Insufficiency Bisoprolol Study (IBIS) (38) study of 641 patients noted a 20% reduction in the primary endpoint of mortality and a 34% reduction in hospitalizations for heart failure. However, the primary endpoint did not reach statistical significance and clearly, in retrospect, this was an underpowered study. This led to the larger CIBIS II study (39) of 2,647 patients. This study was also terminated early by its DSMB for a 34% risk reduction with an accompanying 36% reduction in hospitalization for worsening heart failure.

Studies of Metoprolol

The MDC Metoprolol Dilated Cardiomyopathy Study (40) evaluated 383 patients with Class II–III idiopathic dilated cardiomyopathy with a target dose of 50 to 75 mg twice daily. A reduction in primary endpoint of death or need for transplantation reached borderline significance; however, there was no mortality benefit noted.

The larger MERIT-HF (41) study used the extended-release formulation of metoprolol and studied 3,991 patients with Class II–IV heart failure of mixed etiology. The target dose in the study was 200 mg once daily and the achieved dose in the active group was 159 mg per day. Again, this study was stopped by its DSMB for a 34% reduction in all-cause mortality and this was accompanied by reductions in hospitalization.

Studies of Nevibolol

The SENIORS study (18) evaluated nevibolol in 2,128 patients over 70 years of age versus placebo. SENIORS was different from the earlier placebo-controlled studies in that it not only focused on the elderly but also on patients with diastolic as well as systolic heart failure. The study met its primary endpoint of death or heart failure hospitalization with significantly fewer events in these patients. When analyzed according to systolic or diastolic (dichotomized at an ejection fraction of 35%), there was no heterogeneity in this beneficial response. Nevertheless, neither of these subgroups reached statistical significance as the study was not powered to test these subgroups individually.

Studies of Bucindolol

Bucindolol was evaluated in the Beta-blocker Evaluation of Survival Trial (BEST) (42) study of bucindolol versus placebo in patients with advanced systolic chronic heart failure. The study did not meet its overall primary endpoint and was terminated for futility. A number of subgroup analyses suggested that patients with the most advanced disease (e.g., NYHA Class IV) and African-Americans did not benefit and thus may have contributed to the overall equivocal result. It has also been suggested that because of the beta-2 to beta-1 ratio of bucindolol, there may have been too much sympathoinhibition, leading to a MOXCON-type (43) effect (in the MOXCON study, the potent central sympatholytic moxonidine was associated with increased mortality).

Mortality in Key Subgroups

Because heart failure is associated with a number of significant comorbid conditions, considerable attention has been paid to key subgroups to determine whether these specific patients may also benefit from beta-blocker therapy. In general, subgroups such as patients with diabetes mellitus, patients with advanced age, and gender and race subgroups have all noted a similar (beneficial) response (44–47).

TOLERABILITY OF BETA-BLOCKERS IN HEART FAILURE

The major reason for avoidance of commencement of beta-blockers relates to concerns regarding the tolerability of these agents. These concerns are understandable, given traditional teaching of the importance of increased sympathetic drive in attempting to overcome systolic ventricular dysfunction in the setting of CHF. It is, of course, this sympathetic activation that is blocked by these agents.

Concerns regarding these agents in heart failure include perceived complexity in initiation and uptitration, risk of intolerance and worsening of heart failure symptoms status with initiation, and perceived delay in beneficial effects on outcomes. All of the above are perceived to be especially true in patients with advanced disease (48). In order to dispel these misconceptions, a large database of tolerability of beta-blockers in the management of heart failure can be drawn up on from a variety of sources. These include data from the placebo-controlled clinical trial experience across a broad spectrum of heart failure severity; a large, open-label registry experience from everyday clinical practice; and, most recently, comprehensive analysis of the initiation process of beta-blockers within major trials (48).

Markers of Tolerability of Drug Therapy

There are a number of generic markers of how well a patient is able to tolerate the introduction and maintenance of a prescribed drug. These include the adverse event profile, permanent treatment discontinuation rates, mean achieved dose in relation to the target dose of the drug, and the percent of patients reaching target dose.

Data from Clinical Trials

Tolerability in clinical trials based on percent drug discontinuation can be observed to be less with the beta-blocking agent than with placebo in all of the major trials conducted (35,36,39,41,42,49). Risk ratios range from 0.73 to 1.0. The mean achieved dose in these trials has been found to be of the order of 80% or higher in relation to the target dose (Table 28-1) (48). To put this in perspective, the mean achieved dose in the ACE inhibitor trials was of a lower percentage than this in relation to target dose; we must also remember that the beta-blocker trials were conducted on top of background ACE inhibitor therapy.

Open-Label Experience

There also exists a large open-label experience, particularly with the agent carvedilol. In this experience, tolerability (defined as percent of patients remaining on therapy at the time of evaluation and having been on therapy for at least 3 months) was between 69% and 95% (48). Furthermore, the mean achieved dose among these patients was relatively high, being between 30 and 51 mg per day (48). While these data are not controlled, they are important because these represent the experiences of prescribers in everyday clinical practice, as distinct from the highly motivated investigators and carefully selected patients involved in clinical trial research programs.

Tolerability During Initiation of Therapy

The early initiation experience of two major trials has been reported. In the MERIT-HF trial (50), there was a slight excess of discontinuations with metoprolol compared with placebo over the first 3 months of therapy, in contrast to slightly fewer withdrawals with metoprolol by the end of the study. This early excess of discontinuations was particularly prominent among the more advanced NYHA class III–IV patients. Therefore, these data supported the historical paradigm that there may be poorer tolerability during the initial phase of introduction of beta-blocker.

There was no early excess of permanent withdrawals with carvedilol within the COPERNICUS study (51), an overall more advanced group of heart failure patients. Furthermore, this remained true even when a high-risk subset of 624 patients (with frequent or recurrent hospitalization, very low ejection fraction, and/or need for intravenous therapy) was studied.

There were fewer major cardiovascular events or mortality in the carvedilol group, compared to placebo, in the COPERNICUS study during the first 8 weeks. Interestingly, this was particularly true within the highest-risk subset of patients. The point estimates for the relative risk of these early events was similar to that observed for the overall study, suggesting that the well-demonstrated

TABLE 28-1

KEY TOLERABILITY PARAMETERS IN LARGE-SCALE CHRONIC HEART FAILURE TRIALS OF BETA-BLOCKERS (N >1,000)

Study and Reference	β-blocker studied	Total (n)	NYHA class	Study Duration (mo)	Study Drug Discontinuation (RR)	Mean Achieved Dose as % of Target Dose	% Reaching Target Dose	Serious Adverse Events Excluding Death (RR)
BEST (42)	Bucindolol	2,708	III–IV	24	0.92	152*		
CIBIS II (39)	Bisoprolol	2,647	III–IV	15.6	1	86	57.5	
COMET (49)	Carvedilol vs metoprolol IR	3,029	II–IV	58	1.0	83.6	Carvedilol, 76 Metoprolol IR, 78	0.97†
COPERNICUS (37)	Carvedilol	2,289	III–IV	10.4	0.84	86	74	0.88
MERIT-HF (41)	Metoprolol CR/XL	3,991	II–IV	15	0.9	79.5	64	
US Carvedilol (35)	Carvedilol	1,094	II–IV	7	0.73	90‡	80	

BEST, Beta-Blocker Evaluation of Survival Trial; CIBIS II, Cardiac Insufficiency Bisoprolol Study II; COMET, Carvedilol or Metoprolol European Trial; COPERNICUS, Carvedilol Prospective Randomized Cumulative Study; CR/XL, controlled/extended release; IR, immediate release; MERIT-HF, Metoprolol CR/XL Randomized Intervention Trial in Congestive Heart Failure; NYHA, New York Heart Association; RR, relative risk; US Carvedilol, U.S. Carvedilol Heart Failure Study.

*Based on target of 100 mg/day. However, 200 mg/day target dose in patients weighing >75 kg.

†Carvedilol vs metoprolol.

‡Based on target dose of 50 mg/day. However, 100 mg/day target dose in patients weighing >85 kg.

efficacy and safety of carvedilol over the entirety of the COPERNICUS study were similar to that of the first 8 weeks of therapy. Indeed, it could be argued that much of the benefit of beta-blocker therapy occurred early, which challenges the paradigm that there is a delay in benefit of beta-blocker therapy in advanced heart failure patients.

CHOICE OF BETA-ADRENOCEPTOR-BLOCKER IN CONGESTIVE HEART FAILURE

Beta-adrenoceptor-blocking drugs are a heterogeneous therapeutic group with many individual agents possessing unique pharmacological properties (52) (Table 28-2). Key pharmacological differences among beta-adrenoceptor-blockers include relative selectivity for the beta-1 and beta-2 adrenoceptor, possession of additional vasodilator properties, differential effects on beta-adrenoceptor upregulation, and a variety of ancillary properties. It is unclear which, if any, of these properties may be of substantial clinical significance. However, clinical and laboratory assessment of a number of these agents permit some cautious observations to be made.

The use of a drug that possesses a vasodilator component may be useful in helping overcome the initial negative inotropy of the beta-adrenoceptor-blocking component of the drug. Beta-adrenoceptor-blocker/-vasodilators appear to be better-tolerated than pure beta-adrenoceptor-blockers during initiation (53). It has been suggested by some that the vasodilator component (rather than the beta-adrenoceptor-blocking component) of these drugs underlies the drugs' beneficial effects. This is unlikely, however, as the vasodilating effects of drugs such as carvedilol are relatively modest and acute vasodilation disappears during chronic therapy with alpha-adrenoceptor-blockade and beta-adrenoceptor-blockade when used in combination (54).

A more important pharmacological property may be that agents such as carvedilol are relatively nonselective inhibitors of beta-1 versus beta-2 adrenoceptors. In heart failure, there is *selective* beta-1-adrenoceptor downregulation with relative preservation of beta-2-adrenoceptor density (relative percentages: beta-1 80% versus beta-2 20% in normal subjects compared with beta-1 60% versus beta-2 40% in CHF patients) (3). If beta-adrenoceptor-blockers truly act as a shield against the toxic effects of catecholamines on the myocardium, blockade of beta-2 adrenoceptors assumes greater significance. Transgenic models of beta-2 overexpression are associated with a heart failure phenotype and early mortality, further supporting this concept (54).

In support of this, one of the earliest studies to point toward a beneficial effect of beta-adrenoceptor-blockers in heart failure was the Beta-blocker Heart Attack Trial (BHAT) in postmyocardial infarction patients with heart failure (55). The beneficial effects seen in that study were with the prototype nonselective beta-adrenoceptor-blocker, propranolol. It has been further postulated that, at target heart failure doses, beta-1 selective agents may become nonselective and act pharmacologically more like agents such as carvedilol.

Beta-adrenoceptor upregulation cannot explain the beneficial effects observed with drugs such as carvedilol in heart failure. These drugs appear to possess a unique pharmacological property (guanine nucleotide modulatable binding) that prevents upregulation from occurring (17). Thus, the beneficial effects observed with carvedilol occur in the absence of beta-adrenoceptor upregulation. Even in the presence of drugs that *do* cause adrenoceptor upregulation (e.g., metoprolol), the beta-adrenoreceptor is nearly completely blocked at pharmacological doses of the drug and, therefore, putative improved inotropic effects that may result from upregulation of receptors and postreceptor activation of cAMP would be blocked at the level of the receptor.

Some drugs possess ancillary properties (52) that have been demonstrated in vitro and may turn out to be of clinical relevance. For example, carvedilol possesses both antiproliferative (56) and antioxidant (57) properties that theoretically may play an important role in disease progression in heart failure. Heart failure is a state of increased oxidative stress and this may contribute to disease progression by stimulation of apoptosis (programmed cell death). Furthermore, carvedilol uniquely inhibits endothelin-1 production from cultured endothelial cells, and this appears to be independent of its beta-adrenoceptor-blocking, alpha-adrenoceptor-blocking, and antioxidant effects (58).

TABLE 28-2
PHARMACOLOGICAL PROPERTIES OF BETA-ADRENOCEPTOR BLOCKING AGENTS STUDIED IN HEART FAILURE

	Selectivity as β-Adrenoceptor Antagonist	Direct Vadilator Activity	Activity as α-Adrenoceptor Antagonist	Intrinsic Sympathomimemtic Activity	Ancillary Properties
Bisoprolol	$\beta_1 >> \beta_2$	−	−	−	−
Bucindolol	$\beta_1 = \beta_2$	+	−	−	−
Carvedilol	$\beta_1 = \beta_2$	+	+	−	++
Metoprolol	$\beta_1 >> \beta_2$	−	−	−	−
Nebivolol	$\beta_1 >> \beta_2$	+	−	−	−
Propranolol	$\beta_1 = \beta_2$	−	−	−	−
Xamoterol	$\beta_1 >> \beta_2$	−	−	++	−

The relative contribution of these ancillary properties versus the underlying beta-adrenoceptor-blocking effects of these drugs remains to be elucidated in further clinical studies. All of the above theoretical considerations point to the need for definitive, head-to-head trials to determine which agent is of the greatest benefit.

The COMET study (49) attempted to test this in a head-to-head comparison of 3,029 CHF patients receiving immediate-release metoprolol versus carvedilol. Doses studied were 25-mg, twice-daily of carvedilol and 50 mg, twice-daily of immediate-release metoprolol. The findings were a 17% reduction in mortality with carvedilol in comparison to immediate-release metoprolol; there was no difference in the coprimary endpoint of death or heart failure hospitalization. This study has led to a considerable debate as to the appropriateness of the choice of metoprolol formulation, dose, and dosing interval. In the study of a broad-based adrenergic therapy (carvedilol versus a beta-1 selective agent, metoprolol), it proved critical to match for beta-1-adrenoceptor-blockade. A simple surrogate of this is reduction in resting heart rate. This parameter was similar through most of the study, with the exception of a small number of time points where carvedilol resulted in a lower heart rate. However, this is not quite so simple because (a) heart rate may be determined by differential effects on baroreceptor function and (b) carvedilol possesses vasodilator activity, as demonstrated by a significantly lower systolic and diastolic blood pressure at many time points in COMET. Clearly, a comparison with an agent that had been proven to be of clinical benefit, such as extended-release metoprolol at a target dose of 200 mg per day and/or bisoprolol at a target dose of 10 mg per day, would be the preferred study. However, it is unlikely that such a study will ever be performed.

APPROACH TO MANAGEMENT OF THE HEART FAILURE PATIENT WITH BETA-ADRENOCEPTOR-BLOCKERS

Two decades of administration of beta-adrenoceptor-blockers to patients with heart failure has taught us much about how to safely administer these agents to these patients. It is clear that the major difficulties with the use of these agents tend to occur during the initiation and uptitration phases of treatment.

Overall, about 50% of patients report worsening symptoms during the uptitration phase (48), although this figure may be exacerbated by the concerns of the treating physician. Nevertheless, it is worth persisting with strategies to achieve target doses of beta-adrenoceptor-blockers, as patients who experience difficulties during uptitration are eventually conferred long-term clinical benefits similar to those who had no problems during initiation (59).

Problems during initiation include worsening of underlying heart failure and, particularly in patients receiving vasodilating beta-adrenoceptor-blockers, symptomatic postural hypotension. In order to minimize the possibility of these problems occurring, it is important to ensure that before initiation is attempted, patients are stable clinically and on stable doses of their concomitant medication. A beta-adrenoceptor-blocking drug should not be administered to patients with unstable or decompensated heart failure.

Very low doses of beta-adrenoceptor-blocker should be used at commencement (e.g., 3.125 mg carvedilol or 1.25 mg bisoprolol or 23.75 mg extended-release metoprolol), then uptitrated on a twice-weekly basis. Patients can generally be initiated in an out-patient setting and there is increasing data on the safety and utility of in-patient initiation during the index heart failure hospitalization.

Postural hypotension, if it is to occur, is generally seen early in patients receiving vasodilating beta-adrenoceptor-blockers . This can usually be effectively managed by temporarily reducing the dose of concomitant ACE inhibitor and/or diuretic to permit establishment and uptitration of the beta-adrenoceptor-blocker. Another useful modification to therapy is to separate the beta-adrenoceptor-blocker and ACE inhibitor dosage time by 3 hours or more to allow the vasodilator effects of one drug to wear off before the next drug is administered. If worsening heart failure occurs with beta-adrenoceptor-blocker initiation, this can generally be treated by an increase in diuretic dose, which usually permits stabilization of the condition. If necessary, a delay in scheduled uptitration of beta-adrenoceptor-blocker may be required.

Atrioventricular block is another potential adverse effect of beta-blockade. This is less likely to be a problem in the current era of cardiac resynchronization therapy (CRT) pacemakers, but needs to be monitored carefully in non-paced patients, especially during the establishment phase.

Can we predict which patients will tolerate beta-adrenoceptor-blockers during initiation? It would be expected that patients most reliant upon sympathetic activation to maintain cardiac output (i.e., patients with severe chronic heart failure) would be those with the greatest difficulties during initiation. However, it has not as yet been definitively demonstrated how systolic blood pressure, high plasma urea, and advanced age were identified as independent factors for nontolerability of carvedilol in the Carvedilol Open-Label Assessment (COLA) I study (60). Therefore, extremely elderly patients as well as patients with borderline hypotension and renal impairment require close supervision during initiation of therapy.

It has now been determined that in-patient commencement of therapy is safe and leads to lower withdrawal rates from therapy, provided the patient has been clinically stabilized prior to beta-blocker initiation (61).

UNANSWERED QUESTIONS WITH BETA-BLOCKERS IN HEART FAILURE

Unexplored Indications with Beta-Blockers

There are two groups of CHF patients who have not been well characterized with regard to beta-blockers, despite the extensive database already accumulated with these agents. First, patients with asymptomatic left ventricular systolic dysfunction have not been prospectively studied as a group, remote from myocardial infarction. This study would be analogous to the SOLVD-Prevention trial conducted in the late 1980s with the ACE inhibitor enalapril (62). Most studies would be composed of patients who were symptomatic of their systolic dysfunction at one point but rendered asymptomatic with the use of diuretics and ACE inhibitors.

There is, as mentioned, very little data within this group of patients. A subgroup (30%) of the Australia-New Zealand carvedilol study (36) of patients with ischemic cardiomyopathy were asymptomatic at time of entry. Their response to beta-blocker therapy appeared to be similar to that of the symptomatic patients. However, formal prospective trial data are needed in this setting. Patients in the *immediate* post-MI period have already been adequately addressed in the Carvedilol Post-Infarct Survival Control in LV Dysfunction (CAPRICORN) study (63).

The second group of patients not well-studied is composed of those with preserved systolic function (or diastolic) heart failure. Diastolic heart failure encompasses a large group of increasingly well-recognized patients (64). In this setting, systolic ventricular function is usually either normal or even supernormal and, thus, diagnosis is somewhat difficult, reliant on exclusion of other contributors to heart failure symptoms (primarily respiratory), as well as often subtle evidence of impaired cardiac relaxation on echocardiography. Perhaps because of this difficulty in defining a (pure) diastolic heart failure population, there have been very few placebo-controlled therapeutic clinical trials within this setting.

Mechanistically, beta-blockers would be expected to substantially benefit diastolic heart failure patients. This is because ventricular dysfunction in this setting is often contributed to by myocardial ischemia, impaired diastolic filling, and poor control of systemic hypertension. A recent 6-month, placebo-controlled trial of carvedilol in the setting of diastolic dysfunction demonstrated a borderline significant improvement in the E wave to A wave (E/A) ratio, a key marker of diastolic dysfunction, but no change in relevant ventricular dimensions (65). More recently, the SENIORS trial (18) demonstrated a similar trend toward reduced mortality/heart failure hospitalization in patients above/below an ejection fraction of 35%. Longer-term trials assessing clinical outcome are urgently needed for beta-blockers (as well as other putative agents) in the specific setting of diastolic heart failure.

Which Agent (Beta-Blocker or ACE Inhibitor) to Use First in Heart Failure?

A key question in CHF therapeutics is the order in which life-saving drugs should be prescribed. The conventional approach has been to initially use an ACE inhibitor, with a beta-blocker then given if the patient remains symptomatic. Although this is a very effective therapeutic strategy (more than halving all-cause mortality in meta-analyses of major clinical trials), this order is purely historical and without any real scientific justification. It is explained by ACE inhibitors having been available and proven as a beneficial CHF therapy before beta-blockers were first used for this indication. A key question, therefore, is whether these drugs would be just as beneficial (if not more so) given the other way around (i.e., a beta-blocker first, followed by an ACE inhibitor), as required. Mechanistic arguments as to why beta-blocker therapy may be a preferred first-line neurohormonal agent in HF include:

- Sympathetic activation occurs ahead of renin-angiotensin activation in the heart failure process.
- The magnitude of LV remodeling regression appears to be greater with beta-blockers than ACE inhibitors in placebo-controlled trials.
- Beta-blockers powerfully inhibit renin release via blockade of renal sympathetic activation.

The CARMEN study (66) examining the impact of these agents on ventricular remodeling has provided interesting surrogate data regarding this issue. In CARMEN, patients were randomized to receive a beta-blocker (carvedilol), an ACE inhibitor (enalapril), or both, with left ventricular remodeling parameters after 18 months of therapy as the primary endpoint of the trial. The results suggest that beta-blockers as monotherapy are as effective, if not more so, than ACE inhibitors at improving ventricular dimensions (reverse remodeling), with both drugs given together being most effective and seemingly safe. These observations are consistent with those made in earlier trials of beta-blockade, in which the magnitude of the improvement in ventricular remodelling by beta-blockers appeared greater than that observed with ACE inhibitors, even though they were given in addition to background ACE inhibitor treatment.

Remodeling is, however, a surrogate endpoint and more definitive trials are required before a change in treatment strategy can be advocated within CHF guidelines. Such a trial is currently being conducted (CIBIS III) (67). In this study, patients are being randomized to receive bisoprolol or ACE inhibitor monotherapy for a period of up to 6 months. The alternative drug class can be added at the investigator's discretion, as clinically necessary; however, this constitutes a study secondary endpoint. After 6 months, patients are mandated to receive the alternative agent if they have not already done so. Major events (e.g., death, hospitalization) over 12 months of total therapy is the primary endpoint of this study.

Pharmacogenomics of Beta-Blockers in Heart Failure

The coming revolution of pharmacogenomics promises to impact the use of beta-blocker therapies in the treatment of CHF. There are specific beta-adrenoceptor polymorphisms (both β_1 and β_2) that may impact the utility of beta-blockers both in terms of adverse effects and clinical efficacy. In addition, the ACE insertion (I)/deletion (D) polymorphism may influence the benefits of beta-blocker therapy. Specifically, among patients with the DD genotype (associated with greatest renin-angiotensin system activation and worst prognosis) there is a beneficial impact of beta-blocker therapy on prognosis (68). However, in II or ID patients there is no additional prognostic benefit observed with beta-blocker therapy. These data suggest a potentially important genetic influence on sympathetically mediated disease progression in human heart failure. Large-scale studies are required to determine the benefits (or otherwise) of guiding therapy based on the above polymorphisms.

Interactions with Novel Heart Failure Therapies

Another key issue for beta-blockers is their use with novel therapies for the treatment of heart failure. For example, biventricular pacing appears to be an important advance in therapy in selected CHF patients. Clearly, we need to know whether there is an incremental benefit of this therapy additional to patients optimally treated with ACE inhibitors and beta-blockers. Although such subgroup analyses have been performed from the biventricular pacing studies, perhaps now is the time for a formal study with beta-blocker and ACE inhibitor therapy mandated in all patients as an entry criterion for these studies.

Similarly, use of stem cell therapies promises a revolution in the treatment of heart failure. Most of the preliminary work in animal models, however, has occurred in the absence of standard, background heart failure therapies. The magnitude of the ventricular function improvements with stem cell therapies is not dissimilar to that observed with drug therapies. Therefore, the question arises (both in these experimental studies and ultimately in human patients) as to whether a substantial and clinically important increment can be observed over and above standard pharmacological therapies, including beta-blockers.

CONCLUSIONS

Beta-blockers have been a major advance in the pharmacological management of the heart failure patient and are a tribute to the persistence and mechanistic mind-set of an early group of Swedish pioneers. Beta-blockers have, however, been slow to be embraced by physicians, particularly because of what could be called the baggage of the past regarding perceived contraindications in this setting. Furthermore, there remain fears surrounding the tolerability and adverse effects of initiation of these agents, which have largely been put to rest by increasingly robust safety data, even toward the more severe end of the heart failure disease spectrum.

The challenge over the next few years is to ensure that all appropriate patients receive these agents; that currently unexplored indications are evaluated in properly conducted clinical trials; and that the place of these agents is clearly defined in the new arena of devices and cell-based therapies.

REFERENCES

1. Packer M. The neurohormonal hypothesis: a theory to explain the mechanism of disease progression in heart failure. *J Am Coll Cardiol.* 1992;20:248–254.
2. Francis GS, Goldsmith SR, Olivari MT, et al. The neurohormonal axis in congestive heart failure. *Am Intern Med.* 1984;101:370–377.
3. Bristow MR, Hershberger RE, Port JD, et al. β-adrenergic pathways in nonfailing and failing human ventricular myocardium. *Circulation.* 1990;82(Suppl I):12–25.
4. Hasking GJ, Esler MD, Jennings GI, et al. Norepinephrine spillover to plasma in patients with congestive heart failure: evidence of increased overall and cardiorenal sympathetic nervous activity. *Circulation.* 1986;73:615–621.
5. Chidsey CA, Braunwald E, Morrow AG. Catecholamine excretion and cardiac stores of norepinephrine in congestive heart failure. *Am J Med.* 1965;39:442–451.
6. Mann DL, Kent RL, Pardons B, et al. Adrenergic effects on the biology of the adult mammalian cardiocyte. *Circulation.* 1992;85:790–804.
7. Hasenfuss G, Holubarsch C, Blanchard EM, et al. Influence of isoproterenol on myocardial energetics. Experimental and clinical investigations. *Basic Research Cardiol.* 1989;84(Supp 1):147–155.
8. Meredith IT, Eisenhofer G, Lambert GW, et al. Cardiac sympathetic nervous activity in congestive heart failure: evidence for increased neuronal norepinephrine release and preserved neuronal uptake. *Circulation.* 1993;88:136–145.
9. Yates JC, Beamish RE, Dhalla NS. Ventricular dysfunction and necrosis produced by adrenochrome metabolite of epinephrine. Relation to pathogenesis of catecholamine cardiomyopathy. *Am Heart J.* 1981;102:210–221.
10. The Xamoterol in Severe Heart Failure Study Group. Xamoterol in severe heart failure. *Lancet.* 1990;336:1–6.
11. Packer M, Carver JR, Rodeheffer RJ, et al. Effect of oral milrinone on mortality in severe chronic congestive heart failure. *N Engl J Med.* 1991;325:1468–1475.
12. Krum H, Liew D. New and emerging drug therapies for the management of acute heart failure. *Intern Med J.* 2003;11:515–520.
13. Cohn JN, Levine B, Olivari MT, et al. Plasma norepinephrine as a guide to prognosis in patients with chronic congestive heart failure. *N Engl J Med.* 1984;311:819–823.
14. Kaye DM, Lefkovits J, Jennings GL, et al. Adverse consequences of high sympathetic nervous activity in the failing human heart. *J Am Coll Cardiol.* 1995;26(5):1257–1263
15. Fowler MB, Laser JA, Hopkins GL, et al. Assessment of the β-adrenergic receptor pathway in the intact failing human heart: progressive receptor downregulation and subsensitivity to agonist response. *Circulation.* 1986;74:1290–1302.
16. Fowler MB. Controlled trials with beta blockers in heart failure: metoprolol as the prototype. *Am J Cardiol.* 1993;71:45C–53C.
17. Bristow MR, Larabee P, Muller-Beckmann, et al. Effect of carvedilol on adrenergic pharmacology in human ventricular myocardium and lymphocytes. *Clin Invest.* 1992;70:S105–S113.
18. Flather MD, Shibata MC, Coats AJ, et al., SENIORS Investigators. Randomized trial to determine the effect of nebivolol on mortality and cardiovascular hospital admission in elderly patients with heart failure (SENIORS). *Eur Heart J.* 2005;26:215–225.
19. Andreka P, Aiyar N, Olson LC, et al. Bucindolol displays intrinsic sympathomimetic activity in human myocardium. *Circulation.* 2002;105:2429–2434.
20. Hershberger RE, Wynn JR, Sundberg L, et al. Mechanism of action of bucindolol in human ventricular myocardium. *J Cardiovasc Pharmacol.* 1990;15:959–967.
21. Cohn JN, Goldstein SO, Greenberg BH, et al. A dose-dependent increase in mortality with vesnarinone among patients with severe heart failure. Vesnarinone Trial Investigators. *N Engl J Med.* 1998;339 (25):1810–1816.
22. Moe GW, Rouleau JL, Charbonneau L, et al. Neurohormonal activation in severe heart failure: relations to patient death and the effect of treatment with flosequinan. *Am Heart J.* 2000;139(4): 587–595.
23. Girbes AR, Zijlstra JG. Ibopamine and survival in severe congestive heart failure: PRIME II. *Lancet.* 1997;350(9071):147–148.
24. Swedberg K. Initial experience with beta blockers in dilated cardiomyopathy. *Am J Cardiol.* 1993;71:30C–38C
25. Waagstein F, Hjalmarson A, Varnauskas E, et al. Effect of chronic beta adrenergic receptor blockade in congestive cardiomyopathy. *Br Heart J.* 1975;37:1022–1026.
26. Swedberg K, Hjalmarson A, Waagstein F, et al. Prolongation of survival in congestive cardiomyopathy by beta-receptor blockade. *Lancet.* 1979;i:1374–1376.
27. Currie PJ, Kelly MJ, McKenzie A, et al. Oral beta-adrenergic blockade with metoprolol in chronic severe dilated cardiomyopathy. *J Am Coll Cardiol.* 1984;3:203–209.
28. Anderson JL, Lutz JR, Gilbert EM, et al. A randomized trial of low-dose beta blockade therapy for idiopathic dilated cardiomyopathy. *Am J Cardiol.* 1985;55:471–475.
29. Krum H, Sackner-Bernstein JD, Goldsmith R, et al. Double-blind, placebo-controlled study of the long-term efficacy of carvedilol in severe chronic heart failure. *Circulation.* 1995;92:1499–1506.

30. Engelmeier RS, O'Connell JB, Walsh R, et al. Improvement in symptoms and exercise tolerance by metoprolol in patients with dilated cardiomyopathy: a double-blind, randomized, placebo-controlled trial. *Circulation.* 1985;72:536–546.
31. Gilbert EM, Anderson JL, Deitchman D, et al. Long-term β-blocker vasodilator therapy improves cardiac function in idiopathic dilated cardiomyopathy: a double-blind, randomized study of bucindolol versus placebo. *Am J Med.* 1990;88:223–229.
32. Woodley SL, Gilbert EM, Anderson JL, et al. β-blockade with bucindolol in heart failure caused by ischemic versus idiopathic dilated cardiomyopathy. *Circulation.* 1991;84:2426–2441.
33. Krum H, Gu A, Wilshire-Clement M, et al. Changes in plasma endothelin-1 levels reflect clinical response to β-blockade in chronic heart failure. *Am Heart J.* 1996;131:337–341.
34. Goldsmith RL, Bigger JT, Bloomfield DM, et al. Long-term carvedilol therapy increases parasympathetic nervous system activity in chronic congestive heart failure. *Am J Cardiol.* 1997;80: 1101–1104.
35. Packer M, Bristow MR, Cohn JN, et al. The effect of carvedilol on morbidity and mortality in patients with chronic heart failure. *N Engl J Med.* 1996;334:1349–1355.
36. Australia-New Zealand Heart Failure Research Collaborative Group. Randomized, placebo-controlled trial of carvedilol in patients with congestive heart failure due to ischemic heart disease. *Lancet.* 1997;349:375–380.
37. Packer M, Coats AJ, Fowler MB, et al. Effect of carvedilol on survival in severe chronic heart failure. *N Engl J Med.* 2001;344: 1651–1658.
38. CIBIS Investigators and Committees. A randomised trial of β-blockade in heart failure. The Cardiac Insufficiency Bisoprolol Study (CIBIS). *Circulation.* 1994;90:1765–1773.
39. CIBIS II Investigators and Committees. The Cardiac Insufficiency Bisoprolol Study (CIBIS II): a randomised trial. *Lancet.* 1999;353: 9–13.
40. Waagstein F, Bristow MR, Swedberg K, et al. Beneficial effect of metoprolol in idiopathic dilated cardiomyopathy. *Lancet.* 1993; 342:1441–1446.
41. Metoprolol CR/XL Randomised Intervention Trial in Congestive Heart Failure (MERIT-HF) Study Group. Effect of metoprolol CR/XL in chronic heart failure. *Lancet.* 1999;353:2001–2007.
42. Beta-Blocker Evaluation of Survival Trial Investigators. A trial of the beta-blocker bucindolol in patients with advanced chronic heart failure. *N Engl J Med.* 2001;344:1659–1667.
43. Cohn JN, Pfeffer MA, Rouleau J, et al., MOXCON Investigators. Adverse mortality effect of central sympathetic inhibition with sustained-release moxonidine in patients with heart failure (MOXCON). *Eur J Heart Fail.* 2003;5:659–667.
44. Ghali JK, Pina IL, Gottlieb SS, et al. Metoprolol CR/XL in female patients with heart failure: analysis of the experience in Metoprolol Extended-Release Randomized Intervention Trial in Heart Failure (MERIT-HF). *Circulation..* 2002;105: 1585–1591.
45. Yancy CW, Fowler MB, Colucci WS, et al. Race and the response to adrenergic blockade with carvedilol in patients with chronic heart failure. *N Engl J Med.* 2001;344(18):1358–1365.
46. Dulin BR, Haas SJ, Abraham WT, et al. Do elderly systolic heart failure patients benefit from beta blockers to the same extent as the non-elderly? Meta-analysis of >12,000 patients in large-scale clinical trials. *Am J Cardiol.* 2005;95:896–898.
47. Haas SJ, Vos T, Gilbert RE, et al. Are beta-blockers as efficacious in patients with diabetes mellitus as in patients without diabetes mellitus who have chronic heart failure? A meta-analysis of large-scale clinical trials. *Am Heart J.* 2003;146:848–853.
48. Krum H. Tolerability of carvedilol in heart failure: clinical trials experience. *Am J Cardiol.* 2004;93(9A):58B–63B.
49. Poole-Wilson PA, Swedberg K, Cleland JG, et al., Carvedilol Or Metoprolol European Trial Investigators. Comparison of carvedilol and metoprolol on clinical outcomes in patients with chronic heart failure in the Carvedilol Or Metoprolol European Trial (COMET): randomised controlled trial. *Lancet.* 2003;362:7–13.
50. Gottlieb SS, Fischer ML, Kjekshus J, et al. MERIT-HF: tolerability of β-blocker initiation NYHA II, III, & IV CHF *Circulation.* 2000;102(Suppl II):II-778 [Abstract].
51. Krum H, Roecker EB, Mohacsi P, et al., Carvedilol Prospective Randomized Cumulative Survival (COPERNICUS) Study Group. Effects of initiating carvedilol in patients with severe chronic heart failure: results from the COPERNICUS Study. *JAMA.* 2003;289: 712–718.
52. Krum H. Beta-adrenoceptor blockers in chronic heart failure—a review. *Br J Clin Pharmacol.* 1997;44:111–118.
53. Eichhorn EJ. The paradox of β-adrenergic blockade for the management of congestive heart failure. *Am J Med.* 1992;92:527–538.
54. Du XJ, Gao XM, Wang B, et al. Age-dependent cardiomyopathy and heart failure phenotype in mice overexpressing beta (2)-adrenergic receptors in the heart. *Cardiovasc Res.* 2000;48:448–454.
55. Chadda K, Goldstein CK, Byington R, et al. Effect of propranolol after acute myocardial infarction in patients with heart failure. *Circulation.* 1986:73:503–510.
56. Ohlstein EH, Douglas SA, Sung CP, et al. Carvedilol, a cardiovascular drug, prevents vascular smooth muscle cell proliferation, migration and neointimal formation following vascular injury. *Proc Natl Acad Sci USA.* 1993;90:6189–6193.
57. Yue T-L, Cheng H-Y, Lysko PG, et al. Carvedilol, a new vasodilator and beta adrenoceptor antagonist, is an antioxidant and free radical scavenger. *J Pharmacol Exp Ther.* 1992;263:92–98.
58. Ohlstein EH, Arleth AJ, Storer B, et al. Carvedilol inhibits endothelin-1 biosynthesis in cultured human coronary artery endothelial cells. *J Mol Cell Cardiol.* 1998;30:167–173.
59. Sackner-Bernstein J, Krum H, Goldsmith RL, et al. Should worsening heart failure early after initiation of beta-blocker therapy for chronic heart failure preclude long-term treatment? *Circulation.* 1995;92(Suppl I):I-395. [Abstract].
60. Krum H, Ninio D, MacDonald P. Baseline predictors of tolerability to carvedilol in patients with chronic heart failure. *Heart* 2000;84:615–619.
61. Gattis WA, O'Connor CM, Gallup DS, et al., IMPACT-HF Investigators and Coordinators. Predischarge initiation of carvedilol in patients hospitalized for decompensated heart failure: results of the Initiation Management Predischarge: Process for Assessment of Carvedilol Therapy in Heart Failure (IMPACT-HF) trial. *J Am Coll Cardiol.* 2004;43:1534–1541.
62. The SOLVD Investigators. Effect of enalapril on mortality and the development of heart failure in asymptomatic patients with reduced left ventricular ejection fractions. *N Engl J Med.* 1992;327:685–691.
63. Dargie HJ. Effect of carvedilol on outcome after myocardial infarction in patients with left-ventricular dysfunction: the CAPRICORN randomised trial. *Lancet.* 2001;357(9266): 1385–1390.
64. Vasan RS. Diastolic heart failure. *BMJ.* 2003;327:1181–1182.
65. Bergstrom A, Andersson B, Edner M, et al. Effect of carvedilol on diastolic function in patients with diastolic heart failure and preserved systolic function. Results of the Swedish Doppler-Echocardiographic Study (SWEDIC). *Eur J Heart Fail.* 2004;6: 453–461.
66. Remme WJ, Riegger G, Hildebrandt P, et al. The benefits of early combination treatment of carvedilol and an ACE-inhibitor in mild heart failure and left ventricular systolic dysfunction. The carvedilol and ACE-inhibitor remodelling mild heart failure evaluation trial (CARMEN). *Cardiovasc Drugs Ther.* 2004;18:57–66.
67. Willenheimer R, Erdmann E, Follath F, et al., CIBIS-III Investigators. Comparison of treatment initiation with bisoprolol vs. enalapril in chronic heart failure patients: rationale and design of CIBIS-III. *Eur J Heart Fail.* 2004;6:493–500.
68. McNamara DM, Holubkov R, Janosko K, et al. Pharmacogenetic interactions between beta-blocker therapy and the angiotensin-converting enzyme deletion polymorphism in patients with congestive heart failure. *Circulation.* 2001;103: 1644–1648.

Inotropic Agents

29

Ozlem Soran *Arthur M. Feldman*

ORAL AND INTRAVENOUS INOTROPIC AGENTS

As noted elsewhere in this text, the primary hemodynamic abnormality in patients with congestive heart failure (CHF) secondary to the presence of a dilated cardiomyopathy is systolic dysfunction. Although dilated cardiomyopathic hearts also demonstrate some degree of diastolic dysfunction, it is the inability to maintain an appropriate cardiac output during stress or at rest that is responsible, in large part, for the symptoms of shortness of breath, edema, and fatigue that characterize patients with this disease. For this reason, physicians turned to inotropes—pharmacologic agents that augment ventricular function—as important therapeutic agents in the management of patients with both acute and chronic congestive heart failure.

Although these agents would intuitively be expected to improve cardiac output and, in so doing, ameliorate both the signs and symptoms of congestive heart failure, their use has been associated with long-standing controversy. Initially, investigators proposed that the use of an inotropic agent would be analogous to flogging a dead horse, as it was generally believed that the contractile apparatus could not be further stimulated because of irreversible structural and biological damage. More recently, the use of inotropic agents has been associated with increased mortality in a group of large, multicenter, randomized, and placebo-controlled clinical trials. However, it remains unclear as to whether an inotropic agent might have advantageous effects in specific subsets of patients or whether the deleterious effects of the inotropic agents developed to date are primarily caused by their ancillary properties rather than by their inherent ability to improve myocardial contractility.

CLASSIFICATION OF INOTROPIC AGENTS

One dilemma in evaluating inotropic agents and their role in the therapy of CHF has been that all inotropic agents have been viewed in a generic sense. That is, regardless of mechanism of action or ancillary properties, all inotropic agents are thought to be equal. However, over the past two decades it has been clearly shown that myocardial contractility could be enhanced by activating or inhibiting a variety of biochemical pathways within the myocyte. In addition, our understanding of excitation–contraction coupling in both the normal and the failing heart has become far more sophisticated, leading to the identification of new and novel therapeutic targets. Finally, the use of recombinant molecular technology has led to the production of selective human proteins that can modify myocardial contractility. Thus, it now becomes important to classify inotropic agents according to their mechanisms of action and view them selectively rather than generically.

Initially, investigators classified inotropic agents according to their route of delivery (i.e., oral versus intravenous). As will be seen later in this chapter, although this classification was useful in describing existing agents it has not proven useful in classifying the many new and unique agents that have recently been developed. More recently, we proposed a method of classification based on the mechanism of action of the various agents (Table 29-1) (1). This allows the caregiver to correlate basic physiology with clinical actions, helps to clarify the potential synergistic

TABLE 29-1
CLASSES OF INOTROPIC AGENTS BY MECHANISM OF ACTION

Class	Definition
I	Agents that increase intracellular cAMP β-adrenergic agonists Phosphodiesterase inhibitors
II	Agents that affect sarcolemmal ion pumps/channels Digoxin
III	Agents that modulate intracellular calcium mechanisms by either: Release of sarcoplasmic reticulum calcium (IP_3)* Increased sensitization of the contractile proteins to calcium
IV	Drugs having multiple mechanisms of action Pimobendan Vesnarinone

*IP_3, inositol trisphosphate.

effects of some of the inotropic agents, and points out the class effects of some of these agents.

Inotropic Agents that Modulate Ion Channel Activity: the Cardiac Glycosides

Over 200 years ago, William Withering first noted that an extract of the foxglove plant was of benefit in the management of patients with CHF. In his initial report, Withering noted that the foxglove plant decreased edema in over 209 patients with dropsy (congestive heart failure) (2). However, subsequent reports by Bouillaud in 1835 (3) and Lewis in 1919 (4) suggested that digoxin was of benefit only in those patients with atrial fibrillation because of its ability to control heart rate in these patients. In contrast, Mackenzie and Christian (5,6) were early proponents of the use of digoxin in patients with normal sinus rhythm, publishing a review of the available literature in 1920. This controversy persisted into the 1990s and was fueled to some degree by reports noting an increase in mortality in patients receiving digoxin after suffering a myocardial infarction (MI) (7,8), as well as highly disparate reports regarding the clinical efficacy of digoxin (5,9–13). However, as noted later, recent large, multicenter, randomized, and placebo-controlled clinical trials have supported the benefits of digoxin in patients with CHF first noted by Withering two centuries ago.

The first conclusive demonstrations of the inotropic properties of digoxin came in 1927 when Wiggers and Stinson showed that digoxin could evoke a positive inotropic effect in the intact heart when heart rate and afterload were kept constant (14). Similarly, digoxin was shown to increase force generation in isolated cardiac muscle with expected shifts in the force–velocity relationships (15,16). More recently, studies in humans confirmed these initial findings in the laboratory, as digoxin enhanced myocardial contractility and increased stroke volume for a given preload and afterload (5). Of equal significance was that digoxin was also found to have a negative chronotropic effect as a result of parasympathetic activation and enhanced vagal tone, and also that it has anti-adrenergic properties (17,18). The effects of digoxin on cardiac contractility are generally accepted as resulting from increased availability of intracellular calcium (19). This increase in intracellular calcium concentration is secondary to inhibition of the sodium-potassium ATPase with a concomitant increase in cellular calcium transport in order to normalize electrolyte gradients (20). However, cardiac glycosides also have potent autonomic effects that can attenuate impaired arterial and cardiopulmonary baroreflex mechanisms in models of CHF (17).

The controversy surrounding the use of digoxin in the management of patients with CHF resulted partly from an inability to assay serum digoxin levels until 1969 (21). The ability to assay digoxin levels was important in understanding the clinical pharmacology of these products. Oral digoxin is absorbed by the gastrointestinal tract and excreted largely by the kidneys with a serum half-life of approximately 36 hours. Its excretion does not appear to be affected by either renal tubular absorption or secretion. However, approximately 20% to 25% of digoxin is protein-bound and, although digoxin is concentrated in the heart and kidneys, digoxin receptors are also present in skeletal muscle. Thus, patients with cardiac cachexia, the elderly, and those with renal dysfunction are prone to digoxin toxicity as a result of marked increases in digoxin concentrations (22). In addition, a variety of drugs and factors affecting gastrointestinal absorption can also alter the bioavailability of digoxin, including (a) cathartics and antacids (23); (b) severe diarrhea (24); (c) cholesterol-binding agents (25); (d) edema of the bowel wall, as is often seen in patients with right-sided heart failure (26,27); and (e) the presence of the intestinal bacterium *Eubacterium lentum*. Also, a variety of drugs and conditions can alter digoxin levels, including omeprazole (28); antibiotic therapy (29); electrolyte abnormalities including hyperkalemia or hypokalemia and hypernatremia or hyponatremia, indomethacin (30); cyclosporine, spironolactone (31); quinidine (32); verapamil (33); amiodarone (34); and propafenone (35). It is therefore imperative that digoxin doses be adjusted to account for the various pharmacologic and physiological factors that can influence digoxin levels, and that digoxin levels be monitored frequently during therapy.

Because of its relatively long half-life, many textbooks provide algorithms for loading digoxin either intravenously or orally to rapidly raise plasma digoxin levels without toxic effects. However, with the exception of patients in atrial fibrillation with rapid ventricular response, it is generally agreed that loading doses of digoxin are not necessary in the patient with CHF (36). Therefore, many physicians begin treatment empirically with 0.125 mg of digoxin per day with an increase to 0.250 mg per day if initial blood levels are low. Several studies have suggested a dose–response relationship between serum digoxin concentrations and hemodynamic effects (37,38). However, there is general agreement that the beneficial effects of digoxin can be obtained with a relatively low risk of toxicity when the serum level of digoxin is between 1.0 and 1.5 ng/mL (36). Because serum digoxin levels equilibrate approximately 12 hours after an oral dose, many physicians recommend that their patients take their digoxin at night so that morning blood samples will accurately reflect peak drug levels.

The use of digoxin in patients with CHF should always be undertaken with a clear recognition of the potential toxicities associated with its use. Clinically, digoxin toxicity can be divided into three major categories: gastrointestinal, neurologic, and cardiovascular. Gastrointestinal effects may include nausea, anorexia, abdominal pain, diarrhea, and vomiting (39). Neurologic toxicities include fatigue, headache, fatigue, visual changes, confusion, psychosis, and seizures; however, visual changes including halos around lights or enhanced yellow and green hues are almost pathognomonic for digoxin toxicity (40). Cardiovascular toxicities of digoxin are also diverse and may include virtually any type of arrhythmia or conduction disturbance (41). However, suspicion of digoxin toxicity should be heightened by the appearance of regularization of an irregular rhythm or a new bradyarrhythmia or tachyarrhythmia. The recent introduction of digoxin-specific antibody fragments has had a major impact on the therapy of digoxin toxicity (42). In a study of 150 patients with life-threatening digoxin intoxication, the use of digoxin-specific Fab antibody fragments was effective in over 90% of the patients, with adverse effects in fewer than 1% of patients.

A decade ago, a group of clinical studies evaluated the efficacy of digoxin in randomized studies. In a double-blind, placebo-controlled comparison of digoxin and the adrenergic agonist xamoterol (433 patients with chronic heart failure), digoxin was not effective in improving exercise duration, although it was associated with improvement in the tiredness associated with daily life as measured by the Likert scale (43). However, these patients were not well-characterized, as nearly 25% of the patients were in New York Heart Association (NYHA) Class I CHF, and the etiology of heart failure was not defined in a large number of the patients. In the Captopril-Digoxin Multicenter Research Group study, patients receiving diuretics were randomized to receive either captopril or digoxin (44). Digoxin treatment increased ejection fraction compared with captopril and placebo and decreased hospitalizations when compared with placebo. However, only captopril improved NYHA class or exercise time and digoxin was associated with an increase in ventricular ectopy.

Finally, DiBianco et al. compared oral milrinone, digoxin, and their combination in the treatment of patients with chronic heart failure (45). Treatment with digoxin significantly increased treadmill exercise time, reduced the frequency of decompensation from heart failure, and increased ejection fraction. However, it should be noted that a substantial number of patients failed to meet the entry criteria because of an inability to exercise. Although these studies suggested a beneficial effect of digoxin, they were not consistent in terms of either outcomes or patient enrollment. Furthermore, the studies were limited by an absence of therapy with angiotensin-converting enzyme (ACE) inhibitors, agents subsequently shown to improve survival and limit hospitalizations in this patient population (46,47).

Over the past decade, several seminal and large clinical trials have clearly demonstrated the utility of digoxin in the therapy of patients with CHF who were receiving concomitant therapy with an ACE inhibitor. In the RADIANCE study (Randomized Assessment of Digoxin on Inhibitors of the ANgiotensin-Converting Enzyme), patients with Class II or III heart failure and left ventricular ejection fractions of 35% or less who were receiving therapy with an ACE inhibitor and digoxin were randomized to having their digoxin continued or being switched to placebo (48). In these patients who were clinically stable while receiving diuretics, digoxin, and an ACE inhibitor, the withdrawal of digoxin was associated with worsening heart failure, deterioration in functional capacity, worsening quality of life, decreased ejection fractions, and increases in heart rate and body weight. In the most definitive assessment of the role of digoxin in the management of patients with chronic CHF, 6,800 patients with left ventricular ejection fractions of $<45\%$ and signs and symptoms of CHF were randomized to receive either digoxin or placebo (49). Physicians were strongly encouraged to treat patients with ACE inhibitors, and 94% of patients were receiving these medications; 81% of patients were receiving diuretics. When the primary endpoint of mortality was assessed, randomization to active therapy had no effect on survival over 52 months of follow-up. However, the use of digoxin was associated with 6% fewer hospitalizations, fewer hospitalizations for worsening heart failure, and a trend toward a decrease in the risk of death attributable to worsening heart failure ($p = 0.06$). In an ancillary trial, digoxin had similar effects in patients with dilated hearts but with ejection fractions $>45\%$. Thus, the results of this study suggest that in clinical practice digoxin therapy is likely to affect the frequency of hospitalizations without adversely affecting survival.

Several recent studies have strongly influenced our views regarding the role of digoxin in the treatment of heart failure. First, it has been recognized that serum digoxin concentrations in the therapeutic range (up to 2 ng per mL) could be associated with an increased frequency of hospitalizations for cardiovascular events other than heart failure and an increased risk of death due to arrhythmias or MI (50). Thus, physicians now recognize that digoxin doses that had previously been considered to be safe may adversely affect the heart, and some clinicians recommend that the digoxin dose be less than 1 ng per mL (51,52). Furthermore, heightened concern exists that digoxin may be contraindicated in patients who are post-MI and those with ongoing ischemia (53). Finally, a retrospective analysis of the Digoxin Investigation Group (DIG) trial suggested that while digoxin had modest effects in men, it had potentially adverse effects in women (54). Thus, because physicians now have an expanded armamentarium for the treatment of heart failure that includes agents such as β-blockers, ACE inhibitors, and aldosterone antagonists as well as new devices, enthusiasm for the use of digoxin has waned and its use has diminished. However, in patients who remain symptomatic despite optimal pharmacologic therapy, digoxin may still play a role in heart failure management.

It is important to note that digoxin has no beneficial properties in patients with diastolic dysfunction and its role in patients with minimal systolic function remains undefined. In addition, it is unclear whether patients who are asymptomatic but have dilated cardiomyopathies are candidates for receiving digoxin therapy. It should also be recognized that because of its positive inotropic properties, digoxin is contraindicated in patients with symptoms of heart failure secondary to hypertrophic cardiomyopathy, as it can worsen pre-existing outflow tract obstructions and increase left ventricular end-diastolic pressures.

Adrenergic Agonists and the Management of Patients with Congestive Heart Failure

The human myocardium relies on β-adrenergic stimulation to augment contractility when the need arises for increased cardiac output such as during exercise or stress (Fig. 29-1) (55,56). This is in contrast to many laboratory animal species such as the rat and the guinea pig, in which the heart is predominantly β/α_1- or H_2-histaminic, respectively (57–59). In addition, unlike many animal species, the human heart contains a balance of β_1- and β_2-adrenergic receptors that demonstrate marked differences in pharmacologic specificity and regulatory behavior (60,61). The human myocardium also contains a relatively small number of α_1-adrenergic receptors, which mediate inconsistent inotropic effects in isolated tissues (10). However, the α_1-receptors are coupled to myocardial cell growth in model systems and this receptor pathway may play a role in the development of cellular hypertrophy that accompanies the development of cardiac dilation and failure. Recent studies have identified the presence of β_3-adrenergic receptors; however, their role in the regulation of myocardial function has not yet been clearly defined (62–64).

The β-adrenergic receptor-coupled pathways have been extensively studied in both the normal and failing human

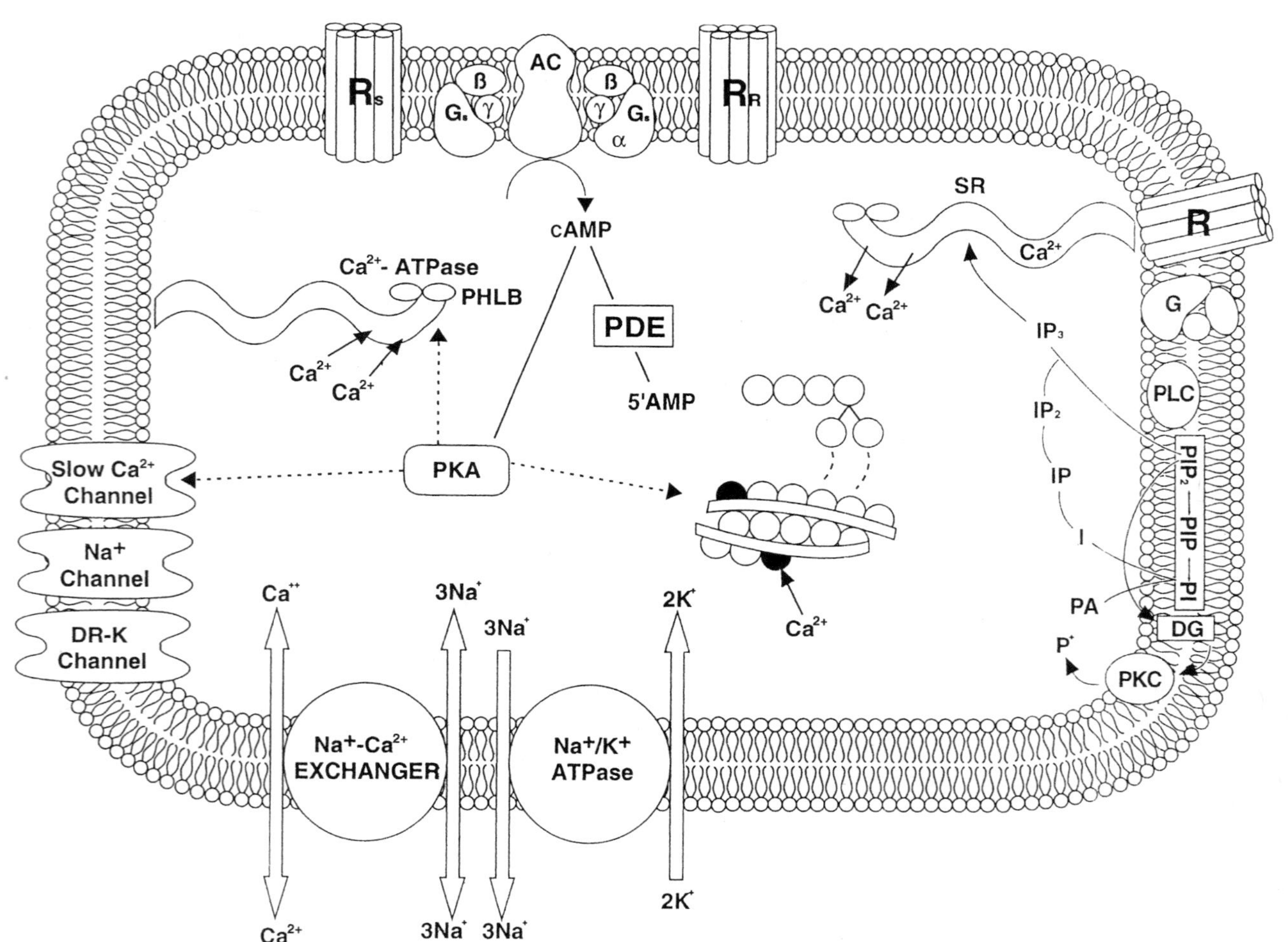

Figure 29-1 Biochemical pathways important in the regulation of cardiac contractility. AC, adenylyl cyclase; ATP, adenosine triphosphate; cAMP, cyclic adenosine monophosphate; DG, diacylglycerol; DR, delayed rectifier; G, guanine nucleotide-binding regulatory proteins that may stimulate (αG_s) or inhibit (αG_i) adenylyl cyclase; I, inositol; IP, inositol phosphate; IP_2, inositol bisphosphate; IP_3, inositol trisphosphate; PDE, phosphodiesterase; PHLB, phospholamban; PI, phosphatidylinositol; PIP, phosphatidylinositol 4-phosphate; PIP_2, phosphatidylinositol 4,5-bisphosphate; PKA, protein kinase A; PKC, protein kinase C; PLC, phospholipase C; R, sarcolemmal receptor; R_i, inhibitory receptor; R_s, stimulatory receptor; SR, sarcoplasmic reticulum; Tn, troponin.

heart over the past two decades (65–67). It is now well-documented that, under normal circumstances, myocardial contractility is augmented through activation of the β-adrenergic–G-protein–adenyl cyclase complex (RGC). This complex serves to identify, transduce, and amplify extracellular signals by increasing the production of the intracellular second messenger cyclic adenosine monophosphate (cAMP). When a ligand interacts with a β-adrenergic receptor, the affinity of the α subunit of the G stimulatory protein ($G_s\alpha$) for guanosine 5′-triphosphate (GTP) is enhanced, facilitating exchange of guanosine 5′-diphosphate (GDP) for GTP. When GDP is released from the guanine nucleotide-binding site of G_s, the G-protein heterotrimer dissociates, releasing free subunits and $G_s\alpha$-GTP. This free $G_s\alpha$ is able to activate the catalytic subunit of adenyl cyclase, resulting in increased production of cAMP. cAMP in turn activates cAMP-dependent protein kinases, which serve as relatively promiscuous phosphorylators that can regulate a variety of cellular proteins including phospholamban, troponin, and the gated calcium channel, resulting in enhanced contraction and relaxation. Alternatively, cAMP can be metabolized to an inactive product by the enzyme phosphodiesterase (PDE). The RGC signal transduction system is under the inhibitory control of the inhibitory guanine nucleotide-binding protein G_i. Activation of G_i inhibits adenylyl cyclase activity not so much by a direct action on the catalytic subunit but, rather, by shifting the stoichiometry of G-protein binding such that there is less free $G_s\alpha$-GTP to activate the catalytic subunit of adenyl cyclase (5).

The RGC complex further modifies cellular function through direct effects of the G-protein subunits on selected ion channels (60). Furthermore, recent studies have demonstrated the importance of other regulatory proteins in the normal functioning of the RGC complex. For example, a family of β-adrenergic receptor kinases (β-ARK) are expressed in the heart and preferentially phosphorylate the agonist-occupied form of the β-adrenergic receptor independent of cAMP (68–70). In so doing, these G-protein-coupled receptors are able to modify the effectiveness of adrenergic agonists by desensitizing the β_1-adrenergic receptors (70). The role of the β-ARKs in cardiac physiology has been validated in transgenic mice overexpressing β-ARK1 (71). These mice express threefold to fivefold more β-ARK1 activity than wild type mice and demonstrate significant attenuation of isoproterenol-induced inotropy.

Further support for the role of the RGC complex in maintaining cardiac function comes from studies using transgenic mice. Overexpression of the β_2-adrenergic receptor results in increased basal myocardial adenyl cyclase activity, enhanced atrial contractility, and increased left ventricular function in vivo, changes that were virtually identical to those seen when wild type mice were exposed to maximal concentrations of adrenergic agonists (72). These mice also demonstrate markedly enhanced relaxation that is associated with a selective reduction in the amount of phospholamban protein (73). Consistent with these findings, transgenic mice overexpressing β-ARK demonstrated attenuation of isoproterenol-stimulated left ventricular contractility, dampening of myocardial adenylyl cyclase activity, and reduced functional coupling of the β-adrenergic receptors, whereas mice expressing the β-ARK inhibitor displayed enhanced cardiac contractility in the presence or absence of isoproterenol (71). In contrast, overexpression of the β_1-adrenergic receptor has been reported to effect the development of a dilated cardiomyopathy. However, the heart failure phenotype does not occur until the mice are well over 1 year of age (M. R. Bristow et al., personal communication). Similarly, overexpression of the α subunit of G_s results in the development of cardiac dilation and diminished left ventricular function (74). However, as noted with β_1-adrenergic receptor overexpression, these changes are seen only in older mice (75).

It is important to note that a characteristic feature of heart failure in humans is the presence of marked and substantial changes in the expression and function of many (if not most) of the key components of the RGC complex. In 1982, Ginsburg et al. first noted that papillary muscle isolated from failing human heart was less responsive to isoproterenol than was heart obtained from nonfailing controls (76). This diminished sensitivity occurred in the presence of increased concentrations of plasma and cardiac norepinephrine (77) and was presumably a result of downregulation of the adrenergic receptors (78). This hypothesis was supported by the seminal study of Bristow et al., who found that heart failure in humans was associated with profound downregulation of the β-adrenergic receptor (79). This downregulation was specific and selective for the β_1-adrenergic receptor, resulting in a shift in the β_1/β_2 receptor ratio (80) and was caused by a diminution in the expression of β_1-adrenergic receptor mRNA rather than by sequestration within the sarcolemma (81). Similar changes in receptor–effector coupling occur in the aged myocardium (82,83). Interestingly, in some patients with idiopathic dilated cardiomyopathy, the extracellular loop of the β_1-adrenergic receptor serves as an autoimmune epitope, which might have physiological implications (84). In addition, heart failure in humans is associated with abnormalities in the functional activity of the G-inhibitory-protein, resulting in diminished receptor–effector coupling (85–88). More recently, investigators have noted altered expression of β-ARK in the failing human heart, suggesting that altered phosphorylation may also play a role in receptor desensitization (89,90).

In view of the marked abnormalities in RGC coupling that characterize the failing human myocardium, it had been proposed that the use of positive inotropic agents having effects through various components of the RGC pathway would have only deleterious consequences. Not only were these pathways less sensitive to adrenergic stimulation, but continued production of cAMP could further compromise function or be cardiotoxic. Although this hypothesis was intuitively reasonable, several findings raised questions as to the potential efficacy of RGC-directed inotropic therapy. First, administration of adrenergic agonists has been associated with abrupt withdrawal of adrenergic drive in patients with symptomatic CHF (91). In addition, when β-receptor density was compared between patients who had received high doses of dobutamine for long periods of time before transplantation and those who had received short periods of dobutamine infusion at relatively low concentrations before transplantation, the higher dose and duration of β-adrenergic therapy were actually associated with higher numbers of β-adrenergic receptors

(59). Finally, when intracellular concentrations of cAMP are increased by inhibiting the function of PDE, there is no associated decrease in β-adrenergic receptor density despite a marked improvement in myocardial contractility (92). When adrenergic drive is relatively low, PDE inhibitors might increase contractility to a limited degree. However, when the RGC complex is activated during exercise or by administration of exogenous catecholamines, the presence of a PDE inhibitor might act synergistically to improve myocardial contractility, as seen in the discussion later.

Clinical Use of Adrenergic Agonists

Dobutamine

Clinicians first used the adrenergic agonist isoproterenol to treat patients with cardiogenic shock in the early 1960s. However, its use was limited because of associated tachycardia, arrhythmias, and diminished vascular resistance (93). In 1975, Tuttle and Mills developed the adrenergic agonist dobutamine by modifying the amino-terminal end of isoproterenol (94). This modification retained the potent inotropic properties of isoproterenol without the associated tachycardia and arrhythmias, although it was useful only as an intravenous preparation. Dobutamine has β_1, β_2, and α_1 effects (95); however, its ability to affect contractility without having positive chronotropic effects may lie in the unique isomeric structure of dobutamine (95,96). Because both β_2- and α_1-receptors are found in the peripheral vasculature, dobutamine elicits a relatively balanced effect on the peripheral vasculature. However, its beneficial effects in patients with CHF might derive from a complex relationship among the various receptors with which it interacts.

There is a general consensus that dobutamine can effect a rapid and relatively robust increase in cardiac contractility in the normal heart as well as in the failing human heart, although the response in patients with CHF is clearly blunted (Table 29-2) (97). Indeed, peak effects can be obtained in as little as 10 minutes and there is a direct correlation between dobutamine dose, plasma concentration, and hemodynamic response (98). The short half-life of dobutamine facilitates its use in clinically unstable patients, as undesirable side effects (including tachyarrhythmias, headaches, anxiety, excessive changes in blood pressure, or increased rates of ventricular response in patients with atrial fibrillation) can be reversed in as little as 10 minutes after discontinuation of intravenous therapy.

In clinical use, dobutamine has been shown to reduce ventricular filling pressures, increase stroke volume, and enhance cardiac output (99–104). Although the continuous use of dobutamine might be associated with receptor downregulation, the efficacy of prolonged therapy remains somewhat controversial. Unverferth et al. demonstrated the development of tolerance in patients receiving dobutamine for over 96 hours (105). However, tolerance could be abrogated by simply increasing infusion rates. More importantly, patients demonstrated an increase in both cardiac output and coronary blood flow that was accompanied by an increase in serum sodium, a decrease in blood urea nitrogen, and an increase in the ATP/creatine phosphate ratio. Furthermore, as mentioned earlier, studies by both Colucci and Bristow noted that the improvements in myocardial function that were effected by continuous infusion of dobutamine actually decreased adrenergic drive and its consequences on adrenergic receptor density.

Although the usefulness of dobutamine in the treatment of patients with acute exacerbation of CHF is well-recognized, several recent reports have questioned whether dobutamine and intravenous diuretics should be the first agents used in these patients, or whether vasodilators in combination with intravenous diuretics are more efficacious (106–108). Furthermore, it is unclear whether patients receiving inotropic and/or intravenous vasodilator therapy should undergo placement of a pulmonary artery catheter to facilitate titration of the medications (109). This important question will be addressed by the upcoming ESCAPE trial under the sponsorship of the National Heart, Lung, and Blood Institute (NHLBI).

Although there has been a general consensus regarding the use of dobutamine in patients with acute heart failure, the usefulness of either intermittent or chronic dobutamine in patients with end-stage heart failure has been a highly contentious issue. Intermittent therapy with dobutamine was based in large part on the finding that the beneficial effects of a 72-hour dobutamine infusion in patients with chronic CHF persisted for up to 4 weeks in over 50% of patients after discontinuation of dobutamine therapy (97). Dobutamine effected a sustained improvement in hemodynamic indexes as well as in biochemical and ultrastructural parameters of the heart, leading investigators to propose that intermittent therapy might provide long-term benefits for patients with

TABLE 29-2
INOTROPES COMMONLY USED FOR HEART FAILURE

Drug	Initial Dose	Target Dose	Major Adverse Reactions
Digoxin	0.125 mg/qd	Serum level ≤1.5 ng/dL	Cardiotoxicity, confusion, nausea, anorexia, visual disturbances
Inotropes	—	(Not to exceed)	Tachycardia, ventricular ectopy, phlebitis, hypotension
Dobutamine (Dobutrex)	1 μg/kg/min	10 μg/kg/min	
Milrinone (Primacor)	0.25 mg/kg/min	0.75 mg/kg/min	
Dopamine	1 μg/kg/min	5 μg/kg/min	

chronic heart failure (105,110). Indeed, a group of investigations in animal models of CHF (111,112) as well as several clinical studies (113,114) supported this hypothesis. Enthusiasm for the use of intermittent dobutamine was dampened, however, with the presentation of a report by Dies that demonstrated an increase in early mortality in patients treated with intermittent dobutamine (115). However, this study was highly flawed in that (a) electrolyte levels were not routinely measured; (b) high concentrations of dobutamine were used throughout the study; and (c) dobutamine concentrations were not titrated for interstudy changes in body weight. Despite this report, several centers have continued to report favorable effects of chronic dobutamine therapy in patients with chronic heart failure (116,117).

Unfortunately, the role of intermittent dobutamine therapy in the management of patients with chronic CHF is further clouded by its use outside the confines of tertiary or quarternary heart failure centers. Because the establishment of outpatient heart failure centers can be highly remunerative, concerns have been raised that patients with NYHA Class II and III symptoms have received intermittent therapy with dobutamine rather than it being reserved for patients who are at end-stage and who have had repeated and frequent hospitalizations requiring inpatient inotropic therapy. It is unlikely that this contentious issue will be resolved until such time as a randomized and placebo-controlled trial having survival and hospitalizations as primary outcomes (and cost as a secondary outcome) is undertaken. Because dobutamine is generic and the patent life of its major competitor in the inotrope marketplace, milrinone, is about to expire, it is unlikely that this type of trial will be undertaken unless governmental agencies such as the NHLBI intervene.

The term chronic therapy with intravenous dobutamine is generally interpreted as meaning regularly scheduled, intermittent therapy. However, it should be kept in mind that many patients require tailored therapy that does not fit into traditional algorithms. For example, some patients require continuous administration of dobutamine outside of a hospital setting. Physicians who care for large numbers of patients with CHF often treat patients who cannot be weaned from intravenous inotropic therapy yet are not candidates for cardiac transplantation because of age or concomitant disease. Rather than remaining hospitalized or dying at home of worsening heart failure after discontinuation of their intravenous therapy, these patients should be treated with chronic and continuous home dobutamine infusion. Although the effects of chronic infusion are undefined, it is clear that it improves quality of life and allows these patients to return to their homes despite their precarious health (117).

Important caveats regarding such therapy include: (a) patients should be maintained on the lowest possible dose of dobutamine; (b) a chronically indwelling catheter such as a peripherally inserted catheter (PIC) line or a Hickman catheter should be utilized for drug delivery in order to diminish the risk of extravascular infiltration; (c) many patients are able to disconnect their catheters when showering or during other activities because the benefits of the infusion will often persist for a period of time after discontinuing therapy; and (d) patients should be assessed by a physician extender at home, on a regular basis, with assessment of weight, a physical examination, and measurement of routine blood chemistries.

Dopamine

Similar to dobutamine, dopamine was first introduced for the treatment of CHF because it was shown to increase cardiac contractility without substantial effects on either blood pressure or heart rate (118,119). However, in contrast with dobutamine, dopamine affects a variety of cardiac and vascular receptors. At low doses (<5 μg/kg per minute), dopamine activates two distinct dopaminergic subtypes (Table 29-3), designated as DA_1 and DA_2 (120,121). DA_1 receptors are located in the vascular smooth muscle of the renal, mesenteric, coronary, and cerebral arteries (122,123) and mediate diuresis and natriuresis (124,125). In addition, DA_1 agonists suppress aldosterone release and vasodilate the splanchnic vasculature (126). Thus, dopaminergic agonists are useful in patients with right-sided heart failure who have markedly elevated levels of aldosterone because of passive liver congestion, as well as in patients with recalcitrant abdominal pain secondary to low cardiac output and diminished splanchnic flow. In contrast, DA_2 receptors are located on postganglionic sympathetic nerves and sympathetic ganglia, and activation of these receptors results in a decrease in norepinephrine release from sympathetic nerve terminals (127,128). Such antiadrenergic effects might also be of benefit in patients with chronic heart failure.

In contrast to the effects of low doses of dopamine, higher concentrations of dopamine (>5 μg/kg per minute) activate both the β_1- and α_1-adrenergic receptors. Although activation of the β_1-adrenergic receptor effects an increase in cardiac contractility (not unlike dobutamine), the activation of the α_1-adrenergic receptors in the peripheral

TABLE 29-3
CELLULAR TARGETS OF COMMONLY USED INOTROPES

Agent	Target	Effect
Digoxin	Inhibition of Na^+, K^+-ATPase	Increased inotropy
Dobutamine	β_1-adrenergic receptor >>> β_2-AR > α_1-AR	Increased inotropy
Dopamine	3–5 μg/kg/min dopaminergic receptors	Increased renal and splanchic perfusion
	>5 μg/kg/min β_1-AR	Increased inotropy (decreased CO)
	>5 μg/kg/min α_1-AR	Increased peripheral resistance (decreased CO)
Milrinone	Phosphodiesterase	Increased inotropy and increased peripheral vasodilatation

vasculature leads to peripheral vasoconstriction. Thus, an increase in myocardial contractility is directly balanced against an increase in afterload, with the net effect being compromised ventricular performance (129). Interestingly, the two receptor-mediated effects can be separated using appropriate receptor antagonists (129,130). Similarly, higher doses of dopamine can be used concomitantly with a vasodilator in order to improve myocardial contractility (131,132), although this combination is generally not utilized in clinical practice. However, the role for higher concentrations of dopamine exists in the treatment of patients with shock secondary to acute volume depletion or sepsis. In this clinical setting, there is a requirement for both enhanced myocardial contractility and peripheral vasoconstriction.

Because of their similar pharmacologic properties, it is important to compare and contrast dobutamine and dopamine (133–135). Dobutamine can best be viewed as a positive inotropic agent having mild vasodilating properties. In contrast, dopamine is both a positive inotrope and a vasopressor. Therefore, dobutamine is most beneficial in patients with cardiac decompensation secondary to diminished left ventricular contractility, whereas dopamine is most useful in cardiovascular decompensation that results from diminished vascular tone. However, these two agents have been found to act synergistically when titrated to appropriate doses. The combination of low doses of dopamine and low doses of dobutamine provides both improved diuresis and enhanced pump function. The efficacy of dopamine appears to be most noticeable in patients with ascites, substantial peripheral edema, and passive liver congestion. In addition, low doses of dopamine are useful in patients with end-stage heart failure who complain of abdominal pain secondary to vasoconstriction in the mesenteric vasculature.

Several recent studies have provided new and interesting information that may have relevance for the clinical use of dopamine in patients with CHF. In the first study, van de Borne et al. demonstrated that dopamine inhibits chemoreflex responses during hypoxic breathing in normal humans, preferentially affecting the ventilatory response more than the sympathetic response (136). However, dopamine also depressed ventilation in normoxic heart failure patients breathing room air. Thus, low-dose dopamine might adversely influence outcome in hypoxic patients and should be used with caution in those patients with heart failure and hypoxia being weaned from respiratory support (137). In a second report, Ouadid et al. suggested the existence of a new type of dopaminergic receptor in the human heart that was positively coupled to adenylyl cyclase (138). Therefore, low doses of dopamine might have inotropic properties over and above those mediated by β_1-adrenergic receptor activation. Finally, a recent study suggests that dobutamine exerts a direct coronary vasodilator effect in patients with idiopathic dilated cardiomyopathy (139). These coronary hemodynamic changes were associated with decreased adrenergic drive and atrial natriuretic factor release, thus providing a novel benefit to dobutamine infusions. However, these intriguing studies require further clarification.

Phosphodiesterase Inhibitors

Because receptor–effector coupling in the failing myocardium is attenuated by a diminished number of β_1-adrenergic receptors, uncoupling of the β_2-adrenergic receptor from adenylyl cyclase, and increased activation of the G-inhibitory-protein, investigators proposed that the contractility of the failing heart could be augmented by increasing cAMP levels independent of receptor–G-protein interactions. One of the first pharmacologic agents that was developed was forskolin. This extract of the Indian coleus plant directly activated adenylyl cyclase through a unique mechanism (140). Although it proved to be a highly potent inotropic agent, its clinical usefulness was limited by its irregular absorption and marked chronotropy.

In 1972, Alousi et al. developed the bipyridine derivative amrinone, which elicited a marked inotropic response and concentration-dependent vasodilatory effects through the inhibition of PDE (141–143). Indeed, the intravenous administration of amrinone increased the cardiac index and decreased left ventricular end-diastolic pressure and pulmonary capillary pressure in patients with chronic CHF without an accompanying change in heart rate (144). These salutary effects of amrinone were associated with improved exercise capacity and decreased anaerobic metabolism (145). Because cAMP and cAMP-dependent mechanisms are ubiquitous, the precise mechanisms by which amrinone increased cardiac contractility remained partially undefined. Initial investigations suggested that amrinone increased cardiac performance by improving left ventricular contractility (146). However, other investigations suggested that the beneficial effects of amrinone on cardiac performance derived from its potent vasodilatory properties (147–150). Because the failing myocardium is deficient in intracellular cAMP because of downregulation of the RGC complex, investigators hypothesized that inhibiting PDE would have little effect, as cAMP is far more avidly bound by cAMP-dependent protein kinases than by the PDEs. However, studies have clearly demonstrated that amrinone increases intracellular cAMP via an inhibition of PDE subfraction III (151,152). Furthermore, physiological effects of amrinone, including enhanced myocardial contraction and relaxation, and augmentation of calcium transport across the sarcolemma, are consistent with a cAMP-mediated event (153,154). An interesting finding was that the myocardial effects of amrinone were species-dependent, as amrinone had minimal effects in rats or rabbits (155).

Although the introduction of amrinone was met with initial enthusiasm, subsequent clinical trials suggested that the intravenous administration of amrinone was associated with numerous side effects, including gastrointestinal irritation, central nervous system complaints, and blood dyscrasias. Furthermore, the long-term use of oral amrinone was not associated with beneficial effects in several randomized and placebo-controlled clinical trials (156,157). In fact, the results of several studies suggested an increased mortality associated with the use of oral amrinone (158).

Despite the failure to identify benefits associated with the use of oral amrinone, a group of other PDE inhibitors were developed for the therapy of chronic CHF, including milrinone, enoximone, and indolidan. None of these agents proved beneficial in long-term studies (45,159) and a large, randomized, and placebo-controlled study assessing the safety and efficacy of oral milrinone in patients with chronic CHF was discontinued because of a marked increase in mortality in those patients randomized to receive milrinone (160). Despite the untoward effects of oral PDE inhibitors, milrinone was developed for use as an intravenous agent. The putative benefits of milrinone were that (a) it could increase intracellular levels of cAMP independent of adrenergic receptor activation; and (b) it provided potent peripheral vasodilation and, in so doing, enhanced cardiac output (156). Indeed, initial studies using intracoronary administration to obviate affects on the peripheral vasculature clearly demonstrated that milrinone exerted both positive inotropic and vasodilator actions (161). Furthermore, milrinone infusion significantly decreased left ventricular end-diastolic pressure, pulmonary wedge pressure, right atrial pressure, and systemic vascular resistance, as well as significantly increasing cardiac index and the peak positive first derivative of left ventricular pressure (162). These beneficial hemodynamic effects were sustained during a 24-hour continuous infusion.

Although the vasodilating properties of milrinone have led some clinicians to prefer it to dobutamine for the therapy of patients with worsening heart failure, there are several limitations to its use: (a) the half-life of milrinone is longer than that of dobutamine, thereby limiting the ability to rapidly discontinue the agent if untoward effects occur; (b) the vasodilatory effects cannot be as precisely titrated as those of a direct-acting vasodilator such as nitroprusside or nitroglycerin compounds; and (c) it is nearly 10 times as expensive as dobutamine.

In view of the potential limitations of therapy with milrinone, it would be important to assess dobutamine and milrinone in a head-to-head comparison. Unfortunately, few studies exist that compare the two agents; those that have been performed must be viewed as largely anecdotal because of their small size. For example, Grose et al. studied the effects of either dobutamine or milrinone on 11 patients in CHF (164). These studies suggested that dobutamine and milrinone could produce similar improvements in cardiac index. However, in contrast with milrinone, dobutamine increased myocardial oxygen consumption and only dobutamine increased the first derivative of left ventricular pressure. Interpretation of these results was limited not just by the small number of patients but also by the fact that dobutamine was infused before the administration of milrinone. However, a second comparison study by Mager et al. provides potentially important information regarding the hemodynamic effects of milrinone (165). They found that milrinone, but not dobutamine, elicited a rapid and marked reduction in pulmonary vascular resistance. However, as with other studies, the total number of patients studied was small and infusions of study drugs were performed sequentially.

In view of the large disparity in costs between these two agents, randomized trials will be required to assess their differences and usefulness. A multicenter, randomized, and controlled trial (OPTIME) is now evaluating the efficacy of milrinone in the management of patients hospitalized for worsening heart failure. Unfortunately, this study is randomizing patients to either milrinone or standard therapy (excluding dobutamine). Therefore, not only will this study not answer the important questions regarding comparison of these two agents, but enrollment has been difficult because of physicians' unwillingness to randomize patients with worsening heart failure to the non-inotrope arm of the study.

Perhaps the most intriguing information regarding the PDE inhibitors has been the recent reports demonstrating the ability of PDE inhibitors to attenuate the production of the proinflammatory cytokine tumor necrosis factor-α (TNF-α). TNF-α is a proinflammatory cytokine that was originally studied because of its important role in the inflammatory response (166). However, within the past decade it was reported by numerous laboratories that TNF-α is a potent negative inotrope (167–170). More recently, studies have demonstrated the ability of exogenously administered TNF-α to increase extracellular matrix turnover, prolong calcium transients, and modulate receptor–effector coupling through enhanced activation of G_i (171). In 1991, Levine et al. first recognized that TNF-α was elevated in the plasma of patients with end-stage dilated cardiomyopathy, and subsequent studies by Mann and others noted that there was a direct correlation between elevations in TNF-α and severity of disease in patients with heart failure (172).

Furthermore, although the normal myocardium does not express TNF-α, the failing heart expresses robust amounts of TNF-α, particularly in the presence of end-stage disease (173). In addition, mice with cardiac-specific overexpression of TNF-α develop cardiac dilation, hypertrophy, diminished adrenergic responsiveness, interstitial infiltrates, fibrosis, and altered calcium homeostasis, and have a 6-month mortality of approximately 25% (174). Importantly, inhibition of the biological effects of TNF-α by the overexpression of TNF-α-soluble receptors abrogates the biological effects of TNF-α (175) and development of the heart failure phenotype (176,177). Thus, agents having anticytokine properties might be expected to have beneficial effects in patients with CHF and, indeed, clinical studies are now under way assessing the efficacy of soluble TNF-α receptors for the therapy of CHF.

The relevance of the TNF-α hypothesis of CHF to inotropic therapy comes from a large number of recent studies demonstrating the potent anticytokine effects of selected PDE inhibitors, including milrinone (178). When peripheral blood mononuclear cells obtained from healthy human subjects were stimulated with lipopolysaccharide, the addition of a PDE inhibitor significantly reduced the ability of the cells to express proinflammatory cytokines (179). Similarly, TNF-α expression by activated mononuclear cells could be abrogated by the combination of a PDE inhibitor and a prostanoid (180). Interestingly, different PDE inhibitors had variable impact on cytokine expression with markedly different ED50s despite identical in vitro concentrations. However, both milrinone and vesnarinone had robust effects in isolated cells (179). Of even greater interest was the finding that neither cAMP derivatives nor adrenergic stimulation could effect similar inhibition of cytokine expression by activated mononuclear cells (181). Therefore, the mechanisms responsible for this potentially important ancillary effect remain undefined.

The clinical relevance of the anticytokine effects of phosphodiesterase inhibitors was first noted in a recent study of the PDE inhibitor pentoxifylline. Pentoxifylline was given to a relatively small group of patients with chronic CHF (182). When compared with placebo, pentoxifylline improved heart failure symptoms, increased left ventricular systolic function, and decreased NYHA classification. However, of even greater interest was the finding that pentoxifylline substantially lowered plasma concentrations of TNF-α while no change was noted in the placebo treatment group. Thus, PDE inhibitors might be useful in the management of patients with CHF if one could avoid the untoward ancillary effects that might have been responsible for the increased mortality seen in patients after long-term oral therapy.

One novel approach to this conundrum has been to combine therapy with an oral PDE inhibitor with a β-blocker in patients with refractory NYHA Class IV heart failure. In a preliminary study of 30 patients, combination therapy with a positive inotrope and a β-blocker appeared to be useful in the treatment of severe heart failure, as patients demonstrated increased ejection fractions, decreased functional classification, and a trend toward fewer hospitalizations (183). This novel strategy requires further investigation (184).

Modulation of Intracellular Calcium Homeostasis

It is well-recognized that the release and reuptake of intracellular calcium are imperative for both normal systolic and diastolic function of the human heart (185). The ability of the heart to regulate calcium homeostasis is dependent on the normal function of a variety of pumps and channels that regulate the transport and storage of calcium. These include (but are certainly not limited to) (a) phospholamban and SR Ca^{2+}-ATPase (SERCA), which together regulate uptake of calcium into the sarcoplasmic reticulum storage pools; (b) the sodium–calcium exchanger, which is important in the mechanism of action of digoxin; (c) the cAMP- and protein kinase-dependent gated calcium channel; and (d) the calcium release channel. Abnormalities in the intracellular handling of calcium are characteristic findings in the failing human heart (186). Indeed, it has been suggested that abnormal intracellular calcium handling is a major cause of systolic and diastolic dysfunction in patients with heart failure (187). These abnormalities are caused in large part by abnormal gating mechanisms of the calcium release channel of the sarcoplasmic reticulum (188) and disturbed intracellular calcium uptake secondary to altered transport by the sarcoplasmic reticulum (189). That these maladaptive changes in myocardial calcium homeostasis are secondary to diminished expression of phospholamban and SERCA has been demonstrated in a number of reports (190–194). In addition, several studies suggest that abnormalities in the expression of the calcium release channel might also contribute to these abnormalities (195) and that enhanced function of the sodium–calcium exchanger may serve to compensate for the depressed sarcoplasmic reticulum function (196).

Interestingly, recent studies have utilized transgenic approaches to demonstrate that alterations in calcium-handling proteins can indeed affect myocardial function and that correction of these defects can normalize function. In several elegant studies, Kranias et al. demonstrated that targeted ablation of the phospholamban gene was associated with markedly enhanced myocardial contractility and loss of β-agonist stimulation (197–199). In a separate group of experiments He et al. demonstrated that overexpression of SERCA in the heart of transgenic mice accelerated calcium transients and improved cardiac relaxation (200). However, recent studies have also demonstrated that depressed sarcoplasmic reticulum function because of decreased expression of SERCA could be normalized by overexpressing SERCA using adenovirus-mediated gene transfer in neonatal rat cardiac myocytes (201). Furthermore, the overexpression of phospholamban in isolated cardiomyocytes could rescue the effects of concomitant gene transfer of SERCA (202). Thus, regulation of calcium-handling proteins in the failing myocardium might have significant and substantial effects on cardiac function.

Unfortunately, pharmacologic agents have not been developed that are able to modulate the actions of the calcium-handling proteins in vivo. Indeed, most existing inotropic agents improve cardiac contractility by either directly or indirectly increasing the levels of free cytosolic calcium (203,204). Although these increases in cytosolic calcium effectively improve myocardial contractility, the rise in intracellular calcium might be associated with undesirable side effects, including ventricular arrhythmias, calcium overload, and cellular necrosis, because reuptake into the storage pools is still abnormal (205–207). Thus, our current approaches to increasing myocardial contractility might be viewed as being counterintuitive because a more appropriate approach would be to increase the uptake of calcium into the storage pools rather than simply increasing concentrations in the cytoplasm.

A second way to alter contractility and obviate the low cytosolic calcium concentrations in the failing heart is to increase the sensitivity of the contractile apparatus to calcium rather than increasing the absolute amount of calcium (208–210). When the sensitivity of the contractile elements to calcium is enhanced, a given force can be obtained by a lower cytosolic calcium concentration, or a higher force can be achieved by the same calcium concentration (205,211). In addition, the increase in developed force would not be at the expense of increased energy needs. Indeed, several investigational agents that increase the sensitivity of the contractile elements to calcium have been associated with improved force-generating states with lower or equivalent metabolic demands (212,213). Although not all of these agents provide an energetic advantage over currently used inotropic agents (213), enhancement of myofibrillar calcium responsiveness represents a novel approach with important theoretical advantages (214). As our knowledge of the molecular mechanisms responsible for modulating cardiac muscle force production increases, we should be able to more appropriately design pharmacologic and molecular strategies for altering the sensitivity of the contractile elements to calcium.

To date, the only agent with calcium-sensitizing effects that has been evaluated in phase II and III clinical trials in the United States has been pimobendan. Unfortunately, clinical trials with this agent were not overwhelmingly successful and its development was discontinued. However, the studies with pimobendan should not inhibit further investigation of calcium sensitizers because it may have been the PDE-inhibiting effects of pimobendan that were responsible for its demise.

A newer calcium sensitizer that is soon to undergo clinical trials in the United States is levosimendan. Like other calcium sensitizers, levosimendan has both calcium-sensitizing and PDE-III inhibitory properties. In investigational animals, levosimendan markedly improved hemodynamic parameters, with effects being greater in animals with impaired left ventricular function than in normal hearts (215). In normal volunteers, levosimendan increased cardiac output by 40% and decreased pulmonary capillary wedge pressure by 40% to 50% in patients with CHF. In patients receiving an ACE inhibitor for therapy of CHF, levosimendan increased mean stroke volume at low doses (but not at high doses) and increased cardiac output, but did not change heart rate (216). A limitation of the clinical use of levosimendan may be the presence of a long-acting active metabolite (217). Therefore, calcium sensitizers intuitively might be useful inotropes in the management of patients with CHF (218); however, experience with levosimendan is very limited and its long-term effects are undefined.

Inotropic Agents Having Multiple Mechanisms of Action

The conundrum regarding the use of inotropic agents in the management of patients with CHF is clearly defined by reviewing the clinical experience with the inotrope vesnarinone. First synthesized in 1983, vesnarinone increased cardiac contractility independent of a change in either heart rate or blood pressure in a variety of animal species except for rats (219). The multiple mechanisms responsible for the inotropic actions of vesnarinone included increased sodium channel open time (220), decreased delayed outward and inward rectifying potassium currents (221), and an increase in whole-cell calcium currents, in part related to an effect on PDE (222). However, in contrast to traditional PDE inhibitors that increase heart rate and shorten the action potential, vesnarinone slowed heart rate and prolonged the action potential (221). Consistent with recent studies of other PDE inhibitors, vesnarinone also demonstrated potent anticytokine properties.

In initial phase I and II studies, short-term therapy with vesnarinone was associated with improvements in cardiovascular hemodynamics and exercise capacity in patients with chronic CHF (217–219). Similarly, several small, randomized, and placebo-controlled clinical trials suggested that vesnarinone had beneficial effects on the combined endpoint of major cardiovascular morbidity and mortality, despite a 2.5% incidence of reversible neutropenia (220,221). In a multicenter, phase II clinical trial, patients were randomized to receive either 120-mg vesnarinone, 60-mg vesnarinone, or placebo (222). The high-dose arm of the study was discontinued upon the advice of the data and safety monitoring committee because of increased mortality; however, 60-mg vesnarinone was associated with a 62% reduction in the risk of dying during the 6-month study period. Similarly, patients randomized to 60-mg vesnarinone had a 50% reduction in the risk of either dying or developing worsening heart failure during the study period. In addition, patients receiving vesnarinone experienced an improvement in quality of life.

In order to validate these initial results, a second phase III study (VesT) was undertaken. In VesT, approximately 3,800 patients were randomized to receive either 30-mg vesnarinone, 60-mg vesnarinone, or placebo for at least 1 year. The study was terminated when a prospectively defined number of deaths had occurred in the placebo arm of the trial. In contrast with earlier studies, the use of 60-mg vesnarinone was associated with a modest and statistically significant increase in mortality and there was a trend toward an increase in mortality in patients receiving 30-mg vesnarinone (223). This increase in mortality was attributable to sudden death rather than to worsening heart failure. Interestingly, patients in the 60-mg vesnarinone group demonstrated a significant improvement in quality of life. However, future development of vesnarinone was terminated because of concerns regarding the increased mortality seen in the VesT trial.

Like so many inotropic agents preceding it, vesnarinone garnered early enthusiasm but was subsequently demonstrated to lack long-term benefit. However, comparison of the various vesnarinone studies provide some interesting lessons regarding the use of inotropic agents. In the earlier multicenter trials, (a) patients were required to exercise on a stationary bicycle before enrollment; (b) digoxin levels were rigidly defined; and (c) patients with renal dysfunction were excluded. Conversely, patients in the VesT trial were not required to exercise, did not have their digoxin levels monitored, could have higher serum creatinines, and were older by design. In addition, the VesT trial had substantially more women than did the earlier vesnarinone studies. Therefore, the patients in VesT were sicker than those in earlier clinical trials. Although we cannot exclude the possibility that chance alone was responsible for the beneficial effects of vesnarinone seen in the earlier clinical trials, we cannot discount the possibility that inotropic agents such as vesnarinone exert more beneficial effects when given earlier in the course of the disease. For example, if the myocardium of patients in the VesT trial had been exposed chronically to elevated levels of proinflammatory cytokines with the resultant development of marked interstitial fibrosis and myofibrillar disarray, it would be unlikely that either anticytokine therapy or inotropic therapy could have a positive impact. More likely, exposing the few remaining viable myocytes to the potassium channel effects of vesnarinone might have resulted in the development of lethal arrhythmias and an increased incidence of sudden death.

Unfortunately, we can only propose explanations for the disappointing results of the VesT trial and hope that our understanding of the pathobiology of CHF will improve and thus allow us to design better therapeutic strategies for improving left ventricular function.

ORAL INOTROPIC AGENTS COMBINED WITH β-BLOCKADE

Enoximone is a novel imidazolone derivative that effects positive inotropy and vasodilation through the selective inhibition of sarcoplasmic reticulum-associated type III PDE (230,231). In patients with chronic heart failure, enoximone's properties appeared to be additive with β-blockers (232) and improved cardiac function without increasing myocardial oxygen demand (233). In two early reports, oral enoximone was beneficial in weaning patients with end-stage heart failure from intravenous dobutamine support (234,235). However, long-term use of enoximone was associated with increased mortality (236). Nevertheless, low doses of enoximone markedly improved exercise capacity and improved symptoms without increased mortality (237).

To further evaluate the effects of enoximone in patients with heart failure, two multicenter, randomized, controlled trials were undertaken. The Oral Enoximone in Intravenous Inotrope-Dependent Subjects (EMOTE) trial assessed the efficacy of enoximone in weaning patients from intravenous inotropic support while the Enoximone Therapy in CHF (ESSENTIAL) trial measured the ability of enoximone when combined with a β-blocker to decrease mortality and hospitalizations and improve functional capacity and quality of life in patients with chronic heart failure (238).

Unfortunately, although the EMOTE trial showed a clinical benefit at 60 days, the 30-day wean rate was not significantly different in the enoximone and placebo treatment groups (239). Similarly, low-dose enoximone when combined with a β-blocker did not demonstrate significant improvement in a population of heart failure patients. Thus, the enoximone development program has been discontinued.

CONCLUSION

In conclusion, the use of inotropic agents in the management of CHF has been marked by great expectations and major disappointments. Despite nearly 200 years of clinical investigations, there are only a handful of approved inotropic agents available in the United States and only one of these agents can be administered orally. Although recent studies suggest that digoxin is not associated with increased mortality and decreases heart failure hospitalizations, its efficacy is far from overwhelming. Furthermore, although both dobutamine and milrinone can provide short-term support during acute exacerbations of worsening heart failure, their long-term use remains highly controversial. However, as pointed out earlier in this discussion, the primary abnormality in the failing human heart is systolic dysfunction and an inability to augment cardiac output during exercise or stress. Therefore, the rationale for using inotropic therapy remains intuitively appealing despite our failure to develop safe and effective inotropic agents. As we continue to delve into the pathobiology of CHF using new and sophisticated molecular and cellular technology, we hope to develop strategies with which to safely and effectively increase the contractile performance of the failing ventricle in order to alleviate the signs and symptoms of this disease.

REFERENCES

1. Feldman AM. A classification system for inotropic agents. *J Am Coll Cardiol.* 1993;22:1223–1227.
2. Wohlfart B, Noble MI. The cardiac excitation-contraction cycle. *Pharmacol Ther.* 1982;16:1–43.
3. Bouillaud J. Traite clinique des maladies du coeur: precede de recherrches nouvelles sur l'anatomie et la physiologie de cet organ. Libraire de l'Academie Royale de Medicine. Paris: J. B. Bailliere; 1841.
4. Lewis T. On cardinal principles in cardiological practice. *Br Med J.* 1919;3072:621.
5. Arnold SB, Byrd RC, Meister W, et al. Long-term digitalis therapy improves left ventricular function in heart failure. *N Engl J Med.* 1980;303:1443–1448.
6. Christian HA. Digitalis effects in chronic cardiac cases with regular rhythm in contrast to auricular fibrillation. *Med Clin North Am.* 1922;5:90.
7. Moss AJ, Davis HT, Conard DL, et al. Digitalis-associated cardiac mortality after myocardial infarction. *Circulation.* 1981;64:1150–1156.
8. Bigger JTJ, Fleiss JL, Rolnitzky LM, et al. Effect of digitalis treatment on survival after acute myocardial infarction. *Am J Cardiol.* 1985;55:623–630.
9. Lee DC, Johnson RA, Bingham JB, et al. Heart failure in outpatients: a randomized trial of digoxin versus placebo. *N Engl J Med.* 1982;306:699–705.
10. Ware JA, Snow E, Luchi PA, et al. Effects of digoxin on ejection fraction in elderly patients with congestive heart failure. *J Am Geriatr Soc.* 1984;32:631.
11. O'Rourke RA, Henning H, Theroux P, et al. Favorable effects of orally administered digoxin on left heart size and ventricular wall motion in patients with previous myocardial infarction. *Am J Cardiol.* 1976;37:708–715.
12. Firth BG, Dehmer GJ, Corbett JR, et al. Effect of chronic oral digoxin therapy on ventricular function at rest and peak exercise in patients with ischemic heart disease. *Am J Cardiol.* 1980;46:481–490.
13. Fleg JL, Gottlieb SH, Lakatta EG. Is digoxin really important in treatment of compensated heart failure? A placebo-controlled crossover study in patients with sinus rhythm. *Am J Med.* 1982;73:244–250.
14. Wiggers CJ, Stinson B. Studies on cardiodynamic action of drugs. III. The mechanism of cardiac stimulation by digitalis and G-strophanthin. *J Pharmacol Exp Ther.* 1927;30:251.
15. Cattell M, Gold H. Influence of digitalis on the force of contraction of mammalian cardiac muscle. *J Pharmacol Exp Ther.* 1938;62:116.
16. Sonnenblick EH, Williams JFJ, Glick G, et al. Studies on digitalis. XV. Effects of cardiac glycosides on myocardial force-velocity relations in the nonfailing human heart. *Circulation.* 1966;34:532–539.
17. Ferguson DW. Digitalis and neurohormonal abnormalities in heart failure and implications for therapy. *Am J Cardiol.* 1992;69:24G–32G.
18. Gomes JA, Kang PS, El-Sherif N. Effects of digitalis on the human sick sinus node after pharmacologic autonomic blockade. *Am J Cardiol.* 1981;48:783–788.
19. Scholz H. Inotropic drugs and their mechanisms of action. *J Am Coll Cardiol.* 1984;4:389–397.
20. Marban E, Smith T. Digitalis. In: Fozzard H, Haber E, Jennings R, eds. *The Heart and Cardiovascular System.* New York: Raven Press; 1986: 1573.
21. Smith TW, Butler VPJ, Haber E. Determination of therapeutic and toxic serum digoxin concentrations by radioimmunoassay. *N Engl J Med.* 1969;281:1212–1216.
22. Johnston GD. Digoxin dose precision: prescribing aids or intuition? *Drugs.* 1980;20:494–499.
23. Brown DD, Juhl RP. Decreased bioavailability of digoxin due to antacids and kaolin-pectin. *N Engl J Med.* 1976;295:1034–1037.
24. Kolibash AJ, Kramer WG, Reuning RH, et al. Marked decline in serum digoxin concentration during an episode of severe diarrhea. *Am Heart J.* 1977;94:806–807.

25. Brown DD, Juhl RP, Warner SL. Decreased bioavailability of digoxin due to hypocholesterolemic interventions. *Circulation.* 1978;58:164–172.
26. Heizer WD, Smith TW, Goldfinger SE. Absorption of digoxin in patients with malabsorption syndromes. *N Engl J Med.* 1971; 285:257–259.
27. Greenberger NJ, Caldwell JH. Studies on the intestinal absorptions of ^{3}H-digitalis glycosides in experimental animals and man. In: Marks BH, Weissler AM, eds. *Basic and Clinical Pharmacology of Digitalis.* Springfield, IL: Charles C Thomas; 1972: 15.
28. Cohen AF, Kroon R, Schoemaker R, et al. Influence of gastric acidity on the bioavailability of digoxin. *Ann Intern Med.* 1991;115:540–545.
29. Lindenbaum J, Rund DG, Butler VPJ, et al. Inactivation of digoxin by the gut flora: reversal by antibiotic therapy. *N Engl J Med.* 1981;305:789–794.
30. Jorgensen HS, Christensen HR, Kampmann JP. Interaction between digoxin and indomethacin or ibuprofen. *Br J Clin Pharmacol.* 1991;31:108–110.
31. Foukaridis GN. Influence of spironolactone and its metabolite canrenone on serum digoxin assays. *Ther Drug Monit.* 1990; 12:82–84.
32. Leahey EBJ, Reiffel JA, Giardina EG, et al. The effect of quinidine and other oral antiarrhythmic drugs on serum digoxin. A prospective study. *Ann Intern Med.* 1980;92:605–608.
33. Klein HO, Lang R, Weiss E, et al. The influence of verapamil on serum digoxin concentration. *Circulation.* 1982;65:998–1003.
34. Nademanee K, Kannan R, Hendrickson J, et al. Amiodarone-digoxin interaction: clinical significance, time course of development, potential pharmacokinetic mechanisms and therapeutic implications. *J Am Coll Cardiol.* 1984;4:111–116.
35. Nolan PEJ, Marcus FI, Erstad BL, et al. Effects of coadministration of propafenone on the pharmacokinetics of digoxin in healthy volunteer subjects. *J Clin Pharmacol.* 1989;29:46–52.
36. Marcus FI, Burkhalter L, Cuccia C, et al. Administration of tritiated digoxin with and without a loading dose. A metabolic study. *Circulation.* 1966;34:865–874.
37. Belz GG, Erbel R, Schumann K, et al. Dose-response relationships and plasma concentrations of digitalis glycosides in man. *Eur J Clin Pharmacol.* 1978;13:103–111.
38. Buch J, Waldorff S. Classical concentration-response relationship between serum digoxin level and contractility indices. *Dan Med Bull.* 1980;27:287–290.
39. Saxena PR, Bhargava KP. The importance of a central adrenergic mechanism in the cardiovascular responses to ouabain. *Eur J Pharmacol.* 1975;31:332–346.
40. Lely AH, Enter CH. Large-scale digitoxin intoxication. *BMJ.* 1970;3:737–740.
41. Smith TW, Antman EM, Friedman PL, et al. Digitalis glycosides: mechanisms and manifestations of toxicity. Part II. *Prog Cardiovasc Dis.* 1984;26:495–540.
42. Antman EM, Wenger TL, Butler VPJ, et al. Treatment of 150 cases of life-threatening digitalis intoxication with digoxin-specific Fab antibody fragments. Final report of a multicenter study. *Circulation.* 1990;81:1744–1752.
43. The German and Austrian Xamoterol Study Group. Double-blind placebo-controlled comparison of digoxin and xamoterol in chronic heart failure. *Lancet.* 1988;1:489–493.
44. The Captopril-Digoxin Multicenter Research Group. Comparative effects of therapy with captopril and digoxin in patients with mild to moderate heart failure. *JAMA.* 1988;259: 539–544.
45. DiBianco R, Shabetai R, Kostuk W, et al., for the Milrinone Multicenter Trial Group. A comparison of oral milrinone, digoxin, and their combination in the treatment of patients with chronic heart failure. *N Engl J Med.* 1989;320: 677–683.
46. Pfeffer MA, Braunwald E, Moye LA, et al, on behalf of the SAVE Investigators. Effect of captopril on mortality and morbidity in patients with left ventricular dysfunction after myocardial infarction. *N Engl J Med.* 1992;327:669–677.
47. The SOLVD Investigators. Effect of enalapril on mortality and the development of heart failure in asymptomatic patients with reduced left ventricular ejection fractions. *N Engl J Med.* 1992;327:685–691.
48. Packer M, Gheorghiade M, Young JB, et al. Withdrawal of digoxin from patients with chronic heart failure treated with angiotensin-converting-enzyme inhibitors. RADIANCE Study. *N Engl J Med.* 1993;329:1–7.
49. The Digitalis Investigation Group [see comments]. The effect of digoxin on mortality and morbidity in patients with heart failure. *N Engl J Med.* 1997;336:525–533.
50. The Digitalis Investigation Group. The effect of digoxin on mortality and morbidity in patients with heart failure. *N Engl J Med.* 1997;336:525–533.
51. Eichhorn EJ, Gheorghiade M. Digoxin. *Prog Cardiovasc Dis.* 2002;44:251–266.
52. Rathore SS, Curtis JP, Wang Y, et al. Association of serum digoxin concentration and outcomes in patients with heart failure. *JAMA.* 2003;289(7):871–878.
53. Leor J, Goldbourt U, Rabinowitz B, et al. Digoxin and increased mortality among patients recovering from acute myocardial infarction: importance of digoxin dose. The SPRINT Study Group. *Cadiovasc Drugs Ther.* 1995;9:723–729.
54. Rathore SS, Wang Y, Krumholz HM. Sex-based differences in the effect of digoxin for the treatment of heart failure. *N Engl J Med.* 2002;347:1403–1411.
55. Robishaw JD, Foster KA. Role of G proteins in the regulation of the cardiovascular system. *Annu Rev Physiol.* 1989;51:229–244.
56. Fleming JW, Wisler PL, Watanabe AM. Signal transduction by G proteins in cardiac tissues. *Circulation.* 1992;85:420–433. [Published erratum appears in *Circulation.* 1992;86:698.]
57. Berridge MJ, Irvine RF. Inositol trisphosphate, a novel second messenger in cellular signal transduction. *Nature.* 1984; 312: 315–321.
58. Landzberg JS, Parker JD, Gauthier DF, et al. Effects of myocardial alpha 1-adrenergic receptor stimulation and blockade on contractility in humans. *Circulation.* 1991;84:1608–1614.
59. Bristow MR, Hershberger RE, Port JD, et al. Beta-adrenergic pathways in nonfailing and failing human ventricular myocardium. *Circulation.* 1990;82:I12–I25.
60. Feldman AM. Experimental issues in assessment of G-protein function in cardiac disease. *Circulation.* 1991;84:1852–1861.
61. Homcy CJ, Vatner SF, Vatner DE. Beta-adrenergic receptor regulation in the heart in pathophysiologic states: abnormal adrenergic responsiveness in cardiac disease. *Annu Rev Physiol.* 1991;53:137–159.
62. Emorine LJ, Marullo S, Briend-Sutren MM, et al. Molecular characterization of the human β3-adrenergic receptor. *Science.* 1989;245:1118–1121.
63. Rohrer D, Schauble E, Chruscinski A, et al. Evaluation of the role of β1-, β2-, and β3-adrenergic receptors in regulating cardiac and peripheral vascular function in knockout mice. *Circulation.* 1997;96:I53.
64. Harding SE. Lack of evidence for β3-adrenoceptor modulation of contractile function in human ventricular myocytes. *Circulation.* 1997;96:I-53.
65. Feldman AM. Modulation of adrenergic receptors and G-transduction proteins in failing human ventricular myocardium. *Circulation.* 1993;87:IV27–IV34.
66. Gaudin C, Ishikawa Y, Wright D, et al. Overexpression of $G_s\alpha$ protein in the hearts of transgenic mice. *J Clin Invest.* 1995; 95:1676–1686.
67. Bristow MR, Hershberger RE, Port JD, et al. β-adrenergic pathways in nonfailing and failing human ventricular myocardium. *Circulation.* 1990;82:I12–I25.
68. Benovic JL, Mayor F, Staniszewski C, et al. Purification and characterization of the β-adrenergic receptor kinase. *J Biol Chem.* 1987;262:9026–9032.
69. Benovic JL, Strasser RH, Caron MG, et al. βadrenergic receptor kinase: identification of a novel protein kinase that phophorylates the agonist-occupied form of the receptor. *Proc Natl Acad Sci USA.* 1986;83:2797–2801.
70. Koch WJ, Milano CA, Lefkowitz RJ. Transgenic manipulation of myocardial G-protein-coupled receptors and receptor kinases. *Circ Res.* 1996;78:511–516.
71. Koch WJ, Rockman HA, Samama P, et al. Cardiac function in mice overexpressing the β-adrenergic receptor kinase or a β-ARK inhibitor. *Science.* 1995;268:1350–1353.
72. Milano CA, Allen LF, Rockman HA, et al. Enhanced myocardial function in transgenic mice overexpressing the β2-adrenergic receptor. *Science.* 1994;264:582–586.

73. Rockman HA, Hamilton R, Jones LR, et al. Enhanced myocardial relaxation *in vivo* in transgenic mice overexpressing the β2-adrenergic receptor is associated with reduced phospholamban protein. *J Clin Invest.* 1996;97:1618–1623.
74. Iwase M, Uechi M, Vatner DE, et al. Cardiomyopathy induced by cardiac $G_s\alpha$ overexpression. *Am J Physiol.* 1997;272:H585–H589.
75. Iwase M, Bishop SP, Uechi M, et al. Adverse effects of chronic endogenous sympathetic drive induced by cardiac $G_s\alpha$ overexpression. *Circ Res.* 1996;78:517–524.
76. Ginsburg R, Bristow MR, Billingham ME, et al. Study of the normal and failing isolated human heart: decreased response of failing heart to isoproterenol. *Am Heart J.* 1983;106:535–540.
77. Hasking G, Esler MD, Jennings GL, et al. Norepinephrine spillover to plasma in patients with congestive heart failure: evidence of increased overall and cardiorenal sympathetic nervous activity. *Circulation.* 1986;73:615–621.
78. Hausdorff WP, Caron MG, Lefkowitz RJ. Turning off the signal: desensitization of β-adrenergic receptor function. *FASEB J.* 1990;4:2881–2889.
79. Bristow MR, Ginsburg R, Minobe W, et al. Decreased catecholamine sensitivity and beta-adrenergic-receptor density in failing human hearts. *N Engl J Med.* 1982;307:205–211.
80. Bristow MR, Ginsburg R, Umans V, et al. Beta 1 and beta 2-adrenergic-receptor subpopulations in nonfailing and failing human ventricular myocardium: coupling of both receptor subtypes to muscle contraction and selective beta 1 receptor down-regulation in heart failure. *Circ Res.* 1986;59:297–309.
81. Bristow MR, Minobe WA, Port JD, et al. Decreased β1-adrenergic receptor mRNA levels in the failing human heart. *J Clin Invest.* 1993;92:2737–2745.
82. White M, Roden RL, Minobe W, et al. Age-related changes in β-adrenergic neuroeffector systems in the human heart. *Circulation.* 1994;90:1225–1238.
83. Schocken DD, Roth GS. Reduced β-adrenergic receptor concentrations in ageing man. *Nature.* 1977;267:856–858.
84. Magnusson Y, Marullo S, Hoyer S, et al. Mapping of a functional autoimmune epitope on the β1-adrenergic receptor in patients with idiopathic dilated cardiomyopathy. *J Clin Invest.* 1990;86:1658–1663.
85. Feldman AM, Cates AE, Veazey WB, et al. Increase of the 40,000-mol wt pertussis toxin substrate (G-protein) in the failing human heart. *J Clin Invest.* 1988;82:189–197.
86. Feldman AM, Cates AE, Bristow MR, et al. Altered expression of α-subunits of G-proteins in failing human hearts. *J Mol Cell Cardiol.* 1989;21:359–365.
87. Feldman AM, Ray PE, Bristow MR. Expression of α-subunits of G-proteins in failing human heart: a reappraisal utilizing quantitative polymerase chain reaction. *J Mol Cell Cardiol.* 1991;23:1355–1358.
88. Feldman AM. Experimental issues in assessment of G-protein function in cardiac disease. *Circulation.* 1991;84:1852–1861.
89. Ungerer M, Bohm M, Elce JS, et al. Altered expression of β-adrenergic receptor kinase and β_1-adrenergic receptors in the failing human heart. *Circulation.* 1993;87:454–463.
90. Ungerer M, Parruti G, Bohm M, et al. Expression of β-arrestins and β-adrenergic receptor kinases in the failing human heart. *Circ Res.* 1994;74:206–213.
91. Colucci WS, Denniss AR, Leatherman GF, et al. Intracoronary infusion of dobutamine to patients with and without severe congestive heart failure. Dose-response relationships, correlation with circulating catecholamines, and effect of phosphodiesterase inhibition. *J Clin Invest.* 1988;81:1103–1110.
92. Lee HR, O'Connell JB, Renlund DG, et al. Use of enoximone in cardiac transplant cadidates: effect on β-adrenergic receptors. *J Am Coll Cardiol.* 1989;13:248A.
93. Smith HJ, Oriol A, Morch J, et al. Hemodynamic studies in cardiogenic shock. Treatment with isoproterenol and metaraminol. *Circulation.* 1967;35:1084–1091.
94. Tuttle RR, Mills J. Dobutamine: development of a new catecholamine to selectively increase cardiac contractility. *Circ Res.* 1975;36:185–196.
95. Ruffolo RRJ, Spradlin TA, Pollock GD, et al. Alpha and beta adrenergic effects of the stereoisomers of dobutamine. *J Pharmacol Exp Ther.* 1981;219:447–452.
96. Schumann HJ, Wagner J, Knorr A, et al. Demonstration in human atrial preparations of alpha-adrenoceptors mediating positive inotropic effects. *Naunyn-Schmiedebergs Arch Pharmacol.* 1978;302:333–336.
97. Unverferth DV, Magorien RD, Lewis RP, et al. Long-term benefit of dobutamine in patients with congestive cardiomyopathy. *Am Heart J.* 1980;100:622–630.
98. Leier CV, Unverferth DV, Kates RE. The relationship between plasma dobutamine concentrations and cardiovascular responses in cardiac failure. *Am J Med.* 1979;66:238–242.
99. Beregovich J, Bianchi C, D'Angelo R, et al. Haemodynamic effects of a new inotropic agent (dobutamine) in chronic cardiac failure. *Br Heart J.* 1975;37:629–634.
100. Akhtar N, Mikulic E, Cohn JN, et al. Hemodynamic effect of dobutamine in patients with severe heart failure. *Am J Cardiol.* 1975;36:202–205.
101. Leier CV, Webel J, Bush CA. The cardiovascular effects of the continuous infusion of dobutamine in patients with severe cardiac failure. *Circulation.* 1977;56:468–472.
102. Bendersky R, Chatterjee K, Parmley WW, et al. Dobutamine in chronic ischemic heart failure: alterations in left ventricular function and coronary hemodynamics. *Am J Cardiol.* 1981;48:554–558.
103. Pozen RG, DiBianco R, Katz RJ, et al. Myocardial metabolic and hemodynamic effects of dobutamine in heart failure complicating coronary artery disease. *Circulation.* 1981;63:1279–1285.
104. Meyer SL, Curry GC, Donsky MS, et al. Influence of dobutamine on hemodynamics and coronary blood flow in patients with and without coronary artery disease. *Am J Cardiol.* 1976;38:103–108.
105. Unverferth DA, Blanford M, Kates RE, et al. Tolerance to dobutamine after a 72-hour continuous infusion. *Am J Med.* 1980;69:262–266.
106. Stevenson LW, Massie BM, Francis GS. Optimizing therapy for complex or refractory heart failure: a management algorithm. *Am Heart J.* 1998;135:S293–S309.
107. Fonarow GC, Stevenson LW, Walden JA, et al. Impact of a comprehensive heart failure management program on hospital readmission and functional status of patients with advanced heart failure. *J Am Coll Cardiol.* 1997;30:725–732.
108. Steimle AE, Stevenson LW, Chelimsky-Fallick C, et al. Sustained hemodynamic efficacy of therapy tailored to reduce filling pressures in survivors with advanced heart failure. *Circulation.* 1997;96:1165–1172.
109. Mueller HS, Chatterjee K, Davis KB, et al. ACC expert consensus document. Present use of bedside right heart catheterization in patients with cardiac disease. *J Am Coll Cardiol.* 1998; 32:840–864.
110. Unverferth DV, Magorien RD, Altschuld R, et al. The hemodynamic and metabolic advantages gained by a three-day infusion of dobutamine in patients with congestive cardiomyopathy. *Am Heart J.* 1983;106:29–34.
111. Liang CS, Tuttle RR, Hood WBJ, et al. Conditioning effects of chronic infusions of dobutamine. Comparison with exercise training. *J Clin Invest.* 1979;64:613–619.
112. Schoemaker RG, Debets JJ, Struyker-Boudier HA, et al. Two weeks of intermittent dobutamine therapy restores cardiac performance and inotropic responsiveness in conscious rats with heart failure. *J Cardiovasc Pharmacol.* 1991;17:949–956.
113. Leier CV, Huss P, Lewis RP, et al. Drug-induced conditioning in congestive heart failure. *Circulation.* 1982;65:1382–1387.
114. Applefeld MM, Newman KA, Grove WR, et al. Intermittent, continuous outpatient dobutamine infusion in the management of congestive heart failure. *Am J Cardiol.* 1983;51:455–458.
115. Dies F. Intermittent dobutamine in ambulatory patients with chronic cardiac failure. *Br J Clin Pract.* 1986;45:37–40.
116. Krell MJ, Kline EM, Bates ER, et al. Intermittent, ambulatory dobutamine infusions in patients with severe congestive heart failure. *Am Heart J.* 1986;112:787–791.
117. Collins JA, Skidmore MA, Melvin DB, et al. Home intravenous dobutamine therapy in patients awaiting heart transplantation. *J Heart Transplant.* 1990;9:205–208.
118. Goldberg LI. Cardiovascular and renal actions of dopamine: potential clinical applications. *Pharmacol Rev.* 1972;24:1–29.
119. Goldberg LI, Volkman PH, Kohli JD. A comparison of the vascular dopamine receptor with other dopamine receptors. *Annu Rev Pharmacol Toxicol.* 1978;18:57–79.
120. Goldberg LI, Kohli JD. Peripheral dopamine receptors: a classification based on potency series and specific antagonism. *Trends Pharmacol Sci.* 1983;4:64.

121. Hilditch A, Drew GM. Peripheral dopamine receptor blockade by SCH 23390 and domperidone *in vitro*. *Eur J Pharmacol*. 1985;116:171–174.
122. Lokhandwala MF, Barrett RJ. Cardiovascular dopamine receptors: physiological, pharmacological and therapeutic implications. *J Auton Pharmacol*. 1982;2:189–215.
123. Goldberg LI, Glock D, Kohli JD, et al. Separation of peripheral dopamine receptors by a selective DA_1 antagonist, SCH 23390. *Hypertension*. 1984;6:I25–I30.
124. Wassermann K, Huss R, Kullmann R. Dopamine-induced diuresis in the cat without changes in renal hemodynamics. *Naunyn-Schmiedebergs Arch Pharmacol*. 1980;312:77–83.
125. Felder RA, Blecher M, Calcagno PL, et al. Dopamine receptors in the proximal tubule of the rabbit. *Am J Physiol*. 1984;247: F499–F505.
126. Hughes JM, Beck TR, Rose CEJ, et al. The effect of selective dopamine-1 receptor stimulation on renal and adrenal function in man. *J Clin Endocrinol Metab*. 1988;66:518–525.
127. Willems JL, Buylaert WA, Lefebvre RA, et al. Neuronal dopamine receptors on autonomic ganglia and sympathetic nerves and dopamine receptors in the gastrointestinal system. *Pharmacol Rev*. 1985;37:165–216.
128. Langer SZ, Arbilla S. Pharmacological significance of pre and postsynaptic dopamine receptors. In: Poste G, Crooke ST, eds. *Dopamine Receptor Agonists*. New York: Plenum Press; 1984: 157.
129. Goldberg LI, Hsieh YY, Resnekov L. Newer catecholamines for treatment of heart failure and shock: an update on dopamine and a first look at dobutamine. *Prog Cardiovasc Dis*. 1977;19:327–340.
130. McNay JL, Goldberg LI. Hemodynamic effects of dopamine in the dog before and after alpha adrenergic blockade. *Circ Res*. 1966;18:I-110.
131. Miller RR, Awan NA, Joye JA, et al. Combined dopamine and nitroprusside therapy in congestive heart failure. Greater augmentation of cardiac performance by addition of inotropic stimulation to afterload reduction. *Circulation*. 1977;55: 881–884.
132. Loeb HS, Ostrenga JP, Gaul W, et al. Beneficial effects of dopamine combined with intravenous nitroglycerin on hemodynamics in patients with severe left ventricular failure. *Circulation*. 1983;68:813–820.
133. Leier CV, Heban PT, Huss P, et al. Comparative systemic and regional hemodynamic effects of dopamine and dobutamine in patients with cardiomyopathic heart failure. *Circulation*. 1978;58:466–475.
134. Stoner JD, Bolen JL, Harrison DC. Comparison of dobutamine and dopamine in treatment of severe heart failure. *Br Heart J*. 1977;39:536–539.
135. Loeb HS, Bredakis J, Gunner RM. Superiority of dobutamine over dopamine for augmentation of cardiac output in patients with chronic low output cardiac failure. *Circulation*. 1977;55: 375–378.
136. van de Borne P, Oren R, Somers VK. Dopamine depresses minute ventilation in patients with heart failure. *Circulation*. 1998;98:126–131.
137. Johnson RLJ. Low-dose dopamine and oxygen transport by the lung. *Circulation*. 1998;98:97–99.
138. Ouadid H, Jdaiaa H, Guilbault P, et al. Possible involvement of a dopaminergic receptor positively coupled to adenylate cyclase in isolated human cardiac cells. *J Physiol*. 1993;467:360P.
139. Dubois-Rande JL, Merlet P, Duval-Moulin AM, et al. Coronary vasodilating action of dobutamine in patients with idiopathic dilated cardiomyopathy. *Am Heart J*. 1993;125:1329–1336.
140. Daly JW. Forskolin, adenylate cyclase, and cell physiology: an overview. *Adv Cyclic Nucleotide Protein Phosphoryl Res*. 1984; 17:81–89.
141. Blinks JR, Olson CB, Jewell BR, et al. Influence of caffeine and other methylxanthines on mechanical properties of isolated mammalian heart muscle. Evidence for a dual mechanism of action. *Circ Res*. 1972;30:367–392.
142. Alousi AA, Farah AE, Lesher GY, et al. Cardiotonic activity of amrinone–Win 40680 [5-amino-3,4′-bipyridine-6(1H)-one]. *Circ Res*. 1979;45:666–677.
143. Millard RW, Dube G, Grupp G, et al. Direct vasodilator and positive inotropic actions of amrinone. *J Mol Cell Cardiol*. 1980; 12:647–652.
144. Benotti JR, Grossman W, Braunwald E, et al. Hemodynamic assessment of amrinone. A new inotropic agent. *N Engl J Med*. 1978;299:1373–1377.
145. Siskind SJ, Sonnenblick EH, Forman R, et al. Acute substantial benefit of inotropic therapy with amrinone on exercise hemodynamics and metabolism in severe congestive heart failure. *Circulation*. 1981;64:966–973.
146. el Allaf D, Cremers S, D'Orio V, et al. Combined haemodynamic effects of low doses of dopamine and dobutamine in patients with acute infarction and cardiac failure. *Arch Int Physiol Biochim*. 1984;92:S49–S55.
147. Wilmshurst PT, Thompson DS, Juul SM, et al. Comparison of the effects of amrinone and sodium nitroprusside on haemodynamics, contractility, and myocardial metabolism in patients with cardiac failure due to coronary artery disease and dilated cardiomyopathy. *Br Heart J*. 1984;52:38–48.
148. Firth BG, Ratner AV, Grassman ED, et al. Assessment of the inotropic and vasodilator effects of amrinone versus isoproterenol. *Am J Cardiol*. 1984;54:1331–1336.
149. Franciosa JA. Intravenous amrinone: an advance or a wrong step? *Ann Intern Med*. 1985;102:399–400.
150. Feldman MD, Copelas L, Gwathmey JK, et al. Deficient production of cyclic AMP: pharmacologic evidence of an important cause of contractile dysfunction in patients with end-stage heart failure. *Circulation*. 1987;75:331–339.
151. Endoh M, Yamashita S, Taira N. Positive inotropic effect of amrinone in relation to cyclic nucleotide metabolism in the canine ventricular muscle. *J Pharmacol Exp Ther*. 1982;221:775–783.
152. Kariya T, Wille LJ, Dage RC. Biochemical studies on the mechanism of cardiotonic activity of MDL 17,043. *J Cardiovasc Pharmacol*. 1982;4:509–514.
153. Gaide MS, Fitterman WS, Wiggins JR, et al. Amrinone relaxes potassium-induced contracture of failing right ventricular muscle of cats. *J Cardiovasc Pharmacol*. 1983;5:335–340.
154. Adams HR, Rhody J, Sutko JL. Amrinone activates K-depolarized atrial and ventricular myocardium of guinea pigs. *Circ Res*. 1982;51:662–665.
155. Siegl PK, Morgan G, Sweet CS. Responses to amrinone in isolated cardiac muscles from cat, rabbit, and guinea pig. *J Cardiovasc Pharmacol*. 1984;6:281–287.
156. DiBianco R, Shabetai R, Silverman BD, et al, with the Amrinone Multicenter Study Investigators. Oral amrinone for the treatment of chronic congestive heart failure: results of a multicenter randomized double-blind and placebo-controlled withdrawal study. *J Am Coll Cardiol*. 1984;4:855–866.
157. Massie B, Bourassa M, DiBianco R, et al. Long-term oral administration of amrinone for congestive heart failure: lack of efficacy in a multicenter controlled trial. *Circulation*. 1985;71:963–971.
158. Packer M, Medina N, Yushak M. Hemodynamic and clinical limitations of long-term inotropic therapy with amrinone in patients with severe chronic heart failure. *Circulation*. 1984;70:1038–1047.
159. Uretsky BF, Jessup M, Konstam MA, et al, for the Enoximine Multicenter Trial Group. Multicenter trial of oral enoximone in patients with moderate to moderately severe congestive heart failure. *Circulation*. 1990;82:774–780.
160. Packer M, Carver JR, Rodeheffer RJ, et al. Effect of oral milrinone on mortality in severe chronic heart failure. The PROMISE Study Research Group [see comments]. *N Engl J Med*. 1991;325:1468–1475.
161. Cody RJ, Muller FB, Kubo SH, et al. Identification of the direct vasodilator effect of milrinone with an isolated limb preparation in patients with chronic congestive heart failure. *Circulation*. 1986;73:124–129.
162. Ludmer PL, Wright RF, Arnold JM, et al. Separation of the direct myocardial and vasodilator actions of milrinone administered by an intracoronary infusion technique. *Circulation*. 1986;73: 130–137.
163. Baim DS, McDowell AV, Cherniles J, et al. Evaluation of a new bipyridine inotropic agent–milrinone–in patients with severe congestive heart failure. *N Engl J Med*. 1983;309:748–756.
164. Grose R, Strain J, Greenberg M, et al. Systemic and coronary effects of intravenous milrinone and dobutamine in congestive heart failure. *J Am College Cardiol*. 1986;7:1107–1113.
165. Mager G, Klocke RK, Kux A, et al. Phosphodiesterase III inhibition or adrenoreceptor stimulation: milrinone as an alternative to dobutamine in the treatment of severe heart failure. *Am Heart J*. 1991;121:1974–1983.

166. Vilcek J, Lee TH. Tumor necrosis factor. *J Biol Chem*. 1991;266: 7313–7316.
167. Finkel MS, Oddis CV, Jacob TD, et al. Negative inotropic effects of cytokines on the heart mediated by nitric oxide. *Science*. 1992;257:387–389.
168. Yokoyama T, Vaca L, Rossen RD, et al. Cellular basis for the negative inotropic effects of tumor necrosis factor-alpha in the adult mammalian heart. *J Clin Invest*. 1993;92:2303–2312.
169. Ungureanu-Longrois D, Balligand JL, Simmons WW, et al. Induction of nitric oxide synthase activity by cytokines in ventricular myocytes is necessary but not sufficient to decrease contractile responsiveness to beta-adrenergic agonists. *Circ Res*. 1995;77:494–502.
170. Schulz R, Panas DL, Catena R, et al. The role of nitric oxide in cardiac depression induced by interleukin-1 beta and tumour necrosis factor-alpha. *Br J Pharmacol*. 1995;114:27–34.
171. Meldrum DR. Tumor necrosis factor in the heart. *Am J Physiol*. 1998;274:R577–R595.
172. Torre-Amione G, Kapadia S, Benedict C, et al. Proinflammatory cytokine levels in patients with depressed left ventricular ejection fraction: a report from the Studies of Left Ventricular Dysfunction (SOLVD). *J Am Coll Cardiol*. 1996;27:1 201–1206.
173. Torre-Amione G, Kapadia S, Lee J, et al. Tumor necrosis factor-alpha and tumor necrosis factor receptors in the failing human heart. *Circulation*. 1996;93:704–711.
174. Kubota T, McTiernan CF, Frye CS, et al. Dilated cardiomyopathy in transgenic mice with cardiac-specific overexpression of tumor necrosis factor-alpha. *Circ Res*. 1997;81:627–635.
175. Kolls J, Peppel K, Silva M, et al. Prolonged and effective blockade of tumor necrosis factor activity through adenovirus-mediated gene transfer. *Proc Natl Acad Sci USA*. 1994;91:215–219.
176. Kapadia S, Torre-Amione G, Yokoyama T, et al. Soluble TNF binding proteins modulate the negative inotropic properties of TNF-alpha *in vitro*. *Am J Physiol*. 1995;268:H517–H525.
177. Bounoutas GS, Kubota T, Miyagishima M, et al. Adenoviral-directed overexpression of soluble tumor necrosis factor receptors reverses myocarditis in transgenic mice with congestive heart failure. *Circulation*. 1998;98:I-737.
178. Matsumori A. The use of cytokine inhibitors. A new therapeutic insight into heart failure. *Int J Cardiol*. 1997;62(Suppl 1): S3–S12.
179. Matsumori A, Ono K, Sato Y, et al. Differential modulation of cytokine production by drugs: implications for therapy in heart failure. *J Mol Cell Cardiol*. 1996;28:2491–2499.
180. Sinha B, Semmler J, Eisenhut T, et al. Enhanced tumor necrosis factor suppression and cyclic adenosine monophosphate accumulation by combination of phosphodiesterase inhibitors and prostanoids. *Eur J Immunol*. 1995;25:147–153.
181. Bergman MR, Holycross BJ. Pharmacological modulation of myocardial tumor necrosis factor alpha production by phosphodiesterase inhibitors. *J Pharmacol Exp Ther*. 1996;279:247–254. [Published erratum appears in *J Pharmacol Exp Ther*. 1997; 280:520.]
182. Sliwa K, Skudicky D, Candy G, et al. Randomised investigation of effects of pentoxifylline on left-ventricular performance in idiopathic dilated cardiomyopathy. *Lancet*. 1998;351:1091–1093.
183. Shakar SF, Abraham WT, Gilbert EM, et al. Combined oral positive inotropic and beta-blocker therapy for treatment of refractory class IV heart failure. *J Am Coll Cardiol*. 1998;31:1336–1340.
184. De Marco T, Chatterjee K. Phosphodiesterase inhibitors in refractory heart failure: bridge to beta-blockade? *J Am Coll Cardiol*. 1998;31:1341–1343.
185. Morgan JP. Abnormal intracellular modulation of calcium as a major cause of cardiac contractile dysfunction. *N Engl J Med*. 1991;325:625–632.
186. Gwathmey JK, Copelas L, MacKinnon R, et al. Abnormal intracellular calcium handling in myocardium from patients with end-stage heart failure. *Circ Res*. 1987;61:70–76.
187. Morgan JP, Erny RE, Allen PD, et al. Abnormal intracellular calcium handling, a major cause of systolic and diastolic dysfunction in ventricular myocardium from patients with heart failure. *Circulation*. 1990;81:III21–III32.
188. D'Agnolo A, Luciani GB, Mazzucco A, et al. Contractile properties and Ca^{2+} release activity of the sarcoplasmic reticulum in dilated cardiomyopathy. *Circulation*. 1992;85:518–525.
189. Pieske B, Sutterlin M, Schmidt-Schweda S, et al. Diminished post-rest potentiation of contractile force in human dilated cardiomyopathy. *J Clin Invest*. 1996;98:764–776.
190. Feldman AM, Ray PE, Silan CM, et al. Selective gene expression in failing human heart. Quantification of steady-state levels of messenger RNA in endomyocardial biopsies using the polymerase chain reaction. *Circulation*. 1991;83:1866–1872.
191. Linck B, Boknik P, Eschenhagen T, et al. Messenger RNA expression and immunological quanitification of phospholamban and SR-Ca^{2+}-ATPase in failing and nonfailing human hearts. *Cardiovasc Res*. 1996;31:625–632.
192. Mercadier JJ, Lompre AM, Duc P, et al. Altered sarcoplasmic reticulum Ca^{2+}-ATPase gene expression in the human ventricle during end-stage heart failure. *J Clin Invest*. 1990;85: 305–309.
193. Ladenson PW, Sherman SI, Baughman KL, et al. Reversible alterations in myocardial gene expression in a young man with dilated cardiomyopathy and hypothyroidism. *Proc Natl Acad Sci USA*. 1992;82:5251–5255.
194. Hasenfuss G, Reinecke H, Studer R, et al. Relation between myocardial function and expression of sarcoplasmic reticulum Ca^{2+}-ATPase in failing and nonfailing human myocardium. *Circ Res*. 1994;75:434–442.
195. Brillantes AM, Allen PD, Takahashi T, et al. Differences in cardiac calcium release channel (ryanodine receptor) expression in myocardium from patients with end-stage heart failure caused by ischemic versus dilated cardiomyopathy. *Circ Res*. 1992;71: 18–26.
196. Studer R, Reinecke H, Bilger J, et al. Gene expression of the cardiac Na^{+}-Ca^{2+} exchanger in end-stage human heart failure. *Circ Res*. 1994;75:443–453.
197. Luo W, Grupp IL, Harrer J, et al. Targeted ablation of the phospholamban gene is associated with markedly enhanced myocardial contractility and loss of β-agonist stiumulation. *Circ Res*. 1994;75:401–409.
198. Hoit BD, Khoury SF, Kranias EG, et al. *In vivo* echocardiographic detection of enhanced left ventricular function in gene-targeted mice with phospholamban deficiency. *Circ Res*. 1995;77: 632–637.
199. Luo W, Wolska BM, Grupp IL, et al. Phospholamban gene dosage effects in the mammalian heart. *Circ Res*. 1996;78: 839–847.
200. He H, Giordano FJ, Hilal-Dandan R, et al. Overexpression of the rat sarcoplasmic reticulum Ca^{2+}-ATPase gene in the heart of transgenic mice accelerates calcium transients and cardiac relaxation. *J Clin Invest*. 1997;100:380–389.
201. Giordano FJ, He H, McDonough PM, et al. Adenovirus-mediated gene transfer reconstitutes depressed sarcoplasmic reticulum Ca^{2+}-ATPase levels and shortens prolonged cardiac myocyte Ca^{2+} transients. *Circulation*. 1997; 96:400–403.
202. Hajjar RJ, Schmidt U, Kang JX, et al. Adenoviral gene transfer of phospholamban in isolated rat cardiomyocytes. *Circ Res*. 1997;81:145–153.
203. Chiu YC, Walley KR, Ford LE. Comparison of the effects of different inotropic interventions on force, velocity, and power in rabbit myocardium. *Circ Res*. 1989;65:1161–1171.
204. Scholz H. Positive inotropic agents: different mechanisms of action. In: Erdmann LK, Greef JC, eds. *Cardiac Glycosides*. Darmstadt: Steinkopff; 1986: 181–188.
205. Katz AM. Potential deleterious effects of inotropic agents in the therapy of chronic heart failure. *Circulation*. 1986;73: III184–III190.
206. Katz AM. Role of the basic sciences in the practice of cardiology. *J Mol Cell Cardiol*. 1987;19:3–17.
207. Kitada Y, Narimatsu A, Matsumura N, et al. Increase in Ca^{2+} sensitivity of the contractile system by MCI-154, a novel cardiotonic agent, in chemically skinned fibers from the guinea pig papillary muscles. *J Pharmacol Exp Ther*. 1987;243:633–638.
208. Brenner B. A new concept for the mechanism of Ca+(+) regulation of muscle contraction. Implications for physiological and pharmacological approaches to modulate contractile function of myocardium. *Basic Res Cardiol*. 1991;86(Suppl 3):83–92.
209. Brenner B. Effect of Ca^{2+} on cross-bridge turnover kinetics in skinned single rabbit psoas fibers: implications for regulation of muscle contraction. *Proc Natl Acad Sci USA*. 1988;85: 3265–3269.

210. Brenner B. Muscle mechanics and biochemical kinetics. In: Squire J, ed. *Molecular Mechanisms of Muscle Contraction*. London: Macmillan; 1990: 77–149.
211. Ferroni C, Spurgeon M, Klockow M, et al. Contractile potentiation without increasing cytosolic calcium in single rat ventricular myocytes. *FASEB J*. 1989;3:4720–4725.
212. Popping S, Mruck S, Fischer Y, et al. Economy of contraction of cardiomyocytes as influenced by different positive inotropic interventions. *Am J Physiol*. 1996;271: H357–H364.
213. Onishi K, Sekioka K, Ishisu R, et al. MCI-154, a Ca^{2+} sensitizer, decreases the oxygen cost of contractility in isolated canine hearts. *Am J Physiol*. 1997;273:H1688–H1695.
214. Lee JA, Allen DG. Calcium sensitisers: mechanisms of action and potential usefulness as inotropes. *Cardiovasc Res*. 1997;36: 10–20.
215. Udvary E, Papp JG, Vegh A. Cardiovascular effects of the calcium sensitizer, levosimendan, in heart failure induced by rapid pacing in the presence of aortic constriction. *Br J Pharmacol*. 1994;114:656–661.
216. Antila S, Eha J, Heinpalu M, et al. Haemodynamic interactions of a new calcium sensitizing drug levosimendan and captopril. *Eur J Clin Pharmacol*. 1996;49:451–458.
217. Antila S, Pesonen U, Lehtonen L, et al . Pharmakinetics of Levosimendor and its active metabolite OR-1896 in rapid and slow acetylators. *Eur J Pharm Sci*. 2004;23:213–222.
218. Lehtonen L, Mills-Owens P, Akkila J. Safety of levosimendan and other calcium sensitizers. *J Cardiovasc Pharmacol*. 1995;26:S70–S76.
219. Tominaga M, Yo E, Ogawa H, et al. Studies on positive inotropic agents. I. Synthesis of 3,4-dihydro-6-[4-(3,4-dimethoxybenzoyl)-1-piperazinyl]-2(1H)-quinolinone and related compounds. *Chem Pharm Bull*. 1984;32: 2100–2110.
220. Lathrop DA, Schwartz A. Evidence for possible increase of sodium channel open time and involvement of Na/Ca exchange by a new positive inotropic drug: OPC-8212. *Eur J Pharmacol*. 1985;19;117:391–392.
221. Iijima T, Taira N. Membrane current changes responsible for the positive inotropic effect of OPC-8212, a new positive inotropic agent, in single ventricular cells of the guinea pig heart. *J Pharmacol Exp Ther*. 1987;240:657–662.
222. Yatani A, Imoto Y, Schwartz A, et al. New positive inotropic agent OPC-8212 modulates single Ca^{2+} channels in ventricular myocytes of guinea pig. *J Cardiovasc Pharmacol*. 1989;13: 812–819.
223. Inoue M, Kim BH, Hori M, et al. Oral OPC-8212 for the treatment of congestive heart failure: hemodynamic improvement and increased exercise capacity. *Heart Vessels*. 1986;2: 166–171.
224. Sasayama S, Inoue M, Asanoi H, et al. Acute hemodynamic effects of a new inotropic agent, OPC-8212, on severe congestive heart failure. *Heart Vessels*. 1986;2:23–28.
225. Feldman AM, Becker LC, Llewellyn MP, et al. Evaluation of a new inotropic agent, OPC-8212, in patients with dilated cardiomyopathy and heart failure. *Am Heart J*. 1988;116:771–777.
226. Author not listed. A placebo-controlled, randomized, double-blind study of OPC-8212 in patients with mild chronic heart failure. OPC-8212 Multicenter Research Group. *Cardiovasc Drugs Ther*. 1990;4:419–425.
227. Feldman AM, Baughman KL, Lee WK, et al. Usefulness of OPC-8212, a quinolinone derivative, for chronic congestive heart failure in patients with ischemic heart disease or idiopathic dilated cardiomyopathy. *Am J Cardiol*. 1991;68:1203–1210.
228. Feldman AM, Bristow MR, Parmley WW, et al. Effects of vesnarinone on morbidity and mortality in patients with heart failure. Vesnarinone Study Group. *N Engl J Med*. 1993;329:149–155.
229. Cohn JN, Goldstein S, Greenberg BH, et al. A dose-dependent increase in mortality with vesnarinone among patients with severe heart failure. Vesnarinone Trial Investigators. *N Engl J Med*. 1998;339:1810–1816.
230. Dage RC, Okerhoim RA. Pharmacology and pharmacokinetics of enoximone. *Cardiology*. 1990;77(Suppl 3):2–13.
231. Movsesian MA, Smith CJ, Krall J, et al. Sarcoplasmic reticulum-associated cyclic adenosine 5′-monophosphate phosphodiesterase activity in normal and failing human hearts. *J Clin Invest*. 1991;88:15–19.
232. Metra M, Nodari 5, D'Aloia A, et al. Beta-blocker therapy influences the hemodynamic response to inotropic agents in patients with heart failure: a randomized comparison of dobutamine and enoximone before and after chronic treatment with metoprolol or carvedilol. *J Am Coll Cardiol*. 2002;40:1248–1258.
233. Baim DS. Effect of phosphodiesterase inhibition on myocardial oxygen consumption and coronary blood flow. *Am J Cardiol*. 1989;63:23A–26A.
234. Lee HR, Hershberger RE, Port JD, et al. Low-dose enoximone in subjects awaiting cardiac transplantation. Clinical results and effects on beta-adrenergic receptors. *J Thorac Cadiovasc Surg*. 1991;102:246–258.
235. Jondeau G, Dubourg O, Delorme G, et al. Oral enoximone as a substitute for intravenous catecholamine support in end-stage congestive heart failure. *Eur Heart J*. 1994;15:242–246.
236. Cowley AJ, Skene AM. Treatment of severe heart failure: quantity or quality of life? A trial of enoximone. Enoximone Investigators. *Br Heart J*. 1994;72:226–230.
237. Lowes BD, Higginbotham M, Petrovich L, et al. Low-dose enoximone improves exercise capacity in chronic heart failure. *J Am Coll Cardiol*. 2000;36:501–508.
238. Lowes BD, Shakar SF, Metra M, et al. Rationale and design of enoximone clinical trials program. *J Cardiac Failure*. In press.
239. Feldman AM, Oren RM, Abraham W, et al. Low dose oral enoximone enhances the ability to wean patients with ultra-advanced heart failure from intravenous inotrope support: results of the oral enoximone in intravenous inotrope-dependent subjects (EMOTE) trial. In submission.

Clinical Approach to Acute and Chronic Heart Failure

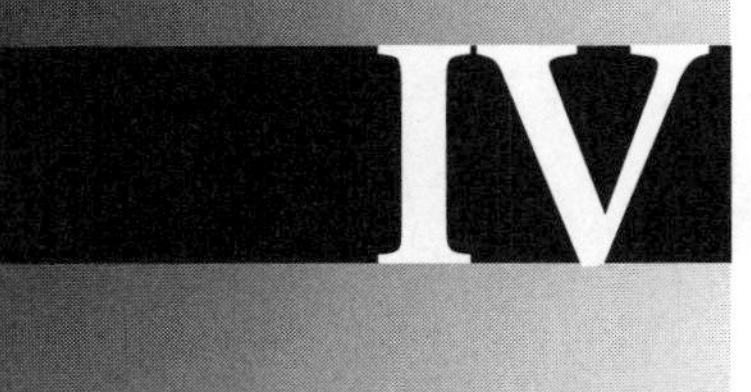

Primary Prevention of Heart Failure

30

David W. Baker *Stephen D. Persell*

The American Heart Association (AHA) estimates that 5 million Americans have symptomatic heart failure (1), and 15 million people are affected worldwide (2). Each year another half-million Americans develop the condition (1). Persons who develop heart failure have markedly impaired quality of life and physical functioning (3), and the majority of patients will die within 5 years of their diagnosis (4,5). Despite tremendous advances in the care of patients with heart failure (6) and improvements in their survival (7,8), their prognosis remains poor. For example, the mortality rate was still approximately 6% to 9% per year in randomized controlled trials of patients with heart failure and moderate to severe left ventricular systolic dysfunction (LVEF $\leq$0.40) who were treated with both an angiotensin-converting enzyme (ACE) inhibitor and a β-blocker (9,10).

While there remain many promising new therapies for heart failure on the horizon, more attention must be given to prevention. The need for emphasis on prevention is underscored by the increasing number of older Americans and the fact that the incidence and prevalence of heart failure increase exponentially with age (11–13). Without improvements in prevention, the prevalence of heart failure and its health and economic consequences will certainly worsen. In recognition of this, the most recent guidelines from the AHA and the American College of Cardiology (ACC) for the evaluation and management of heart failure included a staging system to emphasize the risk factors for heart failure and the need to intervene early to prevent the development of heart failure (Fig. 30-1) (14). Stage A includes patients with risk factors for developing heart failure, including hypertension, coronary artery disease (CAD), diabetes mellitus, previous exposure to cardiotoxic agents, heavy alcohol intake, and possible genetic predisposition to cardiomyopathy (i.e., a family history of idiopathic heart failure). If left untreated, these risk factors will often produce structural heart disease. As individuals develop structural heart disease, patients will usually go through a period when they remain asymptomatic, which is classified as Stage B. Even at this point, it is still possible to intervene to prevent further progression to overt, symptomatic heart failure, which is Stage C.

PRIMARY PREVENTION OF RISK FACTORS FOR HEART FAILURE

Heart failure is a symptom complex that is the final common pathway for a wide array of diseases and pathophysiological processes. Thus, any intervention that reduces cardiovascular disease in a population will ultimately help reduce the incidence of heart failure. In the United States, these key public health targets are prevention of the development of hypertension, diabetes, and ischemic heart disease through lowering average salt intake, increasing intake of fruits and vegetables, increasing physical activity levels, decreasing obesity, reducing tobacco use, and control of dyslipidemias (15–18). Lifestyle and medical therapy to treat hyperlipidemia in accordance with the National Cholesterol Education Program guidelines are aimed primarily at reducing atherosclerotic cardiovascular disease. Controlling hyperlipidemia and preventing myocardial infarctions will ultimately lead to substantial reductions in individuals' subsequent risk of heart failure. Likewise, the use of antiplatelet agents to prevent myocardial infarction would be expected to reduce incident heart failure (19–21).

Prevention of obesity deserves special comment because it is an independent risk factor for hypertension, diabetes,

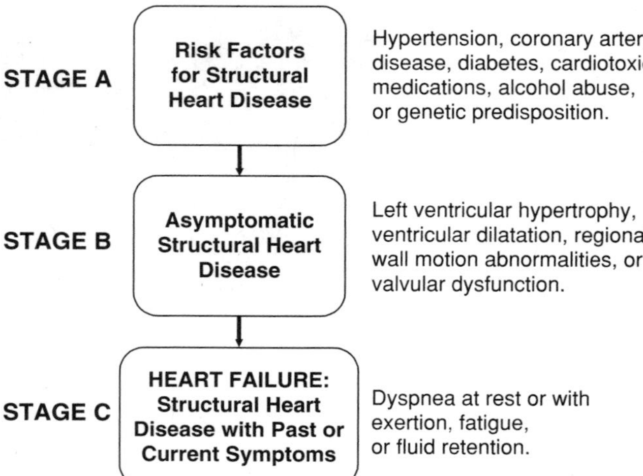

Figure 30-1 Stages of heart failure.

and the lipid abnormalities associated with the metabolic syndrome, and recent studies suggest that obesity may directly increase the risk of developing heart failure (22,23). A full discussion of these public health measures has been reviewed by others and is beyond the scope of this chapter.

In many developing countries, hypertension and ischemic heart disease have become common problems. For example, in India 32% of all deaths in 2000 were due to cardiovascular disease, and the prevalence of hypertension and diabetes is increasing in South Asian countries (24). In these countries, targets for preventing heart failure are similar to those in the United States. However, several other antecedents to heart failure are relevant to specific geographic regions. Heart failure resulting from valvular disease secondary to rheumatic fever remains common among Native Americans in the United States (25) and indigenous peoples in many developing countries (26,27). The incidence of rheumatic fever is related to socioeconomic conditions (25,28). Prevention of heart failure associated with rheumatic fever includes antibiotic treatment of primary streptococcal infections, continuous antibiotic prophylaxis in patients with prior rheumatic fever, and the prevention of infectious endocarditis in persons with rheumatic valvular disease (28,29).

Chagas disease, caused by the protozoa *Trypanosoma cruzi*, remains a common cause of cardiomyopathy in South America (30–33). Chronic Chagas disease occurs predominantly in individuals exposed to the triatomine insect vectors, usually in poor-quality housing, or directly to the *T. cruzi* through blood transfusion. Prevention efforts in South American countries, including the use of insecticides, health education, and surveillance for the insect vectors, have greatly reduced the incidence of Chagas disease since the 1970s (34).

The remainder of this chapter will concentrate on therapies and other strategies to treat the main modifiable risk factors for heart failure in the United States: hypertension (and secondarily, left ventricular hypertrophy [LVH]), CAD (particularly myocardial infarction), diabetes, and valvular heart disease. Improved care for these conditions can substantially reduce the incidence of symptomatic heart failure among patients in stages A and B.

TREATMENT OF HYPERTENSION

Although hypertension is a less-potent risk factor for developing heart failure than myocardial infarction (11), hypertension is so common that it is a major cause of heart failure in the United States. In the 1999–2000 National Health and Nutrition Examination Survey (NHANES), 28.7% of all participants and 65.4% of persons above age 60 had hypertension (35). The Framingham Heart Study estimated that 39% of all heart failure cases in men and 59% of cases in women were attributable to hypertension (36). Uncontrolled hypertension leads to LVH, CAD, and myocardial infarction. Thus, it predisposes patients to heart failure due to both systolic and diastolic dysfunction (37).

Studies have consistently shown that treatment of hypertension dramatically lowers the incidence of heart failure across a wide range of blood pressures (Fig. 30-2) (38–40). The benefits of blood pressure reduction vary across different health outcomes, with an approximately 46% risk reduction for heart failure, a 31% risk reduction for stroke, and a 14% risk reduction for incident coronary

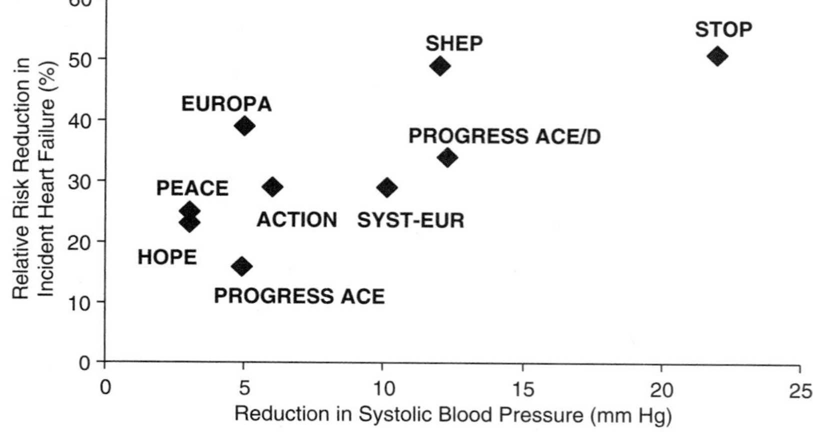

Figure 30-2 Heart failure risk reduction in major, placebo-controlled trials of antihypertensive drugs. ACE, angiotensin-converting enzyme inhibitor; D, diuretic. ACTION, A Coronary Disease Trial Investigating Outcome with Nifedipine GITS (79). EUROPA, European Trial on Reduction of Cardiac Events with Perindopril in Patients with Stable Coronary Artery Disease (76). HOPE, Heart Outcomes Prevention Evaluation Study (77); PEACE, Prevention of Events with Angiotensin-Converting Enzyme Inhibition Trial (75); PROGRESS, Perindopril Protection Against Recurrent Stroke Study (52); SHEP, Systolic Hypertension in the Elderly Program (42); STOP, Swedish Trial in Old Patients with Hypertension (41); SYST-EUR, Systolic Hypertension in Europe Trial (43).

heart disease. The fact that antihypertensive therapy reduces the incidence of heart failure far more than the incidence of coronary heart disease suggests a *direct* effect of lowering blood pressure that is not mediated through a reduction in the rate of myocardial infarction.

Several placebo-controlled studies deserve comment to exemplify the significant health benefits of treating hypertension (Table 30-1). The earliest studies focused on patients with very severe hypertension. The Swedish Trial in Old Patients with Hypertension (STOP-Hypertension) randomized patients with (a) systolic blood pressure 180 to 230 mm Hg and diastolic blood pressure greater than 90 mm Hg, or (b) diastolic blood pressure 105 to 120 mm Hg to receive either a β-blocker (atenolol, metoprolol, or pindolol at the investigator's discretion) or placebo (41). If the blood pressure remained elevated, hydrocholorothiazide could be added. At the end of the trial, the average blood pressure was 167/87 mm Hg in the active treatment group versus 186/96 mm Hg in the placebo group. The risk of developing heart failure was reduced from 4.8% to 2.3%, a 51% relative reduction. The incidence of stroke and cardiovascular mortality were also markedly reduced. Although β-blockers were the first drug initiated in the intervention group, two-thirds of patients were receiving both a β-blocker and hydrocholorothiazide by the study end; therefore, it is not possible to distinguish which drug contributed the most to the blood pressure reduction and the improvements in outcomes.

The Systolic Hypertension in the Elderly Program (SHEP) studied patients with isolated systolic hypertension that was less severe than in STOP (Table 30-1) (42). Patients were eligible if their systolic blood pressure at enrollment was 160 to 219 mm Hg and diastolic blood pressure was less than 90 mm Hg. However, these entry criteria are somewhat misleading. At the time of the first follow-up, the mean blood pressure was 157 mm Hg in the placebo group. Patients randomized to active treatment were first given chlorthalidone with the addition of atenolol as needed for persistently elevated blood pressure (reserpine was used if atenolol was contraindicated). Half of all patients were receiving two agents at the final follow-up visit. At follow-up the difference in the mean pressure between active and control patients in SHEP was only about half of that seen in STOP (Table 30-1). Nevertheless, the benefits in SHEP were strikingly similar to STOP, with the risk of heart failure being cut in half.

The SHEP trial is also noteworthy because investigators conducted stratified analyses for patients with a prior myocardial infarction (by history or electrocardiogram). For this group, the benefits of treating hypertension were even more dramatic, with an 81% reduction in the incidence of heart failure. The enormous benefits of tight blood pressure control for patients with a prior myocardial infarction remain underappreciated, possibly because these results were reported as a subgroup analysis within the main results.

Placebo-controlled trials with dihydropyridine calcium-channel blockers (CCBs) have also been conducted among general hypertensive patient populations (i.e., not restricted to patients with previous cardiovascular disease or diabetes). The Systolic Hypertension in Europe (Syst-Eur) study had similar entry criteria to SHEP (Table 30-1) (43). Patients in Syst-Eur had similar baseline blood pressure to those in SHEP, although their diastolic blood pressure was substantially higher. The active treatment group received nitrendipine initially, which was combined with or replaced by enalapril or hydrochlorothiazide as needed. The blood pressure reduction compared to controls was similar to that in SHEP, and the absolute risk reduction and number needed to treat were nearly identical. However, the relative risk reduction for heart failure was only 29%, substantially less than in STOP and SHEP, and this reduction was not statistically significant. However, a much higher proportion of the placebo group

TABLE 30-1

RELATIVE RISK REDUCTION (RRR) OF INCIDENT HEART FAILURE IN MAJOR PLACEBO-CONTROLLED RANDOMIZED CLINICAL TRIALS OF TREATMENT FOR HYPERTENSION

Study (REF)	Treatment Groups	Mean Age, y	Female (%)	Mean Follow-Up, y	Initial BP, mm Hg	BP Difference,† mm Hg	Incident Heart Failure %	RRR, %	MI, Stroke, or CV Death %	RRR, %
STOP (41)	Atenolol, Metoprolol, or Pindolol (± HCTZ)	76	63	2.1	195/102	22/10	2.3	51	7.1	40
	Placebo	—	—		—	—	4.8	—	11.5	—
SHEP (42)	Chlorthalidone (± Atenolol, ± Reserpine)	72	57	4.5	171/77	12/4	2.3	49*	8.4	33
	Placebo	—	—	—	—	—	4.4	—	12.2	—
Syst-Eur (43)	Nitrendipine ± HCTZ, Enalapril,	70	67	2	174/86	10/5	1.5	29	5.0	31
	Placebo	—	—	—	—	—	2.1	—	7.2	—

REF, Reference; BP, blood pressure; MI, myocardial infarction; CV, cardiovascular; HCTZ, hydrochlorothiazide.
*In SHEP, the relative risk reduction was 81% for patients who had a previous MI and 39% for those who had not previously had an MI.
†Absolute BP difference between the active treatment group and the placebo group at the time of follow-up.

was treated with enalapril or hydrochlorothiazide during the study (60% versus 37% at year 3), which could partially account for the lower than expected reduction in the risk of heart failure. A similar study of nitrendipine conducted in China (Syst-China) found a 58% reduction in heart failure, although the incidence of heart failure was low and the difference in rates again did not reach statistical significance (44).

Thus, treatment of hypertension dramatically reduces the incidence of heart failure, and untreated and uncontrolled hypertension is a major contributor to heart failure in the United States. Even among individuals aged 80 years and older, treatment for hypertension dramatically reduces the incidence of heart failure (45). Older patients have the highest risk of heart failure but they are less likely to have their blood pressure controlled (46). It is never too late to initiate antihypertensive therapy to prevent heart failure.

How Low Is Low Enough?

The studies described above show that modest reductions in blood pressure among patients with mostly stage 1 and 2 hypertension have tremendous benefits. Although we have good data supporting the benefits of reducing systolic blood pressure into the range of 145 mm Hg, we do not know whether the incidence of heart failure can be decreased even more by reducing the blood pressure to the target of <140/90 mm Hg currently recommended by the Seventh Joint National Committee on Prevention, Detection, Evaluation and Treatment of High Blood Pressure (JNC 7) for patients with hypertension who do not have comorbid conditions (47). The Hypertension Optimal Treatment (HOT) trial randomized patients to three different diastolic blood pressure treatment goals: ≤90 mm Hg, ≤85 mm Hg, and ≤80 mm Hg (48). The lowest risk point for major cardiovascular events occurred at 138.5 mm Hg systolic and 82.6 mm Hg diastolic. However, the number of patients who developed heart failure was too small to draw conclusions.

More data are available about the benefits of trying to reach the blood pressure goal of <130/80 mm Hg recommended by JNC for patients with diabetes. The UK Prospective Diabetes Study (UKPDS) found that patients randomized to tighter blood pressure control (mean, 144/82 mm Hg) versus less-tight control (mean, 154/87 mm Hg) had a 60% lower risk of heart failure (95% CI 20% to 80%) (49). The HOT trial found a 51% lower risk of major cardiovascular events among diabetics randomized to a target of ≤80 mm Hg compared to those with a target of ≤90 mm Hg (48). The Appropriate Blood Pressure Control in Diabetes (ABCD) Trial also showed benefits of tighter blood pressure control, including lower rates of myocardial infarction for patients with hypertension randomized to a target diastolic blood pressure of <75 mm Hg versus a target of 80 to 89 mm Hg (50). The ABCD Trial also found lower stroke rates among diabetics without a history of hypertension who were randomized to a target diastolic blood pressure 10 mm Hg below their baseline versus a target of 80 to 89 mm Hg. However, the number of cases of incident heart failure was small in these studies and no conclusions could be drawn.

Patients with hypertension who have suffered a stroke are at high risk for other cardiovascular events, and one study suggests that tight blood pressure control in this group may reduce the risk of heart failure. In the Perindopril Protection Against Recurrent Stroke Study (PROGRESS) patients with prior stroke or transient cerebral ischemia were randomized to placebo or one of two active treatments: the ACE inhibitor perindopril alone or perindopril plus the thiazide diuretic indapamide (51,52). Pretreatment blood pressure was 147/86 mm Hg. Active treatment resulted in a 9/4 mm Hg reduction in blood pressure and a 26% reduction in incident heart failure. The group receiving both the diuretic and the ACE inhibitor had more pronounced blood pressure lowering (12.3/5.0 mm Hg versus 4.9/2.8 mm Hg), and this group had greater reductions in heart failure and major cardiovascular events than did the ACE inhibitor group alone (52,53).

In summary, reducing blood pressure to below 140/90 mm Hg has incremental benefits for reducing heart failure incidence among patients with diabetes and prior stroke. For patients who do not have diabetes or a previous stroke, achieving this blood pressure goal probably reduces cardiovascular disease, although we do not know with certainty whether the incidence of heart failure is also decreased.

Differences Between Antihypertensive Medications

The choice of an antihypertensive agent obviously depends on the drug's ability to reduce overall cardiovascular risk, so choosing an agent because it is best at reducing heart failure risk would make no sense if it is not equally beneficial with respect to other endpoints. The Antihypertensive and Lipid-Lowering Treatment to Prevent Heart Attack Trial (ALLHAT) found that patients treated with the diuretic chlorthalidone, the dihydropyridine CCB amlodipine, and the ACE inhibitor lisinopril had similar rates of cardiovascular events and cardiovascular deaths (54). Meta-analyses have generally reached similar conclusions and other indirect evidence suggests there is a linear relationship between blood pressure reduction and the reduction in cardiovascular events for the most commonly used antihypertensive medications.

Since antihypertensive agents generally result in equivalent rates of cardiovascular events, the antihypertensive drug class that is more successful at preventing heart failure should be preferred over others because of the importance of heart failure as a public health problem. In the ALLHAT study, the 6-year rate of developing heart failure was lowest among patients treated with chlorthalidone (7.7%), intermediate among those treated with lisinopril (8.7%), and highest among those treated with amlodipine (10.2%, $p < 0.001$ for amlodipine and lisinopril compared to chlorthalidone) (54). One meta-analysis that excluded ALLHAT found diuretics to be superior to CCBs for preventing heart failure, but diuretics were not found to be superior compared to ACE inhibitors (39), although other studies have reached different conclusions (55).

β-blockers and adrenergic receptor binders (ARBs) were not included in ALLHAT, so we know much less about these agents. However, a United Kingdom Prospective Diabetes Study (UKPDS) found similar rates of heart failure between the ACE inhibitor captopril and the β-blocker atenolol (56), and the LIFE study found similar rates of heart failure between patients treated with atenolol and the ARB losartan (57). Thus, β-blockers and ARBs are likely to be as beneficial as ACE inhibitors, although their equivalence to diuretics has not been studied.

The ALLHAT trial is the only large, comparative trial of antihypertensive medications that randomized patients to primary treatment with a peripheral α-blocker. The α-blocker arm of the study was terminated early because, compared to treatment with the diuretic cholorthalidone, the group assigned doxazosin had a doubling in heart failure risk as well as a higher risk of stroke (19% increased risk) and combined cardiovascular disease events (25% increased risk) (58). The twofold difference in heart failure observed with doxazosin is comparable in magnitude to the difference seen in early hypertension trials comparing diuretic or β-blocker treatment with placebo. The higher rate of heart failure in the doxazosin group occurred despite only a small blood pressure difference between the diuretic and α-blocker groups (systolic blood pressure 3 mm Hg higher for the doxazosin group). This evidence suggests that blood pressure lowering with a peripheral α-blocker probably has no benefit in reducing heart failure, which is consistent with the results of the VA Cooperative Heart Failure Trial that found the α-blocker prazosin was no more effective than placebo in the treatment of patients with established heart failure (59).

Although debate continues to rage on the optimal first-line antihypertensive, the available evidence suggests that expanding use of thiazide-type diuretics for the treatment of hypertension will help reduce the incidence of heart failure. It is unknown whether diuretics are actually superior at altering the underlying disease processes that lead to ventricular injury and dysfunction, or whether diuretics simply control symptoms of heart failure among patients with early disease. Chlorthalidone and other thiazide-type diuretics appear to achieve similar outcomes for cardiovascular events and mortality but there are no data available for comparative rates of heart failure (60). ACE inhibitors, ARBs, and β-blockers may be somewhat less effective than diuretics, and CCBs and α-blockers are clearly inferior. However, the majority of patients will require more than one drug for blood pressure control, and the optimal therapeutic regimen to prevent heart failure for an individual patient is likely to be the one that lowers blood pressure the most with the least side effects.

Prevention of Heart Failure Among Patients with Left Ventricular Hypertrophy

Poorly controlled hypertension can eventually lead to LVH, a form of asymptomatic left ventricular dysfunction (Stage B, Fig. 30-1). LVH can ultimately cause symptomatic heart failure due to diastolic dysfunction from poor ventricular compliance (Stage C, Fig. 30-1). When present, LVH portends a worse cardiovascular prognosis overall and an increased risk of heart failure (13). Strict control of hypertension is, therefore, extremely important for individuals with LVH. Reduction of left ventricular mass has been observed in patients receiving antihypertensive drug treatment (except for the direct vasodilators) (61,62), and the declining prevalence of severe hypertension and LVH corresponds well with increased use of antihypertensive medications (63). Lifestyle modifications to promote weight loss, reduce salt intake, and increase physical activity also reduce LV mass (64). Furthermore, the regression or lack of development of LVH while taking antihypertensive therapy is a favorable prognostic sign (65,66). There is, however, insufficient clinical evidence to warrant using an individual patient's change in LV mass to guide therapeutic decision making.

It is uncertain whether some antihypertensive medications are better than others for preventing heart failure among patients with LVH. There are theoretical reasons to choose drugs that block the renin-angiotensin-aldosterone system (RAAS) since these agents may have neurohumoral antihypertrophic effects on LV mass that are independent of blood pressure lowering. However, the Treatment of Mild Hypertension Study (TOMHS) does not support this hypothesis. In this trial, individuals with mild hypertension were randomized to placebo, acebutolol, amlodipine, chlorthalidone, doxazosin, or enalapril. All patients received a lifestyle intervention to promote increased physical activity, reduction in salt intake, and weight loss. After 1 year, the groups assigned the thiazide diuretic and the CCB had significantly greater reductions in LV mass than the β-blocker, ACE inhibitor, α-blocker, and placebo groups (64). A meta-analysis of predominantly small studies that excluded TOMHS suggested that LV mass was reduced to a greater extent in patients treated with CCBs, ACE inhibitors, and ARBs compared to β-blockers. Diuretics did not significantly differ from any of the other medication classes (61). In the Losartan Intervention for Endpoint Reduction in Hypertension Study, a large trial in which all participants had LVH by electrocardiogram (ECG) criteria, the ARB losartan reduced LVH more than atenolol and major cardiovascular events were also reduced (57,67). Notably, incident heart failure was similar in both groups. One explanation for this finding is that atenolol slows the heart rate and allows more time in diastole for filling. Thus, even though atenolol had a less-beneficial effect on LVH regression, its other cardiac and neurohormonal effects may have helped prevent heart failure through other pathways, ultimately resulting in equal benefits compared to losartan.

We believe that the debate about which single drug is best for promoting regression of LVH and preventing heart failure is misguided because it directs our attention away from the central clinical problem. Most patients with LVH have blood pressure that is hard to control and will require multiple medications. The main goal for patients with LVH should be to reduce the blood pressure to recommended targets (i.e., <140/90 mm Hg) with whatever combination of medications is effective, tolerated, and affordable for a given patient. We are unaware of any studies that have compared different combinations of drugs to see which are most effective at reducing incident heart failure. Based on the limited amount of data previously described, a reasonable approach would be to start with a combination of a thiazide-type diuretic and either an ACE inhibitor or an ARB and then add a β-blocker or a CCB as needed to reach the appropriate blood pressure target.

PREVENTION STRATEGIES FOR PATIENTS WITH CORONARY ARTERY DISEASE

Ischemic heart disease and myocardial infarction are the predominant causes of heart failure due to left ventricular systolic dysfunction (68). Each year in the United States approximately 1.2 million people are hospitalized with a first (700,000) or recurrent (500,000) infarction (69), and many more have silent myocardial infarctions (1). Approximately 14% of people who suffer a heart attack will develop heart failure over the 5 years after their infarction, and the incidence rises to 22% after 10 years (70). Preventing coronary disease and myocardial infarction is obviously a critical goal if we are to reduce the incidence of heart failure. Although in many cases evidence from randomized, controlled trials is lacking, interventions that successfully reduce the overall risk of CAD and myocardial infarction are all likely to reduce the incidence of heart failure.

This section discusses the importance of treatment of hypercholesterolemia and the use of ACE inhibitors to prevent heart failure. Another important concern for patients with CAD is asymptomatic left ventricular systolic dysfunction (ALVSD). Patients with this condition are at risk for progressive ventricular remodeling and development of heart failure. Because ALVSD is not unique to patients with CAD, treatment of this condition is discussed in the following section.

Treatment of Hypercholesterolemia

Control of hyperlipidemia prevents CAD and myocardial infarction (MI) and in some studies has been proven to reduce the incidence of heart failure. Cholesterol-lowering therapy with a statin in patients with CAD, in addition to the beneficial effects on other cardiovascular events and mortality, has been proven to reduce incident heart failure by 20% in the Scandinavian Simvasatin Survival Study (absolute risk reduction 2% over 5 years) (71). In the A to Z Trial, performed in patients with acute coronary syndromes, high-intensity statin therapy was associated with a 28% reduction in heart failure compared with lower-intensity statin therapy (1.3% absolute risk reduction over 2 years) (72). Reduction in heart failure is not limited to treatment with statins. Use of gemfibrozil in the Veterans' Affairs Cooperative Studies Program High-Density Lipoprotein Cholesterol Intervention Trial reduced the rate of heart failure hospitalization in men with CAD by 22% (2.7% absolute risk reduction over 5.1 years) (73). Several other lipid-lowering medication studies did not show a significant reduction in heart failure events or did not report heart failure as an outcome. However, these reports very likely underestimate the impact of treating hyperlipidemia on heart failure. Since the primary mechanism by which lipid-lowering agents reduce the incidence of heart failure is by reducing the rate of myocardial infarction, demonstration of a significant reduction in heart failure with lipid-lowering drugs may require larger studies with longer follow-up than what is needed to detect reductions in cardiovascular events.

Renin-Angiotensin System Blockade and Reducing Blood Pressure

Patients with established atherosclerotic disease are at increased risk for the development of heart failure. The effects of ACE inhibitors have been tested in patients at high risk of heart failure due to pre-existing cardiovascular disease who had minimal or no elevation in blood pressure. Three large, placebo-controlled trials of ACE inhibitors enrolled predominantly patients with stable CAD without evidence of heart failure (Table 30-2) (74–76). Mean baseline blood pressures for these three

TABLE 30-2
HEART FAILURE AND CARDIOVASCULAR DISEASE OUTCOMES IN TRIALS OF ACE INHIBITORS FOR PATIENTS AT HIGH RISK OF CORONARY DISEASE AND NORMAL OR NEAR-NORMAL BLOOD PRESSURE

Study	Treatment Groups	Patient Population	Mean Age, y	Female (%)	Mean Follow-Up, y	Initial BP, mm Hg	BP Difference at Follow-Up, mm Hg	Incident Heart Failure* %	RRR, %	Primary Composite Endpoint† %	RRR, %
HOPE (11)	Ramipril	CVD or DM and ≥1 CV risk factor	66	27	4.6	139/79	−3/−2	9.0	23	14.0	22
	Placebo							11.5		17.8	
EUROPA (14)	Perindopril	Stable CHD	60	15	4.2	137/82	−5/−2	1.0	39	8.0	20
	Placebo							1.7		9.9	
PEACE (15)	Trandolapril	Stable CHD	64	18	4.8	133/78	−3/−1	2.8	25	21.9	4
	Placebo							3.7		22.5	

ACE, angiotensin-converting enzyme; BP, blood pressure; MI, myocardial infarction; CV, cardiovascular; RRR, relative risk reduction, CHD, coronary heart disease.
*When multiple heart failure outcomes were reported, the outcome with the greatest number of events is shown.
†Primary composite endpoints differ across studies.

trials were 139/79 mm Hg in the Heart Outcomes Prevention Evaluation Study (HOPE), 137/82 mm Hg in the European Trial on Reduction of Cardiac Events with Perindopril in Patients with Stable Coronary Artery Disease (EUROPA) and 133/78 mm Hg in the Prevention of Events with Angiotensin-Converting Enzyme Inhibition Trial (PEACE). Thus, the majority of patients had systolic blood pressure below the recommended target of 140 mm Hg. In these trials, systolic blood pressure was reduced by 3 to 5 mm Hg in the ACE inhibitor groups compared to controls receiving placebo.

ACE inhibitors reduced the risk of major cardiovascular events by 20% to 22% in HOPE and EUROPA but did not reduce risk in PEACE. The lack of a reduction in cardiovascular events in PEACE may have been due to higher rates of lipid-lowering agents, antiplatelet therapy, and coronary artery revascularization prior to study enrollment compared to participants in the other two trials. Although cardiovascular event reduction varied across the studies, all three trials reported similar, statistically significant reductions in incident heart failure with ACE inhibitor treatment, finding relative risk reductions of 23% to 39% compared to placebo (Table 30-2).

Therefore, it appears that ACE inhibitors can reduce the incidence of heart failure among patients with known cardiovascular disease even when their blood pressure is normal or near normal. However, it is not clear whether this beneficial effect is unique to ACE inhibitors. The original report from HOPE claimed that the reduction in outcomes with ramipril was greater than would be expected solely on the basis of the blood pressure reduction seen among treated patients (76). However, this analysis used blood pressures measured in the office. A small subgroup analysis found that ramipril, which was given at bedtime, lowered nighttime blood pressure far more than it reduced office blood pressure (77). Thus, the reduction in the incidence of heart failure in HOPE may have been due solely to the reduction in blood pressure and not due to any unique properties of ACE inhibitors.

It is possible that if these trials had used other antihypertensive agents to lower blood pressure within the normal range, they would have yielded similar benefits to ACE inhibitors. In the case of the ACTION trial (A Coronary Disease Trial Investigating Outcome with Nifedipine GITS), giving long-acting nifedipine to stable coronary disease patients with a mean blood pressure of 137/80 mm Hg reduced blood pressure about 6/3 mm Hg compared to placebo (78). While nifedipine had no effect on the composite endpoint of death, myocardial infarction, refractory angina, debilitating stroke, peripheral revascularization, or overt heart failure was reduced by 29%. The Comparison of Amlodipine versus Enalapril to Limit Occurrences of Thrombosis (CAMELOT) study compared the benefits of treating patients with angiographically-documented CAD and normal or near-normal blood pressure (mean baseline blood pressure 129/78 mm Hg) with amlodipine, enalapril, or placebo (79). At follow-up, blood pressure was about 5.5/3 mm Hg lower in the two active treatment groups than the placebo group. Compared to the placebo group, cardiovascular events were reduced 31% (95% CI 12% to 46%) by amlodipine. Enalapril reduced events by 15% but this did not reach statistical significance. There were too few cases of heart failure in CAMELOT to analyze. Nevertheless, the study shows that the improved outcomes seen in HOPE, EUROPA, and PEACE may have resulted simply from reduced blood pressure and not from a unique effect of ACE inhibitors. Until additional studies are available that test this hypothesis, it is reasonable to add an ACE inhibitor to the regimen of patients with CAD who continue to have high-normal blood pressure despite maximal doses of their current anti-hypertensive medications.

PREVENTION STRATEGIES FOR PATIENTS WITH DIABETES

Diabetes increases the risk of heart failure through multiple pathways. Patients with diabetes have an increased risk of hypertension (80), and their risk of coronary heart disease is so high that the National Cholesterol Program's Adult Treatment Panel III recognized diabetes as a "coronary heart disease equivalent (81)." The 7-year incidence of myocardial infarction is 20.2% among patients with adult-onset (type II) diabetes mellitus compared to only 3.5 % among similar patients without diabetes (82). Patients with ischemic heart disease who have reduced left ventricular ejection fraction (Stage B) are more likely to progress to clinical heart failure (Stage C) if they have comorbid diabetes. Thus, for this extremely high-risk patient population, it is imperative to simultaneously optimize care for hypertension and lipid disorders in addition to glycemic control to prevent cardiovascular events and heart failure.

In a UKPDS analysis, tight blood pressure control (mean blood pressure at follow-up 144/82 mm Hg versus 154/87 for the "less tight control" group) reduced the relative risk of developing heart failure by a dramatic 56% (49). The HOT trial also showed markedly lower rates of cardiovascular events and cardiovascular mortality among diabetics in the group with a treatment goal of a diastolic blood pressure of 80 mm Hg compared to the group with a goal of 85 mm Hg or 90 mm Hg (48). The Appropriate Blood Pressure Control in Diabetes study also found that patients randomized to more aggressive blood pressure goals (a target diastolic blood pressure of 75 mm Hg versus 80 to 89 mm Hg) had a lower incidence of stroke (83). However, heart failure was not reported as an outcome in either trial. A substudy of the HOPE trial found that the relative risk of heart failure among patients with diabetes and nephropathy treated with the ACE inhibitor ramipril was reduced by 20%, although ramipril did not reduce the incidence of severe heart failure requiring hospitalization (84).

Despite evidence that thiazide diuretics and β-blockers worsen hyperglycemia and impair insulin sensitivity, clinical trials show that these medications are safe and effective antihypertensive agents for patients with diabetes. In the ALLHAT trial, chlorthalidone reduced the rate of heart failure among diabetics more than lisinopril, and the rates of other cardiovascular endpoints were similar (54). In a UKPDS study, the rates of heart failure were similar among patients randomized to either atenolol and captopril (56). Although ACE inhibitors have not been shown to reduce rates of heart failure more than other agents among patients with diabetes, ACE inhibitors have a variety of salutary renal and metabolic effects in patients with diabetes, and they remain the first-choice antihypertensive for many experts (80,85). However, to achieve recommended blood pressure goals, many diabetic patients will require treatment with multiple agents. Proper blood pressure control with a regimen that includes a diuretic will dramatically decrease the risk of heart failure, and physicians should not be dissuaded from prescribing low-dose thiazide-type diuretics to patients with diabetes when needed to achieve strict blood pressure control.

Substantial evidence suggests that patients with diabetes have unique pathophysiological processes that injure the heart and predispose patients to heart failure through pathways that are independent of LVH and large vessel atherosclerosis. This so-called diabetic cardiomyopathy is thought to be a direct consequence of hyperglycemia and the buildup of advanced glycosylation end-products. The histology is characterized by prominent interstitial fibrosis, which causes diastolic dysfunction. Although the histological changes have been well-described (86), the pathophysiological changes that lead to this remain unclear. Small-vessel disease was originally thought to play a role (87), but studies using coronary sinus sampling did not find evidence of lactate production during pacemaker-induced tachycardia to suggest functionally significant microvascular disease (88). A variety of metabolic abnormalities have been identified that may lead to decreased contractile function, including decreased myocardial glucose uptake, increased fatty acid oxidation, and abnormalities in cardiomyocyte calcium metabolism (88–91).

Few studies have examined whether tight glycemic control can reduce the incidence of heart failure. Stratton et al. conducted an observational study and found that after adjusting for sex, age, ethnicity, smoking, serum cholesterol and triglyceride levels, albuminuria, and systolic blood pressure, the rate of heart failure increased linearly from 2.3 per 1,000 patient-years for patients with a mean hemoglobin A1c of <6% up to 11.9 per 1,000 patient years for those with a mean glycosylated hemoglobin (hemoglobin A1c) of >10% (92).

Irribaren et al. used population-based data to examine heart failure risk among almost 50,000 patients with type II diabetes. After adjustment for sociodemographic characteristics, cigarette smoking, alcohol consumption, hypertension, obesity, use of β-blockers and ACE inhibitors, type and duration of diabetes, and incidence of interim myocardial infarction, each 1% increase in hemoglobin A1c was associated with an 8% increased risk of heart failure (95% CI 5% to 12%) (93). Compared to patients with a hemoglobin A1c of <7, those with a value of 10 or more had a 56% (95% CI 26% to 93%) higher adjusted relative risk of heart failure (93). Only one clinical trial has examined the benefits of tight glycemic control. The Diabetes Mellitus, Insulin Glucose Infusion in Acute Myocardial Infarction (DIGAMI) study randomized patients within 1 day of acute myocardial infarction to insulin and glucose infusion during hospitalization and then four-times-daily insulin or "usual care." Patients in the aggressive management group had lower mortality, and heart failure was the most common cause of death. However, differences in rates of heart failure were not statistically significant. Thus, the limited data that are available suggest that diabetics are at risk for a unique form of myocardial disease, and physicians and patients with diabetes should be encouraged to strive for tight glycemic control to prevent heart failure.

Thiazolidinediones and Heart Failure

Thus, while there is strong indirect evidence that improving glycemic control will reduce heart failure in patients with diabetes, the best methods to accomplish this goal and also reduce the incidence of heart failure are not known. The thiazolidinediones warrant special comment. The thiazolidinediones pioglitazone and rosiglitazone reduce blood glucose and may have beneficial effects on lipids, blood pressure, and other vascular parameters (94). However, caution is warranted since thiazolidinediones can increase plasma volume and may cause edema. Rarely, overt heart failure has developed. The risk of edema and heart failure appears to be greatest when these drugs are used in combination with insulin. Ongoing clinical trials will better define the cardiovascular risks and benefits of thiazolidinediones in patients with diabetes at increased risk for heart failure (95). It is possible that despite the salutary effects of thiazolidinediones on lipids and other risk factors, they may increase the risk of heart failure among the large population of diabetics at risk for heart failure, especially those with comorbid hypertension and CAD.

PREVENTING PROGRESSION OF ASYMPTOMATIC LEFT VENTRICULAR SYSTOLIC DYSFUNCTION

Many individuals have reduced left ventricular systolic function but no clinical symptoms or signs of heart failure, a condition referred to as asymptomatic left ventricular systolic dysfunction (ALVSD) (96–101). In the ACC/AHA classification system (Fig. 30-1) (14), ALVSD constitutes Stage B: structural heart disease without overt signs or symptoms of heart failure. ALVSD is most commonly seen after a myocardial infarction but it can be found in patients with end-stage hypertensive cardiomyopathy, alcoholic cardiomyopathy, or any of the other processes that can cause ventricular injury. In addition, ALVSD is often found on chest radiographs taken for preoperative evaluation of pulmonary infections, stress echocardiograms performed to evaluate chest pain, and cardiac catheterization (102). Individuals with ALVSD are at risk for developing progressive ventricular dysfunction and overt heart failure (102,103). Several therapies are available that can help prevent this decline.

Renin-Angiotensin System Blockade

In the Studies of Left Ventricular Dysfunction (SOLVD) Prevention trial, enalapril reduced the incidence of heart failure by 37% and hospitalization for heart failure by 36%

among stable, asymptomatic outpatients with LVEF of 35% or less, although mortality was not reduced (102). Among patients 3 to 16 days after myocardial infarction with LVEF of 40% or less but without clinical heart failure in the Survival and Ventricular Enlargement (SAVE) study, captopril reduced the incidence of severe heart failure by 37% and hospitalization for heart failure by 22% (104).

Other studies have shown that ACE inhibitors reduce the incidence of heart failure and prolong survival following myocardial infarction, although the patient populations were more heterogeneous and included patients with symptomatic heart failure as well as ALVSD (105–111). Nevertheless, subgroup analyses of patients who did not have heart failure at the time of randomization suggest that ACE inhibitors reduced the incidence of heart failure. The benefits of ACE inhibitors following myocardial infarction appear greatest among high-risk patients (i.e., reduced LVEF, anterior myocardial infarction, or history of previous myocardial infarction), and individuals in these groups should be treated with an ACE inhibitor unless strong contraindications exist (112).

There are also some data on the benefits of ARBs among patients with ALVSD. In the Valsartan in Acute Myocardial Infarction (VALIANT) trial, participants who had suffered a myocardial infarction within 0.5 to 10 days and had either signs of heart failure or moderate to severe left ventricular systolic dysfunction (average ejection fraction 35%) were randomized to valsartan, captopril, or both (113). Cardiovascular events (including hospitalization for heart failure) were similar in the three groups. Although the VALIANT trial was underpowered to look separately at the subgroup of patients with ALVSD and did not report heart failure as a separate outcome, the study suggests that ARBs are an acceptable alternative to ACE inhibitors for treating ALVSD.

Finally, aldosterone antagonists have been shown to improve survival and decrease the progression of heart failure among patients with severe heart failure (114) and to improve survival and decrease heart failure hospitalization among patients with heart failure following a myocardial infarction (115). However, no trials have examined the use of aldosterone antagonists to prevent the progression from ALVSD to symptomatic heart failure.

β-Adrenergic Blockade

β-adrenergic–blocking agents dramatically improve outcomes for patients with established heart failure (9,10,116–118), including patients with relatively mild heart failure (119). Although no randomized controlled study to date has shown that β-blockers can prevent the development of heart failure among patients with chronic ALVSD, the CAPRICORN trial showed that treating patients with a past history of myocardial infarction and LVEF ≤40% with carvedilol reduced mortality by 33% (120). In addition, a post hoc analysis of the SOLVD study (previously discussed) showed that among patients randomized to enalapril, those who were taking β-blockers at baseline had a 46% lower risk of death from progressive heart failure and a 36% lower risk of death or hospitalization for heart failure (121). It is therefore very likely that prescribing β-blockers for patients with ALVSD should substantially decrease the risk of heart failure, and the recently released ACC/AHA heart failure guideline has made this recommendation (14).

SCREENING FOR ASYMPTOMATIC LEFT VENTRICULAR DYSFUNCTION

The availability of effective therapies to prevent progression of ALVSD raises the question of whether we should screen patients who are at risk for developing heart failure to detect those with presymptomatic disease (100,122–124). If such individuals could be detected early in the course of their disease and treated appropriately, screening for ALVSD could reap important clinical benefits.

Prevalence of ALVSD

ALVSD appears to be relatively common among older patients and those with risk factors for heart failure (125). Mosterd et al. reported that 3% of persons aged 55 or older in a population-based study in Rotterdam had reduced ventricular systolic function (fractional shortening of less than 25%) (98), but it is unclear whether study subjects with a previous history of heart failure were excluded. Morgan assessed patients aged 70 to 84 years from a general practice registry and found 4.8% had reduced left ventricular systolic function (LVEF <48%) with no current symptoms or past history of heart failure using patient questionnaires and chart review (98) Baker et al. studied 482 general internal medicine clinic patients aged 60 and older with either hypertension, diabetes, or CAD and found that 7.9% had an LVEF of ≤45% (100). The prevalence ranged from 5.4% for those with hypertension as a lone risk factor up to 15.4% for those with a prior myocardial infarction. The prevalence was intermediate for patients with diabetes and no history of CAD and those with angina but no prior myocardial infarction. Prior stroke and definite LVH on ECG were independently associated with a higher prevalence of ALVSD (adjusted odds ratios of 2-0 and 3-5, respectively).

Several community-based studies have also reported the prevalence of ALVSD. Among a random sample of men and women aged 25 to 74 in Scotland, 1.4% of participants had a LVEF ≤30% (101). Davies et al. found that 1.8% of a random sample of people aged 45 or older in England had LVEF <40% (97). The prevalence of ALVSD was higher in the Framingham Heart Study (mean age 58 years) (126). A total of 9.3% of men and 2.5% of women had LVEF ≤50% or fractional shortening ≤29% on M-mode echocardiography, 4.1% of men and 0.6% of women had more severe ALVSD with LVEF ≤40% or fractional shortening ≤22%. A community-based study of adults aged 45 and older in Olmstead County, Minnesota found that 10.2% of men and 3.8% of women had LVEF ≤50% and 3.6% of men and 1% of women had LVEF of ≤40% (127). This study also assessed the prevalence of asymptomatic moderate to severe left ventricular diastolic dysfunction based on Doppler echocardiographic flow patterns, and this was even more common (6.6%) than moderate to severe ALVSD. Thus, although studies have used different LVEF cutoffs to classify patients as having ALVSD, the results have consistently shown that approximately 2%

of older adults have ALVSD with LVEF ≤40%, with over three-fourths of these individuals being men. The prevalence of ALVSD increases sharply with advancing age (128).

Prognosis for Individuals with ALVSD

The presence of ALVSD markedly increases the risk of developing overt, symptomatic heart failure. The SOLVD prevention trial (102) included a large number of individuals with an LVEF less than 35% (mean LVEF 28%). Thus, the SOLVD prevention trial only included individuals with moderate to severe ALVSD, and the majority had severe ALVSD. Over 3 years, 30.2% of patients in the placebo group and 20.7% of patients treated with enalapril developed signs or symptoms of heart failure, and 22.5% and 13.9%, respectively, required treatment for heart failure. We know less about the prognosis of individuals with ALVSD and LVEF between 30% to 40% (moderate ALVSD) and LVEF 41% to 50% (mild ALVSD). In the Framingham Study, the rate of developing heart failure was 0.7 and 5.8 per 100 person-years for individuals with and without ALVSD (LVEF ≤50%), and the adjusted rate hazard ratios for developing heart failure were 3.3 for those with mild ALVSD and 7.8 for those with moderate to severe ALVSD (128).

Hypothetical Benefits of Screening for ALVSD

No study has shown that screening for ALVSD improves clinical outcomes (i.e., reduces the rate of incident heart failure) or intermediate outcomes (e.g., reduces the rate of decline in LVEF). However, screening for ALVSD appears to meet recommended criteria to judge whether screening for a disease might be worthwhile (129). First, how great is the burden of suffering from the disease? The prevalence of moderate to severe ALVSD among older adults (approximately 2%) is similar to the proportion of women found to have breast cancer with biannual screening mammography and clinical breast exam over a 10-year period (3.7%) (130) and the proportion of people found to have colorectal cancer with annual or biannual screening with fecal occult blood testing over a 13-year period (2.3%) (131). However, as previously described, the clinical significance and prognosis of patients with mild to moderate ALVSD is not clear. In the Cardiovascular Health Study, of the 553 participants who developed heart failure, only 49 (9%) had depressed LVEF on their baseline echocardiogram (132). Only 4% of the population-attributable risk for heart failure was from decreased left ventricular systolic function at baseline.

Second, is the course of the disease favorably altered by early detection and treatment? In the SOLVD prevention trial (102), treatment of patients with moderate to severe ALVSD (LVEF ≤35%) with an ACE inhibitor substantially reduced the risk of developing heart failure (previously described). The ability of β-blockers to improve cardiac function and decrease the risk of death and progressive disease among patients with overt heart failure offers hope that β-blockers may further decrease the risk of progression from ALVSD to heart failure. Moreover, total mortality was reduced by 19% when patients with ALVSD after myocardial infarction were treated with an ACE inhibitor (104). In contrast, screening for colorectal cancer reduced mortality from colorectal cancer by 33% but did not reduce overall mortality (131). The benefits of treating patients with moderate to severe ALVSD, therefore, compare favorably with those for other diseases targeted by screening programs. However, the majority of people with ALVSD have mild to moderately depressed LVEF, and we know little about the benefits of treating this group. The prognosis of most patients with mild to moderate ALVSD is much better than patients in the SOLVD prevention trial, and the absolute benefits of treatment may be far less.

Possible Screening Tests for ALVSD

The final decision node for determining the utility of screening is whether a simple, reliable, and inexpensive screening test is available. Echocardiography is simple and acceptable to patients, and screening for depressed LVEF alone would be relatively inexpensive if only a brief study was done to estimate LVEF (133). Studies among unselected patient populations have shown that over 80% of patients have echocardiograms that are adequate for quantitative measurements of LVEF (100,134), and interobserver reliability is good. Visual estimation of LVEF has been shown to predict future cardiac events (135), which supports the validity of using this to guide care. Nevertheless, screening echocardiography may be subject to significant numbers of false positive and false negative tests, depending upon the ejection fraction cut-off used to define ALVSD, the interobserver reliability, and the prevalence of ALVSD in the population screened. In addition, if more comprehensive echocardiography measurements were done, the costs would be much higher. A cost-effectiveness analysis of screening for ALVSD found that screening with echocardiography alone (baseline cost estimate $420) was unattractive (more than $100,000 per quality-adjusted life-year gained) (136).

Another possible strategy to screen for ALVSD is to measure serum natriuretic peptides. Inexpensive and reliable clinical assays for brain natriuretic peptide (BNP) are available (137–139). Individuals with elevated levels of natriuretic peptides have a substantially increased risk of developing heart failure (140,141), and elevated levels of natriuretic peptides are sensitive indicators of overt heart failure among patients presenting with dyspnea of unknown etiology (142).

Several studies have examined the accuracy of using BNP to screen for ALVSD (143). Early studies showed strong associations between natriuretic peptides and ALVSD, with BNP generally being more strongly associated with ALVSD than other natriuretic peptides. However, more recent population-based studies have shown that there is only a moderate association between serum BNP levels and ALVSD, especially after taking into account other clinical variables (e.g., blood pressure). In the Framingham Heart Study, the area under the receiver-operator curve (AUC, a measure of predictive accuracy) was 0.79 and 0.85 for detecting LVEF ≤0.40 for men and women, respectively (144). There was no high-risk patient subgroup for whom serum BNP levels appeared to have higher predictive value. BNP testing was more strongly associated with moderate to severe ALVSD in a community-based study in Minnesota, with AUC of 0.89 and 0.92 for detecting LVEF ≤0.40 for men and women, respectively (145). The reasons for the better performance of BNP in the latter study are not clear.

Using data from the Framingham Heart Study, a recent cost-effectiveness analysis found that screening a general population of asymptomatic individuals aged 60 and older for ALVSD with a serum BNP test followed by echocardiography for patients with an elevated BNP (>24 mg/dL for mean and 34 mg/dL for women using the Shionogi BNP assay) was attractive (less than $50,000 per quality-adjusted life-year gained) if the prevalence of ALVSD was 1% or more (136). This result is somewhat surprising in light of the modest predictive value of BNP in the Framingham Heart Study and probably results from the very low cost of the BNP test (baseline estimate $32). In addition, the accuracy of the BNP testing in Framingham was lower than in a community-based study in Minnesota. Therefore, the cost-effectiveness of screening could be even better (i.e., lower cost per quality-adjusted life-year gained) than estimate by their baseline model.

However, some assumptions in this cost-effectiveness model may have favored screening. The model estimated the prognosis and the benefits of treating ALVSD using data from the SOLVD prevention trial, which enrolled patients with moderate to severe ALVSD. The majority of patients with ALVSD have mild to moderate disease, so the model's assumptions may overestimate the benefits of treatment. Moreover, they assumed that patients with ALVSD were not already receiving therapy. In fact, many patients with ALVSD are already receiving ACE inhibitors or β-blockers for hypertension or other conditions, so the benefits of screening would be less in these individuals. Despite these uncertainties, the results suggest that screening patients with a 1% or higher prevalence of having an LVEF of ≤40% who are not already on therapies to prevent the progression of ALVSD may result in improved health outcomes at an acceptable cost.

PREVENTING PROGRESSION OF ASYMPTOMATIC VALVULAR HEART DISEASE

Several decades ago, valvular heart disease was a common cause of heart failure. As the incidence of rheumatic heart disease declined, hypertension and CAD have dwarfed valvular disease as causes of heart failure (146). However, valvular heart disease remains an important cause of heart failure in the United States and worldwide, and studies have identified several therapies that can prevent development of heart failure among patients with selected types of valve lesions.

Aortic Sclerosis

As our population ages, the prevalence of calcific aortic stenosis is likely to rise, and this will become an increasing important cause of heart failure (147). Among individuals aged 75 and older, 37% have aortic sclerosis and 2.6% have aortic stenosis (148). Aortic sclerosis is a progressive disease. The valve area in patients with untreated aortic stenosis will typically diminish by approximately 0.1 cm^2 per year, with an average increase in the pressure gradient across the valve of 7 mm Hg per year (149–151). The risk factors for developing aortic stenosis are similar to those for atherosclerosis (i.e., male sex, smoking, diabetes mellitus, hypertension, and hyperlipidemia) (147,152,153). The rate of progression of stenosis is almost twice as high among individuals with a serum cholesterol concentration above 200 mg/dL.

Several observational studies have found that patients with aortic sclerosis who are treated with HMG CoA reductase inhibitors have lower rates of decline in their aortic valve area than patients who are not treated with these agents (154–157). For example, Novaro et al. found that patients who were treated with an HMG CoA reductase inhibitor had a rate of decrease in aortic valve area of 0.06 cm^2 per year compared to 0.11 cm^2 per year among those who were not being treated with a statin (157). However, a recent randomized controlled trial found that intensive lipid-lowering therapy did not half the progression of calcific aortic stenosis or induce its regression (158). In contrast, ACE inhibitors do not appear to reduce the rate of progression of aortic stenosis (154). Randomized trials are needed to determine whether the results of these observational studies are valid. Since many of the patients with aortic sclerosis are very elderly and are either not surgical candidates or are not willing to undergo surgery, medical management to prevent progression of aortic stenosis is a vitally important issue.

Aortic Regurgitation

There is also evidence that the use of vasodilators can slow or prevent progressive left ventricular injury from aortic regurgitation (159,160). Scognamiglio et al. randomly assigned 143 asymptomatic patients with isolated, severe aortic regurgitation to nifedipine (20 mg twice daily) or digoxin (0.25 mg daily) (159). After 6 years of treatment, only 15% of patients in the nifedipine group had undergone valve replacement compared to 34% of patients in the digoxin group.

Rheumatic Valvular Disease

The only established method for preventing the progression of rheumatic valvular disease is with prevention of recurrent streptococcal infection (28,29). Patients with a history of rheumatic valvular disease should receive prophylaxis against recurrent streptococcal infection until aged 40 and for at least 10 years after the last attack of rheumatic fever. The most commonly used regimens are either penicillin V 250 mg twice daily or benzathine penicillin 1.2 million units intramuscularly monthly. Individuals with penicillin allergy can be treated with a sulfonamide or erythromycin.

REDUCING THE BURDEN OF HEART FAILURE IN THE UNITED STATES

Our greatest opportunity to improve quality of care and decrease the incidence of heart failure appears to be better control of hypertension. Treatment of hypertension dramatically reduces the incidence of heart failure, even among very elderly patients who have the highest risk for heart failure. Physicians and patients need to be made more aware of the benefits of improved control of hypertension, and policy makers should strive to eliminate financial barriers to compliance with the multiple-drug regimens that are often needed to reach optimal blood pressure reductions. Of the 42 million Americans with hypertension, only 52% are currently receiving treatment and only 23% have their blood pressure controlled to <140/90 mm Hg (46). Almost half of the people in the United States who survive a myocardial infarction have uncontrolled hypertension (161). This is particularly tragic because the SHEP trial showed such dramatic reductions in the incidence of heart failure among the subgroup of patients with previous myocardial infarction. Blood pressure control is most inadequate among the elderly (46), the population at highest risk for heart failure.

Physicians also need to redouble efforts to lower cholesterol to recommended targets among patients with a previous myocardial infarction or known coronary artery disease. Patients who have sustained significant ventricular injury, especially those who have reduced systolic function, should be prescribed ACE inhibitors and β-blockers unless strong contraindications exist. Quality of care for these interventions remains problematic. Among patients who suffer a myocardial infarction, many still do not receive treatment for hypercholesterolemia, and 29% of patients with an LVEF of <40% are not prescribed an ACE inhibitor at the time of hospital discharge (162). The reasons why effective therapies are underused are complex and poorly understood. Although physicians frequently do not prescribe recommended therapies (163), other obstacles [e.g., inability to afford medications (164,165), unwillingness to take additional medications, and noncompliance with prescribed medications (166,167)] are also important. Multifaceted intervention programs are needed to improve the quality of medical care and to increase patients' awareness of the importance of these medications and the need for long-term compliance. Long-term disease management programs for patients at risk for developing heart failure may prove beneficial, although more rigorous studies and cost-effectiveness analyses are needed.

If clinical practice can live up to the potential shown from clinical trials, the suffering and economic toll imposed by heart failure can be dramatically reduced. Primary care physicians are a particularly important group to target for quality improvement efforts, since they form a large part of the first line of defense against the pending heart failure epidemic. Further studies are needed to understand the unique barriers to meeting prevention goals in primary care practice.

REFERENCES

1. American Heart Association Heart Disease and Stroke Statistics—2006 Update. Dallas, Texas: American Heart Association;2006.
2. Young JB. The global epidemiology of heart failure. *Med Clin North Am*. 2004;88:1135–1143.
3. Stewart AL, Greenfield S, Hays RD, et al. Functional status and well-being of patients with chronic conditions: Results from the Medical Outcomes Study. *JAMA*. 1989;262:907–913.
4. Ho KK, Anderson KM, Kannel WB, et al. Survival after the onset of congestive heart failure in Framingham Heart Study subjects. *Circulation*. 1993;88:107–115.
5. Levy D, Kenchaiah S, Larson MG, et al. Long-term trends in the incidence of and survival with heart failure. *N Engl J Med*. 2002;347:1397–1402.
6. Jessup M, Brozena S. Heart failure. *N Engl J Med*. 2003;348: 2007–2018.
7. Baker DW, Einstadter D, Thomas C, et al. Mortality trends for 23,505 Medicare patients hospitalized with heart failure in Northeast Ohio, 1991 to 1997. *Am Heart J*. 2003;146:258–264.
8. Macintyre K, Capewell S, Stewart S, et al. Evidence of improving prognosis in heart failure: trends in case fatality in 66,547 patients hospitalized between 1986 and 1995. *Circulation*. 2000;102: 1126–1131.
9. Hjalmarson A, Goldstein S, Fagerberg B, et al. Effects of controlled-release metoprolol on total mortality, hospitalizations, and well-being in patients with heart failure: the Metoprolol CR/XL Randomized Intervention Trial in congestive heart failure (MERIT-HF). MERIT-HF Study Group. *JAMA*. 2000;283:1295–1302.
10. The Cardiac Insufficiency Bisoprolol Study II (CIBIS-II): a randomised trial. *Lancet*. 1999;353:9–13.
11. Kannel WB. Epidemiology and prevention of cardiac failure: Framingham Study insights. *Eur Heart J*. 1987;8(Suppl F):23–26.
12. Kannel WB, Belanger AJ. Epidemiology of heart failure. *Am Heart J*. 1991;121(3 Pt 1):951–957.
13. Ho KK, Pinsky JL, Kannel WB, et al. The epidemiology of heart failure: the Framingham Study. *J Am Coll Cardiol*. 1993;22(4 Suppl A):6A–13A.
14. Hunt HA, Baker DW, Chin MH, et al. ACC/AHA guidelines for the evaluation and management of chronic heart failure in the adult: executive summary a report of the American College of Cardiology/American Heart Association Task Force on Practice Guidelines (Committee to Revise the 1995 Guidelines for the Evaluation and Management of Heart Failure). *Circulation*. 2001;104:2996–3007.
15. Krousel-Wood MA, Muntner P, He J, et al. Primary prevention of essential hypertension. *Med Clin North Am*. 2004;88:223–238.
16. Klein S, Sheard NF, Pi-Sunyer X, et al. Weight management through lifestyle modification for the prevention and management of type 2 diabetes: rationale and strategies: a statement of the American Diabetes Association, the North American Association for the Study of Obesity, and the American Society for Clinical Nutrition. *Diabetes Care*. 2004;27:2067–2073.
17. Murphy D, Chapel T, Clark C. Moving diabetes care from science to practice: the evolution of the National Diabetes Prevention and Control Program. *Ann Intern Med*. 2004;140:978–984.
18. Williamson DF, Vinicor F, Bowman BA. Primary prevention of type 2 diabetes mellitus by lifestyle intervention: implications for health policy. *Ann Intern Med*. 2004;140:951–957.
19. Lauer MS. Clinical practice. Aspirin for primary prevention of coronary events. *N Engl J Med*. 2002;346:1468–1474.
20. Hayden M, Pignone M, Phillips C, et al. Aspirin for the primary prevention of cardiovascular events: a summary of the evidence for the U.S. Preventive Services Task Force. *Ann Intern Med*. 2002;136:161–172.
21. Aspirin for the primary prevention of cardiovascular events: recommendation and rationale. *Ann Intern Med*. 2002;136:157–160.
22. Massie BM. Obesity and heart failure—risk factor or mechanism? *N Engl J Med*. 2002;347:358–359.
23. Kenchaiah S, Evans JC, Levy D, et al. Obesity and the risk of heart failure. *N Engl J Med*. 2002;347:305–313.
24. Ghaffar A, Reddy KS, Singhi M. Burden of non-communicable diseases in South Asia. *BMJ*. 2004;328:807–810.
25. Schaffer WL, Galloway JM, Roman MJ, et al. Prevalence and correlates of rheumatic heart disease in American Indians (the Strong Heart Study). *Am J Cardiol*. 2003;91:1379–1382.
26. Jose VJ, Gomathi M. Declining prevalence of rheumatic heart disease in rural schoolchildren in India: 2001–2002. *Indian Heart J*. 2003;55:158–160.
27. Soler-Soler J, Galve E. Worldwide perspective of valve disease. *Heart*. 2000;83:721–725.
28. Kumar R. Controlling rheumatic heart disease in developing countries. *World Health Forum*. 1995;16:47–51.
29. Feldman T. Rheumatic heart disease. *Curr Opin Cardiol*. 1996;11:126–130.

30. Campbell DA, Westenberger SJ, Sturm NR. The determinants of Chagas disease: connecting parasite and host genetics. *Curr Mol Med.* 2004;4:549–562.
31. Kirchhoff LV, Weiss LM, Wittner M, et al. Parasitic diseases of the heart. *Front Biosci.* 2004;9:706–723.
32. Barrett MP, Burchmore RJ, Stich A, et al. The trypanosomiases. *Lancet.* 2003;362:1469–1480.
33. Higuchi ML, Benvenuti LA, Martins RM, et al. Pathophysiology of the heart in Chagas' disease: current status and new developments. *Cardiovasc Res.* 2003;60:96–107.
34. Moncayo A. Chagas disease: current epidemiological trends after the interruption of vectorial and transfusional transmission in the Southern Cone countries. *Mem Inst Oswaldo Cruz.* 2003;98: 577–591.
35. Hajjar I, Kotchen TA. Trends in prevalence, awareness, treatment, and control of hypertension in the United States, 1988–2000. *JAMA.* 2003;290:199–206.
36. Levy D, Larson MG, Vasan RS, et al. The progression from hypertension to congestive heart failure. *JAMA.* 1996;275:1557–1562.
37. Vasan RS, Levy D. The role of hypertension in the pathogenesis of heart failure. A clinical mechanistic overview. *Arch Intern Med.* 1996;156:1789–1796.
38. Moser M, Hebert PR. Prevention of disease progression, left ventricular hypertrophy and congestive heart failure in hypertension treatment trials. *J Am Coll Cardiol.* 1996;27:1214–1218.
39. Psaty BM, Lumley T, Furberg CD, et al. Health outcomes associated with various antihypertensive therapies used as first-line agents: a network meta-analysis. *JAMA.* 2003;289:2534–2544.
40. Turnbull F. Effects of different blood-pressure-lowering regimens on major cardiovascular events: results of prospectively-designed overviews of randomised trials. *Lancet.* 2003;362:1527–1535.
41. Dahlof B, Lindholm LH, Hansson L, et al. Morbidity and mortality in the Swedish Trial in Old Patients with Hypertension (STOP-Hypertension). *Lancet.* 1991;338:1281–1285.
42. Kostis JB, Davis BR, Cutler J, et al. Prevention of heart failure by antihypertensive drug treatment in older persons with isolated systolic hypertension. SHEP Cooperative Research Group. *JAMA.* 1997;278:212–216.
43. Staessen JA, Fagard R, Thijs L, et al. Randomised double-blind comparison of placebo and active treatment for older patients with isolated systolic hypertension. The Systolic Hypertension in Europe (Syst-Eur) Trial Investigators. *Lancet.* 1997;350: 757–764.
44. Liu L, Wang JG, Gong L, et al. Comparison of active treatment and placebo in older Chinese patients with isolated systolic hypertension. Systolic Hypertension in China (Syst-China) Collaborative Group. *J Hypertens.* 1998;16:1823–1829.
45. Gueyffier F, Bulpitt C, Boissel JP, et al. Antihypertensive drugs in very old people: a subgroup meta-analysis of randomised controlled trials. INDANA Group. *Lancet.* 1999;353:793–796.
46. Hyman DJ, Pavlik VN. Characteristics of patients with uncontrolled hypertension in the United States. *N Engl J Med.* 2001;345:479–486.
47. Chobanian AV, Bakris GL, Black HR, et al. The seventh report of the joint national committee on prevention, detection, evaluation, and treatment of high blood pressure: the JNC 7 report. *JAMA.* 2003;289:2560–2572.
48. Hansson L, Zanchetti A, Carruthers SG, et al. Effects of intensive blood-pressure lowering and low-dose aspirin in patients with hypertension: principal results of the Hypertension Optimal Treatment (HOT) randomised trial. HOT Study Group. *Lancet.* 1998;351:1755–1762.
49. UK Prospective Diabetes Study Group. Tight blood pressure control and risk of macrovascular and microvascular complications in type 2 diabetes: UKPDS 38. *BMJ.* 1998;317:703–713.
50. Estacio RO, Jeffers BW, Hiatt WR, et al. The effect of nisoldipine as compared with enalapril on cardiovascular outcomes in patients with non-insulin-dependent diabetes and hypertension. *N Engl J Med.* 1998;338:645–652.
51. Randomised trial of a perindopril-based blood-pressure-lowering regimen among 6,105 individuals with previous stroke or transient ischaemic attack. *Lancet.* 2001;358:1033–1041.
52. PROGRESS Collaborative Group. Effects of a perindopril-based blood pressure lowering regimen on cardiac outcomes among patients with cerebrovascular disease. *Eur Heart J.* 2003;24: 475–484.
53. Psaty BM, Weiss NS, Furberg CD. The PROGRESS trial: questions about the effectiveness of angiotensin converting enzyme inhibitors. Perindopril pROtection aGainst REcurrent Stroke Study. *Am J Hypertens.* 2002;15:472–474.
54. ALLHAT Officers and Coordinators for the ALLHAT Collaborative Research Group. Major outcomes in high-risk hypertensive patients randomized to angiotensin-converting enzyme inhibitor or calcium channel blocker vs diuretic: the Antihypertensive and Lipid-Lowering Treatment to Prevent Heart Attack Trial (ALLHAT). *JAMA.* 2002;288:2981–2997.
55. Staessen JA, Wang JG, Thijs L. Cardiovascular protection and blood pressure reduction: a meta-analysis. *Lancet.* 2001;358:1305–1315.
56. UK Prospective Diabetes Study Group. Efficacy of atenolol and captopril in reducing risk of macrovascular and microvascular complications in type 2 diabetes: UKPDS 39. *BMJ.* 1998;317:713–720.
57. Dahlof B, Devereux RB, Kjeldsen SE, et al. Cardiovascular morbidity and mortality in the Losartan Intervention For Endpoint reduction in hypertension study (LIFE): a randomised trial against atenolol. *Lancet.* 2002;359:995–1003.
58. Major cardiovascular events in hypertensive patients randomized to doxazosin vs chlorthalidone: the Antihypertensive and Lipid-lowering Treatment to Prevent Heart Attack Trial (ALLHAT). ALLHAT Collaborative Research Group. *JAMA.* 2000;283: 1967–1975.
59. Cohn JN, Archibald DG, Ziesche S, et al. Effect of vasodilator therapy on mortality in chronic congestive heart failure: results of a Veterans Administration Cooperative Study. *N Engl J Med.* 1986;314:1547–1552.
60. Psaty BM, Lumley T, Furberg CD. Meta-analysis of health outcomes of chlorthalidone-based vs nonchlorthalidone-based low-dose diuretic therapies. *JAMA.* 2004;292:43–44.
61. Klingbeil AU, Schneider M, Martus P, et al. A meta-analysis of the effects of treatment on left ventricular mass in essential hypertension. *Am J Med.* 2003;115:41–46.
62. Fagard R, Lijnen P, Staessen J, et al. Mechanical and other factors relating to left ventricular hypertrophy. *Blood Press Suppl.* 1994; 1:5–10.
63. Mosterd A, D'Agostino RB, Silbershatz H, et al. Trends in the prevalence of hypertension, antihypertensive therapy, and left ventricular hypertrophy from 1950 to 1989. *N Engl J Med.* 1999;340:1221–1227.
64. Liebson PR, Grandits GA, Dianzumba S, et al. Comparison of five antihypertensive monotherapies and placebo for change in left ventricular mass in patients receiving nutritional-hygienic therapy in the Treatment of Mild Hypertension Study (TOMHS). *Circulation.* 1995;91:698–706.
65. Verdecchia P, Angeli F, Borgioni C, et al. Changes in cardiovascular risk by reduction of left ventricular mass in hypertension: a meta-analysis. *Am J Hypertens.* 2003;16:895–899.
66. Mathew J, Sleight P, Lonn E, et al. Reduction of cardiovascular risk by regression of electrocardiographic markers of left ventricular hypertrophy by the angiotensin-converting enzyme inhibitor ramipril. *Circulation.* 2001;104:1615–1621.
67. Okin PM, Devereux RB, Jern S, et al. Regression of electrocardiographic left ventricular hypertrophy by losartan versus atenolol: the Losartan Intervention for Endpoint reduction in Hypertension (LIFE) Study. *Circulation.* 2003;108:684–690.
68. Massie BM, Shah NB. Evolving trends in the epidemiologic factors of heart failure: rationale for preventive strategies and comprehensive disease management. *Am Heart J.* 1997;133:703–712.
69. American Heart Association. Heart Disease and Stroke Statistics—2004 Update. 2004.
70. Kannel WB, Sorlie P, McNamara PM. Prognosis after initial myocardial infarction: the Framingham study. *Am J Cardiol.* 1979;44:53–59.
71. No authors listed. Randomised trial of cholesterol lowering in 4444 patients with coronary heart disease: the Scandinavian Simvastatin Survival Study (4S). *Lancet.* 1994;344:1383–1389.
72. de Lemos JA, Blazing MA, Wiviott SD, et al. Early intensive vs. a delayed conservative simvastatin strategy in patients with acute coronary syndromes: phase Z of the A to Z trial. *JAMA.* 2004;292:1307–1316.
73. Rubins HB, Robins SJ, Collins D, et al. Gemfibrozil for the secondary prevention of coronary heart disease in men with low levels of high-density lipoprotein cholesterol. Veterans Affairs High-Density Lipoprotein Cholesterol Intervention Trial Study Group. *N Engl J Med.* 1999;341:410–418.

74. Braunwald E, Domanski MJ, Fowler SE, et al. Angiotensin-converting-enzyme inhibition in stable coronary artery disease. *N Engl J Med*. 2004;351:2058–2068.
75. Fox KM. Efficacy of perindopril in reduction of cardiovascular events among patients with stable coronary artery disease: randomised, double-blind, placebo-controlled, multicentre trial (the EUROPA study). *Lancet*. 2003;362:782–788.
76. Yusuf S, Sleight P, Pogue J, et al. Effects of an angiotensin-converting-enzyme inhibitor, ramipril, on cardiovascular events in high-risk patients. The Heart Outcomes Prevention Evaluation Study Investigators. *N Engl J Med*. 2000;342:145–153.
77. Svensson P, de Faire U, Sleight P, et al. Comparative effects of ramipril on ambulatory and office blood pressures: a HOPE Substudy. *Hypertension*. 2001;38:E28-E32.
78. Poole-Wilson PA, Lubsen J, Kirwan BA, et al. Effect of long-acting nifedipine on mortality and cardiovascular morbidity in patients with stable angina requiring treatment (ACTION trial): randomised controlled trial. *Lancet*. 2004;364:849–857.
79. Nissen SE, Tuzcu EM, Libby P, et al. Effect of antihypertensive agents on cardiovascular events in patients with coronary disease and normal blood pressure: the CAMELOT study: a randomized controlled trial. *JAMA*. 2004;292:2217–2225.
80. Srikanthan P, Hsueh W. Preventing heart failure in patients with diabetes. *Med Clin North Am*. 2004;88:1237–1256.
81. Expert Panel on Detection, Evaluation, and Treatment of High Blood Cholesterol in Adults. Executive Summary of the third report of the National Cholesterol Education Program (NCEP) expert panel on detection, evaluation, and treatment of high blood cholesterol in adults (Adult Treatment Panel III). *JAMA*. 2001;285:2486–2497.
82. Haffner SM, Lehto S, Ronnemaa T, et al. Mortality from coronary heart disease in subjects with type 2 diabetes and in nondiabetic subjects with and without prior myocardial infarction. *N Engl J Med*. 1998;339:229–234.
83. Schrier RW, Estacio RO, Esler A, et al. Effects of aggressive blood pressure control in normotensive type 2 diabetic patients on albuminuria, retinopathy and strokes. *Kidney Int*. 2002;61:1086–1097.
84. Heart Outcomes Prevention Evaluation Study Investigators. Effects of ramipril on cardiovascular and microvascular outcomes in people with diabetes mellitus: results of the HOPE study and MICRO-HOPE substudy. *Lancet*. 2000;355:253–259.
85. Moser M. Current recommendations for the treatment of hypertension: are they still valid? *J Hypertens*. 2002;20(Suppl 1):S3–S10.
86. Regan TJ, Lyons MM, Ahmed SS, et al. Evidence for cardiomyopathy in familial diabetes mellitus. *J Clin Invest*. 1977;60:884–899.
87. Rubler S, Dlugash J, Yuceoglu YZ, et al. New type of cardiomyopathy associated with diabetic glomerulosclerosis. *Am J Cardiol*. 1972;30:595–602.
88. Ungar I, Gilbert M, Siegel A, et al. Studies on myocardial metabolism. IV. Myocardial metabolism in diabetes. *Am J Med*. 1955;18:385–396.
89. Petrova R, Yamamoto Y, Muraki K, et al. Advanced glycation end-product-induced calcium handling impairment in mouse cardiac myocytes. *J Mol Cell Cardiol*. 2002;34:1425–1431.
90. Clark RJ, McDonough PM, Swanson E, et al. Diabetes and the accompanying hyperglycemia impairs cardiomyocyte calcium cycling through increased nuclear O-GlcNAcylation. *J Biol Chem*. 2003;278:44230–44237.
91. Pastukh V, Wu S, Ricci C, et al. Reversal of hyperglycemic preconditioning by angiotensin II: role of calcium transport. *Am J Physiol. (Heart Circ Physiol.)* 2005;288:H1965–H1975.
92. Stratton IM, Adler AI, Neil HA, et al. Association of glycaemia with macrovascular and microvascular complications of type 2 diabetes (UKPDS 35): prospective observational study. *BMJ*. 2000;321:405–412.
93. Iribarren C, Karter AJ, Go AS, et al. Glycemic control and heart failure among adult patients with diabetes. *Circulation*. 2001;103: 2668–2673.
94. Parulkar AA, Pendergrass ML, Granda-Ayala R, et al. Nonhypoglycemic effects of thiazolidinediones. *Ann Intern Med*. 2001;134:61–71.
95. Nesto RW, Bell D, Bonow RO, et al. Thiazolidinedione use, fluid retention, and congestive heart failure: a consensus statement from the American Heart Association and American Diabetes Association. *Diabetes Care*. 2004;27:256–263.
96. Davies MK, Hobbs FDR, Davis RC, et al. Prevalence of left-ventricular systolic dysfunction and heart failure in the Echocardiographic Heart of England study: a population based study. *Lancet*. 2001;358:439–444.
97. McDonagh TA. Asymptomatic left ventricular dysfunction in the community. *Curr Cardiol Rep*. 2000;2:470–474.
98. Mosterd A, de Bruijne MC, Hoes AW, et al. Usefulness of echocardiography in detecting left ventricular dysfunction in population-based studies (The Rotterdam Study). *Am J Cardiol*. 1997;79:103–104.
99. Morgan S, Smith H, Simpson I, et al. Prevalence and clinical characteristics of left ventricular dysfunction among elderly patients in general practice setting: cross sectional survey. *BMJ*. 1999;318:368–372.
100. Baker DW, Bahler RC, Finkelhor RS, et al. Screening for left ventricular systolic dysfunction among patients with risk factors for heart failure. *Am Heart J*. 2003;146:736–740.
101. McDonagh TA, Morrison CE, Lawrence A, et al. Symptomatic and asymptomatic left-ventricular systolic dysfunction in an urban population. *Lancet*. 1997;350:829–833.
102. SOLVD Investigators. Effect of enalapril on mortality and the development of heart failure in asymptomatic patients with reduced left-ventricular ejection fractions. *N Engl J Med*. 1992;327:685–691.
103. Vasan RS, Larson MG, Benjamin EJ, et al. Left ventricular dilatation and the risk of congestive heart failure in people without myocardial infarction. *N Engl J Med*. 1997;336:1350–1355.
104. Pfeffer MA, Braunwald E, Moye LA, et al. Effect of captopril on mortality and morbidity in patients with left ventricular dysfunction after myocardial infarction. Results of the survival and ventricular enlargement trial. The SAVE Investigators. *N Engl J Med*. 1992;327:669–677.
105. Swedberg K, Held P, Kjekshus J, et al. Effects of the early administration of enalapril on mortality in patients with acute myocardial infarction. Results of the Cooperative New Scandinavian Enalapril Survival Study II (CONSENSUS II). *N Engl J Med*. 1992;327:678–684.
106. Ambrosioni E, Borghi C, Magnani B. The effect of the angiotensin-converting-enzyme inhibitor zofenopril on mortality and morbidity after anterior myocardial infarction. The Survival of Myocardial Infarction Long-Term Evaluation (SMILE) Study Investigators. *N Engl J Med*. 1995;332:80–85.
107. Kober L, Torp-Pedersen C, Carlsen JE, et al. A clinical trial of the angiotensin-converting-enzyme inhibitor trandolapril in patients with left ventricular dysfunction after myocardial infarction. Trandolapril Cardiac Evaluation (TRACE) Study Group. *N Engl J Med*. 1995;333:1670–1676.
108. van Gilst WH, Kingma JH, Peels KH, et al. Which patient benefits from early angiotensin-converting enzyme inhibition after myocardial infarction? Results of one-year serial echocardiographic follow-up from the Captopril and Thrombolysis Study (CATS). *J Am Coll Cardiol*. 1996;28:114–121.
109. Borghi C, Marino P, Zardini P, et al. Short- and long-term effects of early fosinopril administration in patients with acute anterior myocardial infarction undergoing intravenous thrombolysis: results from the Fosinopril in Acute Myocardial Infarction Study. FAMIS Working Party. *Am Heart J*. 1998;136:213–225.
110. ISIS-4 (Fourth International Study of Infarct Survival) Collaborative Group. ISIS-4: a randomised factorial trial assessing early oral captopril, oral mononitrate, and intravenous magnesium sulphate in 58,050 patients with suspected acute myocardial infarction. *Lancet*. 1995;345:669–685.
111. Gruppo Italiano per lo Studio della Sopravvivenza nell'infarto Miocardico. GISSI-3: effects of lisinopril and transdermal glyceryl trinitrate singly and together on 6-week mortality and ventricular function after acute myocardial infarction. *Lancet*. 1994;343:1115–1122.
112. Pfeffer MA. ACE inhibition in acute myocardial infarction. *N Engl J Med*. 1995;332:118–120.
113. Pfeffer MA, McMurray JJ, Velazquez EJ, et al. Valsartan, captopril, or both in myocardial infarction complicated by heart failure, left ventricular dysfunction, or both. *N Engl J Med*. 2003;349:1893–1906.
114. Pitt B, Zannad F, Remme WJ, et al. The effect of spironolactone on morbidity and mortality in patients with severe heart failure. Randomized Aldactone Evaluation Study Investigators. *N Engl J Med*. 1999;341:709–717.

115. Pitt B, Remme W, Zannad F, et al. Eplerenone, a selective aldosterone blocker, in patients with left ventricular dysfunction after myocardial infarction. *N Engl J Med*. 2003;348:1309–1321.
116. Packer M, Bristow MR, Cohn JN, et al. The effect of carvedilol on morbidity and mortality in patients with chronic heart failure. U.S. Carvedilol Heart Failure Study Group. *N Engl J Med*. 1996;334:1349–1355.
117. Packer M, Coats AJ, Fowler MB, et al. Effect of carvedilol on survival in severe chronic heart failure. *N Engl J Med*. 2001;344:1651–1658.
118. Effect of metoprolol CR/XL in chronic heart failure: Metoprolol CR/XL Randomised Intervention Trial in Congestive Heart Failure (MERIT-HF). *Lancet*. 1999;353:2001–2007.
119. Australia/New Zealand Heart Failure Research Collaborative Group. Randomised, placebo-controlled trial of carvedilol in patients with congestive heart failure due to ischaemic heart disease. *Lancet*. 1997;349:375–380.
120. Dargie HJ. Effect of carvedilol on outcome after myocardial infarction in patients with left-ventricular dysfunction: the CAPRICORN randomised trial. *Lancet*. 2001;357:1385–1390.
121. Exner DV, Dries DL, Waclawiw MA, et al. Beta-adrenergic blocking agent use and mortality in patients with asymptomatic and symptomatic left ventricular systolic dysfunction: a post hoc analysis of the Studies of Left Ventricular Dysfunction. *J Am Coll Cardiol*. 1999;33:916–923.
122. McMurray JV, McDonagh TA, Davie AP, et al. Should we screen for asymptomatic left ventricular dysfunction to prevent heart failure? *Eur Heart. J*. 1998;19:842–846.
123. McDonagh TA. Screening for left ventricular dysfunction: a step too far? *Heart*. 2002;88(Suppl 2):ii12–ii14.
124. Alexander JH, Patel MR. Screening for structural heart disease: time to stop listening and start looking. *Am Heart J*. 2003;146:570–571.
125. Wang TJ, Levy D, Benjamin EJ, et al. The epidemiology of "asymptomatic" left ventricular systolic dysfunction: implications for screening. *Ann Intern Med*. 2003;138:907–916.
126. Vasan RS, Benjamin EJ, Larson MG, et al. Plasma natriuretic peptides for community screening for left ventricular hypertrophy and systolic dysfunction: the Framingham Heart Study. *JAMA*. 2002;288:1252–1259.
127. Redfield MM, Jacobsen SJ, Burnett JC, Jr., et al. Burden of systolic and diastolic ventricular dysfunction in the community: appreciating the scope of the heart failure epidemic. *JAMA*. 2003;289: 194–202.
128. Wang TJ, Evans JC, Benjamin EJ, et al. Natural history of asymptomatic left ventricular systolic dysfunction in the community. *Circulation*. 2003;108:977–982.
129. Fletcher RH, Fletcher SW, Wagner EH. *Clinical Epidemiology*. 2nd ed. Baltimore: Williams & Wilkins; 1988:159–160.
130. Elmore JG, Barton MB, Moceri VM, et al. Ten-year risk of false positive screening mamograms and clinical breast examinations. *N Engl J Med*. 1998;338:1089–1096.
131. Mandel JS, Bond JH, Church TR, et al. Reducing mortality from colorectal cancer by screening for fecal occult blood. *N Engl J Med*. 1993;328:1365–1371.
132. Gottdiener JS, Arnold AM, Aurigemma GP, et al. Predictors of congestive heart failure in the elderly: the Cardiovascular Health Study. *J Am Coll Cardiol*. 2000;35:1628–1637.
133. Murry PM, Cantwell JD, Heath DL, et al. The role of limited echocardiography in screening athletes. *Am J Cardiol*. 1995;76: 849–850.
134. Morgan S, Smith H, Simpson I, et al. Prevalence and clinical characteristics of left ventricular dysfunction among elderly patients in general practice setting: cross sectional survey. *BMJ*. 1999;318:368–372.
135. Watanabe J, Thamilarasan M, Blackstone EH, et al. Heart rate recovery immediately after treadmill exercise and left ventricular systolic dysfunction as predictors of mortality: the case of stress echocardiography. *Circulation*. 2001;104:1911–1916.
136. Heidenreich PA, Gubens MA, Fonarow GC, et al. Cost-effectiveness of screening with B-type natriuretic peptide to identify patients with reduced left ventricular ejection fraction. *J Am Coll Cardiol*. 2004;43:1019–1026.
137. Del Ry S, Giannessi D, Clerico A. Plasma brain natriuretic peptide measured by fully-automated immunoassay and by immunoradiometric assay compared. *Clin Chem Lab Med*. 2001;39:446–450.
138. Murdoch DR, Byrne J, Morton JJ, et al. Brain natriuretic peptide is stable in whole blood and can be measured using a simple rapid assay: implications for clinical practice. *Heart*. 1997;78: 594–597.
139. Jensen KT, Carstens J, Ivarsen P, et al. A new, fast and reliable radioimmunoassay of brain natriuretic peptide in human plasma. Reference values in healthy subjects and in patients with different diseases. *Scand J Clin Lab Invest*. 1997;57:529–540.
140. Davis KM, Fish LC, Elahi D, et al. Atrial natriuretic peptide levels in the prediction of congestive heart failure risk in frail elderly. *JAMA*. 1992;267:2625–2629.
141. Wang TJ, Larson MG, Levy D, et al. Plasma natriuretic peptide levels and the risk of cardiovascular events and death. *N Engl J Med*. 2004;350:655–663.
142. McCullough PA, Nowak RM, McCord J, et al. B-type natriuretic peptide and clinical judgment in emergency diagnosis of heart failure: analysis from Breathing Not Properly (BNP) Multinational Study. *Circulation*. 2002;106:416–422.
143. Silver MA, Maisel A, Yancy CW, et al. BNP Consensus Panel 2004: A clinical approach for the diagnostic, prognostic, screening, treatment monitoring, and therapeutic roles of natriuretic peptides in cardiovascular diseases. *Congest Heart Fail*. 2004;10:1–30.
144. Vasan RS, Benjamin EJ, Larson MG, et al. Plasma natriuretic peptides for community screening for left ventricular hypertrophy and systolic dysfunction: the Framingham Heart Study. *JAMA*. 2002;288:1252–1259.
145. Redfield MM, Rodeheffer RJ, Jacobsen SJ, et al. Plasma brain natriuretic peptide to detect preclinical ventricular systolic or diastolic dysfunction: a community-based study. *Circulation*. 2004;109:3176–3181.
146. Kannel WB, Ho K, Thom T. Changing epidemiological features of cardiac failure. *Br Heart J*. 1994;72:S3–S9.
147. Chan KL. Is aortic stenosis a preventable disease? *J Am Coll Cardiol*. 2003;42:593–599.
148. Stewart BF, Siscovick D, Lind BK, et al. Clinical factors associated with calcific aortic valve disease. Cardiovascular Health Study. *J Am Coll Cardiol*. 1997;29:630–634.
149. Otto CM, Burwash IG, Legget ME, et al. Prospective study of asymptomatic valvular aortic stenosis. Clinical, echocardiographic, and exercise predictors of outcome. *Circulation*. 1997;95: 2262–2270.
150. Otto CM, Pearlman AS, Gardner CL. Hemodynamic progression of aortic stenosis in adults assessed by Doppler echocardiography. *J Am Coll Cardiol*. 1989;13:545–550.
151. Brener SJ, Duffy CI, Thomas JD, et al. Progression of aortic stenosis in 394 patients: relation to changes in myocardial and mitral valve dysfunction. *J Am Coll Cardiol*. 1995;25:305–310.
152. Croft LB, Goldman ME. Calcific aortic stenosis: new pathophysiologic insights and possible new medical therapy. *Curr Cardiol Rep*. 2003;5:101–104.
153. Mohler ER, 3rd. Are atherosclerotic processes involved in aortic-valve calcification? *Lancet*. 2000;356:524–525.
154. Rosenhek R, Rader F, Loho N, et al. Statins but not angiotensin-converting enzyme inhibitors delay progression of aortic stenosis. *Circulation*. 2004;110:1291–1295.
155. Bellamy MF, Pellikka PA, Klarich KW, et al. Association of cholesterol levels, hydroxymethylglutaryl coenzyme-A reductase inhibitor treatment, and progression of aortic stenosis in the community. *J Am Coll Cardiol*. 2002;40:1723–1730.
156. Aronow WS, Ahn C, Kronzon I, et al. Association of coronary risk factors and use of statins with progression of mild valvular aortic stenosis in older persons. *Am J Cardiol*. 2001;88:693–695.
157. Novaro GM, Tiong IY, Pearce GL, et al. Effect of hydroxymethylglutaryl coenzyme-A reductase inhibitors on the progression of calcific aortic stenosis. *Circulation*. 2001;104:2205–2209.
158. Cowell SJ, Newby DE, Prescott RJ, et al. Scottish Aortic Stenosis and Lipid-Lowering Trial, Impact an Regression (SALTIRE) Investigators. *N Eng J Med*. 2005;352:2389–2397.
159. Scognamiglio R, Rahimtoola SH, Fasoli G, et al. Nifedipine in asymptomatic patients with severe aortic regurgitation and normal left ventricular function. *N Engl J Med*. 1994;331:689–694.
160. Scognamiglio R, Fasoli G, Ponchia A, et al. Long-term nifedipine unloading therapy in asymptomatic patients with chronic severe aortic regurgitation. *J Am Coll Cardiol*. 1990;16:424–429.
161. Qureshi AI, Suri MF, Guterman LR, et al. Ineffective secondary prevention in survivors of cardiovascular events in the US population: report from the Third National Health and Nutrition Examination Survey. *Arch Intern Med*. 2001;161:1621–1628.

162. Jencks SF, Cuerdon T, Burwen DR, et al. Quality of medical care delivered to Medicare beneficiaries: a profile at state and national levels. *JAMA*. 2000;284:1670–1676.
163. McGlynn EA, Asch SM, Adams J, et al. The quality of health care delivered to adults in the United States. *N Engl J Med*. 2003;348:2635–2645.
164. Federman AD, Adams AS, Ross-Degnan D, et al. Supplemental insurance and use of effective cardiovascular drugs among elderly Medicare beneficiaries with coronary heart disease. *JAMA*. 2001;286:1732–1739.
165. Tamblyn R, Laprise R, Hanley JA, et al. Adverse events associated with prescription drug cost-sharing among poor and elderly persons. *JAMA*. 2001;285:421–429.
166. McDermott MM, Schmitt B, Wallner E. Impact of medication nonadherence on coronary heart disease outcomes: a critical review. *Arch Intern Med*. 1997;157:1921–1929.
167. Avorn J, Monette J, Lacour A, et al. Persistence of use of lipid-lowering medications: a cross-national study. *JAMA*. 1998;279: 1458–1462.

Physical Examination in Heart Failure

31

Kanu Chatterjee

The goals of physical examination in patients with suspected or established heart failure are as follows:

1. To determine the potential cause of heart failure
2. To assess the severity of heart failure
3. To determine the hemodynamic profile
4. To assess prognosis
5. During follow-up evaluation, to assess response to therapy

During clinical evaluation of a patient with suspected heart failure, it is desirable to establish a systematic approach every time a patient is examined. These various steps and sequences of physical examination are variable and depend on the examiner's preference; however, if the same sequences are repeated every time the patient is examined, the chances of missing valuable information that can be obtained by physical examination can be minimized. I prefer the following steps:

1. General inspection
2. Examination of arterial pulse
3. Examination of venous pressure and pulse
4. Palpation of precordium and the epigastrum
5. Auscultation of heart sounds and murmurs
6. Examination of abdomen
7. Examination of the inferior extremities
8. Examination of the lungs
9. Recording of blood pressure and respiratory rate
10. Special examinations when indicated, such as fundoscopic examination and the Valsalva maneuver

GENERAL INSPECTION

During evaluation of a patient with suspected or established heart failure, the presence or absence of respiratory distress, and types of altered respiration should be observed. Labored and uncomfortable breathing can be of cardiac or noncardiac origin. However, inability to lie down or associated dry, irritating cough with dyspnea in the supine position usually indicates pulmonary venous congestion. Typical Cheyne-Stokes respiration usually indicates severe heart failure. Although the mechanism of Cheyne-Stokes respiration is not entirely clear, it is associated with decreased chemoreceptor sensitivity. Although it occurs more frequently during sleep, Cheyne-Stokes respiration can occur when the patient is awake. Cheyne-Stokes respiration should be differentiated from Biot respiration. Bitot respiration is characterized by equal amplitude of inspiration during respiratory phase following apnea. Cheyne-Stokes respiration is characterized by gradually increasing amplitude of inspiration during the hyperpneic phase following phases of apnea. Sleep apnea may be obstructive or central, and both types of sleep apnea have been observed in patients with chronic heart failure. Biot respiration is usually associated with neurologic disorders, whereas Cheyne-Stokes respiration is more frequently observed in patients with heart failure.

During inspection, changes in skin color are also observed. A bluish discoloration of the skin usually indicates cyanosis. When cyanosis is observed, a distinction between central and peripheral cyanosis should be made.

Peripheral cyanosis is detected only in exposed skin, such as the lips, nose, earlobes, and extremities. Peripheral cyanosis usually indicates impaired peripheral perfusion due to low cardiac output or marked vasoconstriction. Central cyanosis is associated with a bluish discoloration of the tongue, uvula, and buccal mucous membrane and indicates either intrapulmonary or intracardiac right to left shunt resulting in increased proportion of desaturated hemoglobin greater than 3 g. The distribution of cyanosis can also provide a clue to the diagnosis of the underlying mechanism. If cyanosis along with clubbing is observed only in the inferior extremities and not in the upper extremities, Eisenmenger syndrome associated with patent ductus arteriosus should be suspected.

Bronze- or slate-colored pigmentation of the skin suggests hemochromatosis, which may be associated with restrictive or dilated cardiomyopathy. Patients on chronic amiodarone therapy also develop similar discoloration of the skin, particularly following exposure to sunlight. This discoloration of the skin also may be seen in patients with carcinoid heart disease, another cause of heart failure. Acrosclerosis with thickened edematous and taut skin with or without sclerodactyly suggests systemic sclerosis, a syndrome that may be associated with pulmonary hypertension, pericarditis, right heart failure, systemic hypertension, restrictive cardiomyopathy, and dilated cardiomyopathy. Malar flush indicates the presence of severe pulmonary hypertension, regardless of the cause.

In patients with heart failure, nutritional status should be observed. The presence of cardiac cachexia or marked loss of skeletal muscle mass is usually evident from bitemporal wasting and indicates the presence of severe heart failure. However, hemodynamic abnormalities such as degree of reduction in cardiac output or in elevation of pulmonary venous pressure do not correlate with the presence or absence of cardiac cachexia. Cardiac cachexia in patients with heart failure is associated with a severe abnormality of neuroendocrine profile characterized by marked elevation of angiotensin II and cytokines such as tumor necrosis factor-α. Ascites and peripheral edema that also can be observed during inspection may indicate severe right heart failure or constrictive pericarditis; however, these findings also may be seen in other conditions such as cirrhosis of the liver and nephrotic syndrome.

The clinician should observe the patient for abnormal movement of the head and neck because such movement may yield information about the etiology or severity of heart failure. Lateral movements of the earlobes with each cardiac cycle strongly suggest severe tricuspid regurgitation. Bobbing of the head coincident with each heart beat is usually associated with severe aortic regurgitation. Finally, abnormalities of the eyes such as exophthalmus, lid-lag, stare, or periorbital edema may suggest the presence of thyroid abnormalities or another systemic disease.

EXAMINATION OF THE ARTERIAL PULSE

During initial evaluation, all accessible arterial pulses should be examined. In the superior extremities, both brachial and radial and, if necessary, axillary pulses should be examined. In the inferior extremities, dorsalis pedis, posterior tibial, and femoral pulses should be examined bilaterally. In adult patients, an absent or diminished dorsalis pedis pulse may indicate atherosclerotic peripheral vascular disease that is associated with increased incidence of coronary artery disease. Loss of or decreased femoral pulse unilaterally or bilaterally most frequently indicates local obstructive lesions in adult patients. The radial femoral delay in young patients may indicate coarctation of the aorta. In adult patients, however, it most frequently suggests local obstructive peripheral vascular disease. Rarely in adult patients, severe pseudo-coarctation of the aorta may cause significant radial femoral delay.

In a patient with suspected heart failure, peripheral arterial pulses are examined to detect any abnormalities of the character of the arterial pulse. Pulsus alternans is suspected when strong- and weak-amplitude pulses are appreciated with alternate beats in the presence of a regular pulse (Fig. 31-1). Pulsus alternans can be confirmed by measuring systolic blood pressure by sphygmometer. The phase I Korotkoff sound, which indicates peak systolic blood pressure, is higher with the stronger beats than with the weaker beats. The difference between the stronger and weaker beats represents the magnitude of the pulsus alternans. In some patients, the pulse with the weaker beat is not palpable, which is defined as total pulsus alternans. The precise mechanisms of pulsus alternans are not clear. However, for clinical purposes, pulsus alternans almost always indicates the presence of impaired left ventricular systolic function. Changes in contractile function, preload, and afterload contribute to persistence of pulsus alternans. Changes in left ventricular diastolic function due to abnormalities of ventricular filling also have been shown to contribute to the development and persistence of pulsus alternans. In the failing heart, however, changes in arterial pressure appear to

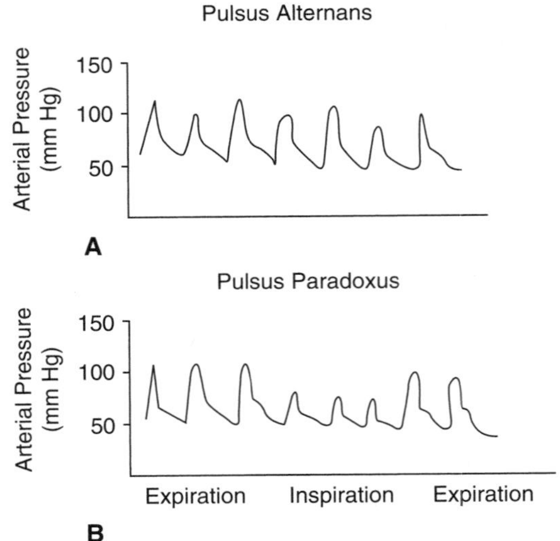

Figure 31-1 Schematic illustrations of pulsus alternans (**A**) and pulsus paradoxus (**B**). Pulsus alternans usually indicates reduced left ventricular systolic function. Pulsus paradoxus is an important sign for the diagnosis of tamponade; however, it can be appreciated in pulmonary disease, marked obesity, and rarely in severe congestive heart failure. (From Chatterjee K. Physical examination. In: Topol EJ, ed. *Textbook of Cardiovascular Medicine*. 1st ed. Vol. 13. Philadelphia: Lippincott-Raven; 1997:285–331.

be the major determinant for the persistence of pulsus alternans. The failing heart is sensitive to altered afterload and resistance to left ventricular ejection. The increased arterial pressure associated with a strong beat increases the resistance to left ventricular ejection for the following beat, which is associated with decreased forward stroke volume and decreased arterial pressure, which reduces the resistance to left ventricular ejection for the following beat, allowing a larger stroke volume and increase in systolic blood pressure.

For clinical purposes, the presence of pulsus alternans indicates depressed left ventricular systolic function and thus allows the diagnosis of systolic ventricular failure. It should be realized, however, that the absence of pulsus alternans does not indicate the absence of impaired left ventricular systolic function. It is of interest to note that with improved left ventricular ejection fraction and increased stroke volume, pulsus alternans may resolve. In some patients with severe left ventricular failure with markedly reduced left ventricular stroke volume and relative hypotension, pulsus alternans may not be obvious. Furthermore, in some conditions such as hypertrophic cardiomyopathy or aortic valve stenosis, arterial pulsus alternans may not be apparent even when left ventricular pressure pulsus alternans is present. In clinical practice, however, if one can detect pulsus alternans it is likely that left ventricular ejection fraction is reduced and further evaluation should be undertaken to confirm the diagnosis of systolic left ventricular failure.

A substantial decrease in the amplitude of the arterial pulse during the inspiratory phase of respiration indicates the presence of pulsus paradoxus (Fig. 31-1). The pulsus paradoxus should be confirmed by measuring systolic blood pressure during the expiratory and inspiratory phases of respiration. A decrease in arterial pressure greater than 12 to 15 mm Hg during inspiration is regarded as pulsus paradoxus and is usually detectable by palpation of the peripheral pulses. The obvious pulsus parodoxus is an important physical finding for the diagnosis of cardiac tamponade. The inspiratory decrease in arterial pressure in tamponade results from the marked inspiratory decline of left ventricular stroke volume due to a decreased end-diastolic volume. During inspiration, there is an increase in venous return to the right atrium and the right ventricle. Due to increased intrapericardial pressure, the intraventricular septum shifts toward the left ventricle during inspiration (reversed Bernheim effect). This diastolic shift of the intraventricular septum toward the left ventricle decreases left ventricular preload, causing a reduction in its stroke volume and, therefore, systolic blood pressure. It should be appreciated, however, that pulsus paradoxus is frequently observed in patients with chronic obstructive pulmonary disease. Pulsus paradoxus is also occasionally observed in patients with pulmonary embolism, pregnancy, marked obesity, and partial obstruction of the superior vena cava. It is rarely encountered in patients with constrictive pericarditis. In hypertrophic obstructive cardiomyopathy, arterial pressure occasionally increases during inspiration (i.e., reversed pulsus paradoxus). The precise mechanism for this phenomenon is not clear.

Analysis of the contour of the carotid pulse and peripheral arterial pulse can provide a useful indication regarding the etiology of left ventricular failure (Fig. 31-2).

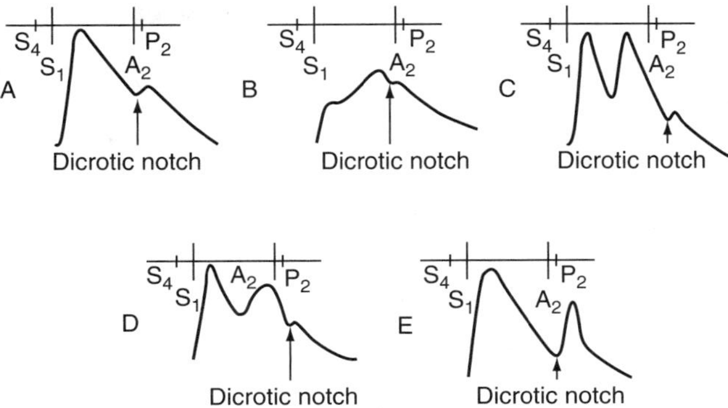

Figure 31-2 Schematic illustrations of carotid arterial pulse characters. Heart sounds are also illustrated. **(A)** Normal. **(B)** Anacrotic pulse with delayed upstroke and peak indicating aortic stenosis. **(C)** Pulsus bisferiens with increased amplitude of both percussion and tidal waves as appreciated in patients with aortic regurgitation. **(D)** Pulsus bisferiens as appreciated in obstructive hypertrophic cardiomyopathy. **(E)** Dicrotic pulse as appreciated in some patients with severe heart failure. (From Chatterjee K. Physical examination. In: Topol EJ, ed. *Textbook of Cardiovascular Medicine*. 1st ed. Vol. 13. Philadelphia: Lippincott-Raven; 1997: 285–331.) S_4, fourth heart sound; S_1, first heart sound; A_2, aortic component of the second heart sound; P_2, pulmonary component of the second heart sound.

The delayed upstroke of the arterial pulse with anacrotic character and delayed peak is most frequently associated with hemodynamically significant aortic valve stenosis. It should be appreciated, however, that in elderly subjects, in whom vascular compliance is reduced, absence of the anacrotic pulse, decreased arterial pulse volume, or delayed peak of the carotid pulse does not necessarily indicate absence of significant aortic stenosis. The pulsus bisferiens character of the arterial pulse indicates predominant aortic regurgitation, although it can be appreciated in patients with obstructive hypertrophic cardiomyopathy. The pulsus bisferiens character is also observed in patients with mixed aortic stenosis and aortic regurgitation. However, when this finding is present, aortic regurgitation is usually the more dominant lesion. The dicrotic arterial pulse is difficult to differentiate at the bedside from pulsus bisferiens. The dicrotic pulse is appreciated in some patients with severe heart failure due to dilated cardiomyopathy and is usually associated with low cardiac output and increased systemic vascular resistance. On the other hand, a dicrotic pulse contour is also appreciated in patients with septic shock who have high cardiac output and low systemic vascular resistance. A dicrotic pulse can be present after aortic valve replacement and usually indicates depressed left ventricular ejection fraction postoperatively. However, in such patients echocardiographic evaluation is desirable to exclude aortic regurgitation due to the malfunction of the prosthetic valve causing pulsus bisferians, which can be misinterpreted as a dicrotic pulse.

During examination of the arterial pulse, it is desirable to evaluate the presence of arrhythmias, although the diagnosis of arrhythmias should always be confirmed by electrocardiography. The incidence of atrial fibrillation can be as high as 20% in patients with chronic congestive heart failure. Atrial fibrillation can be diagnosed at the bedside by noting an irregular pulse. It should be emphasized, however, that atrial flutter or supraventricular tachycardia with variable atrioventricular block also may produce an irregular pulse. Differentiation between these arrhythmias needs to be made by electrocardiography. It is important to determine the heart rate and pulse rate in patients with atrial fibrillation to assess the magnitude of pulse deficit. It has been established that patients with systolic ventricular failure with reduced left ventricular ejection fraction may develop worsening heart failure due to rapid ventricular response, which may not be appreciated by examining the arterial pulse alone. The rapid ventricular response not only impairs left ventricular filling and produces worsening hemodynamics, but also can cause further depression of left ventricular contractile function (inverse force–frequency relationship). In a patient with atrial fibrillation with variable R-R cycle length, it is also desirable to assess the changes in the amplitude of the arterial pulse with changes in the preceding R-R intervals. If there is little or no change in the arterial pulse volume following a long R-R cycle length and a short R-R cycle length, diminished preload and contractile reserve should be suspected.

In patients with established systolic ventricular failure not resulting from chronic left ventricular outflow tract obstruction or aortic regurgitation, the character of the arterial pulse is usually noninformative. The presence of pulsus alternans is the only finding that can suggest impaired left ventricular systolic and diastolic function. It should be also emphasized that absence of pulsus alternans does not exclude systolic ventricular failure, and it can be absent even in patients with severe left ventricular systolic dysfunction with hypotension and reduced stroke volume.

EXAMINATION OF CENTRAL VENOUS PRESSURE AND PULSE

The central venous pressure is usually examined with patients in a 45-degree semirecumbent position. However, when the venous pressure is low, it may be necessary to examine the patient lying supine or even in the Trendelenburg position. When the venous pressure is very high, it is sometimes necessary to examine the patient in the sitting position or in the standing position. It is preferable to examine both right and left internal jugular venous pulse and pressure. In elderly subjects, external jugular veins may be compressed by platisma muscle, which will cause spuriously high readings of venous pressure. In elderly patients, the left internal jugular venous pulse pressure can be higher than that of the right internal jugular vein because of the partial obstruction of the left innominate vein by an unfolded (ectatic) aorta. With inspiration and descent of the diaphragm, this partial obstruction may be relieved and pressures in both right and left internal jugular veins become equal.

The venous pressure is determined by adding 5 cm to the height of the venous column. It should be emphasized that to assess right atrial pressure, it is desirable to note first that there is a transmitted pulsation to the neck veins. In the era of cardiac transplantation when frequent biopsy is performed using the right internal jugular vein, partial right internal jugular venous obstruction can occur so that no pulsation of this vein is observed. At the bedside, venous pulsation is differentiated from carotid artery pulsation by inspection. The venous pulse is characterized by a sharp inward movement, whereas the arterial pulse is characterized by a sharp outward movement. When a patient is in sinus rhythm, inspection of the venous pulse demonstrates a double undulation character that is, however, lost in atrial fibrillation. The double positive waves that are observed in the venous pulse are A and V waves. In clinical practice, the inward movement or negative wave that is observed in the venous pulse is the *y* descent. It is difficult to recognize the *x* descent at the bedside. The venous pulsation also can be differentiated from the arterial pulsation with compression at the root of the neck, which obliterates the venous pulse but not the carotid pulse.

After recognizing the venous pulse and estimating the venous pressure, the character of the venous pulse is analyzed. If an unusually prominent A wave that precedes the carotid pulse upstroke is appreciated, conditions that increase resistance to right atrial emptying during atrial systole should be considered. Tricuspid valve obstruction is relatively uncommon in clinical practice. Right ventricular hypertrophy with or without right ventricular failure is a more important cause of a prominent A wave. In adult patients, a prominent A wave is frequently observed in the presence of a noncompliant right ventricle due to right ventricular hypertrophy, usually due to pulmonary hypertension. However, right ventricular hypertrophy due to right ventricular outflow tract obstruction may also increase resistance to right atrial emptying and, hence, a prominent A wave.

A prominent V wave usually indicates tricuspid regurgitation. However, in some patients with a noncompliant right atrium and increased right atrial venous return, the normal V wave may be accentuated even in the absence of tricuspid regurgitation. Severe tricuspid regurgitation is characterized not only by the presence of a prominent V wave, but also by a sharp *y* descent. Once tricuspid regurgitation is suspected, this diagnosis should be confirmed by auscultation, which reveals an early systolic or pansystolic regurgitant murmur along the lower left sternal border, which may radiate to the right side of the sternum or over the epigastrum. The murmur also increases in intensity during inspiration. Severe tricuspid regurgitation is frequently associated with systolic hepatic pulsation. After the diagnosis of tricupsid regurgitation has been confirmed, it is desirable to assess the intensity of the pulmonic component of the second heart sound to distinguish between primary and secondary tricuspid regurgitation. For clinical purposes secondary tricuspid regurgitation is defined if it is associated with pulmonary hypertension that can be diagnosed if the intensity of the pulmonic component of the second heart sound is increased.

When the venous pressure is elevated without a prominent *x* or *y* descent or only with obvious *x* descent, cardiac tamponade should be excluded. Cardiac tamponade is also associated with quiet precordium and occasionally distant heart sounds and no evidence of pulmonary hypertension. If the venous pulse demonstrates a sharp *y* descent along with elevated mean pressure, restrictive cardiomyopathy or constrictive pericarditis should be considered. In both constrictive pericarditis and restrictive cardiomyopathy, the Kussmaul sign (a lack of decrease or increase in systemic venous pressure during inspiration) is observed. It needs to be appreciated that the Kussmaul sign also may be present in primary right ventricular failure such as right ventricular infarction, pulmonary embolism, and chronic tricuspid regurgitation. Restrictive cardiomyopathy can be associated with mitral and tricuspid valve regurgitation and pulmonary hypertension. The presence of tricuspid and mitral regurgitation with pulmonary hypertension favors the diagnosis of restrictive cardiomyopathy rather than constrictive pericarditis. However, further invasive and noninvasive investigations are necessary for the differentiated diagnosis of constrictive pericarditis and restrictive cardiomyopathy.

In patients with suspected congestive heart failure with or without elevated resting venous pressure, it is desirable to perform the hepatojugular reflux test (abdominal jugular reflux). The positive hepatojugular reflux is defined when there is a rapid increase in jugular venous pressure that remains elevated by 4 cm or more during abdominal compression, lasting for more than 10 seconds (Fig. 31-3). In adult patients a positive hepatojugular reflux is most frequently observed in congestive heart failure resulting from dilated cardiomyopathy. In these patients, a sustained elevation of right ventricular and right atrial pressure probably reflects decreased right ventricular and right atrial compliance resulting from the constraining effect of the pericardium in the presence of a dilated left ventricle. It should be noted, however, that a positive hepatojugular reflux can also be observed in patients with isolated right heart failure due to precapillary pulmonary hypertension or right ventricular infarction.

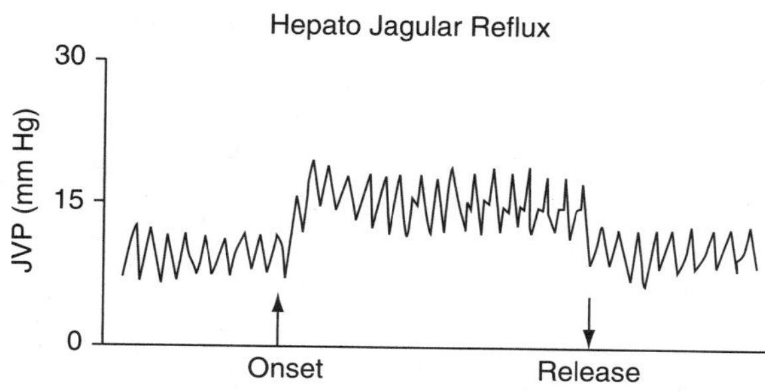

Figure 31-3 Schematic illustration of an example of a positive hepatojugular reflux. Jugular venous pressure (JVP) increases with the beginning of abdominal compression (↑) and remains elevated until it is released (↑). Positive hepatojugular reflux is appreciated frequently in patients with heart failure due to dilated cardiomyopathy. (From Chatterjee K. Physical examination. In: Topol EJ, ed. *Textbook of Cardiovascular Medicine*. 1st ed. Vol. 13. Philadelphia: Lippincott-Raven; 1997:285–331.)

EXAMINATION OF PRECORDIAL PULSATIONS

In patients with suspected or established heart failure, the character of the outward movement of the left ventricular apical impulse is assessed to determine whether it is normal, hyperdynamic, or sustained (Fig. 31-4). The normal apical impulse and the hyperdynamic apical impulse have brief duration and simultaneous palpation of the outward movement, and the carotid pulse gives the impression of asynchrony. When the carotid pulse and the outward movement of the left ventricular apical impulse are synchronous, one should suspect a sustained apical impulse. The most frequent cause of sustained apical impulse in adults is reduced left ventricular ejection fraction. However, severe left ventricular hypertrophy may also produce sustained apical impulse in the presence of normal left ventricular ejection fraction. Severe hypertrophy causing a sustained impulse usually results from hypertrophic cardiomyopathy or severe aortic stenosis. To distinguish between sustained impulse due to hypertrophy or reduced ejection fraction, noninvasive evaluation (preferably with echocardiography) should always be considered. One caveat to the examination of the apical impulse is that in thin subjects the left ventricular apical impulse in the left lateral decubitus position may appear sustained even when

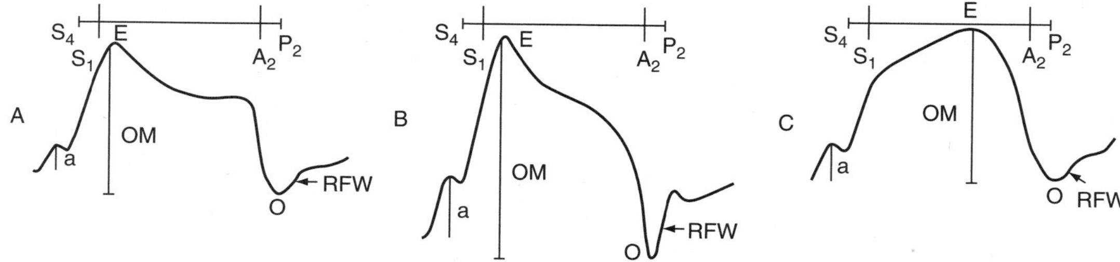

Figure 31-4 Schematic illustration of normal, hyperdynamic, and sustained left ventricular impulses. Heart sounds are also illustrated. **(A)** Normal apical impulse indicates preserved left ventricular ejection fraction. **(B)** Hyperdynamic left ventricular apical impulse is usually appreciated in the volume-overloaded left ventricle, such as in primary mitral regurgitation. Left ventricular ejection fraction is usually preserved. **(C)** Sustained left ventricular impulse indicates depressed left ventricular ejection fraction in absence of severe left ventricular hypertrophy. (From Chatterjee K. Physical examination. In: Topol EJ, ed. *Textbook of Cardiovascular Medicine*. 1st ed. Vol. 13. Philadelphia: Lippincott-Raven; 1997:285–331.) S_4, fourth heart sound; S_1, first heart sound; A_2, aortic component of the second heart sound; P_2, pulmonic component of the second heart sound; A, presystolic wave; OM, outward movement; E, beginning of ejection; O, opening of mitral valve; RFW, rapid filling wave.

the ejection fraction is normal. It should be emphasized that although examination of apical impulse can provide useful information about the presence or absence of depressed ejection fraction, physical examination alone is inadequate to assess the degree of depression of the left ventricular ejection fraction.

When the left ventricular apical impulse is analyzed in the left lateral decubitus position, a double impulse and occasionally a triple impulse can be appreciated. A double impulse usually indicates an accentuated presystolic or A wave along with the outward movement. The palpable A wave usually reflects elevated left ventricular end-diastolic pressure. A palpable S_3 can be appreciated in many patients with heart failure as a late extra hump. It is almost always associated with increased left ventricular diastolic pressure.

The right ventricular impulse can be appreciated by palpation of the lower left parasternal area. A sustained and prolonged left parasternal impulse extending throughout the ejection phase is abnormal and reflects right ventricular failure or right ventricular hypertrophy. Severe mitral regurgitation also may be associated with a systolic left parasternal impulse resulting from left atrial expansion due to mitral regurgitation. Thus, at the bedside, before the diagnosis of right ventricular failure or right ventricular hypertrophy is suspected, it is necessary to exclude significant mitral regurgitation. In patients with right ventricular hypertrophy and failure, a sustained epigastric impulse is also appreciated. A prominent diastolic left parasternal impulse is sometimes observed in patients with constrictive pericarditis; the mechanism of such inward movement is not clear. However, it coincides with the pericardial knock. In constrictive pericarditis, the precordium is usually quiet. In patients with Ebstein anomaly, the precordium also may be quiet. In some patients with Ebstein anomaly, a right parasternal systolic outward movement resulting from a large ventricularized right atrium is occasionally appreciated. In patients with severe chronic pulmonary hypertension with enlargement of the pulmonary artery, the pulmonary artery pulsation is occasionally palpable in the left second interspace and it is frequently associated with a high-frequency vibration representing an accentuated pulmonic component of the second heart sound.

AUSCULTATION OF HEART SOUNDS AND MURMURS

Analysis of the intensity of the first and second heart sounds provides useful hemodynamic information in patients with suspected or established heart failure. An unusually loud first heart sound is distinctly uncommon in heart failure except when it is precipitated by mitral valve obstruction. The Wolf-Parkinson-White syndrome with short PR interval may be associated with increased intensity of the first heart sound. In patients with heart failure in whom dual-chamber (DDD) pacemaker therapy is used with a short PR interval, the intensity of the first heart sound also increases despite an elevated left ventricular end-diastolic pressure. In most patients with heart failure, however, the intensity of the first heart sound is decreased. The intensity of the first heart sound is determined by the rate of closure of the mitral valve. The intensity is decreased when the PR interval is longer, as in patients with first-degree atrioventricular block. Increased left ventricular diastolic pressure also reduces the intensity of the first heart sound. Decreased isovolumic developed pressure/isovolumic contraction time (*dP/dt*), which partly determines the rate of closure of the mitral valve, also may be contributory to reduced intensity of the first heart sound in systolic left ventricular failure. In clinical practice, if the intensity of the first heart sound is markedly reduced in the presence of normal PR interval, elevated left ventricular diastolic pressure should be strongly suspected. The intensity of the first heart sound also can decrease in patients with chronic obstructive pulmonary disease, obesity, and pericardial effusion due to decreased conduction of heart sounds through the chest wall. Under these circumstances, however, all the heart sounds appear soft and distant.

A variable intensity of the first heart sound is common in atrial fibrillation and atrial flutter with variable block. However, these arrhythmias can be diagnosed from analysis of the arterial pulse. Auscultatory alternans characterized by varying intensity of the first heart sound with alternate beat (soft and loud) is a rare finding. When it is associated with pulsus paradoxus, cardiac tamponade is the diagnosis. When it is associated with pulsus alternans, a beat-to-beat alteration in left ventricular *dP/dt* appears to be the mechanism and therefore suggests systolic left ventricular failure.

A decrease in the intensity of the second heart sound does not appear to have any hemodynamic significance. For example, when the intensity of the aortic component of the second heart sound is decreased in patients with aortic stenosis or aortic regurgitation, it does not correlate with hemodynamic severity of these lesions. Similarly, decreased intensity of the pulmonic component of the second heart sound (P_2) correlates poorly with the severity of pulmonary insufficiency or pulmonary stenosis. However, the intensity of P_2 is always decreased in the presence of significant valve or subvalve pulmonary stenosis. An increase in intensity of the second heart sound, both of the aortic (A_2) and pulmonic component (P_2), reflects the degree of deceleration of retrograde flow of the blood column in the aorta and pulmonary artery when the maximum tensing of these valve leaflets occurs. The increased intensity of the pulmonic component of the second heart sound (P_2) indicates pulmonary hypertension irrespective of its etiology. When there is a substantial increase in the intensity of P_2, it can also be heard at the cardiac apex. It is uncommon for P_2 to be transmitted to the cardiac apex in the absence of pulmonary hypertension. In only approximately 5% of normal subjects and only when they are young (i.e., under 20 years of age) can P_2 be recorded by phonocardiography over the cardiac apex. However, when the cardiac apex is occupied by the right ventricle—as in patients with large atrial septal defects and primary tricuspid regurgitation, and rarely in patients with right bundle branch block—P_2 can be heard at the cardiac apex in the absence of pulmonary hypertension.

In patients with suspected or established heart failure, increased intensity of P_2 should be regarded as a manifestation of pulmonary arterial hypertension. Once the diagnosis of pulmonary hypertension is suspected, it is desirable to search for the underlying cause. For practical clinical purposes, pulmonary hypertension is categorized into two types: postcapillary pulmonary hypertension (which results primarily from elevation of pulmonary capillary wedge pressure) and precapillary pulmonary hypertension (when pulmonary arterial pressure is increased due to increased pulmonary vascular resistance). In the latter case, pulmonary capillary wedge pressure remains normal. During evaluation of causes of pulmonary hypertension, conditions that increase pulmonary venous pressure are considered. Postcapillary pulmonary hypertension can result from mitral valve obstruction, which causes elevation of left atrial pressure. In this setting, left ventricular diastolic pressure remains normal. Primary mitral regurgitation, aortic stenosis and aortic regurgitation, primary myocardial dysfunction such as ischemic or nonischemic dilated cardiomyopathy, hypertrophic cardiomyopathy, and restrictive cardiomyopathy all can increase pulmonary venous pressure passively due to increase in left ventricular diastolic and left atrial pressure. In all of these cases, left ventricular diastolic pressure will be elevated when these conditions are excluded, precapillary pulmonary hypertension, including primary pulmonary hypertension, is suspected.

If central cyanosis and clubbing are appreciated, the presence of Eisenmenger syndrome physiology should be suspected. The analysis of the second heart sound can provide a clue to the diagnosis of the etiology of the Eisenmenger syndrome. If the second heart sound is widely split and fixed and the intensity of P_2 is markedly increased, Eisenmenger syndrome with atrial septal defect should be suspected. If there is differential cyanosis and clubbing and the second heart sound is physiologically split with increased intensity of P_2, Eisenmenger syndrome associated with patent ductus arteriosis should be considered. If the second heart sound is single and there is evidence of right ventricular hypertrophy, Eisenmenger syndrome associated with ventricular septal defect should be suspected.

Analysis of the character of the second heart sound may provide important diagnostic information. When the second heart sound is widely split during expiration with inspiratory delay of P_2, right bundle branch block should be suspected, particularly if there are no other abnormal findings. In the presence of a pulmonary ejection sound, a short ejection systolic murmur, and a short, early diastolic murmur localized over the left second intercostal space and associated with wide physiological splitting of the second heart sound, mild pulmonary valve stenosis or idiopathic dilatation of the pulmonary artery should be suspected. A longer ejection systolic murmur with or without a pulmonary ejection sound and decreased intensity of the P_2 with wide splitting of the second heart sound are the findings associated with right ventricular outflow tract obstruction. Increased intensity of the P_2 with or without an ejection systolic murmur and evidence of right ventricular hypertrophy or failure, along with wide physiological splitting of the second heart sound, is the characteristic finding of pulmonary hypertension. Wide, fixed splitting of the second heart sound is a characteristic finding of atrial septal defect, complete atrioventricular canal, or common atrium.

Ancillary investigations including electrocardiogram, chest x-ray, and echocardiogram are essential for the differential diagnosis of these various conditions. A paradoxical splitting of the second heart sound is observed most frequently in patients with left bundle branch block. Right ventricular pacing and accessory pathway with right ventricular pre-excitation also produce paradoxical splitting. Aortic stenosis, obstructive hypertrophic cardiomyopathy, and severe hypertension are other causes of paradoxical splitting of the second heart sound. Severe tricuspid regurgitation is a rare cause of paradoxical splitting. In patients with systolic left ventricular failure, paradoxical splitting is occasionally appreciated in the absence of left bundle branch block. In this case, delayed closure of the aortic valve is due to prolongation of left ventricular emptying.

Both the third and fourth heart sounds are of relatively lower frequency and pitch and are related to early and late diastolic filling of the ventricles, respectively. When these sounds occur in pathological conditions, they are termed gallop sounds. The third heart sound is commonly heard in children and adolescents but it is abnormal when it is heard in an older age group. A left ventricular S_3 gallop is best appreciated over or just medial to the cardiac apex. The presence of an S_3 gallop in patients with aortic valve disease, coronary artery disease, and cardiomyopathy usually indicates significant elevation of left ventricular end diastolic pressure. In patients with chronic aortic regurgitation, the presence of an S_3 gallop can be observed with normal systolic function. It is seen more frequently, however, when left ventricular ejection fraction is also reduced. In patients with primary mitral regurgitation or in volume-overloaded conditions, an S_3 gallop may not be associated with an increase in left ventricular end-diastolic pressure or reduced ejection fraction. A pathological third sound is almost invariably recognized in patients with restrictive cardiomyopathy. A third heart sound (pericardial knock) is a common finding in patients with constrictive pericarditis. The pericardial knock or third heart sound associated with restrictive cardiomyopathy may occur earlier and soon after A_2 and may be confused with opening snap. A pathological S_4 or S_3, or both, is also associated with elevated B-type natriuretic peptide (BNP), which is frequently increased in patients with both systolic and diastolic heart failure.

The fourth heart sound is related to ventricular filling during atrial systole and therefore is absent in patients with atrial fibrillation. In elderly subjects, an audible S_4 is not always associated with hemodynamic abnormality. A palpable S_4, however, almost always indicates elevated left ventricular end-diastolic pressure. The common pathological conditions in which a prominent left-sided S_4 is recognized are systemic hypertension, aortic valvular stenosis, and hypertrophic cardiomyopathy, the conditions that produce significant left ventricular hypertrophy. Pulmonary hypertension and pulmonary valvular stenosis, which produce right ventricular hypertrophy, are associated with a right-sided S_4. In patients with left ventricular aneurysm or nonischemic dilated cardiomyopathy, fourth heart sounds are often associated with a pathological S_3 producing a quadruple rhythm. More commonly, however, a gallop rhythm (horse's gallop) or summation gallop is appreciated particularly in the presence of tachycardia.

Evaluation of heart murmurs may provide clues about the etiology of heart failure. If an ejection systolic murmur along the left sternal border, over the cardiac apex, and over the right second intercostal space is recognized along with decreased carotid pulse amplitude, anacrotic pulse, and delayed peak of the carotid pulse, aortic stenosis should be suspected. In elderly patients who develop aortic stenosis due to calcification of a tricuspid valve, radiation of the murmur to the cardiac apex rather than the carotids is common. The systolic murmur in these cases takes on a raspy quality likened to wood being sawed against the grain. The timing of the murmur offers important clues to the severity of the disease, with early-peaking murmurs indicating less severe and late-peaking murmurs more severe degrees of aortic stenosis. An ejection systolic murmur or a late systolic murmur along the lower left sternal border with sharp carotid pulse upstroke may suggest hypertrophic cardiomyopathy, and appropriate maneuvers should be performed at the bedside to establish the diagnosis. During phase II of the Valsalva maneuver (i.e., the holding phase), if the murmur increases in intensity with decreased or no change in the amplitude of the carotid pulse, obstructive hypertrophic cardiomyopathy should be suspected and appropriate investigations should be undertaken. In elderly patients, a short, superficial ejection systolic murmur (particularly with a scratchy quality) usually indicates aortic sclerosis. However, a superficial, scratchy murmur also can be observed in patients with pericarditis, Ebstein anomaly, and thyrotoxicosis (i.e., the Means-Lerman sign).

Primary mitral regurgitation causing heart failure is almost always associated with either a pansystolic murmur or an early systolic crescendo/decrescendo murmur. In patients with low cardiac output and cardiogenic shock, the mitral regurgitation murmur may be inaudible due to the low flow state. In patients with primary or secondary tricuspid regurgitation with or without clinical overt heart failure, a pansystolic or early systolic murmur is appreciated along the lower left sternal border. This murmur frequently radiates to the right side of the sternum or epigastrum. Characteristically, the murmur of tricuspid regurgitation increases in intensity during inspiration.

In patients with dilated cardiomyopathy, secondary mitral regurgitation is frequently present. The murmur of secondary mitral regurgitation characteristically has poor radiation. Most frequently it is accompanied by evidence of increased left ventricular diastolic pressure, such as S_3 gallop and postcapillary pulmonary hypertension. The murmur of secondary tricuspid regurgitation with or without right heart failure is accompanied by increased intensity of the pulmonic component of the second heart sound.

When mitral stenosis is the mechanism of heart failure, the physical findings of mitral valve obstruction are usually obvious. These auscultatory findings are characterized by a loud first heart sound, a narrow A_2 opening snap interval, and a long or a pandiastolic rumble. The findings of pulmonary hypertension frequently accompany signs of mitral stenosis. A tumor ejection sound and a tumor plop sound, similar to the opening snap, may suggest mitral valve obstruction due to left atrial myxoma. For the differential diagnosis, echocardiography is mandatory.

Chronic aortic regurgitation also can produce heart failure; the characteristic auscultatory finding of chronic aortic regurgitation is an early diastolic murmur. The early diastolic murmur of aortic regurgitation may be best heard along the lower left sternal border or over the cardiac apex. The duration of the murmur is extremely variable. The more severe the heart failure, the more likely it is that the duration of the diastolic murmur will be shorter because pressures within the aorta and left ventricle approach the same level earlier during diastole. In patients with acute aortic regurgitation associated with heart failure, the early diastolic murmur may be very short or may even be absent. In patients with aortic regurgitation, the decreased intensity of the first heart sound or absent first heart sound indicates severe elevation of left ventricular diastolic pressure and is regarded as an indication for emergent surgical intervention.

Pulmonary insufficiency alone seldom produces severe right heart failure. However, long-standing pulmonary insufficiency following corrective surgery of right ventricular outflow tract obstruction may produce right heart failure. In these circumstances, an early diastolic murmur that increases in intensity during inspiration is appreciated. The intensity of P_2 is decreased or P_2 may be absent. The Graham-Steell murmur is the pulmonary insufficiency murmur associated with pulmonary hypertension, and in these circumstances, P_2 is markedly increased in intensity. When a continuous murmur is appreciated in a patient with heart failure, patent ductus arteriosus, coronary artery-venous fistulas, and atrioventricular fistulas should be suspected. However, in adult cardiology patients, these causes for heart failure are extremely uncommon.

EXAMINATION OF THE LUNGS

In patients with suspected or established heart failure, examination of the lungs is performed to determine the presence of pulmonary venous hypertension and pleural effusion. Unilateral or bilateral rales may indicate alveolar edema associated with pulmonary venous hypertension. It should be emphasized, however, that alveolar edema can result from permeability pulmonary edema with normal pulmonary capillary wedge pressure. Expiratory wheeze is occasionally observed in patients with cardiac asthma. However, wheeze is relatively uncommon in patients with chronic congestive heart failure. It should also be emphasized that in patients with chronic left ventricular failure due to ischemic or nonischemic dilated cardiomyopathy, the lungs may be clear and rales or wheezes may be absent even when the pulmonary capillary wedge pressure exceeds 25 mm Hg due to the development of compensatory changes in the pulmonary vascular bed and lymphatic drainage. Right or bilateral pleural effusions associated with basal dullness and diminished breath sounds are a frequent finding in patients with advanced heart failure. Bilateral pleural effusion almost always indicates elevation of both right atrial and pulmonary venous pressures. It should be appreciated, however, that pleural effusions may persist after normalization of systemic and pulmonary venous pressures with diuretic therapy. Thus, at the time of follow-up evaluations, pleural effusions do not necessarily indicate persistently elevated systemic and pulmonary venous pressures.

ABDOMINAL SIGNS

Examination of the abdomen is performed primarily to determine the presence or absence of ascites, hepatosplenomegaly, and a pulsatile liver. Decreased bowel sounds or ileus are almost never manifestations of heart failure. If ascites is detected, one should evaluate systemic venous pressure. If systemic venous pressure is normal, ascites is not related to cardiac failure or constrictive pericarditis. Splenomegaly is a rare finding of heart failure. In cardiac cirrhosis or in subacute bacterial endocarditis, splenomegaly can be present. Hepatomegaly, however, is extremely common in patients with chronic congestive heart failure. If there is a pulsatile liver, one should determine whether hepatic pulsation occurs before or during ventricular systole. Presystolic pulsation suggests tricuspid stenosis and systolic pulsation indicates tricuspid regurgitation. It should be emphasized that absence of pulsatile liver does not exclude tricuspid regurgitation.

SYSTEMIC SIGNS

In patients with suspected or established heart failure, evaluation for the presence of dependent edema is essential. In ambulatory patients edema is usually localized in the inferior extremities. In patients who are maintained at bed rest, the edema can be localized in the sacral and presacral regions. If edema is appreciated, it is desirable to assess the degree of elevation of systemic venous pressure. If the systemic venous pressure is persistently normal, the edema is more likely due to capillary leak rather than due to an increase in hydrostatic pressure. It is also desirable to determine the presence or absence of cachexia. If cachexia is attributable to heart failure, severe neuroendocrine abnormalities (including elevated cytokines) should be suspected. Unusual systemic signs such as arthritis or skin rash may indicate specific etiology of heart failure. However, arthritis and skin rash are not manifestations of heart failure and usually reflect complications of therapy.

PHYSICAL FINDINGS THAT HELP ASSESS THE HEMODYNAMIC PROFILE IN HEART FAILURE

1. Reduced ejection fraction: sustained left ventricular apical impulse, paradoxical splitting of the second heart sound (in absence of left bundle branch block, left ventricular outflow tract obstruction, severe hypertension, and severe tricuspid regurgitation), pulsus alternans, and hepatojugular reflux.
2. Elevated left ventricular diastolic pressure: pathological left ventricular S_3 gallop sound, palpable S_4 or presystolic wave, reduced intensity of the first heart sound in the presence of normal PR interval.
3. Elevated right ventricular diastolic pressure: elevated systemic venous pressure in absence of tricuspid valve obstruction, palpable or audible right ventricular S_3 gallop.
4. Pulmonary hypertension: increased intensity of the pulmonic component of P_2, and audible P_2 over the cardiac apex.
5. Low cardiac output: small-amplitude carotid pulse (in absence of local carotid disease) in patients with left ventricular outflow obstruction and depressed left ventricular systolic function or severe mitral regurgitation (decreased pulse pressure with elevated left ventricular diastolic pressure may also indicate decreased stroke volume).
6. Increased systemic vascular resistance: cold clammy skin, tachycardia, and disproportionately increased diastolic pressure.

It should be appreciated that in patients with chronic heart failure, these physical findings may not always reflect the expected changes in hemodynamics. In patients with chronic heart failure due to dilated cardiomyopathy, however, in addition to a sustained apical impulse and reverse splitting of the second heart sound, a positive hepatojugular reflux strongly indicates reduced left ventricular ejection fraction. Pulsus alternans in patients with suspected or established heart failure almost always indicates reduced left ventricular ejection fraction. Similarly, a gallop rhythm indicates abnormal hemodynamics characterized by elevated left ventricular diastolic pressure and depressed left ventricular systolic function. It should be emphasized that physical examination can only provide qualitative assessment of ventricular function and hemodynamics. Invasive and noninvasive investigations should be entertained to confirm the diagnosis and to assess the severity of the hemodynamic abnormalities in patients with heart failure.

DIAGNOSIS OF HEART FAILURE

The physical signs that suggest congestive heart failure include a gallop sound, pulmonary rales, elevated jugular venous pressure, and peripheral edema. Findings of pulmonary hypertension and tricuspid regurgitation that indicate secondary right ventricular failure are frequently present in patients with chronic, severe left ventricular systolic failure.

It should be appreciated that physical examination is not always sensitive for the diagnosis of heart failure. In patients with chronic, stable systolic left ventricular failure, many of these abnormal physical findings are absent. The interobserver and intraobserver variability in the detection and interpretation of the physical findings of heart failure is also considerable. A number of clinical criteria have been proposed for the diagnosis of chronic heart failure and to maintain a standardization and uniformity in clinical assessment. In the Framingham Heart Study, various symptoms and signs were incorporated for the diagnosis of heart failure; these are summarized in Table 31-1. It is apparent from the

TABLE 31-1
CRITERIA OF CONGESTIVE HEART FAILURE USED IN THE FRAMINGHAM HEART STUDY

Major Criteria	Minor Criteria	Major or Minor Criteria
Paroxysmal nocturnal dyspnea or orthopnea	Ankle edema, night cough, dyspnea on exertion	Weight loss >4.5 kg in 5 days in response to treatment
Neck-vein distension	Hepatomegaly	
Rales	Pleural effusion	
Cardiomegaly	Vital capacity decreased one-half from maximal capacity	
Acute pulmonary edema		
S_3 gallop	Tachycardia (rate of >120/min)	
Increased venous pressure >6 cm H_2O		
Circulation time >25 s		
Hepatojugular reflux		

For establishing a definite diagnosis of congestive heart failure in this study, two major or one major and two minor criteria had to be present concurrently.

table that it is difficult to estimate all the criteria suggested in this study. For example, measurements of circulation time and vital capacity are seldom performed in the clinical practice. In another study (Boston Criteria), a point score system was proposed for the diagnosis of chronic heart failure using various symptoms and abnormal physical and radiological findings (Table 31-2). The diagnosis of heart failure was classified as definite with a score of 8 to 12 points; possible with a score of 5 to 7 points; and unlikely with a score of 4 points or less. Application of such a scoring system in clinical practice is not easily accomplished.

It is essential to determine left ventricular ejection fraction for the diagnosis of systolic ventricular failure and to distinguish systolic from diastolic left heart failure. For practical purposes, when left ventricular ejection fraction is preserved (i.e., >45%), diastolic heart failure is diagnosed if there are clinical signs of heart failure. However, when the ejection fraction is reduced to <45% (usually <40%), left ventricular systolic heart failure is diagnosed when the same signs and symptoms of heart failure are present. Although the presence of physical findings of heart failure and cardiomegaly in chest radiography can identify patients with reduced left ventricular ejection fraction, 30% to 50% of patients diagnosed with congestive heart failure by the conventional clinical criteria may have normal left ventricular ejection fraction estimated by radionuclide ventriculography. Furthermore, patients with significantly reduced left ventricular ejection fraction may not have clinical symptoms and signs of congestive heart failure at the time of evaluation of left ventricular systolic function. Thus, it is essential to assess left ventricular ejection fraction by noninvasive techniques such as by echocardiography in all patients with suspected or established heart failure.

TABLE 31-2
BOSTON CRITERIA FOR CONGESTIVE HEART FAILURE

Criteria	Point Value
Category I: History	
Rest dyspnea	4
Orthopnea	4
Paroxysmal nocturnal dyspnea	3
Dyspnea on walking on level ground	2
Dyspnea on climbing	1
Category II: Physical Examination	
Heart rate abnormality (if 91–110 beats/min, 1 point; if >110 beats/min, 2 points)	1–2
Jugular venous pressure elevation (if >6 cm H_2O plus hepatomegaly or edema, 3 points)	2–3
Lung crackles (if basilar, 1 point; if more than basilar, 2 points)	1–2
Wheezing	3
Third heart sound	3
Category III: Chest Radiography	
Alveolar pulmonary edema	4
Interstitial pulmonary edema	3
Bilateral pleural effusion	3
Cardiothoracic ratio >0.50 (posteroanterior projection)	3
Upper zone flow redistribution	2

FOLLOW-UP CLINICAL EVALUATION

During follow-up clinical evaluation, it is not always necessary to perform invasive or noninvasive evaluations to assess the results of therapeutic intervention. Symptomatic improvement and changes in functional class can be assessed without further investigations. A reduction in the heart rate, resolution of pulsus alternans and gallop rhythm, reduction in the severity of secondary mitral regurgitation, disappearance of S_3 gallop, maintenance of arterial pressure, increase in pulse pressure, and decrease in systemic venous pressure all indicate improvement in cardiac performance. Reduced heart size on chest radiography usually indicates decrease in right heart volume and may not indicate improvement in left ventricular systolic function or decrease in left ventricular dimension. Similarly, absence of clinical and radiological findings of pulmonary venous congestion may not necessarily indicate a reduction in pulmonary venous pressure in patients with chronic heart failure because these findings may not have been present in the first place.

It must also be emphasized that changes in the intensity of the pulmonic component of the second heart

TABLE 31-3
BEDSIDE DIAGNOSIS OF HEART FAILURE AND ITS CAUSES

1. a. Pulsus alternans, sustained and displaced left ventricular impulse, gallop rhythm indicate dilated cardiomyopathy.
   b. Elevated jugular venous pressure, secondary tricuspid regurgitation, sustained left parasternal lift, secondary mitral regurgitation indicate significant hemodynamic abnormalities including postcapillary pulmonary hypertension, elevated right ventricular diastolic pressures, and elevated left ventricular diastolic pressures.
   c. Cheyne-Stokes respiration indicates severe heart failure with lower cardiac output.
   d. Cardiac cachexia indicates severe heart failure with severe neuroendocrine abnormalities, including increased angiotensin, catecholamines, and tumor necrosis factor-α levels in blood.
2. a. Anacrotic radial or carotid pulse, delayed upstroke and delayed peak of carotid pulse, ejection systolic murmur: suspect aortic stenosis.
   b. Pulsus bisferiens and early diastolic murmur: suspect aortic regurgitation.
   c. Pulsus bisferiens or sharp or normal carotid pulse upstroke, long ejection systolic murmur with or without mitral regurgitation murmur, paradoxical splitting of S_2 in absence of left bundle branch block: suspect obstructive hypertrophic cardiomyopathy.
   d. Small volume, carotid pulse with normal upstroke in pressure of findings of heart failure: suspect dilated cardiomyopathy after exclusion of silent aortic and mitral valve disease.
3. a. Elevated jugular venous pressure with nondescript changes in the character with venous pulse, negative Kussmaul sign, quiet precordium, distant heart sounds, with or without auscultatory alternans and pulsus paradoxus: suspect tamponade.
   b. Elevated jugular venous pressure with sharp *y* descent, positive Kussmaul sign, quiet precordium, lack of findings of pulmonary hypertension, nonpulsatile hepatomegaly with or without ascites or peripheral edema: suspect constrictive percarditis.
   c. Elevated jugular venous pressure with sharp *y* descent, positive Kussmaul sign, a sustained left parasternal lift, findings of pulmonary hypertension with or without tricuspid regurgitation, pulsatile hepatomegaly with or without ascites or peripheral edema: suspect restrictive cardiomyopathy.
   d. Elevated jugular venous pressure with prominent V wave and sharp *y* descent with or without positive Kussmaul sign, a sustained left parasternal lift, pulsatile hepatomegaly, parasternal systolic murmur increasing in intensity with inspiration indicate primary or secondary tricuspid regurgitation.
   e. Elevated jugular venous pressure with prominent A wave with or without prominent V wave or *y* descent, increased intensity of the pulmonic component of the second heart sound, with or without secondary signs of pulmonary hypertension, left ventricular S_3 or S_4 gallop, gallop rhythm, findings of aortic or mitral valve disease or sustained left ventricular impulse: suspect postcapillary pulmonary hypertension and right heart failure.
   f. Elevated jugular venous pressure with prominent A wave with or without prominent V wave or *y* descent, increased intensity of the pulmonic component of the second heart sound, with or without secondary signs of pulmonary hypertension and absence of aortic and mitral valve disease, absence of left ventricular S_3 or S_4 gallop and normal left ventricular impulse: suspect precapillary pulmonary hypertension.

sound (P_2) do not correlate to changes in pulmonary artery pressure. The intensity of P_2 may still be increased when there is a substantial decrease in pulmonary artery pressure. The reduction in systemic venous pressure or peripheral edema also does not correlate well with changes in right ventricular volume and pressure. However, improved exercise tolerance, increased pulse pressure along with increase in systolic blood pressure and decreased frequency of S_3 gallop, and absence of secondary mitral and tricuspid regurgitation almost always indicate improved hemodynamics. Nevertheless, it is desirable to perform noninvasive investigations such as echocardiography or radionuclide ventriculography for more precise assessment of changes in left ventricular function during follow-up evaluation. In specific circumstances such as in patients with precapillary or postcapillary pulmonary hypertension, assessment of changes in pulmonary hypertension and pulmonary vascular resistance should be performed by hemodynamic monitoring rather than by clinical examination.

In conclusion, careful physical examination is essential to suspect the etiology of heart failure and to determine the appropriate investigations to confirm the etiology (Table 31-3). Physical examination is helpful to assess left ventricular systolic function and for the diagnosis of systolic and diastolic left ventricular failure. During follow-up evaluation, physical findings are helpful in assessing the results of therapy. However, noninvasive and invasive investigations are required when precise diagnosis of the degree of left ventricular systolic dysfunction, hemodynamic abnormalities, and response to therapy are needed for specific reasons.

SELECTED READINGS

Braunwald E. The physical examination in heart disease. In: Braunwald E, ed. *Heart Disease: A Textbook of Cardiovascular Medicine*. Philadelphia: WB Saunders; 1984: 14.

Chatterjee K. Bedside evaluation of the heart: physical examination. In: Parmley W, Chatterjee K, eds. *Cardiology*. 1st ed. Philadelphia: JB Lippincott; 1997.

Chatterjee K. Physical examination. In: Topol EJ, ed. *Textbook of Cardiovascular Medicine*. 1st ed. Philadelphia: Lippincott-Raven; 1997: 285–331.

Chatterjee K. Systolic ventricular failure. In: Parmley WW, Chatterjee K, eds. *Cardiology*. Vol. 1. Philadelphia: JB Lippincott; 1997: 1–44.

Harvey PW. Gallop sounds, clicks, snaps, whoops, honks and other sounds. In: Hurst JW, ed. *The Heart*. 4th ed. New York: McGraw-Hill; 1978: 255.

Leatham A. The first and second heart sounds. In: Hurst JW, ed. *The Heart*. 4th ed. New York: McGraw-Hill; 1978: 237.

O'Rourke RA, Silverman ME, Sellant RC. General examination of the patient. In: Schlant RC, Alexander RW, eds. *Hurst's the Heart*. 8th ed. New York: McGraw-Hill; 1994: 217–251.

Wood P. Physical signs. In: Wood P, ed. *Diseases of the Heart and Circulation*. London: Eyre & Spottiswoode; 1956.

Natriuretic Peptides as Biomarkers to Detect, Risk-Stratify, and Manage Patients with Heart Failure

32

Susan Isakson ***Alan Maisel***

Cardiac disease is a leading cause of death around the world, accounting for almost 50% of deaths each year (1). Sixty-one million Americans are living with heart disease (1) and almost 4.7 million of them suffer from symptomatic congestive heart failure (CHF) (2). The cost of managing these patients is significant. An estimated $56 billion per year is spent on diagnosing and treating patients with CHF, 70% of which is due to hospitalization (3). In-hospital mortality and readmission rates of heart failure patients are extremely high (4). Echocardiography, while considered to be the gold standard for the diagnosis of heart failure, is a time-consuming and expensiveprocess, and would delay onset of treatment if routinely relied upon as a major diagnostic tool in the acute setting. As such, there has been considerable interest in the development of reliable biomarkers for use in the diagnosis and treatment of heart failure.

Natriuretic peptides (NPs) have become increasingly important markers for evaluation of the dyspneic patient and treatment of CHF.

While NPs are primarily used as a tool for diagnosing or ruling out acute CHF in the dyspneic patient, recent work suggests a much broader application for NPs. B-type natriuretic peptide (BNP) is not only a useful adjunct for diagnosing and monitoring patients with heart failure (stage C and D), but studies now suggest that BNP provides independent prognostic information with respect to the risk of death or rehospitalization. In addition, BNP may have a role in screening high-risk patients for the presence of underlying cardiac dysfunction (stages A and B) (5). BNP has been shown to have significant diagnostic and prognostic value in patients with heart failure and is becoming increasingly important in the management of both in-patients and out-patients.

PHYSIOLOGY OF NATRIURETIC PEPTIDES

Natriuretic peptides play an important role in the maintenance of fluid balance in patients with CHF. Atrial natriuretic peptide (ANP) and BNP are proteins with a 17-amino-acid ring structure that are produced in the myocardium. C-type NP (CNP) is another member of the natriuretic peptide family but is secreted primarily from the vascular endothelium, has little influence on fluid status in the setting of heart failure, and has little clinical utility as a biomarker in CHF. ANP and BNP are synthesized in the form of precursors. The precursor of BNP, preproBNP, is cleaved into the signal peptide sequence and proBNP upon release stimulation. ProBNP is further cleaved by a membrane-bound serine protease into the active C-terminal 32-amino-acid BNP molecule and the N-terminal proBNP (NTproBNP) fragment. NPs are released from the ventricles in response to increased pressure inside the heart due to fluid overload and subsequent stretching of the myocytes. ANP is also released in response to stress and volume overload but, unlike BNP, is released from the atria as well as the ventricles (6).

Primary response genes are activated by stretching of the ventricular walls, causing a rapid upregulation of the production of NPs. The body's response to increased fluid volume and initiation of NP production is rapid; therefore, NP levels accurately reflect the fluid status of the patient. Because NPs are more stable than ANP and because they are primarily secreted by the ventricles, they appear to be more sensitive to left ventricular (LV) dysfunction than are ANP and other neurohormones (7). Unlike ANP, BNP is not released in response to increased activity levels or exercise and is therefore a more accurate indicator of the body's fluid state. In addition, NPs have a relatively short half-life (22 minutes for BNP and 120 minutes for NTproBNP), making them a valuable tool for monitoring and optimizing the treatment of acutely decompensated heart failure patients (1). NPs have therefore emerged as the marker of choice for diagnosis and management of CHF.

The main physiological function of the natriuretic peptides is to maintain fluid homeostasis in the body. BNP exerts powerful natriuretic, diuretic, and vasodilatory effects on the body. The target sites of BNP and ANP molecules are three natriuretic peptide receptors in the kidneys: NPR-A, NPR-B, and NPR-C. Activated NPR-A and NPR-B catalyze the conversion of guanosine triphosphate to cyclic guanosine monophosphate (cGMP) (Fig. 32-1). In this setting, cGMP is strongly vasodilatory and thereby relieves some of the hemodynamic stress on the heart.When activated, the NP receptors in the kidneys stimulate salt and water excretion and increase the glomerular filtration rate. Reduction of the total fluid volume in the body relieves some of the pressure on the heart and improves hemodynamics. Under normal conditions, the renin-angiotensin-aldosterone system (RAAS) can increase stress on heart and oppose vasodila-tory and diuretic efforts (1). BNP counteracts the sodium-conserving, vasoconstrictive, and volume retention effects of the RAAS. Together, BNP and the RAAS counterbalance each other to regulate fluid volume and arterial pressure. BNP also inhibits the synthesis of catecholamines, angiotensin II, aldosterone, and endothelin 1.

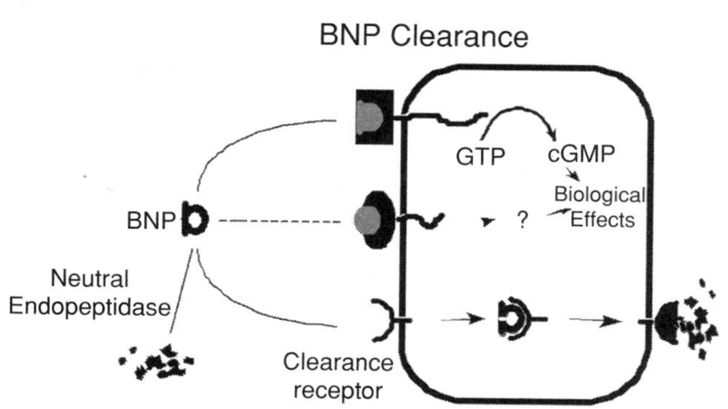

Figure 32-1 The two distinct mechanisms of BNP clearance: endocytosis and enzymatic degradation by endopeptidases. GTP, guanosnine triphosphate.

NATRIURETIC PEPTIDE ASSAYS

The first assay available for use was the Triage Point-of-Care BNP test, approved by the U.S. Food and Drug Administration (FDA) in the fall of 2000. Since that time, a number of assays for both BNP and NTproBNP have been approved and are in clinical use around the world. Table 32-1 is a comparison of the assays and characteristics of BNP and NTproBNP. While it is not within the scope of this chapter to debate the positives and negatives regarding individual molecules and assays, data suggest that both BNP and NTproBNP offer considerable value to the clinician. Thus, it is likely that the final decision as to which biomarker, BNP or NTproBNP, will be used will not necessarily be based on the differences between the two peptides but, rather, on the presence of the pre-existing laboratory equipment necessary to run the assay as well as the perceived need of point-of-care devices versus large laboratory platforms.

One thing can be said with certainty in this regard: The two molecules are not interchangeable. In other words, it would be dangerous for a hospital laboratory to switch from running BNP to NTproBNP, or vice versa, without first making sure the clinicians using the test were aware of

TABLE 32-1
BNP VERSUS NTproBNP ASSAY FORHEART FAILURE

Characteristic	BNP	NTproBNP
Analyte detected	$BNP_{(77-108)}$	$NTproBNP_{(1-76)}$
Molecular weight	3.5 Kd	8.5 d
Hormonally active	Yes	No, inactive peptide
Genesis	Cleavage from proBNP	Cleavage from proBNP
Half-life	2 min	120 min
Major clearance mechanism	Natriuretic peptide receptors	Renal clearance
Increases with normal aging	+	++
Approved cut-off(s) for CHF diagnosis	100 pg/mL	Age <75: 125 pg/mL Age ≥75: 450 pg/mL
Available at the point-of-care	Yes	No
Entry on U.S. market	November 2000	December, 2002

the differences (especially in terms of absolute values), since NTproBNP tends to be about ten-fold more expensive than BNP. In the United States, about 80% to 90% of current NP testing involves BNP (CAP surveys), while in Europe NTproBNP testing is more commonly used. Since BNP testing was the first peptide to be clinically available, experience with its use as well as the development of accepted algorithms have accounted for its increased use in the United States.

DIAGNOSIS OF CONGESTIVE HEART FAILURE

Diagnosing acute heart failure is often difficult. Many patients do not exhibit the typical signs and symptoms of heart failure, such as elevated jugular venous pressure (JVP), S_3 heart sound, rales, and edema. In addition, many of these symptoms are present in other diseases that can often mimic a CHF exacerbation in patients who present with dyspnea. Incorrect treatment can often worsen the patient's condition. For example, treatment with sympathomimetic amines and beta-agonists can induce angina and arrythmias in patients with heart failure (8).

Diagnostic tests in the emergency setting, such as routine laboratory tests, chest x-rays, and electrocardiograms, lack the accuracy to make the appropriate diagnosis. Use of echocardiography, the gold standard test for diagnosis of heart failure, is not always practical in the emergency setting because of the duration of the study and the need for a sonographer to perform the test. In addition, it may be very difficult for the patient to remain still long enough to obtain accurate results. In order to avoid the increased morbidity and mortality that parallels delayed and incorrect diagnoses, it is necessary to have a tool with which to differentiate these diseases and make a rapid and accurate diagnosis.

Several studies have established the role of BNP in the clinical diagnosis of CHF. In a study by Dao et al., 250 patients presenting to the emergency department (ED) with dyspnea were evaluated using BNP values (9). Physicians were blinded to the BNP values and were asked to assess the probability that the patients' dyspnea was caused by an acute CHF exacerbation. BNP values were shown to be the strongest predictors of acute heart failure, being both sensitive to and specific for diagnosing CHF. The mean BNP level in patients found to have CHF was higher than in patients without CHF (1,076 pg/mL versus 38 pg/mL, $p < 0.001$).

These findings provided a foundation for the Breathing Not Properly multinational study, a prospective study that used BNP levels to evaluate the causes of dyspnea. In this study of 1,586 emergency room patients with acute dyspnea, BNP levels were measured upon arrival. Physicians were asked to assess the probability of heart failure. Later, two cardiologists blinded to BNP values were given the clinical data to review and produce a gold standard diagnosis for each patient. BNP levels were found to be more accurate predictors of CHF than any history, physical findings, or lab values (5). A BNP cut-off value of 100 pg/mL had a sensitivity of 90% and a specificity of 76% for differentiating CHF from other causes of dyspnea, and a cut-off level of 50 pg/mL had a negative predictive value of 96% (Fig. 32-2) (5). A BNP level of >230 pg/mL was associated with a relative risk of 7.0 for a CHF-related event in the absence of a correct diagnosis by the physician (5). Physicians in the ED had a 43% rate of indecision when trying to make a diagnosis in dyspneic patients. BNP levels, had they been available to clinicians, would have reduced the rate of indecision to 11%. Incorporation of BNP into the clinical evaluation of the dyspneic patient was found to increase the absolute diagnostic accuracy by 10% (Fig. 32-3) (10).

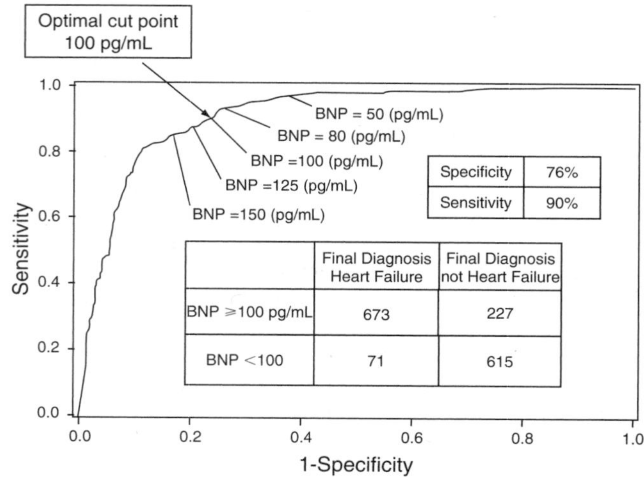

Figure 32-2 Decision statistics from the Breathing Not Properly multinational study. A cut-off point of 100 pg/mL was determined to be the optimal level for distinguishing between decompensated heart failure and other causes of dyspnea. (Adapted from Maisel AS, Krishnaswamy P, NowakRM, et al. Rapid measurement of B-type natriuretic peptide in the emergency diagnosis of heart failure. *N Engl J Med.* 2002;347:161–167.)

Differentiation between causes of dyspnea is a great challenge faced by ED physicians. It is often very difficult to evaluate whether dyspnea is due to pulmonary disease or CHF. In a study of 321 patients with dyspnea who presented to the ED, BNP distinguished between heart failure (mean BNP 759 ± 798 pg/mL) from pulmonary disease (61 ± 10 pg/mL) and other clinical presentations with a high specificity and sensitivity. The mean BNP values of patients with different pulmonary diseases are shown in Figure 32-4. Moreover, when patients who had a history of heart failure but whose dyspnea was due to chronic obstructive pulmonary disease (COPD) (mean BNP 47 ± 23 pg/mL) were compared with patients who had a history of COPD but whose dyspnea was due to heart failure (731 ± 764 pg/mL), a BNP value of 94 pg/mL yielded a sensitivity and specificity of 86% and 98%, respectively, and differentiated heart failure from lung disease with an accuracy of 91% (11). BNP has therefore emerged as a strong diagnostic and prognostic indicator of LV dysfunction and heart failure.

Acute respiratory distress syndrome (ARDS) may also present as dyspnea in the emergency setting and can contribute to the difficulty in making accurate diagnoses in the ED. BNP levels were obtained from 35 patients with ARDS and 42 patients hospitalized with a diagnosis of heart failure. The mean BNP value for those with ARDS was 123 pg/mL, significantly lower than the mean BNP value of 773 pg/mL for patients with CHF (Fig. 32-5). A cut-off

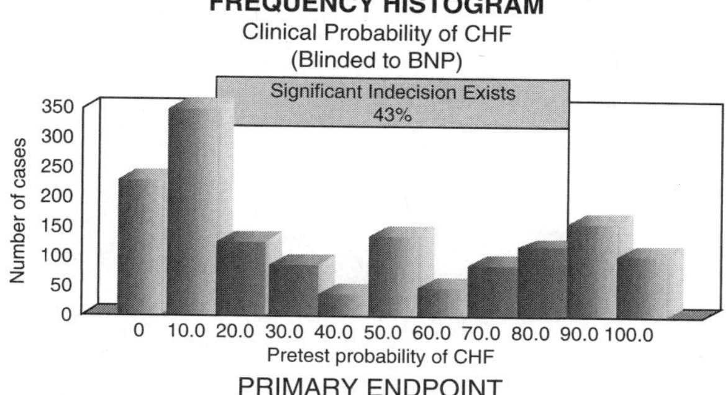

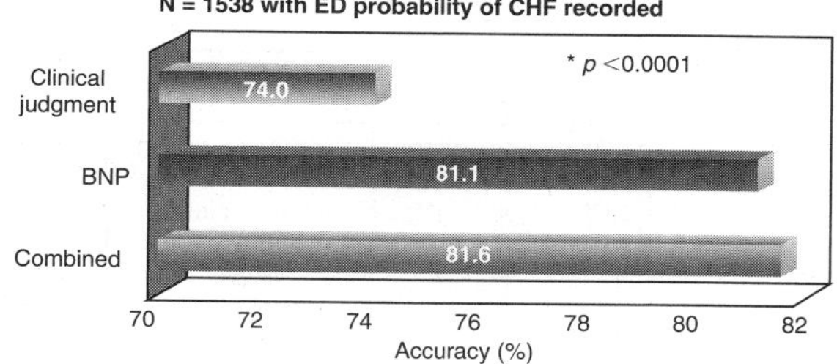

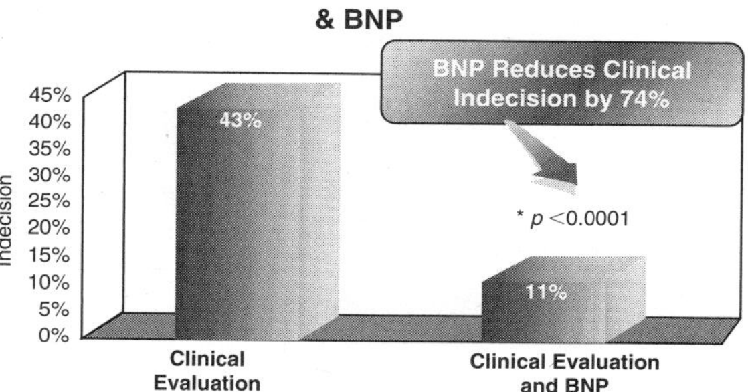

Figure 32-3 Inclusion of BNP levels in the decision-making process significantly reduces the level of clinical indecision in the emergency setting. (Adapted from McCullough PA, Nowak RM, McCord J, et al. B-type natriuretic peptide and clinical judgment in emergency diagnosis of heart failure. Analysis from Breathing Not Properly (BNP) multinational study. *Circulation.* 2002;106:416–422.)

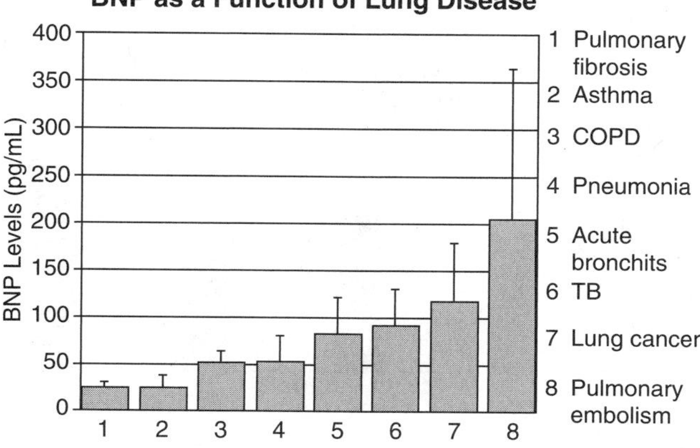

Figure 32-4 BNP levels of patients with different pulmonary diseases. COPD, chronic obstructive pulmonary disease; TB, tuberculosis. (Adapted from Morrison LK, Harrison A, Krishnaswamy P, et al. Utility of a rapid B-natriuretic peptide assay in differentiating congestive heart failure from lung disease in patients presenting with dyspnea. *J Am Coll Cardiol.* 2002;39:202–209.)

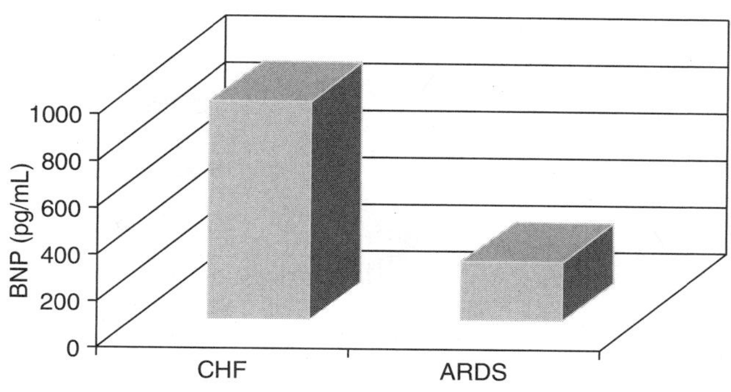

Figure 32-5 Median BNP level in patients with CHF as compared to patients with ARDS. (Adapted from Berman B, Spragg R, Maisel AS. B-type natriuretic peptide (BNP) levels in differentiating congestive heart failure from acute respiratory distress syndrome (ARDS). Abstracts from the 75th Annual Scientific Meeting of the American Heart Association. *Circulation.* 2002;106:S3191.)

point of 360 pg/mL was determined to have a sensitivity of 90%, specificity of 86%, 89% positive predictive value, and 94% negative predictive value for differentiating between ARDS and CHF (6).

Although NP levels can be elevated in patients with pulmonary disease, NP levels are not usually elevated to the extent that they are in patients with heart failure. Secondary analysis of the Breathing Not Properly multinational study found that measurement of BNP levels can expose underlying CHF in patients with bronchospastic diseases such as asthma or COPD (12). Out of 417 patients studied who had a history of asthma or COPD and no history of CHF, 87 (20.9%) were found to have a final diagnosis of CHF. The mean BNP levels for patients with and without a history of CHF were found to be 587.0 and 108.8 pg/mL, respectively. Therefore, routine BNP testing in patients with a history of asthma or COPD may increase the rate of new diagnosis of heart failure by as much as 20% (12).

Nevertheless, utilization of BNP for the diagnosis CHF is not always straightforward. A gray zone exists in which median levels of BNP are more difficult to interpret and use for making clinical diagnoses. An algorithm developed by Maisel et al. that is now in use at the Veterans Administration Medical Center in San Diego, California and many other institutions is illustrated in Figure 32-6. This algorithm provides guidelines for symptomatic and asymptomatic patients and the likelihood of CHF at different BNP values. For symptomatic patients, a BNP value below 100 pg/mL suggests that the symptoms are not likely due to heart failure. In the range of 100 to 400 pg/mL, the algorithm suggests considering alternative diagnoses such as myocardial infarction, pulmonary embolism, or pneumonia, and clinical correlation is strongly recommended. For patients with existing LV dysfunction, underlying cor pulmonale, or acute pulmonary embolism (PE), a diagnosis of CHF with a BNP in the range of 100 to 400 pg/mL is less likely than for patients without any of these factors (25% likelihood of CHF versus 75% likelihood of CHF). Using this algorithm,

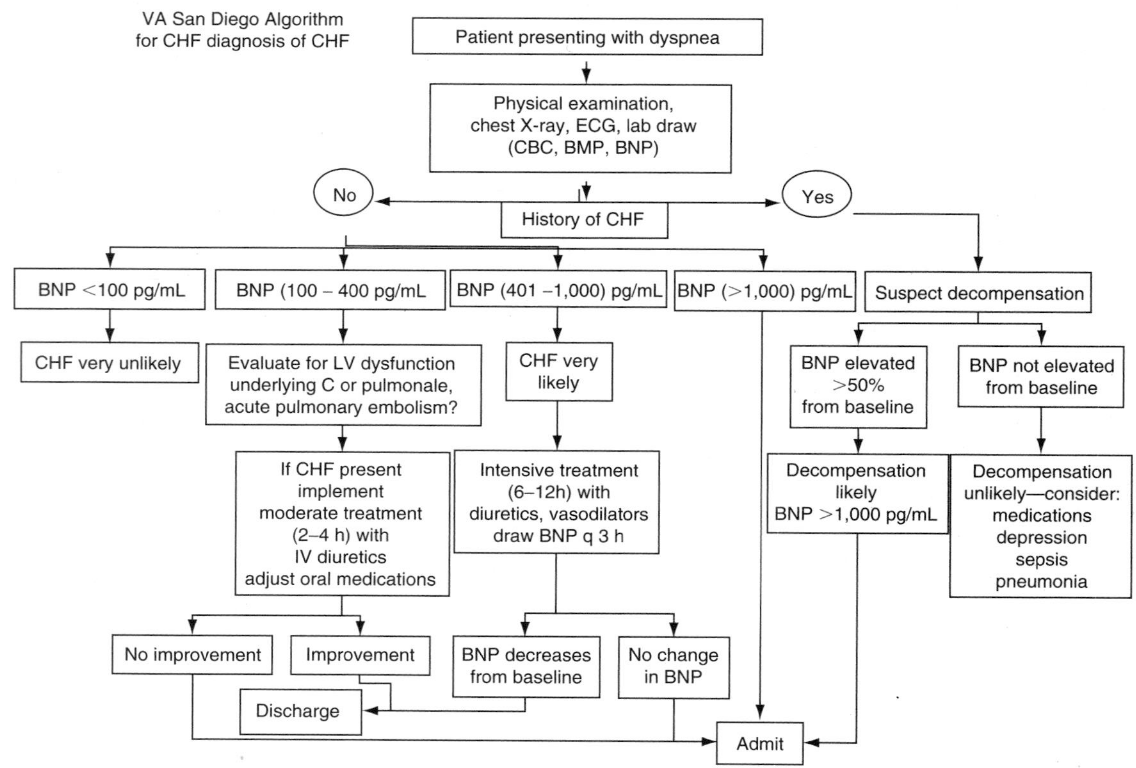

Figure 32-6 San Diego, California, Veterans Administration algorithm for interpreting BNP levels. (Adapted from Maisel, AS. *Critical Pathways in Cardiology.* 2000;I(2):68–73.)

BNP values above 400 pg/mL would be considered highly suggestive of heart failure (13).

CAVEATS OF NATRIURETIC PEPTIDE TESTING

Renal Insufficiency

In patients with renal insufficiency, NP levels cannot be used independently as diagnostic tools. Increased left ventricular hypertrophy and wall tension resulting from the volume overload associated with renal insufficiency is believed to be responsible for increased levels of plasma BNP in chronic kidney disease (CKD) (14). Therefore, a new set of optimal cut-off points has been developed to account for the physiological differences between patients with and without CKD. In patients with CHF and an estimated glomerular filtration rate (eGFR) of <60 mL/min/1.73 m^2, BNP levels have been observed to be significantly higher than in patients with CHF but normal renal function (Fig. 32-7). Data from the Breathing Not Properly study suggests that in CKD patients with eGFR <60, 200 pg/mL is an appropriate cut-off point for BNP in the diagnosis of CHF (14). In a study of BNP levels in hemodialysis patients, some change was noted between predialysis and postdialysis samples, suggesting that it may be a useful marker of fluid volume status and LV wall tension in patients with advanced renal disease (15). The mean BNP before dialysis was 738 pg/mL, while the post-dialysis levels decreased to a mean value of 555 pg/mL. The mean decrease in BNP levels after dialysis approached 22% (15).

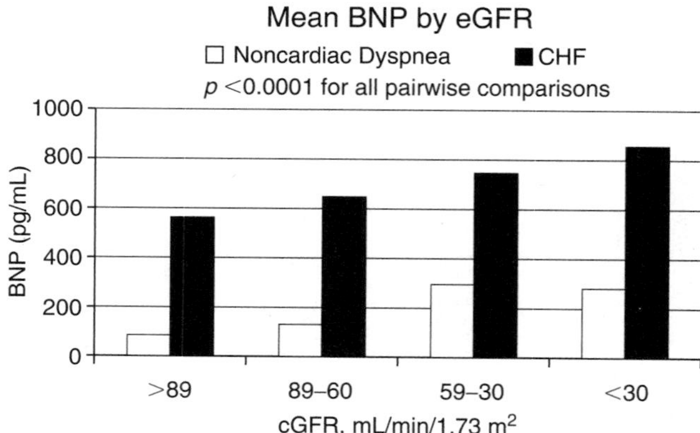

Figure 32-7 BNP levels in patients with and without CHF across different stages of chronic kidney disease. (Reprinted from McCullough PA, Duc P, Omland T, et al. B-type natriuretic peptide and renal function in the diagnosis of heart failure. An analysis from the Breathing Not Properly multinational study. *Am J Kidney Dis.* 2003;41:571–579, with permission.)

Obesity

Obesity, a known risk factor for cardiac disease, has recently been implicated as a more direct risk factor for development of heart failure due to the increased plasma volume and increased cardiopulmonary volume in obese patients (16). Since obese patients are a large subgroup of patients with heart failure, it is important to recognize that BNP levels in obese patients are typically much lower than in nonobese patients. Caution must be taken when interpreting BNP results in obese patients, as the BNP levels themselves may not accurately reflect the fluid status and/or severity of heart failure in these patients (6).

Several studies have demonstrated an inverse relationship between body mass index (BMI) and BNP levels in patients with heart failure. Mehra et al. found that BNP levels were significantly lower in obese versus nonobese patients (16). In patients younger than 65 years of age, obese patients were found to have BNP levels 40% lower than those of nonobese patients when compared to others in the same functional class (16). Additional findings from the Breathing Not Properly study showed that 50% of nonobese patients presenting to the ED with heart failure had BNP values >1,000 pg/mL, while only 8% to 24% of obese patients presenting with heart failure had BNP values >1,000 pg/mL (17) (Fig. 32-8).

There have been several suggested explanations for these findings. NP receptors have been discovered in adipose tissue (18); therefore, it is thought that there is impaired expression of BNP and more rapid degradation of BNP in obese patients (16). Another proposed explanation arises from a condition associated with severe heart failure. Cardiac cachexia in patients with advanced heart failure provides a link between severity of disease and low body weight, and therefore explains the observed trend of higher BNP levels in patients with lower BMIs (17).

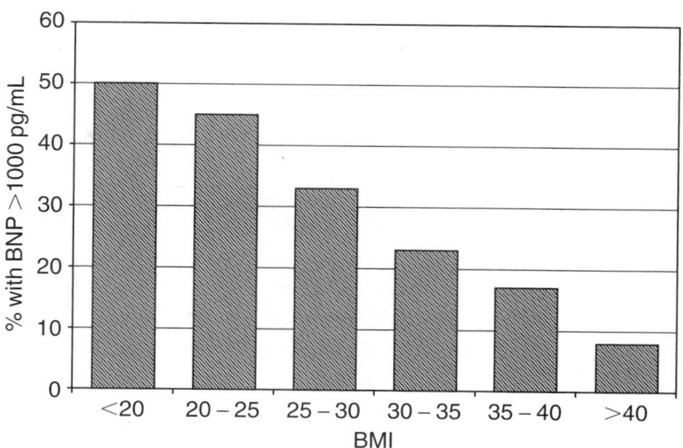

Figure 32-8 Mean BNP levels have been shown to decrease with increasing body mass index. (Adapted from McCord J, Mundy BJ, Hudson MP, et al. Relationship between obesity and B-type natriuretic peptide levels. *Arch Intern Med.* 2004;164:2247–2252.)

Diastolic Dysfunction

Diastolic dysfunction is the cause of heart failure in many patients who present to the ED with dyspnea. Although BNP levels are elevated in patients with diastolic dysfunction, they are not typically as high as in patients with systolic dysfunction (Fig. 32-9). Data from the Breathing Not Properly study suggest that the BNP levels in patients with diastolic dysfunction are roughly half of those in patients with systolic dysfunction (19). Lubien et al. measured BNP in patients who had undergone echocardiographic testing and found that the mean BNP for patients with diastolic dysfunction was 286 pg/mL, whereas the mean BNP for patients with normal LV function was only 33 pg/mL. A cut-off point of 62 pg/mL had a sensitivity of 85%, a specificity of 83%, and an accuracy of 84% for detection of diastolic dysfunction in the setting of normal LV systolic function (20). In addition, patients with different types of diastolic dysfunction exhibited significantly different BNP values. The mean BNP for restrictive filling dysfunctions (determined by echocardiography) was 408 pg/mL, while the mean BNP for impaired relaxation was only 202 pg/mL. Lubien et al. also found that of patients with diastolic dysfunction, those who were symptomatic had higher BNP levels than did those who were asymptomatic (20).

NATRIURETIC PEPTIDES FOR TRIAGING PATIENTS WITH CONGESTIVE HEART FAILURE

BNP is a useful tool in the assessment of patients presenting to the ED with dyspnea. The Rapid Emergency Department Heart Failure Outpatient Trial (REDHOT) examined the relationship between perceived severity of disease by physicians and severity as indicated by BNP levels. Physicians were informed whether the BNP level was greater or less than 100 pg/mL but were not given the actual value. Surprisingly, the patients who were discharged from the hospital had higher BNP levels than those admitted for treatment. The median BNP level for discharged patients was 976 pg/mL, compared with a mean BNP of 766 pg/mL for patients who were admitted to the hospital. Patients with BNP levels <200 pg/mL had an excellent prognosis, with a mortality of 0% at 30 days

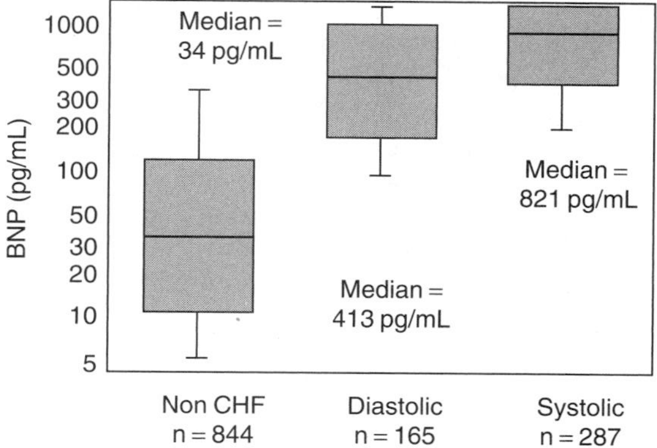

Figure 32-9 Comparison of BNP levels in patients with systolic and diastolic dysfunction. (Adapted from Maisel AS, McCord J, Nowak RM, et al. Bedside B-type natriuretic peptide in the emergency diagnosis of heart failure with reduced or preserved ejection fraction. Results from the Breathing Not Properly multinational study. *J Am Coll Cardiol.* 2003;41:2010–2017.)

and only 2% at 90 days. Therefore, BNP levels improve the accuracy of diagnoses of dyspneic patients made in the ED and can be used as guidelines to assess severity of the disease in individual patients (21).

The inclusion of BNP in clinical decision making has been shown to be cost-effective and to improve quality of care in the emergency and hospital settings. The B-Type Natriuretic Peptide for Acute Shortness of Breath Evaluation (BASEL) study in Switzerland explored the cost-effectiveness of using the BNP tests an adjunct to the standard clinical tools. Patients enrolled in the study were randomized to one of two groups: to receive or not to receive a BNP blood test upon arrival in the ED. Participating physicians were advised that a BNP level below 100 pg/mL made a heart failure diagnosis unlikely, while a BNP level above 500 pg/mL was highly indicative of heart failure. Patients who received a BNP test upon presentation were shown to have 10% fewer admissions, decreased length of hospital stay by a mean of 3 days, and lower mean total cost of treatment. This suggests that use of BNP in evaluating acute dyspnea improves both the cost and quality of care (22).

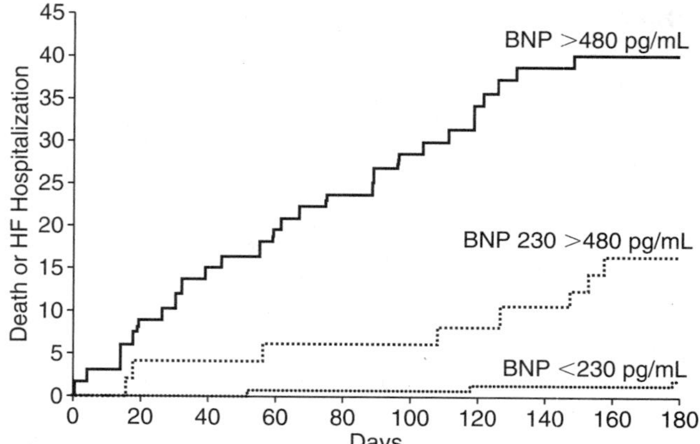

Figure 32-10 Relationship of BNP levels in the emergency department to subsequent cardiac morbidity and mortality. (Reprinted from Harrison A, Morrison LK, Krishnaswamy P, et al. B-type natriuretic peptide predicts future cardiac events in patients presenting to the emergency department with dyspnea. *Ann Emerg Med.* 2002;39:131–138, with permission.)

NATRIURETIC PEPTIDES AND PROGNOSIS

Prognosis and risk stratification appear to be a valuable application of NP testing. Cardiac events have been correlated with NP levels in almost any setting that has been looked at, including in the ED, during hospitalizations and discharge, and during out-patient follow-up. They may also be valuable as a risk predictor in patients with no clinical heart failure.

The reason BNP levels in the emergency setting can be used to triage patients effectively is that they have been shown to be highly prognostic (previously discussed). In a study of 325 patients presenting with dyspnea to the ED, patients with BNP levels >480 pg/mL had a 51% cumulative probability of death (cardiac and noncardiac), hospital admissions (cardiac), or repeat ED visits over the next 6 months. In contrast, only 2.5% of patients with BNP levels <230 pg/mL suffered one of these events (23).

Changes in BNP levels during hospitalizations are important prognostic indicators of a patient's health during the months following a heart failure admission. Only 16% of patients with a fall in BNP levels during hospitalization had a subsequent cardiac event, while 52% of those with rising BNP levels during treatment had either readmission or cardiac death. Patients whose discharge BNP levels fell below 430 pg/mL had a relatively low likelihood of not being readmitted within the following 30 days (Fig. 32-10) (24). These data were supported by a recent study by Bettencourt et al., who found that failure of BNP levels to fall over the hospitalization predicted death or rehospitalization, and that discharge levels <250 pg/mL predicted event-free survival (25).

Cardiac troponins, although primarily used in the diagnosis of coronary disease and acute myocardial infarction, play a role in heart failure, as well. Measurement of troponin levels in addition to BNP levels contributes to the ability of the clinician to properly risk-stratify patients presenting with acute decompensated heart failure. It is not uncommon for patients with heart failure to exhibit a slight elevation of troponin I (cTnI). This minor increase could represent ongoing myocyte injury in response to increased wall tension in the myocardium. Necrosis and apoptosis are two common processes that occur in chronic heart failure and could also be responsible for increased cTnI levels. Activation of the RAAS, adrenergic pathways, inflammatory cytokines, nitric oxide, and oxidative stress have also been implicated as possible triggers of myocyte injury and cTnI elevations (26). These elevations of cTnI in heart failure patients, though small, have significant implications in the risk stratification of these patients. Elevated cTnI was found by Horwich et al. (26) to be significantly correlated with elevated BNP levels and cardiac filling pressures. Elevated cTnI levels were independently associated with higher mortality rates. In patients admitted to the hospital with New York Heart Association (NYHA) Class III or IV heart failure, the risk of death was found to be significantly higher in patients with an admission cTnI level of >0.033 μg/L. When both BNP and troponin were elevated, the risk of death was increased 12-fold above baseline (26).

BNP levels in stable out-patients were found to be independent predictors of sudden death. In a study by Berger et al., BNP levels above 130 pg/mL were shown to be associated with higher risk of sudden death than were levels below 130 pg/mL. Patients with BNP levels below 130 pg/mL only had a 1% incidence of sudden death, while patients with higher BNP levels had a 19% incidence of sudden death (27). The identification of patients at higher risk for sudden death allows earlier, more focused treatment and extended survival. In the Valsartan Heart Failure Trial (Val-HeFT), changes in BNP over time induced by pharmacologic therapy were shown for the first time to correlate with morbidity and mortality (8).

Patients with no heart failure were studied to determine the prognostic value of BNP in a nonselected population. Wang et al. found that in this group, BNP levels were predictive of heart failure, atrial fibrillation, stroke, transient ischemic attack (TIA), and death. The patients with BNP levels in the top 20% of those measured (above 20 pg/mL for men and 23.3 pg/mL for women) were shown to be at higher risk of the events listed above. Relative risks for this group were 1.62 for death, 1.99 for stroke or TIA, 1.91 for atrial fibrillation, and 3.07 for heart failure (28). No association was found, however, between high BNP levels and increased risk of coronary artery disease. The BNP values associated with increased risk in the general population are lower than the accepted values. This study showed that BNP levels begin to increase prior to the onset of symptoms or other clinical signs. It may thus be possible in this population to diagnose heart failure in the earliest stages and initiate treatment before the patient becomes symptomatic.

PEPTIDES FOR SCREENING OF LEFT VENTRICULAR DYSFUNCTION

Another significant challenge faced by clinicians is early detection and diagnosis of heart failure in asymptomatic patients. Screening of the general population for LV dysfunction has become a focus point in the effort to reduce costs of care of heart failure. The prevalence of asymptomatic depressed LV function is high. In fact, in one series, 5% of patients over 55 years of age were found to have decreased ejection fractions. Of these patients, almost one-half were asymptomatic, thus demonstrating a potential need to search for an accurate screening procedure that might be used to screen populations with a high prevalence of LV dysfunction (29).

Screening for asymptomatic LV dysfunction in the general population meets many of the criteria for a successful screening program: it is an important health problem with serious consequences, and the natural history of the disease is such that there is a presymptomatic stage which, when treated, may alter the natural history of the disease. The cornerstone of any screening program is the availability of a suitable diagnostic test. Because of the relative inaccessibility and expense of echocardiography, several studies have evaluated the role of BNP in screening for ventricular dysfunction.

Heidenreich et al. performed a formal cost-effectiveness analysis using computer modeling based on a population prevalence of LV systolic dysfunction of 1%. A screening strategy of BNP testing and, if abnormal, echocardiography, was associated with a cost of $22,300 per quality-adjusted live year (QALY) in men and $77,000 per QALY in women. The authors concluded that this screening strategy was economically attractive in men and possibly in women (29). A study by Nielsen et al. identified 8 pg/mL as a highly sensitive value for detection of LV systolic dysfunction (LVSD). In addition to significantly reducing costs of screening, the use of BNP in screening the general population was useful in detecting LVSD with high sensitivities of 83% to 94%, based on whether the patient was classified as low-risk or high-risk (factors for this decision included past medical history and other clinical findings) (30). Undoubtedly, such a low cut-off of 8 pg/mL may not confer much specificity, but when used purely as a screening test it may still provide a significant reduction in the cost of screening (18). Atisha et al. recently reported that BNP levels under 20 pg/mL were associated with only minor cases of diastolic dysfunction and no cases of major systolic dysfunction (31). Using these and other studies, a potential outpatient algorithm has been established that uses BNP levels as a trigger for subsequent testing, such as echocardiography (Fig. 32-11).

USING NATRIURETIC PEPTIDES IN THE MANAGEMENT OF HEART FAILURE

In-Patient Management

Accounting for over 1 million hospitalizations each year, heart failure admissions have become extremely costly. The readmission rate of these patients is surprisingly high, estimated to be 44% at 6 months in the Medicare population (32). Therapy for decompensated CHF aims at the reduction of filling pressures needed to produce adequate cardiac output; however, patient symptomatology may not accurately reflect underlying hemodynamics, and thus is likely responsible for the high readmission rate. Clinicians must be able to determine the severity of heart disease in hospitalized patients and distinguish between those patients who can be discharged early and those who need more aggressive therapy. Gold standard measurements of filling pressures include either pulmonary catheter-guided pressure measurements or, less optimally, estimates based on Doppler echocardiography. However, the routine performance of these procedures is not practical in most patients. As such, much attention has been focused on finding biomarkers that can estimate left ventricular end-diastolic pressure (LVEDP) for the tailoring of heart failure therapy.

Because BNP is released mainly in response to LV stretch from volume overload, levels would be expected to closely correlate with pulmonary capillary wedge pressure (PCWP) measurements (33). Indeed, in a study by Kazanegra et al. patients admitted for decompensated CHF had BNP levels and hemodynamic measurements taken every 2 hours for the first 24 hours and every 4 hours for the next 24 to 48 hours. PCWP showed a decrease from 33 to 25 mm Hg over the first 24 hours, while BNP levels decreased in parallel from 1,472 to 670 pg/mL. In addition, there was a correlation between rate of change of BNP levels and rate of change of PCWP (34). Thus, in the absence of acute mitral regurgitation and flash pulmonary edema, BNP levels can be a useful indicator of PCWP (as shown in Figure 32-12), a finding that has been replicated by several groups. It should be emphasized that although high filling pressure in the left ventricle is the strongest stimulus for increased BNP levels, it is not the only culprit that causes elevated BNP in hospitalized patients; as such, failure of the BNP to fall is not an absolute indicator of treatment failure. Other possible causes of elevated BNP levels, as described earlier, include right heart failure and

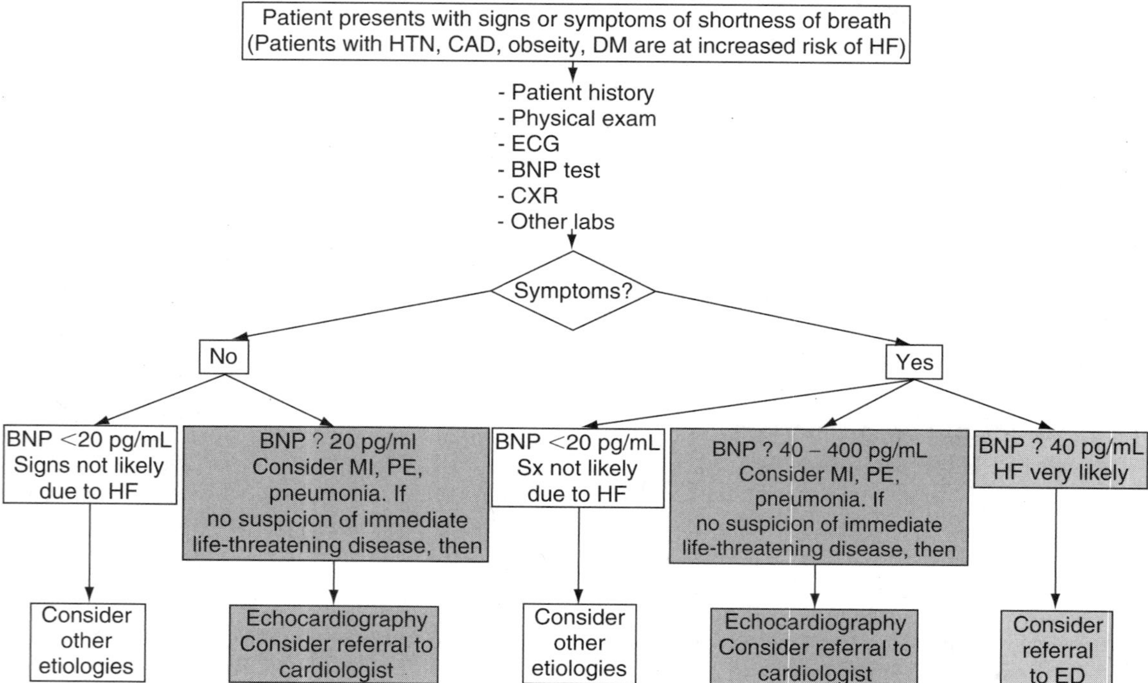

Figure 32-11 An algorithm developed for use of BNP in primary care. (Reprinted from Maisel, AS. Updated algorithms for using B-type natriuretic peptide (BNP) levels in the diagnosis and management of congestive heart failure. *Critical Pathways in Cardiology.* 2004;3(3):1–6, with permission.)

cor pulmonale, pulmonary embolism, and renal failure. BNP levels may also lag behind drops in PCWP if a very rapid decrease in PCWP from high doses of diuretics and or vasodilators (6) is accomplished.

Comparison measurements of cardiac filling pressures by Doppler echocardiography and BNP measurements have also been found to be strongly correlated, suggesting

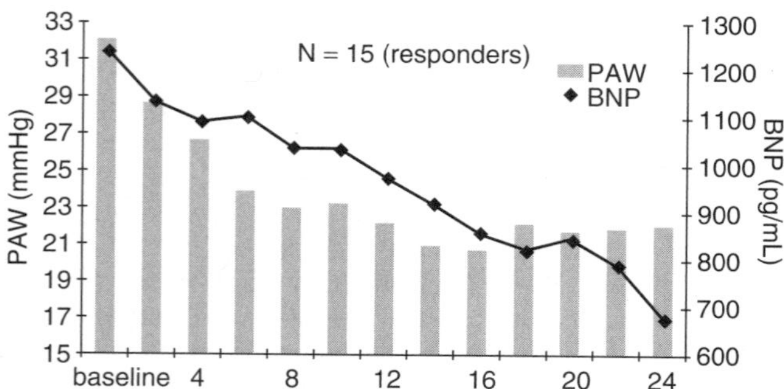

Figure 32-12 The relationship between BNP and pulmonary artery wedge pressure during 24 hours of inpatient treatment. (Adapted from Kazanegra R, Cheng V, Garcia A, et al. A rapid test for B-type natriuretic peptide correlates with falling wedge pressures in patients treated for decompensated heart failure. A pilot study. *J Card Fail.* 2001;7:21–29.)

that BNP can be used in place of costly echocardiography to monitor the patient's progress. BNP has been shown to decrease only in patients whose cardiac filling pressures decreased significantly during their admissions. Patients whose BNP levels do not fall with treatment may suffer from higher rates of subsequent adverse events. Patients with at least a 10% decrease in BNP levels during the first 24 hours of treatment seem to experience the most favorable 60-day outcomes (35).

BNP measurements during hospitalization should probably be obtained (at the very least) on admission and discharge. BNP levels taken 24 hours after the initiation of treatment have proven to be useful in determining whether the patient is in need of more aggressive treatment. In addition, treatment of patients without invasive hemodynamic monitoring (such as Swan-Ganz catheters) can be optimized by using BNP measurements every 2 to 4 hours. BNP levels should not be drawn during infusion of nesiritide or for 2 hours after the infusion is stopped, since the result will include exogenous as well as endogenous BNP.

BNP levels can be used to aid in distinguishing between compensated and decompensated heart failure. Heart failure patients in the euvolemic state have an elevated, but moderately stable, so-called dry BNP level. A significant increase in BNP is seen in these patients in the setting of acute volume overload. BNP levels <200 to 300 pg/mL are likely representative of a true euvolemic state. It is important to establish a patient's dry BNP level at discharge for the purpose of tailoring treatment to reach an optimal condition and for subsequent out patient monitoring of volume status.

In patients whose BNP levels fail to fall with treatment, several possible causes should be considered. Patients with NYHA functional Class IV heart failure do not respond to treatment as readily as patients with Class I, II, and III heart failure. These patients may have very high dry BNP levels, and thus high BNP levels may not necessarily reflect acute volume overload (6). Patients with significant peripheral edema and/or severe ascites may not show an immediate decrease in BNP. A BNP decrease may only be seen in these patients after several liters of urine output. This effect is due to mobilization and excretion of third-space volume prior to any direct reduction in PCWP. When a BNP level does not fall with treatment, it is also possible that the primary cause of symptoms is not acute decompensated heart failure and further differential diagnoses should be considered. Worsening renal function during diuresis can also cause paradoxically increased BNP levels.

Treatment of patients after a heart failure hospitalization is just as important as management during the hospital stay. It is often difficult to determine the stability of patients upon discharge. Postdischarge treatment must be tailored based upon risk stratification from a combination of clinical assessments, lab values, and in-hospital procedures such as echocardiography. High discharge BNP levels have been associated with increased risks of readmission and/or death resulting from subsequent decompensations. BNP has been shown to be more useful in risk stratification of patients admitted for decompensated heart failure than both LV ejection fraction and clinical evaluation (36).

Tailoring treatment and postdischarge clinic visits based on discharge BNP levels is now a common practice. Logeart et al. found that patients discharged with BNP levels above 350 pg/mL were at much higher risk of adverse events than those with lower BNPs. In addition, patients with discharge BNP levels greater than 700 pg/mL had a 31% prevalence of death or heart failure readmission after 1 month. This prevalence increased to 93% after 6 months (36).

Natriuretic Peptides and Out-Patient Treatment Titration

Considering how we modulate diseases like hypertension, diabetes, and lipid abnormalities, it is a wonder that CHF is one of the few disease states that has no current surrogate by which to titrate medication. NPs have a number of characteristics that suggest they can be viable surrogate markers. These include their correlation with NYHA class and LVEDP, their excellent negative predictive values, their relative ease of use, and their low cost.

Several studies have investigated the potential role of BNP as a means to guide titration of out-patient treatment. Murdoch et al. evaluated the utility of BNP-guided angiotensin-converting enzyme (ACE) inhibitor titration compared to clinically guided titration in a small, randomized trial. At the study conclusion, the ACE inhibitor dose was significantly reduced in the BNP group compared to the clinically guided group. These authors concluded that a BNP-tailored approach to vasodilator titration was safe and well-tolerated (37). Troughton et al. conducted a randomized clinical pilot study comparing NTproBNP-guided treatment titration with clinically guided treatment in 69 CHF out-patients. In this study, NTproBNP-guided treatment was associated with a significant reduction in the composite endpoint of admission, cardiovascular death, or worsening CHF (38). The above trials were small in nature but certainly suggest the need for larger trials. These trials are currently under way.

CONCLUSION

Natriuretic peptides have become increasingly important markers for evaluation of the dyspneic patient and treatment of CHF. While NPs are primarily used as a tool for diagnosing or ruling out acute CHF in the dyspneic patient, recent work suggests a much broader application for NPs. This includes triaging patients with acute CHF, screening for asymptomatic LV dysfunction, optimizing patients who are hospitalized for CHF exacerbation, and prognosticating patients with all stages of the disease. NPs are not stand-alone tests and there is a learning curve associated with their use. Further research is likely to help elucidate and refine our understanding and clinical use of the NP levels.

REFERENCES

1. Bhalla V, Willis S, Maisel AS. B-type natriuretic peptide. The level and the drug-partners in the diagnosis and management of congestive heart failure [review]. *Congest Heart Fail.* 2004;10(1 Suppl 1):3–27. (Erratumin *Congest Heart Fail.* 2005;11[3]:161.)
2. Rich MW. Epidemiology, pathophysiology, and etiology of congestive heart failure in older adults. *J Am Geriatr Soc.* 1997;45:968–974.
3. Vinson JM, Rich MW, Sperry JC, et al. Early readmission of elderly patients with congestive heart failure. *J Am Geriatr Soc.* 1990;38:1290–1295.
4. Cohn JN, Levine TB, Olivari MT, et al. Plasma norepinephrine as a guide to prognosis in patients with chronic congestive heart failure. *N Engl J Med.* 1984;311:819–823.
5. Maisel AS, Krishnaswamy P, Nowak RM, et al. Rapid measurement of B-type natriuretic peptide in the emergency diagnosis of heart failure. *N Engl J Med.* 2002;347:161–167.
6. Silver MA, Maisel A, Yancy CW, et al. BNP Consensus Panel 2004: a clinical approach for the diagnostic, prognostic, screening, treatment monitoring, and therapeutic roles of natriuretic peptides in cardiovascular diseases. *Congest Heart Fail.* 2004;10:1–30.
7. Yasue H, Yoshimura M, Sumida H, et al. Localization and mechanism of secretion of B-type natriuretic peptide in comparison with those of A-type natriuretic peptide in normal subjects and patients with heart failure. *Circulation.* 1994;90:195–203.
8. Wuerz RC, Meador SA. Effects of prehospital medications on mortality and length of stay in congestive heart failure. *Ann Emerg Med.* 1992;21:669–674.
9. Dao Q, Krishnaswamy P, Kazanegra R, et al. Utility of B-type natriuretic peptide in the diagnosis of congestive heart failure in an urgent-care setting. *J Am Coll Cardiol.* 2001;37:379–385.
10. McCullough PA, Nowak RM, McCord J, et al. B-type natriuretic peptide and clinical judgment in emergency diagnosis of heart failure. Analysis from Breathing Not Properly (BNP) multinational study. *Circulation.* 2002;106:416–422.
11. Morrison LK, Harrison A, Krishnaswamy P, et al. Utility of a rapid B-natriuretic peptide assay in differentiating congestive heart failure from lung disease in patients presenting with dyspnea. *J Am Coll Cardiol.* 2002;39:202–209.

12. McCullough PA, Hollander JE, Nowak RM, et al. Uncovering heart failure in patients with a history of pulmonary disease. Rationale for the early use of B-type natriuretic peptide in the emergency department. *Acad Emerg Med.* 2003;10:198–204.
13. Maisel AS. The diagnosis of acute congestive heart failure. Role of BNP measurements. *Heart Fail Rev.* 2003;8:327–334.
14. McCullough PA, Duc P, OmLand T, et al. B-type natriuretic peptide and renal function in the diagnosis of heart failure. An analysis from the Breathing Not Properly multinational study. *Am J Kidney Dis.* 2003;41:571–579.
15. Wahl HG, Graf S, Renz H, et al. Elimination of the cardiac natriuretic peptides B-type natriuretic peptide (BNP) and N-terminal proBNP by hemodialysis. *Clin Chem.* 2004;50:1071–1074.
16. Mehra MR, Uber PA, Park MH, et al. Obesity and suppressed B-type natriuretic peptide levels in heart failure. *J Am Coll Cardiol.* 2004;43:1590–1595.
17. McCord J, Mundy BJ, Hudson MP, et al. Relationship between obesity and B-type natriuretic peptide levels. *Arch Intern Med.* 2004;164:2247–2252.
18. Sarzani R, Dessi-Fulgheri P, Paci VM, et al. Expression of natriuretic peptide receptors in human adipose and other tissues. *J Endocrinol Invest.* 1996;19:581–585.
19. Maisel AS, McCord J, Nowak RM, et al. Bedside B-type natriuretic peptide in the emergency diagnosis of heart failure with reduced or preserved ejection fraction. Results from the Breathing Not Properly multinational study. *J Am Coll Cardiol.* 2003;41:2010–2017.
20. Lubien E, DeMaria A, Krishnaswamy P, et al. Utility of B-natriuretic peptide in detecting diastolic dysfunction. comparison with Doppler velocity recordings. *Circulation* 2002;105:595–601.
21. Maisel A, Hollander JE, Guss D, et al. Primary results of the Rapid Emergency Department Heart Failure Outpatient Trial (REDHOT). A multicenter study of B-type natriuretic peptide levels, emergency department decision making, and outcomes in patients presenting with shortness of breath. *J Am Coll Cardiol.* 2004;44:1328–1333.
22. Mueller C, Scholer A, Laule-Kilian K, et al. Use of B-type natriuretic peptide in the evaluation and management of acute dyspnea. *N Engl J Med.* 2004;350:647–654.
23. Harrison A, Morrison LK, Krishnaswamy P, et al. B-type natriuretic peptide predicts future cardiac events in patients presenting to the emergency department with dyspnea. *Ann Emerg Med.* 2002;39:131–138.
24. Cheng V, Kazanagra R, Garcia A, et al. A rapid bedside test for B-type peptide predicts treatment outcomes in patients admitted for decompensated heart failure. A pilot study. *J Am Coll Cardiol.* 2001;37:386–391.
25. Bettencourt P, Ferreira S, Azevedo A, et al. Preliminary data on the potential usefulness of B-type natriuretic peptide levels in predicting outcome after hospital discharge in patients with heart failure. *Am J Med.* 2002;113:215–219.
26. Horwich TB, Patel J, MacLellan WR, et al. Cardiac troponin I is associated with impaired hemodynamics, progressive left ventricular dysfunction, and increased mortality rates in advanced heart failure. *Circulation.* 2003;108:833–838.
27. Berger R, Huelsman M, Strecker K, et al. B-type natriuretic peptide predicts sudden death in patients with chronic heart failure. *Circulation.* 2002;105:2392–2397.
28. Wang TJ, Larson MG, Levy D, et al. Plasma natriuretic peptide levels and the risk of cardiovascular events and death. *N Engl J Med.* 2004;350:655–663.
29. Heidenreich PA, Gubens MA, Fonarow GC, et al. Cost-effectiveness of screening with B-type natriuretic peptide to identify patients with reduced left ventricular ejection fraction. *J Am Coll Cardiol.* 2004;43:1019–1026.
30. Nielsen OW, McDonagh TA, Robb SD, et al. Retrospective analysis of the cost-effectiveness of using plasma brain natriuretic peptide in screening for left ventricular systolic dysfunction in the general population. *J Am Coll Cardiol.* 2003;41:113–120.
31. Atisha D, Bhalla MA, Morrison LK, et al. A prospective study in search of an optimal B-natriuretic peptide level to screen patients for cardiac dysfunction. *Am Heart J.* 2004;148:518–523.
32. Krumholz HM, Parent EM, Tu N, et al. Readmission after hospitalization for congestive heart failure among Medicare beneficiaries. *Arch Intern Med.* 1997;157:99–104.
33. Maeda K, Tsutamoto T, Wada A, et al. Plasma brain natriuretic peptide as a biochemical marker of high left ventricular end-diastolic pressure in patients with symptomatic left ventricular dysfunction. *Am Heart J.* 1998;135:825–832.
34. Kazanegra R, Cheng V, Garcia A, et al. A rapid test for B-type natriuretic peptide correlates with falling wedge pressures in patients treated for decompensated heart failure. A pilot study. *J Card Fail.* 2001;7:21–29.
35. Gackowski A, Isnard R, Golmard JL, et al. Comparison of echocardiography and plasma B-type natriuretic peptide for monitoring the response to treatment in acute heart failure. *Eur Heart J.* 2004;25:1788–1796.
36. Logeart D, Thabut G, Jourdain P, et al. Predischarge B-type natriuretic peptide assay for identifying patients at high risk of re-admission after decompensated heart failure. *J Am Coll Cardiol.* 2004;43:635–641.
37. Murdoch DR, McDonagh TA, Byrne J, et al. Titration of vasodilator therapy in chronic heart failure according to plasma brain natriuretic peptide concentration. Randomized comparison of the hemodynamic and neuroendocrine effects of tailored versus empirical therapy. *Am Heart J.* 1999;138:1126–1132.
38. Troughton RW, Frampton CM, Yandle TG, et al. Treatment of heart failure guided by plasma aminoterminal brain natriuretic peptide (N-BNP) concentrations. *Lancet.* 2000;355:1126–1130.

Noninvasive Imaging Techniques for the Assessment of the Patient with Heart Failure

33

Swaminatha V. Gurudevan *Peng Li* *Mani A. Vannan* *Jagat Narula*

A variety of noninvasive imaging modalities are available to the clinician in the assessment of patients with congestive heart failure. These include echocardiography, radionuclide imaging, and cardiovascular magnetic resonance imaging (CMRI). These methods offer insight into the structural characteristics of the left ventricle (LV) that can impact patient prognosis and guide the treatment of patients with congestive heart failure. They are also helpful in evaluating the structure and disease progression in patients with coexistent valvular heart disease. The progression of left ventricular remodeling and subsequent reverse remodeling after initiation of medical therapy can both be evaluated with these methods. Most importantly, these techniques offer insight into the etiology of ventricular dysfunction and can guide the clinician in selecting the most optimal treatment strategy.

EVALUATION OF STRUCTURAL CARDIAC ABNORMALITIES

Left Ventricular Size and Mass

Measurement of LV cavity size and LV mass provides vital information regarding the etiology, pathophysiology, and prognosis of a patient's heart failure syndrome. Patients with congestive heart failure with a dilated left ventricle represent a subset of individuals who should be identified early and managed aggressively. Data from the SOLVD and SAVE trials (1,2) show that LV dilatation is associated with a significantly higher mortality in patients presenting with clinical evidence of congestive heart failure. Table 33-1 illustrates the data from SOLVD. In addition, dilation of the LV is associated with an increase in overall cardiovascular events following myocardial infarction (MI) (3) and a higher incidence of lethal ventricular arrhythmias post-MI (4). LV size can be followed serially and correlated with clinical improvement during the course of reverse remodeling in response to medical therapy. Successful reduction of LV size with medical therapy is associated with an improvement in mortality as shown in the SAVE trial, illustrated in Figure 33-1.

Echocardiography is the most commonly used method to evaluate the size of the LV cavity. Both two-dimensional and M-mode echocardiography are commonly used to generate measurements of LV end-diastolic diameter (LVEDD) and LV end-systolic diameter (LVESD). The excellent temporal resolution of M-mode echocardiography enables precise measurements of these parameters. Normal LVEDD at our institution ranges from 42 to 55 mm, while normal LVESD ranges from 25 to 36 mm. With the progressive LV enlargement that occurs with dilated cardiomyopathy, both LVEDD and LVESD rise; both variables fall following institution of successful medical therapy (6). This has major prognostic implications, as patients with massive LV enlargement (LVEDD >75 mm or LVESD >60 mm) are at high risk for adverse events, including sudden death (7). Figure 33-2 shows a parasternal long-axis two-dimensional and M-mode echocardiogram in a normal patient and a patient with dilated cardiomyopathy.

LV mass and wall thickness can also be assessed using M-mode echocardiography. Wall thickness is typically measured in the parasternal imaging plane with measurement of the interventricular septal wall thickness (IVST) and posterior wall thickness (PWT). Using the assumption that the LV is spherically shaped, the internal dimensions can be cubed and subtracted from the external dimensions

TABLE 33-1

DATA FROM SOLVD TRIAL: LEFT VENTRICULAR MASS, LEFT VENTRICULAR END-SYSTOLIC DIMENSION AND LEFT ATRIAL DIMENSION AS STRONG PREDICTORS OF MORTALITY IN PATIENTS WITH SYMPTOMATIC HEART FAILURE

	All-Cause Mortality		CV Hospitalization	
	Risk Ratio*	p Value	Risk Ratio*	p Value
LV mass	2.75 (1.62, 4.66)	0.0002	1.81 (1.39, 2.36)	0.0001
LV end-systolic dimension	2.73 (1.43, 5.20)	0.003	NS	NS
LA dimension	1.84 (1.08, 3.15)	0.03	1.37 (1.05, 1.78)	0.02

*Above versus below the mean group comparison adjusted for age, NYHA class, ischemic etiology, and EF.
From Quinones MA, Greenberg BH, Kopelen HA, et al. Echocardiographic predictors of clinical outcome in patients with left ventricular dysfunction enrolled in the SOLVD registry and trials: significance of left ventricular hypertrophy. Studies of Left Ventricular Dysfunction. *J Am Coll Cardiol.* 2000;35:1237–1244, with permission.

to determine the volume of the LV myocardium. This volume is then multiplied by the specific gravity of muscle (1.05 g/cm^3), yielding a value of LV mass (8). Normal values of LV mass indexed to height using this method have been reported at 79.1 ± 19.2 g/m in men and 66.7 ± 15.7 g/m in women (9). These and other normal values for standard M-mode echo measurements are shown in Table 33-2.

LV mass carries significant prognostic implications for the survival of patients with congestive heart failure (10). In the Framingham Heart Study, LV mass calculated using this method was associated with a higher cardiovascular death rate and a higher all-cause mortality, independent of conventional risk factors (11). In addition, the investigators found a relative risk of cardiovascular disease of 1.49 for each incremental increase of 50 g/m in LV mass. These data are shown in Figure 33-3.

Real-time three-dimensional echocardiography is now commercially available and provides a powerful means to evaluate LV cavity size and mass. Using a pyramidal phased-array ultrasound transducer, a full-volume data set acquisition can be performed on four cardiac cycles. This volume is analyzed off-line to determine precise measurements of LVEDD, LVESD, IVST, PWT, and LV mass. When compared with two-dimensional echo, three-dimensional echo has better reproducibility and less test–retest variability (12). It is also less dependent on LV geometric assumptions. This method holds significant promise for the future assessment of LV mass and dimensions. As the technique is relatively new, long-term prognostic data are not yet avail-

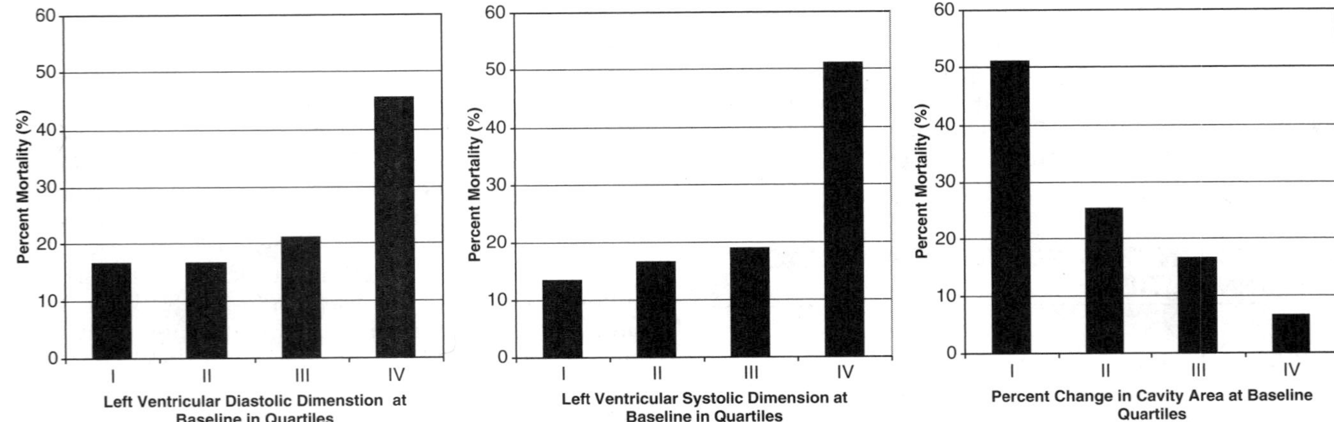

Figure 33-1 Data from the SAVE trial, in which 512 patients were randomized to placebo versus captopril therapy post-myocardial infarction and underwent echocardiography at baseline and at 1 year postinfarction. Patients are divided into quartiles based on dimensions with I representing the quartile of patients with the smallest dimensions or change in dimensions and IV representing quartile of patients with the largest dimensions or change in dimensions. **Left graph** shows increasing mortality with increasing initial LV diastolic dimension with mortality. **Center graph** shows similar mortality increase with increasing LV systolic dimension. **Right graph** shows decreasing mortality with larger percentage change in cavity area at 1 year. (From St. John Sutton M, Pfeffer MA, Plappert T, et al. Quantitative two-dimensional echocardiographic measurements are major predictors of adverse cardiovascular events after acute myocardial infarction. The protective effects of captopril. *Circulation.* 1994;89:68–75, with permission.)

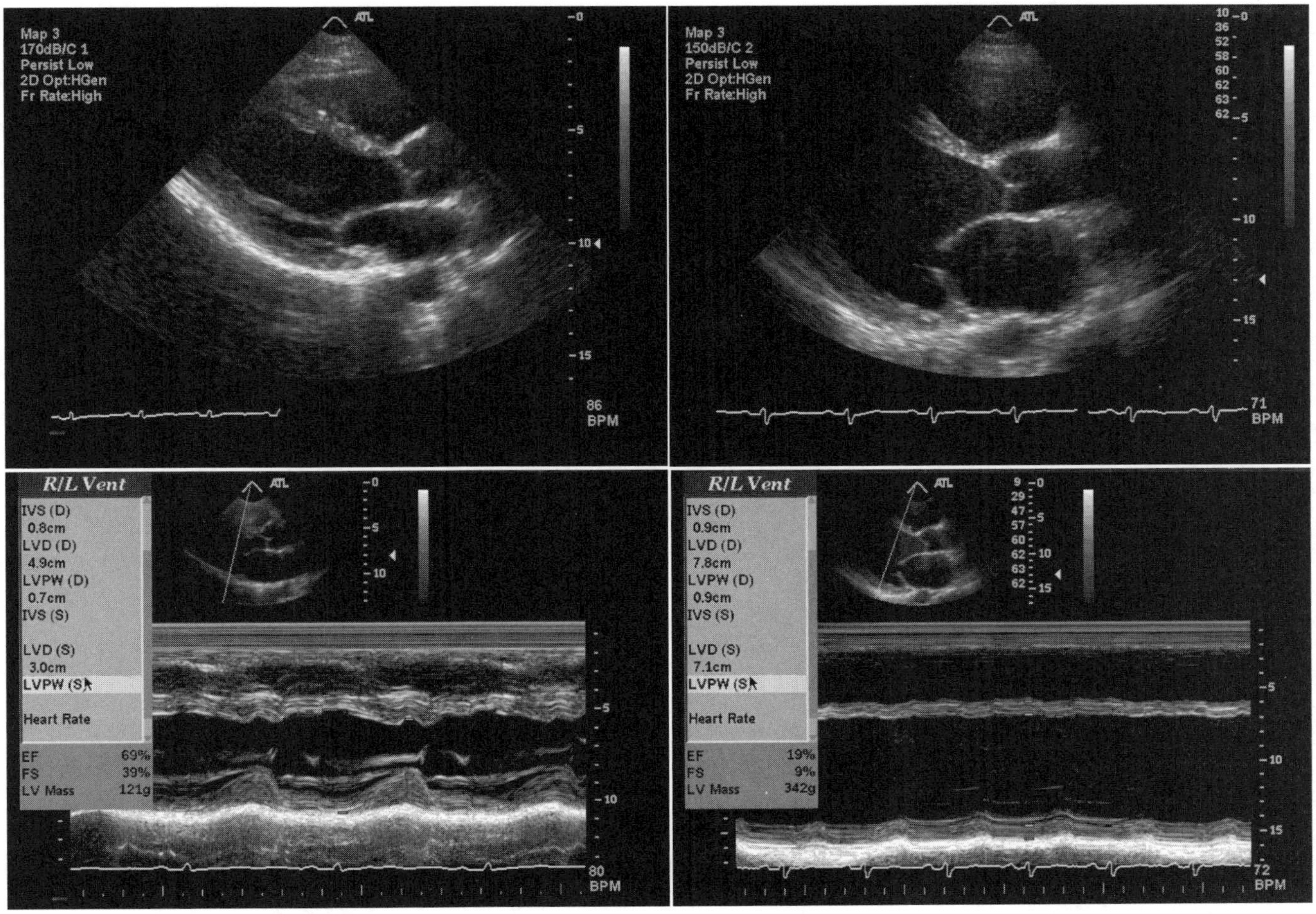

Figure 33-2 Parasternal long-axis two-dimensional and M-mode echocardiogram images from a normal patient (**left**) and a patient with dilated cardiomyopathy (DCM) (**right**). Note the marked increase in LV chamber size and LV mass along with a marked reduction in LV fractional shortening and EF in the patient with DCM.

TABLE 33-2

NORMAL VALUES FOR STANDARD M-MODE ECHOCARDIOGRAPHIC VARIABLES FOR MEN AND WOMEN

Measurement	Range (Male)	Range (Female)
Aorta (cm)	2.6–3.7	2.1–3.4
Left atrium (cm)	2.9–4.2	2.5–3.9
Right atrium (cm)	1.4–2.6	1.5–2.6
Interventricular septum (cm)	0.6–1.1	0.6–1.1
Posterior wall (cm)	0.6–1.1	0.6–1.1
LV end-diastolic dimension (cm)	4.3–5.7	3.8–5.4
LV end-systolic dimension (cm)	2.5–3.6	2.3–3.6
Fractional shortening (%)	30.6–46.5	27.7–44.5
Ejection fraction (%)	57.8–76.3	53.4–75.8
LV mass (g)	78.2–211.8	71.8–154.9
LV mass/BSA (g/m^2)	48.0–102.2	44.0–89.3
LV mass/height (g/m)	49.8–117.4	44.9–91.1

From Schvartzman PR, Fuchs FD, Mello AG, et al. Normal values of echocardiographic measurements. A population-based study. *Arq Bras Cardiol*. 2000;75:107–114, with permission.

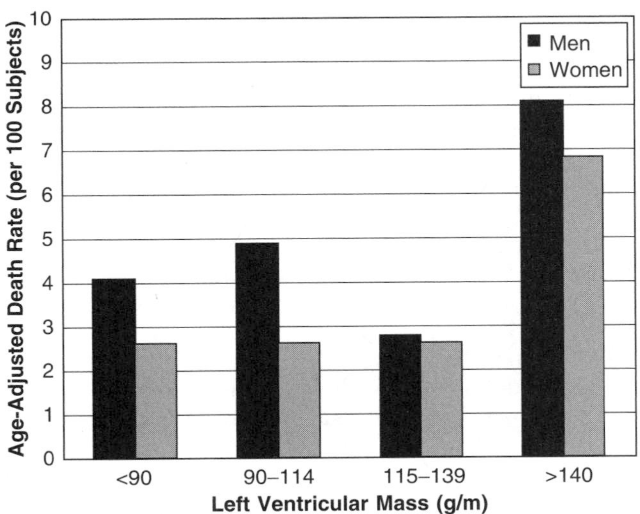

Figure 33-3 Data from the Framingham Heart Study showing age-adjusted death rate based on LV mass, adjusted to patient height. Dark bars represent men and gray bars represent women. (From Levy D, Garrison RJ, Savage DD, et al. Prognostic implications of echocardiographically determined left ventricular mass in the Framingham Heart Study. *N Engl J Med*. 1990;322:1561–1566, with permission.)

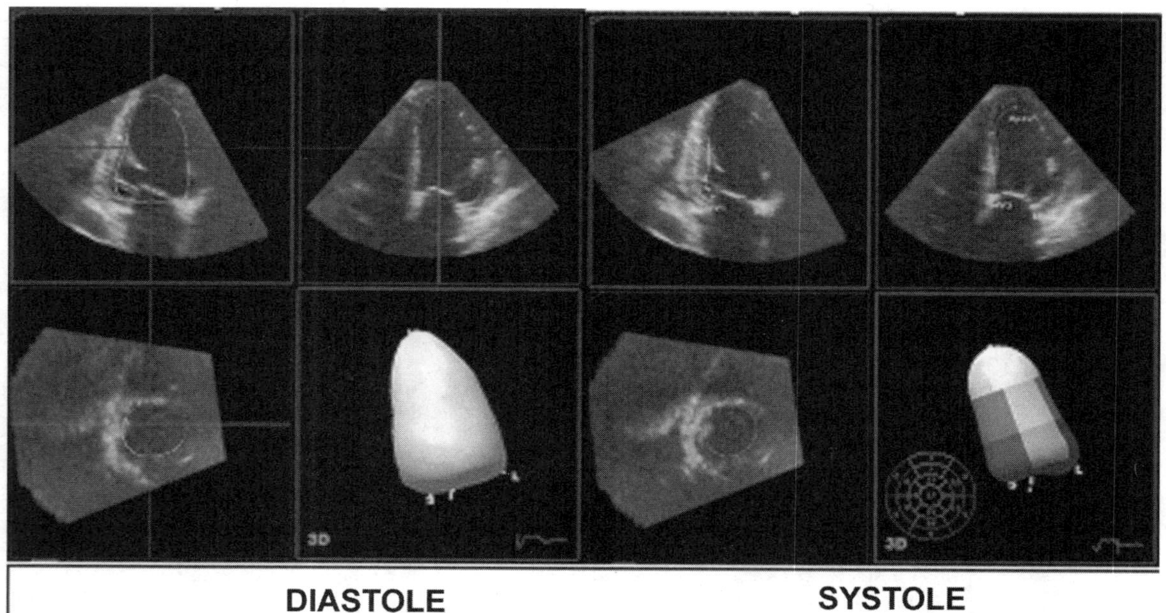

Figure 33-4 Real-time three-dimensional echocardiographic calculation of LV volume at end-diastole (**left**) and end-systole (**right**). Three-dimensional echocardiography enables a derivation of the true geometric shape of the LV, resulting in highly accurate, reproducible measures of LV volumes.

able for three-dimensional measurements. Figure 33-4 shows a real-time three-dimensional echocardiographic analysis of LV volumes and ejection fraction (EF).

While radionuclide ventriculography was originally developed in the 1970s as a method to quantify EF, two methods can be used to determine LV volumes: the first-pass method and the multiple ECG gated acquisition (MUGA) method. The first involves imaging Tc-99-sestamibi- or Tc-99-tetrofosmin-labeled red blood cells with a high temporal sampling rate during their initial transit through the central circulation and is known as the first-pass method. This method is limited to a single acquisition and is typically done in the right anterior oblique view (13). The gated method involves identifying a specific portion of the cardiac cycle by ECG and averaging the measured LV volumes during systole and diastole over several cardiac cycles (14). A quantitative assessment of radionuclide counts can then be obtained during systole and diastole and absolute LV volumes can be derived. Figure 33-5 shows a gated radionuclide assessment of LV volumes and EF.

Radionuclide ventriculography is advantageous as it has a high degree of reproducibility and has a low intraobserver and interobserver variability and analysis can be done independent of LV geometry or abnormalities in regional wall motion (16). Several studies have documented that LV volumes assessed using this method can be followed serially and correlate well with clinical improvement with medical therapy (17). In the SOLVD trial, patients treated with enalapril showed a significant reduction in LV volumes as measured by radionuclide ventriculography, while placebo patients had an increase in LV volumes. These changes in LV volumes correlated with the marked reduction in mortality seen with enalapril therapy (18).

Cardiovascular magnetic resonance imaging (CMRI) has experienced a significant technological evolution during the past 5 years and has emerged as a powerful method to assist the clinician in the assessment of LV volumes (19,20). CMRI provides a three-dimensional data set at multiple levels and phases throughout the cardiac cycle and can thus be performed independent of the geometric characteristics of the LV. Volumes are obtained in the long-axis, short-axis, four-chamber, and two-chamber imaging planes (19). Image acquisition is typically performed during a breath hold in expiration (19). CMRI has the advantages of having a high degree of temporal and spatial resolution and providing simultaneous structural and functional information. Due to their high degree of precision and reproducibility, CMRI measurements of LV mass are often used as the gold standard in living patients for the evaluation of two-dimensional and three-dimensional echo measurements of LV mass (19,20).

Image analysis with CMRI is usually performed offline, with calculation of LVEDV, LVESV, and LV mass. Disadvantages of CMRI include its lack of portability and accessibility to acutely ill patients, the need for breath-hold imaging which may limit utility in patients with heart failure, patient claustrophobia, and operator dependence on specific pulse sequences to achieve optimal image quality.

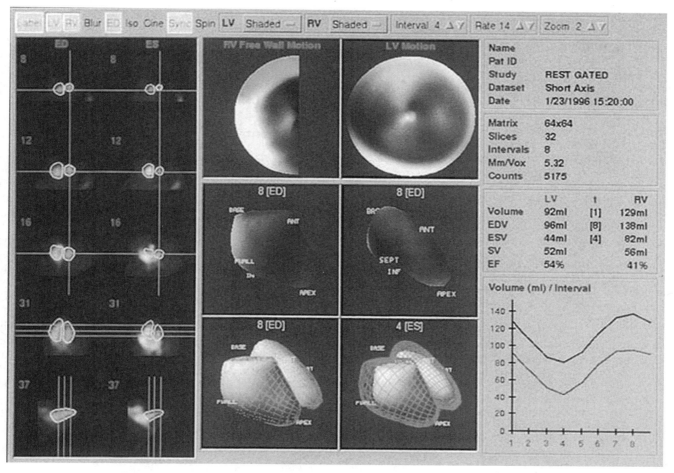

Figure 33-5 Gated blood pool SPECT with use of Tc-99-sestamibi to determine LV and RV volumes and EF. The calculations are based on the number of counts detected at end-systole and end-diastole and are therefore more quantitative and highly reproducible. (From Dilsizian VN, J, ed. *Atlas of Nuclear Cardiology*. Philadelphia: Current Medicine, Inc.; 2003, with permission.)

Left Atrial Size and Volume

Left atrial (LA) volume has been recognized as a powerful indicator of LV diastolic function. During diastole the LA is directly exposed to LV pressures, and LA volume thus reflects the severity and duration of increased LV filling pressure (21). Due to intrinsic variability in atrial size that occurs based on patient size and gender, LA volume is indexed based on body surface area and is often reported as left atrial volume index (LAVI), which is expressed in units of mL/m^2. Normal LAVI has been previously reported as 20 $\pm$ 6 mL/m^2 (22).

There are recent data from patients with nonischemic cardiomyopathy that suggest that an LAVI >68.5 mL/m^2 is associated with a three- to fourfold lower survival free of cardiac transplantation (23). Even modest elevations in LAVI are associated with adverse outcomes: following acute MI, patients with an LAVI >32 mL/m^2 had a sixfold higher mortality than those with LAVI (24). In this patient population, mortality rose progressively as LAVI increased, as shown in Figure 33-6.

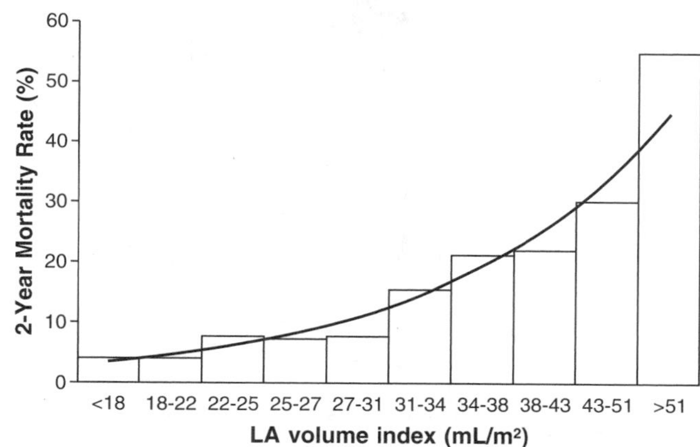

Figure 33-6 Relationship between LA volume index and 2-year mortality in 314 patients who underwent two-dimensional echocardiography following acute myocardial infarction. (From Moller JE, Hillis GS, Oh JK, et al. Left atrial volume: a powerful predictor of survival after acute myocardial infarction. *Circulation*. 2003; 107:2207–2212, with permission.)

Echocardiography is the most common imaging modality used to assess LA size. Linear measurement of LA size is typically performed using M-mode echocardiography in the parasternal window. This measurement is performed at end-systole, just before mitral valve opening, during maximal LA volume. However, this technique is limited by its lack of spatial orientation.

There are two methods of assessing LA volume using two-dimensional echocardiography, as shown in Figure 33-7. The first involves the planimetry of the LA area in the apical four-chamber and apical two-chamber views, along with the measurement of the length of the LA from the mitral annulus to the posterior wall in the four-chamber view. LA volume is then calculated as:

$$\text{LA volume} = 0.85 \times (\text{four-chamber area}) \times (\text{two-chamber area})/(\text{atrial length})$$

LA volume can also be calculated by treating the LA as a prolate ellipse and measuring the anteroposterior length in the parasternal long-axis view and the two orthogonal lengths in the apical four-chamber view, and using the formula:

$$\text{LA volume} = \pi/6 \times (\text{anteroposterior diameter from parasternal view}) \times (\text{anteroposterior diameter from apical four-chamber view}) \times (\text{medial-lateral diameter from apical four-chamber view}).$$

CMRI can also be used to obtain a very accurate assessment of LA volume. Patients are imaged with a breath hold and the LA volume is calculated using the modified Simpson's rule. This method involves considering the LA as a prolate ellipse and dividing it into 10-mm-thick slices. These slices are summed to determine LA volume. Both cine-MR and contrast-enhanced MR have been used with this method to evaluate LA volume, with excellent spatial resolution (25,26).

Right Ventricular Size and Function

Assessment of right ventricular (RV) size and systolic function provides additional prognostic information to the clinician caring for a patient with heart failure. Recent data have shown that RV function has a strong association with a patient's functional capacity, short-term clinical outcome, and long-term survival (27). In a study by de Groote et al. of 205 patients with New York Heart Association (NYHA) Class II or III heart failure, RV ejection fraction (RVEF) derived from radionuclide ventriculography was the only significant independent predictor of event-free survival from cardiovascular mortality and urgent transplantation in this patient population (28).

Imaging of the RV with echocardiography is technically more challenging due to its unique pyramidal shape. When determining RV volume, certain assumptions about the geometric shape of the RV must be made which may not be accurate. The most common echo method employed to assess RV function is the planimetry of the RV fractional area in the apical four-chamber view. In this sin-

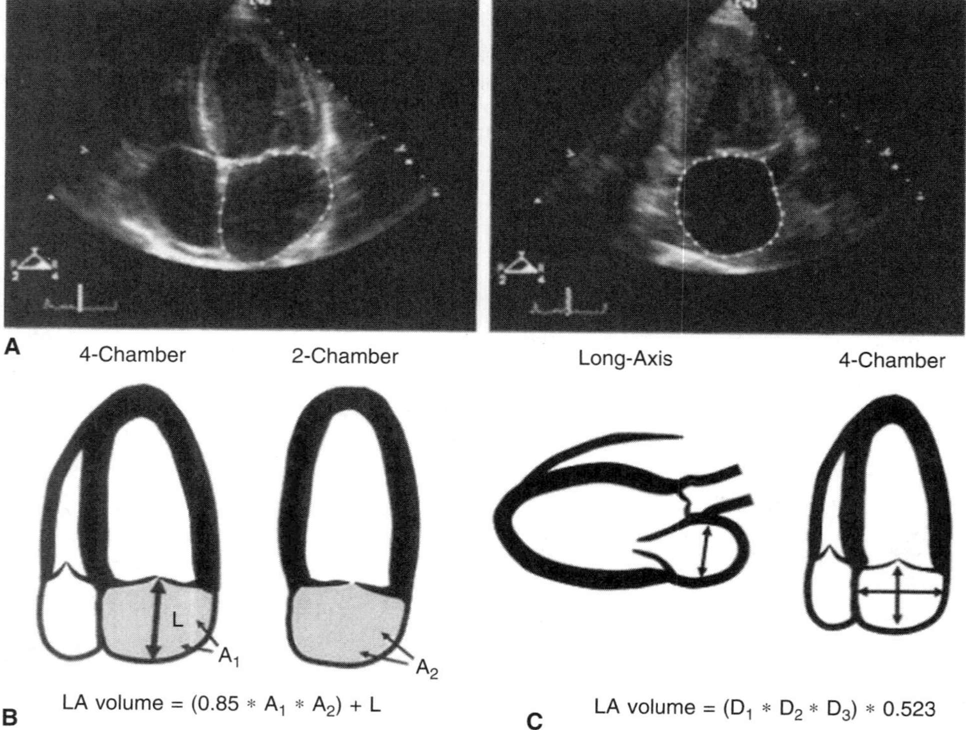

Figure 33-7 Two techniques for the measurement of LA volume by two-dimensional echocardiography. The first method involves planimetry of the LA area in the four-chamber and two-chamber views, while the second involves measurement of the three linear dimensions of the LA and multiplying by $\pi/6$. (From Feigenbaum H, Armstrong WF, Ryan T. *Feigenbaum's Echocardiography*. 6th ed. Philadelphia: Lippincott Williams & Wilkins; 2005, with permission.)

gle plane, end-systolic area is subtracted from end-diastolic area and the result is divided by the end-diastolic area to yield the fractional area change (8).

In the SAVE trial, on univariate analysis of 414 patients who were enrolled post-MI, RV fractional area change (FAC) was a predictor of mortality, cardiovascular mortality, and heart failure. RV dysfunction as indicated by an FAC less than 0.32 predicted a 31.2% event rate, compared with 12.7% in patients without RV dysfunction. In fact, each 5% decrease in RV FAC was associated with a 16% increased odds of cardiovascular mortality (29). Other methods of assessment of RV function include assessment of tricuspid annular plane systolic excursion and linear assessment of RV shortening (30). These methods are summarized in Figure 33-8.

The advent of three-dimensional echocardiography has significantly impacted our ability to assess RV function, as the assumptions about the shape of the RV are no longer necessary; a complete echocardiographic rendering of the RV cavity can be recorded and analyzed, with a more accurate assessment of RV volumes than is possible with two-dimensional echocardiography. This is demonstrated in Figure 33-9.

Radionuclide ventriculography is an established method for determination of RV volumes and EF. It can be performed using both first-pass and equilibrium-gated measurement of radionuclide counts in the right ventricle. It has been considered the traditional gold standard for quantitative assessment of RV volumes and EF (31). CMRI also enables accurate assessment of RV volumes and EF and may become the gold standard for RV volumetric assessment due to its high degree of temporal and spatial resolution. Its reproducibility for RV volume measurements is poorer than for LV volume measurements but is still superior to echocardiographic methods (32).

Pulmonary Artery Pressures

Pulmonary artery pressure and pulmonary vascular resistance are important hemodynamic parameters in patients with chronic heart failure. Increased pulmonary artery pressure is a marker of poor prognosis in patients with LV dysfunction and is associated with a poor outcome following cardiac transplantation (33). Pulmonary hypertension may result from *postcapillary* pulmonary hypertension from chronically elevated LV and LA pressures, or from *precapillary* pulmonary hypertension that can occur secondary to remodeling of the pulmonary arterial tree (34).

Pulmonary artery (PA) pressures are typically assessed during right heart catheterization but can be accurately estimated using Doppler echocardiography. This is performed by measuring the peak velocity of tricuspid regurgitation (V_{TR}) and the application of the modified Bernoulli equation, which states:

$$\text{Pulmonary artery pressure} = \text{right atrial pressure} + 4 \times V_{TR}^2$$

Right atrial (RA) pressure can often be estimated by clinical exam and is assumed to be 5 to 7 mm Hg in a euvolemic patient. The use of tricuspid regurgitation velocity to estimate PA pressure is shown in Figure 33-10, taken from one patient with mild pul-monary hypertension and another with severe pulmonary hypertension.

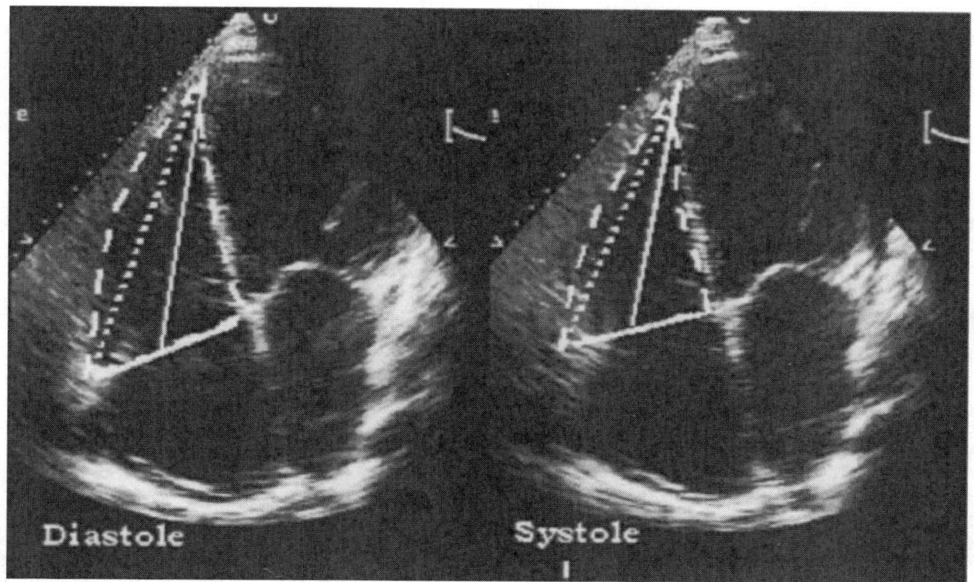

Figure 33-8 Methods of assessment of RV function using two-dimensional echocardiography. The dashed line (- - - - -) demonstrates planimetry of the fractional area during diastole and systole, the solid line (——) demonstrates assessment of tricuspid annular plane excursion, and the dotted line (●●●●●●●●) demonstrates assessment of RV shortening. (Adapted from Thohan V. Prognostic implications of echocardiography in advanced heart failure. *Curr Opin Cardiol.* 2004;19:238–249, with permission.)

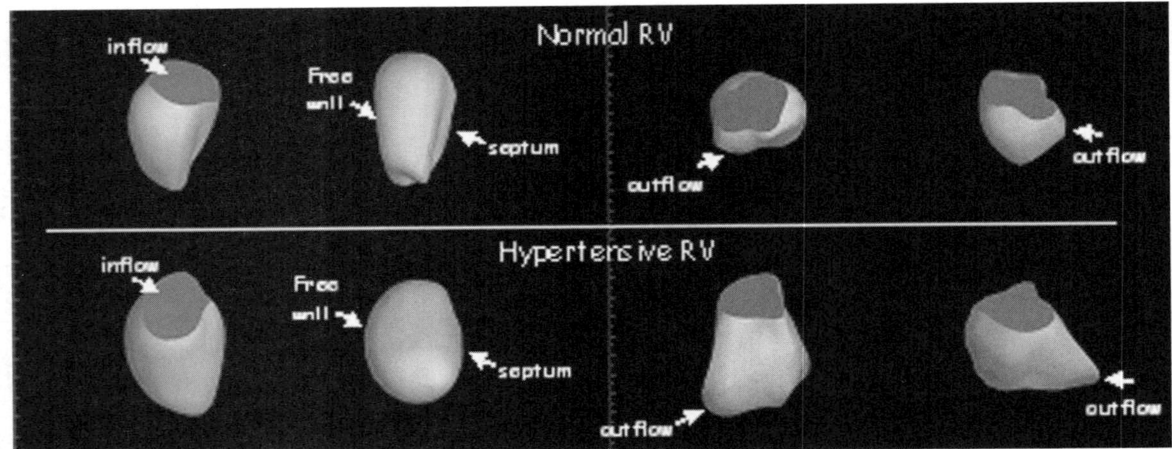

Figure 33-9 Three-dimensional echocardiographic reconstruction of RV volumes in a normal and hypertensive patient. The geometric shape of the RV can be more accurately rendered using three-dimensional echocardiography. (Image courtesy of Peng Li, M.D., University of California, Irvine Division of Cardiology.)

EVALUATION OF LEFT VENTRICULAR FUNCTION

Left Ventricular Systolic Function: Importance of Ejection Fraction

In patients with congestive heart failure, there is no prognostic indicator more important than LV systolic function. The most widely accepted standard for assessing LV systolic function is measurement of LVEF (8). EF depends not only on LV contractility but also on preload and afterload (30). Nonetheless, it remains a simple yet powerful predictor of outcome in all subgroups of patients with congestive heart failure and has a strong influence on the clinician's treatment paradigm. In virtually every large-scale clinical trial that examined patients with systolic dysfunction (SOLVD, CONSENSUS, SAVE, V-HeFT), LVEF was a strong negative predictor of mortality; low EF predicted a higher incidence of recurrent cardiovascular events, ventricular arrhythmias, and cardiovascular death (3,6,35,36). In fact, in stable patients with coronary artery disease (CAD), EF is a stronger predictor of mortality than is the number of diseased vessels (37). In patients with ischemic cardiomyopathy, EF has a strong influence on mortality from sudden death and ventricular arrhythmias (38). Those patients with an EF less than 30% have a significant mortality benefit from implantable cardioverter defibrillator (ICD) therapy, as shown in the MADIT-II trial (39). Figure 33-11 shows data from the V-HeFT VA cooperative studies group that demonstrates improved survival following fractional improvements in ejection fraction with effective medical therapy of heart failure.

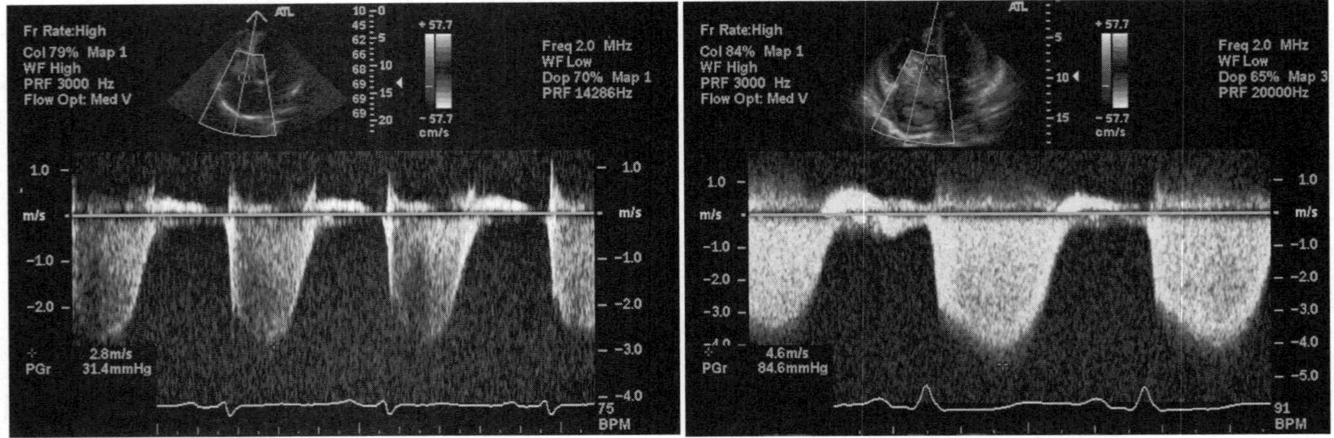

Figure 33-10 Assessment of pulmonary artery pressures using Doppler echocardiography in a patient with mild pulmonary hypertension (**left**) and severe pulmonary hypertension (**right**). The peak velocity of the tricuspid regurgitation jet is estimated using continuous-wave Doppler and the modified Bernoulli equation.

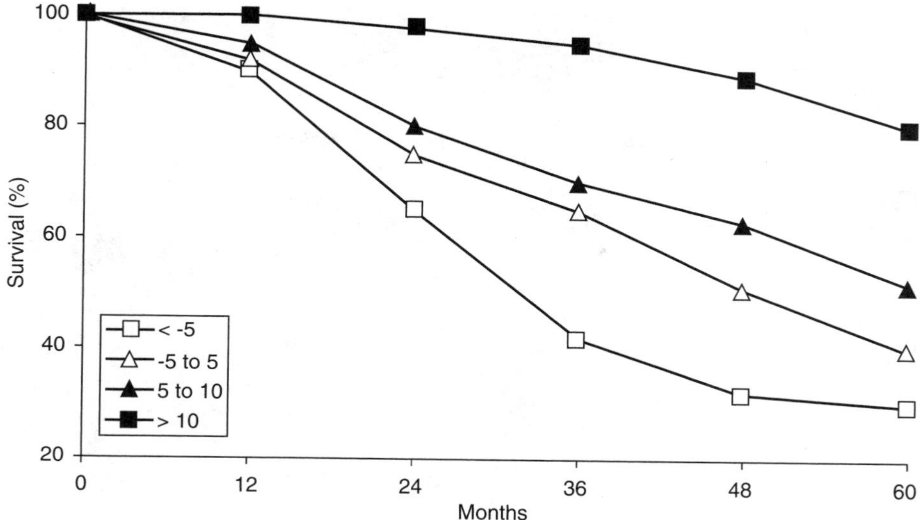

Figure 33-11 Data from V-HeFT VA Cooperative Studies Group demonstrating the impact of improvements in LVEF on mortality in patients with symptomatic heart failure. Patients underwent echocardiography at baseline after a 1-year follow-up with documentation of the interval change in LV systolic function and assessment of outcome at 60 months of follow-up. Survival strongly correlated with each stratum of LVEF change, with the greatest benefit occurring in those individuals who improved their LVEF by more than 10%. (Adapted from Cintron G, Johnson G, Francis G, et al. Prognostic significance of serial changes in left ventricular ejection fraction in patients with congestive heart failure. The V-HeFT VA Cooperative Studies Group. *Circulation.* 1993;87:VI17–V123, with permission.)

The most common method used today to assess LV volume and EF is echocardiography. The most common algorithm used is the biplane Simpson's rule. This treats the LV cavity as a truncated ellipse and calculates the volume in the apical four-chamber and apical two-chamber views as the summed volume of sequential stacked discs. Volumes are then calculated in systole and diastole, with stroke volume divided by end-diastolic volume representing the EF. This is shown in Figure 33-12. Compared to other modalities such as radionuclide ventriculography and CMRI, echocardiography tends to underestimate EF (16).

Hemodynamic assessment of cardiac output and LV contractility can also be accomplished using Doppler ultrasound. Through measurement of velocity and computation of the velocity-time integral (VTI) across the LV outflow tract, LV stroke volume can be determined (8). Multiplying by heart rate yields the cardiac output. As previously discussed, three-dimensional echocardiography holds similar promise as a method to noninvasively quantify LV volumes and compute global and regional EF. Novel methods such as strain rate imaging and velocity vector imaging are emerging techniques that hold promise as load-independent methods of assessing LV contractility and LV torsion. Figure 33-13 demonstrates a two-dimensional echo image of velocity vector imaging.

The use of radionuclide ventriculography for quantification of LV volumes and EF was covered earlier, and this discussion will not be repeated. CMRI is an emerging technique that has evolved considerably in the past decade and holds significant promise in quantifying LV volumes and EF. Gadolinium contrast is typically administered to improve endocardial border detection using automated detection algorithms that are available on most MRI scanners (41). Novel techniques of myocardial tagging with radio frequency pulses (42) or stimulated echo (43) using cine-MRI imaging enable quantification of three-dimensional myocardial strain. Figure 33-14 demonstrates cine-MR assessment of LV volumes and representative four-chamber and two-chamber still images, as well as a tagged MRI LV short-axis image.

Left Ventricular Diastolic Function

A growing number of patients diagnosed with clinical congestive heart failure have evidence of preserved LV systolic function with a normal EF. These patients are presumed to have a disorder of LV diastolic function. Indeed, the prevalence of heart failure with preserved systolic function is increasing considerably. A study by Senni et al. (44) showed a 5.9% prevalence of heart failure with preserved systolic function among 2,042 randomly selected residents of Olmsted County, Minnesota, who underwent echocardiography. The prognosis for patients with isolated LV diastolic dysfunction is more favorable than for patients with combined systolic and diastolic dysfunction. However, when compared with age- and gender-matched normal subjects, the mortality risk is increased fourfold (45,46).

Much of what we understand today about LV diastolic dysfunction we owe to Doppler echocardiography. Diastolic filling of the normal LV is characterized by a larger mitral flow velocity during the early rapid filling phase (E wave) with a smaller phase related to atrial contraction (A wave). Pulmonary venous Doppler shows a systolic-predominant filling pattern. Tissue velocity imaging of the mitral annulus can further assist in the classification of LV diastolic function. It involves the

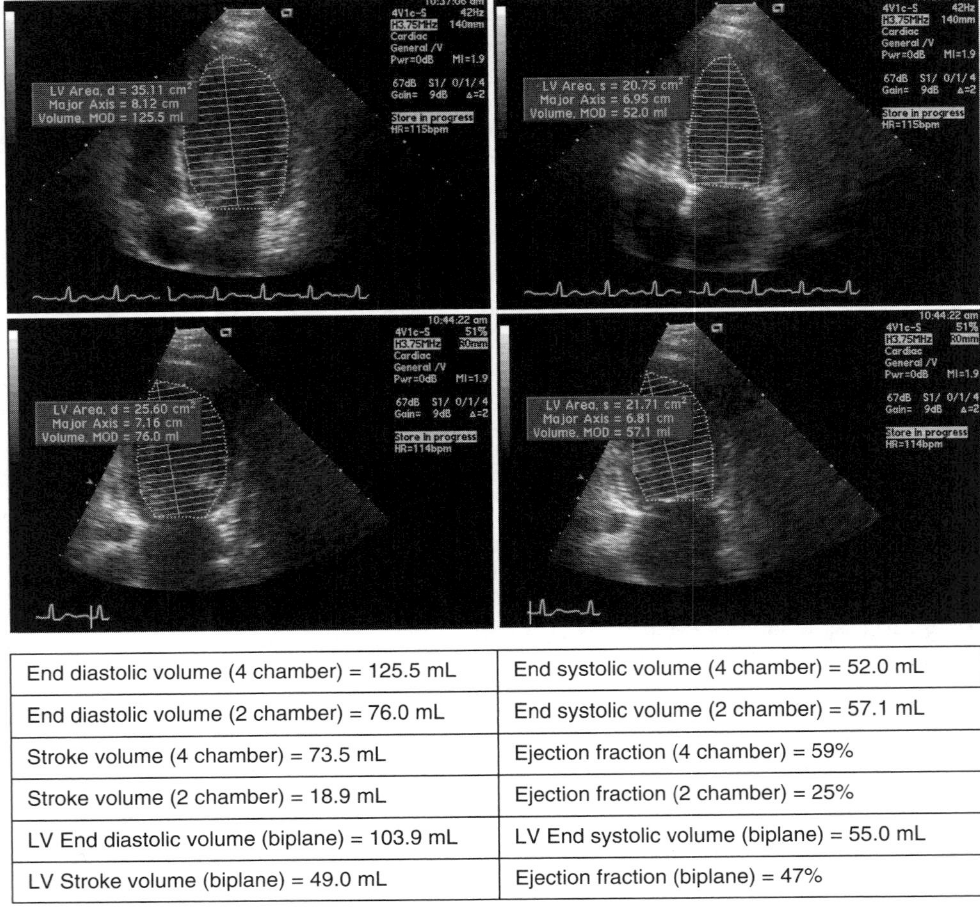

End diastolic volume (4 chamber) = 125.5 mL	End systolic volume (4 chamber) = 52.0 mL
End diastolic volume (2 chamber) = 76.0 mL	End systolic volume (2 chamber) = 57.1 mL
Stroke volume (4 chamber) = 73.5 mL	Ejection fraction (4 chamber) = 59%
Stroke volume (2 chamber) = 18.9 mL	Ejection fraction (2 chamber) = 25%
LV End diastolic volume (biplane) = 103.9 mL	LV End systolic volume (biplane) = 55.0 mL
LV Stroke volume (biplane) = 49.0 mL	Ejection fraction (biplane) = 47%

Figure 33-12 Calculation of EF using two-dimensional echocardiography and the biplane Simpson's rule method. The ventricle is considered as a prolate ellipse. In both the four-chamber and two-chamber planes, the ventricular volume is divided into a series of discs and the volume of each disc is summed up to yield a total cavity volume in systole and diastole.

placement of a sample volume at the septal and lateral portions of the mitral annulus in the apical four-chamber view with application of a low-pass filter to yield tissue velocities rather than blood velocities. As diastolic dysfunction increases in severity, tissue velocities decline predictably (47).

Diastolic dysfunction is typically divided into three phases based on transmitral, pulmonary venous, and tissue Doppler characteristics, as shown in Figure 33-15. The first stage of diastolic dysfunction is characterized by impaired relaxation and a shift from E-wave-dominant passive filling to an A-wave-dominant filling pattern (45). A normal systolic-predominant pulmonary venous flow pattern is maintained and tissue velocities are normal. The second stage, termed pseudonormalization, is characterized by an increase in LV filling pressures with a normal-appearing transmitral filling pattern and a diastolic-predominant pulmonary venous flow signal (45). Tissue velocities begin to decline in this stage. With continued progression of diastolic dysfunction, eventually a restrictive filling pattern is seen. This phase is characterized by brief early diastolic filling driven by markedly elevated LA pressures and a significantly diminished atrial contribution to filling. Pulmonary venous flow is mainly diastolic with a large a-reversal pattern evident in late diastole and tissue velocities are markedly diminished.

The echo variables just described can also be measured using CMRI. Delayed and impaired relaxation can be measured accurately by CMRI blood velocity encoding, and tissue velocities can be similarly measured. Tagged MRI also enables quantification of LV twisting and untwisting, which is believed to be the first characteristic to become altered in early diastolic dysfunction (48). The clinical application of these MRI techniques is still under development and there is currently no accepted standard.

EVALUATION OF THE ETIOLOGY OF HEART FAILURE

Determining the etiology of a patient's congestive heart failure syndrome is one of the most important challenges that a clinician faces. When faced with a patient

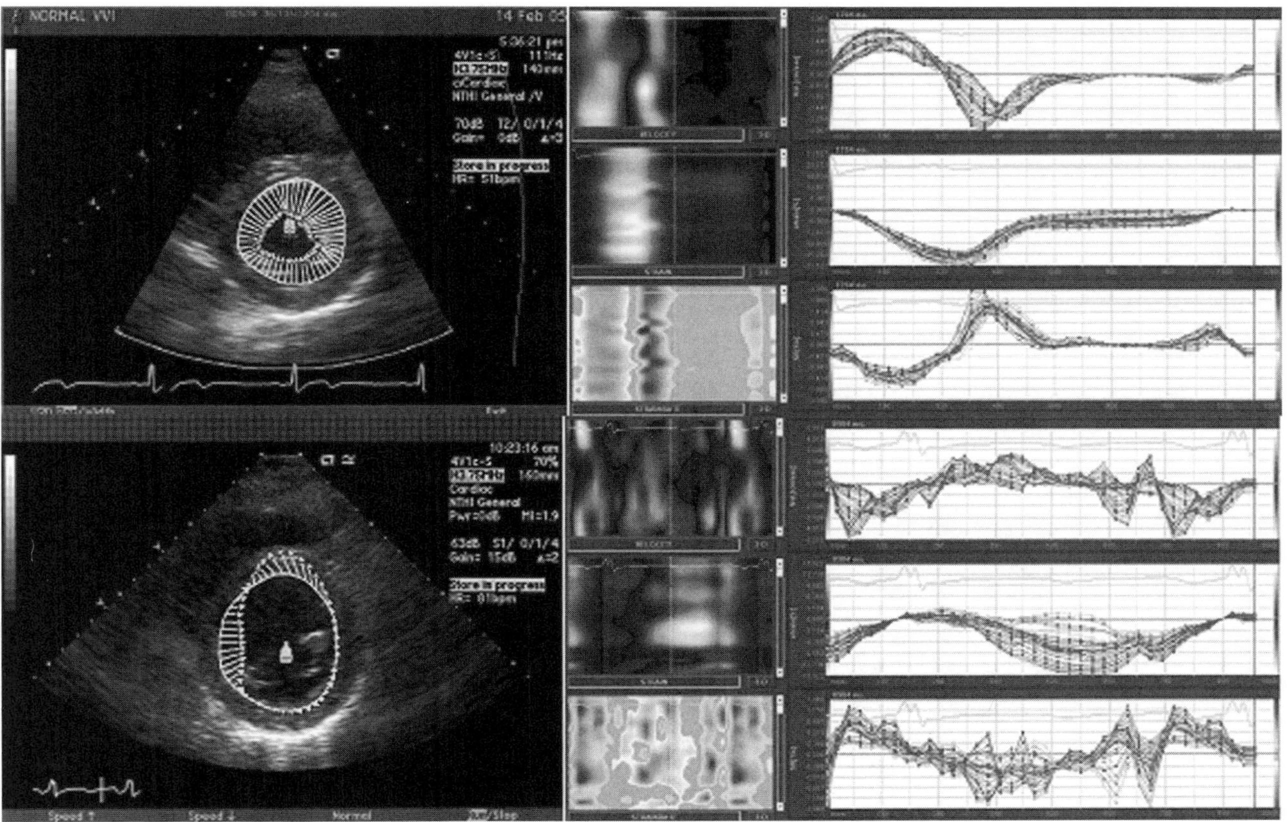

Figure 33-13 Velocity vector imaging of ventricular forces using Doppler echocardiography in a normal patient (**top panel**) and a patient with dilated cardiomyopathy (**bottom panel**). Normal ventricular systole leads to an increase in ventricular torsion as well as longitudinal and radial strain. In the patient with cardiomyopathy, these parameters are diminished. (Image courtesy of Peng Li, M.D., University of California, Irvine Medical Center Division of Cardiology.)

with heart failure, it is crucial for the clinician to ask "Why?" Too often patients are simply treated with diuretics with no push to determine the etiology of heart failure. Once valvular heart disease has been excluded, there are several imaging modalities that may assist the clinician in distinguishing ischemic cardiomyopathy from nonischemic cardiomyopathy. These techniques can also assist in identifying those patients with viable myocardium who are most likely to benefit from revascularization therapy.

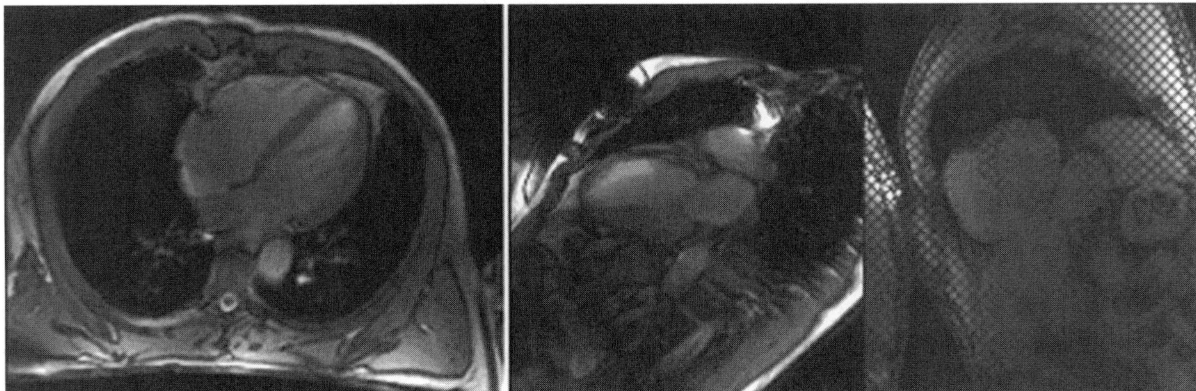

Figure 33-14 CMRI representation of the LV in four-chamber and two-chamber views. Gadolinium contrast appears as a bright white signal while the myocardium appears dark. The **right panel** shows a tagged CMRI representation of the LV. A crosshatched pattern is assigned to each pixel representing the myocardium, which enables study of the several parameters that describe the contractile mechanics of the LV, including LV strain, LV strain rate, and torsion.

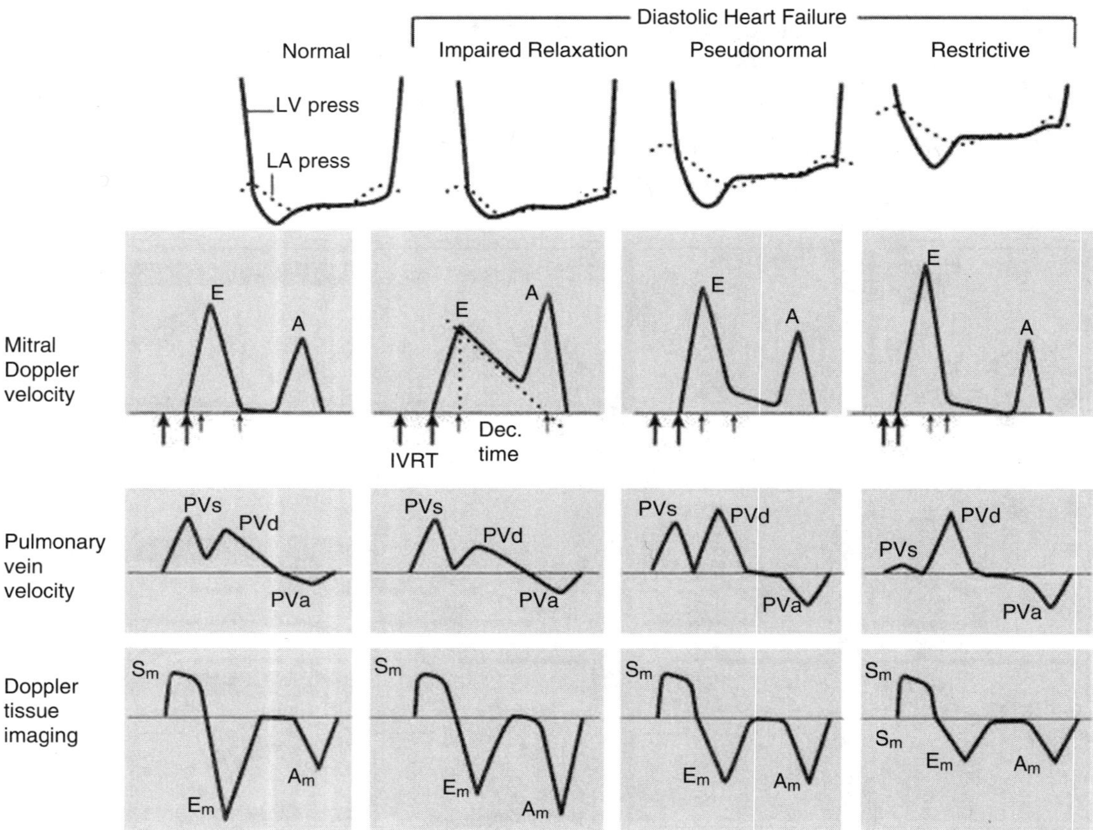

Figure 33-15 Stages of diastolic dysfunction as assessed by Doppler echocardiography. The first stage is characterized by impaired relaxation, and reversal of the E and A signal on the mitral inflow Doppler is seen. As LA pressures rise with worsening diastolic function, the pattern shifts to one of pseudonormalization, where the E/A ratio normalizes. Pulmonary venous Doppler shifts to a diastolic predominant pattern. With severe diastolic dysfunction, a restrictive filling pattern is seen in which the E/A ratio is markedly elevated, and tissue velocities decline as well. Pulmonary venous filling is diastolic-predominant. (Reprinted from Zile MR, Brutsaert DL. New concepts in diastolic dysfunction and diastolic heart failure. Part I: diagnosis, prognosis, and measurements of diastolic function. *Circulation.* 2002;105:1387–1393, with permission.)

Valvular Heart Disease

Every patient presenting with signs and symptoms of congestive heart failure should undergo evaluation for possible valvular heart disease. This is most often done using two-dimensional echocardiography with color flow interrogation of all cardiac valves. The hemodynamic status of the patient can also be evaluated.

Aortic Valve Disease

Aortic stenosis can manifest with congestive heart failure as its presenting syndrome. When patients with severe aortic stenosis present with heart failure symptoms, their prognosis is dismal, with an average unoperated survival of 11 months (49,50). Figure 33-16 shows the mortality in unoperated patients with aortic stenosis presenting with congestive heart failure.

Echocardiography is essential in all patients with suspected aortic stenosis. The most important measurements that the echocardiogram provides are the assessment of the

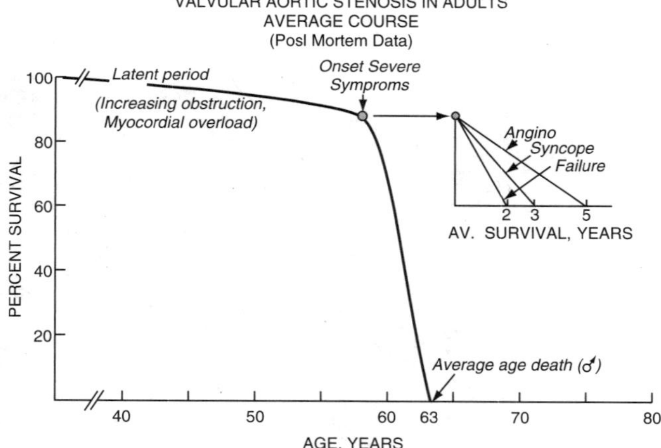

Figure 33-16 Natural history of severe aortic stenosis in unoperated patients. With the onset of symptoms which include there is a progressive, dramatic rise in mortality. Heart failure symptoms are the most ominous, with a median survival of 2 years. (From Ross J Jr., Braunwald E. Aortic stenosis. *Circulation.* 1968;38:61–67, with permission.)

LV systolic function, the estimation of the peak and mean LV-to-aortic gradients, and the evaluation of the aortic valve area (AVA) using the continuity equation, which relates flow through a stenotic orifice to the velocity of blood flow through that orifice and is based on the principle of conservation of mass:

$$A1 \times V1 = A2 \times V2.$$

Substituting the values of the left ventricular outflow tract (LVOT) and AVA and the respective maximum velocities yields the following equation:

$$A_{LVOT} \times V_{LVOT} = AVA \times V_{Ao},$$

where V_{Ao} is the peak veloacity across the aortic valve obtined by continuous wave Doppler.

Solving for AVA yields:

$$AVA = A_{LVOT} \times V_{Ao} / V_{LVOT}.$$

The peak and mean gradients can also be calculated using the modified Bernoulli equation, which relates the peak and mean velocity across the aortic valve to the pressure gradient from left ventricle to aorta.

Echocardiography has been shown to have good accuracy when compared with cardiac catheterization and invasive determination of aortic valve gradient, with a standard error of the estimate of the mean gradient of 10 mm Hg at the best laboratories (51). The accuracy of AVA determination is also quite accurate using echocardiography, with values within 0.3 cm^2 usually obtained (51). Echocardiography can thus provide a noninvasive assessment of hemodynamics and can help guide the clinician's decision to refer for aortic valve replacement. Figure 33-17 shows a continuous-wave Doppler assessment of aortic valve velocity in a patient with severe aortic stenosis.

In patients with severely depressed LV function, echocardiography may underestimate the aortic valve gradient while still showing a very small calculated AVA. In this situation, the calculated AVA may be small due to severe LV dysfunction and inadequate valve opening, or the valve may be truly stenotic. To help clarify this, these patients often require repeat echocardiography during a provocative test, which is usually a dobutamine infusion. Dobutamine increases LV contractility and can unmask a significant gradient (52). In patients with severe aortic stenosis, dobutamine will increase the gradient but will not change the AVA, whereas in those with mild aortic stenosis both the gradient and the AVA will increase.

Magnetic resonance imaging can be of some utility in patients with aortic stenosis. In addition to providing data on LV systolic function, wall thickness, and mass, MRI can be used to precisely determine AVA through planimetry of the aortic valve orifice. Friedrich et al. (53) examined 31 patients with aortic stenosis, comparing measurement of AVA using CMRI, echocardiography, and invasive cardiac catheterization. They found a fair correlation of CMRI measurements with echo measurements ($r = 0.52$) and a better correlation with invasive measurements ($r = 0.78$). Caruthers et al. found similar results while using velocity-encoded CMRI to study 24 patients with aortic stenosis (54). They found a stronger correlation between CMRI velocity-derived AVA and echo-derived AVA ($r = 0.83$). John et al. found similar results with planimetry of the aortic valve (55). Figure 33-18 is an example of the planimetric measurement of orifice area taken from their study.

Aortic regurgitation is frequently asymptomatic in its early stages, but eventually patients present with typical symptoms of LV volume overload and congestive heart failure. The timing of aortic valve replacement is dependent primarily on the presence of symptoms and the degree of LV dilatation. Echocardiography is the primary imaging modality used to quantify the degree of valvular regurgitation.

Mitral Valve Disease

Mitral regurgitation is very common in patients presenting with congestive heart failure. The regurgitation in some cases may be the cause of LV dysfunction, through progres-

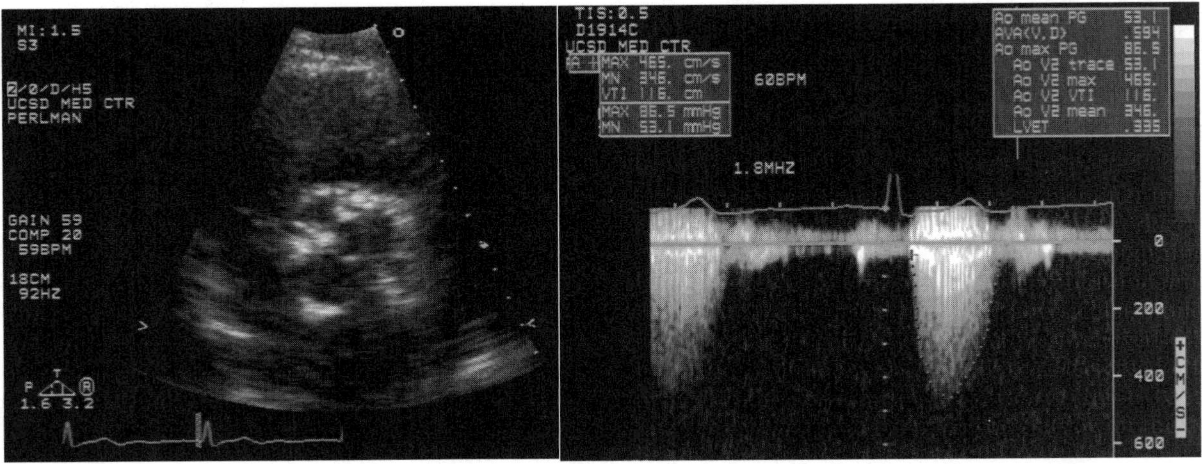

Figure 33-17 Two-dimensional echo images of a patient with severe aortic stenosis. The **left panel** shows a parasternal short-axis image through the aortic valve demonstrating severe calcification of all three cusps. The **right panel** shows a markedly elevated peak velocity of 4.6 m per second across the aortic valve by continuous-wave Doppler, consistent with a peak gradient of 86 mm Hg, a mean gradient of 53 mm Hg, and an aortic valve area of 0.6 cm^2.

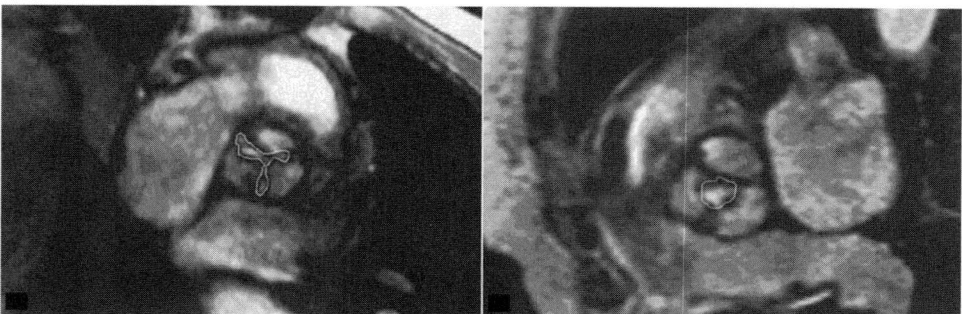

Figure 33-18 CMRIs of a stenotic aortic valve with planimetry of the aortic valve orifice area. The left panel shows a moderately stenotic aortic valve with the white line representing the margin of aortic valve opening. The three-dimensional nature of CMRI enables accurate estimation of aortic valve area with good agreement with echo and catheterization data. (From John AS, Dill T, Brandt RR, et al. Magnetic resonance to assess the aortic valve area in aortic stenosis: how does it compare to current diagnostic standards? *J Am Coll Cardiol.* 2003;42:519–526, with permission.)

sive LV volume overload from the regurgitant lesion. In other instances, remodeling that occurs in patients with pre-existing LV dysfunction can lead to distortion of the papillary muscle apparatus and can result in mitral regurgitation. Mitral stenosis is most commonly caused by rheumatic heart disease and may be amenable to percutaneous balloon valvulotomy or surgical replacement of the mitral valve. Transthoracic and transesophageal echocardiography are the most commonly employed imaging modalities to evaluate mitral stenosis and regurgitation.

Mitral stenosis is best evaluated with transthoracic echocardiography first, with assessment of valve anatomy and functional assessment of the peak and mean gradient. Planimetry of the mitral valve orifice can also be performed. An echo scoring system has been devised to determine suitability of the patient for percutaneous balloon mitral valvulotomy (PBMV) (56). A higher score implies that the patient is a poorer candidate for PBMV. The scoring system, developed by Weyman and Wilkins, is shown in Table 33-3.

The most important echo parameters to evaluate in a patient with mitral regurgitation are LVEDD, LVESD, LA size, and EF. Surgery is often considered when symptoms occur (irrespective of EF) or in an asymptomatic patient when the LVEF is <60% and the LVESD is >45 mm (57). A variety of other methods have been developed to quantify the severity of mitral regurgitation. These include measurement of the vena contracta, calculation of the proximal isovelocity surface area (PISA), assessment for pulmonary venous systolic flow reversal, and measurement of the mitral regurgitant envelope using continuous-wave Doppler (58). Transesophageal echocardiography provides

TABLE 33-3
ECHOCARDIOGRAPHIC SCORING SYSTEM FOR RHEUMATIC MITRAL STENOSIS

Grade	Leaflet Mobility	Subvalvular Thickening	Leaflet Thickening	Leaflet Calcification
0	Normal	Normal	Normal	None
1	Highly mobile valve with only leaflet tips restricted	Minimal thickening just below the mitral leaflets	Leaflets near normal in thickness (4 to 5 mm)	A single area of increased echo brightness
2	Leaflet mid and base portions have normal mobility	Thickening of the chordal structures extending up to one-third of the chordal length	Mid-leaflets normal, considerable thickening of the margins (5 to 8 mm)	Scattered areas of brightness confined to leaflet margins
3	Valve continues to move forward in diastole, mainly from the base	Thickening extending to the distal third of the chords	Thickening extending through the entire leaflet (5 to 8 mm)	Brightness extending into the mid-portion of the leaflets
4	No or minimal forward movement of the leaflets in diastole	Extensive thickening and shortening of all chordal structures extending down to the papillary muscles	Considerable thickening of all leaflet tissue (>8 to10 mm)	Extensive brightness throughout much of the leaflet tissue

Each category is given a score from 0 to 4 and the individual scores are summed to obtain a total score of 0 to 16.
Patients with a valve score of 8 or less tend to have superior outcomes following percutaneous balloon mitral valvulotomy.
Adapted from Wilkins GT, Weyman AE, Abascal VM, et al. Percutaneous balloon dilatation of the mitral valve: an analysis of echocardiographic variables related to outcome and the mechanism of dilatation. *Br Heart J.* 1988;60:299–308, with permission.

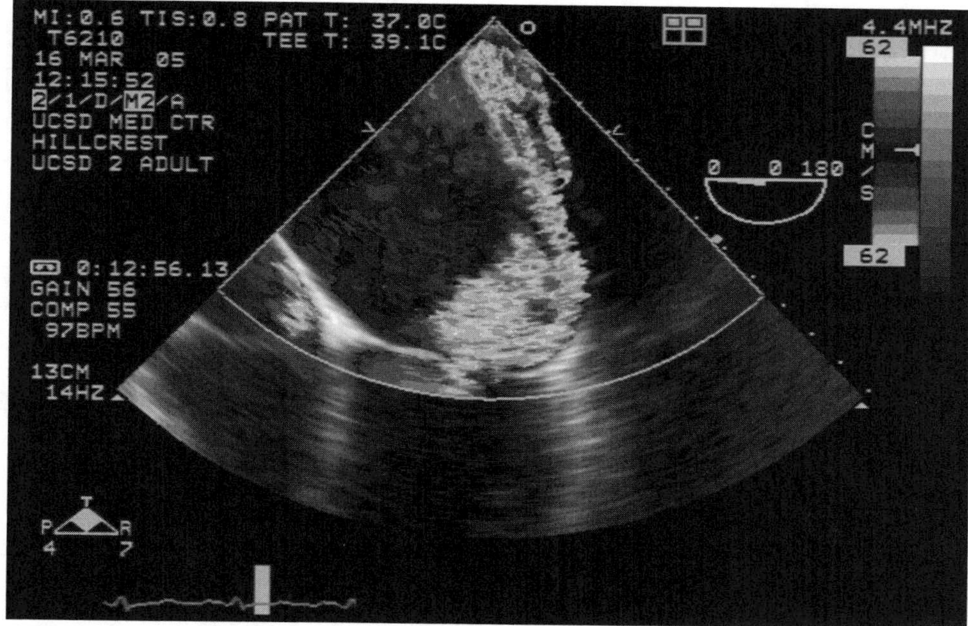

Figure 33-19 Transesophageal echocardiographic color Doppler image of a patient with severe mitral regurgitation. A high-velocity eccentric mitral regurgitant jet is seen tracking posteriorly along the lateral wall of the left atrium into the left superior pulmonary vein. There is marked LA enlargement and a large regurgitant jet diameter.

superior image quality and can be helpful in determining the suitability of the valve for repair, especially if transthoracic images are of inadequate resolution (59). Figure 33-19 shows an image of a transesophageal echocardiogram performed on a patient with severe mitral regurgitation.

Evaluation of Ischemic Heart Disease

One of the earliest assessments that should be made in a patient with new-onset heart failure is the evaluation of significant CAD as the etiology. As described earlier, patients with depressed LV systolic function have the highest mortality from ischemic heart disease, have a higher incidence of ventricular arrhythmias, and benefit the most from revascularization therapy (60,61). The Coronary Artery Surgery Study (CASS) was one of the earliest trials that examined the benefit of bypass surgery over medical therapy in symptomatic patients with CAD (37). In CASS, the benefit of bypass surgery on mortality was the greatest in patients with depressed LV systolic function, defined as an angiographic EF less than 50%. Similar findings were determined in the Veterans Administration cooperative study and European Coronary Surgery Study (62).

Several modalities are available to the clinician for the determination of ischemia, including nuclear scintigraphy, stress echocardiography, and CMRI. These modalities can also be used to detect myocardial viability. This is a critical parameter that must be assessed in patients with heart failure, as patients with significant CAD and viable myocardium are more likely to benefit from revascularization, whereas those with extensive scar and nonviable fibrous tissue are less likely to benefit (63).

Nuclear scintigraphy, in addition to providing volumetric and LV functional assessment in patients with congestive heart failure, also helps to evaluate for ischemic segments and is the most commonly used noninvasive imaging modality to evaluate for the presence of CAD. A radiopharmaceutical (usually Tc-99-sestamibi, Tc-99-tetrofosmin, or Tl-201) is administered to patients at rest and with either mechanical or pharamacologic stress (64). There is differential distribution of the radiopharmaceutical based on coronary stenoses; regions with impaired perfusion are visualized as so-called cold spots with myocardial SPECT imaging. In addition to the evaluation of ischemic burden, nuclear scintigraphy can provide information regarding myocardial viability. As viable myocardium takes up Tl-201 whereas nonviable myocardium does not, 24-hour-delayed imaging can be performed to detect regions of so-called hibernating myocardium. The information provided has diagnostic as well as prognostic value, as patients without scintigraphic evidence of ischemia have a lower incidence of cardiovascular events and mortality than do those with provokable ischemia (65). Figure 33-20 shows an example of a rest-redistribution thallium study in which delayed thallium uptake is clearly seen.

Positron emission tomography (PET) scanning can be of great value in assessing myocardial viability. First, perfusion is assessed using N-13-ammonia, and perfusion defects similar to those obtained using Tl-201 or Tc-99 can be identified. Next, using [18F]-fluorodeoxyglucose (FDG, a metabolic marker for glucose uptake that tracks the transmembrane exchange and phosphorylation of glucose), specific regions of myocardial metabolism can be identified. FDG is taken up by all living myocardial cells and its

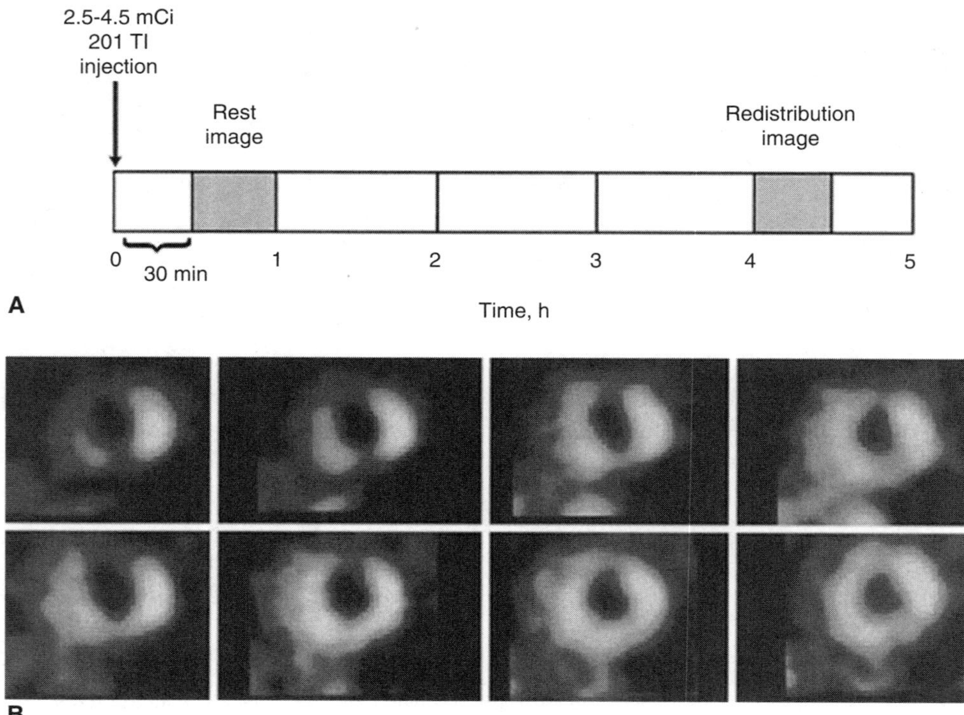

Figure 33-20 Tl-201 image in a patient, demonstrating region of hibernating myocardium in a patient with advanced heart failure. There is a small region in the apical septum that shows redistribution on redistribution thallium imaging. (Adapted from Dilsizian VN, J, ed. *Atlas of Nuclear Cardiology*. Philadelphia: Current Medicine, Inc.; 2003, with permission.)

uptake is therefore a reflection of myocardial viability (64). When used in conjunction with N-13-ammonia imaging, regions of match and mismatch can be identified. As myocardium that is viable yet severely ischemic will not take up N-13 but will take up FDG, these mismatched areas represent regions of viable myocardium that may benefit from revascularization. Figure 33-21 shows an example of a mismatched PET scan, in which a large region of hibernating myocardium can be appreciated.

The resting two-dimensional echocardiogram may provide some clues as to the presence or absence of CAD. The presence of regional wall motion abnormalities such as hypokinesis or akinesis may suggest underlying CAD, especially if they fall in a particular epicardial coronary artery distribution (66). Dobutamine stress echocardiography can also be used to evaluate for an ischemic etiology of LV dysfunction and has powerful prognostic ability in the assessment of patients with heart failure (67–69). In one study, high-dose (40 μg/kg per minute) dobutamine stress echocardiography was successful in identifying patients with CAD when there were two or more myocardial segments with an ischemic response or a scar, with 100% sensitivity and 86% specificity. The presence of more than six akinetic or dyskinetic segments raises the specificity to 96% for an ischemic etiology of the cardiomyopathy (70). Myocardial viability can be assessed by starting the protocol with low-dose dobutamine (5 μg/kg per minute). Viable myocardial segments can show a biphasic response to dobutamine, with improvement in contraction with low-dose dobutamine and a worsening of contraction with high-dose dobutamine (71). The impact of viability assessment by dobutamine stress-echocardiography on the mortality benefit of revascularization is shown in Figure 33-22.

CMRI has emerged as a powerful imaging modality to evaluate the etiology of heart failure and evaluate for myocardial ischemia and viability. Ischemia assessment is done through dobutamine stress-MRI, in which a patient undergoes a staged protocol similar to dobutamine stress echocardiography (72). Cine-MR images are taken at baseline and during the peak heart rate achieved with dobutamine. The presence of stress-induced wall motion abnormalities represents a positive test. In preliminary studies, the sensitivity of dobutamine stress-MRI has ranged from 86% to 91% (72–75).

Viability assessment is performed using delayed gadolinium-enhanced contrast MRI, which is effective in identifying regions of scarred, nonviable myocardium. In one study examining patients with known ischemic or dilated cardiomyopathy, MRI was very effective in identifying patients with CAD, with a 100% sensitivity (76). Another study used delayed-contrast MRI prospectively to evaluate patients with heart failure of unknown etiology with no history of CAD. Overall, there was a sensitivity of 81%, a specificity of 91%, and a diagnostic accuracy of 87% in determining the presence of obstructive CAD (77).

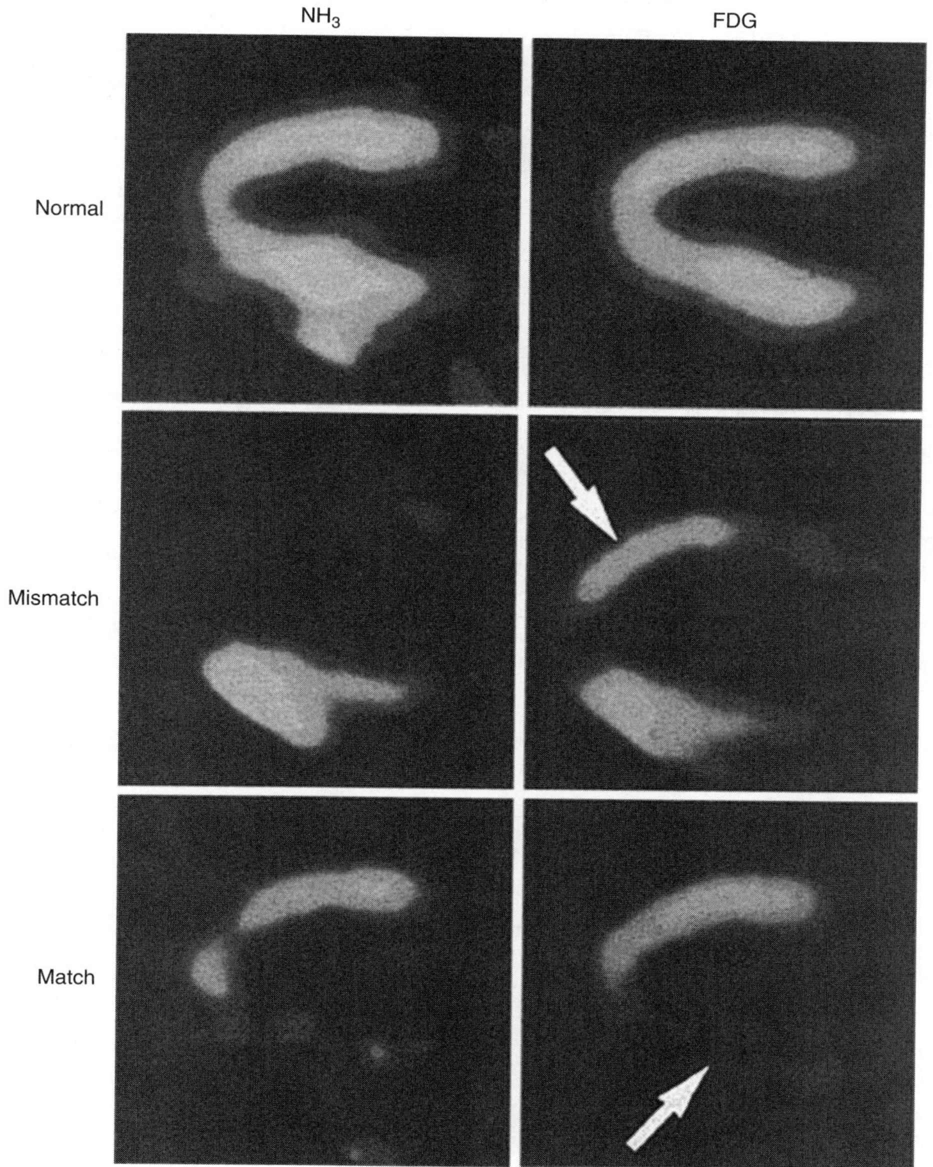

Figure 33-21 Positron emission tomography (PET) scan in three patients, two of whom had SPECT perfusion defects. Top panels shows normal perfusion and metabolism, with normal uptake of NH3 and FDG. Middle panels show anterior NH3 perfusion defect with intact FDG metabolism (arrow), a metabolism-perfusion mismatch suggestive of viable and hibernating myocardium. Lower panels show marched defects in perfusion and metabolism in the inferior wall (**arrow**) suggestive of nonviable scar. (Adapted from Dilizian VN, Narula J, eds. *Atlas of Nuclear Cardiology*. Philadelphia: Current Medicine, Inc., 2003, with permission.)

Perhaps the greatest utility of CMRI is in the assessment of myocardial viability. In patients undergoing revascularization, the presence of segmental hyperenhancement makes it less likely that a given segment of myocardium will recover contractile function if revascularized (78). Figure 33-23 presents the results of a study by Kim et al. (79), which shows an incremental decline in contractile recovery following revascularization with increasing degrees of hyperenhancement. Figure 33-24 shows representative contrast-MRI images of a patient with extensive delayed hyperenhancement involving the septum and anterior wall.

Inflammatory/Infiltrative Heart Disease

Myocarditis

A third category of diseases that can lead to progressive ventricular dysfunction is the inflammatory and infiltrative cardiomyopathies. Acute myocarditis is the prototypical inflammatory cardiomyopathy and can lead to rapidly progressive ventricular dysfunction and death. Coxsackie virus has been implicated in its etiology and pathogenesis (81). Echocardiography can demonstrate ventricular systolic

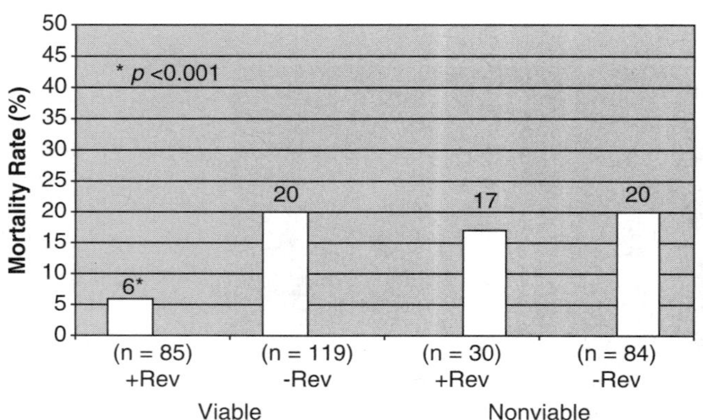

Figure 33-22 Effect of viability assessed by dobutamine-stress echocardiography on mortality rate following subsequent revascularization. Patients with viable myocardium who underwent revascularization had a substantially lower mortality than those who were managed medically, whereas patients with nonviable myocardium had similar outcomes regardless of therapy. (Modified from Afridi I, Grayburn PA, Panza JA, et al. Myocardial viability during dobutamine echocardiography predicts survival in patients with coronary artery disease and severe left ventricular systolic dysfunction. *J Am Coll Cardiol.* 1998;32:921–926, with permission.)

dysfunction that occurs as a result of this disease but lacks the specificity to readily distinguish between acute and chronic ventricular decompensation. Molecular imaging techniques to image the antigen-antibody complexes, such as antimyosin antibody imaging, have shown promise in identifying patients with endomyocardial biopsy-proven myocarditis (82). Figure 33-25 shows an example of antimyosin antibody imaging.

Recent data have also shown that CMRI is useful in the diagnosis of acute myocarditis. Abdel-Aty et al. have shown that an increase in T2 signal intensity coupled with an increased global relative early enhancement (gRE) and an increase in areas of late gadolinium enhancement (LGE) is highly specific for myocarditis (83). The technique had a 76% sensitivity, 95.5% specificity, and 85% diagnostic accuracy for the detection of clinically proven myocarditis. CMRI has also shown promise in distinguishing acute myocardial infarction from myocarditis in patients presenting with chest pain (84).

Restrictive Cardiomyopathy

Restrictive cardiomyopathy is a rare but important cause of heart failure with preserved systolic function. Cardiac

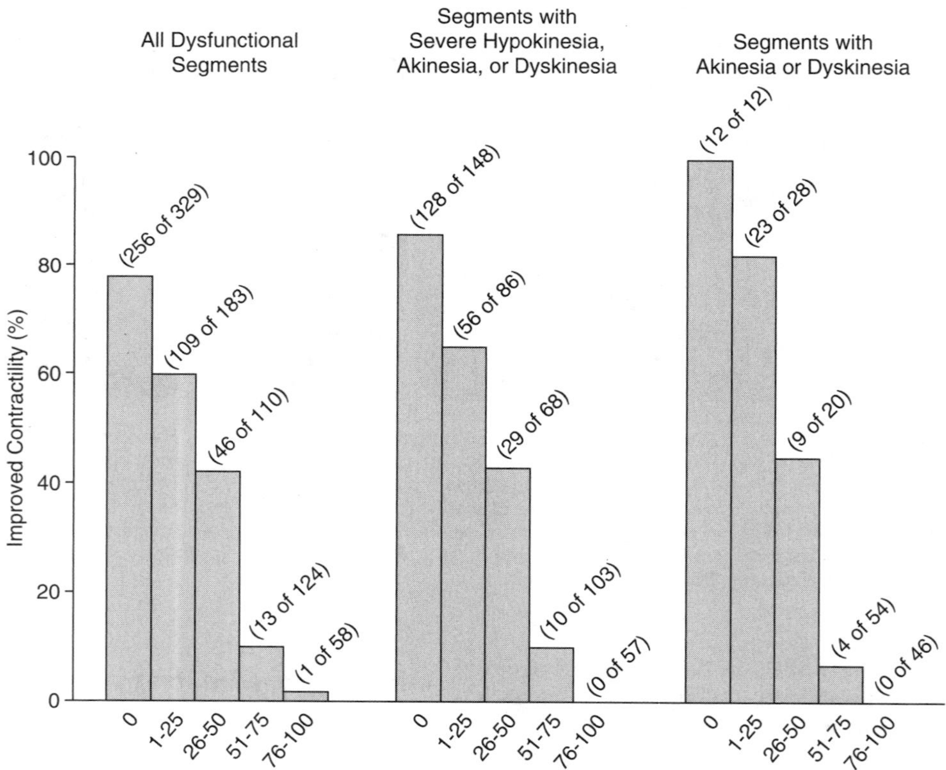

Figure 33-23 Relationship between preoperative transmural extent of hyperenhancement and postoperative functional contractile recovery in 50 patients referred for surgical or percutaneous revascularization. The degree of hyperenhancement was inversely related to the degree of functional recovery, establishing CMRI as a powerful means of assessing myocardial viability. (From Kim RJ, Wu E, Rafael A, et al. The use of contrast-enhanced magnetic resonance imaging to identify reversible myocardial dysfunction. *N Engl J Med.* 2000;343:1445–1453, with permission.)

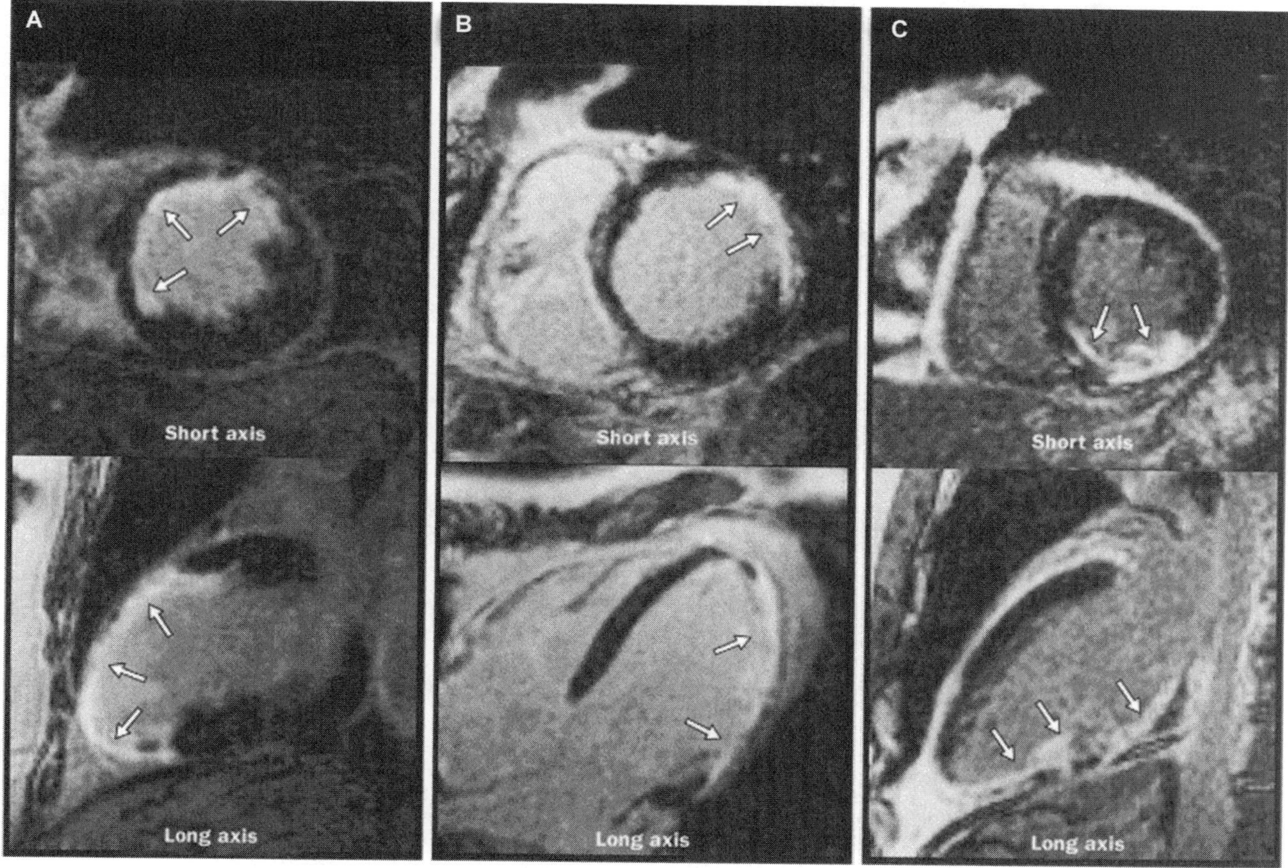

Figure 33-24 Contrast-MRI images of three patients with large anterior (**left panel**), lateral (**middle panel**), and inferior (**right panel**) myocardial infarcts. Delayed-enhancement imaging delineates the regions of scar, which appear bright white. (From Wu E, Judd RM, Vargas JD, et al. Visualisation of presence, location, and transmural extent of healed Q-wave and non-Q-wave myocardial infarction. *Lancet.* 2001;357:21–28, with permission.)

amyloidosis is the prototypical form of restrictive cardiomyopathy. It is caused by a systemic paraproteinemia and the resultant intramyocardial deposition of protein light chains (85). Clinical heart failure is a late finding and is characterized by severe diastolic dysfunction and initially preserved systolic function. Echocardiography in cardiac amyloidosis and other infiltrative disorders typically reveals ventricular hypertrophy with a speckled appearance of the myocardium (86). There is usually preserved LV systolic function with markedly impaired diastolic function. Transmitral Doppler usually reveals a restrictive filling pattern and tissue Doppler imaging shows poor movement of the mitral annulus during ventricular diastole (87,88). There are distinct findings on CMRI that may help identify patients with cardiac amyloidosis. In a recent study by Maceira and Pennell, patients with cardiac amyloidosis had a characteristic pattern on CMRI of global subendocardial late enhancement as well as abnormal myocardial and blood-pool gadolinium kinetics (89). Figure 33-26 shows a CMRI of a patient with cardiac amyloidosis.

Imaging of Associated Pathogenetic Phenomena

Norepinephrine (NE), a vital neurotransmitter in both the central and peripheral nervous systems, is produced in the cytoplasm of sympathetic neurons by dopamine beta-hydroxylase (DBH)-mediated oxidation of dopamine and is stored in vesicles via the action of vesicular monoamine transporter (90). In heart failure, it is believed that both increased neuronal release of NE and decreased efficiency of neuronal NE transporters contribute to decreased myocardial NE content, which correlates with the decrease in LVEF that is seen clinically (91–94).

The diminished NE uptake that occurs in human heart failure can be imaged using iodine-131-meta-iodobenzylguanidine (MIBG), a radiopharmaceutical that is also a functional NE analog. MIBG imaging involves a two-step protocol, with early imaging after MIBG injection followed by delayed imaging in 4 or more hours. The late images are specific for the relative distribution of sympathetic nerve terminals, while the washout rate represents the neuronal function.

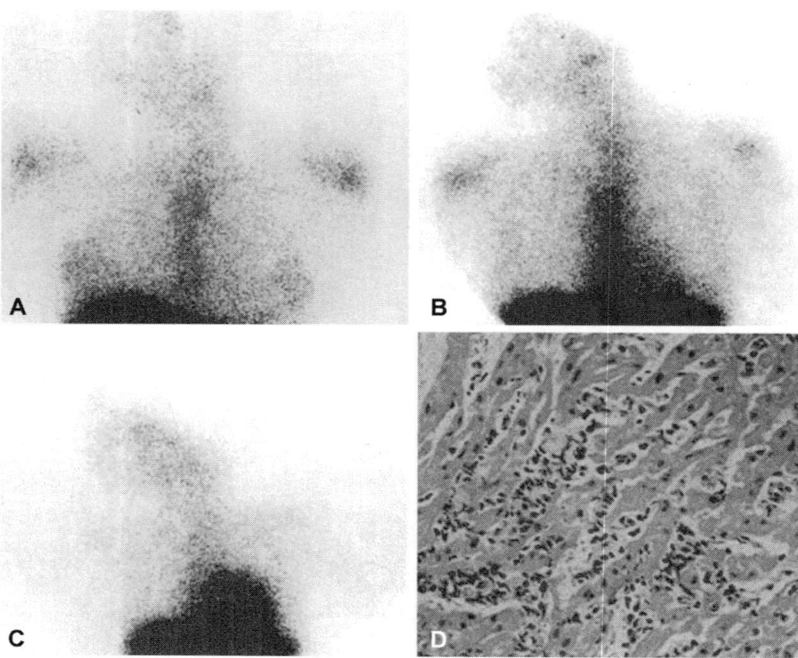

Figure 33-25 Antimyosin antibody imaging in three patients with suspected myocarditis. Patient A shows the absence of myocardial antimyosin uptake in a scan with normal findings. Patient B shows moderate myocardial antimyosin uptake, consistent with myocarditis, while Patient C shows intense myocardial antimyosin uptake; this patient had biopsy-proven myocarditis. **(D)** is the RV endomyocardial biopsy showing a central focus of necrotic myocytes surrounded by a lymphocytic infiltrate that is diagnostic of myocarditis. (From Martin ME, Moya-Mur JL, Casanova M, et al. Role of noninvasive antimyosin imaging in infants and children with clinically suspected myocarditis. *J Nucl Med.* 2004;45:429–437, with permission.)

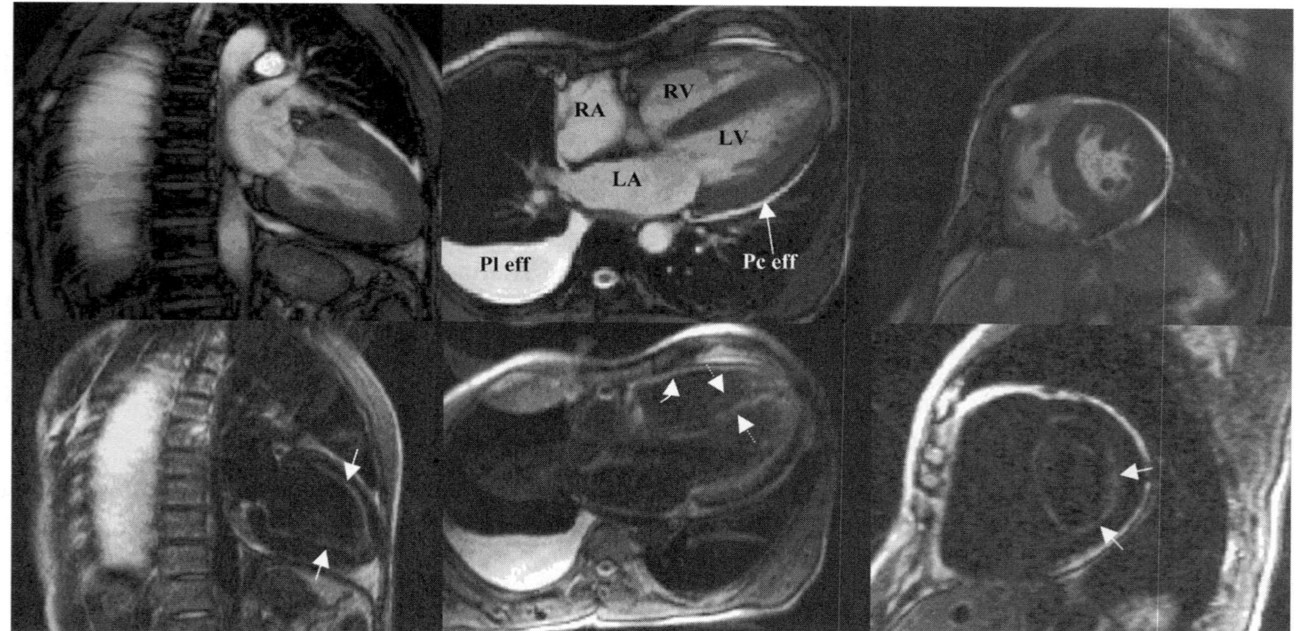

Figure 33-26 CMRI of a patient with systemic light chain (AL) amyloidosis. **Top row** shows vertical long-axis, horizontal long-axis, and short-axis views from diastolic cine frames. The LV is thickened with evidence of pleural and pericardial effusions. The **bottom row** shows late gadolinium enhancement in the same planes. A thin rim of subendocardial delayed enhancement is seen and is thought to be the region of cardiac amyloid infiltration. (From Maceira AM, Joshi J, Prasad SK, et al. Cardiovascular magnetic resonance in cardiac amyloidosis. *Circulation.* 2005;111:186–193, with permission.)

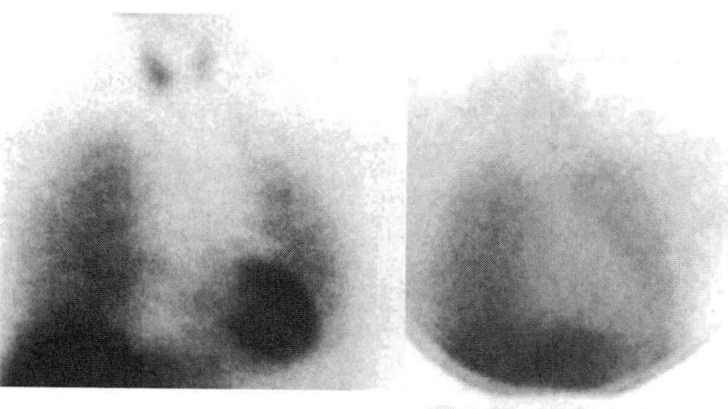

Figure 33-27 Conventional I-123 planar MIBG imaging. Comparison of MIBG uptake in normal myocardium (**left**) with failing myocardium (**right**). There is a marked reduction in MIBG uptake in precordial region in the failing heart. Decline in MIBG uptake correlates with mortality and increases in MIBG uptake correlate with improvements on medical therapy.

Multiple studies have demonstrated that impaired cardiac sympathetic innervation, assessed by MIBG uptake, has valuable potential for predicting adverse clinical outcome, including ventricular arrhythmia and mortality in heart failure patients (95–97). It has been further shown that MIBG uptake improves in response to effective treatment of heart failure (98–100). Figure 33-27 shows an MIBG imaging study in both a normal patient and one with advanced heart failure.

REFERENCES

1. Pouleur HG, Konstam MA, Udelson JE, et al. Changes in ventricular volume, wall thickness and wall stress during progression of left ventricular dysfunction. The SOLVD Investigators. *J Am Coll Cardiol.* 1993;22:43A–48A.
2. St. John Sutton M, Pfeffer MA, Plappert T, et al. Quantitative two-dimensional echocardiographic measurements are major predictors of adverse cardiovascular events after acute myocardial infarction. The protective effects of captopril. *Circulation.* 1994;89:68–75.
3. Pfeffer MA, Braunwald E, Moye LA, et al. Effect of captopril on mortality and morbidity in patients with left ventricular dysfunction after myocardial infarction. Results of the Survival and Ventricular Enlargement trial. The SAVE Investigators. *N Engl J Med.* 1992;327:669–677.
4. Popovic AD, Neskovic AN, Pavlovski K, et al. Association of ventricular arrhythmias with left ventricular remodelling after myocardial infarction. *Heart.* 1997;77:423–427.
5. Quinones MA, Greenberg BH, Kopelen HA, et al. Echocardiographic predictors of clinical outcome in patients with left ventricular dysfunction enrolled in the SOLVD registry and trials: significance of left ventricular hypertrophy. Studies of Left Ventricular Dysfunction. *J Am Coll Cardiol.* 2000;35: 1237–1244.
6. Konstam MA, Rousseau MF, Kronenberg MW, et al. Effects of the angiotensin converting enzyme inhibitor enalapril on the long-term progression of left ventricular dysfunction in patients with heart failure. SOLVD Investigators. *Circulation.* 1992;86:431–438.
7. Hayakawa M, Yokota Y, Kumaki T, et al. Clinical significance of left ventricular hypertrophy in dilated cardiomyopathy: an echocardiographic follow-up of 50 patients. *J Cardiogr.* 1984;14:115–123.
8. Feigenbaum H, Armstrong WF, Ryan T. *Feigenbaum's Echocardiography.* 6th ed. Philadelphia: Lippincott Williams & Wilkins; 2005.
9. Schvartzman PR, Fuchs FD, Mello AG, et al. Normal values of echocardiographic measurements. A population-based study. *Arq Bras Cardiol.* 2000;75:107–114.
10. Casale PN, Devereux RB, Milner M, et al. Value of echocardiographic measurement of left ventricular mass in predicting cardiovascular morbid events in hypertensive men. *Ann Intern Med.* 1986;105:173–178.
11. Levy D, Garrison RJ, Savage DD, et al. Prognostic implications of echocardiographically determined left ventricular mass in the Framingham Heart Study. *N Engl J Med.* 1990;322:1561–1566.
12. Jenkins C, Bricknell K, Hanekom L, et al. Reproducibility and accuracy of echocardiographic measurements of left ventricular parameters using real-time three-dimensional echocardiography. *J Am Coll Cardiol.* 2004;44:878–886.
13. Germano G, Kiat H, Kavanagh PB, et al. Automatic quantification of ejection fraction from gated myocardial perfusion SPECT. *J Nucl Med.* 1995;36:2138–2147.
14. Iskandrian AE, Germano G, VanDecker W, et al. Validation of left ventricular volume measurements by gated SPECT 99mTc-labeled sestamibi imaging. *J Nucl Cardiol.* 1998;5:574–578.
15. Dilsizian VN, Narula J, ed. *Atlas of Nuclear Cardiology.* Philadelphia: Current Medicine, Inc.; 2003.
16. Anand IS, Florea VG, Solomon SD, et al. Noninvasive assessment of left ventricular remodeling: concepts, techniques, and implications for clinical trials. *J Card Fail.* 2002;8:S452–S464.
17. Sharir T, Germano G, Kavanagh PB, et al. Incremental prognostic value of post-stress left ventricular ejection fraction and volume by gated myocardial perfusion single photon emission computed tomography. *Circulation.* 1999;100:1035–1042.
18. The SOLVD Investigators. Effect of enalapril on survival in patients with reduced left ventricular ejection fractions and congestive heart failure. *N Engl J Med.* 1991;325:293–302.
19. Ostrzega E, Maddahi J, Honma H, et al. Quantification of left ventricular myocardial mass in humans by nuclear magnetic resonance imaging. *Am Heart J.* 1989;117:444–452.
20. Sakuma H, Fujita N, Foo TK, et al. Evaluation of left ventricular volume and mass with breath-hold cine MR imaging. *Radiology.* 1993;188:377–380.
21. Matsuda M, Matsuda Y. Mechanism of left atrial enlargement related to ventricular diastolic impairment in hypertension. *Clin Cardiol.* 1996;19:954–959.
22. Wang Y, Gutman JM, Heilbron D, et al. Atrial volume in a normal adult population by two-dimensional echocardiography. *Chest.* 1984;86:595–601.
23. Rossi A, Cicoira M, Zanolla L, et al. Determinants and prognostic value of left atrial volume in patients with dilated cardiomyopathy. *J Am Coll Cardiol.* 2002;40:1425.
24. Moller JE, Hillis GS, Oh JK, et al. Left atrial volume: a powerful predictor of survival after acute myocardial infarction. *Circulation.* 2003;107:2207–2212.
25. Raman SV, Ng VY, Neff MA, et al. Volumetric cine CMR to quantify atrial structure and function in patients with atrial dysrhythmias. *J Cardiovasc Magn Reson.* 2005;7:539–543.
26. Sievers B, Kirchberg S, Addo M, et al. Assessment of left atrial volumes in sinus rhythm and atrial fibrillation using the biplane area-length method and cardiovascular magnetic resonance imaging with TrueFISP. *J Cardiovasc Magn Reson.* 2004;6:855–863.
27. Di Salvo TG, Mathier M, Semigran MJ, et al. Preserved right ventricular ejection fraction predicts exercise capacity and survival in advanced heart failure. *J Am Coll Cardiol.* 1995;25:1143–1153.
28. de Groote P, Millaire A, Foucher-Hossein C, et al. Right ventricular ejection fraction is an independent predictor of survival in patients with moderate heart failure. *J Am Coll Cardiol.* 1998;32:948–954.
29. Zornoff LA, Skali H, Pfeffer MA, et al. Right ventricular dysfunction and risk of heart failure and mortality after myocardial infarction. *J Am Coll Cardiol.* 2002;39:1450–1455.
30. Thohan V. Prognostic implications of echocardiography in advanced heart failure. *Curr Opin Cardiol.* 2004;19:238–249.
31. Rajappan K, Livieratos L, Camici PG, et al. Measurement of ventricular volumes and function: a comparison of gated PET and cardiovascular magnetic resonance. *J Nucl Med.* 2002;43:806–810.
32. Grothues F, Moon JC, Bellenger NG, et al. Interstudy reproducibility of right ventricular volumes, function, and mass with cardiovascular magnetic resonance. *Am Heart J.* 2004;147: 218–223.
33. Costard-Jackle A, Fowler MB. Influence of preoperative pulmonary artery pressure on mortality after heart transplantation: testing of potential reversibility of pulmonary hypertension with nitroprusside is useful in defining a high risk group. *J Am Coll Cardiol.* 1992;19:48–54.

34. Enriquez-Sarano M, Rossi A, Seward JB, et al. Determinants of pulmonary hypertension in left ventricular dysfunction. *J Am Coll Cardiol.* 1997;29:153–159.
35. Cohn JN, Johnson GR, Shabetai R, et al. Ejection fraction, peak exercise oxygen consumption, cardiothoracic ratio, ventricular arrhythmias, and plasma norepinephrine as determinants of prognosis in heart failure. The V-HeFT VA Cooperative Studies Group. *Circulation.* 1993;87:VI5–V16.
36. Edner M, Bonarjee VV, Nilsen DW, et al. Effect of enalapril initiated early after acute myocardial infarction on heart failure parameters, with reference to clinical class and echocardiographic determinants. CONSENSUS II Multi-Echo Study Group. *Clin Cardiol.* 1996;19:543–548.
37. Coronary Artery Surgery Study (CASS): a randomized trial of coronary artery bypass surgery. Comparability of entry characteristics and survival in randomized patients and nonrandomized patients meeting randomization criteria. *J Am Coll Cardiol.* 1984;3:114–128.
38. Solomon SD, Zelenkofske S, McMurray JJ, et al. Sudden death in patients with myocardial infarction and left ventricular dysfunction, heart failure, or both. *N Engl J Med.* 2005;352:2581–2588.
39. Moss AJ, Zareba W, Hall WJ, et al. Prophylactic implantation of a defibrillator in patients with myocardial infarction and reduced ejection fraction. *N Engl J Med.* 2002;346:877–883.
40. Cintron G, Johnson G, Francis G, et al. Prognostic significance of serial changes in left ventricular ejection fraction in patients with congestive heart failure. The V-HeFT VA Cooperative Studies Group. *Circulation.* 1993;87:VI17–V123.
41. Carr JC, Simonetti O, Bundy J, Li D, et al. Cine MR angiography of the heart with segmented true fast imaging with steady-state precession. *Radiology.* 2001;219:828–834.
42. Zerhouni EA, Parish DM, Rogers WJ, et al. Human heart: tagging with MR imaging—a method for noninvasive assessment of myocardial motion. *Radiology.* 1988;169:59–63.
43. Aletras AH, Ding S, Balaban RS, et al. DENSE: Displacement Encoding with Stimulated Echoes in cardiac functional MRI. *J Magn Reson.* 1999;137:247–252.
44. Senni M, Tribouilloy CM, Rodeheffer RJ, et al. Congestive heart failure in the community: a study of all incident cases in Olmsted County, Minnesota, in 1991. *Circulation.* 1998;98:2282–2289.
45. Appleton CP, Firstenberg MS, Garcia MJ, et al. The echo-Doppler evaluation of left ventricular diastolic function. A current perspective. *Cardiol Clin.* 2000;18:513–546, ix.
46. Vasan RS, Larson MG, Benjamin EJ, et al. Congestive heart failure in subjects with normal versus reduced left ventricular ejection fraction: prevalence and mortality in a population-based cohort. *J Am Coll Cardiol.* 1999;33:1948–1955.
47. Zile MR, Brutsaert DL. New concepts in diastolic dysfunction and diastolic heart failure: Part I: diagnosis, prognosis, and measurements of diastolic function. *Circulation.* 2002;105: 1387–1393.
48. Oxenham HC, Young AA, Cowan BR, et al. Age-related changes in myocardial relaxation using three-dimensional tagged magnetic resonance imaging. *J Cardiovasc Magn Reson.* 2003; 5:421–430.
49. Horstkotte D, Loogen F. The natural history of aortic valve stenosis. *Eur Heart J.* 1988;9(Suppl E):57–64.
50. Ross J, Jr., Braunwald E. Aortic stenosis. *Circulation.* 1968;38:61–67.
51. Rahimtoola S. Perspective on valvular heart disease: Update II. In: Knoebel S, ed. *An Era in Cardiovascular Medicine.* New York: Elsevier; 1991: 45–70.
52. Nishimura RA, Grantham JA, Connolly HM, et al. Low-output, low-gradient aortic stenosis in patients with depressed left ventricular systolic function: the clinical utility of the dobutamine challenge in the catheterization laboratory. *Circulation.* 2002;106:809–813.
53. Friedrich MG, Schulz-Menger J, Poetsch T, et al. Quantification of valvular aortic stenosis by magnetic resonance imaging. *Am Heart J.* 2002;144:329–334.
54. Caruthers SD, Lin SJ, Brown P, et al. Practical value of cardiac magnetic resonance imaging for clinical quantification of aortic valve stenosis: comparison with echocardiography. *Circulation.* 2003;108:2236–2243.
55. John AS, Dill T, Brandt RR, et al. Magnetic resonance to assess the aortic valve area in aortic stenosis: how does it compare to current diagnostic standards? *J Am Coll Cardiol.* 2003;42:519–526.
56. Wilkins GT, Weyman AE, Abascal VM, et al. Percutaneous balloon dilatation of the mitral valve: an analysis of echocardiographic variables related to outcome and the mechanism of dilatation. *Br Heart J.* 1988;60:299–308.
57. Otto CM. Timing of surgery in mitral regurgitation. *Heart.* 2003;89:100–105.
58. Keeffe BG, Otto CM. Mitral regurgitation. *Minerva Cardioangiol.* 2003;51:29–39.
59. Irvine T, Li XK, Sahn DJ, Kenny A. Assessment of mitral regurgitation. *Heart* 2002;88(Suppl 4):iv11–iv19.
60. Letsou GV. Selection of appropriate patients with heart failure for aortocoronary bypass surgery. *Curr Opin Cardiol.* 1999;14: 230–233.
61. Nishi H, Miyamoto S, Takanashi S, et al. Complete revascularization in patients with severe left ventricular dysfunction. *Ann Thorac Cardiovasc Surg.* 2003;9:111–116.
62. Bonow RO, Epstein SE. Indications for coronary artery bypass surgery in patients with chronic angina pectoris: implications of the multicenter randomized trials. *Circulation.* 1985;72: V23–V30.
63. Afridi I, Grayburn PA, Panza JA, et al. Myocardial viability during dobutamine echocardiography predicts survival in patients with coronary artery disease and severe left ventricular systolic dysfunction. *J Am Coll Cardiol.* 1998;32:921–926.
64. Hachamovitch R, Berman DS. The use of nuclear cardiology in clinical decision making. *Semin Nucl Med.* 2005;35:62–72.
65. Sharir T, Germano G, Kang X, et al. Prediction of myocardial infarction versus cardiac death by gated myocardial perfusion SPECT: risk stratification by the amount of stress-induced ischemia and the poststress ejection fraction. *J Nucl Med.* 2001;42: 831–837.
66. Medina R, Panidis IP, Morganroth J, et al. The value of echocardiographic regional wall motion abnormalities in detecting coronary artery disease in patients with or without a dilated left ventricle. *Am Heart J.* 1985;109:799–803.
67. Biagini E, Elhendy A, Bax JJ, et al. Seven-year follow-up after dobutamine stress echocardiography: impact of gender on prognosis. *J Am Coll Cardiol.* 2005;45:93–97.
68. Duncan AM, Francis DP, Gibson DG, et al. Differentiation of ischemic from nonischemic cardiomyopathy during dobutamine stress by left ventricular long-axis function: additional effect of left bundle-branch block. *Circulation.* 2003;108: 1214–1220.
69. Liao L, Cabell CH, Jollis JG, et al. Usefulness of myocardial viability or ischemia in predicting long-term survival for patients with severe left ventricular dysfunction undergoing revascularization. *Am J Cardiol.* 2004;93:1275–1279.
70. Vigna C, Russo A, De Rito V, et al. Regional wall motion analysis by dobutamine stress echocardiography to distinguish between ischemic and nonischemic dilated cardiomyopathy. *Am Heart J.* 1996;131:537–543.
71. Armstrong WF, Zoghbi WA. Stress echocardiography: current methodology and clinical applications. *J Am Coll Cardiol.* 2005;45: 1739–1747.
72. Pennell DJ, Underwood SR, Manzara CC, et al. Magnetic resonance imaging during dobutamine stress in coronary artery disease. *Am J Cardiol.* 1992;70:34–40.
73. Baer FM, Voth E, Theissen P, et al. Gradient-echo magnetic resonance imaging during incremental dobutamine infusion for the localization of coronary artery stenoses. *Eur Heart J.* 1994;15: 218–225.
74. Nagel E, Lehmkuhl HB, Bocksch W, et al. Noninvasive diagnosis of ischemia-induced wall motion abnormalities with the use of high-dose dobutamine stress MRI: comparison with dobutamine stress echocardiography. *Circulation.* 1999;99: 763–770.
75. van Rugge FP, van der Wall EE, Spanjersberg SJ, et al. Magnetic resonance imaging during dobutamine stress for detection and localization of coronary artery disease. Quantitative wall motion analysis using a modification of the centerline method. *Circulation.* 1994;90:127–138.
76. McCrohon JA, Moon JC, Prasad SK, et al. Differentiation of heart failure related to dilated cardiomyopathy and coronary artery disease using gadolinium-enhanced cardiovascular magnetic resonance. *Circulation.* 2003;108:54–59.

77. Soriano CJ, Ridocci F, Estornell J, et al. Noninvasive diagnosis of coronary artery disease in patients with heart failure and systolic dysfunction of uncertain etiology, using late gadolinium-enhanced cardiovascular magnetic resonance. *J Am Coll Cardiol.* 2005;45:743–748.
78. Elliott MD, Kim RJ. Late gadolinium cardiovascular magnetic resonance in the assessment of myocardial viability. *Coron Artery Dis.* 2005;16:365–372.
79. Kim RJ, Wu E, Rafael A, et al. The use of contrast-enhanced magnetic resonance imaging to identify reversible myocardial dysfunction. *N Engl J Med.* 2000;343:1445–1453.
80. Wu E, Judd RM, Vargas JD, et al. Visualisation of presence, location, and transmural extent of healed Q-wave and non-Q-wave myocardial infarction. *Lancet.* 2001;357:21–28.
81. Badorff C, Knowlton KU. Dystrophin disruption in enterovirus-induced myocarditis and dilated cardiomyopathy: from bench to bedside. *Med Microbiol Immunol.* (Berlin) 2004;193: 121–126.
82. Martin ME, Moya-Mur JL, Casanova M, et al. Role of noninvasive antimyosin imaging in infants and children with clinically suspected myocarditis. *J Nucl Med.* 2004;45:429–437.
83. Abdel-Aty H, Boye P, Zagrosek A, et al. Diagnostic performance of cardiovascular magnetic resonance in patients with suspected acute myocarditis: comparison of different approaches. *J Am Coll Cardiol.* 2005;45:1815–1822.
84. Laissy JP, Hyafil F, Feldman LJ, et al. Differentiating acute myocardial infarction from myocarditis: diagnostic value of early- and delayed-perfusion cardiac MR imaging. *Radiology* 2005;237(1):75–82.
85. Kholova I, Niessen HW. Amyloid in the cardiovascular system: a review. *J Clin Pathol.* 2005;58:125–133.
86. Bhandari AK, Nanda NC. Myocardial texture characterization by two-dimensional echocardiography. *Am J Cardiol.* 1983;51: 817–825.
87. Oki T, Tanaka H, Yamada H, et al. Diagnosis of cardiac amyloidosis based on the myocardial velocity profile in the hypertrophied left ventricular wall. *Am J Cardiol.* 2004;93: 864–869.
88. Sallach JA, Klein AL. Tissue Doppler imaging in the evaluation of patients with cardiac amyloidosis. *Curr Opin Cardiol.* 2004;19: 464–471.
89. Maceira AM, Joshi J, Prasad SK, et al. Cardiovascular magnetic resonance in cardiac amyloidosis. *Circulation.* 2005;111:186–193.
90. Runkel F, Bruss M, Nothen MM, et al. Pharmacological properties of naturally occurring variants of the human norepinephrine transporter. *Pharmacogenetics.* 2000;10:397–405.
91. Beau SL, Saffitz JE. Transmural heterogeneity of norepinephrine uptake in failing human hearts. *J Am Coll Cardiol.* 1994;23: 579–585.
92. Bohm M, La Rosee K, Schwinger RH, et al. Evidence for reduction of norepinephrine uptake sites in the failing human heart. *J Am Coll Cardiol.* 1995;25:146–153.
93. Rose CP, Burgess JH, Cousineau D. Reduced aortocoronary sinus extraction of epinephrine in patients with left ventricular failure secondary to long-term pressure or volume overload. *Circulation.* 1983;68:241–244.
94. Rose CP, Burgess JH, Cousineau D. Tracer norepinephrine kinetics in coronary circulation. of patients with heart failure secondary to chronic pressure and volume overload. *J Clin Invest.* 1985;76:1740–1747.
95. Merlet P, Benvenuti C, Moyse D, et al. Prognostic value of MIBG imaging in idiopathic dilated cardiomyopathy. *J Nucl Med.* 1999;40:917–923.
96. Merlet P, Valette H, Dubois-Rande JL, et al. Prognostic value of cardiac metaiodobenzylguanidine imaging in patients with heart failure. *J Nucl Med.* 1992;33:471–477.
97. Schofer J, Spielmann R, Schuchert A, et al. Iodine-123 meta-iodobenzylguanidine scintigraphy: a noninvasive method to demonstrate myocardial adrenergic nervous system disintegrity in patients with idiopathic dilated cardiomyopathy. *J Am Coll Cardiol.* 1988;12:1252–1258.
98. Kakuchi H, Sasaki T, Ishida Y, et al. Clinical usefulness of 123I meta-iodobenzylguanidine imaging in predicting the effectiveness of beta blockers for patients with idiopathic dilated cardiomyopathy before and soon after treatment. *Heart.* 1999;81:148–152.
99. Matsui T, Tsutamoto T, Maeda K, et al. Prognostic value of repeated 123I-metaiodobenzylguanidine imaging in patients with dilated cardiomyopathy with congestive heart failure before and after optimized treatments—comparison with neurohumoral factors. *Circ J.* 2002;66: 537–543.
100. Momose M, Kobayashi H, Iguchi N, et al. Comparison of parameters of 123I-MIBG scintigraphy for predicting prognosis in patients with dilated cardiomyopathy. *Nucl Med Commun.* 1999;20:529–535.

Management of Acute and Decompensated Heart Failure

34

Gary S. Francis   W. H. Wilson Tang

The pharmacologic management of acute heart failure has evolved considerably since the last edition of this textbook. We now have more information about the demographics of the syndrome (1), the potential hazards of routine short-term (48-hour) milrinone use (2), the availability of nesiritide to manage these patients in emergency department (ED) and step-down cardiac units (3), and a firm recognition that worsening renal function leads to poor outcomes (4). It is also now widely recognized that the design of clinical trials necessary to support the approval of new drugs for the treatment of acute heart failure is more complex than was previously believed. What outcomes should be measured in these clinical trials and when should they be measured? This has vexed both clinical investigators and regulatory agencies. With the emphasis appropriately placed on clinical outcomes rather than physiological and hemodynamic surrogate measurements, it has become increasingly difficult to successfully gain approval of new drugs for the treatment of acute heart failure. So there is good news and bad news: We know more about patients with acute heart failure but there are few new therapies available to manage these acutely ill patients.

DEMOGRAPHICS

Approximately 1 million patients were hospitalized in 2004 in the United States with acute heart failure, costing more than $14.7 billion (5). About 50% of patients admitted with acute heart failure are readmitted within 6 months (6). Patients admitted to the hospital for acute heart failure have a 12% mortality at 30 days and a 33% mortality at 12 months (7). About 80% of patients hospitalized for heart failure are over 65 years of age (8). The combination of a rapidly expanding elderly population and the precarious financial grounding of many hospitals will continue to challenge us to develop more creative management strategies for patients with acute heart failure. Some EDs have clinical decision units where patients can be treated and stabilized over 24 to 48 hours, occasionally obviating the need for hospitalization or the need for a stay in the intensive care unit. In fact, most patients admitted to the hospital with acute heart failure in 2005 went to telemetry units with only about 15% going to the intensive care unit, according to the large ADHERE (Acute Decompensated Heart Failure National) registry (8).

Despite these demographics, it is estimated that approximately 1 million hospitalizations occur each year in the United States for treatment of acute heart failure (primary diagnosis). Another 2.5 million hospitalizations occur with heart failure as a secondary diagnosis (5). This results in about 6.5 million hospital days per year designated in the United States for acute heart failure. The admissions have increased more than 150% over the past two decades (5), undoubtedly related to growth of the aging population.

The ADHERE registry indicates that the in-hospital mortality for acute heart failure averages about 5% to 8%, with the 1-year mortality rate following hospitalization as high as 40% to 60% (9). Nearly 20% of patients admitted for treatment for acute heart failure are readmitted within 30 days of discharge. Tissue and circulatory congestion are overwhelmingly present in patients admitted with acute heart failure. Many have associated hypertension on admission. In ADHERE, only 3% of admissions have a systolic blood pressure below 90 mm Hg (9). Patients presenting with low-output heart failure are distinctly unusual, whereas preserved left ventricular ejection fration and high blood pressure are common (~40%). The typical patient is about 75 years old, has acute decompensation of previously stable chronic heart failure (~70%), has had a previous hospitalization for heart failure (~50%), and has documented coronary artery disease (57%) and hypertension (73%) (9). About 20% have atrial fibrillation. The median length of hospital stay for acute heart failure in the United States is about 4 days. In ADHERE, a blood urea nitrogen (BUN) >43 mg/dL, blood pressure <115 mm Hg, and a serum creatinine >2.75 mg/dL were independently associated with death during hospitalization (10).

The pathophysiology of heart failure is very complex and is discussed extensively in Part I of this textbook. A fundamental feature of acute heart failure is reduced stroke volume in the setting of increased left ventricular end-diastolic pressure (Fig. 34-1). There is excessive neuroendocrine activation (Fig. 34-2), adding to heightened peripheral vascular resistance, salt and water retention, and impaired cardiac output. The relatively high blood pressure, low cardiac output, and increased resistance are ideal targets for a combination of vasodilator therapy and an intravenous loop diuretic, the usual early therapeutic strategy for patients with acute heart failure. These have remained the cornerstones of therapy but with some new twists added.

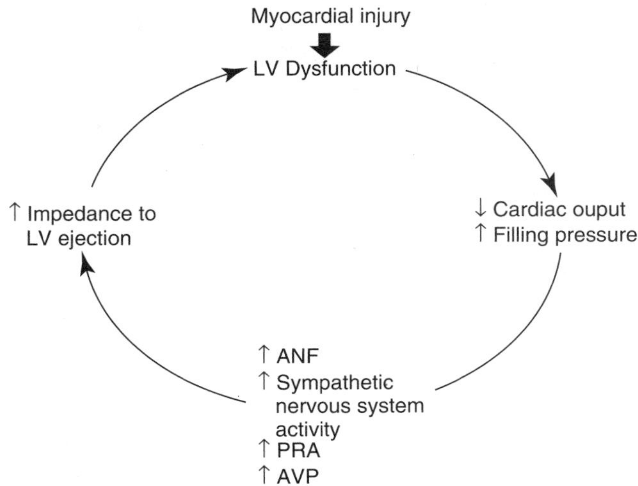

Figure 34-2 Heart failure is a complex clinical syndrome characterized by extensive neuroendocrine activation. The release of neurohormones appears to be in response to reduced cardiac function and a perceived reduction in effective circulatory volume. It is as if neuroendocrine activity is attempting to protect the blood pressure and maintain circulatory homeostasis. Although this may be adaptive early on, chronic neuroendocrine activation leads to peripheral vasoconstriction, left ventricular remodeling, and worsening left ventricular performance, and thus becomes an attractive therapeutic target. Drugs designed to block the exuberant neuroendocrine response, such as ACE inhibitors, have now become the cornerstone of treatment for heart failure.

RECOGNITION OF THE PATIENT IN NEED OF URGENT HOSPITALIZATION: WHAT ARE THE PRECIPITATING FACTORS?

Patients with acute heart failure are invariably short of breath, often to the point where they cannot give a detailed history due to severe dyspnea. The vast majority of patients are congested (i.e., they have findings of acute pulmonary edema, such as tachypnea, desaturation, rales, and abnormal chest X-ray, and often other tissue congestion). However, the differential diagnosis of severe dyspnea is expansive; this symptom can be due to severe asthma or an exacerbation of chronic obstructive pulmonary disease. Thus, establishing the diagnosis of heart failure can be difficult (11). At the time of presentation, usually in the ED, the patient with suspected acute heart failure should have a careful physical examination, a chest X-ray, an electrocardiogram (ECG), and possibly evaluation of plasma B-type natriuretic peptide (BNP) level if the diagnosis is ambiguous. A plasma BNP level <100 pg/mL suggests an alternative diagnosis and unlikely acute heart failure (12,13). BNP as a diagnostic test is most valuable when there is uncertainty about the diagnosis in the ED setting; it is of less value in patients with more chronic, stable heart failure where false negatives may commonly occur (14).

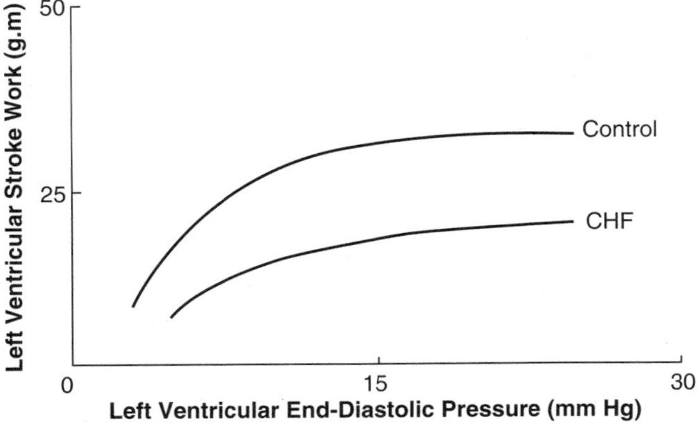

Figure 34-1 The classic manifestation of heart failure remains an inadequate inotropic response to heightened contractile element fiber stretch, usually manifested clinically as a reduced stroke work in response to an increase in left ventricular end-diastolic volume or pressure. For any given preload, the failing ventricle fails to eject a normal stroke volume—Starling's law of the heart. However, our understanding of heart failure has moved well beyond this simple model of pump dysfunction. The diminished stroke volume (and cardiac output) both acutely and chronically activate a series of neuroendocrine responses that remain a powerful force in the long-term prognosis of patients. Incidentally, there is no descending limb operative in the intact circulation because severe mitral regurgitation ensues as left ventricular volume reaches a critical point.

Recently, an assay to the measurement of plasma N-terminal moiety of proBNP (NTproBNP) has also become available as a diagnostic test. The cut-off values are different than for BNP, and individual plasma NTproBNP levels may not necessarily correlate well with plasma BNP levels.

Acute Myocardial Infarction

It is important that physicians caring for patients with heart failure be thoroughly familiar with the factors that

TABLE 34-1
FACTORS LEADING TO ACUTE DECOMPENSATION OF HEART FAILURE

Acute myocardial ischemia
Poorly treated or untreated high blood pressure
New-onset atrial fibrillation or other sustained arrhythmia
Use of negative inotropic drugs such as verapamil, nifedipine, diltiazem, β-adrenergic blockers
Use of nonsteroidal anti-inflammatory drugs (NSAIDs)
Excessive use of alcohol
Endocrine abnormalities (poorly controlled diabetes mellitus, hyperthyroidism, etc.)
Medication and Na^+ noncompliance; lack of information regarding diet, medications, etc.
Concurrent infections such as pneumonia, influenza, etc.

contribute to acute decompensation (Table 34-1). Evidence of acute or intercurrent myocardial ischemia should always be sought. When hospitalization is being considered for such a patient, a 12-lead ECG should always be performed and thoroughly examined with reference to previous ECG tracings when available. Each patient must be carefully queried with regard to possible underlying myocardial ischemia, although this can be a difficult distinction to make clinically.

It may be problematic in the elderly population to make a clear distinction between increased breathlessness from worsening heart failure and increased shortness of breath from acute myocardial ischemia. Older patients are well-known to have more atypical angina and their only manifestation of myocardial ischemia may be shortness of breath. Nevertheless, acute myocardial ischemia is a potentially reversible cause of worsening heart failure and should be investigated and excluded when possible.

Hypertension

Data from the ADHERE registry indicate that the vast majority of patients have severe hypertension on the arrival to the hospital ED with acute heart failure. Low blood pressure is distinctly uncommon. The high blood pressure may be an acute response to severe breathlessness, oxygen desaturation, and to the anxiety of acute pulmonary edema. The massive release of epinephrine and norepinephrine in patients with acute pulmonary edema (personal observations) appears to contribute significantly to the elevation in blood pressure, and diaphoresis, breathlessness, orthopnea, and diaphoresis are the rule. Prompt control of blood pressure is critically important.

Because the failing ventricle is exquisitely sensitive to afterload stress, it is possible that even a modest increase in blood pressure can initiate worsening mitral regurgitation or lead to a direct reduction in myocardial performance. Once severe pulmonary edema ensues, the anxiety and catecholamine excess often produce extreme hypertension, even in the face of what was previously thought to be remarkably reduced left ventricular function. In such cases, aggressive management of hypertension should be initiated as soon as possible. Patients with impending or obvious acute pulmonary edema who manifest breathlessness and hypertension should undergo transfer to an intensive care unit setting where intravenous nitroprusside or another IV vasodilator can be started. One should avoid using short-acting calcium-channel blockers such as sublingual nifedipine to restore normal blood pressure in this setting. Short-acting calcium-channel blockers may cause precipitous hypotension and have been associated with worsening left ventricular function (15,16). The overriding principle is that even modest elevations in blood pressure can lead to acute decompensation of chronic heart failure and therefore should be treated aggressively. In many cases, hospitalization is advised and expeditious, exquisite control of high blood pressure (and mitral regurgitation) with nitroprusside (or even sublingual or chewable nitroglycerin if hemodynamic monitoring is not available) (17) is the preferred strategy. We have less experience with nesiritide in this setting, although other experts in the field advocate its use.

New Onset of Rapid Atrial Fibrillation

New onset of atrial fibrillation is well-known to cause acute cardiac decompensation in a previously stable patient with heart failure (18). Often this is a product of inadequate control of heart rate. In virtually every large study, about 15% to 25% of patients with chronic ambulatory heart failure demonstrate atrial fibrillation (19). Although this may be well-tolerated by patients when it is chronic and the heart rate is well-controlled, the new onset of rapid atrial fibrillation is very often poorly tolerated and represents a medical emergency for some patients. When new-onset, rapid atrial fibrillation is encountered in the out-patient clinic in a patient with heart failure and worsening symptoms, the proper strategy is to transfer the patient to an acute care setting and consider direct-current (DC) cardioversion after precipitating factors such as hypokalemia have been corrected. The temptation to use intravenous diltiazem or digoxin simply to control heart rate in such patients should be avoided (20), as it is clearly more expeditious and definitive to restore normal sinus rhythm with DC cardioversion. The patient should be systemically anticoagulated with heparin, if not already adequately anticoagulated with warfarin. Class I antiarrhythmic agents should be avoided (21), as they have a high failure rate and can worsen left ventricular function. If the patient cannot be easily cardioverted or fails to remain in sinus rhythm, control of heart rate then becomes the primary therapeutic goal. Intravenous digoxin may be helpful in acute rate control (22). For many such patients, amiodarone will become a necessary component of therapy (23). Catheter ablation is also increasingly utilized as a therapeutic strategy for prevention of acute exacerbations in refractory atrial fibrillation (24).

The need to acutely anticoagulate such patients is highly dependent on the urgency of correcting the rapid atrial fibrillation. If the patient has obvious hemodynamic deterioration or severe pulmonary edema, it is more prudent to directly proceed with DC cardioversion than to attempt to optimize the anticoagulant status. Most cardiologists would give intravenous heparin or low-molecular-weight heparin if there are no contraindications (25). In general, it is believed that if the atrial fibrillation is of 48 hours or less in duration, chronic anticoagulation with warfarin may not be necessary (26,27). There is increasing use of transesophageal echocardiography to rule out the presence of thrombus in the left atrial appendage prior to cardioversion in stable patients with atrial fibrillation (28). Nevertheless, a common strategy is to acutely anticoagulate such patients with intravenous heparin and simultaneously employ long-term warfarin therapy, knowing that recurrent atrial fibrillation is a distinct possibility and the presence of heart failure adds to the risk of thromboembolism in the setting of atrial fibrillation (27). Aspirin is not as effective as warfarin in patients with atrial fibrillation (25).

Drug-Induced Heart Failure

A careful drug inventory should be performed in every case of acute decompensation of heart failure. Family members or close friends of the patient are valuable sources of information in this regard. A search should be made for possible recent use or increase in dose of negative inotropic drugs such as verapamil, nifedipine, diltiazem, antiarrhythmics, doxorubicin, or in some cases β-adrenergic blockers. Thiazolidinediones have also been noted to cause fluid retention. Nonsteroidal anti-inflammatory drugs (NSAIDs) are also well-known to provoke worsening heart failure and renal insufficiency (29). They should be considered as possible inciting factors for causing acute decompensation, given their common over-the-counter use by elderly patients. In general, β-adrenergic blockers should be continued at the present dose if the patient is taking them chronically, unless there is a severe low-output state, cardiogenic shock, or a recent increase in dose that may have precipitated worsening heart failure.

Additional Inciting Factors

Excessive alcohol consumption and endocrine abnormalities such as uncontrolled diabetes mellitus, hyperthyroidism, and hypothyroidism should always be excluded or vigorously treated when present. Concurrent infections such as pneumonia and viral illnesses commonly cause acute decompensation of previously stable heart failure and should be ruled out or treated when present. Sodium-laden antibiotics such as imipenem/cilastatin may worsen an already established volume-overloaded state. Sometimes heart failure exacerbations may occur shortly following ventricular arrhythmia, especially after firing of an implantable cardioverter defibrillator (ICD).

Information about medication and dietary compliance should be sought. We now know that many patients do not even fill the prescriptions provided to them by physicians, and drug compliance continues to be a major problem. This is partly due to the high cost and low reimbursement for expensive new therapies. It is not uncommon for patients to fail to renew the prescription for necessary ongoing treatment therapies.

One of the most important safeguards against acute decompensation remains frequent and comprehensive out-patient assessment of the patient by the heart failure team, which should establish a certain degree of bonding and trust between the physician/team and the patient. Such a relationship cannot be assumed after a single visit or two; it requires close and continued surveillance of such fragile patients. Referral to a heart failure program may reduce both symptoms and costs (30–32). Daily weights, measurement of daily dietary sodium intake, and physical activity should be carefully monitored and discussed during clinic visits when the patient is stable and feeling well. Easy access to heart failure nurses and cardiologists is an essential ingredient for keeping potentially decompensated patients out of the hospital.

That being said, there have also been recent studies that challenged the perceived benefits and cost-effectiveness of heart failure disease management clinics (33,34). Most importantly, patients must be continually educated with regard to their diet, activity level, and knowledge of signs and symptoms of decompensation. Even though medical experts may not necessarily agree on criteria of when to admit an individual patient to the hospital for acute decompensation, general principles and guidelines regarding this issue should be discussed beforehand with patients and their families. Patients should be given information about the natural history of the heart failure syndrome and should understand that repeated hospitalizations for acute decompensations may sometimes be necessary.

The importance of dietary sodium restriction cannot be overstated. Often patients are given very little advice about dietary sodium restriction, and salt indiscretion is always a possible consideration as a cause for acute decompensation. For example, the most common cause of diuretic resistance is excessive dietary sodium (34). Because almost half of the patients admitted to the hospital with heart failure will be readmitted in 6 months (36), educational efforts in this regard are likely to have substantial payoff in reducing the need for subsequent hospitalizations for acute decompensation (37). As with most medical disorders, prevention is far and away the best therapeutic strategy when it can be rationally employed. The time for lengthy discussions with patients and their families is not during acute decompensation of a chronic illness but, rather, during the calm of a routine ambulatory clinic visit when the patient is feeling reasonably well. It is at this time that serious discussion regarding diet, medications, prognosis, living wills, resuscitation status, and possible entry into clinical trials studies should be addressed in detail.

WHEN TO HOSPITALIZE THE PATIENT WITH ACUTE HEART FAILURE

The need for hospitalization during acute decompensation of heart failure is always somewhat judgmental and involves close interaction among the attending physician, the heart failure team, the patient, and the patient's family (Table 34-2). The average length of stay for decompensated heart failure in the United States is 4 days (9) but it seems to be trending down. Although hospitalization is clearly the most expensive component of care for patients with heart failure, much of the expense is up-front—in the first few days of hospitalization. Therefore, keeping the patient in the hospital an extra day or two may actually be far more cost-effective than initiating highly expensive home health care to expedite premature discharge from the hospital. Readmission of prematurely discharged patients is more costly than extending the hospital stay slightly to ensure proper clinical stability. Indications for hospitalization of patients with acute decompensation include those described in the following paragraphs.

Clinical or Electrocardiographic Evidence of Acute Myocardial Ischemia or Infarction

Patients who have ECG evidence of acute myocardial ischemia should always be placed in the intensive care unit or coronary care unit. Sequential echocardiograms and serial enzymes or troponin levels should be monitored to exclude acute myocardial necrosis. In some cases, important diagnostic and prognostic information can be gained from coronary arteriography (38). In general, the superimposition of acute myocardial ischemia on severe chronic heart failure will impose an additional intolerable burden, and the possibility of reperfusion therapy (including both percutaneous techniques such as angioplasty and stenting) and coronary artery bypass surgery should always be explored.

TABLE 34-2
WHEN SHOULD PATIENTS BE ADMITTED TO THE HOSPITAL FOR ACUTE DECOMPENSATION OF HEART FAILURE?

Onset of acute myocardial ischemia
Pulmonary edema or increasing respiratory distress
Oxygen saturation below 90% not caused by pulmonary disease
Complicating medical illnesses
Symptomatic hypotension or syncope
Heart failure refractory to out-patient treatment
Anasarca
Inadequate out-patient social support system

Pulmonary Edema or Increasing Respiratory Distress

Patients who are seen in the emergency room, on the hospital ward, or in the out-patient clinic with increasing dyspnea or impending pulmonary edema are candidates to be admitted to the acute care unit. Even in the absence of rales and edema, worsening shortness of breath accompanied by an increase in respiratory rate may be a forewarning of impending pulmonary edema. In some cases, further decompensation fails to develop but, nonetheless, such patients benefit from a thorough investigation as to why their symptoms are changing; they may require changes in their medical therapy. Intimate knowledge of the patient's previous course is obviously very helpful in deciding whether to admit to the hospital.

Hypoxia Independent of Pulmonary Disease

When patients complain of shortness of breath and have hypoxemia with an oxygen saturation less than 90%, hospitalization is usually necessary. Patients with stable, ambulatory heart failure are rarely this hypoxemic during the day unless they have concomitant lung disease. Tachypnea and desaturation are signs of impending pulmonary edema and it seems prudent to admit such patients to the hospital for further care.

Severe Complicating Medical Illnesses

It is not uncommon for patients with chronic heart failure, particularly the elderly, to acutely decompensate with the development of a complicating medical illness. Pneumonia is the classic example, but even a flulike illness may precipitate acute decompensation in a patient with marginally compensated heart failure. Influenza, bacterial infection, and severely decompensated endocrine disorders such as hyperthyroidism and hypothyroidism and diabetes mellitus are all indications to consider hospitalization in patients with heart failure.

Symptomatic Hypotension or Syncope

Patients with heart failure who develop symptomatic hypotension or frank syncope have a poor prognosis, even if it is determined that the symptoms are not directly a consequence of their heart disease (39). This must be distinguished from mildly symptomatic hypotension, which can occur with the use of potent diuretics, angiotensin-converting enzyme (ACE) inhibitors, and β-adrenergic blockers. There is a difference between mild, intermittent lightheadedness and severe lightheadedness or syncope. If the symptoms are mild and are easily attributable to volume depletion and/or ACE inhibitor therapy, it is possible that a reduction in diuretic dose or temporary withdrawal of ACE inhibitor might be sufficient to prevent the need for hospitalization. On the other hand, when it is unclear what the nature of the lightheadedness might be, or if it is severe with the patient nearly passing out or experiencing syncope, the consequences can be serious and the patient should be hospitalized. The risk of sudden death is high in patients with heart failure who have either cardiac or unexplained causes of syncope (40,41), and inpatient electrophysiological evaluation is often indicated. Bradyarrhythmias, tachyarrhythmias, drug-induced hypotension, and vasodepressor syncope need to be considered. In some cases, an ICD should be considered.

Heart Failure Refractory to Out-Patient Treatment

An experienced physician caring for the patient with heart failure can usually determine when the patient is becoming refractory to therapy. Nevertheless, this clinical dilemma can sometimes pose difficulty with regard to the need for hospitalization and whether the patient should be admitted to the general hospital service or requires intensive care. As a general principle, when patients are simply not doing well, are anxious, and one senses apprehension on the part of the patient and the family, it is reasonable to consider hospitalization. The greater the amount of uncertainty as to the precise nature of the problem, the more likely the patient is going to benefit from hospitalization in the intensive care unit with insertion of a pulmonary artery (or Swan-Ganz) catheter and possibly an indwelling arterial catheter. Often patients will tell their physicians that they simply are unable to prevent weight gain or have increasing breathlessness and remain extremely fatigued despite an uptitration of diuretics. In many cases patients will insist that they have been highly compliant with their medications and diet, yet are declining in well-being. Clearly, some patients will benefit from short-term hospitalization, including the temporary use of intravenous vasodilators (e.g., nesiritide or nitroprusside) and/or positive inotropic support.

Often the single most intense complaint of patients with decompensated heart failure is inability to sleep soundly. The insomnia is not necessarily caused by paroxysmal nocturnal dyspnea or orthopnea but, rather, is an inability to fall into a sound and sustained sleep and is accompanied by profound fatigue the following day. Sleep disorders, including central and obstructive apnea, are common in heart failure and can lead to occasional severe oxygen desaturation at night. Nocturnal O_2, continuous positive airway pressure (CPAP), and theophylline have all been used to treat sleep apnea in patients with heart failure. For patients with severe sleep deprivation, hospitalization is advised. Although the precise mechanism of this complaint is sometimes unclear (similar to loss of appetite), it may be a nonspecific response to markedly altered homeostasis and, in our experience, can be associated with impending acute hemodynamic decompensation.

Anasarca

Patients who present with severe peripheral edema and anasarca are generally best treated as in-patients. Continuous intravenous loop diuretics and daily metolazone are sometimes necessary, although the risk of electrolyte disturbances and renal insufficiency heightens with this regimen. In our experience it has been exceedingly difficult to manage such patients in an out-patient setting. They seem to benefit greatly from bed rest, high-dose intravenous diuretics, and temporary vasodilator or inotropic support. Bed rest alone may improve renal blood flow, thereby augmenting the diuretic and vasodilator/inotropic drug effects.

Inadequate Social Support for Safe Out-Patient Management

There are many patients for whom signs and symptoms of heart failure fail to improve because the social support and home situation are simply not suitable. Elderly patients who are unable to care for themselves, patients who cannot weigh themselves, have no access to the telephone, and have no control over their dietary needs are candidates for acute decompensation of chronic heart failure. In many cases, it is best to admit such patients to the hospital and, during the hospitalization, arrange for the patient to have a more structured out-patient support system when possible.

MANAGEMENT OF PATIENTS WITH ACUTELY DECOMPENSATED HEART FAILURE

Patients with severely decompensated heart failure can be difficult to manage. Certain goals of treatment should be considered and patients and their families should be informed of the treatment options. Following admission to the hospital, the precipitating cause of the acute decompensation should be identified and corrected when possible.

Another important goal is to improve hemodynamics. It is not necessary to normalize the hemodynamic profile of the patient with heart failure. In severely ill patients, a pulmonary artery catheter (PAC) should be inserted along with a Foley catheter and, in some cases, an arterial catheter in order to carefully assess the baseline hemodynamic picture. The primary goal should be decongestion of the patient. The results of the Evaluation Study of Congestive Heart Failure and Pulmonary Artery Catheterization Effectiveness (ESCAPE) trial suggest that, while routine use of a PAC is not indicated, there is no incremental risk of using a PAC in critically ill patients admitted for acutely decompensated heart failure (ADHF) (42). Our practice is still to use PACs in patients who are hemodynamically unstable, or in whom the left ventricular filling pressure is uncertain, or in those with oliguria or anuria. Patients in shock should also have a PAC inserted.

Routine laboratory determinations should include hemoglobin, white blood cell count, platelet count, serum electrolytes, blood sugar, liver function tests, BUN, and serum creatinine. A chest X-ray and an EKG should be performed, and usually an echo if there is no prior knowledge of myocardial performance. Depending on the clinical picture, measurement of thyroid function and arterial blood gases (ABGs) should be considered. Patients who are tachypneic or in clinical respiratory distress in whom intubation and ventilatory support are a consideration should have ABGs checked. ABGs should also be measured prior to bilevel positive airway pressure (Bi-PAP) when one anticipates monitoring the response to therapy.

The physical examination may be misleading (43–45), particularly in patients with chronic heart failure. Results from the Candesartan in Heart Failure Assessment of Reduction in Mortality and morbidity (CHARM)-preserved study demonstrate that patients with heart failure and preserved systolic function often have physical findings that are similar to patients with heart failure due to systolic dysfunction. Low blood pressure and a narrow pulse pressure correlate with a low cardiac index, but the presence or absence of rales is not particularly helpful (44). Even when the pulmonary capillary wedge pressure is in excess of 33 mm Hg, rales may be absent in patients with chronic heart failure due to the compensating changes that develop in the lungs over time. Ascites is also difficult to determine at the bedside and ultrasonography is recommended in questionable cases (45).

Diagnostic Considerations

The initial cardiac output and pulmonary capillary wedge pressure in patients admitted with decompensated heart failure are highly variable (Fig. 34-3). In general, one would expect the pulmonary capillary wedge pressure to be in excess of 20 mm Hg in conjunction with a cardiac index less than 2.5 L/min/m^2, but this is not always the case. Many patients demonstrate volume depletion and low cardiac filling pressures. The echo may indicate normal or supernormal ejection-phase indexes, a finding that supports the diagnosis of diastolic heart failure. Patients with diastolic heart failure often have left ventricular hypertrophy or mitral regurgitation (46,47). Elderly women with systemic hypertension and/or diabetes are typical candidates for diastolic heart failure.

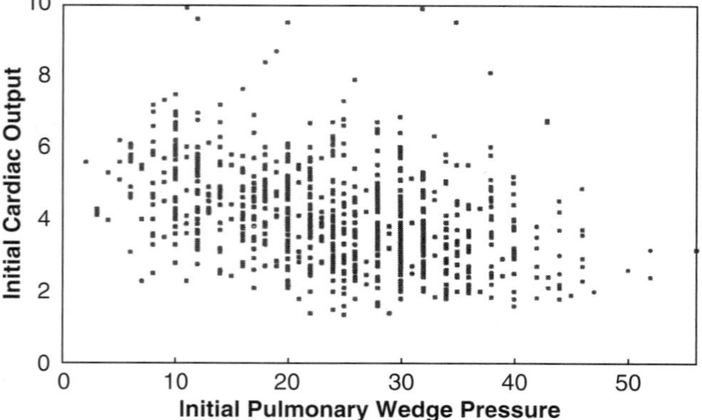

Figure 34-3 These data represent 700 patients referred for possible heart transplantation. The average ejection fraction is 22%. Note the marked heterogeneity in the presenting hemodynamic profile, with a large segment of patients demonstrating a normal pulmonary capillary wedge pressure and some having cardiac outputs between 8 and 10 L per minute. The hemodynamic profile cannot always be easily predicted by the history and physical examination. (From Stevenson LW. Tailored therapy before transplantation for treatment of advanced heart failure: effective use of vasodilators and diuretics. *J Heart Lung Transplant*. 1991;10:468–476, with permission.)

Patients with so-called diastolic heart failure or heart failure with preserved left ventricular function may make up more than one-half of all patients admitted to the hospital with heart failure (48). Differentiating systolic from diastolic heart failure is important, as the treatment and natural history of the two entities may differ somewhat. The echo is the diagnostic test that will most readily differentiate these two forms of heart failure, which not infrequently coexist in patients with acute decompensation.

Initial Hemodynamic Goal

Once the baseline hemodynamic profile is determined, a specific therapeutic plan should be formulated and discussed with the patient and family when appropriate (49). Today, most patients admitted to the hospital with heart failure are already receiving ACE inhibitors, digitalis, and high doses of diuretics; many are also receiving β-adrenergic blockers. When the diagnosis of heart failure is secure and all reversible causes have been excluded, it can be presumed that the current exacerbation is caused by the inexorable progression of heart failure over time. Because patients with decompensated heart failure are almost always tachypneic and short of breath, the primary goal should be to reduce pulmonary capillary filling pressure. This is normally done with an intravenous loop diuretics with or without an intravenous vasodilator such as nitroprusside or nesiritide.

Diuretics

High doses of intravenous loop diuretics are indicated (50) because oral absorption may be impaired in decompensated heart failure (51). Both venodilator (52) and direct vasoconstrictor (53) vascular effects of intravenous furosemide may be observed, but in most instances sodium and water excretion is the dominant effect of diuretic therapy. The choice of the loop diuretic varies substantially among physicians. Furosemide (40 to 120 mg intravenously), bumetanide (0.5 to 2 mg intravenously as a bolus), or torsemide (20 to 40 mg intravenously) may be preferred. When patients are truly refractory to regularly scheduled, high-dose intravenous loop diuretics, it may be prudent to consider giving supplemental intravenous chlorothiazide (500 to 1,000 mg intravenously over 15 minutes) before administering the loop diuretic. This will provide synergy between the diuretics (54,55). As the extracellular volume decreases, a complex array of neuroendocrine changes occur that can stimulate sodium and water reabsorption at sites in the kidney distal to the diuretic action. Following chronic use of loop diuretics, adaptive changes in the distal tubule occur, triggering increased sodium reabsorption. Diuretics such as thiazides or metolazone that are active at the distal tubule may block this compensatory response and may retard the development of distal tubular hypertrophy. These observations form the basis of combination diuretic therapy.

The use of a continuous intravenous furosemide, bumetanide, or torsemide drip may be effective when bolus administration of diuretics does not produce the expected diuresis (56–58). It is possible that the continuous infusion of a loop diuretic may provide more efficient delivery of the diuretic to the nephron, eliminating compensatory sodium retention or rebound that can occur during a diuretic-free interval. The risks of ototoxicity may be less with a continuous intravenous drip of a diuretic, but this is not proven. There may also be less-severe myalgia, a very painful complication that can occur when large doses of intravenous diuretics are given by bolus technique. Considerable uncertainties remain regarding the recommended dose for continuous infusion of diuretics, but furosemide is often given at a dose of 0.1 to 1.0 (or even 2.0) mg/kg per hour (or 10 to 40 mg per hour), and bumetanide as a continuous drip at 0.1 to 0.5 mg per hour. Torsemide is given at 5 to 20 mg per hour. When switching to oral diuretics, torsemide is more rapidly absorbed and has more consistent bioavailability than furosemide (59). Anecdotal information suggests that some patients will spontaneously diurese when either torsemide, bumetanide, or ethacrynic acid is substituted for furosemide, but this phenomenon has not been critically examined. It might be explained by the drugs' varying pharmacokinetics and pharmacodynamics, or may simply be related to higher total dosage of diuretic.

Substituting metolazone (an oral, nonloop diuretic) for intravenous chlorothiazide will help to maintain the synergy between loop and thiazide diuretics (60). Metolazone exerts effects at both the proximal and distal tubules. It should be given about 20 minutes before the loop diuretic (54,55). Because metolazone has a lengthy duration of action (days) and can cause severe volume and electrolyte depletion, it should be prescribed carefully each day on an as-needed basis. Moreover, metolazone's effects can last for days even after discontinuation, leading to severe volume depletion, hypotension, and hypokalemia. To provide a brisk diuresis, metolazone often needs to be titrated to a maximum of 10 mg per day and is sometimes given with an intravenous loop diuretic in a fixed dose of 10 mg per day for 3 days. Once a diuretic response has commenced, the dosing frequency of metolazone should also be decreased to two or three times per week, and eventually discontinued. It is not customary to use metolazone on a daily basis once a diuresis has ensued.

If hypokalemia is modest, oral potassium chloride or intravenous potassium chloride may be sufficient. Occasionally, patients become profoundly hypokalemic following a substantial diuresis and require heroic doses of intravenous potassium chloride to restore serum potassium levels. In such patients it may be prudent to consider an alternative oral potassium-sparing agent such as spironolactone (100 mg per day in divided doses), triamterene (100 mg three times per day), or amiloride (5 mg once per day). When potassium-sparing agents are given with an ACE inhibitor, severe hyperkalemia can sometimes occur. This is particularly true if an NSAID is also being prescribed. In general, NSAIDs should be avoided if at all possible in patients with decompensated heart failure. When spironolactone is continued as daily maintenance therapy, the usual dose is 12.5 to 25 mg per day.

Cardio-Renal Syndrome in Heart Failure

Recently, this term has been applied to patients in whom symptoms of heart failure cannot be relieved (i.e., the patient cannot be diuresed and serum creatinine keeps rising) despite aggressive management with intravenous diuretics, vasodilators, and inotropic drugs (61,62). About 25% of patients undergoing diuresis for acute heart failure will develop worsening renal function. The rising serum creatinine and BUN is associated with a much greater likelihood of readmission and death (63). Inotropic therapy may improve diuresis by increasing renal blood flow and relieve congestion temporarily, but congestion and oliguria may return when inotropic therapy is weaned off. Typically, the BUN and serum creatinine continue to rise and hyperkalemia can become a problem. ACE inhibitors may have to be discontinued and hydralazine and isosorbide dinitrate used in their place.

It is not clear that these patients will have improved renal function when treated with nesiritide (65,66). Not infrequently, this condition is further complicated by worsening hyponatremia. This requires restriction of free water to 1,000 cc per 24 hours, often necessitating concentration of intravenous drips. There is no good evidence that low-dose dopamine increases renal blood flow in this difficult situation. The development of the cardio-renal syndrome during aggressive in-patient treatment bodes poorly for the patient. It seems to occur independent of central hemodynamic status and there is no good evidence that increased cardiac output with positive inotropic agents improves cardio-renal syndrome. In some cases, cessation of an aggressive diuretic regimen at the expense of persistent, mild peripheral edema can stabilize or reverse worsening renal function.

In truly refractory cases, large volumes of excess body water can be removed by ultrafiltration or hemodialysis (67,68). Often blood pressure must be supported with arterial vasoconstrictors such as dopamine or phenylephrine when ultrafiltration or hemodialysis is performed in patients with severe heart failure and very poor left ventricular performance. Intermittent ultrafiltration may sometimes be helpful in preventing patients with stage D heart failure from recurrent hospitalizations (69).

Nitroprusside

It should be remembered that the primary hemodynamic goal in patients with acutely decompensated heart failure is to provide freedom from pulmonary and circulatory congestion. In our experience, this is best accomplished with intravenous diuretics, metolazone, and nitroprusside. Sometimes physicians will express concern that reduction of preload will result in diminished stroke volume. In general, this does not hold true in patients with severe heart failure. In fact, stroke volume is generally maintained as pulmonary capillary wedge pressure is brought into the normal range (Fig. 34-4). Contrary to popular belief, patients with large, dilated hearts and severe chronic and acute heart failure are usually not exquisitely sensitive to reductions in preload. Therefore, attempts to aggressively lower left ventricular filling pressure are nearly always indicated. One reason that a higher stroke volume can be maintained in the face of a reduced filling pressure is that nitroprusside leads to a

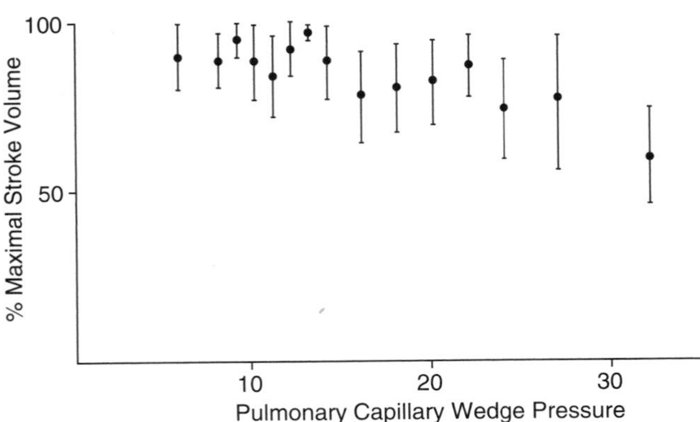

Figure 34-4 Twenty-five patients presenting with advanced heart failure (average LVEF 18%) that had acutely decompensated (average pulmonary capillary wedge pressure 31 ± 5 mm Hg, cardiac index 1.9 L/min/m^2). It is clear that stroke volume can be maintained even when pulmonary capillary wedge pressure is reduced to <15 mm Hg with nitroprusside and diuretics. (From Stevenson LW, Tillisch JH. Maintenance of cardiac output with normal filling pressures in patients with dilated heart failure. *Circulation.* 1986;74:1303–1308, with permission.)

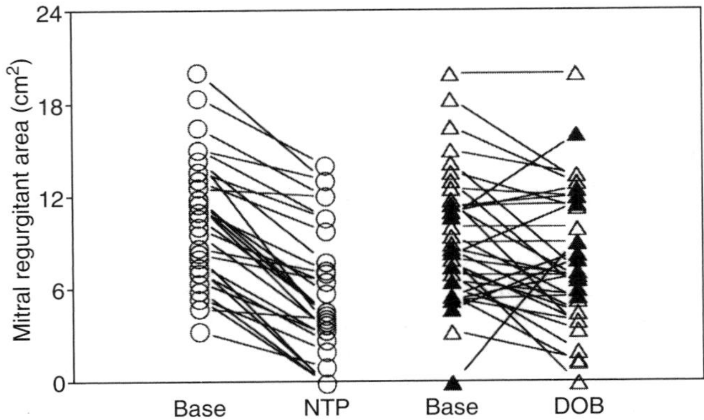

Figure 34-5 Changes in mitral regurgitation after nitroprusside (NTP) and dobutamine (DOB) infusions. Mitral regurgitation decreased in all patients following nitroprusside infusion, whereas the mitral regurgitant response to dobutamine was variable (**open triangles** indicate decrease in mitral regurgitation; **solid triangles** indicate increase in mitral regurgitation). (From Capomolla S, Pozzoli M, Opasich C, et al. Dobutamine and nitroprusside infusion in patients with severe congestive heart failure: hemodynamic improvement by discordant effects on mitral regurgitation, left atrial function, and ventricular function. *Am Heart J.* 1997; 134:1089–1098, with permission.)

redistribution of mitral regurgitant flow out the aorta. An improved stroke volume can be observed even when the pulmonary capillary wedge pressure is reduced to 10 mm Hg, suggesting that it is reasonable to reduce pulmonary capillary wedge pressure to the 10 to 12 mm Hg range whenever possible. A reasonable goal is to initiate nitroprusside at 10 to 20 μg per minute and quickly titrate the drug to allow the systolic pressure (by arterial catheter) to become 90 mm Hg. If blood pressure and perfusion remain adequate, nitroprusside can be increased in dose to achieve a pulmonary capillary wedge pressure of 10 to 12 mm Hg and a right atrial pressure of less than 8 mm Hg.

A subsidiary hemodynamic goal is to improve cardiac index. There is usually no need to normalize cardiac index or raise forward flow dramatically. Although it is popular, there is no clear rationale for targeting a patient to a specific reduction in systemic vascular resistance. Rather, it is important to demonstrate some improvement in cardiac index while reducing pulmonary vascular congestion (70). With nitroprusside, the increase in cardiac index will usually offset the fall in systemic vascular resistance, allowing for either no change or only a slight reduction in systemic blood pressure. Occasionally, patients will demonstrate unwanted or even profound hypotension in response to nitroprusside, in which case positive inotropic support with a drug such as dobutamine (71,72) or milrinone (73–75) might be preferred to nitroprusside. However, nitroprusside is the preferred initial agent because it is safe and simple to titrate, is energetically neutral or even reduces myocardial oxygen demand (76), has no inherent arrhythmogenic or hypokalemic properties, and is rarely toxic (77,78). Nitroprusside also consistently reduces mitral regurgitation, whereas the effects of dobutamine on mitral regurgitation are more variable (Fig. 34-5). Patients with renal insufficiency and/or acidosis who require prolonged infusions of nitroprusside at high doses (in excess of 400 μg per minute) can experience thiocyanate toxicity, and the drug should be used most judiciously in this setting (79).

Nitroglycerin

Although intravenous nitroglycerin can also be used to manage patients with severe congestive heart failure (80,81), large doses are sometimes required to reduce systemic vascular resistance, and tolerance can quickly develop. Headache does not occur with nitroprusside. In patients with underlying severe ischemic heart disease and active myocardial ischemia, there may be a preference for intravenous nitroglycerin over intravenous nitroprusside (82,83). Early reports suggested that nitroprusside has the potential to worsen myocardial ischemia via so-called coronary steal (84), especially in the early setting of acute myocardial infarction (85), although this has rarely been a clinical problem in the management of patients with acutely decompensated chronic heart failure. However, for patients with acute (<48 hours) myocardial infarction or acute myocardial ischemic syndromes and decompensated heart failure, intravenous nitroglycerin may be preferred because of its more favorable effects on coronary blood flow. Intravenous nitroglycerin and nitroprusside can also be used together, although this is rarely seen in clinical practice.

Nesiritide

Diuretics, and in many cases nitroprusside, are clearly beneficial in patients with acute heart failure. In most hospitals, nitroprusside is given only in the intensive care unit, where patients can be carefully monitored with invasive techniques. Nesiritide, a form of recombinant DNA-produced human BNP, is most often given in the ED and on cardiac step-down units, usually without hemodynamic monitoring. Nitroprusside is very inexpensive, while nesiritide is very expensive. Presumably, some of the cost of nesiritide can be offset by avoidance of an expensive intensive care unit stay.

Nesiritide binds to natriuretic peptide receptors (NPR) A and B. Cyclic guanosine monophoshpate (cGMP) is generated, which produces vasodilation along with a modest natriuresis and diuresis. In addition, nesiritide inhibits aldosterone release and renin production, improves coronary blood flow, and may have antiremodeling properties (86). The favorable renal effects are modest relative to loop diuretics and, in one study, were essentially nil when given to patients with chronic heart failure and worsening serum creatinine (65).

Nesiritide clearly reduces pulmonary capillary wedge pressure and improves cardiac output modestly (87). Dyspnea improves (3) but patients are being concomitantly treated with diuretics, so it is difficult to know what the contribution of nesiritide versus diuretics is toward reduction of pulmonary congestion. Studies with nesiritide are ongoing but the dose used by many investigators is 0.01 μg/kg per minute, often after a loading bolus of 2 μg/kg. As we gain more experience with nesiritide, we may be better able to select those patients who will benefit the most. Nesiritide can cause serious, sustained hypotension; this is more likely to occur in patients who have become volume-depleted, usually due to diuretics (88). It would seem prudent not to infuse nesiritide unless one is very confident from clinical evaluation that pulmonary capillary wedge pressure is clearly increased. Nitroprusside can, of course, also cause hypotension, but the half-life is much shorter than nesiritide (seconds versus ~18 minutes). Sustained hypotension rarely occurs with nitroprusside because it can be easily titrated down in dose or stopped.

Recently, two papers by Sackner-Bernstein et al. (65a, 65b) featured the potential for worsening renal function and heightened mortality following nesiritide use for decompensated heart failure. These two meta-analyses have ultimately led to a realization that further studies will be needed to better understand the role of this drug in the management of ADHF. Its role beyond ADHF, such as chronic, intermittent infusions for severe chronic heart failure, is currently under study and cannot be recommended for such until more data are available. Its role in the treatment of ADHF is still emerging but additional data would be most helpful. The use of nesiritide should be limited to patients presenting to the hospital with ADHF who have dyspnea at rest. It should not be used to replace diuretics, to improve renal function, or to enhance diuresis.

Dobutamine

Short-term use of dobutamine is associated with excess mortality (89). Occasionally, adjunctive drugs with positive inotropic properties will become necessary. Although this is to some extent a judgmental issue, when the systolic blood pressure is consistently <85 to 90 mm Hg one should consider adding a positive inotropic agent (such as dobutamine) to nitroprusside. Patients in need of inotropic support who demonstrate renal failure are best treated with dobutamine rather than milrinone, as milrinone is partially excreted by the kidneys and its pharmacokinetics are sensitive to renal function. Moreover, short-term use of milrinone is associated with more sustained hypotension requiring intervention and more new atrial arrhythmias than in placebo (2). The routine use of milrinone as an adjunct to standard therapy for the treatment of acute heart failure is not supported (2).

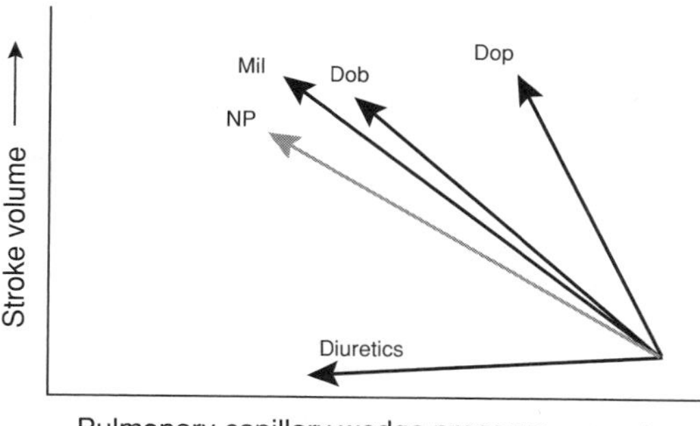

Figure 34-6 Agents commonly used to treat patients with acutely decompensated heart failure include intravenous diuretics, nitroprusside (NP), milrinone (Mil), dobutamine (Dob), and dopamine (Dop). Each has a distinctive hemodynamic profile as well as certain advantages and disadvantages. In general, nitroprusside is preferred because it does not increase myocardial oxygen demand, has an instantaneous onset and offset, and quickly relieves pulmonary vascular congestion. Its major drawback is hypotension, which can usually be offset by adding a small dose of dobutamine or dopamine. Milrinone shares many of the hemodynamic benefits of nitroprusside and probably causes less hypotension. However, milrinone is excreted renally, has a more complex dosing schedule, and is more expensive. Dopamine does not have a primary role in the management of severe heart failure, as it can raise pulmonary capillary wedge pressure. Its proper use is to raise blood pressure and it is the initial agent of choice for patients with shock.

Dobutamine and milrinone have relatively similar hemodynamic profiles (Fig. 34-6). Dobutamine is associated with a small but consistent increase in heart rate, reduction in pulmonary capillary wedge pressure, and increase in cardiac index. Blood pressure is usually only modestly increased with dobutamine, although this is variable. Blood pressure is often slightly reduced by milrinone, especially during the loading dose. Because of hypotension, the conventional loading dose of milrinone is sometimes omitted and patients are simply begun on a maintenance infusion. The effects on pulmonary capillary wedge pressure are variable with both drugs but, in general, there is a more consistent reduction in pulmonary capillary wedge pressure with milrinone than with dobutamine (90). Moreover, milrinone appears to be energetically more favorable than dobutamine (i.e., it produces less myocardial oxygen demand) and therefore might be preferred in patients with underlying ischemic heart disease or active angina pectoris when inotropic support is needed (91).

Milrinone

Short-term routine use of milrinone is waning, as it is associated with an excess mortality (2). Milrinone is a phosphodiesterase inhibitor with potent positive inotropic and vasodilator activity. It has a relatively long half-life and therefore is sometimes given as a loading dose of 50 μg/kg over 10 minutes. The loading dose is then usually followed by an infusion rate of 0.5 μg/kg per minute. Unlike the β-adrenergic agonists (such as dobutamine), milrinone acts to block the phosphodiesterase III enzyme, thus increasing intracellular cyclic adenosine monophosphate (cAMP). It has the theoretical advantage of exerting positive inotropic activity when downregulation of β-adrenergic receptors abrogates the pharmacologic activity of β-agonists such as dobutamine. Unlike the immediate effects of dobutamine, maximal hemodynamic effects of milrinone are observed at 15 minutes after initiation of infusion. Milrinone leads to a more consistent reduction in pulmonary capillary wedge pressure and is associated with a lower oxygen consumption than dobutamine, while producing the same hemodynamic improvement as nitroprusside with less concomitant hypotension (91,92). Therefore, it may be useful in selected patients with severe pulmonary hypertension, coronary disease, and normal renal function.

Milrinone could also be useful in patients who are fully antagonized with β-adrenergic blockers but are in need of temporary hemodynamic support. Because milrinone consistently and sometimes dramatically reduces pulmonary capillary wedge pressure, it can precipitate hypotension when ambient left ventricular filling pressure is low. Therefore, a PAC is recommended when milrinone is used. It is important for physicians to recognize that dopamine, dobutamine, milrinone, and nitroprusside are not interchangeable, and each has rather clear and distinctly different adrenergic and hemodynamic effects (Table 34-3). The use of these drugs for the treatment of patients with acute decompensation of chronic heart failure will vary considerably, depending on one's past training and experience.

Combinations of Dobutamine, Nitroprusside, and Dopamine

The combination of dobutamine and nitroprusside is sometimes used (93), particularly in patients who are modestly hypotensive when receiving nitroprusside alone. Likewise, nitroprusside can be combined with milrinone,

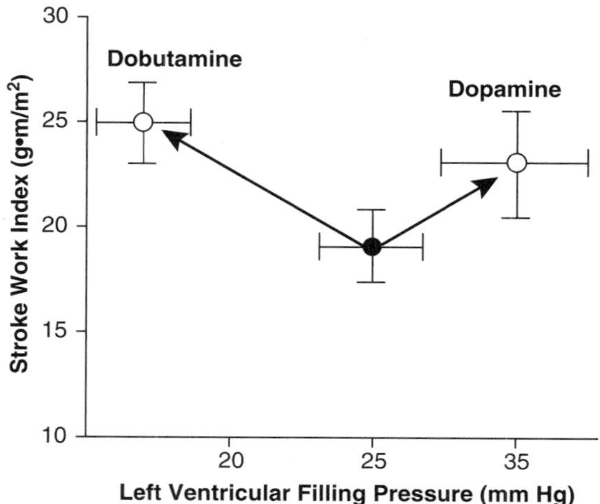

Figure 34-7 A comparison of dobutamine and pressor-dose dopamine on stroke-work index and left ventricular filling pressure in patients with advanced heart failure. Note that dopamine causes an incremental change in left ventricular filling pressure, whereas dobutamine is associated with a reduction in filling pressure. (From Loeb HS, Bredakis J, Gunner RM. Superiority of dobutamine over dopamine for augmentation of cardiac output in patients with chronic low output cardiac failure. *Circulation.* 1977;55:375–378, with permission.)

and milrinone and dobutamine can also be used together. In general, dopamine should be excluded from the therapy of patients with severe congestive heart failure, as it tends to increase systemic vascular resistance in high doses and this can be accompanied by further incremental changes in pulmonary capillary wedge pressure (94) (Fig. 34-7). Instead, dopamine should be reserved for progressive hypotension, where it is often the initial treatment of choice in maintaining blood pressure before insertion of an intra-aortic balloon pump (IABP).

Dobutamine is sometimes used in patients with acute heart failure, low-output syndrome, and low blood pressure. In recent years, heart failure specialists have been accustomed to using smaller doses of dobutamine, usually in the range of 2 to 10 μg/kg per minute. Often patients can be managed with seemingly trivial doses of the drug, even

TABLE 34-3
ADRENERGIC RECEPTOR ACTIVITY AND HEMODYNAMIC PROFILE OF COMMONLY USED POSITIVE INOTROPIC AGENTS AND VASODILATORS

Drug	β_1	β_2	α_1	Vasodilation	Blood Pressure	Filling Pressure	CI	HR	MVo_2
Nitroprusside				++++	→ or ↓	↓↓↓↓	↑↑↑↑	→	→
Dopamine	++++	++	++++	(<3 μg/kg/min)	↑↑↑↑	↑↑	↑↑↑	+++	+++
Dobutamine	++++	+++	+	++	↑	↓↓	↑↑↑	+++	+++
Milrinone				+++	↑↑	↓↓↓	↑↑↑	+++	++
Epinephrine	++++	++	++++	++	↑↑↑↑	±	+++	+++	+++
Norepinephrine	++++	++++	++++		↑↑↑↑	±	++	+++	+++
Nesiritide				+++	→ or ↓	↓↓	↑↑	→	→
NTG (IV)				++	→ or ↓	↓↓↓	↑	→	↓

in the range of 2 to 3 μg/kg per minute. There is no need to drive the cardiac index into the 3 to 5 L/min/m^2 range, as there is no clear added clinical benefit and there is the potential to develop tachycardia, arrhythmias, and precipitation of acute myocardial ischemia when doses of 10 to 40 μg/kg per minute are employed. As with nitroprusside, a specific hemodynamic goal is to reduce the pulmonary capillary wedge pressure to less than 15 mm Hg and the right atrial pressure to less than 8 mm Hg while maintaining a systolic blood pressure ≥80 mm Hg (95) (or mean blood pressure around 65 to 70 mm Hg). These hemodynamic goals should be sustained for at least 48 to 72 hours (96–98).

Dopamine

Dopamine is used primarily for patients with severe hypotension; it is seldom used in our intensive care unit with the availability of other agents. Low-dose dopamine (1 to 3 μg/kg per minute) has primarily dopaminergic effects (99,100) and therefore can dilate specific vascular beds, resulting in a modest reduction in blood pressure (101,102). When dopamine is used in doses of 3 to 10 μg/kg per minute, blood pressure usually rises. Both dobutamine and dopamine have short half-lives, usually measured in minutes.

Epinephrine and Norepinephrine

Patients with profound left ventricular dysfunction awaiting implantation of a left ventricular assist device (LVAD) may sometimes require intravenous epinephrine to maintain circulatory homeostasis. Epinephrine stimulates both β_1- and β_2-adrenergic receptors as well as α_1-receptors in a dose-dependent fashion (Table 34-3). Because of attendant tachycardia and vasoconstriction, it can precipitate acute myocardial ischemia. Nevertheless, epinephrine seems to consistently improve cardiac index in the setting of very severe heart failure and, in some cases, will be life-sustaining before implantation of a mechanical assist device. Adverse effects such as arrhythmias, ST-T wave depression, and chest pain are occasionally seen when infusions are given at a rate above 10 μg per minute. Infusions of epinephrine from 0.1 to 1.0 μg per minute are most effective in restoring cardiac index with an acceptable or minimal increase in heart rate. Clearly, an epinephrine drip is not a routine measure but it can be life-saving in patients who appear to be quickly entering an irreversible downward spiral.

There is a resurgence of interest in using norepinephrine to support blood pressure when patients remain hypotensive while receiving high-dose dopamine. Like epinephrine, norepinephrine has both β_1- and α_1-adrenergic agonist properties, but the lack of β_2-agonist properties allows this drug to raise blood pressure more quickly. The usual dose of norepinephrine is 2 to 4 μg per minute. As with high-dose dopamine or any drug with potent α_1-antagonist properties, care must be taken that necrosis and sloughing of skin do not occur at the site of intravenous injection as a result of extravasation of the drug. The various chemical structures of commonly used catecholamine drugs are depicted in Figure 34-8.

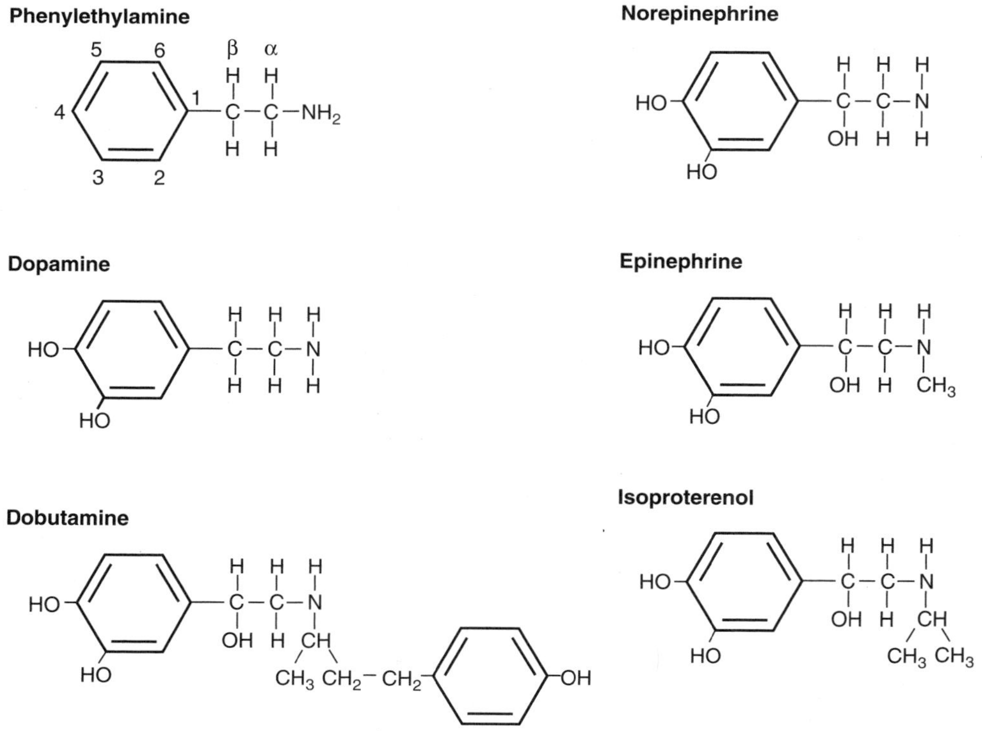

Phenylethylamine

Norepinephrine

Dopamine

Epinephrine

Dobutamine

Isoproterenol

Figure 34-8 The chemical structure of some commonly used catecholamines. Dobutamine is clearly the catecholamine most commonly used to manage patients with acutely decompensated heart failure.

Maintenance of Orally Active Therapy

Unless it is clear that the patient's medications are contributing to worsening heart failure (e.g., first-generation calcium-channel blockers, β-adrenergic blockers, antiarrhythmic drug therapy, NSAIDs), it is prudent to maintain the patient's current oral drug regimen while in the hospital. This includes β-adrenergic blockers. Many patients are receiving digoxin and it is useful to measure the serum digoxin level, as it may be abnormally increased during acute cardiac decompensation (particularly in the setting of worsening renal function). Adjustments of the daily digoxin dose may be necessary in order to maintain a serum level below 1.2 g/mL. Unless substantial and progressive azotemia or hyperkalemia are occurring, ACE inhibitor therapy should be continued. Small doses of short-acting captopril given three to five times per day may be easier to use in the setting of decompensated heart failure, as hypotension (if it occurs) will be of brief duration. Contraindications to ACE inhibitor therapy include hyperkalemia and cardiogenic shock. Modest azotemia (~20% rise in serum creatinine) is not a contraindication to ACE inhibitor therapy.

When the patient is clinically stable, one should titrate the ACE inhibitor to the dose level used in the large clinical trials, such as 10 mg of enalapril twice per day, 20 mg of lisinopril once a day, or 50 mg of captopril three times a day. There is less information about the optimal dose of other less-commonly used ACE inhibitor drugs. It is unclear if increasing the ACE inhibitor dose beyond that recommended by the individual manufacturer is useful. In general, ACE inhibitors have a relatively flat dose–response curve, so that increasing the dose usually results in no meaningful additional hemodynamic improvement. Angiotensin-receptor blockers (ARBs) can be used in lieu of ACE inhibitors in patients with heart failure due to acute myocardial infarction (103).

Adjunctive Medical Therapy

Occasionally, patients will manifest additional clinical improvement when hydralazine and long-acting nitrates are added to conventional therapy (104). This is particularly true when weaning the patient from intravenous therapy or an IABP proves difficult. The typical dose of hydralazine that is effective in severe heart failure is 100 mg four times per day. One usually begins with much smaller doses and titrates up the dose over several days. The typical dose of long-acting isosorbide dinitrate that has been found to be effective in heart failure is 30 to 40 mg three or four times per day. The 5-mononitrates are also widely used in this setting. It is possible that hydralazine offsets nitrate tolerance, thus adding additional support for the combination of nitrates and hydralazine (105,106). A large, randomized, placebo-controlled trial recently confirmed the long-term benefit of adding hydralazine and isosorbide dinitrate to conventional therapy in patients with advanced chronic heart failure (107). This large survival benefit was in an African-American population exclusively but theoretically could be beneficial in a much broader population, especially if blood pressure is somewhat higher than is usually observed in heart failure (as was in this trial).

Electrolyte Depletion and Antiarrhythmic Therapy

Patients with acutely decompensated heart failure are prone to develop life-threatening ventricular arrhythmias (108). Nearly all patients with heart failure have ambient ventricular ectopic beats. As heart failure worsens, it is not unusual for patients to manifest runs of nonsustained ventricular tachycardia or even sustained and symptomatic ventricular tachycardia requiring DC cardioversion. Ventricular fibrillation and severe bradyarrhythmias also occur in patients with advanced heart failure (109). It is important to monitor the serum potassium and serum magnesium levels in such patients, as electrolyte abnormalities are associated with ventricular arrhythmias (110). There appears to be less ventricular ectopy and stabilization of QT prolongation when the serum potassium is kept in the range of 4.5 mEq/L (111). Magnesium should also be replenished when serum levels are low (i.e., 2 mg/dL or less) (112). Hyponatremia is common, can be a poor prognostic sign, and may require restriction of fluids to 1,000 to 1,200 cc per 24 hours (113).

When antiarrhythmic drug interdiction is deemed necessary, it is best to avoid lidocaine (114,115). It has a high frequency of toxicity, particularly in patients with heart failure. If lidocaine is used in the setting of heart failure, the loading dose must be reduced by one-half because of the abnormally contracted volume of distribution. Because many patients with heart failure have passive congestion of the liver and abnormal liver function (116), the metabolism of lidocaine can also be delayed, resulting in higher blood levels and excessive side effects. The toxicity of lidocaine can be frightening and includes convulsions, slurred speech, confusion, mental obtundation, respiratory arrest, and sinus node dysfunction with malignant bradycardia.

Amiodarone

If recurrent, symptomatic, life-threatening arrhythmias persist after correction of serum potassium and serum magnesium levels, intravenous amiodarone should be considered. Amiodarone is a unique antiarrhythmic agent that is now available in both oral and intravenous forms (117–119). Intravenous amiodarone exerts its electrophysiological actions faster than the oral form and is usually preferred in the setting of severe heart failure. Amiodarone inhibits inactivated sodium channels, decreases the frequency of ventricular fibrillation, and may have an important antiadrenergic action (119). Because of its vasodilator properties, it may improve coronary blood flow, reduce afterload, and therefore may also reduce blood pressure. Hypotension occurs in about 25% of patients given intravenous amiodarone. The average fall in blood pressure with intravenous amiodarone is about 20%. A direct, negative inotropic effect has also been suggested, although cardiac output may also improve because of reduction in afterload and improvement in coronary blood flow.

The most frequent adverse effect observed with intravenous amiodarone is hypotension. Proarrhythmic effects are rare but may occur in the form of torsade de pointes. Local phlebitis can occur, particularly when the drug is given in concentrations exceeding 2 mg/mL. To avoid phlebitis, the drug is best given through a central line. It should be mixed in 5% dextrose solution and should be infused with a volumetric pump. The recommended initial intravenous loading dose of amiodarone is 150 mg given over 10 minutes, followed by an intermediate infusion of 1 mg per minute for 6 hours and then 0.5 mg per minute thereafter. Supplemental boluses of 150 mg may be given over 10 to 30 minutes for recurrent arrhythmias but, because of hypotension, a daily dose exceeding 2,000 mg per day should be avoided. Patients who have been receiving intravenous therapy for at least 2 to 3 weeks can be safely started on maintenance oral treatment of amiodarone using 300 to 400 mg per day. After the short-term (less than 1 week) use of intravenous amiodarone, the usual oral loading regimen of 800 mg to 1,400 mg per day can still be given, but an intermediate dose of 400 to 800 mg per day might be suitable in patients who have received at least several days of the drug intravenously.

There is an important interaction between amiodarone and warfarin that can further prolong the international normalized ratio (INR), so smaller doses of warfarin may be necessary if the two drugs are used concurrently. Digoxin levels are also increased by amiodarone use, so the dose of digoxin should be reduced by one-half when amiodarone is prescribed.

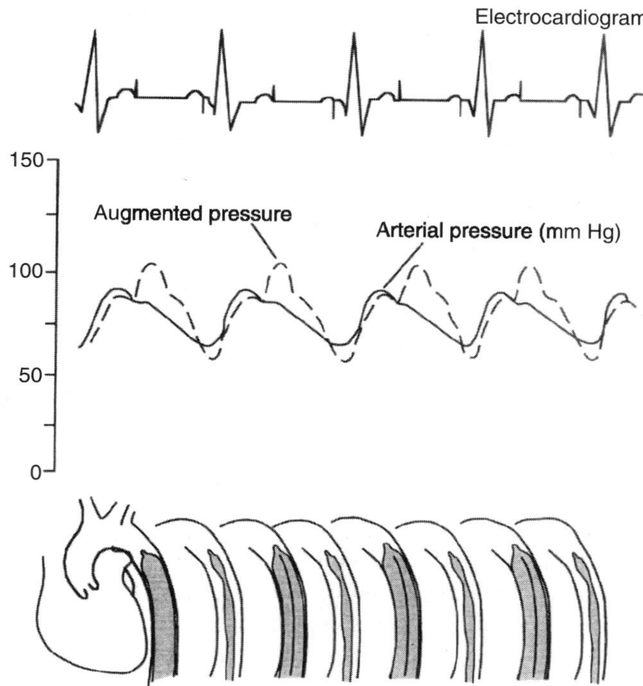

Figure 34-9 The relationships among the electrocardiogram (ECG), the arterial blood pressure, and the intra-aortic balloon pump are depicted. The balloon deflates during systole, which is marked on the ECG by a **downward tic mark**, then inflates during diastole, indicated by the **upward tic mark** at the end of the T wave. The patient's arterial pressure is shown by the **solid line** in the middle panel, whereas the augmented arterial pressure during counterpulsation is depicted by the **dotted line.** (Reproduced from material supplied by St. Jude Medical, Inc., St. Paul, MN.)

MECHANICAL ASSIST DEVICES

Intra-Aortic Balloon Pump

Intra-aortic balloon pumping (IABP) has been available now for nearly a quarter of a century (120). Many changes and refinements in the instrumentation have occurred, making this a safer and more indispensable adjunctive therapy for selected patients. The IABP removes volume from the central aorta before and during left ventricular ejection, thereby reducing aortic impedance. The volume is then returned during diastole, which increases aortic diastolic pressure and probably enhances coronary blood flow (Fig. 34-9). Left ventricular end-diastolic pressure is usually reduced by about 40%, and cardiac output increases by 50%, in most patients following 1:1 augmentation of the circulation by IABP (121,122). Improvement in coronary blood flow is variable but may improve as much as 100%. The dramatic effects of IABP result from a combination of decreased afterload, decreased preload, reduced wall tension, reduced myocardial oxygen demand, and increased coronary blood flow.

The optimal location of the device in the aorta is critical. Augmentation is most adequate when the balloon is as close to the aortic root as practical (123). The proximal tip of the balloon catheter should be placed about 1 cm below the origin of the left subclavian artery. Helium is the optimal gas for the IABP, as it affords faster inflation and deflation and therefore provides for more effective diastolic augmentation. The speed of gas transit is critically important. Balloon leakage or rupture is rare but can occur.

The hemodynamic benefits of IABP are related to the heart rate. It has been suggested that when there is sinus tachycardia the hemodynamic benefits can be improved by assisting every other beat but, in reality, this can reduce what already is suboptimal augmentation. It is generally preferable to pump on every beat, even if there is a sustained tachycardia (124). Atrial fibrillation with a rapid ventricular response, however, will sometimes exceed the ability of the device to maintain timing. In such cases, DC cardioversion may be necessary.

Although there are no clear guidelines as to when to insert an IABP in patients with decompensated heart failure, most heart failure-focused programs have a low threshold to use such devices. When the cardiac index is below 1.5 L/min/m^2 despite pharmacologic support, an IABP is usually employed. The only absolute contraindications include moderate to severe aortic insufficiency and aortic dissection. However, lack of a clear endpoint or definitive therapy for underlying pathology, thoracic or abdominal aneurysm, severe iliofemoral vascular disease, and a clotting disorder are relative contraindications. Peripheral vascular disease is also a relative contraindication for IABP use, and each case must be individualized. The balloon is placed with the guidance of fluoroscopy, and a chest X-ray should be done daily to verify that it is positioned properly. Frequent chest X-rays are necessary in follow-up, as the device may drift within the aorta.

The use of anticoagulation with heparin during IABP is controversial but many centers prefer to give a 5,000-unit bolus of heparin at the onset of pumping and every 4 hours thereafter to maintain the pulse transit time (PTT) between 1.5 and 2 times normal. The leg through which the balloon is inserted must be observed regularly for evidence of ischemia. In addition to vital signs, observations regarding the extremities should be noted by the nursing staff at least once per shift and by the physician as necessary. A mild degree of leg ischemia may be tolerated if the IABP is life-saving. Nevertheless, very close observation is always indicated. If severe leg ischemia is detected the balloon must be removed, although sometimes an attempt is made to insert another balloon through the contralateral femoral artery.

As with pharmacologic support for severe heart failure, it is generally prudent to maintain an IABP for 48 to 72 hours until the cardiac index is consistently greater than 2.2 L/min/m^2 and the pulmonary capillary wedge pressure is less than 18 mm Hg. Weaning of the IABP can be attempted after several days of hemodynamic stability. The purpose of weaning is to allow the heart to gradually take over the circulatory load when the assisted heartbeats are reduced from 1:1 to 1:2, 1:3, 1:4. If weaning results in hemodynamic deterioration, the IABP is resumed and weaning can be initiated 6 to 24 hours later. Heparin administration should be discontinued at least 4 hours before the balloon is removed. Once the balloon is out, the puncture site must be compressed for at least 30 minutes in order to obtain adequate hemostasis. After percutaneous balloon pump removal, patients must lie flat for at least 6 hours and the lower extremities must be observed for signs of ischemia. In many cases, the IABP is used as a bridge to LVAD implantation or even heart transplantation. The successful use of IABP as a bridge to transplantation has become increasingly common. The duration of balloon pump support in most instances has ranged from 1 to 27 days, although support for as long as 327 days has been reported (125). If endotracheal tube extubation is anticipated, it is useful to remove the IABP first, thus allowing the patient to sit up during extubation.

Complications of IABP range from 14% to 45% and are primarily vascular and infectious. Vascular complications include loss of distal pulse, ischemic pain in the leg, thrombosis, emboli, ischemic neuropathy, ischemic foot ulcer, foot drop, amputation, aortic dissection, and false aneurysm formation. Women, particular elderly and small women, have a higher vascular risk. About 25% of patients will develop infectious complications including local infection, bacteremia, and fever, particularly if there is prolonged support. In such cases, blood cultures should be drawn and the balloon may have to be removed if it is considered a possible source of infection. If the patient does not tolerate withdrawal of the IABP, it must sometimes be reinserted in an alternative vascular site.

When to Consider Surgical Intervention

When patients have inadequate perfusion despite aggressive pharmacologic support, consideration should be strongly given to insertion of an IABP. If the patient is a suitable candidate for heart transplantation, it is reasonable to have the LVAD surgical team see the patient at that point. Although not all patients will be candidates for heart transplantation and an LVAD, it is better that the surgeons be apprised of the critically ill nature of the patient before further hemodynamic embarrassment (126,127). Depending on the experience and skill of the LVAD team, physicians should have a relatively low threshold to implant a mechanical assist device if the patient is clearly a transplant candidate. In many cases, the patient fits the cardiac profile for heart transplant candidacy but there is inadequate social, financial, and psychological information because of the sudden and critical nature of the illness. In such cases, it is sometimes reasonable to proceed with the LVAD because mortality without such assistance is very high.

Aortic Flow Augmentation Device

A novel invasive approach for severely decompensated patients utilizes mechanical afterload reduction by a peripherally accessed, external rotary blood pump to enhance blood flow in the descending aorta. A multicenter pivotal study, MOMENTUM (Multicenter trial of the Orqis Medical CRS Enhanced Treatment of CHF, Unresponsive to Medical therapy), is currently in the planning stages to test the safety and efficacy for this aortic flow augmentation device, the Cancion Cardiac Recovery System (Orqis Medical) (130). Preliminary animal and human studies on its hemodynamic efficacies have been promising, albeit very invasive (131–134). As technology for ventricular assist device (VAD) therapy advances, it is likely that smaller and more efficient VADs will be designed specifically for contractile support of the failing heart (135,136).

SUMMARY

The management of acute or decompensated heart failure is complex and requires thorough and careful assessment before a therapeutic plan begins. Such patients are sometimes hospitalized in the intensive care unit or coronary care unit, although they are now increasingly being managed in special care units on the ward. Physicians and nurses familiar with these patients (a heart failure team) have been documented to render improved care. Hemodynamic monitoring is sometimes quite helpful and can be pivotal in guiding pharmacologic therapy. In many cases there is striking clinical benefit, making the care of these patients highly rewarding. However, their care is time-consuming and very expensive, highlighting the fact that prevention of progression of heart failure remains the most important long-term therapeutic strategy.

REFERENCES

1. Francis GS. Acute heart failure: patient management of a growing epidemic. *Am Heart Hosp J*. 2004;2:10–14.
2. Cuffe MS, Califf RM, Adams KF, Jr., et al. Short-term intravenous milrinone for acute exacerbation of chronic heart failure: a randomized controlled trial. *JAMA*. 2002;287:1541–1547.
3. Publication Committee for the VMAC Investigators (Vasodilatation in the Management of Acute CHF). Intravenous nesiritide vs nitroglycerin for treatment of decompensated congestive heart failure: a randomized controlled trial. *JAMA*. 2002;287:1531–1540.

4. Dries DL, Exner DV, Domanski MJ, et al. The prognostic implications of renal insufficiency in asymptomatic and symptomatic patients with left ventricular systolic dysfunction. *J Am Coll Cardiol*. 2000;35:681–689.
5. American Heart Association. *Heart disease and stroke statistics—2005 update*. Dallas, TX: American Heart Association; 2005.
6. Jong P, Vowinckel E, Liu PP, et al. Prognosis and determinants of survival in patients newly hospitalized for heart failure: a population-based study. *Arch Intern Med*. 2002;162:1689–1694.
7. Haldeman GA, Croft JB, Giles WH, et al. Hospitalization of patients with heart failure: National Hospital Discharge Survey, 1985 to 1995. *Am Heart J*. 1999;137:352–560.
8. Fonarow GC. The Acute Decompensated Heart Failure National Registry (ADHERE): opportunities to improve care of patients hospitalized with acute decompensated heart failure. *Rev Cardiovasc Med*. 2003;(4 Suppl 7):S21–S30.
9. Adams KF, Jr., Fonarow GC, Emerman CL, et al. Characteristics and outcomes of patients hospitalized for heart failure in the United States: rationale, design, and preliminary observations from the first 100,000 cases in the Acute Decompensated Heart Failure National Registry (ADHERE). *Am Heart J*. 2005;149:209–216.
10. Fonarow GC, Adams KF, Jr., Abraham WT, et al. Risk stratification for in-hospital mortality in acutely decompensated heart failure: classification and regression tree analysis. *JAMA*. 2005;293:572–580.
11. Cowie MR, Struthers AD, Wood DA, et al. Value of natriuretic peptides in assessment of patients with possible new heart failure in primary care. *Lancet*. 1997;350:1349–1353.
12. Dao Q, Krishnaswamy P, Kazanegra R, et al. Utility of B-type natriuretic peptide in the diagnosis of congestive heart failure in an urgent-care setting. *J Am Coll Cardiol*. 2001;37:379–385.
13. Maisel AS, Krishnaswamy P, Nowak RM, et al. Rapid measurement of B-type natriuretic peptide in the emergency diagnosis of heart failure. *N Engl J Med*. 2002;347:161–167.
14. Tang WH, Girod JP, Lee MJ, et al. Plasma B-type natriuretic peptide levels in ambulatory patients with established chronic symptomatic systolic heart failure. *Circulation*. 2003;108: 2964–2966.
15. O'Mailia JJ, Sander GE, Giles TD. Nifedipine-associated myocardial ischemia or infarction in the treatment of hypertensive urgencies. *Ann Intern Med*. 1987;107:185–186.
16. Grossman E, Messerli FH, Grodzicki T, et al. Should a moratorium be placed on sublingual nifedipine capsules given for hypertensive emergencies and pseudoemergencies? *JAMA*. 1996;276:1328–1331.
17. Mikulic E, Franciosa JA, Cohn JN. Comparative hemodynamic effects of chewable isosorbide dinitrate and nitroglycerin in patients with congestive heart failure. *Circulation*. 1975;52: 477–482.
18. Middlekauff HR, Stevenson WG, Stevenson LW. Prognostic significance of atrial fibrillation in advanced heart failure. A study of 390 patients. *Circulation*. 1991;84:40–48.
19. Stevenson WG, Stevenson LW. Atrial fibrillation and heart failure: five more years. *N Engl J Med*. 2004;351:2437–2440.
20. Falk RH, Leavitt JI. Digoxin for atrial fibrillation: a drug whose time has gone? *Ann Intern Med*. 1991;114:573–575.
21. Stevenson WG, Stevenson LW, Middlekauff HR, et al. Improving survival for patients with atrial fibrillation and advanced heart failure. *J Am Coll Cardiol*. 1996;28:1458–1463.
22. The Digitalis in Acute Atrial Fibrillation (DAAF) Trial Group. Intravenous digoxin in acute atrial fibrillation. Results of a randomized, placebo-controlled multicentre trial in 239 patients. *Eur Heart J*. 1997;18:649–654.
23. Gosselink AT, Crijns HJ, Van Gelder IC, et al. Low-dose amiodarone for maintenance of sinus rhythm after cardioversion of atrial fibrillation or flutter. *JAMA*. 1992;267:3289–3293.
24. Hsu LF, Jais P, Sanders P, et al. Catheter ablation for atrial fibrillation in congestive heart failure. *N Engl J Med*. 2004;351: 2373–2383.
25. Singer DE, Albers GW, Dalen JE, et al. Antithrombotic therapy in atrial fibrillation: the Seventh ACCP Conference on Antithrombotic and Thrombolytic Therapy. *Chest*. 2004;126: 429S–456S.
26. Weigner MJ, Caulfield TA, Danias PG, et al. Risk for clinical thromboembolism associated with conversion to sinus rhythm in patients with atrial fibrillation lasting less than 48 hours. *Ann Intern Med*. 1997;126:615–620.
27. The Stroke Prevention in Atrial Fibrillation Investigators. Predictors of thromboembolism in atrial fibrillation. II. Echocardiographic features of patients at risk. *Ann Intern Med*. 1992;116:6–12.
28. Klein AL, Grimm RA, Murray RD, et al. Use of transesophageal echocardiography to guide cardioversion in patients with atrial fibrillation. *N Engl J Med*. 2001;344:1411–1420.
29. Dzau VJ, Packer M, Lilly LS, et al. Prostaglandins in severe congestive heart failure. Relation to activation of the renin-angiotensin system and hyponatremia. *N Engl J Med*. 1984;310: 347–352.
30. Fonarow GC, Stevenson LW, Walden JA, et al. Impact of a comprehensive heart failure management program on hospital readmission and functional status of patients with advanced heart failure. *J Am Coll Cardiol*. 1997;30:725–732.
31. Reis SE, Holubkov R, Edmundowicz D, et al. Treatment of patients admitted to the hospital with congestive heart failure: specialty-related disparities in practice patterns and outcomes. *J Am Coll Cardiol*. 1997;30:733–738.
32. Edep ME, Shah NB, Tateo IM, et al. Differences between primary care physicians and cardiologists in management of congestive heart failure: relation to practice guidelines. *J Am Coll Cardiol*. 1997;30:518–526.
33. Galbreath AD, Krasuski RA, Smith B, et al. Long-term healthcare and cost outcomes of disease management in a large, randomized, community-based population with heart failure. *Circulation*. 2004;110:3518–3526.
34. DeBusk RF, Miller NH, Parker KM, et al. Care management for low-risk patients with heart failure: a randomized, controlled trial. *Ann Intern Med*. 2004;141:606–613.
35. Ellison DH. Diuretic therapy and resistance in congestive heart failure. *Cardiology*. 2001;96:132–143.
36. Krumholz HM, Parent EM, Tu N, et al. Readmission after hospitalization for congestive heart failure among Medicare beneficiaries. *Arch Intern Med*. 1997;157:99–104.
37. Rich MW, Beckham V, Wittenberg C, et al. A multidisciplinary intervention to prevent the readmission of elderly patients with congestive heart failure. *N Engl J Med*. 1995;333: 1190–1195.
38. Bart BA, Shaw LK, McCants CB, Jr., et al. Clinical determinants of mortality in patients with angiographically diagnosed ischemic or nonischemic cardiomyopathy. *J Am Coll Cardiol*. 1997;30: 1002–1008.
39. Middlekauff HR, Stevenson WG, Stevenson LW, et al. Syncope in advanced heart failure: high risk of sudden death regardless of origin of syncope. *J Am Coll Cardiol*. 1993;21:110–116.
40. Fruhwald FM, Eber B, Schumacher M, et al. Syncope in dilated cardiomyopathy is a predictor of sudden cardiac death. *Cardiology*. 1996;87:177–180.
41. Middlekauff HR, Stevenson WG, Saxon LA. Prognosis after syncope: impact of left ventricular function. *Am Heart J*. 1993;125: 121–127.
42. Bitanay C, Califf RM, Hasselblad V, et al. Evaluation study of congestive heart failure and palmonary artery catheterization effectiveness: the ESCAPE trial. JAMA. 2005; 294(13): 1625–1633.
43. Badgett RG, Lucey CR, Mulrow CD. Can the clinical examination diagnose left-sided heart failure in adults? *JAMA*. 1997; 277:1712–1719.
44. Stevenson LW, Perloff JK. The limited reliability of physical signs for estimating hemodynamics in chronic heart failure. *JAMA*. 1989;261:884–888.
45. Cattau EL, Jr., Benjamin SB, Knuff TE, et al. The accuracy of the physical examination in the diagnosis of suspected ascites. *JAMA*. 1982;247:1164–1166.
46. Cohen GI, Pietrolungo JF, Thomas JD, et al. A practical guide to assessment of ventricular diastolic function using Doppler echocardiography. *J Am Coll Cardiol*. 1996;27:1753–1760.
47. Nishimura RA, Tajik AJ. Evaluation of diastolic filling of left ventricle in health and disease: Doppler echocardiography is the clinician's Rosetta stone. *J Am Coll Cardiol*. 1997;30:8–18.
48. Dougherty AH, Naccarelli GV, Gray EL, et al. Congestive heart failure with normal systolic function. *Am J Cardiol*. 1984;54: 778–782.
49. Francis GS. Diagnosis and management of acute congestive heart failure in the intensive care unit. *J Intens Care Med*. 1989;4: 84–92.

50. Gerlag PG, van Meijel JJ. High-dose furosemide in the treatment of refractory congestive heart failure. *Arch Intern Med.* 1988;148:286–291.
51. Vasko MR, Cartwright DB, Knochel JP, et al. Furosemide absorption altered in decompensated congestive heart failure. *Ann Intern Med.* 1985;102:314–318.
52. Pickkers P, Dormans TP, Russel FG, et al. Direct vascular effects of furosemide in humans. *Circulation.* 1997;96:1847–1852.
53. Francis GS, Siegel RM, Goldsmith SR, et al. Acute vasoconstrictor response to intravenous furosemide in patients with chronic congestive heart failure. Activation of the neurohumoral axis. *Ann Intern Med.* 1985;103:1–6.
54. Oster JR, Epstein M, Smoller S. Combined therapy with thiazide-type and loop diuretic agents for resistant sodium retention. *Ann Intern Med.* 1983;99:405–406.
55. Ellison DH. The physiologic basis of diuretic synergism: its role in treating diuretic resistance. *Ann Intern Med.* 1991;114: 886–894.
56. Rudy DW, Voelker JR, Greene PK, et al. Loop diuretics for chronic renal insufficiency: a continuous infusion is more efficacious than bolus therapy. *Ann Intern Med.* 1991;115:360–366.
57. Martin SJ, Danziger LH. Continuous infusion of loop diuretics in the critically ill: a review of the literature. *Crit Care Med.* 1994;22:1323–1329.
58. Dormans TP, van Meyel JJ, Gerlag PG, et al. Diuretic efficacy of high dose furosemide in severe heart failure: bolus injection versus continuous infusion. *J Am Coll Cardiol.* 1996;28:376–382.
59. Vargo DL, Kramer WG, Black PK, et al. Bioavailability, pharmacokinetics, and pharmacodynamics of torsemide and furosemide in patients with congestive heart failure. *Clin Pharmacol Ther.* 1995;57:601–609.
60. Mouallem M, Brif I, Mayan H, et al. Prolonged therapy by the combination of furosemide and thiazides in refractory heart failure and other fluid retaining conditions. *Int J Cardiol.* 1995; 50:89–94.
61. Shlipak MG, Massie BM. The clinical challenge of cardiorenal syndrome. *Circulation.* 2004;110:1514–1517.
62. Bongartz LG, Cramer MJ, Doevendans PA, et al. The severe cardiorenal syndrome: 'Guyton revisited.' *Eur Heart J.* 2005;26:11–17.
63. Aronson D, Mittleman MA, Burger AJ. Elevated blood urea nitrogen level as a predictor of mortality in patients admitted for decompensated heart failure. *Am J Med.* 2004;116:466–473.
64. Akhter MW, Aronson D, Bitar F, et al. Effect of elevated admission serum creatinine and its worsening on outcome in hospitalized patients with decompensated heart failure. *Am J Cardiol.* 2004;94:957–960.
65. Wang DJ, Dowling TC, Meadows D, et al. Nesiritide does not improve renal function in patients with chronic heart failure and worsening serum creatinine. *Circulation.* 2004;110:1620–1625.
65a. Sackner-Bernstein JD, Skopicki HA, Aaronson KD. Risk of worsening renal function with nesiritide in patients with acutely decompensated heart failure. *Circulation.* 2005;111:1487–1491.
65b. Sackner-Bernstein JD, Kowalski M, Fox M, et al. Short-term risk of death after treatment with nesiritide for decompensated heart failure. *JAMA.* 2005;293:1900–1905.
66. Cataliotti A, Boerrigter G, Costello-Boerrigter LC, et al. Brain natriuretic peptide enhances renal actions of furosemide and suppresses furosemide-induced aldosterone activation in experimental heart failure. *Circulation.* 2004;109:1680–1685.
67. Agostoni PG, Marenzi GC, Pepi M, et al. Isolated ultrafiltration in moderate congestive heart failure. *J Am Coll Cardiol.* 1993;21:424–431.
68. Sharma A, Hermann DD, Mehta RL. Clinical benefit and approach of ultrafiltration in acute heart failure. *Cardiology.* 2001;96:144–154.
69. Sheppard R, Panyon J, Pohwani AL, et al. Intermittent outpatient ultrafiltration for the treatment of severe refractory congestive heart failure. *J Card Fail.* 2004;10:380–383.
70. Francis GS. Vasodilators and inotropic agents in the treatment of congestive heart failure. *Semin Nephrol.* 1994;14:464–478.
71. Leier CV, Unverferth DV. Drugs five years later. Dobutamine. *Ann Intern Med.* 1983;99:490–496.
72. Sonnenblick EH, Frishman WH, LeJemtel TH. Dobutamine: a new synthetic cardioactive sympathetic amine. *N Engl J Med.* 1979;300:17–22.
73. Baim DS, McDowell AV, Cherniles J, et al. Evaluation of a new bipyridine inotropic agent—milrinone—in patients with severe congestive heart failure. *N Engl J Med.* 1983;309:748–756.
74. Anderson JL, Baim DS, Fein SA, et al. Efficacy and safety of sustained (48 hour) intravenous infusions of milrinone in patients with severe congestive heart failure: a multicenter study. *J Am Coll Cardiol.* 1987;9:711–722.
75. Konstam MA, Cody RJ. Short-term use of intravenous milrinone for heart failure. *Am J Cardiol.* 1995;75:822–826.
76. Hasenfuss G, Holubarsch C, Heiss HW, et al. Myocardial energetics in patients with dilated cardiomyopathy. Influence of nitroprusside and enoximone. *Circulation.* 1989;80:51–64.
77. Palmer RF, Lasseter KC. Drug therapy. Sodium nitroprusside. *N Engl J Med.* 1975;292:294–297.
78. Cohn JN, Burke LP. Nitroprusside. *Ann Intern Med.* 1979;91: 752–757.
79. Rindone JP, Sloane EP. Cyanide toxicity from sodium nitroprusside: risks and management. *Ann Pharmacother.* 1992;26: 515–519.
80. Packer M. New perspectives on therapeutic application of nitrates as vasodilator agents for severe chronic heart failure. *Am J Med.* 1983;74:61–72.
81. Packer M. Mechanisms of nitrate action in patients with severe left ventricular failure: conceptual problems with the theory of venosequestration. *Am Heart J.* 1985;110:259–264.
82. Ludbrook PA, Byrne JD, Kurnik PB, et al. Influence of reduction of preload and afterload by nitroglycerin on left ventricular diastolic pressure-volume relations and relaxation in man. *Circulation.* 1977;56:937–943.
83. Flaherty JT, Magee PA, Gardner TL, et al. Comparison of intravenous nitroglycerin and sodium nitroprusside for treatment of acute hypertension developing after coronary artery bypass surgery. *Circulation.* 1982;65:1072–1077.
84. Chiariello M, Gold HK, Leinbach RC, et al. Comparison between the effects of nitroprusside and nitroglycerin on ischemic injury during acute myocardial infarction. *Circulation.* 1976;54: 766–773.
85. Cohn JN, Franciosa JA, Francis GS, et al. Effect of short-term infusion of sodium nitroprusside on mortality rate in acute myocardial infarction complicated by left ventricular failure: results of a Veterans Administration cooperative study. *N Engl J Med.* 1982;306:1129–1135.
86. Chen HH, Burnett JC. Natriuretic peptides in the pathophysiology of congestive heart failure. *Curr Cardiol Rep.* 2000;2: 198–205.
87. Mills RM, LeJemtel TH, Horton DP, et al. Sustained hemodynamic effects of an infusion of nesiritide (human B-type natriuretic peptide) in heart failure: a randomized, double-blind, placebo-controlled clinical trial. Natrecor Study Group. *J Am Coll Cardiol.* 1999;34:155–162.
88. Tang WH, Militello M, Barcelona R, et al. Hypotension associated with nesiritide infusion in patients with decompensated heart failure is related to large volume diuresis: implications for monitoring and dose adjustments [abstract]. *J Am Coll Cardiol.* 2004;43:192A.
89. O'Connor CM, Gattis WA, Uretsky BF, et al. Continuous intravenous dobutamine is associated with an increased risk of death in patients with advanced heart failure: insights from the Flolan International Randomized Survival Trial (FIRST). *Am Heart J.* 1999;138:78–86.
90. Grose R, Strain J, Greenberg M, et al. Systemic and coronary effects of intravenous milrinone and dobutamine in congestive heart failure. *J Am Coll Cardiol.* 1986;7:1107–1113.
91. Monrad ES, Baim DS, Smith HS, et al. Milrinone, dobutamine, and nitroprusside: comparative effects on hemodynamics and myocardial energetics in patients with severe congestive heart failure. *Circulation.* 1986;73:III168–III174.
92. Monrad ES, Baim DS, Smith HS, et al. Effects of milrinone on coronary hemodynamics and myocardial energetics in patients with congestive heart failure. *Circulation.* 1985;71:972–979.
93. Mikulic E, Cohn JN, Franciosa JA. Comparative hemodynamic effects of inotropic and vasodilator drugs in severe heart failure. *Circulation.* 1977;56:528–533.
94. Loeb HS, Bredakis J, Gunner RM. Superiority of dobutamine over dopamine for augmentation of cardiac output in patients with chronic low output cardiac failure. *Circulation.* 1977;55: 375–378.

95. Stevenson LW. Tailored therapy before transplantation for treatment of advanced heart failure: effective use of vasodilators and diuretics. *J Heart Lung Transplant.* 1991;10:468–476.
96. Liang CS, Sherman LG, Doherty JU, et al. Sustained improvement of cardiac function in patients with congestive heart failure after short-term infusion of dobutamine. *Circulation.* 1984;69:113–119.
97. Leier CV, Webel J, Bush CA. The cardiovascular effects of the continuous infusion of dobutamine in patients with severe cardiac failure. *Circulation.* 1977;56:468–472.
98. Unverferth DV, Magorien RD, Lewis RP, et al. Long-term benefit of dobutamine in patients with congestive cardiomyopathy. *Am Heart J.* 1980;100:622–630.
99. Goldberg LI. Dopamine: clinical uses of an endogenous catecholamine. *N Engl J Med.* 1974;291:707–710.
100. Goldberg LI. Cardiovascular and renal actions of dopamine: potential clinical applications. *Pharmacol Rev.* 1972;24:1–29.
101. MacCannell KL, McNay JL, Meyer MB, et al. Dopamine in the treatment of hypotension and shock. *N Engl J Med.* 1966;275: 1389–1398.
102. Goldberg LI. Use of sympathomimetic amines in heart failure. *Am J Cardiol.* 1968;22:177–182.
103. Pfeffer MA, McMurray JJ, Velazquez EJ, et al. Valsartan, captopril, or both in myocardial infarction complicated by heart failure, left ventricular dysfunction, or both. *N Engl J Med.* 2003;349: 1893–1906.
104. Cohn JN, Archibald DG, Ziesche S, et al. Effect of vasodilator therapy on mortality in chronic congestive heart failure. Results of a Veterans Administration cooperative study. *N Engl J Med.* 1986;314:1547–1552.
105. Bauer JA, Fung HL. Concurrent hydralazine administration prevents nitroglycerin-induced hemodynamic tolerance in experimental heart failure. *Circulation.* 1991;84:35–39.
106. Gogia H, Mehra A, Parikh S, et al. Prevention of tolerance to hemodynamic effects of nitrates with concomitant use of hydralazine in patients with chronic heart failure. *J Am Coll Cardiol.* 1995;26:1575–1580.
107. Taylor AL, Ziesche S, Yancy C, et al. Combination of isosorbide dinitrate and hydralazine in blacks with heart failure. *N Engl J Med.* 2004;351:2049–2057.
108. Francis GS. Development of arrhythmias in the patient with congestive heart failure: pathophysiology, prevalence and prognosis. *Am J Cardiol.* 1986;57:3B–7B.
109. Luu M, Stevenson WG, Stevenson LW, et al. Diverse mechanisms of unexpected cardiac arrest in advanced heart failure. *Circulation.* 1989;80:1675–1680.
110. Dargie HJ, Cleland JG, Leckie BJ, et al. Relation of arrhythmias and electrolyte abnormalities to survival in patients with severe chronic heart failure. *Circulation.* 1987;75:IV98–IV107.
111. Choy AM, Lang CC, Chomsky DM, et al. Normalization of acquired QT prolongation in humans by intravenous potassium. *Circulation* 1997;96:2149–2154.
112. Gottlieb SS, Fisher ML, Pressel MD, et al. Effects of intravenous magnesium sulfate on arrhythmias in patients with congestive heart failure. *Am Heart J.* 1993;125:1645–1650.
113. Leier CV, Dei Cas L, Metra M. Clinical relevance and management of the major electrolyte abnormalities in congestive heart failure: hyponatremia, hypokalemia, and hypomagnesemia. *Am Heart J.* 1994;128:564–574.
114. Gottlieb SS, Packer M. Deleterious hemodynamic effects of lidocaine in severe congestive heart failure. *Am Heart J.* 1989;118: 611–612.
115. Gottlieb SS, Kukin ML, Medina N, et al. Comparative hemodynamic effects of procainamide, tocainide, and encainide in severe chronic heart failure. *Circulation.* 1990;81:860–864.
116. Kubo SH, Walter BA, John DH, et al. Liver function abnormalities in chronic heart failure. Influence of systemic hemodynamics. *Arch Intern Med.* 1987;147:1227–1230.
117. Levine JH, Massumi A, Scheinman MM, et al. Intravenous amiodarone for recurrent sustained hypotensive ventricular tachyarrhythmias. Intravenous Amiodarone Multicenter Trial Group. *J Am Coll Cardiol.* 1996;27:67–75.
118. Desai AD, Chun S, Sung RJ. The role of intravenous amiodarone in the management of cardiac arrhythmias. *Ann Intern Med.* 1997;127:294–303.
119. Kowey PR, Marinchak RA, Rials SJ, et al. Intravenous amiodarone. *J Am Coll Cardiol.* 1997;29:1190–1198.
120. Kantrowitz A. Experimental augmentation of coronary flow by retardation of the arterial pressure pulse. *Surgery.* 1953;34: 678–687.
121. Buckley MJ, Leinbach RC, Kastor JA, et al. Hemodynamic evaluation of intra-aortic balloon pumping in man. *Circulation.* 1970;41:II130–II136.
122. Dilley RB, Ross J, Jr., Bernstein EF. Serial hemodynamics during intra-aortic balloon counterpulsation for cardiogenic shock. *Circulation.* 1973;48:III99–III104.
123. Benn A, Feldman T. The technique of inserting an intra-aortic balloon pump. Indications, contraindications, advice for avoiding complications. *J Crit Illn.* 1992;7:435–445.
124. Sorrentino M, Feldman T. Techniques for IABP timing, use, and discontinuance. Counterpulsation can reduce ischemia and improve hemodynamics. *J Crit Illn.* 1992;7:597–604.
125. Ashar B, Turcotte LR. Analyses of longest IAB implant in human patient (327 days). *Trans Am Soc Artif Intern Organs.* 1981;27: 372–379.
126. Kormos RL, Borovetz HS, Armitage JM, et al. Evolving experience with mechanical circulatory support. *Ann Surg.* 1991;214: 471–476; discussion 476–477.
127. Rao V, Oz MC, Flannery MA, et al. Changing trends in mechanical circulatory assistance. *J Card Surg.* 2004;19:361–366.
128. Stevenson LW, Tillisch JH. Maintenance of cardiac output with normal filling pressures in patients with dilated heart failure. *Circulation.* 1986;74:1303–1308.
129. Capomolla S, Pozzoli M, Opasich C, et al. Dobutamine and nitroprusside infusion in patients with severe congestive heart failure: hemodynamic improvement by discordant effects on mitral regurgitation, left atrial function, and ventricular function. *Am Heart J.* 1997;134:1089–1098.
130. Wasler A, Radovancevic B, Fruhwald F, et al. First use of the Cancion cardiac recovery system in a human. *Asaio J.* 2003;49: 136–138.
131. Tuzun E, Conger J, Gregoric ID, et al. Evaluation of a new cardiac recovery system in a bovine model of volume overload heart failure. *Asaio J.* 2004;50:557–562.
132. Czerska B, Oren RM, Bohm M, et al. Orqis Cancion Cardiac Recovery System: hemodynamic effects of a novel minimally invasive approach to cardio-renal support in severe acute heart failure. Heart Failure Society of America, 7th Annual Scientific Session. Toronto, Ontario; 2004.
133. Oren RM, Czerska B, Bohm M, et al. Cancion Cardiac Recovery System: effects on renal, echocardiographic, and health status parameters during and following treatment with a novel, minimally invasive approach to cardio-renal support in severe acute heart failure. Heart Failure Society of America, 7th Annual Scientific Session. Toronto, Ontario; 2004.
134. Zile M. Continuous aortic flow augmentation using Orqis Cancion cardiac recovery system in patients with severe heart failure: determinants of the hemodynamic response. American College of Cardiology, 2005 Scientific Session. Orlando, FL; 2005.
135. Pennington DG, Smedira NG, Samuels LE, et al. Mechanical circulatory support for acute heart failure. *Ann Thorac Surg.* 2001;71:S56–S59; discussion S82–S85.
136. Entwistle JW, 3rd. Short- and long-term mechanical ventricular assistance towards myocardial recovery. *Surg Clin North Am.* 2004;84:201–221.

35

The Medical Management of Chronic Heart Failure in Patients with Systolic Dysfunction

Barry H. Greenberg

Since publication of the first edition of this book, substantial changes in the medical management of heart failure have profoundly altered the clinical course of patients with this condition. Although our ability to define exactly the mechanism by which a treatment affects the natural history of heart failure is more limited than we sometimes imagine, new approaches to therapy have generally been based on improved understanding of the underlying pathophysiology of heart failure. Well-designed clinical trials have been the testing ground for new therapies and, as such, their results form the basis for most of the recommendations presented in this chapter. Ironically, as we learn more about heart failure and the patients who suffer from this condition, we have come to realize that clinical trial results may have limited applicability. This is due to the fact that the heart failure population is extremely heterogeneous and that many important groups of patients, most notably females, the very elderly and, in particular, patients with significant comorbidities, are underrepresented in clinical trials. Nonetheless, well-designed clinical trials provide proof of concept and they remain the ultimate rationale for changes in treating heart failure. Based on the results of these trials, there is much reason for optimism for patients with this condition since there is compelling evidence to indicate they have enjoyed substantial gains in both the quantity and quality of their lives due to these new therapies.

The goal of this chapter is to provide an integrated approach to the medical management of patients with heart failure due to systolic dysfunction. The treatment of patients who develop heart failure with preserved ejection fraction (EF) is reviewed in a separate chapter devoted to this entity alone. Since heart failure patients may or may not have signs and symptoms of fluid overload, the term *chronic heart failure* rather than congestive heart failure will be used throughout. Other chapters in this text include extensive reviews of the pathophysiology, prognosis, and drugs used to treat chronic heart failure, and this chapter will focus on selected aspects of these topics only as they relate to a rational and integrated approach to therapy. Medical management requires an understanding of the pathophysiological framework, and the chapter begins with a brief overview of mechanisms involved in the development and progression of heart failure. It is followed by a review of the drugs (diuretics, angiotensin-converting enzyme inhibitors, β-blockers, digoxin) that are the cornerstones of therapy as well as other agents for which information demonstrating efficacy has become available over the past few years (aldosterone antagonists, angiotensin receptor blockers, and the combination of hydralazine and isosorbide dinitrate).

Another major addition to this chapter is the discussion of the role of device therapy in the treatment of patients with chronic heart failure. Advances in this area have been substantial since the last edition of the text and it is imperative that these new approaches to treating heart failure be considered in the context of the pharmacologic therapies to which they are added in order to maximize their benefits. The results of recent clinical trials will be emphasized since information derived from these studies drives the new directions in management of heart failure patients that are outlined in this chapter. Practical aspects of therapy will also be covered and recommendations for the treatment of patients with varying stages of heart failure will be presented.

PATHOPHYSIOLOGY

In order to effectively approach the many issues related to the treatment of the chronic heart failure patient, it is first necessary to define the condition. This task has become progressively more difficult as increased sophistication of the various disciplines and exigencies of funding have widened the chasm between basic researchers and practicing clinicians. Nonetheless, the heart failure phenotype that develops in genetically modified mice and other experimental animal models is not so different from what the clinician encounters when faced with the patient who presents with a large, poorly contracting ventricle, rales, and pedal edema. A working definition that might satisfy both constituencies is that chronic heart failure is a syndrome in which the inability of the heart to provide adequate amounts of oxygenated blood to vital tissue at normal levels of ventricular filling pressure provokes a widespread and progressive response that affects the structure and function of the heart and other organs throughout the body. One key aspect of this definition is that chronic heart failure is a syndrome that develops as the end result of a variety of different disease processes. Some of these diseases may not even primarily affect the heart. Furthermore, this definition calls attention to the fact that chronic heart failure is a dynamic and progressive process that eventually alters the physiology of the entire organism.

As outlined in Table 35-1, heart failure can be attributed to both cardiac and noncardiac causes. Among the cardiac etiologies, myocardial dysfunction is the most common. Myocardial abnormalities that primarily affect systolic function and those that predominantly alter diastolic function can both give rise to the syndrome of heart failure. Most commonly, however, systolic and diastolic dysfunction exist in the same patient. Valvular heart disease, congenital or acquired structural abnormalities, and pericardial disease are all primarily nonmyocardial causes of heart failure. In each of the latter, however, secondary changes in myocardial structure and function are usually involved and may continue to cause chronic heart failure, even after the primary structural abnormality is corrected.

The pathogenesis and management of heart failure on the basis of diastolic myocardial dysfunction, as well as extracardiac and nonmyocardial causes, are covered in Chapters 19, 20, and 22. Recognition of the fact that heart failure is a syndrome with multiple etiologies, however, brings up one of the most important principles of management. That is, in order to decide on a rational course of therapy, it is essential to define as best as possible the cause of the syndrome and to determine whether or not there is a treatable (and even potentially reversible) etiology. Clearly, the approach to the patient with chronic heart failure due to long-standing severe anemia or on the basis of mitral stenosis will be dramatically different than in a patient who develops progressive cardiac dysfunction due to remodeling after myocardial infarction (MI) or as consequence of doxorubicin myocardial toxicity.

A characteristic of chronic heart failure due to myocardial systolic dysfunction is that at some point, either at rest or during exercise, there is a reduction in the capacity of the heart to pump blood. Regardless of the etiology, the resulting reduction in blood pressure and/or cardiac output stimulates a pathophysiological response involving the heart and multiple other organs throughout the body. The primary goal of the compensatory changes, which are summarized in Table 35-2, is to augment the delivery of oxygenated blood to vital organs such as the heart and brain. It is extremely important to recognize that, in addition to providing (mostly short-term) support for the failing heart, these compensatory changes are also associated with effects whose deleterious nature become apparent over time. For instance, retention of salt and water and venoconstriction serve the important function of increasing blood return to the heart. This helps maximize stretch of cardiac sarcomeres. The resulting increase in shortening of these contractile units will augment stroke volume. The increases in left ventricular (LV) filling pressure and volume that occur, however, contribute to the development of conges-

TABLE 35-1
CONDITIONS RESULTING IN THE SYNDROME OF CHRONIC HEART FAILURE

I. Noncardiac disease (e.g., anemia, hemoglobinopathy, AV fistula, thyroid disease, renal disease)
II. Cardiac disease
  A. Structural (due to intracardiac shunts, valvular lesions, or pericardial abnormalities)
    1. Congenital
    2. Acquired
  B. Myocardial (can involve systolic and/or diastolic functions)
    1. Genetic
      a. Systemic (e.g., hemochromatosis)
      b. Cardiac (such as familial hypertrophic or dilated cardiomyopathy)
      c. Both (e.g., various muscular dystrophies)
    2. Acquired
      a. Ischemic
      b. Abnormal loading conditions (e.g., left heart valvular regurgitation, aortic stenosis, hypertension)
      c. Toxic (e.g., alcohol, doxorubicin, methamphetamines)
      d. Infiltrative (e.g., amyloidosis)
      e. Viral
      f. Other

AV, arteriovenous.

TABLE 35-2
COMPENSATORY CHANGES IN CHRONIC HEART FAILURE

Compensation	Mechanism(s)	Beneficial Effects	Adverse Effects
1. Increased chronotropy 2. Increased inotropy	Sympathetic nervous system	Increased CO (CO = HR × SV)	a. Enhanced myocardial ischemia due to increased MVO_2 b. Proarrhythmic c. Long-term deterioration in myocardial function
3. Increased intravascular volume	a. Salt and water retention by the kidney b. Neurohormonal activation	Increased SV by the Frank-Starling mechanism	a. Pulmonary and systemic congestion b. LV hypertrophy and dilation secondary (or 2°) to increased loading conditions c. Increased wall stress d. Increased myocardial oxygen consumption (MVO_2)
4. Peripheral vasoconstriction	a. Neurohormonal (sympathetic nervous system, renin-angiotensin system, arginine vasopressin, endothelin) b. Structural changes in blood vessels c. Local pathways (e.g., ↓ NO production)	a. Increased SV by Frank-Starling mechanism due to venoconstriction b. Increased arterial pressure (BP = CO × SVR)	a. Decreased stroke volume due to high afterload b. Decreased blood flow to some vascular beds c. LV dilatation and hypertrophy secondary (or 2°) to increased loading conditions
5. LV dilation/ hypertrophy	a. Increased loading conditions b. Neurohormonal factors (sympathetic nervous system, renin-angiotensin system, endothelin, cytokines)	a. Increased SV b. Dilation allows increased LV volume at reduced pressure c. Hypertrophy helps normalize wall stress	a. Enhanced myocardial ischemia b. Long-term deterioration in myocardial function c. Predisposition to arrhythmia d. Secondary mitral regurgitation

CO, cardiac output; HR, heart rate; SV, stroke volume; LV, left ventricle; NO, nitric oxide; BP, blood pressure; SVR, systemic vascular resistance.

tive symptoms. They also increase LV wall stress. In addition to increasing myocardial oxygen demands, the increase in wall stress activates mechanoreceptors and stimulates local neurohormonal release, both of which promote cardiac remodeling (1–6). In this manner, fluid retention ultimately leads to both symptoms of heart failure and progression of the underlying abnormalities in cardiac structure and function.

An aspect of heart failure that is now well recognized is the fact that once myocardial damage occurs, changes in cardiac structure and function are not static. Even when the process is initiated by a discrete event such as an MI, there is convincing evidence that deterioration in myocardial systolic function is progressive (7–10). This is due to the process of cardiac remodeling which occurs in response to injury and/or to alteration in global and regional myocardial loading conditions. In these settings neurohormonal systems are activated throughout the body as well as in the heart itself (11–16). There is convincing evidence that many of these neurohormonal systems promote maladaptive cardiac remodeling. Moreover, we now recognize that by blocking the renin-angiotensin system (RAS), aldosterone, and the sympathetic nervous system we can prevent (or reverse) LV remodeling and systolic dysfunction, relieve symptoms, improve quality of life, and significantly reduce heart failure morbidity and mortality.

DRUGS USED IN THE TREATMENT OF CHRONIC HEART FAILURE

Until recently, diuretics, digoxin, and the angiotensin-converting enzyme (ACE) inhibitors were considered to be the three cornerstones of therapy for heart failure. Information collected over the past decade has allowed β-blockers to enter into this therapeutic pantheon. In addition, there is now information that (at least) selected groups of patients may also greatly benefit by the addition of an aldosterone antagonist, an angiotensin receptor blocker, or the combination of hydralazine and isosorbide dinitrate to their therapeutic regimen.

Diuretics

Because patients with heart failure almost always present with signs and symptoms of pulmonary or systemic congestion, diuretic agents play an integral role in the therapeutic approach to this syndrome. Although there is only limited evidence from clinical trials to document their efficacy (17,18) and no clinical trials demonstrating that they improve survival, the obvious impact of diuretic agents on the signs and symptoms of heart failure has confirmed their therapeutic value in a manner analogous to the use of penicillin in treating pneumococcal pneumonia.

Although diuretics are an essential component of the therapeutic approach to chronic heart failure, it is important to recognize that they are effective primarily as a means of removing excess salt and water. As indicated in Table 35-2, patients with chronic heart failure retain fluid in order to increase LV stroke volume. This response, however, is excessive in most instances. As shown in Figure 35-1, the high levels of LV end-diastolic volume that are usually seen in chronic heart failure are no longer effective in enhancing cardiac output because the patient is positioned on the flat portion of the LV function curve. The accompanying increase in LV filling pressure, however, leads to the development of the signs and symptoms of congestion. The predominant impact of diuretic therapy is to reduce filling pressure and relieve congestion. In this case, the patient moves from point A to point B in the figure. In some instances, diuretic therapy also may increase cardiac output (19,20). This is depicted in Figure 35-1 by movement to point D on a new curve that is positioned upward and to the left. There are several mechanisms through which this can occur. Perhaps the most important is that patients with secondary mitral regurgitation (on the basis of dysfunction of the subvalvular apparatus) may experience a considerable improvement in valvular competence as LV volumes are reduced. Cardiac output also can be increased on the basis of a reduction in wall stress (i.e., afterload) due to a decrease in chamber radius or when relief of pulmonary congestion leads to diminished neurohormonal activation and a consequent reduction in peripheral vasoconstriction (19). Finally, reductions in wall stress help reduce myocardial oxygen demands. In situations where myocardial ischemia is present, the favorable effect that this would have on the balance between myocardial oxygen supply and demand would tend to improve LV contractile performance and increase cardiac output.

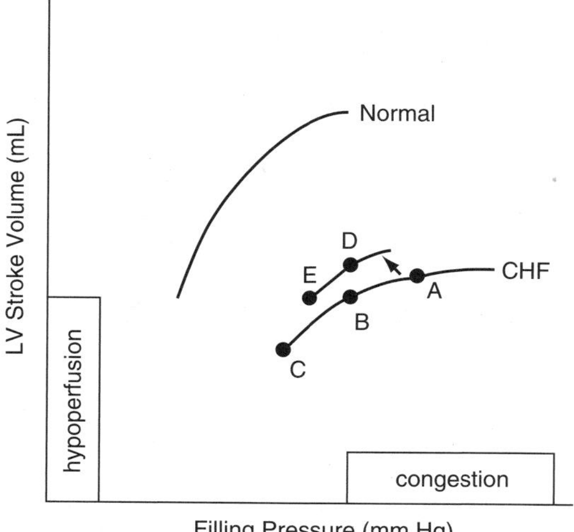

Figure 35-1 Representative LV function curves from a normal subject and a patient with heart failure.

Excessive use of diuretics, however, can lead to a reduction in cardiac output. This is depicted in Figure 35-1 by movement to point C or point E and is related to the fact that diuretics can move the patient from the flat portion of the LV function curve to the ascending portion. In this position, stroke volume is again responsive to the preload stretch of the sarcomeres, and as filling volume is further decreased, cardiac output is reduced. This situation tends to occur when the patient is being aggressively diuresed. Overdiuresis also can be seen as an insidious late occurrence in patients whose LV systolic dysfunction improves over time either spontaneously or in response to therapy. It also tends to occur not infrequently in warm and humid environments when the amount of insensible fluid loss increases. When hypoperfusion due to excessive diuresis occurs, it can be recognized clinically by the complaints of increased weakness and fatigue, signs and symptoms of postural hypotension, or an increase in blood urea nitrogen (BUN) that is out of proportion to increases in serum creatinine (i.e., the BUN/creatinine ratio is increased). When this occurs, reduction in the dose of diuretic is required.

As a result of their potency, relatively low side effect profile, and ability to affect water and solute loss even at low levels of glomerular filtration, loop diuretics such as furosemide, bumetanide, and torsemide are most commonly used for the treatment of heart failure (21,22). Diuretics that act on other portions of the nephron may be used in association with one of the loop diuretics to accomplish specific purposes. For instance, a thiazide diuretic such as metolazone, which acts on the distal collecting tubule, can be used with a loop diuretic to help enhance diuresis in otherwise resistant patients (23,24). In other instances, a potassium-sparing diuretic can be used with a loop diuretic when potassium supplementation proves inadequate to maintain serum levels within the normal range. As will be discussed, the use of an aldosterone antagonist in this setting is particularly appealing since it is associated with a significant reduction in mortality, at least in patients with post-MI left ventricular dysfunction or with advanced heart failure symptoms.

The goal of diuretic therapy is to relieve the signs and symptoms of salt and water retention. In most cases diuretic therapy is initiated along with recommendations to reduce daily sodium intake to the range of 2 g. Even greater reductions to 1.5 g of sodium may be necessary in some clinically tenuous patients. Once patients achieve the euvolemic state, diuretics still need to be continued. The dose, however, may need to be lowered to avoid overdiuresis. Diuretic unresponsiveness can occur owing to a variety of causes, the most common being a deterioration in heart or kidney function; bowel edema, which alters drug absorption; or the use of drugs such as nonsteroidal anti-inflammatory agents, which inhibit the natriuretic effects of loop diuretics (25,26). Diuretic resistance should be treated by first defining the cause. The use of combined diuretic therapy (as described above) or the temporary administration by the intravenous route may be needed to overcome diuretic resistance. In some instances when this condition is due to a reduction in cardiac output and/or renal perfusion pressure, inotropic support with dobutamine or milrinone or the use of ultrafiltration may be necessary to effectively diurese an otherwise refractory patient.

Although diuretics are of unquestionable value in patients who have signs and symptoms of volume overload, their impact on the overall clinical course has been called into question. A post hoc analysis of the Studies of Left Ventricular Dysfunction (SOLVD) database found that compared with patients not taking any diuretic, the risk of hospitalization or death due to worsening HF in patients taking non-potassium-sparing diuretics (PSDs) alone was significantly increased (risk ratio [RR] = 1.31, 95% CI 1.09–1.57; $p = 0.0004$); this was not observed in patients taking PSDs with or without a non-PSD (RR = 0.99, 95% CI 0.76–1.30; $p = 0.95$) (27). Whether this effect was related to a direct action of the diuretic or to other factors that were not adequately controlled for in the course of the analysis cannot be known for certain.

However, these results raise the possibility that loop diuretics might have opposite effects in heart failure patients by relieving symptoms while at the same time adversely affecting long-term prognosis. The latter possibility could be due to diuretic induced electrolyte abnormalities, enhanced neurohormonal stimulation, or an increase in cardiac fibrosis. While the validity of this hypothesis remains uncertain, it does serve as a reminder that diuretic agents should not be given except to help remove accumulated salt and water or to lower elevated blood pressure in the heart failure patient. It is prudent to periodically reassess the need for diuretics and to reduce their dose or even discontinue in stable euvolemic patients. When the latter is being considered, it is important to establish the patient's reliability in recognizing signs and symptoms of volume overload and their ability to restart the diuretic if necessary.

Diuretic agents should never be used as monotherapy in patients with heart failure. As mentioned previously in this chapter, the predominant effect of these drugs is to relieve congestive symptoms. When and if improvements in cardiac function occur, they tend to be modest. Diuretic agents do not alter the natural progression of cardiac dysfunction due to remodeling. Moreover, diuretics activate neurohormonal systems (particularly, the RAS) that have been implicated as causative factors in the progression of disease (28). Thus, diuretics would not be expected to halt or reverse cardiac remodeling and they always must be given in association with neurohormonal blocking agents, as outlined later.

Diuretic agents are associated with a variety of important side effects. The metabolic and electrolyte abnormalities that occur, particularly those involving renal function or serum potassium levels, are a major concern and require careful clinical attention as well as the judicious use of blood chemistry analyses in the follow-up management of patients. Hypokalemia is an important concern because of its association with ventricular arrhythmias (29,30). Thus, use of supplemental potassium is an important adjunct to diuretic therapy in most patients. The use of ACE inhibitors, angiotensin receptor blockers, or aldosterone antagonists tends to decrease the likelihood of hypokalemia, whereas the use of metolazone in association with a loop diuretic tends to increase the likelihood of hypokalemia. The dose of potassium supplementation often needs to be modified when one of these agents is used. Addition of a potassium-sparing diuretic or correction of hypomagnesemia may be needed when refractory hypokalemia occurs.

Digitalis Glycosides

It remains one of the great oddities of clinical medicine that it has taken over two centuries to determine whether the digitalis glycosides are effective therapy for chronic heart failure. The debate has had temporal aspects, with enthusiasm for the drug running high during certain eras but not in others, and there have been geocultural factors leading to widespread acceptance in countries such as Germany and profound skepticism in England. It would seem to be a relatively straightforward process to determine if a particular agent or class of agents does or does not improve the well-being of patients with chronic heart failure. After all, these very issues were decided in relatively short order for the ACE inhibitors (which are helpful) and for oral milrinone (which is not). Since the late 1980s, several small and one large-scale clinical trial, the Digitalis Investigation Group (DIG) study, have helped resolve many of the questions about the clinical efficacy of the digitalis glycosides. In the remainder of this chapter, I will refer to digoxin alone because this is the most widely used of the digitalis preparations.

Digoxin has well-documented inotropic effects (31,32) and it can block impulse transmission across the atrioventricular node. Atrial fibrillation occurs in up to 20% of patients with chronic heart failure, and the use of digoxin is probably least controversial in this setting. The fact that digoxin has only modest positive inotropic effects has been used to argue against its use in chronic heart failure patients who are in normal sinus rhythm. The rebuttal to this argument is that whatever inotropic effect is present, it is enough to produce clinical benefits. In fact, one could argue from the opposite perspective that more intense long-term inotropic support of the heart may actually have deleterious effects in patients with chronic heart failure (33,34). It appears, however, that the noncardiac effects of digoxin, such as enhancing baroreceptor sensitivity (which is diminished in chronic heart failure), are related to clinical efficacy. Digoxin inhibits peripheral sympathetic nervous system activity in patients with chronic heart failure (35). The effects on sympathetic nerve traffic appear to be due to an intrinsic property of the drug rather than to withdrawal of reflex sympathetic stimulation because a comparable improvement in cardiac performance with dopamine does not have the same effect on sympathetic activity. This, of course, raises the question of whether or not digoxin would still have beneficial effects if it were given on top of therapy, which already includes a β-blocking agent.

Although several small clinical trials published in the 1980s suggested that digoxin might be of value in patients with chronic heart failure who were in sinus rhythm (36,37), it was not until somewhat later that this point was established. One of the first trials to demonstrate the value of digoxin compared its effects to those of captopril (an ACE inhibitor) and placebo (38) in patients who had mostly mild [New York Heart Association (NYHA) functional Class I and II symptoms] heart failure and were stable on diuretics alone (after digoxin was withdrawn). Compared with placebo- and captopril-treated patients, the digoxin-treated group demonstrated a significant increase in LV ejection fraction. The captopril-treated patients experienced a significant increase in treadmill exercise time and NYHA class compared with the placebo group. Despite the relatively stable condition of the patients on entry into the study, the brief duration of the trial, and small numbers involved, there was a significant reduction in chronic heart failure-related clinical events in both the captopril and digoxin groups. These results show that in patients with mild chronic heart failure symptoms, both digoxin and captopril are effective therapy and that diuretics alone are not sufficient.

The RADIANCE trial evaluated the effects of digoxin withdrawal in 178 patients with NYHA Class I to III chronic heart failure (39). Patients were required to have an EF below 35%, to be in normal sinus rhythm, and to have been clinically stable on a regimen of digoxin, diuretics, and ACE inhibitors for a period of 8 weeks prior to randomization. During 12 weeks of follow-up, clinical deterioration occurred more frequently in patients who had digoxin withdrawn (28%) than in patients who had digoxin continued (6%). Digoxin withdrawal was associated with a significantly higher likelihood of an increase in diuretic dose, need for emergency room care, or hospitalization for chronic heart failure (25% versus 5% in the group that continued digoxin, $p \leq 0.001$). Patients who had digoxin withdrawn also experienced a significant reduction in treadmill exercise time, distance covered during a 6-minute walk test, and in LV ejection fraction. A similar study conducted in patients who were not receiving ACE inhibitors reported comparable findings (40).

The effects of digoxin on mortality were evaluated in the large-scale DIG trial, in which 6,800 patients with mild to moderate heart failure were randomized to continue digoxin or have it withdrawn from their medical regimen (41). The results showed quite conclusively the absence of any survival benefit with digoxin. A 28% reduction in hospitalizations due to worsening heart failure ($p < 0.001$) confirmed the beneficial effects with digoxin seen in smaller trials. The overall reduction in all-cause hospitalization was 6%. The DIG study also reported an insignificant but nonetheless disquieting increase in sudden death in patients receiving the drug.

The results of these clinical trials justify the use of digoxin in treating patients in sinus rhythm. They also provide evidence for guiding its administration. Digoxin is useful mainly for treating signs and symptoms of heart failure but it has no demonstrable effects on either the progression of LV dysfunction or on survival (41). Therefore, the use of digoxin should be reserved for those chronic heart failure patients who either require rate control of atrial fibrillation or those in sinus rhythm who remain symptomatic after optimization of other first-line therapies.

One of the advantages of digoxin is that it is relatively easy to use and can be given only once a day. Although the drug is not innocuous, the incidence of toxicity in clinical practice is certainly very far below the estimated 15% level that was reported in hospitalized patients in the early 1970s (42). This is likely due to multiple factors, including the avoidance of longer-acting digitalis glycosides, a higher degree of alertness to the signs and symptoms of digoxin toxicity on the part of practicing clinicians, increased recognition of the conditions in which digoxin toxicity is likely to occur, the availability of other agents to treat chronic heart failure both acutely and chronically (thus minimizing the need to "push dig" in patients who are doing poorly), greater attention to electrolyte abnormalities that could potentiate digoxin toxicity, the widespread availability of an assay to determine levels of digoxin in the blood, and general recognition that a low dose of digoxin is all that is necessary for treating heart failure patients (43).

The use of digoxin in the acute management of patients with decompensated chronic heart failure is much less common than in the past because other more potent inotropic and/or vasodilator agents that are rapidly acting and can be carefully titrated are now available. In stable patients, a maintenance dose of digoxin, ranging from 0.125 to 0.25 mg daily, is usually begun. A stable concentration in blood is usually obtained within 5 to 7 days and, when there are concerns about clearance, confirmed by measurement of the serum digoxin level. Continuous measurement of digoxin levels in stable patients is not needed. Even in situations where digoxin levels may be altered by concurrent therapy or worsening renal disease, most physicians simply reduce the dose of the drug. In some cases measuring digoxin levels is an important indicator of the overall compliance of the patient to the medical regimen and it can help sort out the cause of an episode of decompensation. Because there is little evidence that high-dose digoxin offers significant clinical benefit over low-dose therapy (44,45), the use of digoxin levels to titrate the dose of drug has little validity.

Angiotensin-Converting Enzyme Inhibitors

As mentioned in the section on pathophysiology and in other chapters of this text, activation of the RAS plays an important role in the pathogenesis of chronic heart failure. In general, elevations in plasma renin activity correlate with the severity of the condition (46). A reduction in cardiac output and renal perfusion appears to be a major factor in this process (46,47). Patients with asymptomatic LV dysfunction, however, may have increased levels of plasma renin activity, particularly if they are being treated with diuretic agents (28). The local, tissue-based RAS also appears to be upregulated in the setting of LV dysfunction and it appears to play a major role in the progression of the disease by promoting cardiac remodeling (15,16,48,49).

As summarized in Table 35-2, the adverse consequences of activation of the RAS provide a rationale for the use of ACE inhibitors in the treatment of chronic heart failure. The ACE inhibitors, however, may also have other actions that could account for their demonstrated clinical efficacy. Converting enzyme, in addition to blocking the breakdown of angiotensin I to angiotensin II, are also involved in the inactivation of bradykinin, substance P, and other vasoactive compounds (50). The effects on bradykinin may be of particular importance because this substance can stimulate endothelial cells to release prostacyclin (51) and nitric oxide (NO) (52), both of which have vasodilatory properties. Thus, ACE inhibitor potentiation of bradykinin could promote vasodilation through pathways unrelated to the RAS (53). Bradykinin also may have antigrowth effects that could contribute to the effects of ACE inhibitors in preventing cardiac remodeling (54).

As a result of their ability to dilate peripheral vessels and to unload the heart, the ACE inhibitors have been shown to improve cardiac function (55–57). Initially, there is little impact on exercise capacity despite an increase in cardiac output and a reduction in ventricular filling pressures. However, over a period of weeks to months, exercise duration improves in patients with mild to moderate chronic heart failure (38,58,59). Symptomatic improvement also becomes manifest over time. The reasons for the temporal disparity between the acute cardiac and long-term clinical effects of the ACE inhibitors are uncertain. Enhanced peripheral vasodilation and tissue oxygen extraction during chronic (but not acute) therapy have been demonstrated (60,61). This could be related to alterations in tissue mechanisms for oxygen extraction, structural changes in blood vessels, or better conditioning (as cardiac function improves). ACE inhibitors also have been shown to enhance NO production in an experimental model of chronic heart failure (62), and this factor could account for the improved peripheral vasodilation and clinical benefits seen during long-term therapy.

One of the most important goals of the management of patients with chronic heart failure is to prevent further myocardial dysfunction. There is evidence that the LV undergoes progressive change in size, structure, and function over time following MI (7–9). Patients who survive an MI with more than mild myocardial damage experience progressive increases in chamber size and muscle mass (8,9). Both LV dilation and hypertrophy, unfortunately, are strongly related to both late deterioration in LV systolic function and to decreased survival (63–67). The fact that ACE inhibitors favorably affect both mechanical and neurohormonal factors that promote remodeling provided the rationale for evaluating their effects following MI. Initial studies demonstrated that ACE inhibitors prevented post-MI increases in LV chamber size (10,68). SAVE and other well-designed, large-scale clinical trials which evaluated the effects of ACE inhibitors on the clinical course of MI survivors have demonstrated that they are associated with prolonged survival and a lower likelihood of developing heart failure or hospitalization (69–75)—effects that likely are associated with their ability to inhibit post-MI cardiac remodeling.

The effects of ACE inhibitors on survival in patients with LV dysfunction have been studied extensively (76–79). Some of the key features of trials evaluating ACE inhibitors are summarized in Table 35-3. Although ejection fraction cut-offs and other entry criteria varied somewhat between the trials, all patients had moderate to severe LV systolic dysfunction. Functional impairment ranged from the asymptomatic state to NYHA Class IV heart failure. The results provide conclusive evidence that ACE inhibitor therapy improves survival in a broad spectrum of patients with LV dysfunction (76–79). Moreover, they show that ACE inhibitors are effective in most subgroups of patients and that the benefits are not dependent on factors such as age, gender, etiology of chronic heart failure, serum sodium level, or treatment with β-blockers. ACE inhibitors appear to be more effective in reducing mortality in more severely ill patients (e.g., NYHA functional Class IV in CONSENSUS [74]) than in less symptomatic patients (e.g., NYHA functional Class I–II in the SOLVD Prevention arm [78]). There is also some evidence that efficacy of the ACE inhibitors is greater in those patients with more severe depression of LV ejection fraction (77,78) but that their beneficial effects may be attenuated when patients are receiving aspirin (80,81).

The effects of ACE inhibitors on cardiac remodeling in patients with LV dysfunction were evaluated in a subgroup of the SOLVD population (82). Although these patients had evidence of considerable LV dilation and hypertrophy at the time of randomization, patients assigned to placebo demonstrated progressive increases in LV volumes and muscle mass over the 12-month follow-up period, thereby indicating the relentless nature of cardiac remodeling. Further increases in LV volumes and mass, however, were prevented in the enalapril-treated patients. These results from a representative subgroup of the SOLVD study population suggest that the clinical benefits of the ACE inhibitors are related to their favorable effects on the remodeling process. They also show that the opportunity to prevent further increases in muscle mass and chamber volume even after considerable remodeling has occurred.

The side effects associated with ACE include hypotension, hyperkalemia, dizziness and syncope, taste disturbances, worsening renal function, cough, and angioneurotic edema. A reduction in blood pressure is expected with the initiation of therapy, and in most instances it is of little consequence. Patients at increased risk of developing clinically important hypotensive symptoms can be identified by the presence of advanced functional class (i.e., Class IV); recent aggressive therapy with diuretics; use of non-ACE inhibitor vasodilators; presence of low serum sodium levels (i.e., serum Na $<$130 mm L/L) (83); and borderline blood pressure at the time when therapy is initiated. Because many of these patients fall into categories that are most likely to benefit from ACE inhibitor therapy, the greater incidence of hypotension should not be considered a contradiction to initiating treatment. Experience from SOLVD and other trials demonstrates quite clearly that only a small number of patients with LV dysfunction could not be continued on ACE inhibitors because of hypotension or other side effects (74–79).

ACE inhibitor therapy should be initiated at a low dose which is uptitrated over a period of days to weeks depending on the clinical situation. Hospitalized patients in whom dose of drug can be increased in a controlled setting often reach the target dose within a matter of days, while uptitration of ACE inhibitors in the outpatient setting is usually more gradual. Patients should be educated about the possibility of hypotension, and a blood chemistry screen to assess renal function and serum potassium levels should be obtained at 1 week after initiation, following each increase in dose, and when the target dose has been

TABLE 35-3

EFFECTS OF ACE INHIBITOR THERAPY ON SURVIVAL OF PATIENTS WITH LEFT VENTRICULAR DYSFUNCTION

Trial	Population	n	Study Drugs	EF Entry Criteria	NYHA Class	Mean Duration	Reduction in Mortality
1. CONSENSUS	General	253	Enalapril vs. placebo	None	IV	188 days	40%[a]
2. Ve-HFT II	Male U.S. service veterans	804	Enalapril vs. hydralazine-isosorbide dinitrate	≤45%	II–III	30.0 mo	28%[b]
3. SOLVD-Treatment	General	2,569	Enalapril vs. placebo	≤35%	II–III	41.4 mo	16%
4. SOLVD-Prevention	LV dysfunction not requiring CHF therapy	4,228	Enalapril vs. placebo	≤35%	I–II	37.4 mo	8%
5. SAVE	Survivors of recent myocardial infarction	2,231	Captopril vs. placebo	≤40%	I–III	42 ± 10 mo	19%

[a]At 6 months.
[b]At 2 years.
CHF, congestive heart failure; LV, left ventricular.

reached. Many candidates for ACE inhibitors have evidence of mild to moderate renal dysfunction prior to the initiation of therapy. A small bump in BUN or creatinine levels is common and should not cause undue concern. Sustained increases in BUN greater than 15 to 20 mg/dL or in creatinine greater than 0.2 to 0.5 mg/dL can often be successfully treated by adjusting therapy. In patients receiving diuretics or other non-ACE inhibitor vasodilators, a reduction in the dose of these drugs is often sufficient to correct the abnormality. If this tactic fails, one can consider reducing the dose of the ACE inhibitor. However, because the changes in BUN and creatinine are reversible, reduction in dose or discontinuation of ACE inhibitors should be undertaken only after careful consideration of the risk/benefit ratio of doing this.

Cough is a frequent complaint in patients with chronic heart failure (84). However, ACE inhibitor-related cough must be differentiated from cough due to a myriad of other causes (including worsening pulmonary congestion). The problem is highlighted by results from the treatment arm of the SOLVD study, where it was found that although 37% of patients treated with enalapril complained of cough, this symptom was also noted in 31% of placebo-treated patients (77). Thus, while cough due to ACE inhibitors is a real problem, its actual incidence is relatively low. A careful search for other causes of cough should always be undertaken before discontinuing ACE inhibitor therapy. There is no convincing evidence that one ACE inhibitor is more likely to provoke cough than another, and changing the ACE inhibitor is rarely successful in solving the problem. When cough does not resolve after the drug is stopped, one can conclude that the problem is not due to the ACE inhibitor, which should then be restarted while the real cause is sought.

There is a tendency for potassium levels to increase when ACE inhibitors are initiated. As evidenced in both arms of SOLVD (77,78), the change is small and of little or no clinical consequence in most instances. However, in patients with underlying renal dysfunction and in patients receiving potassium-sparing diuretics or large amounts of potassium supplementation, the increase in serum potassium level can on occasion be life-threatening. The condition can be treated by reducing either the non-ACE inhibitor factor (e.g., K^+ supplement) or the ACE inhibitor itself. Vigilance on the part of the physician is necessary, however, to detect hyperkalemia.

An interesting but regrettable phenomenon that has developed with the use of the ACE inhibitors in patients with chronic heart failure is that they tend to be used at lower doses than were used in the studies that provided evidence of efficacy. The obvious reason for this strategy is the desire to avoid side effects. However, SOLVD and other large-scale clinical trials provide strong evidence that the ACE inhibitors tend to be well-tolerated (76–79). It is uncertain whether the same clinical benefits that were noted in the clinical trials will be present when the drugs are used at lower doses. In fact, the ATLAS study showed that high doses of ACE inhibitors are associated with greater improvement in the clinical course (85) and that they are well-tolerated (86). Thus, the use of target doses of ACE inhibitors (e.g., ramipril at 10 mg per day, enalapril or lisinopril at 20 to 40 mg per day, and captopril at 150 mg per day) is strongly recommended.

ANGIOTENSIN RECEPTOR BLOCKERS

Over the past 5 years angiotensin receptor blockers (ARBs) have gained an increasingly important role in the management of patients with heart failure. Their initiation into the treatment regimen was delayed largely because of the earlier availability of ACE inhibitors. However, ARBs are now recognized as being quite useful alternatives to ACE inhibitors in the management of patients with post-MI LV dysfunction and in patients with heart failure due to systolic dysfunction. There is also evidence that their addition to an ACE inhibitor can improve the clinical course of heart failure patients.

ARBs compete with angio-tensin II for occupancy of the type 1 angiotensin II receptor (AT1R) on cells throughout the body. Since most adverse cardiovascular effects of angiotensin II (such as salt and water retention, peripheral vasoconstriction, cardiac myo-cyte hypertrophy, and fibroblast activation) are mediated through the AT1R, blockade of this receptor should be protective. Moreover, ARBs block the effects of angiotensin II regardless of whether it is generated by the usual pathway involving ACE or through alternative pathways. In the heart an alternative pathway involving chymase that is released from mast cells is believed to be particularly important in the generation of angiotensin II (87). An added benefit of the ARBs may be related to so-called shunting of angiotensin II from the AT1R to type 2 angiotensin receptor (AT2R), which is believed to mediate antigrowth effects. There is also evidence that ARBs increase the expression of a homologue of ACE termed ACE2 (88). Activity of this enzyme may be cardioprotective in that it acts to break down angiotensin II while generating Ang-(1–7). This heptapeptide has been shown to have both vasodilatory, antiproliferative, and antigrowth properties that are mediated by activation of a novel non-AT1 or AT2 receptor (89–91).

The efficacy of ARBs in treating patients with post-MI LV dysfunction was demonstrated in the VALIANT study in which the effects of valsartan were compared to captopril (92). This particular ACE inhibitor was chosen as the active comparator in VALIANT based on its proven efficacy in treating patients with post-MI LV dysfunction in the SAVE study. An additional arm of the VALIANT study included patients treated with a combination of captopril and valsartan. The results demonstrated that valsartan was equally as effective as captopril in reducing cardiovascular morbidity and mortality but that the combination was associated with increased adverse events without improving outcomes. In VALIANT (as in previous studies), baseline echocardiographic parameters were shown to be powerful predictors of all major outcomes. Treatment with captopril, valsartan, or the combination of captopril plus valsartan resulted in similar changes in cardiac volume, EF, and infarct segment length between baseline and 20 months after MI, indicating relative equivalence in protection against adverse cardiac remodeling. Based on these results the use of an ARB has been accepted as an alternative to an ACE inhibitor in the treatment of patients with post-MI LV dysfunction.

The effects of an ARB in ACE inhibitor-intolerant patients were assessed in the CHARM-Alternative study (93). This trial included more than 2,000 ACE inhibitor-intolerant patients (due to cough in 72%, symptomatic hypotension in 13%, and renal dysfunction in 12%) with symptomatic heart failure due to LV systolic dysfunction who were randomized to receive treatment with either candesartan or placebo. The primary outcome was the composite of cardiovascular death or hospital admission for heart failure. As shown in Figure 35-2 during a median follow-up of 33.7 months, candesartan was associated with a 23% risk reduction for the combined endpoint ($p = 0.0004$). Each component of the primary outcome was reduced, as was the total number of hospital admissions for CHF. Study-drug discontinuation rates were similar in the candesartan (30%) and placebo (29%) groups. These results were further substantiated by a prior analysis of a group of patients in the Val-HeFT study who were not receiving an ACE inhibitor and in whom valsartan significantly reduced mortality (94).

The results of the CHARM-Alternative and Val-HeFT subgroup analysis provide persuasive evidence of the beneficial effects of ARBs as a treatment for heart failure due to systolic dysfunction in ACE inhibitor-intolerant patients. Previous comparison between the two approaches in the ELITE-2 study, however, indicated that the use of an ARB did not offer benefits that were superior to those of an ACE inhibitor (95). Thus, ARBs remain an alternative for use in heart failure patients who are ACE-intolerant. They could also be continued if the patient was receiving an ARB for a pre-exisiting condition such as hypertension at the time that he or she developed heart failure.

The fact that ACE inhibitors and ARBs have distinct pharmacologic profiles raises the possibility that their combined effects have incremental benefits in heart failure patients. This hypothesis was tested in two large-scale trials, Val-HeFT and CHARM-Added. In Val-HeFT, valsartan was added to standard therapy, which in most cases included an ACE inhibitor. The results demonstrated a significant 13% reduction in the combined primary endpoint of morbidity and mortality (96). This reduction was due largely to a reduction in heart failure hospitalizations and there was no significant impact on mortality. Post hoc analysis of the Val-HeFT database also raised the possibility that the addition of the ARB to patients already receiving an ACE inhibitor and β-blocker might be associated with an increase in mortality. In CHARM-Added, 2,548 patients with NYHA functional Class II–IV CHF and LVEF 40% or lower who were being treated with ACE inhibitors were randomly assigned to either candesartan or placebo (97). After 41 months of follow-up, the composite of cardiovascular death or hospital admission for heart failure was reduced by 15% ($p = 0.011$). Candesartan reduced each of the components of the primary outcome significantly, as well as the total number of hospital admissions for heart failure. Of the patients enrolled in CHARM-Added, 55% were receiving a β-blocker at the time of randomization. Analysis of outcomes in this predefined subgroup failed to detect any evidence of a negative impact of adding the ARB to existing therapy, suggesting that the adverse interaction seen in Val-HeFT was likely a statistical artifact. Based on the results of these studies, the possibility of adding an ARB to standard therapy (including an ACE inhibitor and β-blocker) in heart failure patients who remain symptomatic despite treatment with an ACE inhibitor and β-blocker should be considered.

The side effects of the ARBs are similar to those of the ACE inhibitors except for the absence of cough and a much lower likelihood of angioneurotic edema. The recommendations for uptitration and dosing of the ARBs and for following laboratory assessment of renal function and serum electrolytes are the same as those given for the ACE inhibitors in the previous section. The likelihood of worsening renal function, hyperkalemia, and hypotension is significantly greater with the combination of an ACE inhibitor and ARB than with either drug alone. Vigilance is required when the combination is used in order to avoid untoward consequences.

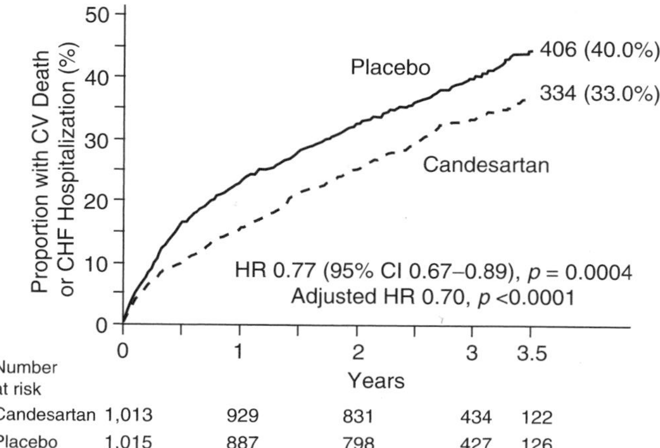

Figure 35-2 Results from the CHARM-Added study demonstrating a reduction in the primary end-point of cardiovascular death or heart failure hospitalization. (From Granger CB, McMurray JJV, Yusuf S, et al. Effects of candesartan in patients with chronic heart failure and reduced left-ventricular systolic function intolerant to angiotensin-converting-enzyme inhibitors: the CHARM-Alternative trial. *Lancet*. 2003; 362:772–776.)

β-ADRENERGIC RECEPTOR ANTAGONISTS

Activation of the sympathetic nervous system is one of the most important factors responsible for the progression of heart failure. Sympathetic activation occurs early in the course (28) and it provides circulatory support by increasing heart rate and contractility and by constricting peripheral blood vessels (Table 35-2). Levels of circulating catecholamines increase in patients with chronic heart failure in proportion to the severity of the disease (28). Norepinephrine has a number of deleterious effects on the adult mammalian cardiomyocyte (98). Catecholamines promote myocyte growth, increase cell death by inducing both necrosis and apoptosis, desensitize β-adrenergic receptors, cause peripheral vasoconstriction, enhance arrhythmias, augment renin release, and impair sodium excretion from the kidney (99–106). Not surprisingly, there is a strong association between high sympathetic nervous activity and an unfavorable prognosis in patients with chronic heart failure (107).

These observations suggest that drugs that interfere with β-adrenergic activation should be useful in the management of patients with chronic heart failure. For many years, however, β-blockers were thought to be harmful in heart failure because of their negative inotropic properties and possible short-term adverse effects. Controlled clinical trials with a number of different β-blockers helped dispel this notion by showing that sustained β-blocker therapy could reduce chronic heart failure symptoms and improve LV systolic function (108–117). Although numerous small- to medium-sized clinical trials as well as retrospective analysis of the use of β-blockers post-MI (118,119) strongly suggested important clinical benefits in heart failure, this promise was not borne out until the results of several large-scale clinical trials became available.

The results of pivotal clinical trials demonstrating the efficacy of β-blockers in the treatment of heart failure are summarized in Figure 35-3. In each of these trials the β-blocker was added to standard treatment which included an ACE inhibitor in the vast majority of patients. Overall, these studies demonstrate that the addition of a β-blocker reduces all-cause mortality risk (in the range of 35%) and they offer a compelling rationale for strongly recommending their use in heart failure patients.

The U.S. Carvedilol Clinical Trials Program was the first to present convincing data of the clinical efficacy of β-blockers in the treatment of chronic heart failure (120). Carvedilol is a nonspecific β-blocker with effects on both the β_1 and β_2 adrenergic receptor (121). It also is an α_1-adrenergic receptor blocker, a property that results in peripheral vasodilation, and it has antioxidant and other potentially beneficial effects (122). Patients enrolled in the four component trials of the U.S. program all had heart failure on the basis of systolic dysfunction as evidenced by an LV ejection fraction of ≥35% (120). Most patients had symptoms of mild to moderate heart failure and were clinically stable on standard therapy that included an ACE inhibitor. The composite data from the four trials demonstrated that patients treated with carvedilol experienced a 65% reduction in mortality (7.8% placebo versus 3.2% carvedilol; $p = 0.0001$). Heart failure hospitalization was also significantly reduced.

The effects of carvedilol in patients with more advanced heart failure were assessed in the COPERNICUS trial (123). This study is of particular importance in that it enrolled patients who were at higher risk than in previous studies based on inclusion criteria that mandated more severe symptoms and lower ejection fraction. The severity of heart failure in the COPERNICUS patients was clearly manifest by the nearly 20% mortality after 1 year in the patients assigned to placebo. Nonetheless, the addition of carvedilol to the medical regimen reduced the primary endpoint of all-cause mortality by 35% ($p = 0.0014$). A significant reduction in hospitalizations was also seen in this study. Differences in outcome in favor of carvedilol were noticeable as early as 2 to 3 weeks after the initiation of treatment. Moreover, carvedilol was generally well-tolerated in this high risk population. Worsening heart failure was the only serious adverse event (with a frequency greater than 2%) and was reported with similar frequency in the placebo and carvedilol groups (6.4% versus 5.1%).

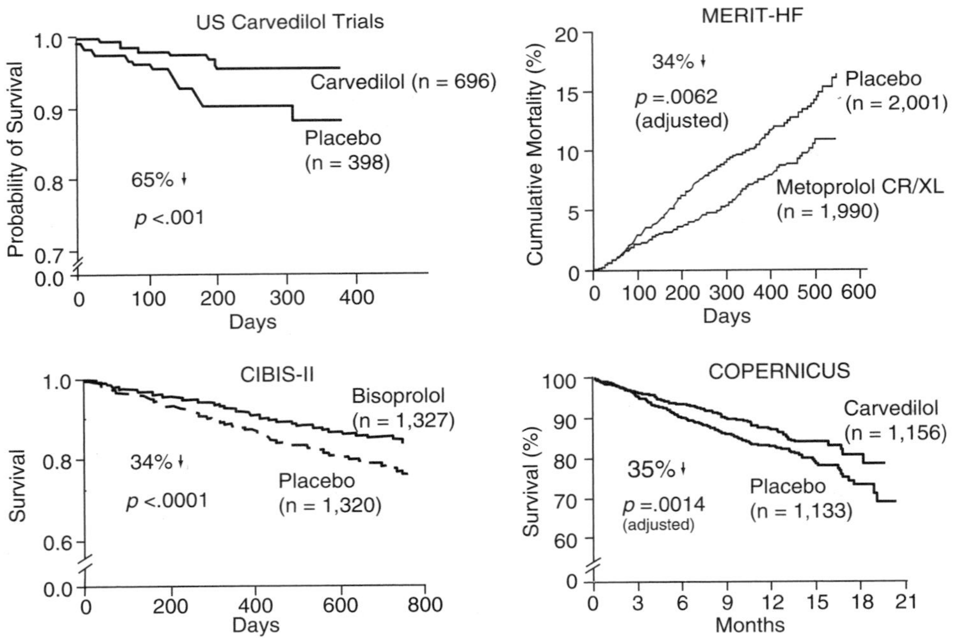

Figure 35-3 Clinical trial results provide incontrovertible evidence that β-blockers improve survival in patients with heart failure. Patients included in these studies had symptomatic heart failure due to LV systolic dysfunction. The results show that the addition of β-blockers to optimal medical therapy that includes an ACE inhibitor reduces mortality risk in the range of 35% compared to placebo. (Packer M, Bristow MR, Cohn JN, et al. The effect of carvedilol on morbidity and mortality in patients with chronic heart failure. *N Engl J Med.* 1996;334: 1349–1355. MERIT-HF Study Group. *Lancet.* 1999;253:2001–2007. CIBIS-II Investigators and Committees. The Cardiac Insufficiency Bisoprolol Study II (CIBIS-II): a randomised trial. *Lancet.* 1999;353:9–13. Packer M, Fowler MB, Roecker EB, et al. *N Eng J Med.* 2001; 344:1651-1658.)

CIBIS II evaluated the effects of bisoprolol, a selective β_1 antagonist, in 2,647 patients with heart failure due to systolic dysfunction (124). Although the patients were classified as NYHA functional Class III and IV, the relatively low annual mortality rate of 12% in the placebo group suggested that these patients may have had less-advanced heart failure. The results showed that the all-cause mortality rate was significantly lowered with bisoprolol by a 34% reduction ($p < 0.0001$). In CIBIS-II sudden death was reduced by 44% and hospitalization for heart failure was decreased by 30% ($p = 0.0005$). The Metoprolol Randomized Intervention Trial in Congestive Heart Failure (MERIT-HF) evaluated the effects of metoprolol succinate, also a β_1 selective agent, in 3,991 patients with predominantly NYHA functional Class II and III heart failure (125). The results showed metoprolol succinate reduced all-cause mortality by 35% ($p < 0.001$). A reduction in sudden cardiac death was also seen.

Overall, these studies demonstrate that β-blocker therapy using either carvedilol, bisoprolol, or metoprolol succinate can favorably affect the clinical course of patients with heart failure and that treatment with these drugs is associated with substantial reductions in both morbidity and mortality. Based on the consistency of the results and the magnitude of the effects on the clinical course that were demonstrated, β-blockers have now emerged as a standard therapy of patients with heart failure due to systolic dysfunction. The results of these studies indicate that β-blockers are of value across a wide spectrum of patients with left LV systolic dysfunction ranging from patients with mild symptomatic impairment to those with severe impairment (e.g., late NYHA functional Class III to early Class IV).

Although the database for β-blockers in patients with asymptomatic LV dysfunction is less robust than in patients with symptomatic heart failure, their use is nevertheless recommended in these patients based on the following considerations: (a) improved outcomes with carvedilol in the Australia–New Zealand study, which included a substantial number of patients with ischemic cardiomyopathy who were without heart failure symptoms (126); (b) evidence of early sympathetic nervous system activation and involvement in the progression of cardiac dysfunction (a situation that is parallel to that seen for the RAS) (28); (c) many of these patients will have conditions such as coronary artery disease and/or hypertension for which β-blockers are already indicated; and (d) recent evidence that metoprolol succinate can prevent adverse remodeling in a population of patients with asymptomatic LV systolic dysfunction.

Because β-blockers were used in patients who were already receiving ACE inhibitors in the clinical trials described above (120,123–126), it appears that the effects of these two classes of drugs are additive. Furthermore, these findings demonstrate the value of blocking neurohormonal activation at more than one point alone. Although there has been some debate on which class of agent to begin first (and some data to suggest that starting the β-blocker initially may be preferable) (127,128), the issue is usually moot in clinical practice. The identification of systolic dysfunction and the initiation of neurohormonal blocking agents usually are triggered by an episode of decompensated heart failure. In this setting the often volume-overloaded patient is treated with a diuretic. At that point it is prudent to also initiate an ACE inhibitor, which by virtue of its vasodilatory properties may help unload the heart and also counteract the activation of the RAS that occurs when diuretics are given. Initiation of a β-blocker is then begun after the patient achieves the euvolemic state. In situations where the patient does not have evidence of volume overload and is a candidate for both classes of agents, it is my usual practice to first start and uptitrate a β-blocker.

The β-blockers that have been shown to be clinically effective in treating heart failure patients include carvedilol, bisoprolol, and metoprolol succinate. The former provides broad-spectrum blockade of adrenergic receptor subtypes while the latter two agents are selective β_1-adrenergic blocking agents. Based on the efficacy demonstrated with these three agents, one can ask the question whether this indicates the presence of a class effect with the implication that all β-blockers could provide essentially the same amount of protection and benefit. Ergo, even agents that were not tested in large-scale clinical trials could be used to treat heart failure patients. The wisdom of this approach, however, has been strongly challenged by the publication of a meta-analysis demonstrating little (if any) cardioprotective effect of atenolol, a commonly prescribed agent (129).

Results from clinical trials also support the concept of clinically important differences between β-blockers. The BEST study evaluated the effects of bucindolol in patients with advanced heart failure (130). Bucindolol is a nonselective β-blocker with vasodilatory properties, a profile that would seem ideal for use in the heart failure population. This clinical trial, however, was stopped prematurely when it became apparent that the effects of bucindolol were considerably less favorable than those of other β-blockers. The reasons for the differences between the effects of bucindolol and other agents remain controversial. While they could be due to inclusion of a larger number of African-Americans or sicker patients in BEST than in the other trials, it is more likely that they were related to the pharmacologic profile of bucindolol, including possible intrinsic sympathomimetic activity (131) and/or its effect in producing more profound early reduction in circulating catecholamine levels than other agents (132).

Further evidence against equal efficacy of all β-blockers is available from the COMET study, which was a head-to-head comparison between carvedilol and metoprolol tartrate (the short-acting preparation of metoprolol) in patients with symptomatic heart failure due to LV systolic dysfunction (133). The results showed that carvedilol 25 mg twice daily was superior to metoprolol tartrate 50 mg twice daily, since patients treated with carvedilol had a 17% risk reduction in all-cause mortality, the primary end-point in the study. The reduction in mortality in favor of carvedilol was seen for death due to pump failure as well as sudden cardiac death. Carvedilol also reduced the risk for MI compared to metoprolol tartrate. These results provide convincing evidence that not all β-blockers are equally effective in reducing cardiovascular risk in heart failure patients. Thus, the strong recommendation is that only the three drugs cited above that were shown in large-scale clinical trials to favorably affect outcomes should be used in the heart failure population.

Recommendations for the initiation of β-blockers include their use only in clinically stable patients who are not volume-overloaded or receiving intravenous diuretics, vasodilators, or inotropic agents to treat decompensated heart failure. Because of the possibility of reducing EF initially, these agents should be started only in stable patients and at a low dose of drug (134). For instance, therapy is usually initiated with 3.125 mg carvedilol twice daily, 1.25 mg of bisoprolol once daily, or 12.5 or 25 mg of metoprolol succinate once daily. Patients should be cautioned that they may experience a worsening in their symptoms such as increased fatigue, more pronounced shortness of breath with or without weight gain, and signs and symptoms of hypotension. Well-defined instruction for adjusting concurrent medication and/or contacting the physician's office should be given to patients at the time that β-blockers are initiated. Patients should be monitored on a regular basis for signs of worsening chronic heart failure, fluid retention, hypotension, and bradycardia during the titration period. In general, the dose of the β-blocker is doubled every 2 weeks in patients who are tolerating therapy. Although the database is limited, it does appear that the more complete the β-blockade, the greater the likelihood of clinical benefit (116,135). Therefore, β-blockers should be gradually titrated upward to the doses found effective in the clinical trials previously described.

Patients who develop signs and symptoms of fluid retention should be treated with increased dose of diuretics (134). Symptomatic hypotension can be treated in a number of different ways. Perhaps the easiest (and most effective) is to temporarily separate the time of administration of the β-blocking agent from the other drugs that the patient is taking. After the condition is stabilized and the β-blocker has been fully titrated upward, the patient can then again try taking all medications at the same time for convenience. Because the β-blockers can slow heart rate, both in patients in normal sinus rhythm and those in atrial fibrillation, there is some concern about provocation of bradyarrhythmias. Patients who become symptomatically bradycardic should have the dose of β-blocker reduced. In some instances, however, physicians have recommended pacemaker support to allow initiation and titration of β-blocker therapy. However, there is no evidence of the overall benefit of this approach and it should be undertaken only after careful consideration of the risk/benefit and cost analysis of such therapy.

Aldosterone Antagonists

The role of aldosterone blockade in the treatment of heart failure has been largely clarified by studies carried out over the past decade. Although it was recognized that aldosterone levels were elevated in patients with heart failure as part of the so-called neurohormonal storm that characterized this condition and that aldosterone stimulated a host of unfavorable effects in cells and tissue throughout the body, the possibility of using aldosterone antagonists to treat heart failure was not seriously considered for many years, despite the availability of agents that could accomplish this. One reason for not pursuing this avenue of therapy was related to the belief that since aldosterone release is stimulated by angiotensin II, the use of ACE inhibitors and ARBs made targeting aldosterone unnecessary. Although angiotensin II is certainly an important regulator of aldosterone production and release, it is now recognized that other factors such as catecholamines, potassium levels, serotonin, NO, and adrenocorticotropic hormone (ACTH) also modulate aldosterone release from the adrenal glands (135). Furthermore, aldosterone can be produced in other organs including the kidneys, blood vessels, and in the heart. Results from the RESOLVD pilot study demonstrating that neither ACE inhibitors, ARBs, nor their combination resulted in sustained suppression of aldosterone were an important clue to the potentially beneficial effects that might accrue from the use of direct-acting aldosterone antagonists (137).

The benefits of adding an aldosterone antagonist to standard medical therapy of patients with heart failure was demonstrated in the RALES trial, which randomized 1,633 patients with severe heart failure to either spironolactone 25 mg daily or to placebo (138). The trial was discontinued early after a mean follow-up of only 24 months when the impact of spironolactone treatment became evident. Administration of this agent resulted in a 30% risk reduction in all-cause mortality, the primary endpoint of the study. This was due to a reduction in the risk of dying from both progressive heart failure and from sudden cardiac death. Hospitalization risk was also reduced significantly (by 35%) in the spironolactone-treated patients, and patients who received the aldosterone antagonist experienced significant improvement in symptoms of heart failure. Although serious hyperkalemia was uncommon in the spironolactone and placebo groups, active therapy was associated with a 10% incidence of gynecomastia in male patients compared to 1% in placebo-treated patients.

In EPHESUS the effects of eplerenone, a selective aldosterone antagonist, were assessed in patients following an acute MI complicated by LV dysfunction and evidence of heart failure (139). The 3,313 patients in EPHESUS were randomized to receive either eplerenone titrated to a maximum of 50 mg daily or placebo in addition to standard medical therapy which included an ACE inhibitor or ARB in 87% and a β-blocker in 75% of patients. The addition of eplerenone to the medical regimen was associated with a 15% risk reduction in all-cause mortality ($p = 0.008$). The other primary endpoint, which was death from cardiovascular causes or cardiovascular hospitalization, was also significantly reduced by eplerenone. There was also a 21% risk reduction for sudden cardiac death. The rate of serious hyperkalemia was 5.5% in the eplerenone group and 3.9% in the placebo group ($p = 0.002$), whereas the rate of hypokalemia was 8.4% in the eplerenone group and 13.1% in the placebo group ($p < 0.001$). As would be expected since eplerenone (unlike spironolactone) does not activate sex hormone receptors, gynecomastia was not significantly increased by eplerenone in patients in the EPHESUS study. Further analysis of the EPHESUS results indicated that the beneficial effects of eplerenone on mortality and sudden cardiac death were already manifest by 30 days post-MI (140), supporting the notion that early initiation of this drug would be protective in the early post-MI period.

The results of RALES and EPHESUS provide convincing evidence that the use of an aldosterone antagonist is beneficial in the post-MI population with evidence of LV dysfunction and manifestations of heart failure, and in patients with severe heart failure (138,139). Although it is likely that an aldosterone antagonist would also be effective in improving outcomes in patients with milder degrees of heart failure than was seen in RALES, this concept has yet to be addressed in a clinical trial and there are no conclusive data to support this possibility. The use of aldosterone antagonist should not be considered as a substitute for another neurohormonal blockers (e.g., an ACE inhibitor or ARB and a β-blocker), which are recommended in these patient groups; rather, aldosterone antagonist should be considered as an addition to these other drugs. In the clinical trials, patients were carefully screened for entry and excluded from the trials if serum creatinine exceeded 2.5 mg/dL or the potassium was greater than 5 mmol/L. Furthermore, both renal function and electrolyte levels were carefully followed with lab examinations at regular intervals after the initiation of drug. Failure to adhere to entry criteria or to rigorously follow-up patients has been associated with increased incidence of serious hyperkalemia and an increase in mortality (141,142). Thus, the need for appropriate selection of patients for this therapy and careful follow-up evaluation cannot be overemphasized.

Hydralazine/Isosorbide Dinitrate

The combination of hydralazine and isosorbide dinitrate was first studied in the treatment of heart failure during the 1970s. Whereas the initial studies focused on the effects of this regimen on cardiac performance in patients with systolic dysfunction and/or left sided valvular regurgitation, the V-HeFT study demonstrated that the combination improved survival in heart failure patients as well (143). The use of the hydralazine/isosorbide combination for the treatment of heart failure, however, was soon overshadowed by the arrival of ACE inhibitors. In V-HeFT II, these agents proved superior to the hydralazine/isosorbide combination in reducing mortality risk despite the fact that the latter improved LV ejection to a significantly greater extent (144). Based on these results and evidence of tachyphylaxis with continued nitrate use, the combination was relegated to a second- or third-line approach for treating heart failure.

Although nitrate tachyphylaxis is a well-described phenomenon, carefully done studies in both experimental animal preparations and heart failure patients have now demonstrated that it is inhibited by co-administration of hydralazine, presumably on the basis of the oxygen radical scavenging properties of the drug (145–147). Furthermore, post hoc evaluation of the V-HeFT results suggested that African-American patients might not have derived as much benefit from ACE inhibitors as non-African-Americans and that the hydralazine/isosorbide combination appeared to be particularly effective in this subgroup (148). Although this possibility has been disputed, an increased prevalence of polymorphisms in genes that regulate NO production has been reported in African-Americans (149–152), an observation that could provide a theoretical basis for why African-Americans might be particularly responsive to the beneficial effects of a drug regimen that works by increasing NO delivery.

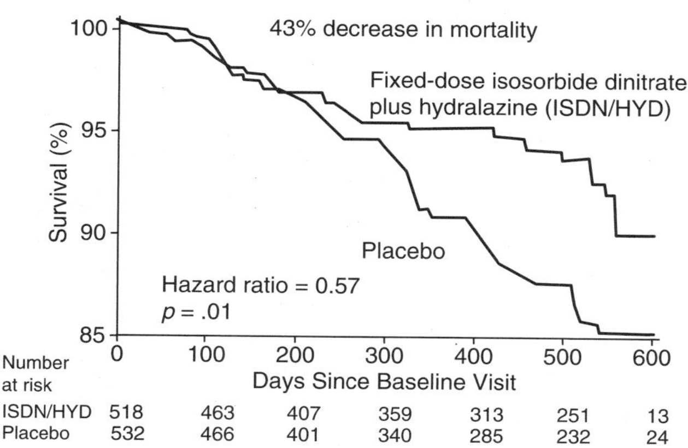

Figure 35-4 Mortality results of A-HeFT demonstrate that administration of fixed-dose isosorbide dinitrate plus hydralazine improves survival in African-American patients with heart failure due to systolic dysfunction. (Adapted from Taylor AL, Ziesche S, Yancy C, et al. Combination of isosorbide dinitrate and hydralazine in blacks with heart failure. *N Engl J Med.* 2004;351:2049–2057.)

In A-HeFT, a total of 1,050 African-American patients who had NYHA Class III or IV heart failure with dilated ventricles were randomly assigned to receive a fixed dose of isosorbide dinitrate plus hydralazine or placebo in addition to standard therapy for heart failure (Fig. 35-4) (153). The study was prematurely terminated due to a significantly higher mortality rate in the placebo group than in the group given isosorbide dinitrate plus hydralazine (10.2% versus 6.2%, $p = 0.02$). Patients receiving active therapy also experienced a 43% reduction in the rate of death from any cause (hazard ratio, 0.57; $p = 0.01$), 33% relative reduction in the rate of first hospitalization for heart failure ($p = 0.001$), and an improvement in quality of life ($p = 0.02$). Overall, 68% of patients in the treatment group reached the target dose of 225 mg of hydralazine/40 mg of isosorbide dinitrate daily in divided doses (thrice daily). There were small but significant reductions in systolic and diastolic blood pressures in the patients receiving the combination compared to patients who got placebo. Altough headache and dizziness were more common in the treated patients, this group experienced significantly lowered likelihood of developing worsening heart failure. Based on the results of A-HeFT, the fixed-dose combination of hydralazine/isosorbide has been approved by the U.S. Food and Drug Administration (FDA) for use in African-American patients. Whether or not this approach will offer similar benefits to non-African-Americans already receiving good neurohormonal blocking therapy is, as of yet, unproven.

Cardiac Resynchronization Therapy

Dyssynchrony between chambers and within the left ventricle itself is an important determinant of systolic and diastolic function of the heart. It also contributes to the severity of mitral regurgitation. The presence of mechanical dyssnchrony is often heralded on the surface electrocardiogram by prolongation of the QRS complex >120 msec. However, this relationship is not absolute and mechanical dyssynchrony can be present in patients without QRS prolongation, while patients with a wide QRS complex may not have extensive mechanical dyssynchrony. Nonetheless, the strong association between the two allows the surface ECG to be used to identify patients at high risk of having mechanical dyssynchrony. In general, about 25% of patients with heart failure due to systolic dysfunction have a QRS >120 msec on their ECG. This prevalence tends to increase with the severity of heart failure. Moreover, as the QRS widens, the natural history of patients gets progressively worse and the risk of mortality goes up considerably (154–156).

The use of cardiac resynchronization therapy (CRT) has emerged as an important adjunct for the treatment of heart failure over the past several years. In most cases CRT involves the placement of pacing leads in the right atrium, right ventricle, and left ventricle. Although the LV lead is introduced using a transvenous approach through the coronary venous system in most cases, surgical placement on the epicardial surface of the heart is occasionally required. Early results with CRT demonstrated that in selected patients it could increase exercise capacity, relieve symptoms, and improve quality of life (157–159). There were also indications that CRT was associated with improvement in cardiac function and reversal of LV remodeling (159–162). Moreover, a meta-analysis of early randomized, controlled trials showed that CRT reduced death from progressive heart failure (163).

The CARE-HF trial evaluated the effects of CRT on morbidity and mortality in patients with NYHA Class III or IV heart failure due to LV systolic dysfunction and cardiac dyssynchrony who were receiving standard pharmacologic therapy (164). As shown in Figure 35-5, in this study CRT reduced the primary endpoint of death from any cause or an unplanned hospitalization for a major cardiovascular event by 37% ($p < 0.001$). Death from any cause, the principal secondary endpoint, was reduced by 36%, an effect that was also highly significant ($p < 0.002$). In addition, there were significant reductions in interventricular mechanical delay, end-systolic volume index, and the area of the mitral regurgitant jet as well as increases in LVEF and improved symptoms and the quality of life ($p < 0.01$ for all comparisons). These results provide persuasive evidence of the benefits of CRT when added to appropriate therapy in patients with NYHA Class III–IV heart failure and QRS prolongation.

Overall, placement of the leads in all three chambers is accomplished in about 90% of cases when the procedure is carried out by a skilled operator. Side effects, which include infection, bleeding and hematoma, diaphragmatic stimulation, perforation of the coronary vein, and provocation of ventricular arrhythmias, occur in approximately 10% of patients (157–164). Of note is the fact that the average QRS duration of most patients in the initial studies of CRT was in the range of 150 msec or more and that entry into CARE-HF for patients with QRS between 120 and 150 msec required echocardiographic confirmation of the presence of mechanical synchrony (164). Tables 35-4 and 35-5 list indications for use CRT as well as conditions in which the efficacy is either less certain or remains unproven.

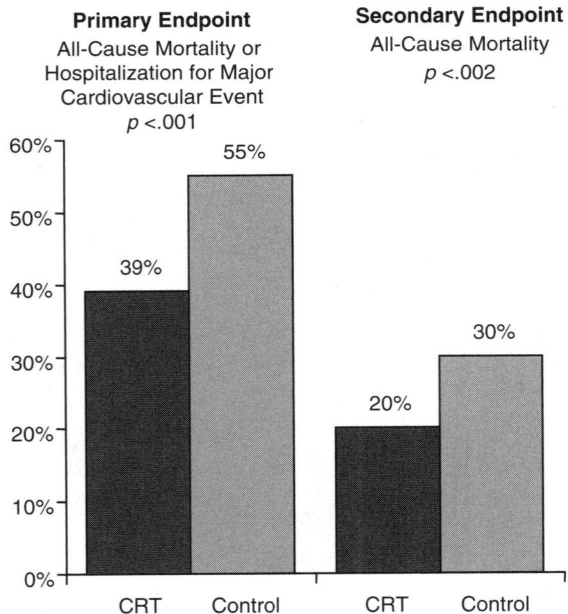

Figure 35-5 Primary and secondary end-point results from CARE-HF demonstrating the incremental benefits of CRT in improving survival in patients already receiving optimal medical therapy. (Adapted from Cleland JG, Daubert JC, Erdmann E, et al. The effect of cardiac resynchronization on morbidity and mortality in heart failure. *N Engl J Med.* 2005;352:1539–1549.)

Implantable Cardioverter/Defibrillators

Sudden cardiac death is a feared complication of heart failure and it is believed to be the cause of death in approximately half of the patients with this condition (125,165,166). Sudden cardiac death is proportionally more common in patients with milder degrees of heart failure than in patients with more severe heart failure. Attempts at reducing sudden death risk by the use of antiarrhythmic agents have proved to be unsuccessful (167). However, recent evidence indicates that placement of an implantable cardioverter/defibrillator (ICD) can significantly reduce this feared complication of heart failure. In MADIT-II patients with a prior myocardial infarction and a LVEF 30% or less were randomly assigned in a 3:2 ratio to receive an implantable defibrillator (742 patients) or conventional medical therapy (490 patients) (168). During an average follow-up of 20 months, the mortality rates were 19.8% in the conventional-therapy group and 14.2% in the defibrillator group, a risk reduction of 31% ($p = 0.016$).

TABLE 35-4

CRITERIA FOR SELECTING PATIENTS FOR CARDIAC RESYNCHRONIZATION THERAPY

1. NYHA functional Class III (or early Class IV) symptoms of heart failure despite optimal medical therapy.
2. Left ventricular ejection fraction ≥35%.
3. QRS duration >120 msec (preferably with evidence of mechanical dyssynchrony in patients with QRS duration between 120 and 150 msec).

TABLE 35-5
CONDITIONS IN WHICH EFFICACY OF CARDIAC RESYNCHRONIZATION THERAPY IS UNCERTAIN

1. QRS prolongation associated with RBBB pattern.
2. Atrial fibrillation.
3. QRS duration between 120 and 150 msec.
4. NYHA functional Class II symptoms.

In SCD-HeFT, patients with NYHA Class II or III heart failure symptoms and an LVEF ≤35% were randomized to conventional therapy plus placebo (847 patients), conventional therapy plus amiodarone (845 patients), or conventional therapy plus an ICD (829 patients) (169). For the primary endpoint of all-cause mortality compared to placebo, amiodarone was associated with a similar risk of death while ICD therapy was associated with a 23% reduction in risk of death ($p = 0.007$). Patients randomized in SCD-HeFT were almost equally divided between those with an ischemic or a nonischemic etiology of heart failure, and the risk reduction with an ICD did not vary according to underlying etiology. The results of these two studies provide compelling evidence of the efficacy of an ICD in improving outcomes in symptomatic heart failure patients due to systolic heart failure regardless of whether or not they have ischemic disease.

MANAGEMENT OF PATIENTS WITH CHRONIC HEART FAILURE

The goals for medical management of patients with chronic heart failure are relatively straightforward. They include providing symptomatic relief, increasing exercise capacity and sense of well-being, avoiding hospitalization, preventing progression of LV dysfunction (and reversal of deleterious remodeling), and prolonging life. There is evidence that, to a certain extent, medical therapy is now able to accomplish these goals. Information summarized in this chapter as well as in many other chapters in this text provide evidence for (and in some cases against) the use of the various agents that are available to treat chronic heart failure. What follows, then, are guidelines for therapy of chronic heart failure patients that are directed toward achieving the goals previously outlined. This approach is summarized in Figure 35-6. Certain basic principles that pertain to all patients with chronic heart failure will first be discussed.

Because chronic heart failure is a syndrome that can develop on the basis of a variety of diseases, it is essential

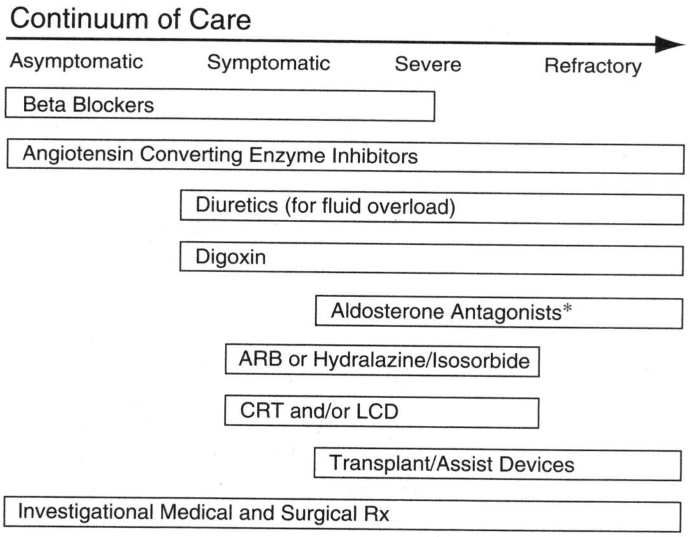

Figure 35-6 Continuum of care for heart failure. This schematic depicts the timing for initiation of therapy according to the symptomatic status of the patient. Diuretics and digoxin are used mainly for relief of symptoms, whereas the neurohormonal blockers such as ACE inhibitors and β-blockers are used to prevent progression of disease. Patients who remain symptomatic despite optimal management would be considered candidates for the addition of either an aldosterone antagonist, an angiotensin receptor blocker (ARB), or a combination of isosorbide dinitrate and hydralazine. The use of cardiac resynchronization therapy (CRT) improves outcomes in symptomatic patients, with evidence of dyssynchrony and implantable cardioverter-defibrillator devices (ICDs) improve survival in systolic dysfunction regardless of whether or not there is an ischemic etiology. Patients who remain refractory should be considered for cardiac transplantation or an assist device if they are otherwise candidates for this procedure. Although not shown on the figure, nonpharmacologic therapy, including salt and water restriction and exercise training, is an important component of the therapeutic regimen. Since the morbidity and mortality of heart failure remain unacceptably high, new approaches for the management of patients at all symptomatic levels are needed. Consideration for patients with heart failure in clinical trials designed to assess medical and surgical approaches is an important part of the therapeutic armamentarium.

to investigate the etiology. If, as in most instances, the cause of chronic heart failure is cardiac, differentiation between structural or mechanical problems and muscle disease is necessary. Whether muscle disease is due to ischemic or nonischemic causes should also be determined. The possibility of revascularization should be considered in patients with ischemic cardiomyopathy and evidence of potentially viable but dysfunctional myocardium (as evidenced by thallium redistribution scan, PET scan, MRI or low-dose dobutamine echocardiogram). Although identification of the cause of many of the dilated nonischemic cardiomyopathies is often not possible, a search for some of the reversible processes is worthwhile if there are clues that one of these conditions may be present. Examples are cardiomyopathy due to thyroid disease, incessant tachycardia, and hemochromatosis. A carefully performed medical history and examination combined with a chest X-ray and electrocardiogram are integral parts of the diagnostic process. Some measurement of LV function is essential in order to both confirm the presence and quantitate the extent of myocardial dysfunction. An echocardiogram is often used for this purpose because it provides information about chamber size, the condition of the heart valves and other structures, as well as an assessment of systolic function. The echocardiogram can also be helpful in defining the etiology of chronic heart failure. Distinct segmental wall motion abnormalities, when present, suggest the presence of coronary artery disease, whereas a hypertrophic LV with a typical ground glass appearance but normal systolic function suggests a diagnosis of amyloidosis. The accompanying Doppler study can be useful in defining abnormal LV filling patterns that are characteristic of diastolic dysfunction (170).

A carefully performed medical history and physical examination will also help determine if medical conditions that exacerbate chronic heart failure or complicate the therapeutic approach are present. The clinical course of chronic heart failure can be quite variable, and in any given patient, it often defies prediction. One survey pointed out that worsening chronic heart failure can often be ascribed to preventable causes (171). Some of these causes are listed in Table 35-6. In a surprisingly large number of cases, patients are found to be doing poorly because of noncompliance. This is a particular problem in elderly patients (172,173). Because chronic heart failure occurs predominately in older patients, the issue of noncompliance and how to deal with it effectively are of considerable importance. The reasons for noncompliance on the part of the patient are multiple, ranging all the way from simple error in adhering to the therapeutic regimen, forgetfulness, physical incapacity limiting the patient's ability to obtain medications, lack of insurance or funding source, to contrary behavior on the part of the patient. The reason for noncompliance may also reside with the physician or other members of the health care team who have not clearly explained to the patient why and how to take the medications. The need for careful explanations to the patient regarding the rationale for the use of various drugs, description of how frequently they should be taken, and what side effects might be expected both initially and during follow-up visits cannot be overemphasized.

TABLE 35-6
CONDITIONS COMMONLY ASSOCIATED WITH WORSENING CHRONIC HEART FAILURE

Noncompliance
Dietary indiscretion
Uncontrolled hypertension
Concurrent administration of drugs with adverse:
  Cardiac effects (e.g., calcium-channel blockers, antiarrhythmics)
  Systemic effects (e.g., nonsteroidal anti-inflammatory drugs)
Alcohol and/or drug abuse
Abnormalities in impulse formation/conduction (i.e., chronotropic incompetence)
Atrial or ventricular arrhythmias
Infection
Anemia
Pulmonary disease (e.g., chronic obstructive pulmonary disease, pulmonary emboli)
Thyroid disease, either hypothyroidism or hyperthyroidism
Stress
Environmental conditions
Pregnancy

Prevention

The best way, by far, to treat heart failure is to prevent its occurrence. Because a substantial portion of all heart failure patients have either coronary artery disease, hypertension, and/or diabetes as the etiology, the treatment of these conditions offers opportunities to successfully intervene before LV dysfunction becomes manifest. Treatment of risk factors for coronary disease has been shown to reduce the future likelihood of developing chronic heart failure. For instance, administration of simvastatin, a cholesterol-reducing agent, to patients with clinically apparent coronary artery disease in the Scandinavian Simvastatin Survival Study (4S) not only reduced overall mortality by 30% ($p = 0.0003$) (174), but also lowered the risk of developing heart failure by 20% ($p = 0.015$) (175). Treatment of hypertension also has been associated with a reduction in the likelihood of developing heart failure. Elderly patients with systolic hypertension experienced a 49% reduction in heart failure in the Systolic Hypertension in the Elderly Program (SHEP) when they received adequate anti-hypertensive therapy (176). The HOPE study enrolled patients at high risk for cardiovascular events based on the presence of atherosclerosis or diabetes and an additional cardiovascular risk factor (177). As depicted in Figure 35-5, the addition of the ACE inhibitor ramipril to the medical regimen of this patient population significantly reduced virtually all cardiovascular endpoints, including a 23% reduction in the risk of developing heart failure (178).

Patients with Asymptomatic Left Ventricular Dysfunction

The goal in this group of patients is to prevent future events and further deterioration in LV performance. Acute intervention such as thrombolysis and/or angioplasty can prevent future likelihood of heart failure in MI patients. As discussed in Chapter 17, revascularization can stabilize or reverse LV systolic dysfunction in selected patients with coronary artery disease.

The use of ACE inhibitors in MI survivors and in patients with asymptomatic LV dysfunction is also an effective preventive measure (68–75,78). A summary of some of the relevant trials and their results is given in Table 35-7. The consistent and highly significant favorable impact of ACE inhibitors on mortality and future likelihood of heart failure in MI survivors with either symptoms of heart failure and/or reduced EF argues strongly for their use in these populations. ACE inhibitor therapy also appears to be effective in inhibiting post-MI cardiac remodeling (82,179). Although the SOLVD prevention arm failed to demonstrate a significant reduction in mortality, there was a 20% reduction in the combined endpoint of death or hospitalization in the enalapril-treated group ($p < 0.001$) (78). Moreover, the favorable trend in survival in the enalapril group, the increasing divergence of mortality curves late in the study, and the highly significant impact of ACE inhibitor on reducing the onset of clinically apparent heart failure all argue in favor of the use of ACE inhibitor in patients with asymptomatic LV dysfunction, regardless of whether or not that the patient has had an MI in the past. Thus, the point that emerges from these studies is that treatment of LV dysfunction with ACE inhibitors at a relatively early stage has beneficial effects on the subsequent clinical course. Results from the VALIANT study demonstrated that the use of valsartan was equally effective as an ACE inhibitor in patients with post-MI LV dysfunction. Whether substituting an ARB for an ACE inhibitor in patients with nonischemic asymptomatic LV dysfunction would give comparable results to those seen with an ACE inhibitor is, however, less certain since these patients have not been studied in a clinical trial.

A question that is often raised in the postinfarction patient is the optimal timing for initiating therapy. Results of the GISSI-3 and ISIS-4 studies show that early administration of ACE inhibitors within the first days post-MI is associated with improved short-term survival (180,181). For instance, the 5-week post-MI mortality rate was reduced by 7% (from 7.69% to 7.19%; $p = 0.02$) with captopril in the ISIS-4 study (181). Although these studies also reported a small excess in hypotension and renal dysfunction in patients treated with ACE inhibitors, in general, the drugs were well-tolerated. Based on these results, the recommendation is to initiate ACE inhibitors in most MI survivors unless there is a contraindication to their use.

Although β-blockers are recommended for the treatment of patients following an MI (182,183), their value in treating patients with post-MI LV dysfunction has been uncertain since this high-risk group (as well as patients with heart failure) was largely excluded from the earlier post-MI trials. In addition, important therapies that were either not available or not used in the earlier β-blocker studies (e.g., revascularization, ACE inhibitors, aspirin, statins) are now routinely administered to patients following an MI. The fact that all these therapies significantly improve the clinical course of patients post-MI has raised the question of whether or nor the addition of a β-blocker would still be of value in these patients. In the CAPRICORN study the addition of carvedilol to patients with post-MI LV dysfunction who received many therapies that were not used in the earlier studies resulted in both improved survival and a reduced likelihood of recurrent MI (184). The beneficial effects of carvedilol were seen in patients regardless of whether or not symptoms of heart failure were present. It was also detected in the subgroup that had undergone post-MI coronary revascularization. These results provide a strong rationale for the use of carvedilol in patients with post-MI LV dysfunction (185). Based on evidence that the likelihood of being maintained on a β-blocker is considerably greater if it is started in-hospital compared to the outpatient setting (186), the recommendation is to initiate therapy post-MI prior to discharge unless there is a contraindication to the use of a β-blocker.

Although clinical trials assessing the effects of β-blockers on clinical endpoints in patients with asymptomatic LV dysfunction have not been performed, the results of the REVERT study presented at the annual scientific session of the HFSA in 2005 help provide a rationale for their use in this setting. In this study, patients with asymptomatic LV dysfunction were randomized to receive either placebo or metoprolol succinate in doses of either 50 mg or 200 mg daily in addition to standard therapy that included an ACE inhibitor. The results showed stepwise reductions in end-systolic (primary endpoint) and end-diastolic volumes as well as increases in EF with the two doses of drug compared to placebo. These results, along with evidence that sympathetic nervous system activation precedes the onset of symptoms in patients with LV dysfunction (16), provide ample justification for recommending the use of a β-blocker along with an ACE inhibitor—a recommendation that is analogous to that given for the use of ACE inhibitors in this population.

The question of whether additional neurohormonal blockade would add further benefits beyond ACE inhibitors (or ARBs) and carvedilol in patients with post-MI LV dysfunction was addressed in the EPHESUS trial, a study that included patients with post-MI LV dysfunction who also had evidence of heart failure (139). Despite treatment with an ACE inhibitor in 87% and a β-blocker in 75% of the patients enrolled in the study, the addition of eplerenone, an aldosterone antagonist, significantly reduced long-term mortality by 15% and sudden cardiac death by 21%. The timing of initiation of an aldosterone antagonist was addressed in a further analysis of the EPHESUS trial data (140). Evidence that reductions in mortality and sudden cardiac death could be demonstrated during the first 30 days post-MI suggests that eplerenone should be started during the MI hospitalization. This strategy seems particularly rational in view of the fact that ICD placement in MADIT II was not considered until at least 30 days post-MI and, in fact, was not performed until several months after the event. In the DINAMIT trial, ICD placement during the first 30 days post-MI did not convey a survival benefit since protection from sudden cardiac death was more than counterbalanced by an increase in risk from death from other causes, with the net effect being no significant improvement in survival (187).

Although calcium-channel blocking agents may be useful in some groups of post-MI patients, their routine use in patients with LV dysfunction is discouraged. This caution is based on their known negative inotropic effects and the

TABLE 35-7
ACE INHIBITOR THERAPY OF MYOCARDIAL INFARCTION SURVIVORS AND PATIENTS WITH ASYMPTOMATIC LEFT VENTRICULAR DYSFUNCTION

Trial	n	Duration	EF	HF Symptoms	ACE Inhibitor, Dose	Reduction in Mortality	Reduction in Development of HF
SAVE	2,231	42	$<$40%	Minimal	Captopril, 150 mg/day	19%	22%
AIRE	2,006	15	—	Present	Ramipril, 5 mg/day	27%	23%
TRACE	1,749	24–50	$<$35%	±	Trandolapril, 4 mg/day	22%	29%
SOLVD (Prevention)	4,228	38	$\leq$35%	Minimal	Enalapril, 20 mg/day	8%[a]	36%

[a] p = NS; all other reductions in morbidity/mortality were $p < 0.05$.
EF, ejection fraction; HF, heart failure.

results of a trial in which diltiazem was compared with placebo in a group of patients during the postinfarction period (188). Overall, the study showed no significant difference between the patients treated with active drug and those treated with placebo. However, in the subgroup of patients with evidence of more severe LV dysfunction, mortality was significantly increased in patients receiving diltiazem. Furthermore, analysis of patients with LV dysfunction followed over a period of 1 year in the SOLVD Registry showed that calcium-channel blocker was associated with significantly increased risk of fatal or nonfatal MI (189). One possible explanation for these findings may be that diltiazem and other calcium blockers used during the SOLVD era have pharmacologic profiles that are unfavorable for a population with LV dysfunction and that the use of calcium-channel blockers that are more specific for the peripheral vasculature or those that are less potent stimulators of the RAS may have some beneficial effects in this population. However, convincing data from well-designed clinical trials supporting this concept are still lacking.

Digoxin and the diuretic agents have been found to be useful only in relieving symptoms. There is no evidence that they favorably affect remodeling or prolong survival (41). Therefore, there is no indication for their use in the truly asymptomatic patient with LV dysfunction.

Symptomatic Left Ventricular Dysfunction

Clinically stable patients with signs and symptoms of fluid retention should be treated with a loop diuretic to relieve congestion. It is also the practice of the author to add digoxin to the medical regimen of such patients, particularly when atrial fibrillation is present. As emphasized in previous sections of this chapter, therapy with digoxin and diuretics should be initiated to relieve symptoms, improve exercise capacity, and reduce the likelihood of hospitalization. Neither inhibition or reversal of cardiac remodeling nor improved survival should be expected. In contrast, ACE inhibitors have been shown to inhibit adverse cardiac remodeling, prevent hospitalizations, and prolong survival as well as increase exercise capacity and relieve symptoms (76–79,82). An ACE inhibitor should be initiated as part of the standard regimen as early as possible unless there is a contraindication to its use, such as intractable cough (with good evidence that it is due to the ACE inhibitor) or a history of ACE inhibitor-related angioedema. The use of an ARB is an acceptable alternative in patients who are ACE-intolerant or who were being treated with an agent in this class at the time they developed heart failure. Based on incontrovertible evidence that β-blockers (when given in addition to ACE inhibitors or ARBs) further inhibit (and even reverse) cardiac remodeling, improve survival in the range of 35% above that seen with ACE inhibitors alone, and reduce hospitalizations (120,124,125), these drugs are considered as first-line therapy in symptomatic heart failure due to LV systolic dysfunction. The magnitude of effect of β-blockade in improving the natural history of heart failure patients far exceeds that of any other treatment, and it is recommended that this therapy be at the very core of the therapeutic regimen. Thus, a β-blocker should be initiated and uptitrated as soon as the patient is clinically stable (e.g., not receiving IV diuretics, vasodilators, or inotropic agents). The 35% improvement in survival with carvedilol in the COPERNICUS study supports the use of β-blockers in patients with more advanced heart failure (123). As noted previously in this chapter, evidence that pharmacologic differences between β-blockers are related to differences in outcomes; therefore, it is strongly recommended that only the three β-blockers (i.e., carvedilol, metoprolol succinate, and bisoprolol) shown to be effective in large-scale clinical trials be used in heart failure patients.

Finally, there is evidence that further inhibition of the widespread neurohormonal activation that is so characteristic of heart failure will be advantageous. Addition of low doses of spironolactone, an aldosterone inhibitor, in the RALES study was shown to improve survival significantly (138). The drug was generally well-tolerated, with the main side effect being development of painful gynecomastia in 8% to 9% of male patients. This problem can be overcome in virtually all cases by switching to eplerenone. Problems with hyperkalemia with aldosterone antagonists may arise when these drugs are started in patients with renal dysfunction or serum potassium levels greater than that allowed in the relevant clinical trials. It is recommended that the "rule of ones" be followed if an aldosterone antagonist is being considered. This involves measurement of renal function and potassium "one day" before and "one day," "one week," and "one month" after initiation of therapy. These measurements should also be repeated periodically thereafter.

As noted previously, neither ACE inhibitors nor β-blockers produce evidence of clinical improvement until after they have been given for several weeks. If at that time the patient remains symptomatic and the blood pressure permits, a sometimes helpful approach is to add a non-ACE inhibitor vasodilator to the regimen. The addition of hydralazine and isosorbide dinitrate in this setting has been shown to produce incremental hemodynamic responses (190), and this combination was shown in the Vasodilator in Heart Failure Trial I (V-HeFT I) to improve survival (79). Nitrates themselves improve exercise tolerance in heart failure patients (191). Recent evidence suggests that the beneficial effects of hydralazine in this combination may be related to its ability to prevent nitrate tolerance by scavenging free oxygen radicals (192). More recently, the addition of a fixed-dose combination of hydralazine and isosorbide dinitrate to standard medical therapy has been shown to provide significant benefits, including a reduction in mortality risk in African-American patients with heart failure (153). Whether or not such benefits would be present in other patients, however, remains uncertain.

Another approach is the use of an ACE inhibitor and an ARB in the treatment of heart failure patients. This combination was shown to reduce combined morbidity/mortality endpoints in the range of 13% to 15% in both the Val-HeFT and CHARM-Added studies (96,97). In the latter, significant reductions in cardiovascular mortality were also noted (77). Earlier concerns that the ACE inhibitor and ARB combination might increase risk in patients already receiving β-blockers have been alleviated by the results of the CHARM-Added study, which reported the lack of any negative interaction of combined therapy with β-blocker use (97).

Definitive criteria for deciding which (if any) additional therapies to use beyond an ACE inhibitor (or ARB) and β-blocker are lacking at present. However, in patients who remain symptomatic despite standard therapy it is worth considering adding either an aldosterone antagonist, the hydralazine/isosorbide combination, or combining treatment with an ACE inhibitor and an ARB. In determining between these approaches, factors such as severity of symptoms, underlying renal function, serum potassium levels, blood pressure, and race are most helpful in deciding which approach would be most appropriate in an individual patient. For instance, one might add an aldosterone antagonist in a patient with normal renal function and serum potassium who is late NYHA functional Class III or early Class IV. Alternatively, the selection would tend toward the use of the hydralazine/isorbide combination in an African-American patient.

The addition of device therapy to the management of patients with heart failure has evolved considerably since the last edition of this text. Since sudden cardiac death is so common in patients with LV systolic dysfunction (126), implantation of an ICD should be considered in symptomatic patients regardless of the underlying etiology. In patients with either an ischemic and nonischemic etiology it is advisable to allow some time (usually a minimum of 30 days from an MI or the diagnosis of heart failure) before recommending an ICD based on the results of the DINAMIT study in post-MI patients (187). Clinical experience suggests that the severity of LV dysfunction often improves in the immediate post-MI period as hibernating and stunned myocardium recovers and in response to the initiation of medical therapy as previously outlined. Substantial improvement in cardiac function may occur in many cases and, when present, the patient may no longer fulfill criteria for an ICD.

The use of CRT has also evolved as an important modality of therapy in patients who continue to have NYHA Class III or early Class IV symptoms in the presence of a wide QRS complex, particularly when there is a left bundle branch block pattern present. These patients have been shown to benefit with an improvement in exercise capacity, relief of symptoms, and a reduction in mortality risk when CRT is initiated (157–164).

For both ICD and/or CRT it is important to emphasize that patients be optimized on medical therapy before a device is considered. In many cases, either symptoms and/or cardiac function will improve with drug therapy alone, obviating the need for device placement and its attendant costs and risks to the patient.

Advanced or Refractory Heart Failure

Patients who continue to do poorly even after these therapies have been initiated present a difficult therapeutic problem to the clinician. After it has been determined that all prescribed medications are being taken correctly, daily sodium intake has been minimized, and none of the myriad factors that are known to exacerbate chronic heart failure are present, several steps can be considered. Patients with predominantly congestive symptoms that are refractory to therapy can often be successfully managed by using a combination of diuretics that affect the nephron at different places. A loop diuretic, such as furosemide, and an agent that acts at the level of the distal tubule, such as metolazone, are often used in conjunction for this purpose (23,24). This is an extremely potent combination, and care should be taken to avoid problems related to overdiuresis and, in particular, the induction of hypokalemia when these two drugs are used together. A trial of intravenous diuretics also can be considered. However, in truly refractory patients, the administration of diuretics in association with an intravenous inotropic agent (to help increase blood flow to the kidney) may be the best way to achieve satisfactory control of fluid balance. Often patients who are successfully treated in this way re-equilibrate to their previous level and can be subsequently managed without the need for continuous intravenous inotrope support. Patients who fail to improve should be considered for cardiac transplantation and/or an LV assist device (LVAD).

OTHER DRUGS

Intravenous Positive Inotropic Agents and Nesiritide

Inotropic agents can be valuable additions to the medical regimen of patients with severe LV systolic dysfunction and refractory heart failure. They are particularly helpful in patients with acute decompensation and evidence of low cardiac output who are refractory to IV diuretics. Intravenous positive inotropic agents can also be considered for patients who become refractory to standard therapy, even after this has been optimized and all other causes of decompensation have been excluded (193). In this setting a short course of treatment with dobutamine or milrinone can be quite helpful in allowing a refractory patient to return to the previous, more stable state (194,195).

The use of outpatient intermittent or continuous inotropic therapy has recently emerged as a possible therapy for end-stage heart failure (196,197). Intermittent administration of nesiritide in an outpatient infusion center or clinic has also been advocated (198). Although anecdotal and noncontrolled data attest to the benefits of outpatient inotropic therapy (199), there is little convincing evidence from well-designed clinical trials to support this approach. Furthermore, the possibility of worsening underlying cardiac function or promoting potentially lethal ventricular arrhythmias with inotropic agents and worsening renal function and survival with nesiritide is of great concern (200,201). Consequently, the recommendation is that intravenous inotropic agents be given only to truly refractory heart failure patients who either could not otherwise be discharged from the hospital or who continue to be readmitted on a regular basis despite optimization of all other therapeutic approaches. The use of outpatient nesiritide is not recommended in any setting at this time.

Antiarrhythmic Drugs

Approximately 50% of patients with chronic heart failure die suddenly, and the presumed cause of death is a ventricular dysrhythmia (125,165,166). Although the ACE inhibitors have been shown to reduce mortality in patients with chronic heart failure, their major impact appears to be on death due to progressive pump failure. Despite the fact that β-blockers have been shown to favorably impact on both death due to progressive pump failure as well as sudden cardiac death (120,124), the latter remains a problem (202). Patients with chronic heart failure have frequent ventricular ectopic beats, and runs of ventricular tachycardia are also common (203,204). As noted elsewhere in this text, although these events do appear to be associated with subsequent mortality and are significant predictors of survival in populations with LV dysfunction, they offer little in the way of information in individual patients (203–206). Although antiarrhythmic agents may successfully treat the ventricular ectopy, there is no convincing evidence that any of the available agents improves survival in patients with chronic heart failure. As shown in the CAST study, drugs that successfully suppress premature ventricular contractions (PVCs) had an unfavorable effect on survival (167). In addition, antiarrhythmic agents tend to have a higher side effect profile, are more likely to be proarrhythmic (207,208), and may precipitate worsening chronic heart failure in patients with LV dysfunction (209). Thus, their routine use in this population is not indicated.

Amiodarone, an agent with multiple pharmacologic properties, including Class III antiarrhythmic effects (210), has been evaluated in patients with heart failure. Although there was a significant improvement associated with amiodarone administration in the GEISICA trial (211), a similar favorable effect was not seen in the STAT study (212). The difference in results between the trials may have been due to the higher proportion of patients with an ischemic etiology in chronic heart failure-STAT. Nonetheless, there is little convincing evidence that amiodarone reduces either overall mortality or sudden cardiac death in patients with LV dysfunction. In SCD-HeFT mortality in the amiodarone-treated group did not differ significantly from that of patients on standard medical therapy alone, and was significantly greater than in the patients who received an ICD (169). Thus, the present recommendation is to treat high-risk post-MI patients (213), patients with symptomatic ventricular rhythm disturbances, and patients with LVEFs of 30% to 35% or below with an ICD.

Anticoagulants

Patients with LV dysfunction are prone to develop embolic complications (214–216). The risk appears to increase with increasing severity of LV dysfunction and in patients with large MIs, particularly when there is evidence of an LV aneurysm. The presence of thrombus in the LV also helps identify patients at risk for future events (217). Patients with previous embolic events and those with atrial fibrillation appear to be at the highest risk. There is virtually no information from well-designed clinical trials evaluating the effects of anticoagulant therapy in patients with chronic heart failure. However, uncontrolled data collected from the SOLVD study suggest that anticoagulation is effective in improving survival in chronic heart failure patients (218). The ongoing WATCH study is designed to assess the efficacy of various forms of anticoagulation in patients with chronic heart failure. Until the results are available, it is difficult to enthusiastically recommend intensive warfarin therapy in patients other than those at high risk, as previously described.

CONCLUSION

There have been enormous strides in the field of clinical and basic research that have affected the way that patients with chronic heart failure are managed. A large body of data from well-designed clinical trials that can be used to guide decision making in patients seen in clinical practice is now available. This information has enabled us to forge a rational basis of therapy for patients with chronic heart failure of varying degrees of severity. We are presently on much firmer ground in our approach to the medical management of chronic heart failure than we were in the past, and it is certain that the recent changes in therapy have resulted in the improved quality and quantity of life of our patients. It must be remembered, however, that chronic heart failure remains a common and extremely lethal disease and there is much work yet to be done.

REFERENCES

1. Mercadier J-J, Lompre A-M, Wisnewsky C, et al. Myosin isoenzymic changes in several models of rat cardiac hypertrophy. *Circ Res.* 1981;49:525–532.
2. Schwartz K, Carrier L, Mercadier J-J, et al. Molecular phenotype of the hypertrophied and failing myocardium. *Circulation.* 1993;87(Suppl VII):VII5–VII10.
3. Chien KR, Knowlton KU, Zhu H, et al. Regulation of cardiac gene expression during myocardial growth and hypertrophy: molecular studies of an adaptive physiologic response. *FASEB J.* 1991:5:3037–3046.
4. Vandenburgh H. Mechanical forces and their second messengers in stimulating cell growth *in vitro*. *Am J Physiol.* 1992;31: R350–R355.
5. Feldman AM, Ray PE, Silan CM, et al. Selective gene expression in failing human heart: quantification of steady-state levels of messenger RNA in endomyocardial biopsies using the polymerase chain reaction. *Circulation.* 1991;83: 1866–1872.
6. Rockman HA, Knowlton KU, Ross J Jr., et al. *In vivo* murine cardiac hypertrophy: a novel model to identify genetic signaling mechanisms that activate an adaptive physiological response. *Circulation.* 1993;87(Suppl VIII):14–21.
7. Pfeffer JM, Pfeffer MA, Fletcher PJ, Braunwald E. Progressive ventricular remodeling in rat with myocardial infarction. *Am J Physiol.* 1991;260:H1046–H1414.
8. Jeremy RW, Allman KC, Bautovich G, et al. Patterns of left ventricular dilation during the six months after myocardial infarction. *J Am Coll Cardiol.* 1989;13:304–310.
9. Eaton LW, Weiss JL, Bulkley BH, et al. Regional cardiac dilatation after acute myocardial infarction: recognition by two-dimensional echocardiography. *N Engl J Med.* 1979;300:57–62.
10. Pfeffer MA, Lamas GA, Vaughan DE, et al. Effect of captopril on progressive ventricular dilatation after anterior myocardial infarction. *N Engl J Med.* 1988;319:80–86.
11. Sadoshima J-I, Xu Y, Slayter HS, et al. Autocrine release of angiotensin II mediates stretch-induced hypertrophy of cardiac myocytes *in vitro*. *Cell.* 1993;75:977–984.
12. Urata H, Healy B, Stewart RW, et al. Angiotensin II-forming pathways in normal and failing human hearts. *Circ Res.* 1990;66:883–890.
13. Francis GS, Benedict C, Johnston DE, et al. Comparison of neroendocrine activation in patients with left ventricular

dysfunction with and without congestive heart failure: a substudy of the Studies of Left Ventricular Dysfunction (SOLVD). *Circulation.* 1990;82:1724–1729.
14. Hirsch AT, Talsness CE, Schunkert H, et al. Tissue-specific activation of cardiac angiotensin converting enzyme in experimental heart failure. *Circ Res.* 1991;69:475–482.
15. Dostal DE, Baker KM. Evidence for a role of an intracardiac renin-angiotensin system in normal and failing hearts. *Trends Cardiovasc Med.* 1993;3:7–74.
16. Francis GS, McDonald KM, Cohn JN. Neurohumoral activation in preclinical heart failure. *Circulation.* 1993;87(Suppl IV): 90–96.
17. Hutcheon D, Nemeth E, Quinlan D. The role of furosemide alone or in combination with digoxin in the relief of symptoms of congestive heart failure. *J Clin Pharmacol.* 1980;20:59–68.
18. Dzau VJ, Hollenberg NK. Renal response to captopril in severe heart failure: role of furosemide in natriuresis and reversal of hyponatremia. *Ann Intern Med.* 1984;100:777–782.
19. Stampfer M, Epstein SE, Beiser GD, et al. Hemodynamic effects of diuresis at rest and during intense upright exercise in patients with impaired cardiac function. *Circulation.* 1968;37:900–911.
20. Wilson JR, Reichek N, Dunkman WB et al. Effect of diuresis on the performance of the failing left ventricle in man. *Am J Med.* 1981;70:234–239.
21. Brater DC. Diuretic therapy. *N Engl J Med.* 1998;339:387–395.
22. Vargo DL, Kramer WG, Block PK, et al. Bioavailability, pharmacokinetics, and pharmocodynamics of torsemide and furosemide in patients with congestive heart failure. *Clin Pharmacol Ther.* 1995;57:601–609.
23. Ghose RR, Gupta SK. Synergistic actions of metolazone with loop diuretics. *BMJ.* 1981;812:1432–1433.
24. Ellison DH. The physiologic basis for duiretic synergism: its role in treating diuretic resistance. *Ann Intern Med.* 1991;114: 886–894.
25. Herchuelz A, Derenne F, Deger F, et al. Interaction between nonsteroidal anti-inflammatory drugs and loop diuretics: modulation by sodium balance. *J Pharmacol Exp Ther.* 1989;248: 1175–1181.
26. Heerkink ER, Leufkins HG, Herings RM, et al. NSAIDS associated with increased risk of congestive heart failure in elderly patients taking diuretics. *Arch Intern Med.* 1998;158: 1108–1112.
27. Domanski M, Norman J, Pitt B, et al. Diuretic use, progressive heart failure, and death in patients in the Studies of Left Ventricular Dysfunction (SOLVD). *J Am Coll Cardiol.* 2003;42:705–708.
28. Francis GS, Benedict C, Johnstone DE, et al. Comparison of neurodenocrine activation in patients with left ventricular dysfunction with and without congestive heart failure: a substudy of the Studies of Left Ventricular Dysfunction (SOLVD). *Circulation.* 1990;82:1724–1729.
29. Steiness E, Oleson KH. Cardiac arrhythmias induced by hypokalemia and potassium loss during maintenance digoxin therapy. *Br Heart J.* 1976;38:167–172.
30. Packer M. Potential role for potassium as a determinant of morbidity and mortality in patients with hypertension and chronic heart failure. *Am J Cardiol.* 1990;65:45E–51E.
31. Sonnenblick EH, Williams JF, Glick G, et al. Studies on digitalis XV. Effects of cardiac glycosides on myocardial force-velocity relations in the non-failing human heart. *Circulation.* 1966;34: 532–539.
32. Arnold SB, Byrd RC, Meister W, et al. Long-term digitalis therapy improves left ventricular function in heart failure. *N Engl J Med.* 1980;303:1443–1448.
33. Parker M, Carver J, Rodeherrer R, et al. Effect of oral milrinone on mortality in severe heart failure. *N Engl J Med.* 1991;325: 1468–1475.
34. German-Austrian Xamoterol Study Group. Double blind placebo-controlled comparison of digoxin and xamoterol in chronic heart failure. *Lancet.* 1988;1:489–493.
35. Ferguson DW, Berg WJ, Sanders JS, et al. Sympathoinhibitory responses to digitalis glycosides in heart failure patients: direct evidence from sympathetic neural recordings. *Circulation.* 1989;80:65–77.
36. Lee DC-S, Johnson RA, Behgham JB, et al. Heart failure in outpatients. A randomized trial of digoxin versus placebo. *N Engl J Med.* 1982;306:699–705.
37. Guyatt GH, Sullivan MJJ, Fallen EL et al. A controlled trial of diagoxin in congestive heart failure. *Am J Cardiol.* 1988; 61:371–375.
38. The Captopril-Digoxin Multicenter Research Group Comparative effects of therapy with captopril and digoxin in patients with mild to moderate heart failure. *JAMA.* 1988;259:539–544.
39. Packer M, Gheorghiade M, Young JB, et al. Withdrawal of digoxin from patients with chronic heart failure treated with angiotensin converting enzyme inhibitors: Radiance Study Group. *N Engl J Med.* 1993;329:1–7.
40. Uretsky BF, Young JB, Shahidi FE, et al on behalf of the PROVED Investigative Group. Randomized study assessing the effect of digoxin withdrawal in patients with mild to moderate congestive heart failure. Results of the PROVED trial. *J Am Coll Cardiol.* 1993;22:955–962.
41. The Digitalis Investigation Group. The effect of digoxin on mortality and morbidity on patients with heart failure. *N Engl J Med.* 1997;336:525–533.
42. Smith TW. Digitalis:mechanisms of action and clinical use. *N Engl J Med.* 1988;318:358–365.
43. Adams KF Jr, Patterson JH, Gattis WA, et al. Relationship of serum digoxin concentration to mortality and morbidity in women in the Digitalis Investigation Group: a retrospective analysis. *J Am Coll Cardiol.* 2005;46:497–504.
44. Gheorghiade M, Hall VB, Jacobsen G, et al. Effects of increasing maintenance dose of digoxin on left ventricular function and neurohormones in patients with chronic heart failure treated with diuretics and angiotensin-converting enzyme inhibitors. *Circulation.* 1995;92;1801–1807.
45. Slatton MC, Ikrani WN, Hall SA, et al. Does digoxin provide additional hemodynamic and autonomic benefit at higher doses in patients with mild to moderate heart failure and normal sinus rhythm? *J Am Coll Cardiol.* 1997;29:1206–1213.
46. Dzau VJ, Colucci WS, Hollinberg NK, et al. Relation of the renin-angiotensin-aldosterone system to clinical state in congestive heart failure. *Circulation.* 1981;63:645–651.
47. Francis GS, Goldsmith SR, Levine TB, et al. The neurohormonal axis in congestive heart failure. *Ann Intern Med.* 1984;101:370–377.
48. Paul M, Wagner J, Dzau V. Gene expression of the renin-angiotensin system in human tissues: quantitative analysis by the polymerase chain reaction. *J Clin Invest.* 1993;91:2058–2064.
49. Urata H, Boehm KD, Philip A, et al. Cellular localization and regional distribution of an angiotensin II-forming chymase in the heart. *J Clin Invest.* 1993;91:1269–1281.
50. Erdos EG. The angiotensin I converting enzyme. *Fed Proc* 1977;36:1760–1765.
51. Barrow SSE, Dollery CT, Heavey DJ, et al. Effect of vasoactive peptides on prostacyclin synthesis in man. *Br J Pharmacol.* 1986;87:243–247.
52. O'Kane KPH, Webb DJ, Collier JG, et al. Local L-N (G-monomethyl-arginine attenuates the vasodilator actions of bradykinin in the human forearm. *Br J Clin Pharmacol.* 1994;38:311–315.
53. Gainer JV, Morrow JD, Loveland A, et al. Effect of bradykinin-receptor blockade on the response to angiotensin-converting-enzyme inhibitor in normotensive and hypertensive subjects. *N Engl J Med.* 1998;339:1285–1291.
54. Lenz W, Scholkens BA. A specific β_2-bradykinin receptor antagonist HOE 140 abolishes the antihypertrophic effect of ramipril. *Br J Pharmacol.* 1992;105:771–772.
55. David R, Ribner HS, Keung E, et al. Treatment of chronic congestive heart failure with captopril, an oral inhibitor of angiotensin converting enzyme. *N Engl J Med.* 1979;301:117–121.
56. Ader R, Chatterjee K, Ports T, et al. Immediate and sustained hemodynamic and clinical improvement in chronic heart failure by angiotensin-converting enzyme inhibitors. *Circulation.* 1980;61:931–937.
57. Levine TB, Franciosa JA, Cohn JN. Acute and long-term response to an oral converting enzyme inhibitor, captopril in chronic heart failure: a rest and exercise hemodynamic study. *Circulation.* 1983;67:807–816.
58. Kramer BL, Massie BM, Topic N. Controlled trial of captopril in chronic heart failure: a rest and exercise hemodynamic study. *Circulation.* 1983;67:807–816.
59. Captopril Multicenter Research Group. A placebo-controlled trial of captopril in refractory chronic congestive heart failure. *J Am Coll Cardiol.* 1983;2:755–763.

60. Mancini DM, Davis L, Wexler JP, et al. Dependence of enhanced maximal exercise performance on increased peak skeletal muscle perfusion during long-term captopril therapy in heart failure. *J Am Coll Cardiol.* 1987;10:845–850.
61. Drexler H, Banhardt U, Meinhertz, et al. Contrasting peripheral short-term and long-term effects of converting enzyme inhibition in patients with congestive heart failure. A double-blind, placebo controlled trial. *Circulation.* 1989;79:491–502.
62. Ontkean M, Gay R, Greenberg B. ACE inhibition with captopril improves EDRF activity in an experimental model of chronic heart failure. [Abstract] *J Am Coll Cardiol.* 1992;19:207A.
63. Hammermeister KE, DeRouen TA, Dodge HT. Variables predictive of survival in patients with coronary disease: selection by univariate and multivariate analyses from the clinical, electrocardiographic, exercise, arteriographic and quantitative angiographic evaluations. *Circulation.* 1979;59:421–430.
64. Norris RM, Barnaby PF, Brandt PWT, et al. Prognosis after recovery from first acute myocardial infarction: determinants of reinfarction and sudden death. *Am J Cardiol.* 1984;53: 408–413.
65. White HD, Norris RM, Brown MA, et al. Left ventricular end-systolic volume as the major determinant of survival after recovery from myocardial infarction. *Circulation.* 1987;76:44–51.
66. Levy D, Garrison RJ, Savage DD, et al. Prognostic implications of echocardiographically determined left ventricular mass in the Framingham Heart Study. *N Engl J Med.* 1990;322: 1561–1566.
67. Quinones MA, Weiner DH, Shelton BJ, et al. for the SOLVD Investigators. Echocardiographic predictors of one-year clinical outcome in the Study of Left Ventricular Dysfunction (SOLVD) Trial and Registry. An analysis of 1,172 patients. *J Am Coll Cardiol.* 2000;35:1237–1244.
68. Sharpe N, Murphy J, Smith H, et al. Treatment of patients with symptomless left ventricular dysfunction after myocardial infarction. *Lancet.* 1988;1:255–259.
69. Pfeffer MA, Braunwald EB, Moye LA, et al. Effect of captopril on mortality and morbidity in patients with left ventricular dysfunction after myocardial infarction. Results of the survival and ventricular enlargement trial. *N Engl J Med.* 1992;327: 669–677.
70. The Acute Infarction Ramipril Efficacy (AIRE) Study Investigators. Effect of ramipril on mortality and morbidity of survivors of acute myocardial infarction with clinical evidence of heart failure. *Lancet.* 1993;342:821–828.
71. Ambrosioni E, Borghi C, Magnani B for the Survival of Myocardial Infarction Long-Term Evaluation (SMILE) study investigators. The effect of the angiotensin-converting-enzyme inhibitor zofenopril on mortality and morbidity after anterior myocardial infarction. *N Engl J Med.* 1995;332: 80–85.
72. Koker L, Torp-Pedersen C, Carlsen JE, et al. A clinical trial of the angiotensis-converting-enzyme inhibitor trandolapril in patients with left ventricular dysfunction after myocardial infarction. *N Engl J Med.* 1995;333:1670–1676.
73. Borghi C, Marino P, Zardini P, et al. for the FAMIS Working Party Bologna, Verona, and Rome, Italy. Short- and long-term effects of early fosinopril administration in patients with acute anterior myocardial infarction undergoing intravenous thrombolysis: results from the Fosinopril in Acute Myocardial Infarction Study. *Am Heart J.* 1998;136:213–225.
74. Latini R, Maggioni AP, Flather M, et al. ACE inhibitor use in patients with myocardial infarction: summary of evidence from clinical trials. *Circulation.* 1995;92:3132–3137.
75. ACE Inhibitor Myocardial Infarction Collaborative Group. Indications for ACE inhibitors in the early treatment of acute myocardial infarction: systematic overview of individual data from 100,000 patients in randomized trials. *Circulation.* 1998;97:2202–2212.
76. The CONSENSUS Trial Study Group. Effects of enalapril on mortality in severe congestive heart failure. Results of the Cooperative North Scandinavian Enalapril Survival Study (CONSENSUS). *N Engl J Med.* 1987;316:1429–1435.
77. The SOLVD Investigators. Effects of enalapril on survival in patients with reduced left ventricular ejection fractions and congestive heart failure. *N Engl J Med.* 1991;325:293–302.
78. The SOLVD Investigators. Effect of enalapril on mortality and the development of heart failure in asymptomatic patients with reduced left ventricular ejection fractions. *N Engl J Med.* 1992;327:685–691.
79. Cohn JN, Johnson G, Zilsche S, et al. A comparison of enalapril with hydralazine-isosorbide dinitrate in the treatment of chronic congestive heart failure. *N Engl J Med.* 1991;325:303–310.
80. Hall D, Zeitler, Rudolf W. Counteraction of the vasodilator effects of enalapril by aspirin in severe heart failure. *J Am Coll Cardiol.* 1992;20:1549–1555.
81. Spaulding C, Charbonnier B, Cohen-Solal A, et al. Acute hemodynamic interaction of aspirin and ticlopidine with enalapril: results of a double-blind, randomized comparative trial. *Circulation.* 1998;98:757–765.
82. Greenberg B, Quinones MA, Koilpillai C, et al. Effects of long-term enalapril therapy on patients with left ventricular dysfunction: results of the SOLVD echocardiography substudy. *Circulation.* 1995;91:2573–2581.
83. Packer J, Medena N, Yushak M. Relationship between serum sodium concentrations and the hemodynamic and clinical response to converting enzyme inhibition with captopril in severe heart failure. *J Am Coll Cardiol.* 1984;3:1035–1043.
84. Israils ZH, Hall WD. Cough and angioneurotic edema associated with angiotensin-converting enzyme inhibitor therapy: a review of the literature and pathophysiology. *Ann Intern Med.* 1992; 11:234–242.
85. Consensus recommendations for the management of chronic heart failure. On behalf of the membership of the advisory council to improve outcomes nationwide in heart failure. *Am J Cardiol.* 1999;83:1A–38A.
86. Massie BM, Armstrong PW, Cleland JGF, et al. Excellent tolerability of high doses of lisinopril in the ATLAS trial. *Circulation.* 1998;98:I-82.
87. Jin D, Takai S, Yamada M, et al. Impact of chymase inhibitor on cardiac function and survival after myocardial infarction. *Cardiovasc Res.* 2003;60:413–420.
88. Ishiyama Y, Gallagher PE, Averill DB, et al. Upregulation of angiotensin-converting enzyme 2 after myocardial infarction by blockade of angiotensin II receptors. *Hypertension.* 2004;43: 970–976.
89. Mendes ACR, Ferreira AJ, Pinheiro SVB, Santos RAS. Chronic infusion of angiotensin-(1–7) reduces angiotensin II level in rats. *Regulatory Peptides* 125;2005:29–34.
90. Langeveld B, van Gilst WH, Tio RA, et al. Angiotensin-(1–7) attenuates neointimal formation after stent implantation in the rat. *Hypertension.* 2005;45:138–141.
91. Tallant EA, Ferrario CM, Gallagher PE. Angiotensin-(1–7) inhibits growth of cardiac myocytes through activation of the mas receptor. *AJP–Heart* 2005;289:1560–1566.
92. Pfeffer MA, McMurray JJV, Velazquez EJ, et al. for the Valsartan in Acute Myocardial Infarction Trial Investigators. Valsartan, captopril, or both in myocardial infarction complicated by heart failure, left ventricular dysfunction, or both. *N Engl J Med.* 2003; 349:1893–1906.
93. Granger CB, McMurray JJV, Yusuf S, et al, for the CHARM Investigators and Committees. Effects of candesartan in patients with chronic heart failure and reduced left-ventricular systolic function intolerant to angiotensin-converting-enzyme inhibitors: the CHARM-Alternative trial. *Lancet.* 2003;362: 772–776.
94. Maggioni AP, Anand I, Gottlieb SO, et al. Effects of valsartan on morbidity and mortality in patients with heart failure not receiving angiotensin-converting enzyme inhibitors. *J Am Coll Cardiol.* 2002;40:1414–1421.
95. Pitt B, Poole-Wilson PA, Segal R, et al. Effect of losartan compared with captopril on mortality in patients with symptomatic heart failure: randomized trial—the Losartan Heart Failure Survival Study ELITE II. *Lancet.* 2000;355:1582–1587.
96. Cohn JN, Tognoni G. A randomized trial of the angiotensin-receptor blocker valsartan in chronic heart failure. *N Engl J Med.* 2001;345:1667–1675.
97. McMurray JJ, Ostergren J, Swedberg K, et al. Effects of candesartan in patients with chronic heart failure and reduced left-ventricular systolic function taking angiotensin-converting-enzyme inhibitors: the CHARM-Added trial. *Lancet.* 2003;362:767–771.

98. Mann DL, Kent RL, Parsons B, Cooper G III. Adrenergic effects on the biology of the adult mammalian cardiocyte. *Circulation.* 1992;85:790–804.
99. Knowlton KU, Michel MC, Itani M, et al. The alpha 1A-adrenergic receptor subtype mediates biochemical, molecular, and morphologic features of cultured myocardial cell hypertrophy. *J Biol Chem.* 1993;268:15374–15380.
100. Communal C, Singh K, Pimental DR, et al. Norepinephrine stimulates apoptosis in adult rat ventricular myocytes by activation of the β-adrenergic pathway. *Circulation.* 1998; 98: 1329–1334.
101. Smith KM, Macmillan JB, McGrath JC. Investigation of alpha$_1$-adrenoreceptor subtypes mediating vasoconstriction in rabbit cutaneous resistance arteries. *Br J Pharmacol.* 1997;122:825–832.
102. Elhawary AM, Pang CC. Alpha 1β-adrenoceptors mediate renal tubular sodium and water reabsorption in the rat. *Br J Pharmacol.* 1994;111:819–824.
103. Simons M, Donwing SE. Coronary vasoconstriction and catecholamine cardiomyopathy. *Am Heart J.* 1985;109:297–304.
104. Molina-Viamonte V, Anyukhovsky EP, Rosen MR. An α-adrenergic receptor subtype is responsible for delayed after-depolarizations and triggered activity during simulated ischemia and reperfusion of isolated canine Purkinje fibers. *Circulation.* 1991;84:1732–1740.
105. Kaumann AJ, Sanders I. Both beta 1- and beta 2-adrenoceptors mediate catecholamine-evoked arrhythmias in isolated human atrium. *Naunyn Schmiedebergs Arch Pharmacol.* 1993;348: 536–540.
106. Muntz KH, Zhao M, Miller JC. Downregulation of myocardial β-adrenergic receptors: receptor subtype selectivity. *Circ Res.* 1994;74:369–375.
107. Kaye DM, Lefkovits J, Jennings GL, et al. Adverse consequences of high sympathetic nervous activity in the failing human heart. *J Am Coll Cardiol.* 1995;26:1257–1263.
108. Heilbrunn SM, Shah P, Bristow MR, et al. Increased β-receptor density and improved hemodynamic response to catecholamine stimulation during long-term metoprolol therapy in heart failure from dilated cardiomyopathy. *Circulation.* 1989;79: 483–490.
109. Nemanich JW, Veith RC, Abrass IB, et al. Effects of metoprolol on rest and exercise cardiac function and plasma catecholamines in chronic congestive heart failure secondary to ischemic or idiopathic cardiomyopathy. *Am J Cardiol.* 1998; 66:843–848.
110. Waagstgein F, Caidaho K, Wallentin I, et al. Long-term β-blockade in dilated cardiomyopathy: effects of short- and long-term metoprolol treatment followed by withdrawal and readministration of metoprolol. *Circulation.* 1989;80:551–563.
111. Gilbert EM, Anderson JL, Deitchman D, et al. Long-term β-blocker vasodilator therapy improves cardiac function in idiopathic dilated cardiomyopathy: a double-blind, randomized study of bucindolol versus placebo. *Am J Med.* 1990;88: 223–229.
112. Anderson JL, Gilbert EM, et al. Long-term (2 year) beneficial effects of beta-adrenergic blocked with bucindolol in patients with idiopathic dilated cardiomyopathy. *J Am Coll Cardiol.* 1991;17:1373–1381.
113. Woodley SL, Gilbert EM, Anderson JL, et al. β-blockade with bucindolol in heart failure caused by ischemic versus idiopathic dilated cardiomyopathy. *Circulation.* 1991;84:2426–2441.
114. Waagstein F, Bristow MR, Swedberg K, et al. Beneficial effects of metoprolol in idiopathic dilated cardiomyopathy. *Lancet.* 1993;342;1441–1446.
115. Fisher ML, Gottlieb SS, Plotnick GD, et al. Beneficial effects of metoprolol in heart failure associated with coronary artery disease: a randomized trial. *J Am Coll Cardiol.* 1994;23: 943–950.
116. Bristow MR, O'Connell JB, Gilbert EM, et al. Dose-response of chronic β-blocker treatment in heart failure from either idiopathic dilated or ischemic cardiomyopathy. *Circulation.* 1994; 89:1632–1642.
117. Olsen SL, Gilbert EM, Renlund DG, et al. Carvedilol improves left ventricular function and symptoms in chronic heart failure: a double-blind randomized study. *J Am Coll Cardiol.* 1995; 25:1225–1231.
118. Chadda K, Goldstein S, Byington R, Curb JD. Effect of propranolol after acute myocardial infarction in patients with congestive heart failure. *Circulation.* 1986;73:503–510.
119. Gottlieb SS, McCarter RJ, Vogel RA. Effect of beta-blockade on mortality among high-risk and low-risk patients after myocardial infarction. *N Engl J Med.* 1998;339:489–497.
120. Packer M, Bristow MR, Cohn JN, et al. The effect of carvedilol on morbidity and mortality in patients with chronic heart failure. *N Engl J Med.* 1996;334:1439–1455.
121. Ruffolo RR, Gallai M, Hieble JP, et al. The pharmacology of carvedilol. *Eur J Clin Pharmacol.* 1990;38(Suppl):82–88.
122. Yue T-L, Cheng H-Y, Lyske PG, et al. Carvedilol: a new vasodilator and beta adrenoreceptor antagonist is an antioxidant and free radical scavenger. *Pharmacol Exp Ther.* 1992;263:92–98.
123. Packer M, Fowler MB, Roecker EB, et al. Effect of carvedilol on the morbidity of patients with severe chronic heart failure: results of the carvedilol prospective randomized cumulative survival (COPERNICUS) study. *Circulation.* 2002;106:2194–2199.
124. CIBIS-II Investigators and Committees. The Cardiac Insufficiency Bisoprolol Study II (CIBIS-II): a randomised trial. *Lancet.* 1999;353:9–13.
125. MERIT-HF Study Group. Effect of metoprolol CR/XL in chronic heart failure: Metoprolol CR/XL Randomized Intervention Trial in Congestive Heart Failure (MERIT-HF). *Lancet.* 1999;353: 2001–2007.
126. Australia/New Zealand Heart Failure Research Collaborative Group. Randomised, placebo-controlled trial of carvedilol in patients with congestive heart failure due to ischaemic heart disease. *Lancet.* 1997;349:375–380.
127. Sliwa K, Norton GR, Kone N, et al. Impact of initiating carvedilol before angiotensin-converting enzyme inhibitor therapy on cardiac function in newly diagnosed heart failure. *J Am Coll Cardiol.* 2004;44:1825–1830.
128. Cleland JG, Coletta AP, Lammiman M, et al. Clinical trials update from the European Society of Cardiology meeting 2005: CARE-HF extension study, ESSENTIAL, CIBIS-III, S-ICD, ISSUE-2, STRIDE-2, SOFA, IMAGINE, PREAMI, SIRIUS-II, and ACTIVE. *Eur J Heart Fail.* 2005;7:1070–1075.
129. Carlberg B, Samuelsson O, Lindholm LH. Atenolol in hypertension: is it a wise choice? *Lancet.* 2004;364:1684–1689.
130. Beta-Blocker Evaluation of Survival Trial Investigators. A trial of the beta-blocker bucindolol in patients with advanced chronic heart failure. *N Engl J Med.* 2001;344:1659–1667.
131. Willette RN, Aiyar N, Yue TL, et al. In vitro and in vivo characterization of intrinsic sympathomimetic activity in normal and heart failure rats. *J Pharmacol Exp Ther.* 1999;289:48–53.
132. Bristow MR, Krause-Steinrauf H, Nuzzo R, et al. Effect of baseline or changes in adrenergic activity on clinical outcomes in the beta-blocker evaluation of survival trial. *Circulation.* 2004; 110:1437–1442.
133. Poole-Wilson PA, Swedberg K, Cleland JG, et al. Comparison of carvedilol and metoprolol on clinical outcomes in patients with chronic heart failure in the Carvedilol Or Metoprolol European Trial (COMET): randomized controlled trial. *Lancet.* 2003;362:7–13.
134. Eichhorn EJ, Bristow MR. Practical guidelines for initiation of beta-adrenergic blockade in patients with chronic heart failure. *Am J Cardiol.* 1997;79:794–797.
135. Bristow MR, Gilbert EM, Abraham WT, et al. Carvedilol produces dose-related improvements in left ventricular function and survival in subjects with chronic heart failure. *Circulation.* 1996;94:2807–2816.
136. Rajagopalan S, Pitt B. Aldosterone as a target in congestive heart failure. *Med Clin North Am.* 2003;87:441–457.
137. McKelvie RS, Yusuf S, Pericak D, et al. Comparison of candesartan, enalapril, and their combination congestive heart failure: randomized evaluation of strategies for left ventricular dysfunction (RESOLVD) pilot study. The RESOLVD Pilot Study Investigators. *Circulation.* 1999;100:1056–1064.
138. Pitt B, Zannad F, Remme WJ, et al. for the Randomized Aldactone Evaluation Study Investigators. The effect of spironolactone on morbidity and mortality in patients with severe heart failure. *N Engl J Med.* 1999;341:709–717.
139. Pitt B, Remme W, Zannad F, et al. Eplerenone, a selective aldosterone blocker, in patients with left ventricular dysfunction after myocardial infarction. *N Engl J Med.* 2003;348:1309–1321.
140. Pitt B, White H, Nicolau J, et al. Eplerenone reduces mortality 30 days after randomization following acute myocardial infarction in patients with left ventricular systolic dysfunction and heart failure. *J Am Coll Cardiol.* 2005;46:425–431.

141. Bozkurt B, Agoston I, Knowlton AA. Complications of inappropriate use of spironolactone in heart failure: when an old medicine spirals out of new guidelines. *J Am Coll Cardiol.* 2003;41:211–214.
142. Juurlink DN, Mamdani MM, Lee DS, et al. Rates of hyperkalemia after publication of the Randomized Aldactone Evaluation Study. *N Engl J Med.* 2004;351:543–551.
143. Cohn JN, Archibald DG, Ziesche S, et al. Effect of vasodilator therapy on mortality on chronic congestive heart failure. Results of a Veterans Administration Cooperative Study. *N Engl J Med.* 1986;314:1547–1552.
144. Cohn JN, Johnson G, Ziesche S, et al. A comparison of enalapril with hydralazine-isosorbide dinitrate in the treatment of chronic congestive heart failure. *N Engl J Med.* 1991;325:303–310.
145. Gogia H, Mehra A, Parikh S, et al. Prevention of tolerance to hemodynamic effects of nitrates with concomitant use of hydralazine in patients with chronic heart failure. *J Am Coll Cardiol.* 1995;26:1575–1580.
146. Munzel T, Kurz S, Rajagopalan S, et al. Hydralazine prevents nitroglycerin tolerance by inhibiting activation of a membrane-bound NADH oxidase. A new action for an old drug. *J Clin Invest.* 1996;98:1465–1470.
147. Daiber A, Mulsch A, Hink U, et al. The oxidative stress concept of nitrate tolerance and the antioxidant properties of hydralazine. *Am J Cardiol.* 2005;96:25i-36i.
148. Carson P, Ziesche S, Johnson G, et al. Racial differences in response to therapy for heart failure: analysis of the vasodilator-heart failure trials. Vasodilator-Heart Failure Trial Study Group. *J Card Fail.* 1999;5:178–187.
149. Tanus-Santos JE, Desai M, Flockhart DA. Effects of ethnicity on the distribution of clinically relevant endothelial nitric oxide variants. *Pharmacogenetics.* 2001;11:719–725.
150. Chen W, Srinivasan SR, Bond MG, et al. Nitric oxide synthase gene polymorphism (G894T) influences arterial stiffness in adults: the Bogalusa Heart Study. *Am J Hypertens.* 2004; 17:553–559.
151. Lapu-Bula R, Quarshie A, Lyn D, et al. The 894T allele of endothelial nitric oxide synthase gene is related to left ventricular mass in African Americans with high-normal blood pressure. *J Natl Med Assoc.* 2005;97:197–205.
152. Marroni AS, Metzger IF, Souza-Costa DC, et al. Consistent interethnic differences in the distribution of clinically relevant endothelial nitric oxide synthase genetic polymorphisms. *Nitric Oxide.* 2005;12:177–182.
153. Taylor AL, Ziesche S, Yancy C, et al. Combination of isosorbide dinitrate and hydralazine in blacks with heart failure. *N Engl J Med.* 2004;351:2049–2057.
154. Iuliano S, Fisher SG, Karasik PE, et al. QRS duration and mortality in patients with congestive heart failure. *Am Heart J.* 2002; 143:1085–1091.
155. Kalahasti V, Nambi V, Martin DO, et al. QRS duration and prediction of mortality in patients undergoing risk stratification for ventricular arrhythmias. *Am J Cardiol.* 2003;92:798–803.
156. Bode-Schnurbus L, Bocker D, Block M, et al. QRS duration: a simple marker for predicting cardiac mortality in ICD patients with heart failure. *Heart.* 2003;89:1157–1162.
157. Auricchio A, Kloss M, Trautmann SE, et al. Exercise performance following cardiac resynchronization therapy in patients with heart failure and ventricular conduction delay. *Am J Cardiol.* 2002;89:198–203.
158. Abraham WT, Fisher WG, Smith AL, et al. Cardiac resynchronization in chronic heart failure. *N Engl J Med.* 2002;346:1845–1853.
159. Abraham WT, Young JB, Leon AR, et al. Effects of cardiac resynchronization on disease progression in patients with left ventricular systolic dysfunction, an indication for an implantable cardioverter-defibrillator, and mildly symptomatic heart failure. *Circulation.* 2004;110:2864–2868.
160. Auricchio A, Spinelli JC, Trautmann SI, et al. Effect of cardiac resynchronization therapy on ventricular remodeling. *J Card Fail.* 2002;8:S549–S555.
161. Yu CM, Fung WH, Lin H, et al. Predictors of left ventricular reverse remodeling after cardiac resynchronization therapy for heart failure secondary to idiopathic dilated or ischemic cardiomyopathy. *Am J Cardiol.* 2003;91:684–688.
162. St. John Sutton MG, Plappert T, Abraham WT, et al. Effect of cardiac resynchronization therapy on left ventricular size and function in chronic heart failure. *Circulation.* 2003;107:1985–1990.
163. Bradley DJ, Bradley EA, Baughman KL, et al. Cardiac resynchronization and death from progressive heart failure: a meta-analysis of randomized controlled trials. *JAMA.* 2003;289: 730–740.
164. Cleland JG, Daubert JC, Erdmann E, et al. The effect of cardiac resynchronization on morbidity and mortality in heart failure. *N Engl J Med.* 2005;352:1539–1549.
165. Goldstein S. The changing epidemiology of sudden death in heart failure. *Curr Heart Fail Rep.* 2004;1:93–97.
166. Saxon LA. Sudden cardiac death: epidemiology and temporal trends. *Rev Cardiovasc Med.* 2005;6:S12–S20.
167. Echt DS, Liebson PR, Mitchell LB, et al. Mortality and morbidity in patients receiving encainide, flecainide, or placebo. The Cardiac Arrhythmia Suppression Trial. *N Engl J Med.* 1991;324:781–788.
168. Moss AJ. MADIT-II. MADIT-II: substudies and their implications. *Card Electrophysiol Rev* 2003;7:430–433.
169. Bardy GH, Lee KL, Mark DB, et al. Amiodarone or an implantable cardioverter-defibrillator for congestive heart failure. *N Engl J Med.* 2005;352:225–237.
170. Nishimura RA, Tajik AJ. Evaluation of diastolic filling of left ventricle in health and disease: Doppler echocardiography is the clinician's Rosetta Stone. *J Am Coll Cardiol.* 1997;30:8–18.
171. Ghali JK, Kadakia S, Cooper R, et al. Precipitating factors leading to decompensation of heart failure. *Arch Intern Med.* 1988; 148:2013–2016.
172. Vinson JM, Rich MW, Sperry JC, et al. Early readmission of elderly patients with congestive heart failure. *J Am Geriatr Soc* 1990;38:1290–1295.
173. Monane M, Bohn RL, Gurwitz JH, Glynn RJ, Avorn J. Noncompliance with congestive heart failure therapy in the elderly. *Arch Intern Med.* 1994;154:433–437.
174. Scandinavian Simvastatin Survival Study Group. Randomised trial of cholesterol lowering in 4,444 patients with coronary heart disease: the Scandinavian Simvastatin Survival Study (4S). *Lancet.* 1994;344:1383–1389.
175. Kjekshus J, Pedersen TR, Olsson AG, et al. The effects of simvastatin on the incidence of heart failure in patients with coronary heart disease. *J Cardiac Failure.* 1997;3:249–254.
176. Kostis JB, Davis BR, Cutler J, et al. for the SHEP Cooperative Research Group. Prevention of heart failure by antihypertensive drug treatment in older persons with isolated systolic hypertension. *JAMA.* 1997;278:212–216.
177. Yusuf S, Sleight P, Pogue J, et al. Effects of an angiotensin-converting-enzyme inhibitor, ramipril, on cardiovascular events in high-risk patients. The Heart Outcomes Prevention Evaluation Study Investigators. *N Engl J Med.* 2000;342: 145–153.
178. Arnold JM, Yusuf S, Young J, et al. Prevention of heart failure in patients in the Heart Outcomes Prevention Evaluation (HOPE) Study. *Circulation.* 2003;107:1284–1290.
179. St. John Sutton M, Pfeffer MA, Plappert T, et al. Quantitative two-dimensional echocardiographic measurements are major predictors of adverse cardiovascular events after acute myocardial infarction: the protective effects of captopril. *Circulation.* 1994;89:68–75.
180. Gruppo Italiano perlo Studio della Sopravvivenza nell infarto Miocardio. G1551–3: effects of lisinopril and transdermal glyceryl and trinitrate singly and together on 6-week mortality and ventricular function after acute myocardial infarction. *Lancet.* 1994;343:1115–1122.
181. ISIS-4 (Fourth International Study of Infarct Survival) Collaborative Group. ISIS-4: a randomised factorial trail assessing early oral captopril, oral mononitrate, and intravenous magnesium sulphate in 58,050 patients with suspected acute myocardial infarction. *Lancet.* 1995;345: 669–685.
182. Beta Blocker Heart Attack Trial (BHAT) Investigators. A randomized trial of propranolol in patients with acute myocardial infarction. I. Mortality results. *JAMA.* 1982;247: 1707–1714.
183. Pedersen TR. The Norwegian Multicenter Study Of Timolol after Myocardial Infarction. *Circulation.* 1983;67:I49–53.
184. Dargie HJ. Effect of carvedilol on outcome after myocardial infarction in patients with left-ventricular dysfunction: the CAPRICORN randomized trial. *Lancet.* 2001;357:1385–1390.

185. Adler A, Greenberg BH. Use of beta blockers in patients with post-MI left ventricular dysfunction. *Curr Treat Options Cardiovasc Med*. 2004;6:335–343.
186. Butler J, Arbogast PG, BeLue R, et al. Outpatient adherence to beta-blocker therapy after acute myocardial infarction. *J Am Coll Cardiol*. 2002;40:1589–1595.
187. Hohnloser SH, Kuck KH, Dorian P, et al. Prophylactic use of an implantable cardioverter-defibrillator after acute myocardial infarction. *N Engl J Med*. 2004;351:2481–2488.
188. Moss AJ, Oakes D, Benhorin J, et al. Interaction between diltiazem and left ventricular function after myocardial infarction. *Circulation*. 1989;80(Suppl IV):102–106.
189. Kostis JB, Lacy CR, Cosgrove NM, Wilson AC. Association of calcium channel blocker use with increased rate of acute myocardial infarction in patients with left ventricular dysfunction. *Am Heart J*. 1997;133:550–557.
190. Massie BM, Packer M, Hanlon JT, et al. Combined captopril and hydralzaine therapy for refractory heart failure. *J Am Coll Cardiol*. 1983;2:338–345.
191. Leier CV, Huss P, Magorien RD, et al. Improved exercise capacity and differing arterial and venous tolerance during chronic isosorbide dinitrate. *Circulation*. 1983;67:817–822.
192. Gorgia H, Mehra A, Parekh S, et al. Prevention of tolerance to hemodynamic effects of nitrates with concomitant use of hydralazine in patients with chronic heart failure. *J Am Coll Cardiol*. 1995;26:1575–1580.
193. Stevenson LW, Massie BM, Francis GS. Optimizing therapy for complex or refractory heart failure: a management algorithm. *Am Heart J*. 1998;135(Suppl):293–309.
194. Steimle AE, Stevenson LW, Chelimsky-Fallick C, et al. Sustained hemodynamic efficacy of therapy tailored to reduce filling pressures in survivors with advanced heart failure. *Circulation*. 1997;30:725–732.
195. Unverferth DV, Magorien RD, Altschuld R, et al. The hemodynamic and metabolic advantages gained by a three-day infusion of dobutamine in patients with congestive cardiomyopathy. *Am Heart J*. 1983;106:29–34.
196. Krell MJ, Kline EM, Bates ER, et al. Intermittent ambulatory dobutamine infusions in patients with severe congestive heart failure. *Am Heart J*. 1986;112:787–791.
197. Collins JA, Skidmore MA, Melvin DB, et al. Home intravenous dobutamine therapy in patients awaiting heart transplantation. *J Heart Transplant*. 1990;9:205–208.
198. Yancy CW, Burnett JC, Jr., Fonarow GC, et al. Decompensated heart failure: is there a role for the outpatient use of nesiritide? *Congest Heart Fail*. 2004;10:230–236-
199. Cesario D, Clark J, Maisell A. Beneficial effects of intermittent home administration of the inotrope/vasodilator milrinone in patients with end-stage congestive heart failure: a preliminary study. *Am Heart J*. 1998;135:121–129.
200. Sackner-Bernstein JD, Skopicki HA, et al. Risk of worsening renal function with nesiritide in patients with acutely decompensated heart failure. *Circulation*. 2005;111:1487–1491.
201. Sackner-Bernstein JD, Kowalski M, Fox M, et al. Short-term risk of death after treatment with nesiritide for decompensated heart failure: a pooled analysis of randomized controlled trials. *JAMA*. 2005;293:1900–1905.
202. Heidenreich PA, Lee TT, Massie BM. Effect of beta-blockade on mortality in patients with heart failure: a meta-analysis of randomized clinical trials. *J Am Coll Cardiol*. 1997;30:27–34.
203. Wilson JR, Schwartz S, St. John Sutton M, et al. Prognosis in severe heart failure: relation to hemodynamic measurements and ventricular ectopic activity. *J Am Coll Cardiol*. 1983;2:403–410.
204. Maskin CS, Siskind SJ, Lejemtel TH. High incidence of nonsustained ventricular tachycardia in severe congestive heart failure. *Am Heart J*. 1984;14:564–590.
205. Gradman A, Deedwania, Cody R, et al. Predictors of total mortality and sudden death in mild to moderate heart failure. *J Am Coll Cardiol*. 1989;14:564–590.
206. Schultz RA, Strauss HW, Pitt B. Sudden death in the year following myocardial infarction. Relation to ventricular premature contractions in the late hospital phase and left ventricular ejection fraction. *Am J Med*. 1997;62:192–199.
207. Slater W, Lambert SL, Podrid PJ, et al. Clinical predictors of arrhythmia worsening by antiarrhythmic drugs. *Am J Cardiol*. 1988;61:349–353.
208. Morganroth J, Anderson JL, Gentzkow GD. Clarification of type of ventricular arrhythmia predicts frequency of adverse cardiac events from flecainide. *J Am Coll Cardiol*. 1986:8:607–615.
209. Podrid PJ, Schoeneberger A, Lown B. Precipitation of congestive heart failure by oral disopyramide. *N Engl J Med*. 1980; 302:614–617.
210. Mason JW. Amiodarone. *N Engl J Med*. 1987;316:455–466.
211. Doval HC, Nul DR, Crancelli HO, et al. Randomised trial of low-dose amiodarone in severe congestive heart failure. *Lancet*. 1994;344:493–498.
212. Singh SN, Fletcher RD, Fisher SD, et al. Amiodarone in patients with congestive heart failure and asymptomatic ventricular arrhythmia. *N Engl J Med*. 1995;333:77–82.
213. The Antiarrhythmics Versus Implantable Defibrillators (AVID) Investigators. A comparison of antiarrhythmic-drug therapy with implantable defibrillators in patients resuscitated from near-fatal ventricular arrhythmias. *N Engl J Med*. 1997;337:1576–1583.
214. Fuster V, Gersh BJ, Guiliani ER, et al. The natural history of idiopathic dilated cardiomyopathy. *Am J Cardiol*. 1981;47: 525–531.
215. Meltzer RS, Visser CA, Fuster V. Intracardiac thrombi and systemic embolization. *Ann Intern Med*. 1986;104:689–690.
216. Cioffi G. Pozzoli M, Forni G, et al. Systemic thromboembolism in chronic heart failure. A prospective study in 406 patients. *Eur Heart J*. 1996;17:1381–1389.
217. Stratton JR, Resnick AD. Increased embolic risk in patients with left ventricular thrombi. *Circulation*. 1987;75:1004–1011.
218. Al-Khadra AS, Salem DN, Rand WM, et al. Warfarin anticoagulation and survival: a cohort analysis from the Studies of Left Ventricular Dysfunction. *J Am Coll Cardiol*. 1998;31:749–753.

Biventricular Pacing in Congestive Heart Failure

36

William T. Abraham

Electrophysiological disturbances, including arrhythmias and conduction disorders, are common in the setting of congestive heart failure. For example, approximately 30% to 40% of unselected heart failure patients with reduced or preserved left ventricular (LV) systolic function exhibit atrial fibrillation (1–3). Nearly one-half of total mortality in heart failure patients with reduced LV ejection fractions may be attributable to ventricular tachyarrhythmias (4,5). About one-third of patients with systolic heart failure have a delay in ventricular conduction when defined as a QRS duration greater than 120 milliseconds (6,7). In this latter instance, the abnormality in ventricular conduction may result in an irregular or dysynchronous pattern of LV contraction, which may further impair the pumping ability of the already failing heart (8–11). Specifically, LV dysynchrony may cause suboptimal ventricular filling, prolonged duration of mitral regurgitation, and a reduction in LV *dP/dt*. Ventricular dysynchrony has also been associated with increased morbidity and mortality in heart failure patients (12–15).

Over the past 10 years, techniques have been developed to correct the mechanical and clinical manifestations of ventricular dysynchrony through the use of atrial-synchronized biventricular pacing, now known as cardiac resynchronization therapy. This technique involves simultaneous pacing of both the right and left ventricles with the goal of improving the ventricular contraction pattern and, ultimately, patient outcomes. Substantial evidence supports the routine use of cardiac resynchronization therapy in congestive heart failure patients with ventricular dysynchrony. More than 4,000 patients have been evaluated in randomized, controlled trials of cardiac resynchronization and several thousand additional patients have been assessed in observational studies and in registries. Results of these studies have consistently demonstrated the safety and efficacy of biventricular pacing in New York Heart Association (NYHA) Class III and IV heart failure patients. In such patients, cardiac resynchronization therapy has been shown to significantly improve LV structure and function, NYHA functional class, exercise tolerance, quality of life, and morbidity and mortality. Given the benefits of biventricular pacing, recent evidence-based guidelines and consensus statements strongly support the use of this therapy in all eligible heart failure patients (16,17). This chapter reviews the history, proposed mechanisms of action, clinical trials evidence, guidelines recommendations, and limitations of cardiac resynchronization therapy, and concludes with a look at future directions for biventricular pacing.

HISTORY OF BIVENTRICULAR PACING FOR CONGESTIVE HEART FAILURE

Cardiac resynchronization therapy was not the first pacing approach evaluated as a treatment for heart failure. Standard right-sided, dual-chamber (DDD) pacing, right ventricular outflow tract/His bundle pacing, and multisite right ventricular pacing were studied and produced inconsistent results on clinical outcomes in heart failure patients (18–23). Hochleitner et al. (18,19) were the first to suggest that right-sided DDD pacing might help correct the conduction disturbances seen in advanced heart failure and improve cardiac function. Expanding on this work, Brecker et al. (20) evaluated the effects of changing the atrial-ventricular (AV) interval during acute DDD pacing in patients with dilated cardiomyopathy and short ventricular filling times due to mitral and/or tricuspid regurgitation. While initially encouraging, the results of these early studies were not confirmed by later studies conducted by other investigators (21–23). Similarly, studies of multisite right ventricular pacing produced generally disappointing results. Considering this limited potential for right-sided pacing in systolic heart failure, attention turned to studies of biventricular pacing.

The evolution of biventricular pacing for the management of heart failure progressed rapidly following the first reported case in 1994 (24). Cazeau et al. (24) applied four-chamber pacing in a 54-year-old man with NYHA Class IV heart failure and several conduction abnormalities, including a QRS duration of 200 milliseconds, a PR interval of 200 milliseconds, and an interatrial conduction time of 90 milliseconds. Standard transvenous pacing leads were placed in the right atrium and right ventricle (RV), the left atrium was paced by a lead placed in the coronary sinus, and the LV was paced by an epicardial lead located on the LV free wall. After 6 weeks of pacing, the patient's clinical status markedly improved to NYHA Class II. Thus, with this single-case experience, the era of biventricular pacing for congestive heart failure was born.

Of course, it took many additional studies and several years to confirm the benefits of biventricular pacing before it could be recommended as a routine therapy for heart failure (16,17). Following Cazeau's initial report, other mechanistic and observational studies provided additional proof of concept supporting the benefits of biventricular pacing in heart failure (10,25–32). The first randomized, controlled trials designed to evaluate the effects of resynchronization therapy on quality of life, functional status, exercise capacity, pathological ventricular remodeling, and morbidity were then begun in the late 1990s. These studies affirmed that biventricular pacing, delivered using a wholly transvenous approach for right atrial, RV, and LV lead placement, was safe and confirmed the benefits seen in earlier uncontrolled experiences (33–40). Finally, randomized, controlled trials to assess the effects of biventricular pacing on morbidity and mortality were initiated. These trials demonstrated unequivocally the effects of cardiac resynchronization therapy, with or without an implantable cardioverter-defibrillator, to reduce morbidity and mortality in patients with moderate to severe heart failure (41–44).

PROPOSED MECHANISMS OF ACTION OF CARDIAC RESYNCHRONIZATION THERAPY

The mechanism of benefit of biventricular pacing remains incompletely understood. In this regard, it is important to note that the underlying target of therapy—ventricular dysynchrony—occurs at three levels within the heart (45). Interventricular dysynchrony describes a mismatch in timing between RV and LV contraction, usually measured as a difference in the onsets of pulmonary and aortic flow. Intraventricular dysynchrony is seen as a loss in the normal contraction pattern of the LV, generally associated with normal (early) activation of the septum and delayed (late) activation of the LV free wall, particularly in the setting of left bundle branch block. The hallmark of LV dysynchrony is paradoxical septal wall motion, where the septum moves away from the LV free wall during systole. Because of the abnormal septal motion, LV end-systolic diameter is increased and regional septal ejection fraction (EF) is decreased. Finally, intramural dysynchrony may affect both the mechanics and biology of the heart.

Early studies of biventricular pacing provided important insight into the potential mechanisms of action of cardiac resynchronization. The hemodynamic improvement seen with atrial-synchronized, biventricular pacing appears related to its ability to increase LV filling time, decrease septal dyskinesis, and reduce mitral regurgitation in the failing heart. Over time, these effects of resynchronization therapy result in improvements in ventricular geometry and function, compatible with reverse remodeling of the heart.

Acutely and chronically, cardiac resynchronization therapy increases LV filling time. In the presence of a long AV delay and/or an interventricular conduction delay (IVCD), LV activation is delayed but atrial activation is not. Thus, both early passive LV filling and the so-called atrial kick may occur simultaneously, resulting in decreased total transmitral blood flow and diminished preloading of the LV (46). These events are often seen as a fusion of the E and A waves on Doppler echocardiogram of transmitral blood flow. With atrial-synchronized biventricular pacing, both ventricles are activated simultaneously; thus, the LV is able to complete contraction and begin relaxation earlier, which increases filling time. The effect of resynchronization therapy can be seen by the return of normal E and A wave separation on Doppler echocardiogram of transmitral blood flow (Fig. 36-1).

Biventricular pacing also decreases septal dyskinesis, resulting in an improved contraction pattern and thus stroke volume. While LV activation and contraction are delayed in the presence of an IVCD, septal activation and contraction are not. This timing mismatch results in septal dyskinesis or paradoxical septal wall motion, in that the septum moves away from the LV free wall during systole. This paradoxical septal wall motion impairs mitral valve function by increasing mitral regurgitation and reduces the septum's contribution to LV stroke volume (47). With biventricular pacing, the ventricles are activated simultaneously, allowing ventricular ejection to occur prior to relaxation of the septum, resulting in decreased mitral regurgitation and increased LV stroke volume (34).

In addition, in the presence of a long PR interval and/or an IVCD, mitral valve closure may not be complete, since atrial contraction is not followed by a properly timed ventricular systole. If the time lag is long enough, a ventricular-atrial pressure gradient may develop and cause diastolic mitral regurgitation (48). By resynchronizing AV activation and contraction, normal mitral valve timing is restored and regurgitation is potentially reduced or eliminated. Serial evaluations in large numbers of heart failure patients with ventricular dysynchrony have confirmed a marked reduction in mitral regurgitant flow following the application of cardiac resynchronization therapy (38).

While there are numerous mechanical benefits of cardiac resynchronization therapy as previously noted, chronic biventricular pacing results in changes in LV structure, function, and gene expression that are compatible with

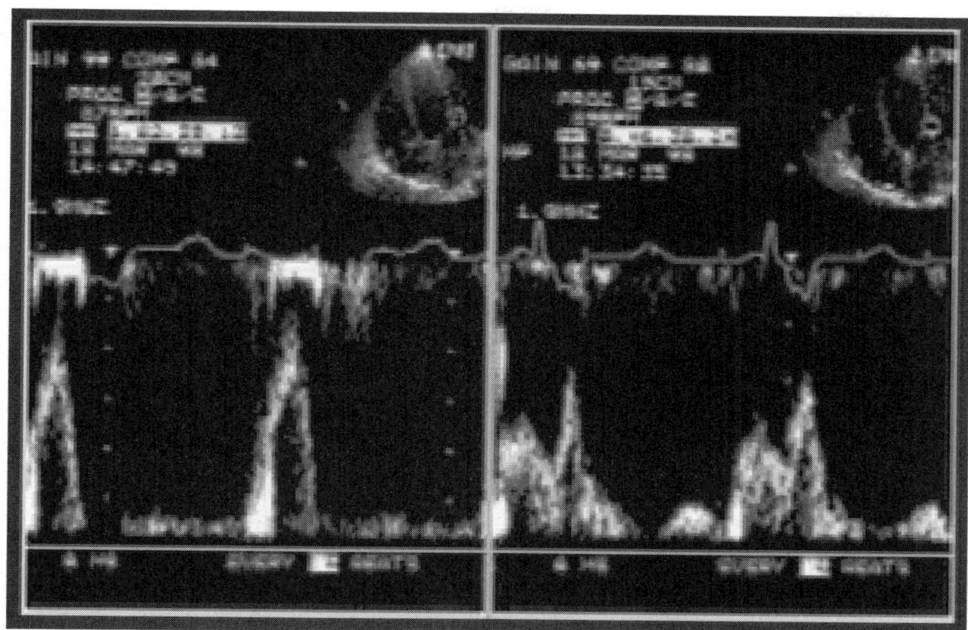

Figure 36-1 Effect of cardiac resynchronization therapy on left ventricular filling. Ventricular dyssynchrony produces fusion of the E and A waves on Doppler echocardiogram of transmitral blood flow (**left panel**), indicating a shortening of diastolic filling time. Cardiac resynchronization therapy increases LV filling time, as seen by the return of normal E and A wave separation on Doppler echocardiogram of transmitral blood flow (**right panel**).

reverse remodeling of the failing heart. In support of this notion are the following observations: (a) cardiac resynchronization therapy improves echocardiographic measures of ventricular remodeling; (b) there are a gradual onset and offset to these changes beyond the acute mechanical effects of biventricular pacing; and (c) changes in myocardial gene expression during chronic resynchronization therapy are compatible with true reverse remodeling. These improvements are similar to that seen with drug treatment of heart failure, particularly with beta-blockade (49–51).

Yu et al. (52) demonstrated the time course of reverse remodeling with biventricular pacing. They evaluated 25 NYHA Class III or IV heart failure patients with baseline EFs less than 40% and QRS durations greater than 140 milliseconds treated with biventricular pacing therapy. Subjects were assessed serially during 3 months of pacing and after pacing had been withheld for 4 weeks. During cardiac resynchronization therapy, there was a progressive improvement in ventricular structure and function. At 3 months, significant improvements were noted in EF, *dP/dt*, myocardial performance index, and mitral regurgitation. LV end-diastolic and end-systolic volumes were significantly reduced. Withholding pacing resulted in a progressive but not immediate loss of effect that occurred over the 4-week period of pacing withdrawal.

These effects of resynchronization therapy on ventricular remodeling have been confirmed in large, randomized, controlled trials. In the Multicenter InSync Randomized Clinical Evaluation (MIRACLE), serial Doppler echocardiograms were obtained at baseline, 3 months, and 6 months in 323 optimally treated NYHA Class III and IV heart failure patients (38,53). Cardiac resynchronization therapy for 6 months was associated with reduced end-diastolic and end-systolic volumes, reduced LV mass, increased EF, reduced mitral regurgitant blood flow, and improved myocardial performance index as compared with control subjects (Fig. 36-2). Similar to Yu's observations, the beneficial effects of biventricular pacing on these parameters were progressive over time.

Finally, preliminary results from Iyengar et al. (54) demonstrate changes in myocardial gene expression that correlate with echocardiographic improvements in cardiac structure, similar to those seen during reverse remodeling with beta-blockade (50,51).

CLINICAL TRIALS EVIDENCE SUPPORTING BIVENTRICULAR PACING

Numerous randomized, controlled trials support the use of cardiac resynchronization therapy. Among these studies are the Pacing Therapies in Congestive Heart Failure (PATH-CHF) trial (33–35), the Multisite Stimulation in Cardiomyopathy (MUSTIC) studies (36), the MIRACLE trial (37,38), MIRACLE ICD (55), the VENTAK CHF/CONTAK CD trials (39), the Cardiac Resynchronization—Heart Failure (CARE-HF) trial (43,44), and the Comparison of Medical Therapy, Pacing and Defibrillation in Heart Failure (COMPANION) trial (41,42). Several of these trials are reviewed next to demonstrate the beneficial effects of resynchronization therapy. Close attention should be paid to the inclusion and exclusion criteria of these trials (Table 36-1), as they define the current indications for cardiac resynchronization therapy.

MUSTIC Trial

Begun in March 1998, the MUSTIC trial was designed to evaluate the safety and clinical efficacy of cardiac resynchronization in patients with severe heart failure (36). MUSTIC was really two studies. The first study involved 58 randomized patients with NYHA Class III heart failure, normal sinus rhythm, and QRS duration of at least 150 milliseconds. All patients were implanted with a device and, after a run-in period, patients were randomized in a

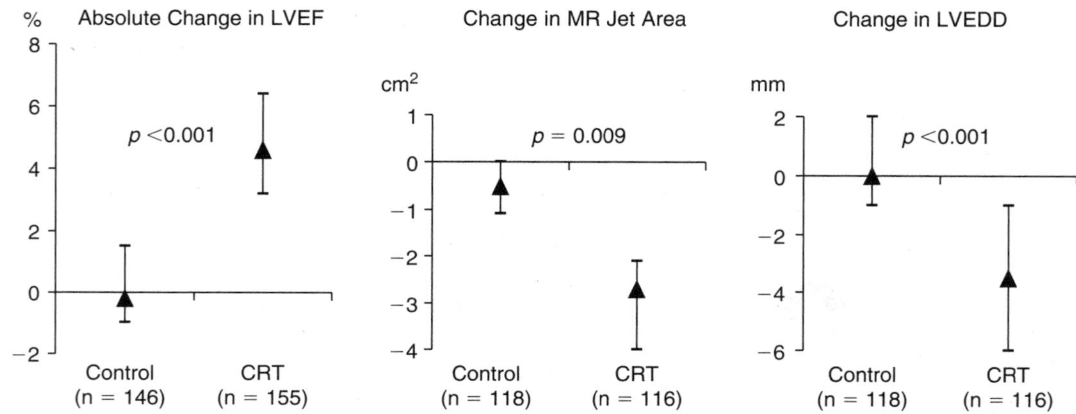

Figure 36-2 Reverse remodeling associated with chronic biventricular pacing. Resynchronization therapy significantly improves LV structure and function, as indicated by an increase in LVEF and reductions in mitral regurgitation and LV dimensions. Paired median changes from baseline at 6 months are shown. Error bars are 95% CI. (Adapted from St. John-Sutton MG, Plappert T, Abraham WT, et al. Effect of cardiac resynchronization therapy on left ventricular size and function in chronic heart failure. *Circulation*. 2003;107:1985–1990, with permission.)

single-blind fashion to receive either active pacing or no pacing. After 12 weeks, patients were crossed-over and remained in the alternate study assignment for 12 weeks. After completing this second 12-week period, the device was programmed to the patient's preferred mode of therapy.

The second MUSTIC study involved few patients (only 37 completers) with atrial fibrillation and slow ventricular rates (either spontaneously or from radio frequency ablation). A VVIR biventricular pacemaker and leads for each ventricle were implanted and the same randomization procedure previously described was applied. However, biventricular VVIR pacing versus single-site right ventricular VVIR pacing, instead of no pacing, were compared in this group.

The primary endpoints for MUSTIC were exercise tolerance (assessed by measurement of peak VO_2 or the 6-minute hall walk test) and quality of life (assessed using the Minnesota Living with Heart Failure questionnaire). Secondary endpoints included rehospitalizations and/or drug therapy modifications for worsening heart failure. Results from the normal sinus rhythm arm of MUSTIC showed that during the active pacing phase, the mean distance walked in 6 minutes was 23% greater than during the inactive pacing phase ($p < 0.001$) (36). Significant improvement was also seen in quality of life and NYHA class. Fewer hospitalizations occurred during active resynchronization therapy, as well.

TABLE 36-1
CHARACTERISTICS OF PATIENTS ENROLLED IN MAJOR TRIALS OF CARDIAC RESYNCHRONIZATION THERAPY*

	NYHA Class	QRS	RHYTHM	ICD?
MIRACLE	III, IV	≥130	normal	no
MUSTIC SR	III	>150	normal	no
MUSTIC AF	III	>200	AF	no
PATH-CHF	III, IV	≥120	normal	no
CONTAK CD	II–IV	≥120	normal	yes
MIRACLE ICD	II–IV	≥130	normal	yes
PATH CHF II	III, IV	≥120	normal	no
CARE-HF	III, IV	≥120	normal	no
COMPANION	III, IV	≥120	normal	no

*All trials required a left ventricular ejection fraction of ≤35% and left ventricular dilation for inclusion.
Normal, normal sinus rhythm; AF, atrial fibrillation;
ICD, implantable cardioverter defibulator.

MIRACLE Trial

MIRACLE was the first prospective, randomized, double-blind, parallel-controlled clinical trial adequately powered and designed to validate the results from previous cardiac resynchronization studies and to further evaluate the therapeutic efficacy and identify mechanisms of potential benefit of cardiac resynchronization therapy (37,38). Primary endpoints were NYHA class, quality of life score (using the Minnesota Living with Heart Failure questionnaire), and 6-minute hall walk distance. Secondary endpoints included assessments of a composite clinical response, cardiopulmonary exercise performance, neurohormone and cytokine levels, QRS duration, cardiac structure and function, and a variety of measures of worsening heart failure and combined morbidity and mortality.

The MIRACLE trial began in October 1998 and was completed late in 2000. Four hundred and fifty-three patients with moderate to severe symptoms of heart failure associated with an LVEF ≤35% and a QRS duration of at least 130 milliseconds were randomized (double-blind) to either cardiac resynchronization (n = 228) or to a control group (n = 225) for 6 months, while conventional therapy for heart failure was maintained (38). Compared with the control group, patients randomized to cardiac resynchronization demonstrated a significant improvement in quality of life score (−18.0 versus −9.0 points, $p = 0.001$), 6-minute walk distance (+39 versus +10 meters, $p = 0.005$), NYHA functional class ranking (−1.0 versus 0.0 class, $p < 0.001$), treadmill exercise time (+81 versus +19 seconds, $p = 0.001$), peak VO_2 (+1.1 versus 0.1 mL/kg per minute, $p < 0.01$), and LVEF (+4.6% versus −0.2%, $p < 0.001$). Cardiac resynchronization therapy patients demonstrated a highly significant improvement in the composite clinical heart failure response endpoint as compared to control subjects, suggesting an overall improvement in heart failure clinical status. Also, when compared with the control group, fewer patients in the resynchronization therapy group required hospitalization (8% versus 15%) or intravenous medications (7% and 15%, respectively) for the treatment of worsening heart failure (both $p < 0.05$). This 50% reduction in hospitalization for the cardiac resynchronization group was accompanied by a significant reduction in length of stay, resulting in a 77% decrease in total days hospitalized over 6 months compared to the control group. Implantation of the device was successful in 92% of patients. The results of this trial led to the U.S. Food and Drug Administration (FDA) approval of the first cardiac resynchronization therapy device in August 2001.

COMPANION Trial

Begun in early 2000, COMPANION was a multicenter, prospective, randomized, controlled clinical trial designed to compare drug therapy alone to drug therapy in combination with cardiac resynchronization in patients with dilated cardiomyopathy, an IVCD, NYHA Class III or IV heart failure, and no indication for a device (41,42). COMPANION randomized 1,520 patients into one of three treatment groups in a 1:2:2 allocation: Group I (308 patients) received optimal medical care only, Group II (617 patients) received optimal medical care and the Guidant CONTAK TR (biventricular pulse generator), and Group III (595 patients) received optimal medical care and the CONTAK CD (combined heart failure/bradycardia/tachycardia device). The primary endpoint of the COMPANION trial was a composite of all-cause mortality and all-cause hospitalization (measured as time to first event) beginning from time of randomization. Secondary endpoints included all-cause mortality and a variety of measures of cardiovascular morbidity. When compared to optimal medical therapy alone, the primary endpoint was significantly reduced (by approximately 20%) in both the cardiac resynchronization therapy and resynchronization therapy plus defibrillator arms. The combined endpoint of mortality or heart failure hospitalization was reduced by 35% for patients receiving resynchronization therapy and 40% for patients receiving biventricular pacing plus a defibrillator (both $p < 0.001$). For the mortality endpoint alone, cardiac resynchronization therapy patients had a 24% risk reduction ($p = 0.060$) and patients with a combined device experienced a risk reduction of 36% ($p < 0.003$) when compared to optimal medical therapy. COMPANION confirmed the results of earlier cardiac resynchronization therapy trials in improving symptoms, exercise tolerance, and quality of life for heart failure patients with ventricular dysynchrony. In addition, COMPANION showed the impact of cardiac resynchronization plus defibrillator therapy in reducing mortality.

CARE-HF Trial

The Cardiac Resynchronization—Heart Failure (CARE-HF) trial was designed to evaluate the effects of resynchronization therapy without a defibrillator on morbidity and mortality in patients with NYHA Class III or IV heart failure and ventricular dysynchrony (43,44). Eight hundred and nineteen patients with LVEFs of 35% or less and ventricular dysynchrony defined as a QRS duration ≥150 milliseconds or a QRS duration between 120 milliseconds and 150 milliseconds with echocardiographic evidence of dysynchrony were enrolled in this randomized, unblinded, controlled trial and followed for an average of 29.4 months (44). Four hundred and four patients were assigned to receive optimal medical therapy alone and 409 patients were randomized to optimal medical therapy plus resynchronization therapy alone. The risk of death from any cause or unplanned hospitalization for a major cardiac event (the primary endpoint analyzed as time to first event) was significantly reduced by 37% in the treatment group compared to control subjects (HR 0.63; 95% CI 0.51–0 .77; $p < 0.001$) (Fig. 36-3). In the cardiac resynchronization therapy group, 82 patients (20%) died during follow-up compared to 120 patients (30%) in the medical group, yielding a significant 36% reduction in all-cause mortality with resynchronization therapy (HR 0.64; 95% CI 0.48–0.85; $p < 0.002$). Resynchronization therapy also significantly reduced the risk of unplanned hospitalization for a major cardiac event by 39%, all-cause mortality plus heart failure hospitalization by 46%, and heart failure hospitalization by 52%.

GUIDELINES RECOMMENDATIONS FOR CARDIAC RESYNCHRONIZATION THERAPY

The 2005 American College of Cardiology/American Heart Association (ACC/AHA) heart failure guideline proposes

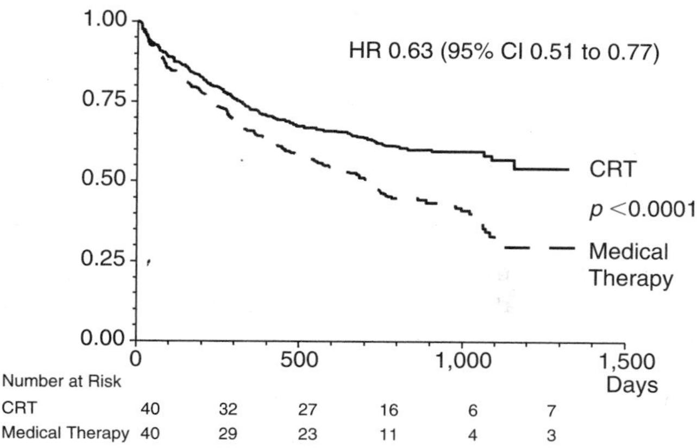

Figure 36-3 Reduction in morbidity and mortality with cardiac resynchronization therapy, without an implantable cardioverter defibrillator. Figure shows event-free survival for the combined endpoint of all-cause mortality and hospitalization for adjudicated major cardiovascular event. (From Cleland JGF, Daubert J-C, Erdmann E, et al., for the Cardiac Resynchronization—Heart Failure (CARE-HF) Study Investigators. The effect of cardiac resynchronization on morbidity and mortality in heart failure. *N Engl J Med.* 2005;352:1539–1549, with permission.)

cardiac resynchronization therapy as a Class I Indication (Level of Evidence: A):

> "Patients with LVEF ≤35%, sinus rhythm, and NYHA functional Class III or ambulatory Class IV symptoms despite recommended optimal medical therapy and who have cardiac dysynchrony, which is currently defined as a QRS ≥120 msec, should receive CRT, unless contraindicated." (16)

According to this guideline recommendation and the evidence base, the criteria for selecting patients for cardiac resynchronization therapy are primarily determined by the inclusion/exclusion criteria of randomized, controlled trials. While echocardiography appears to be a promising way to define ventricular dysynchrony, nearly all randomized, controlled trials performed to date used an electrocardiographic means to define dysynchrony. Thus, the guideline recommendation is carefully worded so as to promote the current use of QRS duration but also to anticipate a possible change in the way ventricular dysynchrony is defined in the future. In general, patients with chronic, moderate to severe (NYHA Class III–IV) heart failure despite optimal standard medical therapy, an LVEF ≤35%, LV end-diastolic diameter of at least 55 to 60 mm, QRS duration of at least 120 milliseconds, and with or without an indication for an ICD benefit from cardiac resynchronization therapy.

LIMITATIONS OF CARDIAC RESYNCHRONIZATION THERAPY

The success rate for placement of a transvenous cardiac resynchronization system has ranged from about 88% to 92% in clinical trials. This means that many patients undergoing an implant procedure will not receive a functioning system using this approach. Patients with failed implants must then settle for either another attempt at transvenous placement of the LV lead or epicardial placement of the lead, or they must resign themselves to no cardiac resynchronization therapy. Implant-related complications are similar to those seen with standard pacemaker and defibrillator technologies, with the additional risk of dissection or perforation of the coronary sinus. While rare, this event may lead to substantial morbidity and even mortality in heart failure patients.

While most patients respond favorably to biventricular pacing, some do not respond. The nonresponder rate for cardiac resynchronization therapy appears to be about 25%, a rate that is similar to the nonresponder rate for heart failure drug therapies. Suboptimal LV lead placement, suboptimal AV and ventricular-ventricular (VV) timing, ventricular scar, heart failure disease progression, and a variety of other factors have been proposed as contributing to the nonresponder rate associated with resynchronization therapy. Ongoing and future studies may facilitate a better understanding of the limitations of cardiac resynchronization therapy and aid in better patient selection.

One identifiable cause of poor response is loss of resynchronization. This may be manifested as frank worsening of heart failure, or it may be more occult and appear as vague weakness or fatigue. A specific programming sequence should be performed in the clinic to determine capture thresholds and document that LV capture is present. Lead dislodgement or a change in capture threshold may result in the loss of LV and thus biventricular pacing. It is also possible that LV lead placement and pacing thresholds are fine but resynchronization is lost for other reasons (56). Anything that frequently or consistently inhibits LV stimulation can effectively inhibit resynchronization therapy. If the AV interval is too long and the patient's intrinsic PR conduction inhibits biventricular pacing, deterioration may occur. The AV interval may have been programmed appropriately but accelerated intrinsic AV conduction could result in loss of effective biventricular pacing. This is commonly seen when atrial fibrillation occurs, resulting in a rapid ventricular response competing with biventricular pacing. Frequent premature ventricular contractions may also inhibit ventricular pacing output. Follow-up of the device itself and battery life are similar to that seen for contemporary dual-chamber pacemakers and defibrillators and are generally managed by an implanting physician; however, heart failure specialists, general cardiologists, and primary care providers must also possess the knowledge required to recognize the aforementioned limitations of resynchronization therapy and troubleshoot them.

FUTURE DIRECTIONS FOR CARDIAC RESYNCHRONIZATION THERAPY

Although initially studied in patients with moderate to severe heart failure, the beneficial effects of biventricular pacing may extend to those with mild heart failure or even to patients with asymptomatic LV dysfunction. Results of a pilot study, the MIRACLE-ICD II trial, support the potential efficacy of resynchronization therapy in Class II heart failure (57). In this study, cardiac resynchronization therapy resulted in significant improvements in ventricular remodeling indices, specifically LV diastolic and systolic volumes ($p = 0.04$ and $p = 0.01$, respectively), and LVEF ($p = 0.02$). Resynchronization therapy patients also showed statistically significant improvements in $\dot{V}E/\dot{V}CO_2$ ($p = 0.01$), NYHA class ($p = 0.05$), and a heart failure clinical composite response ($p = 0.01$). The safety and efficacy of cardiac resynchronization therapy in NYHA Class I and II patients are being further evaluated in the REVERSE (58) and MADIT-CRT trials. Both are randomized, controlled trials evaluating the effects of biventricular pacing on disease progression and outcomes.

Other studies are evaluating potential predictors of response to cardiac resynchronization therapy, which may change the definition of ventricular dysynchrony from an electrocardiographic one (i.e., QRS duration) to an echocardiographic definition. One such trial, the PROSPECT study (59), recently completed its targeted enrollment of 450 patients. This study is prospectively evaluating a variety of echocardiographic measures of ventricular dysynchrony as potential predictors of response.

In this regard, echocardiography has identified evidence of dysynchrony in some patients with QRS durations less than 120 milliseconds. Whether or not these patients benefit from resynchronization therapy remains to be seen and is currently under investigation. In addition, the optimal pacing strategy for heart failure patients with bradycardia or heart block but no evidence of ventricular dysynchrony remains controversial. RV pacing produces LV dysynchrony and may worsen heart failure. This observation was confirmed by the DAVID trial (60). Ongoing studies are evaluating the effects of biventricular pacing versus right-sided pacing in narrow QRS heart failure patients with a brady-pacing indication.

SUMMARY

Cardiac resynchronization therapy is a proven therapeutic modality for patients with ventricular dysynchrony and moderate to severe heart failure. Experience has shown it to be safe and effective, with patients demonstrating significant improvement in clinical symptoms, measures of functional status and exercise capacity, and echocardiographic parameters. Cardiac resynchronization therapy with or without a defibrillator has been shown to substantially reduce the risk of morbidity and mortality in heart failure patients. Ongoing and future clinical trials should help to further define the ideal patient for cardiac resynchronization, limit the nonresponder rate, change the definition of ventricular dysynchrony, and potentially expand the indication to patients with asymptomatic or minimally symptomatic heart failure.

REFERENCES

1. Adams KF, Fonarow GC, Emerman CL, et al. Characteristics and outcomes of patients hospitalized for heart failure in the United States: rationale, design, and preliminary observations from the first 100,000 cases in the Acute Decompensated Heart Failure National Registry (ADHERE). *Am Heart J.* 2005;149: 209–216.
2. Cleland JGF, Swedberg K, Follath F, et al. The EuroHeart Failure survey programme: a survey on the quality of care among patients with heart failure in Europe. Part 1: patient characteristics and diagnosis. *Eur Heart J.* 2003;24:442–463.
3. Fonarow GC, Abraham WT, Albert NM, et al, OPTIMIZE-HF Investigators and Coordinators. Initial hospital, patient, and performance measure characteristics of the Organized Program to Initiate Lifesaving Treatment in Hospitalized Patients with Heart Failure (OPTIMIZE-HF). *J Cardiac Fail.* 2004;10:S112.
4. The MERIT HF Investigators. Effect of metoprolol CR/XL in chronic heart failure: Metoprolol CR/XL Randomised Intervention Trial in Congestive Heart Failure (MERIT HF). *Lancet.* 1999;353:2001–2007.
5. Uretsky BF, Sheehan RG. Primary prevention of sudden cardiac death in heart failure: will the solution be shocking? *J Am Coll Cardiol.* 1997;30:1589–1597.
6. Farwell D, Patel NR, Hall A, et al. How many people with heart failure are appropriate for biventricular resynchronization? *Eur Heart J.* 2000;21:1246–1250.
7. Aaronson KD, Schwartz JS, Chen TM, et al. Development and prospective validation of a clinical index to predict survival in ambulatory patients referred for cardiac transplant evaluation. *Circulation.* 1997;95:2660–2667.
8. Xiao HB, Brecker SJ, Gibson DG. Effects of abnormal activation on the time course of the left ventricular pressure pulse in dilated cardiomyopathy. *Br Heart J.* 1992;68:403–407.
9. Littmann L, Symanski JD. Hemodynamic implications of left bundle branch block. *J Electrocardiol.* 2000;33(Suppl):115–121.
10. Saxon LA, Kerwin WF, Cahalan MK, et al. Acute effects of intraoperative multisite ventricular pacing on left ventricular function and activation/contraction sequence in patients with depressed ventricular function. *J Cardiovasc Electrophysiol.* 1998;9:13–21.
11. Kerwin WF, Botvinick EH, O'Connell JW, et al. Ventricular contraction abnormalities in dilated cardiomyopathy: effect of biventricular pacing to correct interventricular dyssynchrony. *J Am Coll Cardiol.* 2000;35:1221–1227.
12. Xaio HB, Roy C, Fujimoto S, et al. Natural history of abnormal conduction and its relation to prognosis in patients with dilated cardiomyopathy. *Int J Cardiol.* 1996;53:163–170.
13. Unverferth DV, Magorien RD, Moeschberger ML, et al. Factors influencing the one-year mortality of dilated cardiomyopathy. *Am J Cardiol.* 1984;54:147–152.
14. Shamim W, Francis DP, Yousufuddin M, et al. Intraventricular conduction delay: a prognostic marker in chronic heart failure. *Int J Cardiol.* 1999;70:171–178.
15. Brophy JM, Deslauriers G, Rouleau JL. Long-term prognosis of patients presenting to the emergency room with decompensated congestive heart failure. *Can J Cardiol.* 1994;10:543–547.
16. Hunt SA, Abraham WT, Chin MH, et al. ACC/AHA 2005 guideline update for the diagnosis and management of chronic heart failure in the adult. *Circulation.* 2005;112:1825–1852.
17. Strickberger AS, Conti J, Daoud EG, et al. Patient selection for cardiac resynchronization therapy. *Circulation.* 2005;111:2146–2150.
18. Hochleitner M, Hortnagl H, Ng CK, et al. Usefulness of physiologic dual-chamber pacing in drug-resistant idiopathic dilated cardiomyopathy. *Am J Cardiol.* 1990;66:198–202.
19. Hochleitner M, Hortnagl H. Long-term efficacy of physiologic dual-chamber pacing in the treatment of end-stage idiopathic dilated cardiomyopathy. *Am J Cardiol.* 1992;70:1320–1325.
20. Brecker SJ, Xiao HB, Sparrow J, et al. Effects of dual-chamber pacing with short atrioventricular delay in dilated cardiomyopathy. *Lancet.* 1992;340:1308–1312.
21. Innes D, Leitch JW, Fletcher PJ. VDD pacing at short atrioventricular intervals does not improve cardiac output in patients with dilated heart failure. *PACE.* 1994;17:959–965.
22. Linde C, Gadler F, Edner M, et al. Results of atrioventricular synchronous pacing with optimized delay in patients with severe congestive heart failure. *Am J Cardiol.* 1995;75:919–923.
23. Gold MR, Feliciano Z, Gottlieb SS, Fisher ML. Dual-chamber pacing with a short atrioventricular delay in congestive heart failure: a randomized study. *J Am Coll Cardiol.* 1995;26: 967–973.
24. Cazeau S, Ritter P, Bakdach S, et al. Four chamber pacing in dilated cardiomyopathy. *PACE.* 1994;17:1974–1979.
25. Foster AH, Gold MR, McLaughlin JS. Acute hemodynamic effects of atrio-biventricular pacing in humans. *Ann Thorac Surg.* 1995;59:294–300.
26. Bakker P, Meijburg H, de Vries J, et al. Biventricular pacing in end-stage heart failure improves functional capacity and left ventricular function. *J Interv Card Electrophysiol.* 2000;4:395–404.
27. Cazeau S, Ritter P, Lazarus A, et al. Multisite pacing for end-stage heart failure: early experience. *Pacing Clin Electrophysiol.* 1996;19:1748–1757.
28. Blanc JJ, Etienne Y, Gilard M, et al. Evaluation of different ventricular pacing sites in patients with severe heart failure: results of an acute hemodynamic study. *Circulation.* 1997;96:3273–3277.
29. Leclercq C, Cazeau S, Le Breton H, et al. Acute hemodynamic effects of biventricular DDD pacing in patients with end-stage heart failure. *J Am Coll Cardiol.* 1998;32:1825–1831.
30. Kass DA, Chen CH, Curry C, et al. Improved left ventricular mechanics from acute VDD pacing in patients with dilated cardiomyopathy and ventricular conduction delay. *Circulation.* 1999;99:1567–1573.
31. Gras D, Mabo P, Tang T, et al. Multisite pacing as a supplemental treatment of congestive heart failure: preliminary results of the Medtronic Inc. InSync Study. *Pacing Clin Electrophysiol.* 1998;21:2249–2255.
32. Gras D, Leclercq C, Tang A, et al. Cardiac resynchronization therapy in advanced heart failure: the multicenter InSync clinical study. *Eur J Heart Fail.* 2002;4311–4320.
33. Auricchio A, Stellbrink C, Sack S, et al. The Pacing Therapies for Congestive Heart Failure (PATH-CHF) study: rationale, design, and endpoints of a prospective randomized multicenter study. *Am J Cardiol.* 1999;83:130D–135D.

34. Auricchio A, Stellbrink C, Block M, et al., for the Pacing Therapies for Congestive Heart Failure Study Group. Effect of pacing chamber and atrioventricular delay on acute systolic function of paced patients with congestive heart failure. *Circulation.* 1999;99:2993–3001.
35. Auricchio A, Klein H, Spinelli J. Pacing for heart failure: selection of patients, techniques, and benefits. *Eur J Heart Fail.* 1999;1:275–279.
36. Cazeau S, Leclercq C, Lavergne T, et al., for the Multisite Stimulation in Cardiomyopathies (MUSTIC) Study Investigators. Effects of multisite biventricular pacing in patients with heart failure and intraventricular conduction delay. *N Engl J Med.* 2001;344:873–880.
37. Abraham WT, on behalf of the Multicenter InSync Randomized Clinical Evaluation (MIRACLE) Investigators and Coordinators. Rationale and design of a randomized clinical trial to assess the safety and efficacy of cardiac resynchronization therapy in patients with advanced heart failure: the Multicenter InSync Randomized Clinical Evaluation (MIRACLE). *J Card Fail.* 2000;6:369–380.
38. Abraham WT, Fisher WG, Smith AL, et al., for the Multicenter InSync Randomized Clinical Evaluation (MIRACLE) Investigators and Coordinators. Double-blind, randomized controlled trial of cardiac resynchronization in chronic heart failure. *N Engl J Med.* 2002;346:1845–1853.
39. Higgins SL, Hummel JD, Niazi IK, et al. Cardiac resynchronization therapy for the treatment of heart failure in patients with intraventricular conduction delay and malignant ventricular tachyarrhythmias. *J Am Coll Cardiol.* 2003;42:1454–1459.
40. Linde C, Leclercq C, Rex S, et al., on behalf of the Multisite Stimulation In Cardiomyopathies (MUSTIC) Study Group. Long-term benefits of biventricular pacing in congestive heart failure: results from the Multisite Stimulation In Cardiomyopathy (MUSTIC) study. *J Am Coll Cardiol.* 2002;40:111–118.
41. Bristow MR, Feldman AM, Saxon LA, for the COMPANION Steering Committee and COMPANION Clinical Investigators. Heart failure management using implantable devices for ventricular resynchronization: Comparison of Medical Therapy, Pacing, and Defibrillation in Chronic Heart Failure (COMPANION) trial. *J Card Fail.* 2000;6:276–285.
42. Bristow MR, Saxon LA, Boehmer J, et al. Cardiac-resynchronization therapy with or without an implantable defibrillator in advanced chronic heart failure. *N Engl J Med.* 2004;350: 2140–2150.
43. Cleland JGF, Daubert JC, Erdmann E, et al. The CARE-HF study (Cardiac Resynchronization in Heart Failure study): rationale, design and end-points. *Eur J Heart Fail.* 2001;3:481–489.
44. Cleland JGF, Daubert J-C, Erdmann E, et al., for the Cardiac Resynchronization—Heart Failure (CARE-HF) Study Investigators. The effect of cardiac resynchronization on morbidity and mortality in heart failure. *N Engl J Med.* 2005;352:1539–1549.
45. Auricchio A, Abraham WT. Cardiac resynchronization therapy. Current state of the art: cost versus benefit. *Circulation* 2004;109:300–307.
46. Nishimura RA, Hayes DL, Holmes DR, Jr., et al. Mechanism of hemodynamic improvement by dual-chamber pacing for severe left ventricular dysfunction: an acute Doppler and catheterization hemodynamic study. *J Am Coll Cardiol.* 1995;25:281–288.
47. Grines CL, Bashore TM, Boudoulas H, et al. Functional abnormalities in isolated left bundle branch block. The effect of interventricular asynchrony. *Circulation.* 1989;79:845–853.
48. Panidis IP, Ross J, Munley B, et al. Diastolic mitral regurgitation in patients with atrioventricular conduction abnormalities: a common finding by Doppler echocardiography. *J Am Coll Cardiol.* 1986;7:768–774.
49. Bristow MR, Gilbert EM, Abraham WT, et al. The third-generation beta-blocking agent carvedilol produces dose-related improvements in left ventricular function and survival in subjects with chronic heart failure. *Circulation.* 1996;94:2807–2816.
50. Lowes BD, Gilbert EM, Abraham WT, et al. Myocardial gene expression in dilated cardiomyopathy treated with beta-blocking agents. *N Engl J Med.* 2002;346:1357–1365.
51. Abraham WT, Gilbert EM, Lowes BD, et al. Coordinate changes in myosin heavy chain isoform gene expression are selectively associated with alterations in dilated cardiomyopathy phenotype. *Mol Med.* 2002;8:750–760.
52. Yu CM, Chau E, Sanderson JE, et al. Tissue Doppler echocardiographic evidence of reverse remodeling and improved synchronicity by simultaneously delaying regional contraction after biventricular pacing therapy in heart failure. *Circulation.* 2002;105:438–445.
53. St. John-Sutton MG, Plappert T, Abraham WT, et al. Effect of cardiac resynchronization therapy on left ventricular size and function in chronic heart failure. *Circulation.* 2003;107: 1985–1990.
54. Iyengar S, Haas G, Lamba S, et al. Effect of cardiac resynchronization therapy on myocardial gene expression in patients with non-ischemic cardiomyopathy. *J Cardiac Fail.* 2005;11:S97.
55. Young JB, Abraham WT, Smith AL, et al. Safety and efficacy of combined cardiac resynchronization therapy and implantable cardioversion defibrillation in patients with advanced chronic heart failure. The Multicenter InSync ICD Randomized Clinical Evaluation (MIRACLE ICD) trial. *JAMA.* 2003;289: 2685–2694.
56. Wang PL, Kramer A, Estes NAM, et al. Timing cycles for biventricular pacing. *PACE.* 2002;25:62–75.
57. Abraham WT, Young JB, Leon AR, et al. Effects of cardiac resynchronization on disease progression in patients with left ventricular systolic dysfunction, an indication for an implantable cardioverter defibrillator, and mildly symptomatic chronic heart failure. *Circulation.* 2004;110:2864–2868.
58. Linde C, Gold M, Abraham WT, et al. Rationale and design of a randomized controlled trial to assess the safety and efficacy of cardiac resynchronization therapy in patients with asymptomatic left ventricular dysfunction with previous symptoms or mild heart failure: The REsynchronization reVErses Remodeling in Systolic left vEntricular dysfunction (REVERSE) study. *Am Heart J.* 2006;151:288–294.
59. Yu C-M, Abraham WT, Bax J, et al. Predictors of response to cardiac resynchronization therapy (PROSPECT) study design. *Am Heart J.* 2005;149:600–605.
60. Wilkoff BL, Cook JR, Epstein AE, et al. Dual-chamber pacing or ventricular backup pacing in patients with an implantable defibrillator: the Dual Chamber and VVI Implantable Defibrillator (DAVID) Trial. *JAMA.* 2002;288:3115–3123.

The Heart Failure Clinic

37

Marc A. Silver

We are currently witnessing enormous changes in how health care is designed, delivered, and reimbursed. The management of heart failure, because of its prevalence and economic impact in our society, is being affected by many of these changes. Despite an estimated 1.2 million annual primary admissions to acute care facilities in the United States, most of the care for patients with heart failure is delivered outside hospitals, predominantly in physician offices and clinics. The estimated 3.4 annual primary office visits for each patient with heart failure cost approximately $14.7 billion (1). In most areas of medicine, including the management of heart disease in general and of heart failure specifically, the focus has shifted away from inpatient hospital admissions toward an outpatient approach. What has readily become apparent is the large gap that exists between what can usually be offered in most physician offices or clinics and what services are routinely available during an in-patient stay.

What has been born of this gap is the concept of the heart failure clinic. This chapter discusses the rationale and scope of the heart failure clinic, in addition to some of the unique features it offers to patients and those who care for them and pay for their care. Also discussed are some current observational and outcome-based data relevant to the operation of a heart failure clinic and a few practical aspects of implementing this approach.

HEART FAILURE CLINIC: DESCRIPTION

To understand what the term *heart failure clinic* means in most settings, it is necessary to understand what the goals are in setting up such clinics. Often, the motivation for their development has been an awareness of the frequency of hospitalization and subsequent repeated hospitalizations for many patients with heart failure. These hospitalizations frequently involve patients within a capitated reimbursement structure. Care within an academic medical center and the frequent presence of other diseases in patients with advanced heart failure predispose to longer hospital stays and increased costs, which are further increased by the fact that illness is often severe and patients are generally older. The heart failure clinic, then, is often the outgrowth of an institutional task force concerned with the costs of caring for patients with a chronic disease. Targeted activities for the heart failure clinic are straightforward and include, as a baseline, patient education (2) and optimal utilization of standard medical therapy (3). On rarer occasions, the heart failure clinic is developed as part of a prospective approach to offering comprehensive care for a specific disease or population. Regardless of the approach used to initiate a heart failure clinic, they are all similar in structure and function. Typically, a nurse is selected as the initial team member to investigate or initiate development; on occasion, the initial facilitator is a physician.

HEART FAILURE CLINIC: STRUCTURE

An extremely wide variety of approaches have been utilized throughout the United States. This is a reflection of the varied needs and resources available to individual institutions and practices. Therefore, the term heart failure clinic means different things to different people. The spectrum of services that may be offered in a heart failure clinic or program are listed in Table 37-1. Utilization of a

TABLE 37-1
PARTIAL LISTING OF SERVICES OFFERED IN HEART FAILURE CLINICS

Education for patients and families
Education for primary care physicians and cardiologists
Nurse telemanagement
Telephone triage
Critical pathway (hospital) and guideline development
Outpatient inotropic drugs and intravenous diuretics
β-blocker and ACE inhibitor titration programs
Rehabilitation and exercise training
Heart transplantation evaluation
Clinical research

ACE, angiotensin-converting enzyme.

protocol often facilitates the upward titration of drugs such as β-blockers and enhances the ability to attain target doses. For example, by using the protocol set forth in Appendix I, we successfully initiated carvedilol treatment in several hundred patients and target doses were attained in more than 90% of them within a 60-day period. Careful attention to protocol details and the availability of nurses skilled in drug titration allowed for successful titration with a minimum of adverse events. Often, the patients were referred to the heart failure clinic only for the titration period.

Perhaps because of the difficulty of educating elderly patients who frequently have age-associated cognitive deficits or who are ill during a short hospitalization, education remains one of the critical services a heart failure clinic provides most patients (4).

No accurate count of the number of heart failure clinics within the United States is available; however, the current number has been estimated to be more than 150. Some detailed information about 59 of these clinics has been obtained by survey (5). Nearly half have been functional for more than 5 years and new clinics are being developed each year. These are predominantly multidisciplinary clinics with primary involvement of a nurse and a cardiologist. The average clinic manages approximately 150 patients and is staffed by three nurses along with ancillary personnel. Generally, the nurse is the primary organizer and developer of the clinic. Usually, after a brief fact-finding period and a review of the financial impact of heart failure on an institution, a decision is made and resources are allocated to the development of a clinic. Depending on an institution's experiences and resources, the clinic is usually based in an out-patient setting, although this is not always the case. Some institutions may allocate telemetry beds in a hospital unit or even bays in an emergency department to administer intravenous diuretics to decompensated patients, with the goal of preventing repeated admissions. One commonly administered treatment, as yet unproven by randomized clinical research trials, is out-patient inotropic therapy. In fact, 68% of surveyed heart failure clinics utilize infusions of inotropic agents as an approach to the treatment of patients with heart failure (5). The focus of a heart failure clinic might affect its location and facilities. Usually, however, there is an area in or adjacent to the hospital where patients may come on an elective basis for education, dietary instruction, exercise, and supervision. Clinics usually are the outgrowth of an area of expertise and interest, such as cardiac or pulmonary rehabilitation, that already exists within an institution, a cardiac support group, or a physician's office.

Physical requirements similarly vary, and clinics may consist of little more than a telephone or may include an entire suite dedicated to heart failure-related activities. Generally, office space is needed for record storage and telephone communication along with clinical space for the evaluation and treatment of patients. Ideally, there should also be space reserved for patient education, conferences, and lectures as well as private patient-family meetings. Access to a library of heart failure-related materials and internet access are also extremely useful.

IDENTIFICATION OF PATIENTS

Because the average hospital has more than 500 primary heart failure admissions annually, perhaps one of the most difficult tasks is identifying which patients should be targeted for the heart failure clinic. Ideally, some strategy should be directed at improving the outcome of all patients with heart failure as well as those with asymptomatic left ventricular dysfunction and those at risk for the development of heart failure. However, at present most clinics focus on the patient with overt, symptomatic, and usually advanced heart failure. An obvious method to identify patients at highest risk for repeated in-patient admissions and resource utilization has been simply to consider those patients recently hospitalized with heart failure. Increasingly, patients admitted to a hospital with heart failure have very advanced symptoms and poor prognostic markers and, hence, are likely to be readmitted (6). In fact, readmission rates for these patients at 30 and 60 days approach 30% to 50% (7–9). Also, because databases of financial information are found predominantly within medical institutions, outcomes regarding hospital length of stay and readmission are often the easiest to track. However, many other patients may be suitable for enrollment in a heart failure clinic (Table 37-2). Some heart failure clinics are able to work closely with emergency departments (which are the source of most hospital admissions for heart failure) so that in some cases triage, treatment, and release are arranged by the heart failure clinic. This is obviously a good opportunity to enroll patients into the clinic population.

Once the target population has been identified and the services or scope of the heart failure clinic have been determined, the next issue is how to provide these services to the patient population. One of the most common ways to manage heart failure patients is through direct contact, predominantly by standard telephone communications; however, increased use of in-home video and internet connections can be anticipated. Nearly half of the surveyed clinics in the United States reported telephone contact as the primary method of patient management (5). Such contact can be initiated either by the staff of the heart failure clinic or by the patient. In the former case, an initial call is

TABLE 37-2

POTENTIAL PATIENTS SUITABLE FOR ENROLLMENT IN A HEART FAILURE CLINIC

Elderly patients with diagnosis of heart failure (systolic and diastolic)
Patients with one or more hospital admissions for heart failure
Patients with advanced functional status
Patients with chronic comorbidities (e.g., diabetes, COPD)
Patients (and families) whose medical care is fragmented or lacks continuity
Patients (and families) whose medical care suffers because of educational deficits, or patients who have been noncompliant with medical and dietary prescriptions
Patients with asymptomatic LV dysfunction
Patients at risk for heart failure (e.g., after myocardial infarction and after myocardial revascularization)
Patients who can benefit from the clinic services (e.g., education, rehabilitation, drug initiation)
Patients initially triaged from the emergency department

COPD, chronic obstructive pulmonary disease; LV, left ventricular.

usually made to patients soon after a hospital discharge, with the goals being determination of stability, understanding of medication changes, and cooperation with the current medical regimen. Obviously, this entails a transfer of information from the in-patient physicians and nursing staff to the heart failure clinic personnel. In some situations, the heart failure clinic nurses actually visit in-patients so they will be able to provide the continuity required for transition into the out-patient setting.

Beyond the initial phone call, the role of the heart failure clinic often varies considerably. Sometimes a telephone call is made at fixed intervals and patient weight, symptoms, and problems are noted. These are often then relayed to the appropriate physician for further action. In some instances, the nurses and physicians have developed treatment algorithms or orders to be followed in various common clinical scenarios, such as weight gain or leg edema. This usually depends on the teamwork and experience of the heart failure clinic staff.

Another, more recent development in telephone management has been computerized screening for patients at risk for further decompensation. In these systems, daily phone calls may be initiated by the patient; often, contact is initiated when a set of vital signs such as weight, blood pressure, heart rate, and oxygen saturation are measured at home, or even when the cap of a bottle of medication is opened. Regardless of the initial trigger, the home actions are transmitted via the patient's phone line, usually to a central monitoring station. Limits for the various measurements are preset and deviation usually triggers direct patient contact or notification of the heart failure clinic personnel for further action.

MEASUREMENT OF SUCCESS

Regardless of the methods utilized in identifying, communicating with, and treating patients with heart failure, some indicators of the success of interventions are required. As previously mentioned, financial outcomes are frequently the easiest to obtain and measure. However, other types of information can be obtained. As shown in Table 37-3, 72% of heart failure clinics employ outcome measures other than financial data for their patients (5). In addition, quality of life is measured in 58% of patients attending heart failure clinics, as this is perceived to be an important goal of a program treating patients with advanced disease.

Perhaps one of the most important requirements of a heart failure clinic is a suitable medical information system to allow tracking of key measurement parameters. The data set should also serve as an electronic medical record capable of monitoring frequent changes in medications and adverse reactions, which are common in patients with advanced heart failure. A reporting feature of the software is also important to provide an up-to-date summary of information and testing in case the patient should present to the emergency department or require hospital admission. Remote access enhances the value of the data set, particularly when the clinic personnel are limited. Few of the commercially available electronic records are ideal for the management of chronic heart failure but this will probably change as the need becomes more apparent.

TABLE 37-3

POTENTIAL OUTCOME MEASUREMENTS THAT CAN BE USED TO MEASURE SUCCESS OF A HEART FAILURE CLINIC

Financial impact (measure of impact on decreasing use of in-patient resources)
- Hospital length of stay
- Readmission rates
- Hospital cost-to-charge ratio
- Hospital cost and reimbursement rate
- Utilization of intensive care beds
- Utilization of drugs, diagnostic tests

Mortality
Impact on comorbidities and admissions for other than heart failure
Need for heart transplant
Total health care resource utilization
Medication compliance
Quality of life, patient satisfaction scores, depression scores
Exercise tolerance
- Walk time
- Peak oxygen consumption

Prognostic surrogates
- Functional status
- LV, RV ejection fraction
- Serum sodium
- Neurohormones (PNE, TNF-α, BNP)
- Hemodynamics

LV, left ventricular; RV, right ventricular; PNE, plasma norepinephrine; TNF-α, tumor necrosis factor-α; BNP, brain natriuretic peptide.

PERSONNEL AND CHAMPIONS

Perhaps one of the critical features of a successful heart failure clinic is a core of professionals who are champions of the concept and will work diligently to maintain the goal of enhanced quality of life for their patients. There are no requisite backgrounds for these people, nor is any specific number needed to initiate a successful clinic. However, commitment is pivotal and results are usually best when clinic development is part of a plan of care that includes support by administration, nurses, physicians, ancillary personnel, and even local insurers (Table 37-4).

OUTCOMES WITH HEART FAILURE CLINICS

Experience with the heart failure clinic model is increasing and both case-control and randomized trials demonstrate the efficacy of this approach. One of the initial studies to look prospectively at such an approach was conducted by Rich et al. (10). Although the patients in this study were identified within the hospital setting, much of their specialized treatment was carefully coordinated by nurses, who provided telephone contact or home visits. With this approach, survival of the patients discharged alive was improved and there was also a 56% reduction in subsequent readmissions to the hospital. Multiple readmissions were prevented and, although not significant in this population, readmission for causes not related to heart failure was also reduced. Not only have an improvement in symptoms, quality of life, and exercise tolerance and a decrease in hospitalizations been attributed to effective management in heart failure clinics (10–12), but a reduction in the cost of caring for these patients has also been described (10,13,14).

TABLE 37-4
HEART FAILURE CLINIC PERSONNEL

Nurses
Staff nurses
Advanced practice nurses
Nurse clinicians/clinical specialists/nurse educators
Care/case managers
Research nurses
Rehabilitation nurses
Home care nurses
Physicians
Physician champion
Cardiologist/internist/primary care physician
Heart failure specialist
Geriatrician
Other personnel
Administrators
Dietitians
Physical and occupational therapists
Social worker/psychologist/support group facilitator
Data management technician
Research technicians
Clerical staff

West et al. (15) at Stanford University recently described their experience with home-based comprehensive disease management for 51 patients with symptomatic heart failure. Their program, which was based on a system applied to risk factor modification for coronary artery disease (16), was supervised by physicians and implemented by nurses; goals were guideline-driven and clinical monitoring was accomplished via telephone contact. Through this approach, the investigators demonstrated a decreased intake of dietary sodium (38%), enhanced dosing of oral medication, and improved functional status and exercise tolerance. With the heart failure program, they also were able to reduce the number of general out-patient visits, emergency room visits, and hospital admissions.

FUTURE OF HEART FAILURE CLINICS

One of the problems threatening the long-term success of heart failure clinics is that despite an appreciation of the value of this form of disease management, there is currently no mechanism of reimbursement for some of the services rendered. Although reimbursement is increasingly available for extended nursing visits or home care, it is more difficult to obtain reimbursement for the management of complex disease (especially if focused on a single problem), extended teaching, and the required frequent telephone contact. For this reason, thus far it is the so-called at-risk managed care organizations which appreciate the economic benefit of utilizing specialized services to manage heart failure. Within a larger span of capitated reimbursement, the utilization of heart failure clinics will perhaps increase. Also anticipated might be a merging with facilities set up for the treatment of other chronic disease processes (e.g., diabetes and renal insufficiency) that are closely related to heart failure, both medically and educationally. Because these other conditions are so common in patients with heart failure, the heart failure clinic might well expand to become a clinic for the management of a broader range of chronic diseases.

Finally, patients with chronic diseases have shown the greatest interest in the utilization of complementary and alternative medical approaches. Because of the generally less-technological and more hands-on approach of the heart failure clinic, this might be the logical setting in which to scientifically explore the value and potential benefit of some of these complementary approaches.

SUMMARY

Because of the growing number of patients with symptomatic heart failure and the economic impact of this illness on society, we have witnessed an expansion of programs aimed at attenuating this disease. One of the outgrowths of this effort has been the development of the heart failure clinic. These variably structured and focused clinics usually employ a multidisciplinary approach, including patient and family education, drug initiation and titration, telemanagement, data collection, and research. There is evidence that a variety of these approaches have been successful in attenuating disease severity and reducing utilization of expensive inpatient resources. The growth and further refinement of the heart failure clinic will continue for years to come.

REFERENCES

1. O'Connell JB, Bristow MR. The economic impact of heart failure in the United States: time for a different approach. *J Heart Lung Transplant*. 1994;13:S107–S112.
2. Silver MA. Patient knowledge of fundamentals in chronic heart failure. *Congest Heart Fail*. 1996;2:11–13.
3. McDermott MM, Lee P, Mehta S, et al. Patterns of angiotensin-converting enzyme inhibitor prescriptions, educational interventions, and outcomes among hospitalized patients with heart failure. *Clin Cardiol*. 1998;21:261–268.
4. Silver MA. *Success with Heart Failure. Help and Hope for the Millions with Congestive Heart Failure*. 2nd ed. New York: Plenum Publishing; 1998.
5. *Congestive Heart Failure Clinics. Market Research Report. Heart Failure Management*. Minneapolis: Medtronic, Inc.; July, 1997.
6. Stevenson WG, Stevenson LW, Middlekauff HR, et al. Improving survival for patients with advanced heart failure: study of 737 consecutive patients. *J Am Coll Cardiol*. 1995;26:1417–1423.
7. Gooding J, Jette AM. Hospital readmissions among the elderly. *J Am Geriatr Soc*. 1985;33:595–601.
8. Rich MW, Freedland KE. Effect of DRGs on three-month readmission rate of geriatric patients with congestive heart failure. *Am J Public Health*. 1988;78:680–682.
9. Vinson JM, Rich MW, Sperry JC, et al. Early readmission of elderly patients with congestive heart failure. *J Am Geriatr Soc*. 1990;38:1290–1295.
10. Rich MW, Beckham V, Wittenberg C, et al. A multidisciplinary intervention to prevent the readmission of elderly patients with congestive heart failure. *N Engl J Med*. 1995;333:1190–1195.
11. Smith LE, Fabbri SA, Pai R, et al. Symptomatic improvement and reduced hospitalization for patients attending a cardiomyopathy clinic. *Clin Cardiol*. 1997;20:949–954.
12. Hanumanthu S, Butler J, Chomsky D, et al. Effect of a heart failure program on hospitalization frequency and exercise tolerance. *Circulation*. 1997;96:2842–2848.
13. Chapman DB, Torpy J. Development of a heart failure center: a medical center and cardiology practice join forces to improve care and reduce costs. *Am J Managed Care*. 1997;3:431–437.
14. Fonarow GC, Stevenson LW, Walden JA, et al. Impact of a comprehensive heart failure management program on hospital readmission and functional status of patients with advanced heart failure. *J Am Coll Cardiol*. 1997;30:725–732.
15. West JA, Miller NH, Parker KM, et al. A comprehensive management system for heart failure improves clinical outcomes and reduces medical resource utilization. *Am J Cardiol*. 1997;79:58–63.
16. DeBusk RF, Miller NH, Superko R, et al. A case management system: coronary risk factor modification following acute myocardial infarction. *Ann Intern Med*. 1994;120:721–729.

APPENDIX I. SAMPLE HEART FAILURE CLINIC PROTOCOL

Heart Failure Institute, Carvedilol Titration Protocol

1. Tell patient to allow 3 hours for the initial visit; subsequent visits should be 2 hours.
2. Review procedures of heart failure center and show patient-education video on carvedilol and β-blocker therapy.
3. Review goals and potential adverse events with patient and family. Provide question-and-answer session.
4. Make sure patient takes angiotensin-converting enzyme (ACE) inhibitor or other vasoactive drug 2 hours before initial carvedilol dose.
5. Initiate dosing as follows:
   Week 1: 3.125 mg
   If tolerated, continue with 3.125 mg orally twice daily.
   Week 3: 6.25 mg
   If tolerated, continue with 6.25 mg orally twice daily.
   Week 5: 12.5 mg
   If tolerated, continue with 12.5 mg orally twice daily.
   Week 7: 25 mg
   If tolerated, continue with 25 mg orally twice daily.
   (For patients weighing more than 85 kg, titrate to 50 mg twice daily at week 9.)
6. Monitor heart rate and blood pressure and check for signs and symptoms of heart failure at 30, 60, and 120 minutes after each test dose.
7. Consider decrease in diuretic dose for hypotension.
8. Consult heart failure cardiologist for adjustment in other medications.
9. Do not give next-highest dose without consulting a heart failure cardiologist if the patient's heart failure has worsened.
10. Obtain laboratory tests as required.

38

Exercise and Rehabilitation in Congestive Heart Failure

Donna M. Mancini ***Rebecca P. Streeter***

The clinical syndrome of congestive heart failure (CHF) results in changes in the skeletal muscles, peripheral vasculature, and lungs that are a consequence of a chronically decreased cardiac output. Exercise training may be an effective therapeutic modality to retard or reverse the maladaptive changes that develop in the periphery during CHF (1). In this review, we summarize the central and peripheral adaptations encountered in CHF and discuss the prognostic use of exercise testing and the therapeutic potential of exercise training in patients with heart failure.

CARDIAC AND PERIPHERAL DERANGEMENTS IN HEART FAILURE

In the presence of a reduced cardiac output, the heart depends on three principal compensatory mechanisms to maintain normal function (2). First, the Frank-Starling mechanism increases preload to sustain cardiac stroke volume. Second, myocardial hypertrophy develops to increase the mass of contractile tissue. Third, the sympathetic nervous system is activated to augment myocardial contractility. In the short term, these compensatory mechanisms serve to preserve cardiac output. However, eventually these compensatory mechanisms become detrimental, contributing to the progression of the disease process.

In normal subjects, the primary limitation to maximal physical performance is the cardiac-output response (2,3). Patients with heart failure exhibit reduced cardiac-output responses to exercise in comparison with normal subjects. The decreased exercise capacity of patients with heart failure has been attributed to a decreased cardiac-output response, which leads to inadequate perfusion of skeletal muscle and intramuscular lactic acidosis (4,5). In 1981, Weber et al. (6) measured the hemodynamic and ventilatory responses of 40 patients with heart failure during progressive treadmill exercise. This first large application of the measurement of peak oxygen consumption (VO_2) in patients with heart failure demonstrated the usefulness of this technique as a noninvasive method for characterizing cardiac reserve and functional status. Weber et al. demonstrated a significant correlation between cardiac-output response and VO_2 (Fig. 38-1) and were able to classify patients into groups with disease of increasing severity on the basis of this noninvasive technique.

Although peak exercise capacity clearly depends on the cardiac-output response to exercise, this is not the sole determinant of exercise performance in patients with heart failure. The exercise capacity of patients with severely reduced ejection fractions varies widely. Furthermore, therapeutic interventions aimed at acutely increasing cardiac output, such as administration of dobutamine, do not significantly increase peak VO_2 (7,8). This discrepancy between enhanced cardiac output and fixed peak VO_2 can be explained on the basis of the peripheral, vascular, and skeletal muscle derangements in CHF. Because of regional vascular or skeletal abnormalities, the augmented cardiac output cannot be utilized by the exercising muscle beds and, therefore, peak VO_2 is not altered.

Peripheral Vascular Changes in Heart Failure

Experimental evidence suggests that the peripheral circulation undergoes substantial transformations during the progression of CHF, with an alteration of regional vascular control. The alterations occur both at the level of the vascular endothelium (an important modulator of vascular tone) and at the level of the vascular smooth muscle.

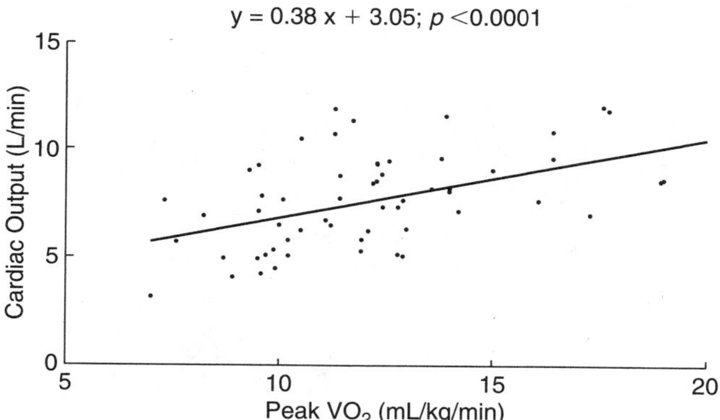

Figure 38-1 Correlation of peak exercise cardiac output with peak VO_2.

In both animal and human models of CHF, the responses to endothelium-mediated vasodilation are blunted. Endothelium-dependent dilation is reduced in the aorta of rats with ischemic cardiomyopathy (9). Kubo et al. (10) demonstrated that endothelium-dependent vasodilation is attenuated in patients with heart failure. Changes in sheer stress are an important determinant of endothelial function. In normal vasculature, the changes in sheer stress on the endothelial cells that accompany alterations in blood flow serve to enhance vasodilation via release of nitric oxide and prostaglandins (11,12). Endothelial dysfunction appears to be a time-dependent alteration. With an increasing severity of CHF, the endothelial vascular function deteriorates. In rats with early stages of heart failure, vascular endothelial function was preserved, whereas in more severe stages an impairment was noted (13). Circulating cytokines such as tumor necrosis factor-α (TNF-α) are elevated in severe heart failure. TNF-α impairs the stimulated release of endothelium-derived relaxing factor (EDRF). Plasma levels of TNF in patients with heart failure are correlated with the degree of endothelial dysfunction assessed by infusion of acetylcholine (14). Chronically decreased perfusion of skeletal muscle, increased angiotensin-converting enzyme (ACE) activity in tissues, increased formation of oxygen free radicals, and increased levels of endothelial vasoconstrictive agents are other potential mechanisms involved in the development of endothelial dysfunction in these patients.

In conjunction with endothelial dysfunction, experimental evidence demonstrates a dysfunction of the vascular smooth muscle in heart failure. Zelis et al. (15–17), in a series of elegant studies, demonstrated that fluid and sodium retention can impair arteriolar vasodilation in humans. Using a canine model of heart failure produced by rapid ventricular pacing, Zelis et al. (16) also measured the arterial sodium content in the aorta and femoral artery in animals with heart failure and in controls. A significant increase in arterial sodium content was demonstrated in the animals with heart failure. Zelis et al. postulated that arteriolar stiffness as a consequence of increased salt and water content results in an abnormal vasodilation response in heart failure.

During exercise, peripheral vasoconstriction is increased to prevent systemic hypotension in patients with heart failure, given their blunted rise in cardiac output (18). Tissue hypoxia and enhanced sympathetic and angiotensin activation are two proposed mechanisms mediating abnormal peripheral vasoconstriction in CHF (19). Institution of sympathetic and renin-angiotensin blockade does not completely reverse the peripheral derangements seen in CHF, although it modifies it.

Regional specificity of the changes in the peripheral circulation has been demonstrated in patients with CHF. Comparison of peak reactive hyperemia in the forearm and calf musculature of these patients revealed diminished hyperemia only in the leg (20). Correlations with peak VO_2 were observed only with peak reactive hyperemia in the calf. Selective deconditioning may be responsible for these regional differences.

Skeletal Muscle Changes in Heart Failure

The metabolic behavior of limb muscles during exercise in patients with heart failure has been examined. Abnormal skeletal muscle metabolism (i.e., reduced oxidative metabolism with earlier shift to glycolytic metabolism) has been demonstrated in patients with heart failure by means of phosphorus 31 magnetic resonance spectroscopy (^{31}P-MRS) (21–27). These abnormalities appear to be independent of total limb perfusion (22,26,27), histochemical changes (24), muscle mass (25), or severe tissue hypoxia (28).

The kinetics of recovery of skeletal muscle oxygenation are prolonged. At comparable levels of exercise, both VO_2 kinetics and muscle oxygenation kinetics were prolonged during recovery in the CHF patients, and the delay worsened with increasing cardiac dysfunction as assessed by peak VO_2. A significant correlation between VO_2 recovery kinetics and metabolic changes assessed with magnetic resonance spectroscopy has been described (29).

A variety of histochemical changes have been reported in muscle biopsy studies from patients with heart failure. These include fiber atrophy, a decrease in oxidative enzymes, and a shift in fiber composition of the muscle with a significant decrease in fatigue resistant oxidative type I fibers and significant increase in the percentage of glycolytic, fast-twitch, easily fatigable type IIb fibers. Mitochondrial changes, including a decrease in the volume and surface density of cristae, were described by Drexler et al. (30). The vascularity of skeletal muscles has been assessed by means of capillary-to-fiber ratios, with some investigators reporting a decrease in all measures of capillary density (30,31) and others reporting no change from normal (32).

Additional histochemical evidence of skeletal muscle change is provided by the demonstration of apoptosis in 47% of skeletal muscle biopsies from patients with CHF versus none in healthy volunteers. Peak oxygen consumption was significantly reduced in patients with apoptosis as compared to patients without (12.0 ± 3.7 mL/kg per minute versus 18.2 ± 4.4 mL/kg per minute; $p = 0.0005$). Apoptosis-positive patients were also found to have a significantly longer history of illness. Intriguingly, a higher level of inducible nitric oxide synthase (iNOS) expression and a lower level of the oncogene bcl-2 expression were also demonstrated in apoptosis-positive biopsies, suggesting possible regulatory mechanisms of apoptosis in the skeletal muscles of these patients. Apoptosis in skeletal muscles may thus contribute to the reduced exercise capacity in CHF patients (33).

To further clarify the role of skeletal muscle iNOS, as well as reduced phosphocreatine resynthesis in exercise intolerance in CHF, vastus lateralis muscle biopsies and bicycle cardiopulmonary tests were compared between 38 male CHF patients and 8 age-matched controls. The investigators found iNOS expression to be significantly higher in CHF patients. This increased iNOS expression correlated with increased nitric oxide production. Mitochondrial creatine kinase (mi-CK), a key enzyme for transfer of high-energy phosphates, was found to be significantly reduced in CHF patients. Importantly, iNOS expression was negatively correlated with maximal oxygen uptake and mi-CK expression. Taken together, the study findings suggest that iNOS expression may attenuate mitochondrial energy transfer in the skeletal muscle of CHF patients, thereby contributing to the metabolic derangements seen in the myocytes and resulting in the characteristically decreased exercise capacity and increased fatigue in this group of patients (34).

In addition to histochemical changes, patients also exhibit generalized muscle atrophy. Anthropomorphic measurements performed in 62 heart failure patients demonstrated evidence of significant muscle loss in 60% of those patients. Muscle volume assessed using magnetic resonance imaging and muscle mass measurements using DEXA scans revealed reduced muscle volume and mass in patients with heart failure compared to normal subjects (35).

This reduction in muscle mass impacts on peak VO_2. Jondeau et al. (36) contrasted peak VO_2 during combined upper arm and maximal leg exercise. In normal subjects the addition of more muscle mass via arm exercise did not increase peak exercise performance and VO_2 remained unchanged. Thus, cardiac-output response to exercise, rather than amount of exercising muscle, appears to determine peak VO_2. However, in patients with severe CHF the addition of upper arm exercise significantly increased peak VO_2. The importance of skeletal muscle mass in limiting peak VO_2 is suggested by this study.

Intrinsic skeletal muscle changes may represent the primary determinant of exercise performance in a subset of patients with heart failure. Wilson et al. (37) measured exercise hemodynamics and leg blood flow in 34 patients with heart failure and 6 normal subjects. All patients exhibited a reduced exercise capacity, with a peak VO_2 of less than 18 mL/kg per minute; however, approximately 25% had normal leg blood flow. Despite normal leg blood flow, lactate release was abnormal in these patients, which implies that their exercise limitation is most probably a consequence of intrinsic skeletal muscle changes rather than a limited cardiac-output response.

In summary, exercise capacity in patients with heart failure is limited not only by changes that affect the ability to increase cardiac output but also by changes in the blood vessels, muscles, and lungs that are a consequence of their disease (Fig. 38-2).

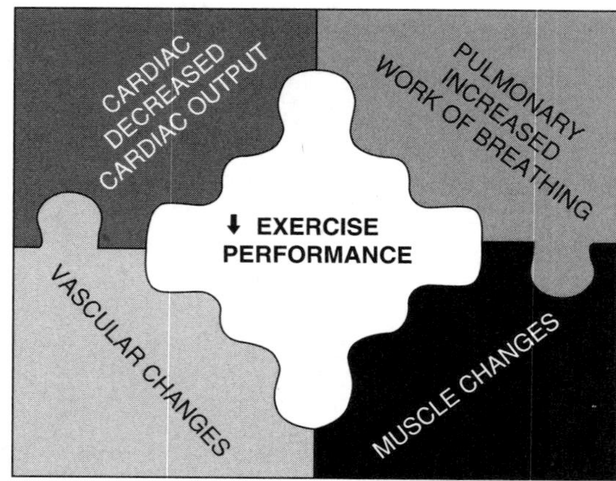

Figure 38-2 Exercise limitations in heart failure arise from a complex interplay of factors, including decreased cardiac output and disease-related changes in the skeletal muscles, peripheral vasculature, and lungs.

SAFETY OF EXERCISE TESTING

Bed rest was formerly a recommended therapy for heart failure, with physical activity discouraged in this patient population. Exercise testing was not used in the diagnosis and management of patients with heart failure because of safety concerns. In the Veterans Heart Failure Trial (VHeFT-1) (38), low-level exercise was used to test 607 patients with moderately advanced heart failure (mean peak VO_2, 14.5 ± 3.9 mL/kg per minute). This was the first large, multicenter trial to use metabolic stress testing to assess disease severity and response to therapy. Patients underwent two graded, symptom-limited tests of bicycle exercise. The safety of exercise testing in patients with moderate to severe heart failure was demonstrated in that the initial stress test was terminated in only 10 patients (1.6%) for arrhythmias, and in only one patient for hypotension (38). Holter monitoring during and for a period of 4 hours after exercise revealed a 5.7% prevalence of asymptomatic ventricular tachycardia during exercise and a 28.8% prevalence during the rest of the monitoring period. The low incidence of adverse events associated with exercise stress testing in patients with CHF demonstrates that those whose condition is stable can safely exercise in a well-supervised setting.

The safety of repeated exercise in CHF was demonstrated in several small training studies of patients with a reduced left ventricular ejection fraction (LVEF). Subsequent exercise testing (39) and exercise training studies in patients with mild to moderate heart failure symptoms also demonstrated no significant ischemic or arrhythmic complications during training.

PROGNOSTIC IMPLICATIONS OF EXERCISE TESTING

Measurement of exercise peak VO_2 has been found to be extremely useful in the risk stratification of patients with heart failure. Indeed, use of peak VO_2 in candidate selection for cardiac transplantation has become standard practice. In a prospective study of 114 ambulatory patients with CHF referred to the University of Pennsylvania for cardiac transplantation, a VO_2 of less than 14 mL/kg per minute was used as a criterion for acceptance for cardiac transplantation (40). Patients were divided into three groups based on the results of their cardiopulmonary stress tests. Patients with a peak VO_2 below 14 mL/kg per minute were accepted as transplant candidates whereas transplant was deferred for patients with a peak VO_2 above 14 mL/kg per minute. A third group included patients with a peak VO_2 below 14 mL/kg per minute who had a significant comorbidity that precluded transplant. Age, LVEF, and resting hemodynamic parameters were similar. One-year survival was 94% in patients with a VO_2 above 14 mL/kg per minute. Accepted transplant candidates with a VO_2 below 14 mL/kg per minute had a 1-year survival of 70%, whereas the patients with a significant comorbidity and reduced VO_2 had a 1-year survival of 47% (Fig. 38-3). Patients accepted for transplant had a falsely elevated survival because all transplants were treated as a censored observation. If urgent transplant was counted as death, the 1-year survival fell to 48%. With this approach, we were able to identify the candidates whose transplant could be deferred. We subsequently developed a predictive model to stratify ambulatory transplant candidates according to risk. Peak VO_2 was a key parameter in the derivation of the survival score (41). Several recent studies have reaffirmed the prognostic utility of VO_2 in the era of beta-blockade and biventricular pacing (42,43).

EFFECTS OF EXERCISE TRAINING

Exercise training has long been advocated as a means to improve quality of life in normal persons and those with disease. Aerobic training results in several beneficial hemodynamic, morphologic, and metabolic changes in humans (44) (Table 38-1).

Many of the central and peripheral changes induced by aerobic training may be particularly effective in patients with heart failure. Demonstrated advantages of training in heart failure include central hemodynamic benefits such as an increase in stroke volume; alteration of autonomic tone with a decrease in sympathetic stimulation; improved endothelial and vascular responsiveness with a decrease in peripheral vascular resistance; and muscle enzymatic changes with an increased oxidative capacity and a decrease in lactate production (Table 38-2).

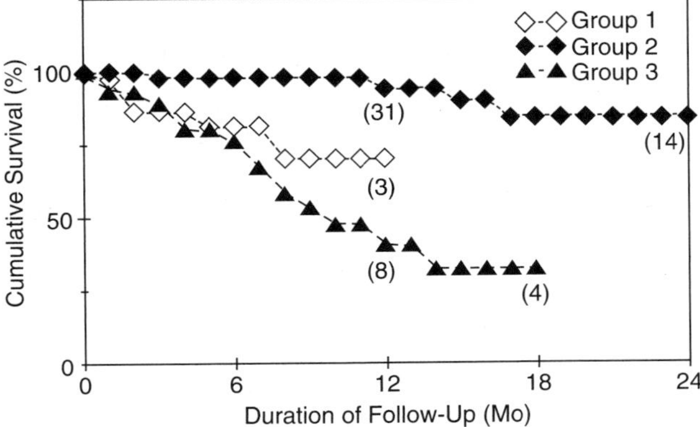

Figure 38-3 One-year survival of patients with CHF based on their maximal VO_2. Group 1 (n = 35): patients with a peak VO_2 below 14 mL/kg per minute were accepted as transplant candidates. Group 2 (n = 52): patients with a peak VO_2 above 14 mL/kg per minute. Group 3 (n = 27): patients with peak VO_2 below 14 mL/kg per minute and significant comorbidity precluding transplant.

Effects of Training on the Heart

Animal models have been used to investigate the effects of exercise training on the failing heart. Using an ischemic rat model of heart failure, Musch et al. (45) studied the effects of endurance training. Fifty rats underwent thoracotomy. In 25 rats, the left anterior descending artery was ligated; the remainder of the animals underwent a sham procedure. These groups were then randomized to sedentary activity versus a training protocol. The training protocol consisted of 60-minute sessions of treadmill exercise 5 days a week for 10 to 12 weeks. Parameters studied included VO_2; heart rate and blood pressure response; rest and exercise hemodynamic measurements; succinate dehydrogenase activity in the soleus and plantaris muscles; and lactate levels and regional perfusion of the skeletal muscle, renal, and splanchnic beds. Following the training program, VO_2 was higher, succinate dehydrogenase activity was increased, and lactate levels were lower during submaximal exercise in the rats with heart failure. No differences were observed in regional perfusion or in hemodynamic measurements. In this rat model of heart failure, all the benefits of training were derived from peripheral mechanisms. Central cardiac function was not altered.

Todaka et al. (46), using a pacing-induced model of CHF in dogs, demonstrated both central and peripheral effects of training. In this study, 12 dogs underwent instrumentation for cardiac pacing and hemodynamic recording. All hearts were then rapidly paced for 4 weeks. Six of the dogs received daily treadmill exercise (4.4 km per hour for 2 hours); the other dogs remained sedentary. At 4 weeks, the maximum rate of pressure rise was higher (2,540 ± 440 mm hg per second versus 1,720 ± 300 mm hg per second;

TABLE 38-1
BENEFITS OF AEROBIC TRAINING

Morphological
↑ Myocardial mass
↑ LV end-diastolic volume
↑ Diameter of coronary arteries
↑ Skeletal muscle capillary-to-fiber ratio
Skeletal muscle
↑ Capillary density
↑ Mitochondrial volume and cristae
↑ Enzymes, citric acid cycle, and electron transport chain
↑ Use of free fatty acids
↑ Local $(A–V)O_2$
Hemodynamic
↓ Heart rate at rest and throughout exercise
↓ Double product at submaximal work loads
↑ Stroke volume
↑ Maximum cardiac output
↑ Maximum VO_2

LV, left ventricular; $(A–V)O_2$, arterial-venous oxygen difference; VO_2, oxygen consumption.

TABLE 38-2
DEMONSTRATED ADVANTAGES OF TRAINING IN HEART FAILURE

Investigator (Reference)	No. of Patients (CHF Etiology)	Ejection Fraction (%)	Training Time (mo)	Training Effects
Coats et al. (47)	11 (CAD)	19	2	↑VO_2, ↓HR
Sullivan et al. (48)	12 (CAD/IDC)	24	4–6	↑VO_2, ↑$(A–V)O_2$ ↓HR, ↓lactate, ↑peak mbf
Hambrecht et al. (55)	22 (CAD/IDC)	26	6	↑VO_2, ↑AT, ↑WC, ↑OX
Letac et al. (67)	8 (CAD)	<45	2	↑WC, ↓HR, ↓BP
Lee et al. (68)	18 (CAD)	<40	12–42	↑WC, ↓HR
Williams et al. (69)	6 (CAD)	<35	6	↓HR
Cohn et al. (70)	10 (CAD)	<27	12	↑VO_2
Wilson et al. (71)	32 (CAD/IDC)	23	12	↔VO_2, ↔AT
Belardinelli et al. (72)	27 (CAD/IDC)	30	2	↑VO_2, ↑OX, ↓lactate, ↓catecholamines
Demopoulos et al. (73)	16 (CAD/IDC)	<30	12	↑VO_2, ↓endothelial function

CHF, congestive heart failure; CAD, coronary artery disease; IDC, idiopathic dilated cardiomyopathy; WC, work capacity; HR, heart rate; BP, blood pressure; AT, anaerobic threshold; VO_2, maximal oxygen consumption; $(A–V)O_2$, arterial-venous oxygen difference; mbf, muscle blood flow; OX, oxidative capacity.

$p < 0.05$) and LV end-diastolic pressure was lower (9 ± 5 mm Hg versus 19 ± 4 mm Hg; $p < 0.05$) in the exercised versus the sedentary dogs. Subsequent in vitro analysis of cardiac function revealed similarly depressed systolic functions in both groups. However, the diastolic myocardial stiffness constant was elevated only in the sedentary group (32 ± 3 in sedentary dogs, 21 ± 3 in exercised dogs, 20 ± 4 in otherwise normal dogs). Thus, daily exercise training preserved hemodynamic measurements in vivo and measures of diastolic stiffness in vitro. In this canine pacing model of CHF, the intrinsic changes in heart function contributing to the overall beneficial hemodynamic effects of exercise training manifested as significant changes in diastolic properties.

In humans with CHF, results of studies on hemodynamic adaptations to exercise have been inconsistent. Minimal hemodynamic changes have been observed in response to training (47,48), while an increase in peak cardiac output has also been observed (49). Some investigators have suggested that high-intensity training may provoke deleterious effects (50). However, subsequent randomized trials have demonstrated no adverse effects of exercise on left ventricular function.

A group of 25 male patients with CHF following myocardial infarction were randomized to an 8-week exercise program consisting of twice-daily outdoor walks and 45-minute stationary cycling sessions four times weekly. The subjects resided in a rehabilitation facility where they received education and were prepared low-fat meals, whereas the control patients lived at home and were instructed not to exert themselves beyond the level of daily living activities. At baseline and at the end of the 8-week study period, respiratory gas exchange and invasive hemodynamic measurements were performed during upright bike exercise. Left ventricular mass, volumes, and ejection fraction were determined by MRI. The subjects who exercised had a significant increase in their exercise capacity (29% increase in VO_{2max}, 19 to 25 mL/kg per minute) that was accompanied by a significant increase in maximal cardiac output (12 to 14 L per minute) and a widening of the maximal (A-V) O_2 difference (13 to 15 mL O_2 per 100 mL). No differences were observed in either group after the study period in pulmonary pressures or left ventricular mass, volume, or function. While the study patients may be atypical given their relatively mild cardiac impairment (mean EF 32%, VO_{2max} 19 mL/kg per minute), there was no evidence for myocardial damage after exercise training (51). Further evidence against deleterious remodeling after exercise training was provided in a follow-up study in the same group of patients who were re-examined with exercise testing and MRI after 1 year. The status of the left ventricle in patients who had undergone training was maintained at 1 year in terms of mass, volume, function, and wall thickness as assessed by MRI. Training had neither a detrimental nor beneficial effect on the remodeling process, yet improvements in exercise capacity were largely maintained (52).

A larger exercise study of 73 men with NYHA Class I–III CHF was also conducted to assess the effect of exercise training on left ventricular function and hemodynamics (53). A minority of these subjects had ischemic heart disease. The exercise intervention was initiated in-hospital for 2 weeks of bicycling 4 to 6 times daily for at minutes at 70% VO_{2max} and continued at home as 20 minutes of bicycling daily for 6 months combined with one weekly session of group exercise (walking, calisthenics, or ball games). Attendance at the group sessions was 60%. At the 6-month follow-up, significant improvements in resting ejection fraction, total peripheral resistance, and stroke volume were noted in the training group.

In another group of 46 patients with ischemic cardiomyopathy, left ventricular function has been assessed by dobutamine stress echocardiography after exercise training (54). Significant improvements in contractile response to dobutamine and thallium activity were observed in subjects who were randomized to exercise three times weekly for 8 weeks at 60% of peak VO_2, while basal contractility remained unchanged. These changes were correlated with the development of collateral coronary circulation in a subset of patients who underwent coronary angiography at the end of the exercise intervention.

Effects of Training on the Periphery

Several studies (47,48,55,56) have attempted to characterize the physiological mechanisms underlying the clinical improvement in patients with heart failure. Sullivan et al. (48) studied 12 patients with heart failure who had a mean VO_2 of 16.3 mL/kg per minute and an ejection fraction of 21%. Aerobic training was performed 3 to 5 hours a week for 6 months. Hemodynamic parameters, skeletal muscle perfusion, VO_2, and LVEF were measured before and after training. With training, peak VO_2 rose 23%, from 16.8 to 20.6 mL/kg per minute. Peak cardiac output, peak arterial-venous oxygen difference (A-V) O_2, and peak leg blood flow also significantly increased. Ejection fraction was unchanged. Training decreased leg lactate production, and leg blood flow during submaximal exercise did not increase, suggesting that the major benefit of training was an increase in oxygen extraction by the skeletal muscles. The largest proportion of the increase in VO_2 was derived from peripheral adaptation, with a possible small central contribution.

Skeletal muscle metabolic abnormalities described in patients with heart failure can be improved with training. Two studies of selective arm training (57,58) and another study of aerobic exercise (59) have demonstrated an improvement but not normalization in the metabolic abnormalities observed during exercise in patients with heart failure. Percutaneous biopsy specimens of the vastus lateralis muscle obtained before and after 6 months of aerobic training in 22 patients demonstrated that training increased the volume density of mitochondria. Staining for cytochrome *c* oxidase-positive mitochondria was used as a qualitative index of oxidative enzyme activity in skeletal muscle. This measurement was also significantly increased with training. Thus, aerobic training in patients with heart failure results in improved oxidative function of skeletal muscle (55). Examination of the vastus lateralis muscle biopsy specimens of the CHF patients by electron microscopy and histochemistry demonstrated a significantly increased surface density of cytochrome *c* oxidase-positive mitochondria, mitochondrial cristae, and mitochondrial inner border membrane. In comparison, there were no significant changes in these characteristics in the control group. After the training period, a significant increase in type I fibers was also noted, as well as a decrease in type II fibers. The changes in mitochondrial ultrastructure and muscle fiber redistribution were significantly correlated with increases in peak oxygen uptake (60).

In CHF patients, alterations in the production of endothelium-derived vasoactive mediators may cause a functional imbalance between vasodilation and vasoconstriction in favor of the constricting factors (61). The effect of exercise training on endothelial-derived mediators, nitric oxide and endothelin-1, in a group of patients with CHF after myocardial infarction has been assessed. Patients with CHF were randomized to an exercise regimen of walking 1 hour twice-daily and riding an exercise bike 45 minutes twice-weekly or to normal activities of daily living. After 8 weeks the urinary nitrate elimination in controls was significantly decreased while it remained unchanged in the exercise group. Given that urinary nitrate elimination is a marker for endogenous nitric oxide production, the results suggest that basal nitric oxide production decreased during the study period in the control group while exercise appeared to attenuate this decrease. Endothelin-1 levels were similar in both groups and did not change. It is unclear why there were no differences in endothelin-1 levels, although multifactorial regulation may be one explanation (62).

The effect of aerobic training on endothelial function has been studied more directly (56). Isolated forearm training with handgrip exercise was carried out for 4 weeks in 12 patients with chronic heart failure. Flow-dependent dilation of the radial artery was assessed with a high-resolution ultrasound system. Measurements were performed at rest; during reactive hyperemia; during an intra-arterial infusion of sodium nitroprusside (an endothelium-independent vasodilator); and following intra-arterial infusion of *N*-monomethyl-L-arginine (L-NMMA) (an inhibitor of endothelial synthesis and release of nitric oxide). The impaired, flow-dependent dilation observed in the patients with heart failure was improved by training. l-NMMA attenuated this improvement, implying that the normalization of flow-dependent dilation during training resulted from enhanced endothelial release of nitric oxide. This is an important finding in that it may indicate that, with training, an improvement in skeletal muscle perfusion occurs.

The effect of systemic training, in contrast to isolated muscle group training, on endothelial function has also been assessed. Hambrecht et al. randomized 20 male patients with NYHA Class II–III CHF to 6 months of regular exercise on a bicycle ergometer at 70% of the heart rate at peak oxygen uptake, or to an inactive nontraining control group. At the end of the study period, leg blood flow as assessed by Doppler wire in the left femoral artery increased significantly in response to acetylcholine, which triggers the release of nitric oxide, in a dose-dependent fashion. The inhibiting effect of L-NMMA, the selective inhibitor of nitric oxide production, was also increased in the exercising subjects. These changes in endothelium-dependent blood flow were correlated with changes in functional work capacity. The study thus suggests that aerobic exercise in patients with CHF can restore endothelial function in skeletal muscle microvasculature (63).

Local muscle group training has been shown to have a systemic effect, as well. Twenty-two males with NYHA Class II–III CHF were randomized to exercise six times per day for 10 minutes on a bicycle ergometer at 70% peak oxygen consumption or to an inactive control group. After 4 weeks of training, high-resolution ultrasound was used to determine radial artery diameter to assess endothelium-dependent vasodilation in response to acetylcholine, endothelium-independent vasodilation in response to nitroglycerin, and flow-dependent vasodilation in response to an occlusion cuff. Endothelium-dependent and flow-dependent vasodilation were found to increase significantly in the training group and these changes were accompanied by a statistically significant 19% increase in oxygen consumption at peak exercise. While local training interventions had been noted to improve local endothelium-dependent vasodilation, importantly in CHF patients, this study suggests that local training can improve systemic endothelial dysfunction as long as a critical muscle mass is trained at a level sufficient to increase shear stress (64).

Modulation of so-called sympathetic overdrive is another mechanism by which exercise training exerts its salutary effects. Evidence of such modulation comes from a study that examined heart rate variability in 20 patients with NYHA Class II–III heart failure before and after training. In this study, training increased the parasympathetically mediated component of heart rate variability and also prolonged exercise duration and increased peak VO_2 (65).

Similarly, Coats et al. (47), in a controlled, crossover, home-based trial of 8 weeks of exercise training in 17 patients with stable, moderate to severe CHF, studied the effect of training on autonomic tone by measuring heart rate variability and spillover of radiolabeled norepinephrine. After training, these measurements demonstrated a shift from sympathetic to enhanced vagal activity. Other investigators have demonstrated a decrease in serum catecholamine levels both at rest and during submaximal exercise following aerobic training (50,55).

Skeletal muscle mass is reduced in chronic heart failure and could lead to early skeletal muscle fatigue and decreased exercise capacity (32). Physical deconditioning may contribute to wasting, especially of the leg muscles. Few studies have demonstrated change in muscle mass in CHF patients undergoing resistance training. In 16 elderly women with NYHA Class I–IV CHF, a randomized trial of high-intensity resistance training to counteract the myopathy of chronic heart failure was conducted. The training group underwent resistance training of large upper and lower body muscle groups at 80% of the maximal weight that could be lifted, 3 days per week for 10 weeks while the control group underwent sham exercise low-intensity stretches. Overall exercise capacity increased significantly in the resistance-trained group, as did strength and endurance gains. However, there was no significant change in total body muscle mass as estimated from a 24-hour urine creatinine collection (66).

What Type of Exercise Training Is Best for Patients with Heart Failure?

Many questions regarding exercise training in patients with heart failure remain unanswered. Indeed, even simple questions such as the best mode of training for these patients is unclear as is the effects of training on long-term morbidity and mortality. Most training studies in patients with reduced LV function (67–70) have demonstrated that moderate-intensity aerobic training is safe in this population and can effect an improvement in work capacity with a concomitant decline in heart rate.

Aerobic training does not invariably result in improved exercise capacity. Compliance with the training regimen is the most frequently cited parameter to predict success. However, studies suggest that the initial cardiac-output response to maximal exercise may determine the response to exercise training. Wilson et al. (71) made hemodynamic measurements during treadmill exercise in 32 patients with heart failure before enrolling them in a rehabilitation program. Patients were divided into a "normal" and "reduced" cardiac-output response to exercise. Patients with a normal cardiac-output response to exercise tolerated training, with many achieving a therapeutic benefit. In contrast, the patients with a reduced cardiac-output response had a high dropout rate during training because of exhaustion, and only one patient benefited from training. This study suggests that exercise training may be beneficial in a certain subset of patients with heart failure.

High-intensity aerobic training may not be sustainable in patients with severe NYHA Class IIIB or IV CHF. Accordingly, a few studies have focused on either low-intensity training or training of specific muscles. Belardinelli et al. (72) investigated the value of low-intensity exercise training in 27 patients with chronic heart failure randomized to training versus control. The exercise prescription included three weekly training sessions of bicycle exercise at 40% of peak VO_2 for 8 weeks. Measurements of peak VO_2, serum catecholamines, and lactate and biopsies of vastus lateralis skeletal muscle were performed before and after training. Peak VO_2 increased and serum lactate and catecholamine levels declined during submaximal exercise, and the volume density of mitochondria was enhanced at the conclusion of the study only in the trained group. Similarly, Demopoulus et al. (73) demonstrated the value of low-intensity training in patients with severe CHF. Using a semirecumbent stationary bicycle, patients trained below 50% of peak VO_2 for 1 hour a day, four times a week, for 3 months. Peak VO_2 rose from 11.5 to 15 mL/kg per minute. Peak reactive hyperemia of the calf but not of the forearm muscle increased with training.

A small, randomized crossover trial of 8 weeks of knee extensor endurance training was conducted in 16 women with CHF. The exercise regimen consisted of bilateral dynamic knee extensions on a knee ergometer with 60 repeats per minute for 15 minutes at 65% of baseline peak work rate three times per week for 4 weeks, followed by exercises at 75% of baseline peak work rate for 4 more weeks. Significant improvements in peripheral oxidative capacity, exercise tolerance, and quality of life were shown. Given the lack of adverse events, the results suggest that this may be a promising mode of rehabilitation in CHF patients (74).

Selective respiratory muscle training has also been applied to patients with CHF. Both the limb and the respiratory muscles are actively recruited during exercise. Reduced resting maximal inspiratory and expiratory mouth pressures have been demonstrated in patients with CHF, consistent with respiratory muscle weakness (75). Selective respiratory muscle training was performed in patients with NYHA Class II–IV CHF (76). Respiratory muscle strength and endurance, in addition to submaximal and maximal exercise capacity, were measured before and after 3 months of training. The protocol combined both endurance and strength training. Following selective respiratory muscle training, respiratory muscle strength and endurance were significantly increased in the trained group. Submaximal and maximal exercise performance was also increased in the patients who completed the training regimen, but not in the comparison group. This study demonstrated that selective respiratory muscle training in patients with heart failure improves exercise capacity and that patients with severe heart failure can complete and benefit from selective muscle training.

The impact of aerobic training on the morbidity and mortality of heart failure remains unclear. Some reports suggest a highly beneficial effect (77). The effects of a moderate-intensity exercise program on hospitalization rate and survival was investigated in 99 subjects with NYHA Class II–IV CHF who were randomized either to thrice-weekly exercise at 60% peak VO_2 for 8 weeks followed by 12 months of twice-weekly exercise at the same intensity, or to a nonexercising control group. A significant improvement in functional capacity was noted after 2 months of exercise training and persisted throughout the study period in the trained group. A significantly lower rate of hospital admission for heart failure was noted (RR 0.29; 95% CI 0.11–0.88; $p = 0.02$), as was a lower cardiac mortality rate (RR 0.37; 95% CI 0.17–0.84; $p = 0.01$) in the trained group. While the results of this study are promising, longer-term, larger-scale studies are needed to definitively the impact of exercise training on mortality. The ACTION-HF trial sponsored by the National Institutes of Health is actively enrolling patients and will hopefully be able to provide an answer to this question in the not-too-distant future.

CONCLUSION

Exercise training appears to have therapeutic benefits for patients with CHF. The beneficial effects appear to be related primarily to peripheral rather than central cardiac mechanisms. Future studies investigating the clinical benefit of low-intensity exercise training and of training regional muscle groups in patients with heart failure appear warranted. The ACTION-HF trial, a multicenter training program examining the long-term effects of exercise training in this patient population, is ongoing and will in the near future answer this important clinical question.

REFERENCES

1. Hornig B, Maier V, Drexler H. Physical training improves endothelial function in patients with heart failure. *Circulation.* 1996;93:210–214.
2. Strobeck JE, Sonnenblick EH. Pathophysiology of heart failure: deficiency in cardiac contraction. In: Cohn JN, ed. *Drug Treatment of Heart Failure*. Secaucus, NJ: Advanced Therapeutics Communications International; 1988: 13–48.
3. Zelis R, Mason DT, Braunwald E. A comparison of peripheral resistance vessels in normal subjects and in patients with congestive heart failure. *J Clin Invest.* 1968;47:960–961.
4. Fardy PS, Yanowitz FG. *Cardiac Rehabilitation, Adult Fitness, and Exercise Testing*. 3rd ed. Baltimore: Williams & Wilkins; 1995: 35–51.
5. Weber K, Janicki J. *Cardiopulmonary Exercise Testing: Physiologic Principles and Clinical Applications*. Philadelphia: WB Saunders; 1986.
6. Weber K, Kinasewitz G, Janicki J, et al. Oxygen utilization and ventilation during exercise in patients with chronic cardiac failure. *Circulation.* 1982;65:1213–1223.
7. Maskin C, Forman R, Sonnenblick E, et al. Failure of dobutamine to increase exercise capacity despite hemodynamic improvement in severe chronic heart failure. *Am J Cardiol.* 1983;51:177–182.
8. Wilson J, Martin J, Schwartz D, et al. Exercise tolerance in patients with heart failure: role of impaired nutritive flow to skeletal muscle. *Circulation.* 1984;69:1079–1087.
9. Yang BC, Khan S, Mehta JL. Blockade of platelet-mediated relaxation in rat aortic rings exposed to xanthine-xanthine oxidase. *Am J Physiol.* 1994;266(6 Pt 2):H2212–H2219.
10. Kubo SH, Rector TS, Bank AJ, et al. Endothelium-dependent vasodilation is attenuated in patients with heart failure. *Circulation.* 1991;84:1589–1596.
11. Katz SD, Biasucci L, Sabba C, et al. Impaired endothelium-mediated vasodilation in the peripheral vasculature of patients with congestive heart failure. *J Am Coll Cardiol.* 1992;19:918–925.
12. Moncada S, Radomski MW, Palmer RMJ. Endothelium-derived relaxing factor. Identification as nitric oxide and role in the control of vascular tone and platelet function. *Biochem Biophys Res Commun.* 1988;37:2495–2501.
13. Koller A, Kaley G. Endothelial regulation of wall shear stress and blood flow in skeletal muscle microcirculation. *Am J Physiol.* 1991;260:H862–H868.
14. Katz SD, Rao R, Berman JW, et al. Pathophysiological correlates of increased serum tumor necrosis factor in patients with congestive heart failure. Relation to nitric oxide-dependent vasodilation in the forearm circulation. *Circulation.* 1994;90:12–16.
15. Teerlink JR, Clozel M, Fischli W, et al. Temporal evolution of endothelial dysfunction in a rat model of chronic heart failure. *J Am Coll Cardiol.* 1993;22:615–620.
16. Zelis R, Mason D, Braunwald E, et al. A comparison of the effects of vasodilator stimuli on peripheral resistance vessels in normal subjects and in patients with congestive heart failure. *J Clin Invest.* 1968;47:960–970.
17. Zelis R, Delea C, Coleman H, et al. Arterial sodium content in experimental congestive heart failure. *Circulation.* 1970;61: 213–216.
18. Jondeau G, Katz SD, Toussaint J-F, et al. Regional specificity of peak hyperemic responses in patients with congestive heart failure. Correlation with peak aerobic capacity. *J Am Coll Cardiol.* 1993;22:1399–1402.
19. Drexler H, Hayoz D, Munzel T, et al. Endothelial function in chronic heart failure. *Am J Cardiol.* 1991;69:1596–1601.
20. Marshall JM. Skeletal muscle vasculature and systemic hypoxia. *News in Physiological Sciences.* 1995;10:274–280.
21. Wilson JR, Fink L, Maris J, et al. Evaluation of energy metabolism in skeletal muscle of patients with heart failure with gated phosphorus-31 nuclear magnetic resonance. *Circulation.* 1985;71: 57–62.
22. Weiner DH, Fink LI, Maris J, et al. Abnormal skeletal muscle bioenergetics during exercise in patients with heart failure: role of reduced muscle blood flow. *Circulation.* 1986;73: 1127–1136.
23. Mancini DM, Ferraro N, Tuchler M, et al. Calf muscle metabolism during leg exercise in patients with heart failure: a ^{31}PNMR study. *Am J Cardiol.* 1988;62:1234–1240.
24. Mancini DM, Coyle E, Coggan A, et al. Contribution of intrinsic skeletal muscle changes to ^{31}P NMR skeletal muscle metabolic abnormalities in patients with heart failure. *Circulation* 1989;80: 1338–1346.
25. Mancini DM, Reichek N, Chance B, et al. Contribution of skeletal muscle atrophy to exercise intolerance and altered muscle metabolism in heart failure. *Circulation.* 1992;85:1364–1373.
26. Massie B, Conway M, Yonge R, et al. Skeletal muscle metabolism in patients with congestive heart failure: relation to clinical severity and blood flow. *Circulation.* 1987;76:1009–1019.
27. Massie B, Conway M, Rajagopalan B, et al. Skeletal muscle metabolism during exercise under ischemic conditions in congestive heart failure: evidence for abnormalities unrelated to blood flow. *Circulation.* 1989;78:320–326,334.
28. Mancini D, Wilson JR, Bolinger L, et al. *In vivo* magnetic resonance spectroscopy measurement of deoxymyoglobin during exercise in patients with heart failure: demonstration of abnormal muscle metabolism despite adequate oxygenation. *Circulation.* 1994;90: 500–508.
29. Cohen-Solal A, Laperche T, Morvan D, et al. Prolonged kinetics of recovery of oxygen consumption after maximal graded exercise in patients with chronic heart failure. *Circulation.* 1995;91:2924–2932.

30. Drexler H, Riede U, Munzel T, et al. Alterations of skeletal muscle in chronic heart failure. *Circulation.* 1992;85:1751–1759.
31. Sullivan M, Green H, Cobb F. Skeletal muscle biochemistry and histology in ambulatory patients with long-term heart failure. *Circulation.* 1990;81:518–527.
32. Mancini DM, Walter G, Reichek N, et al. Contribution of skeletal muscle atrophy to exercise intolerance and altered muscle metabolism in heart failure. *Circulation.* 1992;85:1364–1373.
33. Adams V, Jiang H, Yu J, et al. Apoptosis in skeletal myocytes of patients with chronic heart failure is associated with exercise intolerance. *J Am Coll Cardiol.* 1999;33:959–965.
34. Hambrecht R, Adams V, Gielen S, et al. Exercise intolerance in patients with chronic heart failure and increased expression of inducible nitric oxide synthase in the skeletal muscle. *J Am Coll Cardiol.* 1999;33:174–179.
35. Miyagi K, Asanoi H, Ishizaka S, et al. Importance of total leg muscle mass for exercise intolerance in chronic heart failure. *Jpn Heart J.* 1994;35:15–26.
36. Jondeau G, Katz S, Zohman L, et al. Active skeletal muscle mass and cardiopulmonary reserve. Failure to attain peak aerobic capacity during maximal bicycle exercise in patients with severe congestive heart failure. *Circulation.* 1992;86:1351–1356.
37. Wilson J, Mancini D, Dunkman W. Exertional fatigue due to skeletal muscle dysfunction in patients with heart failure. *Circulation.* 1993;87:470–475.
38. Tristani FE, Hughes CV, Archibald DG, et al. Safety of graded symptom-limited exercise testing in patients with congestive heart failure. *Circulation.* 1987;76:VI54–VI58.
39. Sullivan MJ, Higginbotham MB, Cobb FR. Exercise training in patients with severe left ventricular dysfunction. Hemodynamic and metabolic effects. *Circulation.* 1988;78:506–515.
40. Mancini DM, Eisen H, Kussmaul W, et al. Value of peak exercise oxygen consumption for optimal timing of cardiac transplantation in ambulatory patients with heart failure. *Circulation.* 1991;83:778–786.
41. Aaronson K, Schwartz JS, Chen T, et al. Development and prospective validation of a clinical index to predict survival in ambulatory patients referred for cardiac transplant evaluation. *Circulation.* 1997;95:2660–2667.
42. Lund L, Aaronson K, Mancini D. Predicting survival in ambulatory patients with severe heart failure on beta blocker therapy. *Am J Cardiol.* 2003;92:1350–1354.
43. Koelling TM, Joseph S, Aaronson KD. Heart failure survival score continues to predict clinical outcomes in patients with heart failure receiving beta-blockers. *J Heart Lung Transp.* 2004;23(12): 1414–1422.
44. Wasserman K, Hansen J, Sue D, et al. *Principles of Exercise Testing and Interpretation.* Philadelphia: Lea & Febiger; 1987: 1–45.
45. Musch T, Moore R, Leathers D, et al. Endurance training in rats with chronic heart failure induced by myocardial infarction. *Circulation.* 1986;74:431–441.
46. Todaka K, Wang J, Yi GH, et al. Impact of exercise training on ventricular properties in a canine model of congestive heart failure. *Am J Physiol.* 1997;272:H1382–H1390.
47. Coats AJS, Adamopoulos S, Radaelli A, et al. Controlled trial of physical training in chronic heart failure: exercise performance, hemodynamics, ventillation and autonomic function. *Circulation.* 1992;85:2119–2131.
48. Sullivan MJ, Higginbotham MB, Cobb FR. Exercise training in patients with severe left ventricular dysfunction: hemodynamic and metabolic effects. *Circulation.* 1988;78:506–515.
49. Coats AJS, Adamopoulos S, Meyer TE, et al. Effects of physical training in chronic heart failure. *Lancet.* 1990;335:63–66.
50. Jugdutt B, Michorowski B, Kappagoda C. Exercise training after anterior Q wave myocardial infarction: importance of regional left ventricular function and topography. *J Am Coll Cardiol.* 1988;12:362–372.
51. Dubach P, Myers J, Dzekian G, et al. Effect of high intensity training on central hemodynamic responses to exercise in men with reduced left ventricular function. *J Am Coll Cardiol.* 1997;29: 1591–1598.
52. Myers J, Goebbels U, Dzeikan G, et al. Exercise training and myocardial remodeling in patients with reduced ventricular function: one year follow-up with magnetic resonance imaging. *Am Heart J.* 2000;139:252–261.
53. Hambrecht R, Gielen S, Linke A, et al. Effects of exercise training on left ventricular function and peripheral resistance in patients with chronic heart failure. *JAMA.* 2000;283:3095–3101.
54. Belardinelli R, Georgiou D, Ginzton L, Cianci G, Purcaro A. Effects of moderate exercise training on thallium uptake and contractile response to low-dose dobutamine of dysfunctional myocardium in patients with ischemic cardiomyopathy. *Circulation* 1998;97:553–561.
55. Hambrecht R, Niebauer J, Fiehn E, et al. Physical training in patients with stable chronic heart failure: effects on cardiorespiratory fitness and ultrastructural abnormalities of leg muscles. *J Am Coll Cardiol.* 1995;25:1239–1249.
56. Hornig B, Maier V, Drexler H. Physical training improves endothelial function in patients with heart failure. *Circulation.* 1996;93:210–214.
57. Gaudron P, Hu K, Schamberger R, et al. Effect of endurance training early or late after coronary artery occlusion on left ventricular remodeling, hemodynamics, and survival in rats with chronic transmural myocardial infarction. *Circulation.* 1994;89: 402–412.
58. Giannuzzi P, Tavazzi L, Temporelli PL, et al. Long-term physical training and left ventriuclar remodeling after anterior myocardial infarction: results of the Exercise in Anterior Myocardial Infarction (EAMI) Trial. *J Am Coll Cardiol.* 1993;22:1821–1829.
59. Wilson J, Groves J, Rayos G. Circulatory status and response to cardiac rehabilitation in patients with heart failure. *Circulation.* 1996;94:1567–1572.
60. Hambrecht R, Fiehn E, Yu J, et al. Effects of endurance training on mitochondrial ultrastructure and fiber type distribution in skeletal muscle of patients with stable chronic heart failure. *J Am Coll Cardiol.* 1997;29:1067–1073.
61. Katz SD. The role of endothelium-derived vasoactive substances in the pathophysiology of exercise intolerance in patients with congestive heart failure. *Prog Cardiovasc Dis.* 1995;38:23–50.
62. Callaerts-Vegh Z, Wenk M, Goebbels U, et al. Influence of intensive physical training on urinary nitrate elimination and plasma endothelin-1 levels in patients with congestive heart failure. *J Cardiopul Rehab.* 1998;18 (6):450–457.
63. Hambrecht R, Fiehn E, Weigl C, et al. Regular physical exercise corrects endothelial dysfunction and improves exercise capacity in patients with chronic heart failure. *Circulation.* 1998;98:2709–2715.
64. Linke A, Schoene N, Gielen S, et al. Endothelial dysfunction in patients with chronic heart failure: systemic effects of lower-limb exercise training. *J Am Coll Cardiol.* 2001;37:392–397.
65. Kiilavuori K, Toivonen L, Naveri H, et al. Reversal of autonomic derangements by physical training in chronic heart failure assessed by heart rate variability. *Eur Heart J.* 1995;16:490–495.
66. Pu CT, Johnson MT, Forman DE, et al. Randomized trial of progressive resistance training to counteract the myopathy of chronic heart failure. *J Appl Physiol.* 2001;90:2341–2350.
67. Letac B, Cribier A, Desplances JF. A study of LV function in coronary patients before and after physical training. *Circulation.* 1977;56:375–378.
68. Lee AP, Ice R, Blessey R, et al. Long-term effects of physical training on coronary patients with impaired ventricular function. *Circulation.* 1979;60:1519–1526.
69. Williams RS, McKinnis R, Cobb F, et al. Effects of physical conditioning on left ventricular ejection fraction in patients with coronary artery disease. *Circulation.* 1984;70:69–75.
70. Cohn E, Williams R, Wallace A. Exercise responses before and after physical conditioning in patients with severely depressed left ventricular ejection fraction. *Am J Cardiol.* 1982;49:296–300.
71. Wilson J, Groves J, Rayos G. Circulatory status and response to cardiac rehabilitation in patients with heart failure. *Circulation.* 1996;94:1567–1572.
72. Belardinelli R, Georgiou D, Scocco V, et al. Low intensity exercise training in patients with chronic heart failure. *J Am Coll Cardiol.* 1995;26:975–982.
73. Demopoulos L, Bijou R, Fergus A, et al. Exercise training in patients with severe congestive heart failure: enhancing peak aerobic capacity while minimizing the increase in ventricular wall stress. *J Am Coll Cardiol.* 1997;29:597–603.
74. Tyni-Lenne R, Gordon A, Jansson E, et al. Skeletal muscle endurance training improves peripheral oxidative capacity, exercise tolerance, and health-related quality of life in women with

chronic congestive heart failure secondary to either ischemic cardiomyopathy or idiopathic dilated cardiomyopathy. *Am J Cardiol.* 1997;80:1025–1029.
75. Hammond M, Bauer K, Sharp J, et al. Respiratory muscle strength in congestive heart failure. *Chest.* 1990;98: 1091–1094.
76. Mancini D, Henson D, LaManca J, et al. Benefit of selective respiratory muscle training on exercise capacity in patients with heart failure [Abstract]. *Circulation.* 1995;91:320–329.
77. Belardinelli R, Georgiou D, Cianci G, et al. Randomized, controlled trial of moderate exercise training in chronic heart failure. *Circulation.* 1999;99:1173–1182.

39

Impact and Treatment of Comorbidities in Heart Failure

Tamara B. Horwich   Gregg C. Fonarow

Heart failure is an increasingly common cause of morbidity and mortality. Older age, as well as ischemic heart disease, hypertension, and obesity are risk factors for heart failure. Furthermore, chronic heart failure may predispose to conditions such as anemia, diabetes, depression, and sleep apnea. Thus, heart failure is frequently characterized by comorbid conditions, both cardiovascular and noncardiovascular (Table 39-1). Patients with heart failure have a range of comorbid conditions, with many patients having three or more significant comorbid conditions present. The prevalence of comorbid conditions in patients hospitalized with heart failure enrolled into the ADHERE registry are shown in Table 39-2 (1). The prevalence of comorbid conditions in patients with heart failure enrolled in randomized clinical trials has recently been reviewed by Krum et al. (2).

Comorbidities in heart failure may both contribute to the cause of the disease and have a key role in its progression and response to therapy. Increased burden of comorbidity in heart failure is associated with increased hospitalization rate, increased hospital length of stay, and increased mortality (3,4). There are a multitude of potential comorbidities associated with heart failure; this chapter will focus on diabetes, anemia, obesity, hypercholesterolemia, and chronic obstructive pulmonary disease, with a brief discussion of sleep apnea and depression, as recent investigations have shed new light on the relevance and therapeutic implications of these conditions in heart failure. Other important comorbidities such as coronary artery disease (CAD), atrial fibrillation, and chronic kidney disease are the focus of other chapters in this textbook.

DIABETES AND HEART FAILURE

Diabetes is an important, yet perhaps under-recognized, comorbid condition in heart failure. In clinical trials, diabetes is present in roughly one-quarter of stable outpatients with heart failure and almost one-half of patients hospitalized for heart failure (Table 39-3) (5). Thirty percent of stable, elderly heart failure patients have diabetes, and the prevalence of diabetes rises to 40% in elderly patients hospitalized with heart failure (3,6,7). Conversely, diabetes is frequently complicated by the presence of heart failure, present in 12% of type II diabetics, compared to only 5% of nondiabetics (8).

Several studies have clearly established diabetes as a risk factor for developing heart failure. After myocardial infarction, diabetic patients are more likely than nondiabetic patients to have complicated hospital courses, including the development of heart failure (9). The Framingham Heart Study found that diabetic men had a twofold elevated risk of developing heart failure while diabetic women had a fourfold elevated risk (10). More recent population-based studies have found similarly elevated risk attributable to diabetes (11–13); for example, heart failure incidence was reported at 31 per 1,000 person-years in diabetics compared to 13 per 1,000 person-years in nondiabetics (12). The risk of heart failure is magnified in diabetics with poor glycemic control (14); for each 1% increase in the glycosylated hemoglobin (HbA1c) level, risk of heart failure increases by 8% (15). Diabetes-related risk factors such as hypertension, CAD, and left ventricular hypertrophy all

TABLE 39–1
IMPORTANT COMORBIDITIES IN HEART FAILURE

Cardiovascular
Hypertension
Coronary artery disease
Peripheral vascular disease
Cerebral vascular disease
Hyperlipidemia
Atrial fibrillation
Noncardiovascular
Obesity
Diabetes
Anemia
Chronic kidney disease
Thyroid disorders
Chronic obstructive pulmonary disease
Smoking
Sleep-disordered breathing
Liver disease
Arthritis
Cancer
Depression

independently contribute to the development of heart failure (16,17). Further increasing the risk of heart failure are pathophysiological processes associated with diabetes and insulin resistance, including increased central sympathetic nerve activity (18), endothelial dysfunction (16), and preferential myocardial utilization of fatty acids, which may

TABLE 39–2
COMORBIDITIES IN PATIENTS HOSPITALIZED WITH A PRIMARY DIAGNOSIS OF HEART FAILURE IN THE ADHERE REGISTRY

	Men (n = 41,276)	Women (n = 44,340)
Age (mean)	70.2 ± 13.9	74.6 ± 13.7
LVEF (mean)	32.9 ± 15.7	42.1 ±17.3
EF >40% (%)	28	51
Atrial fibrillation (%)	31	30
Coronary artery disease (%)	64	51
Current smoker (%)	17	10
Diabetes mellitus (%)	44	44
Hyperlipidemia (%)	37	32
Hypertension (%)	69	75
Pacemaker (%)	19	14
Renal insufficiency (%)	33	27
Thyroid disease (%)	11	23
Ventricular tachycardia/ fibrillation (%)	13	5

From Adams KF, Jr., Fonarow G, Emerman C, et al. Characteristics and outcomes of patients hospitalized for heart failure in the United States: rationale, design, and preliminary observations from the first 100,000 cases in the Acute Decompensated Heart Failure National Registry (ADHERE). *Am Heart J.* 2005;149:209–216, with permission.

TABLE 39–3
PREVALENCE OF DIABETES IN PATIENTS WITH HEART FAILURE ENROLLED IN CLINICAL TRIALS

Clinical Trial	Patients with Diabetes, %
SOLVD	25.8
MERIT-HF	24.5
ELITE-II	24.0
Val-HeFT	25.4
COPERNICUS	25.7
OPTIME-CHF (hospitalized)	44.2
VMAC (hospitalized)	47.0

From Fonarow GC. The management of the diabetic patient with prior cardiovascular events. *Rev Cardiovasc Med.* 2003;4(Suppl 6):S38–S49, with permission.

depress myocardial contractility and increase myocardial susceptibility to ischemic injury (19).

Not only does diabetes increase risk of heart failure, but heart failure itself increases the risk of insulin resistance and diabetes (7,20–22). According to one study, the odds of developing diabetes is increased threefold by the presence of heart failure (7) and an additional study found that the risk of diabetes increased with heart failure severity (22). Underlying pathophysiological mechanisms that may directly promote the development of insulin resistance in heart failure include sympathetic nervous system activation and elevated circulating free fatty acids (23).

CAD, hypertension, and a specific diabetic cardiomyopathy are the most common etiologies of heart failure in diabetics, termed by Bell the cardiotoxic triad (24). Hypertension and CAD have consistently been ranked as two of the most important risk factors for development of heart failure in epidemiologic studies (10,11). Diabetes also promotes development of cardiomyopathy independent of CAD or hypertension, via direct effects of hyperglycemia and insulin resistance on the heart. Advanced glycation end-products in the myocardium lead to fibrosis and altered calcium homeostasis, leading to diastolic and systolic dysfunction. Additional cardiotoxic effects of hyperglycemia and insulin resistance include cardiac hypertrophy, endothelial dysfunction, inflammation, and lipotoxicity (25). The relative contribution of diabetes and associated comorbid conditions such as hypertension or CAD is variable.

Diabetes not only predicts development of heart failure but also predicts poor outcomes in patients with established heart failure. Analyses from the Studies of Left Ventricular Dysfunction (SOLVD) trial have shown that diabetes is a risk factor for progression from asymptomatic left ventricular dysfunction to symptomatic heart failure [relative risk (RR) = 1.6] as well as a risk factor for all-cause mortality (RR = 1.4), although this increased risk was observed only in patients with ischemic etiology of heart failure (26,27). Although data from the Beta-blocker Evaluation of Survival Trial (BEST) also linked the diabetes-related mortality risk to ischemic disease (28), others studies have not found the risk to be specific to ischemic heart failure (29–31). In the Danish Investigations on Arrhythmia and Mortality on

Dofetilide (DIAMOND), diabetes predicted mortality (independent of heart failure etiology) in both systolic and diastolic heart failure. The increased mortality risk associated with diabetes has been observed in additional heart failure cohorts, including elderly patients with chronic and new-onset heart failure and advanced heart failure patients in a transplant referral center (3,29,30).

Diabetic heart failure patients derive benefit from standard, life-prolonging heart failure medical therapy. A meta-analysis of six randomized controlled trials of angiotensin-converting enzyme inhibitors (ACEIs) in systolic heart failure, including 2,398 diabetic and 10,188 nondiabetic subjects, found ACEI therapy was associated with a 14% and 15% decreased mortality risk, respectively (Table 39-4) (32). Likewise, subgroup analysis of the Assessment of Treatment with Lisinopril and Survival (ATLAS) study documented a mortality risk reduction of 14% and 6% in those with and without diabetes, respectively (33).

There is also abundant clinical trial evidence supporting the use of beta-adrenergic antagonists to reduce morbidity and mortality in diabetic patients with systolic heart failure (32,34–36). A pooled analysis of three randomized controlled trials, which included 1,883 diabetic and 7,042 nondiabetic heart failure patients, demonstrated a similar magnitude of benefit from beta-blocker therapy in the two cohorts (32). In the Carvedilol or Metoprolol European Trial (COMET), the predefined subgroup of diabetic heart failure patients had improved risk reduction with carvedilol compared to metoprolol, on a similar scale as the nondiabetic cohort (RR 0.85 and 0.82 for diabetics and nondiabetics, respectively) (36).

Beta-blockers may be underutilized in diabetic patients with heart failure or other cardiovascular disease, due to legitimate concerns about worsening of insulin resistance and dyslipidemia, development of hypoglycemic unawareness, or exacerbation of erectile dysfunction. However, severe hypoglycemia is extremely rare in type II diabetes. Furthermore, these undesirable effects are much more common in cardioselective beta-blockers such as metoprolol or atenolol, compared to the nonselective alpha-, beta-blocker carvedilol (37,38). Beneficial effects of the newer vasodilating beta-blockers include improved insulin sensitivity, decreased triglycerides, improved renal blood flow, and reduction of microalbuminuria. These benefits were exemplified in the recent GEMINI trial, which compared carvedilol with metoprolol for hypertension control in 1,235 subjects with type II diabetes mellitus. Although reductions in heart rate and blood pressure were similar, HbA1c and triglycerides were both increased in the metoprolol group compared to unchanged HbA1c and decreased triglycerides in the carvedilol group (39).

Aldosterone antagonists are the third standard, life-prolonging class of drugs essential to heart failure managment (40,41). The Randomized Aldactone Evaluation Study (RALES) trial studied spironolactone in 1,663 patients with NYHA Class III–IV systolic heart failure, finding a 30% reduced mortality risk. However, a diabetic subgroup analysis was not reported (41). The subsequent Eplerenone Post-Acute Myocardial Infarction Heart Failure Efficacy and Survival Study (EPHESUS) study of 3,319 post-myocardial infarction patients with left ventricular dysfunction documented a 15% mortality risk reduction with eplerenone, and risk reduction was consistent in the diabetes (n = 2,122) and nondiabetes subgroups (40). Although the risk of developing hyperkalemia in these trials was low (2% to 5.5%), the frequency of hyperkalemia in patients with diabetes, especially those with renal dysfunction, may be substantially higher (42,43). Prevention of hyperkalemia in higher-risk patients involves lower initiation and maintenance dosing, frequent monitoring of electrolytes and renal function, concomitant loop diuretic therapy, and restricted dietary potassium (43).

TABLE 39–4

EFFECT OF ACE INHIBITORS ON MORTALITY FROM HEART FAILURE IN DIABETIC AND NONDIABETIC PATIENTS

	RR Analysis					
Study Name	**Total N**	**Nondiabetic N**	**Diabetic N**	**RR, Nondiabetic (95% CI)**	**RR, Diabetic (95% CI)**	**RRR (95% CI)**
CONSENSUS	253	197	56	0.64 (0.46–0.88)	1.06 (0.65–1.74)	1.67 (0.93–3.01)
SAVE	2,231	1,739	492	0.82 (0.68–0.99)	0.89 (0.68–1.16)	1.09 (0.79–1.50)
SMILE	1,556	1,253	303	0.79 (0.54–1.15)	0.44 (0.22–0.87)	0.56 (0.25–1.22)
SOLVD-Prevention	4,228	3,581	647	0.97 (0.83–1.15)	0.75 (0.55–1.02)	0.77 (0.54–1.09)
SOLVD-Treatment	2,569	1,906	663	0.84 (0.74–0.95)	1.01 (0.85–1.21)	1.21 (0.97–1.50)
TRACE	1,749	1,512	237	0.85 (0.74–0.97)	0.73 (0.57–0.94)	0.87 (0.65–1.15)
Random effects pooled estimate		10,188	2,398	0.85 (0.78–0.92)	0.84 (0.70–1.00)	1.00 (0.80–1.25)

CONSENSUS, Cooperative North Scandinavian Enalapril Survival Study; SAVE, Survival and Ventricular Enlargement; SMILE, Survival of Myocardial Infarction Long-term Evaluation; TRACE, Trandolapril Cardiac Evaluation.
From Shekelle PG, Rich MW, Morton SC, et al. Efficacy of angiotensin-converting enzyme inhibitors and beta-blockers in the management of left ventricular systolic dysfunction according to race, gender, and diabetic status: a meta-analysis of major clinical trials. *J Am Coll Cardiol.* 2003;41:1529–1538, with permission.

Device therapy for heart failure—implantable cardioverter defibrillators and cardiac resynchronization therapy—has now been established to reduce morbidity and mortality in subsets of heart failure patients. The major device trials have not included analyses stratified by presence of diabetes, yet since there is no evidence to suggest a differential efficacy in diabetes, device therapy is indicated for diabetic heart failure patients who meet established criteria.

The optimal medical regimen for glucose control in diabetics with heart failure is uncertain. Although poor glycemic control has been shown to increase risk of developing heart failure (15), the issue of glycemic control in patients with established heart failure has not been prospectively studied. However, improved glycemic control has potential benefits in heart failure, including improvement of myocardial glucose utilization and decrease of free fatty acids, which may be cardiotoxic (24).

The major classes of diabetes medications have possible adverse effects in heart failure. In a study of 554 advanced heart failure patients, diabetics treated with insulin had a fourfold to fivefold increased mortality risk, while noninsulin-treated diabetics were at similar risk to nondiabetics (29). Although insulin-associated increased risk has not been consistently observed (44), in a large study of elderly post-myocardial infarction patients, insulin-treated diabetics were also at particularly high mortality risk (45). Insulin therapy may merely reflect more advanced disease, but there are also plausible biological mechanisms by which insulin could directly contribute to worsening of heart failure, including increase in sympathetic nervous system activation, promotion of ventricular hypertrophy, and impairment of endothelial function (16,18,46).

Decisions regarding oral antihyperglycemic therapy in heart failure are also not straightforward. According to prescribing information, metformin therapy is contraindicated in heart failure, due to concerns about lactic acidosis (47). Regarding thiazolidinediones (TZDs), the American Heart Association/American Diabetes Assocation consensus statement has recommended that this class of medications be used with caution in NYHA Class I–II heart failure and not used at all in NYHA Class III–IV heart failure, as TZDs have been implicated as causing weight gain, edema, and worsened heart failure (48). However, fluid retention seems to resolve quickly with cessation of TZD therapy (49) and, importantly, TZDs do not adversely affect cardiac structure and function (50). Despite warnings, TZDs and metformin (so-called insulin-sensitizing medications) are used in roughly one-quarter of diabetics with heart failure (51). A recent, large study of Medicare patients has indicated that metformin and TZDs do not worsen heart failure outcomes but, rather, are independently associated with *decreased* mortality risk (13%). Although metformin did not increase risk of lactic acidosis in this cohort, the use of TZDs did increase heart failure hospitalizations (44). Further investigation into medical management of diabetes in heart failure is needed.

ANEMIA

Only recently has anemia been recognized as a prevalent condition in patients with heart failure. The reported prevalence of anemia in heart failure has varied, depending on how anemia is defined and the severity of heart failure in the population studied. Anemia was present in 4% of patients with asymptomatic or mild to moderate heart failure (52) in 17% of a community cohort with new-onset heart failure (53); in 30% of patients with chronic, advanced heart failure (54); and in 49% of patients with acute decompensated heart failure (55).

There are several features of heart failure that have potential to contribute to the development of anemia. Renal insufficiency and hemodilution are present in some but not all heart failure patients with anemia (56,57). The inflammatory cytokine activation of heart failure may engender epogen resistance (58,59). Most recently, ACEIs have been associated with anemia in heart failure (60). The frequency of iron or other deficiencies in heart failure has been reported as low (53,56,61). Understanding the pathophysiology behind anemia in heart failure will require further investigation.

Anemia in heart failure is associated with increased severity of disease; patients with lower hemoglobin (Hb) levels have higher NYHA class, lower exercise capacity, decreased left ventricle ejection fraction (LVEF), an impaired hemodynamic profile (54), as well as increased B-type natriuretic peptide (BNP) and cardiac troponin levels (62). Anemia in heart failure also predicts increased left ventricular mass, as quantified by magnetic resonance imaging, and hypertrophy regresses over time as Hb level improves (63).

In the Framingham study, lower hematocrit (Hct) was associated with increased risk of developing heart failure (64), and anemia in end-stage renal disease has been associated with increased heart failure risk (65). In diverse populations of patients with *established* heart failure, the presence of anemia has clearly been identified as a significant prognosticator of poor outcomes. In a study of 1,061 advanced systolic heart failure patients at a single university referral center, the annual mortality risk increased by 13% for each 1g/dL decrease in Hb, independent of age, gender, CAD, renal function, and hemodynamics. Markedly increased risk was seen with relatively mild degrees of anemia (Hb $<$12.3 g/dL, Fig. 39-1) (54). No elevation of risk was observed at the very highest Hb levels, despite this finding in a subsequent study (66). In an analysis of SOLVD results, with each 1% decrease in Hct, adjusted mortality risk increased by 2.7% (52). Likewise, in acutely decompensated heart failure, an analysis of 906 patients demonstrated a 12% increased risk of death or rehospitalization at 60 days per 1g/dL decrease in Hb (55). In over 12,000 new-onset heart failure patients, anemia conferred an adjusted relative risk of mortality of 1.34 (53), although a smaller study did not find anemia to be a significant prognostic factor in this population (67). Lastly, in heart failure with preserved systolic function (diastolic heart failure), anemia appears to occur with similar frequency and to predict similarly reduced survival (68).

The pathophysiology underlying the association between Hb and impaired heart failure survival deserves further study. Anemia may be a marker of disease severity, reflecting any combination of factors, including inflammatory cytokine activation, volume overload/hemodilution, renal insufficiency, malnutrition, or increased burden of medical comorbidities. On the other hand, anemia

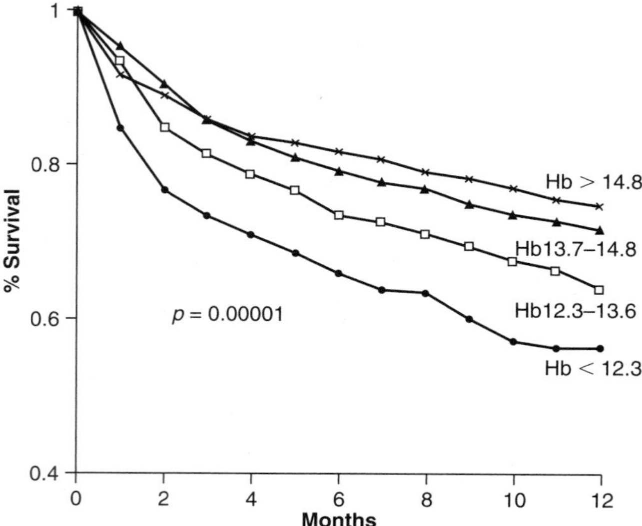

Figure 39–1 Kaplan-Meier survival analysis by quartiles of hemoglobin level. (From Horwich TB, Fonarow GC, Hamilton MA, et al. Anemia is associated with worse symptoms, greater impairment in functional capacity and a significant increase in mortality in patients with advanced heart failure. *J Am Coll Cardiol.* 2002;39:1780–1786, with permission.)

theoretically could contribute to the progression of heart failure, such as increasing the susceptibility of myocardial tissue to hypoxia or ischemia, leading to increased sympathetic nervous system stimulation.

The use of recombinant erythropoietin (EPO) to treat anemia in heart failure patients has been explored in small studies, with promising results. Silverberg et al. conducted a randomized trial of subcutaneous EPO and intravenous iron in 32 heart failure patients with advanced, systolic heart failure and found that the treatment group had significant improvement in NYHA functional class and LVEF, decreased diuretic doses, and fewer hospital days compared to the control group (69), although this study was limited in that it was not blinded or placebo-controlled. A small, randomized, placebo-controlled study by Mancini et al. found increased peak oxygen consumption ($PKVO_2$) on cardiopulmonary exercise testing (11 ± 0.8 to 12.7 ± 2.8 mL/kg per minute) in patients treated with EPO for 3 months compared to a slight decline in $PKVO_2$ in controls. Improved exercise capacity was positively correlated with increased Hb levels (70). Recent preclinical investigation has revealed that EPO may also have beneficial effects in heart failure independent of treating anemia, including decreased myocyte apoptosis and anti-inflammatory activity (71). Of note, in a prior study of patients with end-stage renal disease and heart failure or ischemic heart disease, normalizing Hct (42%) with EPO and intravenous iron compared to maintaining lower Hct levels (30%) was associated with a trend toward increased mortality (72). Thus, the results of randomized trials assessing anemia treatment on exercise capacity (STAMINA-HF) and large-scale, randomized, controlled trials assessing anemia treatment on mortality are needed before treatment of anemia with EPO analogs can be definitively recommended for anemic heart failure patients.

OBESITY

Obesity is an increasingly prevalent condition, present in approximately one-third of the U.S. population (73). Hemodynamic and cardiac structural/functional changes have been documented in obese individuals, even in the absence of clinical cardiac disease. Elevated body mass index (BMI) is associated with increased circulating blood volume and increased cardiac output (74). Compared to normal-weight individuals, echocardiographic studies demonstrate that obesity is associated with morphological cardiac changes, including increased ventricular volume, enlarged atrial area, increased relative wall thickness, and increased left ventricular mass indexed to height. Furthermore, using strain rate imaging, it has been demonstrated that elevated BMI (even in the absence of cardiovascular disease) is associated with both subclinical systolic and diastolic cardiac dysfunction (75–77).

In addition to changes in cardiac structure and function, obesity is associated with multiple cardiovascular risk factors with potential to promote the development of heart failure. Conventional CAD risk factors such as hypertension, diabetes, and dyslipidemia as well as more recently recognized cardiovascular risk factors such as obstructive sleep apnea, inflammation, and atrial fibrillation are clustered in obese individuals (78). It is thus not surprising that elevated BMI is a significant predictor of incident heart failure (13,79). In a Framingham study analysis with a mean follow-up of 14 years, overweight status (BMI ≥ 25 kg/m^2) conferred a 34% increased risk of developing heart failure while obesity (BMI ≥ 30 kg/m^2) conferred a 104% increased risk.

Although overweight and obesity increase the risk for *developing* heart failure, once the heart failure syndrome is established, the epidemiology reverses. Counter to intuition, several studies have demonstrated that elevated BMI is *not* associated with increased risk in chronic heart failure and, in fact, is associated with improved prognosis (54,80–83). This paradoxical relationship was initially described in a study of 1,203 advanced systolic heart failure patients (NYHA III–IV) at a single university referral center (84). Underweight, recommended weight, overweight, and obese patients had similar actuarial 5-year survival and, after adjustment for multiple known prognostic factors, overweight and obese patients had significantly improved survival. A subsequent study, which excluded subjects with cardiac cachexia (unintended weight loss), found that the best 3-year survival rates were seen in the two highest BMI quintile groups (mean BMI of 29 and 34 kg/m2, respectively) (80). The paradoxical relationship between obesity and improved survival has also been extended to patients with mild to moderate heart failure (NYHA I–III) (81). Most recently, analysis of 7,767 stable heart failure patients in the Digitalis Intevention Group Trial adds to the growing body of data on the reverse epidemiology of obesity in heart failure; overweight (BMI 25 to 29.9) and obese (BMI >30) subgroups were at significantly decreased risk for all-cause mortality (0.88 and 0.81, respectively) compared to healthy-weight individuals (BMI 18.5 to 24.9). There was no heterogeneity across subgroups based on ejection fraction, gender, heart failure etiology, and heart failure duration (Fig. 39-2) (83). In patients with left ventricular assist

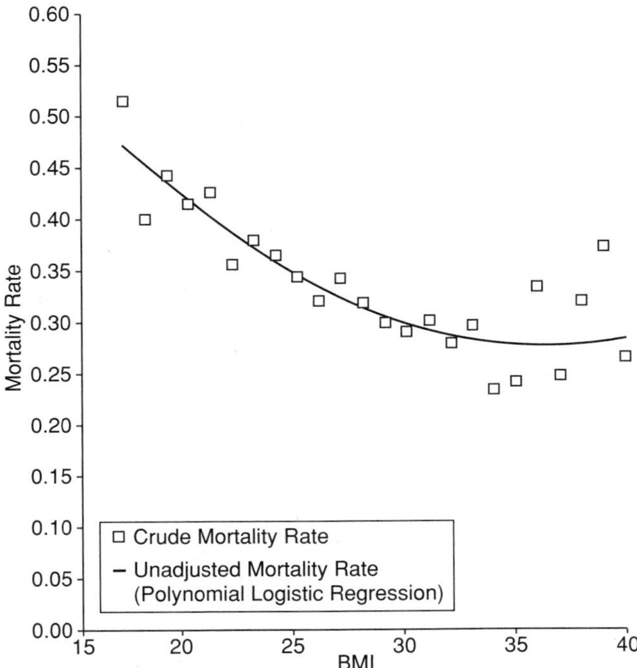

Figure 39–2 Association of body mass index (BMI) as a continuous variable and unadjusted all-cause mortality using polynomial logistic regression. Each point represents the mortality rate associated with a BMI integer. (From Curtis JP, Selter JG, Wang Y, et al. The obesity paradox: body mass index and outcomes in patients with heart failure. (*Arch Intern Med.* 2005;165:55–61, with permission.)

devices, elevated BMI has likewise been associated with improved outcomes (85).

The pathophysiology underlying this paradoxical relationship is incompletely understood but potential explanations have been explored. Obese heart failure patients may simply present at less-advanced stages of disease, due to increased symptoms from excess weight. Alternatively, obese patients may have increased metabolic reserve and less neurohumoral or cytokine activation (86).

Case series suggest that in morbidly obese individuals with heart failure, disease is reversible upon weight loss (87,88). There are no prospective studies on dieting or weight loss programs in heart failure patients who are overweight or obese. Cardiac cachexia is an independent predictor of poor heart failure outcomes (89), reflecting a state of sympathetic activation and catabolic/anabolic imbalance (90). In fact, some investigators have suggested that nutritional supplementation or weight gain as a novel therapeutic goal in heart failure. However, cachexia, as well as obesity, in pre-heart transplant patients have been identified as risk factors for mortality after heart transplantation (91) and, thus, recommendations regarding optimal weight management for patients on the heart transplant waiting list require further investigation.

HYPERCHOLESTEROLEMIA

High cholesterol is a major risk factor for CAD as well as cardiovascular morbidity and mortality (92) and was associated with risk of developing heart failure in the Framingham Heart Study (93). Lipid-lowering therapy has been shown to decrease heart failure incidence in CAD patients (94).

Counter to expectations, high cholesterol levels are *not* associated with increased mortality risk in chronic heart failure. On the contrary, *low* cholesterol has been associated with markedly increased mortality in both ischemic and nonischemic heart failure (95,96). In a study of 1,134 advanced, systolic heart failure patients, low total cholesterol (TC), low- and high-density lipoprotein (LDL and HDL, respectively) cholesterol, and triglycerides were each associated with more severe heart failure symptoms as well as impaired heart failure survival. Five-year survival free from death or need for urgent heart transplantation was less than 25% for patients in the lowest TC quintile (TC <129 mg/dL) compared to greater than 50% for those patients in the two high quintiles (TC >190 mg/dL); 190mg/dL was found to be the best TC cut-off for prediction of mortality by receiver-operator curve (ROC) (97) analysis (95). A similar ROC-derived cut-off for prediction of 1- and 3-year mortality was observed by Raucchhaus et al. in a subsequent study (96).

There are potential explanations for the association between low cholesterol and increased mortality in heart failure. Like obesity, high cholesterol may be reflective of a state of lesser catabolism and greater metabolic reserve. Furthermore, it has been hypothesized that lipoproteins diminish the activation of potentially deleterious inflammatory cytokines in heart failure (98) and, in fact, lipoprotein levels are inversely correlated with cytokines such as tumor necrosis factor (TNF), known to predict mortality in heart failure (96).

Despite the relationship between low cholesterol and increased mortality in heart failure, HMG-CoA reductase inhibitors (statins) have been proposed as a therapy for heart failure. There are also multiple biological mechanisms by which statins could improve symptoms and survival in heart failure. In addition to plaque-stabilizing, anti-ischemic actions, experimental studies provide evidence that statins restore impaired autonomic activation, increase nitric oxide synthesis, improve endothelial function, reverse pathological myocardial remodeling, and decrease inflammatory cytokine activity (97,99–101). However, there are hypothetical risks of statin therapy in heart failure—lowering cholesterol levels and reduction of coenzyme Q levels, which in theory could adversely affect cardiac function and exercise tolerance in heart failure (102).

A growing body of clinical evidence suggests that statin therapy may benefit patients with heart failure. Although patients with clinical heart failure were excluded from most major statin trials, in the Cholesterol and Recurrent Events trial, pravastatin-derived mortality reduction in subjects with left ventricular dysfunction was similar to the risk reduction in subjects with normal systolic function (103). Furthermore, several recent observational studies have found statin therapy to be associated with improved outcomes in heart failure. In a cohort of 551 patients with advanced, systolic heart failure from a single university referral center, statin-treated patients had a 48% decreased risk of all-cause mortality compared to those not treated with statins. The risk reduction was seen in both ischemic and nonischemic cardiomyopathy as well as in patients with both high and low baseline cholesterol levels (104). An analysis of the Prospective Randomized Amlodipine Survival Evaluation (PRAISE) trial also revealed an adjusted RR of 0.48 for heart failure patients on statin therapy (105). Most recently, Ray et al. performed a population-based analysis of elderly individuals hospitalized with newly diagnosed heart failure in Ontario, Canada. Mortality rate was 9.9 per 100 person-years in the statin-treated cohort versus 19.9 per 100 person-years in the nonstatin-treated cohort, translating into a hazard ratio of 0.50 (CI 0.43 to 0.59) (106).

Preliminary experimental data in humans appear promising. In a small, randomized trial of 5 to 10 mg of simvastatin for 14 weeks in 51 patients with systolic dysfunction heart failure (NYHA Class II–III), improvement in LVEF (34% to 41%) occurred in statin-treated subjects compared to no change in LVEF in controls. Furthermore, NYHA class improved in 39% of the statin group compared to 16% in the control group (107). Clearly, larger-scale trials are needed to clarify the role of statins in heart failure, and the results of several trials are currently awaited (102,108).

CHRONIC OBSTRUCTIVE PULMONARY DISEASE

Chronic obstructive pulmonary disease (COPD) and heart failure, with common risk factors such as age and smoking, (109) are frequently coexistent. In studies of the Medicare population, COPD was present in 30% of patients hospitalized with heart failure (6) and 26% of patients diagnosed with chronic heart failure, making COPD the third-most-common noncardiac comorbidity in patients with chronic heart failure, after hypertension and diabetes (3). A non-Medicare-based registry of over 30,000 heart failure hospitalizations in community, tertiary, and academic centers likewise reported a diagnosis of COPD or asthma in nearly one-third of patients (110). Conversely, heart failure is a frequent complicating condition in patients hospitalized with COPD exacerbations (111).

COPD and heart failure may manifest with similar clinical symptoms, such as dyspnea, wheezing, and fatigue. Cardiac auscultation or echocardiography may be difficult in COPD patients, secondary to increased lung volumes (112). Thus, misdiagnosis or failure to recognize overlapping syndromes may occur (113). Fortunately, the advent of the BNP assay presents opportunities for more accurate diagnosis and treatment. In patients presenting with dyspnea, addition of the BNP test to history and physical exam has been shown to differentiate heart failure from pulmonary disease with >90% accuracy (114). Furthermore, in patients with a known diagnosis of COPD or asthma presenting to the emergency department with shortness of breath, using the BNP assay improved detection of newly diagnosed or previously unrecognized heart failure by 20%, compared to using clinical judgment alone (115).

Coexisting COPD and heart failure have a compounding effect in limiting functional capacity, to a greater degree than either syndrome alone. Patients with heart failure have a restrictive ventilatory abnormality as well as reduced lung-diffusing capacity for carbon monoxide (112,116). The restrictive pulmonary defect associated with heart failure may be secondary cardiomegaly, pleural effusions, interstitial edema, or regional lung hypoperfusion resulting in high ventilation/perfusion mismatching (117,118). Patients with heart failure respond to exercise with a greater than normal increase in minute ventilation, but a concomitant COPD-related obstructive ventilatory defect limits this increase in minute ventilation, resulting in severely impaired exercise tolerance. The relative contributions of airway obstruction and lung restriction to pulmonary function in patients with heart failure and COPD have not been thoroughly studied (112).

In addition to magnification of functional impairment, COPD has been associated with worse heart failure outcomes. In a study of 434 patients hospitalized for heart failure, COPD was the single, strongest independent predictor of early readmission (119). In a study of 122,630 elderly, ambulatory heart failure patients, the presence of COPD or bronchiectasis was associated with an increased risk of heart failure hospitalization (40%), any hospitalization (46%), and all-cause mortality (12%) on adjusted analyses (3). In patients hospitalized with heart failure, COPD was identified as a risk factor for 30-day and 1-year mortality in community-based patients in a Canadian study (120) but was not associated with high risk for in-hospital mortality in a large U.S. registry (110).

Patients with heart failure and COPD may not receive optimal, life-prolonging heart failure therapy as a result of physicians' concerns about bronchoconstriction or other adverse effects of beta-blockers (121). Major trials of beta-blockers in heart failure have excluded patients with varying degrees of reactive airway disease or COPD (35,36,112,122). Beta2-adrenergic receptors predominate on bronchial smooth muscle cells and, since beta1 selective (cardioselective) beta-blockers have 20-fold higher affinity for beta1 compared to beta2, risk of bronchoconstriction with cardioselective agents is negligible (123). A meta-analysis of cardioselective beta antagonists in patients with COPD revealed no significant decrease in forced expiratory volume in one second (FEV1) or change in symptoms with initial or long-term therapy, including a subgroup of patients with severe obstruction (124). A meta-analysis of 29 studies of cardioselective beta-blockers in patients with mild to moderate reactive airway disease demonstrated a small, nonclinically significant decrease in FEV1 with initial beta-blocker dose, *but no long-term difference* in symptoms, inhaler use, or FEV1 compared to patients not treated with beta-blockers (125). Beta-blocker dosing in both analyses was in the therapeutic range for heart failure.

It has recently been recognized that noncardioselective beta-blockers such as carvedilol may be superior to previously used beta1 selective antagonists for prolonging survival in systolic heart failure (36). Small studies suggest that carvedilol can be safely utilized in heart failure patients with concomitant COPD. Of 89 Australian heart failure patients who also had COPD or asthma, 85% tolerated carvedilol therapy for at least 3 months, although reasons for intolerance or measures of airway reactivity are unknown (126). Another small study showed an 84% tolerability rate of carvedilol in patients with COPD compared to only 50% in patients with asthma or reversible airway disease (127).

Based on the limited data, experts recommend that beta-blocker therapy *not* be withheld from heart failure patients with COPD. In patients with COPD and no reversible airway disease, cardioselective beta-blockers or carvedilol may be implemented; however, in patients with COPD and reversible airway disease, beta1 selective blockade may be preferred. Because data on the effect of beta-blockers on FEV1 or symptoms during acute COPD exacerbations are unavailable at this time, beta-blocker therapy cannot be recommended during acute exacerbations (112).

Smoking cessation is vitally important for heart failure patients who smoke with or without COPD (128,129). The optimal medical therapy for COPD itself in patients with concomitant COPD and heart failure is not well-defined; inhaled beta-agonists, which alleviate symptoms and improve quality of life in COPD (128), have also been associated with excess cardiovascular risk (130–133). A multicenter, nested case control study of over 13,000 patients followed at seven Veterans Administration Medical Centers (VAMCs) found that in subjects with pre-existing heart failure, inhaled beta-agonist therapy incurred a dose-dependent increased risk of heart failure hospitalizations. There was no increase in heart failure incidence for subjects without pre-existing heart failure (130). A single-center VAMC study of subjects with left ventricular dysfunction demonstrated that inhaled beta-agonist therapy was independently associated not only with heart failure hospitalization but also with increased mortality (131). Although these observational studies do not prove cause and effect, there are potential pathophysiological mechanisms by which beta-agonists may *cause* worsening heart failure, such as downregulation and desensitization of myocardial beta2-adrenergic receptors (134), which may play an important role in progression of heart failure (135).

SLEEP APNEA

Recent studies suggest that 40% to 60% of heart failure patients, whether systolic or diastolic dysfunction heart failure, have the sleep-related breathing disorder obstructive sleep apnea (OSA) (136) or central sleep apnea (CSA) (137–140). Risk factors for CSA include male sex, older age, and atrial fibrillation. Risk factors for OSA include male sex and higher BMI; in women, older age appears to be a strong risk factor (137,138). Furthermore, heart failure itself may predispose to development of sleep apnea via decreased respiratory drive and narrowing of the airways secondary to edema (141).

In addition to causing symptoms of excessive fatigue and daytime drowsiness (142), studies suggest that sleep apnea, particularly CSA, may increase mortality risk in heart failure (143,144). Pathophysiological effects of sleep apnea that potentially contribute to worsening heart failure symptoms and prognosis include hemodynamic changes (145), sympathetic activation (146), inflammatory activation (147), and endothelial dysfunction (148). Preliminary studies show that treatment of sleep apnea with continuous positive airway pressure may have beneficial effects in patients with CSA and OSA, including increased LVEF, improved functional class, and improved survival (149,150). Interestingly, it has also recently been noted that cardiac resynchronization therapy may lead to reduced apnea and hypopnea and better sleep quality in heart failure patients with CSA (151).

DEPRESSION

Depression has a high prevalence in heart failure, ranging from 14% to 37% (152–154) and the incidence of depression in heart failure may be as high as 21% per year (155). Major depression in heart failure has been independently associated with worse heart failure symptoms and quality of life, increased risk of heart failure hospitalization, as well as increased mortality (154,156,157). Social factors such as living alone, the economic burden of medical care, and perceived quality of life predict depression onset in heart failure and thus may help identify at-risk patients (155). Newer pharmacologic antidepressant agents appear to be safe and are recommended for use in heart failure (158); further studies on optimal diagnosis and management of this prevalent heart failure-associated comorbidity are definitely warranted.

REFERENCES

1. Adams KF, Jr., Fonarow G, Emerman C, et al. Characteristics and outcomes of patients hospitalized for heart failure in the United States: rationale, design, and preliminary observations from the first 100,000 cases in the Acute Decompensated Heart Failure National Registry (ADHERE). *Am Heart J.* 2005;149:209–216.
2. Krum H, Gilbert RE. Demographics and concomitant disorders in heart failure. *Lancet.* 2003;362:147–158.
3. Braunstein JB, Anderson GF, Gerstenblith G, et al. Noncardiac comorbidity increases preventable hospitalizations and mortality among Medicare beneficiaries with chronic heart failure. *J Am Coll Cardiol.* 2003;42:1226–1233.
4. Brown AM, Cleland JG. Influence of concomitant disease on patterns of hospitalization in patients with heart failure discharged from Scottish hospitals in 1995. *Eur Heart J.* 1998;19:1063–1069.
5. Fonarow GC. The management of the diabetic patient with prior cardiovascular events. *Rev Cardiovasc Med.* 2003;4(Suppl 6): S38–S49.
6. Havranek EP, Masoudi FA, Westfall KA, et al. Spectrum of heart failure in older patients: results from the National Heart Failure project. *Am Heart J.* 2002;143:412–417.
7. Amato L, Paolisso G, Cacciatore F, et al. Congestive heart failure predicts the development of non-insulin-dependent diabetes mellitus in the elderly. The Osservatorio Geriatrico Regione Campania Group. *Diabetes Metab.* 1997;23:213–218.
8. Nichols GA, Hillier TA, Erbey JR, et al. Congestive heart failure in type 2 diabetes: prevalence, incidence, and risk factors. *Diabetes Care.* 2001;24:1614–1619.
9. Stone PH, Muller JE, Hartwell T, et al. The effect of diabetes mellitus on prognosis and serial left ventricular function after acute myocardial infarction: contribution of both coronary disease and diastolic left ventricular dysfunction to the adverse prognosis. The MILIS Study Group. *J Am Coll Cardiol.* 1989; 14:49–57.
10. Kannel WB. Vital epidemiologic clues in heart failure. *J Clin Epidemiol.* 2000;53:229–235.
11. He J, Ogden LG, Bazzano LA, et al. Risk factors for congestive heart failure in US men and women: NHANES I epidemiologic follow-up study. *Arch Intern Med.* 2001;161:996–1002.
12. Nichols GA, Gullion CM, Koro CE, et al. The incidence of congestive heart failure in type 2 diabetes: an update. *Diabetes Care.* 2004;27:1879–1884.

13. Bibbins-Domingo K, Lin F, Vittinghoff E, et al. Predictors of heart failure among women with coronary disease. *Circulation.* 2004;110:1424–1430.
14. Barzilay JI, Kronmal RA, Gottdiener JS, et al. The association of fasting glucose levels with congestive heart failure in diabetic adults > or = 65 years: the Cardiovascular Health Study. *J Am Coll Cardiol.* 2004;43:2236–2241.
15. Iribarren C, Karter AJ, Go AS, et al. Glycemic control and heart failure among adult patients with diabetes. *Circulation.* 2001;103: 2668–2673.
16. Beckman JA, Creager MA, Libby P. Diabetes and atherosclerosis: epidemiology, pathophysiology, and management. *JAMA.* 2002;287:2570–2581.
17. Ho KK, Pinsky JL, Kannel WB, et al. The epidemiology of heart failure: the Framingham Study. *J Am Coll Cardiol.* 1993;22:6A–13A.
18. Reaven GM, Lithell H, Landsberg L. Hypertension and associated metabolic abnormalities—the role of insulin resistance and the sympathoadrenal system. *N Engl J Med.* 1996;334:374–381.
19. Lopaschuk GD. Metabolic abnormalities in the diabetic heart. *Heart Fail Rev.* 2002;7:149–159.
20. Swan JW, Walton C, Godsland IF, et al. Insulin resistance in chronic heart failure. *Eur Heart J.* 1994;15:1528–1532.
21. Witteles RM, Tang WH, Jamali AH, et al. Insulin resistance in idiopathic dilated cardiomyopathy: a possible etiologic link. *J Am Coll Cardiol.* 2004;44:78–81.
22. Tenenbaum A, Motro M, Fisman EZ, et al. Functional class in patients with heart failure is associated with the development of diabetes. *Am J Med.* 2003;114:271–275.
23. Shah A, Shannon RP. Insulin resistance in dilated cardiomyopathy. *Rev Cardiovasc Med.* 2003;4 (Suppl 6):S50–S57.
24. Bell DS. Heart failure: the frequent, forgotten, and often fatal complication of diabetes. *Diabetes Care* 2003;26:2433–2441.
25. Bell DS. Diabetic cardiomyopathy. *Diabetes Care.* 2003;26: 2949–2951.
26. Dries DL, Sweitzer NK, Drazner MH, et al. Prognostic impact of diabetes mellitus in patients with heart failure according to the etiology of left ventricular systolic dysfunction. *J Am Coll Cardiol.* 2001;38:421–428.
27. Das SR, Drazner MH, Yancy CW, et al. Effects of diabetes mellitus and ischemic heart disease on the progression from asymptomatic left ventricular dysfunction to symptomatic heart failure: a retrospective analysis from the Studies of Left Ventricular Dysfunction (SOLVD) Prevention trial. *Am Heart J.* 2004;148:883–888.
28. Domanski M, Krause-Steinrauf H, Deedwania P, et al. The effect of diabetes on outcomes of patients with advanced heart failure in the BEST trial. *J Am Coll Cardiol.* 2003;42:914–922.
29. Smooke S, Horwich TB, Fonarow GC. Insulin-treated diabetes is associated with a marked increase in mortality in patients with advanced heart failure. *Am Heart J.* 2005;149:168–174.
30. Croft JB, Giles WH, Pollard RA, et al. Heart failure survival among older adults in the United States: a poor prognosis for an emerging epidemic in the Medicare population. *Arch Intern Med.* 1999;159:505–510.
31. Gustafsson I, Brendorp B, Seibaek M, et al. Influence of diabetes and diabetes-gender interaction on the risk of death in patients hospitalized with congestive heart failure. *J Am Coll Cardiol.* 2004;43:771–777.
32. Shekelle PG, Rich MW, Morton SC, et al. Efficacy of angiotensin-converting enzyme inhibitors and beta-blockers in the management of left ventricular systolic dysfunction according to race, gender, and diabetic status: a meta-analysis of major clinical trials. *J Am Coll Cardiol.* 2003;41:1529–1538.
33. Ryden L, Armstrong PW, Cleland JG, et al. Efficacy and safety of high-dose lisinopril in chronic heart failure patients at high cardiovascular risk, including those with diabetes mellitus. Results from the ATLAS trial. *Eur Heart J.* 2000;21:1967–1978.
34. Deedwania PC, Giles TD, Klibaner M, et al. Efficacy, safety and tolerability of metoprolol CR/XL in patients with diabetes and chronic heart failure: experiences from MERIT-HF. *Am Heart J.* 2005;149:159–167.
35. Packer M, Coats AJ, Fowler MB, et al. Effect of carvedilol on survival in severe chronic heart failure. *N Engl J Med.* 2001;344:1651–1658.
36. Poole-Wilson PA, Swedberg K, Cleland JG, et al. Comparison of carvedilol and metoprolol on clinical outcomes in patients with chronic heart failure in the Carvedilol Or Metoprolol European Trial (COMET): randomised controlled trial. *Lancet* 2003;362: 7–13.
37. Bell DS. Advantages of a third-generation beta-blocker in patients with diabetes mellitus. *Am J Cardiol.* 2004;93:49B–52B.
38. Fonarow GC. Managing the patient with diabetes mellitus and heart failure: issues and considerations. *Am J Med.* 2004;116 (Suppl 5A):76S–88S.
39. Bakris GL, Fonseca V, Katholi RE, et al. Metabolic effects of carvedilol vs metoprolol in patients with type 2 diabetes mellitus and hypertension: a randomized controlled trial. *JAMA.* 2004;292:2227–2236.
40. Pitt B, Remme W, Zannad F, et al. Eplerenone, a selective aldosterone blocker, in patients with left ventricular dysfunction after myocardial infarction. *N Engl J Med.* 2003;348:1309–1321.
41. Pitt B, Zannad F, Remme WJ, et al. The effect of spironolactone on morbidity and mortality in patients with severe heart failure. Randomized Aldactone Evaluation Study Investigators. *N Engl J Med.* 1999;341:709–717.
42. Tamirisa KP, Aaronson KD, Koelling TM. Spironolactone-induced renal insufficiency and hyperkalemia in patients with heart failure. *Am Heart J.* 2004;148:971–978.
43. Palmer BF. Managing hyperkalemia caused by inhibitors of the renin-angiotensin-aldosterone system. *N Engl J Med.* 2004;351: 585–592.
44. Masoudi FA, Inzucchi SE, Wang Y, et al. Thiazolidinediones, metformin, and outcomes in older patients with diabetes and heart failure: an observational study. *Circulation.* 2005;111:583–590.
45. Berger AK, Breall JA, Gersh BJ, et al. Effect of diabetes mellitus and insulin use on survival after acute myocardial infarction in the elderly (the Cooperative Cardiovascular Project). *Am J Cardiol.* 2001;87:272–277.
46. Kern W, Peters A, Born J, et al. Changes in blood pressure and plasma catecholamine levels during prolonged hyperinsulinemia. *Metabolism* 2005;54:391–396.
47. Bristol-Myers Squibb. Glucophage prescribing information. Bristol-Myers Squibb, New York; 2004.
48. Nesto RW, Bell D, Bonow RO, et al. Thiazolidinedione use, fluid retention, and congestive heart failure: a consensus statement from the American Heart Association and American Diabetes Association. October 7, 2003. *Circulation.* 2003;108:2941–2948.
49. Tang WH, Francis GS, Hoogwerf BJ, et al. Fluid retention after initiation of thiazolidinedione therapy in diabetic patients with established chronic heart failure. *J Am Coll Cardiol.* 2003;41:1394–1398.
50. St John Sutton M, Rendell M, Dandona P, et al. A comparison of the effects of rosiglitazone and glyburide on cardiovascular function and glycemic control in patients with type 2 diabetes. *Diabetes Care.* 2002;25:2058–2064.
51. Masoudi FA, Wang Y, Inzucchi SE, et al. Metformin and thiazolidinedione use in Medicare patients with heart failure. *JAMA.* 2003;290:81–85.
52. Al-Ahmad A, Rand WM, Manjunath G, et al. Reduced kidney function and anemia as risk factors for mortality in patients with left ventricular dysfunction. *J Am Coll Cardiol.* 2001;38:955–962.
53. Ezekowitz JA, McAlister FA, Armstrong PW. Anemia is common in heart failure and is associated with poor outcomes: insights from a cohort of 12,065 patients with new-onset heart failure. *Circulation.* 2003;107:223–225.
54. Horwich TB, Fonarow GC, Hamilton MA, et al. Anemia is associated with worse symptoms, greater impairment in functional capacity and a significant increase in mortality in patients with advanced heart failure. *J Am Coll Cardiol.* 2002;39:1780–1786.
55. Felker GM, Gattis WA, Leimberger JD, et al. Usefulness of anemia as a predictor of death and rehospitalization in patients with decompensated heart failure. *Am J Cardiol.* 2003;92:625–628.
56. Cromie N, Lee C, Struthers AD. Anaemia in chronic heart failure: what is its frequency in the UK and its underlying causes? *Heart.* 2002;87:377–378.
57. Androne AS, Katz SD, Lund L, et al. Hemodilution is common in patients with advanced heart failure. *Circulation.* 2003;107: 226–229.
58. Deswal A, Petersen NJ, Feldman AM, et al. Cytokines and cytokine receptors in advanced heart failure: an analysis of the cytokine database from the Vesnarinone trial (VEST). *Circulation.* 2001;103:2055–2059.

59. van der Meer P, Voors AA, Lipsic E, et al. Prognostic value of plasma erythropoietin on mortality in patients with chronic heart failure. *J Am Coll Cardiol*. 2004;44:63–67.
60. Ishani A, Weinhandl E, Zhao Z, et al. Angiotensin-converting enzyme inhibitor as a risk factor for the development of anemia, and the impact of incident anemia on mortality in patients with left ventricular dysfunction. *J Am Coll Cardiol*. 2005;45:391–399.
61. Witte KK, Desilva R, Chattopadhyay S, et al. Are hematinic deficiencies the cause of anemia in chronic heart failure? *Am Heart J*. 2004;147:924–930.
62. Ralli S, Horwich TB, Fonarow GC. Relationship between anemia, cardiac troponin I, and B-type natriuretic peptide levels and mortality in patients with advanced heart failure. *Am Heart J*. 2005.In press.
63. Anand I, McMurray JJ, Whitmore J, et al. Anemia and its relationship to clinical outcome in heart failure. *Circulation*. 2004;110:149–154.
64. Kannel WB. Epidemiology and prevention of cardiac failure: Framingham Study insights. *Eur Heart J*. 1987;8(Suppl F):23–26.
65. Foley RN, Parfrey PS, Harnett JD, et al. The impact of anemia on cardiomyopathy, morbidity, and mortality in end-stage renal disease. *Am J Kidney Dis*. 1996;28:53–61.
66. Sharma R, Francis DP, Pitt B, et al. Haemoglobin predicts survival in patients with chronic heart failure: a substudy of the ELITE II trial. *Eur Heart J*. 2004;25:1021–1028.
67. Kalra PR, Collier T, Cowie MR, et al. Haemoglobin concentration and prognosis in new cases of heart failure. *Lancet*. 2003;362:211–212.
68. Brucks S, Little WC, Chao T, et al. Relation of anemia to diastolic heart failure and the effect on outcome. *Am J Cardiol*. 2004;93: 1055–1057.
69. Silverberg DS, Wexler D, Sheps D, et al. The effect of correction of mild anemia in severe, resistant congestive heart failure using subcutaneous erythropoietin and intravenous iron: a randomized controlled study. *J Am Coll Cardiol*. 2001;37: 1775–1780.
70. Mancini DM, Katz SD, Lang CC, et al. Effect of erythropoietin on exercise capacity in patients with moderate to severe chronic heart failure. *Circulation*. 2003;107:294–299.
71. Fiordaliso F, Chimenti S, Staszewsky L, et al. A nonerythropoietic derivative of erythropoietin protects the myocardium from ischemia-reperfusion injury. *Proc Natl Acad Sci USA*. 2005;102: 2046–2051.
72. Besarab A, Bolton WK, Browne JK, et al. The effects of normal as compared with low hematocrit values in patients with cardiac disease who are receiving hemodialysis and epoetin. *N Engl J Med*. 1998;339:584–590.
73. Hedley AA, Ogden CL, Johnson CL, et al. Prevalence of overweight and obesity among US children, adolescents, and adults, 1999–2002. *JAMA*. 2004;291:2847–2850.
74. de Divitiis O, Fazio S, Petitto M, et al. Obesity and cardiac function. *Circulation*. 1981;64:477–482.
75. Wong CY, O'Moore-Sullivan T, Leano R, et al. Alterations of left ventricular myocardial characteristics associated with obesity. *Circulation*. 2004;110:3081–3087.
76. Peterson LR, Waggoner AD, Schechtman KB, et al. Alterations in left ventricular structure and function in young healthy obese women: assessment by echocardiography and tissue Doppler imaging. *J Am Coll Cardiol*. 2004;43:1399–1404.
77. Pascual M, Pascual DA, Soria F, et al. Effects of isolated obesity on systolic and diastolic left ventricular function. *Heart* 2003;89:1152–1156.
78. Schunkert H. Obesity and target organ damage: the heart. *Int J Obes Relat Metab Disord*. 2002;26(Suppl 4):S15–S20.
79. Kenchaiah S, Evans JC, Levy D, et al. Obesity and the risk of heart failure. *N Engl J Med*. 2002;347:305–313.
80. Davos CH, Doehner W, Rauchhaus M, et al. Body mass and survival in patients with chronic heart failure without cachexia: the importance of obesity. *J Card Fail*. 2003;9:29–35.
81. Lavie CJ, Osman AF, Milani RV, Mehra MR. Body composition and prognosis in chronic systolic heart failure: the obesity paradox. *Am J Cardiol*. 2003;91:891–894.
82. Gustafsson F, Kragelund CB, Torp-Pedersen C, et al. Effect of obesity and being overweight on long-term mortality in congestive heart failure: influence of left ventricular systolic function. *Eur Heart J*. 2005;26:58–64.
83. Curtis JP, Selter JG, Wang Y, et al. The obesity paradox: body mass index and outcomes in patients with heart failure. *Arch Intern Med*. 2005;165:55–61.
84. Horwich TB, Fonarow GC, Hamilton MA, et al. The relationship between obesity and mortality in patients with heart failure. *J Am Coll Cardiol*. 2001;38:789–795.
85. Butler J, Howser R, Portner PM, et al. Body mass index and outcomes after left ventricular assist device placement. *Ann Thorac Surg*. 2005;79:66–73.
86. Kalantar-Zadeh K, Block G, Horwich T, et al. Reverse epidemiology of conventional cardiovascular risk factors in patients with chronic heart failure. *J Am Coll Cardiol*. 2004;43:1439–1444.
87. Zuber M, Kaeslin T, Studer T, et al. Weight loss of 146 kg with diet and reversal of severe congestive heart failure in a young, morbidly obese patient. *Am J Cardiol*. 1999;84:955–956, A8.
88. Alpert MA, Terry BE, Mulekar M, et al. Cardiac morphology and left ventricular function in normotensive morbidly obese patients with and without congestive heart failure, and effect of weight loss. *Am J Cardiol*. 1997;80:736–740.
89. Anker SD, Ponikowski P, Varney S, et al. Wasting as independent risk factor for mortality in chronic heart failure. *Lancet*. 1997;349: 1050–1053.
90. Anker SD, Chua TP, Ponikowski P, et al. Hormonal changes and catabolic/anabolic imbalance in chronic heart failure and their importance for cardiac cachexia. *Circulation*. 1997;96:526–534.
91. Lietz K, John R, Burke EA, et al. Pretransplant cachexia and morbid obesity are predictors of increased mortality after heart transplantation. *Transplantation*. 2001;72:277–283.
92. Pekkanen J, Linn S, Heiss G, et al. Ten-year mortality from cardiovascular disease in relation to cholesterol level among men with and without preexisting cardiovascular disease. *N Engl J Med*. 1990;322:1700–1707.
93. Kannel WB, Belanger AJ. Epidemiology of heart failure. *Am Heart J*. 1991;121:951–957.
94. Kjekshus J, Pedersen TR, Olsson AG, et al. The effects of simvatatin on the incidence of heart failure in patients with coronary heart disease. *J Card Fail*. 1997;3:249–254.
95. Horwich TB, Hamilton MA, Maclellan WR, et al. Low serum total cholesterol is associated with marked increase in mortality in advanced heart failure. *J Card Fail*. 2002;8:216–224.
96. Rauchhaus M, Clark AL, Doehner W, et al. The relationship between cholesterol and survival in patients with chronic heart failure. *J Am Coll Cardiol*. 2003;42:1933–1940.
97. Trochu JN, Mital S, Zhang X, et al. Preservation of NO production by statins in the treatment of heart failure. *Cardiovasc Res*. 2003;60:250–258.
98. Rauchhaus M, Coats AJ, Anker SD. The endotoxin-lipoprotein hypothesis. *Lancet*. 2000;356:930–933.
99. Pliquett RU, Cornish KG, Peuler JD, et al. Simvastatin normalizes autonomic neural control in experimental heart failure. *Circulation* 2003;107:2493–2498.
100. Bauersachs J, Galuppo P, Fraccarollo D, et al. Improvement of left ventricular remodeling and function by hydroxymethylglutaryl coenzyme a reductase inhibition with cerivastatin in rats with heart failure after myocardial infarction. *Circulation*. 2001;104:982–985.
101. Tousoulis D, Antoniades C, Bosinakou E, et al. Effects of atorvastatin on reactive hyperemia and inflammatory process in patients with congestive heart failure. *Atherosclerosis*. 2005;178:359–363.
102. Ashton E, Liew D, Krum H. Should patients with chronic heart failure be treated with "statins"? *Heart Fail Monit*. 2003;3:82–86.
103. Sacks FM, Pfeffer MA, Moye LA, et al. The effect of pravastatin on coronary events after myocardial infarction in patients with average cholesterol levels. Cholesterol and Recurrent Events Trial investigators. *N Engl J Med*. 1996;335:1001–1009.
104. Horwich TB, MacLellan WR, Fonarow GC. Statin therapy is associated with improved survival in ischemic and non-ischemic heart failure. *J Am Coll Cardiol*. 2004;43:642–648.
105. Mozaffarian D, Nye R, Levy WC. Statin therapy is associated with lower mortality among patients with severe heart failure. *Am J Cardiol*. 2004;93:1124–1129.
106. Ray JG, Gong Y, Sykora K, et al. Statin use and survival outcomes in elderly patients with heart failure. *Arch Intern Med*. 2005;165: 62–67.

107. Node K, Fujita M, Kitakaze M, et al. Short-term statin therapy improves cardiac function and symptoms in patients with idiopathic dilated cardiomyopathy. *Circulation.* 2003;108:839–843.
108. Tavazzi L, Tognoni G, Franzosi MG, et al. Rationale and design of the GISSI heart failure trial: a large trial to assess the effects of n-3 polyunsaturated fatty acids and rosuvastatin in symptomatic congestive heart failure. *Eur J Heart Fail.* 2004;6:635–641.
109. Viegi G, Scognamiglio A, Baldacci S, et al. Epidemiology of chronic obstructive pulmonary disease (COPD). *Respiration.* 2001;68:4–19.
110. Fonarow GC, Adams KF, Jr., Abraham WT, et al. Risk stratification for in-hospital mortality in acutely decompensated heart failure: classification and regression tree analysis. *JAMA.* 2005;293: 572–580.
111. Scarduelli C, Ambrosino N, Confalonieri M, et al. Prevalence and prognostic role of cardiovascular complications in patients with exacerbation of chronic obstructive pulmonary disease admitted to Italian respiratory intensive care units. *Ital Heart J.* 2004;5:932–938.
112. Sirak TE, Jelic S, Le Jemtel TH. Therapeutic update: non-selective beta- and alpha-adrenergic blockade in patients with coexistent chronic obstructive pulmonary disease and chronic heart failure. *J Am Coll Cardiol.* 2004;44:497–502.
113. Caruana L, Petrie MC, Davie AP, et al. Do patients with suspected heart failure and preserved left ventricular systolic function suffer from "diastolic heart failure" or from misdiagnosis? A prospective descriptive study. *BMJ.* 2000;321:215–218.
114. Morrison LK, Harrison A, Krishnaswamy P, et al. Utility of a rapid B-natriuretic peptide assay in differentiating congestive heart failure from lung disease in patients presenting with dyspnea. *J Am Coll Cardiol.* 2002;39:202–209.
115. McCullough PA, Hollander JE, Nowak RM, et al. Uncovering heart failure in patients with a history of pulmonary disease: rationale for the early use of B-type natriuretic peptide in the emergency department. *Acad Emerg Med.* 2003;10:198–204.
116. Dimopoulou I, Daganou M, Tsintzas OK, et al. Effects of severity of long-standing congestive heart failure on pulmonary function. *Respir Med.* 1998;92:1321–1325.
117. Hosenpud JD, Stibolt TA, Atwal K, et al. Abnormal pulmonary function specifically related to congestive heart failure: comparison of patients before and after cardiac transplantation. *Am J Med.* 1990;88:493–496.
118. Wasserman K, Zhang YY, Gitt A, et al. Lung function and exercise gas exchange in chronic heart failure. *Circulation.* 1997;96: 2221–2227.
119. Harjai KJ, Thompson HW, Turgut T, et al. Simple clinical variables are markers of the propensity for readmission in patients hospitalized with heart failure. *Am J Cardiol.* 2001;87:234–237, A9.
120. Lee DS, Austin PC, Rouleau JL, et al. Predicting mortality among patients hospitalized for heart failure: derivation and validation of a clinical model. *JAMA.* 2003;290:2581–2587.
121. Maggioni AP, Sinagra G, Opasich C, et al. Treatment of chronic heart failure with beta adrenergic blockade beyond controlled clinical trials: the BRING-UP experience. *Heart.* 2003;89:299–305.
122. No authors listed. The Cardiac Insufficiency Bisoprolol Study II (CIBIS-II): a randomised trial. *Lancet.* 1999;353:9–13.
123. Ormiston TM, Salpeter SR. Beta-blocker use in patients with congestive heart failure and concomitant obstructive airway disease: moving from myth to evidence-based practice. *Heart Fail Monit.* 2003;4:45–54.
124. Salpeter SR, Ormiston TM, Salpeter EE, et al. Cardioselective beta-blockers for chronic obstructive pulmonary disease: a meta-analysis. *Respir Med.* 2003;97:1094–1101.
125. Salpeter SR, Ormiston TM, Salpeter EE. Cardioselective beta-blockers in patients with reactive airway disease: a meta-analysis. *Ann Intern Med.* 2002;137:715–725.
126. Krum H, Ninio D, MacDonald P. Baseline predictors of tolerability to carvedilol in patients with chronic heart failure. *Heart.* 2000;84:615–619.
127. Kotlyar E, Keogh AM, Macdonald PS, et al. Tolerability of carvedilol in patients with heart failure and concomitant chronic obstructive pulmonary disease or asthma. *J Heart Lung Transp.* 2002;21:1290–1295.
128. Sutherland ER, Cherniack RM. Management of chronic obstructive pulmonary disease. *N Engl J Med.* 2004;350:2689–2697.
129. Hunt SA, Baker DW, Chin MH, et al. ACC/AHA guidelines for the evaluation and management of chronic heart failure in the adult: a report of the American College of Cardiology/American Heart Association Task Force on Practice Guidelines (Committee to Revise the 1995 Guidelines for the Evaluation and Management of Heart Failure). 2001: American College of Cardiology Web site.
130. Au DH, Udris EM, Curtis JR, et al. Association between chronic heart failure and inhaled beta-2-adrenoceptor agonists. *Am Heart J.* 2004;148:915–920.
131. Au DH, Udris EM, Fan VS, et al. Risk of mortality and heart failure exacerbations associated with inhaled beta-adrenoceptor agonists among patients with known left ventricular systolic dysfunction. *Chest.* 2003;123:1964–1969.
132. Martin RM, Dunn NR, Freemantle SN, et al. Risk of non-fatal cardiac failure and ischaemic heart disease with long acting beta 2 agonists. *Thorax.* 1998;53:558–562.
133. Suissa S, Hemmelgarn B, Blais L, et al. Bronchodilators and acute cardiac death. *Am J Respir Crit Care Med.* 1996;154:1598–1602.
134. Poller U, Fuchs B, Gorf A, et al. Terbutaline-induced desensitization of human cardiac beta 2-adrenoceptor-mediated positive inotropic effects: attenuation by ketotifen. *Cardiovasc Res.* 1998;40:211–222.
135. Liggett SB, Wagoner LE, Craft LL, et al. The Ile164 beta2-adrenergic receptor polymorphism adversely affects the outcome of congestive heart failure. *J Clin Invest.* 1998;102:1534–1539.
136. Giugliano D, Acampora R, Marfella R, et al. Metabolic and cardiovascular effects of carvedilol and atenolol in non-insulin-dependent diabetes mellitus and hypertension. A randomized, controlled trial. *Ann Intern Med.* 1997;126:955–959.
137. Sin DD, Fitzgerald F, Parker JD, et al. Risk factors for central and obstructive sleep apnea in 450 men and women with congestive heart failure. *Am J Respir Crit Care Med.* 1999;160:1101–1106.
138. Javaheri S, Parker TJ, Liming JD, et al. Sleep apnea in 81 ambulatory male patients with stable heart failure. Types and their prevalences, consequences, and presentations. *Circulation.* 1998;97: 2154–2159.
139. Trupp RJ, Hardesty P, Osborne J, et al. Prevalence of sleep disordered breathing in a heart failure program. *Congest Heart Fail.* 2004;10:217–220.
140. Chan J, Sanderson J, Chan W, et al. Prevalence of sleep-disordered breathing in diastolic heart failure. *Chest.* 1997;111:1488–1493.
141. Shamsuzzaman AS, Gersh BJ, Somers VK. Obstructive sleep apnea: implications for cardiac and vascular disease. *JAMA.* 2003;290:1906–1914.
142. Hanly P, Zuberi-Khokhar N. Daytime sleepiness in patients with congestive heart failure and Cheyne-Stokes respiration. *Chest.* 1995;107:952–958.
143. Ancoli-Israel S, DuHamel ER, Stepnowsky C, et al. The relationship between congestive heart failure, sleep apnea, and mortality in older men. *Chest.* 2003;124:1400–1405.
144. Hanly PJ, Zuberi-Khokhar NS. Increased mortality associated with Cheyne-Stokes respiration in patients with congestive heart failure. *Am J Respir Crit Care Med.* 1996;153:272–276.
145. Bradley TD. Right and left ventricular functional impairment and sleep apnea. *Clin Chest Med.* 1992;13:459–479.
146. Somers VK, Dyken ME, Clary MP, et al. Sympathetic neural mechanisms in obstructive sleep apnea. *J Clin Invest.* 1995;96: 1897–1904.
147. Shamsuzzaman AS, Winnicki M, Lanfranchi P, et al. Elevated C-reactive protein in patients with obstructive sleep apnea. *Circulation.* 2002;105:2462–2464.
148. Kato M, Roberts-Thomson P, Phillips BG, et al. Impairment of endothelium-dependent vasodilation of resistance vessels in patients with obstructive sleep apnea. *Circulation.* 2000;102: 2607–2610.
149. Sin DD, Logan AG, Fitzgerald FS, et al. Effects of continuous positive airway pressure on cardiovascular outcomes in heart failure patients with and without Cheyne-Stokes respiration. *Circulation.* 2000;102:61–66.
150. Kaneko Y, Floras JS, Usui K, et al. Cardiovascular effects of continuous positive airway pressure in patients with heart failure and obstructive sleep apnea. *N Engl J Med.* 2003;348:1233–1241.
151. Sinha AM, Skobel EC, Breithardt OA, et al. Cardiac resynchronization therapy improves central sleep apnea and Cheyne-Stokes

respiration in patients with chronic heart failure. *J Am Coll Cardiol.* 2004;44:68–71.

152. Jiang W, Alexander J, Christopher E, et al. Relationship of depression to increased risk of mortality and rehospitalization in patients with congestive heart failure. *Arch Intern Med.* 2001;161: 1849–1856.
153. Koenig HG. Depression in hospitalized older patients with congestive heart failure. *Gen Hosp Psychiatry.* 1998;20:29–43.
154. Rumsfeld JS, Havranek E, Masoudi FA, et al. Depressive symptoms are the strongest predictors of short-term declines in health status in patients with heart failure. *J Am Coll Cardiol.* 2003;42:1811–1817.
155. Havranek EP, Spertus JA, Masoudi FA, et al. Predictors of the onset of depressive symptoms in patients with heart failure. *J Am Coll Cardiol.* 2004;44:2333–2338.
156. Jiang W, Kuchibhatla M, Cuffe MS, et al. Prognostic value of anxiety and depression in patients with chronic heart failure. *Circulation.* 2004;110:3452–3456.
157. Westlake C, Dracup K, Fonarow G, et al. Depression in patients with heart failure. *J Card Fail.* 2005;11:30–35.
158. Guck TP, Elsasser GN, Kavan MG, et al. Depression and congestive heart failure. *Congest Heart Fail.* 2003;9:163–169.

40

Management of Supraventricular Arrhythmias in Patients with Heart Failure

Gregory K. Feld   Doug Gibson   David Krummen

Heart failure is associated with significant morbidity and mortality. Cardiac arrythmias are particularly common in patients with this condition and they appear to increase risk for an event. The greatest risk of mortality is associated with ventricular arrhythmias, which can lead to sudden death. However, supraventricular arrhythmias may also increase morbidity and mortality in heart failure patients (1,2). Of particular concern is the development of atrial fibrillation, which may lead to systemic emboli causing stroke and increased risk of mortality (3–5). Due to the complex mechanisms of supraventricular arrhythmias (Table 40-1) and the potential adverse effects of standard pharmacological therapy in patients with heart failure (Table 40-2), the approach to their diagnosis and treatment (Table 40-3) represents a formidable challenge to the clinician. The diagnosis and management of supraventricular arrhythmias in the patient with heart failure will be addressed in this chapter.

PATHOPHYSIOLOGY OF HEART FAILURE AS IT RELATES TO DEVELOPMENT OF SUPRAVENTRICULAR ARRHYTHMIAS

Supraventricular arrhythmias are more likely to occur in heart failure patients as a result of the associated hemodynamic and electrophysiological abnormalities. Heart failure is typically characterized by increased ventricular diastolic and atrial pressure and, not infrequently, mitral and tricuspid valve regurgitation—abnormalities that may ultimately lead to atrial dilatation and hypertrophy and fibrosis. These hemodynamic and pathophysiological derangements may then lead to abnormalities in atrial electrophysiology, a process called electrical remodeling, with resultant shortening and dispersion of atrial refractoriness and depression of conduction velocity, all of which may predispose to the development of supraventricular arrhythmias (6,7).

Patients with heart failure may also have an abnormally low cardiac output and a compensatory increase in sympathetic nervous system tone, which further increases the risk for development of supraventricular arrhythmias and may make them even more difficult to treat pharmacologically. In addition, since many of the antiarrhythmic drugs used to treat atrial arrhythmias have negative inotropic and chronotropic effects (i.e., they depress contractility and heart rate, respectively), they may worsen heart failure, which, in turn, may reduce their efficacy. Thus, heart failure with its associated hemodynamic and pathophysiological abnormalities creates a favorable electrophysiological milieu for the development of supraventricular arrhythmias and complicates their treatment.

Diagnosis and Treatment of Supraventricular Arrhythmias

Paroxysmal Supraventricular Tachycardia

Supraventricular arrhythmias of any type (Table 40-1), including paroxysmal supraventricular tachycardia (PSVT), may occur in patients with heart failure. The most common forms of PSVT in the general population (8–10) include atrioventricular (AV) nodal re-entrant tachycardia (AVNRT) due to dual AV nodal physiology (Fig. 40-1A,B) and atrioventricular re-entrant tachycardia (AVRT) due to an accessory

TABLE 40-1
SUPRAVENTRICULAR ARRHYTHMIAS

Arrhythmia	Electrophysiologic Mechanism
Sinus node re-entry	Re-entry within or around area of sinus node
Inappropriate sinus tachycardia	Abnormal automaticity in area of sinus node
Interatrial re-entrant tachycardia	Re-entry around scar or area of slow conduction in RA or LA
Focal atrial tachycardia	Abnormal automaticity or triggered activity from a focal area of RA or LA
MAT (multifocal atrial tachycardia)	Abnormal automatcity or triggered activity from multiple foci in RA or LA
Typical (reverse typical) atrial flutter	Macrore-entry circuit in RA, utilizing CTI
Atypical atrial flutter	Functional or anatomical re-entry circuit not utilizing CTI
Paroxysmal atrial fibrillation	Triggered by premature beats originating from the pulmonary veins
Chronic atrial fibrillation	Multiple functional and/or anatomical re-entry circuits in RA and LA
AV nodal re-entry (AVNRT)	Re-entry utilizing and slow AV nodal pathways
Orthodromic AV reentry due to AP	Macrore-entry utilizing AV node antegrade and AP retrograde
Antidromic AV reentry due to AP	Macrore-entry utilizing AP antegrade and AV node retrograde

AP, accessory pathway or accessory atrioventricular connection; AV, atrioventricular; CCW, counterclockwise; CTI, cavo-tricuspid isthmus; CW, clockwise; F-S, fast-slow; LA, left atrium; RA, right atrium; S-F, slow-fast; S-S, slow-slow.

pathway (Fig. 40-2A,B). Although heart failure does not specifically predispose to development of these two forms of PSVT (which are due to underlying abnormal electrophysiological circuits), it may increase the frequency or duration of these arrhythmias as a result of increased circulating serum catecholamine levels and electrical remodeling.

Treatment of PSVT requires not only that the arrhythmia be documented but also that the underlying electrophysiological mechanism be determined if possible (i.e., AVNRT or AVRT), since these two forms of PSVT may respond differently to medical treatment. The underlying mechanism of PSVT can often be delineated by electrocardiogram (ECG) if the arrhythmia can be recorded, especially if during sinus rhythm there is ventricular pre-excitation suggesting Wolff-Parkinson-White (WPW) syndrome. However, in many instances the arrhythmia is nonsustained, making ECG documentation difficult. In such a case, a 24-hour Holter monitor may record a diagnostic ECG if the arrhythmia occurs daily, or a 30-day event monitor (e.g., patient-activated or continuous-loop) may be required if the arrhythmia is less frequent. Once an ECG recording of the arrhythmia has been obtained, a determination of the underlying mechanism can be made in the majority of cases and empiric treatment begun, if indicated.

In some cases, however, documentation of the arrhythmia by ECG fails and the patient must undergo a diagnostic electrophysiology (EP) study. The EP study is a percutaneous, catheterization-based procedure, performed under light sedation, which is guided fluoroscopically or by a three-dimensional electroanatomical (contact or noncontact electrode) mapping system. To perform an EP study, typically two to four multielectrode (i.e., 4 to 20 electrodes) catheters are inserted into the heart, baseline electrical activity is recorded to identify any abnormalities in the electrical conduction system, and the heart is stimulated electrically to induce the clinical arrhythmia. During an EP study, PSVT can be induced in most patients with a history of

TABLE 40-2
TREATMENT OF SUPRAVENTRICULAR ARRHYTHMIAS

Class	Drug Name	Arrhythmias Treated with Drug
IA	Quinidine, disopyramide, procainamide, moricizine	AVRT, AVNRT, AFL, AFIB, IART, AAT
IC$^{\alpha}$	Flecainide$^{\alpha}$, propafenone$^{\alpha}$	AVRT, AVNRT, AFL, AFIB, IART, AAT
II	Beta-blockers (e.g. propranolol, lopressor, metoprolol)	SNRT, IST, AVNRT, AVRT, AAT, AFL, AFIB
III$^{\beta}$	Sotalol, amiodarone	SNRT, IST, AVNRT, AVRT, AAT, IART, AFL, AFIB
IV	AV node blockers (e.g. verapamil, diltiazem)	SNRT, IST, AVNRT, AFL, AFIB
	Digoxin	SNRT, IST, AVNRT, AFL, AFIB

AAT, automatic atrial tachycardia (focal); AVNRT, AV nodal re-entrant tachycardia; AVRT, atrioventricular re-entrant tachycardia (using accessory pathway in antegrade or retrograde direction; AFIB, atrial fibrillation; AFL, atrial flutter; IART, inter atrial re-entrant tachycardia; IST, inappropriate sinus tachycardia; SNRT, sinus node re-entrant tachycardia; α, to be avoided in patients with coronary artery disease, significant ventricular hypertrophy, or heart failure, due to increased risk of mortality as a result of ventricular proarrhythmia associated with their use; β, safer than the Class I drugs in pateints with coronary artery disease, hypertrophy, or heart failure.

TABLE 40-3
DIAGNOSIS OF SUPRAVENTRICULAR ARRHYTHMIAS

Arrhythmia Mechanism	Pharmacological	Nonpharmacological
Sinus node re-entry	Class II, IV, III, or digoxin	RFCA of focal origin near SA node
Inappropriate sinus tachycardia	Class II, IV, III, or digoxin	RFCA of focal origin near SA node
Interatrial re-entrant tachycardia	Class III, IA, IC Class II, IV, digoxin for rate control	RFCA of critical isthmus in circuit demonstrating concealed entrainment
Focal automatic atrial tachycardia	Class II, IC, IA, III Class II, IV, digoxin for rate control	RFCA of focal origin
MAT (multifocal atrial tachycardia)	Class IA, IC, III Class II, IV, digoxin for rate control	AV node ablation with permanent pacemaker implantation
Atrial flutter (Type 1, CCW and CW)	Class III, IA, IC Class II, IV, digoxin for rate control	RFCA of CTI
Atrial flutter (Type 2)	Class III, IA, IC Class II, IV, digoxin for rate control	RFCA of AV node with pacemaker implantation, or AV node modification
Paroxysmal atrial fibrillation	Class IC, IA, III Class II, IV, digoxin for rate control	Curative pulmonary vein isolation, RFCA of AV node with pacemaker implantation, or AV node modification
Chronic atrial fibrillation	Class IA, IC, III Class II, IV, digoxin for rate control	Curative left atrial linear ablation with or without pulmonary vein isolation, RFCA of AV node with pacemaker implantation or AV node modification
AV nodal re-entry (AVNRT)	Class II, IV, digoxin Class IA, IC, III	RFCA of AV nodal slow pathway
AV re-entry due to accessory pathway	Class II, IC, IA, III Avoid Class IV, digoxin	RFCA of accessory pathway

Pharmacological therapy options are listed in order of preferred or most common use. (1), preferred or most common first line treatment, (2), preferred or most common second line treatment

spontaneously occurring arrhythmias, and its underlying mechanism determined. If electrophysiological testing is ultimately required to diagnose the arrhythmia, curative ablation will usually be performed at that time (see following description).

The acute treatment of PSVT, as in a patient presenting to the emergency room in tachycardia, has been made simpler and safer with the development and marketing of adenosine (Adenocard). Adenosine, when given intravenously in a rapid bolus at a dose of 6 to 18 mg, will convert PSVT to sinus rhythm in the majority of patients (11–13). Exogenous adenosine acts by stimulating the adenosine receptor, which, mediated by a G-protein complex, activates the potassium channel IK_{ade}, causing hyperpolarization of the cell membrane and shortening of the action potential duration (14). These effects result in transient AV block that terminates the PSVT. Adenosine is very short-acting due to a half-life of 8 to 10 seconds and, consequently, causes few adverse effects. Side effects related to its use include transient flushing, chest pain, shortness of breath, and precipitation of bronchospasm in patients with a history of asthma (11–13,15). Adenosine may rarely cause atrial fibrillation because it shortens the atrial refractory period by activating the potassium channel IK_{ade} (16). Adenosine-induced atrial fibrillation usually terminates spontaneously in several seconds to minutes, but may (rarely) require cardioversion. In the unusual case where adenosine fails to convert PSVT, a repeat dose may be given; if an underlying WPW syndrome with pre-excitation is not suspected, intravenous verapamil 5 to 10 mg or digoxin 0.25 mg every 30 to 60 minutes up to 1 mg may be given. If WPW syndrome with pre-excitation is suspected or known to be the cause of the PSVT, then intravenous procainamide up to 100 mg per minute, as tolerated hemodynamically, up to a total dose of 1.0 g may be given. If PSVT cannot be converted pharmacologically, or in the event of hemodynamic intolerance of PSVT, direct-current cardioversion under intravenous sedation is usually a safe and very effective alternative.

Following conversion to sinus rhythm and stabilization of the patient, a decision must then be made whether long-term suppression of PSVT is required. In a patient with heart failure, it is important to prevent recurrent PSVT because of the high rate of the tachycardia (often in excess of 150 beats per minute), which may cause rapid and severe hemodynamic deterioration. In those patients with rare or infrequent episodes of PSVT, either no therapy or pharmacologic therapy alone may be appropriate. However, in those with frequent episodes of PSVT or particularly rapid PSVT, and in those who cannot tolerate antiarrhythmic drugs, curative radiofrequency catheter ablation (RFCA) may be performed (17–19).

RFCA involves the endocardial delivery of radiofrequency energy (e.g., 550 kHz) via a large-tip (e.g., 4- to 10-mm) electrode catheter at the location of origin or a critical zone in the electrical circuit of the arrhythmia. Application of radiofrequency energy, at a power of 50 to 100 W to achieve temperatures of 50° to 60°C, produces permanent destruction of the arrhythmogenic tissue by resistive heat-

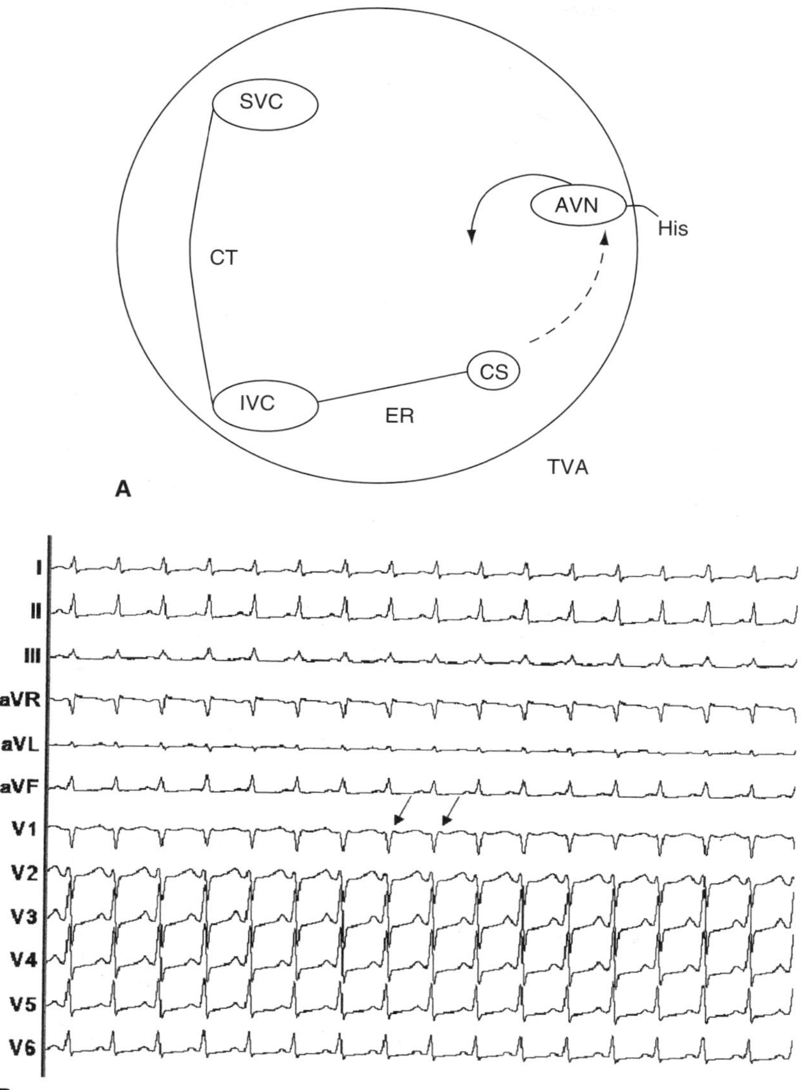

Figure 40-1 **(A)** A schematic diagram of the right atrium demonstrating the putative slow (**dashed line**) and fast (**solid line**) AV nodal pathways and possible re-entrant circuit of the common slow–fast form of AVNRT is shown. As noted by the gap between the head and tail of the activation wavefront, the upper common pathway or atrial turnaround point is controversial. **(B)** A 12-lead ECG of typical slow–fast AV nodal re-entrant tachycardia is shown, in which antegrade AV conduction is over the slow AV nodal pathway and retrograde VA conduction is over the fast AV nodal pathway. Note the narrow QRS complex and absence of an obvious P wave, which is superimposed on the terminal portion of the QRS complex giving rise to a small terminal R′ wave seen in lead V1 (**arrow**). AVN, atrioventricular node; CS, coronary sinus; His, His bundle; ER, eustachian ridge; TVA, trisucpid valve annulus.

ing. The efficacy of RFCA is high (approaching 100% for PSVT) and major complications, including inadvertent AV block requiring pacemaker implantation, are rare, occurring in <1% to 3% of patients. Thus, RFCA has become first-line therapy for most patients with PSVT, particularly in view of the potential for side effects and long-term toxicity from antiarrhythmic drugs.

For patients with PSVT who are not appropriate candidates for RFCA (e.g., due to patient preference or other severe, concurrent illness), antiarrhythmic drugs may be used to prevent recurrences (Tables 40-2 and 40-3). For AVNRT or AVRT due to a concealed accessory pathway (i.e., without pre-excitation on ECG), AV nodal blocking drugs such as digoxin, calcium blockers (e.g., diltiazem or verapamil) or beta-blockers may be effective in preventing arrhythmia recurrence. However, patients with heart failure may not tolerate calcium or beta-blockers due to their negative inotropic and chronotropic effects. Furthermore, in patients with AVRT due to WPW syndrome with ventricular pre-excitation, digoxin and calcium blockers should be strictly avoided due to the potential life-threatening risk of increasing ventricular response to atrial fibrillation. By inhibiting conduction through the AV node, digoxin and calcium blockers may actually increase conduction over the accessory pathway, resulting in an irregular wide-complex ventricular response potentially in excess of 200 beats per minute, which may occasionally lead to ventricular fibrillation.

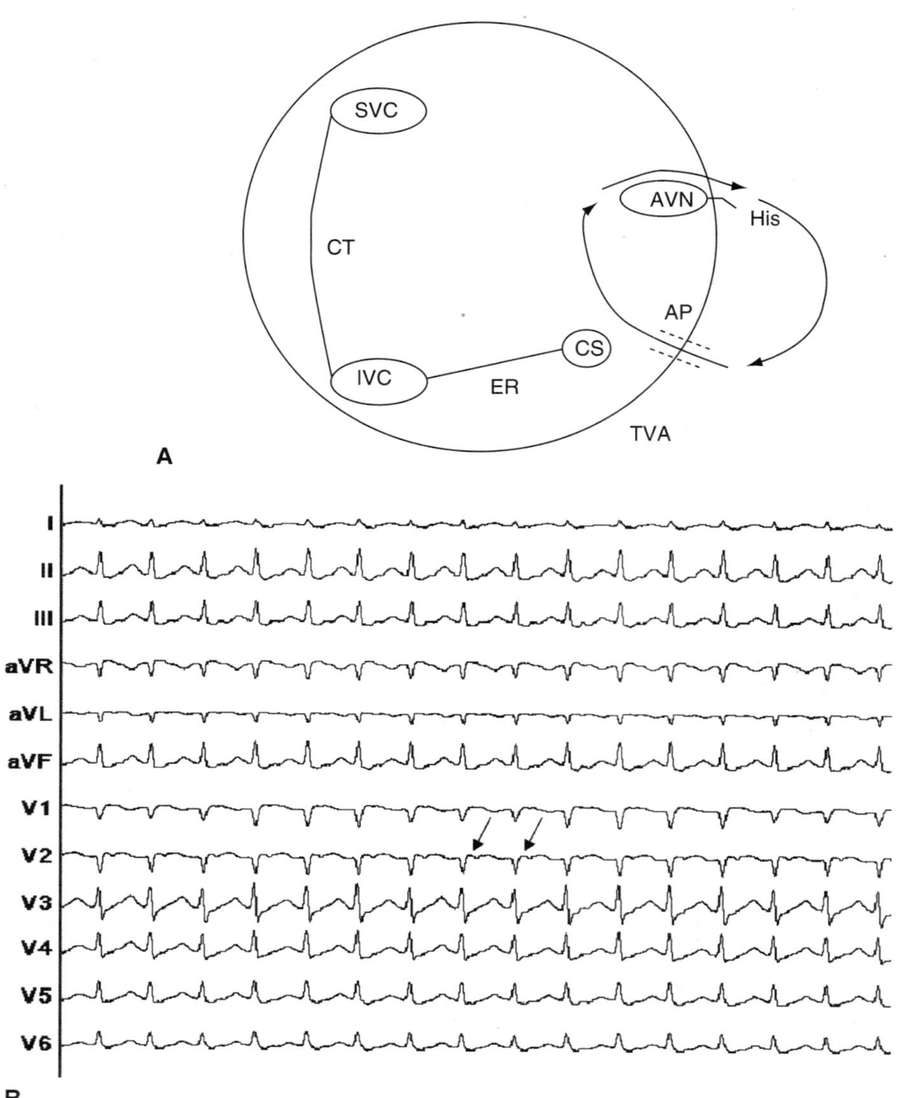

Figure 40-2 **(A)** A schematic diagram of the right atrium demonstrating the re-entry circuit during orthodromic AVRT is shown in a patient with a posteroseptal accessory pathway. Note the antegrade (atrio-ventricular) conduction over the AV node and retrograde (ventriculo-atrial) conduction over the accessory pathway during orthodromic AVRT, with turnaround points in both the atrium and ventricle. **(B)** A 12-lead ECG of orthodromic AV re-entrant tachycardia is shown, in which antegrade AV conduction is over the AV node and retrograde VA conduction is over an accessory pathway. Note the narrow QRS complex, and the P wave visible in the early ST segment (**arrow**).
AP, accessory pathway designated by dotted lines; AVN, atrioventricular node; CS, coronary sinus; His, His bundle; ER, eustachian ridge; TVA, trisucpid valve annulus.

If AV nodal blocking drugs are tolerated but fail to control PSVT, the Class 1 or 3 antiarrhythmic drugs (e.g., flecainide, propafenone, ethmozine, or sotalol and amiodarone) may be effective alone or in combination with AV nodal blocking drugs. However, patients with left ventricular dysfunction and heart failure have a significantly greater risk of mortality due to life-threatening ventricular proarrhythmia from certain antiarrhythmic drugs (20,21). These arrhythmias may include torsade de pointes from Class 1a drugs such as quinidine or Class 3 drugs such as sotalol, and monomorphic ventricular tachycardia from the Class 1c drugs such as flecainide (20,21). Thus, for treatment of atrial arrhythmias in patients with heart failure the risks of antiarrhythmic drugs may outweigh their benefits (22).

If an antiarrhythmic drug is required, amiodarone may be the safest and most effective drug in patients with heart failure since it has only rarely been known to cause ventricular proarrhythmia in the form of torsade de pointes (1,2). Amiodarone, a Class 3 antiarrhythmic drug that combines AV nodal blocking effects, sympatholytic effects, and antiarrhythmic effects, is very effective in preventing recurrence of PSVT (23). Amiodarone has also been shown to have other beneficial effects in patients with heart failure (1,2). For example, amiodarone may reduce mortality in patients with nonischemic cardiomyopathy (1,2). Amiodarone may also improve ejection fraction in some patients, as well as reduce hospitalization for heart failure due to its positive inotropic effects caused by prolongation of ventricular action potential duration (1,2). However, because of its long biological half-life (up to 30 to 90 days) amiodarone must be given initially in a loading dose of 400 to 800 mg (maximum 1,200 mg) per day for several days to 1 to 2 weeks, followed by a maintenance dose of 100 to 200 mg (maximum 400 mg) per day for rapid and continued control of most arrhythmias. The primary limitation of amiodarone is its toxic effects on specific organs, including the thyroid (hyperthyroidism or hypothyroidism), liver (elevation of transaminases), lung (interstitial pneumonitis and fibrosis), skin (hypersensitivity to sun), nervous system (painful peripheral neuropathy), and eye (corneal deposits or optic neuropathy), requiring its discontinuation in up to 20% of patients over time. Due to its long biological half-life, patients being treated with amiodarone must be evaluated for signs of organ toxicity at least every 6 months and the drug discontinued immediately at the sign of any significant toxicity, especially pulmonary toxicity, peripheral neuropathy, or hyperthyroidism.

Atrial Flutter, Re-Entrant Atrial Tachycardia, and Focal Atrial Tachycardia

Atrial flutter, re-entrant atrial tachycardia, and focal atrial tachycardia (Table 40-1) are more common than PSVT in patients with heart failure. In contrast to PSVT, these supraventricular arrhythmias are confined strictly to the atrial myocardium and do not utilize the AV node or an accessory pathway as part of the arrhythmia circuit (24–29). Typical and reverse typical atrial flutter (Fig. 40-3A,B) involve re-entry around the tricuspid valve annulus and are dependent on slow conduction through the cavo-tricuspid isthmus (Fig. 40-4A,B), whereas other forms of re-entrant atrial tachycardia and atypical atrial flutter involve re-entry around anatomical and/or functional obstacles such as the crista terminalis, pulmonary veins, mitral valve annulus, idiopathic or surgical scars, or patches within the atria. Due to their strictly atrial substrate, AV nodal blocking drugs (including adenosine) may slow the ventricular response but an antiarrhythmic drug or electrical cardioversion is usually required to convert these supraventricular arrhythmias to sinus rhythm. However, while the use of adenosine in patients with atrial flutter or atrial tachycardia is rarely therapeutic, it may be diagnostic by transiently blocking AV nodal conduction and allowing one to see the underlying atrial rhythm.

Focal atrial tachycardia differs from re-entrant atrial tachycardia in that it is due to localized automatic or triggered electrical activity that can originate from anywhere in the right or left atrium, but commonly occurs along the crista terminalis, in the coronary sinus or pulmonary veins, or along the atrioventricular valve rings. Automatic atrial tachycardia is uniquely sensitive to adenosine in some cases (30), and thus its conversion to sinus rhythm by adenosine may be both diagnostic and therapeutic. Triggered activity may result from high levels of sympathetic tone commonly seen in patients with heart failure, or from intoxication with digitalis, a drug that is commonly used in patients with heart failure (31).

For the acute pharmacologic conversion of re-entrant atrial tachycardia and atrial flutter, the recently approved antiarrhythmic drug ibutilide (1 or 2 mg over 10 to 20 minutes) has been shown to be very effective (32,36). Ibutilide is a Class 3 antiarrhythmic drug, currently available only in intravenous formulation in the United States. Ibutilide prolongs atrial and ventricular action potential duration predominately by blocking the delayed rectifier potassium channel IK_r (32,33). This compound is effective in converting up to 76% of patients with atrial flutter (34,35). Its serum half-life is approximately 4 hours, during which the patient should be monitored on a hospital telemetry ward or closely in clinic (32–35). Cardiac monitoring is necessary because ibutilide prolongs the QT interval and may cause torsade de pointes ventricular tachycardia in up to 3% to 4% of patients (36). Ventricular proarrhythmia is more common with ibutilide in patients with left ventricular dysfunction (36), even though it produces no adverse hemodynamic effects (37).

Other antiarrhythmic drugs may be used for the acute pharmacologic conversion of atrial flutter and re-entrant atrial tachycardia, including the Class 3 drugs sotalol and dofetilide that have a similar action to ibutilide, the Class 1a drug procainamide (intravenous formulation available), and the Class 1c drugs flecainide and propafenone. However, sotalol is a potent beta-receptor-blocker that may aggravate heart failure, and all the Class 1 drugs may cause ventricular proarrhythmia and are thus usually avoided in patients with heart failure, even for acute use. If antiarrhythmic drugs are contraindicated or there is urgency in converting atrial flutter or re-entrant atrial tachycardia to sinus rhythm due to hemodynamic compromise, direct-current cardioversion is usually highly effective and safe, and may be done using only conscious sedation.

In contrast to atrial flutter and re-entrant atrial tachycardia, the acute pharmacologic conversion of focal atrial tachycardia is often difficult due to its incessant nature. Automatic atrial tachycardia may respond to beta-receptor or calcium-channel blockers, or adenosine (30). Triggered atrial tachycardia due to digitalis toxicity may resolve by simply withholding therapy and/or dose reduction (31). For refractory focal atrial tachycardia, particularly those which may be causing or aggravating heart failure, RFCA may be required (38).

For the long-term suppression of atrial flutter and re-entrant or focal atrial tachycardia (Tables 40-2 and 40-3), the Class 1a and 1c antiarrhythmic drugs are usually avoided in patients with heart failure, due to their potential to cause ventricular proarrhythmia and increase mortality. However, if ventricular dysfunction is not too severe (i.e., left ventricular ejection fraction [LVEF] <20% to 30%) the Class 3 antiarrhythmic drug sotalol may be used with caution in doses of 80 to 160 mg every 12 hours. It is recommended that therapy with sotalol be initiated in the hospital under ECG telemetry monitoring, especially in patients with heart failure, since a small percentage of patients (1.5% to 3.0%) may develop excessive QT prolongation and torsade de pointes ventricular tachycardia. Unfortunately, some patients may not tolerate sotalol due to its potent beta-receptor blocking action, which may aggravate heart failure and cause bradycardia.

Amiodarone may be the preferred antiarrhythmic drug in those patients with heart failure in whom other antiarrhythmic drugs are considered unsafe or ineffective, and, as noted previously, amiodarone may be the safest antiarrhythmic drug from the perspective of ventricular proarrhythmia (1,2). However, while amiodarone may be effective for focal atrial tachycardia (automatic or triggered), it may promote sus-

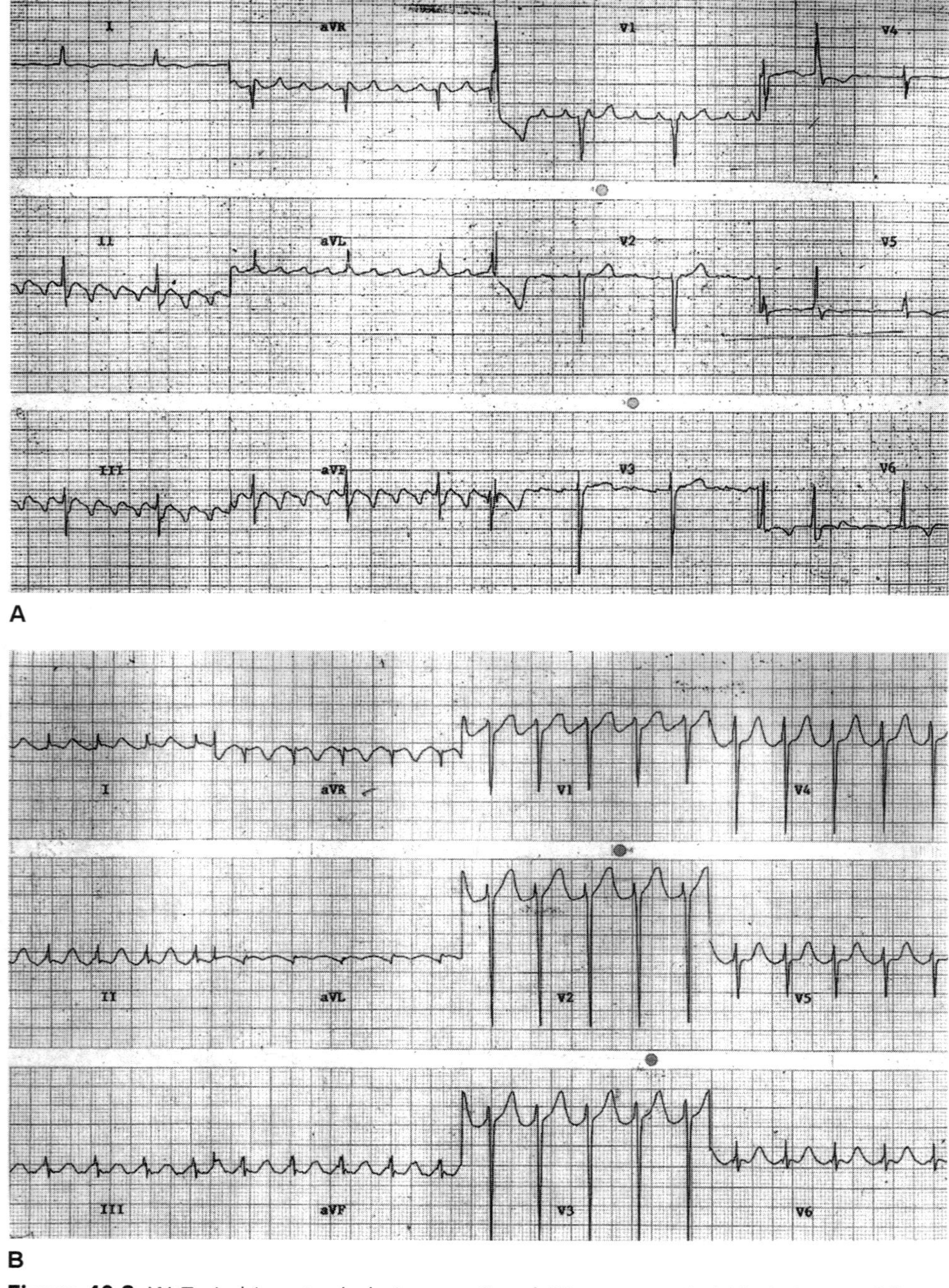

Figure 40-3 **(A)** Typical (counterclockwise type 1) and **(B)** reverse typical (clockwise) atrial flutter are shown in these two 12-lead ECGs. Note the inverted, sawtooth flutter waves in the inferior leads II, III, and aVF in typical AFL, and the sine wave F wave pattern in reverse typical AFL.

tained atrial flutter or atrial tachycardia in some patients due to slowing of atrial conduction velocity. For amiodarone, a loading dose of 400 to 800 mg per day (1,200 mg per day maximum) for several days to 1 to 2 weeks is necessary to reduce the latency of onset of action. This should be followed by a maintenance dose of 100 to 200 mg per day (400 mg per day maximum) for long-term arrhythmia suppression.

In patients with heart failure and atrial flutter or atrial tachycardia, in whom antiarrhythmic drugs are often contraindicated due to side effects or proarrhythmia or are ineffective, RFCA is an effective alternative therapy (26,28,29,39–45). The procedure is performed similarly to that for PSVT, as described earlier in this chapter. In the case of typical or reverse typical atrial flutter, the atrial myocardium between the tricuspid valve annulus and the inferior vena cava (i.e., cavo-tricuspid isthmus) forms a critical zone of slow conduction in the re-entry circuit that, when ablated, will cure the arrhythmia (Fig. 40-5). For other re-entrant or focal atrial tachycardia, an area of slow conduction or the site of earliest atrial activation, respectively, can be identified in the right or left atrium by a process of electrical mapping and, when ablated, will cure the arrhythmia.

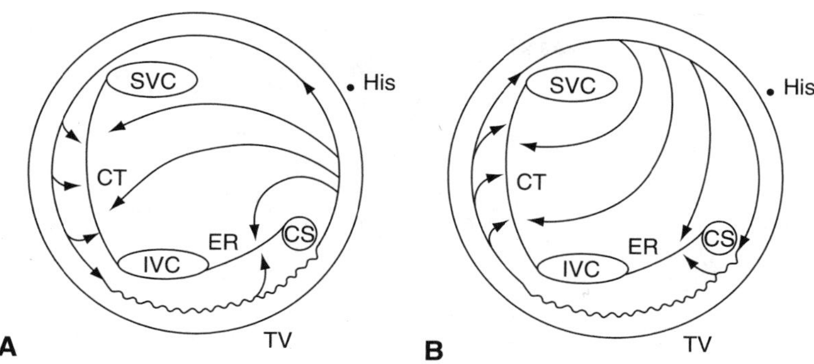

Figure 40-4 Schematic diagrams of typical **(A)** and reverse typical **(B)** AFL are shown. Note the counterclockwise and clockwise re-entry circuits in typical and reverse typical AFL, respectively, with a critical area of slow conduction between the tricuspid valve annulus and inferior vena cava (cavo-tricuspid isthmus).

The initial success rate of RFCA for cure of atrial flutter and re-entrant or focal atrial tachycardia is high, approaching 95% to 100%. However, arrhythmia recurrence is somewhat more frequent after RFCA for atrial flutter and atrial tachycardia than it is for PSVT, ranging from 5% to 10% of patients with an initially successful procedure. Fortunately, it is possible to repeat ablation in most patients with arrhythmia recurrence. The risk of complications during RFCA for atrial flutter and atrial tachycardia is similar to that for PSVT. However, a transseptal catheterization may be required in some patients if the site of origin of the tachycardia is left atrial, which may be associated with a slightly higher risk of complications. Thus, due to its high rate of efficacy and low complication rate, RFCA is now considered a first-line curative therapy for atrial flutter and most re-entrant or focal atrial arrhythmias. In fact, RFCA may be preferred over the use of antiarrhythmic drugs, which are more likely to cause adverse hemodynamic effects and potentially lethal ventricular proarrhythmic effects in patients with heart failure.

Atrial Fibrillation

Atrial fibrillation (Fig. 40-6) occurs with a two- to threefold increased frequency in patients with heart failure, compared to those without structural heart disease (5). This is due in part to the atrial enlargement and electrophysiological abnormalities associated with elevated atrial and ventricular diastolic pressure and atrioventricular valve regurgitation. In patients with heart failure, atrial fibrillation may produce serious adverse hemodynamic effects due to loss of atrial contribution to diastolic filling and a rapid ventricular response, resulting in further hemodynamic deterioration (46,47). Consequently, the sudden onset of atrial fibrillation can cause immediate decompensation of heart failure, which may be life-threatening in some cases. Furthermore, studies have shown that atrial fibrillation independently reduces long-term survival in patients with heart failure (3,4). Atrial fibrillation is also associated with increased risk of systemic embolization due to formation of left atrial thrombi, which may cause stroke and other

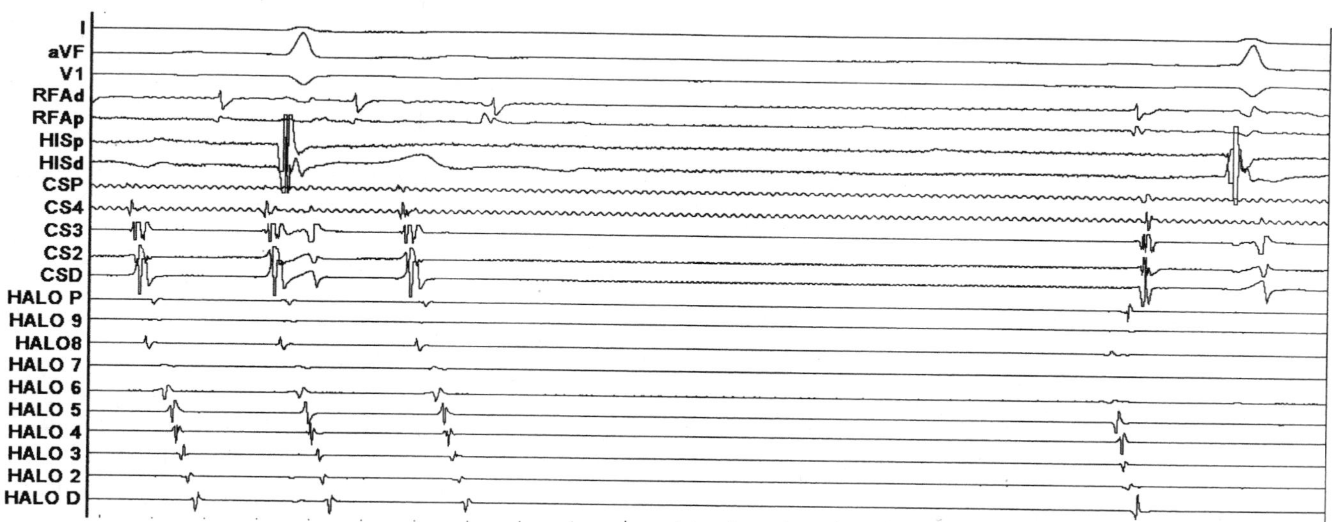

Figure 40-5 Surface ECG leads I, aVF, and V1 and endocardial electrogram recordings from the right atrium (Halo catheter), coronary sinus, His bundle, and radiofrequency ablation catheter during ablation of type 1 atrial flutter. Note that radiofrequency energy application to the region of the CTI (the critical zone of slow conduction in the AFL circuit) results in termination of AFL. This also produces bidirectional CTI conduction block (not shown), resulting in a high long-term cure rate of AFL. $Halo_{D-P}$, distal through proximal electrodes on the 20-pole Halo catheter positioned around the tricuspid valve annulus; CS_{D-P}, distal to proximal electrodes on coronary sinus catheter; His, His bundle catheter electrograms.

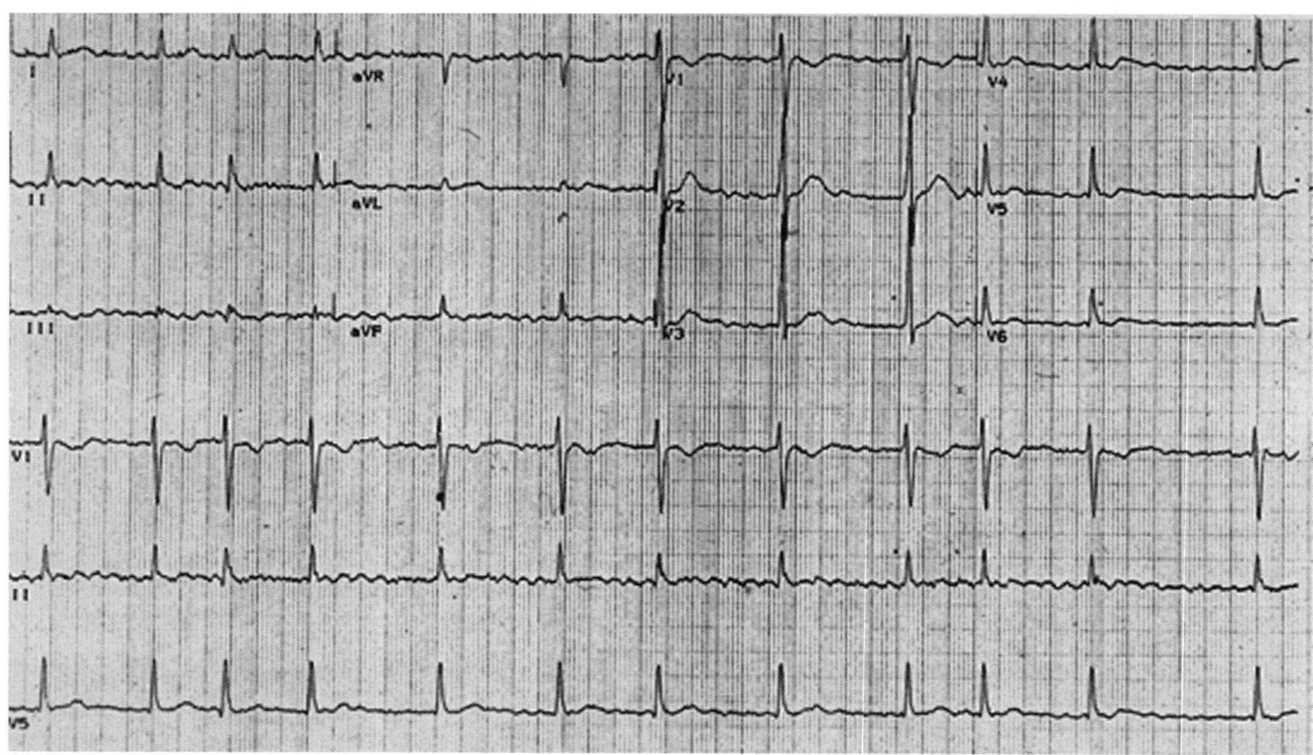

Figure 40-6 A 12-lead ECG of atrial fibrillation is shown. Note the lack of organized P wave activity and the irregularly irregular ventricular response.

embolic complications (5), and this risk is further increased in patients with heart failure (5).

The acute treatment of atrial fibrillation requires a combination of rate control with AV node blocking drugs and anticoagulation with heparin. The acute treatment may also include conversion to sinus rhythm with pharmacologic agents or electrical cardioversion, depending on the hemodynamic status of the patient. Rate control may be achieved acutely with intravenous digoxin (up to 1 mg in 24 hours in four divided doses), or intravenous beta-receptor blockers (e.g., esmolol, metoprolol, or propranolol) or a calcium-channel blocker (e.g., diltiazem or verapamil) if tolerated hemodynamically. Once rate control is achieved, a high percentage of patients (up to 50%) with recent-onset atrial fibrillation will convert spontaneously to sinus rhythm. However, before attempting to convert atrial fibrillation to normal sinus rhythm it is imperative to determine its duration, since the risk of systemic embolization and stroke is significantly increased if an episode has lasted longer than 72 hours. If an episode of atrial fibrillation has lasted longer than 72 hours, rate control, followed by a period of therapeutic anticoagulation (i.e., intravenous heparin acutely followed by oral warfarin with an international normalized ratio [INR] of between 2 or 3 for at least 3 weeks) is recommended before cardioversion. Restoration of sinus may then be best achieved by electrical cardioversion, since the efficacy of antiarrhythmic drugs after 72 hours of sustained atrial fibrillation will be less than 40%. In a patient presenting with atrial fibrillation lasting longer than 72 hours, in whom the hemodynamic effects of the arrhythmia cannot be tolerated for several weeks of anticoagulation, preliminary studies have suggested that the absence of left atrial thrombus on transesophageal echocardiography may allow cardioversion with minimal risk of systemic embolization. However, anticoagulation with heparin and warfarin must be started immediately after conversion and continued for 4 to 12 weeks in order to prevent late embolic events.

In contrast, if an episode of atrial fibrillation has lasted less than 72 hours the risk of embolic events is relatively low and the efficacy of antiarrhythmic drugs will be higher. In this case, following adequate rate control, conversion of atrial fibrillation to sinus rhythm may be achieved by electrical cardioversion or pharmacologically (e.g., ibutilide 1 to 2 mg). The pharmacologic conversion rates for recent-onset atrial fibrillation may reach 70% to 80%, although the risks for ventricular proarrhythmic effects from antiarrhythmic drugs are higher in patients with heart failure. Following conversion of atrial fibrillation to sinus rhythm, chronic treatment may be required with antiarrhythmic drugs.

Chronic treatment of atrial fibrillation in patients with heart failure is often difficult because of its tendency to recur and become chronic. Antiarrhythmic drugs have been extensively used to treat atrial fibrillation (Tables 40-2 and 40-3) and, while effective in a significant percentage of patients, they have been shown to have significant limitations. For example, the efficacy of most antiarrhythmic drugs in preventing recurrence of atrial fibrillation at 6 to 12 months following cardioversion is about 50%, including the Class 1a drugs quinidine, procainamide, and disopyramide, the Class 1c drugs flecainide and propafenone, and the Class 3 drugs sotalol and dofetilide (48–52). Amiodarone may be slightly more effective than other drugs (48–52). Furthermore, most antiarrhythmic drugs have a potential to cause ventricular proarrhythmia and thus actually increase mortality (20–22), with the greatest risk in patients with a history of myocardial infarction or heart failure (21,22).

The Class 1c antiarrhythmic drugs (e.g., flecainide, propafenone) are particularly hazardous in patients with heart failure due to their ventricular proarrhythmic and negative inotropic effects, and thus are generally avoided. The Class 3 antiarrhythmic drugs (e.g., sotalol, dofetilide, amiodarone), although not actually approved for treatment of atrial fibrillation, have similar or slightly greater efficacy compared to the Class 1a and 1c antiarrhythmic drugs in prevention of atrial fibrillation and have a more favorable safety profile in patients with heart failure (1,2,48,50–52). In fact, in the Electrophysiologic Study Versus Electrocardiographic Monitoring (ESVEM) trial, treatment with sotalol was associated with significantly lower mortality compared to that with Class 1 antiarrhythmic drugs in patients with a history of sustained ventricular tachycardia or fibrillation (53). However, because sotalol is a potent beta-blocker it will produce significant negative inotropic effects that may not be tolerated by patients with more severe heart failure; it can also cause life-threatening ventricular proarrhythmia in the form of torsade de pointes ventricular tachycardia in 1% to 3% of patients (50,53,54). Thus, its use is usually restricted to those patients with only mild to moderately severe heart failure and those with normal baseline QT interval and electrolytes.

In contrast, amiodarone in doses of 100 to 200 mg per day has actually been shown to reduce total mortality and the frequency of hospitalization in patients with heart failure of a nonischemic etiology (1,2). Furthermore, amiodarone has not been shown to increase mortality in patients with heart failure due to coronary artery disease (1,2,55,56). This is probably due to the fact that amiodarone has a broad spectrum of hemodynamic and electrophysiological effects, including mild coronary vasodilation and positive inotropic effects, mild calcium channel and beta-receptor blocking activity, moderate sodium channel blocking activity, and potent potassium channel blocking activity (57). It only rarely causes ventricular proarrhythmia in the form of torsade de pointes ventricular tachycardia. Thus, the relatively greater efficacy, neutral to beneficial hemodynamic effect, and low proarrhythmic profile make amiodarone a first-line pharmacologic therapy in patients with atrial fibrillation and heart failure. Unfortunately, its long-term use is associated with potentially serious side effects requiring its discontinuation in up to 15% to 20% of patients (58). The more serious side effects of amiodarone include pulmonary toxicity that manifests as an interstitial inflammation or fibrosis in 4% to 9% of patients, hepatic toxicity with elevation of transaminases in 4% to 9%, hyperthyroidism or hypothyroidism in 1% to 3%, and (rarely) peripheral neuropathy, including optic neuritis (58). Less-serious but relatively frequent side effects include hypersensitivity to sun, causing sunburn in 4% to 9% of patients, corneal deposits causing halo vision in 4% to 9%, neurological symptoms including tremor in 4% to 9%, and gastrointestinal disturbances in 10% to 30%. Using the lowest effective dose (100 to 200 mg per day) can minimize the incidence of side effects, although discontinuation of the drug due to side effects may still be required in a significant percentage of patients.

Dofetilide, a newer Class 3 antiarrhythmic drug, has been shown to have similar efficacy to that of quinidine or sotalol in preventing recurrence of atrial fibrillation (51,52). However, dofetilide may have some advantage over sotalol in that it has no beta-receptor blocking action and thus would not be expected to aggravate heart failure (51,52). Studies of dofetilide in prevention of life-threatening ventricular arrhythmias in postmyocardial infarction patients with an ejection fraction <30% actually demonstrated a neutral effect on all-cause mortality, but reduced mortality when sinus rhythm was restored and maintained and reduced all-cause and heart failure rehospitalization (51,52). This study suggests that dofetilide may be safe for the treatment of atrial fibrillation in patients with heart failure, with less risk of ventricular proarrhythmia than is associated with the Class 1 antiarrhythmic drugs (51,52).

Eventually, if pharmacologic antiarrhythmic therapy fails to maintain sinus rhythm due to inefficacy, side effects, or proarrhythmia, or if a rate control approach with anticoagulation is initially taken, atrial fibrillation may become chronic. In patients with chronic or uncontrolled paroxysmal atrial fibrillation, ventricular rate control is critical. It has been observed that a poorly controlled ventricular response in atrial fibrillation may aggravate pre-existing ventricular dysfunction, and in normal patients may even cause a reversible tachycardia-induced myocardial dysfunction (59). Control of ventricular response may be achieved pharmacologically with the use of AV node blocking drugs such as digoxin, the calcium antagonists, or beta-blockers. However, digoxin alone is often ineffective in controlling ventricular response to atrial fibrillation due to the high sympathetic tone and vagal withdrawal associated with heart failure (60), requiring combined therapy with a calcium antagonist, beta-blocker, or both. Some patients with moderate ventricular dysfunction may tolerate calcium antagonists or beta-blockers, but others may not due to the negative inotropic, chronotropic, and dromotropic effects of these drugs.

In those who do not tolerate calcium antagonists or beta-blockers and in whom AV node blocking drugs are ineffective in controlling ventricular response, ventricular rate control must be achieved by alternative methods. The approach most commonly used is RFCA of the AV node to produce complete AV node block, followed by implantation of a permanent rate-responsive pacemaker (61–63). AV node ablation provides permanent rate control without the need for AV node blocking drugs, and the rate-responsive pacemaker provides a relatively physiologic heart rate (62,63). One limitation of this approach is that the patient is subsequently pacemaker-dependent, and (rarely) this approach is associated with deterioration of ventricular function or sudden death.

As an alternative to AV node ablation with pacemaker implantation, a procedure called AV node modification using RFCA techniques has been developed. In contrast to complete AV node ablation, during AV node modification only the posterior atrial inputs to the AV node are selectively ablated, resulting in slowing of the ventricular response to atrial fibrillation without producing complete AV node block and the need for permanent pacemaker implantation (64–66). This approach is advantageous in that it obviates the need for a pacemaker. However, it is effective in only about 60% to 70% of patients in whom it is attempted, the remainder requiring complete AV node ablation. Furthermore, even in those in whom overall rate control is achieved by AV node modification, symptoms of palpitations may persist due to an irregular ventricular response. However, both AV node ablation with pacemaker implantation and AV node modification have been shown to provide significant short-term and long-term improvement in functional status of the patient and in ventricular function (62,63,66).

Whether one chooses a strategy of rhythm control or rate control combined with anticoagulation for treatment of atrial fibrillation has been the subject of some controversy, but the recently reported Atrial Fibrillation Follow-up Investigation of Rhythm Management (AFFIRM) trial demonstrated in a large population of patients with atrial fibrillation that there was no significant difference in mortality or stroke rates in patients assigned to either strategy (67). The results of this study initially led to a trend to recommend and implement rate control combined with anticoagulation instead of rhythm control. Further recent analysis of data from the AFFIRM trial (68) has shown that maintenance of sinus rhythm is actually associated with reduced mortality (as was warfarin use), whereas antiarrhythmic drug use was associated with increased mortality. Thus, it appears that any benefit derived by rhythm control in the AFFIRM trial may have been negated by the adverse effects of antiarrhythmic drugs used for rhythm control, resulting in no difference in outcome based on an intention-to-treat analysis. These data suggest that if rhythm control could be achieved by a means other than antiarrhythmic drugs, this might reduce mortality. This could be especially important in a population of patients with heart failure, in whom atrial fibrillation increases mortality rates.

In this regard, both surgical and RFCA techniques have been recently developed for the curative treatment of paroxysmal and even persistent atrial fibrillation, although research is still ongoing in this area (69–72). An open heart surgery procedure called the MAZE operation can cure atrial fibrillation (69) but there is a significantly higher mortality risk for this operation in patients with heart failure. Therefore, the MAZE operation is not recommended in these patients unless they are already undergoing cardiac surgery for other reasons such as coronary artery bypass grafting or valve replacement. In such a case, performing a MAZE operation concomitantly with elective surgery may be a reasonable approach to prevent recurrence of atrial fibrillation following surgery (69). Alternatives to the classical "cut and sew" MAZE operation, including cryoablation, microwave ablation, radiofrequency ablation, and ultrasound ablation (which include variably pulmonary vein isolation and/or atrial substrate modification) have been described with variable lesser degrees of long-term success (69).

As an alternative, less-invasive RFCA catheter ablation approaches have been recently developed for treatment of paroxysmal atrial fibrillation, and even persistent atrial fibrillation in some cases (70–72). Paroxysmal atrial fibrillation has been shown in many cases to be triggered by single, premature depolarizations or rapid, sustained electrical activity originating from the pulmonary veins (70–72). The origin of focal atrial tachycardia or premature atrial contractions causing atrial fibrillation is commonly in the orifice of the pulmonary veins, but also occasionally in the right atrium. Patients with focally triggered paroxysmal atrial fibrillation can sometimes be identified on ambulatory ECG monitoring by demonstrating premature atrial contractions or short runs of atrial tachycardia precipitating atrial fibrillation. RFCA of the ostia of the pulmonary veins (segmental or circumferential ablation) can isolate the electrical activity in the pulmonary veins, preventing triggering of atrial fibrillation (Fig. 40-7A,B). In cases with persistent atrial fibrillation, electrical isolation of the pulmonary veins combined with linear ablation designed to mimic the MAZE operation in the left atrium (Fig. 40-8A,B) may also prevent recurrence of atrial fibrillation (70–72).

Recent studies of RFCA in patients with symptomatic atrial fibrillation have actually shown a reduction in all-cause mortality, morbidity due to heart failure and ischemic cerebrovascular events, and improvement in quality-of-life measures (71). Curative RFCA in patients with atrial fibrillation and heart failure has also been shown to improve ventricular function, exercise capacity, and quality of life (71,72). Thus, by restoring sinus rhythm without the use of antiarrhythmic drugs, RFCA may actually reduce morbidity and mortality, and improve quality of life in patients with heart failure and atrial fibrillation. Success rates for RFCA of atrial fibrillation vary from 80% to 95% in patients with paroxysmal atrial fibrillation, to 60% to 80% in patients with persistent atrial fibrillation. In those who initially fail treatment, a second or (rarely) a third procedure may be required to achieve success. RFCA is not without risks, although major complications such as stroke, pulmonary vein stenosis, cardiac perforation and pericardial tamponade requiring pericardiocentesis or surgery, or vascular injury or hemorrhage requiring surgery or transfusion occur in less than 1% to 3% of patients, on average. In the near future, new three-dimensional mapping systems, magnetically or robotically driven catheter systems, and alternative energy sources including cryothermal or microwave energy delivered with long (4- to 6-cm) electrodes will hopefully increase success rates, reduce procedure times, and minimize complications. All of these systems are being tested currently.

In addition to antiarrhythmic drugs and RFCA as rhythm control strategies, pacing and defibrillation therapies are now currently available for patients who are not candidates for either antiarrhythmic drugs or ablation. It has been clearly shown that atrial-based pacing, including single-chamber atrial or dual-chamber pacing, reduces mortality and stroke risk in patients with sick sinus syndrome, many of whom also have atrial fibrillation and in whom heart failure is also common (73,74). Single-chamber ventricular pacing, however, has not demonstrated these benefits in patients with sick sinus syndrome and may even increase mortality and rates of hospitalization for heart failure (73–75). Furthermore, in patients without sick sinus syndrome, pacing has been shown to be only marginally beneficial in suppression of atrial fibrillation, using various types of arrhythmia suppression algorithms (76). However, combined atrial and ventricular defibrillators are currently available that can perform antitachycardia pacing and defibrillation to convert atrial arrhythmias (including atrial fibrillation) to sinus rhythm, in a manner

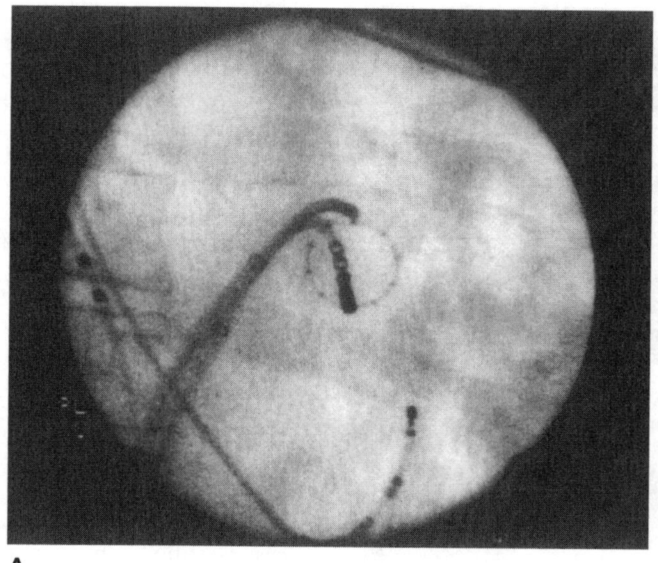

A

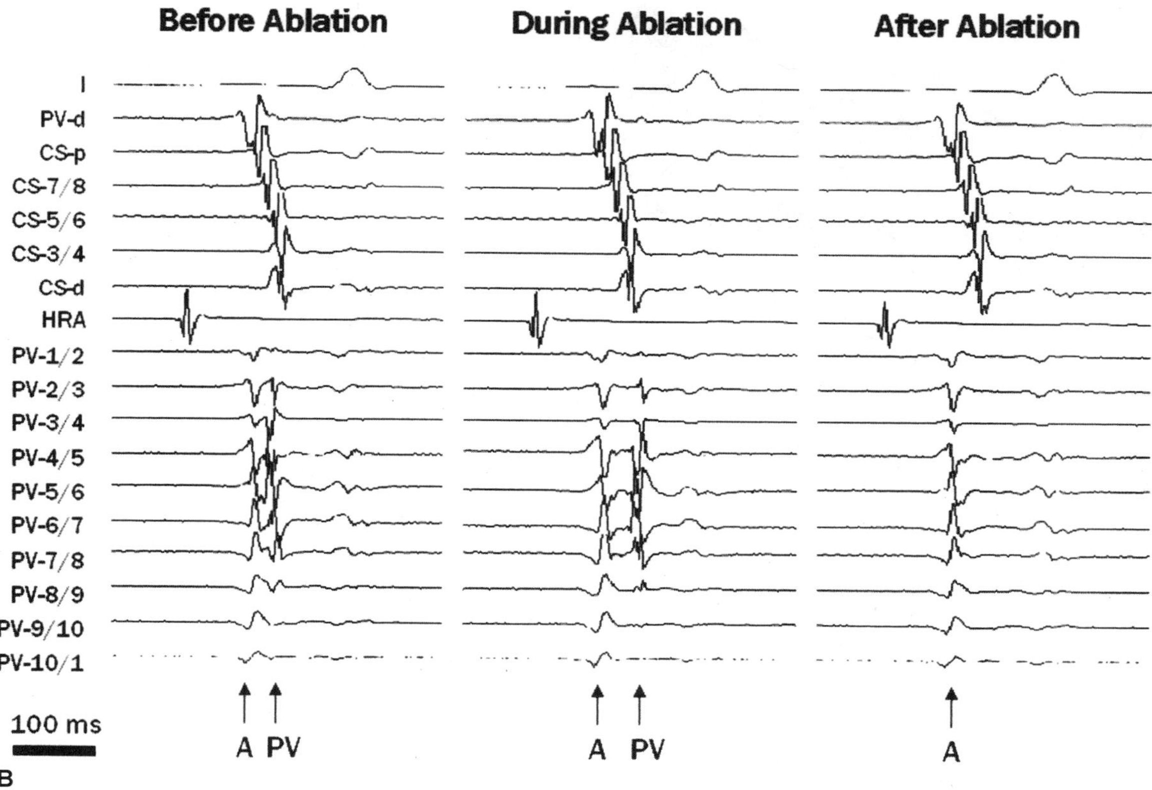

B

Figure 40-7 **(A)** Right anterior oblique fluoroscopic view of Lasso (loop) and ablation catheters positioned in the left lower pulmonary vein for pulmonary vein isolation. **(B)** Radiofrequency PV isolation is shown, demonstrating elimination of PV electrograms from the Lasso catheter during ablation. Note the A and PV potentials before ablation (**left panel**), prolongation of the A and PV potential interval during ablation (**middle panel**), and elimination of the PV potential after ablation (**right panel**). A, atrial potential; PV, PV potential; I, aVF, surface ECG leads; CS_P to CS_D, proximal to distal bipolar coronary sinus electrograms; PV1/2–P10/1, distal to proximal bipolar Lasso catheter electrograms from inside the PV near the ostium; PV-d, bipolar electrogram recorded from ablation catheter positioned in the PV distal to the Lasso catheter; ms, milliseconds.

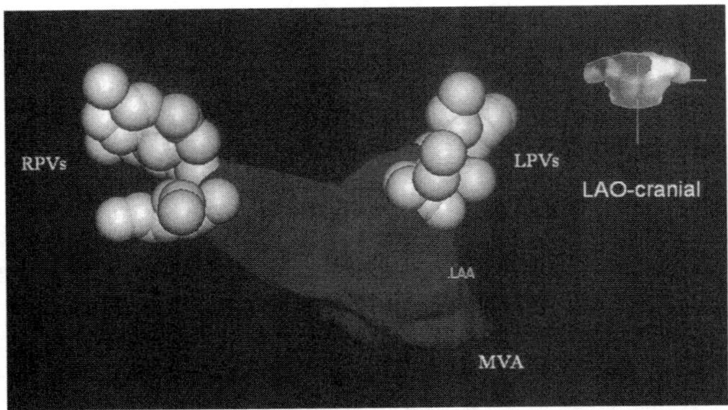

A

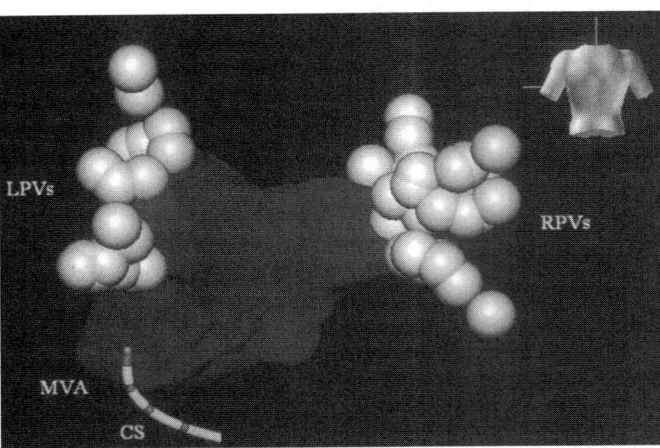

B

Figure 40-8 A three-dimensional anatomical (NAVX) map of the left atrium is shown, demonstrating point-by-point left atrial linear ablation (individual lesions represented by **dots**) for treatment of persistent atrial fibrillation. Note in the anterior **(A)** and posterior **(B)** views that there are two contiguous linear lesions encircling the pulmonary veins, with a line connecting the circular lesions at the roof of the left atrium (i.e., roof line), and the left encircling lesions to the mitral valve annulus (i.e., mitral isthmus line). CS, coronary sinus catheter; MVA, mitral valve annulus; LPVs, left pulmonary veins; RPVs, right pulmonary veins.

similar to that used for life-threatening ventricular arrhythmias (77,78).

While antitachycardia pacing may terminate a majority of atrial tachycardias, including atrial flutter, defibrillation is required to convert atrial fibrillation (77,78). A limitation of current defibrillator technology is the requirement for delivery of energies greater than 2 to 3 joules to convert atrial fibrillation in most cases, and any energy over 2 to 3 joules is typically perceived as painful. Nonetheless, in selected patients with atrial fibrillation (particularly those with heart failure and a reduced ejection fraction) and in whom a ventricular defibrillator is usually recommended for prevention of sudden death due to ventricular arrhythmia, a dual-chamber defibrillator capable of atrial and ventricular antitachycardia pacing and defibrillation may be the treatment of choice.

Regardless of the method used to treat atrial fibrillation, chronic anticoagulation with warfarin is critical to prevent systemic embolization and stroke, particularly since patients with heart failure and atrial fibrillation are at significantly greater risk for embolic complications than are those without heart failure (5,79). It is necessary to maintain an INR in the range of two to three times control in order to reduce the risk of both systemic embolization and hemorrhagic complications. Following a period of 3 to 6 months of suppression of atrial fibrillation, it may be possible to discontinue warfarin in some patients if there are no other indications for its continued use. However, since atrial fibrillation may be asymptomatic in some patients, discontinuing warfarin may pose significant risk of systemic embolization; it may thus be prudent to continue warfarin indefinitely in patients with heart failure and a history of atrial fibrillation.

Using the approaches previously described, including pharmacologic or nonpharmacologic treatments for the suppression of atrial fibrillation, AV nodal blocking drugs or radiofrequency catheter ablation techniques for ventricular rate control, and systemic anticoagulation, the adverse consequences of atrial fibrillation can be prevented or at least mollified in most cases. Clearly, however, an aggressive and systematic approach must be taken to treat atrial fibrillation in patients with heart failure in order to prevent associated complications.

SUMMARY

The treatment of supraventricular arrhythmias has evolved rapidly over the last 10 years, particularly with the development of RFCA techniques, providing important advantages to patients with heart failure. Patients with heart failure are often more symptomatic and have a higher incidence of complications from supraventricular arrhythmias compared to patients without heart disease and normal ventricular function. Thus, in patients with heart failure an aggressive approach for suppression of supraventricular tachycardia using pharmacologic or nonpharmacologic methods is warranted; in the case of atrial fibrillation, effective ventricular rhythm or rate control and anticoagulation are imperative.

REFERENCES

1. Doval HC, Nul DR, Grancelli HO, et al. Randomized trial of low-dose amiodarone in severe heart failure. *Lancet.* 1994;344:493–498.
2. Singh SN, Fletcher RD, Fisher SG, et al. Amiodarone in patients with heart failure and asymptomatic ventricular arrhythmia. *N Engl J Med.* 1995;333:77–82.
3. Stevenson WG, Stevenson LW, Middlekauff HR, et al. Improving survival for patients with atrial fibrillation and advanced heart failure. *J Am Coll Cardiol.* 1996;28:1458–1463.
4. Middlekauf HR, Stevenson WG, Stevenson LW. Prognostic significance of atrial fibrillation in advanced heart failure. A study of 390 patients. *Circulation.* 1991;84:40–48.
5. Risk factors for stroke and efficacy of antithrombotic therapy in atrial fibrillation. *Arch Int Med.* 1994;154:1449–1457.
6. Ravelli F, Allessie M. Effects of atrial dilatation on refractory period and vulnerability to atrial fibrillation in the isolated Langendorff-perfused rabbit heart. *Circulation.* 1997;96:1686–1695.
7. Schoels W, Kuebler W, Yang H, et al. A unified functional/anatomic substrate for circus movement atrial flutter: activation and refractory patterns in the canine right atrial enlargement model. *J Am Coll Cardiol.* 1993;21:73–84.

8. Zipes DP, Jalife J, eds. *Cardiac Electrophysiology: From Cell to Bedside*. Philadelphia: WB Saunders; 1995.
9. Josephson ME, ed. *Clinical Cardiac Electrophysiology: Techniques & Interpretation*. 2nd ed. Philadelphia: Lea & Febiger; 1993.
10. Prystowsky EN, Klein GJ, eds. *Cardiac Arrhythmias: An Integrated Approach for the Clinician*. New York: McGraw-Hill; 1994.
11. Basta M, Klein GJ, Yee R, et al. Current role of pharmacologic therapy for patients with paroxysmal supraventricular tachycardia. *Cardiol Clin*. 1997;15:587–597.
12. Wilbur SL, Marchlinski FE. Adenosine as an antiarrhythmic agent. *Am J Cardiol*. 1997;79:30–37.
13. Ho KY, Wilson NJ, Smith WM. Acute treatment of paroxysmal tachycardia by adenosine. *Australian and New Zealand J Med*. 1994;24:176–181.
14. Wang D, Shryock JC, Belardinelli L. Cellular basis for the negative dromotropic effect of adenosine on rabbit single atrioventricular nodal cells. *Circ Res*. 1996;78:697–706.
15. Drake I, Routledge PA, Richards R. Bronchospasm induced by intravenous adenosine. *Human Exp Toxicol*. 1994;13:263–265.
16. Silverman AJ, Machado C, Baga JJ, et al. Adenosine-induced atrial fibrillation. *Am J Emerg Med*. 1996;14:300–301.
17. Haines DE, Watson DD. Tissue heating during radiofrequency catheter ablation: a thermodynamic model and observations in isolated perfused and superfused canine right ventricular free wall. *PACE*. 1989;12:962–976.
18. Kay GN, Epstein AE, Dailey SM, et al. Selective radiofrequency ablation of the slow pathway for the treatment of atrioventricular nodal reentrant tachycardia. Evidence for involvement of perinodal myocardium within the reentrant circuit. *Circulation* 1992;85:1675–1688.
19. Jackman WM, Wang XZ, Friday KJ, et al. Catheter ablation of accessory AV pathways (Wolff-Parkinson-White) by radiofrequency current. *N Engl J Med*. 1992;324:1605–1611.
20. Coplen SE, Antman EM, Berlin JA, et al. Efficacy and safety of quinidine therapy for maintenance of sinus rhythm after cardioversion. A meta-analysis of randomized control trials. *Circulation*. 1990;82:1106–1116.
21. Cardiac Arrhythmia Suppression Trial Investigators (CAST). Preliminary report: effect of encainide and flecainide on mortality in a randomized trial of arrhythmia suppression after myocardial infarction. *N Engl J Med*. 1989;321:406–412.
22. Flaker GC, Blackshear JL, McBride R, et al. Antiarrhythmic drug therapy and cardiac mortality in atrial fibrillation. The Stroke Prevention in Atrial Fibrillation Investigators. *J Am Coll Cardiol*. 1992;20:527–532.
23. Feld GK, Nademanee K, Weiss J, et al. Electrophysiologic basis for the suppression by amiodarone of orthodromic supraventricular tachycardias complicating pre-excitation syndromes. *J Am Coll Cardiol*. 1984;3:1298–1307.
24. Olgin JE, Kalman JM, Lesh MD. Conduction barriers in human atrial flutter: correlation of electrophysiology and anatomy. *J Cardiovasc Electrophysiol*. 1996;7:1112–1126.
25. Kalman JM, Olgin JE, Saxon LA, et al. Activation and entrainment mapping defines the tricuspid annulus as the anterior barrier in typical atrial flutter. *Circulation*. 1996;94:398–406.
26. Feld GK. Catheter ablation for the treatment of atrial tachycardias. *Prog Cardiovasc Dis*. 1995;38:205–224.
27. Kalman JM, Olgin JE, Karch MR, et al. "Cristal tachycardias": origin of right atrial tachycardias from the crista terminalis identified by intracardiac echocardiography. *J Am Coll Cardiol*. 1998; 31:451–459.
28. Chen SA, Tai CT, Chiang CE, et al. Focal atrial tachycardia: reanalysis of the clinical and electrophysiologic characteristics and prediction of successful radiofrequency ablation. *J Cardiovasc Electrophysiol*. 1998;9:355–365.
29. Chen SA, Chiang CE, Yang CJ, et al. Radiofrequency catheter ablation of sustained intra-atrial reentrant tachycardia in adult patients. Identification of electrophysiological characteristics and endocardial mapping techniques. *Circulation* 1993;88:578–587.
30. Kall JG, Kopp D, Olshansky B, et al. Adenosine-sensitive atrial tachycardia. *PACE*. 1995;18:300–306.
31. Chen SA, Chiang CE, Yang CJ, et al. Sustained atrial tachycardia in adult patients. Electrophysiological characteristics, pharmacological response, possible mechanisms, and effects of radiofrequency ablation. *Circulation*. 1994;90:1262–1278.
32. Yang T, Snyders DJ, Roden DM. Ibutilide, a methanesulfonanilide antiarrhythmic, is a potent blocker of the rapidly activating delayed rectifier K+ current (IKr) in AT-1 cells. Concentration-, time-, voltage-, and use-dependent effects. *Circulation* 1995;91: 1799–1806.
33. Cropp JS, Antal EG, Talbert RL. Ibutilide: a new class III antiarrhythmic agent. *Pharmacother*. 1997;17:1–9.
34. Stambler BS, Wood MA, Ellenbogen KA. Antiarrhythmic actions of intravenous ibutilide compared with procainamide during human atrial flutter and fibrillation: electrophysiological determinants of enhanced conversion efficacy. *Circulation*.1997;96: 4298–4306.
35. Ellenbogen KA, Clemo HF, Stambler BS, et al. Efficacy of ibutilide for termination of atrial fibrillation and flutter. *Am J Cardiol*. 1996;78:42–45.
36. Kowey PR, VanderLugt JT, Luderer JR. Safety and risk/benefit analysis of ibutilide for acute conversion of atrial fibrillation/flutter. *Am J Cardiol*. 1996;78:46–52.
37. Ellenbogen KA, Perry KT, VanderLugt JT. Acute hemodynamic effects of intravenous ibutilide in patients with or without reduced left ventricular function. *Am J Cardiol*. 1997;80: 458–463.
38. Chiladakis JA, Vassilikos VP, Maounis TN, et al. Successful radiofrequency catheter ablation of automatic atrial tachycardia with regression of the cardiomyopathy picture. *PACE*. 1997; 20:953–959.
39. Feld GK, Fleck RP, Chen PS, et al. Radiofrequency catheter ablation for the treatment of human type 1 atrial flutter. Identification of a critical zone in the reentrant circuit by endocardial mapping techniques. *Circulation*. 1992;86: 1233–1240.
40. Cosio FG, Lopez-Gil M, Goicolea A, et al. Radiofrequency ablation of the inferior vena cava-tricuspid valve isthmus in common atrial flutter. *Am J Cardiol*. 1993;71:705–709.
41. Poty H, Saoudi N, Aziz AA, et al. Radiofrequency catheter ablation of type 1 atrial flutter. Prediction of late success by electrophysiologic criteria. *Circulation*. 1995;92:1389–1392.
42. Feld GK, Wharton JM, Plumb V, et al. Radiofrequency catheter ablation of type 1 atrial flutter using large-tip 8mm or 10mm electrode catheters and a high output radiofrequency energy generator: results of a multi-center safety and efficacy study. *J Am Coll Cardiol*. 2004;43:1466–1472.
43. Chen SA, Chiang CE, Yang CJ, et al. Sustained atrial tachycardia in adult patients. Electrophysiological characteristics, pharmacological response, possible mechanisms, and effects of radiofrequency ablation. *Circulation*. 1994;90:1262–1278.
44. Kay GN, Chong F, Epstein AE, et al. Radiofrequency ablation for treatment of primary atrial tachycardia. *J Am Coll Cardiol*. 1993; 21:901–909.
45. Trappe HJ, Paul T, Pfitzner P, et al. Transcatheter ablation of incessant ectopic left atrial tachycardia using radiofrequency current. *J Interven Cardiol*. 1995;8:3–8.
46. Kannel WB, Abbot RD, Savage DD, et al. Epidemiologic features of chronic atrial fibrillation. The Framingham Study. *N Engl J Med*. 1982;306:1018–1022.
47. Ueshima K, Meyers J, Ribisl PM, et al. Hemodynamic determinants of exercise capacity in chronic atrial fibrillation. *Am Heart J*. 1993;125:1301–1305.
48. Gosselink ATM, Crijins HJGM, Van Gelder IC, et al. Low-dose amiodarone for maintenance of sinus rhythm after cardioversion of atrial fibrillation or flutter. *JAMA*. 1992;267:3289–3293.
49. Anderson JL, Gilbert EM, Alpert BL, et al. Prevention of symptomatic recurrences of paroxysmal atrial fibrillation in patients initially tolerating antiarrhythmic therapy. A multi-center, double-blind crossover study of flecainide and placebo with transtelephonic monitoring. *Circulation*. 1989;80: 1557–1570.
50. Juul-Moller S, Edvardsson N, Rehnqvist-Ahlberg N. Sotalol versus quinidine for the maintenance of sinus rhythm after direct current conversion of atrial fibrillation. *Circulation*. 1990;82: 1932–1939.
51. Pedersen OD, Brendorp B, Elming H, et al. Does conversion and prevention of atrial fibrillation enhance survival in patients with left ventricular dysfunction? Evidence from the Danish Investigations of Arrhythmia and Mortality on Dofetilide (DIAMOND) study. *Card Electrophysiol Rev*. 2003;7:220–224.
52. Moller M, Torp-Pedersen CT, Kober L. Dofetilide in patients with heart failure and left ventricular dysfunction: safety aspects and effect on atrial fibrillation. The Danish Investigators of Arrhythmia and Mortality on Dofetilide (DIAMOND) Study Group. *Congest Heart Fail*. 2001;7:146–150.

53. Mason JW, for the Electrophysiologic Study versus Electrocardiographic Monitoring (ESVEM) Investigators. A comparison of electrophysiologic testing with Holter monitoring to predict antiarrhythmic drug efficacy for ventricular tachyarrhythmias. *N Engl J Med*. 1993;329:445–451.
54. Gallik DM, Kim SG, Ferrick KJ, et al. Efficacy and safety of sotalol in patients with refractory atrial fibrillation or flutter. *Am Heart J*. 1997;134:155–160.
55. Cairns JA, Connolly SJ, Roberts R, et al. Randomised trial of outcome after myocardial infarction in patients with frequent or repetitive ventricular premature depolarisations: CAMIAT. Canadian Amiodarone Myocardial Infarction Arrhythmia Trial Investigators. *Lancet*. 1997;349:675–682.
56. Julian DG, Camm AJ, Franglin G, et al. Randomised trial of effect of amiodarone on mortality in patients with left-ventricular dysfunction after recent myocardial infarction: EMIAT. European Myocardial Infarct Amiodarone Trial Investigators. *Lancet*. 1997;349:667–674.
57. Singh BN, Venkatesh N, Nademanee K. The historical development, cellular electrophysiology and pharmacology of amiodarone. *Prog Cardiovasc Dis*. 1989;31:249–280.
58. Vrobel TR, Miller PE, Mostow ND, et al. A general overview of amiodarone toxicity: its prevention, detection, and management. *Prog Cardiovasc Dis*. 1989;31:393–426.
59. Grogan M, Smith HC, Gersh BJ, et al. Left ventricular dysfunction due to atrial fibrillation in patients initially believed to have idiopathic dilated cardiomyopathy. *Am J Cardiol*. 1992;69:1570–1573.
60. Galun E, Flugelman MY, Glickson M, et al. Failure of long-term digitalization to prevent rapid ventricular response in patients with paroxysmal atrial fibrillation. *Chest*. 1991;99:1038–1040.
61. Langberg JJ, Chin MC, Resenqvist M, et al. Catheter ablation of the atrioventricular junction with radiofrequency energy. *Circulation*. 1989;80:1527–1535.
62. Heinz G, Siostrzonek P, Kreiner G, et al. Improvement in left ventricular systolic function after successful radiofrequency His bundle ablation for drug refractory chronic atrial fibrillation and recurrent atrial flutter. *Am J Cardiol*. 1992;69:489–492.
63. Twidale N, Sutton K, Bartlett L, et al. Effects on cardiac performance of atrioventricular node catheter ablation using radiofrequency current for drug-refractory atrial arrhythmias. *Pacing and Clin Electrophysiol*. 1993;16:1275–1284.
64. Feld GK, Fleck RP, Fujimura O, et al. Control of rapid ventricular response by radiofrequency catheter modification of the atrioventricular node in patients with medically refractory atrial fibrillation. *Circulation*. 1994;90:2299–2307.
65. Feld GK. Radiofrequency catheter ablation versus modification of the AV node for control of rapid ventricular response in atrial fibrillation. *J Cardiovasc Electrophysiol*. 1995;6:217–228.
66. Morady F, Hasse C, Strickberger SA, et al. Long-term follow-up after radiofrequency modification of the atrioventricular node in patients with atrial fibrillation. *J Am Coll Cardiol*. 1997;29:113–121.
67. Wyse DG, Waldo AL, DiMarco JP, et al. Atrial Fibrillation Follow-up Investigation of Rhythm Management (AFFIRM) Investigators. A comparison of rate control and rhythm control in patients with atrial fibrillation. *N Engl J Med*. 2002;347(23): 1825–1833.
68. Corley SD, Epstein AE, DiMarco JP, et al. AFFIRM Investigators. Relationships between sinus rhythm, treatment, and survival in the Atrial Fibrillation Follow-Up Investigation of Rhythm Management (AFFIRM) study. *Circulation*. 2004;109:1509–1513.
69. Nitta T. Surgery for atrial fibrillation. *Ann Thorac Cardiovasc Surg*. 2005;11:154–158.
70. Hocini M, Sanders P, Jais P, et al. Techniques for curative treatment of atrial fibrillation. *J Cardiovasc Electrophysiol*. 2004;15: 1467–1471.
71. Pappone C, Rosanio S, Augello G, et al. Mortality, morbidity, and quality of life after circumferential pulmonary vein ablation for atrial fibrillation: outcomes from a controlled nonrandomized long-term study. *J Am Coll Cardiol*. 2003;42:185–197.
72. Hsu LF, Jais P, Sanders P, et al. Catheter ablation for atrial fibrillation in heart failure. *N Engl J Med*. 2004;351:2373–2383.
73. Lamas GA, Orav EJ, Stambler BS, et al. Quality of life and clinical outcomes in elderly patients treated with ventricular pacing as compared with dual-chamber pacing. Pacemaker Selection in the Elderly Investigators. *N Engl J Med*. 1998; 338:1097–1104.
74. Andersen HR, Nielsen JC, Thomsen PEB, et al. Long-term follow-up of patients from a randomized trial of atrial versus ventricular pacing for sick-sinus syndrome. *Lancet*. 1997;350: 1210–1216.
75. Wilkoff BL, Cook JR, Epstein AE, et al. Dual Chamber and VVI Implantable Defibrillator Trial Investigators. Dual-chamber pacing or ventricular backup pacing in patients with an implantable defibrillator: the Dual Chamber and VVI Implantable Defibrillator (DAVID) Trial. *JAMA*. 2002;288:3115–3123.
76. Knight BP, Gersh BJ, Carlson MD, et al. American Heart Association Council on Clinical Cardiology (Subcommittee on Electrocardiography and Arrhythmias); Quality of Care and Outcomes Research Interdisciplinary Working Group; Heart Rhythm Society; AHA Writing Group. Role of permanent pacing to prevent atrial fibrillation: science advisory from the American Heart Association Council on Clinical Cardiology (Subcommittee on Electrocardiography and Arrhythmias) and the Quality of Care and Outcomes Research Interdisciplinary Working Group, in collaboration with the Heart Rhythm Society. *Circulation*. 2005;111:240–243.
77. Schuchert A, Boriani G, Wollmann C, et al. Implantable dual-chamber defibrillator for the selective treatment of spontaneous atrial and ventricular arrhythmias: arrhythmia incidence and device performance. *J Interv Card Electrophysiol*. 2005;12: 149–156.
78. Ricci R, Pignalberi C, Santini M. Efficacy of atrial antitachycardia functions for treating atrial fibrillation: observations in patients with a dual-chamber defibrillator. *Card Electrophysiol Rev*. 2003;7:348–351.
79. Stroke Prevention in Atrial Fibrillation Investigators (SPAF). Stroke prevention in atrial fibrillation: final results. *Circulation*. 1991;84:527–539.

Prevention of Sudden Death in Heart Failure

41

Philip B. Adamson Emilio Vanoli

Sudden cardiac death is defined as death within minutes to hours from the onset of symptoms in a patient who otherwise was clinically stable (1,2). This definition seems simple but, in reality, determining the cause of sudden cardiovascular collapse can be challenging (3). Clinical trials differ about which deaths are considered "sudden," making accurate comparison across trials difficult (4). For example, the Cardiac Insufficiency and Bisoprolol Trial (CIBIS) classified unwitnessed deaths that occurred during sleep as "unknown cause" rather than "sudden," whereas other trials consider overnight deaths as "sudden" (5). Furthermore, the true epidemiology of sudden cardiac death is difficult to quantify, but estimates in the U.S. population range from 300,000 to 500,000 annual deaths that are attributable to sudden cardiac arrest (6–10).

Even with ambiguity of numbers, sudden death (SD) is a major cause of premature mortality in patients who otherwise have stable, even minimally, symptomatic cardiovascular disease. The cardiology community's frustration with SD was clearly stated by Prof. Bernard Lown, who in 1979 considered SD as "the most important challenge facing modern cardiology" (11). Despite significant efforts examining the mechanisms of lethal cardiac arrhythmias over the past 30 years, the syndrome of sudden cardiac death still remains an important challenge facing modern cardiology (12,13). This chapter will focus on the epidemiology of SD in order to identify at-risk patient groups, and will organize available evidence supporting the rationale of pharmacologic arrhythmia suppression and immediate termination strategies when lethal arrhythmias develop. These data will be summarized in a practical approach to provide the currently accepted standard of care for SD prevention in patients with chronic heart failure.

CLINICAL CHARACTERISTICS OF SUDDEN DEATH

Most sudden cardiac deaths result from ventricular tachyarrhythmias, while bradyarrhythmias, great vessel rupture, or pulmonary embolism account for other etiologies of sudden cardiovascular collapse (14–24) (Fig. 41-1). The overwhelming majority of people who develop sustained ventricular tachyarrhythmias outside the hospital die, since immediate electrical therapy is required for any hopes of survival (25,26). For every minute a ventricular arrhythmia is established, the chance of survival is reduced by 10%, so that 10 minutes after cardiovascular collapse, there is virtually no chance of survival (25). The need for immediate therapy helps explain why less than 5% of patients in the United States who have out-of-hospital cardiac arrest survive, even in areas of well-developed rapid response systems. An aspect of SD that is critical to understanding the syndrome is that, by definition, it is not preceded by warning events, even in patients with symptomatic heart failure. A post hoc analysis of the CIBIS-II trial demonstrated that only 20% of the patients who died suddenly during follow-up had worsening heart failure symptoms or warning hospitalization prior to the lethal event (27). In stark contrast, worsening heart failure symptoms and hospitalization preceded almost 90% of the patients who died of pump failure (27). Therefore, since warning symptoms are not present to identify patients at risk for impending sudden cardiovascular collapse, primary prevention of SD must rely on identifying high-risk patients before their fatal event.

Sudden cardiac death generally occurs in the presence of some form of structural heart disease (28–32), such as

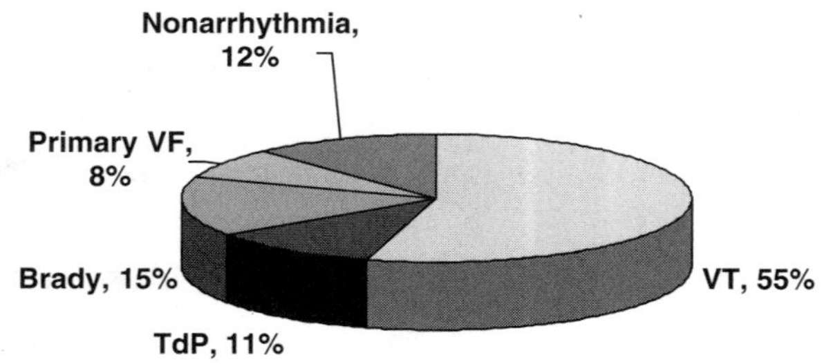

Figure 41-1 Causes of sudden cardiovascular collapse. TdP, torsade du pointes; VT, ventricular tachycardia; VF, ventricular fibrillation; Brady, bradycardia. Nonarrhythmic causes of sudden death include pulmonary embolism, great vessel rupture, and lethal stroke. (Adapted from Bayes de Luna A, Coumel P, Leclercq JF. Ambulatory sudden cardiac death. Mechanisms of production of fatal arrhythmia on the basis of data from 157 cases. *Am Heart J.* 1989;117:151–159.)

myocardial ischemia or infarction (33–35), dilated cardiomyopathy, hypertrophic cardiomyopathy (36), or genetically determined primary electrophysiological abnormalities such as long-QT syndrome (37) or Brugada syndrome (38). Of all the possible associated diseases, ischemic heart disease is the most common underlying pathology that renders the ventricle electrically unstable (33–35,39,40). Thus, SD may occur in profoundly different clinical settings (Fig. 41-2).

The most difficult patients to identify are those who die from lethal arrhythmias as the first manifestation of ischemic heart disease. In contrast to an overall trend toward a reduction in cardiac mortality (10,41), the incidence of sudden arrhythmic death in subjects free of overt ischemic heart disease has remained unaltered over the last 20 years (10,23,32,33). Annually, more than 50,000 Americans die of unheralded SD that is often the first, and last, manifestation of ischemic heart disease. This major public health issue has received little attention, presumably due to the general belief that high-risk individuals cannot be identified with enough predictive accuracy to warrant specific preventive interventions. Indeed, these individuals are usually not under the care of a physician and the unexpected nature of their death precludes any prediction or preparedness.

Autopsy series performed in individuals who died suddenly without prodromal symptoms usually find the presence of significant obstructive coronary artery disease with evidence for a very recent thrombotic event (33). These individuals apparently respond to their first ischemic episode with a lethal arrhythmia, since most autopsy reports fail to actually demonstrate the presence of acute myocardial necrosis, implying that the cardiac arrest occurred immediately in response to the ischemic event. Inherited traits produce familial trends in both risk for SD and autonomic dysfunction that contribute to the overall risk profile of individuals who die suddenly and unexpectedly (21,40).

Those few patients who survive unexpected cardiac arrest without a prior history of cardiovascular disease are characterized by significant cardiac autonomic control system dysfunction resulting in imbalances favoring strong sympathetic input with relatively weak vagal control (42). These findings are supported from experimental evidence in canines at high risk for ventricular fibrillation during their first episode of myocardial ischemia (43–45). High-risk animals respond to acute ischemia with strong sympathetic activation and weak vagal reflexes, which lead to the development of ventricular fibrillation (VF). In contrast,

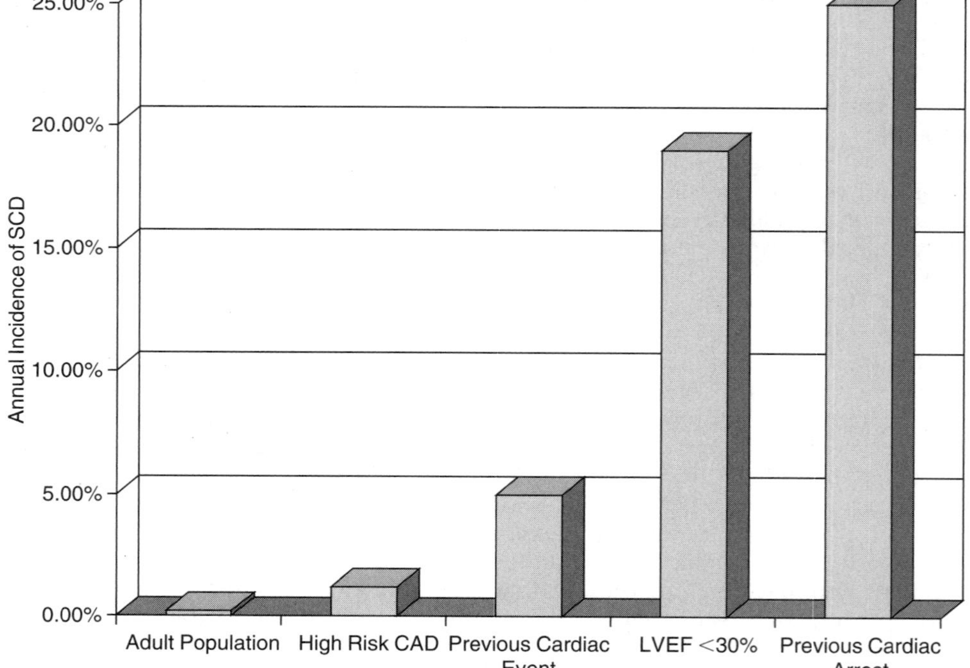

Figure 41-2 Incidence of sudden cardiac death (SCD) in the entire adult population, patients with coronary artery disease (CAD), previous cardiac injury, depressed left ventricular ejection fraction (LVEF), and survivors of cardiac arrest. Note the high incidence of sudden death in patients with left ventricular dysfunction defined as an ejection fraction less than 30%. (Adapted from Larsen MP, Eisenberg MS, Cummins RO, et al. Predicting survival from out-of-hospital cardiac arrest. A graphic model. *Ann Emerg Med.* 1993;22:1652–1658.)

those at low risk for lethal arrhythmias respond to the same ischemic insult with vagal activation and relatively weak sympathetic input, and subsequently have no sustained ventricular arrhythmias. These differences in autonomic response to acute myocardial ischemia, even in the absence of structural heart disease (44,45), are important components of the mechanisms responsible for SD throughout the spectrum of chronic ischemic heart disease, from the first manifestation to end-stage heart failure (46).

The second general condition in which elevated SD risk can be identified is after ventricular injury by myocardial infarction (MI) (Fig. 41-2). The incidence of post-MI sudden cardiac death has decreased over the past 30 years, however, presumably due to early revascularization therapy that restores circulation to the infarct zone (10,46). The incidence of out-of-hospital sudden cardiac arrest is estimated to be 0.8 per 1,000 subject-years in individuals without clinically recognized heart disease. In patients with overt coronary artery disease (CAD), SD incidence is 13.6 per 1,000 subject-years in subjects with prior MI and 21.9 per 1,000 subject-years in subjects with symptomatic heart failure, illustrating that as heart disease progresses, ventricular electrical stability declines over time (Fig. 41-3) (6). The highest risk for SD following MI appears to be in the first 30 days (47,48), but attempting to reduce this risk by using an implantable cardioverter defibrillator was, at least in one population, associated with increased mortality (49).

Minimization of infarct size after MI with early revascularization strategies (50), coupled with prevention of adverse myocardial and electrical remodeling using angiotensin-converting enzyme (ACE) inhibitors (51,52), aldosterone antagonists (53), and beta-blockers (54) routinely after MI, are effective in reducing the incidence of post-MI SD. Less successful approaches to reduce post-MI SD involved using antiarrhythmic drugs in a primary prevention strategy. Trials using this approach with sodium channel (I_{Na}) blockers in post-MI patients from the late 1970s were affected by the change in SD incidence resulting in higher on-treatment mortality compared with placebo, which as a group had an unexpectedly low SD risk (55). Trials investigating antiarrhythmic drug therapy targeting specific ion channels, such as I_{Kr} (56) or using amiodarone (57,58) were associated with either increased mortality on treatment (56) or no effect on overall mortality (57). Further refinements in the treatment of acute coronary syndromes, such as platelet inhibition and routine percutaneous catheter-mediated intervention, seemed to impact short-term SD risk, but only assumptions can be made about long-term (years) benefits.

Following MI, autonomic imbalances favoring the sympathetic nervous system can be detected in patients at high

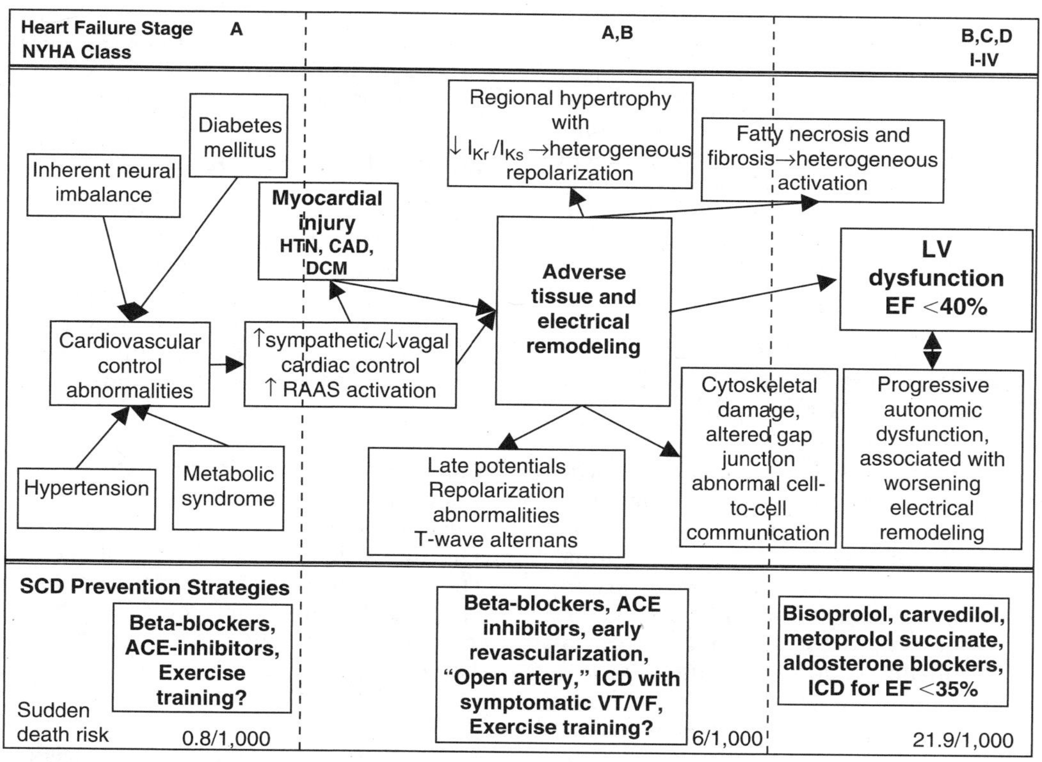

Figure 41-3 An illustration of the proposed mechanisms involved in worsening myocardial and electrophysiologic function as cardiovascular disease progresses from neurohormonal changes associated with risk factors such as hypertension and diabetes, through the development of left ventricular dysfunction. It is important to consider that the outcome of sudden death is the result of tissue and electrophysiologic changes that occur upstream from the clinical arrhythmic event. (Refer to Dinerman JL, Berger R, Haigney MC, et al. Dispersion of ventricular activation and refractoriness in patients with idiopathic dilated cardiomyopathy. *Am J Cardiol.* 1997;79:970–974.)

SD risk as measured by autonomic markers such as heart rate variability (HRV) or baroreflex sensitivity (BRS) (59–61). These markers have Class I consensus recommendation to aid in post-MI risk stratification with a level of evidence A (62). In patients and animals with a healed MI, quantifying vagal reflex activation by relating blood pressure increases with heart rate slowing (the so-called baroreflex sensitivity test) can stratify longitudinal risk for lethal arrhythmias (59,60). Those at high risk for SD have weaker cardiac vagal reflexes, implying that vagal withdrawal, which probably occurs along with sympathetic activation during progressive cardiac disease, is an important component of the mechanisms involved in lethal arrhythmogenesis. Vagal augmentation by electrical stimulation of the cervical sympathovagal trunk significantly reduces the incidence of ventricular fibrillation (VF) when applied to high-risk animals at the time of vulnerability (63). Interestingly, the ventricular arrhythmia suppressive effect of vagal stimulation was, in large part, still present even when heart rate was maintained by atrial pacing.

On the other hand, vagal inhibition by atropine (64) or sympathetic activation by ephedrine (65) also enhances arrhythmic risk and mortality in otherwise low-risk subjects. Patients with conditions such as MI or heart failure, which are characterized by an autonomic control milieu consisting of parasympathetic withdrawal or inherently weak cardiac vagal control coupled with sympathetic activation, have an increased relative risk for lethal arrhythmias.

Patients have an increasing risk for SD as their heart disease progresses from coronary occlusion to heart failure. In this regard, patients with heart failure represent one of the highest-risk groups that are routinely under physicians' care. It is the intent of this chapter to examine potential mechanisms responsible for risk development and provide a basis for primary and secondary prevention SD prevention strategies in patients with chronic heart failure.

LETHAL ARRHYTHMIA SUPPRESSION VERSUS SUDDEN DEATH PREVENTION IN PATIENTS WITH HEART FAILURE

Heart failure pathophysiology is very complex, with regional differences in fibrosis, hypertrophy, infarction, and ischemia that ultimately result in a global decreased force of contraction coupled with a loss of the normal force–frequency relationship. Multiple mechanisms are involved in the development of left ventricular dysfunction but the intimate relationship between cardiac cell excitation and coupling of that excitation with muscle contraction makes it impossible to isolate tissue, structural, and architectural adverse remodeling from the associated changes in cardiac electrophysiology (65–70). The fatal result of these changes (the clinical syndrome of sudden cardiac death) is identified by the presence of lethal arrhythmias (mostly ventricular fibrillation or unstable ventricular tachycardia), but the actual events that lead to arrhythmia development are much more important when considering prevention (Fig. 41-3).

Clinical interventions that effectively reduce the relative risk for SD focus on either the upstream events that eventually lead to the development of lethal arrhythmias, or provide a means for rapid termination of ventricular tachyarrhythmias once they develop. Therefore, SD prevention in patients with chronic heart failure involves two basic mechanisms, each of which will be considered in detail in this chapter.

First, suppressing lethal ventricular tachyarrhythmias can be accomplished by preventing the fixed or functional electrophysiological substrate conducive for arrhythmogenesis and suppressing electrophysiological triggers responsible for initiating a re-entrant circuit. Since the substrate for triggered activity and re-entry is, in large part, dependent on neurohormonal activation in response to injury, it is not surprising that the most effective pharmacologic means to prevent lethal arrhythmias in patients with heart failure is beta-blocker therapy coupled with angiontensin-converting enzyme (ACE) inhibition and aldosterone antagonism. Even with appropriate neurohormonal antagonism, however, the residual risk for SD is still high, which requires inclusion of complementary interventions to effectively reduce overall SD risk.

Along with arrhythmia suppression using appropriate neurohormonal intervention, the second general approach to SD prevention is immediate electrical treatment to terminate potentially lethal ventricular arrhythmias once they are established. This approach is accomplished by use of implantable cardioverter defibrillators designed to deliver either antitachycardic pacing or defibrillation when appropriate arrhythmia sensing occurs. These prevention strategies are synergistic and theoretically produce a >70% relative risk reduction for SD when compared to no intervention (72).

Lethal Arrhythmia Suppression

Cardiac electrophysiology in heart failure patients is the result of complex interactions between local events, such as myocardial ischemia, fibrosis, and replacement of the normal myocardial syncytium, coupled with functional modifications by cardiac control systems primarily arising from the autonomic nervous and renin-angiotensin-aldosterone systems (RAAS). Adverse tissue and architectural remodeling, characteristic of chronic heart failure, is not homogeneous, and this has direct consequences on cardiac electrical properties. In addition to cardiac structural changes, remodeling of cardiac ion channel densities, structure, or function, coupled with alterations in cell-to-cell communication, significantly alter both activation and repolarization. This process, called electrical remodeling, represents the upstream process by which an arrhythmogenic substrate provides risk for lethal tachyarrhythmias (Fig. 41-3, Table 41-1).

Alterations in Activation and Risk for Sudden Death

Cardiac cell activation and conduction of the action potential through the myocardial syncytium depend on availability of appropriate sodium current and cell-to-cell communication through the proper density and distribution

TABLE 41-1

ELECTROPHYSIOLOGICAL CONSEQUENCES OF ADVERSE TISSUE REMODELING LEADING TO A MYOCARDIAL SUBSTRATE AT HIGH RISK FOR SUDDEN CARDIAC DEATH

Remodeling Event	Channel	Activation	Repolarization
Hypertrophy	$\downarrow I_{Ks}$	Delayed	Prolonged
Fibrosis	~	Fractionated	~
Cytoskeletal abnormality	$\downarrow I_{Na}$	Decreased upstroke amplitude	?
Apoptosis	~	Fractionated	?
Infarction/ischemia	$\downarrow I_{Na}$, $\downarrow I_{Kr}$, $\downarrow I_{Ks}$	Fractionated	Prolonged
Dilation	$\downarrow I_{to}$	Delayed	Prolonged

of gap junctions (73–76). Adverse remodeling associated with chronic cardiovascular disease and heart failure can alter activation and conduction by influencing sodium channel (I_{Na}) densities, especially in areas of myocardial ischemia or infarction (75–83). I_{Na} function is also altered in heart failure by changes in cytoskeletal support of the channel (77). Conduction abnormalities can arise from altered I_{Na} or by functional abnormalities imposed by intracellular fibrosis (82) or changes in cell size (83).

These aspects of electrical remodeling can result in a fixed substrate when changes in the ventricular myocardium permanently alter electrophysiological characteristics in the area of change. Examples of fixed electrophysiological abnormalities include fractionated activation across a so-called mottled infarct created by surviving tissue interspersed among necrotic or fibrotic tissue (84–90). Activation fronts encountering areas of patchy fibrosis or fatty necrosis either alter conduction impedance or allow conduction through the zone by way of surviving tissue that forms conduction channels that traverse the area of patchy necrosis. Impulses conducting through channels can exit from the zone of patchy conduction to encounter excitable tissue and give rise to triggers for re-entrant arrhythmias. This combination of delayed activation, unidirectional block, and discontinuous conduction is thought is be the macroscopic mechanisms responsible for re-entrant tachyarrhythmias.

Additional influences on activation electrophysiology include changes in anisotropy or cell-to-cell communication arising from altered gap junctions producing delayed conduction in the affected areas (91). Myocardial ischemia or left ventricular hypertrophy (LVH) results in downregulation of connexin 43 (Cx43), as well as a redistribution of this protein to the lateral aspects of the myocyte (91–93). The stimuli for gap junction remodeling are not completely understood, but likely rely on neural and hormonal control of expression and distribution kinetics.

Activation alterations produce fractionated wavefronts that are detectable in heart failure patients at high SD risk (94). The mechanisms involved in establishing fixed changes in activation involve stimulation of fibrosis and fatty necrosis by angiotensin II, aldosterone, and adrenergic receptor activation. Therefore, neurohormonal intervention is a critical means to prevent permanent changes in the myocardium that produce a fixed substrate for arrhythmias (Fig. 41-3). It is unclear if continued neurohormonal antagonism results in reversal of the electrophysiological substrate for lethal arrhythmias once that substrate is established. What is clear, however, is that altered activation and conduction (especially when coupled with repolarization heterogeneity) are key components of the high-risk substrate (95).

Alterations in Repolarization and Risk for Sudden Death

Prolonged repolarization is characteristic of heart failure pathophysiology, resulting in lengthening of the myocardial monophasic action potential (Fig. 41-4) (69,96). Typically, changes in ventricular function, tissue, and electrical remodeling in heart failure are heterogeneous, which is especially true for repolarization abnormalities (45,97). Repolarization heterogeneity can produce severe repolarization dispersion, which is found in subjects at high risk for lethal arrhythmias (97). Interestingly, lower-risk individuals seem to have much less repolarization heterogeneity compared to their high-risk counterparts. Why some individuals develop severe repolarization heterogeneity is complex, but likely relates to control system responses to injury, such as the degree of sympathetic activation following MI. Abnormal repolarization can be detected in humans and animals at high SD risk by different modalities, including microvolt T wave alternans (98,99), QT interval dispersion, or high-density mapping (97,100–102).

Prolongation of action potential duration may have an adaptive purpose. When the repolarization phase of cardiac tissue prolongs, it increases the likelihood that a re-entrant wavefront may encounter refractory tissue, which would serve to terminate the circuit. With this effect, repolarization prolongation has the potential to be antiarrhythmic, but the prolongation must be global and homogeneous for the effect to prevent an unstable ventricular electrophysiological environment. These conditions are seldom encountered when adverse ventricular remodeling occurs.

Prolonged repolarization in heart failure arises because of changes in expression of functional ion channels responsible for the plateau and rapid repolarization of the monophasic action potential (Fig. 41-4) (66,67,71,103–108). Repolarization abnormalities that contribute to the arrhythmogenic substrate arise from both acute changes in autonomic control (109) and from ion channel remodeling

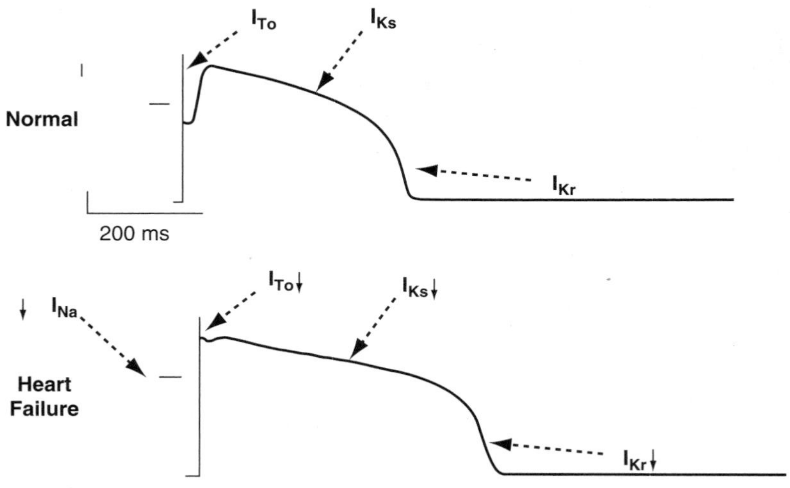

Figure 41-4 Proposed channelopathies involved in activation and repolarization abnormalities in the failing heart. A normal, monophasic action potential is illustrated in the **top panel** and an action potential from a failing ventricle is illustrated in the **bottom panel**. Dysfunction or downregulation of I_{Na}, I_{To}, I_{Kr}, and I_{Ks} are known to occur in the remodeling process involved in progressive cardiovascular disease. While prolongation of the action potential may be initially adaptive, this electrophysiologic abnormality results in a higher risk for re-entrant or triggered arrhythmias.

in the presence of LVH or stretch. Most consistently, downregulation of the transient outward potassium channel, I_{to}, which contributes to the plateau phase of the monophasic action potential, is encountered in cells from most etiologies of heart failure (69,104). Other potassium channel abnormalities that occur in heart failure include reduced delayed rectifier (I_K) current density, coupled with faster deactivation kinetics and slow activation properties, which result in prolongation of the rapid repolarization phase of the monophasic action potential (69,105). LVH results in a significant downregulation of the inward rectifying potassium channel, I_{Ks}, which becomes the predominant channel responsible for myocyte repolarization in states of sympathetic activation (106). Along with changes associated with hypertrophy, cytoskeletal support protein remodeling also influences potassium channel function (110–112). When regional tissue remodeling is present, with areas of compensatory hypertrophy the resulting heterogeneous repolarization kinetics increase the risk for spontaneous ventricular tachyarrhythmias.

Global prolongation of ventricular repolarization in patients with heart failure arises from multiple mechanisms (68), which include potassium channel dysfunction as well as abnormalities in calcium homeostasis (112,113). It must be recognized that calcium handling is a key component that gives rise to decreased force of contraction, but abnormalities in calcium kinetics also have direct electrophysiological ramifications (114). Cells from failing ventricles exhibit a decrease in calcium transient amplitude and its rate of decay. Heterogeneity of calcium transient amplitude and delay when comparing endocardial, midmyocardial, and epicardial regions, as well as global changes associated with regional heterogeneity and ischemia in the failing heart, very likely contribute to ventricular electrophysiological instability (115). Further alterations in the sarcoplasmic reticulum Ca^{2+}-ATPase (SERCA2a), phospholamban, and the sodium-calcium exchanger proteins are described in the failing ventricle and can alter the intracellular calcium concentration. This is associated with ryanodine receptor defects, which when combined with other alterations in calcium homeostasis, increase the risk for calcium-dependent afterdepolarizations (68,116–119). Afterdepolarizations are key elements that form the basis for triggered arrhythmias and sustained polymorphic ventricular tachycardia.

Heterogeneous ventricular repolarization kinetics that result in regional and global prolongation are induced by both acute and chronic changes in neural and hormonal control of the heart. Therefore, fixed repolarization abnormalities can potentially be prevented by neurohormonal intervention when applied early in the adverse remodeling process; however, chronic therapies also have a beneficial effect by preventing functional or momentary abnormalities in repolarization induced by acute neural activation in response to injury or physiological needs. It becomes apparent, then, that neurohormonal blockade, as a means for preventing SD, has a long-term effect by preventing permanent electrical remodeling leading to an arrhythmogenic substrate. It has a short-term effect by preventing momentary electrophysiological alterations that acutely give rise to high arrhythmia risk (Fig. 41-3, Table 41-2). Clinical realities such as patient compliance with medication regimen, bioavailability of ingested medications, and alterations of pharmacokinetics with polypharmacy in patients with heart failure impact the efficacy of neurohormonal interventions intended to prevent SD.

Suppression of Ventricular Arrhythmias by Neurohormonal Intervention

Development of permanent (fixed) electrophysiological substrates can be prevented by early use of neurohormonal interventions including ACE inhibitors, aldosterone antagonism, or antiadrenergic intervention with beta-blockers. Although the direct mechanisms involved in neurohormonal-induced electrical remodeling are not fully characterized, general conclusions can be made from clinical trial observations. For example, ACE inhibitor therapy is less likely to reduce SD risk when started in patients with advanced heart failure (120). However, it reduces mortality primarily by preventing pump failure deaths, presumably by inhibiting progressive architectural changes leading to

TABLE 41-2

HYPOTHESIZED EFFECT OF NEUROHORMONAL INTERVENTION TO PREVENT DEVELOPMENT OF AN ARRHYTHMOGENIC SUBSTRATE OR SUPPRESS ARRHYTHMIA TRIGGERS IN CARDIOVASCULAR DISEASE

Drug Class	Action	Antiarrhythmic Effect	Mortality Reduction	Sudden Cardiac Death Reduction
ACE inhibitors	Antifibrosis	Prevent development of substrate early after injury	↓ 21% heart failure	↓ 20% post-MI, minimal effect in chronic heart failure
Aldosterone antagonism	Antifibrosis	Prevent substrate	↓ 30% NYHA Class III–IV ↓ 15% post-MI LVD	↓ 34% in patients with heart failure
Beta-blockade-bisoprolol-metoprolol succinate-carvedilol	Antiadrenergic, antifibrotic, reduction in hypertrophy, prevention of apoptosis	Prevent substrate and suppress triggers	↓ 34% heart failure ↓ 25% post-MI LVD	↓ 41% in patients with heart failure
Amiodarone	Multiple channel blockade, antiadrenergic	Prevent substrate? Suppress triggers	No effect in patients with heart failure	↓ 18% post-MI

inefficient left ventricular function (120–125). On the other hand, if applied following MI (without the requirement for heart failure), ACE inhibitors seem to reduce the incidence of SD by as much as 20%, as demonstrated by meta-analysis techniques (51).

One can speculate that ACE inhibitor intervention may be effective in reducing SD early after myocardial injury by inhibiting angiotensin II's stimulation of interstitial fibrosis, leading to fractionated activation characteristic of arrhythmogenic substrates (126). It is clear that angiotensin II and aldosterone stimulate proliferation of cardiac fibroblasts, resulting in increased interstitial collagen formation; however, other effects such as promotion of inflammation with the resulting increase in oxygen free radicals and destabilization of atherosclerotic plaques may also increase the risk for ventricular electrical instability (126). In addition to the direct effects on myocardial structure, angiotensin II facilitates adrenergic effects on ventricular electrophysiology by reducing norepinephrine reuptake, increasing the amount of norepinephrine released with each nerve firing, and increasing the firing rate of sympathetic neurons (127–129). Control system interactions operant in the heart failure milieu make it clear that the precise mechanisms involved in the development of lethal arrhythmias are complex and multifactorial. This illustrates that effective SD prevention strategies must account for multiple potential mechanisms requiring the combination of multiple medications and device therapies (Fig. 41-3, Tables 41-1 and 41-2).

Sympathetic Activation and Sudden Death

Sympathetic adrenergic activation in heart failure represents a combination of inherent control system characteristics present before heart disease develops, coupled with how individual systems respond to ventricular injury (45). Sympathetic activation is almost always accompanied by parasympathetic withdrawal, which should be considered when examining how autonomic alterations in heart failure lead to lethal arrhythmias.

Recently, however, these concepts have been applied to an understanding of how cardiac electrophysiology changes when heart failure develops. Evidence from animal studies suggests that individuals may have innate cardiovascular control characteristics with unique responses to injury, which may either protect or predispose them to adverse electrophysiological consequences and SD. Specifically, autonomic markers such as baroreflex sensitivity and heart rate variability can identify a group characterized by imbalanced cardiac autonomic control favoring weak vagal reflexes and strong sympathetic tone even before overt cardiovascular disease occurs (43,44). Immediate responses to myocardial injury in these individuals results in a profound increase in sympathetic activation and vagal withdrawal, which is coupled with a very high SD risk at the time of the first injury or, later, when left ventricular dysfunction occurs. Low-risk subjects are characterized by stronger vagal and weaker sympathetic cardiac control before cardiovascular disease develops, and autonomic control remains relatively quiescent in response to similar myocardial injury. Low-risk subjects have little sympathetic activation even when significant left ventricular dysfunction develops. These data suggest that neurohormonal activation in cardiovascular disease may represent an individual innate characteristic of tonic and reflex cardiac autonomic control, which destines individuals to high or low risk for SD.

In addition to functional changes in global sympathetic outflow to the heart, neural remodeling in the neuroeffector junction can be arrhythmogenic. Sympathetic hypersensitivity in areas of myocardial necrosis alters local cardiac electrophysiology, increasing regional repolarization dispersion and increases risk for lethal arrhythmias (130,131). Myocardial injury can produce regional differences in nerve growth factors, which can stimulate sympathetic nerve sprouting and regionally increase relative sympathetic effect. This phenomenon further destabilizes ventricular electrophysiology and leads to increased risk for SD (132,133).

As opposed to fixed electrophysiological abnormalities that permanently disrupt orderly myocardial activation and repolarization characteristics of the heart, functional abnormalities are temporary and depend on local conditions such as acute sympathetic activation, myocardial ischemia, or inflammation. Functional abnormalities may include changes in local repolarization due to regional increases in sympathetic activation, for example, or may include activation fractionation from conduction delay induced by acute alteration in autonomic tone. Factors such as acute myocardial ischemia or infarction, electrolyte imbalances, or medications can also alter ion channel function, resulting in high risk for functional electrophysiological abnormalities that may lead to SD. Functional abnormalities tend to be difficult to predict and may occur shortly before the initiation of a sustained ventricular arrhythmia.

Since neurohormonal activation leading to adverse tissue and electrical remodeling is so important (134,135), it is logical that beta-blocker therapy, ACE inhibition, and aldosterone antagonism are effective interventions to suppress lethal arrhythmias, thereby reducing the risk for SD in patients with cardiovascular disease. ACE inhibitor therapy is known to reduce SD risk in patients with Stage A and B heart failure, which includes patients with coronary vascular disease or asymptomatic left ventricular dysfunction. However, angiotensin intervention with ACE inhibitors or angiotensin-receptor-blockers has more inconsistent effects on SD risk after heart failure develops. In contrast, beta-blocker therapy (136–139) and aldosterone antagonism (140) consistently reduce the relative risk for SD in patients after MI and in those with heart failure. In this context, CIBIS III documented that beta-blocker therapy can be safely initiated even prior to ACE inhibition (141).

In summary, antagonism of sympathetic activation using beta-blockers coupled with angiotensin-aldosterone intervention using ACE inhibitors and aldosterone antagonists prevents the long-term deleterious effects of neurohormonal activation characteristic of chronic heart failure. The mechanisms of SD prevention with neurohormonal blockade involve prevention of a fixed arrhythmogenic substrate and suppression of functional electrophysiological abnormalities linked to the development of triggered or re-entrant arrhythmias.

Lethal Arrhythmia Termination

It is apparent, then, that lethal arrhythmias occur when a fixed arrhythmogenic substrate develops or if functional electrophysiological changes are significant enough to trigger re-entry. These substrates are highly dependent on neural and hormonal influences, which can change over time depending upon the current cardiovascular milieu. It is understandable, then, that neurohormonal intervention (particularly beta-blocker and aldosterone antagonism therapies) has been shown to be effective in reducing the relative SD risk when evaluated in prospective clinical trials involving patients with heart failure. However, it is also apparent that the ever-changing cardiac electrophysiological substrate is always at some risk for the development of lethal arrhythmias, even in the presence of adequate neurohormonal antagonism.

Compounding this problem is the inevitability of patient noncompliance, which further alters the effects of neurohormonal interventions. This point is illustrated by the mode of death in patients randomized to active therapy in the major beta-blocker trials. Consistently, the relative mortality risk was decreased in the MERIT-HF, CIBIS II, and U.S. Carvedilol trials, but patients on active therapy still died suddenly over 50% of the time. Furthermore, patients more likely to die suddenly were less symptomatic from their heart failure syndrome (Fig. 41-5) (136). This is problematic in medical practice because those heart failure patients at highest relative risk for SD are ones thought to be clinically most stable, which can lead to underutilization of this life-saving technology.

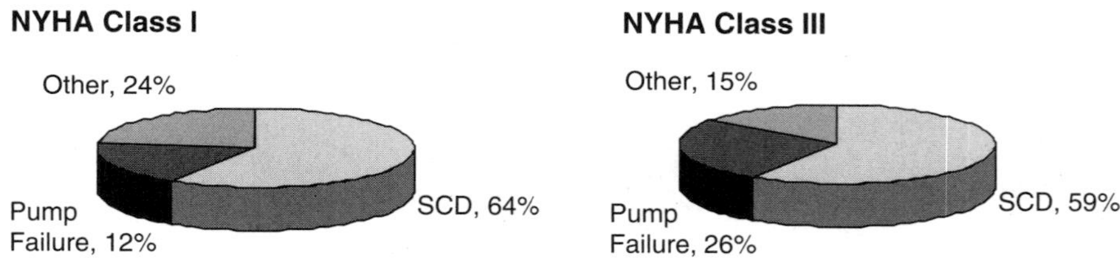

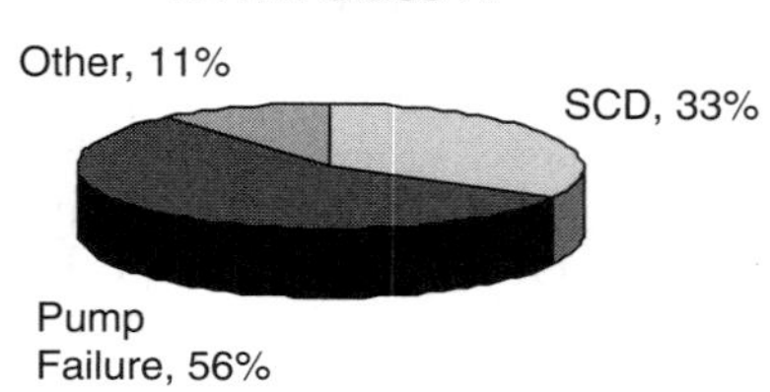

Figure 41-5 Cardiovascular deaths according to NYHA symptom classification from the MERIT-HF trial. Although total mortality was lower in the less-symptomatic group, the percentage of patients dying suddenly was higher. (From Cohn JN. The management of chronic heart failure. *N Engl J Med.* 1996;335:490–498.)

Analyses of when SD occurs also are important to understand prevention, since immediate therapy to terminate lethal arrhythmias is required to have hope for survival. Circadian analyses demonstrate that lethal cardiac events occur more often during the transition from sleep to awake (142). Sleep is an autonomically active condition typically characterized by a surge in vagal activity during non-REM sleep and a decrease in sympathetic activity (143,144). The vagal dominance of nocturnal autonomic cardiac control is generally thought to be associated with lower risk for cardiovascular events, and several studies support this idea. However, approximately 36,000 cases of nocturnal SD occur annually in the United States, representing approximately 15% of all SDs every year. These SDs appear to arise from ventricular tachyarrhythmias, since studies document appropriate implantable cardioverter defibrillator (ICD) discharges in patients with left ventricular dysfunction during sleep (143).

Abrupt control system changes that occur during sleep may serve to destabilize the cardiac electrical system in at-risk patients, which, coupled with the possibility that they may be in the pharmacodynamic trough phase of their beta-blocker effect, may increase the risk for nocturnal SD. In particular, cardiac sympathetic discharges that occur during REM sleep are coupled with a loss of the normal nocturnal vagal surge early after MI (144), and more so in patients with heart failure. This leads to a cardiac autonomic environment conducive for triggered and re-entrant arrhythmias. A post hoc analysis from the CIBIS II study supports this possibility, as it found that 20% of all SDs occurring in patients with heart failure were nocturnal and that bisoprolol reduced the incidence of nocturnal SD in this population. Those who died during sleep while on active therapy, however, were found to have no reduction in heart rate when assessed in the office setting, suggesting that these individuals were nonresponders to the beta-blocker's therapeutic effect. Therefore, neural events that occur during sleep or during the transition from sleep to awake are important components of the milieu conducive for lethal arrhythmias, and some patients are less responsive to beta-blocker therapy than others.

Since SD rates remain high with a significant number occurring at times when no responder would be available, patients at risk for SD (specifically, patients with heart failure) may have long-term benefit from an ICD capable of delivering electrical therapy for lethal arrhythmias immediately upon detection. The strategy of lethal arrhythmia termination using ICD therapy is complementary to that of neurohormonal intervention and now is proven to further reduce cardiovascular mortality in patients with heart failure.

Lethal Arrhythmia Termination Using Implantable Cardioverter Defibrillators—Ischemic Left Ventricular Dysfunction

The potential value of automatic detection of lethal arrhythmias with immediate delivery of electrical defibrillation using an ICD led to intense efforts to identify patients at high enough risk for SD to justify ICD use. Patients with ischemic heart disease and left ventricular dysfunction were the first to be studied, as they represent a group at high risk for arrhythmic death. Several studies enrolled patients with ischemic left ventricular dysfunction in an attempt to risk-stratify groups in need of an ICD.

Early strategies to prevent SD by terminating potentially lethal arrhythmias included the first Multicenter Automatic Defibrillator Implantation Trial (MADIT-I), which attempted to identify a highly selected group of patients based on invasive electrophysiological testing (145). Patients enrolled in MADIT-I had ischemic heart disease, left ventricular dysfunction, nonsustained ventricular tachycardia during ambulatory monitoring, and inducible ventricular tachycardia during invasive electrophysiological testing. Patients in this trial who received an ICD benefited with a significant 54% reduction in total mortality when followed over 2 years. These findings were confirmed by a second long-term, prospective randomized trial with similar design (146).

While mortality reductions were impressive in MADIT-I and MUSTT, the long-term value of electrophysiological testing in predicting SD risk became uncertain when registry findings demonstrated that SD risk in patients without inducible ventricular tachycardia was high (147). It became clear, then, that a more highly selected population, such as those studied in MADIT-I and MUSTT, potentially excluded a large number of at-risk individuals. These paradigm changes led to the hypothesis that appropriate primary SD prevention using ICD therapy would have a greater impact on overall SD incidence if applied to a population with ischemic heart disease and left ventricular dysfunction who had minimal electrophysiological abnormalities.

The second Multicenter Automatic Defibrillator Implantation Trial (MADIT-II) was the first primary prevention trial that examined the hypothesis that ICD therapy may reduce total mortality in patients selected on the presence of ischemic heart disease (previous transmural MI with evidence for obstructive coronary disease and fixed defect on thallium) and left ventricular dysfunction (LVEF <30%) resulting in NYHA Class I–III heart failure symptoms (148). In this trial patients were treated with all standard therapies, some of which were already known to reduce relative SD risks. Patients were then randomized in a prospective manner to continue with maximal medical therapy or receive a prophylactic ICD. MADIT-II was terminated early because of a 31% relative risk reduction for all-cause mortality in the patients randomized to ICD therapy (148). Therefore, primary prevention of SD using arrhythmia termination with an ICD, in addition to maximal medical therapy in patients with ischemic heart disease and significant left ventricular dysfunction, is superior to maximal medical therapy alone.

Lethal Arrhythmia Termination Using Implantable Cardioverter Defibrillators—Nonischemic Left Ventricular Dysfunction

Overall, the reason that ischemic left ventricular dysfunction was thought to be a condition of increased SD risk was due to severe ventricular electrophysiological heterogeneity that developed after MI. It became clear, however, that patients with nonischemic left ventricular injury were also at higher risk for SD and that abnormal cardiac electrophysiology in these patients was not homogeneous.

The Sudden Cardiac Death in Heart Failure Trial (SCD-HeFT) was the first primary prevention trial to include patients with nonischemic left ventricular dysfunction (LVEF <35%). This trial sought to determine which of three strategies is superior for SD prevention: (a) the effects of maximal neurohormonal intervention (beta-blockers, ACE inhibitors and aldosterone antagonists) alone; (b) maximal medical therapy with arrhythmia suppression using amiodarone; or (c) maximal medical therapy coupled with arrhythmia termination using an ICD (149). Total mortality reduction was seen only in the ICD arm, with amiodarone performing similarly to maximal medical therapy alone. The benefits of ICD therapies were seen across all subgroups, except patients with NYHA Class III symptoms. The meaning of this subgroup analysis was unclear because this experience was not corroborated by any other clinical trial. Therefore, the primary outcome of the SCD-HeFT trial established that patients with nonischemic dilated cardiomyopathy (as well as those with ischemic heart disease) resulting in an LVEF <35% had long-term mortality reduction by combining arrhythmia suppression using maximal medical therapy with lethal arrhythmia termination using an ICD.

CLINICAL DECISION MAKING

Device therapy for selected patients with heart failure is designed to reduce the risk for sudden cardiac death using ICDs, or to reduce the chances for progressive pump failure and SD with cardiac resynchronization devices either coupled with or without an ICD (150,151). Recent consensus statements recommend prophylactic defibrillator implantation in patients with chronic heart failure, NYHA Class II–III symptoms, and LVEF <30% from ischemic heart disease who are at least 40 days post-MI (Class I with level of evidence A). Patients without ischemic heart disease and LVEF <30% should also receive ICD therapy for primary prevention of SD if their survival with good functional status is expected to exceed 1 year (Class I with level of evidence B) (152).

According to the recommendations it would be reasonable to offer patients with LVEF between 30% and 35% from any etiology ICD therapy if they have NYHA Class II or III heart failure (Class II, level of evidence B). Again, this recommendation applies to patients whose functional capacity and survival are expected to be stable for longer than 1 year. Recommendations for secondary prevention of SD are not changed. Patients who survive out-of-hospital cardiac arrest or hemodynamically significant ventricular tachycardia in the presence of structural heart disease are best treated with combining medication therapy with an ICD (152).

HEALTH CARE UTILIZATION ISSUES

ICD therapy is an expensive and invasive means to provide primary SD prevention. The effectiveness and economic viability of a therapy can be expressed in costs per quality-of-life-year saved, which is a traditional means to determine the value of a life-saving intervention. Economic calculations based on MADIT-II suggest that costs of ICD therapy in a primary prevention application range from $35,000 to $55,000 per quality-of-life-year saved, depending on the assumptions applied to the calculation algorithm (153). This range of cost per life-year saved is considered acceptable by most medical economic modeling.

Another aspect of ICD use in heart failure patients that impacts value is the fact that the devices only provide acute therapy for sustained, potentially lethal arrhythmias, with little impact on longitudinal heart failure management. In fact, a trend toward increased hospitalizations in patients randomized to receive an ICD in the MADIT-II trial (148) underscores the concept that ICD use prolongs survival but does not influence long-term heart failure management. Recently, however, storage and organization of physiological information derived from the implanted device may transform the therapeutic device into a clinically useful monitoring system (154–156). Autonomic information can be

TABLE 41-3
SELECTED TRIALS ILLUSTRATING THE IMPACT OF DEVICE THERAPY (IMPLANTABLE CARDIOVERTER DEFIBRILLATOR [ICD] AND CARDIAC RESYNCHRONIZATION THERAPY [CRT] USING BIVENTRICULAR PACEMAKERS OR BOTH

Trial (Reference)	Population and Follow-Up	Device	Control Arm Mortality	Mortality Reduction
MADIT-I (145)	LVD, inducible, PVCss/NSVT, 2 years	ICD	38% 27 months	↓ 54%
MADIT-II (148)	Ischemic DCM, NYHA Class II–III CHF, LVEF ≤30%, 9 months	ICD	19.8% 20 months	↓ 31%
SCD-HeFT (149)	All DCM, NYHA Class II–III CHF, LVEF ≤35%, 5 years	ICD	36% 5 years	↓ 23%
COMPANION (150)	All DCM, NYHA Class III–IV CHF, LVEF ≤35%, QRS ≥120 months	CRT CRT-ICD	25% 11.9 months	↓ 34% CRT ↓ 40% CRT/ICD*
CARE-HF (151)	All DCM, NYHA Class III–IV CHF, LVEF ≤35%, QRS ≥120 months	CRT	30% 29.4 months	↓ 36%

All trials required optimal medical therapy prior to enrollment.
*Combined endpoint of death or hospitalization for heart failure.

obtained from continuously measuring heart rate variability, which declines significantly several days before patients develop heart failure symptoms leading to hospitalization (155). Follow-up strategies based on continuously measured heart rate variability may allow risk stratification and triaging of patients based on either absolute values or on changes over time. For example, standard deviation of the median atrial depolarization interval values less than 60 milliseconds are associated with increased hospitalization and mortality risk, whereas a decline in heart rate variability (HRV) over time predicted impending hospitalization with a 70% sensitivity (associated with a 2.4 false positive per patient-year of follow-up) (155).

Additional heart failure status information can be obtained from frequent assessment of intrathoracic impedance measured from the tip of the right ventricular lead to the implanted pulse generator (156). As the lung field in the impedance vector becomes edematous, electrical impedance declines, which appears to be a sensitive means to identify impending heart failure decompensation. The appropriate use of this information in clinical management of patients with heart failure is currently the subject of clinical trials but this promising monitoring feature may prove effective in heart failure disease management (156).

In summary, ICD use is a cost-effective means to achieve primary SD prevention in patients with heart failure from any etiology. The addition of clinically useful physiological monitoring features that are available remotely further improves the overall value of implantable devices that are principally used for therapy delivery. Future iterations of implantable monitors may include long-term, continuous hemodynamic monitoring in addition to already available physiological information (157).

SUMMARY

Sudden cardiac death remains a major challenge to modern cardiology, having multiple potential mechanisms that contribute to lethal arrhythmogenesis. Effective prevention strategies must include suppression of lethal arrhythmias by preventing autonomic-mediated, adverse electrical remodeling using beta-blockers, coupled with prevention of angiotensin- and aldosterone-dependent structural remodeling and fibrosis. Neurohormonal blockade significantly reduces the relative risk for SD but must be coupled with lethal arrhythmia termination strategies using ICDs in patients with depressed left ventricular function (LVEF $<35\%$). This synergy between medical and device therapies is known to be an effective primary prevention strategy in patients with mild to moderate heart failure symptoms (NYHA Class II–III) resulting from left ventricular systolic dysfunction, regardless of etiology. These effective prevention strategies have long-term, cost-effective benefit for patients with chronic heart failure. Heart failure management is complex, requiring expertise in medical and device management of the syndrome. Training programs are evolving to meet the need for specially trained individuals who can fully integrate the skill sets required to provide appropriate medication and device expertise (158).

REFERENCES

1. Hinkle LE, Jr., Thaler HT. Clinical classification of cardiac deaths. *Circulation.* 1982;65:457–464.
2. Zheng ZJ, Croft JB, Giles WH, et al. Sudden cardiac death in the United States, 1989 to 1998. *Circulation* 2001;104:2158–2163.
3. Zipes DP, Wellens HJJ. Sudden cardiac death. *Circulation.* 1998; 98:2334–2351.
4. Narang R, Cleland JG, Erhardt L, et al. Mode of death in chronic heart failure. A request and proposition for more accurate classification. *Eur Heart J.* 1996;17:1390–1403.
5. CIBIS-II Investigators. The Cardiac Insufficiency Bisoprolol Study II (CIBIS-II). A randomized trial. *Lancet.* 1999;353:9–13.
6. American Heart Association. Heart Disease and Stroke Statistics—2005, Update 2005. www.american heart.org.
7. Cobb LA, Fahrenbruch CE, Olsufka M, et al. Changing incidence of out-of-hospital ventricular fibrillation, 1980–2000. *JAMA.* 2002;288:3008–3013.
8. Chugh SS, Jui J, Gunson K, et al. Current burden of sudden cardiac death: multiple source surveillance versus retrospective death certificate-based review in a large U.S. community. *J Am Coll Cardiol.* 2004;44:1268–1275.
9. Fox CS, Evans JC, Larson MG, et al. A comparison of death certificate out-of-hospital coronary heart disease death with physician-adjudicated sudden cardiac death. *Am J Cardiol.* 2005;95: 856–859.
10. Fox CS, Evans JC, Larson MG, et al. Temporal trends in coronary heart disease mortality and sudden cardiac death from 1950 to 1999: the Framingham Heart Study. *Circulation.* 2004;110:522–527.
11. Lown B. Sudden cardiac death: the major challenge confronting contemporary cardiology. *Am J Cardiol.* 1979;43:313–328.
12. Myerburg RJ. Scientific gaps in the prediction and prevention of sudden cardiac death. *J Cardiovasc Electrophysiol.* 2002;13:709–723.
13. Huikuri HV, Makikallio TH, Raatikainen P, et al. Prediction of sudden cardiac death: appraisal of the studies and methods assessing the risk of sudden arrhythmic death. *Circulation.* 2003;108:110–115.
14. Goldman S, Johnson G, Cohn JN, et al. Mechanism of death in heart failure. The Vasodilator-Heart Failure Trials. The V-HeFT VA Cooperative Studies Group. *Circulation.* 1993;87:V124–V131.
15. Bayes de Luna A, Coumel P, Leclercq JF. Ambulatory sudden cardiac death. Mechanisms of production of fatal arrhythmia on the basis of data from 157 cases. *Am Heart J.* 1989;117:151–159.
16. Myerburg RJ, Kessler KM, Castellanos A. Sudden cardiac death. Structure, function and time dependence of risk. *Circulation* 1992;85:12–20.
17. Kempf FC, Jr., Josephson ME. Cardiac arrest recorded on ambulatory electrocardiograms. *Am J Cardiol.* 1984;53:1577–1582.
18. Nikolic G, Bishop RL, Singh JB. Sudden death recorded during Holter monitoring. *Circulation.* 1982;66:218–225.
19. Savage HR, Kissane JQ, Becher EL, et al. Analysis of ambulatory electrocardiograms in 14 patients who experienced sudden cardiac death during monitoring. *Clin Cardiol.* 1987;10:621–632.
20. Gillum RF. Sudden coronary death in the United States: 1980–1985. *Circulation.* 1989; 89:756–765.
21. Jouven X, Desnos M, Guerot C, et al. Predicting sudden death in the population. The Paris Prospective Study I. *Circulation.* 1999;99:1978–1983.
22. Spector PS. Diagnosis and management of sudden cardiac death. *Heart* 2005;27:7–12.
23. Goraya TY, Jacobsen SJ, Kottke TE, et al. Coronary heart disease and sudden cardiac death: a 20-year population-based study. *Am J Epidemiol.* 2003;157:763–770.
24. De Vreede-Swagemakers JJM, Gorgels APM, Dubois-Arbouw WI, et al. Out-of-hospital cardiac arrest in the 1990s: a population-based study in the Maastricht area on incidence, characteristics and survival. *J Am Coll Cardiol.* 1997;30:1500–1505.
25. Larsen MP, Eisenberg MS, Cummins RO, et al. Predicting survival from out-of-hospital cardiac arrest: a graphic model. *Ann Emerg Med.* 1993;22:1652–1658.
26. Lampert S, Lown B, Graboys TB, et al. Determinants of survival in patients with malignant ventricular arrhythmia associated with coronary artery disease. *Am J Cardiol.* 1988;61:791–797.

27. Lechat P, Hulot JS, Escolano S, et al. Heart rate and cardiac rhythm relationships with bisoprolol benefit in chronic heart failure in CIBIS II Trial. *Circulation.* 2001;103:1428–1433.
28. Perper JA, Kuller LH, Cooper M. Arteriosclerosis of coronary arteries in sudden, unexpected deaths. *Circulation.* 1975;52:II27-II33.
29. Solomon SD, Zelenkofske S, McMurray JJ, et al. Sudden death in patients with myocardial infarction and left ventricular dysfunction, heart failure, or both. *N Engl J Med.* 2005;352:2638–2640.
30. El-Sherif N, Turitto G. Risk stratification and management of sudden cardiac death: a new paradigm. *J Cardiovasc Electrophysiol.* 2003;14:1113–1119.
31. Wannamethee G, Shaper AG, Macfarlane PW, et al. Risk factors for sudden cardiac death in middle-aged British men. *Circulation.* 1995; 91:1749–1756.
32. Priori SG, Aliot E, Blomstrom-Lundqvist C, et al. Update of the guidelines on sudden cardiac death of the European Society of Cardiology. *Eur Heart J.* 2003;24:13–15.
33. Schmermund A, Schwartz RS, Adamzik M, et al. Coronary atherosclerosis in unheralded sudden coronary death under age 50. Histo-pathologic comparison with 'healthy' subjects dying out of hospital. *Atherosclerosis.* 2001;155:499–508.
34. Reichenbach DD, Moss NS, Meyer E. Pathology of the heart in sudden cardiac death. *Am J Cardiol.* 1977;39:865–872.
35. Thomas AC, Knapman PA, Krikler DM, et al. Community study of the causes of "natural" sudden death. *BMJ.* 1988;297:1453–1456.
36. McKenna WJ, Firoozi S, Sharma S. Arrhythmias and sudden death in hypertrophic cardiomyopathy. *Card Electrophysiol Rev.* 2002;6:26–31.
37. Schwartz PJ, Priori SG, Spazzolini C, et al. Genotype-phenotype correlation in the long-QT syndrome: gene-specific triggers for life-threatening arrhythmias. *Circulation.* 2001;103:89–95.
38. Antzelevitch C, Brugada P, Borggrefe M, et al. Brugada syndrome: report of the second consensus conference. *Heart Rhythm.* 2005; 2(4):429-40 [Review]. Erratum in: *Heart Rhythm* 2005;2(8):905.
39. Davies MJ, Thomas A. Thrombosis and acute coronary-artery lesions in sudden cardiac ischemic death. *N Engl J Med.* 1984;310:1137–1140.
40. Friedlander Y, Siscovick DS, Weinmann S, et al. Family history as a risk factor for primary cardiac arrest. *Circulation* 1998;97:155–160.
41. Fei L, Anderson MH, Katritsis D, et al. Decreased heart rate variability in survivors of sudden cardiac death not associated with coronary artery disease. *Br Heart J.* 1994;71:16–21.
42. Schwartz PJ, Vanoli E, Stramba-Badiale M, et al. Autonomic mechanisms and sudden death. New insights from analysis of baroreceptor reflexes in conscious dogs with and without a myocardial infarction. *Circulation.* 1988;78:969–979.
43. Schwartz PJ, Billman GE, Stone HL. Autonomic mechanisms in ventricular fibrillation induced by myocardial ischemia during exercise in dogs with healed myocardial infarction. An experimental preparation for sudden cardiac death. *Circulation.* 1984;69:1182–1189.
44. Adamson PB, Huang MH, Vanoli E, et al. Unexpected interaction between beta-adrenergic blockade and heart rate variability before and after myocardial infarction. A longitudinal study in dogs at high and low risk for sudden death. *Circulation.* 1994;90:976–982.
45. Adamson PB, Vanoli E. Early autonomic and repolarization abnormalities contribute to lethal arrhythmias in chronic ischemic heart failure. characteristics of a novel heart failure model in dogs with postmyocardial infarction left ventricular dysfunction. *J Am Coll Cardiol.* 2001;37:1741–1748.
46. Hohnloser SH, Gersh BJ. Changing late prognosis of acute myocardial infarction: impact on management of ventricular arrhythmias in the era of reperfusion and the implantable cardioverter-defibrillator. *Circulation.* 2003;107:941–946.
47. Greenberg H, Case RB, Moss AJ, et al. Analysis of mortality events in the Multicenter Automatic Defibrillator Implantation Trial (MADIT-II). *J Am Coll Cardiol.* 2004;43:1459–1465.
48. Wilber DJ, Zareba W, Hall WJ, et al. Time dependence of mortality risk and defibrillator benefit after myocardial infarction. *Circulation.* 2004;109:1082–1084.
49. Hohnloser SH, Kuck KH, Dorian P, et al. Prophylactic use of an implantable cardioverter-defibrillator after acute myocardial infarction. *N Engl J Med.* 2004;351:2481–2488.
50. Hohnloser SH, Franck P, Klingenheben T, et al. Open infarct artery, late potentials, and other prognostic factors in patients after acute myocardial infarction in the thrombolytic era. A prospective trial. *Circulation.* 1994;90:1747–1756.
51. Domanski MJ, Exner DV, Borkowf CB, et al. Effect of angiotensin converting enzyme inhibition on sudden cardiac death in patients following acute myocardial infarction. A meta-analysis of randomized clinical trials. *J Am Coll Cardiol.* 1999;33:598–604.
52. Garg R, Yusuf S. Overview of randomized trials of angiotensin converting enzyme inhibitors on mortality and morbidity in patients with heart failure. Collaborative Group on ACE inhibitor trials. *JAMA.* 1995;273:1450–1456.
53. Pitt B, Remme W, Zannad F, et al. Eplerenone, a selective aldosterone blocker in patients with left ventricular dysfunction after myocardial infarction. *N Engl J Med.* 2003;348: 1309–1321.
54. Dargie HJ, for The Capricorn Investigators. Effect of carvedilol on outcome after myocardial infarction in patients with left ventricular dysfunction. The CAPRICORN randomized trial. *Lancet.* 2001;357:1385–1390.
55. The Cardiac Arrhythmia Suppression Trial (CAST) Investigators. Preliminary report: effect of encainide and flecainide after myocardial infarction. *N Engl J Med.* 1989;321:406–412.
56. Waldo AL, Camm AJ, deRuyter H, et al., for the SWORD Investigators. Effect of d-sotalol on mortality in patients with left ventricular dysfunction after recent and remote myocardial infarction. *Lancet.* 1996;348:7–12.
57. Julian DG, Camm AJ, Frangin G, et al., on behalf of the EMIAT investigators. The European Myocardial Infarct Amiodarone Trial (EMIAT). The effect of amiodarone on mortality in patients with left ventricular dysfunction surviving a recent myocardial infarction. *Lancet.* 1997;349:667–674.
58. Cairns JA, Connolly SJ, Roberts R, et al., for the Canadian Amiodarone Myocardial Infarction Arrhythmia Trial investigators. Randomised trial of outcome after myocardial infarction in patients with frequent or repetitive ventricular premature depolarisations. CAMIAT. *Lancet.* 1997;349:675–682.
59. La Rovere MT, Bigger JT, Marcus F, et al. ATRAMI (Autonomic Tone and Reflexes After Myocardial Infarction), baroreflex sensitivity and heart-rate variability in prediction of total cardiac mortality after myocardial infarction. *Lancet.* 1998; 351: 478–484.
60. La Rovere MT, Pinna GD, Hohnloser SH, et al. Baroreflex sensitivity and heart rate variability in the identification of patients at risk for life-threatening arrhythmias. implications for clinical trials. *Circulation.* 2001;103:2072–2077.
61. Tsuji H, Larson MG, Venditti FJ, Jr., et al. Impact of reduced heart rate variability on risk for cardiac events. The Framingham Heart Study. *Circulation.* 1996; 94:2850–2855.
62. Priori SG, Alliot E, Blomstrom-Lundqvist C, et al. Task Force on Sudden Cardiac Death of the European Society of Cardiology. *Eur Heart J.* 2001; 22:1374–1450.
63. Vanoli E, De Ferrari GM, Stramba-Badiale M, et al. Vagal stimulation and prevention of sudden death in conscious dogs with a healed myocardial infarction. *Circ Res.* 1991;68:1471–1481.
64. De Ferrari GM, Vanoli E, Stramba-Badiale M, et al. Vagal reflexes and survival during acute myocardial ischemia in conscious dogs with healed myocardial infarction. *Am J Physiol.* 1991;261: H63–H69.
65. Adamson PB, Suarez J, Ellis E, et al. Ephedrine increases ventricular arrhythmias in conscious dogs after myocardial infarction. *J Am Coll Cardiol.* 2004;44:1675–1678.
66. Keefe DL, Schwartz J, Somberg JC. The substrate and the trigger. The role of myocardial vulnerability in sudden cardiac death. *Am Heart J.* 1987;113:218–225.
67. Tomaselli GF, Zipes DP. What causes sudden death in heart failure? *Circ Res.* 2004;95:754–763.
68. Peters NS, Wit AL. Myocardial architecture and ventricular arrhythmogenesis. *Circulation.* 1998;97:1746–1754.
69. Tomaselli GF, Marbán E. Electrophysiological remodeling in hypertrophy and heart failure. *Cardiovasc Res.* 1999;42:270–283.
70. O'Rourke B, Kass DA, Tomaselli GF, et al. Mechanisms of altered excitation-contraction coupling in canine tachycardia-induced heart failure, I. experimental studies. *Circ Res.* 1999;84:562–570.

71. Pogwizd SM, Corr PB. Biochemical and electrophysiological alterations underlying ventricular arrhythmias in the failing heart. *Eur Heart J.* 1994;15(Suppl D):145–154.
72. Adamson PB, Germany R. Therapy interactions in chronic heart failure. Synergies and asynergies of device and medication therapies. *Drug Discovery Today. Therapeutic Strategies.* 2004;1:135–141.
73. Kléber AG, Rudy Y. Basic mechanisms of cardiac impulse propagation and associated arrhythmias. *Physiol Rev.* 2004;84:431–488.
74. Spooner PM, Joyner RW, Jalife J, eds. *Discontinuous Conduction in the Heart.* Armonk, NY: Futura Publishing Co., Inc.; 1997.
75. Smith JH, Green CR, Peters NS, et al. Altered patterns of gap junction distribution in ischemic heart disease. An immunohistochemical study of human myocardium using laser scanning confocal microscopy. *Am J Pathol.* 1991;139:801–821.
76. Spach MS, Miller WT III, Geselowitz DB, et al. The discontinuous nature of propagation in normal canine cardiac muscle. Evidence for recurrent discontinuities of intracellular resistance that affect the membrane currents. *Circ Res.* 1981:48:39–54.
77. Undrovinas AI, Shander GS, Makielski JC. Cytoskeleton modulates gating of voltage-dependent sodium channel in heart. *Am J Physiol.* 1995;269:H203–H214.
78. Sáez JC, Berthoud VM, Brañes MC, et al. Plasma membrane channels formed by connexins: their regulation and functions. *Physiol Rev.* 2003;83:1359–1400.
79. O'Rourke B, Kass DA, Tomaselli GF, et al. Mechanisms of altered excitation-contraction coupling in canine tachycardia-induced heart failure, I: experimental studies. *Circ Res.* 1999;84:562–570.
80. Bouchard RA, Clark RB, Giles WR. Effects of action potential duration on excitation-contraction coupling in rat ventricular myocytes. Action potential voltage-clamp measurements. *Circ Res.* 1995;76:790–801.
81. Luke RA, Saffitz JE. Remodeing of ventricular conduction pathways in healed canine infarct border zones. *J Clin Invest.* 1991;87:1594–1602.
82. Kawara T, Derksen R, de Groot JR, et al. Activation delay after premature stimulation in chronically diseased human myocardium relates to the architecture of interstitial fibrosis. *Circulation.* 2001;104:3069–3075.
83. Spach MS, Heidlage JF, Dolber PC, et al. Changes in anisotropic conduction caused by remodeling cell size and the cellular distribution of gap junctions and Na^+ channels. *J Electrocardiol.* 2001;34(Suppl):69–76.
84. de Bakker JMT, Coronel R, Tasseron S, et al. Ventricular tachycardia in the infarcted, Langendorff-perfused human heart: role of the arrangement of surviving cardiac fibers. *J Am Coll Cardiol.* 1990:15:1594–1607.
85. de Bakker JMT, van Capelle JL, Janse MJ, et al. Slow conduction in the infarcted human heart. 'Zigzag' course of activation. *Circulation.* 1993;88:915–926.
86. Morady F, Frank R, Kou WH, et al. Identification and catheter ablation of slow conduction in the reentrant circuit of ventricular tachycardia in humans. *J Am Coll Cardiol.* 1988;11:775–782.
87. Stevenson WG, Hafzia K, Sager P, et al. Identification of reentry circuit sites during catheter mapping and radiofrequency ablation of ventricular tachycardia late after myocardial infarction. *Circulation.*1993;88:1647–1670.
88. de Bakker JMT, van Capelle FJL, Janse MJ, et al. Reentry as a cause of ventricular tachycardia in patients with chronic ischemic heart disease: electrophysiologic and anatomic correlation. *Circulation.* 1988;77:589–606.
89. de Bakker JMT, van Capelle FJL, Janse MJ, et al. Macroreentry in the infarcted human heart. The mechanism of ventricular tachycardias with a "focal" activation pattern. *J Am Coll Cardiol.* 1991;18:1005–1014.
90. de Bakker JM, Janse MJ. Pathological correlates of ventricular tachycardia in hearts with a healed infarct. In: Zipes DP, Jalife J, eds. *Cardiac Electrophysiology. From Cell to Bedside.* 3rd ed. Philadelphia: WB Saunders; 2000.
91. Peters NS, Green CR, Poole-Wilson PA, et al. Reduced content of connexin43 gap junctions in ventricular myocardium from hypertrophied and ischemic human hearts. *Circulation.* 1993;88: 864–875.
92. Gutstein DE, Morley GE, Tamaddon H, et al. Conduction slowing and sudden arrhythmic death in mice with cardiac-restricted inactivation of connexin43. *Circ Res.* 2001;88:333–339.
93. van Rijen HVM, Eckardt D, Degen J, et al. Slow conduction and enhanced anisotropy increase the propensity for ventricular tachyarrhythmias in adult mice with induced deletion of connexin43. *Circulation.* 2004;109:1048–1055.
94. Dinerman JL, Berger R, Haigney MC, et al. Dispersion of ventricular activation and refractoriness in patients with idiopathic dilated cardiomyopathy. *Am J Cardiol.* 1997;79:970–974.
95. Adamson PB, Barr RC, Callans DJ, et al. The perplexing complexity of cardiac arrhythmias: beyond electrical remodeling. *Heart Rhythm.* 2005;2:650–659.
96. Keating MT, Sanguinetti MC. Molecular and cellular mechanisms of cardiac arrhythmias. *Cell.* 2001;104:569–580.
97. Swann MH, Nakagawa H, Vanoli E, et al. Heterogeneous regional endocardial repolarization is associated with increased risk for ischemia-dependent ventricular fibrillation after myocardial infarction. *J Cardiovasc Electrophysiol.* 2003;14:873–879.
98. Pham Q, Quan KJ, Rosenbaum DS. T-wave alternans: marker, mechanism, and methodology for predicting sudden cardiac death. *J Electrocardiol.* 2003;36:75–81.
99. Bloomfield DM, Steinman RC, Namerow PB, et al. Microvolt T-wave alternans distinguishes between patients likely and patients not likely to benefit from implanted cardiac defibrillator therapy: a solution to the Multicenter Automatic Defibrillator Implantation Trial (MADIT) II conundrum. *Circulation.* 2004;110;1885–1889.
100. Vassallo JA, Cassidy DM, Kindwall KE, et al. Nonuniform recovery of excitability in the left ventricle. *Circulation.* 1988;78:1365–1372.
101. Pinto JM, Boyden PA. Electrical remodeling in ischemia and infarction. *Cardiovasc Res.* 1999;42:284–297.
102. Pak PH, Nuss B, Tunin RS, et al. Repolarization abnormalities, arrhythmia and sudden death tachycardia-induced cardiomyopathy. *J Am Coll Cardiol.* 1997;30:576–584.
103. Kääb S, Nuss HB, Chiamvimonvat N, et al. Ionic mechanism of action potential prolongation in ventricular myocytes from dogs with pacing-induced heart failure. *Circ Res.* 1996;78:262–273.
104. Kääb S, Dixon J, Duc J, et al. Molecular basis of transient outward potassium current downregulation in human heart failure. A decrease in Kv4.3 mRNA correlates with a reduction in current density. *Circulation.* 1998;98:1383–1393.
105. Beuckelmann DJ, Nabauer M, Erdmann E. Alterations of K^+ currents in isolated human ventricle myocytes from patients with terminal heart failure. *Circ Res.* 1993;73:379–385.
106. Volders PGA, Sipido KR, Vos MA, et al. Downregulation of delayed rectifier K+ currents in dogs with chronic complete atriovenricular block and acquired torsades du pointes. *Circulation.* 1999;100:2455–2461.
107. Nerbonne JM, Guo W. Heterogeneous expression of voltage-gated potassium channels in the heart: roles in normal excitation and arrhythmias. *J Cardiovasc Electrophysiol.* 2002;13:406–409.
108. Nerbonne JM, Kass RS. Physiology and molecular biology of ion channels contributing to ventricular repolarization. In: Gussak I, Antzelevitch C, eds. *Contemporary Cardiology. Cardiac Repolarization. Bridging Basic and Clinical Science.* Totowa, NJ: Humana Press; 2003: Chapter 3, 25–62.
109. Volders PGA, Stengl M, van Opstal JM, et al. Probing the contribution of I_{Ks} to canine ventricular repolarization. key role for β adrenergic stimulation. *Circulation* 2003;107:2753–2760.
110. Petrecca K, Miller DM, Shrier A. Localization and enhanced current density of the Kv4.2 potassium channel by interaction with the actin-binding protein filamin. *J Neurosci.* 2000;20: 8736–8744.
111. Wang Z, Eldstrom JR, Jantzi J, et al. Increased focal Kv4.2 channel expression at the plasma membrane is the result of actin depolymerization. *Am J Physiol.* 2004; 286. H749–H759.
112. Yang X, Salas PJ, Pham TV, et al. Cytoskeletal actin microfilaments and the transient outward K^+ current in hypertrophied rat ventriculocytes. *J Physiol.* 2003;541:411–421.
113. Hasenfuss G. Alterations of calcium-regulatory proteins in heart failure. *Cardiovasc Res.* 1998;37:279–289.
114. Gwathmey JK, Copelas L, MacKinnon R, et al. Abnormal intracellular calcium handling in myocardium from patients with end-stage heart failure. *Circ Res.* 1987;61:70–76.
115. Laurita KR, Katra R, Wible B, et al. Transmural heterogeneity of calcium handling in canine. *Circ Res.* 2003;92:668–675.
116. Armoundas AA, Hobai IA, Tomaselli GF, et al. Role of sodium-calcium exchanger in modulating the action potential of ventric-

ular myocytes from normal and failing hearts. *Circ Res*. 2003;93: 46–53.
117. Clark RB, Bouchard RA, Giles WR. Action potential duration modulates calcium influx, Na(+)–Ca2+ exchange, and intracellular calcium release in rat ventricular myocytes. *Ann NY Acad Sci*.1996;779:417–429.
118. Wu Y, Roden DM, Anderson ME. Calmodulin kinase inhibition prevents development of the arrhythmogenic transient inward current. *Circ Res*.1999;84:906–912.
119. Wu Y, MacMillan LB, McNeill RB, et al. CaM kinase augments cardiac L-type Ca2+ current: a cellular mechanism for long Q-T arrhythmias. *Am J Physiol*. 1999;276:H2168–H2178.
120. The CONSENSUS Trial Study Group. Effects of enalapril on mortality in severe congestive heart failure. Results of the Cooperative North Scandinavian Enalapril Survival Study (CONSENSUS). *N Engl J Med*. 1987;316:1429–1435.
121. Hall AS, Murray GD, Ball SG. Follow-up study of patients randomly allocated ramipril or placebo for heart failure after acute myocardial infarction. AIRE Extension (AIREX) Study. Acute Infarction Ramipril Efficacy. *Lancet*. 1997;349:1493–1497.
122. Fletcher RD, Cintron GB, Johnson G, et al. Enalapril decreases prevalence of ventricular tachycardia in patients with chronic congestive heart failure. *Circulation*. 1993;87(Suppl VI):VI49–VI55.
123. Konstam MA, Rousseau MF, Kronenberg MW, et al. Effects of angiotensin converting enzyme inhibitor enalapril on the long-term progression of left ventricular dysfunction in patients with heart failure. *Circulation*. 1992;86:431–438.
124. The SOLVD Investigators. Effect of enalapril on survival in patients with reduced left ventricular ejection fractions and congestive heart failure. *N Engl J Med*. 1991;325:293–302.
125. Yusuf S, Sleight P, Pogue J, et al. Effects of an angiotensin-converting-enzyme inhibitor, ramipril, on cardiovascular events in high-risk patients. The Heart Outcomes Prevention Evaluation Study Investigators. *N Engl J Med*. 2000;342:145–153.
126. Kim S, Iwao H. Molecular and cellular mechanisms of angiotensin II-mediated cardiovascular and renal diseases. *Pharmacol Rev*. 2000;52:11–34.
127. Boadle MC, Hughes J, Roth RH. Angiotensin accelerates catecholamine biosynthesis in sympathetically innervated tissues. *Nature*. 1969;222:987–988.
128. Khairallah PA. Action of angiotensin on adrenergic nerve endings. Inhibition of norepinephrine uptake. *Federation Proceedings*. 1972;31:1351–1357.
129. Farrell DM, Wei CC, Tallaj J, et al. Angiotensin II modulates catecholamine release into interstitial fluid of canine ventricle in vivo. *Am J Physiol*. (*Heart Circ Physiol*.) 2001;281.H813–H822.
130. Inoue H, Zipes DP. Results of sympathetic denervation in the canine heart; sypersensitivity that may be arrhythmogenic. *Circulation*. 1987;75:877–887.
131. Takei M, Sasaki Y, Yonezawa T, et al. The autonomic control of the transmural dispersion of ventricular repolarization in anesthetized dogs. *J Cardiovasc Electrophysiol*. 1999;10:981–989.
132. Cao J-M, Chen LS, KenKnight BH, et al. Nerve sprouting and sudden cardiac death. *Circ Res*. 2000;86:816–821.
133. Chen P-S, Chen LS, Sharifi B, et al. Sympathetic nerve sprouting, electrical remodeling and the mechanisms of sudden cardiac death. *Cardiovasc Res*. 2001;50:409–416.
134. Packer M. The neurohormonal hypothesis: a theory to explain the mechanism of disease progression in heart failure. *J Am Coll Cardiol*. 1992;20:248–254.
135. Cohn JN. The management of chronic heart failure. *N Engl J Med*. 1996;335:490–498.
136. Effect of metoprolol CR/XL in chronic heart failure. Metoprolol CR/XL Randomised Intervention Trial in Congestive Heart Failure (MERIT-HF). *Lancet*. 1999;353;2001–2007.
137. Hjalmarson A, Goldstein S, Fagerberg B, et al. Effects of controlled-release metoprolol on total mortality, hospitalizations, and well-being in patients with heart failure. The Metoprolol CR/XL Randomized Intervention Trial in congestive heart failure (MERIT-HF). MERIT-HF Study Group. *JAMA*. 2000;283:1295–1302.
138. Packer M, Coats AJ, Fowler MB, et al. Effect of carvedilol on survival in severe chronic heart failure. *N Engl J Med*. 2001;344:1651–1658.
139. Swedberg K, Cleland JG, Di Lenarda A, et al. Carvedilol Or Metoprolol European Trial Investigators. Comparison of carvedilol and metoprolol on clinical outcomes in patients with chronic heart failure in the Carvedilol Or Metoprolol European Trial (COMET): randomised controlled trial. *Lancet*. 2003;362:7–13.
140. Pitt B, Zannad F, Remme WJ, et al. The effect of spironolactone on morbidity and mortality patients with severe heart failure. Randomized Aldactone Evaluation Study Investigators. *N Engl J Med*. 1999;341:709–717.
141. Willenheimer R, van Veldhuisen DJ, Silke B, et al. Effect on survival and hospitalization of initiating treatment for chronic heart failure with bisoprolol followed by enalapril, as compared with the opposite sequence. Results of the Randomized Cardiac Insufficiency Bisoprolol Study (CIBIS) III. *Circulation*. 2005;112(16):2426-2435.
142. Lavery C, Murray AM, Mylan C, et al. Nonuniform nighttime distribution of acute cardiac events. A possible effect of sleep states. *Circulation*. 1997;96:3321–3327.
143. Verrier R, Muller JE, Hobson JA. Sleep, dreams, and sudden death: the case for sleep as an autonomic stress test for the heart. *Cardiovasc Res*. 1996;31:181–211.
144. Vanoli E, Adamson PB, Ba-Lin, et al. Heart rate variability during specific sleep stages. A comparison of healthy subjects with patients after myocardial infarction. *Circulation*. 1995;91:1918–1922.
145. Moss AJ, Hall WJ, Cannom DS, et al. Improved survival with an implanted defibrillator in patients with coronary disease at high risk for ventricular arrhythmia. Multicenter Automatic Defibrillator Implantation Trial Investigators. *N Engl J Med*. 1996;335: 1933–1940.
146. Buxton AE, Lee KL, DiCarlo L, et al. A randomized study of the prevention of sudden death in patients with coronary artery disease. *N Engl J Med*. 1999;341:1882–1890.
147. Buxton AE, Lee KL, DiCarlo L, et al. Electrophysiologic testing to identify patients with coronary artery disease who are at risk for sudden death *N Engl J Med*. 2000;342:1937–1945.
148. Moss AJ, Zareba W, Hall WJ, et al. Prophylactic implantation of a defibrillator in patients with myocardial infarction and reduced ejection fraction. *N Engl J Med*. 2002;346:877–883.
149. Bardy GH, Lee KL, Mark DB, et al. Sudden Cardiac Death in Heart Failure Trial (SCD-HeFT) Investigators. Amiodarone or an implantable cardioverter-defibrillator for congestive heart failure. *N Engl J Med*. 2005;352:225–237.
150. Bristow MR, Saxon LA, Boehmer J, et al. Cardiac-resynchronization therapy with or without an implantable defibrillator in advanced chronic heart failure. *N Engl J Med*. 2004;350:2140–2150.
151. Cleland JG, Daubert JC, Erdmann E, et al. The effect of cardiac resynchronization on morbidity and mortality in heart failure. *N Engl J Med*. 2005;352:1539–1549.
152. Hunt SA, Abraham WT, Chin MH, et al. ACC/AHA 2005 guideline update for the diagnosis and management of chronic heart failure in the adult—summary article. A report of the American College of Cardiology/American Heart Association task force on practice guidelines. *J Am Coll Cardiol*. 2005;46: 1116–1143.
153. Al-Khatib SM, Anstrom KJ, Eisenstein EL, et al. Clinical and economic implications of the Multicenter Automatic Defibrillator Implantation Trial-II. *Ann Intern Med*. 2005;142: 593–600.
154. Adamson PB, Kleckner KJ, VanHout WL. Cardiac resynchronization therapy improves heart rate variability in patients with symptomatic heart failure. *Circulation*. 2003;108:266–269.
155. Adamson PB, Smith AL, Abraham WT, et al. Continuous autonomic assessment in patients with symptomatic heart failure: prognostic value of heart rate variability measured by an implanted cardiac resynchronization device. *Circulation*. 2004;110:2389–2394.
156. Yu CM, Wang L, Chau E, et al. Intrathoracic impedance monitoring in patients with heart failure: correlation with fluid status and feasibility of early warning preceding hospitalization. *Circulation*. 2005;112:841–848.
157. Adamson PB, Magalski A, Braunschweig F, et al. Ongoing right ventricular hemodynamics in heart failure: clinical value of measurements derived from an implantable monitoring system. *J Am Coll Cardiol*. 2003;41:565–571.
158. Adamson PB, Abraham WT, Love C, Reynolds DW. The evolving challenge of heart failure management: a call for a new curriculum for training heart failure specialists. *J Am Coll Cardiol*. 2004;1354–1357.

42

Pathogenesis and Therapy of Thrombosis in Patients with Congestive Heart Failure

Jody L. Kujovich *Scott H. Goodnight* *Barry Massie*

During the past decade, substantial progress has been made in the rational use of anticoagulant therapy for thrombosis complicating cardiac disease. However, relatively few clinical investigators have specifically examined the problem of thromboembolism in patients with congestive heart failure. Instead, other diagnostic categories of heart disease, such as acute myocardial infarction (MI), valvular heart disease, atrial arrhythmias, and cardiomyopathies without heart failure have been studied. Patients with heart failure with these associated conditions have sometimes been included in trials of antithrombotic agents and, indeed, the outcomes of these studies have sometimes been inappropriately extrapolated to the broader heart failure population. Only recently has there been a resurgence of interest in heart failure as a specific risk factor for thromboembolic events. Therefore, this chapter will examine the potential role of coagulation abnormalities in the pathophysiology and progression of heart failure and discuss the indications for antithrombotic agents in this condition. We will also discuss the role of anticoagulation in myocardial infarction, left ventricular aneurysm, and atrial fibrillation, since these conditions are often present in patients with heart failure.

PATHOGENESIS OF THROMBOSIS

The equilibrium between factors promoting and inhibiting thrombosis is complex and multifactorial. These dynamics are summarized in Table 42-1. As will be discussed subsequently, these dynamics are often altered significantly in patients with heart failure in a direction favoring thrombosis, raising the question as to whether there may be a broader role for antithrombotic therapies in this setting (1–3).

Vascular Injury

An effective defense against intravascular thrombosis involves a dynamic interplay between the vasculature, platelets, the formation of fibrin, and fibrinolysis (4). Vascular endothelial cells are an essential barrier to thrombosis. For example, the endothelial surface contains a key glycoprotein, thrombomodulin, that supports the activation of protein C, a potent natural anticoagulant. Activated protein C rapidly destroys activated factors V and VIII, major participants in the formation of fibrin. Moreover, the glycosaminoglycan heparan is widely distributed on the endothelial surface and avidly binds antithrombin, another natural anticoagulant. When bound to the endothelial surface, antithrombin rapidly neutralizes the clotting enzyme thrombin, as well as activated factor X and other prothrombotic serine proteases.

Vascular endothelial cells also inhibit platelet adhesion and platelet aggregation. When the endothelium is activated by local injury, inflammation, or other thrombogenic stimuli, prostacyclin (PGI_2), a potent inhibitor of platelet plug formation, is released. Finally, under appropriate circumstances, blood vessels may markedly enhance local fibrinolysis via the synthesis and release of tissue plasminogen activator (t-PA).

Injury to normal vascular endothelium serves as a potent stimulus to thrombosis. For example, in a patient with a transmural MI, endothelial cell damage may develop overlying the ischemic area of endocardium. The loss of the protective endothelium with the exposure of a thrombogenic

TABLE 42-1
COMPARISON OF ANTITHROMBOTIC AND PROTHROMBOTIC PROPERTIES OF BLOOD VESSELS, PLATELETS, AND PLASMA

	Inhibition of Thrombosis	Promotion of Thrombosis
Coagulation	Antithrombin III-activated protein C	Thrombin, factor Xa, factors Va, VIIIa
Platelet reactivity	Prostacyclin (PGI_2)	Thromboxane A_2 (TXA_2)
Fibrinolysis	Tissue plasminogen activator (t-PA)	Plasminogen activator inhibitor (PAI-1)
Vascular tone	Nitric oxide	Endothelin

surface may subsequently culminate in a ventricular thrombus. The ultimate size of the intracavitary clot will be limited by the antithrombotic potential of the surrounding intact endothelium. A similar sequence of events may occur following the rupture of an atherosclerotic plaque within a coronary artery. Platelets and fibrin rapidly accumulate at the area of injury, which may lead to acute coronary artery occlusion and, ultimately, infarction of the myocardium.

Reduced Blood Flow

Sluggish or disturbed blood flow resulting from ventricular failure or atrial fibrillation greatly enhances the likelihood of thrombosis. The supply of coagulation inhibitors such as antithrombin or protein C to an area of local tissue injury is reduced, and activated clotting factors accumulate instead of being flushed into the circulation, where they can be cleared by the liver.

Activated Clotting Factors

Coagulation proteins such as prothrombin or factor X normally circulate in their nonactivated (zymogen) configuration. However, a variety of stimuli may convert them to an activated form, predisposing to thrombosis. Examples include surgical procedures, tissue necrosis following infarction, infections, or inflammatory reactions with the release of thrombogenic cytokines such as interleukin-1 or tumor necrosis factor.

Fibrinolytic Defects

The fibrinolytic balance may be altered in some patients with heart disease, contributing to thrombosis. Plasminogen activator inhibitor (PAI-1), a fibrinolytic inhibitor released from endothelial cells, is the major inhibitor of endogenous t-PA, and high levels may impair the fibrinolytic response, predisposing to coronary thrombosis (5). Elevated PAI-1 levels have been associated with an increased risk for first and recurrent MI in young men in several studies (6,7). A specific allele (4G) of a common polymorphism in the promoter of the PAI-1 gene (4G/5G) is associated with higher PAI-1 activity levels in vitro and in vivo. Molecular studies indicate that the increased PAI-1 activity may reflect differential binding of transcription activators and repressors to the promoter polymorphic site, resulting in a higher basal level of transcription of PAI-1 with the 4G allele (8). The 4G/4G genotype was significantly more prevalent in a group of Swedish men with a first MI before age 45 in comparison with controls, suggesting a twofold increase in coronary risk (8). However the 4G/5G polymorphism was not predictive of arterial or venous thrombosis in a cohort of healthy men in the Physicians' Health Study (9). Elevated levels of D-dimer and t-PA antigen were associated with an increased risk for MI in Physicians' Health Study participants, reflecting activation of the fibrinolytic system (10,11). However, after adjustment for total and high-density lipoprotein (HDL) cholesterol and other atherosclerotic risk factors, these associations were no longer statistically significant, suggesting that elevated t-PA and D-dimer levels may be a consequence rather than the cause of progressive atherosclerotic vascular disease.

Vascular Reactivity

Recent studies demonstrate the importance of vascular tone and its relationship to thrombosis. Intense vasoconstriction appears to promote thrombogenesis, whereas vasodilation may increase blood flow, inhibiting thrombosis. The regulation of vascular tone is complex, and several important mediators are now well characterized. Nitric oxide (NO), previously called endothelium-derived relaxing factor (EDRF), is a free radical product released by vascular endothelial cells in response to a variety of agonists, including thrombin, adenosine diphosphate (ADP), catechols, and various cytokines (12). NO is a potent vasodilator that also inhibits platelet adhesion, activation, secretion, and aggregation, and it promotes platelet disaggregation (13–16).

Endothelins are a family of small peptides produced by several cell types. Endothelin-1, produced by endothelial cells, is the most potent known vasoconstrictor; it increases vascular tone by its local effects on vascular smooth-muscle cells. It is also a mitogen for smooth-muscle cells. Abnormalities in the NO-endothelin system may contribute to endothelial dysfunction in several different types of heart disease (17).

For example, patients with severe heart failure have impaired NO-mediated vasodilation in response to stimuli (18). Plasma endothelin levels are elevated in severe heart failure (19,20) and are thought to contribute to myocardial damage after MI. There are reports of elevated endothelin levels in asymptomatic patients with atherosclerosis and after acute MI (21,22). Pretreatment of rats with anti-endothelin antibodies reduced the degree of myocardial damage induced by MI in an experimental model (23).

Increased Platelet Reactivity

The hypothesis that increased platelet reactivity may contribute to arterial thrombosis has been difficult to test, in part because of the lack of sensitive and specific laboratory assays for platelet activation. Patients with extensive peripheral atherosclerosis have evidence of increased platelet-vascular interactions, based on the excretion of platelet and vascular prostaglandin metabolites in the urine (24). Transient but markedly enhanced platelet reactivity is observed after fibrinolytic therapy for acute coronary thrombosis (25,26). More recently, measurement of platelet surface P-selectin expression by flow cytometry has been used as a marker for platelet activation. One study showed that P-selectin expression increased after the addition of several thrombolytic agents, and suppression of activation required higher doses of aspirin (660 mg per day) (27). Other studies have shown that plasma from patients with acute MI or heart failure enhances platelet aggregation mediated by von Willebrand's factor (28,29). Patients with severe heart failure, rheumatic valvular disease, and atrial fibrillation have elevated levels of platelet-specific proteins (platelet factor 4, β-thromboglobulin) that reflect platelet activation (30–33). There is also evidence of a diurnal variation in platelet reactivity that may contribute to acute coronary occlusion (34–37).

Antiphospholipid Antibodies

Antiphospholipid antibodies (APL Ab) react with epitopes on phospholipid binding proteins. This heterogenous group of antibodies is divided into two major categories based on the laboratory tests used to identify them. Lupus inhibitors, by definition, are antibodies that interfere with phospholipid-dependent coagulation tests in vitro. Anticardiolipin antibodies (ACL Ab) are detected by an immunologic assay in which cardiolipin-coated, enzyme-linked immunosorbent assay (ELISA) plates are used. Patients often have multiple APL Ab, each of which reacts with a specific antigen. Although a number of target proteins have been identified, β_2-glycoprotein-1 and prothrombin are the most common.

APL Ab are strongly associated with both arterial and venous thrombosis, and they have also been linked to a variety of cardiac complications. Cardiac valve abnormalities are found in up to 36% of patients with the primary antiphospholipid antibody syndrome (PAPS) by echocardiography; these usually involve the mitral and aortic valves (38). Leaflet thickening and irregularity and valvular insufficiency are the most common abnormalities. Although these lesions are often clinically silent, they may predispose to thrombosis and increase the risk for systemic embolism. Patients with APL Ab and thrombosis of histologically normal valves have also been reported (39). There are multiple reports of intracardiac mural thrombi involving both atria and ventricles in association with these antibodies (40–43).

MI has also been linked to APL Ab. One study found that a significant proportion of young men with an acute MI had elevated levels of APL Ab that persisted for 2 years (44). Additional thromboembolic complications developed in approximately one-third of these men. More recently, two prospective studies showed that ACL Ab are an independent risk factor for future MI and early death in healthy, asymptomatic middle-aged men (45,46). Another recent prospective study reported that the presence of ACL Ab at the time of acute MI predicted subsequent recurrent MI and thromboembolic events (47). There are also multiple reports of myocardial dysfunction or infarction resulting from thrombotic occlusions of the myocardial microcirculation (48,49).

The mechanisms of thrombosis in patients with APL Ab are still not well understood. Evidence is accumulating that these antibodies may produce an acquired form of resistance to activated protein C (50). Reduced levels of free protein S, which functions as a cofactor for activated protein C (APC), are common in patients with lupus inhibitors, although the mechanism is unknown. The observation that some lupus inhibitors promote increased prothrombin binding to cell and phospholipid surfaces suggests the possibility that accelerated thrombin generation may contribute to thrombosis (51). The addition of APL Ab to cell cultures results in increased tissue factor synthesis by monocytes and endothelial cell expression of adhesion molecules (52,53). APL Ab also bind to oxidized lipoproteins, such as oxidized low-density lipoprotein (LDL), suggesting a potential role in the progression of atherosclerosis and arterial thrombosis (54).

Homocysteine

Homocysteine (HC) is an amino acid generated as a by-product during the metabolism of methionine. Normal plasma contains a small amount of HC (average, 10 μM). Hyperhomocysteinemia is strongly associated with premature atherosclerotic vascular disease and both arterial and venous thrombosis (55,56). Even mildly elevated HC levels significantly increase the risk for MI, stroke, and peripheral vascular disease. In the Physicians' Health Study, the relative risk for MI was increased to 3.4 with HC levels above 15.8 μM (57). Accumulating evidence regarding arterial disease suggests a graded effect on vascular risk rather than a threshold effect, such that the risk would not increase until HC levels exceeded the threshold. A recent meta-analysis concluded that each 5-μM increase in the HC level results in a twofold to fourfold increase in the odds ratio for vascular disease (58). Hyperhomocysteinemia is also an independent risk factor for venous thromboembolism (59).

Hyperhomocysteinemia has several effects that promote atherothrombosis, although the primary mechanism(s) responsible are still unclear. In experimental models, high HC levels have detrimental effects on endothelial cells, platelets, and components of the coagulation and fibrinolytic system that predispose to vascular disease and thrombosis (55,56). There is growing evidence that endothelial injury and dysfunction may be the final common pathogenetic pathway responsible for many of the atherothrombotic effects of HC. HC interferes with the natural antithrombotic properties of endothelium and may impair vascular reactivity by interfering with endothelial cell NO production. High levels also impair fibrinolysis and increase the binding of lipoprotein(a) [Lp(a)] to vascular endothelial cells (60).

Elevated levels of HC result from deficiencies or defects in either the enzymes (cystathionine-β-synthase, N^5,N^{10}-methylenetetrahydrofolate reductase) or the vitamin cofactors (folate, vitamins B_{12} and B_6) involved in the two major metabolic pathways of HC metabolism. There is accumulating evidence that inadequate folate is a major factor contributing to most of the cases of mild to moderate hyperhomocysteinemia in the general population. Vitamin supplementation (folate with or without vitamins B_{12} and B_6) will reduce

HC levels in most cases, although it remains to be shown that lowering HC levels will prevent vascular complications.

Lipoprotein(a)

Lp(a) has been identified as a powerful predictor of premature atherosclerotic vascular disease in several large prospective trials (61). Lp(a) is composed of an LDL-like particle and apolipoprotein(a), a large protein with striking homology to plasminogen. Accumulating experimental and clinical evidence suggests that Lp(a) has both atherogenic and prothrombotic effects. For example, Lp(a) accumulates in atherosclerotic plaque, stimulates smooth-muscle cell proliferation, and promotes cholesterol accumulation (62). The structural homology between apo(a) and plasminogen may enable Lp(a) to interfere with fibrinolysis and act as a procoagulant. Lp(a) has been shown to stimulate the release of plasminogen activator inhibitor (i.e., PAI-1) from endothelial cells and to compete with plasminogen for binding on fibrin on the surface of vascular endothelial cells, inhibiting fibrinolysis (62–64). It also competes with t-PA in converting plasminogen to plasmin. In an experimental model, Lp(a) transgenic mice were resistant to t-PA-mediated thrombolysis of fibrin thrombi (65). HC increases Lp(a) deposition on a fibrin surface, which suggests an adverse synergistic interaction promoting atherothrombosis (60). Elevated Lp(a) levels (defined as >30 mg/dL) are associated with an increased risk for coronary artery, cerebrovascular, and peripheral vascular disease. Thus, it is well established that high levels of Lp(a) are associated with accelerated atherosclerosis and cardiovascular disease, although it is not yet clear whether they also predispose to thrombosis.

CHRONIC ANTICOAGULATION THERAPY

Warfarin, the most commonly used oral anticoagulant in the United States, exerts its antithrombotic effect by inhibiting the vitamin K-dependent γ-carboxylation of a series of glutamic acid residues on clotting factors II, VII, IX, and X (66). These modified amino acid residues are essential for normal functioning of the coagulation proteins and also of the coagulation inhibitors, protein C and protein S. The addition of carboxyl groups to glutamic acid residues allows calcium-mediated binding of the clotting factors to phospholipid surfaces, a process necessary for the formation of fibrin. As a result of pharmacologically induced vitamin K deficiency, warfarin therapy effectively inhibits thrombosis.

A major advance in the safety and efficacy of oral anticoagulation therapy has been the institution of the international normalized ratio (INR) to standardize therapeutic intensities of coumarin antithrombotic therapy throughout the world (67). The INR is a *calculated* prothrombin time (PT) ratio that adjusts for differences in PT reagents and equipment. It is determined by the following simple formula:

$$\text{INR} = \text{PT ratio}^{\text{ISI}}$$

where the ISI is the international sensitivity index of the thromboplastin reagent used for determining the PT. Note that the PT ratio is raised to the *power* of the ISI, which results in an exponential relationship.

The benefits of oral anticoagulation must be carefully balanced against the potential risks for bleeding. One advantage of low-intensity anticoagulation therapy has been a reduction in both major and minor bleeding events. In general, the overall risk for serious bleeding (defined by hospitalization, blood transfusions, and the interruption of anticoagulation therapy) is approximately 1% to 2% a year for a general clinic population. Several studies suggest that these risks are not cumulative but tend to level off after approximately 2 years of therapy (68). Central nervous system hemorrhage is estimated to occur at a rate of approximately 0.1% to 0.2% yearly. About half of these patients will either die or become seriously disabled. Other factors, such as patient reliability, the number and severity of concurrent medical and surgical illnesses, and the availability of anticoagulation clinics with highly trained professional staff or other anticoagulation management systems, may substantially modify the risks for bleeding.

Warfarin can interact with several cardiac medications commonly used in patients with heart failure. For example, amiodarone can substantially increase the anticoagulant effect of warfarin (69). Patients receiving both warfarin and amiodarone or other cardiac medications should have their INR monitored frequently to detect possible pharmacologic interactions.

ANTICOAGULATION AND ANTIPLATELET THERAPY IN PATIENTS WITH CHRONIC HEART FAILURE

Anticoagulation for Chronic Heart Failure

Many patients with heart failure have associated conditions for which antithrombotic therapy is specifically indicated, such as atrial fibrillation, prosthetic heart valves, recent myocardial infarction, and atherosclerotic vascular disease. Warfarin should be standard therapy unless otherwise contraindicated.

The presence of a prothrombotic milieu and the known risk of thromboembolic events in chronic heart failure raise the question of whether broader use of anticoagulation may be indicated. Indeed, several early trials reported improved survival in heart failure patients treated with chronic anticoagulation (70–73).

However, these studies included many patients with primary valvular heart disease and/or atrial fibrillation, as well as others with dilated cardiomyopathies who were managed with prolonged activity limitation or even bedrest. These patients are at higher risk for thromboembolic events than the usual heart failure patient, and thus, generalization of these findings to patients with heart failure due to either ischemic or nonischemic cardiomypathy in sinus rhythm is not appropriate. Nonetheless, a post hoc analysis of the Studies of Left Ventricular Dysfunction (SOLVD) resurrected this question. It reported that in a combined analysis, patients receiving anticoagulation (in a nonrandomized manner) had a 24% lower incidence of death from any cause and an 18% lower risk for hospitalization for worsening heart failure (74).

The mechanism is not immediately obvious, since as will be discussed later, clinically apparent thromboembolic events are relatively uncommon in heart failure patients in sinus rhythm. One potential mechanism is the prevention of so-called silent MIs and their contribution to the progression of heart failure. Indeed, one of the few recent postmortem studies in heart failure patients found that a substantial proportion of patients experiencing both sudden death and death attributed to worsening heart failure had recent, unrecognized MIs (75).

Importantly, several trials have demonstrated that anticoagulation is at least as effective as antiplatelet therapy with aspirin in preventing vascular events during long-term treatment post-MI; this may be the reason for the apparent benefit in heart failure patients (76,77).

Role of Anticoagulation in the Prevention of Embolic Events

Although the routine use of anticoagulation in chronic heart failure patients is not recommended, controversy persists as to whether anticoagulation is indicated for patients considered to be at high risk for embolic events. Intracardiac thrombi are common in patients with dilated cardiomyopathies, and they form in dilated atria as well as ventricles. Mural thrombi have been found in 53% to 75% of patients with nonischemic cardiomyopathies in autopsy studies (78), and multiple thrombi involving more than one cardiac chamber are found in nearly 30% of cases, although these data are several decades old and there is a general perception that thrombi now occur much less frequently in this population. The pathogenesis of thrombosis is in large part related to the marked stasis and aberrant blood flow in the dilated and hypokinetic atrium or ventricle. Once formed, the fibrin clot may remain highly thrombogenic because of the residual thrombin bound to its surface, which is relatively inaccessible to inactivation (79).

Patients with heart failure also have evidence of endothelial injury or dysfunction, which may contribute to activation of platelets and coagulation. Several reports of elevated levels of biochemical markers of platelet activation and thrombin generation suggest that patients with moderate to severe heart failure may have a hypercoagulable or prothrombotic state. In one study, patients with the most severe heart failure (reflected by high plasma catechol levels and a low ejection fraction) were the most likely to have biochemical evidence of platelet and coagulation activation (30). In a follow-up study, high baseline levels of activated coagulation markers were reduced by low-dose warfarin therapy, suggesting that anticoagulation may suppress the prothrombotic state associated with advanced heart failure (80). Patients with advanced heart failure have elevated plasma levels of tumor necrosis factor and other cytokines, which may also activate coagulation (81,82). However, it has not yet been shown that elevated levels of these biochemical markers can be used to identify high-risk patients or predict clinical thromboembolic events.

An echocardiographic study suggested that intraventricular thrombi usually do not change in size or motion profile in the absence of anticoagulation (83). However, thrombi tend to diminish in size gradually or resolve completely within weeks to months when anticoagulants are given. Other studies suggest that a new thrombus will develop in 10% to 20% of patients with a cardiomyopathy during the subsequent 2 years, whereas 10% to 20% of thrombi resolve within the same time period (84).

The rate of clinically apparent systemic cardiogenic emboli is approximately 2% to 3% yearly, from several older studies (85–87). However, these trials are generally retrospective and involve patients referred for echocardiography, in some cases because of suspected intracardiac thrombi. Atrial fibrillation patients were sometimes included. A review of data from the older literature in heart failure patients not receiving anticoagulation reported an average annual incidence of systemic thromboembolism of 1.9%, with a range of 0.9% to 5.5% yearly (88). Prospective data from large clinical trials in the last two decades suggest a rate of systemic embolic events around 1.5% (89,90), although approximately 75% of these are strokes.

The embolic rates in patients with idiopathic dilated cardiomyopathy are similar to those in studies of more heterogeneous populations of heart failure patients, suggesting that thromboembolism results from heart failure itself rather than the specific underlying cause. Although the overall risk for thromboembolism is low, coexisting atrial fibrillation or a history of one or more embolic events in the previous 2 years confers a much higher risk, which approaches 16% to 20% a year (91).

Intuitively, one might think that embolic events occur more frequently in patients with the poorest LV function or the largest left ventricles. However, this has not been confirmed in most analyses. In a retrospective analysis of 6,378 patients enrolled in the SOLVD Prevention and Treatment Trial, no relationship between ejection fraction and embolic risk was observed in men, although in women a 10% reduction in ejection fraction was associated with a 53% increase in thromboembolism (92). One trial in which a significant relationship was observed was the Survival and Ventricular Enlargment (SAVE) trial, which enrolled 2,231 patients with LV dysfunction early after MI (93). There was an 18% increase in stroke risk for each 5% reduction in ejection fraction, and patients with an ejection fraction of 28% or less had a twofold higher risk for stroke than did patients with an ejection fraction of 35% or more. However, this relationship was probably more related to the size of the recent MI than to the severity of LV dysfunction and cannot be extrapolated to chronic heart failure.

Patients with dilated cardiomyopathy are also at risk for pulmonary emboli, with a reported frequency of 5% to 11% (94), and these events are often underdiagnosed. In the analysis of data from the SOLVD trial, pulmonary emboli accounted for 24% and 14% of the total thromboembolic events in women and men, respectively (92). Although right ventricular thrombi are relatively rare, there have been several case reports of biventricular thrombi complicated by pulmonary emboli (95,96).

Recent Trials of Anticoagulation in Heart Failure Patients

Several recent and ongoing trials have sought to evaluate the benefit of warfarin anticoagulation in patients with sinus rhythm. The Warfarin and Aspirin Study in Heart

Failure (WASH) randomized 279 patients to warfarin, aspirin, or placebo (97). There were no significant differences in death or other outcomes between the warfarin and placebo group, although the trial was underpowered and embolic events were rare. The Warfarin and Antiplatelet Therapy in Chronic Heart Failure trial (WATCH) was a much larger, three-arm trial comparing warfarin, aspirin, and clopidogrel in 1,587 patients with heart failure and LV ejection fractions ≤35% who were in sinus rhythm (3). Although the final results of this trial await publication, there were no significant differences in the primary endpoints of death and nonfatal MI or nonfatal stroke, and there appeared to be fewer strokes in the warfarin-treated patients (98). One further trial, the National Institutes of Health (NIH)-sponsored trial is evaluating warfarin and aspirin in patients with heart failure, ejection fractions ≤35% who are in sinus rhythm, with endpoints of death and stroke (99).

Recommendations for the Use of Anticoagulation in Heart Failure Patients

Thus, there are no conclusive outcome data from the modern era to support the routine use of anticoagulation in chronic heart failure patients, either to improve overall outcomes or to prevent embolic events. Therefore, current guidelines do not recommend routine anticoagulation in the general heart failure population (90,100–102).

However, there are groups of heart failure patients in whom anticoagulation is indicated because of associated conditions. These are numerated below.

Recommendations

1. Anticoagulation is not recommended for patients with chronic heart failure without specific indications.
2. Patients with heart failure and atrial fibrillation are at higher risk for thromboembolism (≥5% annually) and should receive long-term anticoagulation with warfarin (INR, 2.0 to 3.0).
3. Patients with heart failure and prior systemic or pulmonary emboli should receive long-term anticoagulation.
4. Patients with a history of recurrent venous thrombosis, and possibly those with a single episode without another specific precipitating factor, should receive long-term anticoagulation.
5. Patients with heart failure and a recent large MI (especially involving the LV anterior wall) should receive anticoagulation for 3 to 4 months.
6. Patients with incidentally detected LV thrombi may be considered for long-term anticoagulation, especially if these are protruding, large, and noncalcified.
7. The target INR for patients with heart failure is 2.0 to 3.0.

Antiplatelet Therapy in Chronic Heart Failure

In considering whether to treat heart failure patients with antithrombotic agents, most clinicians have focused on the risk of systemic embolic events. However, as noted above, there is a broader rationale for considering antithrombotic drugs in this population (3). Many of the adverse outcomes, including sudden death and worsening heart failure, may represent unrecognized coronary events (75). Both antiplatelet drugs and, as discussed in the previous section, anticoagulation have been shown to prevent both recurrent vascular events and death in patients with coronary disease, the most frequent cause of heart failure (103–105).

In the combined SOLVD trials, patients taking antiplatelet agents (primarily aspirin) experienced an 18% lower risk of death (HR 0.82; 95% CI 0.73–0.92; $p = 0.005$) and a 19% lower risk of death or hospital admission for heart failure (HR 0.81; CI 0.74–0.89; $p < 0.0001$) (106).

Both aspirin and anticoagulation were associated with lower risks of sudden death and fatal MI, but only warfarin was associated with a significant reduction in death from worsening heart failure.

Is There an Adverse Effect of Aspirin in Heart Failure Patients?

However, an additional intriguing finding that emerged from the SOLVD analyses was a suggestion of an interaction between aspirin and enalapril that reduced the benefit provided by angiotensin converting enzyme (ACE) inhibitors (106). Although aspirin was associated with an 18% lower hazard of death in the entire study population (HR 0.82; 95% CI 0.73–0.92; $p = 0.0006$), this was entirely due to a 32% lower hazard in the placebo arm, whereas aspirin had no impact on mortality risk in those randomized to enalapril. Conversely, enalapril reduced mortality by 23% (HR 0.77; 95% CI 0.67–0.87) in patients not taking aspirin at baseline, but was associated with a trend toward higher mortality compared to placebo treatment (HR 1.10; CI 0.93–1.30) in those taking aspirin. When this aspirin–enalapril interaction was tested in the Cox regression model in the combined SOLVD trials, it was a significant predictor of all-cause mortality ($p = 0.0005$).

The possible interaction between aspirin and ACE inhibitors has been widely discussed, and this issue is unresolved because of the limitations of the data and the post hoc analyses (107–111).

An overview of several post-infarction ACE inhibitor trials did not demonstrate similar results, suggesting that aspirin probably does not substantially interfere with ACE inhibitors in the early post-infarction period (112). However, a different result was found in a second overview that incorporated several trials of *long-term* ACE inhibitor therapy, including SOLVD, SAVE, the Acute Infarction Ramipril Efficacy trial (AIRE), the trandolapril in patients with reduced left ventricular function trial (TRACE), and the Heart Outcomes Prevention Evaluation (HOPE) (113).

A significant interaction between aspirin and ACE inhibitors was noted for mortality ($p = 0.04$), with patients taking aspirin exhibiting a smaller risk reduction from ACE inhibitor therapy. The authors appropriately emphasize that, with the exception of SOLVD and CONSENSUS II, ACE inhibitors were effective in reducing mortality and other vascular events in patients taking aspirin, as well as in patients not taking aspirin. Nonetheless, the lesser benefit observed in the aspirin-using patients raises the possibility that an alternative antithrombotic agent may be preferable, at least in patients with heart failure or LV dysfunction.

Two studies cited earlier have prospectively evaluated aspirin in heart failure patients. In the WASH trial, aspirin was associated with a significantly higher rate of hospitalizations for heart failure than either warfarin or no treatment, although the number of events was small (97). The same finding was observed in the larger WATCH trial, with a significant 27% fewer patients being hospitalized for heart failure on aspirin compared to warfarin, resulting in 31% fewer hospital admissions (98).

The likely mechanism for this interaction, if it is confirmed, is aspirin-mediated inhibition of prostaglandin synthesis, which is stimulated by ACE inhibitors and may play a role in their beneficial effects. Several lines of evidence support a significant contribution of this bradykinin-prostaglandin pathway in heart failure patients. Aspirin and other nonsteroidal anti-inflammatory drugs reduce or completely prevent the ACE inhibitor-mediated vasodilation and other beneficial effects (114,115).

Importantly, similar inhibition is not seen with ticlopidine, an antiplatelet agent that acts by inhibiting ADP receptors rather than by cyclo-oxygenase inhibition (116).

Although some studies suggest that low doses of aspirin can achieve platelet inhibition by inhibiting thromboxane synthesis without interfering with the vasodilating effects of ACE inhibitors (117,118), others have demonstrated similar hemodynamic effects of aspirin when given at 75-mg or 325-mg doses (119).

Recommendations for the Use of Antiplatelet Drugs in Heart Failure Patients

There are no data from prospective randomized controlled trials demonstrating a benefit for antiplatelet therapy in the broad heart failure population. On the other hand, it is generally accepted that aspirin prevents death and reinfarction following acute MI (103), but few patients with heart failure have been included in these trials and these have not been analysed separately. Aspirin is also widely used long term for secondary prevention in patients with atherosclerotic vascular disease. On the other hand, the evidence for an adverse effect of aspirin in heart failure patients, although provocative and hypothesis-generating, remains inconclusive. Clopidogrel is at least as effective as aspirin for secondary prevention in patients with atherosclerotic vascular disease (120), but data in heart failure patients are relatively limited. Therefore, it is important to weigh the evidence as to whether and in whom aspirin should be recommended in heart failure patients. Based on a review of the literature and current guidelines (90,100–102), the following recommendations can be made.

1. Aspirin is recommended for secondary prevention in heart failure patients with coronary artery disease and cerebrovascular disease.
2. Antiplatelet therapy is not recommended in patients with heart failure due to nonischemic cardiomyopathy or patients considered to be at low risk for vascular events.
3. Anticoagulation or clopidogrel may be considered as alternatives to aspirin in patients with recurrent hospitalizations for heart failure or persistent symptoms.

MYOCARDIAL INFARCTION

Thromboembolic complications develop in a substantial proportion of patients who have an acute MI (94,121,122). LV thrombi develop as the result of a combination of stasis, endocardial injury, and a possible systemic hypercoagulable state associated with acute MI. Stasis occurs in areas of akinesis or dyskinesis, which may be particularly severe in the apical region. Virtually all patients in whom LV thrombi develop have abnormalities of wall motion on echocardiographic examination. The endocardial injury resulting from a transmural infarction exposes subendocardial components, which activate platelets and the coagulation system, and the associated inflammatory reaction also has a prothrombotic effect. Elevated levels of a variety of markers of coagulation activation have been measured during acute MI, suggesting a generalized hypercoagulable state. For example, increased levels of prothrombin fragment 1+2 and fibrinopeptide A reflect accelerated thrombin generation in vivo (123), and increased plasma levels of tissue factor pathway inhibitor (TFPI) in the acute setting suggest activation of the tissue factor-factor VII pathway (124). The myocardium may be the source of a variety of proinflammatory cytokines during ischemia and after reperfusion (125). Once formed, the surface of a fresh thrombus is itself thrombogenic, as a result of fibrin-bound thrombin and factor Xa, which are protected against inactivation by antithrombin.

LV thrombi develop in approximately 30% of patients with acute MI, although the incidence varies significantly depending on the particular population studied. LV thrombi are found predominantly in patients with MI of the anterior wall. For example, pooled echocardiographic data suggest that in the absence of anticoagulation, mural thrombi develop in more than 50% of patients with large antero-apical infarctions, compared with only 2% of patients with MI involving other locations. The extent of the infarct (reflected by peak enzyme levels) correlates with the risk for thrombosis. Increased LV volumes, global LV dysfunction, and severe abnormalities of wall motion (akinesis or hypokinesis) are also risk factors for LV thrombosis. Most LV thrombi develop during the first week after acute MI, although a very few form within the first 24 hours (122). Fresh endocardial injury and inflammation and the early systemic hypercoagulable state may in part explain why the thromboembolic risk is highest during this period.

More recent studies suggest that the prevalence of mural thrombi may be lower than previously reported, as a result of modern strategies of early reperfusion and preservation of LV function. In a prospective echocardiographic study of participants in HEART, 90% of whom received reperfusion therapy (either systemic thrombolysis or primary angioplasty), LV thrombi were detected in 0.6% of patients on day 1, 3.7% on day 14, and 2.5% on day 90 after acute anterior MI (126). The cumulative prevalence was 6.3% by the time of the third echocardiographic examination. Eighty-five percent of LV thrombi present on echocardiograms on day 1 or 14 had resolved by day 90, indicating that complete resolution occurs frequently. Although there is some evidence that resolution is more common with warfarin, several studies have reported a high frequency of thrombus resolution even in the absence of anticoagulation (127).

The current evidence also suggests that anticoagulation prevents the formation of LV thrombi. At least six randomized trials have compared moderate-dose heparin with either placebo or low-dose heparin, and four of these demonstrated a benefit of the higher doses of heparin. In two large, randomized trials, moderate doses of subcutaneous heparin (12,500 U twice daily) reduced the incidence of LV thrombi by 52% in comparison with placebo and by 66% in comparison with low-dose heparin (5,000 U twice daily) (128,129). In the latter study, the frequency of LV thrombi was reduced from 32% to 11%, and the reduction was correlated with the plasma heparin level. An analysis of the pooled data from four studies also concluded that heparin significantly reduces the incidence of mural thrombi after MI (130). More recently, LMWH (dalteparin) was also reported to reduce the formation of mural thrombi significantly (131). Thus, the combined data from multiple studies suggest that the early use of heparin reduces the frequency of LV thrombi by more than 50%.

The average incidence of stroke from any cause after acute MI is 2.9%, but it ranges from 6% in patients with anterior infarctions to only 1% of those with inferior MI. The risk is higher with larger infarcts in most but not all studies. Several studies suggest that systemic emboli occur in approximately 18% of patients with an LV thrombus after acute MI, compared with only 2% of patients without thrombi (132). An analysis of pooled data from 11 studies estimated that patients with echocardiographically detected mural thrombi after MI have a fivefold increased risk for embolic complications in comparison with patients without LV thrombi (130). The risk for embolism is highest during the first 3 months after acute MI, especially the first 10 days, but it may persist indefinitely in patients with LV dysfunction after MI (93). Mural thrombi that either protrude into the LV cavity or are mobile appear to have greater embolic potential. Left atrial (LA) thrombi in patients in whom atrial fibrillation develops are another potential source of emboli after acute MI.

Several studies have shown that anticoagulation is effective in reducing the risk for systemic embolization after acute MI. Three large clinical trials performed within the last 20 years showed that heparin followed by oral anticoagulation reduces the rate of cerebral embolism from approximately 3% to 1%. More recently, several analyses of pooled data from multiple studies each concluded that anticoagulation reduces the risk for embolic complications by approximately 70% in patients with echocardiographically detected LV thrombi after acute MI (130,132,133).

The results from several studies suggest that thrombolytic therapy or other forms of reperfusion may reduce the incidence of LV thrombi after acute MI. Five of six studies addressing the efficacy of thrombolytic therapy suggested a lower frequency of mural thrombi, although the difference was significant in only three of the studies (134–139). Interpretation of these data is limited by the fact that none of the studies was randomized in design, and in most cases, patients who did not qualify for thrombolytic therapy served as the control group. Analysis of the pooled data from these studies also suggested that thrombolytic therapy may prevent LV thrombi (130). One small, randomized trial concluded that streptokinase does not reduce the formation of LV thrombi, based on echocardiography performed at an average of 8 weeks after MI (140). However, the study included only 29 patients with anterior MI, who were randomized relatively late in the acute course, and there was also no improvement of regional or global LV function with thrombolysis. Although thrombolytic agents may reduce the incidence of mural thrombi by several potential mechanisms, the beneficial effect most likely results from limitation of infarct size and preservation of myocardial function rather than from a direct lytic effect.

The optimal antithrombotic regimen for the management of acute MI remains unclear. Previous studies of heparin in patients who did not routinely receive aspirin or fibrinolytic therapy suggest a small but significant benefit. An overview of 21 randomized trials of early anticoagulation in patients with acute MI concluded that in the absence of aspirin and fibrinolytic therapy, heparin reduces mortality by approximately 25%, which corresponds to the prevention of 35 deaths per 1,000 patients treated (141). Heparin also reduces the incidence of stroke and pulmonary emboli by 50%, which corresponds to 10 fewer strokes and 19 fewer pulmonary emboli per 1,000 patients treated. These potential benefits must be weighed against a small excess of major complications of bleeding with the higher-dose heparin regimens (13/1,000 patients). These older studies may no longer be relevant in light of the well-established beneficial effects of aspirin and fibrinolytic therapy, which have now been incorporated into current practice. The more important question of whether the addition of heparin to aspirin and thrombolytic therapy results in clinical benefit is still unresolved. The rationale for the use of heparin is based on the approximately 10% risk for acute coronary reocclusion after successful thrombolysis, the persistent stimulus for thrombosis after plaque rupture, and the observed paradoxical increase in thrombin activity after thrombolytic therapy. There is also some evidence that adjunctive heparin may at least attenuate, if not completely suppress, thrombin generation after thrombolytic therapy (142).

Most of the data on the effects of heparin in combination with aspirin and thrombolytic therapy are found in two large trials, in which a total of 62,000 patients were randomized to different thrombolytic agents and then further assigned to subcutaneous heparin or no other treatment (143–145). In both trials, the 35-day mortality rates were similar with and without heparin, but the patients who received heparin had a significantly higher rate of major bleeding. There is also no evidence that higher-dose intravenous heparin regimens reduce mortality or rates of reinfarction or stroke in patients receiving aspirin and thrombolytic therapy (146). The recent overview of all randomized trials estimated that the addition of heparin would prevent approximately five deaths, three reinfarctions, and one pulmonary embolus for every 1,000 patients treated (141). There was no further reduction in stroke risk beyond the 50% reduction achieved with aspirin alone, but the higher-dose heparin regimens increased the risk for major bleeding (approximately three excess major episodes of bleeding per 1,000 patients). Taken together, the available data suggest marginal clinical benefit from the addition of heparin in patients already receiving aspirin and a thrombolytic agent. The overview analysis and several recent reviews each concluded that the current evidence does not justify the routine use of heparin in the management of acute MI (147,148). Despite the lack of conclusive data, in the United States, intravenous heparin is used in the vast majority of patients with acute MI who receive thrombolytic therapy (149).

Oral anticoagulation with warfarin is effective for secondary prevention of cardiovascular morbidity and mortality after acute MI. In two large, placebo-controlled, randomized trials, oral anticoagulation (INR, 2.8 to 4.8) reduced the rate of reinfarction after acute MI (150,151). The mortality rate and risk for nonhemorrhagic stroke were also significantly reduced in one of the trials (150). Two randomized clinical trials comparing long-term oral anticoagulation with aspirin after acute MI reported no significant difference in mortality or reinfarction rates (152,153). More recently, the Aspirin versus Coumadin Trial (APRICOT) randomized patients to aspirin (325 mg per day) or heparin followed by warfarin (INR, 2.8 to 4.0) after successful thrombolysis (154). After 3 months of follow-up, there was no significant difference in reocclusion, reinfarction, or mortality rates between the warfarin or aspirin groups. Thus, the current evidence suggests that long-term warfarin and aspirin are equally effective in reducing cardiovascular morbidity and mortality after MI. The Coumadin Aspirin Reinfarction Study (CARS) evaluated the effectiveness of combined low fixed doses of warfarin and aspirin versus aspirin monotherapy for secondary prevention after MI (155). The study was terminated prematurely after an interim analysis found no benefit of low-dose coumadin (1 or 3 mg per day; INR, 1.19 to 1.50) plus 80 mg of aspirin per day versus 160 mg of aspirin per day in terms of risk for reinfarction, ischemic stroke, or cardiovascular death. The ongoing Cardiac Hospitalization Atherosclerosis Management Program (CHAMP) trial comparing low-dose Coumadin (INR, 1.5 to 2.5) plus 80 mg of aspirin with 160 mg of aspirin monotherapy may clarify whether low-dose Combination therapy provides additional benefit. However, at present there is no evidence to support combined aspirin and warfarin after acute MI.

Despite the large number of trials of antithrombotic therapy, several important questions remain unanswered. For example, the optimal intensity of warfarin anticoagulation after acute MI is still unclear. The majority of the randomized trials of warfarin versus placebo or aspirin used a target INR range of 2.8 to 4.8, and a recent consensus panel recommended an INR range of 2.5 to 3.5. An analysis of data from the Atrial Septal Pacing Efficacy Clinical Trial (ASPECT) resulted in the conclusion that the optimal INR range (defined as the lowest combined outcome of both thromboembolism and hemorrhage) lies between 2.0 and 4.0, with a trend favoring 3.0 to 3.5 (156). The role, dose, and duration of heparin therapy in patients receiving aspirin and thrombolytic therapy are also controversial. Several recent studies suggest that PTT values above 70 seconds are associated with an unacceptably high rate of intracerebral and other major bleeding (157,158), and recently published guidelines recommend a PTT range of 50 to 75 seconds when intravenous heparin is administered after thrombolytic therapy (159). The question of whether the recommendations for heparin depend on the specific thrombolytic agent used, as recently suggested (159), is unresolved. There have also been several reports suggesting a rebound increase in hypercoagulability after abrupt withdrawal of both intravenous heparin and warfarin after MI (160,161), but it remains to be determined whether tapering anticoagulation will improve outcome.

Recommendations

1. Patients with a large, anterior, transmural MI should receive full-dose heparin; administration should be started promptly at the time of admission. Warfarin may be started simultaneously and should be continued for 3 months (INR, 2.0 to 3.0), after which aspirin can be substituted.
2. Patients with persistent risk factors for systemic embolism (e.g., severe LV dysfunction, atrial fibrillation) after 3 months should be considered for long-term anticoagulation.
3. All patients with acute MI should receive at least low-dose subcutaneous heparin (7,500 U twice daily) or LMWH until they are fully ambulatory unless there is a specific contraindication.
4. Although at present there is inadequate evidence to support the routine use of heparin in patients receiving thrombolytic therapy, heparin is recommended for patients with other indications for anticoagulation, such as large, anterior MI, atrial fibrillation, or congestive heart failure.
5. Aspirin is the preferred agent for secondary prevention after MI. However, warfarin should be considered for patients who are intolerant of aspirin or have recurrent events despite aspirin, and for those at high risk for thromboembolism because of mural thrombi or severe LV dysfunction.

LEFT VENTRICULAR ANEURYSM

Left ventricular aneurysms develop in approximately 5% to 10% of all patients with acute MI, most commonly involving the apex and anterior wall. An LV aneurysm is a risk factor for the development and persistence of mural thrombi during the period immediately after infarction, and it is also associated with a fourfold increased risk for the formation of new or recurrent LV thrombi during the subsequent months after acute MI (136). Systemic embolization occurs in approximately 5% of patients with an intraaneurysmal thrombus, in most cases during the initial weeks after acute infarction (162).

LV thrombi are found in up to 50% of patients with chronic LV aneurysms at autopsy or at the time of surgery. However, patients with chronic LV aneurysms, in contrast to those with acute MI, rarely have systemic emboli (163). In

TABLE 42-2
INCIDENCE OF THROMBOSIS BY DISEASE

Disease	Approximate Yearly Incidence (%)
Cardiomyopathy with prior emboli	2–3
	10–20
Acute MI	
with mural thrombus	18–20
without mural thrombus	2
Chronic LV aneurysm	
with global LV dysfunction	2–3
without LV dysfunction	≤1
Atrial fibrillation	5

MI, myocardial infarction; LV, left ventricular.

one study, systemic embolization occurred in only 1 of 69 patients followed for 288 patient-years without anticoagulation, for an annual incidence of 0.3% (164). The infrequency of embolic complications probably reflects both intra-aneurysmal thrombus morphology and the limited exposure to ventricular blood flow. In contrast to the fresh, friable, and often mobile mural thrombi that develop during the acute phase of infarction and often protrude into the ventricle, thrombi found in chronic LV aneurysms are typically organized, laminated, and sequestered from the circulation. However, in patients with an LV aneurysm and persistent global LV dysfunction, the risks approximate those of patients with dilated cardiomyopathy, approaching 2% to 3% yearly. If the thrombus protrudes into the LV cavity or is mobile, the embolic risk is even higher.

Recommendations

1. In patients with chronic LV aneurysm after acute MI but with good LV function, anticoagulation may be stopped after 3 months, as the risk for hemorrhage probably outweighs the potential benefit of long-term warfarin. This recommendation also applies to patients with an intra-aneurysmal thrombus in the absence of specific features predicting a high risk for embolization.
2. Patients with chronic LV aneurysms and severe global LV dysfunction, protruding or mobile thrombi, or a history of systemic embolism are candidates for long-term anticoagulation.

ATRIAL FIBRILLATION

Atrial fibrillation is a common arrhythmia complicating heart disease and accounts for nearly one-half of all cardiogenic emboli (94,165,166). When atrial fibrillation develops in patients with rheumatic mitral valve disease, the thromboembolic risk increases 6-fold to 18-fold. The rate of systemic embolism in unselected patients with atrial fibrillation is approximately 5% yearly, corresponding to an overall fivefold increase in risk, although the rate varies widely between different patient subgroups.

The primary mechanism of systemic embolism in atrial fibrillation is presumed to be cardioembolism from thrombi that develop as a result of stasis in a dilated and poorly contractile LA. Most thrombi form in the LA appendage, where the velocity of blood flow is reduced, also predisposing to stasis. Elevated plasma levels of various markers of activated coagulation measured in these patients suggest that atrial fibrillation is associated with a prothrombotic state (167,168).

The incorporation of transesophageal echocardiography into clinical practice has increased the detection of LA thrombi and has helped to unravel their pathogenesis. In one study, nearly 45% of patients with atrial fibrillation and acute thromboembolism had evidence of residual LA thrombi, implicating them as a likely source of a substantial proportion of systemic emboli (169). "Spontaneous echocardiographic contrast," thought to reflect local stasis and hypercoagulability, is seen in 90% of patients with atrial fibrillation and atrial thrombi, and it is predictive of embolization in some but not all studies (170). Several prospective studies confirm that LA thrombi are associated with a high risk for subsequent thromboembolism, even in patients receiving anticoagulation (171,172). In a transesophageal echocardiographic study of high-risk participants in the recent Stroke Prevention in Atrial Fibrillation (SPAF) III trial, patients with LA thrombi at the time of enrollment who were randomized to adjusted-dose warfarin had a rate of thromboembolism of 18% yearly (171). Complex atherosclerotic plaque in the thoracic aorta was also a strong independent predictor of subsequent embolism in these high-risk patients (173). The common location of atherosclerotic plaque distal to the origin of the cerebral vessels suggests that this finding may be a marker for an extracardiac mechanism of thromboembolism.

Six randomized, controlled clinical trials published during the last decade have clearly shown that oral anticoagulation significantly reduces the risk for systemic embolism in patients with atrial fibrillation (174–179). Despite varying target INR ranges and primary endpoints, warfarin therapy consistently reduced the rate of thromboembolism in comparison with placebo or control, and the difference was highly significant in five of the six studies. In the Copenhagen Atrial Fibrillation, Aspirin, and Anticoagulation (AFASAK) study, the yearly thromboembolic rate was reduced from 5.5% to 2%, which correlated with a risk reduction of 85% (174). In the original SPAF trial, the annual embolic rate was reduced from 7.4% to 2.3%, a risk reduction of 67% (175). The Boston Area Anticoagulation Trial for Atrial Fibrillation (BAATAF) reported that the rate of embolization was reduced from 2.98% to 0.41% yearly, a risk reduction of 86% (176). The European Atrial Fibrillation Trial (EAFT) differed from the other studies in that it included only patients with a recent transient ischemic attack or stroke, but it reported a remarkably similar 66% relative reduction in risk for stroke (177). Analysis of the pooled data indicates that oral anticoagulation reduces the stroke risk by approximately 68%.

Three of the original studies (AFASAK, SPAF I, and EAFT) also included an aspirin arm, with conflicting results. Aspirin reduced the risk for systemic embolism by 44% in comparison with placebo in SPAF, in contrast to a smaller, nonsignificant risk reduction in the other two studies. An analysis of the pooled data from these three studies concluded that aspirin therapy reduces the annual stroke rate from 8.1% to 6.3% yearly, corresponding to an overall 21% risk reduction in comparison with placebo (180). SPAF II was designed to compare warfarin directly with aspirin in patients of two age groups (181). Patients 75 years old or younger had annual rates of systemic embolism of 1.3% and 1.9% with warfarin and aspirin, respectively, a nonsignificant reduction in risk. In patients older than 75 years, warfarin was associated with a similar small reduction in the embolic rate in comparison with aspirin (3.6% and 4.8% yearly, respectively), at the cost of a significantly higher rate of major hemorrhagic complications (1.6% versus 4.2% yearly).

More recently, the two SPAF III studies evaluated the role of aspirin in patients with atrial fibrillation stratified on the basis of four thromboembolic risk factors: prior history of thromboembolism, systolic blood pressure above 160 mmHg, impaired LV function, and female sex and age over 75 years. The high-risk trial compared the combination of fixed-dose, low-intensity warfarin (INR, 1.2 to 1.5; maximum dose, 3 mg) plus 325 mg of aspirin per day with adjusted-dose warfarin (INR, 2.0 to 3.0) in patients with one or more risk factors, and it was terminated early because of a significantly higher rate of systemic embolism with combined therapy (7.9% versus 1.9% yearly) (182).

In the low-risk trial, a cohort of low-risk patients with atrial fibrillation, defined by the absence of all four thromboembolic risk factors, was treated with aspirin and followed prospectively (183). After an average of 2 years of follow-up, the overall annual embolic rate was 2.2%. Patients with a history of hypertension who received aspirin had a higher annual rate of embolism (3.6%) than did those with no history of hypertension (1.1%), whose annual stroke rate was similar to that of the general population in this age range.

Except for the low-risk SPAF III, most of these trials enrolled variable numbers of patients with heart failure in addition to atrial fibrillation, ranging from 19% in the original SPAF to 50% in the AFASAK. The early randomized trials comparing warfarin with placebo or control did not include subgroup analyses. However, in SPAF II, a planned secondary analysis found that patients with one or more thromboembolic risk factors (including recent heart failure) who received aspirin had a significantly higher rate of systemic embolism (2.9% yearly) than did patients without these risk factors (0.5% yearly) (181). A similar difference in outcome was observed in older (>75 years) patients who received aspirin (7.2% versus 4.2% yearly), suggesting that aspirin is ineffective prophylaxis for the subgroup of patients with congestive heart failure.

More recent multivariate analyses and prospective echocardiographic studies have identified LV dysfunction or heart failure as an important independent thromboembolic risk factor in patients with atrial fibrillation. For example, an analysis of the patients assigned to aspirin in SPAF I and II identified impaired LV function as one of four high-risk features predictive of stroke in this population (184). This analysis was the basis for the risk stratification scheme used to recruit high-risk and low-risk patients for SPAF III. Forty-five percent of the patients randomized to the high-risk SPAF III had clinical or echocardiographic evidence of impaired LV function in addition to atrial fibrillation. The substantially higher event rate with combined therapy in this subgroup (4.2% yearly) also suggests that patients with heart failure have a higher risk for systemic embolism (182).

A recent analysis of echocardiographic and clinical data pooled from three randomized trials (SPAF I, SPINAF, and BAATAF) concluded that LV dysfunction is a strong independent risk factor for stroke in patients with atrial fibrillation (185). Moderate to severe LV dysfunction was associated with a 2.5-fold increase in the relative risk for stroke, even after adjustment for all other clinical risk factors. Thus, patients with heart failure and atrial fibrillation appear to have a higher risk for thromboembolism, and most require adjusted-dose warfarin therapy.

The initial randomized trials in patients with atrial fibrillation used variable target therapeutic ranges for warfarin. For example, high-intensity warfarin (INR, 2.8 to 4.2) was used in AFASAK, intermediate-intensity (INR, 2.0 to 4.5) in SPAF I, and low-intensity (INR, 1.5 to 2.7) in BAATAF. More recent studies have attempted to define the optimal intensity of anticoagulation for patients with atrial fibrillation. A study of the INR-specific incidence rates for both ischemic stroke and major hemorrhage in EAFT found the highest rates of cerebral ischemia at INR values below 2.0 (18% yearly) (186). An INR range of 2.0 to 2.9 was associated with the lowest rate of both ischemia and hemorrhagic complications in this analysis. In SPAF III, low-dose warfarin at a target INR of 1.2 to 1.5 was ineffective prophylaxis in high-risk patients, even when combined with aspirin. Secondary analysis of the event rate at varying levels of anticoagulation suggested a marked increase in risk for systemic embolism at an INR between 1.2 and 1.5 (7.5% yearly) in comparison with an INR of 2.0 or higher (1.6% yearly) (182). These results are consistent with a recent case-control study of anticoagulated patients with atrial fibrillation, which reported a sharp increase in risk for ischemic stroke at INR levels below 2.0 (187). The risk was increased twofold at an INR of 1.7, threefold at an INR of 1.5, and sevenfold at an INR of 1.3. These findings are supported by several reports that warfarin suppresses elevated levels of activated platelet and coagulation markers only at full therapeutic doses (188,189). The consistent results from the randomized trials and retrospective studies support the current consensus recommendation for long-term oral anticoagulation at a target INR range of 2.0 to 3.0 for high-risk patients with atrial fibrillation.

Recommendations

1. Long-term oral anticoagulation (INR, 2.0 to 3.0) is recommended for patients with nonvalvular atrial fibrillation and one or more risk factors (e.g., prior history of thromboembolism, hypertension).
2. Patients with heart failure or echocardiographic evidence of significant LV dysfunction have a higher risk for thromboembolism and should receive warfarin anticoagulation.

3. Patients with contraindications to anticoagulation or who refuse it should receive 325 mg of aspirin per day. Aspirin may also be effective for patients with only mild cardiac disease and no other thromboembolic risk factors.

SUMMARY AND CONCLUSIONS

The role of antithrombotic therapy for patients with heart failure has fluctuated over the last 60 years. Heart failure patients were commonly anticoagulated in the 1950–1970 period, based on trials that often included patients with concomitant valvular disease, atrial fibrillation, cardiomyopathies, and recent MIs. The primary goal was to prevent thromboembolic events, which occurred frequently in these populations.

Over the following decades, the use of anticoagulation declined substantially, in part because a growing proportion of patients suffered from ischemic cardiomyopathy and because new therapies such as ACE inhibitors and β-blockers prolonged survival and diluted the impact of embolic events. Indeed, these were found to be quite uncommon in patients in sinus rhythm, and the risk–benefit ratio of anticoagulation was recognized to be relatively unfavorable. The advent of echocardiography demonstrated that LV thrombi were far less common than had been assumed. At the same time, antiplatelet therapy with aspirin became widely used in the majority of patients with underlying coronary disease and even in those without evident atherosclerotic disease.

However, large trials in the last two decades identified subgroups of heart failure patients in whom anticoagulation was beneficial, such as those with concomitant atrial fibrillation and recent MI. Indeed, anticoagulation was found to be at least as effective as antiplatelet therapy following MI, though the complexity of its use has continued to make aspirin the usual antithrombotic therapy in this group. In this regard, post hoc analyses of several trials have raised concern about potential adverse effects of aspirin in chronic heart failure, although there is no consensus on this question.

Current guidelines recommend anticoagulation and antiplatelet agents primarily for patients with specific indications for this therapy.

REFERENCES

1. Cleland JGF. Anticoagulant and antiplatelet therapy in heart failure. *Curr Opin Cardiol.* 1997;12:276–287.
2. Lip GYH, Gibbs CR. Does heart failure confer a hypercoagulable state? Virchow's triad revisited. *J Am Coll Cardiol.* 1999;33: 1424–1426.
3. Massie BM, Krol W, Ammon S, et al. The Warfarin and Antiplatelet Trial in Chronic Heart failure. Rationale, design, and baseline characteristics. *J Cardiac Fail.* 2004;10:101–112.
4. Harker LA. Disorders of hemostasis: thrombosis. In: Williams WJ, Beutler E, Erslev AJ, et al., eds. *Hematology.* New York: McGraw-Hill; 1990:1559–1569.
5. Wiman B. Plasminogen activator inhibitor 1 (PAI-1) in plasma: its role in thrombotic disease. *Thromb Haemost.* 1995;74:71–76.
6. Hamsten A, Winman B, de Faire U, et al. Increased plasma levels of a rapid inhibitor of tissue plasminogen activator in young survivors of myocardial infarction. *N Engl J Med.* 1985;313: 1557–1563.
7. Hamsten A, Walldius G, Szamosi A, et al. Plasminogen activator inhibitor in plasma: risk factor for recurrent myocardial infarction. *Lancet.* 1987;2:3–9.
8. Eriksson P, Kallin B, Van't Hooft FM, et al. Allele-specific increase in basal transcription of the plasminogen-activator inhibitor 1 gene is associated with myocardial infarction. *Proc Natl Acad Sci USA.* 1995;92:1851–1855.
9. Ridker PM, Hennekens CH, Lindpaintner K, et al. Arterial and venous thrombosis is not associated with the 4G/5G polymorphism in the promoter of the plasminogen activator inhibitor gene in a large cohort of U.S. men. *Circulation.* 1997;95:59–62.
10. Ridker PM, Vaughan DE, Stampfer MJ, et al. Endogenous tissue-type plasminogen activator and risk of myocardial infarction. *Lancet.* 1993;341:1165–1168.
11. Ridker PM, Hennekens CH, Cerskus A, et al. Plasma concentration of cross-linked fibrin degradation product (D-dimer) and the risk of future myocardial infarction among apparently healthy men. *Circulation.* 1994;90:2236–2240.
12. Loscalzo J, Welch G. Nitric oxide and its role in the cardiovascular system. *Prog Cardiovasc Dis.* 1995;38:87–104.
13. Cines DB, Pollak ES, Buck CA, et al. Endothelial cells in physiology and in the pathophysiology of vascular disorders. *Blood.* 1998;91:3527–3561.
14. Vanhoutte PM, Shimokawa H. Endothelium-derived relaxing factor and coronary vasospasm. *Circulation.* 1989;80:1–9.
15. Hogan JC, Lewis MJ, Henderson AH. *In vivo.* EDRF activity influences platelet function. *Br J Pharmacol.* 1988;94:1020–1022.
16. Sneddon JM, Vane JR. Endothelium-derived relaxing factor reduces platelet adhesion to bovine endothelial cells. *Proc Natl Acad Sci USA.* 1988;85:2800–2804.
17. Baig MK, Mahon H, McKenna WJ, et al. The pathophysiology of advanced heart failure. *Am Heart J.* 1998;135:S216–S230.
18. Drexler H, Hayoz D, Munzel T, et al. Endothelial function in congestive heart failure. *Am Heart J.* 1993;126:761–764.
19. Wei CM, Lerman A, Rodeheffer RJ, et al. Endothelin in human congestive heart failure. *Circulation.* 1994;89:1580–1586.
20. Pacher R, BerglerKlein J, Globits S, et al. Plasma big endothelin-1 concentrations in congestive heart failure patients with or without systemic hypertension. *Am J Cardiol.* 1993;71: 1293–1299.
21. Mathew V, Hasdai D, Lerman A. The role of endothelin in coronary atherosclerosis. *Mayo Clin Proc.* 1996;71:769–777.
22. Kurihara H, Yamaoki K, Nagai R, et al. Endothelin: a potent vasoconstrictor associated with coronary vasospasm. *Life Sci.* 1989;44:1937–1943.
23. Watanabe T, Suzuki N, Shimamoto N, et al. Endothelin in myocardial infarction. *Nature.* 1990;344:114.
24. FitzGerald GA, Smith B, Pedersen AK, et al. Increased prostacyclin biosynthesis in patients with severe atherosclerosis and platelet activation. *N Engl J Med.* 1984;310:1065–1068.
25. Fitzgerald DJ, Wright F, FitzGerald GA. Increased thromboxane biosynthesis during coronary thrombolysis: evidence that thromboxane A_2 modulates the response to tissue-type plasminogen activator *in vivo. Circ Res.* 1989;65:83–94.
26. Leopold JA, Loscalzo J. Platelet activation by fibrinolytic agents: a potential mechanism for resistance to thrombolysis and reocclusion after successful thrombolysis. *Coron Artery Dis.* 1995;6: 923–929.
27. Kawano K, Aoki I, Aoki N, et al. Human platelet activation by thrombolytic agents: effects of tissue-type plasminogen activator and urokinase on platelet surface P-selectin expression. *Am Heart J.* 1998;135:268–271.
28. Goto S, Sakai H, Ikeda Y, et al. Arterial thrombosis in heart failure. *Lancet.* 1998;351:1558–1559.
29. Goto S, Sakai H, Ikeda Y, et al. Acute myocardial infarction plasma augments platelet thrombus growth in high shear rates. *Lancet.* 1997;349:543–544.
30. Jafri SM, Ozawa T, Mammen E, et al. Platelet function, thrombin and fibrinolytic activity in patients with heart failure. *Eur Heart J.* 1993;14:205–212.
31. Heppell RM, Berkin KE, McLenachan JM, et al. Haemostatic and haemodynamic abnormalities associated with left atrial thrombosis in nonrheumatic atrial fibrillation. *Heart.* 1997;77: 407–411.

32. Sohara H, Amitani S, Kurose M, et al. Atrial fibrillation activates platelets and coagulation in a time-dependent manner: a study in patients with paroxysmal atrial fibrillation. *J Am Coll Cardiol.* 1997;29:106–112.
33. Tse HF, Lau CP, Cheng G. Relation between mitral regurgitation and platelet activation. *J Am Coll Cardiol.* 1997;30:1813–1818.
34. Hirsh J. Hyperreactive platelets and complications of coronary artery disease. *N Engl J Med.* 1987;316:1543–1544.
35. Tofler GH, Brezinski D, Schafer AI, et al. Concurrent morning increase in platelet aggregability and the risk of myocardial infarction and sudden cardiac death. *N Engl J Med.* 1987;316: 1514–1518.
36. Trip MD, Cats VM, van Capelle FJL, et al. Platelet hyperreactivity and prognosis in survivors of myocardial infarction. *N Engl J Med.* 1990;322:1549–1554.
37. McCall NT, Tofler GH, Schafer AI, et al. The effect of enteric-coated aspirin on the morning increase in platelet activity. *Am Heart J.* 1991;121:1382–1388.
38. Galve E, Ordi J, Barquinero J, et al. Valvular heart disease in the primary antiphospholipid syndrome. *Ann Intern Med.* 1992; 116:293–298.
39. Nickele GA, Foster PA, Kenny D. Primary antiphospholipid syndrome and mitral valve thrombosis. *Am Heart J.* 1994;128: 1245–1247.
40. Plein D, Van Camp G, Efira A, et al. Intracardiac thrombi associated with antiphospholipid antibodies. *J Am Soc Echocardiogr.* 1996;9:891–893.
41. Day SM, Rosenzweig BP, Kronzon I. Transesophageal echocardiographic diagnosis of right atrial thrombi associated with the antiphospholipid syndrome. *J Am Soc Echocardiogr.* 1995;8: 937–940.
42. O'Hickey S, Skinner C, Beattie J. Life-threatening right ventricular thrombosis in association with phospholipid antibodies. *Br Heart J.* 1993;70:279–281.
43. Leventhal LJ, Borofsky MA, Bergey PD, et al. Antiphospholipid antibody syndrome with right atrial thrombosis mimicking an atrial myxoma. *Am J Med.* 1989;87:111–113.
44. Hamsten A, Norberg R, Bjorkholm M, et al. Antibodies to cardiolipin in young survivors of myocardial infarction: an association with recurrent cardiovascular events. *Lancet.* 1986;1: 113–115.
45. Vaarala O, Mänttäri M, Manninen V, et al. Anticardiolipin antibodies and risk of myocardial infarction in a prospective cohort of middle-aged men. *Circulation.* 1995;91:23–27.
46. Wu RH, Nityanand S, Berglund L, et al. Antibodies against cardiolipin and oxidatively modified LDL in 50-year-old men predict myocardial infarction. *Arterioscler Thromb Vasc Biol.* 1997;17: 3159–3163.
47. Zuckerman E, Toubi E, Shiran A, et al. Anticardiolipin antibodies and acute myocardial infarction in nonsystemic lupus erythematosus patients: a controlled prospective study. *Am J Med.* 1996;101:381–386.
48. Kattwinkel N, Villanueva AG, Labib SB, et al. Myocardial infarction caused by cardiac microvasculopathy in a patient with the primary antiphospholipid syndrome. *Ann Intern Med.* 1992;116: 974–976.
49. Murphy JJ, Leach IH. Findings at necropsy in the heart of a patient with anticardiolipin syndrome. *Br Heart J.* 1989;62:61–64.
50. Rao LVM. Mechanisms of activity of lupus anticoagulants. *Curr Opin Hematol.* 1997;4:344–350.
51. Rao LVM, Hoang AD, Rapaport SI. Mechanism and effects of the binding of lupus anticoagulant IgG and prothrombin to surface phospholipid. *Blood.* 1996;88:4173–4182.
52. Kornberg A, Blank M, Kaufman S, et al. Induction of tissue factor-like activity in monocytes by anticardiolipin antibodies. *J Immunol.* 1994;153:1328–1332.
53. Simantov R, LaSala JM, Lo SK, et al. Activation of cultured vascular endothelial cells by antiphospholipid antibodies. *J Clin Invest.* 1995;96:2211–2219.
54. Horkko S, Miller E, Dudl E, et al. Antiphospholipid antibodies are directed against epitopes of oxidized phospholipids. *J Clin Invest.* 1996;98:815–825.
55. D'Angelo A, Selhub J. Homocysteine and thrombotic disease. *Blood.* 1997;90:111.
56. Welch GN, Loscalzo J. Homocysteine and atherothrombosis. *N Engl J Med.* 1998;338:1042–1050.
57. Stampfer MJ, Malinow R, Willett WC, et al. A prospective study of plasma homocysteine and risk of myocardial infarction in U.S. physicians. *JAMA.* 1992;268:877–881.
58. Boushey CJ, Beresford SAA, Omenn GS, et al. A quantitative assessment of plasma homocysteine as a risk factor for vascular disease. *JAMA.* 1995;274:1049–1057.
59. den Heijer M, Koster T, Blom HJ, et al. Hyperhomocysteinemia as a risk factor for deep-vein thrombosis. *N Engl J Med.* 1996; 334:759–762.
60. Harpel PC, Chang VT, Borth W. Homocysteine and other sulfhydryl compounds enhance the binding of lipoprotein(a) to fibrin: a potential biochemical link between thrombosis, atherogenesis, and sulfhydryl compound metabolism. *Proc Natl Acad Sci USA.* 1992;89:10193–10197.
61. Rosenson RS. Beyond low-density lipoprotein cholesterol. A perspective on low high-density lipoprotein disorders and Lp(a) lipoprotein excess. *Arch Intern Med.* 1996;156: 1278–1284.
62. Hajjar KA, Nachman RL. The role of lipoprotein(a) in atherogenesis and thrombosis. *Annu Rev Med.* 1996;47:423–442.
63. Hajjar KA, Gavish D, Breslow JL, et al. Lipoprotein(a) modulation of endothelial cell surface fibrinolysis and its potential role in atherosclerosis. *Nature.* 1989;339:303–305.
64. Etingin OR, Hajjar DP, Hajjar KA, et al. Lipoprotein (a) regulates plasminogen activator inhibitor-1 expression in endothelial cells. A potential mechanism in thrombogenesis. *J Biol Chem.* 1991;266:2459–2465.
65. Palabrica TM, Liu AC, Aronovitz MJ, et al. Antifibrinolytic activity of apolipoprotein(a) *in vivo*: human apolipoprotein(a) transgenic mice are resistant to tissue plasminogen activator-mediated thrombolysis. *Nat Med.* 1995;1:256–259.
66. Hirsh J, Dalen JE, Deykin D, et al. Oral anticoagulants. Mechanism of action, clinical effectiveness, and optimal therapeutic range. *Chest.* 1995;108:231S–246S.
67. Hirsh J, Poller L, Deykin D, et al. Optimal therapeutic range for oral anticoagulants. *Chest.* 1989;95:5S–11S.
68. Gurwitz JH, Goldberg RJ, Holden A, et al. Age-related risks of long-term oral anticoagulant therapy. *Arch Intern Med.* 1988;148:1733–1736.
69. O'Reilly RA, Trager WF, Rettie AE, et al. Interaction of amiodarone with racemic warfarin and its separated enantiomorphs in humans. *Clin Pharmacol Ther.* 1987;42:290–294.
70. Anderson GM, Hull G. The use of dicumarol as an adjunct to the treatment of congestive heart failure. *South Med J.* 1948;41; 365–372.
71. Wishart JH, Chapman CB. Dicumarol therapy in congestive heart failure. *N Engl J Med.* 1948;239:702–704.
72. Harvey WP, Finch CA. Dicumarol prophylaxis of thromboembolic disease in congestive heart failure. *N Engl J Med.* 1950;242:208–211.
73. Griffith GC, Stragnell R, Levinson DC. A study of the beneficial effects of anticoagulant therapy in congestive heart failure. *Ann Intern Med.* 1952;37:867–887.
74. Ritchie JL, Cheitlin M, Eagle KA, et al. ACC/AHA Task Force Report. Guidelines for the evaluation and management of heart failure. Report of the American College of Cardiology/American Heart Association Task Force on Practice Guidelines (Committee on Evaluation and Management of Heart Failure). *J Am Coll Cardiol.* 1995;26:1376–1398.
75. Uretsky BF, Thygesen K, Armstrong PW, et al. Acute coronary findings at autopsy in heart failure patients with sudden death: results from the Assessment of Treatment with Lisinopril and Survival (ATLAS) trial. *Circulation.* 2000;102:611–616.
76. Hurlen M, Abdelnoor M, Smith P, Erikssen J, Arnesen H. Warfarin, aspirin, or both after myocardial infarction. *N Engl J Med.* 2002;347:969–974.
77. Van Es RF, Jonker JJ, Verheught FW, Decers JW, Grobee DE. Aspirin and Coumadin after acute coronary syndromes. *Lancet.* 2002;320:109–113.
78. Roberts WC, Seigel RJ, McNanus BM. Idiopathic dilated cardiomyopathy: analysis of 152 necropsy patients. *Am J Cardiol.* 1987;60:1340–1365.
79. Weitz JI, Hudoba M, Massel D, et al. Clot-bound thrombin is protected from inhibition by heparin-antithrombin III but is susceptible to inactivation by antithrombin III-independent inhibitors. *J Clin Invest.* 1990;86:385–391.

80. Jafri SM, Mammen EF, Masura J, et al. Effects of warfarin on markers of hypercoagulability in patients with heart failure. *Am Heart J*. 1997;134:27–36.
81. Levine B, Kalman J, Mayer L, et al. Elevated circulating levels of tumor necrosis factor in severe chronic heart failure. *N Engl J Med*. 1990;323:236–241.
82. Blum A, Miller H. Role of cytokines in heart failure. *Am Heart J*. 1998;135:181–186.
83. Stratton JR, Nemanich JW, Johannessen KA, et al. Fate of left ventricular thrombi in patients with remote myocardial infarction or idiopathic cardiomyopathy. *Circulation*. 1988;78: 1388–1393.
84. Falk RH, Foster E, Coats MH. Ventricular thrombi and thromboembolism in dilated cardiomyopathy: a prospective follow-up study. *Am Heart J*. 1992;123:136–142.
85. Cioffi G, Pozzoli M, Forni G, et al. Systemic thromboembolism in chronic heart failure. A prospective study in 406 patients. *Eur Heart J*. 1996;17:1381–1389.
86. Katz SD, Marantz PR, Biasucci L, et al. Low incidence of stroke in ambulatory patients with heart failure: a prospective study. *Am Heart J*. 1993;126:141–146.
87. Natterson PD, Stevenson WG, Saxon LA, et al. Risk of arterial embolization in 224 patients awaiting cardiac transplantation. *Am Heart J*. 1995;129:564–570.
88. Baker DW, Wright RF. Management of heart failure: IV. Anticoagulation for patients with heart failure due to left ventricular systolic dysfunction. *JAMA*. 1994;272:1614–1618.
89. Dunkman WB, Johnson GR, Carson PE, et al. Incidence of thromboembolic events in congestive heart failure. *Circulation*. 1993;87(Suppl VI):VI-94–VI-101.
90. Harrington RA, Becker RC, Ezekowitz M, et al. Antithrombotic therapy for coronary artery disease. The Seventh ACCP Conference on Antithrombotic and Thrombolytic Therapy. *Chest*. 2004:126:513S–548S.
91. The Stroke Prevention in Atrial Fibrillation Investigators. Predictors of thromboembolism in atrial fibrillation: I. Clinical features of patients at risk. *Ann Intern Med*. 1992;116:1–5.
92. Dries DL, Rosenberg YD, Waclawiw MA, et al. Ejection fraction and risk of thromboembolic events in patients with systolic dysfunction and sinus rhythm: evidence for general differences in the Studies of Left Ventricular Dysfunction trials. *J Am Coll Cardiol*. 1997;29:1074–1080.
93. Loh E, St John Sutton M, Wun CCC, et al. Ventricular dysfunction and the risk of stroke after myocardial infarction. *N Engl J Med*. 1997;336:251–257.
94. Schussheim AE, Fuster V. Thrombosis, antithrombotic agents, and the antithrombotic approach in cardiac disease. *Prog Cardiovasc Dis*. 1997;40:205–238.
95. Minor RL, Oren RM, Stanford W, et al. Biventricular thrombi and pulmonary emboli complicating idiopathic dilated cardiomyopathy: diagnosis with cardiac ultrafast CT. *Am Heart J*. 1991;122:1477–1481.
96. Missault L, Koch A, Colardyn F, et al. Biventricular thrombi in dilated cardiomyopathy: massive simultaneous pulmonary and systemic embolisation. *Eur Heart J*. 1994;15:713–714.
97. Cleland JGF, Findlay I, Jafri S, et al. The Warfarin/Aspirin Study in Heart Failure (WASH): a randomized trial comparing antithrombotic therapies for patients with heart failure. *Am Heart J*. 2004;148:157–164.
98. Cleland JG, Ghosh J, Freemantle N, et al. Clinical trials update and cumulative meta-analyses from the American College of Cardiology: WATCH, SCD-HeFT, DINAMIT, CASINO, INSPIRE, STRATUS-US, RIO-Lipids and cardiac resynchronisation therapy in heart failure. *Eur J Heart Fail*. 2004;6:501–508.
99. Pullicino P, Thompson JL, Barton B, et al. Warfarin versus aspirin in patients with reduced cardiac ejection fraction (WARCEF): rationale, objectives, and design. *J Card Fail*. 2006;12:39–46.
100. Heart Failure Society of America. Executive summary: HFSA 2006 Comprehensive Heart Failure Practice Guideline. *J Card Fail*. 2006;12:10–38.
101. Hunt SA, Abraham WT, Chin MH, et al. ACC/AHA 2005 guideline update for the diagnosis and management of chronic heart failure in the adult: summary article: a report of the American College of Cardiology/American Heart Association Task Force on Practice Guidelines. *J Am Coll Cardiol*. 2005;46:1116–1143.
102. Swedberg K, Cleland J, Dargie H, et al. Guidelines for the diagnosis and treatment of chronic heart failure: executive summary (update 2005): the Task Force for the Diagnosis and Treatment of Chronic Heart Failure of the European Society of Cardiology. *Eur Heart J*. 2005;26(11):1115–1140.
103. Sixth ACCP Consensus Conference on Antithrombotic Therapy. *Chest* 2001;119(Suppl):1S-370S. Antiplatelet Trialists Collaboration. Collaborative meta-analysis of randomised trials of antiplatelet therapy for prevention of death, myocardial infarction, and stroke in high-risk patients. *BMJ*. 2002;324: 71–86.
104. Van Es RF, Jonker JJ, Verheugt FW, et al. Aspirin and Coumadin after acute coronary syndromes (the ASPECT-2 study): a randomised controlled trial. *Lancet*. 2002;360:109–113.
105. Hurlen M, Abdelnoor M, Smith P, et al. Warfarin, aspirin, or both after myocardial infarction. WARIS I and ASPECT I. *N Engl J Med*. 2002;347:969–974.
106. Al-Khadra AS, Salem DN, Rand WM, et al. Antiplatelet agents and survival: a cohort analysis from the Studies of Left Ventricular Dysfunction (SOLVD) trial. *J Am Coll Cardiol*. 1998; 31:419-425.
107. Massie BM, Teerlink JR. Interaction between aspirin and angiotensin-converting enzyme inhibitors: real or imagined. *Am J Med*. 2000;109:431–433.
108. Guazzi M, Brambilla R, Reina G, et al. Aspirin-angiotensin-converting enzyme inhibitor co-administration and mortality in patients with heart failure. A dose-related adverse effect of aspirin. *Arch Intern Med*. 2003;163:1574–1579.
109. Hall D. The aspirin-angiotensin-converting enzyme inhibitor tradeoff: to halve and halve not. *J Am Coll Cardiol*. 2000;35: 1808–1812.
110. Mahé I, Meune C, Diemer M, et al. Interaction between aspirin and ACE inhibitors in patients with heart failure. *Drug Safety*. 2001;24:167–182.
111. Stys T, Wawson WE, Smaldone GC, et al. Does aspirin attenuate the beneficial effects of angiotensin-converting enzyme inhibition in heart failure? *Arch Intern Med*. 2000;160:1409–1413.
112. Latini R, Tognoni G, Maggioni AP, et al. Clinical effects of early angiotensin-converting enzyme inhibitor treatment for acute myocardial infarction are similar in the presence and absence of aspirin. *J Am Coll Cardiol*. 2000;35:1801–1807.
113. Teo KK, Yusuf S, Pfeffer M, et al. Effects of long-term treatment with angiotensin-converting-enzyme inhibitors in the presence or absence of aspirin: a systematic review. *Lancet*. 2002;360: 1037–1043.
114. Dzau VJ, Packer M, Lilly LS, et al. Prostaglandins in severe congestive heart failure. Relation to activation of the renin-angiotensin system and hyponatremia. *N Engl J Med*. 1984;310:347–352.
115. Hall D, Zeitler H, Rudolph W. Counteraction of the vasodilator effects of enalapril by aspirin in severe heart failure. *J Am Coll Cardiol*. 1992;20:1549–1555.
116. Spaulding C, Charbonnier B, Cohen-Solal A, et al. Acute hemodynamic interaction of aspirin and ticlopidine with enalapril. *Circulation*. 1998;98:757–765.
117. Baur LH, Schipperheyn JJ, van der Laarse A, et al. Combining salicylate and enalapril in patients with coronary artery disease and heart failure. *Br Heart J*. 1995;73:227–235.
118. Jeserich M, Pape L, Just H, et al. Effect of long-term angiotensin inhibition on vascular function in patients with chronic congestive heart failure. *Am J Cardiol*. 1995;76:1079–1082.
119. Davie AP, Love MP, McMurray JJ. Even low-dose aspirin inhibits arachidonic acid-induced vasodilation in heart failure. *Clin Pharmacol Ther*. 2000;67:530–537.
120. CAPRIE Steering Committee. A randomised, blinded, trial of Clopidogrel versus Aspirin in Patients at Risk of Ischaemic Events (CAPRIE). *Lancet* 1996;348:1329–1339.
121. Fuster V, Verstraete M. Hemostasis, thrombosis, fibrinolysis, and cardiovascular disease. In: Braunwald E, ed. *Heart Disease. A Textbook of Cardiovascular Medicine*. Philadelphia: WB Saunders; 1997: 1809–1840.
122. Cairns JA, Lewis HDJ, Meade TW, et al. Antithrombotic agents in coronary artery disease. *Chest*. 1995;108:380S–400S.
123. Merlini PA, Bauer KA, Oltrona L, et al. Persistent activation of coagulation mechanism in unstable angina and myocardial infarction. *Circulation*. 1994;90:61–68.

124. Kamikura Y, Wada H, Yamada A, et al. Increased tissue factor pathway inhibitor in patients with acute myocardial infarction. *Am J Hematol.* 1997;55:183–187.
125. Neumann FJ, Ott I, Gawaz M, et al. Cardiac release of cytokines and inflammatory responses in acute myocardial infarction. *Circulation.* 1995;92:748–755.
126. Greaves SC, Zhi G, Lee RT, et al. Incidence and natural history of left ventricular thrombus following anterior wall acute myocardial infarction. *Am J Cardiol.* 1997;80:442–448.
127. Mooe T, Teien D, Karp K, et al. Long-term follow-up of patients with anterior myocardial infarction complicated by left ventricular thrombus in the thrombolytic era. *Heart.* 1996;75:252–256.
128. SCATI Group. Randomised controlled trial of subcutaneous calcium-heparin in acute myocardial infarction. *Lancet.* 1989; 2:182–186.
129. Turpie AGG, Robinson JG, Doyle DJ, et al. Comparison of high-dose with low-dose subcutaneous heparin to prevent left ventricular mural thrombosis in patients with acute transmural anterior myocardial infarction. *N Engl J Med.* 1989;320:352–357.
130. Vaitkus PT, Barnathan ES. Embolic potential, prevention and management of mural thrombus complicating anterior myocardial infarction: a meta-analysis. *J Am Coll Cardiol.* 1993;22:1004–1009.
131. Kontny F, Dale J, Abildgaard U, et al. Randomized trial of low molecular weight heparin (Dalteparin) in prevention of left ventricular thrombus formation and arterial embolism after acute anterior myocardial infarction: the Fragmin in Acute Myocardial Infarction (FRAMI) Study. *J Am Coll Cardiol.* 1997;30:962–969.
132. van Dantzig JM, Delemarre BJ, Bot H, et al. Left ventricular thrombus in acute myocardial infarction. *Eur Heart J.* 1996;17:1640–1645.
133. Israel DH, Fuster V, Ip JH, et al. Intracardiac thrombosis and systemic embolization. In: Colman RW, Hirsh J, Marder VJ, Salzman EW, eds. *Hemostasis and Thrombosis: Basic Principles and Clinical Practice.* Philadelphia: JB Lippincott Co.; 1994: 1452–1468.
134. Eigler N, Maurer G, Shah PK. Effect of early systemic thrombolytic therapy on left ventricular mural thrombus formation in acute anterior myocardial infarction. *Am J Cardiol.* 1984; 54:261–263.
135. Bhatnagar SK, Al-Yusuf AR. Effects of intravenous recombinant tissue-type plasminogen activator therapy on the incidence and associations of left ventricular thrombus in patients with a first acute Q wave anterior myocardial infarction. *Am Heart J.* 1991; 122:1251–1256.
136. Keren A, Goldberg S, Gottleib S, et al. Natural history of left ventricular thrombi: their appearance and resolution in the post-hospitalization period of acute myocardial infarction. *J Am Coll Cardiol.* 1990;15:790–800.
137. Held AC, Gore JM, Paraskos J, et al. Impact of thrombolytic therapy on left ventricular mural thrombi in acute myocardial infarction. *Am J Cardiol.* 1988;62:310–311.
138. Lupi G, Domenicucci S, Chiarella F, et al. Influence of thrombolytic treatment followed by full-dose anticoagulation on the frequency of left ventricular thrombi in acute myocardial infarction. *Am J Cardiol.* 1989;64:588–590.
139. Natarajan D, Hotchandani RK, Nigam PD. Reduced incidence of left ventricular thrombi with intravenous streptokinase in acute anterior myocardial infarction: prospective evaluation by cross-sectional echocardiography. *Int J Cardiol.* 1988;20:201–207.
140. Stratton JR, Speck SM, Caldwell JH, et al. Late effects of intracoronary streptokinase on regional wall motion, ventricular aneurysm and left ventricular thrombus in myocardial infarction: results from the Western Washington Randomized Trial. *J Am Coll Cardiol.* 1985;5:1023–1028.
141. Collins R, MacMahon S, Flather M, et al. Clinical effects of anticoagulant therapy in suspected acute myocardial infarction: systemic overview of randomised trials. *BMJ.* 1996;313:652–659.
142. Granger CB, Becker R, Tracy RP, et al. Thrombin generation, inhibition and clinical outcomes in patients with acute myocardial infarction treated with thrombolytic therapy and heparin: results from the GUSTO-I Trial. *J Am Coll Cardiol.* 1998;31: 497–505.
143. Gruppo Italiano per Lo Studio Della Sopravvivenza Nell'Infarto Miocardico. GISSI2: a factorial randomised trial of alteplase versus streptokinase and heparin versus no heparin among 12,490 patients with acute myocardial infarction. *Lancet.* 1990;336: 65–71.
144. The International Study Group. In-hospital mortality and clinical course of 20,891 patients with suspected acute myocardial infarction randomised between alteplase and streptokinase with or without heparin. *Lancet.* 1990;336:71–75.
145. ISIS3 Collaborative Group. ISIS3: a randomised comparison of streptokinase vs tissue plasminogen activator vs anistreplase and of aspirin plus heparin vs aspirin alone among 41,299 cases of suspected acute myocardial infarction. *Lancet.* 1992;339:753–770.
146. Mahaffey KW, Granger CB, Collins R, et al. Overview of randomized trials of intravenous heparin in patients with acute myocardial infarction treated with thrombolytic therapy. *Am J Cardiol.* 1996;77:551–556.
147. Hennekens CH, O'Donnell CJ, Ridker PM. Current and future perspectives on antithrombotic therapy of acute myocardial infarction. *Eur Heart J.* 1995;16(Suppl D):2–9.
148. Collins R, Peto R, Baigent C, et al. Aspirin, heparin, and fibrinolytic therapy in suspected acute myocardial infarction. *N Engl J Med.* 1997;336:847–860.
149. Rogers WJ, Bowlby LJ, Chandra NC, et al. Treatment of myocardial infarction in the United States (1990 to 1993). Observations from the National Registry of Myocardial Infarction. *Circulation.* 1994;90:2103–2114.
150. Smith P, Arnesen H, Holme I. The effect of warfarin on mortality and reinfarction after myocardial infarction. *N Engl J Med.* 1990;323:147–152.
151. ASPECT Research Group. Effect of long-term oral anticoagulant treatment on mortality and cardiovascular morbidity after myocardial infarction. *Lancet.* 1994;343:499–503.
152. Lerman A, Holmes DR, Bell MR, et al. Endothelin in coronary endothelial dysfunction and early atherosclerosis in humans. *Circulation.* 1995;92:2426–2431.
153. EPSIM Research Group. A controlled comparison of aspirin and oral anticoagulants in prevention of death after myocardial infarction. *N Engl J Med.* 1982;307:701–708.
154. Meijer A, Verheugt FWA, Werter CJPJ, et al. Aspirin versus Coumadin in the prevention of reocclusion and recurrent ischemia after successful thrombolysis: a prospective placebo-controlled angiographic study: results of the APRICOT Study. *Circulation.* 1993;87:1524–1530.
155. CARS Investigators. Randomised double-blind trial of fixed low-dose warfarin with aspirin after myocardial infarction. *Lancet.* 1997;350:389–396.
156. Azar AJ, Cannegieter SC, Deckers JW, et al. Optimal intensity of oral anticoagulant therapy after myocardial infarction. *J Am Coll Cardiol.* 1996;27:1349–1355.
157. Granger CB, Hirsh J, Califf RM, et al. Activated partial thromboplastin time and outcome after thrombolytic therapy for acute myocardial infarction. Results from the GUSTO-1 Trial. *Circulation.* 1996;93:870–878.
158. GUSTO IIa Investigators. Randomized trial of intravenous heparin versus recombinant hirudin for acute coronary syndromes. *Circulation.* 1994;90:1631–1637.
159. Ryan TJ, Anderson JL, Antman EM, et al. ACC/AHA guidelines for the management of patients with acute myocardial infarction. A report of the American College of Cardiology/American Heart Association Task Force on Practice Guidelines (Committee on Management of Acute Myocardial Infarction). *J Am Coll Cardiol.* 1996;28:1328–1428.
160. Granger CB, Miller JM, Bovill EG, et al. Rebound increase in thrombin generation and activity after cessation of intravenous heparin in patients with acute coronary syndromes. *Circulation.* 1995;91:1929–1935.
161. Grip L, Blomback M, Schulman S. Hypercoagulable state and thromboembolism following warfarin withdrawal in post-myocardial-infarction patients. *Eur Heart J.* 1991;12: 1225–1233.
162. Reeder GS, Lengyel M, Tajik AJ, et al. Mural thrombus in left ventricular aneurysm. Incidence, role of angiography, and relation between anticoagulation and embolization. *Mayo Clin Proc.* 1981;56:77–81.
163. Meltzer RS, Visser CA, Fuster V. Intracardiac thrombi and systemic embolization. *Ann Intern Med.* 1986;104:689–698.
164. Lapeyre ACI, Steele PM, Kazmier FJ, et al. Systemic embolism in chronic left ventricular aneurysm: incidence and the role of anticoagulation. *J Am Coll Cardiol.* 1985;6:534–538.
165. Laupacis A, Albers G, Dalen J, et al. Antithrombotic therapy in atrial fibrillation. *Chest.* 1995;108:352S–359S.

166. Orsinelli DA. Current recommendations for the anticoagulation of patients with atrial fibrillation. *Prog Cardiovasc Dis.* 1996;39:1–20.
167. Mitusch R, Siemens HJ, Garbe M, et al. Detection of a hypercoagulable state in nonvalvular atrial fibrillation and the effect of anticoagulant therapy. *Thromb Haemost.* 1996;75:219–223.
168. Black IW, Chesterman CN, Hopkins AP, et al. Hematologic correlates of left atrial spontaneous echo contrast and thromboembolism in nonvalvular atrial fibrillation. *J Am Coll Cardiol.* 1993;21:451–457.
169. Manning WJ, Silverman DI, Waksmonski CA, et al. Prevalence of residual left atrial thrombi among patients with acute thromboembolism and newly recognized atrial fibrillation. *Arch Intern Med.* 1995;155:2193–2197.
170. Manning WJ. Role of transesophageal echocardiography in the management of thromboembolic stroke. *Am J Cardiol.* 1997; 80(4c):19D–28D.
171. The Stroke Prevention in Atrial Fibrillation Investigators Committee on Echocardiography. Transesophageal echocardiographic correlates of thromboembolism in high-risk patients with nonvalvular atrial fibrillation. *Ann Intern Med.* 1998; 128:639–647.
172. Leung DY, Davidson PM, Cranney GB, et al. Thromboembolic risks of left atrial thrombus detected by transesophageal echocardiogram. *Am J Cardiol.* 1997;79:626–629.
173. Zabalgoitia M, Halperin JL, Pearce LA, et al. Transesophageal echocardiographic correlates of clinical risk of thromboembolism in nonvalvular atrial fibrillation. *J Am Coll Cardiol.* 1998; 31:1622–1626.
174. Petersen P, Godtfredsen J, Boysen G, et al. Placebo-controlled, randomised trial of warfarin and aspirin for prevention of thromboembolic complications in chronic atrial fibrillation. The Copenhagen AFASAK Study. *Lancet.* 1989;1:175–179.
175. Stroke Prevention in Atrial Fibrillation Investigators. Stroke Prevention in Atrial Fibrillation Study. Final results. *Circulation.* 1991;84:527–539.
176. The Boston Area Anticoagulation Trial for Atrial Fibrillation Investigators. The effect of low-dose warfarin on the risk of stroke in patients with nonrheumatic atrial fibrillation. *N Engl J Med.* 1990;323:1505–1511.
177. EAFT (European Atrial Fibrillation Trial) Study Group. Secondary prevention in nonrheumatic atrial fibrillation after transient ischaemic attack or minor stroke. *Lancet.* 1993;342:1255–1262.
178. Ezekowitz MD, Bridgers SL, James KE, et al. Warfarin in the prevention of stroke associated with nonrheumatic atrial fibrillation. *N Engl J Med.* 1992;327:1406–1412.
179. Connolly SJ, Laupacis A, Gent M, et al. Canadian Atrial Fibrillation Anticoagulation (CAFA) Study. *J Am Coll Cardiol.* 1991;18:349–355.
180. The Atrial Fibrillation Investigators. The efficacy of aspirin in patients with atrial fibrillation. Analysis of pooled data from three randomized trials. *Arch Intern Med.* 1997;157: 1237–1240.
181. Stroke Prevention in Atrial Fibrillation Investigators. Warfarin versus aspirin for prevention of thromboembolism in atrial fibrillation: Stroke Prevention in Atrial Fibrillation II Study. *Lancet.* 1994;343:687–691.
182. Stroke Prevention in Atrial Fibrillation Investigators. Adjusted-dose warfarin versus low-intensity, fixed-dose warfarin plus aspirin for high-risk patients with atrial fibrillation: Stroke Prevention in Atrial Fibrillation III randomised clinical trial. *Lancet.* 1996;348:633–638.
183. The SPAF III Writing Committee for the Stroke Prevention in Atrial Fibrillation Investigators. Patients with nonvalvular atrial fibrillation at low risk of stroke during treatment with aspirin. Stroke Prevention in Atrial Fibrillation III Study. *JAMA.* 1998;279:1273–1277.
184. SPAF Investigators. Risk factors for thromboembolism during aspirin therapy in patients with atrial fibrillation. *J Stroke Cerebrovasc Dis.* 1995;5:147–157.
185. Atrial Fibrillation Investigators. Echocardiographic predictors of stroke in patients with atrial fibrillation: a prospective study of 1,066 patients from three clinical trials. *Arch Intern Med.* 2006. In press..
186. The European Atrial Fibrillation Trial Study Group. Optimal oral anticoagulant therapy in patients with nonrheumatic atrial fibrillation and recent cerebral ischemia. *N Engl J Med.* 1995; 333:5–10.
187. Hylek EM, Skates SJ, Sheehan MA, et al. An analysis of the lowest effective intensity of prophylactic anticoagulation for patients with nonrheumatic atrial fibrillation. *N Engl J Med.* 1996;335:540–546.
188. Feinberg WM, Cornell ES, Nightingale SD, et al. Relationship between prothrombin activation fragment F1.2 and international normalized ratio in patients with atrial fibrillation. *Stroke.* 1997; 28:1101–1106.
189. Lip GYH, Lip PL, Zarifis J, et al. Fibrin D-dimer and β-thromboglobulin as markers of thrombogenesis and platelet activation in atrial fibrillation. Effects of introducing ultra-low-dose warfarin and aspirin. *Circulation.* 1996;94:425–431.

Ultrafiltration Therapies for Congestive Heart Failure

43

Maria Rosa Costanzo

Traditional diuretic therapies for congestion in heart failure patients are simultaneously ineffective and expensive. Approximately 1 million hospitalizations, with an estimated cost of $23 billion, occur annually in the United States due to decompensated heart failure (1,2). With an average hospital cost of $5,905 and reimbursement of $4,617, U.S. hospitals lose approximately $1,300 per heart failure admission (2–4). Data from the Acute Decompensated Heart Failure National Registry (ADHERE) show that the majority of heart failure hospitalizations are due to fluid overload in patients who have failed treatment with oral diuretics (5). Despite use of intravenous diuretics in 90% of patients, the average length of stay for a heart failure patient is 4.3 days and 42% of the patients are discharged without complete resolution of symptoms. With current treatment strategies, 50% of the patients lose ≤5 pounds from admission weight and 20% gain weight during the heart failure hospitalization (5). The failure to effectively resolve congestion and reduce weight may contribute to readmission rates, which may be as high as 50% at 6 months (6).

Although many heart failure patients can be successfully treated with diuretics, 25% to 30% of patients develop diuretic resistance, defined as reduced diuresis and natriuresis before resolution of congestion (7). Causes include functional renal failure, hyponatremia, altered diuretic pharmacokinetics, and neurohormonally mediated sodium retention. In salt-restricted patients, fractional excretion of sodium decreases with continued exposure to loop diuretics, the braking phenomenon, and intermittent diuretic administration causes postdiuretic sodium retention (8). Therapies to ameliorate diuretic resistance, including fluid and sodium restriction, increased angiotensin-converting enzyme inhibitors (ACEIs) doses, use of diuretic combinations, and changes in the timing and route of diuretic administration, have limited success (9–13).

Finally, hospital stay may be inappropriately prolonged when aggressive use of intravenous diuretics leads to worsening renal function (14,15). Renal insufficiency and diuretic resistance worsen outcomes as well as hospital length of stay and cost of heart failure patients (16–24). A Study of Left Ventricular Dysfunction (SOLVD) analysis indicates that even mild renal insufficiency in patients with left ventricular systolic dysfunction independently predicts all-cause and pump failure mortality and the combined endpoint of death and heart failure hospitalizations (25,26). An increase of serum creatinine of >0.3 mg/dL, which occurs in nearly one-third of heart failure patients, is associated with poorer prognosis and longer hospitalization (11,27). Recently, the safety of diuretics in heart failure patients has been questioned (28,29). In 1,153 heart failure patients enrolled in the Prospective Randomized Amlodipine Evaluation (PRAISE), high diuretic doses independently increased mortality, sudden death, and pump failure death, associating diuretic resistance with a poor prognosis in heart failure patients (30). Intravenous diuretic use can decrease cardiac output, increase pulmonary capillary wedge pressure and total systemic vascular resistance, and reduce renal blood flow and glomerular filtration rates (31,32). The results of recently published studies have confirmed the association of high diuretic doses with worsening renal function in heart failure patients (33).

PATHOPHYSIOLOGY OF SODIUM AND WATER RETENTION IN HEART FAILURE

The data previously summarized are sobering, but not surprising, because in heart failure patients hemodynamic abnormalities and neurohormonal activation lead to progressive deterioration of renal function. Knowledge of the processes linking cardiac and renal dysfunction is critical for the understanding of the effects of mechanical fluid removal by ultrafiltration in patients with heart failure (Fig. 43-1) (34).

In heart failure, arterial underfilling produced by a decrease in cardiac output is the primary determinant of renal sodium and water retention. Because approximately 85% of the plasma volume resides in the low-pressure venous side and only 15% in the arterial side of the circulation, an expansion of total blood volume can occur in the venous system and yet arterial underfilling causes the kidney to increase reabsorption of sodium and water. The unloading of high-pressure baroreceptors in the left ventricle, carotid sinus, and aortic arch, resulting from arterial underfilling, is an afferent signal that decreases vagal and glossopharyngeal inhibitory tone in the central nervous system. This leads to activation of the sympathetic nervous system, which mediates an initially compensatory but later detrimental increase in peripheral and renal vascular resistance and increase in renin release from the kidney (35). Renin then activates angiotensin II, which stimulates secretion of aldosterone from the adrenal cortex, leading to renal sodium and water retention.

In addition, activation of the sympathetic nervous system stimulates the supra-aortic and paraventricular nuclei in the hypothalamus, which results in nonosmotic release of vasopressin and subsequent aquaporin 2-mediated renal water retention. As the left ventricle fails, the increase in left atrial and ventricular pressures stimulates release of natriuretic peptides, which mediate both vasodilatation and renal sodium excretion (36). Eventually, however, vasoconstrictive and volume-retaining mechanisms overwhelm the effects of natriuretic peptides. Initially, glomerular filtration rate is maintained by the increase in efferent arteriolar resistance and capillary hydrostatic pressure. Ultimately, however, renal blood flow decreases to the point where glomerular filtration rate cannot be maintained and renal dysfunction becomes progressive (37).

Salt and water retention in heart failure is further augmented by the development of diuretic resistance (7–9). The magnitude of natriuresis decreases after each diuretic dose (braking phenomenon). A decline in effective intravascular volume, by reducing the amount of sodium chloride (NaCl) that is filtered and by increasing that which is reabsorbed, is key to the occurrence of the braking phenomenon. When given *acutely*, thiazide diuretics reduce NaCl absorption in the proximal tubule by inhibiting carbonic anhydrase (38). In contrast, intravascular volume contraction due to *chronic* administration of thiazide

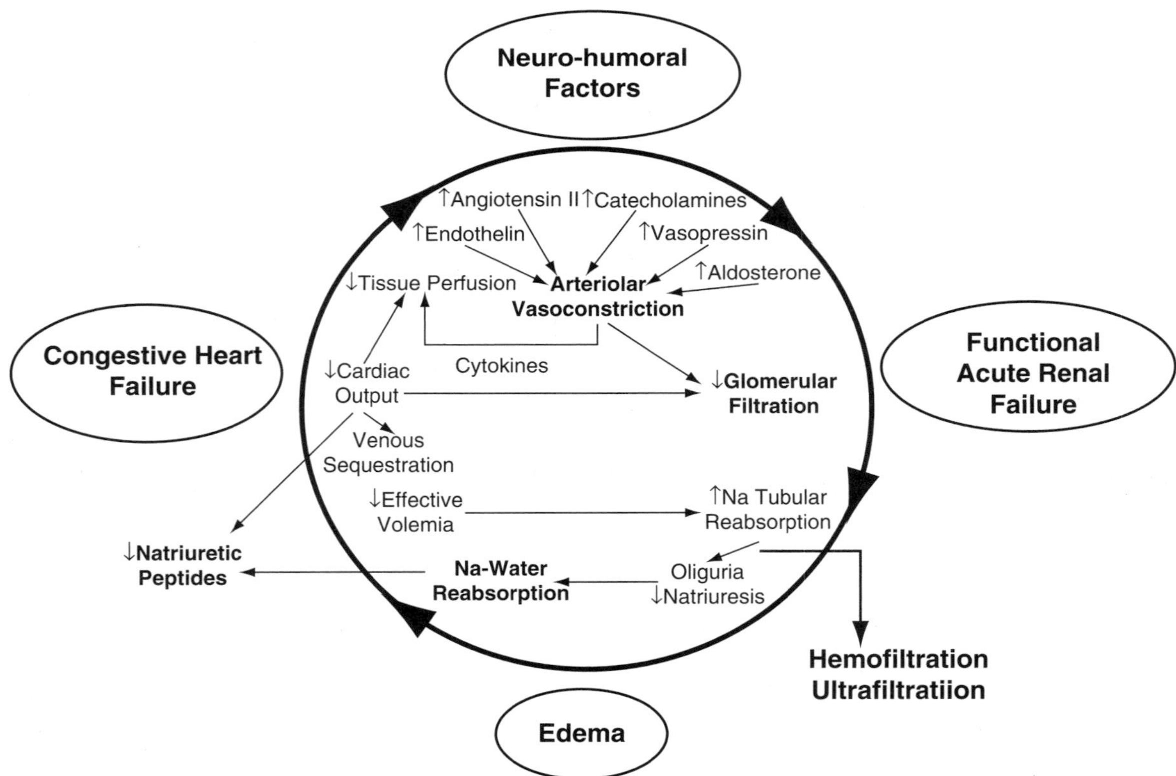

Figure 43-1 Schematic representation of the vicious circle linking heart failure and renal failure and of the possible role of ultrafiltration in interrupting it. (Adapted from Canaud B, Leblanc M, Leray-Moragues H, et al. Slow continuous ultrafiltration for refractory congestive heart failure. *Nephrol Dial Transplant.* 1998;13 (Suppl 4):51–55, with permission.)

diuretics increases NaCl reabsorption both in the proximal tubule due to increased filtration fraction and decreased renal interstitial pressure, and in the distal tubule due to reduced delivery of NaCl (38).

In addition, increased efferent sympathetic nerve activity reduces urinary NaCl excretion by reducing renal blood flow, by stimulating renin release at the macula densa, by enhancing tubular NaCl reabsorption, and by interacting with hormonal modulators of NaCl transport. Loop diuretics stimulate renin secretion by inhibiting NaCl uptake into the macula densa cells and by enhancing renal production of prostacyclin. Furthermore, chronic administration of loop diuretics induces distal tubular epithelial cells hypertrophy and hyperplasia due to increased solute delivery to the distal tubule (39,40).

In the milieu of heart failure and diuretic resistance, an attractive alternative to diuretics is removal of excess fluid with ultrafiltration, a therapy which does not cause prolonged intravascular volume contraction or stimulation of macula densa-mediated neurohormonal activation.

ULTRAFILTRATION

The Process

The process of ultrafiltration consists of the production of plasma water from whole blood across a semipermeable membrane (hemofilter) in response to a transmembrane pressure gradient (Fig. 43-2) (41). The pressure gradient across ultrafiltration membranes is generated by the classic Starling forces, which include the hydrostatic pressures in the blood and in the filtrate compartments, and the oncotic pressure generated by plasma proteins. Hydrostatic pressure is determined by the blood pressure in the filtering device, generated by either the patient's endogenous blood pressure or by an extracorporeal pump plus the siphoning effect of suction occurring in the ultrafiltrate compartment. The sum of these pressures generates the transmembrane pressure, driving the plasma water through the hemofilter exactly as Starling forces operate in a capillary bed (41). The correlation between ultrafiltration rates and transmembrane pressure gradient describes the filtering membrane's hydraulic permeability (Kf) (Fig. 43-3). The correlation is linear within a certain range of pressures, beyond which it flattens due to the coating of the blood side of the membrane by plasma proteins (42,43).

Ultrafiltration Membranes

Ultrafiltration membranes can be characterized according to different parameters. The polymeric structure can be of natural (cellulosic) or synthetic origin. Cellulosic membranes are homogeneous and hydrophilic, whereas synthetic membranes have a finely porous structure. These characteristics result in specific interactions with electrically charged solutes or hydrophilic–hydrophobic molecules and influence the membrane's hemocompatibility. Finally, membranes can be divided into "low-flux" or "high-flux" according to their hydraulic permeability. For extracorporeal ultrafiltration, synthetic high-flux membranes (made of polysulfone, polyamide, polymethylmethacrylate, or polyacrylonitrile) are generally employed because of their excellent permeability (Kf >20 mL/hour $\times$ mm Hg $\times$ m^2) and biocompatibility (43).

Hemofilters also vary according to the ultrafiltration technique for which they are employed. While standard hemofilters are used for ultrafiltration accompanying hemodialysis, clotting-resistant minifilters providing ultrafiltration rates between 2 to 10 mL/minute are used for isolated or slow, continuous ultrafiltration (SCUF) (44). When hydrostatic pressure exceeds oncotic pressure, the ultrafiltrate, consisting of water and nonprotein-bound low- and middle-molecular–weight solutes, passes through the semipermeable membrane into the ultrafiltrate space, while macromolecules (mostly proteins and cells) are retained. With isolated ultrafiltration, the solute is passively removed by accompanying the solvent flow (convective transport) (45,46).

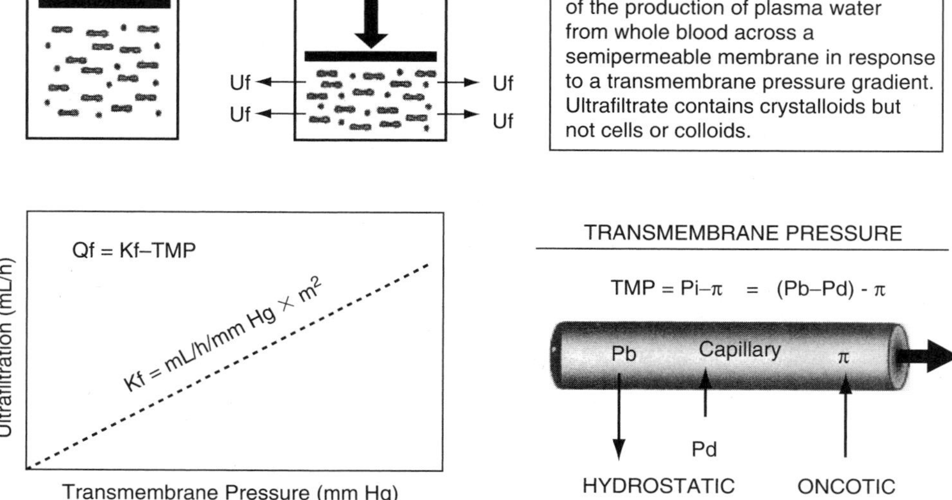

Figure 43-2 Description of the physical process of ultrafiltration and graphic representation of the ultrafiltration coefficient of a membrane as a function of ultrafiltration rate and applied pressure. Kf, ultrafiltration coefficient; Qf, ultrafiltration rate; Pb, blood hydrostatic pressure; Pd, ultrafiltrate hydrostatic pressure; Pi, hydrostatic pressure; TMP, transmembrane pres- sure; π, oncotic pressure. (From Ronco C, Ricci Z, Bellomo R, Bedogni F. Extracorporeal ultrafiltration for the treatment of overhydration and congestive heart failure. *Cardiology.* 2001:96:155–168, with permission.)

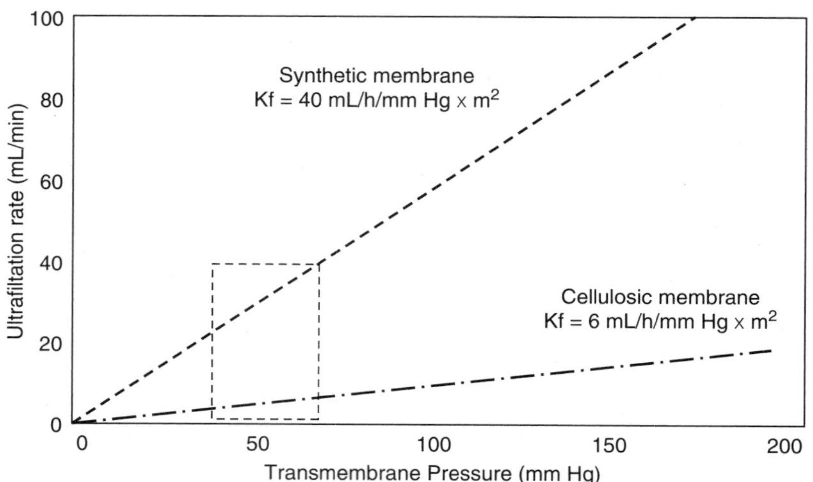

Figure 43-3 Ultrafiltration coefficients of different dialysis membranes. Kf, ultrafiltration coefficient; TMP, transmembrane pressure; Uf, ultrafiltration. (From Ronco C, Ricci Z, Bellomo R, Bedogni F. Extracorporeal ultrafiltration for the treatment of overhydration and congestive heart failure. *Cardiology.* 2001:96:155–168, with permission.)

In contrast, solute removed by dialysis diffuses down a concentration gradient. Small solutes readily move through membrane pores by diffusion or convection, whereas larger molecules can pass very slowly through membranes only by diffusion. Convection actually helps direct larger molecules through the pores so that with convection the transport rates for small- and middle-sized molecules are similar. In convective transport, the solute concentration in the ultrafiltrate is essentially equal to the solute concentration in the water component of the plasma on the blood side of the membrane (46). The sieving coefficient, which is the ratio between the concentration of the solute in the filtrate and in the blood, represents the permeability of the solute for that membrane. Ultrafiltration membranes have pores with molecular size cut-off so that molecules larger than the pores cannot pass through the membrane, even with convection. A sieving coefficient of zero indicates that the solute is completely rejected by the membrane (macromolecules and proteins), whereas a sieving coefficient of 1 indicates that the solute readily passes through the membrane. The sieving coefficient of sodium is essentially 1, indicating that the ultrafiltrate has a sodium concentration similar to that of the plasma. Protein-bound molecules, such as drugs, are retained by all membranes except for those used in plasmapheresis procedures (45–47). Therefore, the sieving coefficient of a drug is that of the fraction of the drug which is not bound to plasma proteins (47,48). Albumin, a negatively charged macromolecule, creates a Gibbs-Donnan effect at the blood–membrane interface, slightly decreasing the sieving of small cations and increasing that of small anions.

Vascular Access and Extracorporeal Pumps

The process of ultrafiltration is performed on blood extracted from the patient after cannulation of an artery or vein. The blood is then returned to the patient via a separate access to the venous circulation (41). While in end-stage renal disease ultrafiltration is performed with the puncture of an arterial–venous fistula, graft, or permanent catheter, in patients with volume overload ultrafiltration is carried out with a temporary access to the circulation. With arterial–venous access, an extracorporeal blood pump is unnecessary because the pressure gradient between the arterial and venous circulations is a force sufficient to drive the blood to the surface of the ultrafiltration membrane. For the arterial–venous approach, the femoral artery and vein are percutaneously cannulated with large-bore, low-resistance catheters to achieve the maximal blood flow for a given arterial–venous pressure gradient.

Because in the Hagen-Poiseuille equation blood flow is the dependent variable, any constriction in the extracorporeal circuit increases resistance and lowers blood flow. If an extracorporeal pump is used, a double lumen venous catheter is placed in the femoral or jugular vein, allowing extraction and return of blood with minimal recirculation. With this approach, pressure is the dependent variable, while flow is maintained constant by the pump (Fig. 43-4) (49).

Thus, production of ultrafiltrate can be modified by several methods. Techniques to manipulate hydrostatic pressure

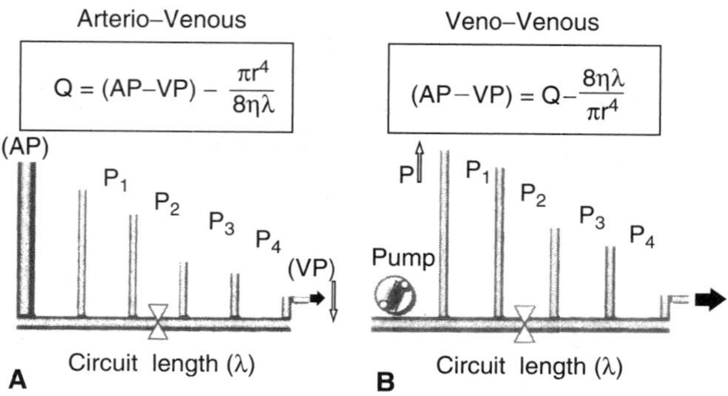

Figure 43-4 Description of pressure–flow relationship in a spontaneous arterial–venous-driven circuit **(A)** and in a pump-driven circuit **(B)**. While in the first circuit a constriction may cause a decrease in flow, in the second a constriction creates a change in pressure profile. AP, arterial pressure; P, local pressure; Q, flow; VP, venous pressure. (From Ronco C, Ricci Z, Bellomo R, Bedogni F. Extracorporeal ultrafiltration for the treatment of overhydration and congestive heart failure. *Cardiology.* 2001:96:155–168, with permission.)

on the blood side of the membrane include increasing systemic blood pressure, lowering resistance in the blood pathway, and inserting a blood pump proximally to the filter. Alternatively, suction (negative pressure) can be generated on the filtrate side to draw plasma water through the membrane. Mechanical fluid removal methods can be divided in isolated ultrafiltration techniques, hemofiltration, and ultrafiltration in conjunction with dialysis. While pure ultrafiltration is only a fluid-controlling method, all the others can simultaneously achieve some degree of blood purification. In blood-cleansing techniques, as ultrafiltration occurs the ultrafiltrate is replaced with clean fluid that dilutes solute concentration in the blood not yet driven through the filter. Based on frequency and duration, ultrafiltration techniques can be classified as acute or isolated, intermittent or continuous. With appropriate ultrafiltration rates, the extracellular fluid gradually refills the intravascular space and blood volume is maintained. If the ultrafiltration rate is too high, blood volume may decrease because intravascular volume depletion exceeds reabsorption of fluid from the interstitium into the vascular space.

Therefore, the three key factors for the removal of an adequate amount of fluid without hemodynamic compromise include accurate determination of the amount of fluid to be removed, optimization of fluid removal rate, and maintenance of circulating blood volume (50). To facilitate appropriate amounts and rates of fluid removal, instruments that monitor blood volume changes can be inserted into extracorporeal circuits during treatment (e.g., Crit Line, produced by Hemametrics, Inc., Salt Lake City, Utah). With online blood volume monitors, ultrafiltration can be slowed or arrested until complete intravascular refill has taken place (51). In peritoneal dialysis, an osmotically active substance, such as glucose, creates a hypertonic dialysate. This hypertonicity is the driving force for the ultrafiltration of plasma water from peritoneal capillaries across the peritoneal membrane into the peritoneal cavity, from which it is eventually drained away.

KEY DIFFERENCES IN FLUID REMOVAL WITH DIURETICS, ULTRAFILTRATION, AND DIALYSIS

To understand the differential effects of diuretics, ultrafiltration, and dialysis on hemodynamic and neurohormonal abnormalities occurring in heart failure, it is critical to recognize the distinctive characteristics of fluid removal with these three therapies. The fluid removed with diuretics has a sodium concentration lower than that of the plasma. In contrast, the ultrafiltrate is essentially isoosmotic and isonatric compared with plasma, except for minimal differences due to the Gibbs-Donnan effect produced by albumin. Therefore, for any amount of fluid withdrawn, more sodium is removed with ultrafiltration than with diuretics (41). With diuretics, natriuresis drives water excretion and, therefore, sodium and water removal cannot be dissociated (38).

With hemofiltration techniques the ultrafiltrate is similar to plasma water, but total body sodium can be manipulated by adjusting sodium concentration in the replacement solution. The ability to dissociate sodium and water removal permits the normalization of electrolyte levels in both extracellular and intracellular compartments (41). With diuretics, intravascular volume contraction is prolonged and inhibition of NaCl uptake in the macula densa, coupled with augmented release of prostacyclin, enhances renal secretion of renin (41). These effects augment neurohormonal activation which, in turn, promotes sodium and water retention, ultimately reducing the diuretics' ability to relieve the signs and symptoms of circulatory congestion (35–47).

In contrast, ultrafiltration does not stimulate macula densa-mediated neurohormonal activation, nor does it produce prolonged intravascular volume contraction because ultrafiltration removes fluid from the blood at the same rate at which fluid is reabsorbed from the edematous interstitium (Fig. 43-5) (52). In fact, changes in plasma volume (ΔPV) during ultrafiltration can be estimated from changes in hematocrit(Ht) according to the following formula:

$$\Delta PV = 100/(100 - Ht_{pre}) \times [100\ (Ht_{pre} - Ht_{post})]/Ht_{post}$$

where "pre" and "post" are the two time points considered. Plasma refilling rate (PRR, mL per minute), which represents a measurement of the fluid volume transport from the interstitium into the vascular space during ultrafiltration, is filtrate volume/time, where time is the duration of ultrafiltration if ΔPV = 0. When PRR equals the ultrafiltration rate, blood volume stability is preserved.

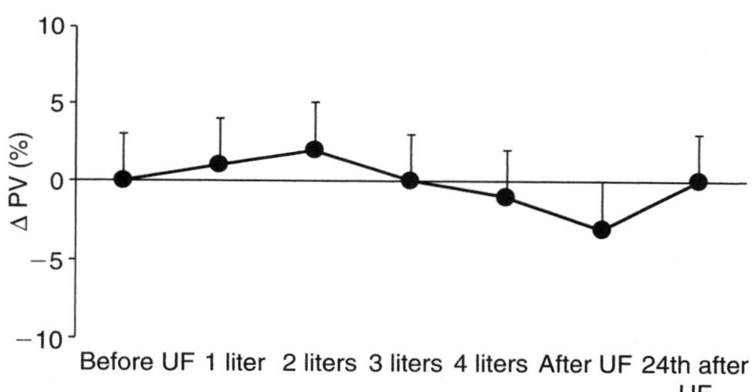

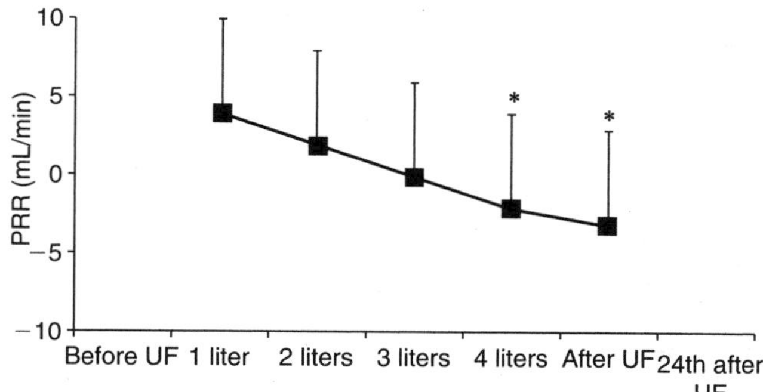

Figure 43-5 Percent change in plasma volume (PV) **(upper panel)** and plasma refilling rate (PRR) **(lower panel)** during isolated veno–venous ultrafiltration (UF) in 24 NYHA Class IV heart failure patients. (From Marenzi GC, Lauri G, Grazi M, et al. Circulatory response to fluid overload removal by extracorporeal ultrafiltration in refractory congestive heart failure. *J Am Coll Cardiol.* 2001;38:963–968, with permission.)
*$p < 0.01$ versus 1 L.

Ultrafiltration performed in conjunction with dialysis results in hypotonia or hypertonia because water removal is linked to that of other solutes such as urea and electrolytes, which are removed in proportions dependent upon the technique used. Diffusion removes solute osmoles preferentially from the vascular space and extracellular fluid. Because cells become hypertonic compared to extracellular fluid, water moves from extracellular fluid into the cells. Because dialysis also results in fluid removal across the dialyzer, extracellular fluid volume depletion and hypotension can occur. Because with filtration the osmolality of cells and extracellular fluid remains the same, as extracellular water and solutes are removed by the filter, cellular fluids and solutes quickly replenish the extracellular fluid space (53–55). Thus, the basis for maintenance of cardiovascular stability during ultrafiltration relates to many factors, including minimal osmolar shifts, appropriate neurohormonal sympathetic responses, and rapid redistribution of volume. These responses have been observed with nearly all continuous or intermittent ultrafiltration techniques (56–77).

The following description of individual techniques will be preceded by an overview of the effects of ultrafiltration in patients with varying acuity and severity of congestive heart failure.

RATIONALE FOR THE USE OF ULTRAFILTRATION IN HEART FAILURE

The facts previously summarized indicate that the unique feature of ultrafiltration is the ability to remove excess fluid from the extravascular space without significantly affecting circulatory volume (Table 43-1). Thus, ultrafiltration techniques appear ideally suited to interrupt the vicious circle of volume overload, neurohormonal activation, and worsening renal dysfunction occurring in heart failure (34,62,64–67,78–82). In patients with both acute and chronic heart failure, ultrafiltration has been consistently shown to improve the symptoms of congestion, lower right atrial and pulmonary arterial wedge pressures, improve cardiac output, decrease neurohormone levels, correct hyponatremia, restore diuresis, and reduce diuretics requirements (Figs. 43-6 and 43-7) (69,83–86).

TABLE 43-1
RATIONALE FOR THE USE OF ULTRAFILTRATION IN HEART FAILURE

Rationale	Therapeutic Goal
Fluid regulation	Relieve pulmonary edema
	Reduce ascites and/or peripheral edema
	Hemodynamic stabilization
	Improve oxygenation
	Facilitate blood product replacement without excess volume
	Enable parenteral nutritional support without excess volume
Solute regulation	Correct acid–base balance
	Correct serum sodium content
	Eliminate "myocardial depressant factor" or known toxins
	Correct uremia
	Correct hyperkalemia and other electrolyte disturbances
Establish homeostasis	Reset water omostat
	Restore diuretic responsiveness
	Reduce neurohormonal activation

Ultrafiltration in Moderate Heart Failure

The use of ultrafiltration in patients with only moderate heart failure has shed significant light on the mechanisms by which ultrafiltration improves hemodynamics and functional capacity and attenuates neurohormonal activation. Patients with moderate heart failure can have radiographic evidence of pulmonary congestion in the absence of peripheral edema. This pulmonary overhydration significantly contributes to decreased functional capacity and to mutually detrimental heart–lung interactions (87,88). Thus, a therapy that improves patients' functional capacity by reducing pulmonary overhydration is attractive in patients with moderate heart failure.

In a controlled study in which 36 NYHA Class II and III heart failure patients were randomly assigned to either a single veno–venous ultrafiltration session removing 1,880 ± 174 mL of fluid, or no treatment, ultrafiltrated patients had significant reduction of right atrial pressure (from 8 ± 1 mm Hg to 3.4 ± 0.7 mm Hg; p <0.001) and pulmonary artery wedge pressure (from 18 ± 2.5 mm Hg to 10 ± 1.9 mm Hg; p <0.001); decreased radiographic lung water score (from 15. 2 ± 2.2 mm Hg to 8.1 ± 1.0 mm Hg; p <0.001); as well as improvement in peak exercise oxygen consumption (VO_{2max}) (from 15.5 ± 1 mL/kg per minute to 17.6 ± 0.9 mL/kg per minute; p <0.001). These changes were associated with increased maximal voluntary ventilation (from 110 ± 4 L/minute to 128 ± 9 L/minute; p <0.01) and tidal volume, and reduced dead space to tidal volume ratio at peak exercise (89). The improvement in exercise performance was associated with decreased norepinephrine levels at rest, a downward shift in norepinephrine kinetics at submaximal exercise (suggesting normalization of neurohormonal responses during exercise), and an increase in norepinephrine levels during orthostatic tilt (suggesting normalization of circulatory responses to orthostatic hypotension) (89,90).

These favorable functional and neurohormanal changes persisted, on average, for 6 months after treatment. These data suggest that the observed benefit of ultrafiltration in patients with moderate congestive heart failure is attributable to decreased pulmonary stiffness resulting from a reduction in lung water content (89,91). This clearly improves lung mechanics, as suggested by changes in spirometry values both at rest and during exercise (87,89,92–94). Of 17 patients who underwent removal of 1,777 ± 35 mL of ultrafiltrate, compared to 8 patients without significant functional improvement, the 9 patients with a >10% increase in VO_{2max} had a greater reduction in right and left ventricular filling pressures for a given cardiac output; increase in peak exercise ventilation due to

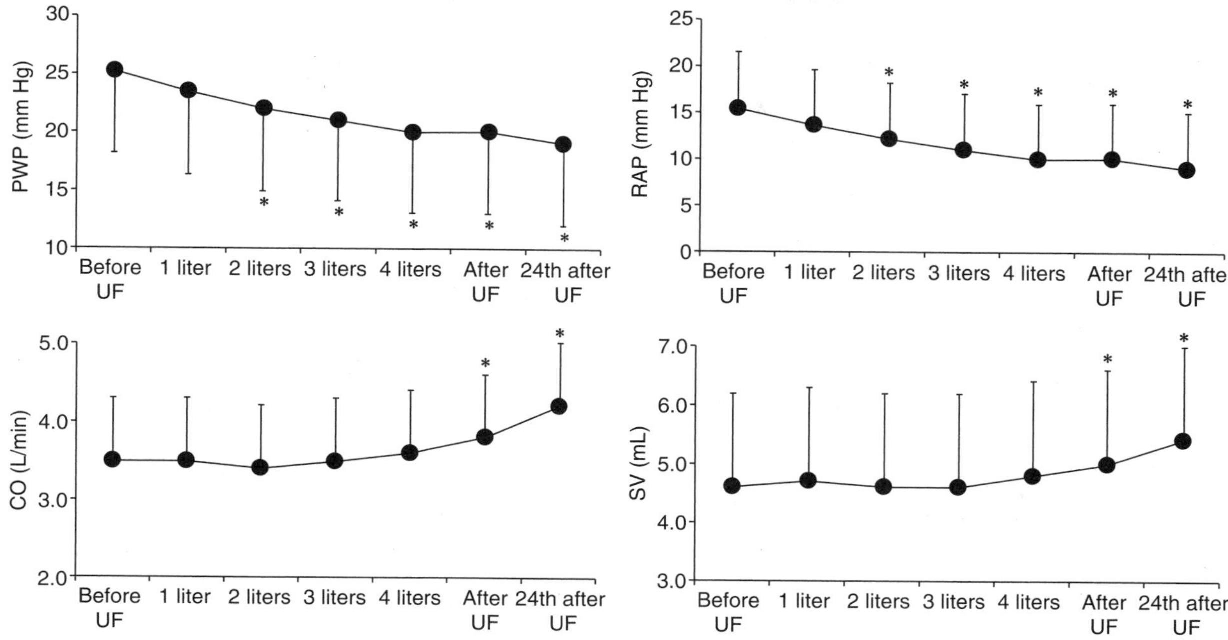

Figure 43-6 Mean pulmonary artery wedge pressure (PWP), mean right atrial pressure (RAP), cardiac output (CO), and stroke volume (SV) before, during, and after isolated veno–venous ultrafiltration in 24 NYHA Class IV heart failure patients. (From Marenzi GC, Lauri G, Grazi M, et al. Circulatory response to fluid overload removal by extracorporeal ultrafiltration in refractory congestive heart failure. *J Am Coll Cardiol.* 2001;38:963–968, with permission.)
*p <0.01 versus before ultrafiltration.

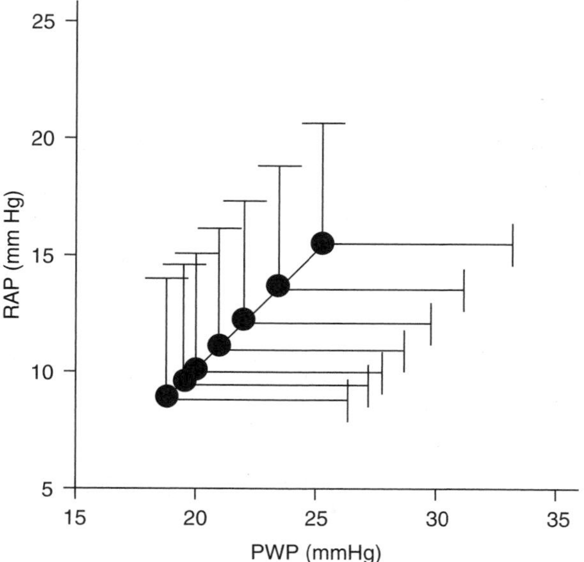

Figure 43-7 Right atrial pressure (RAP) versus pulmonary artery wedge pressure (PWP) during isolated veno–venous ultrafiltration in 24 NYHA Class IV heart failure patients. Mean [black circle] ± SD [bar]) are, from right to left, data obtained before ultrafiltration, and after 1 L, 2 L, 3 L, and 4 L of ultrafiltrate, at the end, and 24 hours after ultrafiltration. A 1:1 reduction of right and left atrial pressures suggests lowering of extracardiac constraint. (From Marenzi GC, Lauri G, Grazi M, et al. Circulatory response to fluid overload removal by extracorporeal ultrafiltration in refractory congestive heart failure. *J Am Coll Cardiol.* 2001;38:963–968, with permission.)

increased tidal volume and decreased dead space to tidal volume ratio; lower esophageal pressure swing (end expiratory–end inspiratory pressure) for a given tidal volume; and increased peak exercise dynamic lung compliance, defined as the ratio of changes in volume to changes in pressure over a tidal breath (from 0.10 ± 0.05 L/mm Hg to 0.14 ± 0.03 L/mm Hg; p <0.01) (87).

Thus, after ultrafiltration, ventilation not only increases but it also becomes more efficient. The pulmonary restrictive pattern commonly present in heart failure has been shown to result from increased extravascular fluid content, pulmonary blood volume, dead space to tidal volume ratio, and heart size (93,94–96). After ultrafiltration, reduction in intrathoracic pressure and removal of the constraining effect exerted on the heart by the overhydrated lungs decrease the external work of the heart (87,93,94). Improvement in pulmonary mechanics leads to a reduction in heart size and improvement of diastolic relaxation abnormalities. In 24 patients undergoing single veno–venous ultrafiltration of 1,976 ± 760 mL, reduction in filling pressures and extravascular lung water and improvement of VO_{2max} were associated with decreased Doppler echocardiography signs of restriction, including a reduction in early to late filling ratio in both ventricles (mitral valve from 2 ± 2 to 1.1 ± 1.1; p <0.001, and tricuspid valve from 1.3 ± 1.3 to 0.69 ± 0.18; p <0.001) and an increase in the deceleration time of mitral and tricuspid flows, reflecting a redistribution of ventricular filling to late diastole. Change in ventricular filling patterns, lung water content, and functional performance persisted at 3 months.

These results suggest that reduction of interstitial lung water is the mechanism whereby ultrafiltration modified the pattern of ventricular filling and increased functional capacity. After ultrafiltration, the right and left ventricular Starling curves during exercise show a definite reduction in filling pressures for a given cardiac output. It seems likely that the overhydrated lungs exert a constraining effect on the heart and that normalization of lung water content can indirectly improve heart dynamics. The ultrafiltration-induced increase in dynamic lung compliance during exercise may have contributed to improvement of exercise performance by reducing the cost of breathing and to the fall of the external work of the heart, an organ which during its rhythmic action pulls and pushes against the lungs (97). These mechanisms are closely interrelated with reduction in lung water content, increase in dynamic lung compliance, and improvement in right and left ventricular Starling curves and exercise capacity. They provide a unified explanation why, after ultrafiltration-induced changes in the mechanical characteristics of the intrathoracic milieu, the heart functions in more favorable conditions and improvement lasts beyond the duration of treatment.

In heart failure patients, maximal flow–volume loops do not increase after exercise and functional residual capacity decreases at the onset of exercise and increases thereafter (98). It is possible that ultrafiltration may also improve these aspects of lung function. Lung diffusing capacity is strictly related to exercise capacity and is frequently impaired in patients with heart failure. Ultrafiltration does not improve lung diffusion (93). These data suggest that in chronic heart failure, impairment of alveolar capillary diffusion capacity is not due to lung water accumulation but to accumulation of cells and connective tissue along the alveolar capillary membrane. Because these changes are irreversible, changes in lung diffusion capacity are unreliable indicators of the efficacy of ultrafiltration.

The result of another study showed that the favorable hemodynamic, neurohumoral, and ventilatory responses to ultrafiltration occurring in stable chronic heart failure patients were not observed in patients who received only a continuous diuretic infusion matched to achieve equivalent fluid removal. Sixteen NYHA Class II and III heart failure patients were randomly allocated to receive either a single ultrafiltration treatment (n = 8) or intravenous furosemide (n = 8, mean furosemide dose = 248 mg) to remove approximately 1,600 mL of fluid (92). Soon after fluid withdrawal by either method, biventricular filling pressures and body weight were reduced and plasma renin, norepinephrine, and aldosterone levels were increased. After furosemide, neurohormones levels remained elevated for the next 4 days and during this period patients had positive water balance, recurrent elevation of filling pressures, and lung congestion without improvement of VO_{2max}. In contrast, after ultrafiltration, neurohormones levels fell below baseline within 48 hours, whereas water metabolism was equilibrated at a new set point (less fluid intake and diuresis without weight gain) (Fig. 43-8). Favorable circulatory and neurohormonal changes were correlated with lung water reabsorption, which was increased only in ultrafiltration-treated patients. Improvement was sustained at 3 months after ultrafiltration (Figs. 43-9 and 43-10) (92).

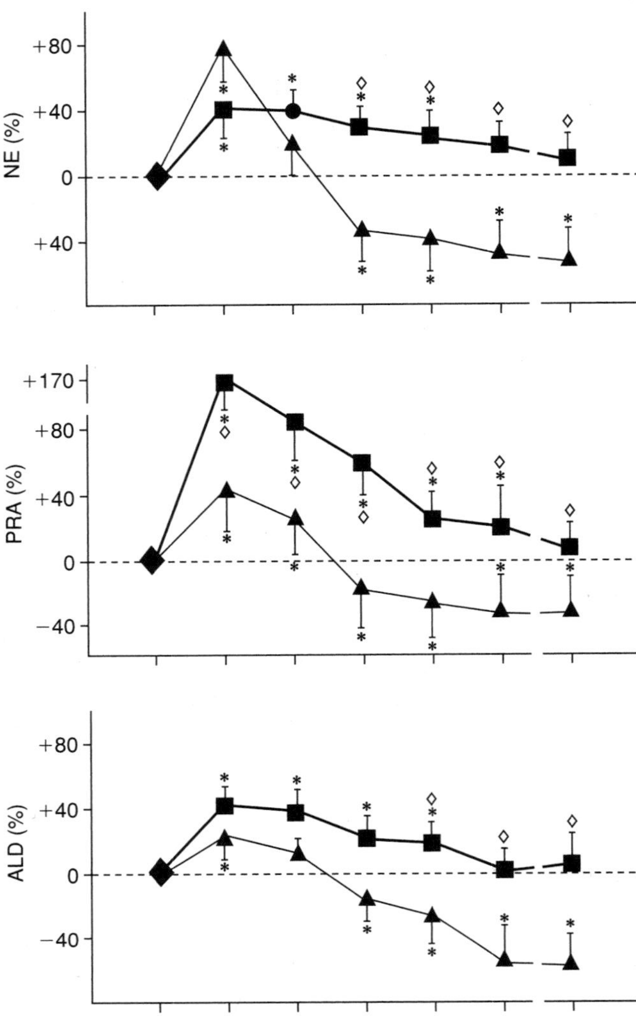

Figure 43-8 Average percent changes from baseline (b) of circulating norepinephrine (NE), plasma renin activity (PRA), and aldosterone (ALD) immediately after (0) ultrafiltration (black triangles) or intravenous furosemide (black squares) and 1, 2, 3, 4 days (d) and 3 months later. Differences from baseline (asterisks) are significant at $p < 0.01$; differences from the corresponding value in the other group (diamonds) are significant at $p < 0.01$. (From Agostoni PG, Marenzi GC, Lauri G, et al. Sustained improvement in functional capacity after removal of body fluid with isolated ultrafiltration in chronic cardiac insufficiency: failure of furosemide to provide the same result. *Am J Med.* 1994;96:191–199, with permission.)

These data indicate that while ultrafiltration and furosemide are equally effective in terms of acute volume of fluid removed and resolution of congestive symptoms, their long-term effects are significantly different. Specifically, the effects of ultrafiltration on pulmonary water metabolism and neurohormone levels are due to mechanisms not occurring with diuretics. The fluid removed by ultrafiltration has different sodium content compared to the fluid removed with diuretics. Indeed, ultrafiltration removes fluid with a sodium concentration similar to that of plasma, so that approximately 150 mmol of sodium are withdrawn with each liter of ultrafiltrate. In contrast, the urine of heart failure patients is hypotonic compared with

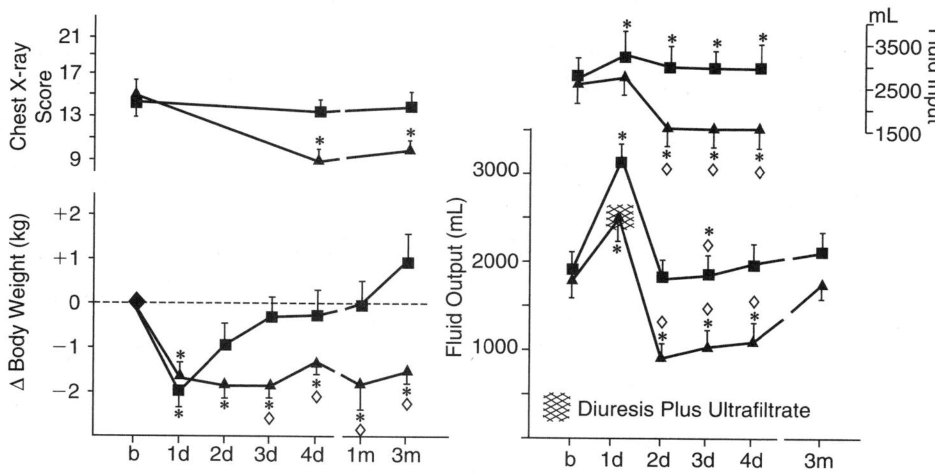

Figure 43-9 Chest X-ray lung water score, changes in body weight, fluid input and output at various periods after isolated veno–venous ultrafiltration (black triangles) or intravenous furosemide (black squares). Data are presented as means ± SEM. Differences from baseline (asterisks) are significant at $p < 0.01$; differences from the corresponding value in the other group (diamonds) are significant at $p < 0.01$. B, baseline; d, day; m, month. (From Agostoni PG, Marenzi GC, Lauri G, et al. Sustained improvement in functional capacity after removal of body fluid with isolated ultrafiltration in chronic cardiac insufficiency: failure of furosemide to provide the same result. *Am J Med.* 1994;96:191–199, with permission.)

plasma and the 50 mmol of sodium usually present in 1 L of urine increases to only 100 mmol with furosemide administration (99). As a consequence, ultrafiltration provides the greatest possible amount of sodium elimination per unit of fluid removed. It is possible that the different amounts of sodium removed with similar amounts of fluid account for the differential effects of ultrafiltration and diuretics on neurohormonal responses, which in turn, will result in different renal sodium and water reabsorption.

It should be noted that ultrafiltration's clinical benefits are amplified and sustained over time in patients receiving ACEI. In one study, ACEI-treated patients maintained the weight reduction achieved after ultrafiltration, whereas weight returned to pre-ultrafiltration values in patients not taking ACEI (100). Improvement of exercise capacity and reduction in pulmonary interstitial fluid scores lasted longer after ultrafiltration in patients treated versus those not treated with ACEI. In chronic heart failure patients, the body's defense reaction against hypovolemic stimuli is maintained, albeit blunted, by the renin-angiotensin system (101). Withdrawal of excess of fluid by ultrafiltration produces greater benefit when combined with ACEI because these drugs will block the neurohormonally mediated increase in renal sodium and water reabsorption occurring in response to forced dehydration. Indeed, it is well-known that ACEI action is optimal when the renin-angiotensin system is maximally activated (102). By inducing transient hypovolemia with the resulting transient activation of the renin-angiotensin system, ultrafiltration creates the ideal condition for ACEIs to exert their favorable hemodynamic and renal effects. This indicates that fluid balance is readjusted at a different set point in patients receiving ACEI.

Ultrafiltration in Decompensated Heart Failure

Ultrafiltration has been consistently shown to improve signs and symptoms of congestion, increase diuresis, lower diuretic requirements, and correct hyponatremia also in patients with advanced heart failure (69). Among 32 NYHA Class II–IV heart failure patients with varying degrees of hypervolemia, the baseline 24 hour diuresis and natriuresis were inversely correlated with neurohormone levels and renal perfusion pressure (mean aortic pressure–mean arterial pressure). The response to ultrafiltration ranged from neurohormonal activation and reduction of diuresis in patients with the mildest hypovolemia and urine output >1,000 mL per 24 hours to neurohormonal inhibition and potentiation of diuresis and natriuresis in those with the most severe volume overload and urine output <1,000 mL per 24 hours (69).

In the majority of cases, the decrease in norepinephrine level was proportional to the potentiation of diuresis. This finding suggests that subtraction of total body water uncovers enough cardiac reserve to increase cardiac output and attenuate neurohormonal activation. These benefits are then maintained because the resulting enhancement of diuresis leads to improved norepinephrine clearance from the circulation (84). As in moderate heart failure, it is possible that also in advanced heart failure the earliest effect of ultrafiltration is the reduction of the extravascular pulmonary fluid, with a subsequent decrease in pulmonary extravascular resistance, improvement of ventilation and gas exchange, and a decrease in hypoxia-induced vasoconstriction. Ultrafiltration itself via baroreceptor-mediated reflexes may reset neurohormonal activation, which, in turn, may explain the intermediate- and long-term benefits observed after ultrafiltration (84).

The removal of myocardial depressant factors (85) has also been invoked as an explanation for the clinical benefits associated with ultrafiltration. A myocardial depressant substance has been extracted from the ultrafiltrate obtained from patients with congestive heart failure and acute renal failure (37,103). In 36 patients with acutely decompensated heart failure, ultrafiltration was associated with an increased cardiac index and oxygenation status, decreased pulmonary artery pressure and vascular resistance, as well as reduced requirement for inotropic support (104). SCUF or daily ultrafiltration has also been shown to effectively control volume in patients with severe congestive heart failure regardless of concomitant renal function (34). It is not known if the clinical benefits of ultrafiltration translate into improved survival.

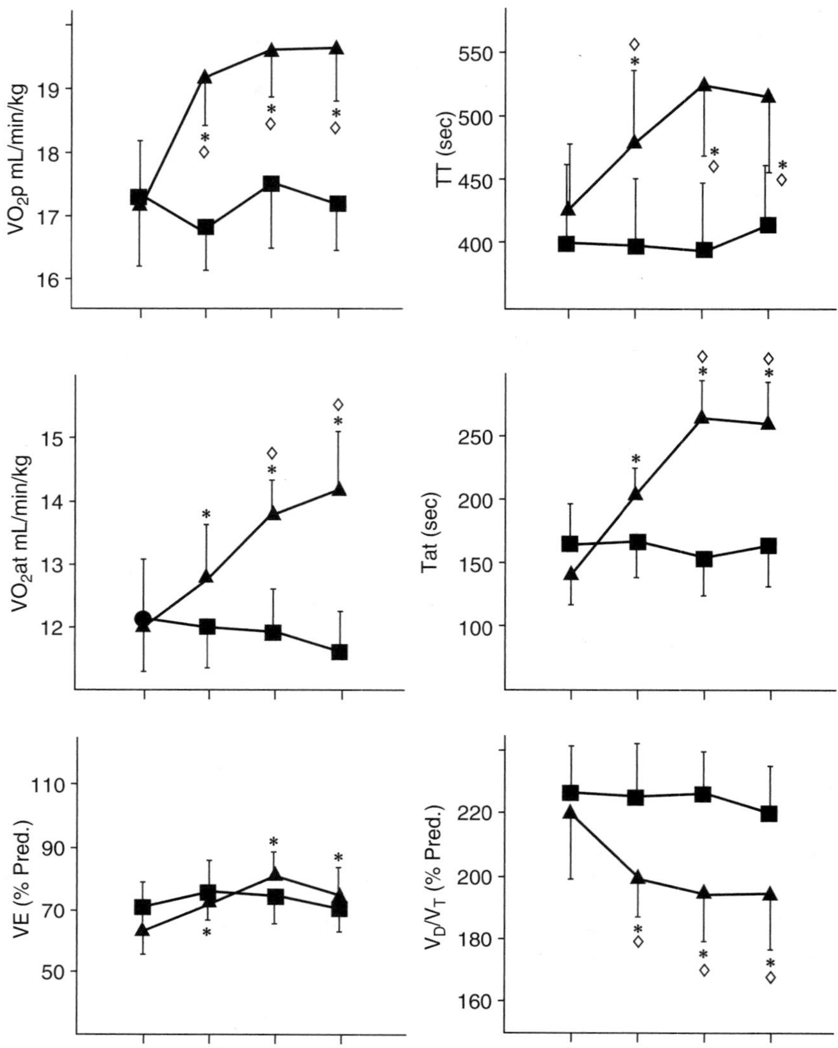

Figure 43-10 Peak oxygen consumption (VO_2p), exercise tolerance time (TT), oxygen consumption at anaerobic threshold (VO_2at), time to anaerobic threshold (Tat), maximal voluntary ventilation (% of predicted value; V_E), dead space/tidal volume ratio at peak exercise (% of predicted value; V_D/V_T) at baseline (b), 4 days (d), 1 month (m) and 3 months after isolated veno–venous ultrafiltration (black triangles) or intravenous furosemide (black squares). Data are presented as means ± SEM. Differences from baseline (asterisks) are significant at $p < 0.01$; differences from the corresponding value in the other group (diamonds) are significant at $p < 0.01$. (From Agostoni PG, Marenzi GC, Lauri G, et al. Sustained improvement in functional capacity after removal of body fluid with isolated ultrafiltration in chronic cardiac insufficiency: failure of furosemide to provide the same result. *Am J Med.* 1994;96:191–199, with permission.)

Acute heart failure, which is most commonly due to decompensation of chronic heart failure, can also occur in the setting of circulatory collapse complicating myocardial infarction, hypertension, pericardial disease, cardiomyopathy, myocarditis, pulmonary embolus, or arrhythmias or after cardiac surgery (105–107). In these clinical settings ultrafiltration has been used predominantly after diuretics have failed or in the presence of acute renal failure. However, the results of some studies suggest that earlier utilization of ultrafiltration can expedite and maintain compensation of acute heart failure by simultaneously reducing volume overload without causing intravascular volume depletion and re-establishing acid–base and electrolyte balance (39).

The use of ultrafiltration in patients with advanced heart failure has also highlighted the risks associated with mechanical fluid removal. Overly aggressive ultrafiltration in patients with decompensated heart failure can convert nonoliguric renal dysfunction into oliguric failure by increasing neurohormonal activation and decreasing renal perfusion pressure, with minimal opportunity of recovery of renal function. Patients with this outcome become permanently dependent on dialysis. In addition, permanent renal loss can eliminate the option of heart transplantation in patients with end-stage heart failure. Prior to initiating a treatment course with extracorporeal therapies, the clinician must clearly explain the risk and potential pitfalls of this technique. It is generally disastrous to add a chronic need for dialysis to an already decompensated cardiac status. In some cases a trial of ultrafiltration can be offered for a limited time to evaluate potential benefits. However, there must be a clearly delineated plan to withdraw support if predefined parameters of improvement are not achieved (108–115). Severity of renal dysfunction influences the type and intensity of ultrafiltration approach. Heart failure patients without overt renal impairment may benefit from isolated ultrafiltration. In patients with moderate to severe renal dysfunction, stabilization of cardiac and metabolic functions can only be achieved with hemofiltration (108).

ROLE OF ULTRAFILTRATION IN HEART FAILURE PATIENTS UNDERGOING OPEN HEART SURGERY

Open heart surgery is usually associated with hypervolemia because of the 3 to 4 L of crystalloids and colloids typically infused during cardiopulmonary bypass (CPB), including CBP pump prime, cardioplegia, and fluid administered to reverse intraoperative hypotension. In addition, patients may undergo heart surgery in conditions that may induce or worsen pre-existing heart failure. Regardless of the circumstances, fluid overload aggravates postoperative hypoxemia and organ edema, which, in turn, delays recovery and worsens outcomes (116). Furthermore, perioperative hypervolemia is augmented by the inflammatory response induced by CPB (117). In this setting, reduced postoperative anemia, thrombocytopenia, and hypoalbuminemia (observed after removal of 3 to 4 L of fluid by hemofiltration) have been attributed to the resulting hemoconcentration (118). Preservation of colloidal osmotic pressure by hemofiltration have also been shown to reduce the incidence of postoperative pleural effusions requiring invasive chest drainage (116). Experimental and clinical evidence has also shown that hemofiltration can remove by convective clearance myocardial depressant factors such as tumor necrosis factor-α (TNF-α) and interleukin-1β (IL-1β) (119). In one study in which patients with postoperative inflammation underwent high-volume (6 L per hour) hemofiltration, hemodynamic improvement was associated with significant reduction of C3a and C5a anaphylatoxins (116). In inotrope-dependent heart surgery patients, vasoactive drugs were removed by hemofiltration at rates only slightly higher than by endogenous clearance (120). In early studies in which hemofiltration was applied late (>8 days) and at rates (≤1 L per hour) to treat postoperative hypervolemia, mortality rates after treatment have ranged between 52% and 87.5% (121–123). In contrast, early and intensive application of hemofiltration in heart surgery patients with volume overload and renal dysfunction was associated with lower posttreatment mortality rates ranging from 40% to 60% (116,124).

CONTINUOUS ULTRAFILTRATION TECHNIQUES

The continuous ultrafiltration techniques include continuous hemofiltration in the arterial–venous (CAVH) or veno–venous mode (CVVH); SCUF in the arterial–venous or veno–venous mode; continuous hemodialysis in the arterial–venous (CAVHD) or veno–venous (CVVHD) modes continuous hemodiafiltration in the arterial–venous (CAVHDF) or veno–venous mode (CVVHDF); continuous high-flux dialysis in the arterial–venous (CAVHFD) or veno–venous (CVVHFD) mode: and continuous plasmafiltration-adsorption (108). The individual characteristics of these ultrafiltration modalities are shown in Figure 43-11.

Continuous dialysis without the use of extracorporeal blood pumps, first suggested in 1960, did not become clinically applicable until the introduction, more than a decade later, of hemodiafiltration membranes more permeable than typical hemodialysis membranes. Although originally designed for chronic intermittent hemofiltration, in the mid 1970s the new technology was shown to be feasible in the setting of acute circulatory congestion (71,125). Using a large-bore catheter inserted into the femoral artery and the patient's own blood pressure, arterial blood is delivered to a hemofilter. Systemic blood pressure provides the driving force to achieve sufficient blood flow. When hydrostatic pressure exceeds oncotic pressure, ultrafiltrate is generated. Ultrafiltrate drains by gravity through tubing into a collection bag, creating mild negative pressure in the blood chamber of the filter, favoring further ultrafiltration. Because blood cells and proteins remain in the blood chamber and are returned to the femoral vein, the filter allows efficient removal of plasma water and dissolved solutes from the vascular space while conserving blood cells and large plasma proteins.

This type of CAVH was originally designed as a renal replacement therapy. Large volumes of uremic ultrafiltrate are removed and cleaned, and a replacement solution is administered in volumes determined by the desired net fluid gain or loss. When the replacement fluid volumes are large, both chemical and clinical manifestations of uremia can be adequately controlled. The procedure has been subsequently modified to remove excess fluid in the setting of diuretic unresponsive oliguria, with or without uremia (125).

With SCUF, replacement volumes are much lower than with CAVH. The most recent advance in this area has been the reintroduction of extracorporeal blood pumps (70,73). Because the blood flow provided by the pump eliminates the need for an arterial–venous pressure gradient, the technique does not require arterial cannulation and can be performed with veno–venous vascular access (CVVH). Both SCUF and CVVH are ideally suited for hemodynamically unstable patients unable to tolerate the rapid fluid volume shifts occurring with intermittent isolated ultrafiltration or home peritoneal dialysis because of abdominal or respiratory problems. Thus, until the introduction of simplified intermittent *peripheral* veno–venous ultrafiltration techniques, CVVH and SCUF were the recommended therapies for the more critically ill, hypotensive patients with congestive heart failure (70–73).

Because CVVH requires an extracorporeal blood pump, air embolism and blood loss can occur. In contrast with SCUF, which is driven only by the patient's arterial–venous pressure gradient, air embolism is uncommon and blood loss is self-limited. On the other hand, extracorporeal blood pumps, by producing a constant blood flow, can provide, without an arterial puncture, ultrafiltration rates not achievable with SCUF.

All continuous therapies require anticoagulation. Volume depletion can be avoided by careful clinical management. No prospective studies have compared SCUF with CVVH for the treatment of congestion. Published reports suggest that complication rates are acceptable (126–128). Both CVVH and SCUF can reduce congestion without causing hypotension because the fluid removed with these techniques is isotonic with plasma (46,71,74–77,129–132). Several studies have shown that

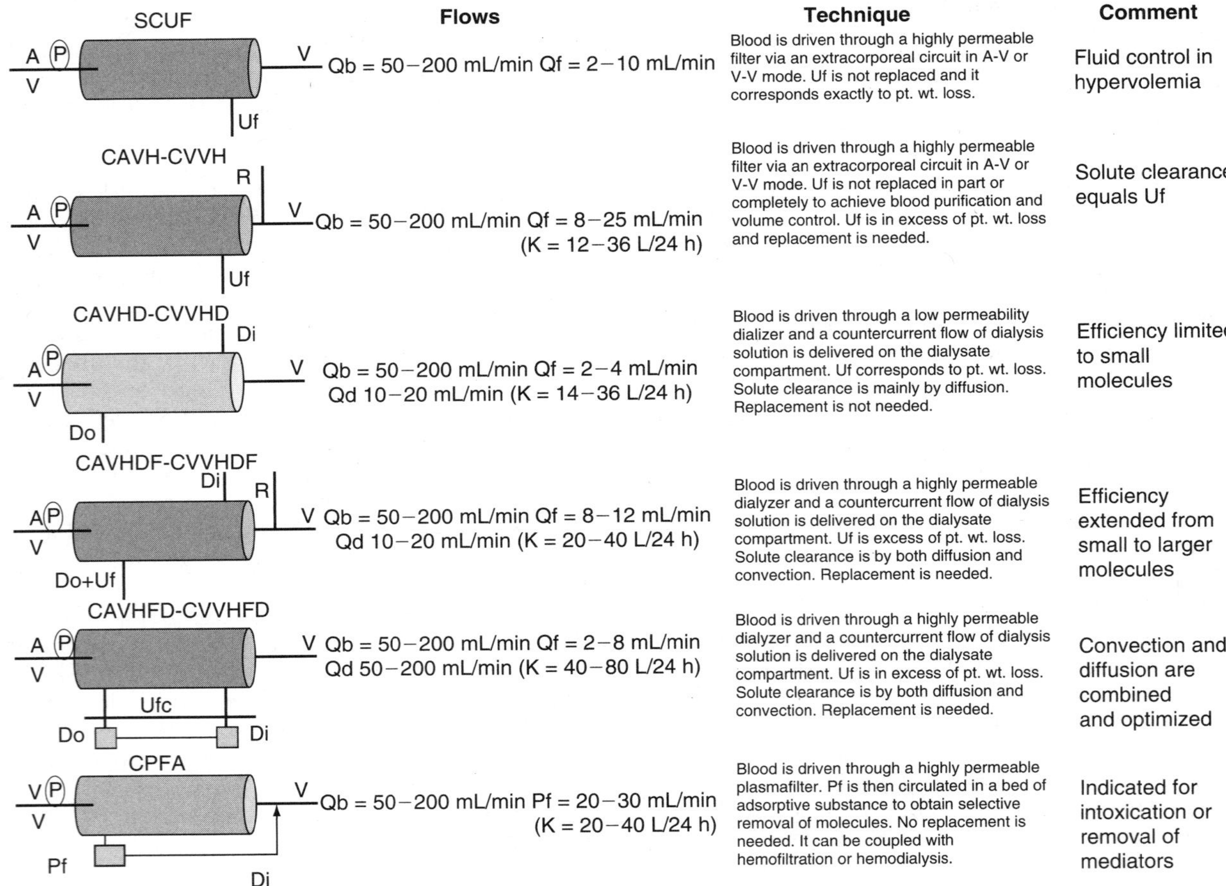

Figure 43-11 Schematic representation and definition of the different continuous ultrafiltration therapies. A, artery; V, vein; Qb, blood flow; Qd, dialysate flow; Qf, ultrafiltration rate; Pf, plasma filtration rate; Di, dialysate inlet; Do, dialysate outlet; Uf, ultrafiltrate; P, pump (dotted circle indicates that the pump is used only in the veno–venous mode); Ufc, ultrafiltration control system; K, clearance; R, replacement fluid; dark grey, high-flux membrane; light grey, low-flux membrane. (Adapted from Ronco C, Bellomo R. Continuous renal replacement therapy: evolution in technology and current nomenclature. *Kidney Int.* 1998:66(Suppl):S160–S164.)

as plasma water is removed by ultrafiltration it is rapidly replaced by interstitial and cellular water. Hypotension complicating chronic intermittent hemodialysis is caused (in most cases) by rapid changes in osmolality (133–136). In patients studied at separate sessions with each procedure, hemofiltration, unlike hemodialysis, was associated with either unchanged or increased systemic vascular resistance, leading to preservation of blood pressure (57–59). Furthermore, autonomic dysfunction has been documented in patients undergoing hemodialysis but not in those treated with hemofiltration (57,58,60).

Preservation of venous and arterial tone partially explains why hypotension seldom occurs during hemofiltration (59,61). Several investigators believe that convection removes circulating myocardial depressants that are not removed by diffusion (53,137–139). The differential characteristics of the fluid removed by hemofiltration versus dialysis have been outlined in the corresponding paragraph in this chapter. When SCUF is technically successful, ultrafiltration rate can vary from 0 to 20 mL per minute with a practical goal of about 5 mL per minute. The clinical urgency will dictate the ultrafiltration rate, which can be easily adjusted. For CVVH, an ultrafiltration rate of 40 mL per minute can be achieved.

With continuous ultrafiltration techniques, even low ultrafiltration rates can produce significant dehydration. Thus, based on the severity of volume overload, a time frame for fluid removal and ultrafiltration rate should be determined prospectively. For ultrafiltration to occur, there must be a transmembrane pressure gradient from blood to the ultrafiltration compartment. The major determinants of transmembrane pressure are the blood's hydrostatic pressure produced by either systemic blood pressure or an extracorporeal blood pump; the negative hydrostatic pressure in the ultrafiltration compartment produced by gravity siphon effect of the filtrate line or by a suction device; and the plasma oncotic pressure (140). As plasma water is ultrafiltered, blood concentrates because cells and proteins are retained during transit through the device. Thus, plasma oncotic pressure rises toward the distal end of the filter. Increased viscosity reduces ultrafiltration and increases the risk of filter clotting. During CAVH or SCUF the hydrostatic pressure in the blood compartment is roughly balanced by the opposing oncotic pressure (76). Thus, the net transmembrane pressure is essentially generated by the siphon or vacuum suction effect of the ultrafiltration compartment. The transmembrane pressure generated by the column of ultrafiltration is equal to the vertical distance from the filter to the ultrafiltrate collector (cm × 0.75 mm Hg/cm H_2O). Thus, a 40-cm column will generate a transmembrane pressure of 40 cm H_2O × 0.75 mm Hg/cm H_2O = 29.6 mm Hg. Vacuum suction can be achieved with a hemodialysis machine, a portable vacuum machine, or wall suction. In these circumstances, the gauges on the devices are generally accurate to within 10% (140).

In the absence of an extracorporeal blood pump, the vascular access must guarantee an adequate arterial–venous gradient. Thus, catheters must transmit the arterial pressure to the filter with minimal pressure loss due to the resistance within the access itself. The placement of large-bore percutaneous catheters requires specific technical skills (127,128). Special catheters for CAVH have been designed that meet the requirements specified earlier (83,141). While in vitro there is a direct relationship between pressure and flow for a given catheter length and diameter, in vivo blood flow in the circuit is reduced by the resistances of the extracorporeal circuit components (74,142,143). According to the Hagen-Poiseuille law, the larger the catheter in the same blood vessel is, the greater is the flow at the same pressure. Because the filter itself is the major resistance in the extracorporeal circuit, the small catheter lumen does not jeopardize performance but enhances safety (74). A short access of 13 gauge or larger appears to be adequate.

External shunts such as the Quinton-Scribner require surgical placement and distal ligation of the artery. Although adequate CAVH can often be achieved with external shunts, the blood flow generated with this vascular access is inferior to the flows generated by the percutaneous catheters (74,128,144). Thus, percutaneous access for CAVH has become the first choice for most clinicians. External shunts may be preferable in the presence of severe femoral vascular atherosclerosis or prosthetic femoral vascular material, or the desire to maintain leg mobility, or when the risk of hemorrhage from a blind arterial puncture is unacceptable. The long-term thrombosis rates are similar for percutaneous catheters and external shunts. At a given blood pressure, filtration rates are higher with a large-bore catheter because more of the arterial pressure is transmitted to the filter (74).

The clinician must weigh all these arguments in deciding the appropriate access for an individual patient. There are multiple resistances in the extracorporeal circuit of CAVH, including the vascular accesses, the blood lines, and the filters themselves. The relative resistances are highest in the filter compared to the lines and vascular accesses (145). Nonetheless, the resistances along the entire extracorporeal circuit are additive and no component should be ignored. Resistances can be lowered by altering the shape of the blood pathway. According to the Hagen-Poiseuille law, shortening the length and increasing the radius will reduce resistances in each component of the circuit. Because in CVVH the extracorporeal blood pump generates an adequate net transmembrane pressure, vacuum suction is rarely needed and the type of vascular access or blood lines are less important than in SCUF (146). In CVVH the extracorporeal blood pump produces flow rates of 100 to 150 mL per minute. The veno–venous double lumen catheters can be placed in the internal jugular, subclavian, or femoral veins. The extracorporeal blood pump system includes a roller pump, arterial pressure sensor, air detector, and venous pressure alarms. Use of this equipment requires instruction from trained hemodialysis personnel. The ultrafiltration rate can be controlled directly by a pump on the ultrafiltration line or indirectly by altering blood flow. Alternatively, venous pressure can be raised by placing a screw clamp on the venous blood line or negative pressure can be applied by suction to the ultrafiltrate compartment.

Problem Solving with Arterial–Venous Slow Continuous Ultrafiltration

In the first few minutes of SCUF or CAVH, an ultrafiltration rate >10 mL per minute is optimal, 5 to 10 mL per minute is acceptable, and <5 mL per minute is inadequate. In the latter case, line kinking or occlusion must be excluded, the patient's blood pressure checked, and the vertical distance between the filter and the ultrafiltrate collector measured. Because filter clotting is unlikely immediately after initiation of treatment, hemoconcentration must be excluded when ultrafiltration rates are <10 mL per minute despite a systolic blood pressure >90 mm Hg. Filtration fraction (the ratio between ultrafiltration rate and plasma flow rate) is calculated with the following formula:

$$\text{Filtration Fraction} = (1 - (\text{Hct}_{in}/\text{Hct}_{out})/(1 - \text{Hct}_{in})$$

where Hct "in" and "out" refer, respectively, to the hematocrit in the inlet and outlet lines (147). A filtration fraction of >20% is adequate, whereas a filtration fraction of 35% to 40% is maximally efficient (74).

When arterial protein concentration and hematocrit are normal, the higher the filtration fraction is, the greater is the risk for fiber clotting. In conditions in which the ultrafiltration rate is low despite a high filtration fraction, replacement fluid should be prediluted. Conditions in which filtration fraction is <20% because of a low transmembrane pressure gradient include hypotension, insufficient negative pressure in the ultrafiltrate compartment, and loss of hydrostatic pressure in the blood lines. Measures that increase ultrafiltration fraction include maximizing the vertical distance between the filter and the ultrafiltrate collector and institution of suction-assisted ultrafiltration (148). The ultrafiltration line is air seal connected to wall suction, and gradually the suction pressure is raised to bring the ultrafiltration rate to a desirable rate.

Wall suction above 200 mm Hg is not recommended. With ongoing suction, blood pressure no longer controls ultrafiltration rate and significant blood loss can occur if there is a blood leak in the ultrafiltrate compartment. Routinely, no blood detection alarms are present in the system; therefore, frequent evaluation will be necessary. If ultrafiltration rate drops later during treatment, 50 mL of saline can be rapidly injected in the arterial sleeve with the arterial blood line briefly occluded proximally to observe the condition of the filter itself. Clots will appear as streaks along the filter fibers. If significant clotting has occurred (to the point of limiting ultrafiltration rates), the filter and tubing must be changed.

Problem Solving with Continuous Ultrafiltration in the Veno–Venous Mode

Causes of CVVH ultrafiltration rates lower than the rate set on the filtrate pump controller include inadequate blood flow; failure to deliver fresh, water-rich blood to the filter; a high filtrate compartment pressure overcoming the blood pump-generated transmembrane pressure; or frank filter fiber occlusion. If filter tubing occlusion is excluded, 50 to 100 mL of 0.9% saline can be injected to determine the fibers' patency. If occluded, the filter must be replaced. If the filter fibers are patent, the ultrafiltration rate can be augmented by increasing the blood flow rate. When the blood flow rate is too low for a set ultrafiltration rate, the filtration fraction increases to the point of impairing ultrafiltration because it increases the oncotic pressure on the blood side of the membrane. For optimal veno-venous ultrafiltration, the filtration fraction should be less than 40%. Increases in blood flow rate to 200 to 300 mL per minute will increase transmembrane pressure and lower the filtration fraction. Plasma water becomes the filtrate, so plasma-rich water is necessary for ideal function. Increases in plasma flow rate by addition of water prevent excessive rise of the oncotic pressure of the retained plasma and cleanse the inner surface of the membrane where cells, platelets, and large proteins accumulate, retarding filtration. Loss of filter fibers due to either blood clotting or membrane coating by platelets reduces the operating surface area. Corrective measures include saline flushing, augmented anticoagulation, or replacement of the filter.

An excessively high ultrafiltration rate due to high transmembrane pressure generated by the blood pump can be lowered by correcting the filtrate roller occlusion or by increasing the ultrafiltration rate to at least 1,200 mL per hour. An increase in the pressure measured with the venous drip chamber may be caused by any occlusion of venous return, including the venous return vascular access or, more frequently, by clotting in the drip chamber. This is a very convenient and predictable warning of system clotting. A decrease in the pressure measured within the venous drip chamber indicates inadequate blood delivery to the drip chamber, most commonly from clotting within the filter or from occlusion of the blood pathway proximal to the drip chamber. An increase in the arterial pressure proximal to the pump is secondary to any occlusion distal to the measuring site. A decrease in the arterial pressure proximal to the pump is caused by inadequate delivery of blood to the blood pump, generally from occlusion of the vascular access or collapse of the blood vessel. If pressures are measured in the arterial position distal to the pump, the pattern parallels that of the arterial pre-pump position and the problem-solving approach is the same.

CVVH can be associated with insertion complications, thrombosis, or infection. Insertion complications include atrial and ventricular arrhythmias, arterial laceration, hemothorax, pneumothorax, air embolism, pericardial tamponade, central vein or cardiac chamber perforation, and malpositioning. Antiarrhythmic medications or cardioversion are needed in less than 1% of all central vein catheterizations. Femoral and carotid artery puncture are easily treated with 20 minutes of direct pressure. Bleeding from subclavian artery puncture can be significant but it is usually self-limited. The use of heparin in this circumstance should be avoided. Hemothorax or pneumothroax, albeit rare, usually occurs with cannulation of the subclavian vein. Air embolism results from accidental introduction of air through the introducer needle, dilator, or catheter. Vascular or myocardial perforation can result in life-threatening pericardial tamponade or hemothorax. Hypotension, especially during dialysis, is a sign of pericardial tamponade. Malpositioned or kinked lines can be pulled back or rotated. Urokinase (5,000 U per mL) or streptokinase (2,500 U per mL) can be injected once or twice into a clotted catheter with a dwell time ranging from 30 minutes to several hours, followed by aspiration of luminal contents. The process can be repeated if the clot does not dissolve. Line replacement is an option. Femoral vein cannulation is associated with the greatest risk of infection.

Intermittent Isolated Ultrafiltration with Central Veno–Venous Access

Intermittent isolated ultrafiltration is an extracorporeal dehydrating procedure in which blood is pumped through a filter by an extracorporeal blood pump aided either by suction applied to the ultrafiltrate compartment (negative pressure) or from resistance induced in the venous line (positive pressure). Because of the extracorporeal blood pump, a dual lumen veno–venous catheter will generate a blood flow of 500 to 1,000 mL per hour. Hemodynamic tolerance is the limiting factor of ultrafiltration rate. Tolerance is usually related to the rapidity of fluid removal. Most adult patients will tolerate for a short time ultrafiltration rates of 500 to 1,000 mL per hour, which are technically achievable with intermittent ultrafiltration (67,68). Slower ultrafiltration rates over longer periods of time improve hemodynamic tolerance. Because patient intolerance is rate-limiting, it advisable to avoid any major therapeutic manipulations or diagnostic procedures while ultrafiltration is being performed. The skin exit site must be cleaned and sterilized daily, lumina must be flushed with heparin to maintain their patency, and use of the catheters for other intravenous infusions must be avoided. Infusion of blood or lipid-containing products through the ultrafiltration catheters shortens their patency and increases infectious complications. Injection of 5,000 U per mL of urokinase for 1 to 8 hours usually reverses occlusion due to intraluminal thrombosis.

Ultrafiltration can occur in the presence or absence of dialysate. When dialysate is present, in addition to fluid and solute removal by ultrafiltration (convective transport of solute), there also is solute removal by diffusion. When diffusion occurs, the ultrafiltrate is hypotonic relative to intracellular water. In the absence of dialysate, intracellular water, plasma water, and ultrafiltration have the same osmolality. The sodium content of ultrafiltration is essentially equal to that of plasma water (45,46). Patients tolerate isotonic ultrafiltration much better than they do hypotonic ultrafiltration (57–61,67,80,131,132). Intermittent isolated ultrafiltration is effective in removing salt and water in overhydrated patients with moderate and severe congestive heart failure (56,62,67–69,80,81,89,91,149–151).

Many patients regain responsiveness to diuretics after one or more ultrafiltration treatments, suggesting that untapped cardiac functional reserve is recruited by ultrafiltration (56). In addition, ascites, peripheral edema, and respiratory compromise may dramatically improve. Serum sodium concentration normalizes without worsening of renal function. As expected, plasma volume falls and plasma oncotic pressure rises (65). Ultrafiltration increases the colloid osmotic pressure of plasma and the transcapillary gradient (152). The increase in plasma oncotic pressure is maximal in the first 60 minutes of ultrafiltration and then levels off as refilling occurs. After ultrafiltration, the decreased venous pressure further enhances the net transcapillary pressure gradient change, favoring interstitial fluid reabsorption. The descriptions of the hemodynamic responses to intermittent ultrafiltration in these patients are relatively consistent and are similar to those of chronic dialysis patients undergoing ultrafiltration (57–59,153).

Most reports note that heart rate does not change and that blood pressure or systemic vascular resistance does not fall if the ultrafiltration rate is limited to 500 to 1,000 mL per hour for only a few hours (64,67–69,83,99,149, 150,154). Cardiac output either rises or is stable (64,67, 68). Pulmonary capillary wedge pressure is unchanged or decreased (64). Right atrial pressure and pulmonary vascular resistance fall (65–68). An improved ejection fraction and a decrease radiographic cardiothoracic ratio have also been described (10).

Advantages of intermittent isolated ultrafiltration include the avoidance of an arterial puncture and the short exposure to systemic anticoagulation. Disadvantages include the need for specialized dialysis equipment and personnel, which may limit the feasibility of the procedure, and the removal of large amounts of fluid in one limited session per day. Thus, the extracellular fluid space may be filling and emptying in a nonphysiological manner. Slower, more protracted ultrafiltration minimizes these problems. The complications of intermittent isolated ultrafiltration are similar to those observed in hemodialysis but without the unique complications, such as electrolyte disturbances, associated with diffusion. However, hemorrhage from anticoagulation and extracorporeal blood pump complications, such as air embolism, can occur; trained dialysis personnel are required to minimize these complications. Intermittent isolated ultrafiltration has been described in more than 100 NYHA Class IV heart failure patients who have failed aggressive vasodilator, diuretic, and inotropic therapy (62,69,80,81). Of 52 such patients treated with slow isolated ultrafiltration, 13 died less than 1 month after treatment (nonresponders), 24 had both cardiac and renal improvement (responders) for either <3 months (n = 6) or for >3 months (n = 18), and 15 (partial responders) had hemodynamic improvement but worsening renal function requiring either long-term weekly ultrafiltration (n = 8), continuous ambulatory peritoneal dialysis (n = 1), or intermittent high-flux hemofiltration or hemodiafiltration (n = 6). Adequate diuresis was restored in 1 month in 24 of the 39 responders and partial responders. Four of the 15 partial responders had sufficient recovery of renal function to undergo heart transplantation 3 to 9 months after isolated ultrafiltration.

Thus, intermittent ultrafiltration can be used as a nonpharmacologic approach for the treatment of congestive heart failure refractory to maximally tolerated medical therapy. Restoration of diuresis and natriuresis after intermittent ultrafiltration identified patients with recoverable cardiac functional reserve. Intermittent isolated ultrafiltration is valuable in partial responders because it improves quality of life and may be used as a bridge to heart transplantation.

The high short-term mortality in this and in another study (in which 23 of 86 patients [27%] died within 2 months after ultrafiltration) is consistent with the poor prognosis associated with advanced heart failure.

Simplified Intermittent Isolated Ultrafiltration with Peripheral Veno–Venous Access

All ultrafiltration techniques described earlier require cannulation of a central vein for fluid withdrawal, blood return, or both. Recently, a new device (Aquadex System 100, CHF-Solutions, Minneapolis, MN) has become clinically available that permits both withdrawal of fluid and blood return through peripheral veins (Fig. 43-12). However, central venous access remains an option with

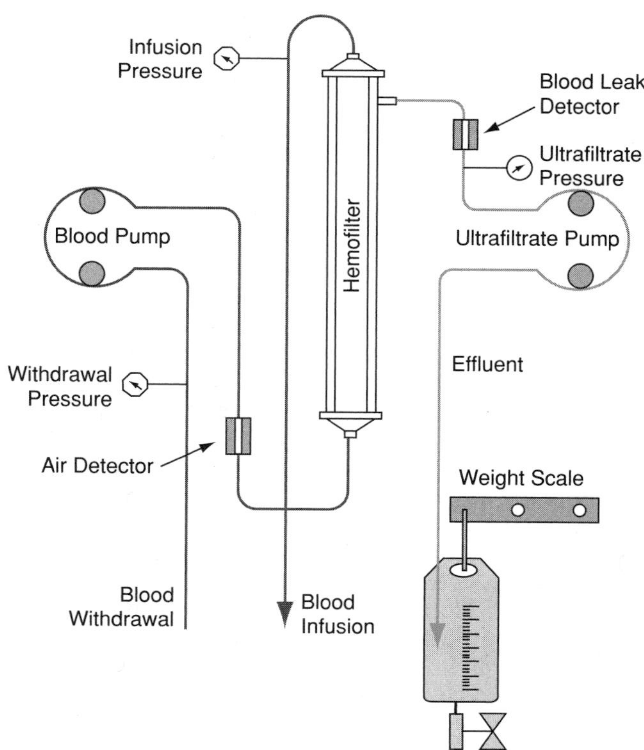

Figure 43-12 The Aquadex System 100 peripheral veno–venous system (CHF-Solutions, Minneapolis, MN).

this device. Fluid removal can range from 10 to 500 mL per hour, blood flow can be set at 10 to 40 mL per minute, and total extracorporeal blood volume is only 33 mL. The device consists of a console, an extracorporeal blood pump, and venous catheters. The console controls the rate at which blood is removed from the patient and extracts ultrafiltrate at a user-set maximum rate. The device is designed to monitor the extracorporeal blood circuit and to alert the user to abnormal conditions. The device has one user setting that determines the rate of ultrafiltrate removal. Liquid removed during treatment drains into an ultrafiltrate bag. When the bag is full, the ultrafiltration pump stops and alarms until the bag is emptied; the blood pump continues to operate. Blood is withdrawn from a vein through the withdrawal catheter. Tubing connects the withdrawal catheter to the blood pump. Blood passes through the withdrawal pressure sensor just before it enters the blood pump tubing loop. During operation, the pump loop is compressed by rotating rollers that propel the blood through the tubing.

After exiting the blood pump, blood passes through the air detector and enters the hemofilter. The hemofilter is bonded to a clip-on cartridge that mounts onto the ultrafiltrate pump raceway on the side of the console. Blood enters the filter through a port on the bottom, exits through the port at the top of the filter, and passes through the infusion pressure sensor before returning to the patient. Inside the hemofilter, there is a bundle of hollow fibers. The ultrafiltrate passes through the fiber walls, fills the space between the fibers inside the filter case, and exits the filter through a port near the top of the filter case. After exiting the filter, ultrafiltrate passes through a blood leak detector.

Ultrafiltrate sequentially passes through the ultrafiltrate pressure sensor, the ultrafiltrate pump, and the collecting bag that is suspended from the weight scale. The device is very simple to use and requires minimal supervision and programming. Setup of the device takes less than 10 minutes. Treatment can be performed by any nurse trained in the use of the device and does not require specialized dialysis personnel.

To date, three clinical trials of intermittent peripheral veno–venous ultrafiltration have been completed. In the first study, of 21 fluid-overloaded patients, removal of an average of 2,611 ± 1,002 mL (range 325 to 3,725 mL) over 6.43 ± 1.47 hours reduced weight from 91.9 ± 17.5 kg to 89.3 ± 17.3 kg ($p < 0.0001$), and also reduced signs and symptoms of pulmonary and peripheral congestion without associated changes in heart rate, blood pressure, electrolytes, or hematocrit (155).

The aim of the second study was to determine if ultrafiltration with this same Aquadex System 100 before intravenous diuretics in patients with decompensated heart failure and diuretic resistance results in euvolemia and hospital discharge in 3 days, without hypotension or worsening renal function. Ultrafiltration was initiated within 4.7± 3.5 hours of hospitalization and before intravenous diuretics in 20 heart failure patients with volume overload and diuretic resistance (age 74.5 ± 8.2 years; 75% ischemic disease; ejection fraction 31% ± 15%), and continued until euvolemia. Patients were evaluated at each hospital day, at 30 days, and at 90 days. An average of 8,654 ± 4,205 mL was removed with 2.6 ± 1.2 8-hour ultrafiltration courses. Twelve patients (60%) were discharged in ≤3 days. One patient was readmitted in 30 days and two patients in 90 days. Weight ($p = 0.006$), Minnesota Living with Heart Failure scores ($p = 0.003$), and Global Assessment ($p = 0.00003$) were improved after ultrafiltration, at 30 days and 90 days. B-type natriuretic peptide levels were decreased after ultrafiltration (from 1,236 ± 747 pg/mL to 988 ± 847 pg/mL) and at 30 days (816 ± 494 pg/mL; $p = 0.03$. Blood pressure, renal function, and medications were unchanged. The results of this study suggest that in heart failure patients with volume overload and diuretic resistance, early ultrafiltration before intravenous diuretics effectively and safely decreases length of stay and readmissions. Clinical benefits persisted at 3 months after treatment (156).

The aim of the third study was to compare the safety and efficacy of ultrafiltration with the Aquadex System 100 device versus those of intravenous diuretics in patients with decompensated heart failure. Compared to the 20 patients randomly assigned to intravenous diuretics, the 20 patients randomized to a single, 8-hour ultrafiltration session had greater median fluid removal (2,838 mL versus 4,650 mL; $p = 0.001$) and median weight loss (1.86 kg versus 2.5 kg; $p = 0.24$). Ultrafiltration was well-tolerated and not associated with adverse hemodynamic renal effects. The results of this study show that an initial treatment decision to administer ultrafiltration in patients with decompensated congestive heart failure results in greater fluid removal and improvement of signs and symptoms of congestion than those achieved with traditional diuretic therapies (157).

INTERMITTENT HEMODIALYSIS

Intermittent hemodialysis is the most-utilized form of chronic dialysis (158). Widespread availability and familiarity with the technique are clearly the major advantages. Although home hemodialysis is now feasible, end-stage heart failure patients are not appropriate candidates for home intermittent hemodialysis until newer techniques become available. (159). In the United States patients with advanced heart failure can receive hemodialysis only if they meet criteria for end-stage renal disease because there is no approved reimbursement for hemodialysis for indications other than end-stage renal disease.

Chronic hemodialysis requires repeated access to the circulation. Generally, this involves creation of an arterial–venous fistula that creates blood flows ranging from several hundred milliliters to 2 L per minute. Such flow requires compensation by an increase in cardiac output. Consequently, the creation of these fistulas can be associated with exacerbation or development of congestive heart failure in patients with underlying cardiac dysfunction (160). In these patients, permanent venous catheters are the preferred vascular access for hemodialysis. Tunneled, cuffed, silicone catheters such as the double lumen Permacath or the double catheter Duocath are inserted percutaneously into the internal jugular vein, providing an adequate vascular access for ultrafiltration or hemofiltration for several years with a reduced risk of complications including infections (161,162). These venous catheters can be used within minutes of insertion and their blood flow does not increase cardiac workload as much as arterial–venous fistulas. In addition, with venous catheters the venous capacitance system is preferentially emptied while effective intravascular volume is preserved.

However, even with intravenous catheters, hemodialysis is the most poorly tolerated type of dehydration procedure by heart failure patients because large amounts of fluid are rapidly removed in 3 to 6 hours once to three times per week. Patients with heart failure have better hemodynamic tolerance to daily hemodialysis approaches. In most cases, one 4-hour hemodialysis session can lower the blood urea nitrogen (BUN) by at least 60%, remove 50 to 150 mEq of potassium, and remove 3 L of fluid by ultrafiltration.

PERITONEAL DIALYSIS

This past decade has seen tremendous progress in unraveling the mechanisms of ultrafiltration with peritoneal dialysis (PD). Recent studies have confirmed the three-pore model hypothesis, and the detection of aquaporin-1 in the peritoneum has clarified the concept of sodium sieving (163–170). Dextrose has traditionally been used as an osmotic agent to generate ultrafiltration during PD, as it is cheap and easy to use.

Once the PD solution is instilled into the peritoneal cavity, three simultaneously occurring processes determine the magnitude of net ultrafiltration: a convective transfer of fluid into the peritoneal cavity (transcapillary ultrafiltration); a diffusive transfer of fluid from the peritoneal cavity into the bloodstream; and a convective flow of fluid into the lymphatic channels (171). Only one of these processes, transcapillary ultrafiltration, is modifiable. The other two, diffusive reabsorption and lymphatic absorption, occur at a constant rate. This transcapillary ultrafiltration is dependent upon the osmotic force generated by the dextrose present in the PD fluid. The osmotic force is maximal at the time of the installation of peritoneal fluid so that the rate of ultrafiltration is maximal at time zero. Because osmotic force is dependent upon the concentration of dextrose, the more hypertonic the dialysate is, the greater are the initial and subsequent rates of ultrafiltration (172,173).

If the goal of PD is the removal of fluid for rapid alleviation of congestive symptoms, short dwell duration would ensure the continuous presence of fresh dialysate and maintain a near maximal rate of ultrafiltration. This is most easily achieved with automated PD via the use of a cycler. Since glucose is absorbed into the bloodstream during the period of dwell, the osmotic gradient dissipates over time, leading to a decrease in the rate of ultrafiltration (174,175). The rate of absorption of glucose is dependent upon the transport characteristics of the peritoneum, a patient-specific factor that can be measured with the standardized peritoneal equilibration test (175). Knowledge of the patient's transport type is probably not relevant during the management of acute volume overload. However, it is critical to determine the optimal duration of dwell for maximum ultrafiltration during the long-term management of any patient with PD.

In addition to using hypertonic dialysate and an optimal duration of dialysate dwell, ultrafiltration can be enhanced by increasing the volume of instilled dialysate (172). There are probably two mechanisms by which an increase in the volume of dialysate increases the rate of ultrafiltration. First, a larger amount almost always means an increase in the amount of instilled dextrose. Second, and perhaps more important, the larger volume results in an increase in the effective peritoneal surface area and, hence, in the recruitment of large number of capillaries that participate in the process of ultrafiltration. However, unlike the tonicity of the dialysate and the duration of dwell, the volume of instilled dialysate is limited by patient tolerance. This may be particularly true in individuals with congestive heart failure, in whom a large volume of dialysate may further compromise ventilatory function by elevating the diaphragm.

PERITONEAL DIALYSIS IN HEART FAILURE

In the presence of congestive heart failure and/or inadequate renal perfusion, PD can be a life-saving method for removing fluid and stabilizing hemodynamics. Acute PD is the oldest dialysis-type dehydrating procedure and, arguably, is the simplest to perform technically (176–178). The first drainage and ultrafiltration can occur within 1 hour. Furthermore, the facilities, equipment, and skills required are readily available. Because of these favorable factors, the complication rate is low, especially if acute PD lasts ≤48 hours (179,180).

Acute PD can be performed on an intermittent basis with repeated puncturing of the peritoneum for catheter placement. The dialysate exchange rate is rapid and the dialysis is fairly aggressive in order to keep the duration of the procedure short, which reduces the rate of infectious complications. Alternatively, a permanent PD catheter can be placed and the PD can be performed intermittently or continuously on a chronic basis. Continuous PD is referred to as continuous equilibration peritoneal dialysis (CEPD) when performed in the hospital setting, or as continuous ambulatory peritoneal dialysis (CAPD) when carried out in the out-patient setting (181). Automated PD (APD) can be performed in the home during the night with the use of machines designed for this specific purpose. With continuous PD, the dialysate exchange rate is slower than with acute peritoneal dialysis. In CEPD the patient usually requires admission and the nursing staff performs the CEPD. Whereas CEPD requires hospitalization and specialized nursing personnel, CAPD or APD can be performed at home by either the patient or family members.

All of these techniques are simple and permit slow, gentle removal of fluid. If the PD system functions properly, the amount of fluid that can be removed is regular and predictable. Advantages of PD include avoidance of the electrolyte abnormalities (e.g., hypokalemia, hyponatremia, hypochloremia, and metabolic alkalosis) commonly caused by diuretics, and decreased requirements for sodium and water restriction.

Depending on the dextrose concentration, the osmolality of clinically available peritoneal dialysates ranges from 346 to 485 mmol/kg. The sugar is the source of the dialysates' hypertonic activity because the electrolyte content of the dialysate generally resembles that of plasma water. Water diffuses down its concentration gradient from the extracellular fluid spaces bathing the peritoneal cavity into the hypertonic peritoneal dialysate. This process begins as soon as the dialysate comes in contact with the vascular peritoneal membranes. Thus, ultrafiltration occurs immediately after initiation of PD and before any drainage has occurred. Because dextrose is gradually absorbed and diluted by the incoming ultrafiltrate, ultrafiltration declines over time (176–184). There is a fairly high and constant ultrafiltration rate for about 2 hours. Because it takes time to fill the peritoneal cavity enough to expose the entire functional surface, exchanges lasting less than 1 hour exploit high ultrafiltration rates but leave the peritoneal cavity partially empty and thus are less efficient (184).

In contrast to early high complications rates, improved PD techniques are associated with a modest risk of hypernatremia and hyperglycemia. Peritonitis, abdominal wall infection, and hydrothorax are rare in acute PD. They occur most frequently in CAPD and are intermediate in APD. Filling of the peritoneal cavity with dialysate can reduce venous return by increasing abdominal pressure but this benefit can be negated by compromise of inspiratory vital capacity, resulting from elevation of the diaphragm (180–186). This problem can be minimized by reducing dialysate volumes and increasing the exchange rate.

The disadvantages of PD may vary depending on the clinical situation. Abnormal abdominal conditions, such as an ileus or the presence of drains, prosthetic material such as vascular grafts, adhesions, or recent incisions are relative contraindications for PD. The discomfort associated with PD is mild. The major disadvantage of PD is that success is not always predictable. Failure is frequently caused by mechanical or technical problems such as improper drainage. Inadequate drainage has been reported in 38% of patients and it can become a serious problem in one-third of the cases (179). When the system drains properly, ultrafiltration is adequate to dehydrate the patient. However, the rate of fluid removal cannot always be accurately predicted, even when drainage is satisfactory.

Since the first description of PD in the management of refractory congestive heart failure (187), the course of over 60 patients treated with PD has been described (188–198). Most cases are NYHA Class III heart failure patients who also have renal failure, or NYHA Class IV patients unresponsive to diuretics, inotropes, and vasodilators. If the results of these studies are pooled, overall survival rates at 1 and 2 years are, respectively, 37% and 15%. The magnitude of the physiological changes induced by PD cannot be accurately predicted. At 1 month and 1 year, respectively, systolic blood pressure may drop by 10 and 7 mm Hg and diastolic blood pressure by 7 and 3 mm Hg (199). The greater fall in blood pressure with PD compared with hemodialysis can be partially attributed to impairment in venous return to the heart from increased intra-abdominal pressure due to the presence of peritoneal fluid (192,200). This may have distinct advantages for patients with severe heart failure. However, other predictable physiological changes may be detrimental.

Pulmonary complications of PD include increase of alveolar oxygen gradient in the supine position due to the presence of peritoneal dialysate, decrease in functional residual capacity, rise in mean inspiratory pressure, and pulmonary restriction (201–204). Furthermore, peritonitis, a fairly common complication of CAPD, exacerbates these pulmonary abnormalities (202).

PD can be used for the treatment of congestion in heart failure patients because it induces a net fluid loss into the dialysate. Dialysate that contains 1.5% dextrose can induce an average ultrafiltration rate of up to 5 mL per minute. This usually requires an inflow volume of at least 2 L. A 2-L, 1.5% dextrose exchange over 1 hour will remove an extra 200 mL of fluid. A similar volume and duration of exchange with 4.25% dextrose can generate an average ultrafiltration rate of 12 mL per minute, resulting in a net loss of >600 mL per hour. Exchanges of 2.5% dextrose will produce intermediate fluid losses. Because the presence of ascites or residual dialysate precludes an accurate estimate of hourly fluid losses, these should be averaged over 6 to 12 hours.

Acute Peritoneal Dialysis

Catheter placement and initial dialysate exchange can be completed in 1 hour. Hence, ultrafiltration can occur immediately. Trocar or guidewire techniques for PD catheter placement are routinely utilized in most critical care centers. Initial use of 2 L of 4.25% dextrose dialysate may generate an ultrafiltration rate of 800 mL per hour. Use of less hypertonic dialysate or prolongation of the dwell time of the dialysate in the peritoneum will slow the ultrafiltration rate. Effective ultrafiltration requires that dialysate be in contact with the peritoneal membrane. Time can be wasted with ineffectual drainage. The fluid should flow in as fast as the gravity feed will allow it with the feed raised as high as practical. The dialysate should not be pumped or forced into the peritoneum. The drain time should also be as rapid as possible. Setting an upper limit to drain time is reasonable, but the next exchange should be promptly initiated if drainage appears complete before the end of the set time. Drainage appears complete when the drainage stream changes from a rapid to a slow dribble. If only a fraction of the initial exchange returns and drainage was transiently rapid (few minutes), the next exchange should be promptly initiated with the aim, depending on patient tolerance, to repeat the exchange after 1 to 2 L of additional volume. Thus, when acute PD is used in patients with refractory heart failure, improvement of signs and symptoms of congestion can be best achieved by using maximally tolerated dwell volumes, hypertonic dialysate, and short dwell times with a cycler.

Because aggressive ultrafiltration is planned in acute PD, hypotension and electrolyte abnormalities are more likely than with continuous PD. Thus, vitals signs, weight, electrolytes, and glucose should be frequently measured during acute PD. Hypernatremia can occur because water diffuses into the dialysate faster than sodium (205). Hyperglycemia can result from the use of high-dextrose-concentration dialysates regardless of the presence of glucose intolerance or diabetes. Regular monitoring of dialysate white blood cell counts permits early detection of peritonitis. Hypokalemia can be prevented by placing appropriate amounts of KCl in the dialysate before inflow.

Long-Term Peritoneal Dialysis

Permanent PD catheters are required for CEPD, APD, and CAPD and can be placed at the bedside under local anesthesia (206). Patient tolerance, physician acceptance, and overall results are excellent. Because both CEPD and CAPD utilize long dwell times, ultrafiltration and solute and electrolyte shifts occur more slowly and require less-intense monitoring. Unlike acute PD, CEPD, CAPD, and APD require the input of a nephrologist. Improvement of signs and symptoms of volume overload can be expected with PD because currently available PD solutions permit fluid removal rates of 67 to 568 mL per hour (178,189,207–212). These rates are similar to those obtainable with continuous extracorporeal therapies.

Several investigators have studied the effect of PD on hemodynamic variables of the systemic and renal circulations. As expected, fluid removal results in reduction in plasma volume (188,189), improvement in hyponatremia, and reduction in pulmonary capillary arterial wedge pressure (188,189,191). The frequently observed improvement in diuretic responsiveness is attributable to improved renal hemodynamics, as documented by an increase in insulin and para-amino hippurate clearances and reduction in the filtration fraction (212).

At least 111 patients with chronic congestive heart failure treated by long-term PD have been reported to date. In about half of these patients, PD was initiated solely for the management of congestive heart failure as renal dysfunction was not severe enough to require dialysis (193–197,213–219). Hence, the therapy was modified to achieve adequate ultrafiltration. These studies demonstrate that in such patients one to three hypertonic exchanges daily with short dwell times will maintain euvolemia. However, the reduction in the daily number of exchanges is clearly attractive to patients and has the potential to decrease the incidence of peritonitis from touch contamination.

Icodextrin-based PD solutions are now available in many parts of the world (220). The ability of icodextrin to generate sustained ultrafiltration over long periods of dwell may be especially advantageous under such circumstances (220–222). A significant proportion of patients may be able to maintain euvolemia with only one overnight exchange with icodextrin-based solutions with or without the need for additional exchanges with glucose-based solutions.

A major concern regarding the use of PD in patients with advanced heart failure has been that the morbidity from congestive heart failure may be replaced by PD-related complications. This concern is less compelling today with significant declines in peritonitis rates in CAPD-treated patients. Moreover, more than 90% of patients reported in the literature have functional improvement (196,197,215,217,218). Except for one study, a significant reduction in hospitalization rates after initiation of CAPD has been reported (197,218,219). Thus, CAPD may improve functional capacity and quality of life in select patients with advanced heart failure refractory to maximally tolerated medical therapy. The effects of PD on survival rates are not known.

ANTICOAGULATION

Anticoagulation is recommended with any extracorporeal circuit to avoid filter clotting (223). Adequate extracorporeal anticoagulation can be achieved with the infusion of heparin at 10 IU/kg per hour into the arterial blood line without excessive systemic anticoagulation (224,225). However, in one study, use of this heparin dose was associated with bleeding complications in high-risk patients. In another study in which heparin dose was adjusted to achieve a 50% increase in whole blood PTT, bleeding complications occurred in 20% of the patients (226). No set heparin dose regimen will be universally successful in nonuremic patients because heparin half-life varies from 45 minutes to 4 hours and it is not closely correlated with weight, surface area, clotting time, or heparin dose (227). In most cases, however, heparin half-life lengthens with increasing doses (228). Thus, there is great intrapatient and interpatient variability.

Depending on the clinical condition, in patients with normal coagulation a heparin bolus of 10 to 20 IU/kg should be administered intravenously 2 to 3 minutes before allowing blood to pass through the filter, followed by a maintenance dose of 10 IU/kg per hour with the goal to achieve a PTT of approximately 90 seconds in the extracorporeal circuit and 45 seconds in the systemic circulation. Another recommendation is to titrate the heparin dose to keep the peripheral venous PTT 20 to 30 seconds above control (229). In one study, while heparin doses of 1,000 U per hour were associated with minimal filter clotting, with doses of 500 IU per hour filters had to be changed daily due to clotting. Patients with thrombocytopenia require lower heparin doses. Filter clotting is usually a gradual process. If clotting is detected, the filter must be expeditiously replaced to prevent extension of the clot into the blood lines or vascular access.

Alternative anticoagulation therapies have been proposed for patients undergoing CVVH and SCUF. Substitution of heparin with prostacyclin is limited by hypotension and inability to monitor effects and inhibition (for at least 12 hours beyond treatment) of platelets' function, which is correctable only with platelet transfusion (230–233). Citrate anticoagulation can be used instead of heparin during conventional diffusion dialysis because the citrate–calcium complex is removed from the circulation by the dialyzer (234–236). In procedures without concurrent diffusive solute removal, citrate anticoagulation is considered experimental (237). Regional heparinization refers to infusion of protamine at 1 mg per hour into the venous limb of the extracorporeal circuit for each 100 IU per hour of heparin administered in the arterial sleeve to keep extracorporeal PTT >150 seconds and PTT of returning venous blood at 50 to 60 seconds. The use of regional heparinization in CAVH reportedly did not significantly extend filter patency (238–240).

Low-molecular-weight heparin (LMWH) has also been studied as an alternative to unfractionated heparin in patients undergoing hemofiltration or dialysis. In a 12-month randomized study of 70 patients starting dialysis, those treated with LMWH required fewer erythrocyte concentrates, had constant factor VIII activity, stable triglyceride levels, and decreased postheparin lipolytic activity (241). A randomized crossover trial in 21 chronic hemodialysis patients of LMWH versus nadroparin showed that the two anticoagulants were similar in terms of biocompatibility and dialyzer function (242). Divided LMWH doses induce less systemic anticoagulation than a bolus dose. Using measurements of dialyzer fiber bundle volume and urea clearance (both of which are reduced by fiber clotting), one study showed that a LMWH dose 125 aXa UICKg is associated with a 3% fiber bundle volume reduction, whereas with doses of 150, 175, and 200 there was no reduction in fiber bundle volume or urea clearance (244). Variable kinetics are the main limitations to the use of LMWH in CAVH (241,244). Some investigators propose that more adequate mixing of heparin, by infusing it early in the arterial line and mounting the venous end of the filter upright and increasing dilution (2.5 to 10 IU per mL), will reduce dose requirements while improving local anticoagulation (245). In CVVH the increased risk of filter clotting due to the hemoconcentration induced by high flow rates is balanced by the decreased risk of clotting due to less stasis of blood and constant washing of the membranes by CVVH's high flow rates.

SUMMARY

Of the ultrafiltration approaches described, the most practical are veno–venous ultrafiltration techniques in which isotonic plasma is propelled through the filter by an extracorporeal pump. These approaches avoid an arterial puncture, remove a predictable amount of fluid, are not associated with significant hemodynamic instability, and, in the case of peripheral veno–venous ultrafiltration, do not require specialized dialysis personnel and can be performed in the out-patient setting.

Ultrafiltration techniques have been used in patients with decompensated heart failure and volume overload refractory to diuretic therapy. These patients generally have pre-existing renal insufficiency (calculated creatinine clearance 30 to 90 mL per minute) and, despite daily oral diuretic doses, develop signs of pulmonary and peripheral congestion. Ultrafiltration and diuretic holiday may restore diuresis and natriuresis.

In patients whose renal function declines while they are hospitalized for decompensated heart failure, life-saving medications such as ACEIs are stopped and diuretic doses are reduced, despite persistent volume overload. Inotropic agents are often initiated in the hope that increases in cardiac output and renal perfusion will reverse renal dysfunction. This strategy, however, has been associated with increased morbidity and mortality. Based on the well-documented relationship between increases of right atrial pressure and diuretic use and reductions of glomerular filtration rate, a strategy of temporarily holding diuretics and reducing volume excess with ultrafiltration seems logical in these patients.

Some patients with volume overload refractory to all available intravenous vasoactive therapies have had significant improvements of symptoms, hemodynamics, and renal function following ultrafiltration.

The ADHERE documents that 50% of patients hospitalized with volume overload loss ≤5 kg from their admission weight, despite use of intravenous diuretics. A strategy of *early* ultrafiltration and diuretic holiday can result in more effective weight reduction and can shorten hospitalization.

Patients with severe cardiac dysfunction undergoing cardiovascular surgery are at increased risk of developing volume overload during CPB and cardioplegia. In many of these patients diuretics do not produce sufficient sodium and water diuresis. In these patients ultrafiltration can produce more effective reduction of volume overload and reduce morbidity and mortality.

Patients should not be considered for ultrafiltration if the following conditions exist: venous access cannot be obtained; hematocrit is ≥40%; there is a hypercoagulable state; systolic blood pressure is <85 mm Hg or there are signs or symptoms of cardiogenic shock; patients require intravenous pressors to maintain an adequate blood pressure; or there is end-stage renal disease, as documented by a requirement for dialysis approaches.

Intermittent hemodialysis should not be used for removal of excess fluid because large fluid shifts in short periods of time may lead to hemodynamic instability and worsening of the overall clinical status. Intermittent hemodialysis should be instituted when patients meet criteria for end-stage renal disease. The role of PD for short-term management of refractory heart failure is limited to situations in which extracorporeal ultrafiltration is either impossible or unavailable. For the long-term management of refractory volume overload in patients with advanced heart failure, PD may be a viable option. However, further investigation of the efficacy and safety of this approach is needed before specific recommendations can be made on the use of PD in patients with advanced heart failure.

REFERENCES

1. American Heart Association. Heart Disease and Stroke Statistics—2006 Update. Dallas, Tex as: American Heart Association; 2006. http.//circ.ahajournals.org/cgi/reprint/circulationaha.105.17160001. Date accessed:1/22/2006.
2. Redfield MM. Heart Failure—an epidemic of uncertain proportions. *N Engl J Med.* 2002;347:1442–1444.
3. Haldeman, GA, Croft JB, Giles WH, et al. Hospitalization of patients with heart failure: National Hospital Discharge Survey, 1985–1995. *Am Heart J.* 1999;137:352–360.
4. Massie BM, Shah NB. Evolving trends in the epidemiologic risk factors of heart failure: rationale for preventive strategies and comprehensive disease management. *Am Heart J.* 1997; 133:703–712.
5. Adams KF, Fonarow GC, Emerman CL, et al. Characteristics and outcomes of patients hospitalized for heart failure in the United States: Rationale, design, and preliminary observations from the first 100,000 cases in the Acute Decompensated Heart Failure National Registry (ADHERE). *Am Heart J.* 2005;149: 209–216.
6. Aghababian RV. Acutely decompensated heart failure: opportunities to improve care and outcomes in the emergency department. *Rev Cardiovasc Med.* 2002;3(Suppl. 4):S3–S9.
7. Ferguson JA, Sundablad KJ, Becker PK, et al. Role and duration of diuretic effect in preventing sodium retention. *Clin Pharmacol Ther.* 1997;62:203–208.
8. Ellison DH. Diuretic therapy and resistance in congestive heart failure. *Cardiology.* 2001;96:132–143.
9. Brater DC. Diuretic therapy. *N Engl J Med.* 1998;339:387–395.
10. Kittleson M, Hurwitz S, Shah MR, et al. Development of circulatory-renal limitations to angiotensin-converting enzyme inhibitors identifies patients with severe heart failure and early mortality. *J Am Coll Cardiol.* 2003;41:2029–2035.
11 Weinfeld MS, Chertow GM, Stevenson LW. Aggravated renal dysfunction during intensive therapy for advanced chronic heart failure. *Am Heart J.* 1999;138:285–290.

12. Pitt B, Zannad F, Remme WJ, Cody R, et al. for the Randomized Aldosterone Evaluation Study Investigators. The effect of spironolactone on morbidity and mortality in patients with severe heart failure. *N Engl J Med.* 1999;341:709–717.
13. Juurlink, DN, Mamdani MM, Lee DS, et al. Rates of hyperkalemia after publication of the Randomized Aldactone Evaluation Study. *N Engl J Med.* 2004;351:543–551.
14. Mehta RL, Pascual MT, Soroko S, et al. for the PICARD Study Group. Diuretics, mortality and non recovery of renal function in acute heart failure. *JAMA.* 2002;288:2547–2553.
15. Philbin EF, Cotto M, Rocco TA, Jr., Jenkins PL. Association between diuretic use, clinical response and death in acute heart failure. *Am J Cardiol.* 1997;80:519–522.
16. Sarnak MJ, Levey AS, Schoolworth AC, et al. Kidney disease as a risk factor for the development of cardiovascular disease. A statement from the American Heart Association Councils on Kidney in Cardiovascular Disease, High Blood Pressure Research, Clinical Cardiology, and Epidemiology and Prevention. *Circulation.* 2003;108:2154–2169.
17. Fried LF, Shlipak MG, Crump C, et al. Renal insufficiency as a predictor of cardiovascular outcomes and mortality in elderly individuals. *J Am Coll Cardiol.* 2003;41:1364–1372.
18. Mahon NG, Blackstone EH, Francis GS, et al. The prognostic value of estimated creatinine clearance alongside functional capacity in ambulatory patients with chronic congestive heart failure. *J Am Coll Cardiol.* 2002;40:1106–1113.
19. Mann JFE, Gerstein HC, Pogue J, et al.; for the HOPE Investigators. Renal insufficiency as a predictor of cardiovascular outcomes and the impact of ramipril: the HOPE randomized trial. *Ann Intern Med.* 2001:134:629–636.
20. Mcclellan WM, Flanders WD, Langston RD, et al.; Anemia and renal insufficiency are independent risk factors for death among patients with congestive heart failure admitted to community hospitals: a population-based study. *J Am Soc Nephrol.* 2002;13:1928–1936.
21. Ahmad A, Rand WM, Manjunath G, et al. Reduced kidney function and anemia as risk factors for mortality with left ventricular dysfunction. *J Am Coll Cardiol.* 2001;38:955–962.
22. Chae CU, Albert CM, Glynn RJ, et al. Mild renal insufficiency and risk of congestive heart failure in men and women ≥ 70 years of age. *Am J Cardiol.* 2003;92:682–686.
23. Hillege HL, Girbes ARJ, de Kam PJ, et al. Renal function, neurohormonal activation, and survival in patients with chronic heart failure. *Circulation.* 2000;102:203–210.
24. Krumholz HM, Chen YT, Vaccarino V, et al. Correlates and impact on outcomes of worsening renal function in patients ≥ 65 years of age with heart failure. *Am J Cardiol.* 2000;85:1110–1113.
25. Dries DL, Exner DV, Domanski MD, et al. The prognostic implications of renal insufficiency in asymptomatic and symptomatic patients with left ventricular systolic dysfunction. *J Am Coll Cardiol.* 2000;35:681–689.
26. Knight EL, Glynn RJ, McIntyre KM, et al. Predictors of decreased renal function in patients with heart failure during angiotensin-converting enzyme inhibitor therapy: results from the Studies of Left Ventricular Dysfunction (SOLVD). *Am Heart J.* 1999; 138:849–855.
27. Butler J, Forman DE, Abraham WT, et al. Relationship between heart failure treatment and development of worsening renal function among hospitalized patients. *Am Heart J.* 2004;147:331–338.
28. Domanski M, Norman J, Pitt B, et al. Diuretic use, progressive heart failure, and death in patients in the Studies Of Left Ventricular Dysfunction (SOLVD). *J Am Coll Cardiol.* 2003;42:705–708.
29. Cooper HA, Dries DL, Davis CE, et al. Diuretics and risk of arrhythmic death in patients with left ventricular dysfunction (SOLVD). *Circulation.* 1999;100:1311–1315.
30. Neuberg GW, Miller AB, O'Connor CM, et al. for the PRAISE Investigators. Prospective Randomized Amlodipine Survival Evaluation. Diuretic resistance predicts mortality in patients with advanced heart failure. *Am Heart J.* 2002;144:31–38.
31. Francis GS, Benedict C, Johnstone DE, et al., Comparison of neuroendocrine activation in patients with left ventricular dysfunction with and without congestive heart failure. A substudy of the Studies Of Left ventricular Dysfunction (SOLVD). *Circulation.* 1990;82:1724–1729.
32. Gottlieb SS, Brater DC, Thomas I, et al. BG9719 (CVT-124), an A_1 adenosine receptor antagonist, protects against the decline in renal function observed with diuretic therapy. *Circulation.* 2002;105:1348–1353.
33. Hawkins RG, Houston MC. Is population-wide diuretic use directly associated with the incidence of end-stage renal disease in the United States? *Am J Hypertens.* 2005;18:744–749.
34. Canaud B, Leblanc M, Leray-Moragues H, et al. Slow continuous ultrafiltration for refractory congestive heart failure. *Nephrol Dial Transplant.* 1998;13(Suppl 4):51–55.
35. Cadnapaphornchai MA, Gurevich AK, Weinberger HD, et al. Pathophysiology of sodium and water retention in heart failure. *Cardiology.* 2001;96:122–131.
36. Schrier RW, Abraham WT. Hormones and hemodynamics in heart failure. *N Engl J Med.* 1999;341:577–585.
37. Bellomo R, Ronco C. The kidney in heart failure. *Kidney Int.* 1998;53(Suppl 66):S58–S61.
38. Walter SJ, Shirley DG. The effect of chronic hydrochlorothiazide administration on renal function in the rat. *Clin Sci.* 1986;70:379–387.
39. Ellison DH, Velazquez H, Wright FS. Adaptation of the distal convoluted tubule of the rat: structural and functional effects of dietary salt intake and chronic diuretic infusion. *J Clin Invest.* 1989;83:113–126.
40. Loon NR, Wilcox CS, Unwin RJ. Mechanism of impaired natriuretic response to furosemide during prolonged therapy. *Kidney. Int.* 1989:36:682–689.
41. Ronco C, Ricci Z, Bellomo R, Bedogni F. Extracorporeal ultrafiltration for the treatment of overhydration and congestive heart failure. *Cardiology.* 2001:96:155–168.
42. Clark WR, Macias WL, Molitoris BA, et al. Plasma protein adsorption to highly permeable hemodialysis membranes. *Kidney Int.* 1995;48:481–488.
43. Clark WR, Hamburger RJ, Lysaght MJ. Effect of membrane composition and structure on solute removal and biocompatility in hemodialysis. *Kidney Int.* 1999;56:2005–2015.
44. Ronco C, Ghezzi P, Bellomo R, et al. New perspectives in the treatment of acute renal failure. *Blood Purif.* 1999;17:166–172.
45. Paganini EP, Flague J, Whiman G, et al. Amino acid balance in patients with oliguric renal failure undergoing slow continuous ultrafiltration (SCUF). *Trans Am Soc Artif Intern Org.* 1982;28:615–620.
46. Kaplan AA, Longnecker RE, Folkert VW. Continuous venous hemofiltration—a report of six months' experience. *Ann Intern Med.* 1984;100:358–367.
47. Golper TA, Wedel SK, Kaplan AA, et al. Drug removal during continuous arteriovenous haemofiltration: theory and clinical observations. *Int J Artif Org.* 1985;8:307–312.
48. Golper TA. Drug removal during continuous hemofiltration. *Contrib Nephrol.* 1991;93:110–116.
49. Ronco C, Bellomo R. *Critical Care Nephrology.* Dodrecht: Kluwer Academic; 1998.
50. Metha RL. Fluid management in CRRT. *Contrib Nephrol.* 2001;132:335–348.
51. Ronco C, Brendolan A, Dan M, et al. Machines for continuous renal replacement therapy. *Contrib Nephrol.* 2001;132: 323–334.
52. Marenzi GC, Lauri G, Grazi M, et al. Circulatory response to fluid overload removal by extracorporeal ultrafiltration in refractory congestive heart failure. *J Am Coll Cardiol.* 2001;38:963–968.
53. Teo KK, Basile C, Ulan RA, et al. Effects of hemodialysis and hypertonic hemodiafiltration on cardiac function compared. *Kidney Int.* 1987;32:399–407.
54. Schuenemann B, Borghardt J, Falda Z, et al. Reactions of blood pressure and body spaces to hemofiltration treatment. *Trans Am Soc Artif Org.* 1978;24:687–689.
55. Kimura G, Irie A, Kuroda K, et al. Absence of transcellular fluid shift during haemofiltration. *Proc Eur Dialysis Tranplant Assoc.* 1980;17:192–196.
56. Dileo M, Pacitti A, Bergerone S, et al. Ultrafiltration in the treatment of refractory heart failure. *Clin Cardiol.* 1988;11: 449–459.
57. Quellhorst E, Schuenemann B, Hidebrand U, et al. Response of the vascular system to different modification of ultrafiltration. *Proc Eur Dialysis Tranplant Assoc.* 1980;17:197–204.

58. Baldamus CA, Ernst W, Frei U, et al. Sympathetic and haemodynamic response to volume removal during different forms of renal replacement therapy. *Nephron*. 1982;31:324–332.
59. Paganini EP, Fouad F, Tarazi RC, et al. Hemodynamics of isolated ultrafiltration in chronic hemodialysis patients. *Trans Am Soc Artif Intern Org*. 1979;25:422–425.
60. Zucchelli P, Santoro A, Sturani A, et al. Effects of hemodialysis and hemofiltration on the autonomic control of circulation. *Trans Am Soc Artif Intern Org*. 1984;30:163–167.
61. Chen WT, Chaignon M, Omvik P, et al. Hemodynamic studies in chronic hemodialysis patients with haemofiltration/ultrafiltration. *Trans Am Soc Artif Intern Org*. 1978;24:682–686.
62. Asaba H, Bergstrom J, Furst P, et al. Treatment of diuretic resistant fluid retention with ultrafiltration. *Acta Med Scand*. 1978;204:145–149.
63. Morgan SH, Mansell MA, Thompson FD. Fluid removal by haemofiltration in diuretic resistant cardiac failure. *Br Heart J*. 1985;55:218–219.
64. Simpson IA, Rae AP, Simpson K, et al. Ultrafiltration in the management of refractory congestive heart failure. *Br Heart J*. 1986;55:344–347.
65. Fauchauld P, Forfang K, Amlie J. An evaluation of ultrafiltration as treatment of therapy resistant cardiac edema. *Acta Med Scand*. 1986;219:47–52.
66. Donato L, Biagini A, Contini C, et al. Treatment of end-stage congestive heart failure by extracorporeal ultrafiltration. *Am J Cardiol*. 1987;59:379–380.
67. Rimondini A, Cipolla CM, Della Bella P, et al. Hemofiltration as short-term treatment for refractory congestive heart failure. *Am J Med*. 1987;83:43–48.
68. L'Abbate A, Emdin M, Piacenti M, et al. Ultrafiltration: a rational treatment for heart failure. *Cardiology*. 1989;76:384–390.
69. Cipolla CM, Grazi S, Rimondini A, et al. Changes in circulating norepinephrine with hemofiltration in advanced congestive heart failure. *Am J Cardiol*. 1990;66:987–994.
70. Canaud B, Cristol JP, Klouche K, et al. Slow continuous ultrafiltration: a means of unmasking myocardial functional reserve in end stage cardiac disease. *Contrib Nephrol*. 1991;93:79–85.
71. Kramer P, Kaufhold G, Grone HJ, et al. Management of anuric intensive care patients with arteriovenous hemofiltration. *Int J Artif Org*. 1980;3:225–230.
72. Paganini EP, Nakamoto S. Continuous ultrafiltration in oliguric renal failure. *Trans Am Soc Artif Intern Org*. 1980;26:201–204.
73. Lepape A, Bene B, Pedrix JP, et al. Double pump driven continuous haemofiltration (CVVH). In: Siebert HG, Mann H, eds. *Continuous Arteriovenous Haemofiltration*. Basel: S Karger; 1985: 53–58.
74. Lauer A, Sacaggi A, Ronco C, et al. Continuous arteriovenous hemofiltration in critically ill patients. *Ann Intern Med*. 1983;99:455–460.
75. Henderson AW, Donald LL, Levin NW. Clinical use of Amicon Diafilter. *Dialysis Transplant*. 1983;12:523–525.
76. Synhaivsky A, Kurtz SB, Wochos DN, et al. Acute renal failure treated by slow continuous ultrafiltration: preliminary report. *Mayo Clin Proc*. 1983;58:729–733.
77. van Geelen JA, Vincent HH, Schalekamp MADH. Continuous arteriovenous haemofiltration and haemodiafiltration in acute renal failure. *Nephrol Dialysis Transplant*. 1988;2:181–186.
78. Kramer BK, Schweda F, Riegger GAJ. Diuretic treatment and diuretic resistance in heart failure. *Am J Med*. 1999;106:90–96.
79. Bayliss J, Norell M, Canepa-Anson R, et al. Marked activation of the renin angiotensin aldosterone system by loop diuretics. *Br Heart J*. 1987:57:17–22.
80. Silverstein ME, Ford CA, Lysaght MJ, et al. Treatment of severe volume overload by ultrafiltration. *N Engl J Med*. 1974; 291:747–751.
81. Gerhardt RE, Abdulla AM, Mach SJ, et al. Isolated ultrafiltration in the treatment of fluid overload in cardiogenic shock. *Arch Intern Med*. 1979;139:358–359.
82. Simpson RA, Simpson K, Rae AP, et al. Ultrafiltration in diuretic-resistant cardiac failure. *Ren Fail*. 1987;10:115–119.
83. Marenzi G, Grazi S, Lauri G, et al. Interrelation of humoral factors, hemodynamics and fluid and salt metabolism in congestive heart failure: effects of extracorporeal ultrafiltration. *Am J Med*. 1993;94:49–56.
84. Bergerone S, Golzio PG, Pacitti A. Atrial natriuretic factor and concomitant hormonal, hemodynamic and renal function changes after slow continuous ultrafiltration. *Int J Cardiol*. 1992;36:305–307.
85. Blake P, Hasewaga Y, Khosla MC, et al. Isolation of "myocardial depressant factor(s)" from the ultrafiltrate of heart failure patients with acute renal failure. *ASAIO J*. 1996;42:M911–M915.
86. Burchardi H. History and development of continuous renal replacement techniques. *Kidney Int*. 1998;66(Suppl):S120–S124.
87. Agostoni PG, Marenzi GC, Sganzerla P, et al. Lung-heart interaction as a substrate for the improvement in exercise capacity following body fluid volume depletion in moderate congestive heart failure. *Am J Cardiol*. 1995;76:793–798.
88. Agostoni PG, Butler J. Cardiopulmonary interaction in exercise. In: Whipp BJ, Wasserman K, eds. *Exercise: Pulmonary Physiology and Pathophysiology*. New York: Dekker; 1991: 221–252.
89. Agostoni PG, Marenzi GC, Pepi M, et al. Isolated ultrafiltration in moderate heart failure. *J Am Coll Cardiol*. 1993;21:424–431.
90. Marenzi GC, Agostoni PG, Guazzi MD, et al. The noradrenaline plasma concentration and its gradient across the lung. *Eur J Clin Invest*. 2000;30:660–667.
91. Marenzi GC, Lauri G, Guazzi MD, et al. Ultrafiltration in moderate heart failure: exercise oxygen uptake as a predictor of the clinical benefit. *Chest*. 1995;108:94–98.
92. Agostoni PG, Marenzi GC, Lauri G, et al. Sustained improvement in functional capacity after removal of body fluid with isolated ultrafiltration in chronic cardiac insufficiency: failure of furosemide to provide the same result. *Am J Med*. 1994;96:191–199.
93. Agostoni PG, Guazzi M, Bussotti M, et al. Lack of improvement of lung diffusing capacity following fluid withdrawal by ultrafiltration in chronic heart failure. *J Am Coll Cardiol*. 2000;36:1600–1604.
94. Agostoni PG, Marenzi GC, Pepi M, et al. Changes in the physical characteristics of the lung can account for the improvement observed after ultrafiltration in patients with moderate heart failure. *Cardiologia*. 1993;38:425–429.
95. Marenzi GC, Grazi M, Susini G, et al. Intra- and extravascular volumes in congestive heart failure and their redistribution following extracorporeal ultrafiltration. *Cardiologia*. 1998; 43:1193–1200.
95. Wasserman K, Zhang Y, Gitt A, et al. Lung function and exercise gas exchange in chronic heart failure. *Circulation*. 1997;96: 2221–2227.
96. Agostoni PG, Cattadori G, Guazzi M, et al. Cardiomegaly as a possible cause of lung dysfunction in patients with heart failure. *Am Heart J*. 2006;140:E24–E28.
97. Agostoni PG, Marenzi GC. Sustained benefit from ultrafiltration in moderate congestive heart failure. *Cardiology*. 2001;96: 183–189.
98. Johnson BD, Beck KC, Olson LJ, et al. Ventilatory constraints during exercise in patients with chronic heart failure. *Chest*. 2000;117:321–332.
99. Canaud B, Leray-Moragues H, Garred, et al. Slow isolated ultrafiltration for the treatment of congestive heart failure. *Am J Kidney Dis*. 1996;28(Suppl):S67–S73.
100. Agostoni PG, Marenzi GC, Guazzi M. Influence of ACE inhibition on fluid metabolism in chronic heart failure and its pathophysiologic relevance. *J Cardiovasc Pharmacol Ther*. 1996;1: 279–286.
101. Marenzi GC, Lauri G. Assanelli E. The influence of ACEI inhibitors on urinary electrolyte secretion and the response to transitory hypovolemia in chronic heart failure. *Cardiologia*. 1997;42:1277–1283.
102. Cody RJ, Laragh JH. Use of captopril to estimate renin-angiotensin-aldosterone activity in the pathophysiology of chronic heart failure. *Am Heart J*. 1982;104:1184–1189.
103. Blake P, Paganini EP. Refractory congestive heart failure: overview and application of extracorporeal ultrafiltration. *Adv Ren Replac Ther*. 1996;166–173.
104. Coraim FI, Wolner E. Continuous hemofiltration for the failing heart. *New Horiz*. 1995;3:725–731.
105. Bellomo R, Ronco C. Indications and criteria for initiating renal replacement therapy in the intensive care unit. *Kidney Int*. 1998;66(Suppl):S106–S109.

106. Schetz MRC. Classical and alternative indications for continuous renal replacement therapy. *Kidney Int.* 1998;66(Suppl): S129–S132.
107. Manns M, Siglar MH, Teehan BP. Continuous renal replacement therapies: an update. *Am J Kidney Dis.* 1998;32:185–207.
108. Ronco C, Bellomo R. Continuous renal replacement therapy: evolution in technology and current nomenclature. *Kidney Int.* 1998:66(Suppl):S160–S164.
109. Bellomo R, Farmer M, Parkin G, et al. Severe acute renal failure: a comparison of acute continuous hemodiafiltration and conventional dialytic therapy. *Nephron.* 1995;71:59–64.
110. Ronco C. Continuous renal replacement therapies in the treatment of acute renal failure in intensive care patients. 2. Clinical indications and prescription. *Nephrol Dial Transplant.* 1994;9(Suppl 4):201–209.
111. Bellomo R, Metha RL. Acute renal replacement in the intensive care unit: now and tomorrow. *New Horiz.* 1995;3:761–767.
112. Bellomo R, Ronco C. Continuous versus intermittent renal replacement therapy in the intensive care unit. *Kidney Int.* 1998;66(Suppl):S125–S128.
113. Schetz M. Non-renal indications for continuous renal replacement therapy. *Kidney Int.* 1999;72(Suppl):S88–S94.
114. Meyer MM. Renal replacement therapies. *Crit Care Clin.* 2000;16:29–58.
115. Bellomo R, Ronco C. Renal dysfunction in patients with cardiac disease and after cardiac surgery. *New Horiz.* 1999;7: 524–532.
116. Bellomo R, Raman J, Ronco C. Intensive care unit management of critically ill patients with fluid overload after open heart surgery. *Cardiology.* 2001;96:169–176.
117. Boyle EM, Prohlman TH, Johnson MC, et al. Endothelial cell injury in cardiovascular surgery: the systemic inflammatory response. *Ann Thorac Surg.* 1997;63:277–284.
118. Journois D, Pouard P, Greeley WJ, et al. Hemofiltration during cardiopulmonary bypass in pediatric cardiac surgery. Effects on hemostasis, cytokines and complement components. *Anesthesiology.* 1994;81:1181–1189.
119. Bellomo R, Tipping P, Boyce N. Continuous veno-venous hemofiltration with dialysis removes cytokines from the circulation of septic patients. *Crit Care Med.* 1993;21:522–526.
120. Bellomo R, McGrath B, Boyce N. Effect of continuous veno-venous hemofiltration with dialysis on hormone and catecholamine clearance in critically ill patients with acute renal failure. *Crit Care Med.* 1994;22:833–837.
121. Bouduin SV, Wiggins, Keogh BF, et al. Continuous veno-venous hemofiltration following cardio-pulmonary bypass. Indications and outcome in 35 patients. *Intensive Care Med.* 1993;19: 290–293.
122. Levy B, Clavey M, Burtin P, et al. Continuous veno-venous hemofiltration after cardiac surgery. A retrospective study in 16 patients with multiple organ failure. *Ann Fr Anesth Reanim.* 1992;11:436–441.
123. Tsang GMK, Dar M, Clayton D, et al. Hemofiltration in a cardiac intensive care unit: time for a rational approach. *ASAIO J.* 1996;42:M710–M713.
124. Bent P, Tan HK, Bellomo R, et al. Early and intensive continuous hemofiltration for severe renal failure after cardiac surgery. *Ann Thorac Surg.* 2001;71:832–837.
125. Kramer P, Wigger W, Rieger J, et al. Arteriovenous haemofiltration: a new and simple method for treatment of overhydrated patients resistant to diuretics. *Klin Wochenschr.* 1977;55: 1121–1122.
126. Kramer P, Buhler J, Kehr A, et al. Intensive care potential of continuous arteriovenous hemofiltration. *Trans Am Soc Artif Intern Org.* 1982;28:28–32.
127. Grone HJ, Kramer P. Puncture and long term cannulation of the femoral artery and vein in adults. In: Kramer P, ed. *Arteriovenous Hemofiltration.* Berlin: Springer-Verlag; 1985: 35–47.
128. Olbricht CJ, Schurek HJ, Stolte H, et al. The influence of vascular access mode on the efficiency of CAVH. In: Sieberth HG, Mann H, eds. *Continuous Arteriovenous Hemofiltration.* Basel: S Karger; 1985: 14–24.
129. Darup J, Bleese N, Kalmar P, et al. Hemofiltration during extracorporeal circulation (ECC). *Thorac Cardiovasc Surg.* 1979; 27:277–230.
130. Paganini EP, O'Hara P, Nakamoto S. Slow continuous ultrafiltration in hemodialysis resistant oliguric acute renal failure patients. *Trans Am Soc Artif Intern Org.* 1984;30:173–177.
131. Ing TS, Asbach DL, Kanter A, et al. Fluid removal with negative-pressure hydrostatic ultrafiltration using a partial vacuum. *Nephron.* 1975:14:451–455.
132. Bergstrom J, Asaba H, Furst P, et al. Dialysis, ultrafiltration and blood pressure. *Proc Eur Dialysis Transplant Assoc.* 1976;13: 293–305.
133. Henrich WL, Woodard TD, Blachley JD, et al. Role of osmolality in blood pressure stability after dialysis and ultrafiltration. *Kidney Int.* 1980;18:480–488.
134. Swartz RD, Somermeyer MG, Hsu CH. Preservation of plasma volume during hemodialysis depends on dialysate osmolality. *Am J Nephrol.* 1982;2:189–194.
135. Fleming SJ, Wilkinson JS, Greenwood RN, et al. Effect of dialysate composition on intercompartment fluid shift. *Kidney Int.* 1987;32:267–273.
136. Fleming SJ, Wilkinson JS, Greenwood RN, et al. Blood volume changes during isolated ultrafiltration and combined ultrafiltration-dialysis. *Nephrol Dialysis Transplant.* 1988;32:272–276.
137. Lazarus JM, Henderson LW, Kjellstrand CM, et al. Panel conference: cardiovascular instability during hemodialysis. *Trans Am Soc Artif Intern Org.* 1982;28:656–665.
138. Henderson LW. Symptomatic hypotension during dialysis. *Kidney Int.* 1980;17:571–576.
139. Keshaviah P, Shapiro FL. A critical examination of dialysis-induced hypotension. *Am J Kidney Dis.* 1982;2:290–301.
140. Golpert A, Kaplan AA, Narashiman N, et al. Transmembrane pressure generated by filtrate line suction maneuvers and predilution fluid replacement during in vitro continuous arteriovenous hemofiltration. *Int J Artif Org.* 1987;10:41–46.
141. Scribner BH, Caner JEZ, Buri R, et al. The technique of continuous hemodialysis. *Trans Am Soc Artif Intern Org.* 1960;6: 88–103.
142. Ronco C, Brendolan A, Bragantini L, et al. Studies on blood flow dynamic and ultrafiltration kinetics during continuous arteriovenous hemofiltration. *Blood Purif.* 1986;4:220.
143. Ronco C, Brendolan A, Bragantini L, et al. Continuous arteriovenous hemofiltration. *Contrib Nephrol.* 1985;48:70–88.
144. Olbricht CJ, Schurek HJ, Tytul S, et al. Comparison between Scribner shunt and femoral catheters as vascular access for continuous arteriovenous hemofiltration. In: Kramer P, ed. *Arteriovenous Hemofiltration.* Berlin: Springer-Verlag; 1985: 57–66.
145. Pallone TL, Peterson J. Continuous arteriovenous hemofiltration: an in vitro simulation and mathematical model. *Kidney Int.* 1988;33:685–698.
146. Ronco C, Bosch JP, Lew S, et al. Technician and clinical evaluation of a new hemofilter for CAVH: theoretical concepts and practical application of a different flow geometry. In: Fabris LA, Ronco C, eds. Proceedings of the international symposium on continuous arteriovenous hemofiltration. Milan: Witchig Editore; 1986: 55–61.
147. Bosh JP, Geronemus R, Glabman S, et al. High flux hemofiltration. *Artif Org.* 1978;2:339–342.
148. Kaplan AA, Longnecker RE, Folkert VW. Suction-assisted continuous arteriovenous hemofiltration. *Trans Am Soc Artif Intern Org.* 1983;29:408–413.
149. Iorio L, Simonelli R, Nacca R, et al. Daily hemofiltration in severe heart failure. *Kidney Int.* 1997;51:S62–S65.
150. Dormans T, Huige R, Gerlag P. Chronic intermittent haemofiltration and haemodialysis in end stage chronic heart failure refractory to high dose furosemide. *Heart.* 1996;75:349–351.
151. Pepi M, Marenzi GC, Agostoni PG, et al. Sustained cardiac diastolic changes elicited by ultrafiltration in patients with moderate congestive heart failure: pathophysiological correlates. *Br Heart J.* 1993;70:135–140.
152. Kishore K, Yagi N, Paganinini E. Renal replacement therapy in congestive heart failure. *Semin Dialysis.* 1997;10:259–266.
153. Wehle B, Asaba H, Castenfors J, et al. Haemodynamic changes during sequential ultrafiltration and dialysis. *Kidney Int.* 1979;15:411–418.
154. Guazzi M, Agostoni P, Perego B. Apparent paradox of neurohumoral axis inhibition after body fluid volume depletion in

patients with congestive heart failure and water retention. *Br Heart J*. 1994;72:534–539.

155. Jaski BE, Ha J, Denys BG, et al. Peripherally inserted veno-venous ultrafiltration for rapid treatment of volume overloaded patients. *J Card Fail*. 2003;9:227–231.
156. Costanzo MR, Saltzberg MT, O'Sullivan JE, et al. Early ultrafiltration in patients with decompensated heart failure and diuretic resistance *J Am Coll Cardiol*. 2005;46:2047–2051.
157. Bart BA, Boyle A, Bank AJ, et al. Randomized controlled trial of ultrafiltration versus usual care for hospitalized patients with heart failure: relief for acutely fluid overloaded patients with decompensated congestive heart failure. *J Am Coll Cardiol*. 2005;46:2043–2046.
158. United States Renal Data System, Bethesda, MD. U.S. Department of Health and Human Services, Public Health Service, National Institutes of Health, 2000.
159. Kjellerstrand C, Ting G. Daily hemodialysis for the next century. *Adv Ren Repl Ther*. 1998;5:267–274.
160. Anderson CB, Codd JR, Graff RA. Cardiac failure and upper extremity arteriovenous dialysis fistulas. *Arch Intern Med*. 1976;136:292–297.
161. Pourchez T, Moriniere P, Fournier A, et al. Use of Permacath (Quinton) catheter in uraemic patients in whom creation of conventional vascular access for haemodialysis is difficult. *Nephron*. 1989;53:297–302.
162. Leblanc M, Bosc JY, Paganini EP, et al. Central venous dialysis catheter dysfunction. *Adv Renal Repl Ther*. 1997;4:377–389.
163. Rippe B, Stelin G. Simulations of peritoneal solute transport during CAPD. Application of two-pore formalism. *Kidney Int*. 1989;35:1234–1244.
164. Rippe B, Stelin G, Haraldsson B. Computer simulations of peritoneal fluid transport in CAPD. *Kidney Int*. 1991;40:315–325.
165. Pannekeet MM, Mulder JB, Weening JJ, et al. Demonstration of aquaporin-CHIP in peritoneal tissue of uremic and CAPD patients. *Perit Dial Int*. 1996;16(Suppl):S54–S57.
166. Devuyst O, Nielsen S, Cosyns JP, et al. Aquaporin-1 and endothelial nitric oxide synthase expression in capillary endothelia of human peritoneum. *Am J Physiol*. 1998;275:H234–H242.
167. Yang B, Folkesson HG, Yang J, et al. Reduced osmotic water permeability of the peritoneal barrier in aquaporin-1 knockout mice. *Am J Physiol*. 1999;276:C76–C81.
168. Henderson LW. Peritoneal ultrafiltration dialysis: enhanced urea transfer using hypertonic peritoneal dialysis fluid. *J Clin Invest*. 1966;45:950–955.
169. Nolph HD, Hano JE, Teschan PE. Peritoneal sodium transport during hypertonic peritoneal dialysis. Physiologic mechanisms and clinical implications. *Ann Intern Med*. 1969;70:931–941.
170. Chen TW, Khanna R, Moore H, et al. Sieving and reflection coefficients for sodium salts and glucose during peritoneal dialysis in rats. *J Am Soc Nephrol*. 1991;2:1092–1100.
171. Nolph KD, Mactier R, Khanna R, et al. The kinetics of ultrafiltration during peritoneal dialysis:the role of lymphatics. *Kidney Int*. 1987;32:219–226.
172. Twardowski ZJ, Khanna R, Nolph KD. Osmotic agents and ultrafiltration in peritoneal dialysis. *Nephron*. 1986;42:93–101.
173. Imholz Al, Koomen GC, Struijk DG, et al. Effect of dialysate osmolarity on the transport of low molecular weight solutes and proteins during CAPD. *Kidney Int*. 1993;43:1339–1346.
174. Heimburger O, Waniewski J, Werynski A, et al. A quantitative description of solute and fluid transport during peritoneal dialysis. *Kidney Int*. 1992;41:1320–1332.
175. Twardowski ZJ, Nolph KD, Khanna R. Peritoneal equilibration test. *Perit Dial Bull*. 1987;7:138–147.
176. Frank HA, Seligman AM, Fine J. Treatment of uremia after acute renal failure by peritoneal dialysis. *JAMA*. 1976;130:703–705.
177. Odel HM, Ferris DO, Power H. Peritoneal lavage as an effective means of external excretion. *Am J Med*. 1950;9:63–77.
178. Maxwell MH, Rockney RE, Kleeman CR, et al. Peritoneal dialysis. 1. Technique and application. *JAMA*. 1959;170:917–924.
179. Vaamonde CA, Michael YF, Metzger RA, et al. Complications of acute peritoneal dialysis. *J Chron Dis*. 1975;28:637–659.
180. Miller RB, Tassistro CR. Peritoneal dialysis. *N Engl J Med*. 1969;281:945–949.
181. Steiner RW. Continuous equilibrium peritoneal dialysis in acute renal failure. *Perit Dial Int*. 1989;9:5–7.
182. Smeby LC, Wideroe TE, Orstad S. Individual differences in water transport during continuous peritoneal dialysis. *Am Soc Artif Intern Org*. 1981;4:17–27.
183. Rubin J, Nolph KD, Popovich RP, et al. Drainage volume during continuous ambulatory peritoneal dialysis. *Am Soc Artif Intern Org*. 1979;2:54–60.
184. Rubin J, Adair C, Barnes T, et al. Dialysate flow rate and peritoneal clearance. *Am J Kidney Dis*. 1984;4:260–267.
185. Gotlib L, Mines M, Garmizo L, et al. Hemodynamic effects of increasing intra abdominal pressure in peritoneal dialysis. *Perit Dialysis Bull*. 1981;1:41–43.
186. Blumberg A, Keller R, Marti HR. Oxygen affinity of erythrocytes and pulmonary gas exchange in patients on continuous ambulatory peritoneal dialysis. *Nephron*. 1984;38:248–252.
187. Schneierson SJ. Continuous peritoneal irrigation in the treatment of intractable edema of cardiac origin. *Am J Med Sci*. 1949;218:76–79.
188. Mailloux LU, Swartz CD, Onesti G, et al. Peritoneal dialysis for refractory congestive heart failure. *JAMA*. 1967:199:873–878.
189. Cairns KB, Porter GA, Kloster FE, et al. Clinical and hemodynamic results of peritoneal dialysis for severe cardiac failure. *Am Heart J*. 1968;76:227–234.
190. Raja RM, Krasnoff SO, Moros JG, et al. Repeated peritoneal dialysis in treatment of heart failure. *JAMA*. 1970:213:2268–2269.
191. Malach M. Peritoneal dialysis for intractable heart failure in acute myocardial infarction. *Am J Cardiol*. 1972;29:61–63.
192. Shapira J, Lang R, Jutrin I, et al. Peritoneal dialysis in refractory congestive heart failure I: Intermittent peritoneal dialysis. *Perit Dialysis Bull*. 1983;3:130–132.
193. Robson M, Bira A, Knobel B, et al. Peritoneal dialysis in refractory congestive heart failure. 2. Continuous ambulatory peritoneal dialysis. *Perit Dial Bull*. 1983;3:133–134.
194. Weinrauch LA, Kaldany A, Miller DG, et al. Cardiorenal failure treatment of refractory biventricular failure by peritoneal dialysis. *Uremia Invest*. 1984;8:1–8.
195. Kim D, Khanna R, Wu G, et al. Successful use of peritoneal dialysis in refractory heart failure. *Perit Dial Bull*. 1985;5: 127–130.
196. Mc Kinnie JJ, Bourgeois RJ, Husserl FE. Long term therapy for heart failure with continuous ambulatory peritoneal dialysis. *Arch Intern Med*. 1985;145:1128–1129.
197. Rubin J, Ball R. Continuous ambulatory peritoneal dialysis as treatment for severe congestive heart failure in the face of chronic renal failure. Report of eight cases. *Arch Intern Med*. 1986;146:1533–1535.
198. Konig PS, Lhotta K, Kronenberg F, et al. CAPD: a successful treatment in patients suffering from therapy-resistant congestive heart failure. *Adv Perit Dial*. 1991;7:97–101.
199. Stablein DM, Hamburger RJ, Linblad AS, et al. The effect of CAPD on hypertension control: a report of the national CAPD registry. *Perit Dial Int*. 1988;8:141–144.
200. Cannata JB, Isles CG, Briggs JD, et al. Comparison of blood pressure control during hemodialysis and CAPD. *Dialysis Transplant*. 1986;15:674–679.
201. Berlyne GM, Lee HA, Ralston AJ, Woodcock JA. Pulmonary complications of peritoneal dialysis. *Lancet*. 1966;3:75–78.
202. Taveira Da Silva AM, Davis WB, Winchester JE, et al. Peritonitis, dialysate infusion and lung function in continuous ambulatory peritoneal dialysis (CAPD). *Clin Nephrol*. 1985;24;79–83.
203. Epstein SW, Inouye T, Robson M, et al. Effect of peritoneal dialysis fluid on ventilatory function. *Perit Dialysis Bull*. 1982;2:120–122.
204. Gomez-Fernandez P, Sanchez-Agudo L, Calatrave JM, et al. Respiratory muscle weakness in uremic patients under continuous ambulatory peritoneal dialysis. *Nephron*. 1984;36:219–223.
205. Gault MH, Ferguson EL, Sidhu JS, et al. Fluid and electrolyte complications of peritoneal dialysis. *Ann Intern Med*. 1971;75:253–262.
206. Ash SR, Handt AE, Bloch R. Peritoneoscopic placement of the Tenckoff catheter: further clinical experience. *Perit Dialysis Bull*. 1983;3:8–12.
207. Burns RO. Peritoneal dialysis: clinical experience. *N Engl J Med*. 1962;267:1060–1064.
208. Barry KG, Schwartz FD. Peritoneal dialysis: current status and future applications. *Pediatr Clin North Am*. 1964:11:593.

209. Lund HG, Hughes RK. Peritoneal dialysis before cardiac surgery. *Ann Thorac Surg.* 1967:4:470–473.
210. Rae AI, Hopper J, Jr. Removal of peripheral oedema fluid by peritoneal dialysis. *Br J Urol.* 1968;40:336–343.
211. Chopra MP, Gulati RB, Portal RW, et al. Peritoneal dialysis for pulmonary oedema after acute myocardial infarction. *Br Med J.* 1970;3:77–80.
212. Shilo S, Slotki IN, Iaina A. Improved renal function following acute peritoneal dialysis in patients with intractable congestive heart failure. *Isr J Med Sci.* 1987;23:821–824.
213. Mousson C, Tanter Y, Chalopin JM, et al. Treatment of refractory congestive cardiac insufficiency by continuous peritoneal dialysis. Long term course. *Press Med.* 1988;17:1617–1620.
214. McLigeyo SO. Intermittent peritoneal dialysis in the management of refractory heart failure. *Centr Afr J Med.* 1992;38: 421–424.
215. Stegmayr BG, Banga R, Lundberg L, et al. PD treatment for severe congestive heart failure. *Perit Dial Int.* 1996;16(Suppl): S231–S235.
216. Torney V, Conlon PJ, Farrell J, et al. Long term successful management of refractory congestive cardiac failure by intermittent ambulatory peritoneal ultrafiltration. *QJM.* 1996;89:681–683.
217. Ryckelnck JP, Lobbedez T, Valette B, et al. Peritoneal ultrafiltration and treatment-resistant heart failure. *Nephrol Dial Transplant.* 1998;13(Suppl 4):56–59.
218. Elhalel-Dranittzki M, Rubinger D, Moscovici A, et al. CAPD to improve quality of life in patients with refractory heart failure. *Nephrol Dial Transplant.* 1998;13:3041–3042.
219. Freida P, Ryckelnck JP, Potier J, et al. Place de l'ultrafiltration peritoneale dans le traitment medical de l'insuffisance cardiaque au stade IV de la NYHA. *Bull Dial Perit.* 1995;5:7–18.
220. Gokal R. Newer peritoneal dialysis solutions. *Adv Ren Replace Ther.* 2000;7:302–309.
221. Pannekeet MM, Shouten M, Langendijk MJ, et al. Peritoneal transport characteristics with glucose polymer dialysate. *Kidney Int.* 1996;0:979–986.
222. Rippe B, Levin L. Computer simulations of ultrafiltration profiles with icodextrin-based peritoneal fluid in CAPD. *Kidney Int.* 2000;57:2546–2556.
223. Smith D, Paganini EP, Suhoza K, et al. Nonheparin continuous renal replacement therapy. In: Noel Y, Kjellstrand C, Ivanovich P, eds. *Progress in Artificial Organs.* Cleveland: ISAO Press; 1986: 226–230.
224. Kramer P, Schrader J, Bohnsack W, et al. Continuous arteriovenous hemofiltration: a new kidney replacement therapy. *Proc Eur Dialysis Transpl Assoc.* 1981;18:743–749.
225. Schrader J, Scheler F. Coagulation disorders in acute renal failure and anticoagulation during CAVH with standard heparin and with low molecular weight heparin. In: Sieberth HG, Mann H, eds. *Continuous Arteriovenous Hemofiltration.* Basel: S Karger; 1985: 25–36.
226. Olbricht C, Mueller C, Schurek HJ. Treatment of acute renal failure by continuous spontaneous hemofiltration. *Trans Am Soc Artif Intern Org.* 1982;28:33–37.
227. Bull BS, Korpman RA, Huse WM, et al. Heparin therapy during extracorporeal circulation. I. Problems inherent in existing heparin protocols. *J Thorac Cardiovasc Surg.* 1975;69: 674–684.
228. Bjornsson TD, Wolfran KM, Kitchell BB. Heparin kinetics determined by three assay methods. *Clin Pharmacol Ther.* 1982;31: 104–113.
229. Ossenkopple GJ, van der Muellen J, Bronsveld W, et al. Continuous haemofiltration as an adjunctive therapy for septic shock. *Crit Care Med.* 1985;13:102–104.
230. Zusman RM, Rubin RH, Cato AE, et al. Hemodialysis using prostacyclin instead of heparin as the sole antithrombotic agent. *N Engl J Med.* 1981;304:934–939.
231. Smith MC, Danviriyasup K, Crow JW, et al. Prostacyclin substitution for heparin in long term hemodialysis. *Am J Med.* 1982;73:669–678.
232. Canaud B, Mion C, Arujo A, et al. Prostacyclin (epoprostenol) as the sole antithrombotic agent in postdilutional haemofiltration. *Nephron.* 1988;48:206–212.
233. Ota K, Kawaguchi H, Takahashi K, et al. A new prostacyclin analogue: an anticoagulant applicable to hemodialysis. *Trans Am Soc Artif Intern Org.* 1983;12:419–424.
234. Pinnick RV, Wiegmann TB, Diederich DA. Regional citrate anticoagulation for hemodialysis in the patient at high risk for bleeding. *N Engl J Med.* 1983;308:268–261.
235. Flanigan MJ, Von Brecht J, Freeman RM, et al. Reducing the hemorrhagic complications of hemodialysis: a controlled comparison of low dose heparin and citrate anticoagulation. *Am J Kidney Dis.* 1983;9:147–153.
236. Metha RL, McDonald BR, Aguilar MM, et al. Regional citrate anticoagulation for continuous arteriovenous hemodialysis in critically ill patients. *Kidney Int.* 1990;38:976–981.
237. Ahmad S, Yeo KT, Jensen WM, et al. Citrate anticoagulation during in vivo simulation of slow hemofiltration. *Blood Purif.* 1990;8:170–182.
238. Kaplan AA, Petrillo R. Regional heparinization for continuous arteriovenous hemofiltration. *Trans Am Soc Artif Intern Org.* 1987;33:312–315.
239. Milne B, Rodgers K, Cervenko F, et al. Hemodynamic effects of intra-aortic administration versus intravenous administration of protamine for reversal of heparin in man. *Can Anaesth Soc.* 1983;30:347–351.
240. Ellison N, Beatty P, Blake DR, et al. Heparin rebound. *J Thorac Cardiovasc Surg.* 1974;67:723–729.
241. Schrader J, Stibbe W, Armstrong V, et al. Comparison of low molecular weight heparin in hemodialysis/hemofiltration. *Kidney Int.* 1988;33:890–896.
242. Janssen M, Deegens J, Kapinga T, et al. Citrate compared to low molecular weight heparin anticoagulation in chronic hemodialysis patients. *Kidney Int.* 1996;49:806–813.
243. Lai K. Wang A, Ho K, et al. Use of low dose low molecular weight heparin in hemodialysis. *Am J Kidney Dis.* 1996;28:721–726.
244. Hory B, Cachoux A, Toulemonde F. Continuous arteriovenous hemofiltration with low molecular weight heparin. *Nephron.* 1985;41:125.
245. Scurek HJ, Biela D. Continuous arteriovenous hemofiltration: improvement in the handling of fluid balance and heparinization. *Blood Purif.* 1983;1:189–196.

44

Surgical Approaches to Patients with Chronic Congestive Heart Failure

Edwin C. McGee, Jr. *Kathleen L. Grady* *Patrick M. McCarthy*[*]

Heart failure afflicts almost 5 million Americans and more than 500,000 new cases are diagnosed annually (1). About 300,000 deaths annually are attributed to heart failure as either a primary or contributory cause. With an estimated 1-year mortality of 50%, survival is dismal for medically treated New York Heart Association (NYHA) Class IV, or stage D heart failure patients. Medical treatment with angiotensin-converting enzyme (ACE) inhibitors, beta-blockers, and resynchronization therapy are cornerstones of care. Heart failure unresponsive to maximal medical therapy occurs in 60,000 patients each year (2).

Heart transplantation is successful surgical treatment for end-stage heart failure. Due to a limited pool of suitable donors, the number of heart transplants performed annually has been fairly static at just over 2,000 per year in the United States (Fig. 44-1) (3). About 500 to 1,000 patients die each year while on the United Network for Organ Sharing (UNOS) waiting list (4). In addition, end-stage heart failure patients may have comorbid conditions that preclude transplantation, or patients on the list may develop complications that preclude transplantation.

Interest in alternative surgical therapies for patients with advanced heart failure has increased. Some surgical therapies may delay listing for a heart transplant or preclude the need for transplantation altogether. Many individuals with heart failure stemming from ischemic or valvular lesions can potentially be helped by conventional surgical procedures such as coronary revascularization and valve repair or replacement. Furthermore, certain individuals with stage D heart failure are candidates for more advanced surgical therapies such as transplantation and mechanical assistance. Some potential candidates for conventional surgery need mechanical assistance as a backup strategy in case difficulty is encountered during weaning from bypass. The determination of the best treatment for any particular patient is not always straightforward and is best made by a multidisciplinary team led by cardiologists and surgeons who have specific interest and training in the management of patients with heart failure. In this chapter we will outline the approach we take when thinking of surgical options for patients with heart failure.

CONVENTIONAL SURGICAL PROCEDURES

Coronary Artery Disease

Ischemic Cardiomyopathy

Ischemic heart disease remains the leading cause of congestive heart failure (CHF) in the United States and the developed world, accounting for 40% to 70% of cases (5,6). The randomized Coronary Artery Surgery Study (CASS) and VA trials included patients with left ventricular (LV) dysfunction (7,8). Both demonstrated improved survival for surgical versus medical therapy in patients with coronary artery disease and LV dysfunction. A second randomized VA study of patients with unstable angina demonstrated improved survival for patients with LV dysfunction who underwent surgical revascularization (9). The CASS registry, a nonrandomized portion of the CASS trial, demonstrated a lower rate of sudden cardiac death in patients with LV dysfunction who had been revascularized (10). However, patients with a left ventricular ejection fraction (LVEF) <35% were included in none of these studies, as they were felt to be too high-risk to undergo coronary revascularization.

* We wish to acknowledge the editorial assistance of Brandi Carr and Linda Flores-Huerta.

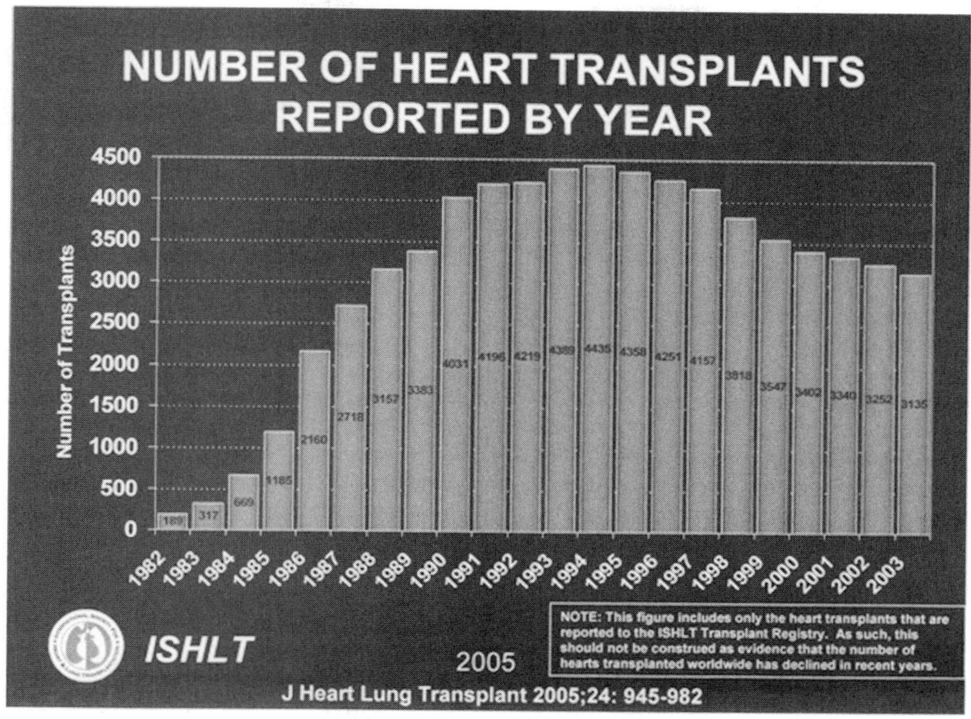

Figure 44-1 Number of heart transplants in the United States by year (International Society of Heart and Lung Transportation).

Even with modern, state-of-the-art pharmacotherapy, survival is poor for medically treated patients with ischemic cardiomyopathy (11–17). The Assessment of Treatment with Lisinopril and Survival (ATLAS) trial studied the effect of high- and low-dose lisinopril in 2,035 patients with ischemic cardiomyopathy. The high-dose group had an 8% decrease in mortality after 4 years when compared to the low-dose group, but mortality was still 44% (18). In ATLAS, acute coronary events were the cause of death in 54% of patients. The Studies of Left Ventricular Dysfunction (SOLVD) database examined the effect of enalapril on survival in 5,410 patients with LVEF <35%. In SOLVD, patients who had undergone surgical revascularization within 2 years of study entry had improved survival and a lower rate of sudden cardiac death when compared to patients who had not undergone revascularization (19). Numerous retrospective studies (20), summarized in Table 44-1, have shown that coronary artery bypass in individuals with LVEFs <25% can be accomplished with operative mortality rates ranging from 2% to 8%. Improvement in EF after revascularization has also been demonstrated (20) and is summarized in Table 44-2.

Viability testing is of paramount importance in discriminating which patients with multivessel coronary artery disease and LV dysfunction will benefit from revascularization. A recent meta-analysis of 24 studies examined the impact that myocardial viability has on survival after revascularization for ischemic cardiomyopathy. A clear benefit of revascularization for patients with viability was demonstrated (21). This study involved 3,022 patients with an average LVEF of 32%. Follow-up was 25 months. Revascularized patients with viability had a 3.2% annual mortality rate as compared to a 16% annual mortality rate in patients with viability who did not undergo revascularization. Although the results were not statistically significant, patients without viability who underwent revascularization fared worse than those who were managed medically, with annual mortalities of 7.7% and 6.2%, respectively (21). Magnetic resonance imaging (MRI) is our preferred method for discerning viability. In addition to providing information on viability, MRI also clearly defines anatomy for possible ventricular reconstruction. Positron emission tomography (PET) or other nuclear imaging is reserved for those individuals who cannot undergo MRI because of pacing or automatic internal cardiac defibrillator (AICD) hardware.

LV dysfunction is a risk factor for coronary artery bypass, and individuals with uncompensated heart failure have a very high operative mortality. Although outcomes were better than those in the medical arm, the operative arm of the randomized Should We Revascularize Occluded Coronaries in Cardiovascular Shock (SHOCK) trial had a very high event rate, with 30-day and 1-year mortality rates of 42% and 56%, respectively (22).

Although no randomized trials comparing outcomes of medical and surgical therapy for ischemic cardiomyopathy have been completed, it is apparent that most people with ischemic cardiomyopathy die from ischemia, and much evidence exists to support the beneficial effect of surgery. For individuals with compensated heart failure, revascularization leads to improved long-term survival and can be safely performed in patients with viability despite severely comprised ventricular function (23).

TABLE 44-1
RESULTS OF CORONARY ARTERY BYPASS GRAFT FOR SEVERE LEFT VENTRICULAR DYSFUNCTION

First Author	Points	Years	Ejection Fraction	Perioperative Mortality (%)	Late Mortality (yr)
Vlietstra	10	1966–1972	<0.25	–	60% (2)
Manley	183	1968–1971	mean 0.22	16.0	43% (5)
Yatteau	24	1968–1972	<0.25	42	50% (2)
Oldham	11	1969–1972	≤0.25	55	–
Zubiate	140	1969–1975	<0.20	22	41.6% (6)
Faulkner	46	1969–1975	mean 0.21	4.0	17% (2)
Mitchel	9	–	<0.20	0.0	11% (1)
Fox	7	1971–1974	<0.20	0.0	14%
Jones	41	1973–1977	<0.20	2.5	10% (1)
Alderman	82	1975–1979	≤0.25	8.0	37% (5)
Mochtar	62	1975–1983	mean 0.25	4.8	30% (5)
Zubiate	93	1976–1981	<0.20	5.0	50% (5)
Hochberg	51	1976–1982	0.20–0.24	12.0	42% (3)
Hochberg	41	1976–1982	<0.20	37.0	85% (3)
Sanchez	23	1982–1989	mean 0.28	9.0	24% (2)
Kron	39	1983–1988	<0.20	2.6	17% (3)
Blakeman	20	1984–1988	mean 0.18	15.0	30% (1)
Wong	22	1986–1989	mean 0.25	9.0	23% (3)
Christakis	487	1982–1990	<0.20	9.8	–
Hammermeister	251	1987–1990	<0.20	9.2	–
Louie	22	1984–1990	mean 0.23	13.6	28% (3)
Milano	118	1981–1991	<0.25	11	42% (5)
Shapira	74	1986–1991	<0.30	–	13.5% (5)
Anderson	203	1983–1992	mean 0.34	6.0	41% (5)
Hausmann	265	1986–1992	mean 0.24	7.6	13% (3)
Kaul et al	210	1987–1992	≤0.20	10.0	27% (5)
Mickleborough	79	1982–1993	<0.20	3.8	32% (5)
Langenburg	96	1983–1993	≤0.25	8.3	–
Elefteraides	135	1986–1994	≤0.30	5.2	29% (4.5)
Iskandrian	269	1991–1994	≤0.35	7.1	–
Kawachi	50	1982–1995	≤0.30	8.0	26% (5)
Moshkovitz	75	1991–1994	≤0.35	2.7	27% (4)
Trachiotis	156	1981–1995	<0.25	3.8	35% (5)
Baumgartner	61	1990–1996	<0.25	8.0	–
Cimochowski	111	1992–1996	<0.35	1.8	–
Argenziano [CABG Patch]	454 no CHF 443 CHF	1993–1996	≤0.35	3.5 no CHF 7.7 CHF	–
DeCarlo	80	1994–1996	≤0.30	6.3	18% (2)
Luciani	116	1991–1998	≤0.30	1.7	25% (5)

TABLE 44-2
IMPROVEMENT IN EJECTION FRACTION AFTER CORONARY ARTERY BYPASS GRAFT FOR SEVERE LEFT VENTRICULAR DYSFUNCTION IN RECENT SERIES

First Author	Preoperative EF (Mean ±SD)	Postoperative EF (Mean ± SD)	Patients with EF Increase (%)	Interval to Postoperative EF	*p*
Milano	0.21	0.27	N/A	N/A	<0.005
Shapira	0.24	0.36	73% (>0.07)	5.8 mo	<0.0001
Elefteraides	0.24	0.34	70% (≥0.05)	4.6 mo	<0.0001
De Carlo	0.27 ± 0.04	0.38 ± 0.08	N/A	N/A	<0.001
Luciani	0.28 ± 0.05	0.38 ± 0.09	N/A	N/A	<0.001

Left Ventricular Reconstruction

Surgical reconstruction of a dyskinetic aneurysm or akinetic scar to produce a more efficient ventricle is referred to as left ventricular reconstruction (LVR). For patients with ischemic cardiomyopathy and an area of discrete ventricular scar, combined coronary revascularization and LVR is an attractive option. The first ventricular reconstructions consisted of linear aneurysm repairs that removed the thin-walled scar lateral to the left anterior descending artery. In the 1980s, more complete reconstructions (including the septum) were described by Cooley et al., Dor et al., and Jatene (24–26).

Theoretical, mathematical, and observational data exist demonstrating the beneficial effects of LVR. Mathematical modeling predicts that resection of a dyskinetic scar will lead to a net improvement in cardiac function and a reduction in ventricular wall stress (27). After LVR, improvements are seen both in myocardial oxygen consumption and myocardial efficiency which lead to an improvement in the neurohormonal milieu of heart failure (28–33).

Indications for Left Ventricular Reconstructive Surgery in Ischemic Cardiomyopathy

Most patients undergo LVR because of other operative indications, such as left main coronary artery disease, three vessel diseases with positive viability studies, or severe mitral regurgitation. The Reconstructive Endoventricular Surgery returning Torsion Original Radius Elliptical (RESTORE) study is a multicenter registry that looked at the results of 1,198 postinfarction patients who underwent LVR (34). Ninety-five percent of patients underwent concomitant coronary artery bypass surgery (CABG) and 22% underwent concomitant mitral valve repair. Sixty-six percent of patients had LVR or akinetic segment, whereas 34% had LVR for a dyskinetic segment. Thirty-day mortality was 5.3%. Five-year survival was 80% for patients who underwent LVR for a dyskinetic segment versus 65% for those who underwent LVR for an akinetic segment (Fig. 44-2). The average improvement in LVEF was 10%, mean NYHA functional class improved from 3.0 to 1.9, and the 5-year readmission rate for heart failure was 15% (34).

In our practice, reconstruction is performed if there is a discrete thin-walled aneurysm that collapses with venting the left heart. If there is diffuse scar mixed with muscle in all three coronary territories, revascularization without reconstruction is undertaken. We do not reconstruct areas that are thick-walled without visible scar or without scar that is apparent by MRI. As viability studies are only 80% to 90% accurate, we do not reconstruct areas that are, upon direct inspection in the operating room, thick-walled muscle even though preoperative studies indicated nonviable scarred myocardium. If there is any question as to viability, we err on the side of revascularization and forego reconstruction. Most often, reconstruction is performed for a true dyskinetic aneurysm, but we will reconstruct thin akinetic scar.

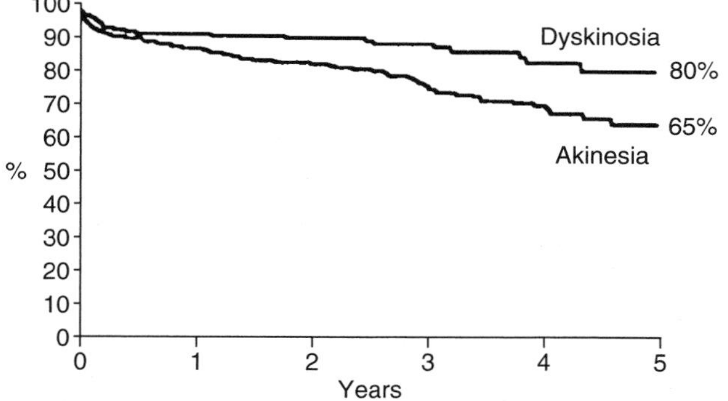

Figure 44-2 Left ventricular reconstruction.

The Surgical Treatment of Ischemic Heart Failure (STITCH) trial is a multicenter prospective randomized trial designed to study the effect of ventricular reconstruction on survival. Patients with ischemic cardiomyopathy (LVEF <35%) and who are NYHA Class III or IV, with an akinetic or dyskinetic segment, are randomized to optimal medical therapy or surgery. The patients in the surgical arm are further randomized to revascularization alone or revascularization plus LVR. The estimated date of study completion is 2008.

Valvular Heart Disease

Mitral Valve

Nearly 50% of patients with an LVEF <35% have 3+ or 4+ mitral regurgitation (MR), and almost 35% have 3+ to 4+ tricuspid regurgitation (TR) (35). Patients with significant mitral regurgitation have been shown to be statistically more likely to die than those without MR following medical therapy (35) post-MI (36) or post-percutaneous coronary intervention (37). Historically, mitral valve surgery in this group of patients with low LVEF was thought to be hazardous and the operative risk prohibitive if the LVEF <40% (38). It was thought that surgical correction of MR in this group removed the so-called pop-off mechanism which allowed the LV to decompress into the low-pressure left atrium. However, this high mortality was more likely related to the state of the art of cardiac surgery in the 1970s and 1980s.

Two mechanisms typically lead to MR in heart failure patients. Annular dilatation (Carpentier type I) predominates in dilated cardiomyopathy, and posterior leaflet restriction (Carpentier type IIIb) predominates in ischemic cardiomyopathy (39). In advanced ischemic disease, a mixture of the two pathologies often exists. It is important to understand that in both mechanisms the underlying valvular and subvalvular apparatus appear normal. Bolling et al. (40) were the first to show that mitral valve repair can be performed on patients with severe LV dysfunction and MR with a low operative mortality. Other authors have demonstrated a similar low operative mortality in patients undergoing mitral valve surgery (41–43). Intermediate survival, functional class, and ventricular functional changes (improved LVEF, decreased sphericity, and decreased ventricular volumes) have been demonstrated to be improved in patients undergoing mitral valve repair (40,41).

Historically, patients with chronic ischemic mitral regurgitation (IMR) have been dealt with by coronary revascularization alone; many groups still support this strategy (44–46). Other groups have shown that even more moderate amounts of MR in patients undergoing coronary artery bypass do not resolve following coronary bypass alone (47,48) and may reduce survival of patients compared to those without MR (47). Some have also indicated that adding mitral valve repair to this group of patients with 2+ to 3+ MR will improve late survival (49).

Adding mitral valve repair to coronary artery bypass to improve survival and late functional class remains controversial. Some reports have failed to show any benefit (44–46) and others have demonstrated that recurrent MR following repair of functional MR secondary to IMR is common (50,51). Three concepts explain the recurrence of IMR. First, work from D. C. Miller's laboratory has indicated that fixing the septal lateral dimension (AP dimension) is the most important maneuver to effect competence of the valve (52,53). Second, several recent papers indicate that intertrigonal dilatation does occur in patients with ischemic cardiomyopathy (54–57). Both of these concepts indicate that a complete rigid ring would be preferable to partial bands or suture annuloplasties. Third, several studies confirm the asymmetric nature of IMR with a jet that occurs primarily at the medial commissure (P3 region) (58) and is secondary to tethering of the posteromedial papillary muscle. As such, we believe that the best way to deal with IMR is a complete ring that takes into account the asymmetric dilation at P3.

Is there ever a role for outright valve replacement in IMR? Calafiore et al. have shown that mitral valve coaptation depth (the distance between the mitral valve annular plane and the coaptation point of the mitral leaflets) is a strong predictor of recurrent MR after annuloplasty alone (59). An increased coaptation depth is associated with a more spherical ventricle and, in their series, Calafiore et al. reported that values greater than 10 mm were at high risk of recurrent MR after repair with a non-ring suture annuloplasty. In the Cleveland Clinic series that looked at repair versus replacement for IMR, repair was associated with improved survival except in the sickest subset of patients (60). In individuals with severe heart failure and extensive leaflet tethering we consider proceeding directly to chordal-sparing mitral valve replacement utilizing a bioprosthetic valve. We agree with Miller that in these patients with limited long-term survival there is no role for a mechanical prosthesis which exposes the patient to the morbidity of warfarin (52).

Does mitral valve repair extend the life of patients with severe LV dysfunction? No randomized trials have yet been performed. Several studies have demonstrated improvements in NYHA functional class, EF, and rate of rehospitalization (40,41). However, one retrospective study indicated no difference in 5-year survival (61). It is time for a prospective randomized trial to study the effects of mitral valve surgery in patients with low EF. Perhaps with a combination of patient selection and the utilization of new repair techniques we will be able to create stable freedom from recurrent MR and improve long-term survival.

Aortic Valve

Aortic stenosis is a highly correctable cause of heart failure with a very predictable natural history. Aortic valve replacement is indicated for symptomatic patients and for asymptomatic individuals with evidence of severe aortic stenosis. Decision making in such patients is straightforward. Patients with aortic stenosis who have a low cardiac output and LV dysfunction are described as having low-gradient aortic stenosis, as their ventricles are too compromised to generate a pressure gradient across the aortic valve. Further complicating matters is the fact that the severity of aortic stenosis can be difficult to quantify in patients with profound LV depression and low cardiac output using the standard echocardiographic formulae. Right and left heart catheterization and dobutamine echocardiography are useful tests for confirming the severity of aortic stenosis in these patients.

It has recently been shown that with current myocardial protection strategies, aortic valve replacement can be done with low risk, even in those patients who until recently were felt to be inoperable. A series from the Cleveland Clinic reported outcomes of three groups of patients with aortic stenosis managed from 1990–1998 (62). Group I consisted of 68 patients who underwent aortic valve replacement for aortic value area <0.75 cm^2, LVEF <35%, and mean gradient <30 mm Hg. Group II had aortic valve replacement for an aortic valve area <0.75cm^2, LVEF <50%, and mean gradient of 35 mm Hg. Group III included 89 patients who were not operated on and had an aortic valve area of 0.75 cm^2, gradient <30 mm Hg, and LVEF <35%. Operative mortality was 5.9% and 4.0% for groups I and II, respectively. One- and 4-year survival were 82%/75% and 92%/82% for groups I and II, respectively. One-year survival for the medically managed Group III was 20% (Fig. 44-3).

Balloon valvuloplasty should be mentioned because it occasionally can play an important role in the treatment of aortic stenosis (63). We reserve its use for the patient with critical aortic stenosis presenting with low-output-induced renal failure. Balloon valvuloplasty allows some of these patients to be optimized so they may undergo valve replacement with lower morbidity. Valvuloplasty as stand-alone therapy is not associated with good long-term results (63).

An aggressive approach can also be utilized when dealing with aortic insufficiency. As with aortic stenosis, modern myocardial protection strategies and improved operative and perioperative care have extended the limits of who can benefit from valve replacement. A series from

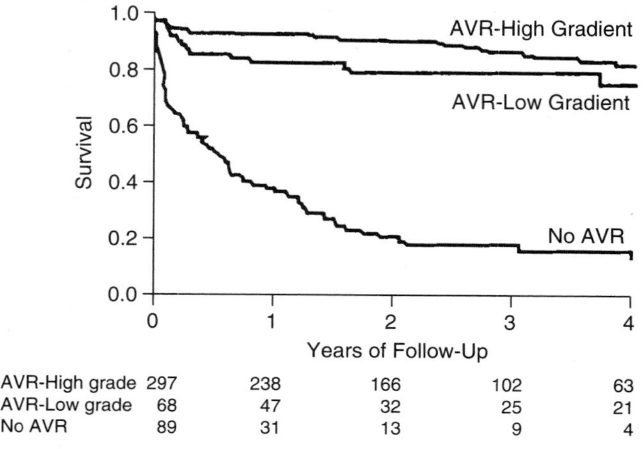

Figure 44-3 Survival curve of patients with aortic stenosis and decreased injection fraction.

the Cleveland Clinic looked at patients with aortic insufficiency and LV depression (LVEF <30%), a group previously thought of as inoperable. Thirty-day mortality was 0% and 5-year survival was 84% for the group that underwent aortic valve replacement after 1990 (64).

Tricuspid Valve

Until recently, the tricuspid valve has been largely ignored in the treatment of individuals with heart failure. Consistent repair of the tricuspid valve has been elusive. Numerous suture annuloplasties have been described but long-term durability is lacking. A recent report from the Cleveland Clinic (65) described the outcomes of 790 tricuspid repairs performed from 1990–1999 (65). Eighty-nine of patients had a mitral valve procedure. Operative mortality was 8% and 5-year survival was 65%. Repair with a rigid ring provided the best long-term freedom from recurrent TR. The authors concluded that formal ring annuloplasty of the tricuspid valve should be undertaken for TR deemed to be greater than 2+ by preoperative transthoracic echocardiogram. Other groups have demonstrated similar encouraging results. Kuwaki et al. (66) reported a hospital mortality of 8.9% and 10-year survival of 84% in their series of 260 patients (97% NYHA Class III or IV) undergoing tricuspid repair. Improvement in RV function has also been demonstrated after tricuspid repair (67).

Atrial Fibrillation

Atrial fibrillation commonly coexists with mitral valvular pathology and heart failure, and has been shown to be an independent predictor of mortality (68,69). The gold standard therapy for atrial fibrillation is the Cox-Maze III operation. Over 90% of patients who undergo the Cox-Maze III are cured of atrial fibrillation (70). In addition, patients with atrial fibrillation can have a tachycardia-induced cardiomyopathy which can improve when the causative tachycardia is treated, and some groups have demonstrated an overall improvement in LVEF in patients who have undergone the Maze procedure (70). While highly effective, the classic Maze has failed to become established in the cardiac surgery community because of its complexity. There has been a recent influx of new technology that can create full-thickness atrial lesions and precludes the need for surgical incisions and subsequent suture repair (71). The simplest lesion set, consisting of a pulmonary vein isolation and stapling of the left atrial appendage, can be done quickly, is highly effective (71), and can be done safely in the sickest of patients.

Epicardial Pacing Wires

Resynchronization

Cardiac resynchronization is an important therapy for patients with heart failure and intraventricular conduction delay. Several trials have shown improvements in ventricular function and quality of life for patients with CHF and a prolonged QRS who undergo placement of a biventricular pacemaker (72–75). The fact that biventricular pacemakers are often placed concurrently with AICDs makes the procedure even more attractive. The majority of these procedures can be accomplished percutaneously in the electrophysiology lab, with the LV lead being placed in a lateral wall coronary vein. However, certain patients do not have venous anatomy amenable to coronary sinus lead placement, and early and late failure rates are 12% and 10%, respectively (76). Historically, these patients had to undergo open thoracotomy for LV epicardial lead placement. More recently, minimally invasive techniques have been described for epicardial lead placement (76). It has become our policy to routinely place LV leads any time we operate on patients with a QRS >120 ms. At the end of the procedure we simply tunnel them to the left infraclavicular fossa and place them in a subcutaneous pocket to facilitate future biventricular pacing.

Dilated Cardiomyopathy

Although many procedures and devices have been investigated for treating patients with dilated cardiomyopathy, none is currently approved by the U.S. Food and Drug Administration (FDA). Several of these procedures have received considerable attention in the literature (medical and lay), and the following section is intended to bring the reader up to date on their status.

Partial Left Ventriculectomy (The Batista Procedure)

Randas Batista, a cardiac surgeon practicing in Brazil, was frustrated by the lack of therapy for patients with Chagas disease and dilated cardiomyopathy (77). Knowing about the success of LV aneurysm surgery, and reasoning that ventricular dilatation itself decreased efficiency, he embarked upon a series of operations to remove a portion of the ventricular wall in patients with dilated cardiomyopathy. The operation was designed to reduce the ventricular radius and thereby decrease ventricular wall stress through the Law of LaPlace. The myocardial resection was typically undertaken in the lateral wall between the papillary muscles. The heart was then smaller, had less wall stress, and had better systolic function.

Cardiac surgeons in the United States heard of this approach when Dr. Batista spoke about this approach during the discussion of a lung volume reduction paper (78). In 1995, U.S. and British centers began performing the Batista procedure with mixed results. The results of the Cleveland Clinic experience have been extensively reported. Two patients died, resulting in a hospital mortality of 3.2% (81), 11 patients (18%) received a left ventricular assist device (LVAD) as rescue therapy, and 32 patients returned to Class IV heart failure. Three-year survival was 60% and LVEF increased from 16% ± 7.6% to 31.5% ± 10.9% ($p \leq 0.0001$). Changes in ventricular volume and EF were relatively stable over time. Increased pulmonary artery systolic pressure was a predictor of poor survival. Reduced maximum exercise oxygen consumption predicted a rapid return to Class IV heart failure, and higher left atrial pressure was associated with a lower event-free survival. Preoperative MR was not a risk factor for any outcome after the Batista procedure.

The procedure was largely abandoned in 1998 because it was unpredictable. Mathematical modeling and finite element analysis showed a leftward shift of pressure–volume loops, but at the expense of a counteracting effect in diastole, leading to significant diastolic dysfunction (88–90). The Batista procedure improved systolic function but worsened diastolic function, with a net effect of little benefit on overall LV pumping capacity (89–91). The heterogeneity of diastolic dysfunction may be related to underlying ventricular fibrosis and could explain why some patients demonstrate a clinical benefit and others showed no improvement or even worsened after surgery.

Acorn CorCap Cardiac Support Device

Increased understanding of ventricular remodeling and the hypothesis that LV remodeling may independently contribute to disease progression in heart failure have contributed to the development and evaluation of several innovative surgical approaches which have attempted to prevent or reverse LV remodeling. The earliest notion that passive containment of the ventricle may contribute to reverse remodeling was reported in studies of cardiomyoplasty (92). Although both cardiomyoplasty and the Batista procedure have generally been abandoned due to relatively poor and inconsistent outcomes, the search for a surgical means to provide passive LV constraint and remodeling has continued. In response to this search, the Acorn CorCap has been developed and a clinical trial has recently been completed in advanced heart failure patients (94).

The Acorn CorCap is a mesh-like polyester jacket that is surgically wrapped around a dilated left ventricle to provide passive LV constraint and thereby counteract deleterious changes that occur with LV remodeling (94). Preclinical studies of the CorCap in animal models have demonstrated decreased end-systolic and end-diastolic volumes (95); improved diastolic function, reduced chamber sphericity, and decreased wall stress (96); and increased EF and fractional shortening (97).

The Acorn Pivotal Trial, a prospective, randomized, unblinded evaluation of the CorCap cardiac support device, was recently completed to evaluate safety and efficacy in NYHA Class III and IV heart failure patients (18 to 80 years of age) on optimal medical therapy (94). Enrolled patients were randomized to the CorCap device with optimal medical therapy or optimal medical therapy alone. Some patients demonstrated modest improvement, and approval by the FDA is under review.

Myocor Myosplint

The theory behind the Batista procedure was based on the law of LaPlace with the idea that a reduction of the ventricular radius would lead to a reduction in ventricular wall stress (98). The Myocor Myosplint was designed to change the shape of the ventricle into a bilobed configuration, with each lobe having a reduced radius and therefore reduced wall stress. Since the ventricular wall is not removed (as with the Batista procedure), the effects upon diastolic dysfunction should be less marked. Finite element analysis indicates that the net effect of the shape change induced by the Myosplint should lead to an improvement in cardiac function and an improvement in stroke volume (99). Computational model analysis of the same concept came to similar conclusions (100).

Three-dimensional echocardiography performed in a porcine heart failure model with the Myosplint showed there is reduced end-diastolic and end-systolic volume, improved EF, and decreased wall stress, and that the changes were sustained after 1 month of pacing (98). In this animal model, however, there were no associated changes in cardiac output or end-diastolic pressure. A phase I study was initiated in the United States and Germany. Changes in ventricular volume and EF from initial patients showed the expected changes. However, the company developed a new product, Coapsys, that is designed to achieve off-pump mitral valve repair along with some ventricular volume reduction; it is currently in clinical trials. The fate of the Myosplint device is therefore uncertain and the device may be set aside in favor of the device more focused on the reduction of MR.

Advanced Surgical Therapy

Transplantation

A full discussion of orthotopic cardiac transplantation is beyond the scope of this chapter. Needless to say, it remains the standard by which all other surgical therapies for heart failure are measured. With current triple-drug immunosuppressive regimens and standardized management protocols, excellent quality of life and long-term survival are possible, with 1-, 5-, and 10-year survival rates ≥80%, 65%, and 45%, respectively (101). However, transplantation continues to have limited applicability not only because of the shortage of donor organs but also because of the hesitancy of transplant surgeons and physicians to accept less than ideal but still usable donor hearts. Recent interest in the resuscitation of donor hearts has led to the development of protocols with the goal of increasing utilization of these so-called marginal donor hearts (102).

Three techniques exist for orthoptopic cardiac transplantation: biatrial, bicaval, and total. As originally described by Lower and Shumway (95) and modified by Barnard (96), the biatrial technique leaves recipient cuffs of both the right and left atrium which are subsequently anastomosed to the donor atrial cuffs. The bicaval technique, with separate anastomosis for the superior and inferior venae cavae, was introduced in 1991 (105) and is thought to be advantageous in terms of improved atrial geometry. The technique of total orthotopic transplantation (106) carries this concept one step further, with the donor left atrium being anastomosed to recipient pulmonary vein cuffs. Although theoretically more appealing, the total technique is more time-consuming and creates inaccessible suture lines which are potentially problematic in terms of hemostasis. Several retrospective and prospective series have looked at outcomes after bicaval and bi-trial transplants (107–111). Only one study has shown improved survival with utilization of the bicaval technique, and this study has been criticized due to an inordinately high mortality in the biatrial group

(112). A recent survey of cardiac transplant centers demonstrated that 38% of centers use the bicaval technique exclusively, 13% use the biatrial technique exclusively, 4.5% use the total technique exclusively, and 44% use a combination of techniques (113).

Long-term outcomes after heart transplantation are limited by allograft vasculopathy, infection, and other sequelae of long-term rejection. Right heart failure can also be a significant source of morbidity after heart transplantation and is often exacerbated by TR, which is usually secondary to high recipient pulmonary vascular resistance. Even though the incidence of TR is seen less frequently with the bicaval technique than with the standard biatrial technique, it can still be problematic. Some groups now advocate that donor tricuspid annuloplasty be performed with every cardiac transplant (114).

It should also be emphasized that for patients to receive a transplant they must first be referred for a transplant evaluation. It is unfortunate that many physicians still look upon transplantation as experimental and either do not refer patients at all or wait until after significant end-organ dysfunction has developed.

Mechanical Assistance

Bridge to Transplant

Circulatory support devices [ventricular assist devices (VADs) and total artificial hearts (TAHs)] have been under development since the 1960s, encouraged by grant support from the National Institutes of Health, National Heart Lung and Blood Institute (115). Four decades later, a number of VADs are currently approved by the FDA for use as a bridge to heart transplantation (116). The first use of TAH to bridge a patient to transplant was in 1969 (117) and the first use of a VAD was in 1978 (118). Numerous studies have shown comparable outcomes after transplantation between bridged and nonbridged patients (119–122). A bridge strategy allows for critically ill patients to be stabilized and receive a heart in a more optimal condition and has allowed numerous patients to survive a long wait for a heart. Several devices are currently FDA-approved as a bridge to transplantation. These include devices with the capability for short- and long-term support and those that can be configured for uni-ventricular and biventricular support (Figs. 44-4 and 44-5).

The Cardiowest total artificial heart received FDA support in 2004 as a bridge to a transplant (123). Most consider implantable VADs to be preferable to total heart replacement at this time, given that with VADs home discharge is more readily feasible and that native heart function can often provide a safety net should device failure occur.

Bridge to Recovery

Recovery of native ventricular function after mechanical assistance has been demonstrated by several groups. The largest series is from the Berlin Heart Institute that reported 13 out of 23 patients exhibiting stable cardiac recovery after LVAD explantation (124). The group from Harefield (125) has established a protocol using the drug clenbuterol, a selective beta2-receptor agonist, to promote physiological myocardial hypertrophy and subsequent ventricular recovery. Recovery has been demonstrated most frequently in patients suffering from myocarditis (126).

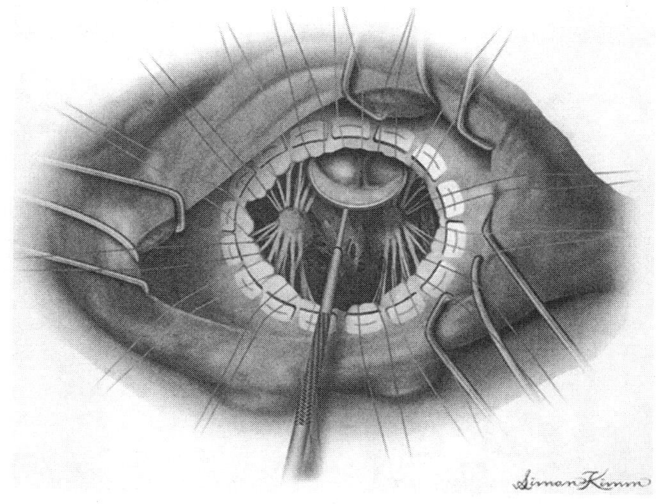

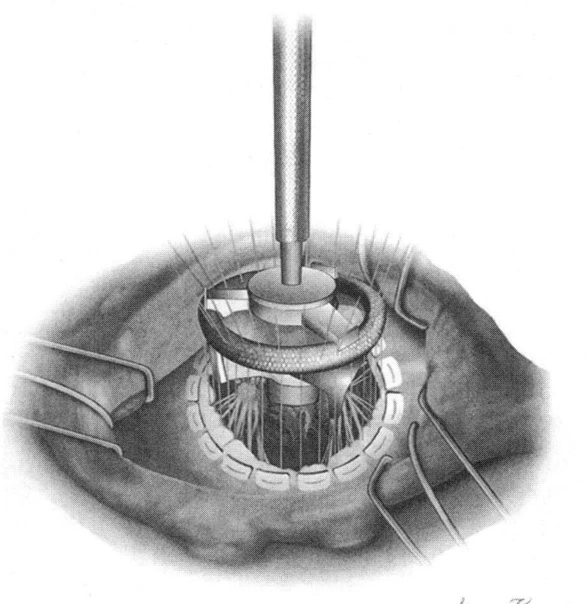

Figure 44-4 Chordal sparing mitral valve replacement. (From Periera JJ, Laure MS, Bashir M, et al. Survival after aortic valve replacement for severe aortic stenosis with low transvalvular gradients and severe left ventricular dysfunction. *J Am Coll Cardiol.* 2002;39:1356–1363.)

Destination Therapy (Permanent Ventricular Assistance)

In 2002, the HeartMate XVE LVAD was approved as destination therapy for end-stage heart failure patients who are not candidates for heart transplantation, based on the results of the pivotal Randomized Evaluation of Mechanical Assistance for the Treatment of Congestive Heart Failure (REMATCH) trial (Fig. 44-6) (127).

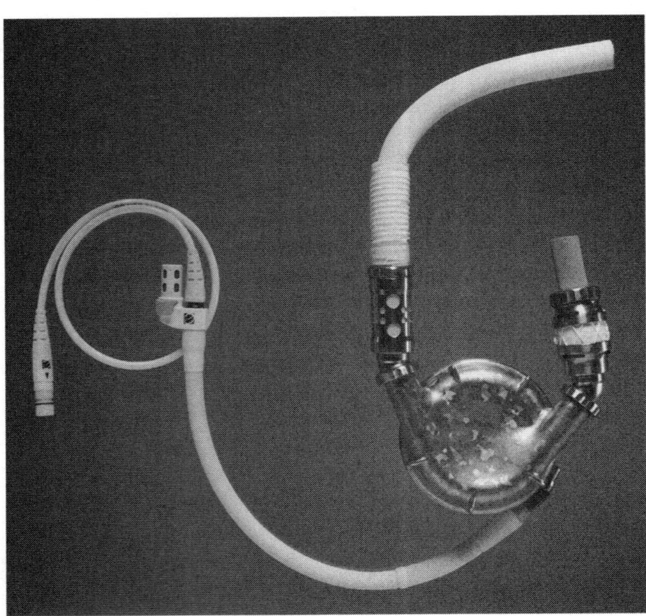
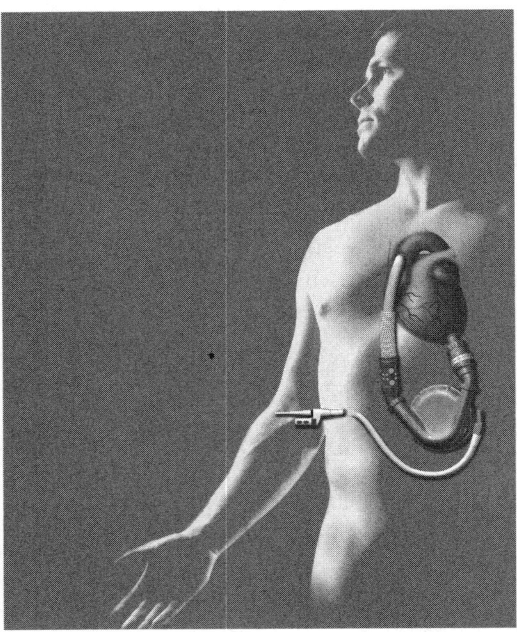

Figure 44-5 Novacor left ventricular assist device (printed with permission from Thoratec©).

REMATCH compared outcomes of patients randomized to optimal medical therapy versus implantation of the HeartMate XVE LVAD. Superior survival and quality of life in patients randomized to the HeartMate XVE LVAD were demonstrated (127). A similar pulsatile pump with a long history in the bridge to transplant arena, the Novacor LVAD, is currently under study in the Randomized Evaluation of Novacor LVAD in a Non-Transplant Population (RELIANT) trial (Fig. 44-7). Second-generation LVADs with axial flow technology, such as the Heartmate II (Thoratec) (Fig. 44-8), Debakey VAD (MicroMed), and the Jarvik 2000 are currently undergoing clinical trials in both the bridge to transplant and destination therapy arenas (128–130). It is hoped that their smaller size will help lessen device-related complications. TAHs are not yet commercially available as destination therapy.

Patients who are considered for VAD implantation as destination therapy typically have advanced age and comorbid conditions that preclude transplantation. They have long-standing stage D, NYHA Class IV heart failure despite maximal medical therapy and cardiac resynchro-

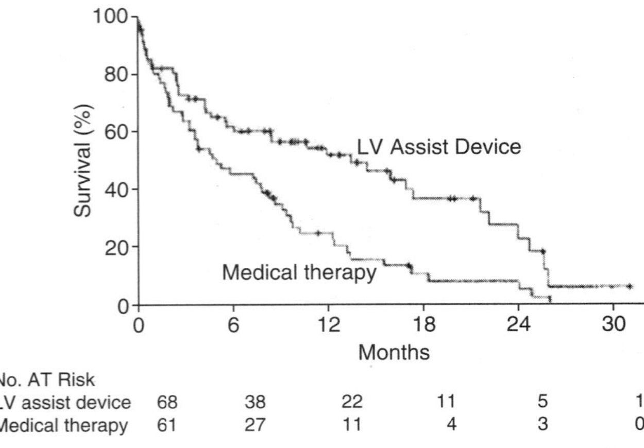

Figure 44-6 Survival of non-transplant candidates receiving optimal medical therapy versus mechanical assistance (From Rose EA, Gelijns AC, Moskowitz AJ, et al. Long-term use of a left ventricular device for end-stage heart failure. *N Engl J Med.* 2001;345: 1435–1443, with permission).

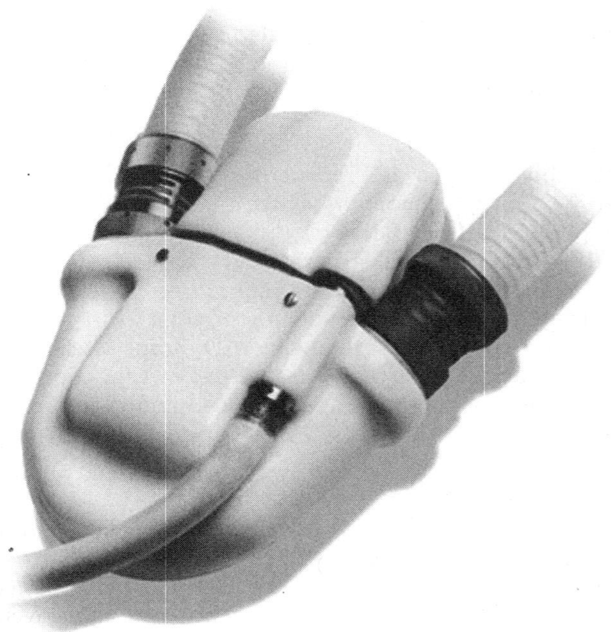

Figure 44-7 Novacor left ventricular assist device (printed with permission from WorldHeart©).

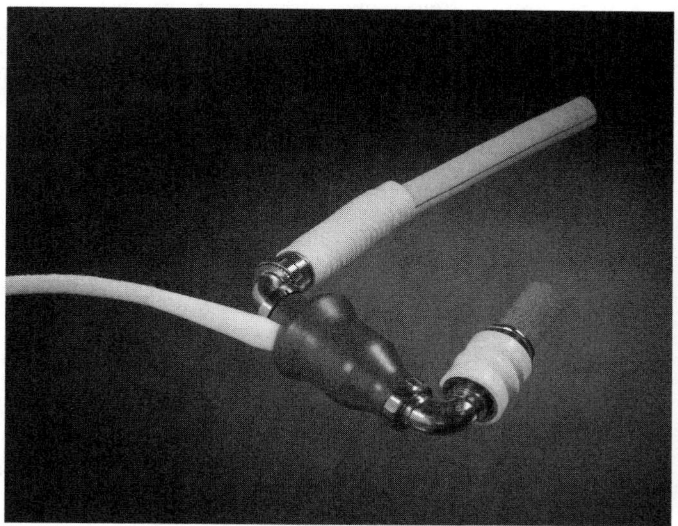

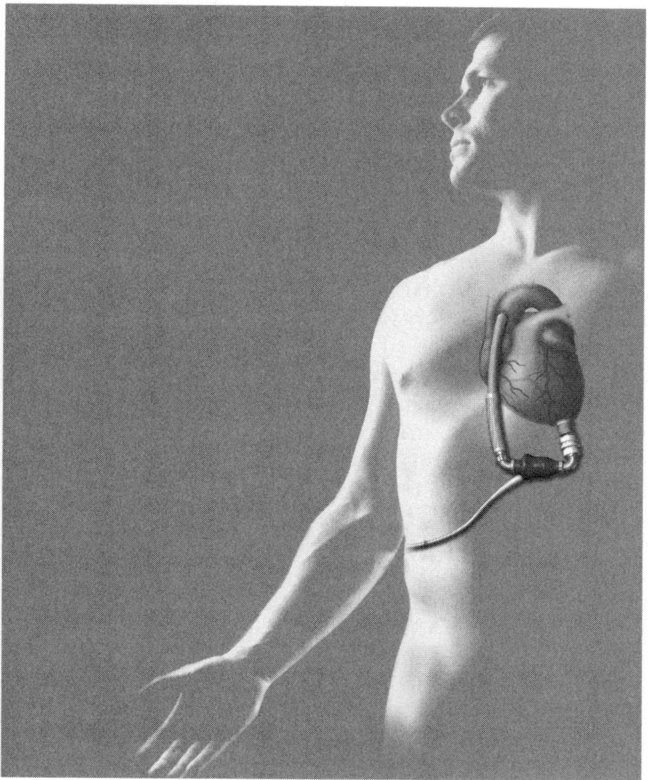

Figure 44-8 Heartmate II LVAD (printed with permission from Thoratec©).

nization. These patients have hemodynamic compromise (systolic blood pressure <80 mm Hg, pulmonary capillary wedge pressure >20 mm Hg, cardiac index <2 L/min/m^2, systemic vascular resistance >2,100 dynes/sec/cm^3, and prerenal azotemia) despite the presence of inotropic and/or intra-aortic balloon pump support (131).

Complications of mechanical assistance include sepsis, multiorgan failure, RV failure (sometimes requiring biventricular support), bleeding, infection, thromboembolism, neurologic dysfunction, and device malfunction or failure. It is hoped that design modifications of these devices and development of future-generation devices will eventually reduce the incidence of device complications. Of the more than 4,000 VADs and approximately 500 TAHs implanted worldwide, only 250 LVADs have been implanted as destination therapy (personal communication, Jerry Heatley, Thoratec Corp). Destination therapy is an underutilized therapy for certain select patients who are not transplant candidates.

SUMMARY

While medical treatment with ACE inhibitors, beta-blockade, and resynchronization therapy are cornerstones of medical care for advanced heart failure patients, many individuals with heart failure stemming from ischemic and valvular lesions can be improved by conventional surgical procedures such as coronary revascularization and valve repair or replacement. A recent paper from the Cleveland Clinic foundation reported the results of conventional surgery in patients initially referred for transplantation (131). With the exception of patients undergoing the Batista procedure, survival was equivalent in patients (who were initially referred for transplantation) who underwent high-risk conventional surgery and those who underwent transplantation (Fig. 44-9). The

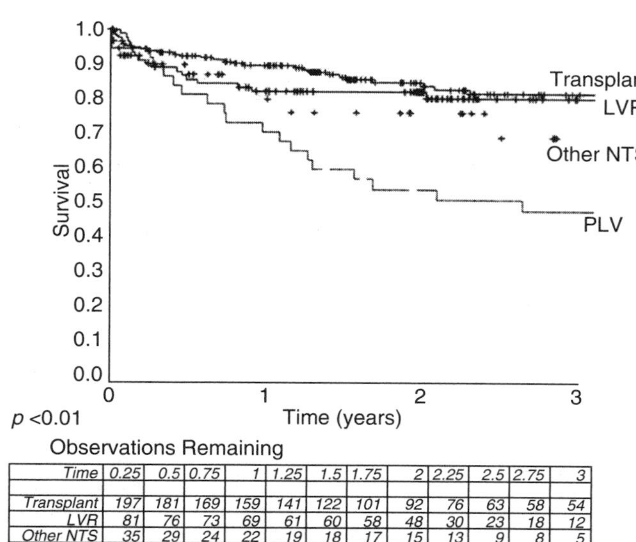

Time	0.25	0.5	0.75	1	1.25	1.5	1.75	2	2.25	2.5	2.75	3
Transplant	197	181	169	159	141	122	101	92	76	63	58	54
LVR	81	76	73	69	61	60	58	48	30	23	18	12
Other NTS	35	29	24	22	19	18	17	15	13	9	8	5
PLV	35	31	28	26	24	21	19	17	17	16	16	15

Figure 44-9 Survival of patients initially referred for transplant who underwent conventional surgery. (From, Mahon NG, O'Neill JO, Young JB, et al. Contemporary outcome of outpatients referred for cardiac transplantation evaluation to a tertiary heart failure center: impact of surgical alternatives. *J Card Fail.* 2004;10(4) 273–277, with permission).

contraindications to conventional surgery for heart failure are severe uncompensated, inotrope-dependent heart failure. Such patients usually do not benefit from conventional surgical approaches. We think that if major comorbidities do not exist, these patients are best served by transplantation or ventricular assistance as destination therapy. Some patients fall in a grey zone. It is not always clear if these individuals will tolerate or improve with surgery. These patients are best managed with conventional surgery with mechanical assistance as a backup strategy in case difficulty is encountered during weaning from cardiopulmonary bypass.

Heart failure does not have to be a death sentence. Many therapies, both medical and surgical, exist for patients with this disabling condition. The determination of the most appropriate treatment for any particular patient is not always straightforward and is best made by a multidisciplinary team led by cardiologists and surgeons who have specific interest and training in the management of patients with heart failure and who individualize treatment for each patient. The majority of individuals can be managed by conventional surgical procedures such as coronary revascularization and valve repair or replacement. A certain subset of patients with ischemic cardiomyopathy benefit from LV reconstruction. For those individuals with advanced heart failure, transplantation and mechanical assistance offer the hope of prolonged survival and enhanced quality of life.

REFERENCES

1. American Heart Association heart disease and stroke statistics — 2005 Update. http://www.american-heart.org/presenter.jhtml/?identifier=1200026
2. Funk D. Epidemiology of end-stage heart disease. In: Hogness JR, Van Antwerp M, eds. *The Artificial Heart: Prototypes, Policies, and Patients*. Committee to Evaluate the Artificial Heart Program of the National Heart, Lung, and Blood Institute. Washington, D.C.: National Academy Press; 1991:251–261.
3. Taylor DO, Edwards LB, Boucek MM, et al. The Registry of the International Society for Heart and Lung Transplantation: twenty-first official adult heart transplant report. *J Heart Lung Transplant*. 2004;23:796–803.
4. Kauffman HM, McBride MA, Schield CF, et al. Determinants of waiting time for heart transplants in the United States. *J Heart Lung Transplant*. 1999;18:414–419.
5. McMurray JJ, Stewart S. Epidemiology, etiology, and prognosis of heart failure. *Heart*. 2000;83:596–602.
6. Sutton GC. Epidemiological aspects of heart failure. *Am Heart J*. 1990;120:1538–1540.
7. Kaiser GC, Davis KB, Fisher LD, et al. Survival following coronary artery bypass grafting in patients with severe angina pectoris (CASS). An observational study. *J Thorac Cardiovasc Surg*. 1985;89:513–524.
8. The VA Cooperative Study Group. Eighteen-year follow-up in the Veterans Affairs Cooperative Study of coronary artery bypass surgery for stable angina. *Circulation*. 1992;86:121–130
9. Sharma GV, Deupree RH, Khur SF, et. Al. Coronary bypass surgery improves survival in high risk unstable angina. Results of a Veteran Administration Cooperative Study with an 8-year follow-up. Veterans Administration Unstable Angina Cooperative Study Group. *Circulation*. 1991;84(Suppl 3): 260–267.
10. Myers WO, Gersh BJ, Fisher LD, et al. Medical versus early surgical therapy in patients with triple-vessel and mild angina pectoris: a CASS registry study of survival. *Ann Thorac Surg*. 1987;44:471–486.
11. Faulkner SL, Stoney WS, Alford WC, et al. Ischemic cardiomyopathy: Medical versus surgical treatment. *J Thorac Cardiovasc Surg*. 1977;74:77–82.
12. Franciosa JA, Wilen M, Ziesche S, et al. Survival in men with severe chronic left ventricular failure due to either coronary heart disease or idiopathic dilated cardiomyopathy. *Am J Cardiol*. 1983;51:831–836.
13. Harris PJ, Lee KL, Harrell FE, et al. Outcome in medically treated coronary artery disease. Ischemic events: nonfatal infarction and death. *Circulation*. 1980;62:718–726.
14. Manley JC, King JF, Zeft HJ, et al. The "bad" left ventricle: results of coronary surgery and effect on late survival. *J Thorac Cardiovasc Surg*. 1976;72:841–847.
15. Vlietstra RE, Assad-Morell JL, Frye RL, et al. Survival predictors in coronary artery disease: medical and surgical comparisons. *Mayo Clinic Proc*. 1977;52:85–90.
16. Yatteau RF, Peter RH, Behar VS, et al. Ischemic cardiomyopathy: the myopathy of coronary artery disease, natural history, and results of medical versus surgical treatment. *Am J Cardiol*. 1974;34:520–525.
17. Zubiate P, Kay JH, Dunne EF. Myocardial revascularization for patients with ejection fraction of 0.2 or less: 12 years' results. *West J Med*. 1984;140:745–749.
18. Uretsky BF, Thygesen K, Armstrong PW, et al. Acute coronary findings at autopsy in heart failure patients with sudden death. Results from the assessment of treatment with lisinopril and survival (ATLAS) trial. *Circulation*. 2000;102:611–616.
19. Veenhuyzen GD, Singh SN, McAreavey D, et al. Prior coronary artery bypass surgery and risk of death among patients with ischemic left ventricular dysfunction. *Circulation*. 2001;104: 1489–1493.
20. Kumpati GS, McCarthy PM, Hoercher KJ. Surgical treatments for heart failure. *Cardiol Clin*. 2002;19(4):669–681.
21. Allman KC, Shaw LJ, Hachamovitch R, et al. Myocardial viability testing and impact of revascularization on prognosis in patients with coronary artery disease and left ventricular dysfunction: a meta-analysis. *J Am Coll Cardiol*. 2002;39:1151–1158.
22. Hochman JS, Sleeper LA, Webb JG, et al. Early revascularization in acute myocardial infarction complicated by cardiogenic shock. *New Engl J Med*. 1999;341:625–634.
23. Lytle BW. The role of coronary revascularization in the treatment of ischemic cardiomyopathy. *Ann Thorac Surg*. 2003;75(6)(Suppl 1):S2–S5.
24. Cooley DA, Collins HA, Morris GC, et al. Ventricular aneurysm after myocardial infarction. Surgical excision with the use of temporary cardiopulmonary bypass. *JAMA*. 1958;167:557–560.
25. Dor V, Kreitmann P, Jourdan J, et al. Interest of physiological closure (circumferential plasty on contractile areas) of left ventricle after resection and endocardectomy for aneurysm or akinetic zone. Comparison with classical technique about a series of 209 left ventricular resections. *J Cardiovasc Surg*. 1985;26:73.
26. Jatene AD. Left ventricular aneurysmectomy. Resection or reconstruction. *J Thorac Cardiovasc Surg*. 1985;89:321–331.
27. DiDonato M, Sabatier M, Toso A, et al. Regional myocardial performance of non-ischemic zones remote from anterior wall left ventricular aneurysm. *Eur Heart J*. 1995;16:1285–1292.
28. Dang AB, Guccione JM, Zhang P, et al. Effect of ventricular size and patch stiffness in surgical anterior ventricular restoration: a finite element model study. *Ann Thorac Surg*. 2005;79:185–193.
29. Artrip JH, Oz MC, Burkoff D. Left ventricular volume reduction surgery for heart failure: a physiologic perspective. *J Thorac Cardiovasc Surg*. 2001;122:775–782.
30. DiDonato M, Sabatier M, Dor V, et al. Effects of the Dor procedure on left ventricular dimension and shape and geometric correlates of mitral regurgitation one year after surgery. *J Thorac Cardiovasc Surg*. 2001;121:9125.
31. Buckberg GD. Early and late results of left ventricular reconstruction in thin-walled chambers: is this our patient population? *J Thorac Cardiovasc Surg*. 2004;128:21–26.
32. Schenk S, McCarthy PM, Starling RC, et al. Neurohormonal response to left ventricular reconstruction surgery in ischemic cardiomyopathy. *J Thorac Cardiovasc Surg*. 2004;128:38–43.
33. Dor V. Left ventricular reconstruction: the aim and the reality after twenty years. *J Thorac Cardiovasc Surg*. 2004;128: 17–20.

34. Athanasuleas CL, Buckberg GD, Stanley AW, et al., RESTORE group. Surgical ventricular restoration in the treatment of congestive heart failure due to post-infarction ventricular dilation. *J Am Coll Cardiol*. 2004;44:1439–1445.
35. Koelling TM, Aaronson KD, Cody RJ, et al. Prognostic significance of mitral regurgitation and tricuspid regurgitation in patients with left ventricular systolic dysfunction. *Am Heart J*. 2002;144:524–529.
36. Grigioni F, Enriquez-Sarano M, Zehr KJ, et al. Ischemic mitral regurgitation: long-term outcome and prognostic implications with quantitative Doppler assessment. *Circulation*. 2001;103: 1759–1764.
37. Ellis SG, Whitlow PL, Raymond RE, et al. Impact of mitral regurgitation on long-term survival after percutaneous coronary intervention. *Am J Cardiol*. 2002;89:315–318.
38. Braunwald E. Valvular heart disease. In: *Heart Disease: A Textbook of Cardiovascular Medicine*. Philadelphia: WB Saunders; 1980.
39. Carpentier A. Cardiac valve surgery—the "French correction." *J Thorac Cardiovasc Surg*. 1983;86:323–337.
40. Bolling SF, Pagani FD, Deeb GM, et al. Intermediate-term outcome of mitral reconstruction in cardiomyopathy. *J Cardiovasc Surg*. 1998;115:381–386.
41. Bishay ES, McCarthy PM, Cosgrove DM, et al. Mitral valve surgery in patients with severe left ventricular dysfunction. *Eur J Cardiothoracic Surg*. 2000;17:213–221.
42. Rothenburger M, Rukosujew A, Hanmmel D, et al. Mitral valve surgery in patients with poor left ventricular function. *Thorac Cardiovasc Surg*. 2002;50:351–354.
43. Gummert JF, Rahmel A, Bucerius J, et al. Mitral valve repair in patients with end-stage cardiomyopathy: who benefits? *Eur J Cardiothorac Surg*. 2003;23:1017–1022; discussion, 1022.
44. Diodato MD, Moon MR, Pasque MK, et al. Repair of ischemic mitral regurgitation does not increase mortality or improve long-term survival in patients undergoing coronary artery revascularization: a propensity analysis. *Ann Thorac Surg*. 2004;78: 794–799.
45. Trichon BH, Glower DD, Shaw LK, et al. Survival after coronary revascularization, with and without mitral valve surgery, in patients with ischemic mitral regurgitation. *Circulation*. 2003;108(Suppl II): II-103–II-110.
46. Duarte IG, Shen Y, MacDonald MJ, et al. Treatment of moderate mitral regurgitation and coronary disease by coronary bypass alone: late results. *Ann Thorac Surg*. 1999;68:426–430.
47. Lam BK, Gillinov AM, Blackstone EH, et al. Importance of moderate ischemic mitral regurgitation. *Ann Thorac Surg*. 2005;79:462–470.
48. Aklog L, Filsoufi F, Flores KQ, et al. Does coronary artery bypass grafting alone correct moderate ischemic mitral regurgitation? *Circulation*. 2001;104(Suppl I): I-68–I-75.
49. Prifti E, Bonacchi M, Frati G, et al. Ischemic mitral valve regurgitation grade II–III correction in patients with impaired left ventricular function undergoing simultaneous coronary revascularization. *J Heart Valve Dis*. 2001;10:754.
50. McGee EC, Jr., Gillinov AM, McCarthy PM, et al. Recurrent mitral regurgitation after annuloplasty for functional ischemic mitral regurgitation. *J Thorac Cardiovasc Surg*.. 2004;128:916–924.
51. Bhudia SK, McCarthy PM, Smedira NG, et al. Edge-to-edge (Alfieri) mitral repair: results in diverse clinical settings. *Ann Thorac Surg*. 2004;77:1598–1606.
52. Miller DC. Ischemic mitral regurgitation redux—to repair or to replace? *J Thorac Cardiovasc Surg*. 2001;122:1059–1062.
53. Timek TA, Lai DT, Tibayan FA, et al. Septal-lateral annular cinching ('SLAC') reduces mitral annular size without perturbing normal annular dynamics. *J Heart Valv Dis*. 2002;11:2–9; discussion, 10.
54. Hueb AC, Jatene FB, Moreira LFP, et al. Ventricular remodeling and mitral valve modifications in dilated cardiomyopathy: new insights from anatomic study. *J Thorac Cardiovasc Surg*. 2002; 124:1216–1224.
55. McCarthy PM. Does the intertrigonal distance dilate? Never say never. *J Thorac Cardiovasc Surg*. 2002;124:1078–1079.
56. Tabayan FA, Rodriguez F, Langer F, et al. Annular remodeling in chronic ischemic mitral regurgitation: ring selection implications. *Ann Thorac Surg*. 2003;76:1549–1555.
57. Gorman JH III, Gorman RC, Jackson BM, et al. Annuloplasty ring selection for chronic ischemic mitral regurgitation: lesson from the ovine model. *Ann Thorac Surg*. 2003;76:1556–1563.
58. Kwan J, Shiota T, Agler DA, et al. Geometric differences of the mitral apparatus between ischemic and dilated cardiomyopathy with significant mitral regurgitation. *Circulation*. 2003;107:1135–1140.
59. Calafiore AM, Gallina S, Di Mauro M, et al. Mitral valve procedure in dilated cardiomyopathy: repair or replacement?, *Ann Thorac Surg*. 2001;71:1146–1153.
60. Gillinov AM, Wierup PN, Blackstone EH, et al. Is repair preferable to replacement for ischemic mitral regurgitation? *J Thorac Cardiovasc Surg*. 2001;122:1125–1141.
61. Wu A, Aaronson KD, Bolling SF, et al. Impact of mitral valve annuloplasty on mortality risk in patients with mitral regurgitation and left ventricular systolic dysfunction. *JACC*. 2005;45:381–387.
62. Periera JJ, Laure MS, Bashir M, et al. Survival after aortic valve replacement for severe aortic stenosis with low transvalvular gradients and severe left ventricular dysfunction. *J Am Coll Cardiol*. 2002;39:1356–1363.
63. Smedira NG, Ports TA, Merrick SH, et al. Balloon aortic valvuloplasty as a bridge to aortic valve replacement in critically ill patients. *Ann Thorac Surg*. 1993;55(4):914–916.
64. McCarthy PM, Kumpati GS, Blackstone EH, et al. Aortic valve surgery for chronic aortic regurgitation with severe LV dysfunction: time for a reevaluation? *Circulation*. 2001;104(Suppl): II-684.
65. McCarthy PM, Bhudia SK, Rajeswaran J, et al. Tricuspid valve repair: durability and risk factors for failure. *J Thorac Cardiovasc Surg*. 2004;127(3):674–685.
66. Kuwaki K, Morishita K, Tsukamoto M, et al. Tricuspid valve surgery for functional tricuspid valve regurgitation associated with left-sided valvular disease. *Eur J Cardiothorac Surg*. 2001;20:577.
67. Mukherjee D, Nader S, Olano A, et al. Improvement in right ventricular systolic function after surgical correction of isolated tricuspid regurgitation. *J Am Soc Echocardiogr*. 2000;13(7): 650–654.
68. Lloyd-Jones DM, Wang TJ, Leip EP, et al. Lifetime risk for development of atrial fibrillation: the framing study. *Circulation*. 2004;110(9):1042–1046.
69. Quader MA, McCarthy PM, Gillinov AM, et. Al. Does preoperative atrial fibrillation reduce survival after coronary artery bypass grafting? *Ann Thorac Surg*. 2004;77:1514–1522; discussion, 1522–1524.
70. Schaff HV, Dearani JA, Daly RC, et al. Cox-Maze procedure for atrial fibrillation: Mayo Clinic experience. *Semin Thorac70. Cardiovasc Surg*. 2000;(1):30–37.
71. Gillinov MA, McCarthy PM. Advances in the surgical treatment of atrial fibrillation. [Review] *Cardiol Clin*. 2004;22(1): 147–57.
72. Ansalone G, Giannantoni P, Ricci R, et al. Doppler myocardial imaging to evaluate the effectiveness of pacing sites in patients receiving biventricular pacing. *J Am Coll Cardiol*. 2002; 39(3):489–499.
73. Young JB, Abraham WT, Smith Al, et al. Combined cardiac resynchronization and implantable cardioversion defibrillation in advanced chronic heart failure. The MIRACLE ICD Trial. *JAMA*. 2003;289:2685–2694.
74. Auricchio A, Stellbrink C, Sack S, et al. Long-term clinical effect of hemodynamically optimized cardiac resychronization therapy in patients with heart failure, and ventricular function delay. *J Am Coll Cardiol*. 2002;39:2026–2033.
75. Linde C, Braunschweig F, Gadler F, et al. Long-term improvements in quality of life by biventricular pacing in patients with chronic heart failure: results from the Multisite Stimulation in Cardiomyopathy Study (MUSTIC). *Am J Cardiol*. 2003;91: 1090–1095.
76. Navia JL, Atik FA. Minimally invasive surgical alternatives for left ventricle epicardial lead implantation in heart failure patients. *Ann Thorac Surg*. 2005;80(2):751–754.
77. Batista RJ, Santos JL, Takeshita N, et al. Partial left ventriculectomy to improve left ventricular function in end-stage heart disease. *J Card Surg*. 1996;11:96–98.
78. Miller JI Jr., Lee RB, Mansour KA. Lung volume reduction surgery: lessons learned. *Ann Thorac Surg*. 1996;61(5):1464–1469.

79. Franco-Cerceda A, McCarthy PM, Starling RC, et al. Partial left ventriculectomy. *J Thorac Cardiovasc Surg.* 1997;114: 755–765.
80. Dickstein ML, Spotnitz HM, Rose EA, et al. Heart reduction surgery: an analysis of the impact on cardiac function. *J Thorac Cardiovasc Surg.* 1997;113:1032–1040.
81. Ratcliffe MB, Hong J, Salahieh A, et al. The effect of ventricular volume reduction surgery in the dilated, poorly contractile left ventricle: a simple finite element analysis. *J Thorac Cardiovasc Surg.* 1998;116:566–577.
82. Burkhoff D. New heart failure therapy: the shape of things to come? *J Thorac Cardiovasc Surg.* 2003;125:S50–S52.
83. Schreuder JJ, Steendijk P, van der Veen FH, et al. Acute and short-term effects of partial left ventriculectomy in dilated cardiomyopathy: assessment by pressure-volume loops. *J Am Coll Cardiol.* 2000;36:2104–2114.
84. Kass DA, Baughman KL, Pak PH, et al. Reverse remodeling from cardiomyoplasty in human heart failure. External constraint versus active assist. *Circulation.* 1995;91:2314–2318.
85. Batista R. Partial left ventriculectomy—the Batista procedure. *Eur J Cardiothorac Surg.* 1999;15(Suppl I):S12–S19.
86. Mann DL, Acker MA, Jessup M, et al. Rationale, design, and methods for a pivotal randomized clinical trial for the assessment of a cardiac support device in patients with New York Heart Association Class III-IV heart failure. *J Cardiac Fail.* 2004;10(3):185–192.
87. Saavedra FW, Tunn R, Mishima T, et al. Reverse remodeling and enhanced adrenergic reserve from a passive external ventricular support in experimental dilated heart failure. *Circulation.* 2000;102(Suppl II):II-683.
88. Chaudhry PH, Mishima T, Sharov VG, et al. Passive epicardial containment prevents ventricular remodeling in heart failure. *Ann Thorac Surg.* 2000;70:1275–1280.
89. Power J, Raman J, Byrne M. Passive ventricular constraint is a trigger for a significant degree of reverse remodeling in an experimental model of degenerative heart failure and dilated cardiomyopathy. *Circulation.* 2000;102(Suppl II):II-502.
90. McCarthy PM, Takagaki M, Ochiai Y, et al. Device based change in left ventricular shape: a new concept for the treatment of dilated cardiomyopathy. *J Thorac Cardiovasc Surg.* 2001;122: 482–490.
91. Guccione JM, Salahieh A, Moonly SM, et al. Myosplint decrease wall stress without depressing function in the failing heart: a finite element model study. *Ann Thorac Surg.* 2003;76: 1171–1180.
92. Melvin DB. Ventricular radius reduction without resection: a computational analysis. *ASAIO J.* 1999;45:160–165.
93. Taylor DO, Edward, LB, Boucek MM, et al. The Registry of the International Society for Heart and Lung Transplantation: twenty-first official adult heart transplant report. *J Heart Lung Transplant.* 2004;23:796–803.
94. Zaroff JG, Rosengard BR, Armstrong WF, et al. Consensus conference report maximizing use of organs recovered from the cadaver donor: cardiac recommendations. *Circulation.* 2002; 106:836–841.
95. Lower R, Shumway NE. Studies on orthotopic homotransplantation of the canine heart. *Surg Form.* 1960;11:18–19.
96. Barnard CN. What we have learned about heart transplants. *J Thorac Cardiovasc Surg.* 1968;56:457–468.
97. Sievers HH, Weyand M, Kraatz EG, et al. An alternate technique for orthotopic cardiac transplantation, with preservation of the normal anatomy of the right atrium. *Thorac Cardiovasc Surg.* 1991;39:70–72.
98. Dreyfus G, Jebara V, Mihaileanu S, et al. Total orthotopic heart transplantation: an alternative to the standard technique. *Ann Thorac Surg.* 1991;52:1181–1184.
99. Grande AM, Rinaldi M, D'Armini AM, et al. Orthotopic heart transplantation: standard versus bicaval technique. *Am J Cardiol.* 2000;85:1329–1333.
100. Gamel AE, Yonan NA, Grant S, et al. Orthotopic cardiac transplantation: a comparison of standard and bicaval Wythenshawe techniques. *J Thorac Cardiovasc Surg.* 1999;109:721–730.
101. Leyh RG, Jahnke AW, Kraatz EG, et al. Cardiovascular dynamics and dimensions after bicaval and standard cardiac transplantation. *Ann Thorac Surg.* 1995;59:1495–1500.
102. Gamel AE, Deiraniya AK, Rahman AN, et al. Orthotopic heart transplantation hemodynamics: does atrial preservation improve cardiac output after transplantation? *J Heart Lung Transplant.* 1996;15:564–571.
103. Beniaminovitz A, Savoia MT, Oz M, et al. Improved atrial function in bicaval versus orthotopic techniques in cardiac transplantation. *Am J Cardiol.* 1997;80:1631–1635.
104. Copeland JG. Heart transplantation: the standard versus bicaval technique controversy. *Transplant Proceedings* 2000;32(7): 1519–1520.
105. Aziz TM, Burgess MI, El-Gamel A, et al. Orthotopic cardiac transplantation technique: a survey of current practice. *Ann Thorac Surg.* 1999;68(4):1242–1246.
106. Jeevanadum V, Russell H, Mather P, et al. A one-year comparison of prophylactic donor tricuspid annuloplasty in heart transplantation. *Ann Thorac Surg.* 2004;78:759–766.
107. The artificial heart program: current status and history. In: Hogness JR, VanAntewerp M, eds. The Artificial Heart: Prototypes, Policies, and Patients. Washington, D.C.: National Academy Press; 1991:14–25.
108. Helman DN, Rose EA. History of mechanical circulatory support. *Prog Cardiovasc Dis.* 2000;43:1–4.
109. Cooley DA, Liotta D, Hallman GL, et al. Orthotopic cardiac prothesis for two-staged cardiac replacement. *Am J Cardiol.* 1969;24:723–730.
110. Norman JC, Brook MI, Cooley DA, et al. Total support of the circulation of a patient with post-cardiotomy stone-heart syndrome by a partial artificial heart (ALVAD) for 5 days followed by heart and kidney transplantation. *Lancet.* 1978;1: 1125–1127.
111. Frazier OH, Macris MP, Myers TJ, et al. Improved survival after extended bridge to cardiac transplantation. *Ann Thorac Surg.* 1994;57:1416–1422.
112. Oz MC, Argenziano M, Catanese KA, et al. Bridge experience with long-term implantable left ventricular assist devices. Are they an alternative to transplantation? *Circulation.* 1997;95: 1844–1852.
113. Sun BC, Catanese KA, Spanier TB, et al. 100 long-term implantable left ventricular assist devices: the Columbia Presbyterian interim experience. *Ann Thorac Surg.* 1999;68: 688–694.
114. Navia JL, McCarthy PM, Hoercher KJ, et al. Do left ventricular assist device (LVAD) bridge-to-transplantation outcomes predict the results of permanent LVAD implantation? *Ann Thorac Surg.* 2002;74(6):2051–2063.
115. Copeland JG, Smith RG, Arabia FA, et al. Cardiac replacement with a total artificial heart as a bridge to transplantation. *N Engl J Med.* 2004;351(9):859–867.
116. Hetzer R, Muller JH, Weng YG, et al. Midterm follow-up of patients who underwent removal of a left ventricular assist device after cardiac recovery from end-stage dilated cardiomyopathy. *J Thorac Cardiovasc Surg.* 2000;128:843–855.
117. Hon JKF, Yacoub MH. Bridge to recovery with the use of left ventricular assist device and clenbuterol. *Ann Thorac Surg.* 2003;75:S36–S41.
118. Grinda JM, Chevalier P, D'Attellis N, et al. Fulminant myocarditis in adults and children: bi-ventricular assist device for recovery. *Eur J Cardiothorac Surg.* 2004;(6):1169–1173.
119. Rose EA, Gelijns AC, Moskowitz AJ, et al. Long-term use of a left ventricular device for end-stage heart failure. *N Engl J Med.* 2001;345:1435–1443.
120. Frazier OH, Meyers TJ, Gregoric ID, et al. Initial clinical experience with the Jarvik 2000 implantable axial-flow left ventricular assist system. *Circulation.* 2002;105:2855–2860.
121. Noon GP, Morley DL, Irwin S, et al. Clinical experience with the MicroMed DeBakey ventricular assist. *Ann Thorac Surg.* 2001;71:S133–S138.
122. Frazier OH, Delgado RM, Kar B, et al. First clinical use of the redesigned HeartMate II left assist system in the United States. *Tex Heart Inst J.* 2004;31(2):157–159.
123. Williams MR, Oz MC. Indications and patient selection for mechanical ventricular assistance. *Ann Thorac Surg.* 2001;71:S86–S91.
124. Mielniczuk L, Mussivand T, Davies R, et al. Patient selection for left ventricular assist devices. *Artif Organs.* 2004;28(2): 152–157.

125. Kukuy EL, Oz MC, Haka Y. Long-term mechanical circulatory support. In: Cohen LH, Edmunds LH Jr., eds. *Cardiac Surgery in the Adult*. New York: McGraw-Hill; 2003:1491–1506.
126. Deng MC, Edwards LB, Hertz MI, et al. Mechanical circulatory support device data base of the International Society for Heart and Lung Transplantation: second annual report—2004. *J Heart Lung Transplant*. 2004;23(9):1027–1034.
127. Miller LW. Patient selection for the use of ventricular assist devices as a bridge to transplantation. *Ann Thorac Surg*. 2003;75:S66–S71.
128. Minami K, El-Banayosy A, Sezai A, et al. Morbidity and outcome after mechanical ventricular support using Thoratec, Novacor, and HeartMate for bridging to heart transplantation. *Artif Organs*. 2000;24:421–426.
129. Frazier OH. Mechanical cardiac assistance: historical perspectives. *Sem Thorac Cardiovasc Surg*. 2000;12:207–219.
130. Copeland JG, Arabia FA, Tsau PH, et al. Total artificial hearts: bridge to transplantation. *Cardiol Clin*. 2003;21:101–113.
131. Mahon NG, O'Neill JO, Young JB, et al. Contemporary outcome of outpatients referred for cardiac transplantation evaluation to a tertiary heart failure center: impact of surgical alternatives. *J Card Fail*. 2004;10(4) 273–277.

45 Use of Mechanical Devices in Treating Heart Failure

Timothy J. Myers Reynolds M. Delgado, III O. H. Frazier

Congestive heart failure (CHF) is the most common cause of death in the industrialized world. Current medical therapy can relieve its symptoms (1) and can even prolong life in some cases (2,3). Unfortunately, the relentless nature of the underlying disease process means that CHF almost always proves fatal in the end. When conventional therapy fails to alleviate end-stage heart failure, mechanical circulatory support (MCS) is a possible option. During the past several decades, MCS has become an effective means of saving many patients who would otherwise die of progressive CHF.

Today physicians can choose from a wide range of MCS systems, depending on the desired degree of support, length of support, and extent of postoperative mobility. Short-term MCS may be used to maintain patients who develop acute, reversible heart failure after a myocardial infarction or open heart surgery. Longer-term MCS may be applied to patients with severe acute and chronic heart failure, including those awaiting heart transplantation. With prolonged (>30-day) support, transplant candidates may undergo cardiac rehabilitation, which often reverses cardiac and end-organ dysfunction, improving the patient's operative status (4,5).

MCS has evolved, somewhat in parallel with cardiac transplantation, toward the goal of lowering the morbidity and mortality of CHF. By combining these two interventions, physicians are salvaging many otherwise hopeless cases. MCS is now being used as destination therapy. According to the Institute of Medicine, MCS could benefit some 35,000 to 70,000 Americans per year (6).

After briefly describing the history of MCS systems, this chapter will focus first on the major devices currently being used for short-term support, and then on implantable systems being used for longer-term bridging to transplantation and destination therapy.

HISTORY

Although the use of mechanical devices to support the human heart has become prevalent only within the last decade, the concept of MCS has a long history. Nearly two centuries ago, LeGallois (7) speculated that temporary or permanent support of the failing heart was possible. Since that time, the concept of MCS has continued to unfold, accompanied by advancing insights into cardiovascular physiology.

In the twentieth century, research into organ perfusion and preservation of the circulation was carried out by many investigators, including DeBakey (8), Lindbergh (9), and Gibbon (10), who laid the foundation for today's MCS systems. In 1953, the clinical introduction of cardiopulmonary bypass ushered in the era of open heart surgery and highlighted the need for temporary support of the circulation (10). In a sense, the heart–lung machine may be considered the parent of mechanical assist devices. It fueled the imagination of many cardiovascular specialists and gave rise to 40 years of rapid development in assist-device technology.

A major breakthrough in MCS systems occurred in 1961, when Moulopoulos et al. (11) introduced the intra-aortic balloon pump. This device was not used clinically until 6 years later, when Kantrowitz et al. (12) implanted it in a patient with cardiogenic shock. Since that time, it has been extremely valuable for treating potentially reversible left ventricular dysfunction. Intra-aortic balloon pump support remains the most common form of MCS.

Other early breakthroughs included the first use of a roller pump to assist the left ventricle, by Dennis et al. (13) in 1962. In addition, Spencer et al. (14) used an extracorporeal roller pump to support patients in postcardiotomy cardiogenic shock. In 1963, DeBakey et al. (15–17) implanted a pulsatile pump in three patients who had undergone open heart surgery. This air-driven, tube-type pump, made of Dacron-reinforced Silastic with ball valves at the inflow and outflow ports, was the first ventricular assist device to be implanted clinically. Later, the same group used an extracorporeal ventricular assist device (VAD) in two patients who became long-term survivors.

In 1964, the National Institutes of Health (NIH) had established its Artificial Heart Program, whose goals included the development of both partial and total artificial hearts. At first, the research was multifaceted, using resources from medicine, the basic sciences, engineering, industry, and systems management. Throughout that decade, NIH programs emphasized the separate development of various components of circulatory support and replacement devices. This federal funding source continued the development of MCS for many years.

In 1969, Cooley (18) performed the first clinical bridge-to-transplant operation when he implanted a Liotta total artificial heart (TAH) in a 47-year-old terminally ill man. The pneumatically driven, diaphragm-type, dual-ventricular TAH was positioned orthotopically, replacing the native ventricles. It functioned well, sustaining the patient for 64 hours until a donor heart could be transplanted. Since that time, the TAH has undergone considerable evolution.

In 1982, William DeVries (19) performed the first of five TAH implantations intended to serve as permanent cardiac replacements. In these cases, the TAH was the Jarvik-7 model designed by Robert Jarvik. Although this pump was able to support the total circulation for prolonged periods, patients had to remain hospitalized and tethered to control consoles. In addition, the series was plagued by device-related complications, particularly infection and stroke, and only two of the patients survived for more than a year (20).

After 1970, the direction of government-sponsored research shifted. The NIH institute responsible for the Artificial Heart Program achieved bureau status and became the National Heart, Lung, and Blood Institute (NHLBI); MCS research was performed under the auspices of the Devices and Technology Branch of the Division of Heart and Vascular Diseases. In the mid-1970s, having performed extensive animal and in vitro tests of device safety and reliability, the NHLBI challenged physicians, engineers, and private companies to develop a fully implantable device for the long-term support of CHF patients. As a result, a wide range of VADs were introduced to support patients in postcardiotomy shock (21–26). Most of these devices were pneumatically actuated pulsatile pumps (27,28).

By 1978, the Texas Heart Institute was conducting clinical tests of an abdominally positioned left ventricular assist device (LVAD). That same year, Cooley and Norman (29) used this LVAD as a bridge to transplantation in a patient who had developed stone heart syndrome after undergoing valve replacement. The single-chambered, implantable device supported the patient's circulation for 5 days until a donor heart became available. In 1986, we began testing a fully implantable LVAD, now called the HeartMate (Thoratec Corp., Pleasanton, CA), which was designed for long-term or permanent left ventricular support (30). The original, pneumatically powered version of this device began undergoing clinical testing in bridge-to-transplant patients in 1986 (31). Five years later, an electrically powered, more portable version of the HeartMate entered into clinical trials (32). Both versions of the HeartMate, pneumatic and electric, have completed clinical trials and were commercially approved by the U.S. Food and Drug Administration (FDA) in 1994 and 1998, respectively. The HeartMate electric LVAD was then commercially approved for destination therapy in 2003. Likewise, the Thoratec VAD (Thoratec Corp., Pleasanton, CA) and the Novacor N100 VAS (World Heart Corp., Oakland, CA) systems have also received commercial approval as a bridge to heart transplantation.

In the 1990s, a new generation of potentially more reliable and versatile MCS devices, the rotary pumps, were being developed. Today, axial-flow VADs such as the Jarvik 2000 Heart (Jarvik Heart, Inc., New York, NY) and HeartMate II (Thoratec Corp., Pleasanton, CA) are being tested clinically as bridges to transplant and show potential for use as permanent, long-term therapy. Others are now being applied in the catheterization laboratory and the operating room to cases of acute heart failure.

The clinical use of MCS systems is now widespread. Despite numerous design modifications and refinements, no ideal system has yet evolved. Nevertheless, current systems can salvage many patients with end-stage CHF, providing hope where none had previously existed.

SHORT-TERM CIRCULATORY SUPPORT

Settings in Which Short-Term Mechanical Circulatory Support May Be Useful

Short-term (up to 2-week) MCS is an important strategy for controlling acute, reversible heart failure presenting as cardiogenic shock. Often, this condition is caused by an acute myocardial infarction involving more than 40% of the left ventricular mass (33); in such cases, MCS can support the patient's circulation until his or her condition improves enough for myocardial revascularization to be undertaken. Alternatively, cardiogenic shock may develop after open heart surgery; short-term mechanical support may allow the patient to be weaned from cardiopulmonary bypass and to regain adequate ventricular function. No matter what causes the cardiogenic shock, the chance of death is greater than 80% without MCS (34–38).

Of course, the most familiar form of MCS is cardiopulmonary bypass itself, which permits the heart to be stopped long enough for intricate repairs to be performed on it. Unfortunately, cardiopulmonary bypass and cardiac arrest can produce numerous adverse effects, including additional myocardial ischemic damage necessitating continued MCS (39,40). Today, acute coronary occlusions are usually managed with aggressive interventional procedures in the cardiac catheterization laboratory. In patients who have dissection, rupture, or reocclusion or who are otherwise at high risk, MCS is often used as a bridge to either balloon angioplasty or emergency coronary bypass. Other possible indications for short-term MCS include acute myocarditis and cardiac dysfunction or labile pulmonary hypertension immediately after heart transplantation.

Appropriate Devices for Short-Term Mechanical Circulatory Support

Intra-Aortic Balloon Pump

The world's most widely used MCS system is the intra-aortic balloon pump (IABP), which was introduced during the 1960s by Moulopolous (11) and Kantrowitz (12). The polyurethane balloon is attached to the catheter, which is inserted percutaneously into the common femoral artery and is then advanced to the descending thoracic aorta (Fig. 45-1). Alternatively, if severe peripheral vascular disease is present the balloon may be inserted into the abdominal aorta via a retroperitoneal approach or, during open heart surgery, into the aortic arch via the subclavian artery.

The pump's action depends on several unique but fairly simple physiological principles. At the start of diastole, the balloon inflates and forces blood distal and proximal to the catheter, which augments coronary perfusion by increasing the diastolic pressure in the aortic root. At the beginning of systole, the balloon deflates, producing a lower pressure within the aorta; blood is ejected from the left ventricle with less resistance, increasing the cardiac output by as much as 40% and decreasing the left ventricular stroke work and myocardial oxygen requirements (41). In this manner, the balloon supports the heart indirectly. Although designed to provide short-term MCS, the IABP has occasionally been used in heart transplant candidates for weeks at a time.

The device's limitations include an inability to completely unload the left ventricle. In fact, the IABP will function only if the patient's heart can produce at least some cardiac output and has a regular cardiac rhythm. Adequate IABP function depends on appropriate timing of the balloon cycle and is suboptimal in the presence of arrhythmias. Moreover, patients with this device cannot leave their hospital beds. In up to 43% of cases, the pump must be removed because of peripheral vascular hemorrhagic or thromboembolic complications, which may require surgical intervention (42,43). Despite the device's life-saving capability, IABP recipients have a mortality that ranges from 7% to 86% (44).

ABIOMED BVS 5000 and AB 5000

When short-term uni-ventricular or biventricular support is needed for patients with potentially reversible ventricular dysfunction, the ABIOMED BVS 5000 or AB 5000 (ABIOMED, Inc., Danvers, MA) devices may be used. These externally positioned systems, composed of one or two disposable blood pumps governed by a single console, provide pulsatile flow (Fig. 45-2) (45). Although the BVS 5000 system was introduced clinically in the late 1980s and the

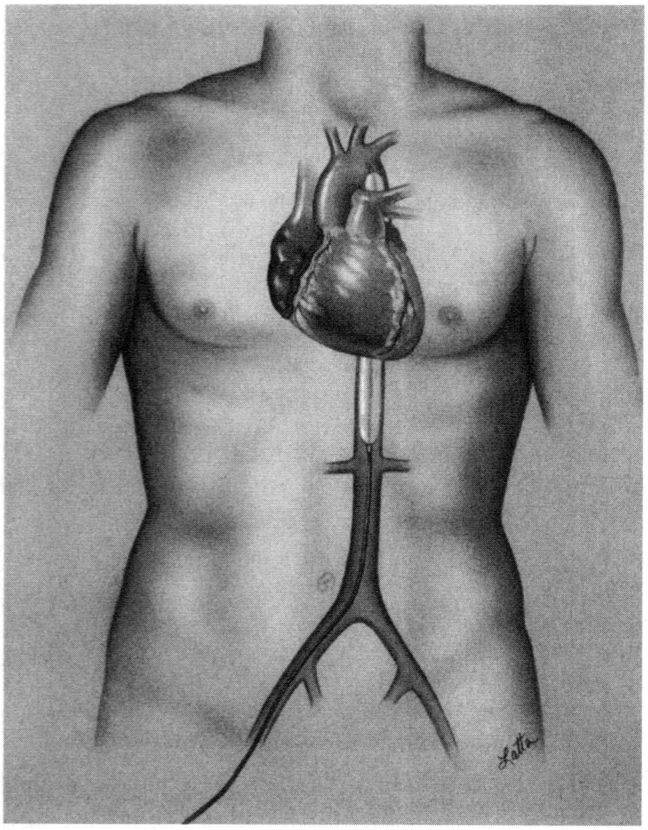

Figure 45-1 Inflated balloon in the thoracic aorta.

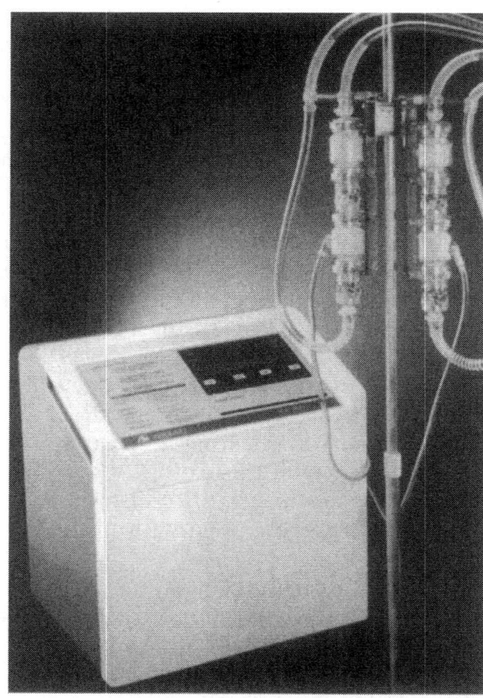

Figure 45-2 ABIOMED BVS 5000 console and blood pumps. (Reproduced from Frazier OH, Short HD, Wampler RK, et al. Mechanical circulatory support in the transplant population. In: Frazier OH, Macris MP, Radovancevic B, eds. *Support and Replacement of the Failing Heart.* Philadelphia: Lippincott-Raven; 1996:156–159, with permission.)

AB 5000 in 2003, both systems are widely used today. Compared with the older technology, however, the AB 5000 provides a higher pump flow of approximately 1.5 L per minute and allows patient ambulation during use.

The BVS 5000 is a dual-chambered, gravity-filled pump that provides approximately 5 L per minute of support (46). Within the pump, one-way flow is ensured by two trileaflet valves, one between the ventricular and atrial chambers and the other in the ventricular outflow tract. All blood-contacting surfaces within the pump are covered with a proprietary polyetherurethane (Angioflex) that is designed to be biocompatible and nonthrombogenic. Depending on the type of circulatory assistance needed, wire-reinforced 46 F inflow cannulas are inserted into the patient's right or left atrium. At the distal end of each wire-reinforced outflow cannula is a 14-mm Angioflex-coated Dacron graft, which is connected to the aorta or pulmonary artery. To prevent infection, each cannula is covered with Dacron velour at its transcutaneous exit site.

The AB 5000 circulatory support system is used to support one or both sides of the heart. Each pneumatically driven, one-chambered pump utilizes the same valves and polyurethane material as the BVS 5000. For left-sided support, blood inflow from the left atrium or ventricle is returned to the thoracic aorta. For right-sided support, inflow from the right atrium returns to the pulmonary artery. Cannulation for the AB 5000 is similar to that for the BVS 5000.

A pneumatic, microprocessor-controlled drive console automatically controls the stroke volume of each pump and monitors filling by means of a driveline connected to the ventricular housing. The console adjusts the left and right blood pumps independently, and it automatically determines pump rates and systolic/diastolic intervals by sensing driveline airflow. Pumping is not synchronized with the heartbeat and the pump rate is increased or decreased depending on the rate at which the pump fills. During weaning, the flow rate is reduced by means of a control knob.

Patients supported by either ABIOMED device often require prolonged intensive care, including multiple intravenous medications, chest tube drainage, and invasive cardiovascular monitoring. Many will have undergone extensive cardiac surgery with cardiopulmonary bypass (47). Because use of either system entails a risk of thromboembolism, patients must take anticoagulants (48). Bleeding and reoperation are the most frequently reported complications. In most cases, ambulation and physical rehabilitation are very difficult. Ambulation with the AB 5000 pump is possible because the pump is vacuum-filled; ambulation with the gravity-filled BVS 5000 pump is not likely. Patients who cannot be weaned from support are considered candidates for implantation of a long-term MCS device.

Over 6,000 patients have been supported with the BVS 5000 and 88 patients have been supported with the AB 5000. Indications for BVS 5000 use have included postcardiotomy cardiogenic shock in 63% of cases, acute myocardial infarction (AMI) cardiogenic shock in 9%, failed heart transplant in 8%, myocarditis in 2%, and other indications in 18%. A similar trend has been noted for the AB 5000, although it has also been used to provide right heart support after LVAD implantation.

Medtronic Perfusion Systems Pump

Another option often used for short-term uni-ventricular or biventricular MCS is the Medtronic Perfusion Systems Bio-Pump (Medtronic, Inc., Minneapolis, MN; formerly miomedicus pump), an extracorporeal centrifugal device available in two disposable models: an 80-mL model for adults (maximal flow, 10 L minute) and a 48-mL model for children. In this device, rotating acrylic cones generate continuous flow according to the constrained vortex principle (Fig. 45-3). The pump is magnetically coupled to an external motor and console where impeller speed is manually adjusted.

Clinicians have acquired considerable experience with the Bio-Pump because it is primarily used for cardiopulmonary bypass and is available in the majority of centers that perform cardiac surgery. Its advantages include simplicity, versatility, and cost-effectiveness. Limitations include the need for specialized personnel to supervise the system and the need for anticoagulation. Moreover, durability or thrombosis problems preclude use of the Bio-Pump for more than 5 days, although this limit is occasionally exceeded. In any case, the pump component should be replaced every 48 to 96 hours. Despite heparin bonding, the pump circuit is susceptible to thrombus formation; systemic heparinization is often necessary, which can intensify bleeding complications (49). The externalized cannulas are also potential sites of infection.

Beyond its cardiopulmonary bypass applications, the Medtronic Perfusion Systems pump is mainly used to provide temporary support in patients with postcardiotomy heart failure (50–52). It has also been used to support children in cardiogenic shock following repair of congenital heart defects (53) and to provide temporary right heart support following heart transplantation or LVAD implantation (54,55). Although more than half of patients supported with the Medtronic Perfusion Systems pump can be weaned from support, the hospital discharge rate is only 22% (56). Frequent and severe complications due to comorbidities are common during support in this population.

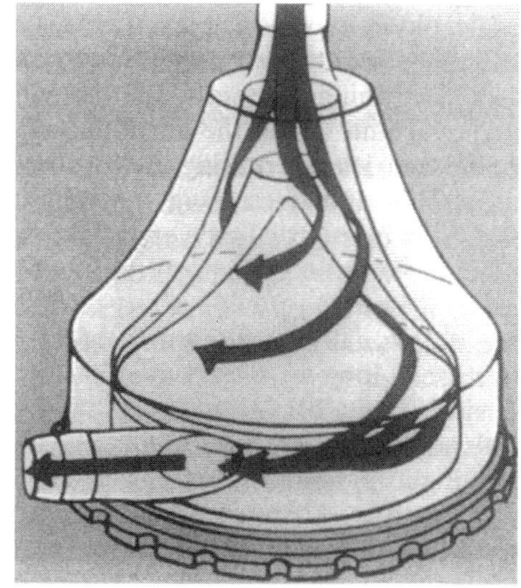

Figure 45-3 Medtronic Perfusion Systems Pump (Biomedicus Pump).

TandemHeart

The TandemHeart percutaneous VAD (Cardiac Assist, Inc., Pittsburgh, PA) is intended for short-term use for up to 14 days in cases of acute heart failure (Fig. 45-4). The TandemHeart is very small, with a priming volume of only 7 mL, but can produce continuous flows of up to 3.5 L per minute. A heparinized bearing lubrication system protects the impeller from wear and helps to prevent thrombosis within the pump, thus minimizing the need for anticoagulants. The device is inserted percutaneously through a femoral vein and advanced across the intra-atrial septum into the left atrium. Blood is withdrawn from the left atrium through a 21-F transseptal cannula and pumped to one or both femoral arteries through 15 or 17 F outflow cannulas.

The TandemHeart has been used to provide support during high-risk percutaneous coronary intervention (PCI), cardiogenic shock following AMI, and postcardiotomy heart failure (57). In most cases of high-risk PCI, the device is removed at the end of the procedure or within a few hours if the postoperative course is uncomplicated. In cases of cardiogenic shock or postcardiotomy heart failure, it is used to support patients until sufficient cardiac recovery occurs or, barring that, until more definitive long-term therapy can be considered.

At present, the clinical experience with the TandemHeart is small (57,58). At our institution, we have applied it with some success in seven cases of high-risk PCI, six cases of bridging to implantation of a long-term VAD, eight cases of cardiogenic shock, and three cases of support during cardiac surgical procedures.

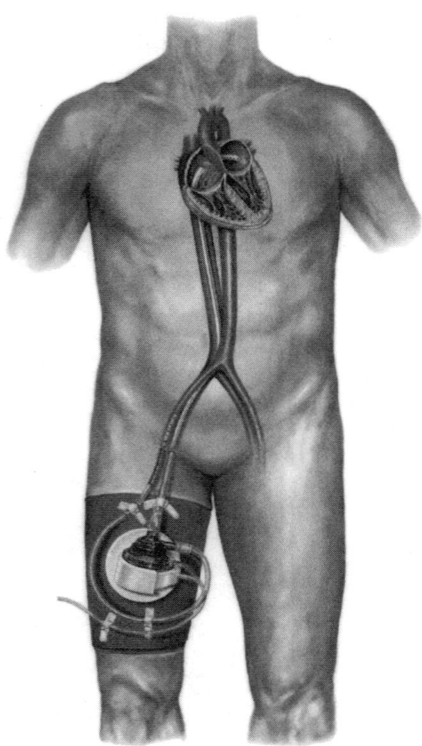

Figure 45-4 TandemHeart percutaneous ventricular assist device.

Investigational Devices for Short-Term Mechanical Circulatory Support

Two promising short-term VAD systems are undergoing clinical trials: the Impella Recover (Impella CardioSystems AG, Aachen, Germany) and Levitronix CentriMag (Levitronix LLC, Waltham, MA). Both have made it through FDA phase I studies and have entered phase II pivotal trials. These new systems are intended to support patients for up to 2 weeks while myocardial function recovers or, in the case of no recovery, until implantation of a long-term VAD. The most frequent indications for their use are AMI and failure to wean from cardiopulmonary bypass.

Impella Recover

The Impella Recover is a miniature catheter-mounted pump that can provide either left or right heart support at flows of 5 to 6 L per minute. The device can be threaded percutaneously through a femoral artery into the ventricle for support during acute heart failure or inserted directly into the ventricle through a sternotomy for support during postcardiotomy heart failure. The Impella Recover has been used extensively in Europe (59,60) and has only recently been introduced in the United States for clinical trials.

The device has been used for circulatory support in more than 350 patients worldwide, including left heart support in the majority, right heart support in 23, and biventricular support in 11. Left heart support is provided by the Recover LD version (Fig. 45-5) and right heart support by the Recover RD (Fig. 45-6). Indications have included support during high-risk percutaneous transluminal coronary angioplasty, support during cardiogenic shock following acute myocardial infarction, and failure to wean from cardiopulmonary bypass. On several occasions, this system has been used as a short-term bridge to heart transplant or for support during off-pump coronary artery bypass procedures.

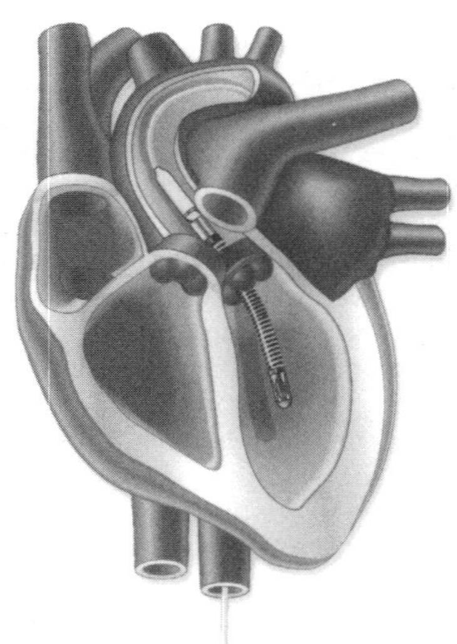

Figure 45-5 Impella Recover LD pump.

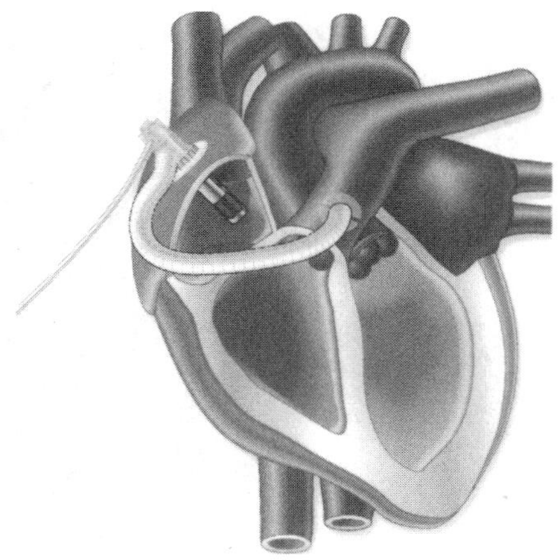

Figure 45-6 Impella Recover RD pump.

Levitronix CentriMag

The Levitronix CentriMag system is designed to provide circulatory support for up to 14 days to patients suffering from severe, acute, but potentially reversible cardiac failure (61). The system, which can be readily adapted to available cannulas and tubing, consists of a blood pump, motor, and drive console (Fig. 45-7). Within the pump's housing, which contains no seals or bearings, a magnetically levitated impeller rotates at speeds of up to 5,500 rpm and can produce a centrifugal flow of 10 L per minute. This contact-free pumping mechanism is intended to enhance biocompatibility and reliability by eliminating the friction and heat that can contribute to hemolysis, thrombosis, and wear.

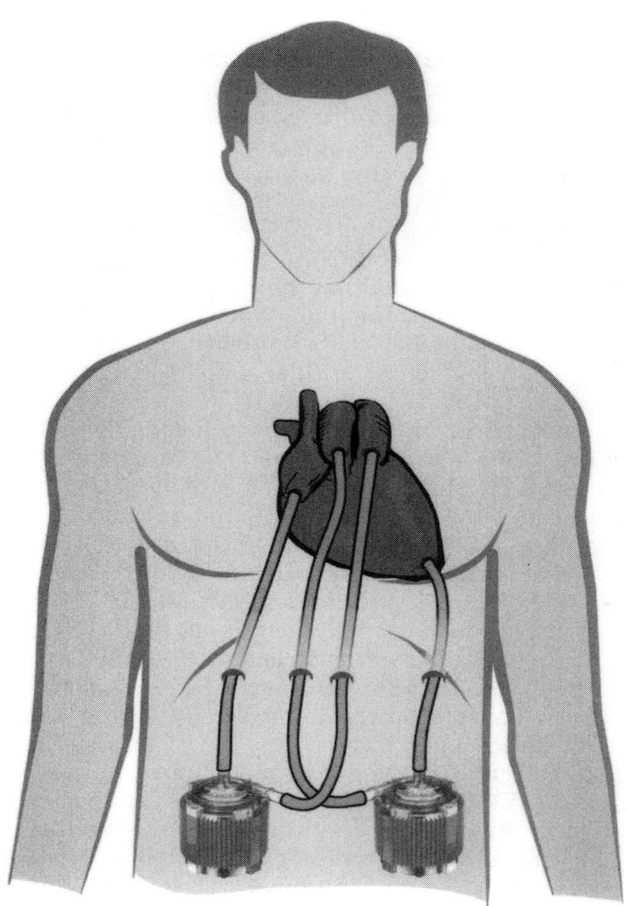

Figure 45-7 Levitronix CentriMag pump.

In Europe, the CentriMag is approved for use as an extracorporeal MCS device for up to 14 days in patients in severe, potentially reversible ventricular failure. In the United States, it is still considered an investigational device but has entered a clinical trial to evaluate its safety and effectiveness in the treatment of postcardiotomy cardiogenic shock under an FDA exemption.

More than 160 patients have been supported by the CentriMag pump for indications including postcardiotomy cardiogenic shock (40%), pretransplantation heart failure (13%), posttransplantation heart failure (13%), and cardiogenic shock following AMI (9%). This apparent versatility may allow its use in a broad range of patients.

BRIDGING TO TRANSPLANTATION

Since the early 1980s, MCS systems have been widely used as bridges to cardiac transplantation, keeping the patient alive until a suitable donor heart can be found. The first patients to receive these systems were confined to the intensive care unit. Today, however, selected patients with implantable MCS systems can leave the hospital and undergo cardiac rehabilitation (62,63). Mechanical assistance reduces the mortality of transplant candidates by 55% (64) and enhances their chance of posttransplant survival (4,5).

Once circulatory support is initiated, it tends to reverse the complex physiologic abnormalities that characterize the body's response to heart failure. Kidney and liver dysfunction is often reversed and neurohormonal activation returns to normal levels (65). Neurohormonal normalization takes about 5 weeks and is usually accompanied by improvements in other organs. By the time a donor heart is found, most long-term MCS recipients who were originally in New York Heart Association (NYHA) class IV will have improved to class I. As a result, they are more likely to survive transplantation and undergo long-term recovery and rehabilitation. For optimal results, MCS should be initiated early, before multiorgan failure occurs.

Patient Selection

In bridge-to-transplant cases, survival largely depends on careful patient selection (66). Bridging to transplantation should be considered for patients whose hemodynamic status deteriorates rapidly despite optimal medical therapy and/or intra-aortic balloon support. Traditional hemodynamic selection criteria include a pulmonary capillary wedge pressure over 20 mm Hg, a cardiac index ≤ 2 L/min/m^2, or a systolic blood pressure no higher than 80 mm Hg. However, these criteria may not hold true for all patients needing mechanical support; medical therapy often improves the hemodynamic values but severe irreversible heart failure remains. Patients with adequate hemodynamic values may be dependent on multiple cardioactive drugs and intra-aortic balloon support, in which case these patients can be reasonable candidates for an implantable VAD. The following conditions render a patient ineligible for MCS: elevated, fixed pulmonary vascular resistance; irreversible kidney or renal failure; respiratory failure; sepsis; or a severe neurological deficit. These conditions are also exclusionary criteria for cardiac transplantation. Although patients older than 60 years and those who require mechanical ventilation for respiratory insufficiency are not necessarily excluded from MCS, they are less likely to have a good outcome. Moreover, the most commonly used long-term pumps are too bulky to fit small patients (body surface area <1.5 m^2).

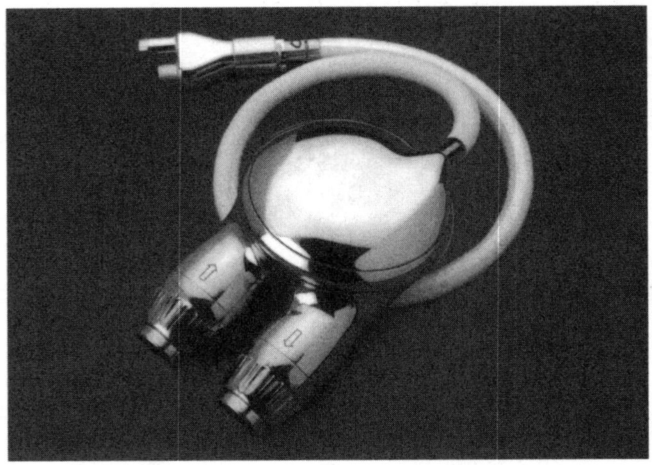

Figure 45-9 Thoratec implantable ventricular assist device.

Appropriate Devices for Bridging to Transplantation

Thoratec Ventricular Assist Device

The Thoratec VAD (Thoratec Corp., Pleasanton, CA) is intended to be used both for bridging to heart transplantation and for myocardial recovery; however, because it has been used primarily as a bridge device, the discussion of this system is included in this section (67). The Thoratec VAD was originally developed as a paracorporeal pump (pVAD) that resided on the anterior abdominal wall and was connected to two cannulas that were externalized subcostally. An implantable version (iVAD) was commercially approved in 2004. The primary difference between the pVAD and the iVAD is the external housing of the pump. The pVAD (Fig. 45-8) has a rigid polycarbonate shell and the iVAD (Fig. 45-9) has a housing constructed from a titanium alloy. Both versions of the pump contain a flexible, seam-free, segmented pump sac and Bjork-Shiley concavo-convex tilting disk valves in the inlet and outlet tracts. The pVAD and iVAD devices have specific cannulas that differ only in length.

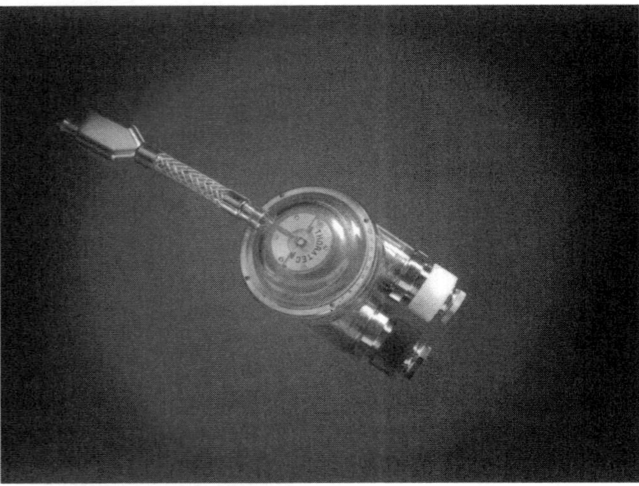

Figure 45-8 Thoratec paracorporeal ventricular assist device.

The pneumatically powered pulsatile pump has a maximal stroke volume of 65 mL and maximal output of 7 L per minute. The conventional dual-drive console or the newer portable console can be used to provide power and control to either pump. Both drive consoles can provide fixed or automatic rate control. Depending on whether one or two pumps are used, the system can provide left, right, or biventricular assistance. When left ventricular support is needed, the inflow cannula is placed in either the left atrium or the apex of the left ventricle. For atrial inflow, a wire-reinforced, right-angled cannula is used. In bridge-to-transplant cases, a large-bore, straight-wire-reinforced cannula may be inserted into the left ventricular apex. Outflow is achieved via a 12-mm, preclotted, woven Dacron graft located at the distal end of each outflow cannula, which is connected to the aorta or pulmonary artery.

In clinical use since 1976 (68), the Thoratec VAD has been valuable for treating reversible postcardiotomy failure or bridging to transplantation. When used as a bridging device in a multicenter study involving 154 patients, this system provided left ventricular support in 22% of the cases and biventricular support in the other 78%. Successful transplantation was performed in 65% of the patients. One year posttransplant, the actuarial survival rate was 82%, which is similar to that of the general heart transplant population. The most common sequelae were hemorrhage (42%) and infection (36%). In another study, involving postcardiotomy patients alone, 37% were weaned from the device and their survival rate was 57%. The most common complications in this series were perioperative myocardial infarction and renal failure (69).

Worldwide, 2,018 Thoratec pumps were used for bridging to transplantation between 1984 and 2005. Biventricular support was necessary in 1,163 cases and isolated left ventricular assistance in 722 cases. Because the Thoratec VAD can provide biventricular support, this device is often the system of choice in cases of profound right ventricular failure and/or elevated pulmonary vascular resistance. Because the pump sac is vulnerable to thrombus formation, continuous anticoagulant therapy is necessary as soon as operative bleeding ceases to be a threat. Anticoagulation is achieved with a combination of dextran, dipyridamole, and heparin or warfarin (70,71).

CardioWest Total Artificial Heart

Originally called the Jarvik-7 or the Symbion TAH, the present CardioWest TAH (SynCardia Systems, Inc., Tucson, AZ) is implanted orthotopically in patients who need biventricular support (Fig. 45-10) (72,73). The CardioWest TAH is a biventricular, implantable bridge-to-transplant system for full cardiac replacement. The system features two pneumatic blood pumps, each with a semirigid, polyurethane polyester (Biomer) outer shell (Ethicon, Inc., Somerville, NJ) and a four-layer flexible Biomer diaphragm. One-way blood flow is ensured by a Medtronic-Hall tilting-disk valve in each pump's inflow and outflow tracts. Whereas the cuffed inflow cannulas are sewn to the atrial remnants of the native heart, the outflow cannulas are attached to the aorta and pulmonary artery by means of Dacron grafts.

The external pneumatic drive console is connected to the blood pumps by means of drivelines brought out through the patient's left flank. At the skin exit sites, the Silastic drivelines are covered with velour to encourage tissue ingrowth to help prevent infection. The console controls the cardiac output by adjusting the pump rate. The operator adjusts the driving pressure, filling vacuum, and systolic time. During diastole, pump filling is aided by vacuum; during systole, blood ejection is caused by the positive air pressure generated by pulses of air from the console. A smaller and more portable drive console is under development and is being tested clinically in Europe. The smaller drive console is intended to allow support of patients outside of the hospital while they await a transplant.

The most common problems associated with the CardioWest TAH are hemorrhage, thromboembolism, device malfunction, and infection (74). Nevertheless, this system can be safely used for prolonged periods as a bridge to transplantation in patients with end-stage heart failure. As of August 2004, clinical trial results with this system included 81 bridge-to-transplant patients who had a 79% survival to transplant (75). The survival to transplant for the control group was only 46%. The positive results of this clinical trial led to commercial approval for use as bridge to heart transplant in October 2004.

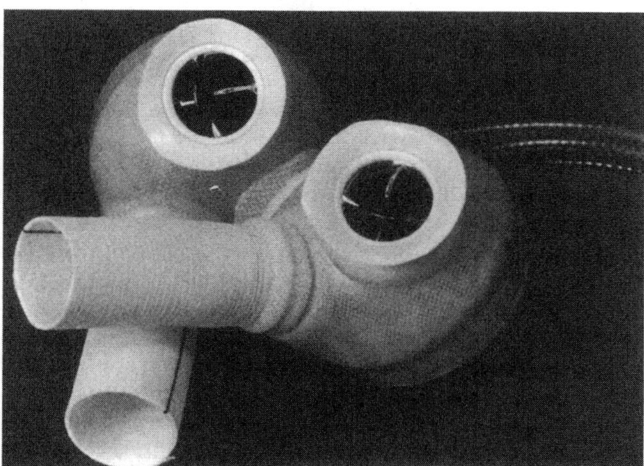

Figure 45-10 SynCardia CardioWest total artificial heart. (Reproduced from Frazier OH, Short HD, Wampler RK, et al. Mechanical circulatory support in the transplant population. In: Frazier OH, Macris MP, Radovancevic B, eds. *Support and Replacement of the Failing Heart*. Philadelphia: Lippincott-Raven; 1996:156–159, with permission.)

Novacor Left Ventricular Assist Device

The pulsatile Novacor left ventricular assist system (LVAS) (World Heart Corp., Oakland, CA) is designed to be used as a bridge to transplant or destination therapy (76). The electromagnetically driven, implantable blood pump (Fig. 45-11) has a seamless polyurethane pump sac that, when actuated by dual pusher plates, produces a maximum stroke volume of 70 mL. The pump is linked to a bedside or wearable external control unit by a percutaneous cable, which not only provides power but also allows external venting. With early Novacor models, the large, heavy drive console limited patient mobility. The newer, battery-powered model now allows some patients to live at home while awaiting a suitable donor heart. The control unit adjusts the flow rate on the basis of signals emitted by transducers within the pump. One-way blood flow is ensured by a 21-mm bioprosthetic valve in the inflow and outflow tracts.

Implantation of the Novacor necessitates a median sternotomy and an extended midline abdominal incision. The pump is placed within the abdominal wall, anterior to

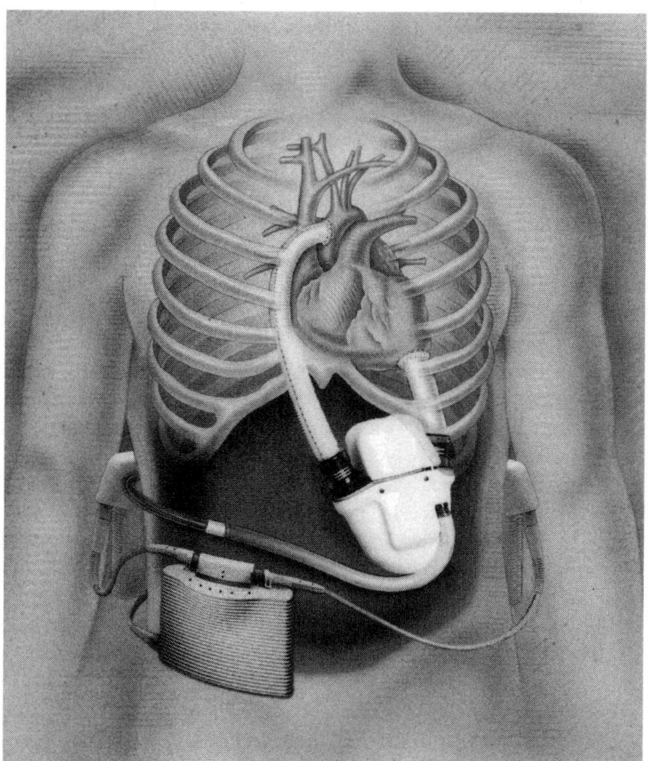

Figure 45-11 Novacor left ventricular assist device. (Reproduced from World Heart Corp., Oakland, CA, with permission.)

the posterior rectus sheath, between the left iliac crest and the costal margin. During placement of the inflow and outflow cannulas, cardiopulmonary bypass is necessary. The percutaneous driveline is externalized through the right lateral portion of the abdominal wall.

The Novacor was first used in 1984 and was modified to be more portable in 1993. The materials used in the inflow and outflow conduits were changed in 1998, which significantly reduced the incidence of thromboembolism (77,78). In bridge-to-transplant trials, the device yielded a 78% survival-to-transplant rate and some patients were supported for over 3 years. Over 1,500 patients have been supported by the Novacor, with no deaths due to device failure. The device was commercially approved in 1998. It has proved to be reliable (76,79) but is still beset by complications including hemorrhage, sepsis, and thromboembolism (79,80).

In 2004, the Randomized Evaluation of the Novacor LVAS in a Non-Transplant Population (RELIANT) trial was initiated to demonstrate equivalency between the Novacor and the HeartMate XVE when used for destination therapy. The trial will be conducted in up to 40 clinical centers and will enroll up to 390 patients. Recipients will be randomized in a 2:1 ratio to receive either the Novacor or the HeartMate as treatment. Patients receiving the HeartMate will serve as controls for the study.

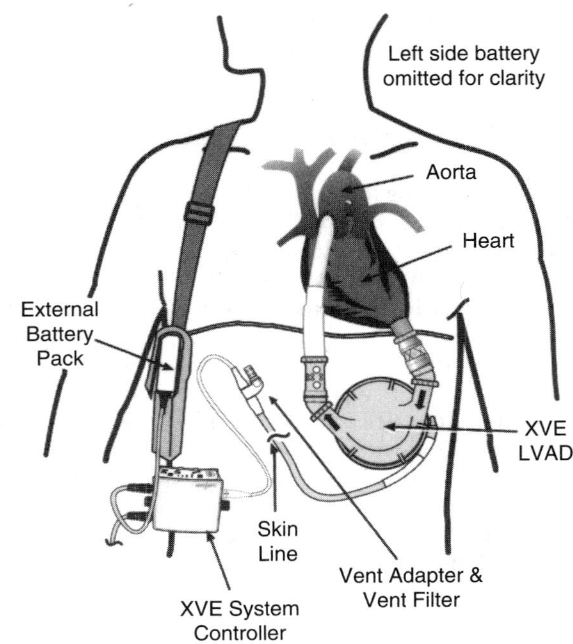

Figure 45-12 HeartMate XVE left ventricular assist device. (Reproduced from Thoratec Corp., Pleasanton, CA, with permission.)

HeartMate Left Ventricular Assist Device

The pulsatile HeartMate XVE LVAS (Thoratec Corp., Pleasanton, CA) (Fig. 45-12) is also designed for long-term use as a bridge to transplant or destination therapy. Originally conceived in 1975, the technology has reached its current state through a number of design iterations. After better immunosuppression made heart transplantation a clinical reality in the early 1980s, an implantable pneumatic (IP) version of the HeartMate entered clinical trials as a bridge to transplant in 1986 and was commercially approved for this indication in 1994 (31). A vented electric version called the HeartMate VE underwent clinical trials as a bridge to transplant from 1991 to 1996 (81) and as destination therapy from 1996 to 2003 (82). The current portable design is now commercially approved for both indications.

The HeartMate XVE blood pump has a flexible polyurethane diaphragm within a titanium alloy shell. The titanium and woven Dacron inflow and outflow cannulas each contain a 25-mm porcine xenograft valve. The outflow cannula is extended by a 20-mm woven Dacron graft, which is trimmed to the proper length at implantation. To encourage the formation of a pseudoneointimal lining and thereby minimize thromboembolism, all blood-contacting surfaces except the valves are specially textured (83,84). The titanium surfaces are covered with sintered titanium spheres and the diaphragm is covered by fibrils that arise from its polyurethane base. Examination of explanted HeartMate blood pumps has shown their blood-contacting surfaces to be lined with a smooth, well-adherent neointima consisting mainly of fibrin and collagen (85). In past studies, the neointima usually contained leukocytes, erythrocytes, and platelets after periods of brief support. After extended support, however, the neointima tended to contain macrophages and smooth muscle cells. In some cases, endothelial cells were also present (86). The pump produces a maximal effective stroke volume of 83 mL with a maximum flow rate of 10 L per minute at a pumping rate of 120 per minute. An electric motor situated within the pump housing is connected to a percutaneous driveline that provides an electrical connection between internal and external components and a means for atmospheric venting. A small system controller and battery pack allow patients almost unlimited physical freedom.

The HeartMate XVE safely provides adequate cardiac output with an acceptable risk of infection, thromboembolism, or other complications (30,87). It also consistently improves the clinical status of bridge-to-transplant patients (30,31). Most patients who are in NYHA Class IV before receiving the HeartMate will return to Class I after 3 to 4 weeks of support. Meanwhile, they are able to move around and exercise. In cases of prolonged (>30-day) support, use of the HeartMate may even improve the outcome of transplantation. The results emphasize the importance of MCS in permitting recovery and rehabilitation before cardiac transplantation is performed (4).

In bridge-to-transplant trials of the pneumatic and electric HeartMates, 71% of LVAD-supported patients versus 34% of untreated controls survived to transplant (64,81). Worldwide, the HeartMate XVE has now supported 4,645 patients as either a bridge to transplant (93%) or as destination therapy (7%). The majority of these patients received minimal or no anticoagulant therapy, with an LVAD-related thromboembolic rate of only 3%. Since market approval of this system, improved patient selection and management has led to improved overall outcomes. The majority of patients who survive the perioperative period undergo rehabilitation and hospital discharge.

Investigational Bridge-to-Transplant Systems

Jarvik 2000 Heart

The Jarvik 2000 Heart (Jarvik Heart, Inc., New York, NY) is an implantable LVAS (Fig. 45-13) that produces continuous blood flow by means of a single, rotating, vaned impeller (88). The system consists of a blood pump, a 16-mm outflow graft, a percutaneous power cable, a speed controller, and a direct-current power supply. The power cable is constructed of pacemaker-type wires that are insulated with polyurethane and partially covered with Dacron. The impeller is composed of a neodymium-iron-boron magnet and hydrodynamic titanium blades, which are held in position by two ceramic bearings. The motor spins the impeller at 8,000 to 12,000 rpm, generating a mean flow of 3 to 6 L per minute.

The pump is implanted within the left ventricle and through a left thoracotomy or sternotomy, and the outflow graft may be placed either on the ascending or descending aorta (89,90). A Silastic sewing cuff, placed on the left ventricular apex, secures the pump within the left ventricle. The percutaneous power cable is externalized through the right side of the abdomen. Also, it can be implanted without cardiopulmonary bypass (91). Power is supplied by either lead-acid or lithium-ion batteries.

In the United States, a phase I clinical trial began in April 2000 and a multicenter pivotal trial began in May 2005. Though used only as a bridge to transplant in the United States, the pump has been used as a bridge to transplant and as destination therapy in Europe. As of May, 2005, there have been 63 bridge cases in the United States and 21 in Europe, with 19 destination therapy cases in Europe. The longest posttransplantation survival time is just over 5 years and the longest destination therapy patient remains on support at almost 5 years (92). The device has been remarkably mechanically reliable and has a low incidence of complications.

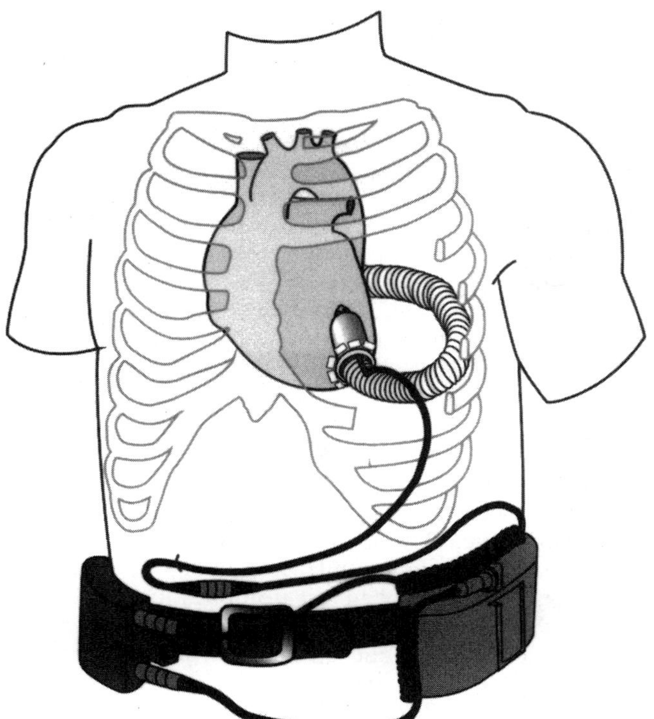

Figure 45-13 Jarvik 2000 Heart left ventricular assist device.

HeartMate II

The HeartMate II LVAS is a new axial-flow pump system designed to be more durable than the conventional intermittent-flow pumps (Fig. 45-14) (93). Like other axial-flow pumps, this small device has one movable part, the impeller, which should lead to enhanced reliability. The size also will allow for implantation in a broader range of patients. The initial European clinical studies with the HeartMate II were discouraging because of pump thrombosis. Design changes to the surfaces of the pump appear to have resolved the problems and there has been no incidence of pump thrombosis in the 36 patients in the phase I clinical trials. As of March 2005, phase II clinical studies are under way to assess the safety and effectiveness of the HeartMate II as a bridge to cardiac transplantation and as destination therapy.

The inflow cannula has a sintered titanium blood-contacting surface and is placed in the left ventricle; the pump is positioned subdiaphragmatically and the outflow graft is anastamosed to the ascending aorta. The impeller rotates on a bearing and is powered by an electromagnetic motor contained within the housing of the pump. The power cable exits the right lower quadrant of the abdomen. The external controller and batteries can be worn by the patient, allowing for full mobility. Operating at speeds of 6,000 to 15,000 rpm, the pump can generate up to 10 L per minute of cardiac output. Pump flow is estimated by a computerized algorithm that uses impeller speed and power consumption. The implantation technique is similar to that used to implant the HeartMate XVE.

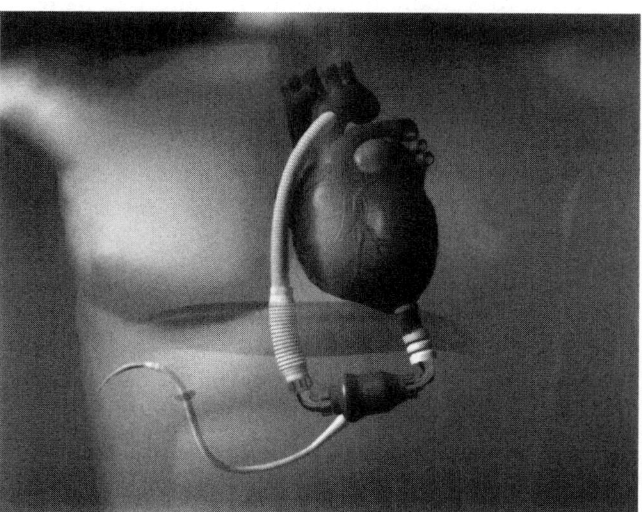

Figure 45-14 HeartMate II left ventricular assist device. (Reproduced from Thoratec Corp., Pleasanton, CA, with permission.)

Since our initial experience with the HeartMate II (94), our center has implanted the device in seven additional patients, with over 50 implants at 12 other U.S. and European centers. To date, the device-related complication rate is minimal and the original problem of pump thrombosis appears to be resolved. The feasibility phase of the clinical trial has been completed and patients are being enrolled in a phase II study with two arms (bridge to transplantation and destination therapy).

MicroMed DeBakey Ventricular Assist Device

The MicroMed DeBakey VAD (MicroMed Cardiovascular, Inc., Houston, TX) is a small, implantable, continuous-flow pump designed for long-term left ventricular support (Fig. 45-15). This small pump weighs 93 g and is 30.5 mm in diameter. The system includes a titanium pump and inlet cannula, a percutaneous power cable, an ultrasonic flow probe, and a Dacron outflow graft. The magnetic impeller is the only moving part of the pump. The impeller spins at 7,500 to 12,500 rpm and is capable of generating blood flow >10 L per minute. The impeller is driven by a brushless, direct-current motor that is contained within the pump housing. The pump is attached to an inlet cannula that is positioned in the left ventricle. The outflow graft from the pump is anastamosed to the ascending aorta.

The MicroMed DeBakey VAD is implanted through a median sternotomy with the use of cardiopulmonary bypass (95). The inflow cannula is inserted into the left ventricle through an apical core and ring. The pump is positioned subdiaphragmatically in a pocket created in the abdominal wall. The percutaneous power cable is externalized through the right side of the abdomen. The final implant step is to anastomose the outflow graft to the ascending aorta.

The external controller operates the pump and displays operating information, including battery charge status. The controller provides audible alerts in the event power is disconnected or any abnormal operating conditions occur. Two batteries will power the VAD for approximately 6 to 8 hours. The controller and two batteries weigh approximately 5 pounds and allow patient mobility. The computerized data acquisition system is used to monitor the patient and to allow for changes in the operating parameters of the VAD. The system provides power to the pump and is used to control the speed of the pump. The data acquisition system monitors pump flow rate, pump speed, and power usage. A portable patient home support system provides primary power to the MicroMed DeBakey VAD while the patient is stationary for long periods or is sleeping. It provides a battery backup and charges up to four batteries simultaneously.

The MicroMed DeBakey VAD has been in clinical trials since November 1998, with 300 implants as of February 2005. Most implants have been for bridging to heart transplantation. In January 2004, the device entered a clinical trial in which patients are randomized to receive either the MicroMed DeBakey VAD or the HeartMate XVE as destination therapy. In March 2004, this device received market approval under a Humanitarian Device Exemption from the FDA for use in children between 5 and 16 years of age. The clinical outcomes and complication rates for this system are similar to those of other implantable VAD systems (96,97).

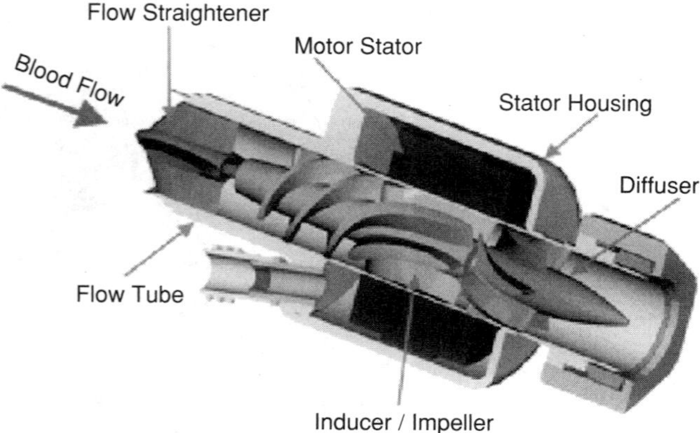

Figure 45-15 MicroMed DeBakey VAD pump. (Reproduced from MicroMed Cardiovascular, Inc., Houston, TX, with permission.)

Perioperative Complications of Bridging to Transplantation

The bridge-to-transplant population is vulnerable to perioperative hemorrhage, sepsis, thromboembolism, renal failure, technical failure, and neurological sequelae (98,99). The most frequent serious problems are hemorrhage and sepsis. Hemorrhage, which occurs in up to 60% of patients, results from liver dysfunction, the implant procedure itself, and the blood trauma caused by cardiopulmonary bypass and blood pump rheology (100). Biventricular MCS is more likely to cause hemorrhage than is univentricular assistance (13). Hemorrhage often leads to reoperation, which then leads to more invasive care and monitoring; the result is a high frequency of infection due to the increased exposure (100). Percutaneous drivelines are also very susceptible to infection. Infection occurs in 30% to 40% of cases, resulting in significant morbidity (101–104). Nevertheless, even frequent infection does not necessarily rule out successful cardiac transplantation (103,105). Patients with comorbid conditions are at the highest risk for severe sepsis. The new axial-flow systems appear to be less susceptible to device-related infection (106,107).

BRIDGING TO RECOVERY

Our first observation of significant myocardial recovery following prolonged LVAS support was a 33-year-old man who received a HeartMate in 1991. He died 503 days later of a neurological thromboembolic complication, while still receiving MCS (4). Before death, the patient had a near-normal ejection fraction and evidence of physiological and anatomic myocardial recovery. Since that time, similar results have been observed, both in HeartMate recipients and in patients with other systems (108,109). The authors have shown that when MCS is continued for more than 30 days it improves not only hemodynamic and functional variables but also histological markers of heart failure (110). Moreover, the phenotype of pathological hypertrophy and fibrosis is also improved (111). As a result of this experience, researchers have proposed the concept of bridging to recovery. In fact, this goal has been accomplished in the United States, Germany, and Japan with removal of the MCS device after 3 to 7 months (112,113). This approach has been successful at this institution and has resulted in sustained NYHA Class I status in most cases after device explantation.

Nevertheless, the number of bridge-to-recovery patients remains small and experts have not yet decided how best to stratify candidates for this treatment with respect to risk. So far, the best candidates appear to be those with nonischemic cardiomyopathy; in these cases, risk stratification should be based on the patient's cardiac functional reserve during minimal MCS support (114). Identifying those patients who will likely recover and determining the adequacy of recovery will require more study (114–116). Other important questions must also be answered. What etiologies of heart failure are reversible? Is recovery sustainable and for how long? What clinical parameters will reliably predict lasting recovery? Should patients be weaned from MCS support and, if so, how? Because the donor heart pool is continuing to decline, bridging to recovery will probably assume increasing importance during the twenty-first century.

DESTINATION THERAPY

As previously mentioned, the HeartMate XVE is the only LVAD system commercially approved for destination therapy. The HeartMate II, Novacor, and MicroMed DeBakey VAD systems are being studied in phase II multicenter pivotal trials that include a 2:1 randomization with the HeartMate XVE for destination therapy. Although the Jarvik 2000 is not presently undergoing a clinical trial for destination therapy in the United States, the European experience for this indication has been very encouraging (117). The continuing disproportion between heart donors and recipients worldwide will lead to further development of VADs for destination therapy.

Destination therapy with implantable VADs came about with the REMATCH trial (82). This randomized, controlled study demonstrated significantly enhanced 1- and 2-year survival for LVAD-supported patients versus those receiving optimal medical therapy. However, the better survival came at the cost of a higher rate of serious adverse events, including bleeding, infection, and device malfunction. Continuous-flow devices now being used and tested clinically show promise for providing reliable long-term support.

CARDIAC REPLACEMENT

AbioCor Total Artificial Heart

The AbioCor implantable replacement heart (ABIOMED, Inc., Danvers, MA) is intended for permanent support

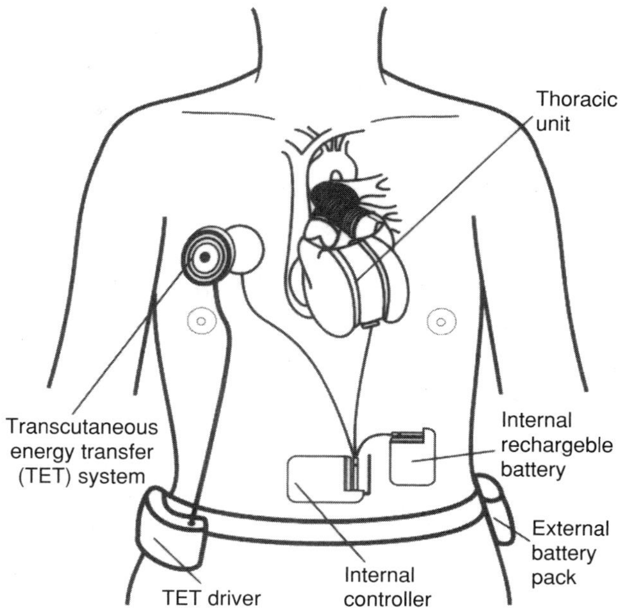

Figure 45-16 AbioCor total artificial heart.

(Fig. 45-16). The AbioCor is a completely self-contained, TAH designed to be portable and to allow a patient to continue an active lifestyle (118). The pump is made of titanium and a polyether-based polyurethane called Angioflex. The pump is powered through transcutaneous energy transfer (TET), and an atrial flow-balancing chamber adjusts for left/right flow balance. The TET system consists of internal and external coils that transmit power across the skin. The balance chamber and the TET system eliminate the need for percutaneous lines, external venting, or an implanted compliance chamber. This unique design allows the AbioCor to be totally implanted within the body. Unlike recipients of other TAHs, AbioCor recipients are not tethered to a large pneumatic console and do not require percutaneous power cables.

The AbioCor system consists of an internal thoracic unit, a rechargeable battery, an electronics package, and an external battery pack. The thoracic unit weighs about 2 pounds and includes two ventricles with valves and a hydraulic pumping system. The implantable electronics unit monitors and controls the pump rate depending on the physiological needs of the patient. The AbioCor operates on both internal and external lithium batteries. The internal battery is recharged from the external console or from an external battery pack. The internal batteries provide approximately one-half hour of power. External battery packs can power the AbioCor system for approximately 4 hours.

The AbioCor is intended for use in patients with end-stage heart failure who are not eligible for heart transplant and are at risk of imminent death despite maximal medical therapy. Candidates for the AbioCor have biventricular failure but whose other vital organs continue to be viable or are potentially recoverable. The AbioCor is indicated for patients who may benefit from heart replacement and who do not meet the criteria for support with an LVAD.

In a phase I trial, 14 patients received the AbioCor as destination therapy. Thromboembolism was a significant adverse event and there were two pump failures in this group of patients. The longest-surviving recipient was supported 512 days, much of that time while outside of the hospital. A smaller system is being developed for application to a broader patient population.

FUTURE MECHANICAL CIRCULATORY SUPPORT SYSTEMS

The MCS systems of the future are presently under development. This next generation of blood pumps is incorporating many of the lessons learned over the past two decades. One such lesson is that reliable pumps need to be simple and have as few moving parts as possible. Another is that the smaller artificial surface areas presented by smaller pumps can enhance biocompatibility. Improved reliability and biocompatibility should enhance long-term survival.

The design of some next-generation pumps involves magnetic levitation of the pump mechanism. In such designs, impeller- or pusher-plate-type pumps can be actuated without friction and, therefore, without wear on pump components. Frictionless pumps do not generate heat and theoretically can be miniaturized without sacrificing their ability to deliver a sufficient volume of blood. This should enhance biocompatibility by minimizing the risk of thrombogenicity and bacterial colonization. These design features should also allow for easy modification of frictionless pumps as artificial hearts or ventricular assist systems.

At our institution, we are working on a TAH that utilizes two axial-flow pumps: one for the pulmonary circulation and one for the systemic circulation. The pumps are attached to the native atria, which serve as reservoirs of blood for the pumps. This system allows for passive pressure and flow equalization, thus avoiding the need for a compliance chamber, external vent, or a balancing mechanism. Preliminary animal studies with this new artificial heart design have been very promising.

Another future concept being developed at our institution is one in which a long-term VAD system is implanted without surgery. This concept involves a small axial-flow pump inserted into the aorta and then anchored to the aortic wall with struts. This device can be implanted with local anesthesia in the cardiac catheterization laboratory. It would be suitable for patients who are too ill for surgery or less-sick patients who need some support to enhance cardiac recovery. This approach may broaden the use of mechanical support to those for whom extensive surgery is a less-than-desirable option.

New short-term devices are being employed in the catheterization laboratory for treatment of cardiogenic shock, bridging to recovery, bridging to revascularization, or bridging to long-term support with an implantable VAD system. One such system now under investigation, the Orqis Cancion cardiac recovery system (Orqis Medical, Lake Forest, CA), is intended to augment aortic blood flow for up to 4 days. Two cannulas are inserted via the femoral vessels, one cannula terminating in the upper aorta and the other in the lower aorta. The cannulas are connected to a centrifugal pump that creates increased flow from the upper aorta to the lower aorta, improving organ function and decreasing cardiac work. This minimally invasive, rapid-access approach may broaden MCS application by treating a less-sick population of patients at an earlier point in their heart failure progression.

CONCLUSION

Over the past four decades, MCS has evolved somewhat sporadically. Cardiopulmonary bypass evolved quickly in the 1960s to become the cornerstone of modern cardiac surgery. Although VADs and TAHs were of interest to some researchers, these technologies did not begin to proliferate until the 1990s. Now, in the early twenty-first century, a variety of devices is available to treat a broad range of heart failure patients; pump systems are smaller, more reliable, and more biocompatible; and clinicians have learned a great deal about patient and MCS device selection and postoperative management. Although improvements are still needed in a number of areas, MCS has an expanding role to play in restoring an increasing number of end-stage heart failure patients to productive, high-quality lives.

REFERENCES

1. Cohn JN. The management of chronic heart failure. *N Engl J Med.* 1996;335:490–498.
2. The SOLVD Investigators. Effect of enalapril on survival in patients with reduced left ventricular ejection fraction and congestive heart failure. *N Engl J Med.* 1991;325:293–302.
3. Packer M, Bristow MR, Cohn JR, et al. The effect of carvedilol on morbidity and mortality in patients with chronic heart failure. *N Engl J Med.* 1996;334:1349–1355.
4. Frazier OH, Macris MP, Myers TJ, et al. Improved survival after extended bridge to cardiac transplantation. *Ann Thorac Surg.* 1994;57:1416–1422.
5. Kormos RL, Murali S, Dew MA, et al. Chronic mechanical circulatory support: rehabilitation, low morbidity, and superior survival. *Ann Thorac Surg.* 1994;57:51–57.
6. Funk D. Epidemiology of end-stage heart disease. In: Committee to Evaluate the Artificial Heart Program of the National Heart, Lung and Blood Institute. *The Artificial Heart: Prototypes, Policies and Patients.* Washington: National Academy Press; 1991: 251.
7. Gallois CJJ. *Experiences on the Principle of Life.* Philadelphia: Charles C. Thomas; 1813. Translation of Le Gallois CJJ. *Experiences sur la Principe de la Vie.* Paris;1812.
8. DeBakey ME. A simple continuous flow blood transfusion instrument. *New Orleans Med Surg J.* 1934;87:386.
9. Lindbergh CA. An apparatus for the culture of whole organs. *J Exp Med.* 1935;62:409.
10. Gibbon JH. Application of a mechanical heart and lung apparatus to cardiac surgery. *Minn Med.* 1954;37:171.
11. Moulopoulos SD, Topaz SR, Kolff WJ. Extracorporeal assistance to circulation and intra-aortic balloon pumping. *Trans Am Soc Artif Intern Organs.* 1962;8:85–89.
12. Kantrowitz LA, Tjonneland S, Freed PS, et al. Initial clinical experience with intra-aortic balloon pumping in cardiogenic shock. *JAMA.* 1968;201:113.
13. Dennis C. Left-heart bypass. In: *Mechanical Devices to Assist the Failing Heart. Publication No. 1283.* Washington: National Academy of Sciences—National Research Council; 1966:27.

14. Spencer FD, Eiseman B, Trinkle JK, et al. Assisted circulation for cardiac failure following intracardiac surgery with cardiopulmonary bypass. *J Thorac Cardiovasc Surg*. 1965;49:56.
15. DeBakey ME, Liotta D, Hall CW. Left heart bypass using an implantable blood pump. In: *Mechanical Devices to Assist the Failing Heart*. Proceedings of a conference sponsored by The Committee on Trauma, September 9–10, 1964. Washington: National Academy of Sciences—National Research Council; 1966: 223.
16. Hall CW, Liotta D, Henly WS, et al. Development of artificial intrathoracic circulatory pumps. *Am J Surg*. 1964;108: 685–692.
17. DeBakey ME. Left ventricular bypass pump for cardiac assistance. Clinical experience. *Am J Cardiol*. 1971;27:3–11.
18. Cooley DA, Liotta D, Hallman GL, et al. Orthotopic cardiac prosthesis for two-staged cardiac replacement. *Am J Cardiol*. 1969;24:723–730.
19. DeVries WC. The permanent artificial heart: four case reports. *JAMA*. 1988;259:849–859.
20. Johnson KE, Liska MB, Joyce LD, et al. Use of total artificial hearts: summary of world experience. 1969–1991. *Am Soc Artif Intern Organs J*. 1992;35:M486.
21. Litwak RS, Koffsky RM, Jurado RA, et al. Use of left heart assist device after intracardiac surgery: technical and clinical experiences. *Ann Thorac Surg*. 1976;21:191–202.
22. Peters JC, McRea JC, Fukumasu H, et al. Recovery of cardiac function with total transapical left ventricular bypass. *Trans Am Soc Artif Intern Organs*. 1980;26:262.
23. Golding LR, Groves LK, Peter M, et al. Initial clinical experience with a new temporary left ventricular assist device. *Ann Thorac Surg*. 1978;29:66.
24. Magovern GJ, Park SB, Maher TD. Use of centrifugal pump without anticoagulants for postoperative left ventricular assist. In: Attar S, ed. *New Developments in Cardiac Assist Devices*. New York: Praeger; 1985: 103.
25. Pennington DG, Merjavy JP, Swartz MR, et al. Clinical experience with a centrifugal pump ventricular assist device. *Trans Am Soc Artif Intern Organs*. 1982;28:93.
26. Norman JC. Mechanical ventricular assistance: a review. *Artif Organs*. 1981;5:103.
27. Bernhard WF, LaFarge CG, Liss RH, et al. An appraisal of blood trauma and the prosthetic interface during left ventricular bypass in the calf and in humans. *Ann Thorac Surg*. 1978;26:427.
28. Norman JC, Duncan JM, Frazier OH, et al. Intracorporeal (abdominal) left ventricular assist devices or partial artificial hearts. *Arch Surg*. 1981;116:1441–1445.
29. Norman JC, Cooley DA, Kahan BD, et al. Total support of the circulation of a patient with postcardiotomy stone heart syndrome by a partial artificial heart (ALVAD) for 5 days followed by heart and kidney transplantation. *Lancet*. 1978;1:1125–1127.
30. Frazier OH, Duncan JM, Radovancevic B, et al. Successful bridge to heart transplantation with a new left ventricular assist device. *J Heart Lung Transplant*. 1992;11:530–537.
31. Frazier OH, Rose EA, Macmanus Q, et al. Multicenter clinical evaluation of the HeartMate. 1000IP left ventricular assist device. *Ann Thorac Surg*. 1992;53:1080–1090.
32. Frazier OH. Chronic left ventricular support with a vented electric assist device. *Ann Thorac Surg*. 1993;55:273–275.
33. Page DL, Caulfield JB, Kastor JA, et al. Myocardial changes associated with cardiogenic shock. *N Engl J Med*. 1971;285:133–137.
34. Parmley W. Cardiac failure. In: Rosen MR, Hoffman BF, eds. *Cardiac Therapy*. Boston: Martinus Nijhoff; 1983: 21.
35. Shoemaker WC, Blanc RD, Appel PL. Therapy of critically ill postoperative patients based on outcome prediction and prospective clinical trials. *Surg Clin North Am*. 1985;65:811–833.
36. Campbell CD, Tolitano DJ, Weber KT, et al. Mechanical support for postcardiotomy heart failure. *J Card Surg*. 1988;3:181–191.
37. Pae WE, Pierce WE. Combined registry for the clinical use of mechanical ventricular assist pumps and the total artificial heart: third official report. *J Heart Transplant*. 1986;5:6–7.
38. Votapka TV, Pennington DG. Circulatory assist devices in congestive heart failure. *Cardiol Clin*. 1994;12:143–154.
39. Edmunds LH, Jr. Why cardiopulmonary bypass makes patients sick: strategies to control the blood-synthetic surface interface. *Adv Card Surg*. 1995;6:131–167.
40. Hammon JW, Jr., Stump DA, Kon ND, et al. Risk factors and solutions for the development of neurobehavioral changes after coronary artery bypass grafting. *Ann Thorac Surg*. 1997;63: 1613–1618.
41. Igo SR, Hibbs CW, Trono R, et al. Intra-aortic balloon pumping: theory and practice. *Artif Organs*. 1978;2:249–256.
42. Alcan KE, Stertzer SH, Wallsh E, et al. Current status of intra-aortic balloon counterpulsation in critical care cardiology. *Crit Care Med*. 1984;12:489–495.
43. Alderman JD, Gabliani GI, McCabe CH, et al. Incidence and management of limb ischemia with percutaneous wire-guided intra-aortic balloon catheters. *J Am Coll Cardiol*. 1987;9: 524–530.
44. Creswell LL, Rosenbloom M, Cox JL, et al. Intra-aortic balloon counterpulsation: patterns of usage and outcome in cardiac surgery patients. *Ann Thorac Surg*. 1992;54:11.
45. Shook BJ. The AbioMed BVS 5000 biventricular support system. System description and clinical summary. In: *Cardiac Surgery: State of the Art Reviews*. Philadelphia: Hanley & Belfus; 1993: 309.
46. Frazier OH, Short HD, Wampler RK, et al. Mechanical circulatory support in the transplant population. In: Frazier OH, Macris MP, Radovancevic B, eds. *Support and Replacement of the Failing Heart*. Philadelphia: Lippincott-Raven; 1996: 156–159.
47. Jett GK. AbioMed BVS 5000: experience and potential advantages. *Ann Thorac Surg*. 1996;61:301–304.
48. Petrofski JA, Patel VS, Russell SD, et al. BVS support after cardiac transplantation. *J Thorac Cardiovasc Surg*. 2003;126:442–447.
49. Dixon CM, Magovern GJ. Evaluation of the Biopump for long term cardiac support without heparinization. *J Extracorp Technol*. 1982;14:331.
50. Noon GP, Ball JW, Jr., Papaconstantinou HT. Clinical experience with BioMedicus centrifugal ventricular support in 172 patients. *Artif Organs*. 1995;19:756–760.
51. Noon GP, Ball JW, Jr., Short HD. Bio-Medicus centrifugal ventricular support for postcardiotomy cardiac failure: a review of 129 cases. *Ann Thorac Surg*. 1996;61:291–295.
52. Pitsis AA, Dardas P, Mezilis N, et al. Temporary assist device for postcardiotomy cardiac failure. *Ann Thorac Surg*. 2004;77: 1431–1433.
53. Undar A, McKenzie ED, McGarry MC, et al. Outcomes of congenital heart surgery patients after extracorporeal life support at Texas Children's Hospital. *Artif Organs*. 2004;28:963–966.
54. Reiss N, El-Banayosy A, Mirow N, et al. Implantation of the Biomedicus centrifugal pump in post-transplant right heart failure. *J Cardiovasc Surg* (Torino). 2000;41:691–694.
55. Weitkemper HH, El-Banayosy A, Arusoglu L, et al. Mechanical circulatory support: reality and dreams experience of a single center. *J Extra Corpor Technol*. 2004;36:169–173.
56. Noon GP, Lafuente JA, Irwin S. Acute and temporary ventricular support with Biomedicus centrifugal pump. *Ann Thor Surg*. 1999;68:650–654.
57. Vranckx P, Foley DP, de Feijter PJ, et al. Clinical introduction of the TandemHeart, a percutaneous left ventricular assist device, for circulatory support during high-risk percutaneous coronary intervention. *Int J Cardiovasc Intervent*. 2003;5: 35–39.
58. Kar B, Butkevich A, Civitello AB, et al. Hemodynamic support with a percutaneous left ventricular assist device during stenting of an unprotected left main coronary artery. *Tex Heart Inst J*. 2004;31:84–86.
59. Jurmann MJ, Siniawski H, Erb M, et al. Initial experience with miniature axial flow ventricular assist devices for postcardiotomy heart failure. *Ann Thorac Surg*. 2004;77: 1642–1647.
60. Martin J, Benk C, Yerebakan C, et al. The new "Impella" intracardiac microaxial pump for treatment of right heart failure after orthotopic heart transplantation. *Transplant Proc*. 2001;33: 3549–3550.
61. Mueller JP, Kuenzli A, Reuthebuch O, et al. The CentriMag: a new optimized centrifugal blood pump with levitating impeller. *Heart Surg Forum*. 2004;7:E477–E480
62. Myers TJ, Catanese KA, Vargo RL, et al. Extended cardiac support with a portable left ventricular assist system in the home. *ASAIO J*. 1996;42:M576–M579.

63. Richenbacher WE, Seemuth SC. Hospital discharge for the ventricular assist device patient: historical perspective and description of a successful program. *ASAIO J*. 2001;47:590–595.
64. Frazier OH, Rose EA, McCarthy P, et al. Improved mortality and rehabilitation of transplant candidates treated with long-term implantable left ventricular system. *Ann Surg*. 1995;222: 327–338.
65. Burnett CM, Duncan JM, Frazier OH, et al. Improved multiorgan function after prolonged univentricular support. *Ann Thorac Surg*. 1993;55:65–71.
66. Scheinin SA. Selection and management of patients undergoing bridge to transplantation. *Heart Failure*. 1995;10:238–250.
67. Farrar DJ, Hill JD, Gray LA, et al. Heterotopic prosthetic ventricles as a bridge to cardiac transplantation. *N Engl J Med*. 1988; 318:333.
68. Pae WE, Jr., Rosenberg G, Donachy JH, et al. Mechanical circulatory assistance for postoperative cardiogenic shock: a three year experience. *Trans Am Soc Artif Intern Organs*. 1980;26:256.
69. Pennington DG, McBride LR, Swartz MT, et al. Use of the Pierce-Donachy ventricular assist device in patients with cardiogenic shock after cardiac operations. *Ann Thorac Surg*. 1989; 47:130.
70. Arabia FA, Smith RG, Rose DS, et al. Success rates of long-term circulatory assist devices used currently for bridge to heart transplantation. *Am Soc Artif Intern Organs J*. 1996;42: M542–M546.
71. Farrar DJ, Hill JD. Univentricular and biventricular Thoratec VAD support as a bridge to transplantation. *Ann Thorac Surg*. 1993;55:276.
72. Olsen DB. ASAIO presidential address. Artificial organs of the future. *Am Soc Artif Intern Organs J*. 1992;38:134.
73. Copeland JG, Levinson MM, Smith R, et al. The total artificial heart as a bridge to transplantation. A report of two cases. *JAMA*. 1986;256:2991–2995.
74. Copeland JG, Smith RG, Arabia FA, et al. Cardiac replacement with a total artificial heart as a bridge to transplantation. *N Engl J Med*. 2004;351:859–867.
75. Copeland JG, Smith RG, Arabia FA, et al. Total artificial heart bridge to transplantation: a 9-year experience with 62 patients. *J Heart Lung Transplant*. 2004;23:823–831.
76. Wheeldon DR, LaForge DH, Lee J, et al. Novacor left ventricular assist system long-term performance: comparison of clinical experience with demonstrated in vitro reliability. *ASAIO J*. 2002;48:546–551.
77. Dagenais F, Portner PM, Robbins RC, et al. The Novacor left ventricular assist system: clinical experience from the Novacor registry. *J Card Surg*. 2001;16:267–271.
78. Murali S. Long-term circulatory support—left ventricular assist system for advanced heart failure. *US Cardiology*. London: Business Briefings, Ltd.; 2004.
79. McCarthy PM, Portner PM, Tobler HG, et al. Clinical experience with the Novacor ventricular assist system. *J Thorac Cardiovasc Surg*. 1991;102:578.
80. Portner PM, Oyer PE, Pennington DG, et al. Implantable electrical left ventricular assist system: bridge to transplantation and the future. *Ann Thorac Surg*. 1989;47:142.
81. Frazier OH, Rose EA, Oz MC, et al. Multicenter clinical evaluation of the HeartMate vented electric left ventricular assist system in patients awaiting heart transplantation. *J Thorac Cardiovasc Surg*. 2001;122:1186–1195.
82. Rose EA, Gelijns AC, Moskowitz AJ, et al. Long-term mechanical left ventricular assistance for end-stage heart failure. *N Engl J Med*. 2002;345:1435–1443.
83. Rose EA, Levin HR, Oz MC, et al. Artificial circulatory support with textured interior surfaces. *Circulation*. 1994;90(5 Pt 2): II87–II91.
84. Graham TR, Dasse KA, Coumbe A, et al. Neo-intimal development of textured biomaterial surfaces during clinical use of an implantable left ventricular device. *Eur J Cardiothorac Surg*. 1990;4:182–190.
85. Dasse DA, Chipman SD, Sherman CN, et al. Clinical experience with textured blood contacting surfaces in ventricular assist devices. *Am Soc Artif Intern Organs Trans*. 1987;33:418–425.
86. Frazier OH, Baldwin RT, Eskin SJ, et al. Immunochemical identification of human endothelial cells on the lining of a ventricular assist device. *Tex Heart Inst J*. 1993;20:78.
87. Myers TJ, McGee MG, Zeluff B, et al. Frequency and significance of infections in patients receiving prolonged LVAD support. *Am Soc Artif Intern Organs Trans*. 1991;37:M425.
88. Frazier OH, Myers TJ, Jarvik RK, et al. Research and development of an implantable, axial-flow left ventricular assist device: the Jarvik 2000 Heart. *Ann Thorac Surg*. 2001;71:S125–S132; discussion S144–S146.
89. Siegenthaler MP, Martin J, Frazier OH, et al. Implantation of the permanent Jarvik 2000 left-ventricular-assist-device: surgical technique. *Eur J Cardiothorac Surg*. 2002;21:546–548.
90. Westaby OH, Frazier DW, Pigott, et al. Implant technique for the Jarvik 2000 heart. *Ann Thorac Surg*. 2002;73:1337–1340.
91. Frazier OH. Implantation of the Jarvik 2000 left ventricular assist device without the use of cardiopulmonary bypass. *Ann Thorac Surg*. 2003;75:1028–1030.
92. Westaby S, Banning AP, Jarvik R, et al. First permanent implant of the Jarvik 2000 Heart. *Lancet*. 2000;356:900–903.
93. Burke DJ, Burke E, Parsaie F, et al. The HeartMate II: design and development of a fully sealed axial flow left ventricular assist system. *Artif Organs*. 2001;25:380–385.
94. Frazier OH, Delgado RM, 3rd, Kar B, et al. First clinical use of the redesigned HeartMate II left ventricular assist system in the United States: a case report. *Tex Heart Inst J*. 2004;31:157–159.
95. Hetzer R, Potapov EV, Weng Y, et al. Implantation of MicroMed DeBakey VAD through left thoracotomy after previous median sternotomy operations. *Ann Thorac Surg*. 2004;77:347–350.
96. Noon GP, Morley DL, Irwin S, et al. Clinical experience with the MicroMed DeBakey ventricular assist device. *Ann Thorac Surg*. 2001;71:S133–S138.
97. Goldstein DJ. Worldwide experience with the MicroMed DeBakey ventricular assist device as a bridge to transplantation. *Circulation*. 2003;108(Suppl 1):II272–II277.
98. Quaini E, Pavie A, Chieco S, et al. The Concerted Action "Heart" European registry on clinical application of mechanical circulatory support systems: bridge to transplant. The Registry Scientific Committee. *Eur J Cardiothorac Surg*. 1997;11:182–188.
99. Mehta SM, Aufiero TX, Pae WE, Jr., et al. Combined Registry for the Clinical Use of Mechanical Ventricular Assist Pumps and the Total Artificial Heart in conjunction with heart transplantation: sixth official report–1994. *J Heart Lung Transplant*. 1995;14:585–593.
100. Livingston ER, Fisher CA, Bibidakis EJ, et al. Increased activation of the coagulation and fibrinolytic systems leads to hemorrhagic complications during left ventricular assist implantation. *Circulation*. 1996;94(Suppl 1):II227–II234.
101. Holman WL, Murrah CP, Ferguson ER, et al. Infections during extended circulatory support: University of Alabama at Birmingham experience. 1989 to 1994. *Ann Thorac Surg*. 1996;61:366–371.
102. McBride LR, Swartz MT, Reedy JE, et al. Device related infections in patients supported with mechanical circulatory support devices for greater than 30 days. *Am Soc Artif Intern Organs Trans*. 1991;37:M258–M259.
103. Springer WE, Wasler A, Radovancevic B, et al. Retrospective analysis of infection in patients undergoing support with left ventricular assist systems. *Am Soc Artif Intern Organs J*. 1996;42:M763–M765.
104. McCarthy PM, Schmitt SK, Vargo RL, et al. Implantable LVAD infections: implications for permanent use of the device. *Ann Thorac Surg*. 1996;61:359–365.
105. Pennington DG, McBride LR, Peigh PS, et al. Eight years experience with bridging to cardiac transplantation. *J Thorac Cardiovasc Surg*. 1994;107:472–481.
106. Siegenthaler MP, Martin J, Pernice K, et al. The Jarvik 2000 is associated with less infections than the HeartMate left ventricular assist device. *Eur J Cardiothorac Surg*. 2003;23:748–755.
107. Frazier OH, Myers TJ, Gregoric ID, et al. Initial clinical experience with the Jarvik 2000 implantable axial-flow left ventricular assist system. *Circulation*. 2002;105:2855–2860.
108. Frazier OH, Myers TJ. Left ventricular assist system as a bridge to myocardial recovery. *Ann Thorac Surg*. 1999;68:734–741.
109. Hetzer R, Muller JH, Weng Y, et al. Bridging-to-recovery. *Ann Thorac Surg*. 2001;71:S109–S113.
110. Frazier OH, Benedict CR, Radovancevic B, et al. Improved left ventricular function after chronic left ventricular unloading. *Ann Thorac Surg*. 1996;62:675–681.

111. Altemose GT, Gritsus V, Jeevanandam V, et al. Altered myocardial phenotype after mechanical support in human beings with advanced cardiomyopathy. *J Heart Lung Transplant.* 1997;16:765–773.
112. Muller J, Wallukat G, Weng YG, et al. Temporary mechanical left heart support. Recovery of heart function in patients with end-stage idiopathic dilated cardiomyopathy. *Herz.* 1997;22:227–236.
113. Entwistle JW, 3rd. Short- and long-term mechanical ventricular assistance towards myocardial recovery. *Surg Clin North Am.* 2004;84:201–221.
114. Reinlib L, Abraham W. Recovery from heart failure with circulatory assist: a working group of the National, Heart, Lung, and Blood Institute. *J Card Fail.* 2003;9:459–463.
115. Hetzer R, Muller J, Weng Y, et al. Cardiac recovery in dilated cardiomyopathy by unloading with a left ventricular assist device. *Ann Thorac Surg.* 1999;68:742–748.
116. Khan T, Delgado RM, Radovancevic B, et al. Dobutamine stress echocardiography predicts myocardial improvement in patients supported by left ventricular assist devices (LVADs): hemodynamic and histologic evidence of improvement before LVAD explantation. *J Heart Lung Transplant.* 2003;22:137–146.
117. Frazier OH, Shah NA, Myers TJ, et al. Use of the Flowmaker (Jarvik 2000) left ventricular assist device for destination therapy and bridging to transplantation. *Cardiology.* 2004;101:111–116.
118. Dowling RD, Gray LA, Jr., Etoch SW, et al. Initial experience with the AbioCor implantable replacement heart system. *J Thoracic Cardiovasc Surg.* 2004;127:131–141.

Cardiac Transplantation

46

Anantharam V. Kalya   Jeffrey David Hosenpud

Over the past 30 years, cardiac transplantation has evolved from a highly experimental procedure performed in a handful of centers to an accepted modality of therapy for the treatment of end-stage heart disease. Cardiac transplantation is now performed on every continent and in over 300 centers worldwide (1). Unfortunately, despite continuing expansion of the criteria for acceptable donor organs, the availability of donor hearts limits the availability of this form of therapy. It is estimated that in the United States alone, over 20,000 patients could benefit from cardiac transplantation yet the number of donor hearts procured is only around 2,500 (2). This chapter reviews the current state of cardiac transplantation, its successes, and the challenges yet to be overcome.

RECIPIENT SELECTION

The basic tenets expressed in the criteria developed by the Stanford group in the early 1970s (3,4) continue to apply today. Cardiac transplantation must be reserved for those patients with disabling symptoms of congestive heart failure (New York Heart Association [NYHA] late functional Class III and IV) whose likelihood of survival is poor over the next 6 to 12 months. There have been, however, several modifications of ancillary inclusion and exclusion criteria over the past 20 years. As a result, cardiac transplantation is now being offered to sicker and higher-risk patients. Table 46-1 outlines the inclusion and exclusion criteria generally agreed-upon by the transplant community. In addition, given the shortage of acceptable organs for heart transplantation, attempts are currently under way to further refine these criteria and ultimately establish uniform listing criteria. One such attempt by the United Network for Organ Sharing (UNOS) has proposed the criteria shown in Table 46-2. Other groups, including the American Heart Association (AHA), have published position papers regarding appropriate listing criteria (5,6).

Age

Based on early data from Stanford showing a 20% decrement in 1-year survival in patients over the age of 50 years, the upper age limit for cardiac transplantation was considered 50 years (3). Several subsequent single-center studies could not demonstrate a mortality increase in patients between the ages of 50 and 65 (7–9). One additional study investigating not only survival, infection, and rejection but also overall hospitalization and noncardiac morbidity demonstrated no major differences in these parameters between those patients above and below the age of 55 (10). A more recent study performing similar analyses in patients above and below the age of 65 did, however, demonstrate that those over age 65 had prolonged hospitalizations, longer rehabilitation, and a trend toward reduced survival that did not reach statistical significance (11).

These single-center experiences have not been confirmed by multicenter or registry data (12). Using multivariate analysis, the joint UNOS/International Society for Heart and Lung Transplantation (ISHLT) Thoracic Registry has consistently shown an independent, linear increased risk with increasing age that is highly statistically significant (1). Despite these data, the standards in the transplant community are to offer heart transplantation up to the age of 65 years, with rare individuals (approximately 2% of all patients) transplanted over the age of 65.

TABLE 46-1
RECIPIENT SELECTION CRITERIA

Inclusion Criteria

Severe, symptom-limiting heart failure (NYHA Class III or IV) on full medical management
At substantial risk for cardiac death within 1 year
No alternative treatment options
Age usually less than 65 years
History of medical compliance/good psychosocial environment

Exclusion Criteria

Irreversible renal or hepatic disease (relative)
Severe pulmonary parenchymal disease (absolute)
Irreversible elevated pulmonary vascular resistance >6 Wood units (absolute)
Diabetes with important end-organ damage (relative)
Peripheral or cerebral vascular disease (relative)
Active systemic or organ parenchymal infection (absolute)
Cardiac involvement as part of systemic disease [e.g., amyloidosis, sarcoidosis (relative)]
Chronic viral infection [e.g., hepatitis B, HIV (absolute)]
High titers of cytotoxic antibodies to multiple HLA antigens (relative)
Active medical noncompliance or substance abuse (absolute)

Pulmonary Vascular Resistance

Severe and irreversible (nonreflex) pulmonary hypertension has consistently been demonstrated to be a risk factor for poor outcome following cardiac transplantation in both single-center (3,13) and multicenter (14) reports. The reason for this is the inability of the transplanted right ventricle to acutely adapt to elevated pulmonary artery pressures. The transplanted right ventricle is usually procured from a donor with normal pulmonary vascular resistance (PVR) and, hence, is of normal thickness. In addition, it is extremely susceptible to preservation injury and perioperative dysfunction from rapid rewarming during the implantation procedure. Potential recipients who have pulmonary artery hypertension on routine cardiac catheterization (a PVR of greater than 3 Wood units) receive intravenous vasodilators (sodium nitroprusside, prostaglandin E, nitric oxide by infusion/inhalation in gradually increasing doses to blood pressure tolerance) to determine whether the elevation in pulmonary pressures is secondary to pulmonary vasoconstriction or irreversible disease.

Frequently, pulmonary artery pressures and resistance will fall into the acceptable range with acute pharmacologic intervention. A small number of patients, however, with truly reversible pulmonary hypertension will require several days of intensive medical management before

TABLE 46-2
LISTING CRITERIA PROPOSED BY THE UNITED NETWORK FOR ORGAN SHARING (UNOS) SUBCOMMITTEE ON UNIFORM LISTING CRITERIA

Indications For Transplant Listing

Cardiogenic shock or low output with reversible end-organ dysfunction requiring mechanical support
Low output of refractory heart failure requiring continuous inotropic support
Advanced heart failure signs and symptoms (NYHA Class III and IV) with objective documentation of marked functional limitation and poor 12-month prognosis despite maximized medical therapy
Recurrent or rapidly progressive heart failure symptoms unresponsive to maximized medical therapy
Severe heart failure caused by restrictive or hypertrophic cardiomyopathy
Refractory angina or arrhythmias

Inadequate Indications for Transplant Listing

Left ventricular ejection fraction (LVEF) <30% with mild to moderate congestive heart failure (CHF)
NYHA Class IV symptoms on suboptimal medical regimen
A prior episode of decompensation with symptoms now well-controlled on medical therapy
A prior need for inotropic support for decompensated CHF with symptoms now well-controlled on medical therapy
Patients with LVEF <20% but peak VO_2 >16 mL/kg/min unless clinically unstable or possessing other known indications (refractory angina, life-threatening arrhythmias)

pulmonary pressures fall. We have observed that selected patients on left ventricular assist devices (LVADs), who had severe pulmonary hypertension and suboptimal response to vasodilators, show significant improvement in their pulmonary pressures and vascular resistance after a few months of LVAD support (15). Those patients who persist in having elevated PVR despite intensive medical management may be candidates for heart-lung transplantation.

Infection

Patients in severe congestive heart failure are at increased susceptibility to infection, especially those waiting in intensive care units for cardiac transplantation. Because of the immediate requirements for immunosuppression following cardiac transplantation, patients must be adequately treated for any recent infection and be free of infection at the time of transplantation. In general, upper respiratory viral infections and uncomplicated bacteria have not been considered a contraindication for proceeding to transplantation.

Noncardiac Organ System Dysfunction

Severe congestive heart failure is frequently associated with prerenal azotemia and passive hepatic congestion (16,17). It is therefore important to separate these abnormalities from intrinsic organ dysfunction, as several of the commonly used immunosuppressive agents have either renal or hepatic toxicity (18,19). Patients with a serum creatinine greater than 2 mg/dL or hepatic enzyme abnormalities greater than twice normal should therefore have careful evaluations to exclude intrinsic organ dysfunction. In addition, severe heart failure frequently impacts pulmonary function. In a series of 17 patients studied with spirometry before and several months following cardiac transplantation, the principal spirometric abnormality was a reduction in lung volumes (restrictive pattern) before transplantation that was completely reversible following transplantation (20). The reduction in lung volumes was strongly correlated to the increase in cardiac volume, and obstructive physiology (if present before transplantation) was unchanged following cardiac replacement and normalization of hemodynamics. These data suggest that severe obstructive pulmonary physiology before transplantation would be unlikely to improve substantially following cardiac transplantation. Therefore, those patients with a forced vital capacity less than 50% of predicted with obstructive physiology would be extremely high-risk for postoperative pulmonary complications and nosocomial infection.

Systemic Diseases and Prior Malignancies

Diabetes had initially been considered a contraindication to cardiac transplantation because of the corticosteroids required as part of the immunosuppressive regimen. With the advent of lower-dose steroid protocols utilizing cyclosporine-based immunosuppression, the inclusion of diabetics as candidates for cardiac transplantation has gradually increased. Diabetics with severe end-organ damage are still, for the most part, excluded as candidates. Otherwise, it appears that patients with controlled diabetes have acceptable outcomes following cardiac transplantation (21).

Although definitive studies have not been performed, patients with prior malignancies who are considered cured are now being considered for and have undergone cardiac transplantation (22). The disease-free interval that is acceptable is obviously highly dependent on the natural history of the underlying malignancy. Several of these patients were treated with doxorubicin and have cardiomyopathy and heart failure on this basis (23). Whether these patients are at a higher risk for the development of recurrent or new malignancies is yet to be determined.

Finally, other systemic diseases such as amyloidosis and sarcoidosis have been traditionally considered contraindications for cardiac transplantation because of the concern that these would recur in the allografted organ. The initial small experience with amyloidosis appeared to be positive, with seven patients having intermediate-term survival equivalent of that of an age- and sex-matched control group (22). A longer follow-up of these patients demonstrated that despite the favorable intermediate prognosis, most patients developed progressive amyloid involvement in major organ systems and ultimately a reduced survival (24). Anecdotal reports of patients with cardiac sarcoidosis undergoing cardiac transplantation are available (25,26). Sarcoid granulomas can, however, recur in the allograft (27).

Medical Compliance, Substance Abuse, and Psychosocial Support

The complexity of the pre-, peri-, and post-operative care in cardiac transplantation necessitates a patient who understands the disease and is willing to comply with the recommendations made by the transplant team. Active substance abuse clearly threatens this compliance. The potential emotional stress in all aspects before and after transplantation may be better coped with if social support is available for the patient. Interestingly, however, it is extremely difficult to predict medical outcome and compliance using standard psychosocial evaluation parameters (28).

RECIPIENT EVALUATION

Table 46-3 outlines the typical evaluation performed for a patient referred for cardiac transplantation. The principal goals of this evaluation are (a) to determine the underlying cardiac disease and, if possible, delineate alternative treatment strategies; (b) to quantify cardiovascular function, degree of symptoms attributable to the cardiac function, and PVR; (c) to determine whether immunological barriers, such as preformed antibodies to histocompatibility leukocyte antigens (HLAs), are present, either precluding transplantation or modifying posttransplant treatment approaches; and (d) to evaluate other organ function and disease that might impact posttransplant outcome.

TABLE 46-3
RECIPIENT EVALUATION

Complete History and Physical Examination

Cardiovascular Evaluation
- Coronary angiography (if indicated)
- Endomyocardial biopsy (to rule out myocarditis, amyloidosis, etc., if indicated)
- Quantitative left ventricular ejection fraction
- Quantitation of pulmonary vascular resistance by catheterization
- Ambulatory electrocardiography (if indicated)
- Lipid studies

Noncardiac Organ Function Evaluation
- Pulmonary function studies
- Chemistries for renal and hepatic function
- Urinalysis
- Hematology
- Coagulation studies
- Peripheral or cerebral vascular studies (if indicated)
- Pregnancy testing

Infection Surveillance Evaluation
- Skin testing for myobacteria and systemic fungi
- Cytomegalovirus serology
- *Toxoplasma gondii* serology
- Bacterial cultures (if indicated)
- Hepatitis B, C serology
- HIV serology

Dental Examination

Systemic Disease Surveillance Evaluation
- Thyroid function
- Rheumatologic screening
- Mammography and PAP screening (if indicated)
- Serum protein electrophoresis
- Stool for hemoglobin

Immunologic Evaluation
- Blood type and screen
- Panel reactive antibody screen (detection of HLA antibody)

Psychosocial Evaluation

THE CARDIAC DONOR

The passage of the Uniform Anatomical Gift Act in 1968 (29), the general acceptance of criteria for brain death (30), and an increasing public awareness have brought about an increase in the number of available organs. However, in the past several years the number of donors and heart transplant operations worldwide has reached a plateau despite expansion of the criteria for an acceptable heart donor, consistent with a reduction in the numbers of what was previously considered the optimal heart donor. This, coupled with expanded recipient criteria, has resulted in a greater donor–recipient number mismatch. Figure 46-1 demonstrates the increase in donor age that has had to be required to maintain the relatively consistent number of transplants being performed worldwide (1). In 1988, the median waiting time for heart transplant candidates was 117 days. In 1996, the time to transplant had increased to 224 days, almost double (2). The median waiting time for heart transplant in 1999 was 502 days, and in 2002 was 392 days (UNOS Organ Procurement and Transplantation Network: Median waiting times for registrations listed between 1997-2002). The reduction in the heart transplant listings from 1999 to 2002 may reflect changes in listing criteria (31). The American College of Cardiologists/American Heart Association (ACC/AHA) guidelines for heart failure management have been more stringent regarding the listing criteria because of improved survival among the heart failure patients on medical management (32).

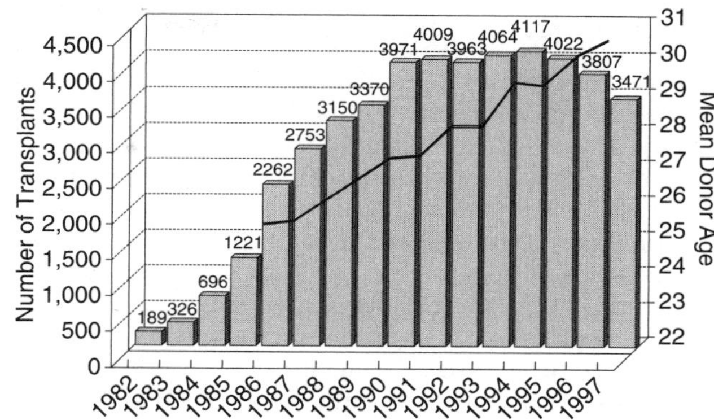

Figure 46-1 Heart transplant volume and mean donor age, by year. (From Hosenpud JD, Bennett LE, Keck BM, et al. The Registry of the International Society for Heart and Lung Transplantation: fifteenth official report—1998. *J Heart Lung Transplant.* 1998; 17:656–668.)

Brain Death

Neither the organ procurement agency nor the transplant teams have any involvement with the patient until brain death is declared and consent for organ donation is obtained. Table 46-4 presents the clinical and laboratory findings in brain death. In general, there is absence of cortical function as assessed by spontaneous movement, response to stimuli, or response to pain. There is absence of brainstem function, including a host of brainstem reflexes and spontaneous respiration. Finally, the electroencephalogram has no activity and, if measured, there is no cerebral blood flow (33,34).

TABLE 46-4
BRAIN DEATH

Absence of Cortical Function
- No spontaneous movement
- No response to external stimuli
- No response to pain

Absence of Brainstem Function
- No spontaneous respirations
- Absent pupillary and corneal reflexes
- Absent occulocephalic reflexes
- Absent vestibulo-occular reflexes

Absence of Activity on Electroencephalogram

Absence of Cerebral Blood Flow

Screening for Organ Donation

Aspects of screening of potential donors can be divided into those required for screening the donor for any and all organ donation and those specific for cardiac donation. Generalized donor screening centers around excluding transmissible diseases such as infections and malignancy. Screening now routinely carried out includes a careful medical and social history to eliminate patients whose exposure or lifestyles might increase the likelihood of viral diseases such as hepatitis B or C or human immunodeficiency virus (HIV); specific serology for hepatitis B and C, HIV, and human T-cell lymphotropic virus 1 (HTLV-1); and surveillance bacterial cultures. Patients with active sepsis are usually not considered for organ donation. Localized infection in the lung or urinary tract may allow for the donation of organs not directly involved. Likewise, despite malignancy being a contraindication for organ donation, patients with localized central nervous system malignancy are generally considered acceptable organ donors.

Once the potential organ donor has been screened for the general contraindications to organ donation, specific issues dealing with cardiac donation can then be addressed. The issues relate primarily to two questions: the function of the heart and the possibility of occult or overt coronary disease. Initially, cardiac donors were strictly age-limited to men aged 30 years or less and women aged 35 years or less, specifically to reduce the likelihood of occult coronary disease (35). With the progressive shortage of donors, this age limit was increased to 40 and 45 years, respectively (36); currently, many centers will consider organ donors age 50 years and beyond, depending on the age and stability of their recipients. The use of an older donor will, however, have an impact on overall posttransplant survival, given the known increase in mortality of the recipient as donor age increases (12). In general, most centers will attempt to obtain coronary angiography on the older donors but in some smaller hospitals this is not always achievable. With the same concerns, insulin-requiring diabetics are generally excluded from cardiac donation unless coronary angiography can be obtained, and those with other coronary risk factors are carefully evaluated. The electrocardiogram can be extremely helpful in this regard if pathological Q waves are present. ST segment shifts, T-wave changes, and arrhythmias are generally not helpful, as all of these are not infrequently associated with brainstem herniation and brain death (37,38).

The first indication of the integrity of cardiac function is the degree of inotropic support required to maintain stable vital signs in the donor. This, however, can be extremely misleading because, before brain death, a goal of the physicians (neurosurgeons or neurologists) caring for the patient is to minimize cerebral edema. This is usually accomplished by aggressive diuresis and fluid restriction. It is not unusual to find a potential organ donor receiving high-dose inotropic and vasopressor support, which can be rapidly weaned with aggressive fluid replacement. Most cardiac transplant programs will further evaluate a potential donor if inotropic support (usually either dobutamine or dopamine) can be reduced to below 10 μg/kg per minute. The echocardiogram (ECG) is now frequently utilized to evaluate cardiac function in the donor. Gilbert et al. demonstrated that echocardiography identified a full 29% of their successful cardiac donors who would have otherwise been excluded using ECG and clinical findings alone (39). Table 46-5 reviews the current screening criteria for cardiac organ donation.

TABLE 46-5
SCREENING CRITERIA FOR CARDIAC DONATION

General Organ Donation Screening
Absence of Infection
Hepatitis B and C, HIV, and HTLV-1 serology
Negative blood cultures
Psychosocial/Lifestyle Screening
Absence of Malignancy (excluding primary CNS tumors)
Screening for Coronary Disease
Age usually less than 55 years
Coronary angiography, if possible:
Men >40 years
Women >45 years
No pathological Q waves on ECG
No history of insulin-requiring diabetes
No other prior cardiac history
Screening for Cardiac Function
No requirement for high-dose inotropic support (after volume replacement)
No prolonged resuscitation
Normal echocardiogram (mild segmental wall motion or mitral prolapse not a contraindication; expanded criteria using moderate wall motion abnormalities if normal coronaries)

THE TRANSPLANT OPERATION

The cardiac transplant operation is, in fact, a multifaceted procedure that involves two operations—myocardial protection and organ transportation. With some modifications, the technical aspects of the cardiac transplant operation are essentially those initially described by Lower and Shumway 45 years ago (40).

Myocardial Preservation

The techniques of cold cardioplegia have been developed in cardiovascular surgery over the past 20 years. There appears to be adequate preservation of the myocardium at temperatures below 20°C. A number of preservation solutions have been employed over the years, with centers gradually moving away from using standard Euro-Collins solution or Stanford University solution to newer solutions such as University of Wisconsin (UW) solution. In a recent survey performed by the University Hospital Consortium, 39% of centers were using Stanford solution, 22% UW solution, and the remainder a variety of preservation solutions. The UW solution has been demonstrated to have a profound effect on both renal and liver preservation for transplantation. Although there are animal studies demonstrating improved cardiac preservation with UW solution (41,42), recent animal studies and one clinical study suggest that UW solution is associated with endothelial cell injury and a higher incidence of allograft vasculopathy (chronic rejection) posttransplantation (42,43).

Ischemic Time

As shown in Figure 46-2 based on data from the joint UNOS/ISHLT Thoracic Registry, it is absolutely clear that ischemic time (the time from aortic cross-clamp in the donor to cross-clamp release and restoration of coronary flow in the recipient) is a strong and independent determinant of early survival (12,44,45). Most centers will, therefore, not exceed 4 hours of ischemic time unless their recipient is extremely unstable. Unfortunately, it is the sicker recipients who generally need a well-functioning allograft in the early posttransplant period. Methods for improving myocardial preservation, thus allowing for greater ischemic times, are currently under active investigation. One would hope that with improved preservation and better immunological matching of donors and recipients, greater use of donated cardiac organs could be achieved.

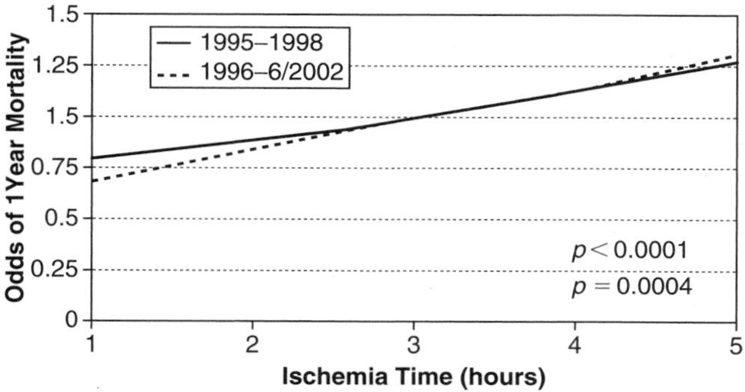

Figure 46-2 Effect of ischemic time on relative risk of mortality. (From Taylor DO, Edwards LB, Boucek MM, et al. The Registry of the International Society for Heart and Lung Transplantation: twenty-first official adult heart transplant report—2004. *J Heart Lung Transplant.* 2004;23:796-803.)

Traditional (Shumway) Donor Cardiectomy

The donor heart is reached through a standard midline sternotomy. The heart is inspected visually to evaluate chamber size and wall motion and palpably to detect the degree of chamber filling and the presence of coronary calcification. Once the heart is considered appropriate for transplantation, the transplant center is notified and the recipient operation begins. While other organs are being harvested, the aorta and pulmonary artery are dissected free and controlled with tapes, as is the superior vena cava. Just before harvest, heparin is administered, the superior vena cava is ligated, the inferior vena cava is cross-clamped, and cold cardioplegic solution is administered into the aorta. The aorta is then cross-clamped and the various cardiac structures are transected in the following order: (a) the superior vena cava (between double ligations); (b) inferior vena cava and right lower pulmonary vein; (c) aorta and pulmonary artery; and finally, (d) the remaining pulmonary veins. The pulmonary veins are connected to form the left atrial cuff and the heart is packaged for transport. Figure 46-3 demonstrates the preparation of the donor heart.

Traditional (Shumway) Recipient Operation

The recipient is brought to the operating room and central venous (or pulmonary artery) and intra-arterial catheters are placed. The operation is via a midline sternotomy, usually started when communication from the donor team indicates the donor heart is suitable for transplantation. After dissection and control of the great veins and arteries, heparin is administered and the patient is cooled and placed on cardiopulmonary bypass (usually not before the donor heart has arrived at the transplant center). The native heart is excised with incisions transecting the various cardiac structures in the following order: (a) the lateral wall of the right atrium, continuing inferiorly and medially to and across the intra-atrial septum; (b) the aorta and pulmonary artery; and, finally, (c) the left lateral wall of the left atrium. The allograft implantation is then carried out using running suture with anastomoses in the following order: (a) left atrial free wall, (b) intra-atrial septum, (c) right atrium, (d) pulmonary artery, and (e) aorta. The early and late stages of the allograft implantation are demonstrated in Figures 46-4 and 46-5, respectively.

Bicaval/Total Recipient Operation

Two more recent variations of this procedure have been undertaken to attempt to reduce injury to the sinus node and to improve atrial transport by avoiding the competing atrial contractions between the recipient and donor atria. The initial bicaval anastomotic approach is shown in Figure 46-6. In this procedure, the recipient right atrium is

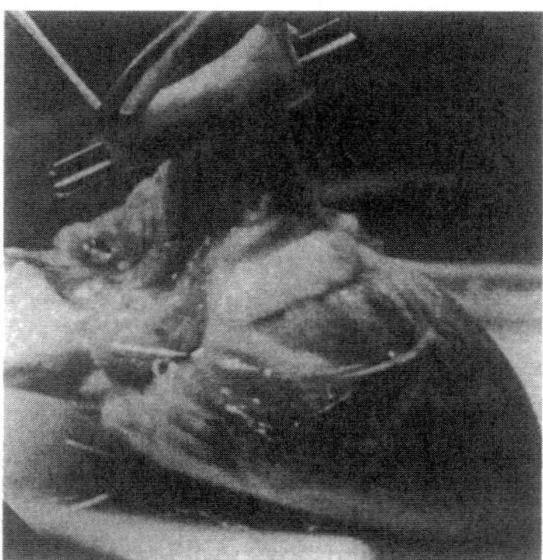

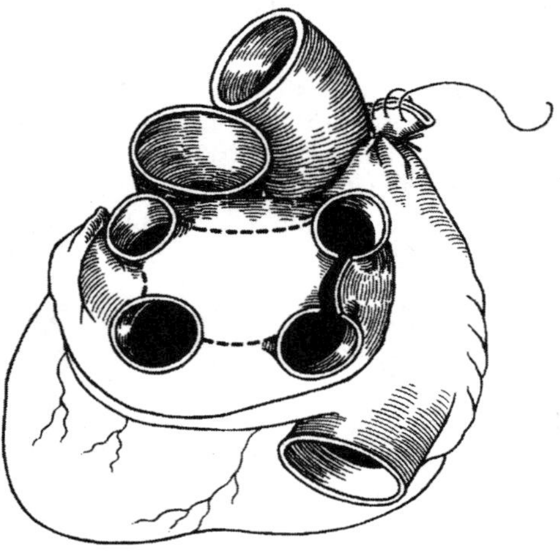

Figure 46-3 Donor heart preparation. (From Cobanoglu Davies RA, Koshal A, Walley V, et al. Temporary diastolic noncompliance with preserved systolic function after heart transplantation. *Transplant Proc.* 1987;19:3444–3447.)

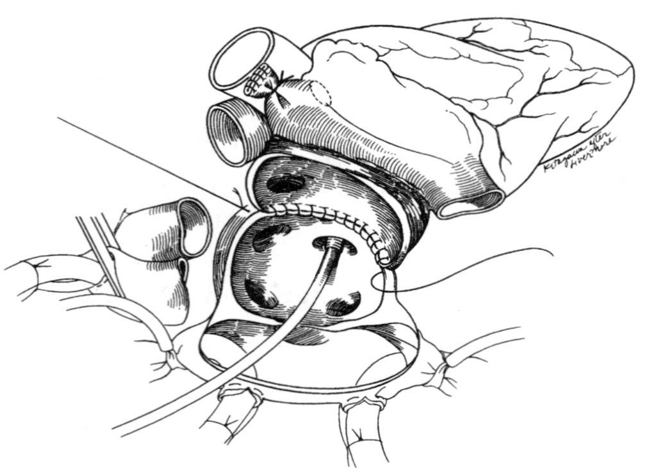

Figure 46-4 Allograft implantation, initial left atrial anastamosis. (From Cobanoglu Davies RA, Koshal A, Walley V, et al. Temporary diastolic noncompliance with preserved systolic function after heart transplantation. *Transplant Proc.* 1987;19:3444–3447.)

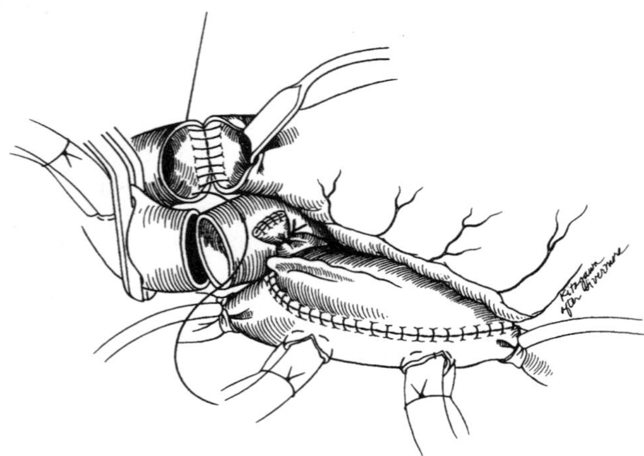

Figure 46-5 Nearly completed allograft implantation. (From Cobanoglu Davies RA, Koshal A, Walley V, et al. Temporary diastolic noncompliance with preserved systolic function after heart transplantation. *Transplant Proc.* 1987;19:3444–3447.)

completely removed and the inferior and superior vena cavae are anastomosed directly to the intact donor atrium. The anastomosis of the left atrium is similar to the traditional approach. A modification this approach described by Dreyfus et al. (46) is to remove the recipient left atrium, leaving only left and right pulmonary vein "buttons," which are directly anastomosed to the intact donor left atrium (not shown). In a small study involving 18 patients, Sievers et al. demonstrated the preservation in atrial size and a reduction in tricuspid regurgitation during exercise in those undergoing the bicaval approach versus the traditional approach, but no difference in exercise capacity could be demonstrated (47). Deleuze et al., in a much larger series, demonstrated that those patients undergoing the newer technique had less delayed sinus node function and initially lower pulmonary artery pressure and higher resting cardiac indeces compared to those undergoing the traditional anastomosis (48). Whether long-term outcomes are different is yet to be determined.

PERIOPERATIVE CARE

Immunosuppression Induction

Although immunosuppression is discussed in depth later in this chapter, a few comments are appropriate at this time. The majority of centers continue to use cyclosporine (4 to 10 mg/kg) and azathioprine (2 to 5 mg/kg) preoperatively and intravenous prednisolone (0.5 to 2 g) intraoperatively. Some centers are using mycophenolate mofetil in place of azathioprine and/or tacrolimus in place of cyclosporine. In contrast to renal transplantation, the use of monoclonal and polyclonal anti-T-cell antibodies routinely as prophylaxis has declined over the past 5 years, primarily because of reports demonstrating an increased rate of infection and malignancy posttransplantation (49,50) and the relative lack of data suggesting improvement in outcomes using these agents (51,52). Monoclonal antibodies, specifically the monoclonal antibody to the T-cell receptor (anti-CD3) OKT3, have been effective in prevent-

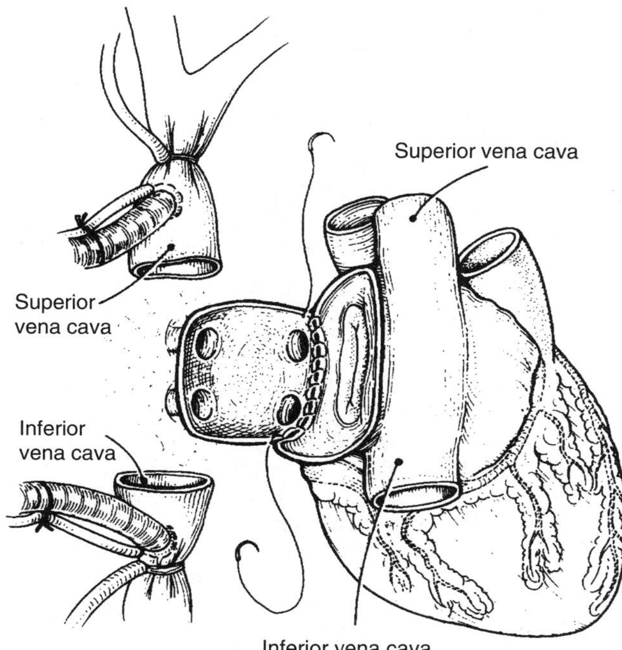

Figure 46-6 The alternative bicaval anastomotic technique for heart transplantation. (From Deleuze et al. Davies RA, Koshal A, Walley V, et al. Temporary diastolic noncompliance with preserved systolic function after heart transplantation. *Transplant Proc.* 1987;19:3444–3447.)

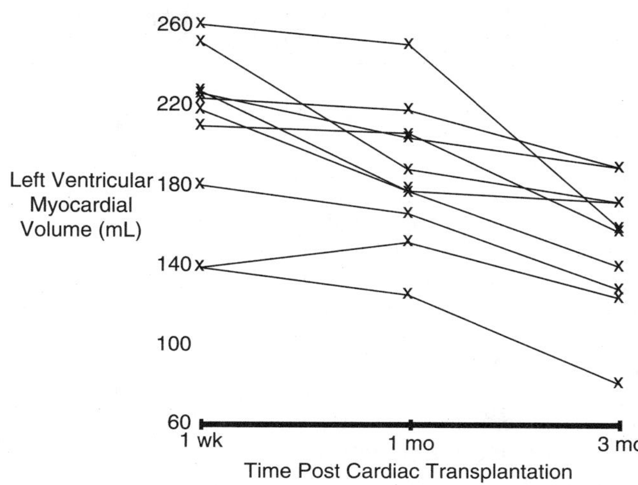

Figure 46-7 Calculated myocardial volumes in 10 patients after cardiac transplantation demonstrating a serial decline in myocardial volume (mass) from 1 week to 3 months. (From Stinson EB, Caves PK, Griepp RB, et al. Hemodynamic observations in the early period after human heart transplantation. *J Thorac Cardiovasc Surg.* 1975;69:264–270.)

ing rejection in the first 14 days if cyclosporine has to be withheld because of early renal dysfunction. Newer monoclonal antibodies such as daclizumab (Zenapax), which is directed against the interleukin-2 (IL-2) receptor, may be similarly efficacious without some of the toxicity associated with OKT3. Polyclonal antibody preparations can also be used in this manner.

Allograft Hemodynamic Support

It is critically important to understand several aspects of allograft physiology early posttransplantation to provide appropriate postoperative support. Despite careful attempts at myocardial preservation and limiting total ischemic times, the allograft is ischemically damaged immediately following transplantation. This, coupled with mild to moderate elevations in PVR in the recipient (53), the denervated state of the allograft (54,55), and the ischemic damage to the sinus node (56), results in the heart and predominantly the right ventricle being in need of support. As one might anticipate, acute right ventricular failure is the most common nonimmunologic cause of perioperative death following cardiac transplantation (57). The ischemic damage to the allograft, in addition to being manifest as reduced systolic function and sinus node activity, is also manifest by a reduction in ventricular compliance associated with myocardial edema, which can be present for up to 3 months following transplantation (58,59).

Figure 46-7 demonstrates that left ventricular myocardial volumes measured by echocardiogram in 10 allograft recipients are still not normal by 1 month following transplantation. Stinson et al. investigated hemodynamics in 10 allograft recipients immediately postoperatively and for the first 7 days (60). Cardiac function was severely depressed initially (cardiac index 1.8 L/min/m^2, stroke volume index 21 mL/m^2) and then gradually improved. Isoproterenol was extremely effective in providing both inotropic as well as chronotropic support and is now, in most centers, the initial catecholamine of choice following transplantation. If additional inotropic support is required, it is important to choose agents that directly stimulate β_1-receptors such as dobutamine or epinephrine or inhibit cyclic adenosine monophosphate (cAMP) breakdown by phosphodiesterase (milrinone, amrinone). Agents that indirectly provide inotropic support by releasing stored norepinephrine (or dopamine) will be effective for the first several hours following transplantation but will lose their effectiveness because of the denervated state. Elevations in PVR exacerbated by the use of blood products can be treated using vasodilators such as sodium nitroprusside or prostaglandin E_2 (61). Most often, inotropic, chronotropic, and vasodilator support can successfully be discontinued between 3 and 5 days following transplantation.

Infection Control

Although early experience had most transplant centers using some form of protective isolation, the efficacy of these measures has never been demonstrated. As a result, the general trend has been to relax these measures to a considerable degree. Most patients receive prophylactic antibacterial agents effective against skin organisms for several days following transplantation. At centers where *Pneumocystis* and cytomegalovirus infections have produced substantial morbidity, patients receive prophylactic hyperimmune globulin and/or ganciclovir or acyclovir (CMV) and trimethoprim-sulfamethoxazole (*Pneumocystis*). The efficacy of these measures, although suggestive, is not clearly proven (62–64).

IMMUNOSUPPRESSION: THE DIAGNOSIS AND TREATMENT OF REJECTION

It is clear to all involved in the field of heart transplantation that with the advances in surgical care, the procedure itself is now only a minor part of the therapy of transplantation. The immunologic barrier between donor and recipient continues to be a substantial challenge. Table 46-6 presents the classification, mechanisms, and manifestations of the various forms of rejection. Hyperacute rejection is secondary to preformed alloantibodies, which are routinely screened for in the initial evaluation (previously discussed). Acute cellular rejection is the focus of the current discussion. Chronic rejection is manifest by an accelerated development of coronary artery disease (CAD), discussed later.

The primary concept of immunosuppression therapy is diagrammed in Figure 46-8. One initially induces an immunosuppressive state. Once induced, immunosuppression intensity is reduced over time, with episodic intensification for isolated episodes of rejection. Figure 46-9 demonstrates a simplified representation of the cellular immune response to alloantigens and the effects on this response by various classes of immunosuppressive agents. As stated previously, the specific immunosuppression protocols used vary substantially from center to center, but most use a combination of agents. Table 46-7 lists the specific agents by class. What follows is a brief description of the more commonly used agents.

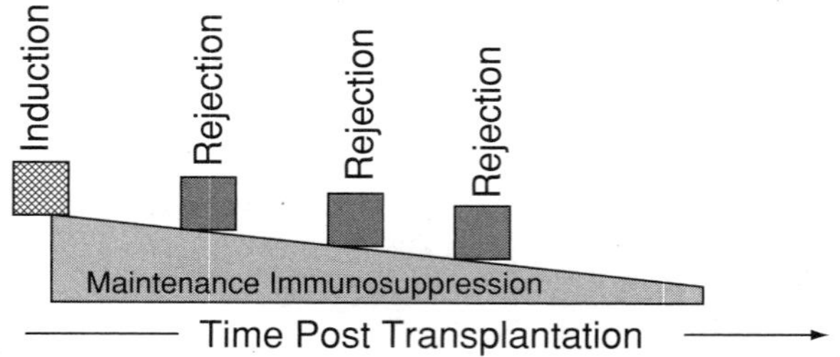

Figure 46-8 Schema approach to long-term immunosuppression following transplantation. Patients are induced with high-dose immunosuppression and then maintained on ever-decreasing intensity of therapy. Immunosuppression is augmented for discrete rejection episodes.

Cyclosporine

This agent has clearly revolutionized the field of transplantation in its 15 years of clinical use. First discovered in 1972 by Jean Borel (65,66) and recognized as a potent inhibitor of T-cell function, it is now the mainstay of cardiac transplant immunosuppression. Cyclosporine is a T-cell-specific drug that inhibits the gene transcription of multiple lymphokines, including interferon-γ, interleukin-2 (IL-2), and probably interleukins 3 through 7 (67,68). These cytokines are extremely important for activation and recruitment of the various components of the immune system. For example, IL-2 is the primary signal for T-cell proliferation and clonal expansion (69). Interferon-γ may be primarily responsible for increasing target cell surface expression of major histocompatibility antigens necessary for recognition by the immune system (68). In clinical use, in most instances, a loading dose of between 5 and 10 mg/kg is administered preoperatively, and the maintenance dose ranges from 3 to 8 mg/kg in divided doses. The specific dose for a given patient is determined by blood or serum levels and can vary considerably from patient to patient and even within a given patient because of the complex metabolism of the drug. In addition, there are several drugs that interact with cyclosporine metabolism, both increasing and decreasing its metabolism (70). Recently, cyclosporine serum level monitoring done 2 hours post-dose has shown better correlation to the drug exposure, reduced renal dysfunction, and no increase in rejection rate (71). The major toxicities of cyclosporine are the induction or exacerbation of hypertension and renal impairment, both of which occur in the majority of patients taking the drug (72). Other less-common side effects include hepatotoxicity, neurotoxicity, seizures, gingival hyperplasia, hirsutism, and hyperglycemia. Most side effects are dose-related and will not preclude its use.

Tacrolimus

This agent was first isolated from *Streptomyces tukubaensis* in 1994 in Japan. The mechanism of action is quite similar to that of cyclosporine but it has a potency approximately 100 times that of cyclosporine. The initial experience with this agent was in liver transplantation, and over the ensuing years it has become the agent of choice in this setting. More recently, tacrolimus has been used in cardiac transplantation and early reports suggest an equivalent efficacy overall (73).

TABLE 46-6
CLASSIFICATION OF REJECTION

Classification	Time Course	Immune Mechanism	Manifestation
Hyperacute	0–3 days	Preformed alloantibody	Acute graft dysfunction vascular injury
Acute	>7 days	T-cell-mediated	Parenchymal inflammation, graft dysfunction
Chronic	>6 months	? T-cell-mediated	Coronary artery disease
Xeno	Hours	Complement/natural antibody	Coagulation necrosis

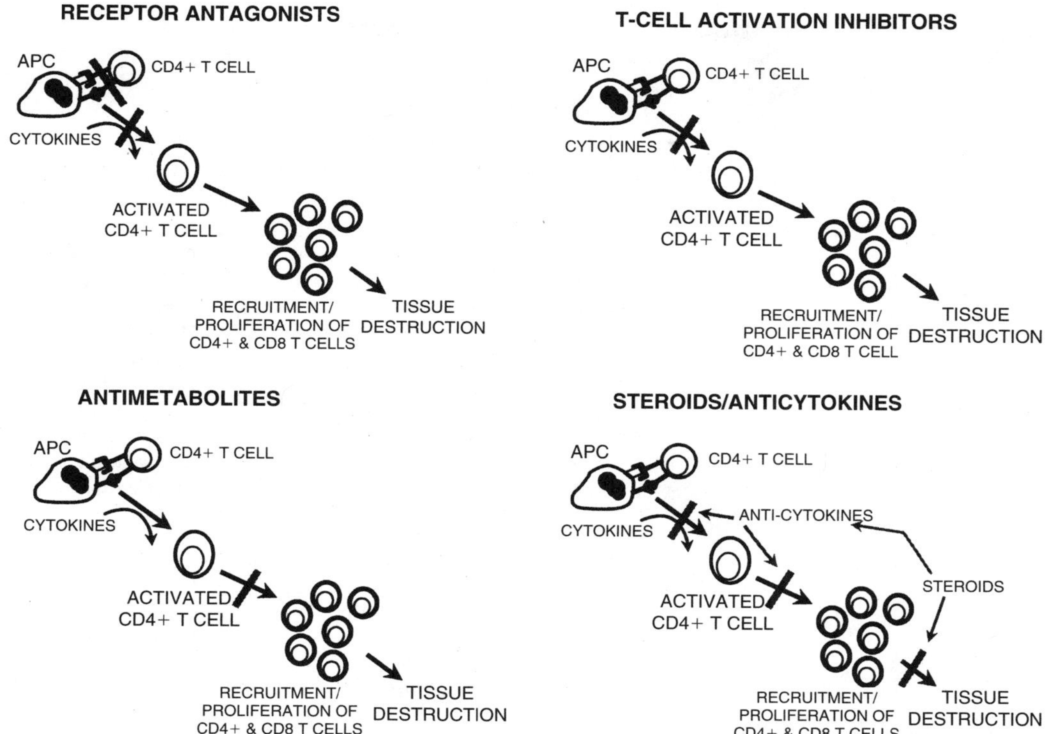

Figure 46-9 A schematic representation of the immune response and the effects of immunosuppressive agents by class.

There are reports of tacrolimus being effective in rescuing patients who have failed cyclosporine immunosuppression (74). Tacrolimus dosing is based on trough serum levels and usually ranges from 0.1 to 0.15 mg/kg per day in divided doses. Tacrolimus is used in place of cyclosporine in many immunosuppressive maintenance regimens, and many centers consider it as the first choice of immunosuppressant over cyclosporine because of apparent lower risk of acute rejection (75). A recent three-arm multicenter trial was done comparing three groups of heart transplant patients with combinations of tacrolimus and sirolimus, tacrolimus and mycophenolate mofetil (MMF), and cyclosporine and MMF immunosuppressive regimens. The tacrolimus and sirolimus group showed a significant decrease in any treated rejection, with fewer patients developing coronary allograft vasculopathy by intravascular ultrasound in the first year posttransplantation (76). Toxicity is also quite similar to that of cyclosporine and, in addition to the renal toxicity, diabetes, and hypertension, there is a higher incidence of neurologic side effects compared to cyclosporine. Interestingly, gingival hypertrophy and hirsutism are much less common (77).

Azathioprine

The initial discovery that the purine analog 6-mercaptopurine (6-MP) was an effective immunosuppressive agent was made by Calne in 1960 in an animal model of renal transplantation (78). The nitroimidazolyl derivative of 6-MP, azathioprine, was synthesized in 1975 and subsequently shown to be effective in clinical renal transplantation (79,80). The mechanism of action of azathioprine is to inhibit de novo purine biosynthesis, which ultimately blocks cell proliferation (81). Although cardiac transplantation went through a period in which azathioprine–prednisone protocols were replaced with cyclosporine–prednisone protocols, the combination of all three agents has been shown to improve outcomes (82).

The usual dose of azathioprine is 1.5 to 2.5 mg/kg. It is not clear whether the immunosuppressive effects of azathioprine relate to the suppression of total white blood count or are independent of the marrow suppression. This has led primarily to two philosophies regarding its dosing: the philosophy of using a standard dose (usually 2 mg/kg) unless toxicity intervenes, or the philosophy that the dose should be increased progressively to reduce total white count to a target level (usually around 5,000 per μL). As one might expect, the principal toxicity of azathioprine is bone marrow suppression. This is readily reversible with reduction of the dose. Other less-common side effects are hepatic toxicity (an unusual form of hepatic veno-occlusive disease) and pancreatitis (17,81). Finally, prolonged use has been associated with the development of malignancy, specifically skin cancers (81). This risk brings into question the philosophy of using higher doses of azathioprine to control total white blood cell counts.

Mycophenolate Mofetil

This metabolite of mycophenolic acid, like azathioprine, is a purine metabolism inhibitor. It is unique in that it is specific for the de novo pathway of purine synthesis. The advantage that this property extends to MMF is that most cells have

TABLE 46-7
IMMUNOSUPPRESSIVE AGENTS

Agent	Mechanism of Action	Status
Receptor Antagonists		
ATG	T-cell cytotoxic/traffic	FDA-approved
OKT3	$CD3^+$ cytotoxic/traffic	FDA-approved
Xomazyme-$CD5^+$	$CD5^+$ cytotoxic/traffic	Clinical trials
Anti-TAC	$CD25^+$ cytotoxic/traffic	FDA-approved
Dab486-IL2	$CD25^+$ cytotoxic/traffic	Clinical trials
Anti-LFA-1	Cellular adhesion	Clinical trials
Anti-ICAM-1	Cellular adhesion	Clinical trials
OKT4a	$CD4^+$ anergy	Clinical trials
Anti-IL-1 receptor	IL-1 receptor blocker	Clinical trials
Soluble HLA	Inhibits Ag presentation	Clinical trials
Antimetabolites		
Azathioprine	Inhibits PRPP amidoransferase	FDA-approved
Methotrexate	Inhibits dihydrofolate reductase	FDA-approved
Mycopheonolate	Inhibits IMP dehydrogenase	FDA-approved
Mizoribine	Inhibits IMP dehydrogenase	Clinical trials
Brequinar	Inhibits DHP dehydrogenase	Clinical trials
T-cell Activation Inhibitors		
Inhibitors		
Early		
Cyclosporine A	Inhibits Ser/Thr phosphatase	FDA-approved
Cyclosporine G	Inhibits Ser/Thr phosphatase	Clinical trials
Tacrolimus	Inhibits Ser/Thr phosphatase	FDA-approved
SDZ Imm 125	Inhibits Ser/Thr phosphatase	Clinical trials
Late		
Rapamycin	Unclear	Clinical trials
Leflunomide	Inhibits tyrosine kinase	Clinical trials
Cytokine Inhibitors		
Anti-IL-6	Neutralizes IL-6	Clinical trials
Anti-TNF	Neutralizes TNF	Clinical trials
Soluble IL-1 receptor	Neutralizes IL-1	Clinical trials
IL-10	Inhibits cytokine synthesis	Preclinical
Suppressor Inducers		
Skf 105685	Unclear	Preclinical
Aldesleukin (IL-2)	Stimulates via IL-2 receptor	Clinical trials
Anti-Ag Presentation		
Deoxyspergualine	Blocks Ag presentation	Clinical trials

IMP, inosine monophosphate; Ser, serine; Thr, threonine; IL, interleukin; Ag, antigen; TNF, tumor necrosis factor; FDA, U.S. Food and Drug Administration.
Adapted from Eisen H, Ross H. Optimizing the immunosuppressive regimen in heart transplantation. *J Heart Lung Transplant.* 2004;23:S207–S213.

both the de novo and salvage pathways of purine synthesis intact. Lymphoid cells, on the other hand, do not contain the salvage pathway, making this agent relatively specific for lymphocytes. As one would expect, the incidence of anemia, thrombocytopenia, and global leukopenia is lower for MMF than for azathioprine. A recent large, multicenter, randomized trial comparing MMF to azathioprine in heart transplantation demonstrated a modest but statistically significant increase in survival and a reduction in hemodynamically significant rejection in the MMF group (83).

The major side effect of MMF is gastrointestinal intolerance but, in general, the agent is very well-tolerated. MMF appears to be a potent inhibitor of B-cell proliferation and antibody production (84). Because of this property, it has been hoped that the incidence of chronic rejection would be lower than with immunosuppressive agents not as effective on the humoral arm. The above-mentioned randomized study has not demonstrated a lower incidence of chronic rejection in MMF-treated patients by 1 year, but 2- and 3-year follow-up is still in progress. A 3-year follow-up study in heart transplant patients, using either azathioprine or MMF along with cyclosporine and steroids, showed that the MMF-treated group had reduced mortality, decreased prevalence of accelerated coronary atherosclerosis, but an increased incidence of nonlethal viral infections (85).

Corticosteroids

The first reported use of adrenocorticotropic hormone (ACTH) in renal allograft recipients in 1960 (86) very shortly led to corticosteroids becoming standard therapy for maintenance immunosuppression. The mechanisms of action of corticosteroids are both immunosuppressive and anti-inflammatory. The specific immunosuppressive activity results from (a) inhibition of the release of the recruiting and inflammatory monokines IL-1 (responsible for initial helper T-cell activation), IL-6, and tumor necrosis factor (87,88) and (b) their direct lymphocytotoxic effects. Their anti-inflammatory effects are mediated by inhibiting the release of inflammatory mediators such as the leukotrienes, anaphalotoxins, and chemotaxins from macrophages (89). Thus, in contrast to cyclosporine, corticosteroids are quite nonspecific in their effects on the alloimmunologic response. Their use clinically in heart transplantation varies from center to center, but almost all transplant programs use intravenous methylprednisolone in the intraoperative and perioperative periods. Once the patient can take oral medications, prednisone is used initially in doses of approximately 0.5 mg/kg and tapered over time. Several centers are now maintaining patients on cyclosporine and azathioprine alone to avoid the many side effects of chronic corticosteroid administration, including obesity, cushingoid features, hyperlipidemia, hyperglycemia, hirsutism, bone demineralization, gastric irritation, and mood changes—all well-known to clinicians. It is not yet clear, however, that the elimination of corticosteroids from maintenance immunosuppression will not have adverse long-term effects for the allograft. There have been reports of higher incidence of acute rejection with early steroid withdrawal; however, the long-term survival of these patients beyond 10 years is improved (90,91). There is the suggestion that incidence of late serious infections may be lower in patients who had successful steroid withdrawal (92).

Antilymphocyte Antibodies

The use of antilymphocyte preparations, either polyclonal or monoclonal, is restricted to either early posttransplant prophylaxis against rejection or to the treatment of acute rejection. Polyclonal antilymphocyte or antithymocyte preparations are produced by inoculating human lymphocytes (or thymocytes) into animals (usually rabbits or horses), allowing a humoral response to occur, and collecting and purifying the antibody fraction from animal serum. These antibodies are by design directed against a whole host of antigens on the human lymphocytes, hence the term polyclonal. The hybridoma technique developed by Kohler and Milstein (93), of fusing a single plasma cell clone to a malignant cell line, led to the development of specific monoclonal antibodies directed at unique antigens. The advantages of polyclonal preparations are their diversity in potentially blocking the immune response at multiple sites, but the disadvantage (given their method of synthesis) is the extreme variability from lot to lot. This is not the case with monoclonal preparations, where specific antibody titers can be controlled. Neither antibody preparation has a role in ongoing maintenance immunosuppression because of the requirement that they be given parenterally and because of the development of host antibodies against the animal protein. A solution to this latter problem may be forthcoming with the development of chimeric or fusion antibodies that are primarily human in structure.

One of the first controlled trials using polyclonal antilymphocyte serum was reported by Sheil et al. in cadaveric renal allograft recipients in 1971 (94). The first available monoclonal antibody directed against the T-cell receptor (CD3 antigen) was OKT3; this was initially studied in renal transplantation for the treatment of acute rejection by Cosimi et al. in 1981 (95). The mechanism of action of both the polyclonal preparations and OKT3 is to deplete T-lymphocytes during the course of their administration; hence, they are extremely effective in halting acute rejection. Despite lymphocyte levels tending to revert to normal shortly after the discontinuation of these agents, it was hoped that if they are administered in the early posttransplant period the immune response would be permanently altered, leading to a greater partial tolerance (96).

Subsequent studies comparing protocols adding antilymphocyte preparations to initial immunosuppression induction have not demonstrated a substantial change in rejection patterns (51,52). In addition, there are now studies suggesting that the prophylactic use of these agents may increase both early infection rates and severity as well as increase the risk of developing malignancy (49,50).

Sirolimus

Sirolimus (rapamycin) is a natural product of actinomycete *Streptomyces hygroscopicus*, isolated from the soil. Its structure resembles tacrolimus; however, the function is different in that it inhibits the "target of rapamycin" (TOR) kinases, crucial in the growth and proliferation of T- and B-lymphocytes and smooth muscle cells. The studies to date have been done primarily in renal transplant patients, where sirolimus treatment has resulted in significantly lower incidences of acute rejection. A prospective, randomized trial involved 46 heart transplant patients with coronary vasculopathy who were assigned to either sirolimus or continued standard care. Over a 2-year follow-up period, three sirolimus patients versus 14 control patients reached the primary endpoint (death; requiring angioplasty or bypass surgery; myocardial infarction; or a 25% worsening of the catheterization score). This study showed that sirolimus is an effective therapy in secondary prevention of ischemic events (97). The major side effects of sirolimus are hypertriglyceridemia, thrombocytopenia, and neutropenia. Sirolimus also potentiates the nephrotoxic effects of calcineurin inhibitors.

Everolimus

Everolimus is a proliferation signal inhibitor, an analog of sirolimus. It inhibits T-cell and nonhematopoietic proliferation, thus decreasing the risk of acute rejection and coronary artery vasculopathy (CAV). It inhibits vascular remodeling and neointimal proliferation, which are both key components of CAV; however, it has shorter half-life and greater bioavailability than sirolimus. In a recent double-blind, randomized trial involving 634 heart transplant patients, everolimus has shown superior efficacy to azathioprine in reducing the severity and incidence of cardiac allograft vasculopathy. There was a significant increase in creatinine in the everolimus group compared to the azathioprine group (98). Myelosuppression and hyperlipidemia have also been seen with everolimus use.

Newer Agents and Immunosuppressive Strategies

A whole host of immunosuppressive agents directed toward unique aspects of the immune response are currently under investigation. These include newer T-cell activation inhibitors such as rapamycin, pyrimidine analogs such as brequinar sodium, and unrelated agents such as deoxyspergualine and prostaglandin analogs. In addition, new monoclonal antibodies directed to specific T-cell subtypes, chimeric molecules, and hybrid molecules coupled to cell toxins are under investigation. Finally, nonpharmacologic mechanisms to alter the immune response, such as lymphoid irradiation and photochemical therapy, may be potential tools in the therapy of allograft recipients. The days of being limited to azathioprine, prednisone, and cyclosporine are rapidly vanishing. Figure 46-10 demonstrates current data from the joint UNOS/ISHLT Thoracic Registry on maintenance immunosuppression use at 1 and 3 years posttransplantation. Mycophenolate mofetil is beginning to be substituted for azathioprine, and tacrolimus for cyclosporine in a smaller number of patients (1).

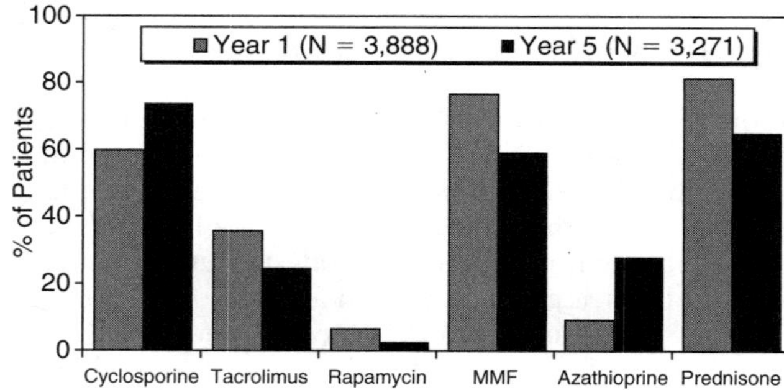

Figure 46-10 Current use of immunosuppressive agents following cardiac transplantation. (From Hosenpud JD, Bennett LE, Keck BM, et al. The Registry of the International Society for Heart and Lung Transplantation: fifteenth official report—1998. *J Heart Lung Transplant*. 1998;17:656–668, with permission.)

Acute Rejection: Diagnosis and Treatment

One of the most important advances in cardiac transplantation, equivalent in import to the development of cyclosporine, was the use of transvenous endomyocardial biopsy for monitoring allograft rejection. The application of this technique to cardiac transplantation was reported by Caves et al. at Stanford in 1973 (99). Until that time, rejection was monitored by changes in ECG volume reflecting myocardial edema, and changes in allograft function. Not only were these early methods at times inaccurate (lacking both sensitivity and specificity) but, in addition, by the time many of these features were manifest, rejection was already advanced. Endomyocardial biopsy monitoring allowed for the early detection of rejection, thus improving the chances for effective therapy. The typical monitoring protocol calls for weekly endomyocardial biopsies for the first 1 to 2 months following transplantation, with the frequency of biopsies declining with increasing time from transplantation. Figure 46-11 demonstrates the actual acute rejection incidence from one large cardiac transplant program. It is most common in the first 3 months posttransplantation and then declines dramatically thereafter. If rejection is present and requires treatment, endomyocardial biopsy is again performed to assess efficacy of treatment (at short intervals) until the rejection episode is completed.

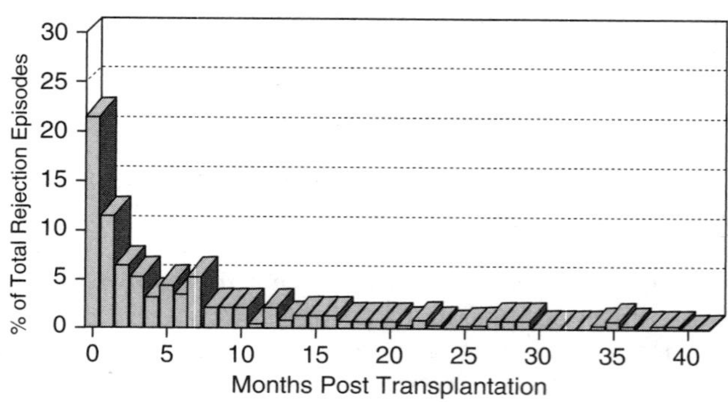

Figure 46-11 The incidence of rejection over time following transplantation from a large cardiac transplant program.

The currently accepted histological grading scale developed and supported by ISHLT is presented in Table 46-8 (100). Figure 46-12 demonstrates an endomyocardial biopsy with moderate acute rejection (ISHLT Grade 3A). Both a multifocal, intense, inflammatory infiltrate and evidence of myocyte damage are present.

The intensity of the rejection response and the proximity of the rejection episode to transplantation usually guides the intensity of antirejection therapy. In general, only rejection grades of moderate or greater are treated with intensification of immunosuppression, because lesser grades may resolve spontaneously (70) or with minor increases in maintenance immunosuppression. The alterations of immunosuppression can include stepwise increases in corticosteroids, courses of antilymphocyte antibodies (monoclonal or polyclonal), or drugs such as methotrexate. Figure 46-13 presents the actual rejection treatment approach used over a 4-year period in one large transplant program.

Chronic Rejection and Cardiac Allograft Vasculopathy

The principal factor limiting long-term survival following cardiac transplantation is a unique form of diffuse, obliterative CAD termed cardiac allograft vasculopathy (CAV). An example of this diffuse process is shown in Figure 46-14. The incidence of the disease (based on surveillance coronary angiography) is as high as 15% per year with a 5-year prevalence as high as 45% (101). Moreover, this incidence is likely underestimated, based on data comparing intravascular ultrasound to diagnostic coronary angiography (102,103). It is most certainly a form of chronic rejection, as the disease is limited solely to the allograft.

Whether humoral or cellular mechanisms are more important is controversial, with evidence supporting both cellular (104,105) and humoral (106,107) arms. In addition, there are emerging data that other factors such donor age (108,109), cytomegalovirus infection (110,111), and serum lipid levels (112) may impact the disease process. Whether these stresses are etiologic or somehow alter the immune response is an area of active investigation.

The histopathology is unique, as well. In contrast to traditional atherosclerosis, which is focal and proximal in nature, CAV is a diffuse process involving the entire length of the coronary tree (101). Only later do the lesions become more complex with differential areas of narrowing (113). There is concentric myointimal proliferation (Fig. 46-15) in CAV, in contrast to the frequently eccentric involvement in traditional CAD. The internal elastic lamina is usually intact and there is rarely calcium deposition until late in the disease (101). Although many lesions are bland without evidence of an inflammatory infiltrate, scattered mononuclear cells can at times be identified throughout the myointima. Libby et al. pointed out the presence and close association of mononuclear cells just below the endothelial layer, suggesting a role for cell-mediated immunity (114). It has been shown from the registry that the risk factors for development of angiographic CAV of any severity during the first 5 to 7 years after transplantation include pretransplant CAD, prior HLA sensitization, history of hypertension in the donor, and rejection severe enough to require hospitalization within 5 years of transplantation (115).

It is ironic that the major late complication following cardiac transplantation is the development of CAV, yet the vast majority of patients (with exceptions) are afferently denervated so they have no chest pain. For this reason, most centers perform routine annual coronary angiography to screen for the development of CAV. Intravascular ultrasound (IVUS) appears to be very sensitive in identifying early CAV. It has been shown that IVUS data may be a surrogate marker for clinical outcomes (patients with >5 mm intimal thickening on IVUS had more events of death, myocardial infarction, and retransplantation) (116,117). Multivessel imaging with IVUS (as opposed to single-vessel imaging) has also been shown to be more sensitive in detecting CAV (118). Use of IVUS has also been successfully utilized to monitor the effectiveness of immunosuppressive and lipid-lowering therapy in treating CAV (97,98).

Unfortunately, because of the diffuse nature of CAV, if it is discovered its treatment cannot be approached by traditional methods such as coronary bypass grafting. Although angioplasty has been attempted for high-grade lesions superimposed on the diffuse disease (119,120), the long-term outcome of this intervention is unknown. A retrospective analysis of 62 patients between 1990 and 2000 with CAV undergoing angioplasty showed that the freedom from

TABLE 46-8
INTERNATIONAL SOCIETY FOR HEART AND LUNG TRANSPLANT (ISHLT) BIOPSY GRADING SCALE

No Rejection
Grade 0, no rejection
Mild Rejection
Grade 1A, focal, perivascular, or interstitial infiltrate without myocyte necrosis
Grade 1B, diffuse, sparse interstitial infiltrate without myocyte necrosis
Moderate Rejection
Grade 2, focal (single) active (lymphoblasts, plasma cells) infiltrate with myocyte necrosis
Grade 3A, multifocal interstitial active infiltrate with myocyte necrosis
Grade 3B, diffuse (involving all areas) active infiltrate with myocyte necrosis
Severe Rejection
Grade 4, diffuse aggressive infiltrate (lymphoblasts, polymorphonuclear cells, and eosinophils) with myocyte necrosis, edema, and hemorrhage

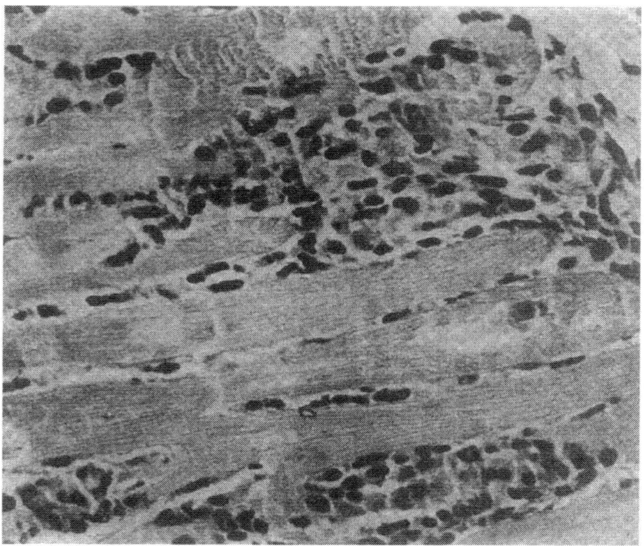

Figure 46-12 Endomyocardial biopsy showing moderate acute rejection with interstitial inflammation and myocyte necrosis (**arrows**). Hemotoxylin-eosin, 675× magnification. (From Ray J, Hosenpud JD. In: Hosenpud JD, Cobanoglu A, Norman DJ, Starr A, eds. *Cardiac Transplantation*. New York: Springer-Verlag; 1991, with permission.)

restenosis was 95% at 1 month, 81% at 3 months, and 57% at 6 months. Predictors of freedom from restenosis were the use of stents, higher antiproliferative immunosuppressant dosing, and the era in which the patients were treated. Despite effectiveness of angioplasty and stenting, the overall survival after development of severe CAV remains poor (121). At this juncture, repeat transplantation is currently the only available treatment option.

MEDICAL COMPLICATIONS FOLLOWING CARDIAC TRANSPLANTATION

The majority of medical complications following cardiac transplantation are a direct result of the immunosuppression required to preserve allograft function. These can be divided into acute and chronic complications, with the common acute complications being infection, acute renal dysfunction, hypertension, diabetes, and neurologic complications. The more chronic complications include malignancy, chronic renal dysfunction, and bone disease.

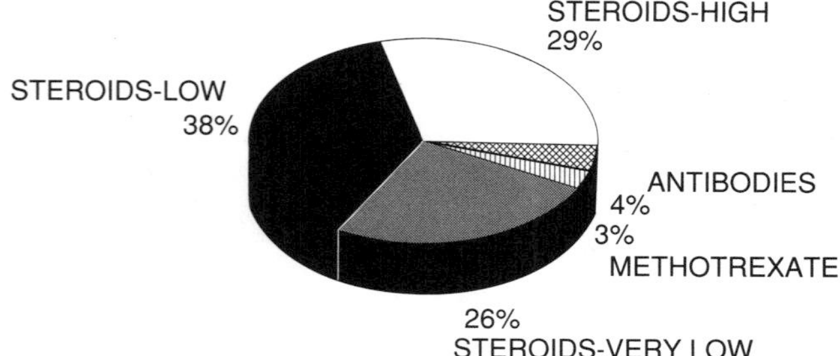

Figure 46-13 Agents used for rejection episode treatment in a large cardiac transplant program over 4 years.

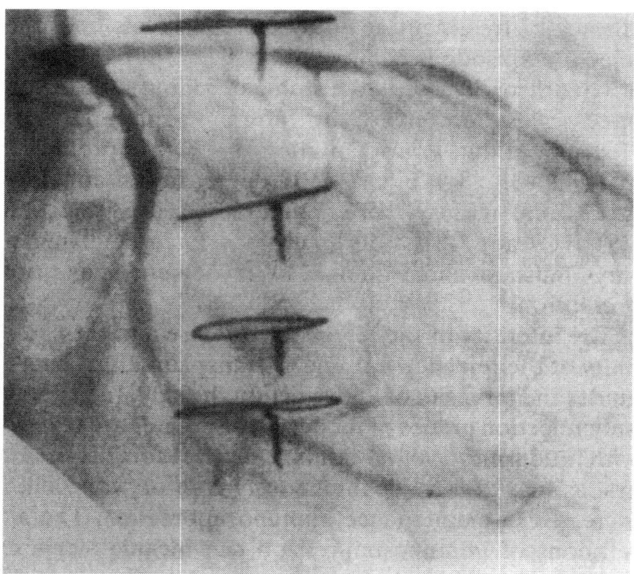

Figure 46-14 Coronary angiography from a patient with cardiac allograft vasculopathy (chronic rejection). (From Ray J, Hosenpud JD. Endomyocordial biopsy: techniques and interpretation of rejection. In: Hosenpud JD, Cobanoglu A, Norman DJ, Starr A, eds. *Cardiac Transplantation*. New York: Springer-Verlag; 1991, with permission.)

Infection

The increased incidence of important infection is directly related to immunosuppression. This is illustrated in Figure 46-16, which demonstrates the highest incidence of infection early, coinciding with the initial higher doses of immunosuppression used coupled with the more frequent augmentation of immunosuppression for acute rejection

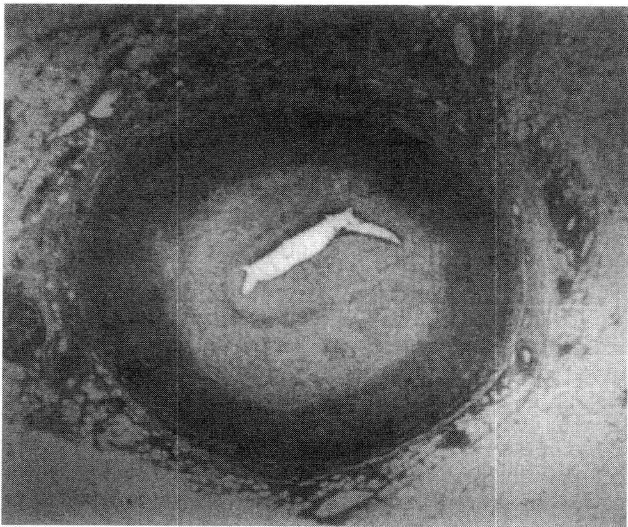

Figure 46-15 Concentric myointimal hyperplasia of cardiac allograft vasculopathy. Hemotoxylin-eosin, 58× magnification. (From Ray J, Hosenpud JD. Endomyocordial biopsy: techniques and interpretation of rejection. In: Hosenpud JD, Cobanoglu A, Norman DJ, Starr A, eds. *Cardiac Transplantation*. New York: Springer-Verlag; 1991, with permission.)

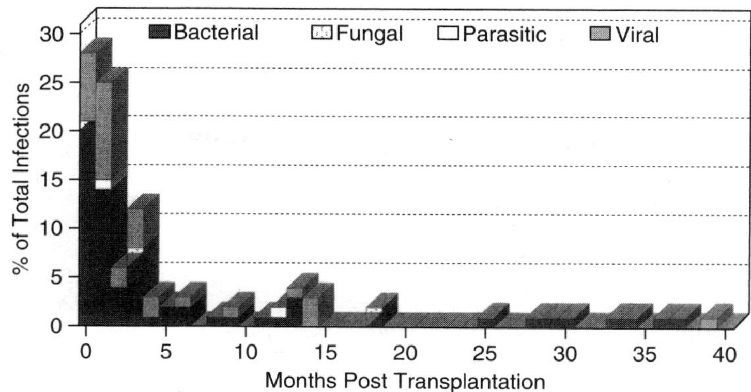

Figure 46-16 The incidence of infection over time following transplantation from a large cardiac transplant program. This parallels the incidence of rejection and results from the requirement to augment immunosuppression.

episodes. In addition, certain infections are more or less likely at certain times posttransplantation. The incidence of serious infection dropped substantially following the introduction of cyclosporine and the reduction of corticosteroids in the maintenance immunosuppression protocols. Hofflin et al. reported a 72% reduction in infectious death in cyclosporine-based immunosuppression compared to azathioprine/prednisone maintenance (122). In a meta-analysis, cyclosporine contributed to a 50% reduction in serious infection and a shift from predominantly bacterial infections to a higher percentage of viral infections in the cyclosporine-treated patients (123).

Bacterial infections continue, however, to be an important problem following cardiac transplantation, with those secondary to surgical complications being most common in the early posttransplant period. Intravascular catheter bacteremias, mediastinitis, and pneumonias account for the majority of these. Frequent changes in vascular access and aggressive pulmonary toileting following early extubation may be helpful. Mediastinitis, fortunately the least-common of these infection sites, requires urgent and aggressive therapy with surgical drainage, debridement, and irrigation. Because of the delayed healing with corticosteroid use and the relatively avascular sternum, plastic procedures such as the use of a skeletal muscle or omentum flap are frequently required (122,123).

Although allograft recipients are susceptible to all of the usual pathogens, serious infection following the transplant hospitalization is not infrequently caused by opportunistic agents. Examples of opportunistic agents transmitted via the donor organ or blood products include cytomegalovirus and *Toxoplasma gondii*. Opportunistic infections transmitted by environmental exposure include organisms such as *Legionella, Pneumocystis, Listeria, Nocardia, Candida,* and *Aspergillus*.

Cytomegalovirus (CMV) is clearly the most common opportunistic infection seen following transplantation. Depending on demographics, up to 80% of the general population has been exposed to CMV. Following transplantation, it is almost exclusively transmitted by the donor organ or is reactivated in a recipient with prior exposure. Those patients with no prior exposure (as evidenced by negative serology for CMV) who receive an organ from a donor who is also CMV seronegative will not develop CMV infection or disease (126). Those patients who are CMV seronegative who receive a heart from a seropositive donor will almost always develop a primary CMV infection, which usually produces the most severe disease. Those with prior CMV exposure, whether or not they receive a heart from a seropositive donor, will likely develop recurrent CMV infection (secondary infection), albeit usually with milder symptoms than those accompanying primary disease (127).

The manifestations of CMV disease are quite variable, ranging from a mononucleosis-like syndrome with viremia to important tissue invasion with pneumonitis, hepatitis, or gastrointestinal invasion. Mortality from tissue-invasive CMV disease and, especially, pneumonia (the most common cause of posttransplant interstitial pneumonia) following transplantation has been reported as high as 80% (127,128). With the introduction of the guanine analog ganciclovir, this mortality has dropped substantially (129,130). Possibly as disturbing as the acute infectious morbidity caused by CMV is the previously mentioned association with the development of CAV. There appears to be an even stronger association with CAV in patients who are persistently culture-positive for CMV (131). The use of prophylactic oral ganciclovir should impact the incidence of this problem.

It is extremely important that the approach to the febrile allograft recipient be an aggressive one. Full evaluation, including bacterial, viral, and fungal blood cultures, should be obtained. If there are respiratory symptoms with or without associated x-ray findings, early adequate pulmonary culturing (usually bronchoscopy with brushings, but with a low tolerance to proceed to lung biopsy) is critical to direct appropriate therapy to the wide range of potential pathogens in this population. In the early postoperative period, computerized tomographic studies of the chest are extremely helpful to evaluate collections of fluid and rule out mediastinitis, which can present much less acutely than in the nonimmunocompromised host. Finally, knowing the possible etiologic agents based on preoperative infection screening (CMV and *Toxoplasma* serology, myobacterial and systemic fungal skin testing, etc.) and the time posttransplantation will also assist in making the appropriate diagnostic and therapeutic decisions in these complex patients.

TABLE 46-9
INCIDENCE OF MALIGNANCY POST-TRANSPLANT

Malignancy/Type		1-Year Survivors	5-Year Survivors	7-Year Survivors
No Malignancy		15,396 (96.8%)	4,697 (83.1%)	1,994 (75.9%)
Malignancy (all types combined)		502 (3.2%)	957 (16.9%)	633 (24.1%)
Malignancy Type	*Skin*	228	639	462
	Lymph	119	105	57
	Other	109	228	157
	Type Not Reported	46	39	15

Malignancy

The most common immunosuppression-related malignancies are skin cancers and lymphoproliferative disorders. As shown in Table 46-9, the overall risk of developing a posttransplant malignancy is between 3.2% at 1 year, 16.9% at 5 years, and up to 24.1% at 7 years based on the joint UNOS/ISHLT Thoracic Registry (1), which is 100-fold greater than in the population at large (132). The lymphomas that develop posttransplantation are unique in several aspects. First, they are generally of B-cell origin, associated with Epstein-Barr virus, and can present as a polyclonal lymphoproliferative disorder or a more traditional monoclonal lymphoma (133,134). Second, they frequently present extranodally, with the central nervous system, the gastrointestinal tract, and the lung being common sites. Finally, chemotherapy does not appear to be beneficial, and aggressive reduction of immunosuppression coupled with local therapy with or without the use of acyclovir has resulted in remissions (134).

Miscellaneous

The majority of other medical complications relate to side effects directly attributable to the specific immunosuppressive agents used posttransplantation. Diastolic hypertension is an almost uniform side effect of cyclosporine and is contributed to by corticosteroids. It is poorly controlled with conventional antihypertensive agents, although calcium antagonists, particularly nifedipine, are reasonably effective. Diabetes and hyperlipidemia are primarily secondary to corticosteroids but are also complications of cyclosporine. Bone disease, particularly compression fractures, are corticosteroid-related and can be especially severe if osteoporosis predates the transplant. A more unusual form of bone disease, also secondary to steroids, is osteonecrosis, most commonly of the hip, followed in frequency by the knees and shoulders. This has a reported incidence as high as 20% in renal allograft recipients (135). Finally, renal dysfunction is a major complication of cyclosporine therapy (72).

PHYSIOLOGY OF THE TRANSPLANTED HEART

Despite certain similarities, there are substantial differences in the function of the transplanted cardiac allograft compared to the normal heart. The factors that can substantially influence allograft function can be divided into three major categories: (a) mechanical, including loss of normal atrial transport, donor-recipient size matching, and preservation injury; (b) denervation and denervation hypersensitivity; and (c) effects of acute and chronic rejection.

Mechanical Factors

Normally, the atrial contribution to total stroke volume is between 15% and 20% (136). As previously described, the reconstruction of the left and right atria as a consequence of the transplant operation results in a larger atrial chamber with both recipient and donor atrial components and usually two sinus nodes. Only the donor sinus node is electrically coupled to the donor ventricle because electrical impulses will not traverse the suture line. Stinson et al. demonstrated that with synchrony of the donor and recipient atria, atrial contraction contributed between 2 and 4 mm Hg to left ventricular filling (56). Unfortunately, this coatrial synchrony is the exception rather than the rule, as demonstrated by Figure 46-17 showing both recipient and donor P waves. In this case, it is unlikely that random recipient atrial contractions have a meaningful contribution to ventricular filling and, when completely out of phase with donor atrial contractions, may actually hinder ventricular filling. As mentioned previously, one of the potential benefits of the newer bicaval anastomotic technique is to eliminate the competition between donor and recipient atria and potentially restore normal atrial function.

Cardiac transplantation is unique in that the heart size is not explicitly matched to the circulation. Most centers use body weights to match a given donor organ to a given recipient and allow for as much as a 30% discrepancy between the two. This donor–recipient mismatch in size can play an important role in allograft function, especially if there are inadequate compensatory changes. If a patient receives a relatively smaller heart, attempts to maintain stroke volume will result in higher filling pressures in order to maintain cardiac output. If stroke volume is inadequate, an increase in heart rate will be required. Conversely, if the recipient receives a relatively larger heart, filling pressures will be lower, stroke volume will be greater, and a slower heart rate will meet cardiac output needs. This is exactly what was demonstrated in 34 allograft recipients studied 3 months following transplantation (137).

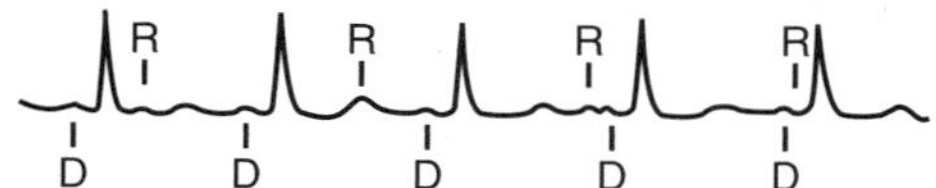

Figure 46-17 Electrocardiogram from a cardiac allogarft recipient demonstrating both recipient (R) and donor (D) P waves. Note that the recipient P wave rate is slower, and the P waves are not associated with the donor QRS complexes.

Denervation

With the transection of the aorta, pulmonary artery, and atria, the donor heart is completely separated from both sympathetic and parasympathetic innervation. The loss of both afferent and efferent autonomic innervation results in a variety of reflexes summarized in Figure 46-18. There is loss of efferent vagal tone to the sinus node, resulting in an increase in resting heart rate and a loss of sympathetic tone to mediate reflex increases in heart rate and contractility brought about by exercise, hemorrhage, or acute vasodilation. A loss of cardiac afferents affects cardiorenal reflexes important in salt and water handling and reflexes that influence peripheral vascular tone (138). Although gross clinical and histological observations had led to the conclusion that reinnervation did not occur in the human allograft, data suggest that partial reinnervation can and does occur (139). Using tyramine-induced release of norepinphrine across the cardiac bed, Wilson et al. demonstrated that late following transplantation, functioning sympathetic neurons are present in the allograft. In the patients with this partial reinnervation, a sympathetic reflex loop can also be demonstrated and many of these patients have a slightly higher heart rate response to exercise (139). We and others have noted that some patients exhibit typical angina in response to ischemia consistent with partial afferent innervation (140). Despite these very interesting findings, the changes noted are subtle; for the most part, patients following cardiac transplantation are functionally denervated.

In the normally innervated heart, resting heart rate is slow because of resting vagal tone. With the onset of exercise, vagal tone is released and heart rate increases rapidly and proportionally to the level of exercise. The increase in cardiac output associated with exercise is primarily related to the increase in heart rate, with stroke volume playing only a minor role (141–143). Stinson et al. defined the exercise response in allograft recipients 1 and 2 years following cardiac transplantation (144). They demonstrated that the allograft heart had a resting heart rate approximately 30% higher than the normally innervated heart. With the onset of exercise, heart rate increased very gradually with a rapid increase in filling pressures. The substantial increase in cardiac output was mediated predominantly via an increase in stroke volume. Subsequent studies demonstrated that the increase in heart rate paralleled an increase in circulating catecholamines (145).

Table 46-10 demonstrates resting and exercise hemodynamics in 23 allograft recipients 1 year following cardiac transplantation, and contrasts these to normal values

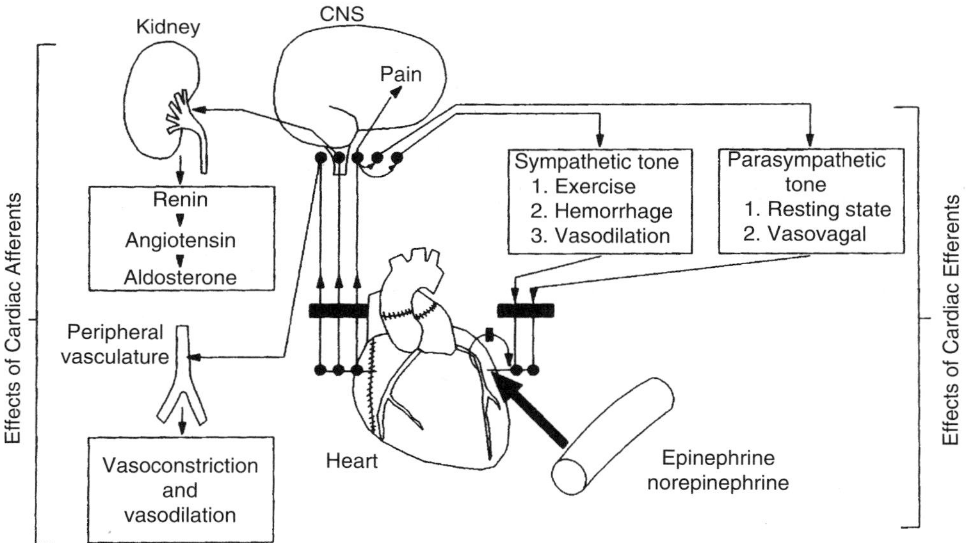

Figure 46-18 The effects of cardiac denervation involve the loss of both the cardiac afferents and efferents. The cardiac afferents have potential roles in salt and water regulation via the renin-angiotensin-aldosterone system, in reflex control of the peripheral vasculature, and in the sensation of cardiac pain. The cardiac efferents are responsible for the rapid changes in heart rate and contractility associated with changes in the physiologic state. In addition, central reflexes are transmitted to the heart via the vagal efferent nerves. Finally, cardiac denervation results in hypersensitivity to circulating catecholamines caused by the lack of adrenergic neuronal uptake. (From Wilson RF, McGinn AL, Laxson DD, et al. Regional differences in sympathetic reinnervation after cardiac transplantation. *Circulation.* 1991;84(Suppl II):489, with permission.)

TABLE 46-10
REST AND EXERCISE HEMODYNAMICS 1 YEAR POSTTRANSPLANTATION

Parameter	Normal	Rest	Exercise
Right atrial (mm Hg)	0–8	6 ± 2	14 ± 7
Pulmonary artery mean (mm Hg)	9–16	18 ± 3	32 ± 9
Pulmonary wedge (mm Hg)	1–10	10 ± 3	20 ± 6
Cardiac output (L/min)	–	5.0 ± 0.9	9.9 ± 1.7
Cardiac index (L/min/m^2)	2.4–4.2	2.5 ± 0.5	5.0 ± 0.8
Stroke volume (mL)	—	55 ± 9	77 ± 13
Stroke index (mL/m^2)	30–56	28 ± 6	39 ± 7
Heart rate (bpm)	—	90 ± 11	122 ± 18
Mean arterial (mm Hg)	70–105	91 ± 12	102 ± 14
SVR (Wood U)	10–19	17.7 ± 4.0	9.3 ± 2.4

(146). One can therefore summarize these data as follows: Individuals with cardiac innervation rely on heart rate primarily to increase cardiac output with exercise. Cardiac allograft recipients rely primarily on stroke volume mediated via the Starling mechanism and pay for this increase with substantial increases in filling pressures. Only with increasing circulating catecholamines does heart rate add to the exercise response.

Another important aspect of allograft denervation is the altered response to commonly used cardiovascular drugs. Some of these are illustrated in Table 46-11. Important examples are digitalis, which has no effect in controlling atrial fibrillation, and atropine, which has no effect on bradycardias; both responses are normally mediated by stimulation and inhibition, respectively, of vagal efferents.

Cardiac Function in Acute Rejection

Before the introduction of cyclosporine, allograft rejection not infrequently led to acute ventricular dysfunction (147,148). The combination of earlier detection and the use of cyclosporine have altered the natural history of rejection in that systolic dysfunction is rare and, if present, is many times a premorbid event (149,150). Several investigators have reported that although systolic function may be normal, abnormalities in diastolic function may be present with rejection. Dawkins et al. demonstrated that mean isovolumic relaxation time fell with progressively severe rejection (149). Paulsen et al. demonstrated that rejection was associated with a prolonged rapid filling period (151). In addition to alterations in allograft function acutely, there may also be alterations that occur over the longer term. In 20 patients followed serially over 3 years following cardiac transplantation, resting and exercise pressures and flows remained fairly stable, with the exception of a gradually falling resting cardiac output. This fall in cardiac output was associated with a gradual fall in left ventricular end-diastolic volume and stroke volume measured by radionuclide ventriculography and was weakly correlated with the total number of rejection episodes over the 3-year period. No other clinical factor was associated with this fall in ventricular volumes. These data suggest that although therapy may reverse the acute alterations in allograft function, repeated rejection episodes can have lasting effects on the allograft.

TABLE 46-11
CARDIOVASCULAR DRUGS AFTER CARDIAC TRANSPLANTATION

Drug	Effect in Recipient	Mechanism
Digitalis	Normal increase in contractility, minimal AV nodal effect	Denervation
Atropine	None	Denervation
Epinephrine	Increased contractility and chronotropy	Denervation hypersensitivity
Norepinephrine	Increased contractility and chronotropy	Denervation hypersensitivity
Isoproterenol	Normal increase in inotropy/chronotropy	No neuronal uptake
Quinidine	No vagolytic effect	Denervation
Verapamil	Normal AV block	Direct effect
Nifedipine	No reflex tachycardia	Denervation
Hydralazine	No reflex tachycardia	Denervation
β-blockers	Increased antagonist effect during exercise	Denervation

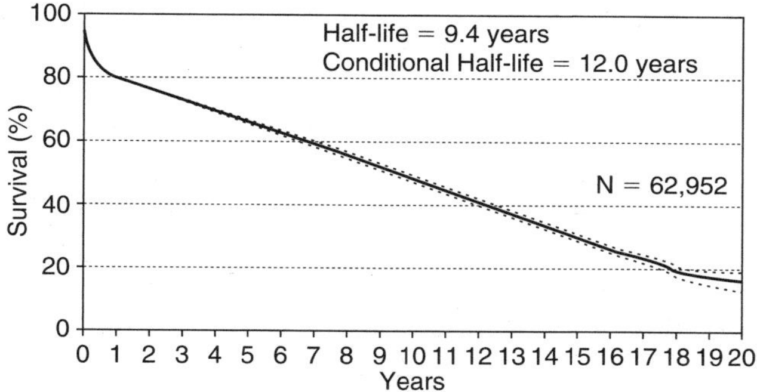

Figure 46-19 Survival following cardiac transplantation. (From Taylor DO, Edwards LB, Boucek MM, et al. The Registry of the International Society for Heart and Lung Transplantation: twenty-first official adult heart transplant report—2004. *J Heart Lung Transplant*. 2004;23:796-803, with permission.)

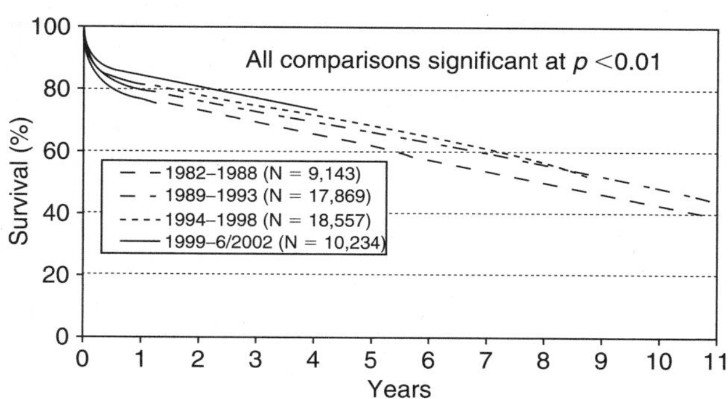

Figure 46-20 Survival following cardiac transplantation by era. (From Taylor DO, Edwards LB, Boucek MM, et al. The Registry of the International Society for Heart and Lung Transplantation: twenty-first official adult heart transplant report—2004. *J Heart Lung Transplant*. 2004;23:796-803, with permission.)

OUTCOMES

Survival

Figure 46-19 demonstrates the overall survival following cardiac transplantation based on close to 41,000 patients followed in the UNOS/ISHLT registry (1). The 1-, 5-, and 10-year survival rates are 79%, 65%, and 45%, respectively. Breaking down this survival into more recent eras, as shown in Figure 46-20, demonstrates steady improvement over time. In the most recent time period, the 1- and 5-year survival rates are 82% and 68%, respectively, compared to 70% and 51%, respectively, for the years 1980 through 1985 (12). These registry data permit a multivariate analysis of risk factors known to impact survival, as shown in Table 46-12 (11). The most powerful risks include repeat transplantation, ventilator or VAD as a bridge to transplantation, recipient and donor age, and ischemic time. Cause of death is shown in Figure 46-21. Early posttransplantation, nonspecific graft failure infection and rejection are

TABLE 46-12
RISK FACTORS FOR 1-YEAR MORTALITY IN ADULT HEART TRANSPLANTATION

	1995–1998 (*N* = 13,523)		1999–June 2002 (*N* = 7,067)	
Factor	**OR**	***p* Value**	**OR**	***p* Value**
Dialysis	2.11	0.0001	2.52	<0.0001
Diagnosis: congenital heart disease	1.97	0.0002	2.66	<0.0001
Ventilator	1.85	0.0002	2.47	<0.0001
Repeat transplant	1.76	<0.0001	1.08	0.7
Intra-aortic balloon pump	1.46	0.002	1.23	0.2
Diagnosis: other (excluding cardiomyopathy)	1.35	0.001	1.42	0.01
Donor history of cancer	1.33	0.21	1.78	0.012
Diagnosis: coronary artery disease	1.31	<0.0001	1.05	0.5
In-hospital (including ICU)	1.26	0.0009	1.42	<0.0001
Infection requiring IV drug therapy within 2 weeks of transplant	1.25	0.05	1.02	0.9
HLA-B mismatches (per mismatch)	1.22	0.0002	1.13	0.11
Prior transfusions	1.21	0.046	1.25	0.06
Donor CMV+/recipient CMV–	1.20	0.001	1.34	0.0003
PRA >10%	1.19	0.13	1.43	0.02
HLA DR mismatches (per mismatch)	1.15	0.001	1.1	0.13
Insulin-dependent diabetes	1.13	0.3	1.41	0.02
Female donor	1.11	0.04	1.07	0.4
Sternotomy	0.86	0.03	1.01	0.9
IV inotropes	0.83	0.005	0.83	0.04

CMV, cytomegalovirus; HLA, human leukocyte antibody; ICU, intensive care unit; IV, intravenous; PRA, panel reactive antibody; OR, odds ratio.
From Taylor DO, Edwards LB, Boucek MM, et al. The Registry of the International Society for Heart and Lung Transplantation: twenty-first official adult heart transplant report—2004. *J Heart Lung Transplant*. 2004;23:796-803, with permission.

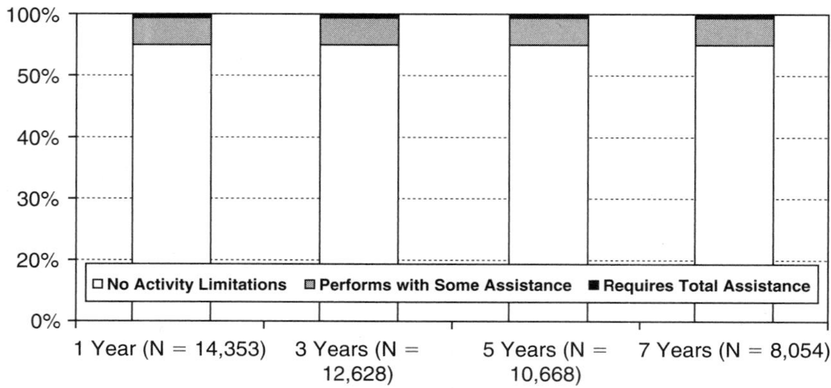

Figure 46-21 Functional ability following cardiac transplantation. (From Taylor DO, Edwards LB, Boucek MM, et al. The Registry of the International Society for Heart and Lung Transplantation: twenty-first official adult heart transplant report—2004. *J Heart Lung Transplant.* 2004;23:796-803, with permission.)

most common. In the intermediate time posttransplantation, deaths are dominated by infection and rejection. As noted previously, late following transplantation, CAV is the most common cause of death (12).

Rehabilitation and Quality of Life

Outcome other than survival has been the topic of several investigations. It is the general perception that most patients are medically rehabilitated following cardiac transplantation and that it is usually social impediments (loss of insurance and disability income, inability to acquire employment because of health risk) that prevent full rehabilitation and return to productive life. Gaudiani et al. reported the Stanford experience, which demonstrated an 86% rehabilitation rate in 143 transplant recipients (152). Lough et al. reported that the principal negative factors following transplantation were related to side effects from immunosuppression; nonetheless, 89% of patients were rehabilitated (153).

In 35 patients following cardiac transplantation, Bunzel et al. evaluated a variety of factors, including physical, emotional, financial, and an overall satisfaction parameter. Based on an improvement scale from 0 to 50, the average overall improvement in the total score was 25 (154). A multicenter study investigating parameters that predicted posttransplant return to work was reported. Those patients who were male, with a good educational background, who felt they were physically able to work, who would not lose health insurance or disability income, and who were at least 6 months posttransplant had the greatest likelihood of returning to gainful employment. The overall return-to-work rate in this series of 250 patients was 45% (155). Data from the UNOS/ISHLT registry are shown in Figure 46-21 (1). Most patients have no activity limitations over the first 3 years posttransplantation.

One can conclude from these data that both survival and quality of life are quite acceptable following cardiac transplantation, with a high percentage of patients being fully rehabilitated and becoming productive members of society.

TABLE 46-13
CAUSE OF DEATH AFTER CARDIAC TRANSPLANTATION

Cause of Death	0–30 Days (N = 2.759)	31 Days–1 Year (N = 2.310)	>1 Year–3 Years (N = 1.737)	>3 Years–5 Years (N = 1.492)	>5 Years (N = 4.009)
CAV	43 (1.6%)	111 (4.8%)	257 (14.8%)	268 (18.0%)	651 (16.2%)
Acute Rejection	188 (6.8%)	288 (12.5%)	165 (9.5%)	63 (4.2%)	43 (1.1%)
Lymphoma	2 (0.1%)	46 (2.0%)	77 (4.4%)	80 (5.4%)	201 (5.0%)
Malignancy, other	2 (0.1%)	49 (2.1%)	181 (10.4%)	281 (18.8%)	763 (19.0%)
CMV	4 (0.1%)	29 (1.3%)	15 (0.9%)	3 (0.2%)	4 (0.1%)
Infection, non-CMV	370 (13.4%)	784 (33.9%)	234 (13.5%)	145 (9.7%)	393 (9.8%)
Primary Failure	747 (27.1%)	186 (8.1%)	119 (6.9%)	68 (4.6%)	200 (5.0%)
Graft Failure	400 (14.5%)	245 (10.6%)	298 (17.2%)	218 (14.6%)	567 (14.1%)
Technical	208 (7.5%)	28 (1.2%)	15 (0.9%)	17 (1.1%)	43 (1.1%)
Other	101 (3.7%)	122 (5.3%)	123 (7.1%)	104 (7.0%)	240 (6.0%)
Multiple Organ Failure	382 (13.8%)	228 (9.9%)	86 (5.0%)	83 (5.6%)	335 (8.4%)
Renal Failure	17 (0.6%)	19 (0.8%)	31 (1.8%)	51 (3.4%)	238 (5.9%)
Pulmonary	116 (4.2%)	77 (3.3%)	77 (4.4%)	60 (4.0%)	163 (4.1%)
Cerebrovascular	179 (6.5%)	98 (4.2%)	59 (3.4%)	51 (3.4%)	168 (4.2%)

CAV, cardiac allograft vasculopathy; CMV, cytomegalovirus.
From Taylor DO, Edwards LB, Boucek MM, et al. The Registry of the International Society for Heart and Lung Transplantation: twenty-first official adult heart transplant report—2004. *J Heart Lung Transplant.* 2004;23:796-803, with permission.

CONCLUSIONS

Cardiac transplantation is now a viable and proven therapy for the treatment of end-stage heart disease. Acute and subacute survival are now at very acceptable levels; however, long-term survival continues to remain a major challenge. This is more evident as infants and children make up an ever-increasing percentage of patients transplanted. In contrast to the adult population, 5- and even 10-year survivals in this population are not considered acceptable.

Despite its current success, the other principal limitation to cardiac allograft transplantation is the restricted ability to apply this therapy to only 10% of patients who could benefit. It is unlikely that there will be much further relaxation of donor acceptability to increase the number of potential organs. Therefore, other technologies must be actively sought, including the use of artificial devices and possibly, ultimately, xenograft transplantation. Only then can the successes in the field of transplantation be fully appreciated.

REFERENCES

1. Hosenpud JD, Bennett LE, Keck BM, et al. The Registry of the International Society for Heart and Lung Transplantation: fifteenth official report—1998. *J Heart Lung Transplant.* 1998;17:656–668.
2. United Network for Organ Sharing. *1997 Annual Report.* Washington, DC: U.S. Department of Health and Human Services, 1997.
3. Baumgartner WA, Reitz BA, Oyer PE, et al. Cardiac transplantation. *Curr Probl Surg.* 1979;16:2–61.
4. Copeland JG, Stinson EB. Human heart transplantation. *Curr Probl Cardiol.* 1979;4:1–51.
5. Costanzo MR, Augustine S, Bourge R, et al. Selection and treatment of candidates for heart transplantation. A statement for health professionals from the Committee on Heart Failure and Transplantation of the Council on Clinical Cardiology, American Heart Association. *Circulation.* 1995;92:3593–3612.
6. Miller LW, Kubo SH, Young JB, et al. Report of the consensus conference of candidate selection for heart transplantation: 1993. *J Heart Lung Transplant.* 1995;14:562–571.
7. Miller LW, Vitale-Noedel N, Pennington DG, et al. Heart transplantation in patients over age 55. *J Heart Transplant.* 1988;7:254–257.
8. Olivari MT, Antolick A, Kaye MP, et al. Heart transplant in elderly patients. *J Heart Transplant.* 1988;7:258–264.
9. Carrier M, Emery RW, Riley JE, et al. Cardiac transplantation in patients over the age of 50 years. *J Am Coll Cardiol.* 1986;8:285–288.
10. Hosenpud JD, Pantely GA, Norman DJ, et al. A critical analysis of morbidity and mortality as it relates to recipient age following cardiac transplantation. *Clin Transplant.* 1990;4:51–54.
11. Heroux AL, O'Sullivan EJ, Kao WG, et al. Should cardiac transplantation be a treatment option after 65 years of age? *J Heart Lung Transplant.* 1992;11:220.
12. Taylor DO, Edwards LB, Boucek MM, et al. The Registry of the International Society for Heart and Lung Transplantation: twenty-first official adult heart transplant report—2004. *J Heart Lung Transplant.* 2004;23:796-803.
13. Griepp RB, Stinson EB, Dong E, et al. Determinants of operative risk in human heart transplant. *Am J Surg.* 1971;122:192–197.
14. Rodheffer RJ, Naftel DC, Stevenson LW, et al. Secular trends in cardiac transplant recipient and donor management in the United States, 1990–1994. *Circulation.* 1996;94:2883–2889.
15. Kalya A, Hosenpud JD, et al. Chronic mechanical left ventricular support improves pulmonary vascular resistance in patients bridged to transplantation. *J Heart Lung Transplant.* 2004;23:S83.
16. Pastan SO, Braunwald E. Renal disorders and heart disease. In: Braunwald E, ed. *Heart Disease.* Philadelphia: WB Saunders; 1988:1828–1835.
17. Kubo SH, Walter BA, John DHA, et al. Liver function abnormalities in chronic heart failure. Influence of systemic hemodynamics. *Arch Intern Med.* 1987;147:1227–1230.
18. Kaplan SR, Calabresi P. Immunosuppressive agents. *N Engl J Med.* 1973;289:1234–1236.
19. Moran M, Tomlanovich S, Myers BD. Cyclosporine-induced chronic nephropathy in human recipients of cardiac allografts. *Transplant Proc.* 1985;17(4 Suppl 1):185–190.
20. Hosenpud JD, Stibolt TA, Atwal K, et al. Abnormal pulmonary function specifically related to congestive heart failure: comparison of patients before and after cardiac transplantation. *Am J Med.* 1990;88:493–496.
21. Rhenman MJ, Rhenman B, Icenogle T, et al. Diabetes and heart transplantation. *J Heart Transplant.* 1988;7:356–358.
22. Armitage JM, Griffith BP, Kormos RL, et al. Cardiac transplantation in patients with malignancy. *J Heart Transplant.* 1989; 8:89.
23. Minow RA, Benjamin RS, Lee ET, et al. Adriamycin cardiomyopathy: risk factors. *Cancer.* 1977;39:1397–1402.
24. Hosenpud JD, Uretsky BF, O'Connell JB, et al. Cardiac transplantation for amyloidosis. Results of a multicenter survey. *J Heart Transplant.* 1990;9:346–350.
25. Hosenpud JD, DeMarco T, Frazier OH, et al. Progression of systemic disease and reduced long-term survival in patients with cardiac amyloidosis undergoing heart transplantation. *Circulation.* 1991;84(Suppl III):III338–III343.
26. Valantine HA, Tazelaar HD, Macoviak J, et al. Cardiac sarcoidosis: response to steroids and transplantation. *J Heart Transplant.* 1987;6:244–250.
27. Oni AA, Hershberger RE, Norman DJ, et al. Recurrence of sarcoidosis in a cardiac allograft: control with augmented corticosteroids. *J Heart Lung Transplant.* 1992;11:367–369.
28. Maricle RA, Hosenpud JD, Norman DJ, et al. The lack of predictive value of preoperative psychologic distress for postoperative medical outcome in heart transplant recipients. *J Heart Lung Transplant.* 1991;10:942–947.
29. Sadler AM, Sadler BL, Statson EB. The Uniform Anatomical Gift Act. *JAMA.* 1968;206:2505–2506.
30. Black PM. Brain death. *N Engl J Med.* 1978;299:338–344.
31. Lewis EF, Tsang SW, Fang JC, et al. Frequency and impact of delayed decisions regarding heart transplantation on long-term outcomes in patients with advanced heart failure. *J Am Coll Cardiol.* 2004;43:794-802.
32. Hunt SA, Baker DW, Chin MH, et al. ACC/AHA guidelines for the evaluation and management of chronic heart failure in the adult: executive summary. *J Heart Lung Transplant.* 2002;21(2):189–203.
33. Pallis C. Prognostic significance of a dead brain stem. *Br Med J.* 1981;286:123–124.
34. Powner DJ, Fromm GH. The electroencephalogram in the determination of brain death. *N Engl J Med.* 1979;300:502.
35. Griepp RB, Stinson EB, Clark DA, et al. The cardiac donor. *Surg Gynecol Obstet.* 1971;133:792–798.
36. Copeland JG. Cardiac transplantation. *Curr Probl Cardiol.* 1988;13:157–224.
37. Fentz V, Gormsen J. Electrocardiographic patterns in patients with cerebrovascular accidents. *Circulation.* 1962;25:22.
38. Novitzky D, Wicomb WN, Cooper KDC, et al. Electrocardiographic, hemodynamic and endocrine changes occuring during experimental brain death in the chacma baboon. *J Heart Transplant.* 1984;4:63.
39. Gilbert EM, Krieger SK, Murray JL, et al. Echocardiographic evaluation of potential cardiac transplant donors. *J Thorac Cardiovasc Surg.* 1988;95:1003–1007.
40. Lower RR, Shumway NE. Studies on orthotopic homotransplantation of the canine heart. *Surg Forum.* 1960;11:18–19.
41. Gott JP, Pan-Chih, Dorsey LMA, et al. Cardioplegia for transplantation: failure of extracellular solution compared with Stanford or UW solution. *Ann Thorac Surg.* 1990;50:348–354.
42. Gott JP, Brown WM, 3rd, Pan-Chih, et al. Cardioplegia for heart transplantation: unmodified UW solution compared with Stanford solution. *J Heart Lung Transplant.* 1992; 11:353–362.

43. Pearl JM, Laks H, Drinkwater DC, et al. Loss of endothelium-dependent vasodilation and nitric oxide release after myocardial protection with University of Wisconsin solution. *J Thorac Cardiovasc Surg*. 1994;107:257–264.
44. Drinkwater DC, Rudis E, Laks H, et al. University of Wisconsin solution versus Stanford cardioplegic solution and the development of cardiac allograft vasculopathy. *J Heart Lung Transplant*. 1995;14:891–896.
45. Heck CF, Shumway SJ, Kaye MP. The Registry of the International Society for Heart Transplantation: sixth official report–1989. *J Heart Transplant*. 1989;8:271–276.
46. Dreyfus G, Jebara V, Mihaileanu S, et al. Total orthotopic heart transplantation: an alternative to the standard technique. *Ann Thorac Surg*. 1991;52:1181–1184.
47. Sievers HH, Leyh R, Jahnke A, et al. Bicaval versus atrial anastomoses in cardiac transplantation. *J Thorac Cardiovasc Surg*. 1994;108:780–784.
48. Deleuze PH, Benvenuti C, Mazzucotelli JP, et al. Orthotopic cardiac transplantation with direct caval anastomosis: is it the optimal procedure? *J Thorac Cardiovasc Surg*. 1995;109: 731–737.
49. Hooks MA, Wade CS, Millikan WJ, Jr., et al. CD-3: a review of its pharmacology, pharmacokinetics, and clinical use in transplantation. *Pharmacotherapy*. 1991;11:26–37.
50. Swinnen LJ, Costanzo-Nordin MR, Fisher SG, et al. Increased incidence of lymphoproliferative disorder after immunosuppression with the monoclonal antibody OKT3 in cardiac-transplant recipients. *N Engl J Med*. 1990;323:1723–1728.
51. Kriett JM, Kaye MP. The registry of the International Society for Heart Transplantation: seventh official report–1990. *J Heart Transplant* 1990;9:323–330.
52. Johnson MR, Mullen GM, O'Sullivan EJ, et al. The risk/benefit ratio of perioperative OKT3 in cardiac transplantation. *J Heart Lung Transplant*. 1992;11:207.
53. Lewin W. Factors in the mortality of closed head injuries. *BMJ*. 1953;1:1239.
54. Cannom DS, Graham AF, Harrison DL. Electrophysiological studies in the denervated transplanted human heart: response to atrial pacing and atropine. *Circ Res*. 1973;32:268–278.
55. Cannom DS, Rider AK, Stinson EB, et al. Electrophysiologic studies in the denervated transplanted human heart. II. Response to norepinephrine, isoproterenol and propranolol. *Am J Cardiol*. 1975;36:859–866.
56. Stinson EB, Schroeder JS, Griepp RB, et al. Observations on the behavior of recipient atria after cardiac transplantation in man. *Am J Cardiol*. 1972;30:615–622.
57. Cobanoglu A. Operative techniques and early postoperative care in cardiac transplantation. In: Hosenpud JD, Cobanoglu A, Norman DJ, Starr A, eds. *Cardiac Transplantation*. New York: Springer-Verlag; 1991: 95–114.
58. Davies RA, Koshal A, Walley V, et al. Temporary diastolic noncompliance with preserved systolic function after heart transplantation. *Transplant Proc*. 1987;19:3444–3447.
59. Hosenpud JD, Norman DJ, Cobanoglu MA, et al. Serial echocardiographic findings early after heart transplantation: evidence for reversible right ventricular dysfunction and myocardial edema. *J Heart Transplant*. 1987;6:343–347.
60. Stinson EB, Caves PK, Griepp RB, et al. Hemodynamic observations in the early period after human heart transplantation. *J Thorac Cardiovasc Surg*. 1975;69:264–270.
61. Pascual JMS, Fiorelli AI, Bellotti GM, et al. Prostacyclin in the management of pulmonary hypertension after heart transplantation. *J Heart Transplant*. 1990;9:644–651.
62. Syndman DR, Werner BG, Heinze-Lacey B, et al. Use of cytomegalovirus immune globulin to prevent cytomegalovirus disease in renal-transplant recipients. *N Engl J Med*. 1987; 317:1049–1054.
63. Balfour HH, Chace BA, Stapleton JT, et al. A randomized, placebo-controlled trial of oral acyclovir for the prevention of cytomegalovirus disease in recipients of renal allografts. *N Engl J Med*. 1989;320:1381–1387.
64. Higgins RM, Bloom SL, Hopkin JM, et al. The risks and benefits of low-dose cotrimoxazole prophylaxis for *Pneumocystis* pneumonia in renal transplantation. *Transplantation* 1989;47: 558–560.
65. Borel JF, Feurer C, Bugler HU, et al. Biological effects of cyclosporin A: a new antilymphocytic agent. *Agents Actions* 1976; 6:468–475.
66. Borel JF, Feurer C, Magnee C, et al. Effects of the new antilymphocytic peptide cyclosporin A in animals. *Immunology*. 1977;32:1017–1025.
67. Cohen DJ, Loertscher R, Rubin MF, et al. Cyclosporine: a new immunosuppressive agent for organ transplantation. *Ann Intern Med*. 1984;101:667–682.
68. Kalman VK, Klimpel GR. Cyclosporin A inhibits the production of gamma interferon (IFN gamma) but does not inhibit production of virus induced IFN alpha/beta. *Cell Immunol*. 1983; 78:122–129.
69. Grey HM, Chestnut R. Antigen processing and presentation to T cells. *Immunol Today*. 1985;6:101–106.
70. Salomon DR, Limacher MC. Chronic immunosuppression and the treatment of acute rejection. In: Hosenpud JD, Cobanoglu A, Norman DJ, Starr A, eds. *Cardiac Transplantation*. New York: Springer-Verlag; 1991: 139–168.
71. Eisen H, Ross H. Optimizing the immunosuppressive regimen in heart transplantation. *J Heart Lung Transplant*. 2004;23:S207–S213.
72. McGiffin DC, Kirklin JK, Naftel DC. Acute renal failure after heart transplantation and cyclosporine therapy. *J Heart Transplant*. 1985;4:396–399.
73. Pham SM, Kormos RL, Hattler BG, et al. A prospective trial of tacrolimus (FK506) in clinical heart transplantation: intermediate-term results. *J Thorac Cardiovasc Surg*. 1996;111:764–772.
74. Jordon ML, Shapiro R, Vivas CA, et al. FK506 rescue for resistant rejection of renal allografts under primary cyclosporine immunosuppression. *Transplantation*. 1994;57:860–865.
75. Rinaldi M, Grimm M, Yonan NA, and the European Tacrolimus Heart Study Group. Risk/benefit evaluation of tacrolimus vs. cyclosporine microemulsion after cardiac transplantation: 18-month results. [abstract] *J Heart Lung Transplant*. 2004; 23:S45–S46.
76. Kobashigawa W, Miller LW, Felker GM, et al. 12-month report of a 3-arm multicenter comparison of tacrolimus (TAC), MMF or TAC/sirolimus (SRL) and steroids vs cyclosporine microemulsion (CYA), MMF and steroids in de novo cardiac transplant recipients. [abstract] *J Heart Lung Transplant*. 2005;24:S61–S62.
77. Przepiorka D. Tacrolimus: preclinical and clinical experience. In: Przepiorka D, Sollinger H, eds. *New Immunosuppressive Drugs*. Glenview, IL: Physicians & Scientists Publishing; 1994:29–50.
78. Calne RY. Rejection of renal homografts: inhibition in dogs by 6-mercatopurine. *Lancet*. 1960;1:417–418.
79. Murray JE, Merrill JP, Harrison JH, et al. Prolonged survival of human kidney homografts by immunosuppressive therapy. *N Engl J Med*. 1963;268:1315–1323.
80. Woodruff MFA, Robson JS, Nolan B, et al. Homotransplantation of kidney in patients treated by preoperative local irradiation and postoperative administration of an antimetabolite (Imuran): report of six cases. *Lancet*. 1963;2:675–682.
81. McCormack JJ, Johns DG. Purine antimetabolites. In: Chabner B, ed. *Pharmacologic Principles of Cancer Treatment*. Philadelphia: WB Saunders; 1982: 213–228.
82. Shumway SJ, Kaye MP. The International Society for Heart Transplantation Registry. In: Terasaki P, ed. *Clinical Transplant 1988*. Los Angeles: UCLA Tissue Typing Laboratory; 1988: 1–5.
83. Kobashigawa JA. Results of randomized trial of mycophenolate mofetil versus azathioprine in heart transplantation. Paper presented at the 17th Annual Meeting and Scientific Sessions of the International Society for Heart and Lung Transplantation, London, April, 1997.
84. Young CJ, Sollinger H. Mycophenolate mofetil (RS-61443). In: Przepiorka D, Sollinger H, eds. *New Immunosuppressive Drugs*. Glenview, IL: Physicians & Scientists Publishing; 1994: 93–110.
85. Dandel M, Lehmkuhl H, Knosalla C, et al. Maintenance immunosuppression with mycophenolate mofetil: long-term efficacy after heart transplantation. [abstract] *J Heart Lung Transplant*. 2005;24:S150.
86. Merrill JP, Murray JE, Harrison JH, et al. Successful homotransplantation of the kidney between nonidentical twins. *N Engl J Med*. 1960;262:1251–1260.

87. Durum SK, Schmidt JA, Oppenheim JJ. Interleukin-1: an immunological perspective. *Annu Rev Immunol.* 1985;3: 263–288.
88. MacDonald HR, Habholz MT. T-cell activation. *Annu Rev Cell Biol.* 1986;2:231–253.
89. Russell SW, Salomon DR. Macrophage effector and regulatory functions. In: Reif AE, Mitchell MS, eds. *Immunity to Cancer.* New York: Academic Press; 1985: 205–216.
90. Ring WS, DiMaio JM, Jessen ME, et al. Steroid withdrawal improves late survival after heart transplantation: 10 year results. *J Heart Lung Transplant.* [abstract] 2002;21:167.
91. Husa R, Cecere R, Cantarovich M, et al. Acute heart transplant rejection associated with late steroid withdrawal. *J Heart Lung Transplant.* [abstract]2002;21:167.
92. Mehra MR, Uber PA, Park MH, et al. Corticosteroid weaning in the tacrolimus and mycophenolate era in heart transplantation: clinical and neurohormonal benefits. *Transplant Proc.* 2004;36: 3152–3155.
93. Kohler G, Milstein C. Continuous cultures of fused cells secreting antibody of predefined specificity. *Nature.* 1975;256: 495–497.
94. Sheil AGR, Kelly GE, Storey BG. Controlled clinical trial of anti-lymphocyte globulin in patients with renal allografts from cadaver donors. *Lancet.* 1971;1:359–363.
95. Cosimi AB, Burton RC, Colvin RB. Treatment of acute renal allograft rejection with OKT3 antibody. *Transplantation.* 1981; 32:535–539.
96. Bristow MR, Gilbert EM, Renlund DG, et al. Use of OKT3 in heart transplantation: review of the initial experience. *Transplant Proc.* 1988;7:1–11.
97. Mancini D, Pinney S, Burkoff D, et al. Use of rapamycin slows progression of cardiac transplantation vasculopathy. *Circulation.* 2003;108:48–53.
98. Eisen HJ, Tuzcu EM, Dorent R, et al. Everolimus for the prevention of allograft rejection and vasculopathy in cardiac transplant recipients. *N Engl J Med.* 2003;349:847–858.
99. Caves PK, Stinson EB, Billingham M, et al. Percutaneous transvenous endomyocardial biopsy in human heart recipients. Experience with a new technique. *Ann Thorac Surg.* 1973; 16:325–336.
100. Billingham ME, Cary NRB, Hammond ME, et al. A working formulation for the standardization of nomenclature in the diagnosis of heart and lung rejection: heart rejection study group. *J Heart Transplant.* 1990;9:587–601.
101. Hosenpud JD, Shipley DG, Wagner CR. Cardiac allograft vasculopathy: current concepts, recent developments, and future directions. *J Heart Lung Transplant.* 1992;11:9–23.
102. St. Goar FG, Fausto JP, Alderman EL, et al. Intracoronary ultrasound in cardiac transplant recipients. *In vivo* evidence of angiographically silent intimal thickening. *Circulation.* 1992;85: 979–987.
103. Ventura HO. Coronary artery imaging with intravascular ultrasound in patients following cardiac transplantation. *Transplantation.* 1992;53:216–219.
104. Liu G, Butany J. Morphology of graft arteriosclerosis in cardiac transplant recipients. *Hum Pathol.* 1992;23:768–783.
105. Hosenpud JD, Everett JP, Wagner CR, et al. Cardiac allograft vasculopathy: association with cell-mediated but not humoral alloimmunity to donor specific vascular endothelium. *Circulation.* 1995;92:205–211.
106. Rose EA, Smith CR, Petrossian GA, et al. Humoral immune responses after cardiac transplantation: correlation with fatal rejection and graft atherosclerosis. *Surgery.* 1989; 106:203–207.
107. Crisp SJ, Dunn MJ, Rose ML, et al. Antiendothelial antibodies after heart transplantation: the accelerating factor in transplant-associated coronary artery disease. *J Heart Lung Transplant.* 1994;13:81–92.
108. McGiffin DC, Savunen T, Kirklin JK, et al. Cardiac transplant coronary artery disease. A multivariate analysis of pretransplantation risk factors for disease development and morbid events. *J Thorac Cardiovasc Surg.* 1995;109:1081–1088.
109. Mehra MR, Ventura HO, Chambers RB, et al. The prognostic impact of immunosuppression and cellular rejection on cardiac allograft vasculopathy: time for reappraisal. *J Heart Lung Transplant.* 1997;16:743–751.
110. Grattan MT, Moreno-Cabral CE, Starnes VA, et al. Cytomegalovirus is associated with cardiac allograft rejection and atherosclerosis. *JAMA.* 1989;261:3561–3566.
111. Koskinen PK, Nieminen MS, Krogerus LA, et al. Cytomegalovirus infection and accelerated cardiac allograft vasculopathy in human cardiac allografts. *J Heart Lung Transplant.* 1993;12:724–729.
112. Eich D, Thompson JA, Daijin K, et al. Hypercholesterolemia in long term survivors of heart transplantation: an early marker of accelerated coronary artery disease. *J Heart Lung Transplant.* 1991;10:45–49.
113. Billingham ME. Cardiac transplant atherosclerosis. *Transplant Proc.* 1987;19(Suppl 5):19–25.
114. Libby P, Salomon RN, Payne DD, et al. Functions of the vascular wall cells related to development of transplantation-associated coronary arteriosclerosis. *Transplant Proc.* 1989;21:3677–3684.
115. Taylor DO, Edwards LB, Boucek MM, et al. The Registry of the International Society for Heart and Lung Transplantation: twenty-first official adult heart transplant report—2004. *J Heart Lung Transplant.* 2004;22:616–624.
116. Mehra MR, Ventura HO, Stapleton DD et al. Presence of severe intimal thickening by intravascular ultrasonography predicts cardiac events in cardiac allograft vasculopathy. *J Heart Lung Transplant.* 1995;14:632–639.
117. Mehra MR, Ventura HO, Uber PA, et al. Is all intimal proliferation created equal in cardiac allograft vasculopathy? The quantity-quality paradox. *J Heart Lung Transplant.* 2003;22:118–123.
118. Kapadia SR, Ziada KM, L'Allier L, et al. Intravascular ultrasound imaging after cardiac transplantation: advantage of multi-vessel imaging. *J Heart Lung Transplant.* 2000;19:167–172.
119. Vetrovec GW, Cowley MJ, Newton CM, et al. Applications of percutaneous transluminal angioplasty in cardiac transplantation. Preliminary results in five patients. *Circulation.* 1988; 78(Suppl III):III83–III86.
120. Halle AA, Wilson RF, Vetrovec GW, for the Cardiac Transplant Angioplasty Study Group. Multicenter evaluation of percutaneous transluminal coronary angioplasty in heart transplant recipients. *J Heart Lung Transplant.* 1992;11:S138–S141.
121. Benza RL, Zoghbi GJ, Tallaj J, et al. Palliation of allograft vasculopathy with transluminal angioplasty: a decade of experience. *J Am Coll Cardiol.* 2004;43:1973–1981.
122. Hofflin JA, Potasman I, Baldwin JC, et al. Infectious complications in heart transplant recipients receiving cyclosporine and corticosteroids. *Ann Intern Med.* 1987;106:209–216.
123. Hosenpud JD, Norman DJ, Pantely GA, et al. Low morbidity and mortality from infection following cardiac transplantation using maintenance triple therapy and low-dose corticosteroids for acute rejection. *Clin Transplant.* 1988;2:201–206.
124. Trento A, Dummer GS, Hardesty RL. Mediastinitis following heart transplantation: incidence, treatment, and results. *Heart Transplant.* 1984;3:336–340.
125. Miller R, Ruder J, Karwande SV, et al. Treatment of mediastinitis after heart transplantation. *J Heart Transplant.* 1986;5:477–479.
126. Chou S, Norman DJ. The influence of donor factors other than serologic status on transmission of cytomegalovirus to transplant recipients. *Transplantation.* 1988;46:89–93.
127. Dummer JS, White LT, Ho M, et al. Morbidity of cytomegalovirus infection in recipients of heart or heart-lung transplants who received cyclosporine. *J Infect Dis.* 1985;152:1182–1191.
128. Smith CB. Cytomegalovirus pneumonia state of the art. *Chest.* 1989;95(Suppl):182S–187S.
129. Watson FS, O'Connell JB, Amber IJ, et al. Treatment of cytomegalovirus pneumonia in heart transplant recipients with 9(1,3-dihydroxy-2-proproxy-methyl)-guanine (DHPG). *J Heart Transplant.* 1988;7:102–105.
130. Keay S, Petersen E, Icenogle T, et al. Ganciclovir treatment of serious cytomegalovirus infection in heart and heart-lung transplant recipients. *Rev Infect Dis.* 1988;10(Suppl 3):S563–S572.
131. Everett JP, Hershberger RE, Norman DJ, et al. Prolonged cytomegalovirus infection with viremia is associated with development of cardiac allograft vasculopathy. *J Heart Lung Transplant.* 1992;11:S133–S137.
132. Penn I. Malignancies associated with immunosuppressive or cytotoxic therapy. *Surgery.* 1978;83:492–502.

133. Cleary ML, Sklar J. Lymphoproliferative disorders in cardiac transplant recipients are multiclonal lymphomas. *Lancet.* 1984;2:491–493.
134. Hanto DW, Gajl-Peczalska KJ, Balfour HH, et al. Acyclovir therapy of Epstein-Barr virus-induced posttransplant lymphoproliferative diseases. *Transplant Proc.* 1985;17:89–92.
135. Ibels LS, Alfrey AC, Huffer WE, et al. Aseptic necrosis of bone after renal transplantation: experience in 194 transplant recipients and review of the literature. *Medicine.* 1978; 57:25–45.
136. Rahimtoola SH, Ehsani A, Sinno MZ, et al. Left atrial transport function in myocardial infarction: importance of its booster pump function. *Am J Med.* 1975;59:686–694.
137. Hosenpud JD, Pantely GA, Morton MJ, et al. Relationship between recipient: donor body size matching and hemodynamics 3 months following cardiac transplantation. *J Heart Transplant.* 1989;8:241–247.
138. Hosenpud JD, Morton MJ. Physiology and hemodynamic assessment of the transplanted heart. In: Hosenpud JD, Cobanoglu A, Norman DJ, Starr A, eds. *Cardiac Transplantation.* New York: Springer-Verlag; 1991: 169–189.
139. Wilson RF, McGinn AL, Laxson DD, et al. Regional differences in sympathetic reinnervation after cardiac transplantation. *Circulation.* 1991;84(Suppl II):489.
140. Vora KN, Hosenpud JD, Ray J, et al. Angina pectoris in a cardiac allograft recipient. *Clin Transplant.* 1991;5:20–22.
141. Thadani U, Parker JO. Hemodynamics at rest and during supine and sitting bicycle exercise in normal subjects. *Am J Cardiol.* 1978;41:52–59.
142. Pflugfelder PW, Purves PD, McKenzie FN, et al. Cardiac dynamics during supine exercise in cyclosporine-treated orthotopic heart transplant recipients: assessment by radionuclide angiography. *J Am Coll Cardiol.* 1987;10:336–341.
143. Ross J, Linhart JW, Braunwald E. Effects of changing heart rate in man by electrical stimulation of the right atrium. Studies at rest, during exercise and with isoproterenol. *Circulation.* 1965; 32:549–558.
144. Stinson EB, Griepp RB, Schroeder JS, et al. Hemodymanic observations one and two years after cardiac transplantation in man. *Circulation.* 1972;45:1183–1193.
145. Pope SE, Stinson EB, Daughters GT, et al. Exercise response of the denervated heart in long-term cardiac transplant recipients. *Am J Cardiol.* 1980;46:213–218.
146. Grossman WH. *Cardiac Catheterization and Angiography.* Philadelphia: Lea & Febiger; 1986.
147. Griepp RB, Stinson EB, Dong E, Jr., et al. Acute rejection of the allografted human heart. *Ann Thorac Surg.* 1971;12:113–126.
148. Leachman RD, Cokkinos DVP, Rochelle DG, et al. Serial hemodynamic study of the transplanted heart and correlation with clinical rejection. *J Thorac Cardiovasc Surg.* 1971;61: 561–569.
149. Dawkins KD, Oldershaw PJ, Billingham ME, et al. Changes in diastolic function as a noninvasive marker of cardiac allograft rejection. *J Heart Transplant.* 1984;3:286–294.
150. Haverich A, Kemnitz J, Fieguth HG, et al. Non-invasive parameters for detection of cardiac allograft rejection. *Clin Transplant.* 1987;1:151–158.
151. Paulsen W, Magid N, Sagar K, et al. Left ventricular function of heart allografts during acute rejection: an echocardiographic assessment. *J Heart Transplant.* 1985;4:525–529.
152. Gaudiani VA, Stinson EB, Alderman E, et al. Long-term survival and function after cardiac transplantation. *Ann Surg.* 1981;194:381–385.
153. Lough ME, Lindsey AM, Shinn JA. Life satisfaction following heart transplantation. *J Heart Transplant.* 1985;4:446–449.
154. Bunzel B, Grundbock, A, Laczkovics A, et al. Quality of life after orthotopic heart transplantation. *J Heart Lung Transplant.* 1991;10:455–459.
155. Paris W, Woodbury A, Thompson S, et al. Return to work after cardiac transplantation. *J Heart Lung Transplant.* 1992;11:195.

Strategies for Gene and Cell Therapy in Heart Failure

47

Shi Yin Foo ***Anthony Rosenzweig***

The advances in cardiovascular care in the last three decades have paradoxically led to an increase in the number of individuals with heart disease, as survival rates from previously fatal myocardial infarctions (MIs) have improved. Consequently, more patients suffer from repeated MIs, congestive heart failure, and clinically significant arrhythmias. Despite progress in pharmacologic and device-based therapies, heart failure remains a growing cause of morbidity and mortality. Most current therapies are aimed at mitigating disease progression rather than reversing the underlying causes. Thus, investigation of novel biological therapies for heart failure is driven by both a clinical need for more effective treatment and a desire to correct fundamental abnormalities in an attempt to reverse the pathology of heart failure.

Genetic therapies provide an opportunity for highly specific manipulation of molecular pathways for which no pharmacologic reagent may exist. Moreover, the ability to manipulate these pathways locally in the myocardium can obviate concerns about systemic side effects inherent in pharmacologic approaches (1). Cell replacement strategies offer an opportunity to restore the number and function of endogenous cell populations, including cardiomyocytes and endothelial cells. However, each of these strategies introduces new concerns not seen with traditional approaches including potentially fatal vector toxicities (2,3) or cell-induced ventricular arrhythmias (4).

Despite these concerns, there is cause for cautious optimism and careful consideration of these approaches is warranted. In this chapter, we describe progress in these growing fields as it relates to heart failure. We consider, in turn, gene- and cell-based strategies under active investigation.

GENE-BASED THERAPY: OVERVIEW

Since heart failure encompasses a wide variety of primary causes, from coronary insufficiency to idiopathic cardiomyopathies, gene therapy strategies may need to be tailored to the specific form of heart failure—one size, or gene, may not fit all. For example, strategies to induce the growth of new blood vessels in specific regions of the heart may make sense for ischemic but not nonischemic cardiomyopathies where effective therapy may require more global, myocyte-targeted therapy. However, common features seen in heart failure of many etiologies, such as myocyte loss and abnormalities of excitation–contraction coupling, are potentially attractive candidates for intervention that might be applicable to a variety of primary disorders. In any context, successful gene therapy will require three critical components appropriate to the disease target at hand: a vector for delivery of the therapeutic genetic material, an appropriate delivery system, and, perhaps most important, a validated molecular target that can be appropriately modulated.

Vectors

There have been significant improvements in the vectors available for gene transfer (5–7) and a growing number have been used in both experimental and clinical gene transfer experiments (Table 47-1). Importantly, some of the most commonly used systems are not applicable to cardiac gene transfer, which requires in vivo gene delivery (as compared to ex vivo gene transfer) to cells that are not generally replicating. Here we focus on vectors most relevant to cardiac gene transfer.

TABLE 47-1
VECTORS FOR GENE DELIVERY

Vector	Efficiency (Maximum Observed)	Expression	Immune Response	Chromosomal Integration	Concerns
Adenovirus	100% in vitro	Onset 6–24 hours Peak 7 days	Robust, can be fulminant	No	Inflammatory myocarditis Cytotoxicity
rAAV	40% at 4 weeks 10% at 1 year In vivo	Slow onset (weeks) Duration lifelong	Moderate to minimal	Yes	Cytotoxicity Neoplastic transformation
Lentivirus	80% in vitro	Onset 12–48 hours Duration lifelong	Minimal	Yes	Neoplastic transformation
Naked DNA	5%–10% in vivo	Onset 1–7 days Duration short-term	Moderate	No	Cytotoxicity Local inflammation
HVJ-liposomes	80% in vitro	Onset 6–24 hours Duration short-term	Moderate	No	Cytotoxicity

Plasmid DNA

Multiple investigators have demonstrated that the heart can internalize and express genes injected directly as plasmid DNA (also termed naked DNA) to indicate the absence of a more elaborate packaging system. Use of plasmids avoids many biosafety concerns associated with viral vectors. However, both the level of transgene expression and the efficiency of gene transfer (percentage of target cells actually expressing the transgene) are generally much lower with unmodified plasmid DNA than with viral vectors or more elaborate chemical packaging systems. Nevertheless, muscle injection of plasmid vectors encoding secreted angiogenic factors has demonstrated significant biological effects in animals models (8–10).

A variety of modifications have been explored in the hope of enhancing the effectiveness of plasmid transfection without invoking the biosafety issues that accompany viral vectors. Liposomal preparations encase a DNA vector core with an artificial lipid bilayer that facilitates fusion with cell membranes (11). In some models, liposomal gene transfer to the heart appears effective despite a relatively low efficiency, perhaps because it evokes less local or inflammatory reaction than do adenoviral vectors (12). Other investigators have used a hybrid liposomal micelle containing envelope components of the HVJ virus (hemagglutinating virus of Japan or Sendai virus) to transfect a variety of cell types, including cardiomyocytes (13). However, transgene expression remains transient.

In another approach, liposomal-DNA micelles are attached to the phospholipid shell of gas-filled microbubbles, similar to those used as echocardiography contrast material. The mixture is injected intravenously and ultrasonography is used to cavitate the microbubbles while in the myocardial circulation. Cavitation causes a local shockwave that appears to enhance cell uptake of the plasmid (14). Newer strategies untested in the heart include peptide-cDNA heteroduplexes, in which the peptide contains a nuclear localization signal to enhance importation of the cDNA (15) and RNA-based peptide aptamers, which target and inhibit specific proteins (16). Finally, proteins that enhance cellular entry of exogenous material (such as the HIV *tat* protein) have been used to enhance both liposomal (12) and viral gene transfer (17).

Adenoviruses

Strategic advantages of recombinant adenoviral vectors for cardiac gene transfer include ease of preparation at extremely high titer and effective transduction of nonreplicating cells, including cardiomyocytes in vivo after direct injection or perfusion approaches (18). However, transient expression of introduced genes and induction of a potent host immune and inflammatory response limit their usefulness. Notably, up to 97% of individuals have pre-existing antibodies to common adenoviral serotypes (19) that can antagonize receptor binding, activate complement, and induce an inflammatory response (20). In addition, adenoviral infection of endothelial cells can upregulate adhesion molecules such as ICAM-1 and VCAM-1, leading to increased local infiltration of leukocytes (21) and the development of neointimal hyperplasia (22). These immune responses are likely responsible for decreasing the efficiency of the initial infection.

Another concern is the virtually unavoidable low-level contamination of recombinant adenoviral preparations with replication-competent adenovirus, likely generated through recombination events (23). This may be of particular concern for cardiac gene transfer since adenovirus has been isolated from cases of myocarditis and idiopathic dilated cardiomyopathy (IDCM) (24). Intriguingly, type 2 and 5 adenoviruses share a common receptor with the coxsackie B viruses (25), a known cause of myocarditis. However, the pathogenic role of adenovirus in myocarditis is unproven and, to date, no cases of myocarditis have been reported after adenoviral cardiac gene transfer. New packaging cell lines that further separate genomic replication components may decrease the likelihood of wild-type virus generation by several orders of magnitude (26).

Cardiac gene transfer with original (*first-generation*) adenoviral vectors in animal models usually effects high-level transgene expression for approximately 1 week in vivo (18,27–29), at which point it is eliminated or markedly diminished by the host cellular immune response. A variety of approaches have been explored to mitigate these responses, including the use of agents such as cyclosporin A (30,31) or soluble CTLA-Ig (32), which inhibits antigen presentation to T cells. However, the potential side effects of long-term immunosuppression dampen enthusiasm for this as a clinical solution. Since some of the host response is directed to viral antigens, considerable effort has been directed at attenuation of adenoviral gene expression by introduction of mutations in additional early adenoviral genes [so-called *second-generation* vectors (33)] or engineered deletion of virtually all viral genes, as in so-called gutless vectors (34). Both of these approaches prolong transgene expression and further decrease the likelihood of recombination-mediated generation of replication competent adenovirus. Interestingly, in some instances retaining specific adenoviral genes can actually reduce the host response (e.g., retention of the E3 region mitigated inflammation and neointima formation after vascular gene transfer in vivo) (35). Currently, little is known about the long-term or clinical effects of second-generation and gutless adenoviral vectors in the cardiovascular system.

Adeno-Associated Viruses

Recombinant adeno-associated viruses (rAAV) appear particularly promising for cardiac gene transfer (5,36,37) for several reasons. They are derived from parvoviruses, which are not known to be pathogenic in humans and generally do not evoke a vigorous cellular immune response. rAAV achieve transgene expression lasting months in many systems (36,38,39). Cardiac injection of rAAV generally produces less initial but more sustained transgene expression in comparison to the adenoviral vectors previously discussed (5,36,37). Thus, rAAV may be the vector of choice for sustained expression of secreted gene products. However, less is known regarding the ability of rAAV to mediate sufficient transgene expression to modulate overall heart function, as reported with adenoviral vectors (40). As with newer-generation adenoviral vectors, the production and purification of sufficient clinical grade rAAV remain challenging.

A growing number of adeno-associated viruses (AAV) serotypes have been isolated (41,42). AAV2 has been the most commonly used AAV vector, although its efficiency for cardiomyocytes appears relatively low, with ~25% of the cardiomyocytes within the area of cardiac injection expressing the transgene at 1 month (43). The efficiency of AAV2 gene transfer can be limited by pre-existing antibodies that result from prior wild-type infection (19). The prevalence of anti-AAV2 antibodies in human serum can be as high as 35% to 80%, depending on the population (44). The adaptive, cell-mediated immune response is also activated by AAV but is much weaker than with adenovirus. This, in combination with the ability of AAV genomes to integrate, likely accounts for the dramatically improved duration of transgene expression after AAV gene transfer.

To enhance tissue specificity, recombinant AAV serotypes have been generated that use the AAV2 genome packaged into the viral capsids of other serotypes (43,45). Of these, recombinant AAV1 vectors carrying the AAV2 internal terminal repeats (ITR) sequences [rAAV1(2) vectors] transduced adult cardiomyocytes both in vitro and in vivo at the highest frequency. In vivo, the efficiency was approximately 40% of cardiomyocytes within a 5-mm radius of the injection site 1 month after injection, but less than 10% at 1 year after intervention (43). This approach may be ideally suited to gene products that initiate a cascade of effects and can act in a paracrine manner. Another advantage of the rAAV1(2) vectors is the relative lack of exposure of humans to the AAV1. In general, human serum lacks neutralizing antibodies to the AAV1 virus. In one study, only 20% of healthy individuals harbored anti-AAV1 antibodies and these antibodies were less potent than anti-AAV2 antibodies in preventing viral infection (46). However, development of a humoral immune response would likely hamper attempts at repeated gene replacement using the same vector.

AAV8 appears to have a robust tropism for striated muscle, including the heart (47). Interestingly, this particular serotype outperforms AAV1 in cardiac muscle transduction after intravenous administration, but not after intramuscular injection in mice, suggesting that an additional barrier to successful gene transfer in vivo is the ability to traverse the blood vessel wall (47).

AAV vectors, in general, mediate a relatively low-level transgene expression that can require weeks to reach its peak. Recently, Samulski et al. have developed AAV vectors encoding a single-stranded, self-complementary DNA strand that substantially accelerates and enhances transgene expression (48). However, the use of AAV is also limited by the small size of the virus, which severely constrains the amount of DNA that can be packaged (<5 kb). Self-complementing AAV, which essentially encode both strands in one molecule, reduce this amount by approximately twofold.

Lentiviruses

Although derived from a family of retroviruses that includes human and feline immunodeficiency viruses, lentiviruses can infect both dividing and nondividing cells, in contrast to other retroviruses which infect only actively replicating cells. This distinction is critical to their ability to transduce cardiomyocytes. Lentiviruses encode an RNA genome, which is converted to DNA and integrated into the host chromosome. Lentiviruses have specific tropisms that restrict their host cell range, but this can be overcome by pseudotyping the viral envelope through incorporation of the envelope from other retroviruses (particularly vesicular stomatitis virus, which has a broad host range). Integration into the host genome enhances the stability of transgene expression but also carries the risk of potentially serious adverse effects. These effects can arise either through insertional mutagenesis or transactivation of neighboring genes, as seen in recent clinical trials of retroviral gene therapy (2,49). Lentiviral gene vectors have been successfully employed in a wide variety of cell types, including cardiomyocytes (50–55).

Advanced-generation lentiviruses achieve gene transfer efficiencies in cardiomyocytes comparable to that of adenoviral vectors. These lentiviruses contain elements of the HIV *pol* gene as a nuclear transport signal and an mRNA-stabilizer from the woodchuck hepatitis virus to increase integration (56). Transduction efficiency in cultured rat cardiomyocytes was over 80%. After delivery of these lentiviral vectors through coronary perfusion to the rat heart after aortic clamping, 85% of cardiomyocytes expressed the reporter transgene at 15 days (56).

Lentiviruses elicit relatively little immune response to intrinsic viral proteins, although the use of lentivirus in vivo may be limited by complement activation acutely (57). The adaptive, cytotoxic immune response that limits long-term expression appears primarily directed against the exogenous transgenes. Complement activation can be mitigated somewhat by using different pseudotypes; vesicular stomatits virus capsid proteins appear particularly prone to complement activation. In some studies, pseudotyping with more exotic envelope proteins, such as those from Ebola and Mokola viruses, allows for higher infection efficiency in cardiomyocytes in vivo (54). However, the immune response to these recombinant vectors has not been fully characterized.

Herpes Virus/Amplicons

Herpes simplex 1 (HSV-1) can infect both dividing and nondividing cells and has a broad host cell range although it has a strong tropism toward neurons. The wild-type virus has a large genome and, thus, vectors derived from HSV-1 can accommodate large transgenes (>35 kb). This feature has been exploited for cardiac gene transfer for large genes such as the ryanodine receptor and titin (58), which would not be feasible with most other vector systems. Two types of HSV-1-based vectors are currently in use. These include vectors produced by inserting exogenous genes into the viral backbone, and HSV amplicon virions that are produced by inserting transgenes into a plasmid carrying the HSV origin of replication and packaging signal.

Toxicity

The previous discussion above and Table 47-1 should make clear that no vector is ideal; each brings limitations and potential toxicities. These toxicities have led to a concerning number of complications in early clinical experience. One of the most widely publicized involved a 17-year-old patient with partial ornithine transcarbamylase (OTC) deficiency, an X-linked defect of the urea cycle which causes a variety of neurologic symptoms including seizures and mental retardation (59). Therapy for the condition relies on alternative substrate administration but mortality rates with the disease are high. Following the administration of an adenoviral vector encoding carrying OTC, this patient developed acute respiratory distress syndrome, ultimately dying of multiple organ failure. This patient developed a systemic inflammatory syndrome with activation of the complement cascade that contributed to his demise (60,61). Thus, the host immune response mounted to viral vectors can have catastrophic consequences. In another instance, ex vivo retroviral gene transfer to bone marrow stem cells led to long-term remission in a small number of children (2) but was complicated by clonal, leukemic T-cell proliferation apparently related to construct insertion inducing aberrant proto-oncogene expression (2). While such insertional effects had always been considered a theoretical possibility with integrating vectors, the surprisingly high frequency of the event [occurring in two of the first 10 treated patients (2)] is obviously of great concern. Approaches to minimizing this risk currently being investigated include targeting viral integration to specific sites in the genome (62), use of chromatin-insulator elements to prevent the nonspecific activation of nearby oncogenes (63), and inclusion of inducible suicide genes to permit targeted destruction of transformed cells (64).

Delivery Methods

Many of the issues concerning delivery are common to both genetic and cell-based therapies and will be addressed together in this section. A variety of systems have been explored in animal models (53,65–69), while clinical experience is more limited. Some techniques successfully employed in animals may not be applicable to the sick cardiac patients most in need of such therapies. As with the choice of vector, the optimal delivery method also depends on disease context and the therapeutic target. The focal transgene expression achieved with direct injection (whether surgical or catheter-based) may be appropriate for angiogenic therapy to hypoperfused myocardial segments in ischemic cardiomyopathy, while delivery of cell-autonomous transgenes to improve cardiomyocyte function in nonischemic cardiomyopathy likely requires more diffuse delivery.

Systemic

In the simplest approach, genes or cells are injected intravenously. However, this approach often suffers from the twin evils of inadequate delivery to the target organ and extraneous, possibly detrimental delivery to unintended tissues. For gene delivery, systemic intravenous delivery usually results in either extremely low or undetectable levels of cardiac transgene expression. In contrast, certain cell populations (such as bone marrow-derived angioblasts) have been shown to home preferentially to areas of ischemic injury (70). Nevertheless, systemic delivery of cells will likely result in delivery of fewer cells to the heart than will direct delivery. Ex vivo expansion of the cell populations could be used to overcome this barrier but may heighten concerns over inappropriate homing to other sites.

Intramyocardial Direct Injection

Direct injection of vectors or cells into the myocardium introduces high concentrations of the therapeutic agent in a highly localized manner. The exposure of the region at risk to these agents is not limited by cell or vector uptake through the vascular system but does, in general, entail more invasive procedures such as transendocardial or transcoronary vein injection during catheterization, or epicardial injection during cardiac surgery (4,71).

Direct injection has several advantages. First, injection can be limited to regions mostly likely to benefit while minimizing adverse effects in other regions or systemically. Second, in patients with coronary stenoses, direct injection provides access to hypoperfused myocardium excluded from artery-based perfusion approaches. Third, intramyocardial delivery obviates concerns in cell-based therapy that coronary infusion could pose an embolic risk in the small-caliber vessels of the heart. These features likely account for the fact that direct injection was one of the first techniques utilized clinically for both genes (72) and cells (73).

The highly focal nature of delivery may necessitate multiple injections to cover the entire region at risk, increasing the risk of mechanical injury or perforation. Direct injection of cells may lead to islands of cells that are isolated from an adequate blood supply and are thus unlikely to survive. In addition, patients most in need of such rescue therapies may be the individuals least likely to do well due to the invasiveness of these procedures. Finally, this approach will generally not be appropriate for conditions and molecular targets that require delivery of therapy to a majority of the heart.

Perfusion-Based approaches

A variety of catheter designs permit cannulation and perfusion of genes or cells down a coronary artery with or without occlusive balloon inflation. Some investigators have reported that myocardial gene delivery with this approach is quite efficient (74–76), although systemic vector delivery can also be substantial. A variation of coronary-mediated delivery is whole-heart perfusion with cross-clamping of the aorta alone or in combination with the pulmonary artery, first performed successfully in rodents (66,77). This approach achieves diffuse, relatively homogeneous myocardial transduction and is capable of modulating the overall intrinsic contractile properties of the heart (66,78). Extrapolation of these studies to human disease could entail perfusion in association with cardiopulmonary bypass (79) or retroperfusion via catheters (80).

Targets for Gene Therapy in Heart Failure

While some approaches to therapeutic gene delivery focus on the underlying cause of heart failure (as in the case of angiogenesis), the diverse etiologies that can contribute to heart failure, as well as the usual long delay between these inciting events and clinical presentation, represent significant challenges to this approach. For these reasons, many strategies have targeted features common to multiple forms of heart failure, including loss of cardiomyocytes through programmed cell death, abnormalities of excitation–contraction coupling and calcium handling, as well as dysfunctional adrenergic signaling (Table 47-2).

Improving Cardiac Perfusion

The most common contributor to heart failure in the United States is ischemic injury related to coronary artery disease (CAD). Therapeutic angiogenesis is directed at improving myocardial perfusion, particularly in patients for whom traditional percutaneous or surgical options have been exhausted. Currently, these efforts have been directed at relieving symptoms of ischemia, although the potential to improve cardiac function has been suggested by animal models, underscoring the close connection between angiogenic pathways and cardiac function (81). In animals, vascular endothelial growth factor (VEGF), fibroblast growth factor-2 (FGF-2), hepatocyte growth factor, or hypoxia-inducible factor-1 (HIF-1) (82) can induce neovascularization. In some animal models, new vessel formation is accompanied by improvements in myocardial contractile function (83,74). Early uncontrolled trials have suggested a reasonable safety profile (84). Although small numbers of patients have improved after direct myocardial delivery of VEGF (72,84), efficacy cannot be inferred in the absence of contemporaneous controls. It seems likely that extrapolation to the heart failure population awaits evidence from large, randomized, placebo-controlled trials.

Cardiomyocyte Loss

Most heart failure is accompanied by cardiomyocyte death. Importantly, in animal models, even low levels of programmed cell death or apoptosis of cardiomyocytes—comparable to that seen in human heart failiure—are sufficient to cause a lethal cardiomyopathy (85). For this reason, a variety of strategies have evolved directed at preventing death of cardiomyocytes through apoptosis or other mechanisms.

Several conceptual obstacles hinder the application of such therapies to heart failure. First, most of these approaches have been tested in models of acute ischemic

TABLE 47-2
TARGETS FOR GENE THERAPY IN HEART FAILURE

Strategy	Target Genes	Disease Application	Concerns
Neovascularization	VEGF, bFGF, HGF, Ang-1, HIF-1a	Chronic myocardial ischemia Ischemic cardiomyopathy	Potentiation of occult malignancies
Cardioprotection	Anti-apoptotic genes: Bcl-2, Akt (overexpression) Bad, p53, Fas ligand (inhibition)	Acute myocardial infarction Chronic ischemia Congestive heart failure	Oncogenic transformation
Preserving contractile function	Calcium regulation: SERCA2a (overexpression) Phospholamban (inhibition)	Congestive heart failure	Long-term effects in humans of increased contractility unclear
	Adrenergic signaling: β_2-adrenergic receptor (overexpression) βAR kinase (inhibition) Type VI adenylyl cyclase	Congestive heart failure	Increased myocardial oxygen demand Long-term effects in humans of increased contractility unclear

injury that provide important validation that specific molecules regulate cardiomyocyte survival in vivo but do not directly test their role in heart failure. Second, inhibition of apoptosis may simply alter the mode of cell death or promote survival of dysfunctional cardiomyocytes, resulting in little clinical benefit. Finally, by the time patients present with clinical heart failure it may be too late for effective prevention of cardiomyocyte loss. Despite these considerations, manipulating apoptotic signaling pathways in animal models suggests substantial benefit not only on cardiomyocyte survival but function, as well (86). Growing evidence suggests this reflects the convergence of signaling pathways that control cardiomyocyte survival and function. This fortuitous finding suggests these strategies may well be worth pursuing.

Bcl-2

Bcl-2 is a mitochondrial-associated protein that regulates cytochrome c release from mitochondria which leads to caspase 9 activation. In many cells, Bcl-2 overexpression inhibits apoptosis and increases proliferation [reviewed in (87)]. In a rabbit model, left ventricular injection of an adenoviral vector encoding Bcl-2 immediately after transient ligation of the circumflex artery reduced cardiomyocyte apoptosis and improved left ventricular fractional shortening as well as whole-heart geometry 6 weeks after ischemic injury (88). Since even low levels of apoptosis can cause dilated cardiomyopathy (85), the observed reduction in apoptosis likely contributes to the favorable remodeling seen after Bcl-2 gene transfer despite similar initial infarcts. Importantly, this study establishes that delivery of vectors in a clinically relevant time frame (after reperfusion) can have substantial benefits. Moreover, ventricular remodeling seen after infarction is a major contributor to heart failure in patients and, thus, targeting anti-apoptotic signaling in this context may be beneficial.

Of more direct relevance to heart failure are studies of genetic deletion (89,90) or inhibition (91) of the ErbB2 receptor, which shed light on herceptin (trastuzumab)-induced cardiomyopathy in patients. Mice in which ErbB2 has been deleted in cardiomyocytes develop a dilated cardiomyopathy (89,90), which can be rescued by neonatal gene transfer of the anti-apoptotic Bcl-protein, Bcl-XL (90). Although one explanation for this benefit would be inhibition of apoptosis, little if any apoptosis was observed (89,90). An alternative model is based on our observations that antibodies to the ErbB2 receptor cause activation of apoptotic signaling, mitochondrial dysfunction, and reduced adenosine triphosphate (ATP) levels in cardiomyocytes in the absence of substantial levels of apoptosis (91). We hypothesize that mitochondrial dysfunction (induced by antibodies or other stimuli) contributes to overall cardiac dysfunction and propose that "interrupted apoptosis" may contribute to heart failure both through compromising the function of surviving cardiomyocytes and by sensitizing cardiomyocytes to future apoptotic stimuli. Consistent with this model, myopathic human hearts demonstrate activation of apoptotic signaling that is much more widespread than the number of apoptotic cardiomyocytes (92). Thus, the benefits of targeting apoptotic signaling pathways are potentially much greater than would be anticipated from the relatively small number of overtly apoptotic cardiomyocytes.

Phosphoinositide 3-Kinase/Akt Signaling

Cantley et al. (93,94) first implicated phosphoinositide 3-kinase (PI 3-kinase) and its downstream effector, the serine-threonine kinase, Akt, as critical determinants of cell survival. A variety of cardioprotective peptides, including hormones, growth factors, and cytokines (e.g., insulin, gp130-dependent cytokines, insulin-like growth factor I [IGF-I]) activate this signaling pathway, which is sufficient to inhibit cardiomyocyte apoptosis (95). Acute activation of Akt also prevents abnormalities of contraction or Ca^{2+}-handling in surviving cardiomyocytes (96), thus promoting meaningful rescue, while Akt inhibition accelerates hypoxia-induced cardiomyocyte dysfunction (96). In vivo acute activation of Akt substantially improves regional and overall cardiac function after ischemia-reperfusion (96). These data are consistent with the model that convergent pathways (downstream of Akt activation) modulate both cardiomyocyte survival and function.

Paradoxically, however, Akt phosphorylation is increased in hearts of chronic heart failure patients (97), raising the possibility that *chronic* Akt activation could become maladaptive. Transgenic mice with cardiac-specific activation of Akt (98–100) have dramatically impaired functional recovery in an isolated heart ischemia-reperfusion model (101). Chronic Akt activation leads to feedback inhibition of upstream signaling with a significant reduction in expression of the insulin receptor substrate (IRS)-adaptor proteins; this precludes activation of PI 3-kinase in response to the usual stimuli (101). Intriguingly, a similar decrease in IRS-1 was seen in cardiac samples from patients with heart failure (101). Multiple pathways downstream of PI 3-kinase (Fig. 47-1) likely work in parallel to control cardiomyocyte survival, including Akt as well as the homologous kinase, serum and glucocorticoid-responsive kinase-1 (SGK1), an important determinant of cardiomyocyte survival (102). Expression of IGF-I itself (1), capable of simultaneously activating all

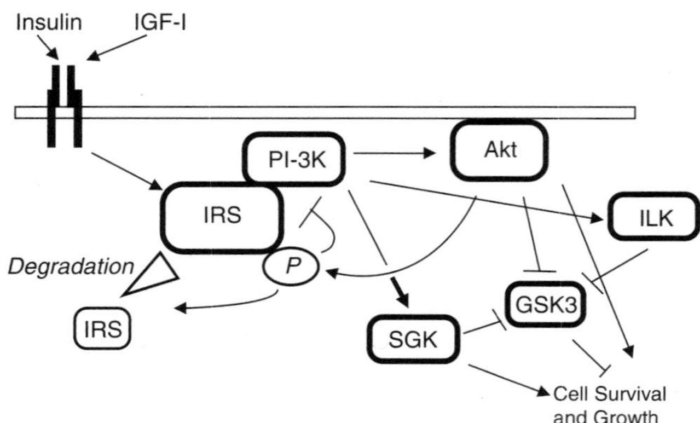

Figure 47-1 Schematic of PI 3K signaling pathways. Multiple PI 3K-dependent pathways modulate cell survival and growth, including Akt, SGK, and integrin-linked kinase (ILK). Chronic activation of Akt leads to feedback inhibition of IRS/PI 3K signaling, resulting in loss of signaling through parallel prosurvival mechanisms.

these downstream pathways, may be one strategy to circumvent these issues. Long-term exogenous expression of both Bcl-2 and Akt also raises the specter of oncogenic transformation (103,104). Feasible approaches to improving the biosafety of such strategies include tissue-specific and/or regulatable promoters to control expression, as well as transient vector systems.

Preserving Cardiomyocyte Function

β-Adrenergic Signaling

β-adrenergic receptors are downregulated in chronic heart failure. In animal models, adenoviral gene transfer of the β_2-adrenergic receptor (β_2-AR) improves left ventricular contractility both at baseline and in response to isoproterenol (105,106). β_2-ARs are also functionally uncoupled after chronic stimulation, at least in part through the action of the βAR kinase (βARK1) (107,108). Inhibition of βARK1 via expression of a peptide inhibitor ('βARKct') maintains β_2-AR density and signaling at normal levels in a rabbit model of MI and failure (108), suggesting that this may correct some of the abnormalities of β-adrenergic signaling seen in heart failure.

Adenylyl Cyclase

Cyclic adenosine monophosphate (cAMP) mediates many of the effects of β-adrenergic signaling. Gene transfer of type VI adenylyl cyclase improves contractility in a pig model of pacing-induced cardiac dysfunction (76). This approach forms the basis for a Phase I/II clinical trial in heart failure (109) currently being initiated.

The long-term consequences of enhancing adrenergic signaling in heart failure patients are unclear and stand in stark contrast to the current clinical standard of care of using β-adrenergic antagonists. Would the increase in contractility come at the expense of increased myocardial oxygen demand and energy expenditure that could have adverse long-term consequences? Clinically, it is conceivable that any improvement in patient morbidity might be offset by an increase in mortality, a scenario not unlike that seen with a variety of pharmacologic heart failure treatments (110).

Calcium Handling

Intracellular calcium currents in the myocardium are tightly regulated via the sarcoplasmic reticulum (SR). During the relaxation phase, the SR calcium adenosine triphosphatase pump (SERCA2a) reaccumulates calcium into the SR. The activity of SERCA2a is, in turn, regulated by the protein phospholamban. SERCA2a and SR Ca^{2+}-ATPase activity are reduced in heart failure (111,112), raising the possibility that restoring SR ATPase activity could improve cardiac function in heart failure.

Adenoviral gene transfer of SERCA2a leads to an increase in SR Ca^{2+}-ATPase activity in normal cardiomyocytes and acceleration of the relaxation phase (113). Moreover, SERCA2a overexpression improves dysfunction in human cardiomyocytes isolated from failing hearts (114). In vivo, cardiac gene delivery of SERCA2a in a rat heart failure model restores both systolic and diastolic function (78). Of note, in contrast to adrenergic signaling, SERCA2a overexpression enhances contractility without increasing cAMP or energy requirements, and survival in animal models is actually improved by this intervention (78,115). The ultimate test of these concepts will require clinical validation. A clinical trial of SERCA2a gene transfer for end-stage heart failure patients requiring ventricular assist devices for support is currently being initiated.

CELL-BASED THERAPY: OVERVIEW

A variety of sources have been considered for cardiac cell replacement, including skeletal myoblasts (4), embryonic stem cells (116), and adult progenitor cell populations, most commonly derived from bone marrow (117). Progenitors from peripheral blood (118) and even fat tissue (119) are also being explored. Proponents suggest that transdifferentiation of donor cells into cardiomyocytes or vascular endothelium could improve cardiac function directly or indirectly, respectively. While improved cardiac function in animal models has often been observed after cell transfer, it remains unclear whether these improvements represent regeneration or secondary effects such as secretion of cardioprotective peptides mediating paracrine benefits (120) or modulation of passive mechanical properties of myocardium. Further complicating analysis, most of these studies use noninvasive, load-dependent measures of contractility and thus may be confounded by alterations in load conditions. In addition, only a few studies employ control cells to demonstrate that use of progenitor cells is necessary for the observed benefits. Understanding the mechanisms underlying observed alterations in function is thus of more than academic interest, for it will help assess the potential of these approaches and guide future work.

Several groups have identified endogenous cells in the adult heart with characteristics of progenitor cells and the ability to give rise to cardiomyocytes (121–123). Importantly, these studies challenge the longstanding dogma that adult cardiomyocytes cannot divide. However, the endogenous regenerative capacity of the adult heart appears insufficient in most clinical settings characterized by myocyte loss. Fully exploiting the observation of endogenous progenitor populations will require learning how to enhance the number or function of these cells in vivo or how to harvest and expand these ex vivo in clinically relevant time frames and quantities. In all of these studies, cell heterogeneity remains a significant issue since no unique cell marker has been identified that specifically identifies cardiac progenitors.

CELL POPULATIONS FOR CARDIAC THERAPY IN HEART FAILURE

Multiple cell sources are currently under investigation for cardiac replacement therapies (Table 47-3). Some are multipotent and thus have the theoretical advantage of being able to differentiate into multiple cell lineages, including endothelium and cardiomyocytes. However, whether substantial transdifferentiation occurs and whether this results in a relative advantage of the use of pluripotent cell populations

TABLE 47-3
PROGENITOR CELL POPULATIONS FOR CELL-BASED THERAPY

Cell Population	Source	Advantages	Disadvantages
Skeletal myoblast	Autologous muscle biopsy (satellite cells)	Ease of harvest and culture Ischemia-resistant	Risk of arrhythmia
Unfractionated bone marrow	Autologous bone marrow	Ease of harvest Multipotent—may give rise to several terminal cell types Genetic manipulation possible	Not fully characterized
Mesenchymal stem cells	Autologous bone marrow	Multipotent—may give rise to several terminal cell types Genetic manipulation possible Secrete various proangiogenic cytokines	Low frequency in bone marrow Not fully characterized
Endogenous resident cardiac stem cells	Autologous heart	Can form electromechanical coupling Amenable to clonal expansion Multipotent—both cardiomyocytes and endothelium	Insufficient characterization Difficult to harvest
Embryonic stem cells	Allogenic blastocyst	Pluripotent Can form electromechanical coupling Genetic manipulation possible	Donor availability Ethical and moral controversy Immune response to allogenic transplant

remain controversial. Moreover, given the heterogeneity of populations being instilled, it remains unclear which subset of the donor cells actually mediates any observed functional effects. Cell populations being considered are listed below.

Endothelial Progenitor Cells

The bone marrow-derived hemangioblast is a common precursor for both endothelial and hematopoietic lineages (124). Endothelial progenitor cells (EPCs) can be identified in bone marrow of numerous species as cells expressing hematopoietic stem cell (HSC) markers such as CD34 or the even more immature HSC marker CD133, and an endothelial marker such as the VEGF receptor-2 (VEGFR2 or Flk-1) (125,126). These populations are maintained at baseline in the bone marrow, although a subset appears to circulate in the adult blood (127). Ischemic tissues secrete cytokines such as vascular endothelial growth factor or stromal cell-derived factor-1 (SDF-1), which mobilize and recruit EPCs (128,129). Because myeloid and endothelial cells share a common progenitor ancestor, EPCs can also be mobilized by administration of granulocyte colony stimulating factor (G-CSF), granulocyte-monocyte colony stimulating factor (GM-CSF), and even erythropoietin (128,130). Other cell types in the bone marrow such as mesenchymal stem cells and the side population compartments can also give rise to cells of the endothelial lineage (131), although intermediaries such as EPCs have not been demonstrated per se for these stem cells.

EPCs circulating (CEPCs) in the peripheral blood (132) may arise from bone marrow hemangioblasts or distinct mesenchymal or multipotential adult progenitor cell compartments in the bone marrow (127). Alternatively, some CEPCs could arise from circulating myeloid or other progenitors, such as CD14+/CD34– myeloid subpopulations, that may transdifferentiate into vascular endothelium (133). CEPCs usually express CD34 and VEGFR2 (125), although CD34 can also be expressed by mature endothelial cells albeit at a lower level (125).

Animal studies suggest that infusion of endothelial progenitors—either directly derived from the bone marrow or cultivated ex vivo—can promote neovascularization and augment capillary density (139). The administration of human bone marrow-derived CD34+ cells into a rat model of MI resulted in the incorporation of these cells into 20% to 25% of the myocardial vascular bed at risk (70). This correlated with decreased apoptosis in the peri-infarct region and sustained improvements in contractile function (70).

EPCs incorporate into normal blood vessels at extremely low rates. However, after tissue injury, incorporation rates as high as 90% have been reported for bone marrow-derived cells (134–137). Engraftment of donor EPCs can be demonstrated in denuded grafts and angioplastied arteries (138,139), suggesting that EPCs may contribute to endothelial repair and regeneration. In addition, EPCs could also promote neovascularization by the secretion of paracrine proangiogenic factors for the migration and proliferation of mature endothelial cells (120). This endogenous repair function may be defective in the patients who need it the most, such as those with risk factors for coronary disease or established CAD (140). If so, this might complicate efforts to harvest and restore EPCs in patients with acute coronary syndromes, as these patients may have fewer or less-functional EPCs available. Nevertheless, clinical trials have begun testing this approach (see Clinical Trials, discussed later, and Table 47-4). Thus far, these trials demonstrate that bone marrow populations can be delivered without major adverse effects. Although cardiac func-

TABLE 47-4

CLINICAL TRIALS FOR CELL-BASED THERAPY IN HEART DISEASE

Disease	Study	N (Treated)	Controls	Timing	Cell Type	Cell# ($\times 10^6$)	EF (Mean)	Endpoints	Follow-Up
Acute MI	Strauer et al.	10	Nonrandomized (10 controls)	8 days after acute MI	BMCs	28	51	LVEF improved 57% to 62%; ESV 82 to 67 mm SPECT: decrease in % infarct area	3 months
Acute MI	TOPCARE-AMI Assmus et al.	29 30	Historical, case-matched (11 controls)	At time of MI 4.3 days after acute MI	BMCs CEPCs	245 10	42 42	LVEF improved 51% to 60% in both groups ESV decreased Reduced infarct size	4 months (MRI at 1 yr)
Acute MI	Fernandez-Aviles et al.	20	Nonrandomized (13 controls)	13.5 days after acute MI	BMCs	78		LVEF improved 51% to 57% ESV 81 to 71 mm	6 months
Acute MI	BOOST Wollert et al.	30	Randomized but not blinded (30 controls)	4.8 days after MI	BMCs		50	LVEF improved 50% to 57%	6 months
Chronic CAD and CHF	Menasche et al.	10	No controls	At CABG	Skeletal myoblasts	871	24	LVEF improved to 32% Improvement in NYHA Class scores	10 months
Chronic CAD	Fuchs et al.	10	No controls	>1 month after MI	BMCs	78.2	47	ECHO: no change in LVEF; angina/QOL scores improved Bruce treadmill test: increased exercise time	3 months
Chronic CAD CABG patients	Stamm et al.	6	No controls	At CABG	CD133+ BMCs	1.5	36	Echocardiographic EF: improved to 49 %	8–16 months
Chronic CAD medically refractory	Tse et al.	8	No controls	Stable angina	BMCs	NR	58	MRI: no change in EF, 11.6% improvement in wall thickening and 3.9% reduction in mass of hypoperfused myocardium	3 months
Chronic CAD and CHF	Perin et al.	14	Nonrandomized, open-label (7 controls)	End-stage ischemic HF (>3 months from MI)	BMCs	25.5	30	ECHO: EF improved from 30% to 36% ESV: 146 to 123 mm VO_{2max}:improvement,17.96 to 23.38 mL/kg/min	4, 6 and 12 months

tion has improved in many patients in these trials, the absence of randomized and blinded controls, as well as long-term follow-up, precludes a rigorous conclusion of efficacy from information available to date.

Myocyte Progenitors

Skeletal Myoblasts

Delivery of cells capable of contraction is intuitively appealing and the first cells used for improvement of contractile function were skeletal muscle myoblasts (4). These progenitors exist as quiescent satellite cells under the basement membrane of mature myocyte fibers and can be readily isolated and expanded in vitro. When implanted into the heart, myoblasts differentiate into myotubes, contract and retain skeletal muscle characteristics but apparently do not couple electromechanically with the surrounding myocardium, potentially leading to contractile dyssynchrony and arrhythmia (141,142). In early uncontrolled clinical experience, delivery of autologous skeletal muscle myoblasts during cardiac bypass surgery was followed not only by cardiac contractile function (143), but also an apparent increase in ventricular arrhythmias (144) necessitating implantable cardioverter defibrillator (ICD) implantation. Ongoing randomized trials are designed to reveal whether the potential benefits of this approach outweigh the risks.

Bone Marrow Progenitors

Whether bone marrow-derived stem cells can transdifferentiate to regenerate cardiomyocytes and other cellular constituents of the myocardium remains highly controversial. Immunohistochemical studies suggested that bone marrow injected into murine hearts after infarction could substantially repopulate multiple lineages in the peri-infarct area (145,146). Similarly, bone marrow progenitors isolated on the basis of their exclusion of Hoechst staining as a side population have also demonstrated benefits in a model of murine coronary artery occlusion (134). In contrast, two groups using a Cre-Lox lineage tracing strategy did not demonstrate a significant contribution of bone marrow-derived cells to myocardium after ischemic injury (147,148).

Mesenchymal Stem Cells

Mesenchymal stem cells (MSCs) represent a distinct bone marrow-derived population that has been reported to acquire a cardiomyocyte phenotype (117,149,150). MSCs and are CD34–/CD133– cells that reside in the bone marrow stroma and are much less abundant than HSCs but appear to have a wide differentiation range, including adipocytes, osteocytes, and chondrocytes (151). Improvement in local contractile function and remodeling after infarction has been reported after MSC transplantation to infarcted hearts (149,150). Dzau et al. reported that bone marrow-derived MSCs transduced with Akt were remarkably able to repair injured myocardium (152), but later found that apparent benefits may result primarily from paracrine effects of secreted factors rather than transdifferentiation (120). MSCs in culture secrete a variety of cytokines and growth factors, including VEGF, basic fibroblast growth factor (bFGF), and transforming growth factor-β (TGF-β) (153) that could contribute to enhanced cardiac function. MSCs may have relatively low immunogenicity, which could be advantageous for allogeneic use clinically and forms the basis of an ongoing Phase I clinical trial (154).

Endogenous Cardiac Progenitors

Several groups have reported evidence for resident progenitor cells in the heart itself (121–123). Although no unique markers of these populations have yet been identified, they are amenable to isolation and clonal expansion (121,122). They appear capable of promoting vascular and cardiomyocyte generation when injected into murine infarct models (121,122). However, the practical hurdles associated with obtaining and expanding these cells from the hearts of ill patients to provide syngeneic donor cells would obviously be substantial.

Embryonic Stem Cells

Totipotent stem cells isolated from the inner cell mass of the developing embryo have also been proposed as a source for cardiac stem cells. Human embryonic stem cell-derived cardiomyocytes appear structurally and functionally like early cardiac cells and can couple electrically with normal myocardium. These cells could, in theory, be expanded indefinitely. However, issues regarding the host responses to allogenic transplantation as well as concerns regarding possible tumorigenicity of these cells remain unresolved. In addition, the generation (let alone clinical application) of these cells is currently the subject of intense debate due to the associated religious and ethical implications of such work.

Adipose Tissue

A variety of other tissues under study appear to have stem cell populations, including adipose tissue. Cells derived from human adipose tissue have been reported to form a number of different cell lineages, including cardiomyocytes, in vitro (119). Therapeutic benefits of application of these cells in in vivo animal models remain to be demonstrated.

CLINICAL TRIALS OF CELL-BASED THERAPY

Multiple groups have initiated and reported early clinical trials of cardiac cell therapy (Table 47-4). Although many have inferred some improvement in cardiac function, it is important to note that most have been either uncontrolled and compared only to baseline measurements, or compared to historical controls. Given the frequent improvement of cardiac function after initial ischemic insult (particularly when accompanied by reperfusion, as in many of these trials), such inferences must be interpreted cautiously. To date, one randomized, controlled trial (155) also reported an improvement in ejection fraction at 6 months after coronary infusion of unfractionated bone marrow cells in acute infarct patients. Of note, in this trial all patients were not subjected to precisely the same treatments (presumably because of ethical concerns regarding risk) and thus the trial could not be fully blinded. Interestingly, the early benefit of cell therapy over standard therapy apparently was not sustained at 1 year. Nevertheless, this important trial provides a significant first step toward rigorously evaluating the potential benefits—and risks—of such therapies. Ongoing randomized, double-blind trials should add to our understanding of the role of cell therapy.

Important conceptual distinctions should be noted in the rationale and design of trials reported to date. Some are directed at improving myocardial perfusion through formation of new vessels. Understandably, this approach has primarily been directed at acute infarct patients, although patients with chronic, intractable ischemia represent another potential target population. Other trials attempt primarily to rescue heart failure through implantation of cells that will restore contractile function, presumably through generation of new cardiomyocytes. As previously noted, the method of delivery in these two types of trials also mirrors disease features. In acute MI, cells are generally infused via the coronaries, often under high pressure with intermittent occlusion of flow. In contrast, intramyocardial injections (for example, in the border zones of chronic infarcts identified by electromechanical mapping) have been used more commonly in treating chronic heart failure.

Progenitor Cell Treatment for Acute MI

Four trials implanting cells have reported intracoronary infusion of progenitor cells after acute MI (118,155–157). Although patients receiving cell therapy demonstrated some improvement in left ventricular ejection fraction and end-systolic volume parameters [most frequently measured with magnetic resonance imaging (MRI)], concerns regarding how these trials were controlled and/or blinded, as well as the short duration of follow-up, preclude definitive conclusions regarding any efficacy. Notably, of the cumulative 119 patients treated, no intracoronary embolic events were reported and the rates of malignant arrhythmias, restenosis, or death appear comparable to rates with standard therapy alone.

Interestingly, despite significant differences in the cell number delivered (three orders of magnitude), timing after MI (from 1 day to 2 weeks), and the cell populations used (unfractionated bone marrow versus circulating EPCs), the magnitude of benefit was remarkably similar. Across the four studies, left ventricular ejection fraction in the treated groups generally improved 6% to 10%, whereas end-systolic volume improved by 15% to 20%. The explanation for this is not clear. It is possible that only a small subpopulation of cells in these injections is actually responsible for the beneficial effect, although one might then expect a lack of effect in trials using too few cells. Alternatively, some other barrier may function as a bottleneck for successful engraftment, such that the number of cells infused is not rate-limiting in these studies. Some recent work has also suggested that a phenomenon of postconditioning may also exist, where intermittent ischemia reflow episodes after re-establishment of luminal patency in acute MI may actually help to preserve myocyte viability (158,159). Current trials cannot exclude the possibility that intracoronary infusion itself (requiring 3 to 15 balloon inflations for 2 to 4 minutes per inflation) might have some biological effect because control patients (when present) were not subjected to this same treatment. Nevertheless, these trials suggest that intracoronary infusion of these cells is relatively safe in the setting of acute MI. Demonstration of true efficacy awaits larger double-blind and randomized controlled trials.

Progenitor Cell Therapy for Chronic Myocardial Ischemia

Trials utilizing cell therapy in chronic ischemic heart disease have used direct intramyocardial injections of cells into the myocardium at infarct border zones. These injections may be done at the time of coronary artery bypass graft (CABG) surgery under direct visualization, or via an intracardiac catheter with adjunctive electromechanical mapping to identify viable regions. As noted earlier, the first cardiomyoplasty used skeletal myoblasts implanted at the time of CABG. Symptoms improved in the 10 treated patients, as did ejection fraction (from 24% to 32%) (4), although, as noted, the absence of a control group precludes conclusions regarding efficacy; the concomitant revascularization obviously confounds the contribution of cell therapy. Four of the 10 patients developed sustained ventricular tachycardia and required implantation of defibrillators. The lack of appropriate electrical coupling between myoblast and cardiomyocyte may lead to spatially distinct calcium currents that, in turn, predispose to arrhythmia. ICDs are currently mandatory in patients undergoing trials of skeletal myoblast stem cell therapy.

After direct intramyocardial injection of unfractionated bone marrow (71,160,161), a decrease in the hypoperfused area and subjective angina scores were noted. The improvement in perfusion per se suggests that the implanted cells may contribute to neovascularization in these contexts, as well. Improvement in cardiac indexes was variable, although studies enrolling patients with lower baseline cardiac function appeared to improve more after treatment as measured by change in ejection fraction or exercise capacity (71,160–162). However, the heterogeneity of the populations treated, as well as absence of randomized, blinded controls in these trials, may confound this analysis. Of note, no increase in ventricular arrhythmias has been reported after transplantation of bone marrow populations, nor have acute mechanical complications of direct injection been reported in these early experiences.

FUTURE DIRECTIONS

The increasing population of patients with congestive heart failure provides a clinical impetus to consider novel therapeutic approaches, including targeted genetic and stem cell therapies. Gene- and cell-based therapies hold great potential for the amelioration of heart failure, and a large number of genes and cell populations have shown promise in animal studies. The transition from preclinical, animal models to human clinical trials must be tempered with caution, however, because of the inherent limitations of such animals models and also because the risks are likely significant and difficult to anticipate fully. Additional research is needed to inform and guide these efforts. Continued improvement in vector systems and promoter elements provides tissue-specific and/or regulated transgene expression; further evaluation and validation of potential targets will be a necessary foundation for successful genetic therapies. Ongoing efforts to better characterize progenitor cell populations and to understand the mechanisms of recruitment, homing, and integration of progenitor cell populations, as well as potential paracrine contributions to repair, will facilitate efforts at cell replacement therapy. As clinical trials proceed in either gene- or cell-based therapies, rigorous controlled trials assessing efficacy on hard clinical endpoints as well as long-term safety will be essential. For each clinical target, potential risks and benefits must be carefully considered in the context of the patient population and available conventional therapeutic options. While it is premature to conclude whether these efforts will ultimately be successful, a combination of rigorous basic and clinical research will at least provide answers to these questions and may open new avenues of therapeutic possibilities.

REFERENCES

1. Chao W, Matsui T, Novikov MS, et al. Strategic advantages of insulin-like growth factor-1 expression for cardioprotection. *J Gene Med.* 2003;5:277–286.
2. Hacein-Bey-Abina S, von Kalle C, Schmidt M, et al. A serious adverse event after successful gene therapy for X-linked severe combined immunodeficiency. *N Engl J Med.* 2003;348:255–256.
3. Marshall E. Gene therapy death prompts review of adenovirus vector. *Science.* 1999;286:2244–2245.
4. Menasche P, Hagege AA, Vilquin JT, et al. Autologous skeletal myoblast transplantation for severe postinfarction left ventricular dysfunction. *J Am Coll Cardiol.* 2003;41:1078–1083.
5. Gao GP, Wilson JM, Wivel NA. Production of recombinant adeno-associated virus. *Adv Virus Res.* 2000;55:529–543.
6. Cemazar M, Sersa G, Wilson J, et al. Effective gene transfer to solid tumors using different nonviral gene delivery techniques: electroporation liposomes and integrin-targeted vector. *Cancer Gene Ther.* 2002;9:399–406.
7. Rosenzweig A, ed. *Vectors for Gene Therapy.* New York: John Wiley & Sons; 2001: 12.10.13–12.18.19.
8. Isner JM. Myocardial gene therapy. *Nature.* 2002;415:234–239.
9. Marban E. Cardiac channelopathies. *Nature.* 2002;415:213–218.
10. Towbin JA, Bowles NE. The failing heart. *Nature.* 2002;415: 227–233.
11. Song YK, Zhang G, Liu D. Cationic liposome-mediated DNA delivery to the lung endothelium. *Methods Mol Biol.* 2004;245:115–124.
12. Sen L, Hong YS, Luo H, et al. Efficiency, efficacy, and adverse effects of adenovirus vs. liposome-mediated gene therapy in cardiac allografts. *Am J Physiol.* (*Heart Circ Physiol.*) 2001;281:H1433–H1441.
13. Shin WS, Kawaguchi H, Liao JK, et al. Toxic action of nitric oxide on myocardial cells: direct evidence from gene transfer in vivo. *J Card Fail.* 1996;2:S149–S153.
14. Korpanty G, Chen S, Shohet RV, et al. Targeting of VEGF-mediated angiogenesis to rat myocardium using ultrasonic destruction of microbubbles. *Gene Ther.* 2005;12(17):1305–1312.
15. Wilson JM, Grossman M, Wu CH, et al. Hepatocyte-directed gene transfer in vivo leads to transient improvement of hypercholesterolemia in low density lipoprotein receptor-deficient rabbits. *J Biol Chem.* 1992;267:963–967.
16. Sullenger BA, White RR, Rusconi CP. Therapeutic aptamers and antidotes: a novel approach to safer drug design. *Ernst Schering Res Found Workshop.* 2003;217–223.
17. Gratton JP, Yu J, Griffith JW, et al. Cell-permeable peptides improve cellular uptake and therapeutic gene delivery of replication-deficient viruses in cells and in vivo. *Nat Med.* 2003;9:357–362.
18. Hajjar RJ, Schmidt U, Matsui T, et al. Modulation of ventricular function through gene transfer in vivo. *Proc Natl Acad Sci USA.* 1998;95:5251–5256.
19. Chirmule N, Propert K, Magosin S, et al. Immune responses to adenovirus and adeno-associated virus in humans. *Gene Ther.* 1999;6:1574–1583.
20. Cichon G, Boeckh-Herwig S, Schmidt HH, et al. Complement activation by recombinant adenoviruses. *Gene Ther.* 2001;8:1794–1800.
21. Rafii S, Dias S, Meeus S, et al. Infection of endothelium with E1(−)E4(+) but not E1(−)E4(−) adenovirus gene transfer vectors enhances leukocyte adhesion and migration by modulation of ICAM-1, VCAM-1, CD34, and chemokine expression. *Circ Res.* 2001;88:903–910.
22. Newman KD, Dunn PF, Owens JW, et al. Adenovirus-mediated gene transfer into normal rabbit arteries results in prolonged vascular cell activation inflammation and neointimal hyperplasia. *J Clin Invest.* 1995;96:2955–2965.
23. Lochmuller H, Jani A, Huard J, et al. Emergence of early region 1-containing replication-competent adenovirus in stocks of replication-defective adenovirus recombinants (delta E1 + delta E3) during multiple passages in 293 cells. *Hum Gene Ther.* 1994;5:1485–1491.
24. Martin AB, Webber S, Fricker FJ, et al. Acute myocarditis. Rapid diagnosis by PCR in children. *Circulation* 1994;90:330–339.
25. Bergelson JM, Cunningham JA, Droguett G, et al. Isolation of a common receptor for coxsackie B viruses and adenoviruses 2 and 5. *Science.* 1997;275:1320–1323.
26. Kim JS, Lee SH, Cho YS, et al. Development of a packaging cell line for propagation of replication-deficient adenovirus vector. *Exp Mol Med.* 2001;33:145–149.
27. del Monte F, Williams E, Lebeche D, et al. Improvement in survival and cardiac metabolism following gene transfer of SERCA2a in a rat model of heart failure. *Circulation.* 2001;104(12):1424–1429.
28. Del Monte F, Butler K, Boecker W, et al. Novel technique of aortic banding followed by gene transfer during hypertrophy and heart failure. *Physiol Genomics.* 2002;9:49–56.
29. del Monte F, Harding SE, Dec GW, et al. Targeting phospholamban by gene transfer in human heart failure. *Circulation.* 2002;105:904–907.
30. Dai Y, Schwarz EM, Gu D, et al. Cellular and humoral immune responses to adenoviral vectors containing factor IX gene: tolerization of factor IX and vector antigens allows for long-term expression. *Proc Natl Acad Sci USA.* 1995;92:1401–1405.
31. Fang B, Eisensmith RC, Wang H, et al. Gene therapy for hemophilia B: host immunosuppression prolongs the therapeutic effect of adenovirus-mediated factor IX expression. *Hum Gene Ther.* 1995;6:1039–1044.
32. Kay MA, Holterman AX, Meuse L, et al. Long-term hepatic adenovirus-mediated gene expression in mice following CTLA4Ig administration. *Nat Genet.* 1995;11:191–197.
33. Engelhardt JF, Ye X, Doranz B, et al. Ablation of E2A in recombinant adenoviruses improves transgene persistence and decreases inflammatory response in mouse liver. *Proc Natl Aca Sci USA.* 1994;91:6196–6200.
34. Kochanek S, Clemens PR, Mitani K, et al. A new adenoviral vector: replacement of all viral coding sequences with 28 kb of DNA independently expressing both full-length dystrophin and beta-galactosidase. *Proc Natl Aca Sci USA.* 1996;93:5731–5736.
35. Wen S, Driscoll RM, Schneider DB, et al. Inclusion of the E3 region in an adenoviral vector decreases inflammation and neointima formation after arterial gene transfer. *Arterioscler Thromb Vasc Biol.* 2001;21:1777–1782.

36. Ng P, Evelegh C, Cummings D, et al. Cre levels limit packaging signal excision efficiency in the Cre/loxP helper-dependent adenoviral vector system. *J Virol.* 2002;76:4181–4189.
37. Gao G, Qu G, Burnham MS, et al. Purification of recombinant adeno-associated virus vectors by column chromatography and its performance in vivo. *Hum Gene Ther.* 2000;11:2079–2091.
38. Ng P, Parks RJ, Cummings DT, et al. A high-efficiency Cre/loxP-based system for construction of adenoviral vectors. *Hum Gene Ther.* 1999;10:2667–2672.
39. Cordier L, Gao GP, Hack AA, et al. Muscle-specific promoters may be necessary for adeno-associated virus-mediated gene transfer in the treatment of muscular dystrophies. *Hum Gene Ther.* 2001;12:205–215.
40. Svensson EC, Marshall DJ, Woodard K, et al. Efficient and stable transduction of cardiomyocytes after intramyocardial injection or intracoronary perfusion with recombinant adeno-associated virus vectors. *Circulation.* 1999;99:201–205.
41. Chao H, Liu Y, Rabinowitz J, et al. Several log increase in therapeutic transgene delivery by distinct adeno-associated viral serotype vectors. *Mol Ther.* 2000;2:619–623.
42. Gao GP, Alvira MR, Wang L, et al. Novel adeno-associated viruses from rhesus monkeys as vectors for human gene therapy. *Proc Natl Acad Sci USA.* 2002;99:11854–11859.
43. Du L, Kido M, Lee DV, et al. Differential myocardial gene delivery by recombinant serotype-specific adeno-associated viral vectors. *Mol Ther.* 2004;10:604–608.
44. Erles K, Sebokova P, Schlehofer JR. Update on the prevalence of serum antibodies (IgG and IgM) to adeno-associated virus (AAV). *J Med Virol.* 1999;59:406–411.
45. Rabinowitz JE, Rolling F, Li C, et al. Cross-packaging of a single adeno-associated virus (AAV) type 2 vector genome into multiple AAV serotypes enables transduction with broad specificity. *J Virol.* 2002;76:791–801.
46. Xiao W, Chirmule N, Berta SC, et al. Gene therapy vectors based on adeno-associated virus type 1. *J Virol.* 1999;73:3994–4003.
47. Wang Z, Zhu T, Qiao C, et al. Adeno-associated virus serotype 8 efficiently delivers genes to muscle and heart. *Nat Biotechnol.* 2005;23:321–328.
48. Fu H, Muenzer J, Samulski RJ, et al. Self-complementary adeno-associated virus serotype 2 vector: global distribution and broad dispersion of AAV-mediated transgene expression in mouse brain. *Mol Ther.* 2003;8:911–917.
49. Check E. Second cancer case halts gene-therapy trials. *Nature.* 2003;421:305.
50. Naldini L, Blomer U, Gallay P, et al. In vivo gene delivery and stable transduction of nondividing cells by a lentiviral vector. *Science.* 1996;272:263–267.
51. Naldini L, Blomer U, Gage FH, et al. Efficient transfer integration and sustained long-term expression of the transgene in adult rat brains injected with a lentiviral vector. *Proc Natl Acad Sci USA.* 1996;93:11382–11388.
52. Sakoda T, Kasahara N, Hamamori Y, et al. A high-titer lentiviral production system mediates efficient transduction of differentiated cells including beating cardiac myocytes. *J Mol Cell Cardiol.* 1999;31:2037–2047.
53. Peng KW, Pham L, Ye H, et al. Organ distribution of gene expression after intravenous infusion of targeted and untargeted lentiviral vectors. *Gene Ther.* 2001;8:1456–1463.
54. MacKenzie TC, Kobinger GP, Kootstra NA, et al. Efficient transduction of liver and muscle after in utero injection of lentiviral vectors with different pseudotypes. *Mol Ther.* 2002;6:349–358.
55. Zhao J, Pettigrew GJ, Thomas J, et al. Lentiviral vectors for delivery of genes into neonatal and adult ventricular cardiac myocytes in vitro and in vivo. *Basic Res Cardiol.* 2002;97:348–358.
56. Bonci D, Cittadini A, Latronico MV, et al. "Advanced" generation lentiviruses as efficient vectors for cardiomyocyte gene transduction in vitro and in vivo. *Gene Ther.* 2003;10:630–636.
57. DePolo NJ, Reed JD, Sheridan PL, et al. VSV-G pseudotyped lentiviral vector particles produced in human cells are inactivated by human serum. *Mol Ther.* 2000;2:218–222.
58. Goins WF, Krisky DM, Wolfe DP, et al. Development of replication-defective herpes simplex virus vectors. *Methods Mol Med.* 2002;69:481–507.
59. Hollon T. Researchers and regulators reflect on first gene therapy death. *Nat Med.* 2000;6:6.
60. Bostanci A. Gene therapy. Blood test flags agent in death of Penn subject. *Science.* 2002;295:604–605.
61. Marshall E. Gene therapy death prompts review of adenovirus vector. *Science.* 1999;286:2244–2245.
62. Goncalves MA, van Nierop GP, Tijssen MR, et al. Transfer of the full-length dystrophin-coding sequence into muscle cells by a dual high-capacity hybrid viral vector with site-specific integration ability. *J Virol.* 2005;79:3146–3162.
63. Recillas-Targa F, Valadez-Graham V, Farrell CM. Prospects and implications of using chromatin insulators in gene therapy and transgenesis. *Bioessays.* 2004;26:796–807.
64. Qasim W, Gaspar HB, Thrasher AJ. T cell suicide gene therapy to aid haematopoietic stem cell transplantation. *Curr Gene Ther.* 2005;5:121–132.
65. Guzman RJ, Lemarchand P, Crystal RG, et al. Efficient gene transfer into myocardium by direct injection of adenovirus vectors. *Circ Res.* 1993;73:1202–1207.
66. Hajjar RJ, Schmidt U, Matsui T, et al. Modulation of ventricular function through gene transfer in vivo. *Proc Natl Acad Sci USA.* 1998;95:5251–5256.
67. Donahue JK, Kikkawa K, Thomas AD, et al. Acceleration of widespread adenoviral gene transfer to intact rabbit hearts by coronary perfusion with low calcium and serotonin. *Gene Ther.* 1998;5:630–634.
68. Fromes Y, Salmon A, Wang X, et al. Gene delivery to the myocardium by intrapericardial injection. *Gene Ther.* 1999;6:683–688.
69. Ikeda Y, Gu Y, Iwanaga Y, et al. Restoration of deficient membrane proteins in the cardiomyopathic hamster by in vivo cardiac gene transfer. *Circulation.* 2002;105:502–508.
70. Kocher AA, Schuster MD, Szabolcs MJ, et al. Neovas cularization of ischemic myocardium by human bone-marrow-derived angioblasts prevents cardiomyocyte apoptosis, reduces remodeling and improves cardiac function. *Nat Med.* 2001;7:430–436.
71. Perin EC, Dohmann HF, Borojevic R, et al. Transendocardial autologous bone marrow cell transplantation for severe chronic ischemic heart failure. *Circulation.* 2003;107:2294–2302.
72. Rosengart TK, Lee LY, Patel SR, et al. Angiogenesis gene therapy: phase I assessment of direct intramyocardial administration of an adenovirus vector expressing VEGF121 cDNA to individuals with clinically significant severe coronary artery disease. *Circulation.* 1999;100:468–474.
73. Hagege AA, Carrion C, Menasche P, et al. Viability and differentiation of autologous skeletal myoblast grafts in ischaemic cardiomyopathy. *Lancet.* 2003;361:491–492.
74. Giordano FJ, Ping P, McKirnan MD, et al. Intracoronary gene transfer of fibroblast growth factor-5 increases blood flow and contractile function in an ischemic region of the heart. *Nat Med.* 1996;2:534–539.
75. Kaspar BK, Roth DM, Lai NC, et al. Myocardial gene transfer and long-term expression following intracoronary delivery of adeno-associated virus. *J Gene Med.* 2005;7:316–324.
76. Lai NC, Roth DM, Gao MH, et al. Intracoronary adenovirus encoding adenylyl cyclase VI increases left ventricular function in heart failure. *Circulation.* 2004;110:330–336.
77. Champion HC, Georgakopoulos D, Haldar S, et al. Robust adenoviral and adeno-associated viral gene transfer to the in vivo murine heart: application to study of phospholamban physiology. *Circulation.* 2003;108:2790–2797.
78. Miyamoto MI, del Monte F, Schmidt U, et al. Adenoviral gene transfer of SERCA2a improves left-ventricular function in aortic-banded rats in transition to heart failure. *Proc Natl Acad Sci USA.* 2000;97:793–798.
79. Davidson MJ, Jones JM, Emani SM, et al. Cardiac gene delivery with cardiopulmonary bypass. *Circulation.* 2001;104:131–133.
80. Boekstegers P, von Degenfeld G, Giehrl W, et al. Myocardial gene transfer by selective pressure-regulated retroinfusion of coronary veins. *Gene Ther.* 2000;7:232–240.
81. Isner JM, Losordo DW. Therapeutic angiogenesis for heart failure. *Nat Med.* 1999;5:491–492.
82. Shyu KG, Wang MT, Wang BW, et al. Intramyocardial injection of naked DNA encoding HIF-1alpha/VP16 hybrid to enhance angiogenesis in an acute myocardial infarction model in the rat. *Cardiovasc Res.* 2002;54:576–583.

83. Mack CA, Patel SR, Schwarz EA, et al. Biologic bypass with the use of adenovirus-mediated gene transfer of the complementary deoxyribonucleic acid for vascular endothelial growth factor 121 improves myocardial perfusion and function in the ischemic porcine heart. *J Thorac Cardiovasc Surg.* 1998;115:168–176; discussion 176–167.
84. Losordo DW, Vale PR, Hendel RC, et al. Phase 1/2 placebo-controlled double-blind dose-escalating trial of myocardial vascular endothelial growth factor 2 gene transfer by catheter delivery in patients with chronic myocardial ischemia. *Circulation.* 2002; 105:2012–2018.
85. Wencker D, Chandra M, Nguyen K, et al. A mechanistic role for cardiac myocyte apoptosis in heart failure. *J Clin Invest.* 2003;111:1497–1504.
86. Matsui T, Tao J, del Monte F, et al. Akt activation preserves cardiac function and prevents injury after transient cardiac ischemia in vivo. *Circulation.* 2001;104:330–335.
87. Cory S, Adams JM. The Bcl2 family: regulators of the cellular life-or-death switch. *Nat Rev Cancer.* 2002;2:647–656.
88. Chatterjee S, Stewart AS, Bish LT, et al. Viral gene transfer of the antiapoptotic factor Bcl-2 protects against chronic postischemic heart failure. *Circulation.* 2002;106:I212–I217.
89. Ozcelik C, Erdmann B, Pilz B, et al. Conditional mutation of the ErbB2 (HER2) receptor in cardiomyocytes leads to dilated cardiomyopathy. *Proc Natl Acad Sci USA.* 2002;99:8880–8885.
90. Crone SA, Zhao YY, Fan L, et al. ErbB2 is essential in the prevention of dilated cardiomyopathy. *Nat Med.* 2002;8:459–465.
91. Grazette LP, Boecker W, Matsui T, et al. Inhibition of ErbB2 causes mitochondrial dysfunction in cardiomyocytes. Implications for herceptin-induced cardiomyopathy. *J Am Coll Cardiol.* 2004; 44:2231–2238.
92. Narula J, Pandey P, Arbustini E, et al. Apoptosis in heart failure: release of cytochrome C from mitochondria and activation of caspase-3 in human cardiomyopathy. *Proc Natl Acad Sci USA.* 1999;96:8144–8149.
93. Franke TF, Cantley LC. Apoptosis. A bad kinase makes good [news]. *Nature.* 1997;390:116–117.
94. Cantley LC. The phosphoinositide 3-kinase pathway. *Science.* 2002;296:1655–1657.
95. Matsui T, Li L, del Monte F, et al. Adenoviral gene transfer of activated phosphatidylinositol 3′-kinase and Akt inhibits apoptosis of hypoxic cardiomyocytes in vitro. *Circulation.* 1999;100: 2373–2379.
96. Matsui T, Tao J, del Monte F, et al. Akt activation preserves cardiac function and prevents injury after transient cardiac ischemia in vivo. *Circulation.* 2001;104:330–335.
97. Haq S, Choukroun G, Lim H, et al. Differential activation of signal transduction pathways in human hearts with hypertrophy versus advanced heart failure. *Circulation.* 2001;103:670–677.
98. Shioi T, McMullen JR, Kang PM, et al. Akt/protein kinase B promotes organ growth in transgenic mice. *Mol Cell Biol.* 2002;22:2799–2809.
99. Condorelli G, Drusco A, Stassi G, et al. Akt induces enhanced myocardial contractility and cell size in vivo in transgenic mice. *Proc Natl Acad Sci USA.* 2002;99:12333–12338.
100. Matsui T, Li L, Wu JC, et al. Phenotypic spectrum caused by transgenic overexpression of activated Akt in the heart. *J Biol Chem.* 2002;277:22896–22901.
101. Nagoshi T, Matsui T, Aoyama T, et al. Phosphoinositide 3-kinase rescues the detrimental effects of chronic Akt activation in the heart during ischemia-reperfusion injury. JCI. 2005;115(8): 2128–2138.
102. Aoyama T, Matsui T, Novikov M, et al. Serum and glucocorticoid-responsive kinase-1 regulates cardiomyocyte survival and hypertrophic response. *Circulation.* 2005;111:1652–1659.
103. Tsujimoto Y, Finger LR, Yunis J, et al. Cloning of the chromosome breakpoint of neoplastic B cells with the t(14;18) chromosome translocation. *Science.* 1984;226:1097–1099.
104. Bellacosa A, Testa JR, Staal SP, et al. A retroviral oncogene, akt, encoding a serine-threonine kinase containing an SH2-like region. *Science.* 1991;254:274–277.
105. Maurice JP, Hata JA, Shah AS, et al. Enhancement of cardiac function after adenoviral-mediated in vivo intracoronary beta2-adrenergic receptor gene delivery. *J Clin Invest.* 1999;104: 21–29.
106. Akhter SA, Skaer CA, Kypson AP, et al. Restoration of beta-adrenergic signaling in failing cardiac ventricular myocytes via adenoviral-mediated gene transfer. *Proc Natl Acad Sci USA.* 1997;94:12100–12105.
107. Akhter SA, Luttrell LM, Rockman HA, et al. Targeting the receptor-Gq interface to inhibit in vivo pressure overload myocardial hypertrophy. *Science.* 1998;280:574–577.
108. Esposito G, Prasad SV, Rapacciuolo A, et al. Cardiac overexpression of a G(q) inhibitor blocks induction of extracellular signal-regulated kinase and c-Jun NH(2)-terminal kinase activity in in vivo pressure overload. *Circulation.* 2001;103:1453–1458.
109. www.wiley.co.uk/genmed. Clinical trials: charts and statistics.
110. Packer M, Carver JR, Rodeheffer RJ, et al. Effect of oral milrinone on mortality in severe chronic heart failure. The PROMISE Study Research Group. *N Engl J Med.* 1991;325:1468–1475.
111. Beuckelmann DJ, Nabauer M, Erdmann E. Intracellular calcium handling in isolated ventricular myocytes from patients with terminal heart failure [see comments]. *Circulation.* 1992;85:1046–1055.
112. Hasenfuss G. Calcium pump overexpression and myocardial function. Implications for gene therapy of myocardial failure [editorial; comment]. *Circ Res.* 1998;83:966–968.
113. Hajjar RJ, Kang JX, Gwathmey JK, et al. Physiological effects of adenoviral gene transfer of sarcoplasmic reticulum calcium ATPase in isolated rat myocytes. *Circulation.* 1997;95:423–429.
114. del Monte F, Harding SE, Schmidt U, et al. Restoration of contractile function in isolated cardiomyocytes from failing human hearts by gene transfer of SERCA2a. *Circulation.* 1999;100: 2308–2311.
115. del Monte F, Williams E, Lebeche D, et al. Improvement in survival and cardiac metabolism after gene transfer of sarcoplasmic reticulum Ca(2+)-ATPase in a rat model of heart failure. *Circulation.* 2001;104:1424–1429.
116. Kehat I, Kenyagin-Karsenti D, Snir M, et al. Human embryonic stem cells can differentiate into myocytes with structural and functional properties of cardiomyocytes. *J Clin Invest.* 2001;108:407–414.
117. Makino S, Fukuda K, Miyoshi S, et al. Cardiomyocytes can be generated from marrow stromal cells in vitro. *J Clin Invest.* 1999;103:697–705.
118. Assmus B, Schachinger V, Teupe C, et al. Transplantation of Progenitor Cells and Regeneration Enhancement in Acute Myocardial Infarction (TOPCARE-AMI). *Circulation.* 2002;106:3009–3017.
119. Rangappa S, Fen C, Lee EH, et al. Transformation of adult mesenchymal stem cells isolated from the fatty tissue into cardiomyocytes. *Ann Thorac Surg.* 2003;75:775–779.
120. Gnecchi M, He H, Liang OD, et al. Paracrine action accounts for marked protection of ischemic heart by Akt-modified mesenchymal stem cells. *Nat Med.* 2005;11:367–368.
121. Beltrami AP, Barlucchi L, Torella D, et al. Adult cardiac stem cells are multipotent and support myocardial regeneration. *Cell.* 2003;114:763–776.
122. Oh H, Bradfute SB, Gallardo TD, et al. Cardiac progenitor cells from adult myocardium: homing differentiation and fusion after infarction. *Proc Natl Acad Sci USA.* 2003;100:12313–12318.
123. Laugwitz KL, Moretti A, Lam J, et al. Postnatal isl1+ cardioblasts enter fully differentiated cardiomyocyte lineages. *Nature.* 2005;433:647–653.
124. Schatteman GC, Awad O. Hemangioblasts angioblasts, and adult endothelial cell progenitors. *Anat Rec A Discov Mol Cell Evol Biol.* 2004;276:13–21.
125. Peichev M, Naiyer AJ, Pereira D, et al. Expression of VEGFR-2 and AC133 by circulating human CD34(+) cells identifies a population of functional endothelial precursors. *Blood.* 2000;95:952–958.
126. Gehling UM, Ergun S, Schumacher U, et al. In vitro differentiation of endothelial cells from AC133-positive progenitor cells. *Blood* 2000;95:3106–3112.
127. Lin Y, Weisdorf DJ, Solovey A, et al. Origins of circulating endothelial cells and endothelial outgrowth from blood. *J Clin Invest.* 2000;105:71–77.
128. Takahashi T, Kalka C, Masuda H, et al. Ischemia- and cytokine-induced mobilization of bone marrow-derived endothelial progenitor cells for neovascularization. *Nat Med.* 1999;5: 434–438.
129. Askari AT, Unzek S, Popovic ZB, et al. Effect of stromal-cell-derived factor 1 on stem-cell homing and tissue regeneration in ischaemic cardiomyopathy. *Lancet.* 2003;362:697–703.
130. Bahlmann FH, De Groot K, Spandau JM, et al. Erythropoietin regulates endothelial progenitor cells. *Blood.* 2004;103:921–926.

131. Reyes M, Dudek A, Jahagirdar B, et al. Origin of endothelial progenitors in human postnatal bone marrow. *J Clin Invest.* 2002;109:337–346.
132. Shi Q, Rafii S, Wu MH, et al. Evidence for circulating bone marrow-derived endothelial cells. *Blood.* 1998;92:362–367.
133. Schmeisser A, Garlichs CD, Zhang H, et al. Monocytes coexpress endothelial and macrophagocytic lineage markers and form cord-like structures in Matrigel under angiogenic conditions. *Cardiovasc Res.* 2001;49:671–680.
134. Jackson KA, Majka SM, Wang H, et al. Regeneration of ischemic cardiac muscle and vascular endothelium by adult stem cells. *J Clin Invest.* 2001;107:1395–1402.
135. Lyden D, Hattori K, Dias S, et al. Impaired recruitment of bone-marrow-derived endothelial and hematopoietic precursor cells blocks tumor angiogenesis and growth. *Nat Med.* 2001;7: 1194–1201.
136. Crosby JR, Kaminski WE, Schatteman G, et al. Endothelial cells of hematopoietic origin make a significant contribution to adult blood vessel formation. *Circ Res.* 2000;87:728–730.
137. Murayama T, Tepper OM, Silver M, et al. Determination of bone marrow-derived endothelial progenitor cell significance in angiogenic growth factor-induced neovascularization in vivo. *Exp Hematol.* 2002;30:967–972.
138. Werner N, Junk S, Laufs U, et al. Intravenous transfusion of endothelial progenitor cells reduces neointima formation after vascular injury. *Circ Res.* 2003;93:e17–24.
139. Walter DH, Rittig K, Bahlmann FH, et al. Statin therapy accelerates reendothelialization: a novel effect involving mobilization and incorporation of bone marrow-derived endothelial progenitor cells. *Circulation.* 2002;105:3017–3024.
140. Hill JM, Zalos G, Halcox JP, et al. Circulating endothelial progenitor cells, vascular function, and cardiovascular risk. *N Engl J Med.* 2003;348:593–600.
141. Leobon B, Garcin I, Menasche P, et al. Myoblasts transplanted into rat infarcted myocardium are functionally isolated from their host. *Proc Natl Acad Sci USA.* 2003;100:7808–7811.
142. Ghostine S, Carrion C, Souza LC, et al. Long-term efficacy of myoblast transplantation on regional structure and function after myocardial infarction. *Circulation.* 2002;106:I131–I136.
143. Menasche P, Hagege AA, Scorsin M, et al. Myoblast transplantation for heart failure. *Lancet.* 2001;357:279–280.
144. Menasche P. Skeletal myoblast for cell therapy. *Coron Artery Dis.* 2005;16:105–110.
145. Orlic D, Kajstura J, Chimenti S, et al. Mobilized bone marrow cells repair the infarcted heart improving function and survival. *Proc Natl Acad Sci USA.* 2001;98:10344–10349.
146. Orlic D, Kajstura J, Chimenti S, et al. Bone marrow cells regenerate infarcted myocardium. *Nature.* 2001;410:701–705.
147. Murry CE, Soonpaa MH, Reinecke H, et al. Haematopoietic stem cells do not transdifferentiate into cardiac myocytes in myocardial infarcts. *Nature.* 2004;428:664–668.
148. Balsam LB, Wagers AJ, Christensen JL, et al. Haematopoietic stem cells adopt mature haematopoietic fates in ischaemic myocardium. *Nature.* 2004;428:668–673.
149. Shake JG, Gruber PJ, Baumgartner WA, et al. Mesenchymal stem cell implantation in a swine myocardial infarct model: engraftment and functional effects. *Ann Thorac Surg.* 2002;73:1919–1925; discussion 1926.
150. Toma C, Pittenger MF, Cahill KS, et al. Human mesenchymal stem cells differentiate to a cardiomyocyte phenotype in the adult murine heart. *Circulation.* 2002;105:93–98.
151. Pittenger MF, Mackay AM, Beck SC, et al. Multilineage potential of adult human mesenchymal stem cells. *Science.* 1999;284:143–147.
152. Mangi AA, Noiseux N, Kong D, et al. Mesenchymal stem cells modified with Akt prevent remodeling and restore performance of infarcted hearts. *Nat Med.* 2003;9:1195–1201.
153. Kinnaird T, Stabile E, Burnett MS, et al. Marrow-derived stromal cells express genes encoding a broad spectrum of arteriogenic cytokines and promote in vitro and in vivo arteriogenesis through paracrine mechanisms. *Circ Res.* 2004;94:678–685.
154. Bhatia R, Hare JM. Mesenchymal stem cells: future source for reparative medicine. *Congest Heart Fail.* 2005;11:87–91; quiz 92–93.
155. Wollert KC, Meyer GP, Lotz J, et al. Intracoronary autologous bone-marrow cell transfer after myocardial infarction: the BOOST randomised controlled clinical trial. *Lancet.* 2004;364: 141–148-
156. Fernandez-Aviles F, San Roman JA, Garcia-Frade J, et al. Experimental and clinical regenerative capability of human bone marrow cells after myocardial infarction. *Circ Res.* 2004;95:742–748.
157. Strauer BE, Brehm M, Zeus T, et al. Repair of infarcted myocardium by autologous intracoronary mononuclear bone marrow cell transplantation in humans. *Circulation.* 2002;106: 1913–1918.
158. Hausenloy DJ, Yellon DM. New directions for protecting the heart against ischaemia-reperfusion injury: targeting the Reperfusion Injury Salvage Kinase (RISK)-pathway. *Cardiovasc Res.* 2004;61:448–460.
159. Tsang A, Hausenloy DJ, Mocanu MM, et al. Postconditioning: a form of "modified reperfusion" protects the myocardium by activating the phosphatidylinositol 3-kinase-Akt pathway. *Circ Res.* 2004;95:230–232.
160. Tse HF, Kwong YL, Chan JK, et al. Angiogenesis in ischaemic myocardium by intramyocardial autologous bone marrow mononuclear cell implantation. *Lancet.* 2003;361:47–49.
161. Fuchs S, Satler LF, Kornowski R, et al. Catheter-based autologous bone marrow myocardial injection in no-option patients with advanced coronary artery disease: a feasibility study. *J Am Coll Cardiol.* 2003;41:1721–1724.
162. Perin EC, Dohmann HF, Borojevic R, et al. Improved exercise capacity and ischemia 6 and 12 months after transendocardial injection of autologous bone marrow mononuclear cells for ischemic cardiomyopathy. *Circulation.* 2004;110: II213–II218.

End-of-Life Considerations

48

Marc A. Silver

"Perfection of tools and confusion of goals are characteristics of our time."

—Albert Einstein

Every other chapter in this text is dedicated to the enhanced diagnosis and treatment of patients who are in the continuum of heart failure stages. This chapter, however, focuses on the situation that occurs when the disease triumphs over the therapies we have to offer and the patient approaches the end of his or her life. Its goal is to help us understand the tools and skills we need, already have, and have yet to acquire to help our patients and their families during the stage of heart failure that leads to death.

DEFINING END-STAGE HEART FAILURE AND IMPAIRED AWARENESS OF ADVANCED DISEASE STATUS

Perhaps the greatest barrier in addressing end-of-life issues for patients with heart failure is the realization of when a patient is at or may be approaching that stage of his or her disease history. The common classification scenarios using clinical signs and symptoms, and even the New York Heart Association functional classification (Class I–IV), have been dysfunctional since clinicians often witness marked status improvements in some patients when therapy is altered. This often leads to an understanding on the part of the patient, the family, and even the treating team of physicians and nurses that the patient is substantially better and has distanced himself or herself from end of life.

One of the major contributions of the recent American College of Cardiology and American Heart Association (ACC/AHA) guidelines for the management of chronic heart failure was the introduction of a series of stages the patient who was initially at risk and subsequently has heart failure passes through (Stages A–D) (1). Several observations underscore the value of the staging approach. The first is that as a patient progresses from one stage to the next the progress proceeds in one direction only. The patient who develops symptomatic heart failure (e.g., Stage C) has forever missed their opportunity to only be at risk (Stage A) or have only asymptomatic ventricular dysfunction (Stage B). We may be creating a few exceptions to this rule with left ventricular mechanical assist, for example, but in general this observation holds true.

The second key observation regarding this staging system is that while the early stages (Stages A and B) may last years or decades, the latter stages (Stages C and D) are typically measured in years and often only months or weeks (Fig. 48-1). Based on these observations it would seem clear to the physicians and nurses, at least, that the patient who developed the signs and symptoms of heart failure should reasonably be considered a patient in an advanced stage of the disease process. Typically, these patients come to medical attention in greatly decompensated states with multiple organ systems impacted by the heart failure syndrome and its consequences, and yet the gravity often goes unnoticed.

There are myriad other indicators, ranging from neurohormonal measurements to actual Medicare hospitalization mortality rates for patients with heart failure, that indicate the advanced state and proximity to death of these patients (Table 48-1) (2). We are also aware of newer, simple clinical tools that use commonly available clinical and laboratory parameters to define in-hospital mortality as high as 20% for a given heart failure hospital admission

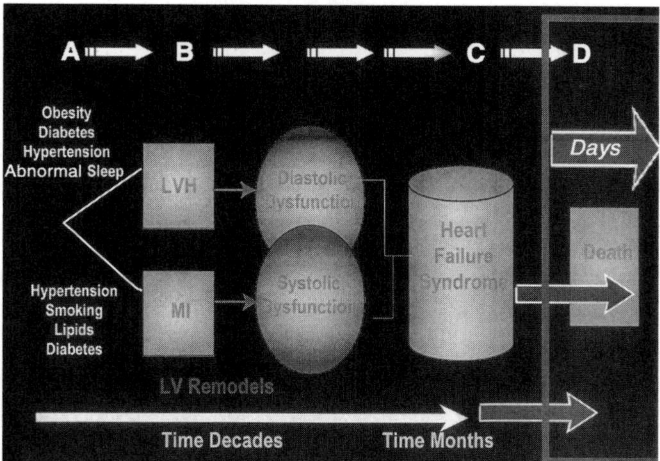

Figure 48-1 Drawing indicating the progression of heart failure according to the ACC/AHA stages of heart failure. The progression depicts a progressively shorter interval between stages as the disease progresses, with end of life coming often within days for patients with Stage D disease.

(3). Despite availability of these tools there has been extremely limited attention to or action focused on end-of-life disease planning. The barriers and gaps that can be identified are discussed later; nevertheless, the awareness of the advanced disease status of such patients may be the initial and most important barrier.

Even when there is an awareness of advanced disease status for patients, what is often communicated to them and their families is the likelihood of a more prolonged survival than typically occurs. In such cases, all involved may miss the opportunity to prepare adequately for end of life. Heart failure patients are not unique in this disparity in disease status and survival expectation. Even in patients with cancer there is frequently a gap between what is the perceived survival by treating physicians, the communicated survival, and the actual survival (4). Overall, a new paradigm must be developed and continued in the years ahead regarding the role of the professional staff and their need to objectify and identify end-of-life status, to communicate this effectively, as well as to provide better options.

OPTIONS FOR END-OF-LIFE CARE FOR HEART FAILURE PATIENTS

There are many options for patients with advanced heart failure, including those near end of life. As with other stages of heart failure, these options are limited by host factors and timing. For the patient hospitalized with cardiogenic shock and end-organ failure, the options may be quite limited. However, for many patients for whom the advanced state of their heart failure (see previous) and the natural trajectory of the disease state are recognized (Fig. 48-2), the options are more wide-ranging.

The possibilities for patients who are judged to be at the end of life range from simple steps that can be taken to limit further suffering and pain, to broad-scale planning of care, coordination of the care, careful discussions with the patient and those he or she chooses to help him or her in the final stages, and, perhaps equally important, the avoidance of additional tests and procedures. Other measures serve mainly to begin to gain patient and family acceptance and awareness of death. Somewhere in this process the caregiver should have begun to talk about the advanced nature of the disease and the options for advanced heart failure, including transplantation, left ventricular assist, and implanted cardiac defibrillators. Often this begins with a discussion of advanced directives.

Many patients at this advanced stage have already received those advanced therapies. For those who have not, however, a discussion of benefit and life objectives should take place prior to moving ahead with those therapies. The discussion that follows presumes prior discussions regarding advanced therapies and determination that these therapies either have already been employed or are not appropriate for the patient. The caregiver needs also to develop a skill set of communication that extends beyond eliciting advanced directives (5).

TABLE 48-1
PARTIAL LISTING OF METRICS FOR ADVANCED HEART FAILURE

Patients in Whom End-of-life Considerations Apply
Recurrent admissions and frailty requiring assistance with two or more activities of daily living
Patients with clinical worsening despite expert evaluation and treatment by a team experienced with advanced heart failure care
Patients unwilling or unable to tolerate more aggressive heart failure care
Patients who have undergone advanced therapies but now wish to deactivate them (e.g., implanted cardiac defibrillators)
NYHA functional status
Elderly age
Race
Comorbidities (e.g., renal insufficiency, hypotension)
Recent defibrillation
Elevated biomarkers (e.g., norepinephrine, B-type natriuretic hormone)

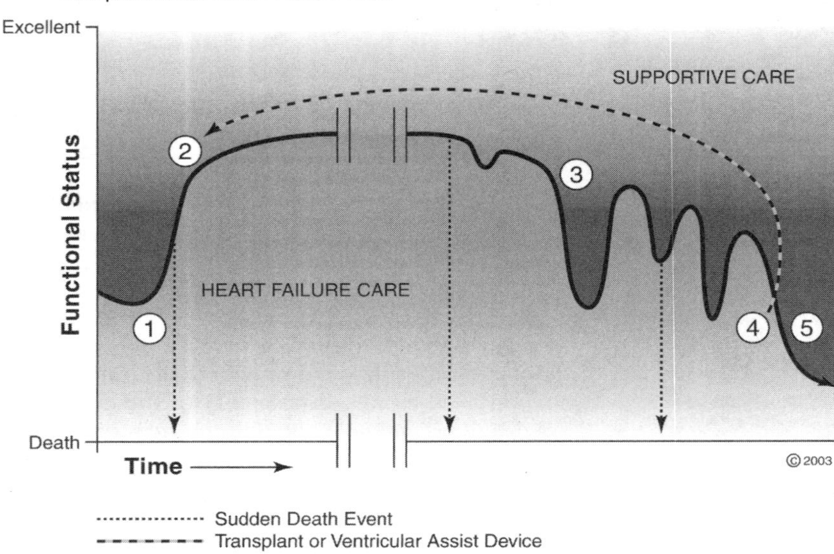

Figure 48-2 Natural trajectory of heart failure, Stages C and D. Note the recurrent periods of decompensation, shorter intervals between episodes of clinical deterioration, and failure to return to improved functional status. (From Goodlin SJ, Hauptman PJ, Arnold R, et al. Consensus statement: palliative and supportive care in advanced heart failure. *J Card Fail* 2004;10:200–209, with permission from Elsevier.)

For the health care provider facing these situations it is best to follow a pattern of discussion so that key information is not presumed by a particular patient or family. In general, these six discussion steps, adopted from Robert Buckman (6), include:

1. *Getting started.* This step involves preparation to make sure you have all the medical facts and have the collaboration of other key team members (other consultants, for example). If you are the primary caregiver as viewed by this patient and family, then this responsibility should not be delegated to anyone else or it will lose its import. Also, you should set aside enough time to have the conversation. The conversation should take place in a conducive environment (private, without interruptions) and should include the patient and whomever else he or she may indicate should be there. Once ready to begin, it is most important to introduce the topic and set goals for the conversation, such as, "Mr. Jones, thanks for allowing all of us to speak openly today. Your heart (renal/liver, etc.) failure is getting much worse and I believe you are nearing the end of your life. We want to talk today about what you know and would like to know, and have you help us make the right decisions for you, according to your preferences. This will be a difficult conversation but we need to start somewhere. At the end we will talk about options and plans and will proceed according to that plan."
2. *What does the patient know?* This is a key step since, due to fear, illness, significant cognitive dysfunction, and/or depression, there is often a gap between what patients may know about their disease severity and what we might expect them to know. I usually sense that patients are keenly aware of their advanced states but a quick reassessment of their status is always in order. It is useful to review recent hospitalizations, procedures, and steps taken to improve their status and to admit when these did not provide the hoped-for improvement.
3. *How much does the patient want to know?* Most caregivers are familiar with the style of interaction they and their patients share, particularly about details regarding their health status. However, it is a good idea to be very clear about which issues are not open for discussion. The patient may make clear that he or she not want to receive certain information (e.g., to not have a discussion about the role of dialysis). The patient may also indicate the desire to pass information on to another family member, thereby not declining the information but, rather, deferring the decisions to someone else. In general, however, most patients will want to hear their current options even if they later defer the decision-making to others. Many other issues impact what patients want to know, including age and culture. We need to assess these special circumstances as they arise.
4. *Sharing the information.* This step, in essence, is a succinct clinical summary of the patient's status, severity of illness, careful assessment of his or her proximity to death, and the background for the discussion that will follow. During this step the provider needs to avoid a long monologue and be alert to understanding—stopping and briefly clarifying questions as they arise.

It is important to maintain eye contact and avoid jargon and euphemisms. Speaking clearly and directly is important to avoid any misinterpretations about the seriousness of the disease state or the conversation. It should be noted that with cancer patients physicians typically overstate their assessment of survival and, indeed, their assessment of survival typically overestimates actual survival. It is acceptable to use brief periods of silence to let the words sink in as well as to check, using visual clues and observing body language, that the message is being assimilated. At the end of this step one can allow for a period of silence; take a brief break and say that you will return in 10 minutes to begin the next discussions. This decision is based on your sense of the patient's level of understanding. Always ask if there are questions anyone wants clarified before moving on to the next stage. Finally, at the end of this stage you might hear responses that alert you to areas of fear or concern that should be addressed before moving on.

5. *Responding to feelings*. If you have done the first steps properly, more likely than not a brief period of emotion (and at the same time, relief) will follow. This will depend on the level of understanding and preparedness the patient and the others in the room have of the advanced disease state. In any case, allow time for these emotions to arise and be aired. You should listen quietly and attentively and encourage all present to verbalize their feelings. Do not expect a recapitulation of the advanced pathophysiology of the patient's heart failure, but simply asking the patient, "John, does all that sound right to you?" may be validating and may open the patient up to begin to say a few words and engage him or her for the next step. Be sure that what the patient can enunciate reflects what you think you have told him or her.
6. *Planning and follow-up*. In this step you need to make clear what the next steps or plans are. This can include a discussion of all the options but this is rarely the final meeting, nor is this a good time to discuss every last issue related to end-of-life care. It is, moreover, a starting point where options can be explored and resources used. For example, one might provide a list of local hospice or palliative care organizations that can be contacted. If there is a palliative care service, you might say that you will place a consult to that service so they can explain more options. It is necessary to be very clear about who will do what steps and when the next planning meeting will take place. Before completing this conversation it is important to assess the patient's (and family's) emotional state and safety. A brief period of silence from the caregiver, supported by an occasional nod of acknowledgment, often provides the assurance the patients and families need that the caregiver understands the emotional impact of the conversation that was just held and will be there, ready to help with the next stages.

A provocative insight into a patient's emotions near the end of life has been offered by Finucane (7), which provides perspectives useful to anyone discussing these issues.

THE KNOWLEDGE BASE AND BARRIERS FOR ADEQUATE HEART FAILURE END-OF-LIFE CARE

There are multiple issues leading to inadequate end-of-life care for patients with heart failure. These include the lack of awareness on the part of patients and caregivers regarding the advanced nature of the disease, as well as discomfort with initiating or having the conversation just described. Few caregivers are specifically trained in giving bad news and, much less, in serving as a central figure in carrying out end-of-life planning. Nevertheless, it is critical for caregivers of heart failure patients to develop and hone these skills and to take ownership for leading these discussions. For most chronic diseases such as heart failure, the doctor and nurse teams become a major part of the patient's existence; to delegate (or, worse) abrogate these responsibilities will certainly imply abandonment and make the end-of-life process more difficult and confusing.

For guidance during the other less advanced stages of heart failure, we often turn to guidelines and consensus statements. These are usually formalized recommendations from expert panels supported by clinical evidence, often in the form of trials or studies. Lacking trial data, the guideline writers, based on experience and insight, often provide a recommendation. Unfortunately, this level of recommendations for the end-stage of heart failure has not been attained.

In an attempt to begin to address these issues, Goodlin et al. convened a panel to explore the current knowledge as well as the gaps in the knowledge base on palliative and supportive care in advanced heart failure (8). This group identified multiple issues but they created succinct recommendations focusing on needs in both the clinical (Table 48-2) and research (Table 48-3) arenas. They also appropriately documented that most clinical trials of patients with advanced heart failure have, to date, underrepresented women, the elderly, and nonwhite racial groups; hence, there are still gaps to overcome (9).

The limited information suggests that common questions and concerns among end-of-life patients include issues of pain and suffering. Nevertheless, some patients indicate a willingness to undergo additional treatments and procedures if there is hope of even short-term survival (10,11). This dichotomy suggests that better methods of communicating are essential in order to enhance patient understanding. Needless to say, an unambiguous statement of patient and family preference is a critical factor in making end-of-life decisions.

Important discords arise when policies and procedures of organizations (e.g., hospices) substantially alter the tempo and intensity of the pattern of care many advanced heart failure patients have received. Many patients with advanced disease receive therapies including home inotropes or have defibrillators, and many hospices to date are willing to and can support these therapies. However,

TABLE 48-2
PARTIAL LISTING OF IMPORTANT CLINICAL GAPS NEEDING TO BE ADDRESSED FOR PATIENTS WITH ADVANCED HEART FAILURE

Subject	Recommendation	Level of Evidence Rated in ACC/AHA Guidelines	Special Considerations	Limitations
Medical management	Diuretics to optimize volume status	Yes	Weight and estimated jugular venous pressure are clinical measures	
	ACE inhibitor or ARB	Yes	Dosage should be titrated to maximal doses in trials	Discontinuation indicated if patient develops a >30% rise in serum creatinine, or hypotension. Hydralazine and nitrates may then be an option
	β-blocker or a,β-blocker	Yes	Patient should be euvolemic before starting medication	Symptoms and quality of life were not reported in trials. Hypotension and negative inotropy may limit use.
	Continuous outpatient support with inotropes	Yes	May allow outpatient care for otherwise seriously ill patients	Increased ventricular actopy reported for all inotropes; increased mortality
	Oral inotropes	No	Study under way—no FDA-approved drugs	Combination with b-blockers may improve mortality soon in older studies
	CPAP for sleep-disordered breathing	No	Improve LV function and reduce norepinephrine levels with apnea or Cheyne-Stokes respiration	Equipment not well-tolerated by all patients; may also palliate fatigue
	Oxygen supplementation for sleep-disordered breathing	No		Recommended when CPAP not tolerated; no published data of effectiveness
Palliation of dyspnea	Oxygen	No	No clear evidence in HF	No physiologic benefit in one study
	Opioids	No	Unstudied in HF	Physiologic effects not known in HF
Palliation of fatigue	Psychostimulants	No	Unstudied in HF; benefit in cancer and HIV	
Treatment of depression	Antidepressants	No	Unstudied in HF	
Advanced technologies	VAD	No	Patients must manage the technology	Few VAD recipients in REMATCH survived beyond 2 years
	Implantable cardioverter defibrillator	No	Tested in patients with prior MI	Quality of life not assessed; uncertainty in patients with intolerable symptoms
	Cardiac resynchronization	No	Uncertain benefit for patients with advanced HF	
Communication	Advance care planning	No	Not tested in HF	Advance directives have no impact on care, symptoms, or quality of life
	Honest communication about the course of HF	No	Not tested in HF	
	Understand patient needs for information and address their concerns	No	Not tested in HF; reduce anxiety in cancer patients	
Interdisciplinary supportive care	Concurrent supportive care and HF disease management	No	Not tested in HF	
Structure of care	Scamiess translations between sites of care	No	Not tested in HF or other diseases	
Hospice care		No	Not tested in HF or other diseases	Variable approaches to care by different agencies

ACC/AHA, American College of Cardiology/American Heart Association; ACE, angiotensin-converting enzyme; ARB, angiotensin receptor blockers; CPAP, continuous positive airway pressure; FDA, U.S. Food and Drug Administration; LV, left ventricular; HF, heart failure; HIV, human immunodeficiency virus; VAD, ventricular assist device; REMATCH; Randomized Evaluation of Mechanical Assistance for the Treatment of Congestive Heart Failure.
Adapted from Goodlin SJ, Hauptman PJ, Arnold R, et al. Consensus statement: palliative and supportive care in advanced heart failure. *J Card Fail.* 2004;10: 200–209, with permission from Elsevier.

TABLE 48-3
PARTIAL LISTING OF IMPORTANT RESEARCH GAPS NEEDED TO BE ADDRESSED FOR PATIENTS WITH ADVANCED HEART FAILURE

Topic	Recommendation	Specific Areas for Research
Prognosis and trajectory of illness in advanced HF	Descriptive, longitudinal study that includes a broad population of patients with advanced HF	1. Nature, severity, and pattern of symptoms in advanced HF 2. Identification of critical turning points in the course of the disease that require re-examination of goals, treatments, and patient preferences 3. Clinical features and psychosocial dynamics that distinguish a patient's course and outcomes with advanced technologies versus medical management or palliative care 4. Issues and needs that are most important to patients and family members, and how these can be assessed in the course of care
Symptom treatment, optimizing quality of life for patients and family members	Studies to identify which interventions are effective in managing specific symptoms and optimizing quality of life Addition to measurement of symptoms and quality of life to all trials in advanced HF	1. Outcome measures to best address patients' quality of life and patient/family needs in advanced HF 2. Use of opioids for dyspnea acutely or long term in persons with advanced HF 3. Interventions to improve fatigue in HF 4. Impact of antidepressants on symptoms of anxiety, depression, and fatigue in HF and on the physiology of HF 5. Aspects of interdisciplinary care that benefit symptoms, quality of life, and patient/family needs in advanced HF
Communication with patients and family members about advanced HF	Studies to identify how best to communicate with patients and family members about the expected course of their illness, their concerns and fears, and dying from HF	1. Patient and family member understanding about disease and its course 2. Information desired by patients and their family about their disease and effective formats for providing this information 3. Communication by primary care physicians, cardiologists, and HF specialists with patients and family members about dying from HF 4. Impact of specific training on communication between practicing physicians and their advanced HF patients
System of care	Studies to identify components of care and systems that positively impact patient and family outcomes, associated costs and cost-effectiveness	1. Treatments, staff skills, and knowledge essential to the provision of care for patients with advanced HF, and integration into hospice care 2. Models of care and payment structures to best meet patient/family needs most cost-effectively

HF, heart failure.
Adapted from Goodlin SJ, Hauptman PJ, Arnold R, et al. Consensus statement: palliative and supportive care in advanced heart failure. *J Card Fail.* 2004;10: 200–209, with permission from Elsevier.

many hospices will not accept patients with intravenous vasoactive therapies and most do not have policies to turn off defibrillators. Other key issues identified by Goodlin et al. (8) include the role of opioids in heart failure care of the advanced-stage patient, which is important since dyspnea may well be perceived as a pain sensation (12).

An important barrier that needs to be recognized is that patients often change their wishes regarding care during various stages of the end of life. In the Study to Understand Prognoses and Preferences for Outcomes and Risks of Treatment (SUPPORT) trial, several issues emerged (13). In addition to low comprehension of discussions regarding resuscitative status during a heart failure hospitalization (25%), many patients (40%) changed their preferences following discharge. Whether this reflects altered perceptions, inadequate communication about disease status, or is truly a decision reversal also needs to be explored. Data suggesting lack of adequate referral to hospice programs for heart failure patients suggest that it is more likely related to poor communication about disease status rather than true decision reversal (14,15).

It is interesting to note that the SUPPORT trial evaluated the effect of an intervention and was found to have effected no increased physician–patient communication. This suggests that, as it was a decade ago, we still have enormous gaps in approaching advanced heart failure patients with good communication skills (16).

SUMMARY AND RECOMMENDATIONS

As our epidemic of heart failure grows, we will increasingly be faced with caring for patients with advanced heart failure who have arrived at the end of life. Our duty is to recognize the arrival of this stage of the disease process and to help our colleagues identify and predict its arrival. We must provide the same level of expertise and evidenced-based medicine for patients with end-of-life needs as we do for all other disease stages in heart failure. A host of resources are available for the interested clinician (17) but it remains the obligation of all who provide care to help identify, learn from, and counsel patients at this stage of their disease.

Against the background of enormous need and even larger gaps in our knowledge base for the ideal approaches to end-of-life care for our patients with advanced heart failure, several issues are clear and several recommendations can be put forward to the caregiver for patients with heart failure. These include:

- Caregivers should apply available prognosticators to identify patients who are approaching end of life. These patients may have short-lived clinical improvements but can be identified by understanding their natural disease trajectory.
- Ongoing education for patients and families should include honest discussion about potential for survival and meaningful functional status. Recognize that there is wide variability in patient preferences for life quality versus survival.
- All patients with heart failure should have advanced directives regarding resuscitative choices; these may vary depending on clinical status. Additional, focused discussions should include preferences and knowledge about hospice and palliative care, relief of pain and suffering, use of continuous inotropes, and deactivation of implanted defibrillators.
- The caregivers (nurses and physicians) are a critical part of the end-of-life discussion and decision-making. Members of these teams should lead these discussions and must not delegate or abrogate these obligations. The discussions should follow a plan that includes a review of disease severity, current knowledge of the patient and family, and clear planning steps.
- Trials that include the range of heart failure patients with advanced disease, including women and all ages and races, should attempt to build a usable and practical database of information from which more specific guidelines can be crafted.
- Heart failure caregivers must take on new roles with hospice and palliative care organizations to promote changes in perceptions of needs of heart failure patients. They should also work to clarify policies that will allow more patients with end-stage heart failure to enter end-of-life care.

REFERENCES

1. Hunt SA, Baker DW, Chin MH, et al. American College of Cardiology/American Heart Association guidelines for the evaluation and management of chronic heart failure in the adult: executive summary. *J Am Coll Cardiol.* 2001;38: 2101–2113.
2. Pantilat SZ, Steimle AE. Palliative care for patients with heart failure. *JAMA.* 2004;291:2476–2482.
3. Fonarow GC, Adams KF, Abraham WT, et al. Risk stratification for in-hospital mortality in acutely decompensated heart failure. *JAMA.* 2005;293:572–580.
4. Lamont EB, Christakis NA. Prognostic disclosure to patients with cancer near the end of life. *Ann Intern Med.* 2001;134: 1096–2000.
5. Tulsky JA. Beyond advanced directives. Importance of communication skills at the end of life. *JAMA.* 2005;294:359–365.
6. Buckman B. How to Break Bad News: a Guide for Health Care Professionals. University of Toronto Press, 1992. Toronto, CA.
7. Finucane TE. Care of patients nearing death: another view. *J Am Geriatr Soc.* 2002;50:551–553.
8. Goodlin SJ, Hauptman PJ, Arnold R, et al. Consensus statement: palliative and supportive care in advanced heart failure. *J Card Fail.* 2004;10:200–209.
9. Heiat A, Gross CP, Krumholz HM. Representation of the elderly, women and minorities in heart failure clinical trials. *Arch Intern Med.* 2002;162:1682–1688.
10. Stanek EJ, Oates MB, McGhan WF, et al. Preferences for treatment outcomes in patients with heart failure: symptoms versus survival. *J Card Fail.* 2000;6:225–232.
11. Lewis EF, Johnson PA, Johnson W, et al. Preferences for quality of life or survival expressed by patients with heart failure. *J Heart Lung Transplant.* 2001;20:1016–1024.
12. Jennings AL, Davies AN, Higgins JPT, et al. A systematic review of the use of opioids in the management of dyspnoea. *Thorax.* 2002;57:939–944.
13. The SUPPORT Investigators. A controlled trial to improve care for seriously ill hospitalized patients. *JAMA.* 1995;274: 1591–1596.
14. Levenson JW, McCarthy EP, Lynn J, et al. The last six months of life for patients with congestive heart failure. *J Am Geriatr Soc.* 2000;48(Suppl 5):S101–S109.
15. Zambroski CH. Hospice as an alternative model for care of older patients with end-stage heart failure. *J Cardiovasc Nurs.* 2004;19: 76–83.
16. Stevenson LW. Rights and responsibilities for resuscitation in heart failure. Tread gently on thin places. *Circulation.* 1998;98:619–622.
17. Kass-Bartelmes BL, Hughes R. Advance care planning. Preferences for care at the end of life. Rockville, MD: Agency for Healthcare Research and Quality; 2003. Research in Action Issue No. 12. AHRQ Pub. No. 03-0018. http://www.ahrq.gov/research/endliferia.htm. Accessed July 15, 2005.

Future Directions

49

Jeffrey David Hosenpud ***Barry H. Greenberg***

Over the 12 years that have elapsed since the publication of the first edition of this text, there have been substantial changes in our understanding of the basic mechanisms that lead to the development of heart failure and in our approach to treating this syndrome. These advances have resulted in striking improvements in the clinical course of heart failure patients. Nonetheless, there is much work still to be done. Morbidity and mortality from heart failure remain unacceptably high. Moreover, the pandemic of heart failure in the population shows no sign of abating. Nor is it likely to diminish as long as the population continues to age and our success in treating underlying etiologies of heart failure such as hypertension and coronary artery disease remains incomplete. There are, however, many promising approaches in both the basic and clinical arenas, and we briefly present some of these in this final chapter of the third edition of *Congestive Heart Failure.*

PREVENTION

Coronary artery disease is now recognized as the major etiologic factor in the development of heart failure in the United States and other developed nations. As the techniques used for percutaneous and surgical revascularization continue to be refined, the ability to protect myocardium from ischemia and/or infarction can only be expected to improve. The realization of very short "door to open vessel" times for acute myocardial infarction (MI) in most metropolitan areas has resulted in substantial myocardial salvage that will, by inference, reduce progressive left ventricular (LV) dysfunction and the development of heart failure. For those with chronic ischemic disease that is not amenable to coronary revascularization, an intriguing possibility is the potential for delivery of growth factors such as vascular endothelium growth factor (VEGF) or basic fibroblast growth factor (bFGF) to jeopardized areas of myocardium. Preliminary studies have indicated that growth factors can promote capillary growth to these areas from other, not critically stenosed, vessels (1,2). A randomized clinical trial directly injecting plasmid DNA for VEGF2 (pVGI.1) into ischemic myocardium (catheter technique) in patients with refractory angina is currently under way. Whether this or similar techniques ultimately produce adequate neovascularization and whether neovascularization ultimately prevents myocardial dysfunction are both critical issues that need to be resolved.

In view of the ongoing heart failure pandemic, treatment of risk factors for coronary artery disease should be a high priority for the health care system over the next decade. The power of preventive measures was made very apparent by the results of the Scandinavian Simvastatin Survival Study (4S) trial in which the use of the HMG-CoA reductase inhibitor simviastatin not only improved survival but also significantly reduced the future risk of developing heart failure (3). Another potentially fertile area is in the treatment of hypertension. Not only is this condition widespread in the United States, but it is estimated that only approximately one in four hypertensive patients is receiving adequate therapy. When hypertension is treated, the impact on preventing heart failure is substantial. In the Systolic Hypertension in the Elderly Program (SHEP), treatment of elderly patients with systolic hypertension resulted in a 49% reduction in the likelihood of developing heart failure (4).

Additional targets that demand increased attention include diabetes and obesity. Both of these conditions are increasing in prevalence at alarming rates and both are important risk factors for heart failure. Parenthetically, the lack of success in treating risk factors and preventing heart failure is somewhat surprising, even given the "crazy quilt" of health care systems that have evolved in the United States. It will take a concerted and sustained effort by numerous concerned parties, including the government, pharmaceutical companies, consumer and physician groups, and enlightened health maintenance organizations, to bring about change in this area. If risk factor management can be improved, however, it will have a substantial effect on the incidence of heart failure and its clinical sequelae.

The syndrome of heart failure is a continuum in which some injurious process activates a coordinated series of structural and functional changes that result in cardiac remodeling. Neurohormones such as angiotensin II, norepinephrine, aldosterone, proinflammatory cytokines, and other mediators are believed to play important roles in this process. There is evidence that early initiation of neurohormonal blockers can be used to successfully inhibit remodeling and help avert progression to heart failure. The successful use of angiotensin-converting enzyme inhibitors (ACEIs) in the post-MI population and in asymptomatic patients with LV dysfunction in the Studies of Left Ventricular Dysfunction (SOLVD) prevention trial provided the initial proof of principle for this approach (5–7). Further evidence has become available with the use of beta-blocking drugs in the Carvedilol Post-Infarct Survival Control In LV Dysfunction (CAPRICORN) study (8).

What is needed, however, is a means of reliably and inexpensively screening a population at risk for early indicators of cardiac dysfunction. Some evidence suggests that the family of natriuretic peptides (i.e., atrial and B-type natriuretic peptides [ANP and BNP, respectively]) that are released from the heart in response to stretch may be useful to detect evidence of incipient heart failure (9). If this proves to be the case, one could envision screening populations at risk (e.g., elderly patients with one or more cardiac risk factors) with a blood test to help select patients for early initiation of neurohormonal blockade.

DIAGNOSIS

Using modern techniques of linkage analysis, investigators have uncovered genetic mutations that result in a number of inherited cardiovascular diseases, including hypertrophic cardiomyopathy. A genetic basis for dilated cardiomyopathy was felt to be rare, with perhaps 1% to 2% of cases being familial. More recently, two reports suggest that a familial component is present in 35% to 48% of cases if LV enlargement is included as a clinical indicator for association (10,11). To date, 16 autosomal genes, two major x-linked gene families (dystrophin and tafazzin), and one family with a troponin I defect have been described (12). Progress in understanding these point mutations and specifically how they lead to dilated cardiomyopathy should help reveal intracellular pathways and mechanisms that give rise to the heart failure phenotype.

Alternatively, in many and probably most cases, the development of heart failure is not caused by a monogenic disorder. Rather, progressive changes in response to injury lead to structural and functional changes that are the cause of heart failure. First, what is the injury, and second, what are the modifiers to that injury? Recent studies have again raised the possibility that viruses are a likely cause of initial injury. In one study, viral genomes were present in biopsy samples of more than 60% of patients with dilated cardiomyopathy (13). In another study, parvovirus B19 was a commonly detected viral pathogen (14).

The likelihood and rapidity of the development of heart failure, as previously suggested, appear to vary greatly among patients, suggesting that there may be genetic modifiers of the rate of progression (15). Polymorphisms in genes encoding receptors, enzymes, as well as structural and contractile proteins could be responsible for these differences among patients. One of the first of these polymorphisms to be recognized as a gene that could affect the progression of heart failure in susceptible populations was the polymorphism in the ACE gene (16). Whether or not individuals homozygous for the deletion mutation and who express higher levels of ACE activity are at increased risk of developing the heart failure phenotype or developing more severe disease, however, is uncertain. Although polymorphisms in a great many other genes could potentially alter the likelihood of development and rate of progression of cardiac dysfunction, reports in the literature have been inconsistent, with some surveys concluding that there is increased risk with a particular polymorphism while others report the absence of any increased risk. Clearly, this is a area that will require increased attention in the future.

ASSESSMENT OF THERAPY AND PROGNOSIS

Over the past 5 years we have laid to rest the controversy of mortality associated with invasive hemodynamic monitoring and can be assured that we are not committing medical homicide by placement of a Swan-Ganz catheter (17). On the other hand, based on the results of the Evaluation Study of Congestive Heart Failure and Pulmonary Artery Catheterization Effectiveness (ESCAPE) trial (17), we are not so sure that we are helping patients when we employ this strategy for directing management of heart failure. Although we have been clearly seduced by a blood test that diagnoses heart failure (BNP) and are ready to embrace its use to follow heart failure therapy (18), the effectiveness of this test in altering long-term outcomes remains uncertain. The use of this diagnostic test would appear to have the greatest value in the emergency room setting, particularly when there is uncertainty about the interpretation of the signs and symptoms that motivated the patient to seek urgent medical attention.

Another intriguing possibility to consider for the long-term monitoring of the status of heart failure patients is the use of implantable hemodynamic monitoring (Chronical, Medtronic Inc., Minneapolis, MN) (19). As we await definitive results of the usefulness of this and other strategies to help follow our patients, it may be premature to relegate the stethoscope to the Smithsonian and declare the death of the physical examination as a means of determining the presence and severity of heart failure. However, it has become painfully apparent that physicians are becoming progressively less adept at examining their patients and interpreting the free information that is readily available to the savvy clinician from physical findings.

MEDICAL TREATMENT

Most of the advances in the medical management of heart failure have utilized the approach of blocking neurohormonal pathways that have been inappropriately activated in the heart failure state. However, this approach has not been uniformly successful. Endothelin is a hormone that mediates many adverse cellular effects and, like other neurohormonal mediators, it is elevated in patients with heart failure (20). Despite evidence of benefits in experimental animal models, the use of endothelin antagonists have not been found to improve outcomes in heart failure patients (19). Paradoxically, there has been considerable interest in the heart failure community in a therapeutic strategy that involves augmenting an already activated neurohormonal system (i.e., administering nesiritide, a preparation of recombinant human BNP, for acutely decompensated heart failure). Enthusiasm for this approach was sparked by evidence of superiority of administration of nesiritide to both standard diuretic therapy and to the use of a fixed dose of nitroglycerin for the treatment of acutely decompensated heart failure in the Vasodilation in the Management of Acute Congestive Heart Failure (VMAC) trial (21). However, re-evaluation of the available database raised concerns that treatment with nesiritide might have negatively impacted renal function and increased mortality (22,23). While these negative effects of nesiritide may be related to the use of higher doses of the drug than are currently recommended, these issues need clearer definition from additional clinical trials in order to determine the role of nesiritide in treating patients with acutely decompensated heart failure.

Two other neurohormonal systems that have been targeted for intervention are the arginine vasopressin and adenosine systems. While there is evidence that blockade of these systems may have beneficial effects, the early results seen in relatively small studies need to be proved by testing the agents in well-designed clinical trials employing relevant endpoints.

DEVICES, SURGICAL APPROACHES, AND REPLACEMENT THERAPY

In the past several years we have witnessed new devices, new surgical and catheter techniques, and improvements on more-established therapies designed to improve or replace cardiac function. It is anticipated that within the next few years the roles of some of these newer techniques will be defined, and some will most certainly be more broadly applied. By and large, these techniques fall into three major categories: (a) attempts to improve or augment intrinsic cardiac function; (b) conventional surgical treatment applied to patients not previously approached or approached percutaneously; and (c) cardiac replacement strategies.

One of the most promising interventions in the first category has been the use of cardiac resynchronization therapy. Not only has this approach improved symptoms and exercise tolerance, but it also appears to improve morbidity and mortality as well as promote reverse remodeling (24). In fact, we devote an entire chapter to this relatively new therapy in this edition of the text. Another new approach that is currently being tested is the use of cardiac contractility modulation (CCM) by electric currents applied during the refractory period. Preliminary evidence indicates that this treatment improves myocardial contractility as well as the clinical status of selected patients with advanced heart failure (25).

The field of cell transplantation for myocardial regeneration continues to evolve. Several clinical studies involving skeletal myoblasts or bone marrow progenitor cells have been now reported using either direct inoculation during surgery, transendocardial inoculation via catheter, or transcoronary venous injection. All of these studies have essentially been feasibility trials with rare numbers of patients showing actual cell engraftment at cardiac explantation (for transplant) or autopsy (26–29). Significant issues regarding the type of cell best suited for transplantation and the mechanism(s) by which these cells improve cardiac function still remain. In addition, given the limited number of patients thus far studied, the safety of the various procedures and treatments also is not well-defined. Nonetheless, this approach to treating heart failure holds considerable promise for the future.

In the second category, there had been substantial enthusiasm for mitral valve repair in patients with severe LV dysfunction and functional mitral insufficiency. Much of this enthusiasm was based upon the initial experience reported by the University of Michigan (30). In a recent report from this same group, however, that included 126 patients with severe LV dysfunction undergoing mitral repair, there did not appear to be any survival benefit from this approach based on comparison with nonoperated patients that were treated over the same time period (31). Although it is possible that mitral repair in this patient population is not beneficial, an alternative explanation is that surgical trauma to an already impaired left ventricle could mask any benefits that are derived from improving mitral insufficiency. It is possible that this question can ultimately be answered with the development of a new percutaneous catheter technique to reduce the amount of mitral insufficiency. This technique employs a catheter to clip the midportion of the anterior mitral leaflet to the midportion of the posterior mitral leaflet, thereby creating a dual orifice that reduces mitral insufficiency. The preliminary trial with this technique has been reported and the results are quite encouraging (32).

Finally, cardiac replacement strategies have continued to evolve and are anticipated to bring new approaches to the treatment of end-stage heart failure. As discussed in Chapter 45, a number of new immunosuppressive agents that are more efficacious, less toxic, or both, have been released for clinical use or are in clinical trials. This renaissance in immunosuppression is likely to continue with the ability to computer-model potential agents and to target specific molecular targets with our greater understanding of the molecular events of immune activation and the cell cycle. Unfortunately, only approximately 2,500 heart transplants are being performed annually in the United States, while the anticipated need for organ replacement is, at minimum, 10 times that number.

The field of xenotransplantation (cross-species transplantation) has largely stalled. While investigation and continued advancement in preventing xenograft rejection have continued in the laboratory, the major concern which has profoundly influenced interest in expanding to clinical trials is the potential transmission of disease from animal to human. The current worldwide concern of the H5N1 virus (commonly referred to as bird flu) will only serve to strengthen these concerns.

In contrast, interest in the use of mechanical ventricular assist devices continues to expand. As discussed in Chapter 43, there are now a number of small axial flow pumps in clinical trials. The advantages of these pumps are their small size and their reduced energy requirements compared to the first- and second-generation pulsatile pumps. The potential disadvantage of this generation of pumps is that they are unlikely to completely replace LV or RV function, so some intrinsic cardiac function will likely be required. On the other hand, adding 3 to 4 L per minute of flow would likely convert 90% of all patients with severe heart failure from New York Heart Association (NYHA) functional Class III or IV to Class I to II.

Economic Trends in Heart Failure Care

Close to 5 million people are afflicted with heart failure in the United States alone, with an annual cost in this country of between $20 and $40 billion (33). These figures are only likely to increase with the increasing age of the population. It is no wonder that there are major efforts underway to impact the care of these patients. We have seen the development of heart failure specialty clinics, primarily in academic medical centers but starting to expand into the community (34). These latter clinics are primarily nurse-run and protocol-driven. Hospitals are developing inpatient heart failure care maps; insurance companies are instituting heart failure management programs and nurse coordinators; and the pharmaceutical industry is sponsoring heart failure symposia, consensus recommendations, advisory boards, and management software. Because of the potential benefits of early diagnosis and therapeutic interventions in the hope of preventing adverse cardiac remodeling, it is not unreasonable to expect major efforts in screening and early intervention in the coming years. One might anticipate this effort to be largely nurse-managed. Finally, with development of expensive new technologies for more advanced heart failure, sophisticated attempts to cost-justify their use are likely to be undertaken, if not by health care professionals, certainly by third-party payers.

SUMMARY

This chapter gives us the opportunity to reflect on the successes and failures that have been experienced in the field of heart failure over the past several years, while also allowing us to gaze into the crystal ball and try to predict the future. As was concluded in this chapter in the first two editions of *Congestive Heart Failure*, changes in the world of heart failure are occurring rapidly. This is true both of our understanding of the pathophysiology and in the way we treat patients. We had hoped that some of the predictions based on early data would have borne fruit by this time, and they yet may do so at some point in time in the future. However, we are still not ready to routinely inject growth factors, stem cells, or myoblasts into the heart. Xenotransplantation remains a long way off and many of the promising pharmaceuticals have not been as helpful as we had predicted. Alternatively, genetic screening for cardiomyopathy and prevention of progression from acute infarction to heart failure are now realizable goals. Catheter interventions continue to replace traditional surgical techniques and new methodologies are being reported on regularly. Mechanical cardiac support continues to advance at a blinding rate. Costs initially will be high but will moderate with more generalized use and should be at least partially buffered by reduced costs in intensive care units and terminal care. We hope that with the next edition, the predictions made here will be substantially further along.

REFERENCES

1. Banai S, Jaklitsch MT, Shou M, et al. Angiogenic-induced enhancement of collateral blood flow to ischemic myocardium by vascular endothelial growth factor in dogs. *Circulation.* 1994;89:2183–2189.
2. Giordano F, Ping P, McKirnan D, et al. Intracoronary gene transfer of fibroblast growth factor-5 increases blood flow and contractile function in an ischemic region of the heart. *Nature Med.* 1996;2:534–539.
3. Kjekshus J, Pedersen TR, Olsson AG, et al. The effects of simvastatin on the incidence of heart failure in patients with coronary heart disease. *J Card Failure.* 1997;3:249–254.
4. Kostis JB, Davis BR, Cutler J, et al. for the SHEP Cooperative Research Group. Prevention of heart failure by antihypertensive drug treatment in older persons with isolated systolic hypertension. *JAMA.* 1997;278:212–216.
5. Pfeffer MA, Braunwald EB, Moye LA, et al. Effect of captorpil on mortality and morbidity in patients with left ventricular dysfunction after myocardial infarction. Results of the survival and ventricular enlargement trial. *N Engl J Med.* 1992;327:669–677.
6. The Acute Infarction Ramipril Efficacy (AIRE) Study Investigators. Effect of ramipril on mortality and morbidity of survivors of acute myocardial infarction with clinical evidence of heart failure. *Lancet.* 1993;342:821–828.
7. The SOLVD Investigators. Effects of enalapril on survival in patients development of heart failure in patients with reduced left ventricular ejection fractions. *N Engl J Med.* 1992; 327: 685–691.
8. The CAPRICORN Investigators. Effect of carvedilol on outcome after myocardial infarction in patients with left-ventricular dysfunction: the CAPRICORN randomised trial. *Lancet.* 2001;(357) 1385–1390.
9. McDonagh TA, Robb SD, Murdoch DR, et al. Biochemical detection of left ventricular systolic dysfunction. *Lancet.* 1998;351:9–13.

10. Grunig E, Tasman JA, Kucherer H, et al. Frequency and phenotypes of familial dilated cardiomyopathy. *J Am Coll Cardiol.* 1998;31:186–194.
11. Baig MK, Goldman JH, Caforio AP, et al. Familial dilated cardiomyopathy: cardiac abnormalities are common in asymptomatic relatives and may represent early disease. *J Am Coll Cardiol.* 1998;31:195–201.
12. Burkett EL, Hershberger RE. Clinical and genetic issues of familial dilated cardiomyopathy. *J Am Coll Cardiol.* 2005;45:969–981.
13. Kuhl U, Pauschinger M, Noutsias M, et al. High prevalence of viral genomes and multiple viral infections in the myocardium of adults with "idiopathic" left ventricular dysfunction. *Circulation.* 2005;111:887–893.
14. Lotze U, Egerer R, Tresselt C, et al. Frequent detection of parvovirus B19 genome in the myocardium of patients with idiopathic dilated cardiomyopathy. *Med Microbiol Immunol.* 2004;193:75–82.
15. Loh E, Rebbeck TR, Mahoney PD, et al. Common variant in *AMPD1* gene predicts improved clinical outcome in patients with heart failure. *Circulation.* 1999;99:1422–1425.
16. Cambien F, Poirier O, Lecerf L, et al. Deletion polymorphism in the gene for angiotensin-converting enzyme is a potent risk factor for myocardial infarction. *Nature.* 1992;359:641–644.
17. Binannay C, Califf RM, Hasselblad V, et al. Evaluation study of congestive heart failure and pulmonary artery catheterization effectiveness in the ESCAPE trial. *JAMA.* 2005;294:1625–1633.
18. Jourdain P, Funck F, Gueffer P, et al. Benefits of BNP plasma levels for optimizing therapy: the systolic heart failure treatment supported by BNP multicenter randomized trial (STARS-BNP). [Abstract] *J Am Coll Cardiol.* 2005;l45(Suppl A):3A.
19. Cleland JG, Coletta AP, Freemantle N, et al. Clinical trials update from the American College of Cardiology meeting: CARE-HF and the remission of heart failure, Women's Health Study, TNT, COMPASS-HF, VERITAS, CANPAP, PEECH and PREMIER. [Congresses] *Eur J Heart Fail.* 2005;7(5):931–936.
20. Lerman A, Kubo S, Tschumperlin LK, Burnett JC. Plasma endothelin concentrations in humans with end-stage heart failure and after heart transplantation. *J Am Coll Cardiol.* 1992;20: 849–853.
21. Publication Committee for the VMAC Investigators. Intravenous nesiritide vs nitroglycerin for treatment of decompensated congestive heart failure: a randomized controlled trial. *JAMA.* 2002;287:1531–1540.
22. Sacjner-Bernstein JD, Skopicki HA, Aaronson KD. Risk of worsening renal function with nesiritide in patients with acutely decompensated heart failure. *Circulation.* 2005;111:1487–1491.
23. Sackner-Bernstein JD, Kowalski M, Fox M, et al. Short-term risk of death after treatment with nesiritide for decompensated heart failure. A pooled analysis of randomized controlled trials. *JAMA.* 2005;293:1900–1905.
24. Cleland JG, Daubert JC, Erdmann E, et al. The effect of cardiac resynchronization on morbidity and mortality in heart failure. *N Engl J Med.* 2005;352:1539–1549.
25. Pappone C, Rosanio S, Burkhoff D, et al. Cardiac contractility modulation by electric currents applied during the refractory period in patients with heart failure secondary to ischemic or idiopathic dilated cardiomyopathy. *Am J Cardiol.* 2002;90: 1307–1313.
26. Schachinger V, Assmus B, Britten MB, et al. Transplantation of progenitor cells and regeneration enhancement I acute myocardial infarction: final one-year results of the TOPCARE-AMI Trial. *J Am Coll Cardiol.* 2004;44:1690–1699.
27. Siminiak T, Fiszer D, Jerzykowska O, et al. Percutaneous transcoronary-venous transplantation of autologous skeletal myoblasts in the treatment of post-infarction myocardial contractility impairment: the POZNAN trial. *Eur Heart J.* 2005;26: 1188–1195.
28. Dohmann HF, Perin EC, Takiya CM, et al. Transendocardial autologous bone marrow mononuclear cell injection in ischemic heart failure: postmortem anatomicopathologic and immunohistochemical findings. *Circulation.* 2005;112:521–526.
29. Dib N, McCarthy P, Campbell A, et al. Feasibility and safety of autologous myoblast transplantation in patients with ischemic cardiomyopathy. *Cell Transplant.* 2005;14:11–19.
30. Bolling SF, Pagani FD, Deeb GM, et al. Intermediate-term outcome of mitral reconstruction in cardiomyopathy. *J Thorac Cardiovasc Surg.* 1998;115(2):381–386.
31. Wu AH, Aaronson KD, Bolling SF, et al. Impact of mitral valve annuloplasty on mortality risk in patients with mitral regurgitation and left ventricular dysfunction. *J Am Coll Cardiol.* 2005; 45:381–387.
32. Feldman T, Wasserman HS, Herrmann HC, et al. Percutaneous mitral valve repair using the edge-to-edge technique: six-month results of the EVEREST phase I clinical trial. *J Am Coll Cardiol.* 2005;46:2134–2140.
33. O'Connell JB, Bristow MR. Economic impact of heart failure in the United States: time for a different approach. *J Heart Lung Transplant.* 1994;13:S107–S112.
34. Rich MW, Beckman V, Wittenberg C, et al. A multidisciplinary intervention to prevent readmission of elderly patients with congestive heart failure. *N Engl J Med.* 1995;333:1190–1195.

Index